Hagberg and Benumof's

AIRWAY MANAGEMENT

Hagberg and Benumof's

AIRWAY MANAGEMENT

5TH EDITION

CARIN A. HAGBERG, MD, FASA

Chief Academic Officer
Division Head
Division of Anesthesiology, Critical Care, and Pain Medicine
Bud Johnson Clinical Distinguished Professor of Anesthesiology
Department of Anesthesiology and Perioperative Medicine
University of Texas MD Anderson Cancer Center
Houston, Texas

CARLOS A. ARTIME, MD

Professor and Clinical Executive Vice Chair
Department of Anesthesiology, Critical Care, and Pain Medicine
McGovern Medical School at University of Texas Health Science Center at Houston
Houston, Texas

MICHAEL F. AZIZ, MD

Professor and Vice Chair for Clinical Affairs
Department of Anesthesiology and Perioperative Medicine
Oregon Health and Science University
Portland, Oregon

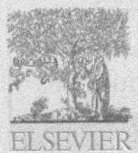

ELSEVIER

Elsevier

1600 John F. Kennedy Blvd.
Suite 1800
Philadelphia, PA 19103-2899

HAGBERG AND BENUMOF'S AIRWAY MANAGEMENT, FIFTH EDITION 978-0-323-79538-8

Previous editions copyrighted 2018, 2013, 2007, and 1996.

Content Strategist: Sarah Barth/Kayla Wolfe
Content Development Manager: Kathryn DeFrancesco
Content Development Specialist: Jennifer Pierce
Publishing Services Manager: Shereen Jameel
Project Manager: Janish Paul/Manikandan Chandrasekaran
Design Direction: Renee Duenow

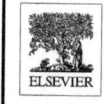
Last digit is the print number: 9 8 7 6 5 4 3 2 1

This book is dedicated to the more than
six million people who died of COVID-19 during
the two years we spent preparing this edition.

We also dedicate this book to healthcare workers
across the globe for their hard work and sacrifice caring
for patients during this once-in-a-century pandemic,
particularly those practitioners involved in airway management,
who placed themselves at great personal risk.

Contributors

Imran Ahmad, MBBS, FRCA
Consultant Anaesthetist
Department of Theatres, Anaesthesia and Perioperative Medicine
Guy's and St Thomas' NHS Foundation Trust
London, England;
Honorary Senior Lecturer
King's College London
London, England

Ronda E. Alexander, MD
Assistant Professor
Department of Otorhinolaryngology – Head & Neck Surgery
University of Texas Medical School at Houston
Houston, Texas;
Director
Texas Voice Performance Institute
Houston, Texas

Carlos A. Artime, MD
Professor and Clinical Executive Vice Chair
Department of Anesthesiology, Critical Care, and Pain Medicine
McGovern Medical School at University of Texas Health Science
    Center at Houston
Houston, Texas

Michael F. Aziz, MD
Professor and Vice Chair for Clinical Affairs
Department of Anesthesiology and Perioperative Medicine
Oregon Health and Science University
Portland, Oregon

Paul A. Baker, MBChB, MD, FANZCA
Associate Professor
Department of Anaesthesiology
University of Auckland
Auckland, New Zealand;
Consultant Anaesthetist
Department of Paediatric Anaesthesia
Starship Children's Health
Auckland, New Zealand

Christine M. Ball, MBBS, MD, FANZCA
Anaesthetist
Department of Anaesthesia and Perioperative Medicine
Alfred Hospital
Prahran, Victoria, Australia;
Adjunct Associate Professor
Department of Anaesthesia and Perioperative Medicine
Monash University, Prahran
Victoria, Australia

Irving Basañez, MD
ENT Section Chief
Department of Surgery
Tennessee Valley Healthcare System
Nashville, Tennessee;
Adjunct Assistant Professor
Department of Otolaryngology – Head & Neck Surgery
Vanderbilt University Medical Center
Nashville, Tennessee

Shawn T. Beaman, MD, FASA
Associate Professor
Chief Anesthesiologist, UPMC Presbyterian
Department of Anesthesiology and Perioperative Medicine
University of Pittsburgh Medical Center
Pittsburgh, Pennsylvania

Elizabeth C. Behringer, MD
Cardiac Surgical Intensivist – Anesthesiologist
Division of Cardiovascular Surgery & Critical Care
Kaiser Permanente Los Angeles
The Kaiser Permanente Bernard J Tyson School of Medicine
Los Angeles, California

Jacqueline A. Bello, MD
Professor
Departments of Radiology and Neurosurgery
Albert Einstein College of Medicine
Director of Neuroradiology
Department of Radiology
Montefiore Medical Center
Bronx, New York

Jonathan L. Benumof, MD
Professor Emeritus
Department of Anesthesia
University of California San Diego
San Diego, California

Lauren C. Berkow, MD, FASA
Professor
Department of Anesthesiology
University of Florida College of Medicine
Gainesville, Florida

Ansgar M. Brambrink, MD, PhD
Emanuel M. Papper Professor of Anesthesiology and Chair
Department of Anesthesiology
Columbia University
New York, New York

Darren Alan Braude, MD, EMT-P
Professor
Department of Emergency Medicine and Anesthesiology
University of New Mexico Health Sciences Center
Albuquerque, New Mexico;
Co-Director, Center for Prehospital Resuscitation
Department of Emergency Medicine
University of New Mexico Health Sciences Center
Albuquerque, New Mexico

Staci D. Cameron, MD
Assistant Professor
Director of Pediatric Pain Service
Department of Anesthesiology, Critical Care, and Pain Medicine
Division of Pediatric Anesthesiology
McGovern Medical School at University of Texas Health Science
    Center at Houston
Houston, Texas

Davide Cattano, MD, PhD, FASA
Professor
Department of Anesthesiology, Critical Care, and Pain Medicine
McGovern Medical School at University of Texas Health Science
    Center at Houston
Houston, Texas

Laura F. Cavallone, MD
Associate Professor
Department of Anesthesiology
Director of ENT Anesthesia
Department of Anesthesia & Critical Care
University of Chicago
Chicago, Illinois

T. Linda Chi, MD
Professor
Department of Diagnostic Radiology
University of Texas MD Anderson Cancer Center
Houston, Texas

Nicholas Chrimes, BSc, MBBS (Hons), FANZCA
Consultant Anaesthetist
Department of Anaesthesia
Monash Medical Centre
Melbourne, Victoria, Australia

Edmond Cohen, MD, FASA
Professor of Anesthesiology and Thoracic Surgery
Director of Thoracic Anesthesia
Department of Anesthesiology, Perioperative and Pain Medicine
Icahn School of Medicine at Mount Sinai
New York, New York

Neal H. Cohen, MD, MPH, MS
Vice Dean
Professor Emeritus
Departments of Anesthesia and Perioperative Care and Medicine
UCSF School of Medicine
San Francisco, California

Tim M. Cook, BA (Cantab), MBBS, FRCA
Consultant in Anaesthesia and Intensive Care Medicine
Department of Anaesthesia and Intensive Care Medicine
Royal United Hospitals Bath
Bath, England

Richard M. Cooper, BSc, MSc, MD, FRCPC
Professor Emeritus
Department of Anesthesiology and Pain Medicine
University of Toronto
Toronto, Ontario, Canada;
Anesthesiologist (Retired)
Department of Anesthesia and Pain Management
University Health Network Toronto General Hospital
Toronto, Ontario, Canada

Pierre Diemunsch, MD, PhD
Chairman
Department of Anesthesiology
Department of Intensive Care and Perioperative Medicine
University Hospital of Hautepierre
Strasbourg, France

D. John Doyle, MD, PhD, DPhil
Professor of Anesthesiology
Anesthesiology Institute
Cleveland Clinic
Cleveland, Ohio

James DuCanto, MD
Staff Anesthesiologist
Department of Anesthesiology
Advocate Aurora Summit Medical Center
Summit, Wisconsin;
Clinical Adjunct Professor
University of Wisconisn School of Medicine
Madison, Wisconsin

Laura V. Duggan, MD, MSc (Clinical Epidemiology), FRCPC
Associate Professor
Department of Anesthesiology and Pain Medicine
University of Ottawa
Ottawa, Ontario, Canada

Richard P. Dutton, MD, MBA
Chief Quality Officer
US Anesthesia Partners;
Adjunct Professor
Texas A&M University College of Medicine;
Staff Anesthesiologist
Baylor University Medical Center
Dallas, Texas

Kariem El-Boghdadly, MBBS, BSc, FRCA, EDRA, MSc
Consultant Anaesthetist
Department of Theatres, Anaesthesia and Perioperative Medicine
Guy's and St Thomas' NHS Foundation Trust
London, England;
Honorary Senior Lecturer
King's College London
London, England

Louise Ellard, MBBS, FANZCA, AdvPTEeXAM, MCL
Deputy Director
Department of Anaesthesia
Austin Health
Melbourne, Victoria, Australia

Jessica L. Feinleib, MD, PhD, FASA
The Veterans Health Administration
Assistant Professor
Department of Anesthesiology
Yale School of Medicine
West Haven, Connecticut

David Z. Ferson, MD
Professor
Department of Anesthesiology and Perioperative Medicine
University of Texas MD Anderson Cancer Center
Houston, Texas

Lorraine J. Foley, MD
Clinical Assistant Professor
Department of Anesthesia
Tufts School of Medicine
Boston, Massachusetts;
Atlantic Anesthesia LLC
Department of Anesthesia
Shields Medford Surgical Ambulatory Surgical Center
Medford, Massachusetts

Luis Gaitini, MD
Professor
Former Director
Anesthesiology Department
Bnai Zion Medical Center
Haifa, Israel

Richard E. Galgon, MD, MS
Staff Anesthesiologist
Department of Perioperative Services
SSM Health Dean Medical Group
Janesville, Wisconsin

Michael Alfred Gibbs, MD, FACEP
Professor and Chairman
Department of Emergency Medicine
Carolinas Medical Center
Charlotte, North Carolina

Robert Greif, MME, FERC
Professor
Department of Anaesthesiology and Pain Medicine
Bern University Hospital and University of Bern
Bern, Switzerland;
School of Medicine
Sigmund Freud University Vienna
Vienna, Austria

Thomas E. Grissom, MD, MSIS, FCCM, FASA
Associate Professor
Department of Anesthesiology
University of Maryland School of Medicine
Baltimore, Maryland

Sara Guzman-Reyes, MD
Associate Professor of Anesthesiology
APD and Director Acute Pain Service Lyndon B. Johnson Hospital;
Department of Anesthesiology, Critical Care, and Pain Medicine
McGovern Medical School at University of Texas Health Science Center at Houston
Houston, Texas

Carin A. Hagberg, MD, FASA
Chief Academic Officer
Division Head
Division of Anesthesiology, Critical Care, and Pain Medicine
Bud Johnson Clinical Distinguished Professor of Anesthesiology
Department of Anesthesiology and Perioperative Medicine
University of Texas MD Anderson Cancer Center
Houston, Texas

Heather K. Hayanga, MD, MPH
Associate Professor
Department of Anesthesiology
West Virginia University
Morgantown, West Virginia

Thomas Heidegger MD, DESA, FEAMS
Head
Department of Anaesthesia
Spital Grabs
Grabs, Switzerland;
Professor
Department of Anaesthesiology and Pain Medicine
Bern University Hospital and University of Bern
Bern, Switzerland

Andy Higgs, MBChB, DA, FRCA, FFICM
Consultant in Anaesthesia & Intensive Care Medicine
Department of Critical Care
Warrington & Halton Hospitals NHS Foundation Trust
Warrington, Cheshire, England

Caleb B. Hodge, DO
Fellow
Department of Trauma Anesthesiology
UMMC - R. Adams Cowley Shock Trauma Center
Baltimore, MD

Orlando Hung, BSc (Pharmacy), MD, FRCPC
Professor
Department of Anesthesia, Surgery, and Pharmacology
Dalhousie University
Halifax, Nova Scotia, Canada

Haitham Ibrahim, MD
Assistant Professor
Anesthesia Department
Yale School of Medicine
New Haven, Connecticut

Narasimhan Jagannathan, MD, MBA
Anesthesiologist-in-Chief
Phoenix Children's Hospital;
Professor
University of Arizona School of Medicine
Phoenix, Arizona

Ranu R. Jain, MDv
Professor
Assistant Division Chief of Pediatric Anesthesia
Program Director
Pediatric Anesthesia Fellowship
Department of Anesthesiology, Critical Care, and Pain Medicine
Division of Pediatric Anesthesiology
McGovern Medical School at University of Texas Health Science
    Center at Houston
Houston, Texas

Liane B. Johnson, MDCM, FRCSC, FACS
Associate Professor
Department of Surgery, Division of Otolaryngology-HNS
Dalhousie University, IWK Health Centre
Halifax, Nova Scotia, Canada

Mark Kastner, MD
Physician
Emergency Medicine
Carolinas Medical Center
Charlotte, North Carolina

Jeffrey P. Keck Jr., MD
Department of Anesthesiology
Southeast Health
Cape Girardeau, Missouri
Jackson, Missouri

P. Allan Klock Jr., MD
Professor and Chairman
Department of Anesthesia and Critical Care
University of Chicago
Chicago, Illinois

Joshua B. Knight, MD, FASE
Assistant Professor
Department of Anesthesiology and Perioperative Medicine
University of Pittsburgh Medical Center
Pennsylvania, Pittsburgh

George Kovacs, MD, MHPE, FRCPC
Professor
Departments of Emergency Medicine
Anaesthesia, Medical Neurosciences & Division of Medical
    Education;
Director
Clinical Cadaver Program
Dalhousie University;
Medical Director
EHS Lifeflight Critical Care Transport Program
Halifax, Nova Scotia, Canada

Michael Seltz Kristensen, MD
Head of Research & Development
Section for Anesthesia for ENT Head Neck and Maxillofacial
    Surgery
Department of Anesthesia
Center of Head and Orthopaedics
Rigshospitalet, University Hospital of Copenhagen
Copenhagen, Denmark

Olivier Langeron, MD, PhD
Professor of Anesthesiology and Critical Care
Head of Department of Anesthesiology and Critical Care
University Hospital Henri Mondor Assistance Publique –
    Hôpitaux de Paris (APHP)
University Paris-Est-Créteil (UPEC)
Creteil, France

Sarah A. Lee, MD
Assistant Professor
Department of Anesthesiology and Pain Medicine
University of Washington Medical Center
Seattle, Washington

Helen A. Lindsay, MBChB
Anaesthetic Specialist
Department of Anaesthesia & Perioperative Medicine
Auckland City Hospital
Auckland, New Zealand

Lynette J. Mark, MD
Associate Professor
Department of Anesthesiology & Critical Care Medicine
Department of Otolaryngology/Head and Neck Surgery
Johns Hopkins University
Baltimore, Maryland

Nathan D. Mark, DO
Staff Anesthesiologist
Department of Anesthesiology
Mercy Regional Medical Center
Durango, Colorado

**Stuart D. Marshall, MBChB, M.HumanFact, PhD, CHIA,
    MAICD, MRCA, FANZCA**
Senior Lecturer
Department of Anaesthesia and Perioperative Care
Monash University
Melbourne, Victoria, Australia;
Honorary Associate Professor
Department of Medical Education
University of Melbourne
Melbourne, Victoria, Australia

Reeba Mathew, MD, FCCP
Associate Professor
Doctor of Internal Medicine
McGovern Medical School at University of Texas Health Science
    Center at Houston
Houston, Texas

Adrian Matioc, MD
Staff Anesthesiologist (retired)
Department of Anesthesiology
William S. Middleton VA Medical Center
Madison, Wisconsin;
Clinical Adjunct Professor (retired)
Department of Anesthesiology
University of Wisconsin School of Medicine and Public Health
Madison, Wisconsin

Andrew C. McClelland, MD, PhD
Assistant Professor
Department of Radiology
Montefiore Medical Center
Bronx, New York

Joseph H. McIsaac III, MD, MS, MBA, CPE, FASA
Chief of Trauma Anesthesia
Department of Anesthesiology
Hartford Hospital
Hartford, Connecticut;
Clinical Professor of Anesthesiology
Department of Anesthesiology
University of Connecticut School of Medicine
Farmington, Connecticut

Alistair F. McNarry, MA, MB, BChir, FRCA
Consultant Anaesthetist
Western General and St John's Hospitals
NHS Lothian
Edinburgh, UK

David M. Mirsky, MD
Pediatric Neuroradiologist
Department of Radiology
Children's Hospital Colorado
Aurora, Colorado;
Assistant Professor
Department of Radiology
University of Colorado
Aurora, Colorado

Basma Mohamed, MBChB
Assistant Professor
Department of Anesthesiology
University of Florida College of Medicine
Gainesville, Florida

Tiffany Sun Moon, MD, FASA
Associate Professor
Department of Anesthesiology & Pain Management
The University of Texas Southwestern Medical Center
Dallas, Texas

Thomas C. Mort, MD
Professor
Department of Anesthesiology & Surgery
University of Connecticut School of Medicine
Farmington, Connecticut;
Associate Director, Surgical ICU
Hartford Hospital
Hartford, Connecticut

Jarrod M. Mosier, MD
Associate Professor of Emergency Medicine
Department of Emergency Medicine
University of Arizona
Tucson, Arizona;
Associate Professor of Medicine
Department of Medicine
Section of Pulmonary, Critical Care, Allergy, and Sleep
University of Arizona
Tucson, Arizona

Sabine Nabecker, MD, PhD, AFAMEE, FHEA
Assistant Professor
Department of Anesthesiology and Pain Management
Sinai Health System
University of Toronto
Toronto, Ontario, Canada

Alexander Nagrebetsky, MD, MSc
Resident
Assistant Professor
Department of Anesthesia, Critical Care, and Pain Medicine
Massachusetts General Hospital
Harvard Medical School
Boston, Massachusetts

Robert Naruse, MD, FASA
Vice Chair & Professor
Department of Anesthesiology
Cedars-Sinai Medical Center
Los Angeles, California

Vladimir Nekhendzy, MD, FASA
Clinical Professor of Anesthesiology
Department of Anesthesiology, Perioperative and Pain Medicine
Stanford University School of Medicine;
Clinical Professor of Otolaryngology (by courtesy)
Otolaryngology–Head and Neck Surgery
Stanford University School of Medicine
Stanford, California

Kevin F. O'Grady, BASc, MHSc, MD, FRCSC
Plastic Surgeon
Private Practice
Richmond Hill, Ontario, Canada

Babatunde Ogunnaike, MD
Professor
Department of Anesthesiology and Pain Management
The University of Texas Southwestern Medical Center
Dallas, Texas

Matthew W. Oh, BS
Medical Student
Department of Anesthesiology and Pain Management
The University of Texas Southwestern Medical Center
Dallas, Texas

Hernando P. Olivar, MD
Clinical Professor
Department of Anesthesiology and Pain Medicine
University of Washington
Seattle, Washington

Irene P. Osborn, MD
Professor
Department of Anesthesiology
Albert Einstein College of Medicine
Bronx, New York

Ellen O'Sullivan, MB BCh, FRCA
Consultant Anaesthetist
St. James Hospital
Dublin, Ireland

Dhamodaran Palaniappan, MBBS, MD
Associate Clinical Professor
Department of Anesthesiology
University of Connecticut School of Medicine
Farmington, Connecticut;
Section Chief–Thoracic Anesthesia
Department of Anesthesiology
Hartford Hospital
Hartford, Connecticut

Matteo Parotto, MD, PhD
Associate Professor
Department of Anesthesiology and Pain Management
Interdepartmental Division of Critical Care Medicine
University of Toronto, Ontario, Canada;
Staff Physician
Department of Anesthesia and Pain Management
Toronto General Hospital
Toronto, Ontario, Canada

Anil Patel, MBBS, FRCA
Consultant Anaesthetist
Department of Anaesthesia
Royal National Throat Nose & Ear Hospital
London, England;
Department of Anaesthesia
University College Hospital
London, England

Bela Patel, MD
Professor of Medicine
Department of Internal Medicine;
Director, Division of Critical Care Medicine
Department of Internal Medicine
McGovern Medical School at University of Texas Health Science
    Center at Houston
Houston, Texas

Alberto G.G. Piacentini, MD
Istituto Mediterraneo Trapianti
Department of Anesthesia and Critical Care
ISMETT UPMC
Palermo, Italy

Oliver J. Poole, MD, RRT
Resident
Department of Anesthesia, Pain Management, and Perioperative
    Medicine
Dalhousie University
Halifax, Nova Scotia, Canada

Paul Potnuru, MD
Assistant Professor
Department of Anesthesiology
McGovern Medical School at University of Texas Health Science
    Center at Houston
Houston, Texas

Joseph J. Quinlan, MD
Professor of Anesthesiology
Department of Anesthesiology
University of Pittsburgh
Pittsburgh, Pennsylvania

Ana Lisa Ramirez-Chapman, MD, BA
Assistant Professor
Program Director, Obstetric Anesthesia Fellowship
Director of Obstetric Anesthesia
Lyndon B. Johnson Hospital
Department of Anesthesiology, Critical Care, and Pain Medicine
McGovern Medical School at University of Texas Health Science
    Center at Houston
Houston, Texas

Fiona Roberts, MB Bch, BAO, FCAI, FJFICMI
Department of Anaesthesiology
Mater Hospital
Dublin, Ireland

William H. Rosenblatt, MD
Professor
Department of Anesthesia
Yale University School of Medicine
New Haven, Connecticut

Christopher Ross, MD, FRCPC, FACEP, FAAEM
Visiting Professor
Department of Surgery
University of Illinois
Rockford, Illinois;
Attending Physician
Department of Emergency Medicine
Mercyhealth
Rockford, Illinois

Soham Roy, MD
Professor and Chief of Pediatric Otolaryngology
Department of Otorhinolaryngology
The University of Texas Health Science Center at Houston
Houston, Texas

Ron E. Samet, MD
Assistant Professor of Anesthesiology
Department of Anesthesiology
R Adams Cowley Shock Trauma Center
University of Maryland School of Medicine
Baltimore, Maryland

Jan-Henrik Schiff, MD, PhD, MPH
Department of Anaesthesiology, Intensive Care Medicine,
    Emergency Medicine and Pain Therapy
Klinikum Stuttgart
Stuttgart, Germany

Bettina U. Schmitz, MD, PhD, MSMS (simulation), DEAA
Professor of Anesthesiology
Director Regional Anesthesia Service
Department of Anesthesiology
Texas Tech University HSC
Lubbock, Texas

Sam R. Sharar, MD
Professor
Department of Anesthesiology and Pain Medicine
University of Washington School of Medicine
Seattle, Washington

Saimir Sharofi, CRT, RRT, MMA
Director of Respiratory Services
Pulmonary Lab/Rehab
Hartford Healthcare
Hartford, Connecticut

Keivan Shifteh, MD
Professor of Clinical Radiology
Department of Radiology
Montefiore Medical Center
Bronx, New York

Maged Soliman, MBBch, MSc
Advanced Airway Fellow
Department of Anesthesiology
Montefiore Medical Center
Bronx, New York

Kathryn Sparrow, BSc, MD, FRCPC, MScHQ
Assistant Professor
Discipline of Anesthesia
Memorial University of Newfoundland
St. John's, Newfoundland and Labrador, Canada

Srikanth Sridhar, MD
Associate Professor
Department of Anesthesiology, Critical Care, and Pain Medicine
McGovern Medical School at University of Texas Health Science Center at Houston
Houston, Texas

Michael Thomas Steuerwald, MD, FACEP, FAEMS
Medical Director
University of Wisconsin Med Flight
Berbee Walsh Department of Emergency Medicine
University of Wisconsin – Madison
Madison, Wisconsin

Tracey Straker, MD, MS, MPH, CBA, FASA
Professor
Department of Anesthesiology
Albert Einstein College of Medicine
Bronx, New York;
Professor, Clinical Medicine
Department of Medicine
CUNY School of Medicine
Manhattan, New York

Sriharsha Subramanya, MD, FRCA(UK)
Department of Anesthesiology and Critical Care
Hartford Hospital
Hartford, Connecticut

Maya S. Suresh, MBBS
Professor
Vice Chair of Faculty Affairs
Department of Anesthesiology, Critical Care, and Pain Medicine
McGovern Medical School at University of Texas Health Science Center at Houston
Houston, Texas

Wendy H. Teoh, MBBS, FANZCA, FAMS
Senior Consultant Anaesthesiologist
Private Anaesthesia Practice
Wendy Teoh Pte. Ltd.
Republic of Singapore

Felipe Urdaneta, MD
Clinical Professor
Department of Anesthesiology
University of Florida
Gainesville, Florida;
Staff Anesthesiologist
Department of Anesthesia
North Florida/South Georgia Veterans Health System
Gainesville, Florida

Sonia Vaida, MD
Professor
Department of Anesthesiology
Penn State Health Milton S. Hershey Medical Center
Hershey, Pennsylvania

Manuel C. Vallejo Jr., MD, DMD
Professor of Anesthesiology, Obstetrics & Gynecology, and Medical Education
West Virginia University
Morgantown, West Virginia

Naveen Vanga, MD
Associate Professor of Anesthesiology
Vice Chair of Education
Department of Anesthesiology, Critical Care, and Pain Medicine
McGovern Medical School at University of Texas Health Science Center at Houston
Houston, Texas

Kathryn K. Walker, MD, MEd
Assistant Professor
Department of Anesthesiology
University of Pittsburgh
Pittsburgh, Pennsylvania

Andreas Walther, MD, MHBA
Professor, Head of Deparrtment
Department of Anesthesiology, Intensive Care, Emergency Medicine and Pain Therapy
Klinikum Stuttgart
Stuttgart, Germany

Mark T. Warner, MD
Assistant Professor
Department of Internal Medicine
Division of Critical Care
McGovern Medical School at University of Texas Houston Medical School
Houston, Texas

David J. Wilkinson, MBBS, FRCA, FCARCSI (Hon)
Retired Consultant Anaesthetist
Boyle Department of Anaesthesia
St. Bartholomew's Hospital
London, England

William C. Wilson, MD, MA
Clinical Professor Emeritus
Department of Anesthesiology and Perioperative Care
University of California Irvine;
Chief Medical Officer, SVP
Clinical Research and Medical Affairs
Masimo
Irvine, California

David T. Wong, MD
Professor
Department of Anesthesiology and Pain Medicine
University of Toronto
Toronto, Ontario, Canada

Mark Zakowski, MD, FASA
Professor of Anesthesiology
Department of Anesthesiology
Cedars-Sinai Medical Center
Los Angeles, California

Marko Zdravkovic, MD, PhD
Assistant Professor
Department of Anaesthesiology, Intensive Care and Pain Management
University Medical Centre Maribor
Maribor, Slovenia;
Faculty of Medicine
University of Ljubljana
Ljubljana, Slovenia

Foreword

Dr. Carin Hagberg, who edited the second, third, and fourth editions of this book, has again achieved her goal with her hard work and dedication. This latest edition confirms its place as the essential resource for *all* practitioners involved in airway management. This includes not only practitioners involved in anesthesia practice but also those involved in airway management in other settings, including the emergency room and the intensive care unit. The COVID-19 pandemic has shed a light on the importance of safe airway management, its multidisciplinary nature, and the need for a unifying approach based on evidence-based guidelines and algorithms. It is, therefore, timely to update this textbook to be the definitive comprehensive resource on this vital topic.

The basic structure and philosophy of the book remain the same and continue to support the original purpose articulated so well by Dr. Jon Benumof: to "encompass and clearly present the knowledge and forethought that will allow the clinician to solve airway problems and avoid complications."

Since the previous edition of the book, there have been many advances in techniques, equipment, and new global airway algorithms. Huge importance has been placed on human factors awareness in safely managing complex airway scenarios, and this has been addressed in a new chapter in this book. Another recent development since the preceding iteration has been the use of combination techniques, and this is also addressed as a new chapter. Further updates include adding a summary box with the key points at the beginning of each chapter and improving the layout with the addition of many more high-quality images and videos.

It is a testament to Dr. Hagberg's dedication and worldwide reputation that she has persuaded such an array of worldrenowned experts in this field, from all over the globe, to contribute to this fifth edition of the book. For airway experts, it provides further insights and sometimes challenges their current thinking. For every airway practitioner, it is an essential resource presented in an easy-to-read style.

On behalf of the airway community as a whole, I would like to congratulate Dr. Hagberg and her co-editors on this latest achievement, producing the most comprehensive book on the topic to date. It has evolved remarkably over the various editions, while keeping its accessible style and ease of navigation. The goal of this book is to improve airway management safety, and I am confident that this fifth edition will help to achieve this.

Ellen O'Sullivan, MB BCh, FRCA

Preface

There have been significant advances in airway management over the past two decades and since the publication of the fourth edition of *Hagberg and Benumof's Airway Management*, edited by Dr. Carin Hagberg, along with two co-editors, Drs. Carlos Artime and Michael Aziz. It is essential that clinicians become familiar with the most recent developments in equipment and scientific knowledge to allow the safe practice of airway management.

In the fifth edition of this book, there are two new chapters: (1) Human Factors and (2) Combination Techniques, both of which are considered important topics in airway management. Four chapters have either been merged with others or deleted. The remaining chapters have been updated to address current thinking and practice. Although many of the authors remain the same, several new authors have added to this edition their expertise in the field of airway management.

To aid the reader in understanding and retaining complex and detailed information, an increased number of video recordings have been included in this edition, which illustrate the use of the different airway devices and techniques currently available to the clinician. Rather than clinical pearls at the end of each chapter, *Key Points* are now highlighted at the beginning of each chapter. Also, as in the previous edition, each chapter includes a summary and selected references.

The basic structure and philosophy of the book have not changed. It is divided into seven parts. The first section (Chapters 1–7) provides basic clinical science considerations of airway management. The second section (Chapters 8–12) presents the development of an airway management plan, as well as global airway algorithms and the new chapter on human factors. The third section (Chapters 13–16) emphasizes patient preparation and preintubation ventilation procedures, as well as techniques for induction of general anesthesia. The fourth section (Chapters 17–30) covers the wide variety of techniques and devices used for airway management. The history of airway management is re-examined, and the many new airway devices and techniques are detailed. The indications for and confirmation of tracheal intubation are provided. The fifth section (Chapters 31–43) covers management of difficult airway situations, such as in pediatric patients and in growing areas of airway management including non-operating room locations, such as radiology and gastroenterology, and the intensive care unit. The sixth section (Chapters 44–48) emphasizes postintubation procedures and discusses such issues as monitoring the airway, extubation, and complications of airway management. The seventh and last section (Chapters 49–53) presents societal considerations of airway management, including airway education, clinical documentation of airway management, conduction of airway research, airway management and outcomes reporting, and the role of the airway community.

The editors of this book are often asked by family, friends, or colleagues with a limited understanding of airway management "Why does one need an entire textbook dedicated to putting in a breathing tube?" A glance at the table of contents of this book can begin to provide clues; however, a short answer is that airway management is a complex skill with multiple variables, a very short time limitation, and life-or-death consequences. Airway practitioners must possess a great deal of knowledge and proficiency in order to save a patient's life when difficulty is encountered.

Improvements in airway management have led to a documented decline in the incidence of airway-related preoperative morbidity. Much of this has been because of the development and widespread implementation of devices designed for management of the difficult airway. Because of the plethora of these devices already available and the fast pace at which new ones are introduced, airway practitioners must understand the *fundamentals* of the practice of airway management in order to optimally utilize the available technology. This book covers in detail the anatomy, physics, and physiology about which mastery is necessary in order to use airway devices to their full potential. It is imperative to understand not only the techniques associated with the various airway devices, but also when their use would be most appropriate in a given situation.

As with many clinical skills, information and study will only go so far in achieving proficiency. It is essential to have experience with techniques in various clinical situations in order to develop expertise. However, because most airways are managed without difficulty, there are limitations to experience with airway management. An in-depth understanding of the concepts presented in this text is vital to the successful management of any encounter with a difficult airway scenario. Expertise also entails ongoing learning, skill maintenance, simulation, advancing research, and self-assessment—all of which are aided with the use of this book.

We are most fortunate to live in this unprecedented era of safe anesthesia practice and should continue to look forward to the future advances that will continue to occur and what research on airway management will unfold. The contributors to this book will undoubtedly be central to this progress, and we look forward to working with them in future editions.

Carin A. Hagberg, MD, FASA
Carlos A. Artime, MD
Michael F. Aziz, MD

Acknowledgments

The preparation of this fifth edition of *Hagberg and Benumof's Airway Management* has required the help and cooperation of many during a challenging time in our history: the COVID-19 pandemic. The authors who contributed to this edition did so while dealing with the profound impacts of the pandemic on both their clinical practices and personal lives. To each individual, we acknowledge a debt of gratitude. It has been both an honor and privilege to have worked with all of the authors from across the world, including expert anesthesiologists, emergency room specialists, intensivists, surgeons, radiologists, and basic scientists.

As we publish the fifth edition of this textbook, we acknowledge the contributions of Jonathan Benumof, MD, who authored and edited the first edition in 1996. Dr. Benumof's impact on advancing the field of airway management in anesthesiology and other medical specialties cannot be overstated.

The staff of Elsevier has contributed in countless ways, with competence, patience, and hard work, particularly Mary Hegeler and Jennifer Pierce, Content Development Specialists, and Sarah Barth, Publisher, who kept us on task and played a vital role in the quality of the final written text.

We especially wish to express our heartfelt thanks to our families, particularly our spouses—Steven Roberts, Kimberly Aziz, and Michelle Artime—without whose understanding, forbearance, and support, this textbook would not have been possible.

Carin A. Hagberg, MD, FASA
Carlos A. Artime, MD
Michael F. Aziz, MD

Contents

Video Contents

PART 1

Basic Clinical Science Considerations

1

Functional Anatomy of the Airway

MARK ZAKOWSKI AND MANUEL C. VALLEJO JR.

CHAPTER OUTLINE

KEY POINTS

- Cricoarytenoid arthritis can lead to airway difficulties in patients with rheumatoid arthritis or systemic lupus erythematosus.
- To diagnose vocal cord dysfunction, it is necessary to examine the position of the vocal cords during inspiration and phonation.
- The recurrent laryngeal and superior laryngeal nerves may be injured during thyroid surgery, leading to severe vocal cord dysfunction.
- Bilateral partial recurrent nerve palsy is more dangerous than complete palsy.

- Neck movement during anesthesia can result in movement of the tip of the endotracheal tube (ETT); neck flexion causes the ETT to advance, while neck extension causes withdrawal.
- New imaging techniques such as virtual endoscopy and multidetector computed tomography (MDCT) are providing added insight into the structure and function of the airways in health and disease.
- Upper airway obstruction in sedated patients occurs at the level of soft palate rather than at the level of the tongue.
- Infections, such as COVID-19, may lead to prolonged anatomic changes in the lung parenchyma.

Introduction

The "airway" is not merely a passive conduit of air; it serves a dynamic and important physiologic role in the human body. The air passages, starting from the nose and ending at the bronchioles, are necessary for the delivery of humidified and filtered respiratory gas to and from the alveoli. During clinical anesthesia, an anesthesiologist uses these air passages to deliver anesthetic gases to the alveoli, while maintaining vital respiratory gas transport. Anesthesiologists and other medical practitioners often gain access to the airway by means of an endotracheal tube (ETT) or other airway devices that are introduced directly into the patient's upper or lower air passages. An understanding of the airway structures is critical for establishing and maintaining the airway.

For the purpose of anatomic description, the airway is divided into the upper airway, which extends from the nose to the glottis or thoracic inlet, and the lower airway, which includes the trachea, the bronchi, and the subdivisions of the bronchi. The upper airway also serves other important functions, such as olfaction,

deglutition, and phonation in addition to humidification and filtering of inspired gases. A detailed anatomic description of all these structures is beyond the scope of this chapter. Structural details as they relate to function in health and disease and some important anesthetic implications are explained here. In addition, some advances in imaging techniques that give insight to functional anatomy are described.

Upper Airway

Nose

Structure

The airway functionally begins at the nares and the mouth, where air first enters the body. In the adult human, the two nasal fossae extend 10 to 14 cm from the nostrils to the nasopharynx. The two fossae are divided mainly by a midline quadrilateral cartilaginous septum together with the two extreme medial portions of the lateral cartilages. The nasal septum is composed mainly of

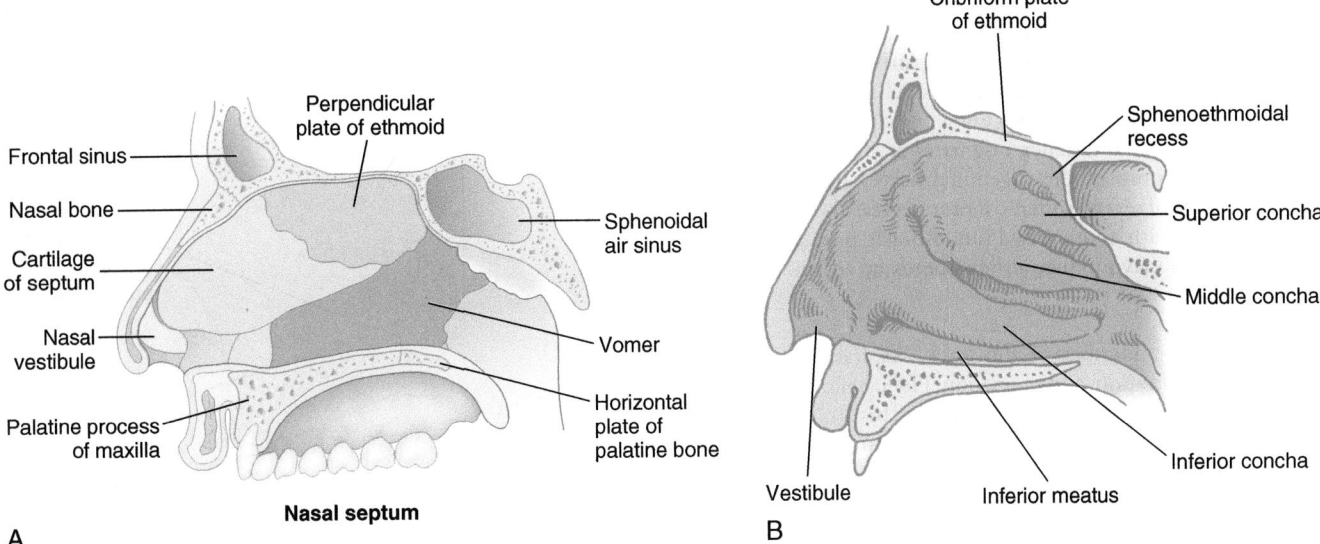

A

Nasal septum

B

• **Fig. 1.1** (A) Medial wall (septum) of the nasal cavity. The sphenoid sinus opens into the sphenoethmoidal recess. The frontal, maxillary, and ethmoidal sinuses open into meatuses of the nose. Notice that the nasal septum contains cartilage in front and bone in the back. (B) Lateral wall of the nasal cavity. The conchae are also known as the *nasal turbinates*. (Modified from Ellis H, Feldman S. *Anatomy for Anaesthetists*. 6th ed. Blackwell Scientific; 1993.)

the perpendicular plate of the ethmoid bone descending from the cribriform plate, the septal cartilage, and the vomer (Fig. 1.1). It is normally a midline structure but can be deviated to one side.[1] Disruption of the cribriform plate secondary to facial trauma or head injury may allow direct communication with the anterior cranial fossa. The use of positive-pressure mask ventilation in this scenario may lead to the intracranial entry of air, bacteria, or foreign material, resulting in meningitis or sepsis. In addition, nasal airways, nasotracheal tubes, and nasogastric tubes may be inadvertently introduced into the subarachnoid space in patients with facial trauma. The posterior portion of the septum is usually midline, but trauma-associated septal deviations and congenital choanal atresia can cause posterior obstruction (Fig. 1.2).

Each nasal fossa is convoluted and provides approximately 60 cm² of surface area on each side for warming and humidifying inspired air.[2] The nasal fossa is bound laterally by inferior, middle, and superior turbinate bones (conchae),[3] which divide the fossa into scroll-like spaces called the *inferior, middle, and superior meatuses* (see Fig. 1.1).[2,4,5] The inferior turbinate usually limits the size of the nasotracheal tube that can be passed through the nose, and damage to the lateral wall may occur as a result of vigorous attempts during nasotracheal intubation. The arterial supply to the nasal cavity is mainly from the ethmoid branches of the ophthalmic artery, the sphenopalatine and greater palatine branches of the maxillary artery, and the superior labial and lateral nasal branches of the facial artery. A confluence of these blood vessels, known as *Kiesselbach's plexus*, is situated in Little's area on the anterior-inferior portion of the nasal septum. This is a common source of clinically significant epistaxis. The turbinates have a rich vascular supply that, depending upon ambient air temperature, affords the nasal airway the ability to expand or contract according to the degree of vascular engorgement. The vascular mucous membrane overlying the turbinates can be easily damaged, leading to hemorrhage, which can be profuse. The paired paranasal sinuses—sphenoid, ethmoid, maxillary, and frontal—drain through apertures termed *ostia* into the lateral wall of the nose.

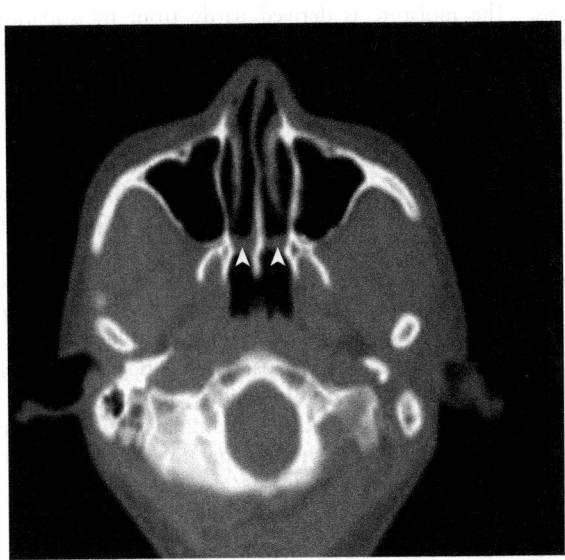

• **Fig. 1.2** Bilateral choanal atresia as seen by computed tomography. Arrows point to the area of posterior obstruction. (From Li X, Cai X, Zhang L, et al. Bilateral congenital choanal atresia and osteoma of ethmoid sinus with supernumerary nostril: a case report and review of the literature. *J Med Case Rep*. 2011;5:583.)

Prolonged nasotracheal intubation may lead to infection of the maxillary sinus due to obstruction of and lack of drainage through the ostia.[6]

The olfactory area is located in the upper third of the nasal fossa and includes the middle and upper septum and the superior turbinate bone. The respiratory portion is located in the lower third of the nasal fossa.[5] The respiratory mucous membrane consists of both ciliated columnar epithelium containing goblet cells and nonciliated columnar epithelium with microvilli and basal cells. The olfactory cells have specialized hairlike processes, called *olfactory hairs*, which are innervated by tendrils of the olfactory nerve.[5]

The nonolfactory sensory nerve supply to the nasal mucosa is derived from the first two divisions of the trigeminal nerve—the anterior ethmoidal and maxillary nerves. Airborne chemical irritants cause firing of the trigeminal nerves, which are presumably responsible for reflexes such as sneezing and apnea.[7] The afferent pathway for the sneezing reflex originates at the histamine-activated type C neurons of the trigeminal nerve, and the efferent pathway consists of several somatic motor nerves. The act of sneezing is associated with an increased intrathoracic pressure of up to 100 mm Hg and may produce airflow speeds up to 100 mph.[7]

Function

The nose serves a number of functions: respiration, olfaction, humidification, filtration, and phonation. Phylogenetically, breathing was intended to occur through the nose. This arrangement not only enables an animal to smell dangers but also permits uninterrupted conditioning of inspired air while feeding. Resistance to airflow through the nasal passages is double that of the mouth; therefore, during exercise or respiratory distress, mouth breathing occurs to facilitate a reduction in airway resistance and increased airflow. The nose is also able to prewarm and condition inspired air to a temperature of 32°C to 34°C over a wide range of ambient temperatures, from 8°C to 40°C.[8]

Approximately 10,000 L of ambient air pass through the nasal airway per day, and 1 L of moisture is added to this air in the process.[9] The moisture is derived partly from transudation of fluid through the mucosal epithelium and partly from secretions produced by glands and goblet cells. These secretions have significant bactericidal properties. Foreign body invasion is further minimized by the actions of the stiff hairs (vibrissae), the ciliated epithelium, and the extensive lymphatic drainage of the area.

The parasympathetic autonomic nerves reach the nasal mucosa from the facial nerve after relay through the sphenopalatine ganglion, and sympathetic fibers are derived from the plexus surrounding the internal carotid artery via the vidian nerve.[10] A series of complex autonomic reflexes controls the blood supply to the nasal mucosa and allows it to shrink and swell quickly. Reflex arcs also connect this area with other parts of the body. For example, the Kratschmer reflex leads to bronchiolar constriction on stimulation of the anterior nasal septum in animals. A demonstration of this reflex may be seen in the postoperative period as a patient becomes agitated when the nasal passage is packed.[10]

Pharynx

Structure

The pharynx provides a common pathway for food and respiratory gases, extending 12 to 15 cm from the base of the skull to the level of the cricoid cartilage anteriorly and the inferior border of the sixth cervical vertebra posteriorly.[11] The widest level occurs at the hyoid bone (5 cm), while the narrowest occurs at the level of the esophagus (1.5 cm), which is the most common site for obstruction with foreign body aspiration. The pharynx is subdivided into the nasopharynx, oropharynx, and laryngopharynx. The nasopharynx, which primarily serves a respiratory function, lies posterior to the termination of the turbinates and nasal septum and extends to the soft palate. The oropharynx has primarily a digestive function and starts below the soft palate, extending to the superior edge of the epiglottis. The laryngopharynx (hypopharynx) lies between the fourth and sixth cervical vertebrae, starts at the superior border of the epiglottis, and extends to the inferior border of the cricoid cartilage, where it narrows

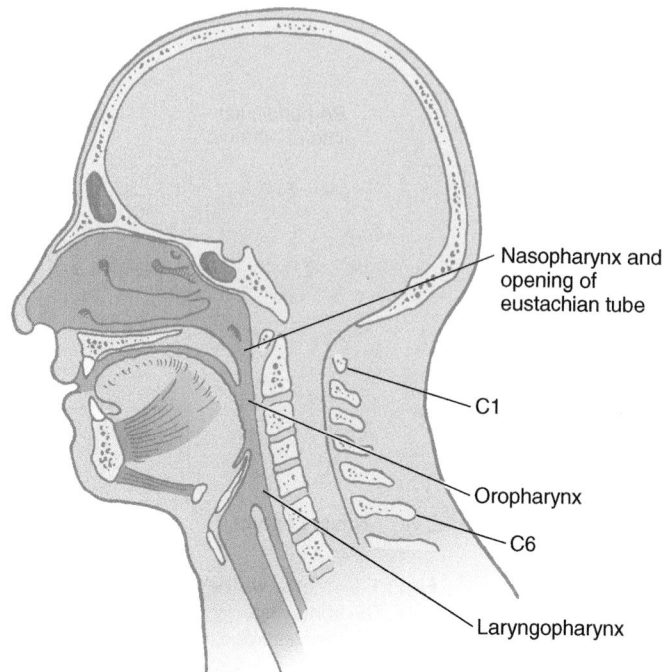

• **Fig. 1.3** Sagittal section through the head and neck showing the divisions of the pharynx. The laryngopharynx is also known as the *hypopharynx*. (Modified from Ellis H, Feldman S. *Anatomy for Anaesthetists*. 3rd ed. Blackwell Scientific; 1993.)

and becomes continuous with the esophagus (Fig. 1.3). The eustachian tubes open into the lateral walls of the nasopharynx.

The lateral walls of the oropharynx contain the tonsillar pillars in the fauces. The anterior pillar contains the glossopharyngeus muscle, and the posterior pillar contains the palatoglossus muscle.[12] The wall of the pharynx consists of two layers of muscles, an external circular layer and an internal longitudinal layer. Each layer is composed of three paired muscles. The stylopharyngeus, salpingopharyngeus, and palatopharyngeus muscles form the internal layer; they elevate the pharynx and shorten the larynx during deglutition. The superior, middle, and inferior constrictors form the external layer; they advance food in coordinated contractions from the oropharynx into the esophagus.

The constrictors of the external layer are innervated by filaments arising from the pharyngeal plexus (formed by motor and sensory branches from the vagus, the glossopharyngeal, and the external branch of the superior laryngeal nerve). The inferior constrictor is additionally innervated by branches of the recurrent laryngeal and external laryngeal nerves. The internal layer is innervated by the glossopharyngeal nerve. The glossopharyngeal nerve may easily be blocked by local anesthetic to the level of the posterior tonsillar pillars to facilitate awake airway management (see Chapter 13).

Patency of the pharynx is vital to the patency of the airway and proper gas exchange in nonintubated patients. Proper placement of an ETT requires an understanding of the distance relationships from the oropharynx to the vocal cords and carina. Complications, such as an ETT cuff leak at the level of the vocal cords or endobronchial intubation, may thus be avoided (Fig. 1.4).

Function

Inhaled particles greater than 10 μm are removed by inertial impaction on the posterior nasopharynx. In addition, smaller

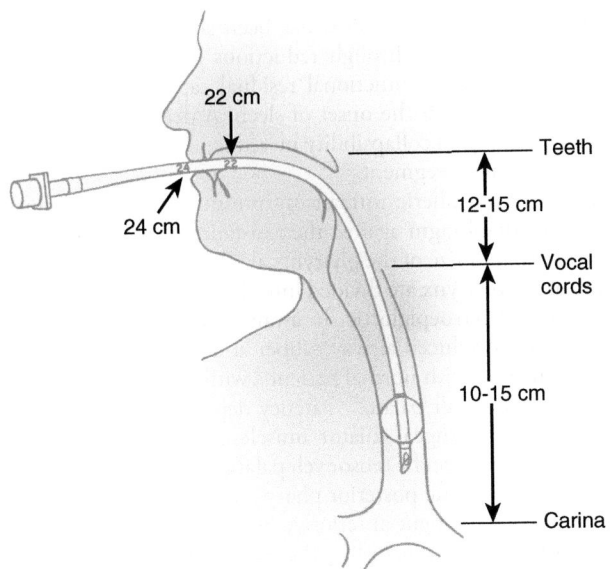

• **Fig. 1.4** Important distances for proper endotracheal tube placement. (From Stone DJ, Bogdonoff DL. Airway considerations in the management of patients requiring long-term endotracheal intubation. *Anesth Analg.* 1992;74:276.)

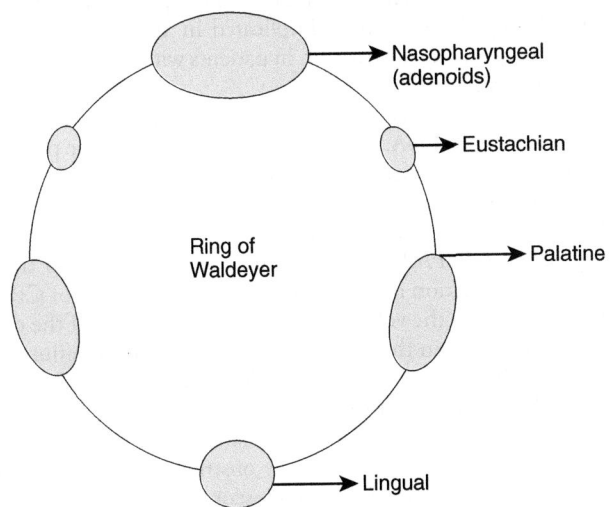

• **Fig. 1.5** The ring of Waldeyer, a collection of lymphoid (tonsillar) tissue that guards against pathogen invasion. (Modified from Hodder Headline PLC, London.)

particles lose momentum and become suspended as a result of the sharp directional change of the inhaled airstream (90 degrees) at the nasopharynx. Being unable to remain suspended, the particles subsequently impact and become trapped by the pharyngeal walls. The body defends against the trapped impacted particles, bacteria, and viruses by the circularly arrayed lymphoid tissue located at the entrance to the respiratory and alimentary tracts, known as the *ring of Waldeyer* (Fig. 1.5). The ring includes masses of lymphoid tissue or tonsils, including the two large palatine, lingual, eustachian tubal, and nasopharyngeal tonsils.

The nasopharyngeal tonsils are also called the *adenoids*.[13,14] These structures occasionally impede the passage of ETTs, especially if they are infected or enlarged. Specifically, enlarged adenoid tissue may impede passage of a nasotracheal tube or nasal airway or may simply obstruct the nasal airway passages. The

lingual tonsils are located between the base of the tongue and the epiglottis. During routine anesthetic evaluation of the oropharynx, the lingual tonsils are typically not visible. Lingual tonsillar hypertrophy, which is usually asymptomatic, has been reported as a cause of unanticipated difficult intubation and fatal upper airway obstruction.[15] In addition, sepsis originating from one of the numerous lymphoid aggregates may lead to a retropharyngeal or peritonsillar abscess, which poses anesthetic challenges.[6]

Ciliary activity also works to clear trapped nonsoluble particles that are held in an outer mucous layer within the nares. This function is influenced by temperature, viscosity of the mucus, and the osmotic properties of the discharge. The ciliary movement can be negatively affected by many factors, such as viral infections or environmental agents, including air pollution and cigarette smoke. The loss or decrease of ciliary function leads to chronic and recurrent infections and can gradually severely injure the respiratory tract, leading to conditions such as chronic bronchitis, sinusitis, and otitis.[8]

Upper Airway Obstruction

Sedation and Anesthesia

Traditionally, upper airway obstruction in patients who are sedated or anesthetized (without an ETT) or who have altered levels of consciousness for other reasons has been understood to be the result of the tongue falling back onto the posterior pharyngeal wall. Specifically, a reduction in genioglossus muscle activity leads to posterior displacement of the tongue with subsequent obstruction.[16]

However, a number of publications offer a different explanation. The velopharyngeal segment of the upper airway adjacent to the soft palate has more recently become the primary focus. This area is particularly prone to collapse and has been found to be the predominant flow-limiting site during sedation and anesthesia,[17] speech disorders, and obstructive sleep apnea (OSA) (Fig. 1.6). Nandi and colleagues, using lateral radiographs in patients under general inhalational anesthesia, showed that obstructive changes in the airway occurred at the level of the soft palate and epiglottis.[18] A magnetic resonance imaging (MRI) study found that patients receiving intravenous sedation for anxiolysis with midazolam had anterior-posterior dimensional changes in the upper airway at the level of the soft palate and epiglottis while sparing the tongue (see Fig. 1.6).[19] In addition, Mathru and colleagues, using MRI to evaluate volunteers receiving propofol anesthesia, found that obstruction occurs at the level of the soft palate and not the tongue.[20] Therefore, it appears that the soft palate and epiglottis may play a more significant role than the tongue in pharyngeal upper airway obstruction.

Obstructive Sleep Apnea

Reduction in the luminal size of the pharynx also serves as a factor in the development of respiratory obstruction in patients with OSA.[21] This problem has been studied with the use of imaging techniques including computed tomography (CT) and MRI, nasopharyngoscopy, fluoroscopy, and acoustic reflection.[22] Structural changes that include tonsillar hypertrophy, retrognathia, and variations in craniofacial structures have been linked to an increased risk of OSA, presumably by increasing upper airway collapsibility. CT and MRI studies in awake subjects have shown increased fatty tissue deposition and submucosal edema in the lateral walls of the pharynx, both of which can narrow the pharyngeal lumen and predispose to obstruction during sleep, when protective neuromuscular mechanisms wane.[23] Obesity, the most

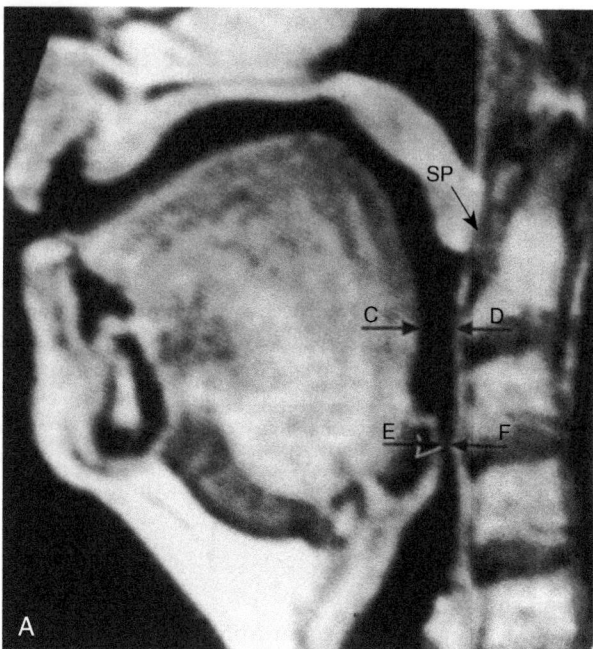

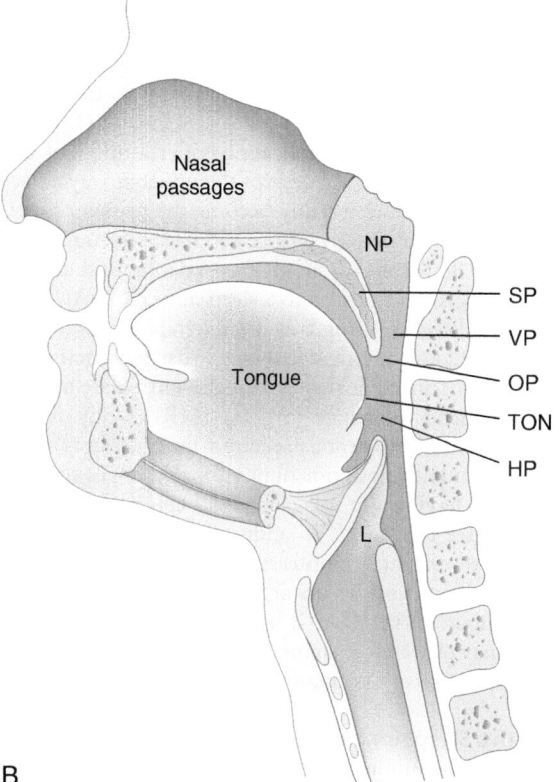

• **Fig. 1.6** (A) Medial sagittal magnetic resonance image of the upper airway showing site of airway obstruction in sedated patients. In the obstructed state, the soft palate *(SP)* is in contact with the posterior pharyngeal wall. *(C–D)* Minimum anteroposterior diameter at level of tongue; *(E–F)* minimum anteroposterior diameter at level of epiglottis. (B) The velopharynx *(VP)* and its relation to the soft palate *(SP)*, nasopharynx *(NP)*, oropharynx *(OP)*, tonsil *(TON)*, hypopharynx *(HP)*, and larynx *(L)*. (From Shorten GD, Opie NJ, Graziotti P, et al. Assessment of upper airway anatomy in awake, sedated and anaesthetized patients using magnetic resonance imaging. *Anaesth Intensive Care.* 1994;22:165.)

common risk factor for OSA, has been shown to increase pharyngeal collapsibility through reductions in lung volumes, particularly decreases in functional residual capacity (FRC), which are accentuated with the onset of sleep. A decrease in FRC may increase pharyngeal collapsibility by reduction of tracheal traction on the pharyngeal segment.[23,24]

The subatmospheric intraairway pressure created by contraction of the diaphragm against the resistance of the nose can lead to a reduction in size of the pharyngeal airway. The collapsible segments of the pharynx are divided into three areas: retropalatal, retroglossal, and retroepiglottic. In awake male patients with OSA, CT revealed a reduced airway caliber at all levels of the pharynx when compared with normal patients, with the narrowest portion posterior to the soft palate.[25] Patency depends on the contractile function of pharyngeal dilator muscles in these segments. The muscles involved are the tensor veli palatini, which retracts the soft palate away from the posterior pharyngeal wall; the genioglossus, which moves the tongue anteriorly; and the muscles that move the hyoid bone forward, including the geniohyoid, sternohyoid, and thyrohyoid muscles.[23,26] In the awake state, genioglossal and tensor veli palatini muscle activity has been observed to be elevated in OSA patients when compared to normal subjects. Observations such as these suggest that increased upper airway dilator muscle activity compensates for a more anatomically narrow upper airway in OSA. Consequently, the reduction in upper airway muscle activity during sleep has been implicated in an increased likelihood of upper airway obstruction in patients with OSA compared with healthy subjects.[23,24]

Studies also show that the configuration of the airway may differ in patients with OSA. Normally, the longer axis of the pharyngeal airway is transverse; however, in OSA patients the anteriorposterior axis is predominant. This orientation may be less efficient and affect upper airway muscle function. Continuous positive airway pressure (CPAP) has been found to be effective in treating airway obstruction in these patients. The application of CPAP appears to increase the volume and cross-sectional area of the oropharynx, especially in the lateral axis.[27] Upper body elevation can improve respiratory mechanics and reduce the risk of OSA.[28]

The velopharynx, an area of the pharynx adjacent to the soft palate, has assumed an increased importance in the understanding of OSA, speech disorders, and airway obstruction under anesthesia (see Fig. 1.6B).[29] Flexible nasoendoscopy and MRI are recommended for studying velopharyngeal dysfunction.[29–31] Six skeletal muscles—the tensor veli palatini, levator veli palatini, musculus uvulae, palatoglossus, palatopharyngeus, and superior pharyngeal constrictor—help form the so-called velopharyngeal sphincter. The proper function of the sphincter is vital to opening and closing of the nasal passages to airflow during deglutition and normal breathing. Recent air pressure measurement studies during sleep have confirmed the velopharynx as the site of significant obstruction in OSA patients.[32]

The same anatomic characteristics associated with OSA can make direct laryngoscopy and intubation more difficult. Patients with a history of severe OSA have a 16% incidence of difficult intubation compared with a 3% risk in the control group.[33]

Larynx

Structure

The larynx, which lies in the adult neck opposite the third through sixth cervical vertebrae,[12] sits at the crossroads between the food and air passages (or conduits) and consists of cartilages forming

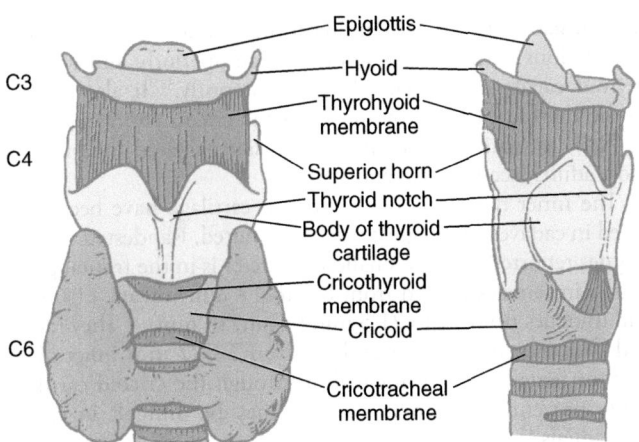

• **Fig. 1.7** External frontal *(left)* and anterolateral *(right)* views of the larynx. Notice the location of the cricothyroid membrane and thyroid gland in relation to the thyroid and cricoid cartilages in the frontal view. The horn of the thyroid cartilage is also known as the *cornu*. In the anterolateral view, the shape of the cricoid cartilage and its relation to thyroid cartilage are shown. (Modified from Ellis H, Feldman S. *Anatomy for Anaesthetists*. 6th ed. Blackwell Scientific; 1993.)

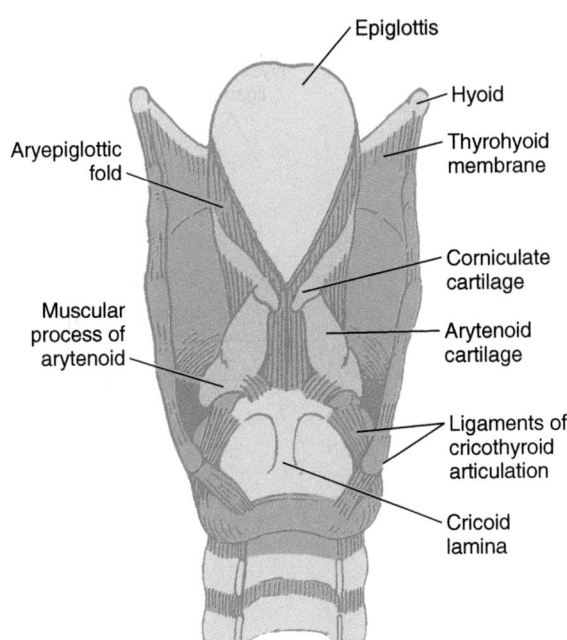

• **Fig. 1.8** Cartilages and ligaments of the larynx seen posteriorly. Notice the location of the corniculate cartilage within the aryepiglottic fold. (Modified from Ellis H, Feldman S. *Anatomy for Anaesthetists*. 6th ed. Blackwell Scientific; 1993.)

the skeletal framework, along with ligaments, membranes, and muscles. The larynx may be located somewhat higher in females and children. Until puberty, no differences in laryngeal size exist between males and females. At puberty, the larynx develops more rapidly in males than in females, almost doubling in the anteroposterior diameter. The female larynx is smaller and more cephalad.[12] The average measurements of the length, transverse diameter, and sagittal diameter of the adult larynx are 44, 36, and 43 mm, respectively, in the male and 41, 36, and 26 mm, respectively, in the female.[34] Most larynxes develop somewhat asymmetrically.[35] The inlet to the larynx is bounded anteriorly by the upper edge of the epiglottis, posteriorly by a fold of mucous membrane stretched between the two arytenoid cartilages, and laterally by the aryepiglottic folds.[10]

Bones of the Larynx

The hyoid bone (Fig. 1.7) participates in the function of speech, respiration, mastication, and swallowing, as well as maintaining the patency of the airway between the oropharynx and the tracheal rings.[36] The hyoid bone suspends and anchors the larynx during respiratory and phonatory movement. Stabilization of the hyoid is important for patency of the airway, serving as a buttress to provide attachment for the anterior neck musculature.[36] With a unique U-shape, the bone derives its name from the Greek word *hyoeides*, meaning "shaped like the letter upsilon." The hyoid bone has a body, 2.5 cm wide by 1 cm thick, and greater and lesser horns (cornua). The hyoid does not articulate with any other bone. It is attached to the styloid processes of the temporal bones by the stylohyoid ligament and to the thyroid cartilage by the thyrohyoid membrane and muscle. Intrinsic tongue muscles originate on the hyoid, and the pharyngeal constrictors are also attached there.[3,12,37]

Cartilages of the Larynx

Nine cartilages provide the framework of the larynx (Fig. 1.8; see also Fig. 1.7). These are the unpaired thyroid, cricoid, and epiglottis and the paired arytenoids, corniculates, and cuneiforms. They are connected and supported by membranes, synovial joints, and ligaments. The ligaments, when covered by mucous membranes,

are called *folds*. The thyroid, cricoid, and arytenoid cartilages consist of hyaline cartilage, whereas the other cartilages are elastic cartilage. Hyaline cartilage tends to ossify in the adult beginning around age 25 and is completely converted into bone by age 65; this process occurs earlier in men than in women.[8]

Thyroid Cartilage. The thyroid cartilage, the longest laryngeal cartilage and the largest structure in the larynx, acquires its shieldlike shape from the embryologic midline fusion of the two distinct quadrilateral laminae.[38] In females, the sides join at an angle of approximately 120 degrees; in males, the angle is closer to 90 degrees. This smaller thyroid angle explains the greater laryngeal prominence ("Adam's apple"), longer vocal cords (anterior-posterior axis), and, thus, lower pitched voice in males.[39] The thyroid notch lies in the midline at the top of the fusion site of the two laminae.[40] On the inner side of this fusion line are attached the vestibular ligaments and, below them, the vocal ligaments (Fig. 1.9). The superior (greater) and inferior (lesser) cornua of the thyroid are slender, posteriorly directed extensions of the edges of the lamina. The lateral thyrohyoid ligament attaches the superior cornu to the hyoid bone, and the cricoid cartilage articulates with the inferior cornu at the cricothyroid joint. The movements of this joint are rotatory and gliding, resulting in changes in vocal cord length.

Cricoid Cartilage. The cricoid cartilage represents the anatomic lower limit of the larynx and helps support it (see Fig. 1.9).[38] The name *cricoid* is derived from the Greek words *krikos* and *eidos*, meaning "shaped like a ring," and has been described as having a signet-ring shape. The cricoid is thicker and stronger than the thyroid cartilage and represents the only complete cartilaginous ring in the airway. For this reason, cautious downward pressure (30 N) on the cricoid cartilage to occlude the esophagus to try to prevent passive regurgitation is possible without subsequent airway obstruction.[41] Traditionally, it has been thought that the pediatric airway was narrowest at the level of the cricoid, and recommendations for ETT size were made based on the size of the cricoid ring. However,

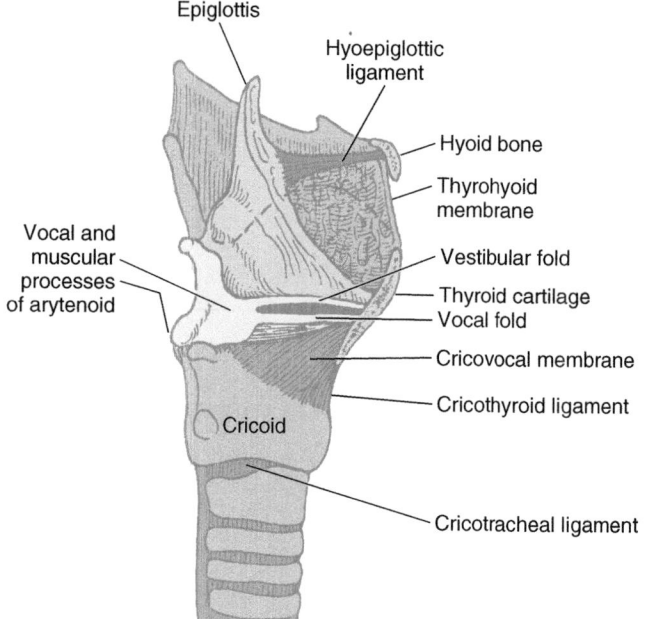

Epiglottis

Hyoepiglottic ligament

Hyoid bone

Thyrohyoid membrane

Vocal and muscular processes of arytenoid

Vestibular fold

Thyroid cartilage

Vocal fold

Cricovocal membrane

Cricothyroid ligament

Cricoid

Cricotracheal ligament

• **Fig. 1.9** Sagittal (lateral) view of the larynx. The vocal and vestibular folds and the thyroepiglottic ligament attach to the midline of the inner surface of the thyroid cartilage. Also note the relationship between the cricovocal membrane (conus elasticus) and the vocal folds. (Modified from Ellis H, Feldman S. *Anatomy for Anaesthetists*. 6th ed. Blackwell Scientific; 1993.)

and muscles. The cricoid lamina forms ball-and-socket synovial articulations with the arytenoids posterosuperiorly and with the thyroid cartilage inferolaterally and anteriorly.[38] It also attaches to the thyroid cartilage by means of the cricothyroid membrane (CTM), a relatively avascular and easily palpated landmark in most adults (see Figs. 1.8 and 1.9).

The inner diameters of the cricoid cartilage have been measured in cadavers, with great variability noted. Randestad and colleagues reported that the smallest diameter is in the frontal plane, which in females ranged from 8.9 to 17 mm (mean, 11.6 mm) and in males from 11 to 21.5 mm (mean, 15 mm).[45] They identified that placement of a standard-size ETT (7 mm inner diameter for females, 8 mm for males) through the cricoid cartilage, while preventing mucosal necrosis, may be difficult in certain individuals.[45]

The CTM represents an important identifiable landmark, providing access to the airway by percutaneous or surgical cricothyrotomy. The dimensions of the CTM have been identified in cadaveric specimens.[46–48] However, the actual methods of obtaining the anatomic measurements varied, making comparisons difficult to interpret. Caparosa and Zavatsky described the CTM as a trapezoid with a width ranging from 27 to 32 mm, representing the actual anatomic limit of the membrane, and a height of 5 to 12 mm.[47] Bennett and colleagues reported the width as 9 to 19 mm and the height as 8 to 19 mm, whereas Dover and colleagues reported a width of 6 to 11 mm and a height of 7.5 to 13 mm, using the distance between the cricothyroid muscles as their horizontal limit. The width and height of the membrane are reported to be smaller in females than in males.[9,50]

Anteriorly, vascular structures overlie the membrane and pose a risk of hemorrhage.[46,48,49] Cadaveric studies have reported the presence of a transverse cricothyroid artery, a branch of the superior thyroid artery, traversing the upper half of the membrane. Therefore, a transverse incision in the lower third of the membrane is recommended. The superior thyroid artery courses along the lateral edge of the membrane, and various branches of the

studies using video bronchoscopy in anesthetized and paralyzed infants have shown that the glottic opening may be narrower than the cricoid region.[42] Therefore, an ETT may cause more damage to the vocal cords than to the subglottic area. Prolonged or excessively large ETT use may cause subglottic stenosis (Fig 1.10).[43,44]

The lamina, the bulky portion of the cricoid, is located posteriorly. The tracheal rings are connected to the cricoid by ligaments

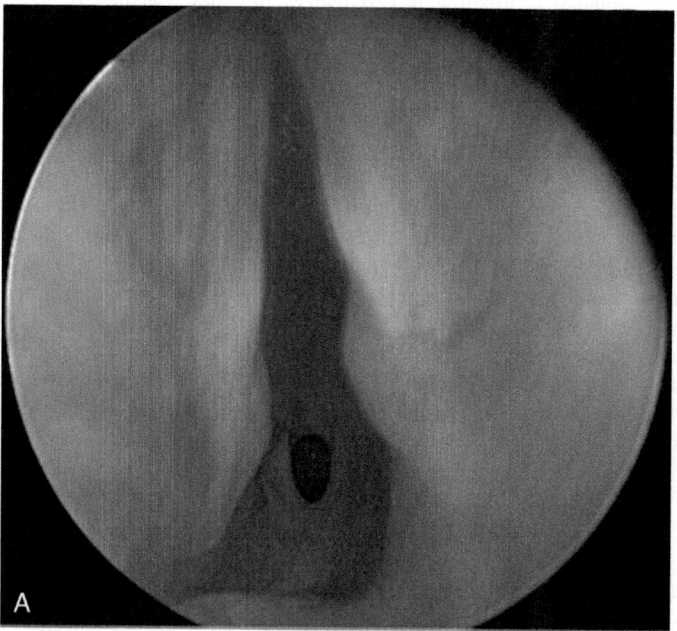

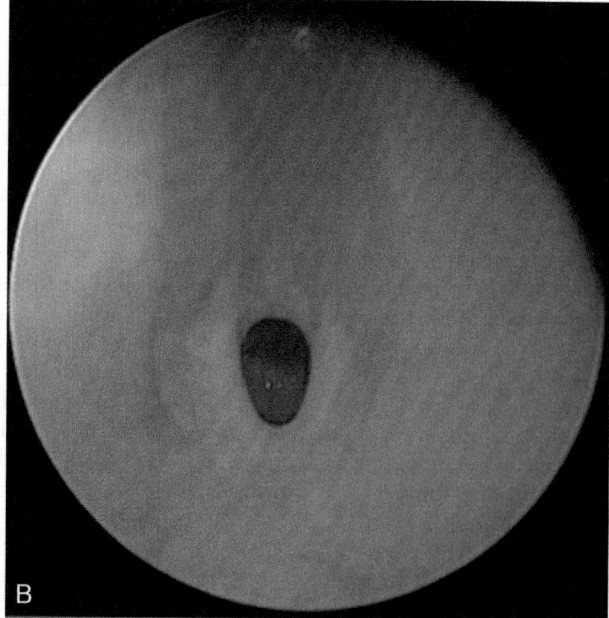

• **Fig 1.10** Direct laryngoscopic view of grade III subglottic stenosis. (A) Glottis and subglottis. (B) Zoomed-in view of the subglottic stenosis. (From Marston AP, White DR. Subglottic stenosis. *Clin Perinatol.* 2018;45:787–804.)

superior and inferior thyroid veins and the jugular veins are also reported to traverse the membrane.

Arytenoids. The two arytenoid cartilages (see Fig. 1.8) are shaped like three-sided pyramids, and they lie in the posterior aspect of the larynx.[50] The arytenoid's medial surface is flat and is covered with only a firm, tight layer of mucoperichondrium.[50,51] The base of the arytenoid is concave and articulates by a true diarthrodial joint with the superior lateral aspect of the posterior lamina of the cricoid cartilage. It is described as a ball-and-socket with three movements—rocking or rotating, gliding, and pivoting—that control adduction and abduction of the vocal cords. All such synovial joints can be affected by rheumatoid arthritis. Cricoarytenoid arthritis is present in the majority of patients with rheumatoid arthritis and can cause life-threatening upper airway obstruction.[52] Cricoarytenoid arthropathy has also been reported as a rare but potentially fatal cause of acute upper airway obstruction in patients with systemic lupus erythematosus.[53]

The lateral extension of the arytenoid base is called the *muscular process*. Important intrinsic laryngeal muscles, the lateral and posterior cricoarytenoids, originate here. The medial extension of the arytenoid base is called the *vocal process*. Vocal ligaments, the bases of the true vocal folds, extend from the vocal process to the midline of the inner surface of the thyroid lamina (see Fig. 1.9). The fibrous membrane that connects the vocal ligament to the thyroid cartilage actually penetrates the body of the thyroid. This membrane is called *Broyles' ligament*. This ligament contains lymphatics and blood vessels and therefore can act as an avenue for extension of laryngeal cancer outside the larynx.[38,54] The relationship between the anterior commissure of the larynx and the inner aspect of the thyroid cartilage is important to otolaryngologists, who perform thyroplasties and supraglottic laryngectomies on the basis of its location. A study of cadavers reported that the anterior commissure of the larynx can usually be found above the midpoint of the vertical midline fusion of the thyroid cartilage ala.[51,55]

Epiglottis. The epiglottis is considered to be vestigial by many authorities.[56] Composed primarily of fibroelastic cartilage, the epiglottis does not ossify and maintains some flexibility throughout life.[38,50,57] It is shaped like a leaf and is found between the larynx and the base of the tongue (see Figs. 1.8 and 1.9).[37,51] The anterior surface of the epiglottis is concave, and this, in combination with laryngeal elevation, aids in airway protection during deglutition.[1] In approximately 1% of the population, the tip and posterior aspect of the epiglottis are visible during a pharyngoscopic view with the mouth opened and tongue protruded; this does not always predict ease of intubation.[58] The upper border of the epiglottis is attached by its narrow tip or petiole to the midline of the thyroid cartilage by the thyroepiglottic ligament (see Fig. 1.9). The hyoepiglottic ligament connects the epiglottis to the back of the body of the hyoid bone.[37,59] The mucous membrane that covers the anterior aspect of the epiglottis sweeps forward to the tongue as the median glossoepiglottic fold and to the pharynx as the paired lateral pharyngoepiglottic folds.[38] In laryngomalacia—the leading cause of stridor in infants affecting 45% to 75% of all infants with congenital stridor—supraglottic tissue collapses onto the glottis during inspiration. Treatment involves surgical excision of the redundant epiglottic tissue.[60] The pouchlike areas found between the median and lateral folds are the valleculae (Fig. 1.11). The tip of a properly placed Macintosh laryngoscope blade rests in this area. The vallecula is a common site of impaction of foreign bodies, such as fish bones, in the upper airway.

The introduction of advanced scanning techniques using contrast-enhanced multidetector computed tomography (MDCT)

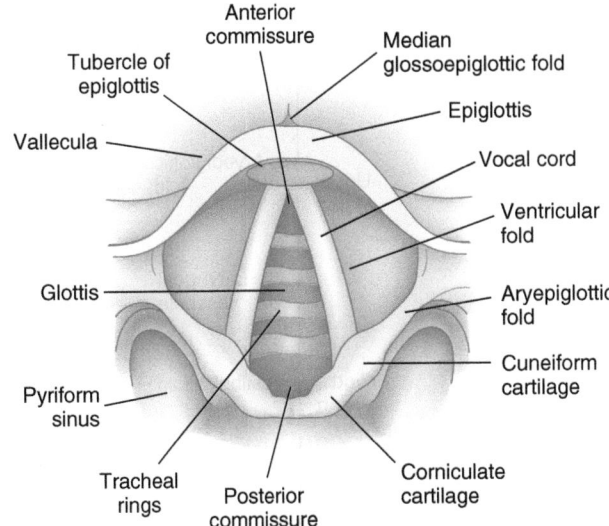

• **Fig. 1.11** Larynx as visualized from the hypopharynx. Note the location of the anterior and posterior commissures of the larynx and the aryepiglottic fold. Elevations in the aryepiglottic folds are the cuneiform cartilages. (Modified from Tucker HM. Anatomy of the Larynx. In Tucker HM, ed. *The Larynx.* 2nd ed. Thieme Medical; 1993:9.)

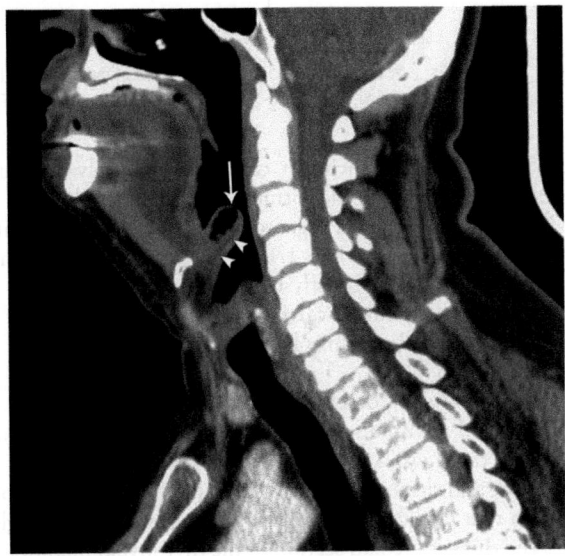

• **Fig. 1.12** Acute epiglottitis with epiglottic abscess formation. Sagittal section of enhanced computed tomography showing an enlarged epiglottis that contains air *(arrow)* anterior to the epiglottic cartilage *(double arrowhead)*. (From Hindy J, Novoa R, Slovik Y, et al. Epiglottic abscess as a complication of acute epiglottitis. *Am J Otolaryngol.* 2013;34:362–365.)

has enabled three-dimensional (3-D) and four-dimensional (4-D) visualization of larger airways. Images of normal and diseased structures can be generated by using special postprocedure CT virtual endoscopy computer software. The presence of air-filled lumens of the upper airways makes it possible for technical staff to build high-quality endoscopy-like images. Similar techniques have been applied to lower airways also. A virtual endoscopic picture of acute epiglottitis can be seen in Fig. 1.12.[61]

Cuneiform and Corniculate Cartilages. The epiglottis is connected to the arytenoid cartilages by the laterally placed aryepiglottic ligaments and folds (see Figs. 1.8 and 1.11). Two sets of paired fibroelastic cartilages are embedded in each aryepiglottic

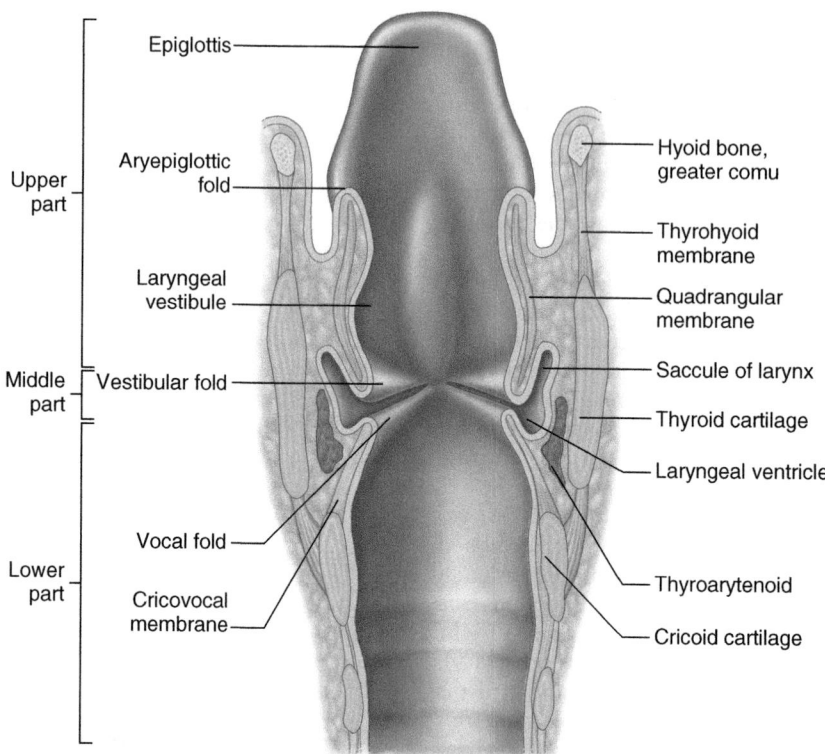

• **Fig. 1.13** Coronal view of the larynx. Note the location of the vestibule, ventricle, and saccule. (Modified from Standring S. *Gray's Anatomy*. 39th ed. Philadelphia: Elsevier; 2005. Fig. 36.9.)

fold.[50] The sesamoid cuneiform cartilage is roughly cylindrical and lies anterosuperior to the corniculate cartilage in the fold. The cuneiform may be seen laryngoscopically as a whitish elevation through the mucosa (see Fig. 1.11). The corniculate is a small, triangular object visible directly over the arytenoid cartilage. The cuneiform and corniculate cartilages reinforce and support the aryepiglottic folds[38,51] and may help the arytenoids move.[12,57]

False and True Vocal Cords

The thyrohyoid membrane (see Figs. 1.7–1.9), attaching the superior edge of the thyroid cartilage to the hyoid bone, provides cranial support and suspension.[12] It is separated from the hyoid body by a bursa that facilitates movement of the larynx during deglutition.[51] The thicker median section of the thyrohyoid membrane is the thyrohyoid ligament, and its thinner lateral edges are pierced by the internal branches of the superior laryngeal nerves.

Beneath the laryngeal mucosa is a fibrous layer containing many elastic fibers, known as the *fibroelastic membrane* of the larynx. Its upper area, the quadrangular membrane, extends in the aryepiglottic fold between the arytenoids and the epiglottis. The lower free border of the membrane is called the *vestibular ligament*; it forms the vestibular folds, or false cords (see Figs. 1.9 and 1.11).[37,39,52]

The CTM joins the cricoid and thyroid cartilages. The thickened median area of this fibrous tissue is the cricothyroid ligament. Laterally, the conus elasticus (or cricovocal membrane) extends up inside the thyroid lamina to the anterior commissure where its free edge thickens to form the vocal ligament. The vocal ligaments, which extend from the vocal processes of the arytenoids to the inner surface of the thyroid cartilage, form the base of the vocal folds, or true vocal cords (see Fig. 1.11).[12,51] The CTM thus connects the cricoid, thyroid, and arytenoid cartilages.[39,52]

Laryngeal Cavity

The laryngeal cavity extends from the laryngeal inlet to the lower border of the cricoid cartilage (Fig. 1.13). When it is viewed laryngoscopically from above, two paired inward projections of tissue are visible in the laryngeal cavity: the superiorly placed vestibular folds, or false cords, and the more inferiorly placed vocal folds, or true vocal cords (see Fig. 1.11). The space between the true cords is called the *rima glottidis*, or the *glottis* (see Fig. 1.12). The glottis is divided into two parts. The anterior intermembranous section is situated between the two vocal folds. The two vocal folds meet at the anterior commissure of the larynx (see Fig. 1.11). The posterior intercartilaginous part passes between the two arytenoid cartilages and the mucosa, stretching between them in the midline posteriorly, forming the posterior commissure of the larynx (see Fig. 1.11).[39] The width and shape of the glottis change with the movements of the vocal folds and arytenoid cartilages during phonation and respiration; however, in the resting state when the structures are uninfluenced by muscular action, such as in quiet respiration, the vocal processes are approximately 8 mm apart. The space extending from the laryngeal inlet down to the vestibular folds is known as the *vestibule* or *supraglottic larynx* (see Fig. 1.13). The laryngeal space from the free border of the cords to the cricoid cartilage is called the *subglottic* or *infraglottic larynx*.

On the basis of cadaver studies, measurements of the subglottis have been characterized.[46,62,63] Understanding the anatomic relationships between the cricothyroid space and the vocal folds is important to minimize complications from cricothyrotomy (Fig. 1.14).[64] Bennett and colleagues reported this distance to be 9.78 mm.[46] The fossa between the vestibular folds and the glottis is termed the *ventricle* or the *sinus* (see Fig. 1.13). The ventricle expands anterolaterally to a pouchlike area called the *laryngeal saccule* (see Fig. 1.13).[38] The saccule contains many lubricating glands

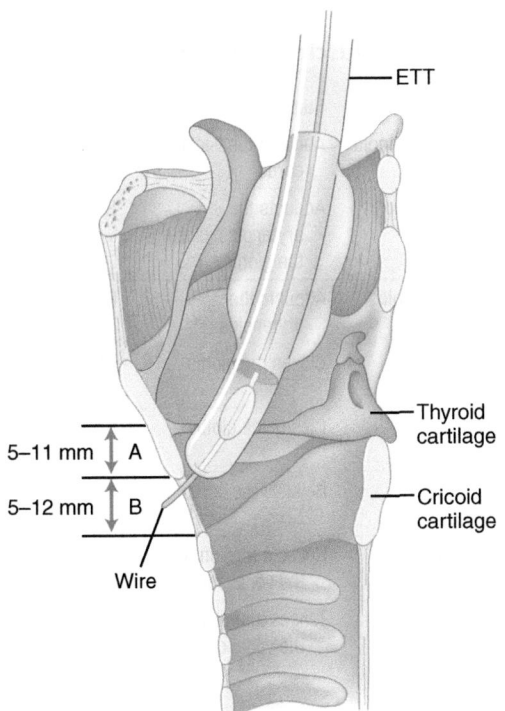

ETT

5–11 mm — A
5–12 mm — B

Wire

Thyroid cartilage

Cricoid cartilage

• **Fig. 1.14** Illustration showing the relationships of the larynx, thyroid, and cricoid cartilages, including the distance (range) from the vocal cords to the anteroinferior edge of the thyroid cartilage (A) and the distance (range) from the anteroinferior edge of the thyroid cartilage to the anterosuperior edge of the cricoid cartilage (B). Also shown is the wire penetrating the cricothyroid membrane for retrograde intubation. *ETT*, Endotracheal tube.
• (From Kuriloff DB, Setzen M, Portnoy W. Laryngotracheal injury following cricothyroidotomy. *Laryngoscope.* 1989;99:125.)

TABLE 1.1 Extrinsic Muscles of the Larynx

Muscle	Function	Innervation
Sternohyoid	Indirect depressor of the larynx	Cervical plexus (C1–C3) Ansa cervicalis
Sternothyroid	Depresses the larynx Modifies the thyrohyoid and aryepiglottic folds	Cervical plexus (C1–C3) Ansa cervicalis
Thyrohyoid	Depresses the larynx Modifies the thyrohyoid and aryepiglottic folds	Cervical plexus (C1) via the hypoglossal nerve
Thyroepiglottic	Mucosal inversion of aryepiglottic fold	Recurrent laryngeal nerve
Stylopharyngeus	Assists folding of thyroid cartilage	Glossopharyngeal nerve
Inferior pharyngeal constrictor	Assists in swallowing	Pharyngeal plexus of the vagus nerve

muscles are the stylohyoid, geniohyoid, mylohyoid, thyrohyoid, digastric, and stylopharyngeus muscles. The infrahyoid muscle group includes the omohyoid, sternothyroid, thyrohyoid, and sternohyoid muscles. These "strap" muscles, in addition to lowering the larynx, can modify the internal relationship of laryngeal cartilages and folds to one another. The inferior constrictor of the pharynx primarily assists in deglutition (Table 1.1).[12,38-40] The function and innervation of the extrinsic muscles are summarized in Table 1.1.

Intrinsic Muscles of the Larynx. The function of the intrinsic musculature is threefold: (1) to close the cords and the laryngeal inlet during deglutition, (2) to open the vocal cords during inspiration, and (3) to alter the tension of the cords during phonation.[12,38,51] The larynx can close at three levels: (1) the aryepiglottic folds by contraction of the aryepiglottic and oblique arytenoid muscles, (2) the false vocal cords by action of the lateral thyroarytenoid muscles, and (3) the true vocal cords by contraction of the cricothyroid, lateral cricoarytenoid, and interarytenoid muscles (Fig. 1.15). The interarytenoid muscles are comprised of the transverse arytenoid and oblique arytenoid muscles. All of the intrinsic muscles of the larynx, except for the transverse arytenoid muscle, are paired.[12]

The cricothyroid muscle has been considered to be both an extrinsic and an intrinsic muscle of the larynx because its actions affect both laryngeal movement and the glottic structures. The paired cricothyroid muscles join the cricoid cartilage and the thyroid cartilage and are the only intrinsic muscles found external to the larynx itself (Fig. 1.16). The muscle has two parts: a larger, ventral section runs vertically between the cricoid and the inferior thyroid border, while the smaller, oblique segment attaches to the posterior inner thyroid border and the lesser cornu of the thyroid. During swallowing, the muscle contracts and the ventral head draws the anterior part of the cricoid cartilage toward the relatively fixed lower border of the thyroid cartilage. The oblique head of the muscle rocks the cricoid lamina posteriorly. Because the arytenoids do not move, the vocal ligaments are tensed and the glottic length is increased 30%.[51,65]

The thick posterior cricoarytenoid muscle originates near the entire posterior midline of the cricoid cartilage. Muscle fibers run superiorly and laterally to the posterior area of the muscular

and is believed to help in voice resonance in apes.[51,56] The pyriform sinus lies laterally to the aryepiglottic fold within the inner surface of the thyroid cartilage (see Fig. 1.11).[51]

The epithelium of the vestibular folds is of the ciliated pseudostratified variety (respiratory), whereas the epithelium of the vocal folds is of the nonkeratinized squamous type.[40] Therefore, the entire interior of the larynx is covered with respiratory epithelium, except for the vocal folds.[10]

The orientation of the true and false cords helps prevent aspiration and enhance airway protection. The false cords are directed inferiorly at their free border. This position can help to stop the egress of air during a Valsalva maneuver. The true cords are oriented slightly superiorly (see Fig. 1.11). This prevents air or matter from entering the lungs. Great pressure is required to separate adducted true cords.[57] Air trapped in the ventricle during closure pushes the false cords and the true cords more tightly together.[15,40,57]

Muscles of the Larynx

The complex and delicate functions of the larynx are made possible by an intricate group of small muscles. These muscles can be divided into extrinsic and intrinsic groups.[56,59] The extrinsic group connects the larynx with its anatomic neighbors, such as the hyoid bone, and modifies the position and movement of the larynx. The intrinsic group facilitates the movements of the laryngeal cartilages against one another and directly affects glottic movement.

Extrinsic Muscles of the Larynx. The suprahyoid muscles attach the larynx to the hyoid bone and elevate the larynx. These

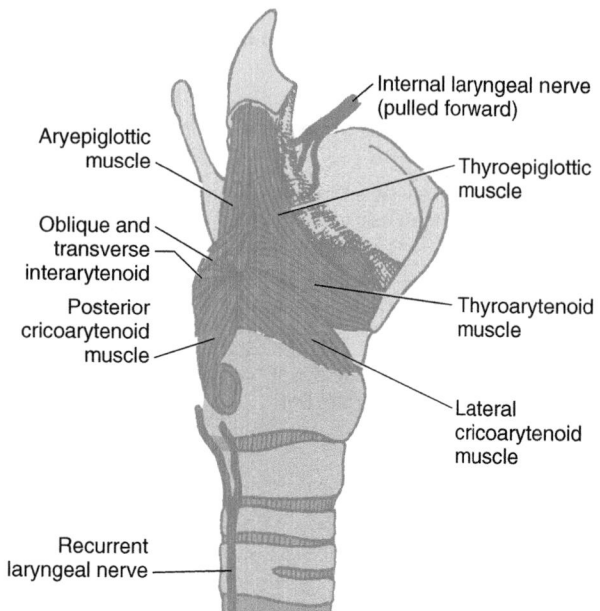

• **Fig. 1.15** Intrinsic muscles of the larynx and their nerve supply. (Modified from Ellis H, Feldman S. *Anatomy for Anaesthetists*. 6th ed. Blackwell Scientific; 1993.)

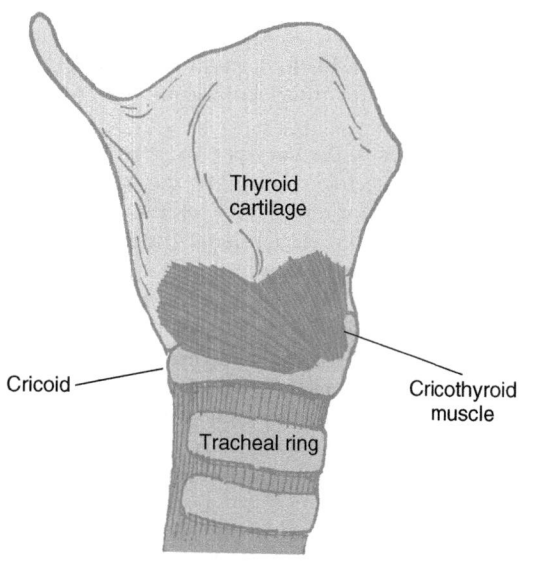

• **Fig. 1.16** The cricothyroid muscle and its attachments. (Modified from Ellis H, Feldman S. *Anatomy for Anaesthetists*. 6th ed. Blackwell Scientific; 1993.)

TABLE 1.2 Intrinsic Muscles of the Larynx

Muscle	Function	Innervation
Posterior cricoarytenoid	Abducts the vocal cords	Recurrent laryngeal nerve
Lateral cricoarytenoid	Adducts the arytenoids, closing the glottis	Recurrent laryngeal nerve
Transverse arytenoid	Adducts the arytenoids	Recurrent laryngeal nerve
Oblique arytenoid	Closes the glottis	Recurrent laryngeal nerve
Aryepiglottic	Closes the glottis	Recurrent laryngeal nerve
Vocalis	Relaxes the cords	Recurrent laryngeal nerve
Thyroarytenoid	Relaxes tension on the vocal cords	Recurrent laryngeal nerve
Cricothyroid	Tenses and elongates the vocal cords	Superior laryngeal (external branch)

process of the arytenoid cartilage.[20] Upon contraction, the posterior cricoarytenoid rotates the arytenoids and moves the vocal folds laterally. The posterior cricoarytenoid is the only true abductor of the vocal folds.[39,50,51,57]

The lateral cricoarytenoid muscle joins the superior border of the lateral cricoid cartilage and the muscular process of the arytenoid. This muscle rotates the arytenoids medially, adducting the true vocal cords.[38] The unpaired transverse arytenoid muscle joins the posterolateral aspects of the arytenoids. This muscle, which is covered anteriorly by a mucous membrane, forms the posterior commissure of the larynx. Its contraction brings the arytenoids together and ensures posterior adduction of the glottis.[38,39,50]

The oblique arytenoids ascend diagonally from the muscular processes posteriorly across the cartilage to the opposite superior arytenoid and help close the glottis (see Fig. 1.15). Fibers of the oblique arytenoid may continue from the apex through the aryepiglottic fold as the aryepiglottic muscle, which attaches itself to the lateral aspect of the epiglottis. The aryepiglottic muscle and the oblique arytenoid act as a purse-string sphincter during deglutition.[51]

The thyroarytenoid muscle is broad and sometimes is divided into three parts (see Fig. 1.15). It is among the fastest-contracting striated muscles.[57] The muscle arises along the entire lower border of the thyroid cartilage. It passes posteriorly, superiorly, and laterally to attach to the anterolateral surface and the vocal process of the arytenoid. The segment of thyroarytenoid muscle that lies adjacent to the vocal ligament (and frequently surrounds it) is called the *vocalis muscle*. The vocalis is the major tensor of vocal fold and can "thin" the fold to achieve a high pitch. Beneath the mucosa of the fold, extending from the anterior commissure back to the vocal process is a potential space called *Reinke's space*. This area can become edematous if traumatized. The more laterally attached fibers of the thyroarytenoid function as the principal adductor of the vocal folds.[51] The most lateral section of the muscle, sometimes called the *thyroepiglottic muscle*, attaches to the lateral aspects of the arytenoids, the aryepiglottic fold, and even the epiglottis. When it contracts, the arytenoids are pulled medially, down, and forward.[38,51] This shortens and relaxes the vocal ligament. Table 1.2 summarizes the intrinsic musculature of the larynx.

Blood Supply of the Larynx

Blood supply to the larynx is derived from the external carotid and subclavian arteries. The external carotid gives rise to the superior thyroid artery, which bifurcates, forming the superior laryngeal artery. This artery courses with the superior laryngeal nerve through the thyrohyoid membrane to supply the supraglottic region. The inferior thyroid artery, derived from the thyrocervical trunk of the subclavian artery, terminates as the inferior laryngeal artery. This vessel travels in the tracheoesophageal groove with the recurrent laryngeal nerve and supplies the infraglottic larynx. There are extensive connections with the ipsilateral superior laryngeal artery and across the midline. A small cricothyroid artery may branch from the superior thyroid and cross the CTM. It most commonly travels near the inferior border of the thyroid cartilage, along the upper third of the CTM.[51]

Function

The primary function of the larynx is to serve as the "watchdog" of the respiratory tract, allowing passage only to air and preventing secretions, food, and foreign bodies from entering the trachea. The larynx has the ability to generate a cough and other reflexive actions that help propel any ingested material out from the respiratory tract. In addition, it functions as the organ of phonation. Finally, the larynx can adduct the vocal folds and create a seal that allows for increased intrathoracic and intraabdominal pressures to be generated for coughing or Valsalva maneuvers.

Innervation of the Larynx

The recurrent laryngeal nerves and the internal and external branches of the superior laryngeal nerves function as the main nerves of the larynx. The external branch of the superior laryngeal nerve supplies motor innervation to the cricothyroid muscle, while all the other laryngeal muscles are controlled by the recurrent laryngeal nerve (see Fig. 1.15). The superior laryngeal and recurrent laryngeal nerves are derivatives of the vagus nerve.

The superior laryngeal nerve usually separates from the main trunk of the vagus nerve off the inferior vagal ganglion, just outside the jugular foramen. At approximately the level of the hyoid bone, it divides into the smaller external and larger internal branches. The external branch travels below the superior thyroid artery to the cricothyroid muscle, giving off a branch to the inferior constrictor of the pharynx along the way. The internal branch travels along with the superior laryngeal artery and passes through the thyrohyoid membrane laterally between the greater cornu of the thyroid and the hyoid. The nerve and artery together pass through the pyriform sinus, where the nerve may be anesthetized by spraying local anesthetic intraorally. The internal laryngeal nerve divides almost immediately into a series of sensory branches that provide sensory innervation for the posterior aspect of the base of the tongue, the surfaces of the epiglottis, the aryepiglottic fold, and the mucous membrane over the back of the larynx. Sensory innervation of the epiglottis is dense, and the true vocal cords are more heavily innervated posteriorly than anteriorly.[57]

The left recurrent laryngeal nerve branches from the vagus in the thorax and courses cephalad after hooking around the arch of the aorta in close relation to the ligamentum arteriosum, at approximately the level of the fourth and fifth thoracic vertebrae. On the right, the nerve loops posteriorly beneath the subclavian artery, at approximately the first and second thoracic vertebrae, before following a cephalad course to the larynx. Both nerves ascend the neck in the tracheoesophageal groove before they reach the larynx. The nerves enter the larynx just posterior to, or rarely anterior to, the cricothyroid articulation. The recurrent laryngeal nerve supplies motor function to all the intrinsic muscles of the larynx except the cricothyroid and the sensory innervation to the larynx below the vocal cords. Parasympathetic fibers to the larynx travel along the laryngeal nerves, and sympathetic fibers from the superior cervical ganglion travel to the larynx with blood vessels. Tables 1.1 and 1.2 summarize the innervation of the laryngeal musculature.

Clinical problems can arise from both the exaggeration and the depression of upper airway reflexes. A heightened reflex response can lead to laryngospasm and prolonged paroxysm of cough, whereas depressed reflexes can increase the risk of aspiration and compromised airway.[66]

Glottic Closure and Laryngeal Spasm

Stimulation of the superior laryngeal nerve endings in the supraglottic region can induce protective closure of the glottis. This short-lived phenomenon is a polysynaptic involuntary reflex.[57] The triggering of other nerves, notably cranial nerves such as the trigeminal and glossopharyngeal, can produce a lesser degree of reflex glottic closure.[67,68] The nerve endings in the mammalian supraglottic area are highly sensitive to touch, heat, and chemical stimuli.[69] This sensitivity is particularly intense in the posterior commissure of the larynx, close to where the pyriform recesses merge with the hypopharynx.[69,70] Complex sensory receptors, similar in structure to lingual taste buds, have been demonstrated here.[71] Instillation of water, saline, acids, or bases has been demonstrated to cause glottic closure in vitro and in vivo.[72] Infants also respond to stimulation with prolonged apnea, although this response disappears later in life.[3]

The term *episodic paroxysmal laryngospasm* has been coined to describe laryngeal dysfunction that may or may not arise as a true episode of respiratory distress.[72,73] Postoperative superior laryngeal nerve injury has been reported to cause paroxysmal laryngospasm associated with stridor and acute airway obstruction. Superior laryngeal nerve blockade may be temporarily effective in some patients.[74]

Laryngospasm occurs when glottic closure persists long after removal of the stimulus.[68,70] This has led to speculation that laryngospasm represents a focal seizure of the adductors innervated by the recurrent laryngeal nerve[75] and may be initiated by repeated superior laryngeal nerve stimulation.[68] The recurrent laryngeal nerve may also be responsible for laryngospasm.[76] Symptoms abate, perhaps through a central mechanism, as hypoxia and hypercarbia worsen.[77]

Vocal Cord Palsies

The recurrent laryngeal nerve may be traumatized during surgery on the thyroid and parathyroid glands.[14,78] Trauma, malignancy or benign process of the neck, pressure from an ETT or a supraglottic airway, or stretching of the neck may also affect the nerve.[10,59,64,79] The left recurrent laryngeal nerve may be compressed by neoplasms in the thorax, aneurysm of the aortic arch, or an enlarged left atrium and may occasionally be injured during ligation of a patent ductus arteriosus.[37] The left nerve is twice as likely as the right one to be injured because of its close relationship to many intrathoracic structures. Damage to the external branch of the superior laryngeal nerve is the most common cause of iatrogenic voice change after thyroidectomy.[80]

Under normal circumstances, the vocal cords meet in the midline during phonation (Fig. 1.17). On inspiration, they move away from each other. They return toward the midline on expiration, leaving a small opening between them. When laryngospasm occurs, both the true and false vocal cords lie tightly in the midline opposite each other. To arrive at a clinical diagnosis, the position of the cords must be examined laryngoscopically during phonation and inspiration (Fig. 1.18; see Fig. 1.17).

The recurrent laryngeal nerve carries both abductor and adductor fibers to the vocal cords. The abductor fibers are more vulnerable, and moderate pressure injury or trauma can cause a pure

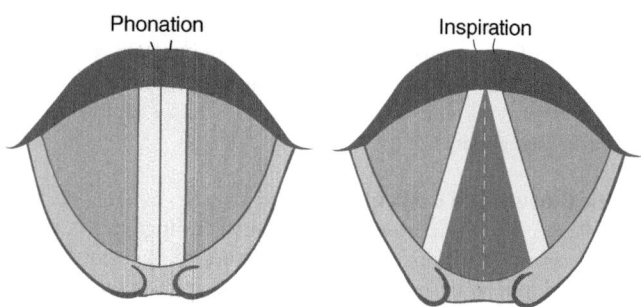

• **Fig. 1.17** Position of the vocal cords during phonation and inspiration. (From Hodder Headline PLC, London.)

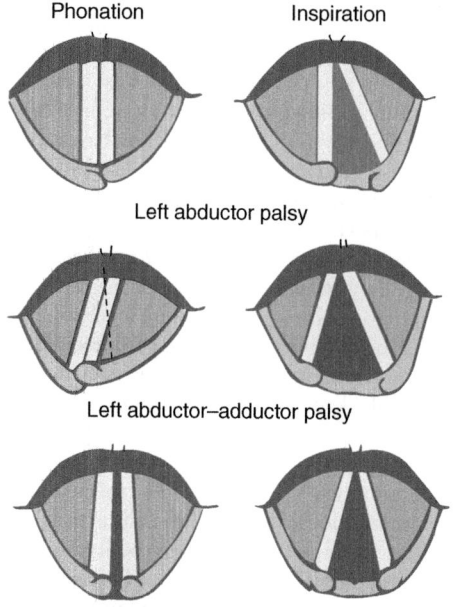

Left abductor palsy

Left abductor–adductor palsy

Bilateral recurrent laryngeal palsy

• **Fig. 1.18** Graphic representation of different types of vocal cord palsies. Notice that in complete bilateral recurrent laryngeal palsy *(bottom)* the vocal cords remain in the abducted position and the glottic opening is preserved. For details see text. (From Hodder Headline PLC, London.)

abductor paralysis (Selmon's law).[81] Severe trauma causes both abductor and adductor fibers to be affected.[10] Pure adductor paralysis does not occur as a clinical entity. In the case of pure unilateral abductor palsy, both cords meet in the midline on phonation (because adduction is still possible on the affected side). However, only the normal cord abducts during inspiration (see Fig. 1.18). In the case of complete unilateral palsy of the recurrent laryngeal nerve, the abductors and adductors are both affected. On phonation, the unaffected cord crosses the midline to meet its paralyzed counterpart, appearing to lie in front of the affected cord (see Fig. 1.18).[10] On inspiration, the unaffected cord moves to full abduction. When abductor fibers are damaged bilaterally (incomplete bilateral damage to the recurrent laryngeal nerve), the adductor fibers draw the cords toward each other, and the glottic opening is reduced to a slit, resulting in severe respiratory distress (see Fig. 1.18).[56,59] However, with a complete palsy, each vocal cord lies midway between abduction and adduction, and a reasonable glottic opening exists. Thus, bilateral incomplete palsy is more dangerous than a complete bilateral palsy.

Damage to the external branch of the superior laryngeal nerve or to the superior laryngeal nerve trunk causes paralysis of

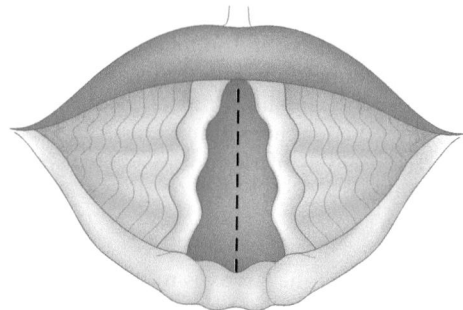

• **Fig. 1.19** Cadaveric position of vocal cords. Notice the wavy appearance of the vocal cords. For details see text. (From Hodder Headline PLC, London.)

the cricothyroid muscle (the tuning fork of the larynx), resulting in hoarseness that improves with time because of increased compensatory action of the opposite muscle. The glottic opening appears oblique during phonation. The aryepiglottic fold on the affected side appears shortened, and the one on the normal side is lengthened. The cords may appear wavy. The symptoms include frequent throat clearing and difficulty in raising the vocal pitch.[65] A complete bilateral paralysis of the vagus nerves affects the recurrent laryngeal nerves and the superior laryngeal nerves. In this condition, the vocal cords assume the open abducted, cadaveric position.[4,10] The vocal cords are relaxed and appear wavy (Fig. 1.19).[10,65] A similar picture may be seen after the use of muscle relaxants.

Topical anesthesia of the larynx may affect the fibers of the external branch of the superior laryngeal nerve and paralyze the cricothyroid muscle, signified by a "gruff" voice. Similarly, a superior laryngeal nerve block may affect the cricothyroid muscle in the same manner as surgical trauma does. These factors must be considered when evaluating postthyroidectomy vocal cord dysfunction after surgery.

Lower Airway

Trachea and Bronchi

Structure

The adult trachea begins at the cricoid cartilage, opposite the sixth cervical vertebra (see Figs. 1.7 and 1.8). It is 10 to 20 cm long and roughly 12 mm in diameter. It is flattened posteriorly and contains 16 to 20 horseshoe-shaped cartilaginous rings; the first and last rings are broader than the rest. Beginning at the sixth ring, the trachea becomes intrathoracic. The lower borders of the last ring split and curve interiorly between the two bronchi to form the carina at the level of the fifth thoracic vertebra (angle of Louis, second intercostal space). The posterior part of the trachea, devoid of cartilage, consists of a membrane of smooth muscle and fibroelastic tissue joining the ends of the cartilages. Fusion of the tracheal cartilages posteriorly is referred to as *stove-pipe trachea* and can present mimicking severe asthma and can lead to difficulty with intubation.[82] The muscle of the trachea is stratified with an inner circular and an outer longitudinal layer. The longitudinal bundles predominate in children but are virtually absent in adults.[50,56] Both the trachea and the proximal airways have extensive submucosal glands beneath the epithelium.[83]

The trachea lengthens during neck extension mainly between the vocal cords and the sternal notch. This explains why an ETT fixed at the mouth ascends on average 2 cm in the trachea with

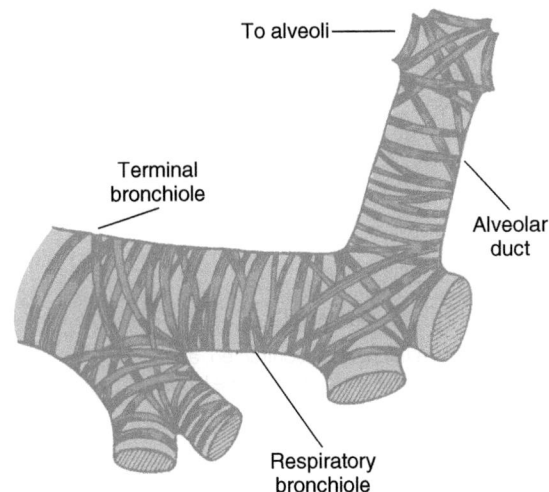

• **Fig. 1.20** Bronchiolar division and geodesic network of muscle layer surrounding the airway. Two smooth muscle spirals run in opposite directions. This arrangement enables the muscles to constrict and shorten the airways at the same time. (Modified from Hodder Headline PLC, London.)

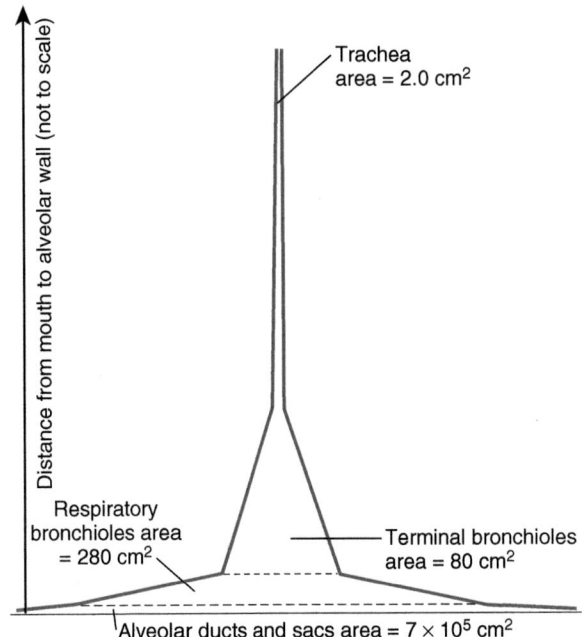

• **Fig. 1.21** Relationship between cross-sectional area and generation of the airway. Notice the abrupt increase in cross-section when the respiratory bronchiole is reached (inverted thumbtack arrangement). For details, see text. (From Hodder Headline PLC, London.)

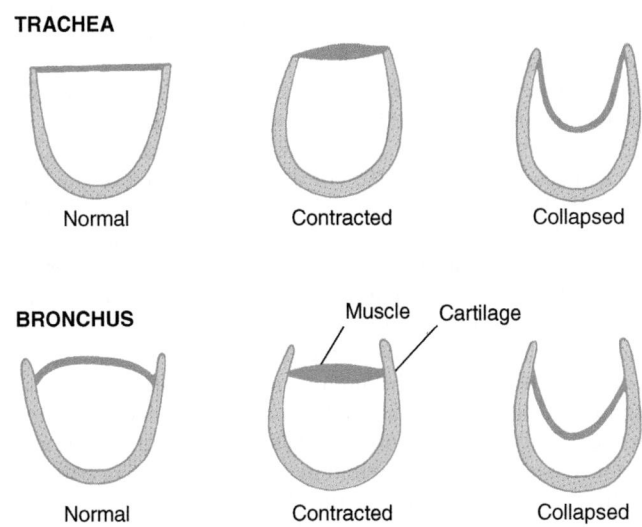

• **Fig. 1.22** Cross-sectional view of trachea and bronchus. Notice the different sites of attachment of the posterior membrane in the tracheal and bronchial sections. Also notice the invagination of the posterior membrane into the lumen in the collapsed state. (From Horsfield K. The relation between structure and function of the airways of the lung. *Br J Dis Chest.* 1974;68:145.)

neck extension.[84] The tip of the tracheal tube moves toward the vocal cords, increasing the chance of accidental extubation. During flexion, an ETT moves approximately 2 cm toward the carina and can enter the mainstem bronchus, depending on the original tube position and the extent of flexion; this occurs in both adults and children.[84–86] Consequently, one should exercise constant vigilance when the neck is moved in intubated patients to detect displacement of the ETT.

In the adult, the right mainstem bronchus is wider and shorter and takes off at a steeper angle than the left mainstem bronchus. Therefore, ETTs, suction catheters, and foreign bodies more readily enter the right bronchial lumen. In children younger than 3 years of age, however, the angulations of the two bronchi are almost equal. The right mainstem bronchus gives rise to three lobar bronchi, and the left to two. Both the main bronchi and the lower lobe bronchi are situated outside the lung parenchyma. The large main bronchi are 7 to 12 mm in diameter; they divide into 20 bronchopulmonary divisions supplying each respective lobule's medium bronchi (4 to 7 mm in diameter) and small bronchi (0.8 to 4 mm in diameter). Bronchioles are bronchi that are smaller than 0.8 mm in diameter, and they do not have any cartilage in their walls.[51] The tracheobronchial airways occupy 1% of the lung volume, with the remaining 99% composed of large vessels and lung parenchyma.[83]

Bronchioles are of two types: terminal and respiratory. The terminal bronchioles do not bear any alveoli and do not have cilia or mucous-producing cells.[87] The terminal bronchioles lead into the alveoli-bearing respiratory bronchioles. Each terminal bronchiole leads to three respiratory bronchioles, and each respiratory bronchiole leads to four generations of alveolar ducts (Fig. 1.20).[51] Although the diameter of each new generation of airway decreases progressively, the aggregate cross-sectional area increases. This is especially true for airways 2 mm or less in diameter, because further branching is not accompanied by concomitant decreases in caliber. The failure of the airway diameter to decrease with subsequent divisions produces the "inverted thumbtack" appearance on a figure depicting increasing surface area as a function of generation of the airway (Fig. 1.21).[6] There are over 300 million alveoli, each lined with pulmonary capillaries, resulting in a net surface area of approximately 70 m² available for blood-gas exchange.[88]

The bronchi are surrounded by irregular cartilaginous rings that are similar in structure to the trachea except that the attachment of the posterior membrane is more anterior (Fig. 1.22).[52] The rings give way to discrete, cartilaginous plates as the bronchi become intrapulmonary at the lung roots (Fig. 1.23). Eventually, even these plates disappear, usually at airway diameters of approximately 0.6 mm.[52]

The rings or plates of the bronchi are interconnected by a strong fibroelastic sheath within which a myoelastic layer consisting of

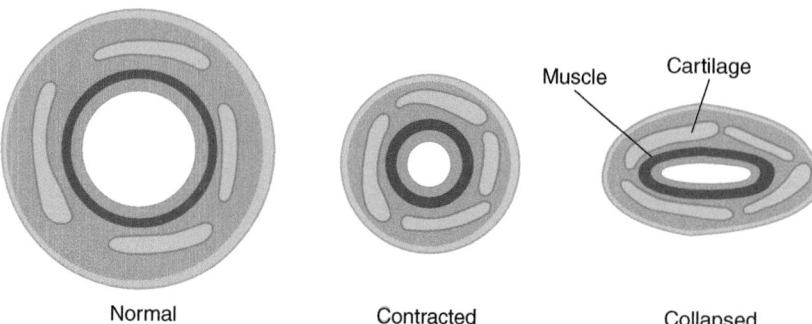

• **Fig. 1.23** Cross-sectional views of medium bronchi (4 to 8 mm diameter) in the normal, contracted, and collapsed states. (From Horsfield K. The relation between structure and function of the airways of the lung. *Br J Dis Chest.* 1974;68:145.)

smooth muscle and elastic tissue is arrayed.[5] The myoelastic band is arranged in a special pattern called a *geodesic network*, representing the shortest distance between two points on a curved surface (see Fig. 1.20). This architectural design serves as the strongest and most effective mechanism for withstanding or generating pressures within a tube without fiber slippage along the length of the outer surface of the tube. The network of smooth muscle runs around the airway in two opposing spirals. This arrangement helps in not only constricting the airway but also shortening it.[89] The primary function of the muscular component is to change the size of the airway according to the respiratory phase. The smooth muscle tone (bronchomotor tone) is predominantly under the influence of the vagus nerve. The elastic layer runs longitudinally but encircles the bronchus at the points of division.[5]

The muscular layer becomes progressively thinner distally, but its thickness relative to the bronchial wall increases. Therefore, the terminal bronchiole with the narrowest lumen has perhaps the thickest muscle at almost 20% of the total thickness of the wall, which lacks cartilaginous support.[51,52] For this reason, smaller bronchioles may be readily closed off by action of the musculature during prolonged bronchial spasm. Such an arrangement may facilitate closure of nonperfused portions of the lung when a ventilation-perfusion mismatch occurs (e.g., pulmonary embolism). The smooth muscles and the glands of the cartilaginous airways are innervated by the autonomic nervous system. They are stimulated by the vagus and inhibited by sympathetic impulses derived from the upper thoracic ganglia. This smooth muscle mass can increase twofold to threefold in patients with severe asthma.[89]

In utero exposure to nicotine has been shown to increase the number of smaller-diameter bronchioles.[90] In mice, cigarette smoke exposure causes a mild inflammatory response and upregulation of genes involved with oxidative stress.[91] With aging, collagen fibers supporting alveolar ducts change, causing alveolar enlargement with reduced alveolar surface tension, leading to greater lung distension.[92] Age and smoking may further alter gene expression, mitochondrial function, and susceptibility to infections in humans.[93] Genetic risk markers have been associated with differences in lung structure, including small airway count and diameter, that are associated with risk of chronic obstructive pulmonary disease (COPD).[94]

Blood Supply

Bronchial arteries supply the bronchi and the bronchioles; the arterial supply extends into the respiratory bronchiole. Arterial anastomoses occur in the adventitia of the bronchiole. The branches enter the submucosa after piercing the muscle layer to form the submucosal capillary plexus. Venules arising from the capillary plexus reach the venous plexus in the adventitia by penetrating the muscle layer. When the muscle layer contracts, the arteries can maintain forward flow to the capillary plexus; however, the capillaries cannot force the blood back into the venous plexus. Therefore, prolonged bronchial spasm can lead to mucous membrane swelling in the small airways.[6] The venous drainage of the bronchi occurs through the bronchial, azygos, hemiazygos, and intercostal veins. Communication between the pulmonary arteries and the bronchiolar capillary plexus leads to normally occurring "anatomic shunting," which typically amounts to approximately 3% of pulmonary blood flow.

Iatrogenic tracheal injury can occur as a complication of prolonged tracheal intubation. The cuff of the ETT, when inflated at a pressure greater than the capillary arterial plexus pressure (typically 10 to 22 mm Hg), can cause tissue ischemia leading to the development of a stricture. This fibrotic narrowing of the trachea usually occurs at the level of the second or third thoracic vertebra and within 3 to 6 weeks after extubation.[95]

Function

Airway Epithelium

The cartilaginous airways are lined by a tall, columnar, pseudostratified epithelium containing at least 13 cell types.[34] This lining produces mucus, an important part of the respiratory defense mechanism. The mucus is steadily propelled toward the outside by the beating of the epithelial cilia, which push mucus and trapped foreign material along like a conveyer belt mechanism. In disease states, mucus clearance may be impaired due to altered cohesive and adhesive properties.[96] Ciliary beating can be depressed by anesthetics and prolonged intubation, leading to an increase in secretions. The large airways have a mucous secretory apparatus that consists of serous and goblet cells and submucosal glands. The submucosal glands empty into secretory tubules, which in turn connect with the larger connecting ducts. Several connecting ducts unite and form the ciliated duct that opens into the airway lumen. No mucous glands are present in the bronchioles.

The most numerous cells of the large airways are the ciliated epithelial cells, which bear 250 cilia per cell.[10,34] The length of the cilia decreases progressively in the smaller airways. On the surface of the cell are found small claws and microvilli. The microvilli probably regulate the volume of secretions through reabsorption, a function that may be shared with the brush cells scattered along the airways. The basal cell, more numerous in the large airways, imparts to the epithelium the pseudostratified appearance. The other cell types, except for the K cell, develop from the basal cell

TABLE 1.3	Types of Tracheobronchial Cells
Cell	**Probable Function**
Epithelial	
Goblet	Mucous secretion
Serous	Mucous secretion
Ciliated	Mucous propulsion–resorption, supportive
Brush	Mucous resorption
Basal	Supportive, parent
Intermediate	Parent
Clara	Supportive, parent
K cell	Neuroendocrine; possible mechanoreceptor, chemoreceptor
Mesenchymal	
"Globule" leukocyte	Immunologic defense
Lymphocyte	Defense

Modified from Jeffrey PK, Reid L. New features of the rat airway epithelium: a quantitative and electron microscopic study. *J Anat.* 1975;120:295.

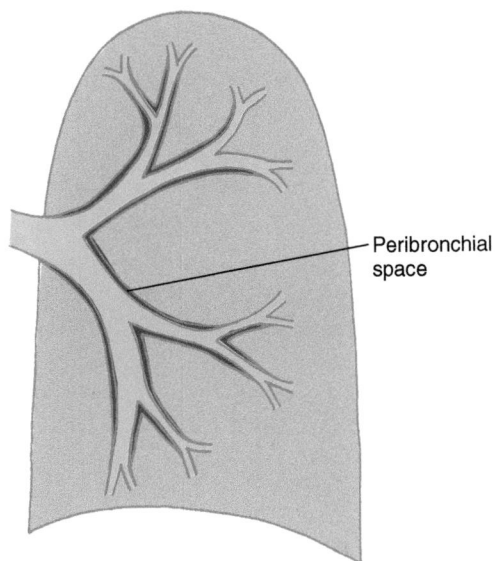

• **Fig. 1.24** Illustration showing formation of the peribronchial space by invagination of the visceral pleura. (From Horsfield K. The relation between structure and function of the airways of the lung. *Br J Dis Chest.* 1974;68:145.)

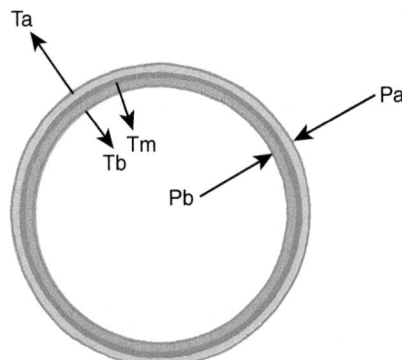

• **Fig. 1.25** Vector diagram showing transmural forces influencing airway caliber: *Pa,* Alveolar gas pressure; *Pb,* barometric pressure; *Ta,* alveolar elastic forces; *Tb,* bronchial elastic forces; *Tm,* bronchial muscular forces. *Arrow* direction indicates the direction of the force. The algebraic sum of these forces determines the size of the airway lumen at any given time. (From Horsfield K. The relation between structure and function of the airways of the lung. *Br J Dis Chest.* 1974;68:145.)

through the intermediate cell. This cell lies in the layer above the basal cell and differentiates into cell types with secretory or ciliary function.[10,34,53] The K cell, or Kulchitsky-like cell, resembles the Kulchitsky cells of the gastrointestinal tract. These cells take up, decarboxylate, and store amine precursors such as levodopa (L-dopa), and therefore they are known as *amine precursor uptake and decarboxylation (APUD) cells.* The functions of the K cells are not definitely known, but proposed roles include mechanoreception (stretch) or chemoreception (carbon dioxide). Globule leukocytes are derived from subepithelial mast cells and interact with them to transfer immunoglobulin E into the secretions and to alter membrane permeability to locally produced or circulating antibodies. The ubiquitous lymphocytes and plasma cells defend against pathogens. Table 1.3 lists important cell types that constitute the airway epithelium.

The nonciliated bronchiolar epithelial cell, or Clara cell, largely makes up the cuboidal epithelium of the bronchioles. The Clara cells assume the role of basal cells as a stem cell in the bronchiole. Only six cell types have been recorded in the human bronchiole: the ciliated, brush, basal, K, and Clara cells; and the globular leukocyte. These cells form a single-layered simple cuboidal epithelium.

Forces Acting on the Airway

Different forces acting on the airway continuously and dynamically alter its morphology. These forces are modified by (1) the location of a given airway segment (intrathoracic or extrathoracic), (2) the phases of respiration, (3) lung volume, (4) gravity, (5) age, and (6) disease.[52,53]

Intrathoracic, intrapulmonary airways such as the distal bronchi and bronchioles are surrounded by a potential space: the peribronchial space (Fig. 1.24). The bronchi are untethered and therefore move longitudinally within this sheath. However, the bronchiolar adventitia is attached by an elastic tissue matrix to the adjoining elastic framework of the surrounding alveoli and parenchyma. Consequently, the bronchioles are subject to transmitted tissue forces, such as those that occur when the lungs expand. The

connective tissue of the parenchyma pulls on the bronchioles, increasing their diameter and decreasing their resistance to the flow of air.[10,48]

Various factors act to modify the airway lumen (Fig. 1.25). The forces that tend to expand the lumen include the pressure of the gas in the bronchioles and the elastic tissue forces of the alveoli. Forces that tend to close the airway include the elasticity of the bronchial wall, which dynamically increases as the lumen expands; the forces of bronchial muscle contraction; and the pressure of the gas in the surrounding alveoli. The algebraic sum of these forces at any given time determines the diameter of the airway.[51,52]

The lower part of the trachea and proximal bronchi are intrathoracic but extrapulmonary; consequently, they are subject to intrathoracic pressure (intrapleural pressure) but not to the tissue elastic recoil forces. The upper trachea is both extrathoracic and extrapulmonary; although it is unaffected by the elastic recoil of

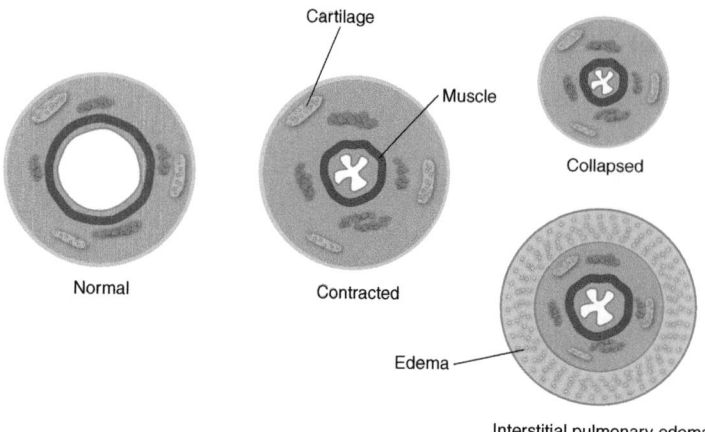

• **Fig. 1.26** Structure of small bronchi (0.8 to 4 mm in diameter). Notice that the mucous membrane is thrown into folds in the contracted and collapsed states, reducing the airway lumen. Also shown is the accumulation of interstitial edema in the peribronchial space. (Modifed from Horsfield K. The relation between structure and function of the airways of the lung. *Br J Dis.* 1974;68:145.)

the lung, it is subject to the effects of ambient pressure and cervical tissue forces.[48,52]

During spontaneous inspiration, the lung expands, which lowers the alveolar pressure more than it does the bronchial pressure, creating a pressure gradient that induces airflow. This increases the elastic retractive forces of the connective tissue and opens the intrathoracic airways. However, extrathoracic intraluminal pressure decreases relative to atmospheric pressure, resulting in a decrease in the diameter of the upper trachea. During expiration, alveolar pressure rises and exceeds the tissue retractive forces, thus decreasing the intrathoracic airway diameter. In this case, the extrathoracic intraluminal pressure rises above the atmospheric pressure, and the upper trachea expands. On forced expiration, alveolar pressure is greatly elevated, further reducing the diameter of the smaller airways.

The dynamic forces are altered by gravity such that the forces tending to expand the lung are greater at the top than at the bottom of the lung regardless of whether the patient is prone, supine, or erect.[54] The diameter and length of the airways of all sizes vary directly by the cube root of the lung volume variation when the lung expands.[55] On expiration below the FRC, the retractive forces gradually decrease the airway size toward the point of closing volume. Because of the effect of gravity, the basal airways close first. The retractive forces of the elastic tissues decrease with aging, which explains why closing volume increases with age. This effect is exaggerated in diseases involving elastic tissue damage (e.g., pulmonary emphysema).

Relationship Between Structure and Function

The extent to which the retractive forces affect airway morphology is related to the specific structure of the airway segment in question. When the fibromuscular membrane of the trachea contracts, the ends of the cartilages are approximated, and the lumen narrows in both the intrathoracic and the extrathoracic trachea. When the radial forces decrease airway diameter, the posterior membrane invaginates into the lumen; however, the rigid cartilaginous hoops prevent luminal occlusion (see Fig. 1.22, collapsed trachea). Extrapulmonary bronchi behave in a similar fashion.

The medium intrapulmonary bronchi within the peribronchial sheath are surrounded by cartilaginous plates. Although these plates add some rigidity to the wall, they do not prevent collapse, so these airways are dependent on the elastic retractive forces of the surrounding tissue (see Fig. 1.25).[52] Therefore forced expiration can collapse many bronchioles in emphysema.

The miniature carinas at small airway bifurcations maintain airway lumens. Intrinsic bronchial muscles reduce the lumen and increase the mean velocity of the airflow during forced expiratory maneuvers, particularly in the peripheral airways with small flow rates. Here, two additional anatomic adaptations contribute to increasing flow rates. First, as the muscular ring contracts, the mucous lining is thrown into accordion-type folds that project into the lumen, further narrowing it (Fig. 1.26).[53] Second, the venous plexus situated between the muscle and the cartilage fills and invaginates into the lumen during muscle contraction. These mechanisms permit bronchoconstriction without distorting the surrounding tissues and minimize the muscular effort required to reduce the airway lumen. The drawback of such an arrangement is that even a small amount of fluid or sputum can result in complete occlusion of the small airways.[52] Therefore it is not surprising that airway resistance is increased tremendously during an asthmatic attack that is characterized by both bronchospasm and increased secretions.[56,57,97] The small airways can also be affected by interstitial pulmonary edema, a condition in which the peribronchial space accumulates fluid, isolating the bronchus from the surrounding retractive forces (see Fig. 1.26).

In severe asthma, thickening of the airway walls occurs due to increases in smooth muscle mass, infiltration with inflammatory cells, deposition of connective tissue, vascular changes, and mucous gland hyperplasia. Such thickening is called *airway remodeling*. Airway remodeling can occur in milder and even asymptomatic cases of asthma. In the past, airway thickening was confirmed with the use of invasive techniques such as biopsy. More recently, scanning techniques have been used to study airway remodeling.[98] MDCT has been used to objectively assess airway remodeling in patients with severe asthma. MDCT used in conjunction with special software can yield reproducible results concerning airway

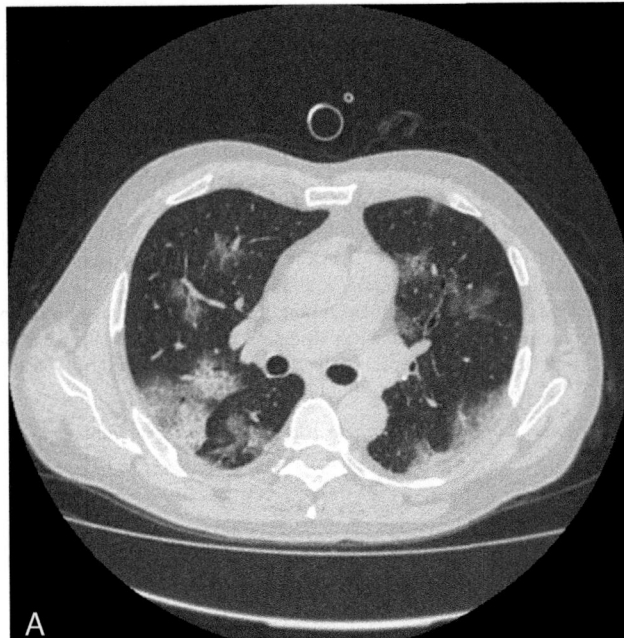

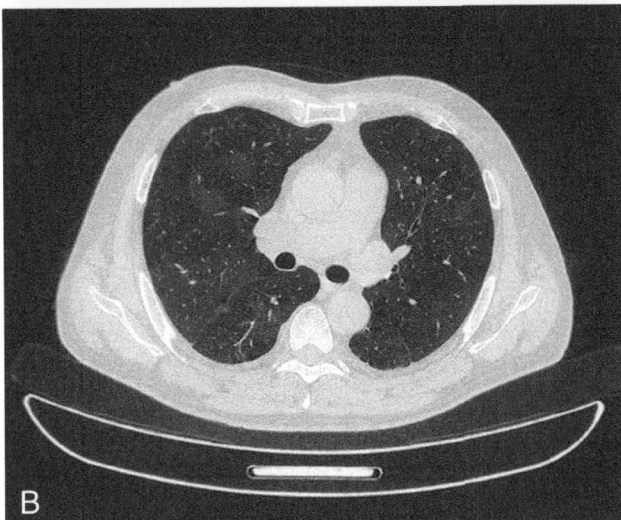

• **Fig. 1.27** Anatomical changes associated with COVID-19 seen on computed tomography at 1 week (A) and 4 months (B), indicating acute and chronic changes. (From Yun Y, Wang Y, Hao Y, Xu L, Cai Q. The time course of chest CT lung changes in COVID-19 patients from onset to discharge. *Eur J Radiol Open.* 2021:8:100305.)

remodeling, and the 3-D airway images allow for correlation of airway function with structural changes.[98] The indices of airway wall thickness measured by MDCT are inversely correlated with changes in the 1-second forced expiratory volume (FEV₁). Noninvasive measurement of airway thickness over a period of time has the ability to show responses to treatment with corticosteroids and bronchodilators.[98,99] Chronic inflammation, ambient particulate matter, smog, and infections can contribute to increased remodeling of the airways.

COVID-19 and the Lower Airways

In December 2019, a contagious disease caused by a novel coronavirus (SARS-CoV-2) was first identified in Wuhan, China. COVID-19, as the disease was named by the World Health

Organization, grew to become a global pandemic in 2020, affecting tens of millions of people. The inhaled SARS-CoV-2 virus binds to nasal and tracheobronchial epithelial cells, resulting in respiratory inflammation. In most patients, COVID-19 disease is mild, but in as many of 5% of patients, it can be severe, leading to respiratory failure, acute cardiac injury, septic shock, multiorgan dysfunction, and death.[100,101] The mortality rate is about 2%, but this rate varies markedly with age and comorbidity.[100]

The virus primarily damages airway epithelium, small intestine epithelium, and vascular endothelium, which are organs with high angiotensin-converting enzyme-2 (ACE2) expression.[100,101] Clinically, the most affected organs are the lungs and the cardiovascular system.[100] Lung inflammation begins with involvement of alveolar type II cells and is mediated by proinflammatory macrophages and granulocytes. Antigen presentation stimulates the body's humoral and cellular immunity, and this immune response is mediated by virus-specific B and T cells.[100] Approximately 20% of infected patients develop pulmonary infiltrates.

Radiographic imaging findings correlate with histopathologic features of other viral pneumonias (e.g., SARS-CoV-1, which was associated with the 2003 SARS outbreak), with diffuse alveolar damage, interstitial lymphocyte infiltration, edema, fibrosis, alveolar hemorrhage, alveolar type II cell hyperplasia, and hyaline tissue formation.[101] On imaging, ground-glass opacities are usually seen during the initial stages of COVID-19 disease (acute phase of diffuse alveolar damage), followed by progression to consolidation and bandlike opacities (parenchymal bands) in the later stages of the disease.[101] Persistent postrecovery changes may include altered pulmonary function (e.g., decreased FEV₁) with functional impairment and CT imaging revealing residual pulmonary opacities and fibrotic bands (Fig. 1.27).[101–103] Lung diffusing capacity (D$_{LCO}$) was reduced by more than 20% and 40% in 51% and 15% of patients, respectively, at 4 months post COVID-19, with physical activity-related functional impairment in 54%.[104] Similarly, at 6 months post COVID-19, 56% of patients requiring ventilation or high-flow nasal cannula and 29% of those simply requiring oxygen had decreased D$_{LCO}$ by >20%.[105] Women were at two- to fourfold higher risk of decreased D$_{LCO}$ in these studies.

An altered sense of smell is a common symptom of COVID-19. The olfactory sensory neurons are structurally supported by sustentacular (SUS) cells, which express ACE2, and damage to SUS cells may be a mechanism for anosmia with disarray of neurons.[106] Recovery of smell can take several weeks; however, smell disturbances can be permanent.

Conclusion

This chapter describes salient features of the human respiratory passages as they relate to their functional anatomy in health and disease relevant to airway management. Practitioners involved in airway management should possess knowledge of the structures that they will frequently use as a passageway to care of patients in their professional career.

Selected References

8. Pohunek P. Development, structure and function of the upper airways. *Paediatr Respir Rev.* 2004;5:2–8.
23. Patil SP, Schneider H, Schwartz AR, Smith PL. Adult obstructive sleep apnea: pathophysiology and diagnosis. *Chest.* 2007;132:325–337.

28. Maeda A, Fujita N, Nagasaka Y. Respiratory and airway considerations in obstetric patients. *Current Anesthesiology Reports.* 2019/03/01 2019;9(1):48–54. doi:10.1007/s40140-019-00309-0

29. Rowe MR, D'Antonio LL. Velopharyngeal dysfunction: evolving developments in evaluation. *Curr Opin Otolaryngol Head Neck Surg.* 2005;13:366–370.

33. O'Dell K. Predictors of difficult intubation and the otolaryngology perioperative consult. *Anesthesiol Clin.* 2015;33:279–290.

52. Kolman J, Morris I. Cricoarytenoid arthritis: a cause of acute upper airway obstruction in rheumatoid arthritis. *Can J Anaesth.* 2002;49:729–732.

61. Thomas BP, Strother MK, Donnelly EF, Worrell JA. CT virtual endoscopy in the evaluation of large airway disease: review. *AJR Am J Roentgenol.* 2009;192:S20–S30.

66. Nishino T. Physiological and pathophysiological implications of upper airway reflexes in humans. *Jpn J Physiol.* 2000;50:3–14.

78. Fewins J, Simpson CB, Miller FR. Complications of thyroid and parathyroid surgery. *Otolaryngol Clin North Am.* 2003;36:189–206.

83. Hyde DM, Hamid Q, Irvin CG. Anatomy, pathology, and physiology of the tracheobronchial tree: emphasis on the distal airways. *J Allergy Clin Immunol.* 2009;124:S72–S77.

87. Patwa A, Shah A. Anatomy and physiology of respiratory system relevant to anaesthesia. *Indian J Anaesth.* Sep 2015;59(9):533–41. doi:10.4103/0019-5049.165849

95. Lawrence D, Branson B, Oliva I, Rubinowitz A. The wonderful world of the windpipe: a review of central airway anatomy and pathology. *Can Assoc Radiol J.* 2015;66:30–43.

101. Salehi S, Reddy S, Gholamrezanezhad A. Long-term pulmonary consequences of coronavirus disease 2019 (COVID-19): what we know and what to expect. *J Thorac Imaging.* Jul 2020;35(4):W87–W89. doi:10.1097/RTI.0000000000000534

All references can be found online at eBooks.Health.Elsevier.com.

2

Radiographic and Cross-Sectional Imaging of the Airway

ANDREW C. McCLELLAND, T. LINDA CHI, DAVID M. MIRSKY, JACQUELINE A. BELLO, DAVID Z. FERSON, AND KEIVAN SHIFTEH

CHAPTER OUTLINE

KEY POINTS

- Airway practitioners should be acquainted with common imaging modalities. A review of available imaging studies should always be included as part of the preoperative assessment of the airway.
- The most useful imaging studies to review include neck, spine, and chest radiographs and cross-sectional imaging studies of the cervical spine or the soft tissue of the neck. A review of the scout image or topogram can provide a more complete assessment of the airway from the nares to the bronchi.
- Computerized tomography (CT) is preferred in acute trauma because of the speed of acquisition, high-resolution imaging, bone detail, and detection of acute blood. The major disadvantage is the delivery of ionizing radiation to patients undergoing CT examination.

- Magnetic resonance imaging (MRI) is the modality of choice for detection of acute stroke. No ionizing radiation is used, but only nonferromagnetic equipment can be used and patients must be carefully screened for a history of implants.
- Assessment of the airway starts at the nose. The presence of septal deviation or bony spurs can affect the ease of nasotracheal or nasogastric tube insertion.
- The presence of macroglossia, retrognathia, and large lingual tonsils at the tongue base may predict difficult intubation.
- The degree of airway narrowing or deviation can be assessed on cross-sectional imaging of the neck.
- The level of the larynx in an adult patient is usually between C4 to C6. Evidence of a low-lying larynx or anterior displacement of the larynx is a potential predictor of difficult intubation.

Introduction

A number of imaging studies may be acquired in the work-up of a patient who presents with a new medical condition. A patient's imaging library can include a chest radiograph, computed tomography (CT) of the chest, and/or CT or magnetic resonance imaging (MRI) of the brain and/or neck that provide some view of the airway, if only a cursory glance. This information about the airway can be aptly used for formulating an anesthetic plan. The main goal of this chapter is to introduce airway practitioners to normal airway anatomy, as visualized on radiography (plain film or digital radiograph) and cross-sectional imaging (e.g., CT and MRI), and to illustrate the anatomic variants and pathologic processes that can compromise the airway. The technology behind the different imaging modalities, as well as their technical differences, is briefly reviewed, with the main emphasis placed on evaluation of the airway using available radiologic studies, which most patients already have as part of their often extensive medical work-up. Familiarity with normal anatomy and its variants is useful to better understand how pathologic processes may affect and compromise the airway in ways that are most relevant to anesthesiologists.

The airway can be regarded as a tubular conduit for air inhaled from the nares to the tracheobronchial tree. The soft tissue structures bordering the airway may affect the integrity of the airway with respect to extrinsic compression, luminal encroachment, or airway displacement. Segmentation of the airway into the head, neck, and chest compartments is artificial but usually done, addressing the pathologies affecting these anatomic regions and for ease of discussion. Different imaging modalities, such as x-ray, CT, and MRI, can evaluate airway structures and the surrounding tissues with different levels of accuracy and spatial resolution. When analyzing these imaging modalities, one must be familiarized with the advantages and disadvantages of each imaging technique. This is especially important when selecting a study that will best depict the anatomic structures and pathologic processes affecting the airway that are of clinical interest.

Imaging Modalities

A brief description of the different imaging modalities is presented here, starting with plain x-ray films and, more currently, digital radiographs. This will enable the reader to develop a good foundation for understanding how different imaging modalities are used in modern diagnostic imaging.

Conventional Radiograph and Digital Radiograph

Wilhelm Conrad Roentgen, a German physicist, discovered x-rays on November 8, 1895, while studying the behavior of cathode rays (electrons) in high-energy cathode ray tubes. By serendipity, he noted that a mysterious ray that escaped the cathode ray tube struck a small piece of paper coated with fluorescent barium platinocyanide on a workbench 3 feet away, causing a faint fluorescent glow. Different objects placed between the cathode ray tube and the fluorescent screen changed the brightness of the fluorescence, indicating that the mysterious ray penetrated objects differently. When Roentgen held his hand between the tube and the screen and saw the outline of the bony skeleton of his hand, he quickly realized the significance of his discovery. For his work, he was awarded the first Nobel Prize for Physics in 1901.[1]

X-rays are a type of electromagnetic radiation, which, as the name implies, transports energy through space as a combination of electric and magnetic fields. In diagnostic radiology, the predominant energy source used for imaging is ionizing radiation, such as alpha particles, beta particles, gamma rays, and x-rays. The science of electromagnetic waves and x-ray generation is very complex and exceeds the scope of this chapter. In principle, x-rays are produced by energy conversion as a fast stream of electrons is suddenly decelerated in an x-ray tube.[2] The x-ray beam produced can be directed toward the part of the body being studied. The final image is dependent on the degree of attenuation of the beam by matter (e.g., soft tissues and bone). Attenuation, the reduction in the intensity of the beam as it traverses matter of different composition, is caused by the absorption or deflection of photons from the beam. The transmitted beam determines the final image, which is represented in shades of gray.[2-5] The lightest or brightest area on the film or image represents the greatest attenuation of the beam by tissue and the least amount of beam transmitted to film. An example would be bone, a high-density material that attenuates much of the x-ray beam; images of bone on radiographs are very bright or white.

Conventional imaging (plain film or x-ray) is obtained using screen film cassette technology in which the film is processed using several chemical "washes" or chemical reactions to produce a two-dimensional image of the body part under examination on a large field of view film.[6] With most radiology departments converting to an all-digital environment, heavily relying on various picture archiving communication systems (PACS) for workflow and archiving of radiologic studies, digital radiography has largely replaced screen film cassette plain film.

Computed Tomography

After the discovery of x-rays, it became apparent that images of the internal structures of the human body could yield important diagnostic information. However, the usefulness of the x-rays is limited by the projection of a three-dimensional object onto a two-dimensional display. With x-rays and radiographs, the details of internal objects are masked by the shadows of overlying and underlying structures. The goal of diagnostic imaging is to bring forth the organ or area of interest in detail and eliminate the unwanted information. Various film-based traditional tomographic techniques were developed, culminating in the creation of CT or computerized axial tomography (CAT).[7,8] The first clinically viable CT scanner was developed by Hounsfield and commercially marketed by EMI (EMI Limited, Middlesex, England) for brain imaging in the early 1970s.[9] Since then, several generations of CT scanners have been developed.

As with conventional plain film or digital radiography, CT technology requires x-rays as the energy source. Whereas conventional radiography employs a single beam of x-rays from a single direction and yields a static image, CT images are obtained by using multiple collimated x-ray beams from multiple angles and the transmitted radiation is counted by a row or rows of detectors. A fan-shaped x-ray source rotates around the patient, who is enclosed in a gantry. The radiation counted by the detectors is analyzed using mathematical equations to localize and characterize the tissues within the imaged section based on density and attenuation measurements. A single cross-sectional image is produced with one rotation of the gantry. The gantry must then "unwind" to prepare for the next slice while the table with the patient moves forward or backward a distance predetermined by slice thickness.

An intrinsic limitation of this technique is the time necessary for movement of the mechanical parts.[7,9]

Introduction of slip-ring technology in the 1990s, along with development of faster computers, high-energy x-ray tubes, and multidetectors, enabled continuous activation of the x-ray source without having to unwind the gantry. With continuous movement of the tabletop, this process is known as the helical CT. Because the information acquired using helical CT is volumetric, as compared with the single slice obtained with conventional CT, the entire thorax or abdomen can be scanned in a single breath-hold. Volumetric information also makes it possible to identify small lesions more accurately and allows better three-dimensional reconstruction.[7] Because of the higher speed of data acquisition, misregistration and image degradation caused by patient motion are no longer significant concerns. This is especially important when scanning uncooperative patients and trauma victims. The absorbed radiation dose used in a multidetector helical CT as compared with a conventional single-detector row CT is dependent on the scanning protocol and varies with the desired high-speed or high-quality study.[10]

CT examination is best for depiction of bone and for detection of calcium and blood. The advantage of CT technology is that data acquisition is very quick, and the acquired data can be used for multidimensional reconstructions, which allow the display of different organs in an anatomic format that can be easily recognized by clinicians.

Magnetic Resonance Imaging

In contrast to radiography and CT, MRI uses no ionizing radiation. Instead, imaging is based on the resonance of the atomic nuclei of certain elements such as sodium, phosphorus, and hydrogen in response to radio waves of the same frequency produced in a static magnetic field environment. Current clinical MRI units use protons from the nuclei of hydrogen atoms to generate images because hydrogen is the most abundant element in the body. Every water molecule contains two hydrogen atoms, and larger molecules, such as lipids and proteins, contain many hydrogen atoms. MRI data are acquired by using powerful electromagnets to create a magnetic field, which influences the alignment of protons in hydrogen atoms in the body. When radio waves are applied, protons are knocked out of natural alignment, and when the radio wave is stopped, the protons return to their original state of equilibrium, realigning to the steady magnetic field and emitting energy, which is translated into weak radio signals. The time it takes for the protons to realign is referred to as a relaxation time and is dependent on the tissue composition and cellular environment.[11,12] The different relaxation times and signal strength of the protons are processed by a computer, which generates diagnostic images. With MRI, the chemical and physical properties of matter are examined at the molecular level. The relaxation times, T1 and T2, for each tissue type are expressed as constants at a given magnetic field strength. Imaging that optimizes T1 or T2 characteristics is referred to as T1-weighted or T2-weighted imaging. Tissue response to pathologic processes usually includes an increase in bound water, or edema, which lengthens the T2 relaxation time and appears as a bright focus on T2-weighted images.[11,12]

MRI is more sensitive, but not necessarily more specific, in detecting pathology than CT, which depicts anatomy with unparalleled clarity. Imaging with MRI provides metabolic information at the cellular level, allowing one to link organ function and physiology to anatomic information. MRI and CT technologies also have other differences: (1) MRI shows poor bony detail, whereas CT provides excellent images of bony structures; (2) hemorrhage, especially acute, is clearly visible on CT scans as bright or white areas, but it may be difficult to diagnose with MRI because the appearance of blood varies temporally depending on the stage of breakdown of hemoglobin; (3) MRI is very susceptible to all types of motion artifacts, ranging from patient movement, breathing, swallowing, and phonation to vascular and cerebrospinal fluid pulsation and flow; and (4) MRI is time consuming—a typical MRI takes 30 to 45 minutes, whereas a CT scan can be performed in less than 1 minute—thus, patients with altered mental status or other difficulties sitting still can be imaged much more easily with CT.

MRI scanners operate in a strong magnetic field environment, and strict precautions must be observed. Because any item containing ferromagnetic substances introduced into the magnetic field environment can become a projectile and result in deleterious consequences for patients, personnel, and the MRI scanner itself, no metal objects should be brought into the MRI suite if one is not absolutely certain about their composition. Only specially designed nonferromagnetic equipment is used in the MRI suite, including anesthesia machines, monitoring equipment, oxygen tanks, intravenous poles, infusion pumps, and stretchers. One must also remove pagers, telephones, computers, credit cards, and analog watches because the strong magnetic field can cause malfunction or permanent damage. Patients must be carefully screened for implantable pacemakers, intracranial aneurysm clips, implants (e.g., cochlear implants, penile implants, or spinal cord stimulators), and other foreign metallic objects before entering the MRI environment. In addition to the risk of ferromagnetic objects acting as projectiles externally, producing unwanted movement internally, or causing equipment malfunction, there is also the risk of heating, which can cause severe thermal injuries to the patient.

Basics of Radiograph Interpretation

The aim of this chapter is to review imaging of the airway. There is, however, useful information from imaging studies of other parts of the body. For example, imaging of the brain can give information regarding intracranial pathology such as masses and mass effect, including brain herniation, hemorrhage, and hydrocephalus. Readily apparent from imaging of the chest are aeration status of each lung; the presence or absence of pneumothorax, mediastinal shifts, or pleural effusion; diaphragm position; heart size; positioning of the endotracheal tube (ETT); and intravascular access catheters. Abdominal imaging provides information regarding the presence or absence of ileus, pneumoperitoneum, and mass effect.

To illustrate the usefulness of radiography in evaluating the airway, we focus our discussion on the interpretation of plain films or digital radiographs of the cervical spine, chest, and neck. These are probably the radiographic studies most frequently ordered in a hospital setting and also are the most relevant to anesthesiologists because a composite of these studies gives a picture of the entire airway. Although these radiologic studies are usually obtained for reasons other than airway evaluation, it is in this group of patients who are "normal" or "cleared for surgery" that one may glean important observations about the airway. In cross-sectional imaging (e.g., CT or MRI), the digital scout view of a neck, cervical spine, or chest study provides a similar image to a digital radiograph of the neck or chest and renders useful airway information. With a dedicated study of the neck or cervical spine, multidimensional reconstructions from those studies allow an excellent view of the airway, usually from the nares to tracheal bifurcation. The anatomy and pathology displayed by these imaging techniques may alert the anesthesiologist to potential difficulties in securing a patient's airway and help him or her to develop an alternative anesthetic plan. The following sections address the basics of imaging interpretation with respect to airway anatomy and pathology.

Cervical Spine Radiography

Radiologic Anatomy

The cervical spine articulates with the occiput cranially and the thoracic vertebrae caudally. The bony elements, muscles, ligaments, and intervertebral discs support and provide protection to the spinal cord. On a lateral radiograph of the cervical spine, one can appreciate the bony morphology of the vertebrae and the disc spaces and assess the alignment of the vertebral column very quickly. This indirectly provides information regarding the integrity of the ligaments, which are crucial in maintaining alignment of the cervical spine. Individual ligaments and muscle groups, however, all have the same or similar attenuation and cannot be differentiated from one another on a radiograph. Soft tissue pathology, including ligamentous injury, is better assessed by MRI. Regardless of the type of imaging study, a systematic approach is recommended to evaluate the spine for alignment, bony integrity, cartilage, joint space, and soft tissue abnormalities.

There are seven cervical vertebrae: C1 through C7. C1 and C2 are different from the other cervical vertebrae and are considered to be more a part of the cervico-cranium. The atlas (C1) is a ring-like vertebra characterized by the absence of a vertebral body. It does not contain pedicles or laminae, as do other vertebrae, and has no true spinous process. It consists of an anterior arch, the anterior tubercle, a lateral mass on each side, and a posterior arch. The anterior and posterior arches are relatively thin, and the lateral masses are heavy and thick structures. Rudimentary transverse processes extend laterally and contain the transverse foramina, through which pass the vertebral arteries.[13] Ossification of the atlas begins with the lateral masses during intrauterine life. At birth, neither the anterior nor the posterior arches are fused. Fusion of the anterior arch is complete between the seventh and tenth years of life. During the second year of life, the center of the posterior tubercle appears, and by the end of the fourth year of life, the posterior arch becomes complete. Nonfusion of the anterior and/or posterior arch exists as a normal variant in adults and should not be mistaken as a fracture (Fig. 2.1).[14]

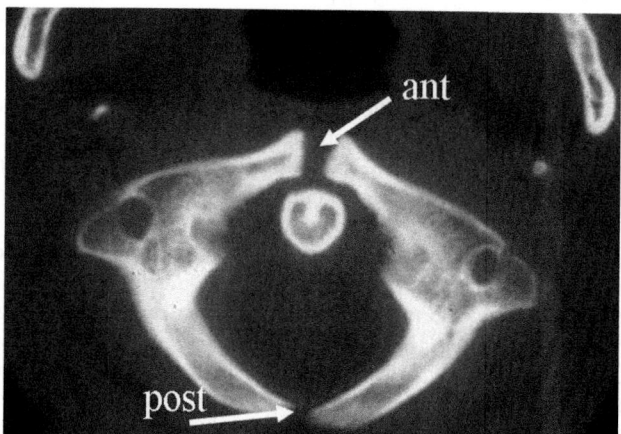

• **Fig. 2.1** Nonfused anterior and posterior arches of C1, normal variant. Axial computed tomography, bone algorithm.

The second cervical vertebra, the axis (C2), is the largest and heaviest cervical segment. The odontoid process (dens) serves as the theoretical body of C1, around which the atlas rotates and bends laterally. In contrast to the other cervical vertebrae, C2 does not have a discrete pedicle. The dens is situated between the lateral masses of the atlas and is maintained in its normal sagittal relationship to the anterior arch of C1 by several ligaments, most important of which is the transverse atlantal ligament. Superiorly, the dentate (apical) ligament extends from the tip of the clivus to the tip of the dens. Alar ligaments secure the tip of the dens to the occipital condyles and to the lateral masses of the atlas. They are the second line of defense in maintaining proper position of the dens. The tectorial membrane is a continuum of the posterior longitudinal ligament from the body of C2 to the upper surface of the occipital bone, anterior to the foramen magnum.

The C2 vertebra arises from five or six separate ossification centers, depending upon whether the vertebral body has one or two centers. The vertebral body is ossified at birth, and the posterior arch is partially ossified. They fuse posteriorly by the second or third year of life and unite with the body of the vertebrae by the seventh year. The dens ossifies from two vertically oriented centers that fuse by the seventh fetal month. Cranially, a central cleft separates the tips of these ossification centers (Fig. 2.2A), which can mimic a fracture when ossification is incomplete. The *ossiculum terminale*, the ossification center for the tip of the dens, may be visible on plain film, conventional tomograms, or CT scans and unites with the body by age 11 or 12 years. Failure of the ossiculum terminale to either develop or unite with the dens may result in a bulbous cleft dens tip. Incomplete fusion of dental ossification centers can result in persistent ossiculum terminale or os odontoideum, which can mimic fractures. (Fig. 2.2B–D).

From C3 to C7, the cervical vertebrae are uniform in shape but increase in size, with the seventh vertebra being the largest and heaviest. All the vertebrae have transverse processes containing the foramen transversarium through which the vertebral arteries pass (Fig. 2.3). The articular masses are dense, heavy, rhomboid-shaped structures bounded by articulating superior and inferior facets. The pedicles are short and posterolaterally oblique in orientation.[14,15]

Cervical Spine Anatomy and Pathology

To answer a specific clinical question, different views of the cervical spine are frequently needed. The most common views are the lateral, anteroposterior (AP), open-mouth odontoid, oblique, and pillar views (Fig. 2.4A–D). A systematic approach is recommended to assess the integrity of the cervical spine. Examination of the cervical spine should include visualization of all seven cervical vertebrae and the first thoracic vertebra (T1). This is especially important for trauma victims because 7% to 14% of fractures are known to occur at the C7 or C7–T1 level.[16] One must evaluate the spine for alignment, bone integrity, cartilage, joint space, and soft tissue abnormalities. The disadvantages of cervical spine x-rays are the limited range of tissue attenuation and the loss of spatial resolution caused by overlapping bone structures.

A normal lateral cervical radiograph should demonstrate normal alignment of the anterior and posterior aspects of the vertebral bodies and intact vertebrae (Fig. 2.4A). The posterior vertebral body line is more reliable than the anterior vertebral body line, which is often encumbered by the presence of anterior osteophytes and must be intact. The facet joints overlap in an orderly fashion, like shingles on a rooftop (Fig. 2.4D). The spinolaminar line is uninterrupted, and the interlaminar and interspinous distances

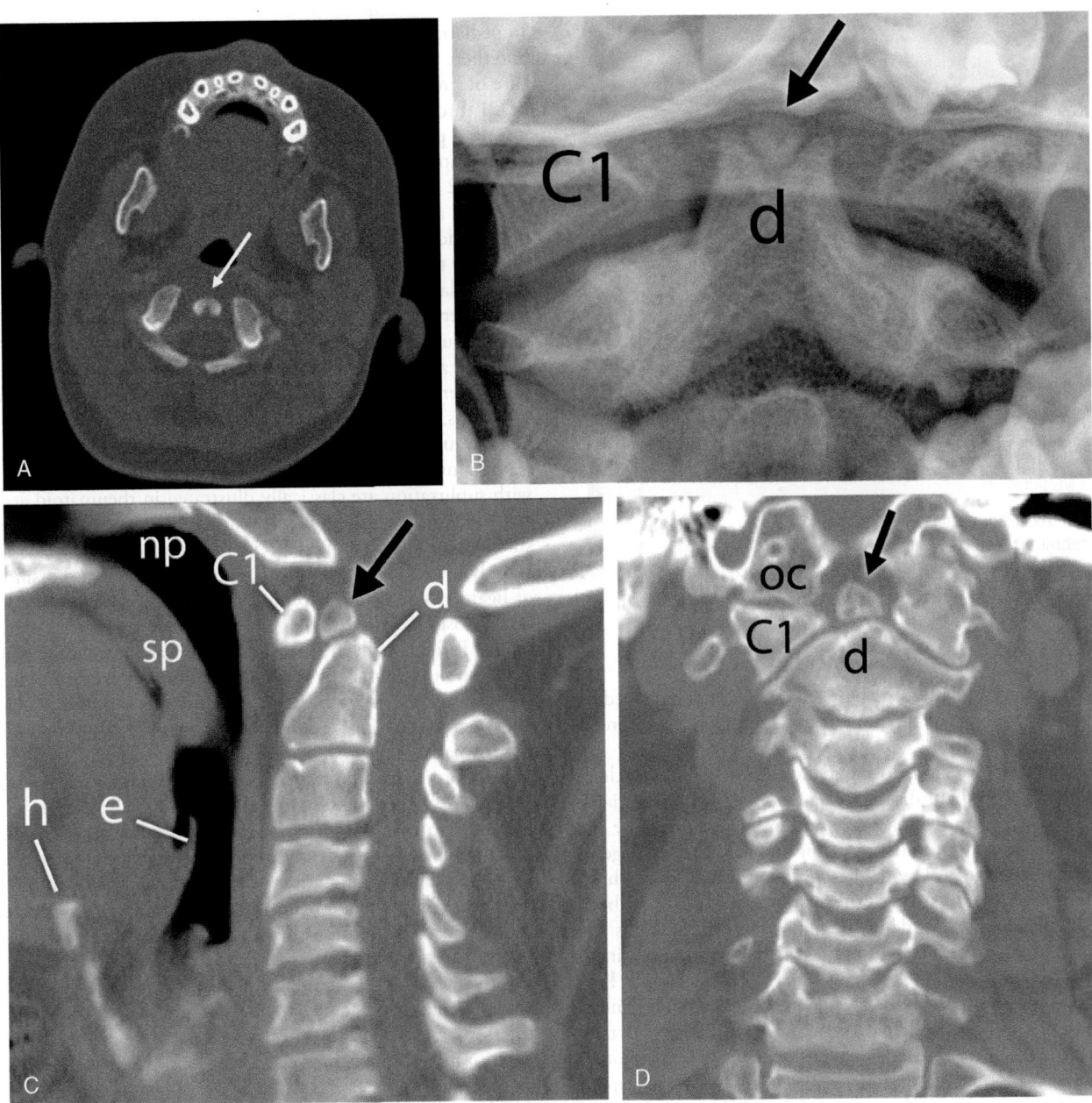

• **Fig. 2.2** Normal variations of the dens. (A) Cleft dens (*arrow*) on axial computed tomography (CT). (B) Frontal radiograph demonstrating a persistent ossiculum terminale (*arrow*), representing a nonunited terminal dental ossification center. (C) Sagittal and (D) coronal CTs, which show a well-corticated ossific density superior to a foreshortened dens, compatible with os odontoideum (*arrow*). There is characteristic secondary hypertrophy of the anterior C1 arch. Congenital and remote traumatic etiologies have been hypothesized. *d*, dens; *C1*, C1 vertebrae; *oc*, occipital condyle; *np*, nasopharynx; *e*, epiglottis; *h*, hyoid; *sp*, soft palate.

are uniform. The spinolaminar line is the dense cortical line representing the junction of the posterior laminae with the posterior spinous process as seen on lateral radiographs. The posterior spinal line is an imaginary line extending from the spinolaminar line of the atlas to C3 (Fig. 2.5A–D).[14] The anatomy and integrity of the craniocervical junction are crucial to the anesthesiologist. To achieve successful and safe endotracheal intubation, the anterior atlantodental interval (AADI), the vertical and anterior-posterior position of the dens, and the degree of extension of the head on the neck must be considered. The anterior arch of C1 bears a constant relationship to the dens (the AADI), or the *predental space*. It is defined as the space between the posterior surface of the

anterior arch of C1 and the anterior surface of the dens. In flexion, because of the physiologic laxity of the cervicocranial ligaments, the anterior tubercle of the atlas assumes a more normal-appearing relationship to the dens, and the AADI increases in width, greater rostrally than caudally. In children and in flexion, the AADI is normally about 5 mm. In adults, it is generally accepted that the AADI should be 3 mm or less (Figs. 2.6A and B).[14] If all the ligaments have been disrupted, AADI can measure 10 mm or more. In atlantoaxial subluxation, the dens is invariably displaced posteriorly (Fig. 2.6C–E), which causes narrowing of the spinal canal and potential impingement of the spinal cord. The space available for the spinal cord is defined as the diameter of the spinal canal as

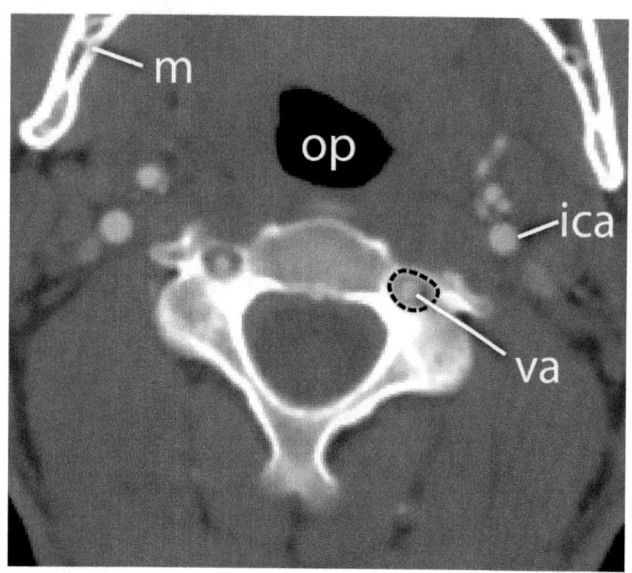

• **Fig. 2.3** Axial computed tomography (CT) angiogram demonstrates the vertebral arteries (*va*) within the transverse foramen (*dashed black outline*) of the C3 vertebra. *ica*, Internal carotid artery; *m*, mandible; *op*, oropharynx.

measured in the AP plane, at the C1 level, that is not occupied by the odontoid process. In the normal spine, this space is approximately 20 mm.[13]

The distance between the occiput and the posterior tubercle of C1, the atlanto-occipital distance (Fig. 2.7A,B), is quite variable from individual to individual. Head extension is limited by the abutment of the occiput to the posterior tubercle of C1. Congenital occipitalization of C1 with the occiput not only limits head extension but also adds stress to the atlantoaxial joint. It has been proposed that a shorter atlanto-occipital distance decreases the effectiveness of head extension and contributes to difficult intubation.[13,17] Nichol and Zuck observed that in patients with limited or no extension possible at the atlanto-occipital joint, general extension of the head actually brings the larynx "anterior," thus limiting the visibility of the larynx on laryngoscopy.[17] Although the majority of head extension occurs at the atlanto-occipital joint, some extension can also occur at C1–C2.[17]

The position and anatomy of the dens with respect to the anterior arch of C1 and the foramen magnum are worthy of attention. Congenital anomalies of the dens, such as hypoplasia, can result in a loss of the buttressing action of the dens during extension and subsequent compression of neural elements. Conditions that are associated with odontoid hypoplasia are Morquio, Klippel-Feil, and Down syndromes; neurofibromatosis; dwarfism; spondyloepiphyseal dysplasia; osteogenesis imperfecta; and congenital scoliosis.[13,18] These patients are predisposed to atlantoaxial subluxation and craniocervical instability, and therefore hyperextension of the head for intubation should be avoided. In addition, congenital fusion of C2 and C3 (Fig. 2.8A–D), whether occurring as an isolated anomaly or as part of Klippel-Feil syndrome, places added stress at the C1–C2 junction.

Pseudosubluxation and *pseudodislocation* are terms applied to the physiologic anterior displacement of C2 on C3 that is frequently seen in infants and young children (Fig. 2.9). Physiologic anterior displacement of C2 on C3 and of C3 on C4 occurs in 24% and 14%, respectively, of children up to the age of 8 years.[15]

In pediatric trauma cases, if C2 is noted to be anteriorly displaced and there are no other signs of trauma, such as posterior arch fracture or prevertebral soft tissue hematoma, the spinolaminar lines of C1 through C3 should have a normal anatomic relationship. In a neutral position, the spinolaminar line of C2 lies upon, or up to 1 mm anterior or posterior to, the imaginary posterior spinal line. If the C2 vertebra is intact, the spinolaminar line of C2 moves 1 to 2 mm anterior to the posterior spinal line in flexion as the C2 body glides forward with respect to C3. Similarly, in extension the posterior translation of the C2 body is mirrored by similar posterior displacement of the spinolaminar line of C2 with respect to the posterior spinal line. In traumatic spondylolisthesis, which is rare in children and more common in adults, the C2 body would translate anteriorly in flexion and posteriorly in extension, and the posterior spinal line would be maintained because of intact ligaments. However, flexion and extension films are not advisable when traumatic spondylolisthesis is suspected.

Inflammatory arthropathies involving the atlantoaxial joint with subluxation are classically illustrated in rheumatoid arthritis and ankylosing spondylitis. The underlying cause of atlantoaxial subluxation is quite different in these two entities. Ankylosing spondylitis is characterized by progressive fibrosis and ossification of ligaments and joint capsules. In rheumatoid arthritis, there is bone erosion, synovial overgrowth, and destruction of the ligaments. Patients with rheumatoid arthritis are not only susceptible to AP subluxation at the C1–C2 junction but are also at risk for vertical subluxation of the dens. Whether this condition is referred to as "cranial settling,"[14] superior migration of the odontoid process, or basilar invagination, the result is the same. The odontoid process protrudes above the foramen magnum, narrowing the available space for the spinal cord and potentially leading to cord compression with the slightest head extension (Fig. 2.10A–C).

In response to the effective foreshortening of the spine secondary to the superior migration of the dens, there is acquired rotational malalignment between the spine and larynx.[19] The larynx and the trachea, because they are semirigid structures and as a result of the tethering effect of the arch of aorta as it passes posteriorly over the left main bronchus, are predictably displaced caudally, deviated laterally to the left, rotated to the right, and anteriorly angulated. The effective neck length can be affected by superior migration of the dens, severe spondylosis with loss of disc space, or iatrogenic causes secondary to surgery. The soft tissues of the pharynx become more redundant, which is attributable to the relative shortening of the neck and further obscures the view of the larynx. On laryngoscopy, the vocal cords are rotated clockwise. The presence of a rotated airway is suspected when the frontal view of the cervical spine demonstrates a deviated tracheal air column.

Historically, bone landmarks other than the spine, appreciated on a lateral cervical spine x-ray study, have been used to preoperatively predict difficult laryngoscopy and endotracheal intubation based on anatomic factors. Mandibular size and the ratios of the various measurements and their relationship to the hyoid bone have been proposed as predictors of difficult laryngoscopy (Fig. 2.11).[20] These measurements are meant to reflect the oral capacity, degree of mouth opening, and the level of larynx.[21,22] It is apparent that the causes of difficult laryngoscopy and endotracheal intubation are multifactorial. Combined with a clinical examination, anatomic measurements and findings assessed by radiography can help to alert the anesthesiologist to a potentially difficult airway. Acute cervical spine injury is often the indication for ordering a cervical spine examination. Although CT and MRI are exceptional in detailing bone and soft tissue abnormalities,

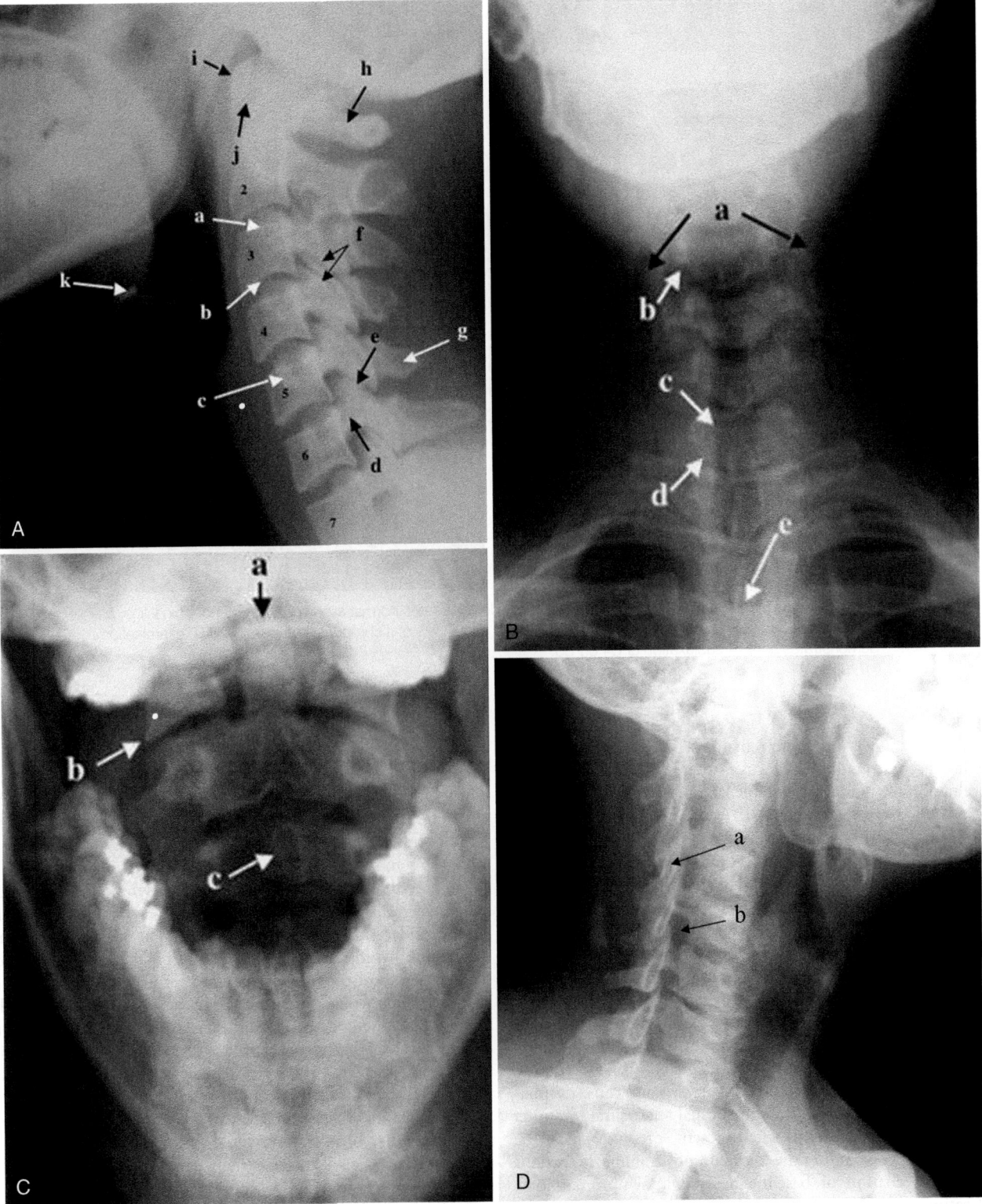

• **Fig. 2.4** Normal cervical spine series. Lateral (A), anteroposterior (B), open-mouth odontoid (C), and oblique (D) views of the cervical spine. (A) *a*, Upper end plate of C3 cervical vertebra; *b*, lower end plate of C3; *c*, transverse process; *d*, pedicle; *e*, facet joint; *f*, articulating facets; *g*, posterior spinous process; *h*, posterior arch of C1; *i*, anterior arch of C1; *j*, atlantoaxial distance; *k*, hyoid bone. (B) *a*, Smoothly undulating cortical margins of the lateral masses; *b*, joint of Luschka; *c*, superior end plate; *d*, inferior end plate; *e*, midline posterior spinous process. (C) *a*, Odontoid tip centered between the lateral masses of the axis; *b*, symmetrical lateral margins of the lateral atlantoaxial joints; *c*, spinous process. (D) *a*, Laminae of the articular masses reflecting the shingling effect; *b*, intervertebral (neural) foramen.

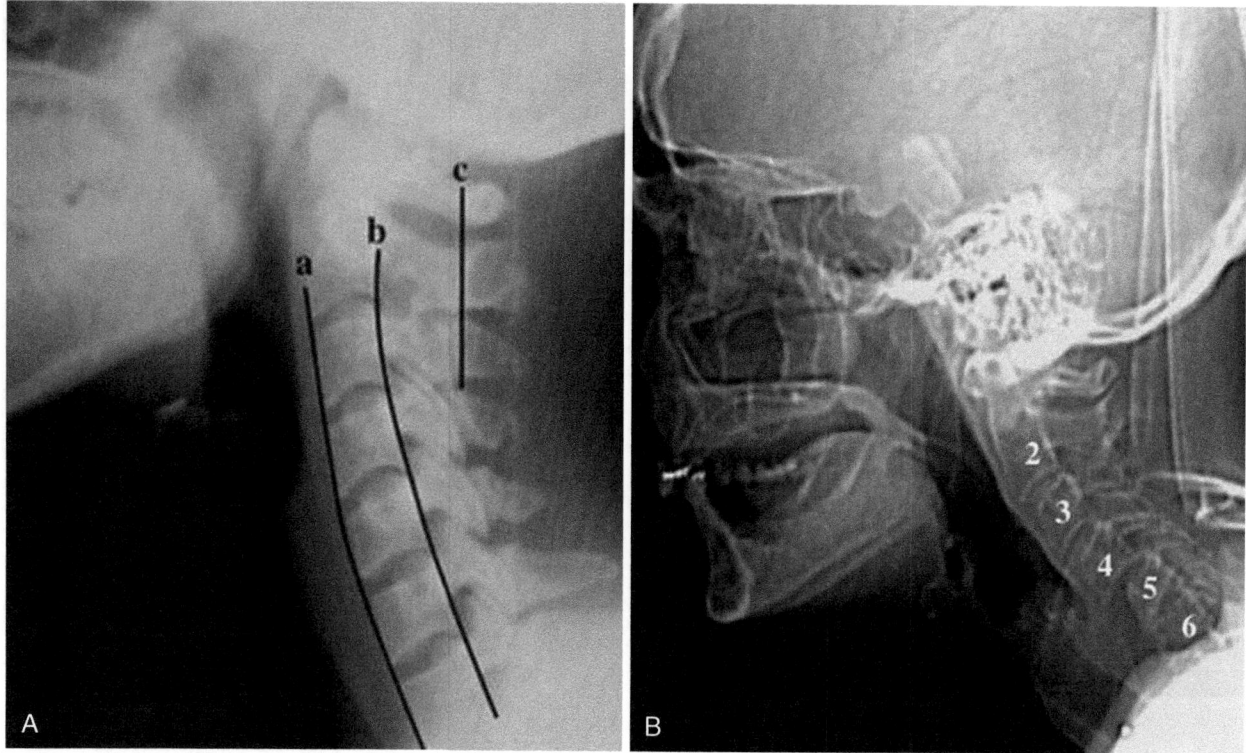

• **Fig. 2.5** (A) Normal lateral cervical spine radiograph demonstrates normal alignment; *a*, anterior spinal line; *b*, posterior vertebral line; *c*, posterior spinal line. (B) Lateral scout view of a computed tomography (CT) examination demonstrates anterior subluxation of C4 on C5.

plain film of the cervical spine remains a good initial screening study. It is useful to tailor and focus further imaging of the spine. For evaluation of trauma, cross-table lateral, AP, and open-mouth odontoid views are recommended. A lateral view reveals most injuries (Fig. 2.12); however, patients who are rendered quadriplegic by severe ligamentous injuries may demonstrate a normal lateral cervical spine x-ray. By adding the AP and open-mouth odontoid views to the cross-table lateral view of the cervical spine, the sensitivity of detecting significant injury is increased from 82% to 93%.[23] Cross-sectional imaging (i.e., CT and MRI of the spine) has become a mainstay in the evaluation of the cervical spine, especially in the setting of acute trauma (Fig. 2.13A–B).

Cervical spine x-rays are also ordered for the evaluation of cervical spondylosis (Fig. 2.14). The hypertrophic bone changes associated with this condition are well depicted on x-ray studies. Large anterior osteophytes that project forward may cause dysphagia and difficult intubation. The spinal canal and neural foramina are assessed for stenosis, and, when present, precautions can be taken when hyperextending the neck and positioning the patient to avoid exacerbation of baseline neurologic symptomatology. Calcification and ossification are well depicted on x-ray examination. Ossification of the anterior longitudinal ligament and diffuse idiopathic skeletal hyperostosis can also lead to large anterior osteophytes that narrow the airway and have been reported as causes of difficult intubation (Fig. 2.15A–C).[24] This can be readily appreciated on plain films. Another condition that also may signal difficult intubation is calcification of the stylohyoid ligament (Fig. 2.16A–E).[25]

Cervical Airway Anatomy and Pathology

The lateral cervical spine radiograph, obtained to evaluate the integrity and alignment of the bony cervical spine, allows an incidental view of the aerodigestive tract and a gross assessment of the overall patency of the airway. Useful bony landmarks of the pharynx and larynx that can be appreciated on the lateral neck x-ray are the hard palate, hyoid bone, thyroid, and cricoid cartilages (Fig. 2.17). The hard palate separates the nasopharynx from the oropharynx. The larynx can be thought of as being suspended from the hyoid bone. Muscles acting on the hyoid bone elevate the larynx and provide the primary protection from aspiration. The largest cartilage in the neck is the thyroid cartilage, which, along with the cricoid cartilage, acts as a protective shield for the inner larynx. The cricoid cartilage is the only complete cartilaginous ring in the respiratory system. It is located at the level where the larynx ends and the trachea begins.

Normal air-filled structures seen on lateral plain film are the nasopharynx, oropharynx, and hypopharynx. Air in the pharynx outlines the soft palate, uvula, base of the tongue, and nasopharyngeal airway (Fig. 2.18). Any sizable soft tissue pathology results in deviation or effacement of the airway. The tongue constitutes the bulk of the soft tissue in the oral cavity and the oropharynx. In children, and sometimes in adults, prominent lymphatic tissues, such as adenoids and palatine tonsils, may encroach on the nasopharyngeal and oropharyngeal airway. Lingual tonsils are located at the base of the tongue above the valleculae, which are air-filled pouches between the tongue base and the free margin of the epiglottis.

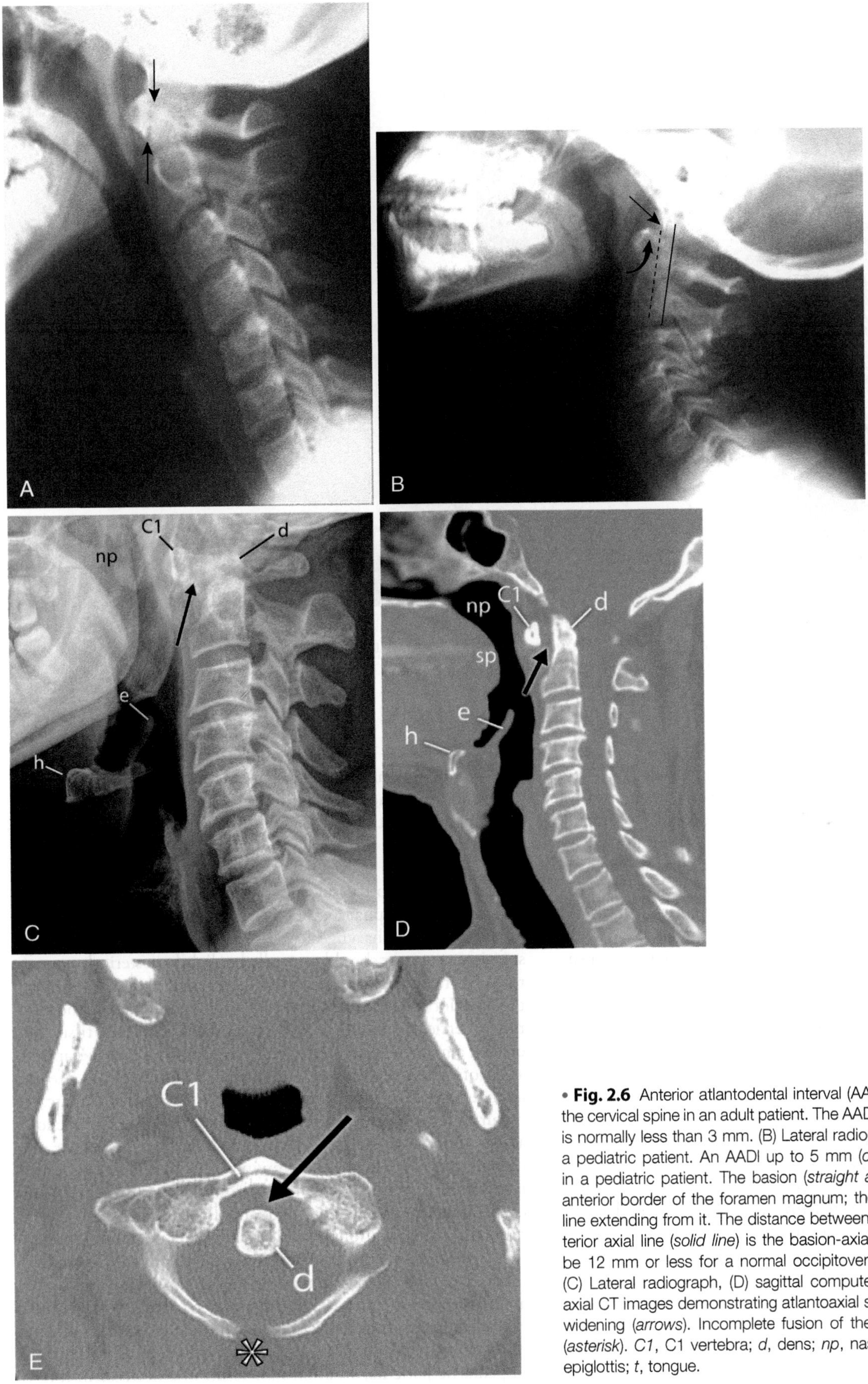

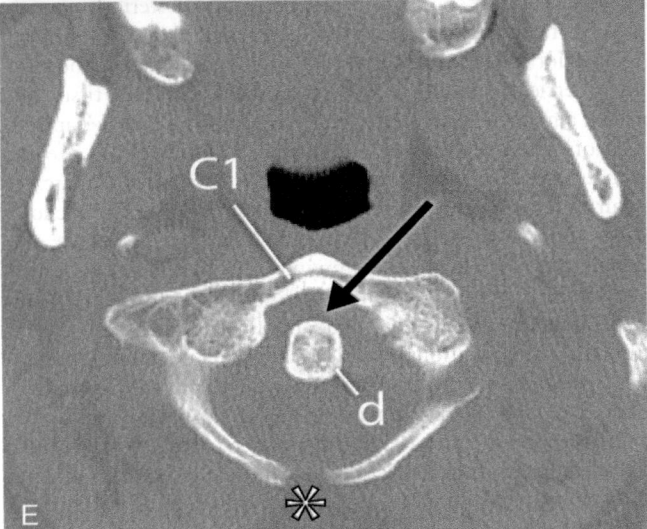

• **Fig. 2.6** Anterior atlantodental interval (AADI). (A) Lateral radiograph of the cervical spine in an adult patient. The AADI or predental space (*arrows*) is normally less than 3 mm. (B) Lateral radiograph of the cervical spine in a pediatric patient. An AADI up to 5 mm (*curved arrow*) can be normal in a pediatric patient. The basion (*straight arrow*) is the midpoint of the anterior border of the foramen magnum; the *dotted line* is an imaginary line extending from it. The distance between the dotted line and the posterior axial line (*solid line*) is the basion-axial interval (BAI), which should be 12 mm or less for a normal occipitovertebral relationship in a child. (C) Lateral radiograph, (D) sagittal computed tomography (CT), and (E) axial CT images demonstrating atlantoaxial subluxation with atlantodental widening (*arrows*). Incomplete fusion of the posterior C1 arch is noted (*asterisk*). *C1*, C1 vertebra; *d*, dens; *np*, nasopharynx; *h*, hyoid bone; *e*, epiglottis; *t*, tongue.

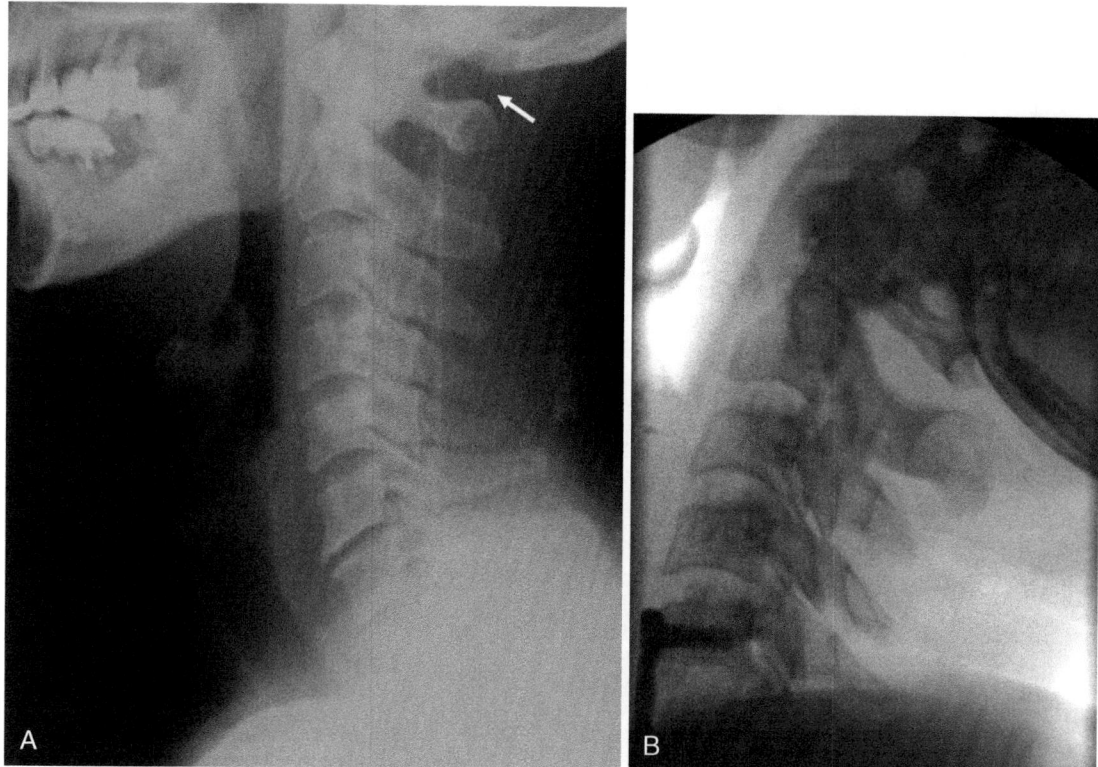

• **Fig. 2.7** Atlanto-occipital distance. (A) Lateral cervical spine in neutral position with the atlanto-occipital distance demarcated (*arrow*). (B) Lateral cervical spine in hyperextension. Head extension is limited by the abutment of the occiput to the posterior tubercle of C1.

The epiglottis is an elastic fibrocartilage in the shape of a flattened teardrop or leaf that tapers inferiorly and attaches to the thyroid cartilage. The epiglottis tends to be more angular in infants than in adults. During the first several years of life, the larynx changes its position in the neck.[26,27] The free edge of the epiglottis in neonates is found at or near the C1 level, and the cricoid cartilage, representing the most caudal portion of the larynx, is at the C4–C5 level. By adolescence, the epiglottis is found at the C2–C3 level, and the cricoid is at C6 level. The adult epiglottis is usually seen at the C3 level, with the cricoid at C6–C7. However, the position of these structures in the normal population varies by at least one vertebral body level. A thin, lucent, air-filled stripe oriented in the AP direction on a lateral view demarcates the position of the laryngeal ventricle at the base of the aryepiglottic folds, just above the true vocal cords (Fig. 2.19A and B). Lateral to the aryepiglottic fold is the pyriform sinus of the hypopharynx. This anterior mucosal recess is between the posterior third of the thyroid cartilage and the aryepiglottic fold. The extreme lower aspect of the pyriform sinus is situated between the mucosa-covered arytenoids and the mucosa-covered thyroid cartilage at the level of the true vocal cords. The air column caudally represents the cervical trachea. On the AP view, the false and true vocal cords above and below the laryngeal ventricles, as well as the subglottic region and the trachea, may be identified. Calcified thyroid cartilage can sometimes be visualized.

The soft tissues dorsal to the airway, the prevertebral tissue, are adherent to the anterior surface of the atlas and the axis

and are the normal soft tissue structures of the posterior pharynx extending from the clivus to the nasopharynx and hypopharynx. The ligaments of the cervicocranium, critical to maintaining stability throughout this region, are directly involved in the range of motion of the cervicocranium and anteriorly contribute to the prevertebral soft tissue shadow. Superimposed on these deep structures are the pharyngeal constrictor muscles and the mucosa of the posterior pharyngeal wall. The cervicocranial prevertebral soft tissue contour should normally be slightly posteriorly concave rostral to the anterior tubercle of C1, anteriorly convex in front of the anterior tubercle, and posteriorly concave caudal to the anterior tubercle, depending on the amount of adenoidal tissue and on the amount of air in the pharynx. Adenoidal tissue appears as a homogeneous, smoothly lobulated mass of varying size and configuration. The anterior surface of the adenoid is demarcated by air anteriorly and inferiorly. The air inferior to the adenoids allows differentiation between adenoids and the presence of a nasopharyngeal hematoma commonly associated with major midface fractures. In infants and young children, the soft tissues of the cervicocranium are lax and redundant. Depending on the phase of respiration and position, the thickness of the prevertebral soft tissues may appear to increase and simulate a retropharyngeal hematoma. This finding may extend to the lower cervical spine. This anomaly becomes normal if imaging is repeated with the neck extended and during inspiration. By 8 years of age, the contour of the soft tissues should resemble that seen in adults.[14] Of note, in pediatric patients, sedation may result in a decrease in the AP

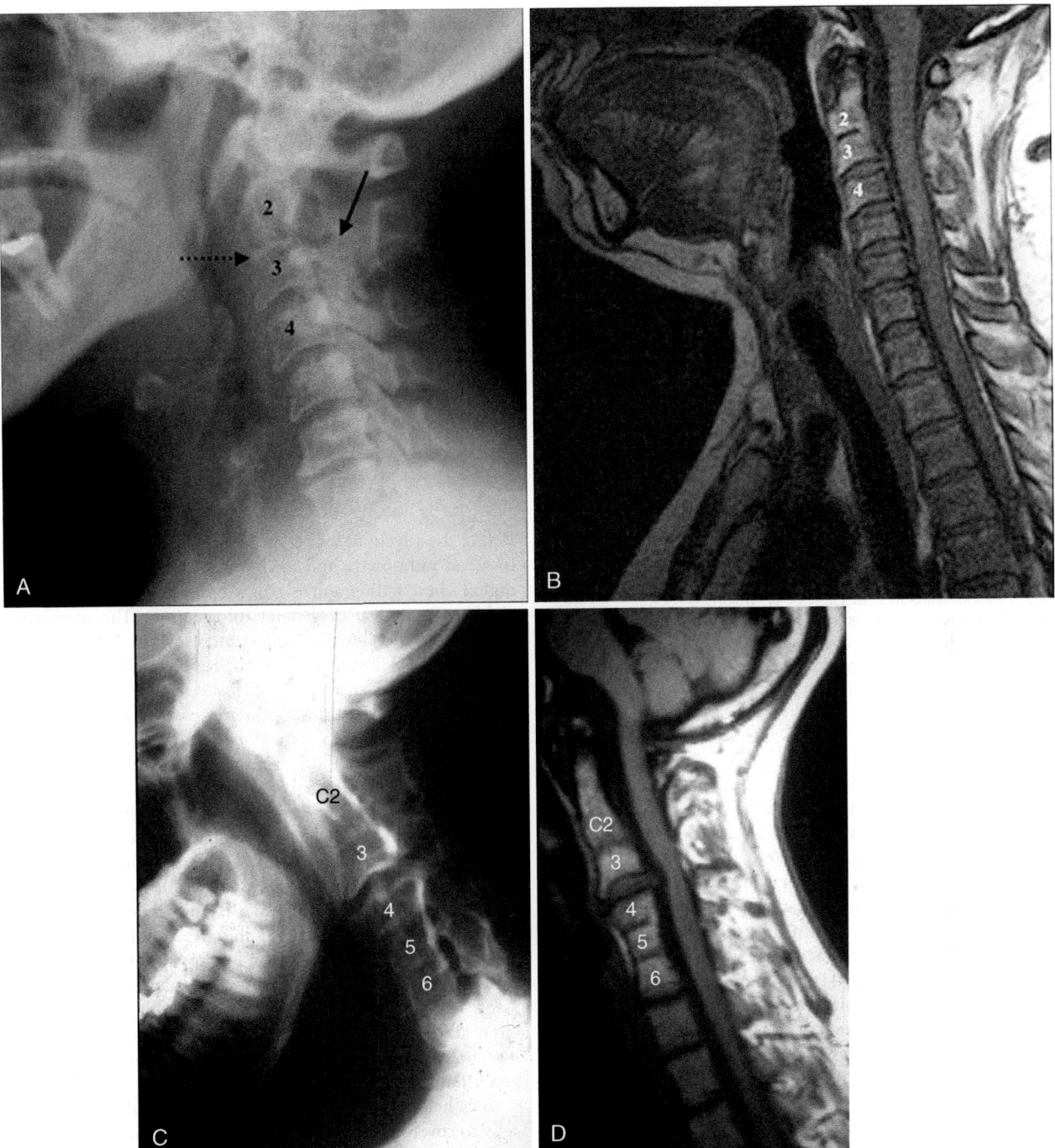

• **Fig. 2.8** Congenital fusion of C2 and C3. (A) Lateral cervical spine radiograph and (B) sagittal T1-weighted magnetic resonance (MR) study demonstrating fusion of C2 and C3 vertebral bodies (*dotted arrow*) and lateral and posterior elements (*arrow*). (C) A lateral radiograph and (D) T1-weighted MR cervical spine of a patient with Klippel-Feil syndrome. There is fusion of C2 to C3 and fusion of C4 to C6. Not surprisingly, a disc herniation is present at the point of greatest mobility at C3–C4.

diameter of the pharynx at the levels of the palatine tonsils, the soft palate, and the epiglottis.

In the lower neck, from C3 to C7, the prevertebral soft tissue shadow differs from that in the cervicocranium because of the beginning of the esophagus and the prevertebral fascial space, which are recognized on the lateral radiograph as a fat stripe. By

standard anatomic description, the esophagus begins at the level of C4; however, the esophageal ostium in vivo may normally be found as high as C3 and as low as C6 and varies with the phase of swallowing and the flexion or extension of the cervical spine.[28] The prevertebral soft tissue thickness—the distance between the posterior pharyngeal air column and the anterior portion of the

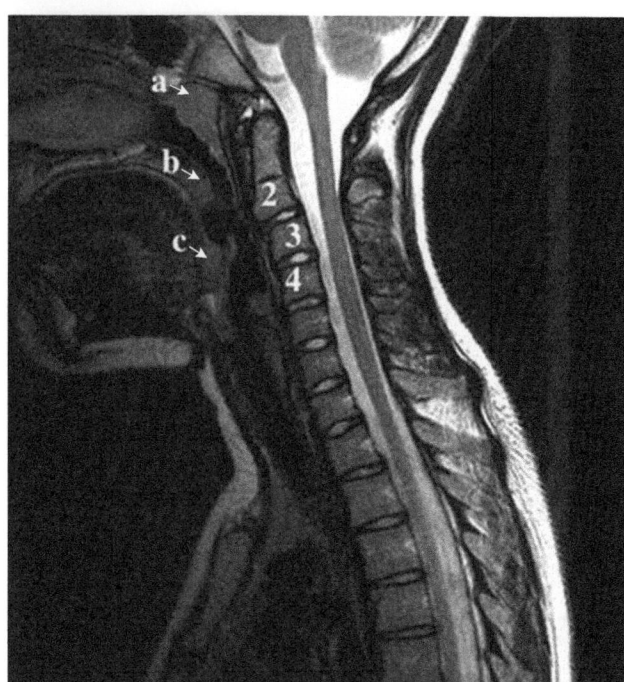

• **Fig. 2.9** Pseudosubluxation at C2–C3. T2-weighted sagittal magnetic resonance (MR) cervical spine study demonstrates physiologic anterior displacement of C2 on C3 in a child. Also seen are normal soft tissue masses encroaching on the airway from adenoids (a), palatine tonsils (b), and lingual tonsils at the base of the tongue (c).

third or fourth vertebra—should not exceed one-half to three-quarters of the diameter of the vertebral body. In the opinion of Harris and Mirvis, only the measurement at C3 is valid, and it should not exceed 4 mm (Fig. 2.20A and B).[14] More caudally, at the cervicothoracic junction, assessment of the prevertebral soft tissues is based on contour rather than actual measurement. This contour should parallel the arch formed by the anterior cortices of the lower cervical and upper thoracic vertebral bodies.

In truth, plain film or digital radiograph diagnosis of upper airway diseases has been supplanted by cross-sectional imaging, except in a few situations in which plain x-ray findings are pathognomonic of the disease. Two classic examples of plain film or digital radiologic diagnosis are acute epiglottitis and croup. In acute epiglottitis, or *supraglottitis*, a more encompassing term, edema and swelling of the epiglottis are present, with or without involvement of the aryepiglottic folds and arytenoids. Historically, the causative organism was usually *Haemophilus influenza*; with the introduction of the Haemophilus vaccine, group A β-hemolytic streptococcus is more commonly responsible for such infections. Airway compromise with a rapidly progressive course requiring emergency tracheostomy is a possibility if the entity goes unrecognized and untreated. In general, the infection is milder in adults than in children. The radiographic findings are swelling or enlargement of the epiglottis. On a lateral radiograph of the neck, thickening of the free edge of the epiglottis can be appreciated and is referred to as the "thumb sign" (Fig. 2.21). The width of the adult epiglottis should be less than one-third of the AP width of the C4 body. Cross-sectional imaging is superfluous; however,

theoretically, the degree of airway compromise can be quantified by three-dimensional reconstruction.

In laryngotracheobronchitis, or croup, the subglottic larynx is involved. It affects younger children and has a less fulminant course than acute epiglottitis. The swelling of the soft tissues in the subglottic neck can be appreciated on an AP view of the neck (Fig. 2.22). There is usually a long, segmental narrowing of the glottis and subglottic airway with loss of the normal angle between the vocal cords and the subglottic airway. The narrowing of the upper trachea has been referred to as the "steeple" sign.[29] The hypopharynx is usually dilated because of the airway obstruction distally.

Cervical spine examination using a soft tissue technique is also useful for the evaluation for the presence of radiopaque foreign bodies, such as a fish bone. Ingested foreign bodies most often lodge at the level of the pyriform sinus (Fig. 2.23A–D).

Chest Radiography

Radiology Overview

Before the advent of CT, chest x-ray (CXR) was routinely ordered to assess pulmonary and cardiovascular status. Today, a CXR or digital chest radiograph is still a cost-efficient examination that yields a great deal of general information. The most common views of the chest are the posteroanterior (PA), AP, and lateral projections (Fig. 2.24A–D). Film cassette-based PA CXR is obtained with the patient's anterior chest closest to the film cassette and the x-ray beam directed from a posterior to anterior direction. Alternatively, the AP chest view is done with the patient's back closest to the film cassette and the x-ray beam directed in the anterior to posterior direction. The part of the chest closest to the film cassette is the least magnified; therefore, the cardiac silhouette is larger on the AP projection. The lateral projection is most often performed with the patient's left chest closest to the film cassette for better delineation of the structures in the left hemithorax, which is more obscured by the heart on a PA projection. Other common projections obtained include oblique, decubitus, and lordotic views. The oblique view is useful for assessing a lesion with respect to other structures in the chest. The decubitus view is helpful to assess whether an apparent elevated hemidiaphragm is due to a large subpulmonic pleural effusion. The lordotic view is useful to look for a suspected small apical pneumothorax, which can also be accentuated on an expiratory phase view.

It is helpful to train one's eyes to analyze the CXR systematically to cover the details of the chest wall, including the ribs, lungs, and mediastinal structures that include the heart and the outline of the tracheobronchial tree. On an adequate inspiratory film, the hemidiaphragms are below the anterior end of the 6th rib, or at least below the 10th posterior rib, and the lung expansion should be symmetrical. The right hemidiaphragm is usually half an interspace higher than the left, which is depressed by the heart (see Fig. 2.24). Without a doubt, the art of CXR interpretation has been supplanted by the advent of CT, which demonstrates chest pathology with unparalleled clarity. However, CXR can still afford a composite survey of the chest at one quick glance. One can easily compare lung volumes, the position of the mediastinum, the presence or absence of major airspace disease, and a gross assessment of cardiac status.

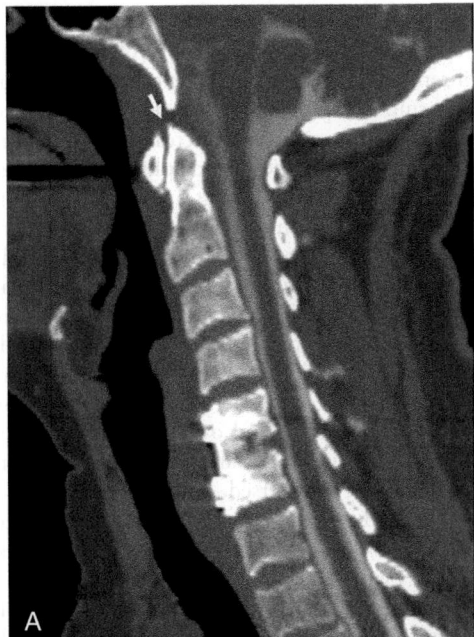

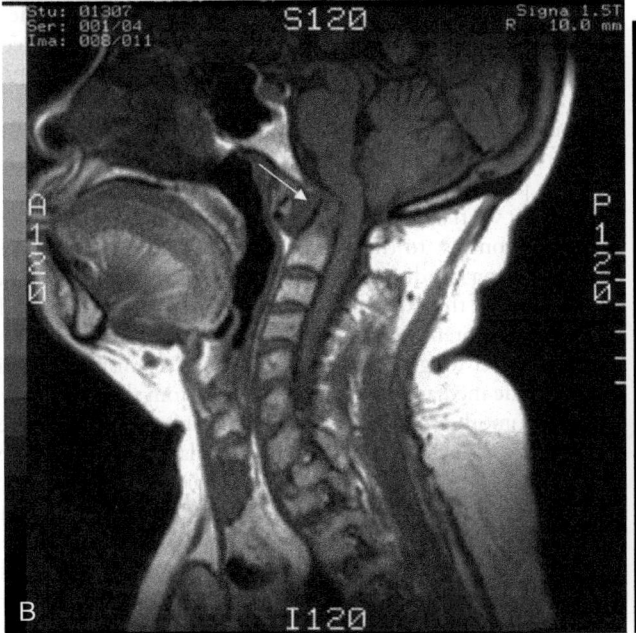

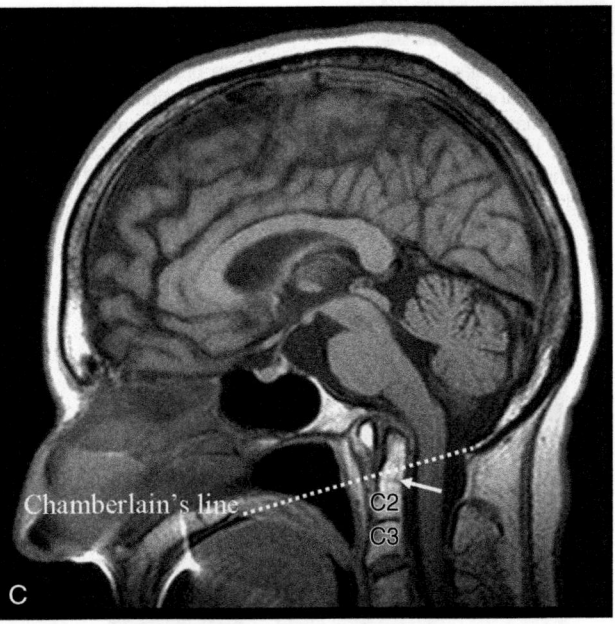

• **Fig. 2.10** (A) Position of the dens in a normal patient, (B) rheumatoid patient, and (C) nonrheumatoid patient with basilar invagination and platybasia. (A) Postmyelogram computed tomography (CT) with sagittal reformation demonstrates normal relationship of the dens with respect to the foramen magnum, brainstem, and anterior arch of C1. Normal atlantoaxial distance (AADI) is seen (*arrow*). (B) T1-weighted sagittal magnetic resonance (MR) study of the cervical spine in a rheumatoid patient with erosion and pannus formation at the atlantoaxial joint resulting in an increased AADI (*arrow*), posterior subluxation of the dens, and brainstem compression. (C) Sagittal MR study of the brain in a nonrheumatoid patient with a normal AADI, but basilar invagination and platybasia result in vertical subluxation of the dens and brainstem compression. The line drawn from the hard palate to the posterior lip of the foramen magnum is Chamberlain's line (*dotted line*); basilar invagination is defined as extension of the odontoid tip 5 mm or above this line. Also, note fusion of the C2 and C3 vertebrae. The small linear dark line at the level of mid-C2 is the subdental synchondrosis (*arrow*).

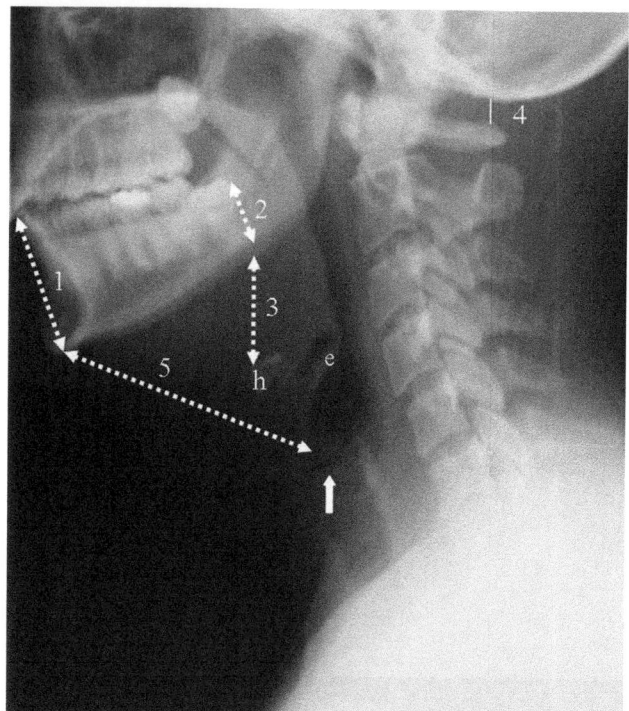

• **Fig. 2.11** Mandibular and hyoid measurements proposed as predictors of difficult laryngoscopy. *1*, Anterior depth of mandible; *2*, posterior depth of mandible; *3*, mandibulohyoid distance; *4*, atlanto-occipital distance; *5*, thyromental distance; *e*, epiglottis; *h*, hyoid bone; *solid arrow*, laryngeal ventricle demarcating the level of the larynx. The true vocal cords are just below the level of the laryngeal ventricle.

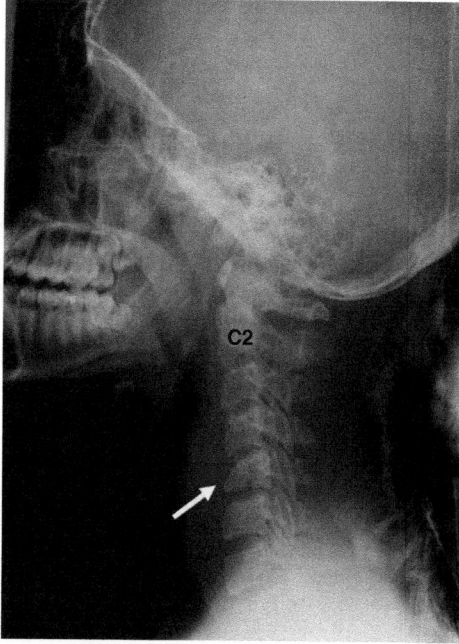

• **Fig. 2.12** Cervical spine fracture. Lateral radiograph of the cervical spine demonstrates a compression fracture of the C5 vertebra (*arrow*).

Chest Anatomy and Pathology

A high hemidiaphragm implies reduced lung volume, which can be caused by phrenic nerve paralysis, thoracic conditions causing chest pain that results in splinting, or extrapulmonic processes such as an enlarged spleen or liver, pancreatitis, or subphrenic abscess. The presumed level of the hemidiaphragm is seen as the edge or transition between aerated lungs and the opacity of the organs in the abdomen. If the thin leaves of the hemidiaphragm are outlined by air, a pneumoperitoneum should be considered (Fig. 2.25). A well-expanded lung should appear radiographically lucent but be traversed by "lung markings"—thin threads of interstitium consisting of septa and arterial, venous, and lymphatic vessels. In most normal individuals, the lungs appear less lucent at the bottom, owing to the distribution of the pulmonary vasculature, the effect of gravity, and overlying soft tissues such as breast tissues. In congestive heart failure or pulmonary venous hypertension, this pattern is reversed, with "cephalization" and engorgement of the pulmonary veins in the upper lung zones (Fig. 2.26; see Fig. 2.24). In general, any process that replaces the airspaces of the lungs with a substance such as fluid, pus, or cells causes the x-ray beam to be more attenuated, allowing less of the beam to be transmitted through the patient to the film, resulting in an image that is less dark or more opaque (white) in the areas affected. A whole host of diseases could be responsible, depending on the clinical picture, including pleural effusion, pulmonary edema, pneumonia, lung mass, lung collapse (atelectasis), lung infarct or contusion, and metastatic disease (Fig. 2.27A–J). The key, from the anesthesiologist's point of view, is not to make the correct pathologic diagnosis but to note the abnormality, which may affect ventilation, and to adjust the anesthetic practice accordingly. In contrast to the increased opacity of the lung caused by the preceding conditions is a hemithorax that appears too lucent and devoid of the expected lung markings. Two entities should be considered. Foremost is a pneumothorax (Fig. 2.28A–C); if large, the collapsed lung is medially positioned against the mediastinum. If the mediastinum is shifted away from the midline, a tension pneumothorax may be present, and emergent management is required. Occasionally, the cause of a unilateral lucent lung is the presence of large emphysematous blebs in patients with chronic obstructive pulmonary disease, which are sometimes difficult to differentiate from a moderate to large pneumothorax. More rare causes include pulmonary oligemia (decreased pulmonary flow) from a thromboembolism of the right or left pulmonary artery, pulmonary neoplasm, or obstructive hyperinflation. Bilateral lucent lungs are more difficult to appreciate. These are usually seen in patients with pulmonary stenosis secondary to cyanotic heart disease and right-to-left shunts. A discussion of the pediatric chest and congenital heart and lung diseases is beyond the scope of this chapter.

Moving centrally in the chest, one encounters the mediastinum, which contains the hila, tracheobronchial tree, heart and great vessels, lymph nodes, esophagus, and thymus. The mediastinum is extrapleural and outlined by air in the adjacent lungs. Except for the air within the trachea and the mainstem bronchi, on conventional chest radiographs the remainder of the mediastinal structures are soft tissues or water density. Therefore, it is extremely difficult to localize a mediastinal lesion. Traditional

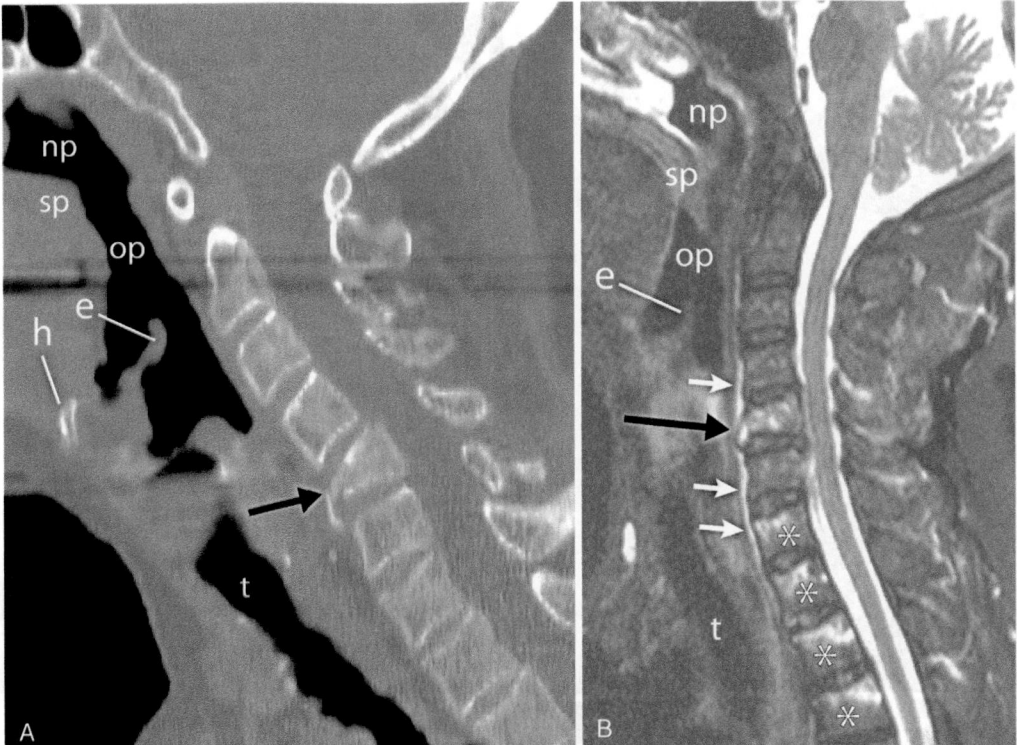

• **Fig. 2.13** (A) Sagittal computed tomography (CT) image shows anterior wedge deformity of the C5 vertebral body with fracture lines (*arrow*). There is bony retropulsion impinging the spinal canal. (B) Sagittal short-tau inversion recovery magnetic resonance (MR) image shows marrow edema associated with C5 fracture (*long black arrow*). There is trace prevertebral edema (*short white arrows*) suggestive of ligamentous injury. Marrow edema (*asterisks*) is seen in additional vertebrae without significant height loss, indicating subtle fractures not clearly evident on CT. *np*, nasopharynx; *sp*, soft palate; *op*, oropharynx; *h*, hyoid bone; *e*, Epiglottis; *t*, trachea.

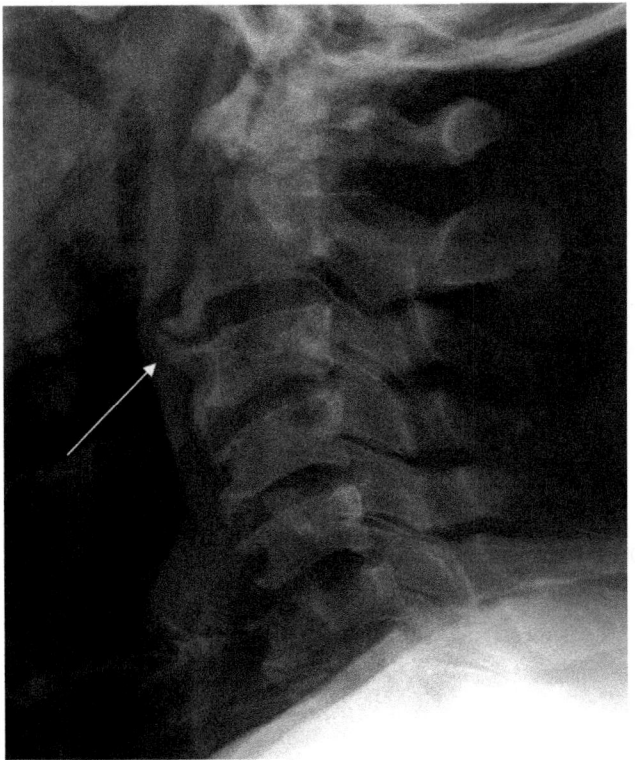

• **Fig. 2.14** Cervical spondylosis. Lateral cervical spine radiograph reveals large anterior osteophytes (*arrow*) that indent the airway and oropharynx.

pleural reflections or vertical lines are described for a frontal CXR that, if deviated, would suggest the presence of mediastinal pathology. Felson has proposed a radiologic approach to subdividing the mediastinum on a lateral radiograph into three compartments: anterior, middle, and posterior.[30] The anterior and middle mediastinum are divided by the line extending along the back of the heart and the front of the trachea. The middle and posterior mediastinal compartments are separated by the line connecting a point on each thoracic vertebra about a centimeter behind its anterior margin (Fig. 2.29).[30]

Conditions that can be found in each of the compartments of the mediastinum are logically based on the anatomic structures found within the compartments. For example, tracheal, esophageal, and thyroid lesions would lie in the middle mediastinum. Neurogenic tumors and spinal problems would be in the posterior mediastinum. Cardiac and thymic lesions would occupy the anterior mediastinum. Certain diseases, such as lymph node disorders, lymphoma, and aortic aneurysms, may arise in any or all three compartments.[30] Many modifications to the divisions of the mediastinum have been proposed.[31]

The great vessels and the heart should be centrally located on the AP view of the mediastinum. The aortic knob is usually on the left, and the cardiothoracic ratio on the AP view should be roughly less than 50%. The hila are composed of the pulmonary arteries and their main branches, the upper lobe pulmonary veins, the major bronchi, and the lymph glands (Fig. 2.30A and B). The positions of the trachea, carina, and mainstem bronchi are outlined by air. The carinal bifurcation angle is typically 60 to

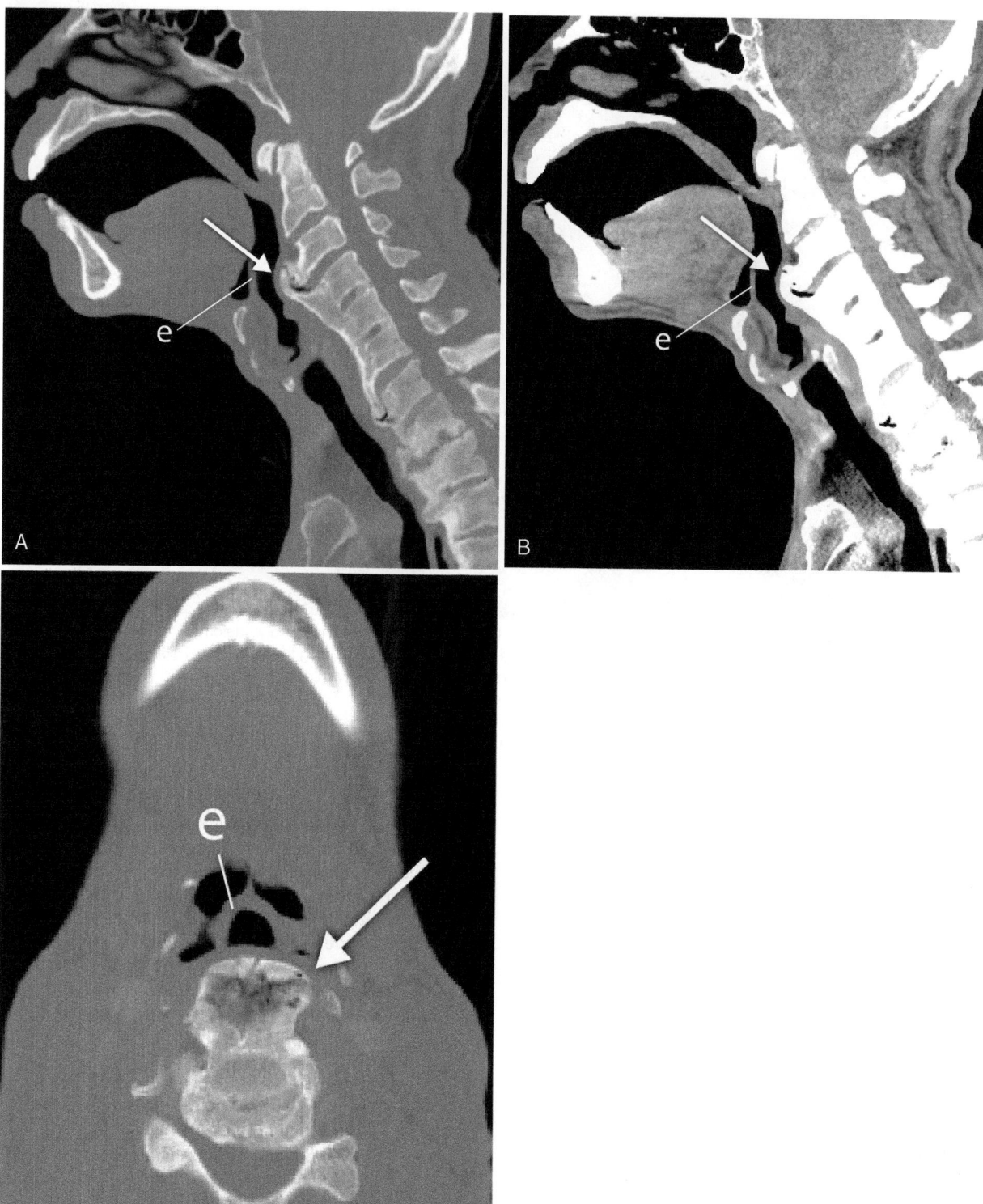

• **Fig. 2.15** Diffuse idiopathic skeletal hyperostosis (DISH). Lateral computed tomography (CT) images in (A) bone and (B) soft tissue algorithm demonstrate multilevel anterior bridging osteophytes of the cervical spine compatible with DISH. A prominent bridging osteophyte at C3–C4 (*arrow*) indents the posterior pharyngeal wall and narrows the airway. (C) Axial CT image at C3–C4 shows effacement of the airway from a prominent osteophyte (arrow). *e*, Epiglottis.

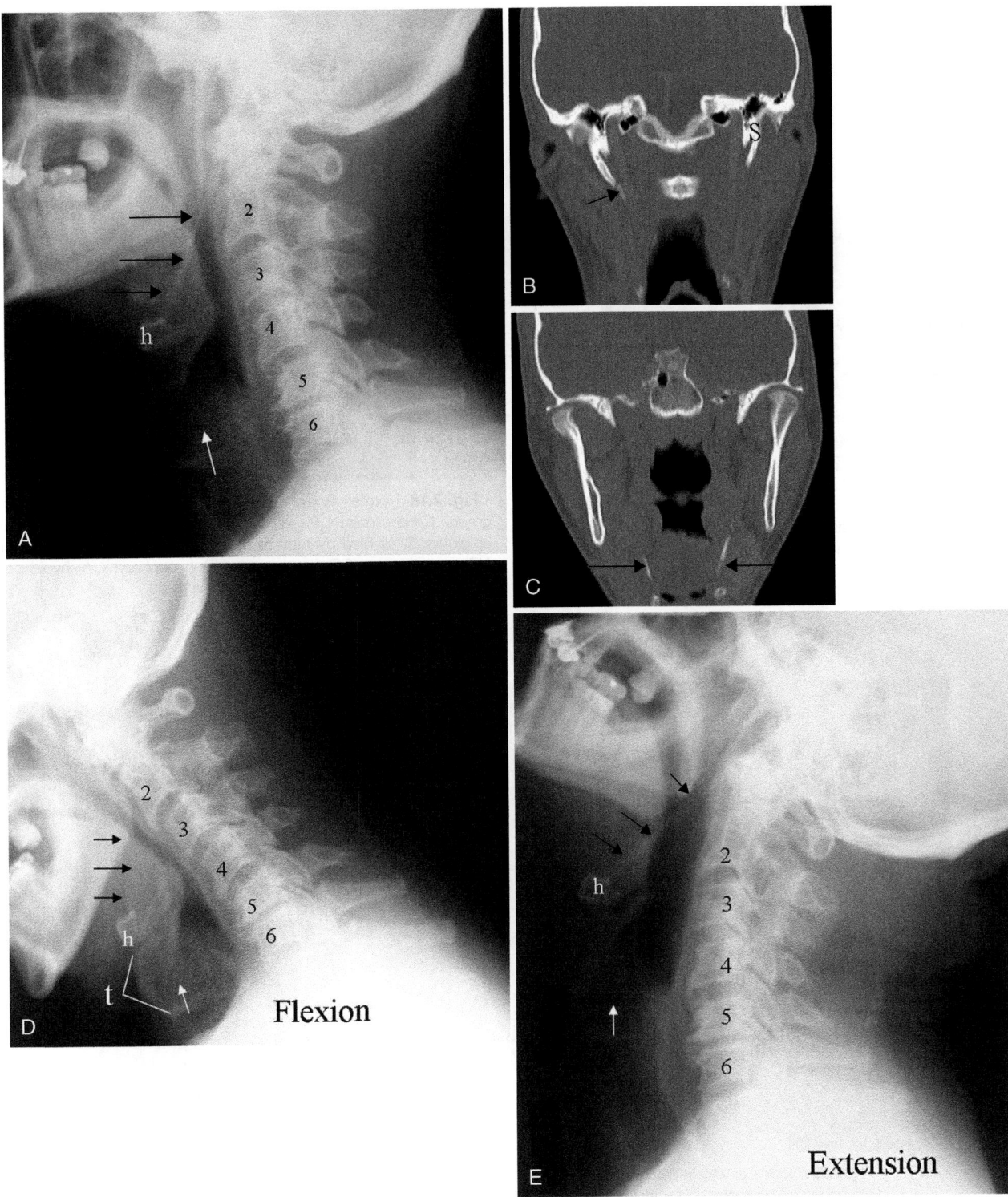

• **Fig. 2.16** Calcified stylohyoid ligament. (A) Lateral cervical spine radiograph. (B and C) Coronal CT, bone algorithm. (D) Lateral cervical spine flexion view. (E) Lateral cervical spine extension view: *black arrows*, calcified stylohyoid ligaments; *white arrows*, laryngeal ventricle at the level of the vocal cords. *h*, Hyoid bone; *s*, styloid process; *t*, calcified thyroid cartilage. Note the change in the level of the hyoid bone and the vocal cords with flexion and extension of the neck.

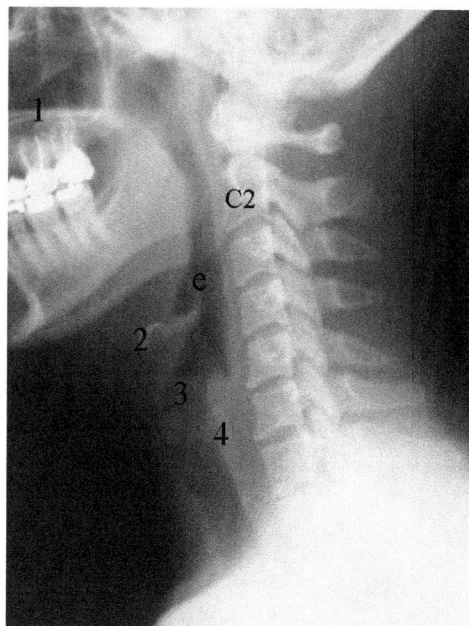

• **Fig. 2.17** Normal bony landmarks on a lateral cervical spine radiograph. *1*, Hard palate; *2*, hyoid bone; *3*, calcified thyroid cartilage; *4*, calcified cricoid cartilage; *e*, epiglottis.

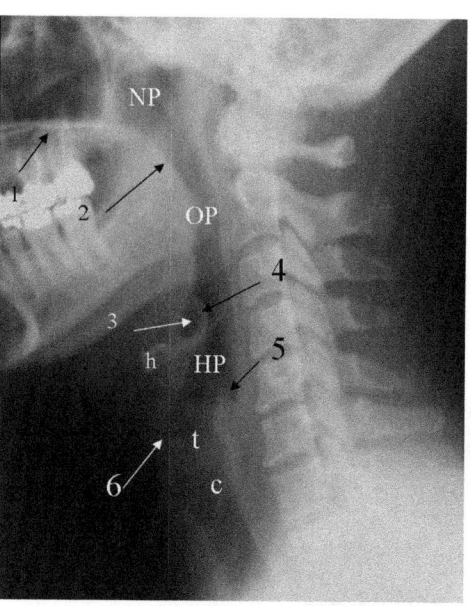

• **Fig. 2.18** Normal airway structures on a lateral cervical spine radiograph. *1*, Hard palate; *2*, soft palate and uvula; *3*, air-filled vallecula; *4*, epiglottis; *5*, air-filled pyriform sinus; *6*, air-filled stripe laryngeal ventricle; *NP*, nasopharynx; *OP*, oropharynx; *HP*, hypopharynx; *h*, hyoid bone; *t*, thyroid cartilage; *c*, noncalcified cricoid cartilage.

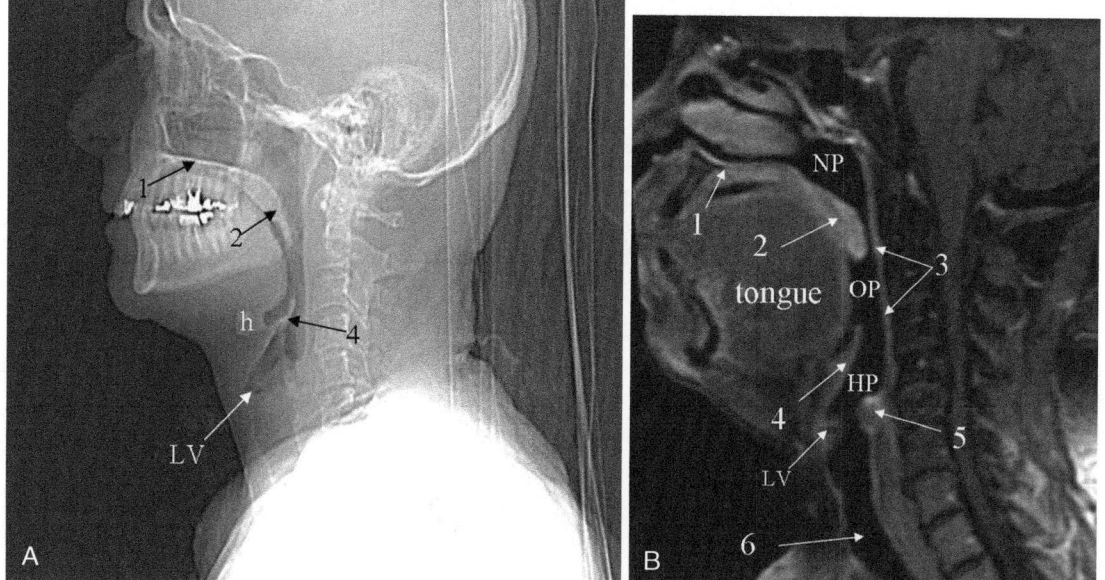

• **Fig. 2.19** Normal airway structures. (A) Computed tomography (CT) lateral scout view. (B) T1-weighted, fat-suppressed postcontrast sagittal magnetic resonance (MR) cervical spine study. *1*, Hard palate; *2*, soft palate and uvula; *3*, retropharyngeal or prevertebral soft tissue; *4*, epiglottis; *5*, arytenoid prominence; *6*, trachea air column; *h*, hyoid bone; *LV*, laryngeal ventricle; *NP*, nasopharynx; *OP*, oropharynx; *HP*, hypopharynx.

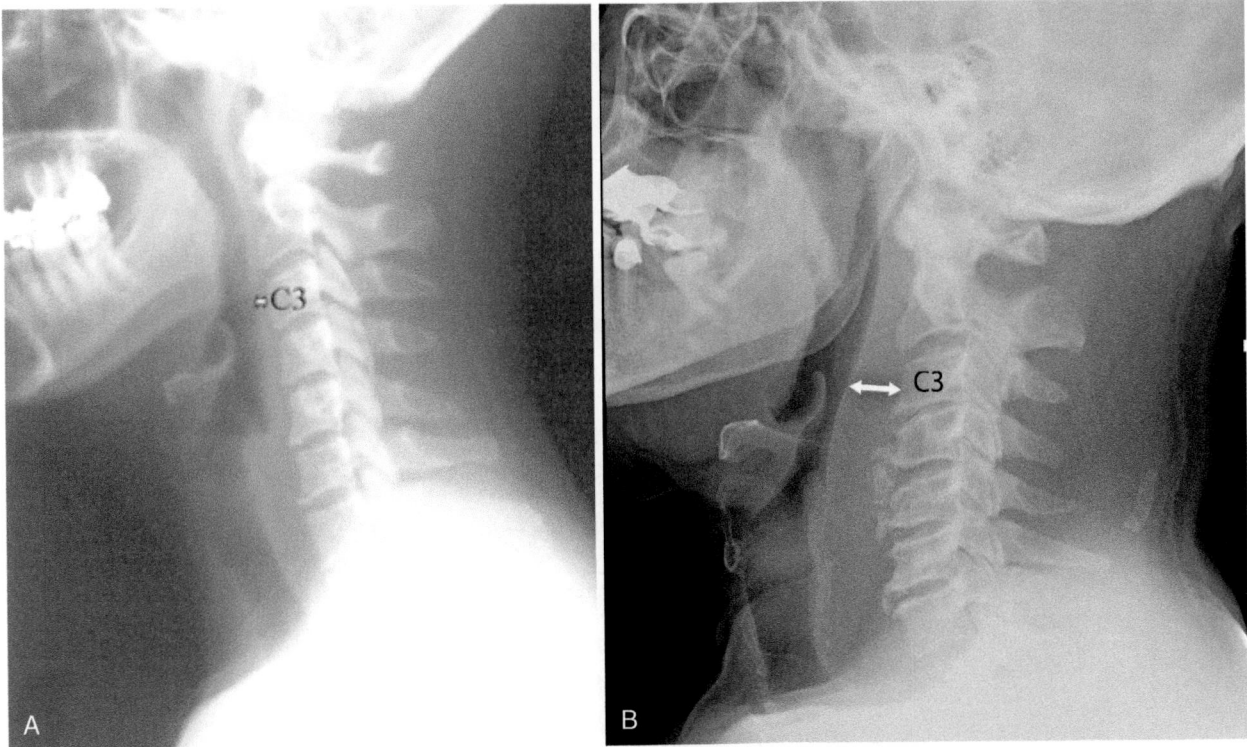

• **Fig. 2.20** Prevertebral soft tissues on lateral cervical spine radiograph. (A) Normal adult. (B) Prominence of prevertebral soft tissue in an adult; the airway is displaced anteriorly.

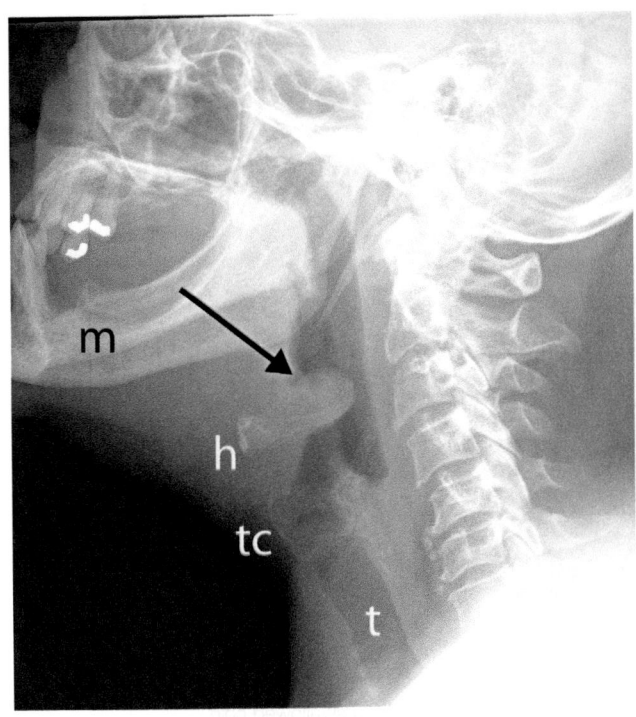

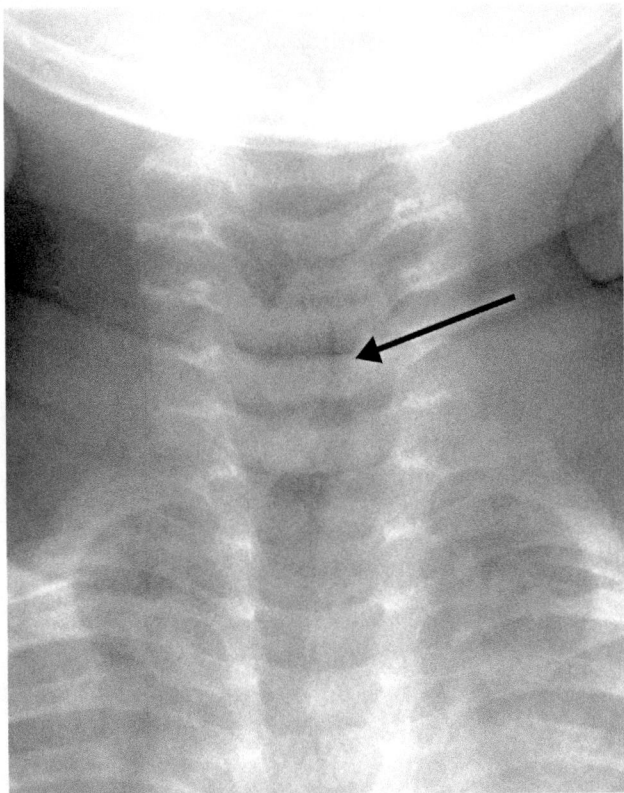

• **Fig. 2.22** Croup. Anteroposterior soft-tissue neck radiograph in an infant. Long segment narrowing of the subglottic airway is present with loss of the normal angle between the vocal cords and the subglottic airway (the "steeple sign") (*arrow*).

• **Fig. 2.21** Epiglottitis. Lateral soft tissue neck radiograph in an adult demonstrating an enlarged and swollen epiglottis (the "thumb sign") (*arrow*). *m*, mandible; *h*, Hyoid; *tc*, tracheal cartilage; *t*, trachea.

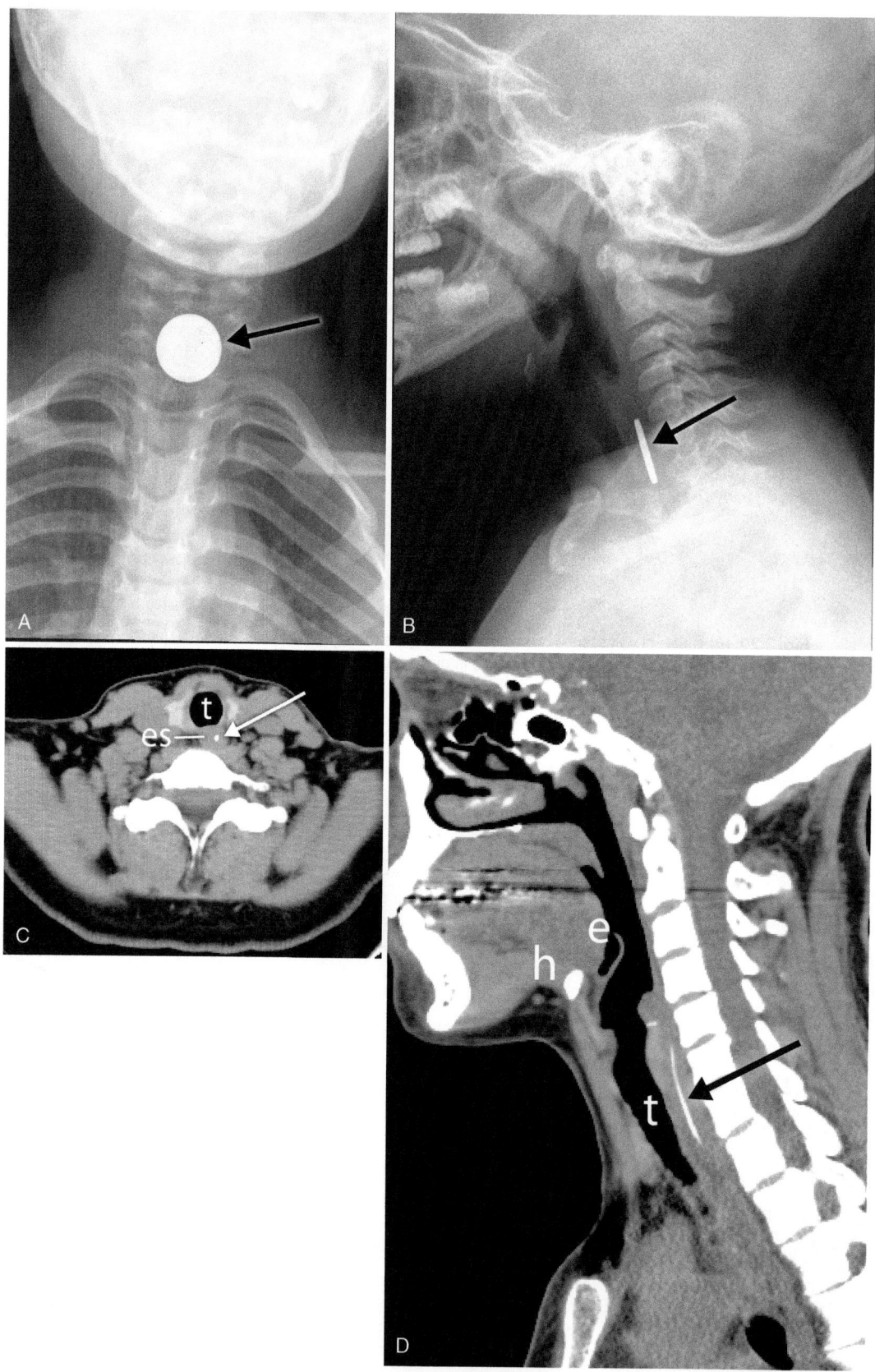

• **Fig. 2.23** Foreign bodies. (A) Frontal and (B) lateral soft tissue neck in a patient with a swallowed coin in the hypopharynx/cervical esophagus (*arrow*). (C) Axial and (D) sagittal computed tomography (CT) of the neck in a different patient with an ingested fish bone (*arrow*). *e,* Epiglottis; *h,* hyoid; *t,* trachea; *es,* esophagus.

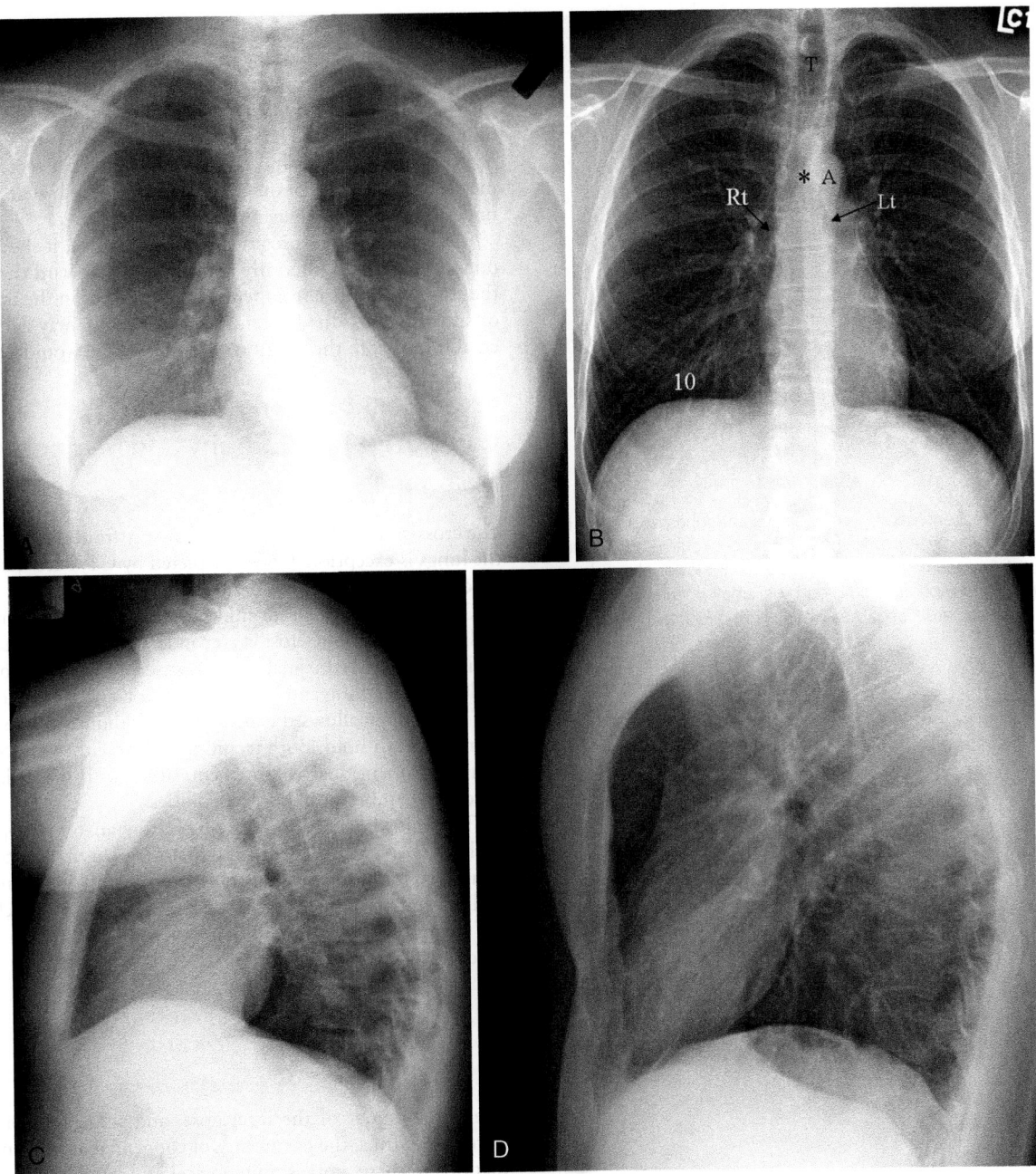

• **Fig. 2.24** Normal chest radiographic studies of the chest. (A) Normal posteroanterior (PA) view of a female with increased density at the lung bases related to overlying breast tissues. (B) PA chest of a male with lucent lungs: *T*, trachea; *A*, aorta; *asterisk*, carina; *Rt*, right main bronchus; *Lt*, left main bronchus; *10*, 10th posterior rib. (C) Normal lateral chest view. (D) Lateral chest view of a patient with chronic obstructive pulmonary disease (COPD) showing barrel-shaped chest with increase in the retrosternal air; note that the lung base appears progressively more lucent overlying the dorsal spine.

75 degrees.[31] The right mainstem bronchus has a steeper angle than the left (see Fig. 2.24); it usually branches off the trachea at 25 to 30 degrees, whereas the left mainstem bronchus leaves the trachea at a 45-degree to 50-degree angle. The trachea is a tubular structure extending from the cricoid cartilage to the carina, which is located at approximately the T5 level. C-shaped hyaline cartilage rings, which can calcify with age, outline the trachea anteriorly; the posterior trachea is membranous. The mean transverse diameter of the trachea is approximately 15 mm for women and 18 mm for men.[31] The trachea in the cervical region is midline, but it is deviated to the right in the thorax.

Adequate positioning of an ETT in an intubated patient is usually documented by obtaining a chest radiograph. The tip should be intrathoracic and at a distance above the carina that

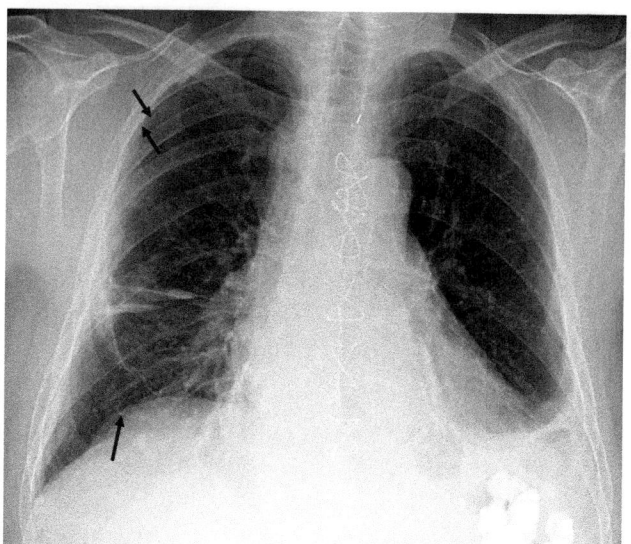

• **Fig. 2.25** Pneumoperitoneum. Postoperative anteroposterior chest in a patient after thoracotomy. *Arrows* in right upper chest outline a thin pleural line defining a tiny pneumothorax. *Arrow* in the right lower chest demarcates the right hemidiaphragm outlined by a small pneumoperitoneum. This patient also has cardiomegaly as well as right midlung and left basilar atelectasis.

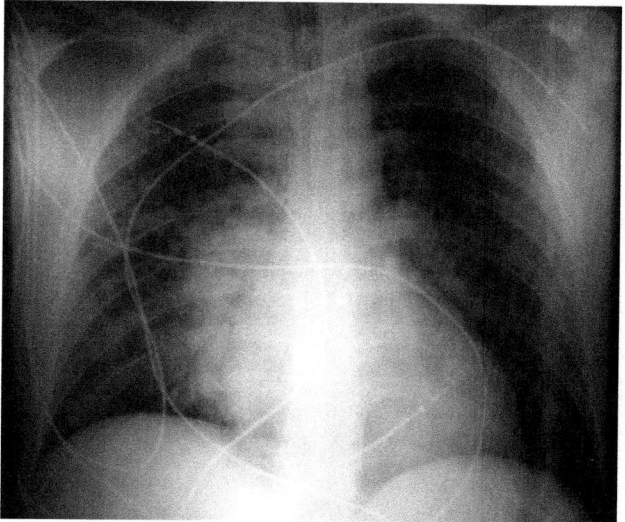

• **Fig. 2.26** Congestive heart failure. Anteroposterior chest radiograph demonstrates engorgement of the perihilar vasculature. An endotracheal tube and nasogastric tube are in place.

ensures equal ventilation to both lungs. One should evaluate the ETT position with the patient's head and neck in a neutral position; however, in an intensive care unit setting, this may not be possible. The tip of the ETT may move up or down by 1 to 2 cm with extension or flexion of the neck, respectively. Rotation of the head and neck usually results in ascent of the tip.[31] The optimum position of the tip of the ETT is approximately 3 to 5 cm above the carina; this allows enough latitude for movement of the patient's head such that the tip does not enter the right main bronchus and the inflated cuff remains below the vocal cords (Fig. 2.31A and B).[32] Malpositioning of the cuff at the level of the vocal cords or pharynx increases the

risk of aspiration. Overinflation of the cuff at the level of the vocal cords may lead to necrosis.[33] The inflated cuff of the ETT should fill the tracheal air column without changing its contour. Overall, the ETT size should be about two-thirds the diameter of the tracheal lumen. If the tip of the ETT extends beyond the carina, intubation of the right main bronchus occurs, which can be detected by asymmetric breath sounds or on CXR. If unrecognized, atelectasis in the underventilated lung may result.

If a nasogastric or orogastric tube is in place, it should be seen on CXR to course inferiorly and to the left, toward the fundus of the stomach in the left upper quadrant, except in the unusual case of situs inversus. Inadvertently, a gastric tube may achieve bronchial intubation; the errant course of the tube would be evident.

Cross-Sectional Anatomy and Pathology: Computed Tomography and Magnetic Resonance Imaging

The cross-sectional anatomy of the airway from the nasal cavity to the lungs is exceptionally well depicted by CT; MRI can be a useful complement in the evaluation of these regions. MRI is superior to CT in evaluating tumor infiltration of soft tissues but lacks the ability to depict bone erosions secondary to tumor because cortical bone gives no MRI signal. MRI is susceptible to motion artifact, including breathing and vascular pulsation artifacts, whereas spiral CT technology allows the entire neck or thorax to be scanned in a single breath-hold. Both techniques allow either direct scanning or three-dimensional volume acquisition with multiplanar postprocessing and reformation capabilities.

The following sections describe airway anatomy applicable to both MRI and CT. Recognizing that the pharynx is a continuous structure, for ease of discussion, the nasopharynx, oropharynx, and hypopharynx are discussed separately. Within each section, the anatomy and pertinent pathology with relevance to anesthetic practice are elaborated.

Nose, Nasal Cavity, and Sinuses

Development and Structure

The development of the face, nose, and sinuses is complex but systematic. Thus, the occurrence of congenital lesions and malformations in these areas is quite logical and predictable, dependent on the time of prenatal insult. Face development, nose development, and sinus development are temporally and spatially related to the development of the optic nerve, globe, and corpus callosum, which accounts for the frequency of concurrent anomalies.

The major features of the face develop in the fourth to eighth week of gestation, owing to the growth, migration, and merging of several processes adjoining the stomodeum, which is a slit-like invagination of the ectoderm that marks the location of the mouth. At the fourth week of gestation, two sets of paired and one set of unpaired prominences, derivatives of the first branchial arch, can be identified bordering the stomodeum. The unpaired median frontonasal prominence is located superiorly, the paired maxillary processes are lateral, and the paired mandibular processes are inferior.[34] The various cleft lip, palate, and face syndromes (Figs. 2.32A–C and 2.33A–G) can be explained by the failure of different processes to grow, migrate, and/or merge properly.[34,35]

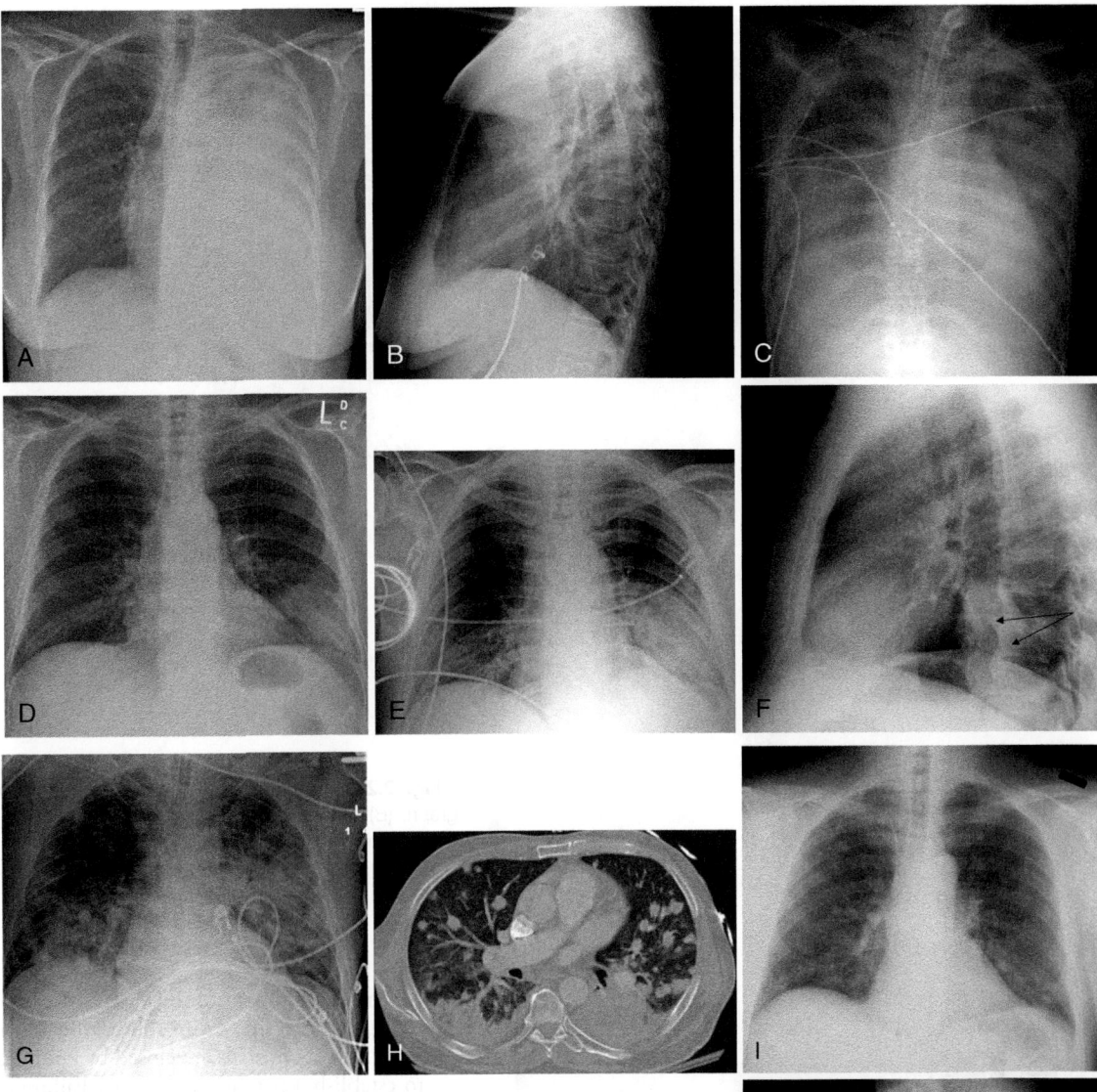

• **Fig. 2.27** (A and B) Left pleural effusion. (A) Posteroanterior (PA) view of the chest shows almost complete whiteout of the left hemithorax and minimal residual aerated left upper lung zone. There is a mass effect with deviation of the trachea to the right. (B) On the lateral view, the pleural effusion is less apparent. The tipoff is the lack of the expected lucency overlying the spine at the base; see Figs. 2.24C and D. (C) Pulmonary edema. Anteroposterior (AP) view of the chest demonstrates bilateral hazy lung fields with air bronchogram. (D–F) A tracheostomy tube is noted. Left lower lung mass. (D) PA and (E) AP radiographs of the chest. Note that although the inspiratory effort is the same on both the PA and AP views (hemidiaphragm below the ninth posterior rib), the cardiac silhouette and the left lower lobe mass appear larger on the AP view because of the film geometry and magnification factor. (F) The lateral view helps to localize the disease process to the lateral segment of the left lower lobe. A mass is noted with postobstructive atelectasis (*arrows*). (G and H) Aspergillosis. (G) AP chest radiograph shows nodular densities in both lungs. The differential includes inflammatory and neoplastic processes. Note that the tip of the endotracheal tube is in a good position, above the carina, and a central line is noted on the right. (H) Axial computed tomography (CT) of the chest better demonstrates the nodular pattern of lung involvement. (I and J) Melanoma metastases to the lungs. (I) PA and (J) lateral radiographs of the chest demonstrate nodular densities in both lungs in a patient with known melanoma. These examples illustrate that radiographic findings are similar when lung parenchyma is infiltrated with inflammatory or neoplastic cells.

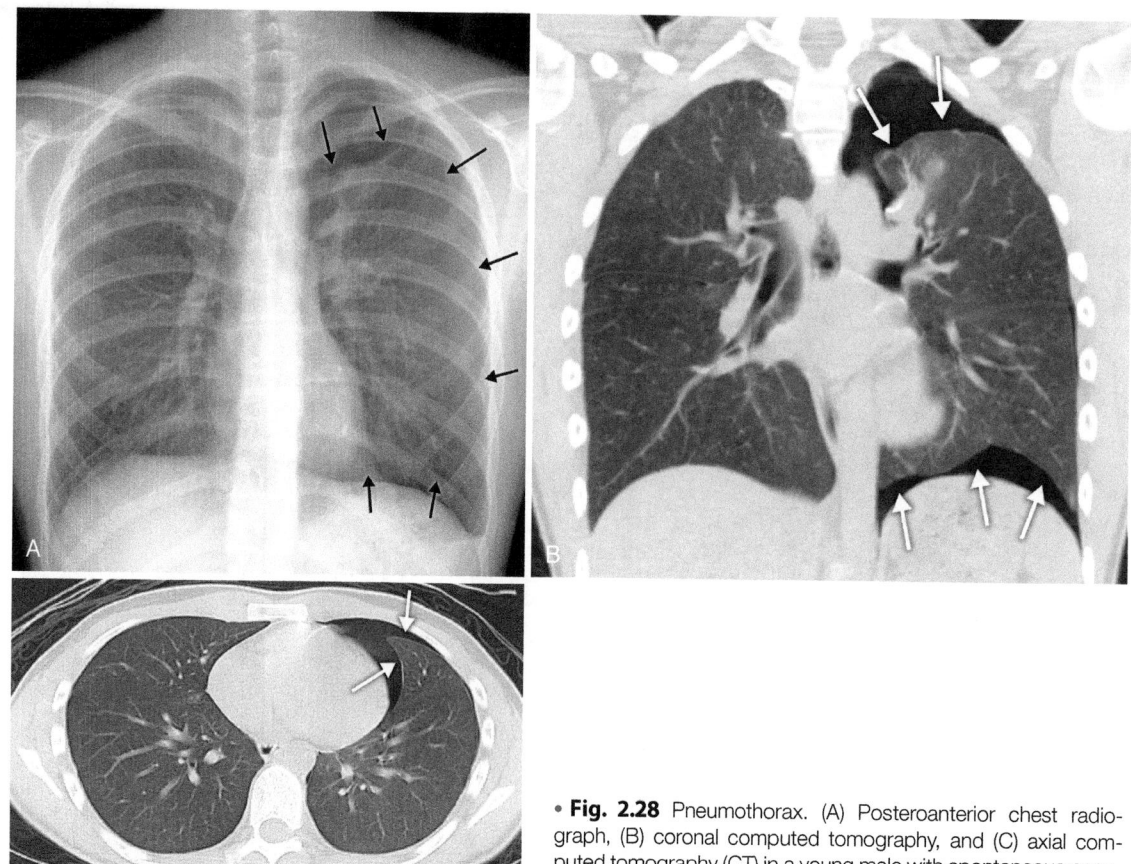

• **Fig. 2.28** Pneumothorax. (A) Posteroanterior chest radiograph, (B) coronal computed tomography, and (C) axial computed tomography (CT) in a young male with spontaneous pneumothorax. A thin pleural line (*arrows*) separates lung parenchyma from air in the pleural space.

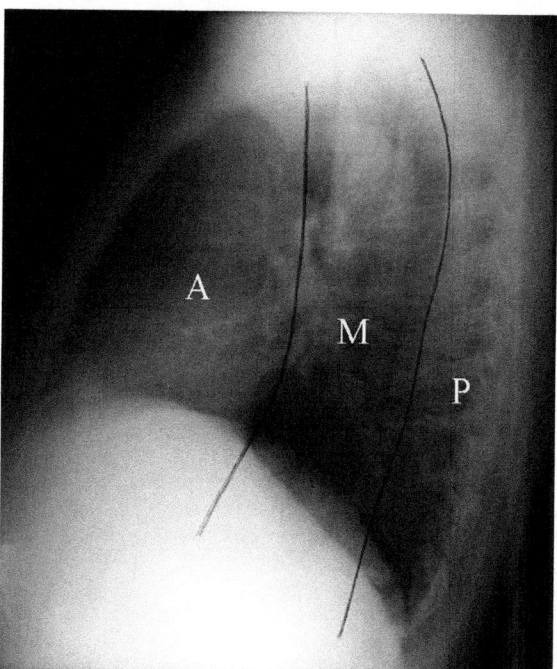

• **Fig. 2.29** Mediastinal compartments. Lateral chest radiograph with imaginary lines drawn on the film to demonstrate the three mediastinal compartments. The anterior (*A*) and middle (*M*) mediastinal compartments are divided by the line extending along the back of the heart and front of the trachea. A line drawn connecting each thoracic vertebra about a centimeter behind its anterior margin separates the middle from the posterior compartment (*P*).

The development of the nasal cavity is complete by the second month of fetal life. From the second to the sixth month of prenatal life, the nostrils are closed by epithelial plugs that recanalize to establish a patent nasal cavity. Failure to do so could account for the congenital stenoses and atresias that cause nasal airway obstruction, which are often seen in conjunction with craniofacial anomalies.[35]

The nose is pyramidal in shape and refers to both the external feature and the nasal cavity. It is one of the two gateways to the aerodigestive tract. Most of the airflow to the lungs occurs through the nasal cavity. Mouth breathing is not physiologic; it is a learned action. The three physiologic functions of the nose are respiration, defense, and olfaction.[36] In respiration, airflow is modified by nasal resistance at the level of the nares and the nasal valves to allow efficient pulmonary ventilation. A major portion of the nasal airflow passes through the middle meatus. The passage of inspired air through the nasal cavity allows humidification and warming.[36]

Imaging Anatomy and Pertinent Pathology

Cross-sectional imaging of the nose and paranasal sinuses allows examination of the airway from the nares to the nasopharynx. A dedicated examination of the nose and sinuses yields detailed information about this region (Fig. 2.34A–J). Incidental imaging of the sinuses and airway on a routine brain or spine study often allows general assessment of the airway that may be useful in the overall preoperative assessment of a patient (Fig. 2.35A–D). Not only is anatomy well defined by cross-sectional imaging, but it can

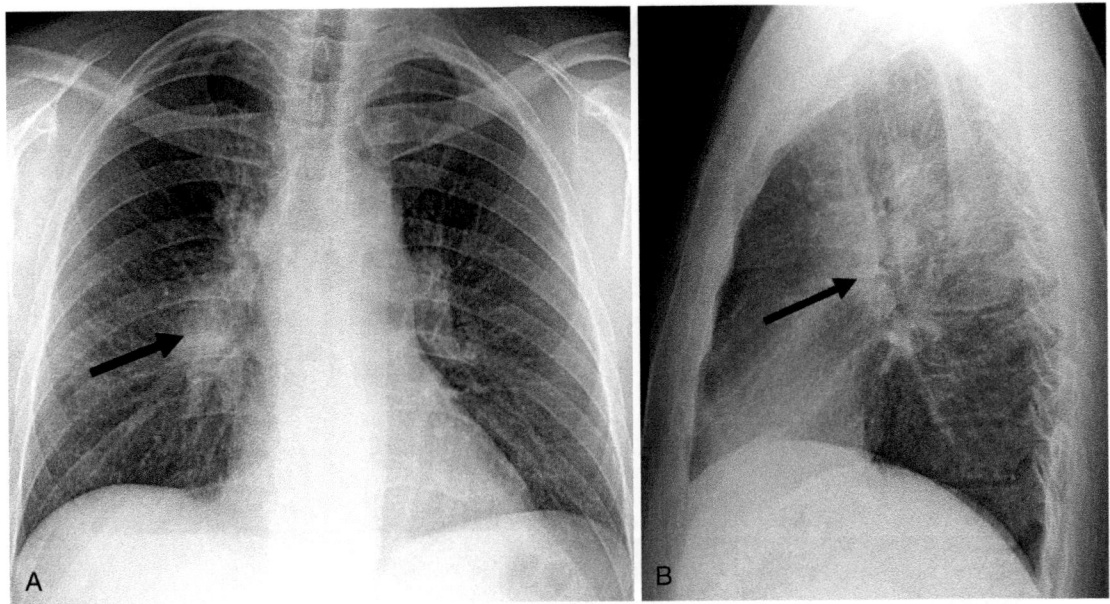

• **Fig. 2.30** Right hilar mass and nodes (*arrows*). (A) Posteroanterior and (B) lateral chest radiographs.

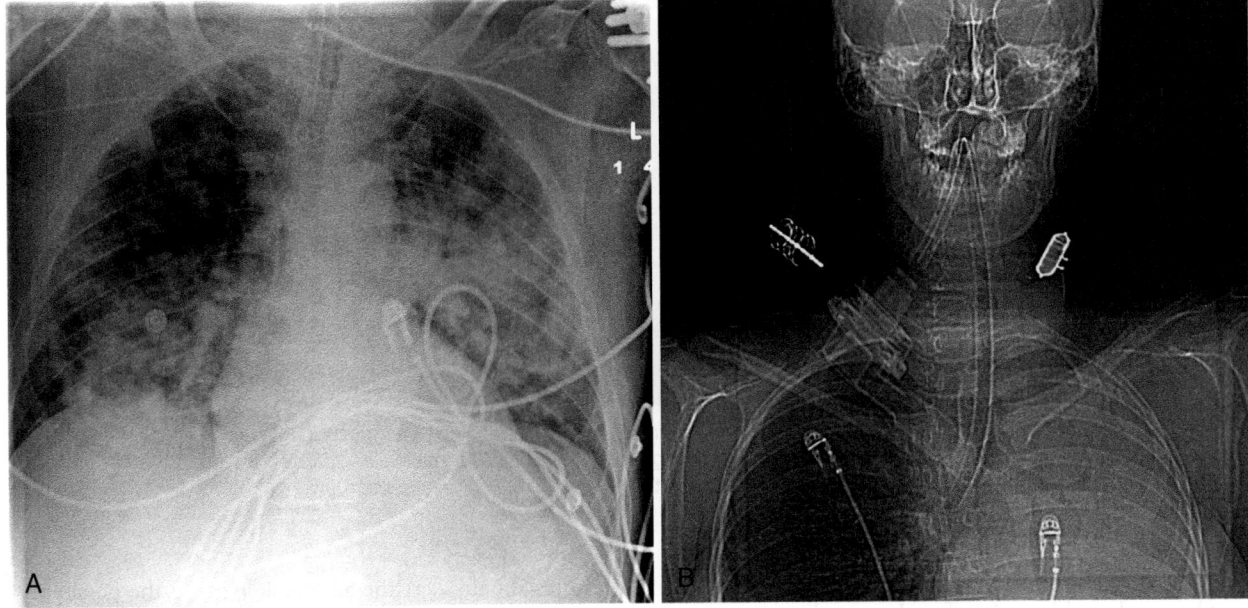

• **Fig. 2.31** (A) Anteroposterior (AP) portable chest radiograph. Most chest examinations in the intensive care unit are done with a portable x-ray machine in the AP projection. Note the acceptable position of the endotracheal tube (ETT) above the carina. A right subclavian central venous line is present with the tip in the superior vena cava. Multiple cables attached to monitors are noted crossing the chest. (B) An AP computed tomographic (CT) scout view obtained for a soft tissue neck study reveals an errant ETT in the right main bronchus resulting in nonaeration of the left lung.

also be a window to viewing physiologic function, in particular the nasal cycle (the cyclic variation in the thickness of the mucosa of the nasal cavity), which occurs every 20 minutes to 6 hours.[36,37] This physiologic change is manifested as an alternating side-to-side swelling of the turbinates.

The bony housing of the nose and nasal cavities is well depicted by CT; by changing the viewing windows and level, the soft tissue

component can be better appreciated. The nasal cavity is divided into two cavities separated by the nasal septum. The roof of the nasal cavity is formed by the cribriform plate of the ethmoid bone; the hard palate serves as the floor. Protruding into the nasal cavity along the lateral wall of each nasal cavity are mucosa-covered scroll-like projections of bone called *turbinates* or *conchae*. They are named the inferior, middle, superior, and supreme turbinates;

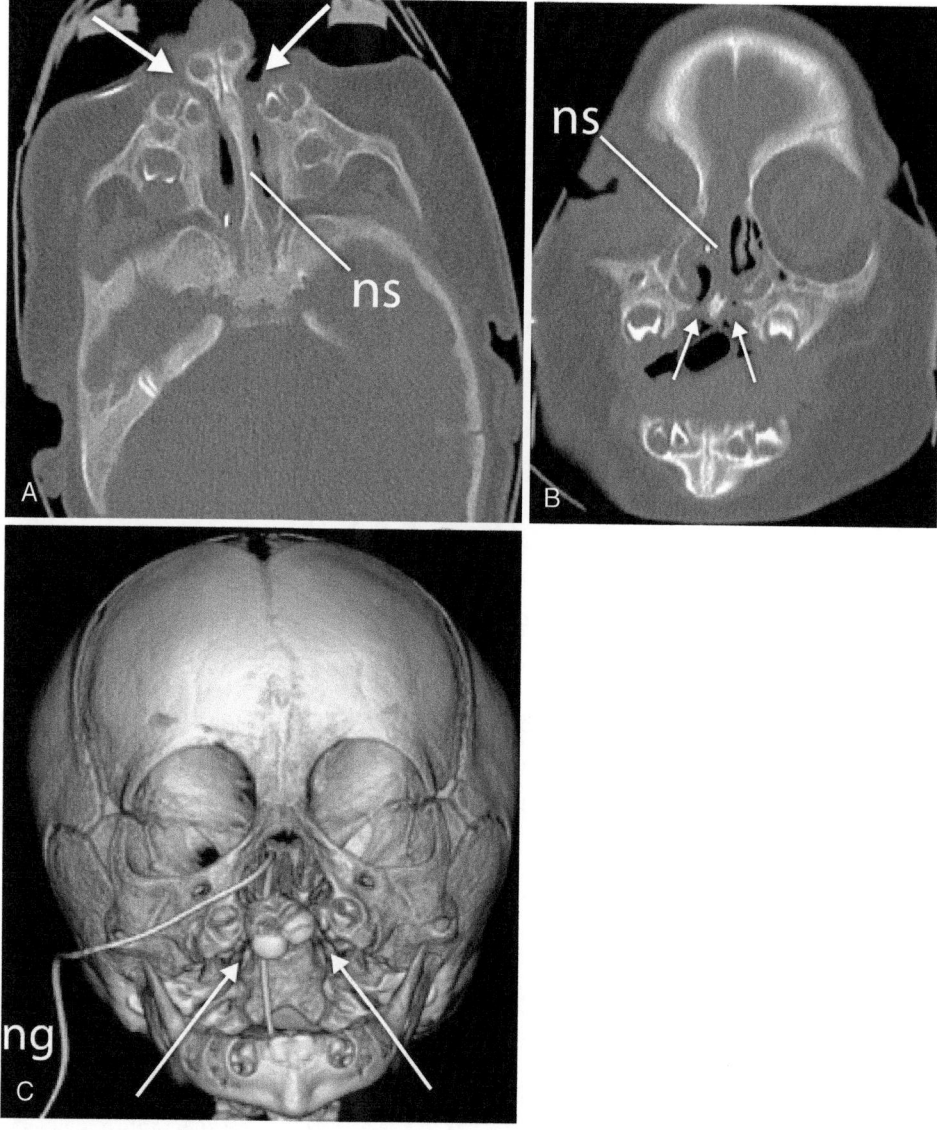

• **Fig. 2.32** Cleft lip and palate (*arrows*). (A) Axial and (B) coronal computed tomography (CT) images with (C) three-dimensional reconstruction demonstrating bilateral cleft of the lip, maxilla, and palate. This results in communication between the nasal and oral cavities (*arrows in B*). *ns*, Nasal septum.

the latter is seen only in 60% of people.[36] The airspace beneath and lateral to each turbinate is referred to as the meatus, into which the paranasal sinuses drain.

Congenital Anomalies

Relevant to anesthetic practice is an awareness that the midline craniofacial dysraphisms can be categorized into two groups: an inferior group, in which the clefting primarily affects the upper lip, with or without the nose; and a superior group, in which the clefting primarily affects the nose, with or without involvement of the forehead and upper lip (see Fig. 2.32). It is the inferior group that is associated with basal encephalocele (i.e., sphenoidal, sphenoethmoid, and ethmoid encephaloceles), callosal agenesis, and optic nerve dysplasia. The superior group is characterized by hypertelorism, a broad nasal root, and a median cleft nose, with or without a median cleft upper lip. The superior group is also associated with an increased incidence of frontonasal and intraorbital encephaloceles (see Fig. 2.33).[35] The presence of these phenotypic

features should alert the anesthesiologist to the possibility of an encephalocele intruding into the nasal cavity, and caution can be exercised when inserting a nasogastric tube or nasal airway.

Congenital nasal airway obstruction most commonly occurs in the posterior nasal cavity, secondary to choanal atresia (Fig. 2.36). The atresia may be bony, membranous, or both. At birth, severe respiratory difficulty and the inability to insert a nasogastric tube more than 3 to 4 cm into the nose despite the presence of air in the trachea and the lungs suggest the diagnosis of bilateral choanal atresia. Most atresias, however, are unilateral and may remain undetected until late in life. Stenosis of the posterior nasal passages (choanae) is more common than true atresia. Approximately 75% of children with bilateral choanal stenosis or atresia have other congenital abnormalities, including Apert, Treacher Collins, and fetal alcohol syndromes. Because the pathology is usually manifested as bony overgrowth, CT is the imaging modality of choice. The major feature of choanal atresia is an abnormal widening of the vomer (Fig. 2.37A and B).

The nasal capsule, which is the cartilage around the developing nasal cavity of the embryo, serves as the foundation of the upper part of the face. During development, this cartilage eventually becomes ossified or atrophied; all that remains in adults is the anterior part of the nasal septum and the alar cartilages that surround the nostrils. The midline septal cartilage is continuous with the cartilaginous skull base. At birth, the lateral masses of the ethmoid are ossified, but the septal cartilage and the cribriform plates are still cartilaginous. Another ossification center appears in the septal cartilage anterior to the cranial base and becomes the perpendicular plate of the ethmoid. In about the third to sixth year, the lateral masses of the ethmoid and perpendicular plates become united across the roof of the nasal cavity by ossification of the cribriform plate, which unites somewhat later with the vomer below. Growth of the septal cartilage continues for a short time after craniofacial union is complete, which probably accounts for what is commonly seen as a deviated nasal septum.[34] There are acquired etiologies of a deviated septum, such as secondary to trauma, and there are varying degrees of septal deviation. In most cases, septal deviation is not problematic for nasogastric tube or nasal airway insertion, but having prior knowledge of anatomy of the nasal cavity allows one to choose the path of least resistance.

Rhinosinusitis and Polyps

In general, no imaging is required for work-up of uncomplicated rhinosinusitis. Views of the sinus are included in a routine CT study of the brain. The air within the sinuses abuts the bony sinus wall and appears black on both CT and MRI. To assess the bony structures, CT is preferred; however, MRI is extremely useful to differentiate inflammatory disease from tumor. Inflammatory sinus disease is characterized by increased water content; therefore, an increased T2 signal (i.e., a bright signal) is produced on T2-weighted imaging. Common inflammatory sinus disease

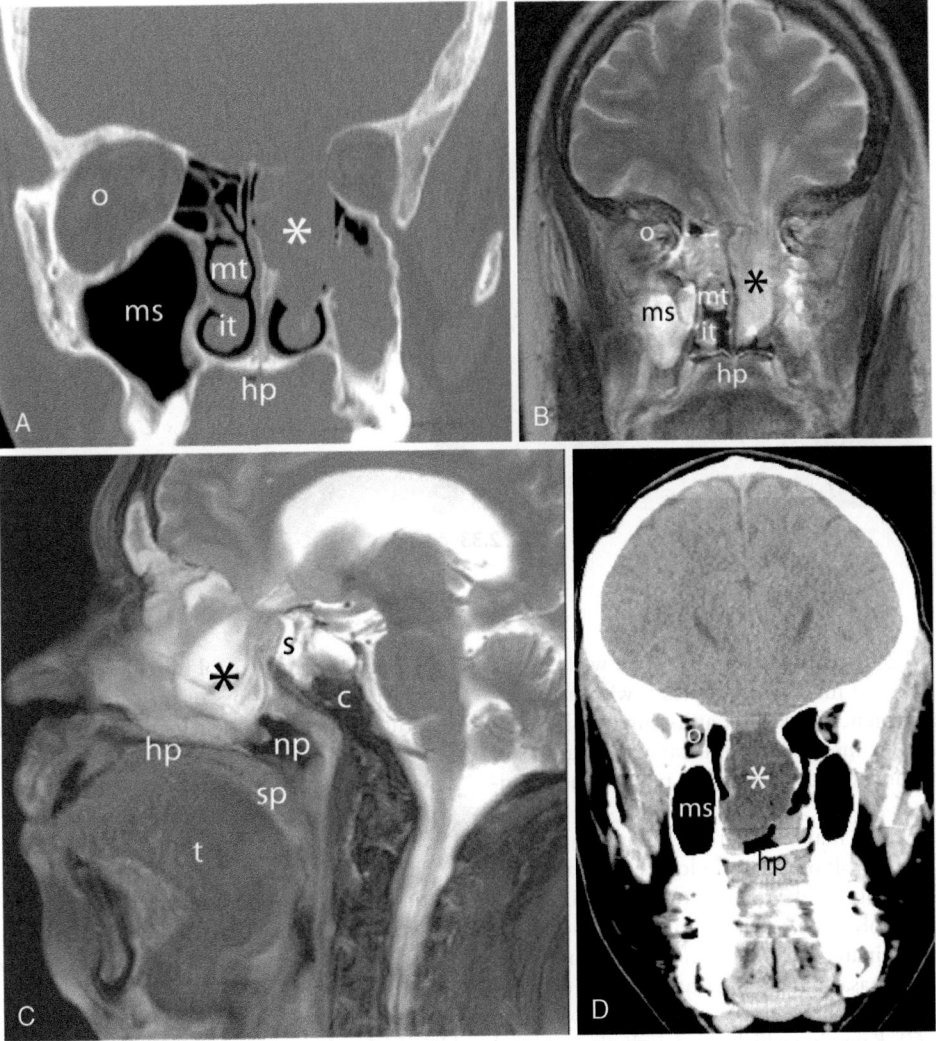

• **Fig. 2.33** Encephalocele (*asterisk*) in two patients. Patient 1: (A–C) Frontoethmoidal encephalocele: (A) coronal computed tomography (CT); (B) coronal T2-weighted; and (C) sagittal T2-weighted magnetic resonance (MR) imaging demonstrates a defect in the left fovea ethmoidalis with herniation of meninges and brain parenchyma into the nasal cavity. Patient 2: (D–G) Sphenoidal encephalocele: (D) coronal CT, (E) sagittal CT, (F) coronal CT, and (G) sagittal T2-weighted MRI demonstrate a defect in the planum sphenoidale with meninges and brain parenchyma extending into the nasal cavity. *mt*, middle turbinate; *it*, inferior turbinate; *o*, orbit; *ms*, maxillary sinus; *s*, sphenoid sinus; *hp*, hard palate; *sp*, soft palate; *c*, Clivus; *np*, nasopharynx; *t*, tongue.

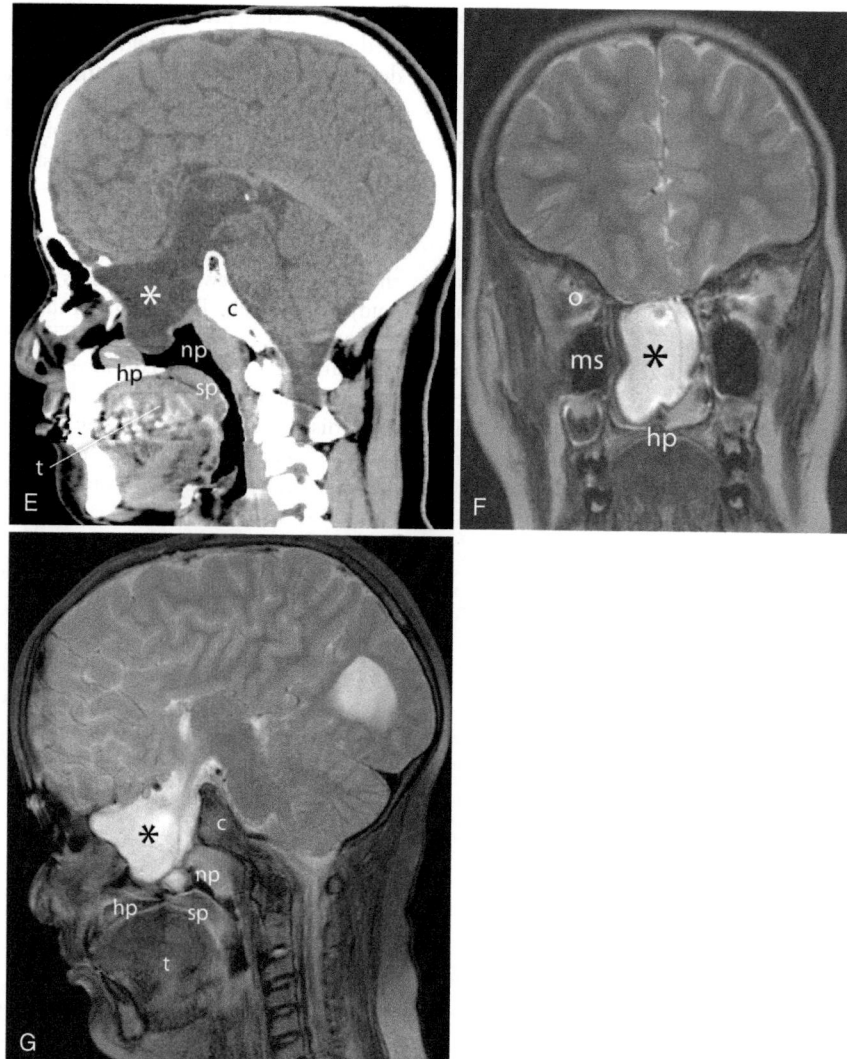

• **Fig. 2.33** cont'd

is most often seen as T2 hyperintense lining of the walls of the sinus representing thickened mucosa. In contrast, with increased cellularity, tumor masses generally exhibit an isointense signal on T2-weighted imaging. The most common local complications of inflammatory sinusitis are swollen turbinates, polyps, and retention cysts.

Nasal airway obstruction may result from rhinitis and turbinate hypertrophy. Common sinonasal pathologies that can affect the airway are easily recognizable on cross-sectional imaging. Examples include nasal polyps or a concha bullosa, which is an enlarged and aerated turbinate, most often the middle turbinate. Sensibly, the presence of nasal polyps or polyposis may discourage an anesthesiologist from attempting nasal intubation (Figs. 2.38A–C and 2.39A–C). Knowing which nasal cavity is narrowed by the presence of a concha bullosa helps to guide the selection of which nasal cavity to cannulate (Fig. 2.40A and B).

Trauma

Facial fractures are often classified using the Le Fort system and its variants. This system is based on experiments predicting the course of fractures based on lines of weakness in the facial skeleton. Of all

the facial fractures, nasal fractures are the most common and may involve the nasal bones or the cartilaginous structures. If the nasal septum is fractured and a hematoma results, the vascular supply to the cartilage may be compromised, leading to cartilage necrosis. If the septal hematoma is not recognized and treated, it becomes an organized hematoma, causing thickening of the septum that can result in impaired breathing (Fig. 2.41A–E). Without a doubt, CT is the modality of choice for evaluating trauma to the facial structures. Three-dimensional reconstruction and surface rendering can also be performed to better highlight fracture deformities. Even if all the details of a complex facial fracture are not known, an oral airway is preferable to a nasal airway, except in the case of mandibular fracture (Fig. 2.42A–C), where a nasal approach to intubation is preferred.

Tumors and Other Pathology

Malignant tumors of the nasal cavity and paranasal sinuses are rare and have a poor prognosis because they are frequently diagnosed in an advanced stage. They are often accompanied by inflammatory disease. MRI is superior to CT in differentiating tumor from inflammatory disease; therefore, it is useful for delineating

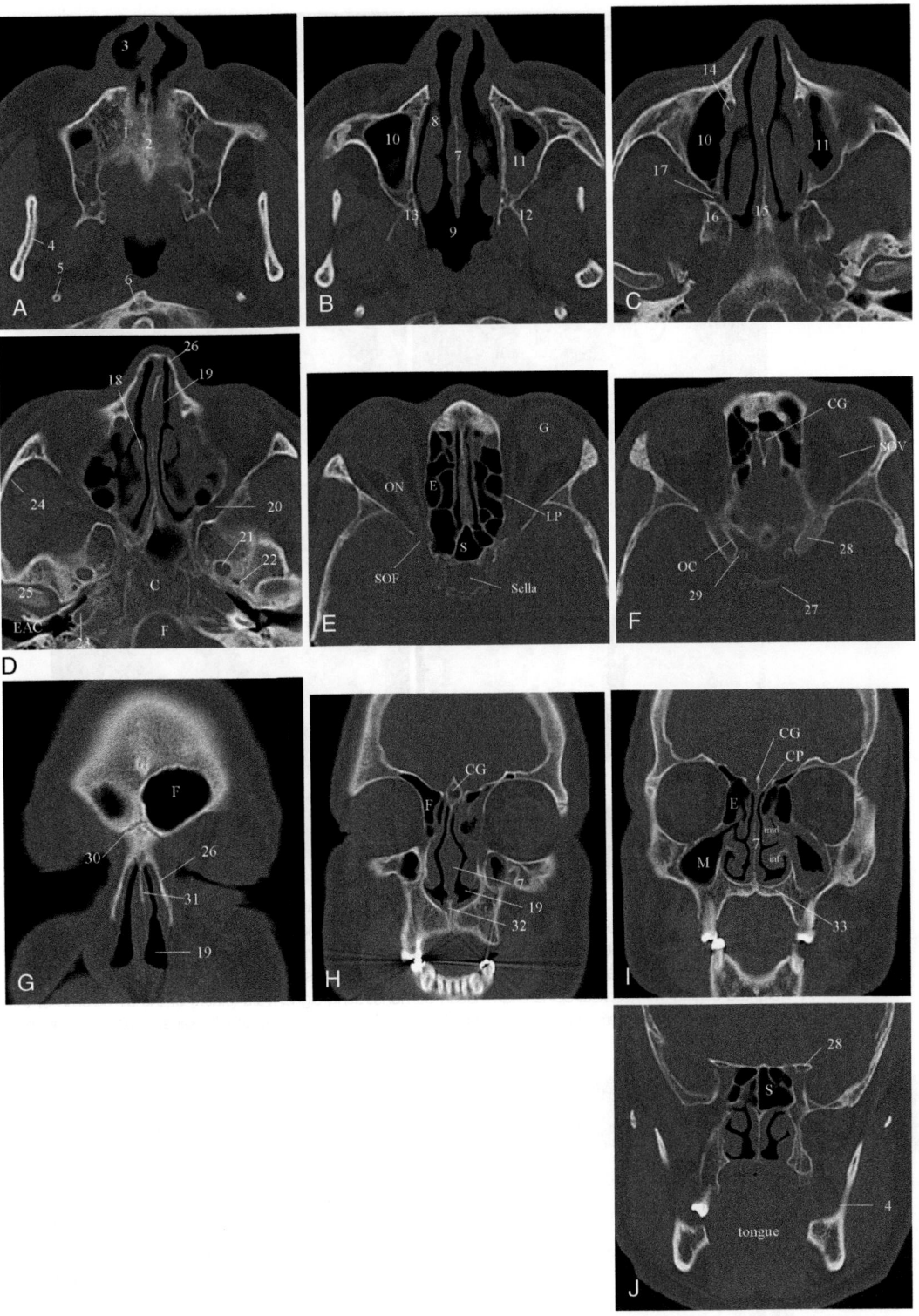

• **Fig. 2.34** (A–F) Axial computed tomography (CT) showing anatomy of the sinonasal cavity. (G–J) Coronal CT showing anatomy of sinonasal cavity. *1,* Hard palate; *2,* base of nasal septum; *3,* nostril; *4,* ramus of mandible; *5,* styloid process; *6,* anterior arch of C1; *7,* nasal septum; *8,* inferior turbinate; *9,* nasopharynx; *10,* right maxillary sinus; *11,* left maxillary sinus with inflammatory mucosal disease; *12,* lateral pterygoid plate; *13,* medial pterygoid plate; *14,* nasolacrimal duct; *15,* rostrum sphenoid; *16,* pterygoid process; *17,* pterygopalatine fossa; *18,* middle turbinate; *19,* nasal cavity; *20,* inferior orbital fissure; *21,* foramen ovale; *22,* foramen spinosum; *23,* carotid canal; *24,* zygomatic arch; *25,* mandibular head; *26,* nasal bone; *27,* dorsum sella; *28,* anterior clinoid; *29,* calcified carotid artery; *30,* nasofrontal suture; *31,* perpendicular plate of ethmoid; *32,* vomer; *33,* hard palate; *C,* clivus; *CG,* crista galli; *E,* ethmoid sinus; *EAC,* external auditory canal; *F,* foramen magnum; *G,* globe; *inf,* inferior turbinate; *mid,* middle turbinate; *OC,* optic canal; *ON,* optic nerve; *S,* sphenoid sinus; *SOF,* superior orbital fissure; *SOV,* superior ophthalmic vein.

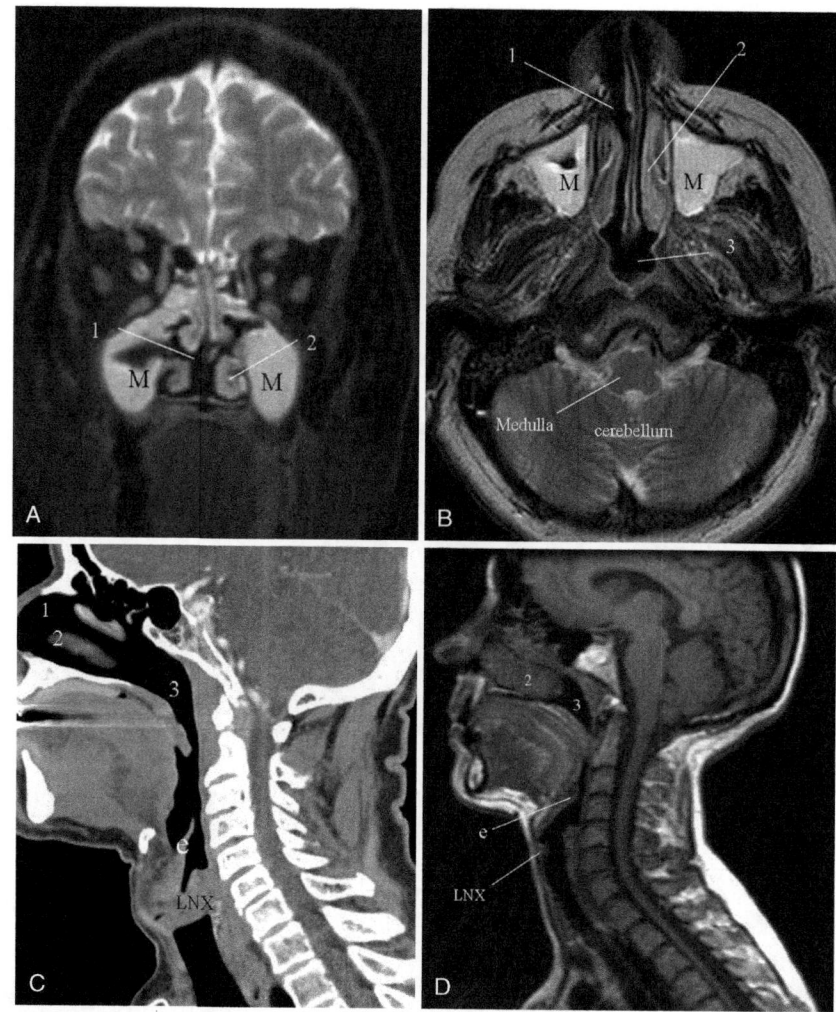

• **Fig. 2.35** Airway as seen on routine studies. (A) T2-weighted coronal magnetic resonance (MR) imaging of the brain demonstrates hyperintense inflamed thickened mucosa of the maxillary sinuses. (B) T2-weighted axial MR imaging of the brain demonstrates sinus disease with a clear nasal cavity and nasopharynx. (C) Sagittal reformation from computed tomography (CT) neck examination demonstrates a clear airway from nose to trachea. (D) T1-weighted sagittal MR cervical spine examination demonstrating signal void (*black*) of the air column of the airway. *1,* Nasal cavity; *2,* inferior turbinate; *3,* nasopharynx; *M,* maxillary sinus with thickened mucosa; *e,* epiglottis; *LNX,* larynx.

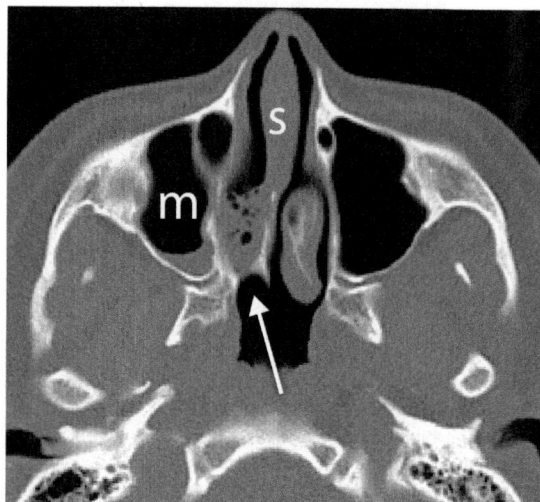

• **Fig. 2.36** Choanal atresia. Axial computed tomography (CT) image demonstrates choanal stenosis on the right (*arrow*). *s,* nasal septum; *m,* Maxillary sinus.

the tumor boundary from the often associated inflammatory component. Inflammatory diseases involve a high water content; therefore they have high T2-weighted intensity and appear bright on MRI. Nasal and paranasal tumors are generally cellular and have an intermediate-intensity signal on T2-weighted imaging (Fig. 2.43A–D).[38,39] CT, on the other hand, is useful for assessing bone involvement. The histology of a tumor can sometimes be suggested by the way in which the bone is affected: Aggressive bone destruction is usually seen in squamous cell carcinoma, esthesioneuroblastoma, sinonasal undifferentiated carcinoma, metastatic lung and breast cancers, sarcomas, and rare fibrous histiocytomas (Fig. 2.44A–D).

Juvenile nasopharyngeal angiofibroma is a benign but locally aggressive hypervascular tumor of the sinonasal cavity found almost exclusively in young adolescent males. The most common presenting signs are unilateral nasal obstruction and spontaneous epistaxis. It usually arises at the sphenopalatine foramen at the lateral nasopharyngeal wall and is locally destructive over time.[38] The imaging characteristics consist of a mass in the nasal cavity and nasopharynx, a widened pterygopalatine fossa,

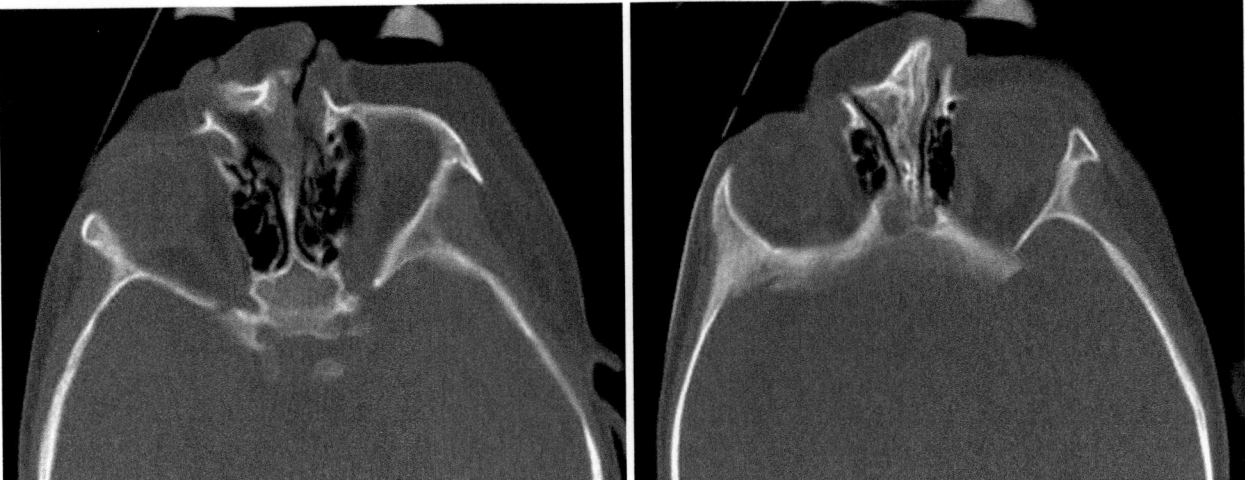

• **Fig. 2.37** Congenital nasal deformity. Axial computed tomography (CT) scans demonstrate abnormal nasal bone architecture with a soft tissue cleft and impact on nasal airways.

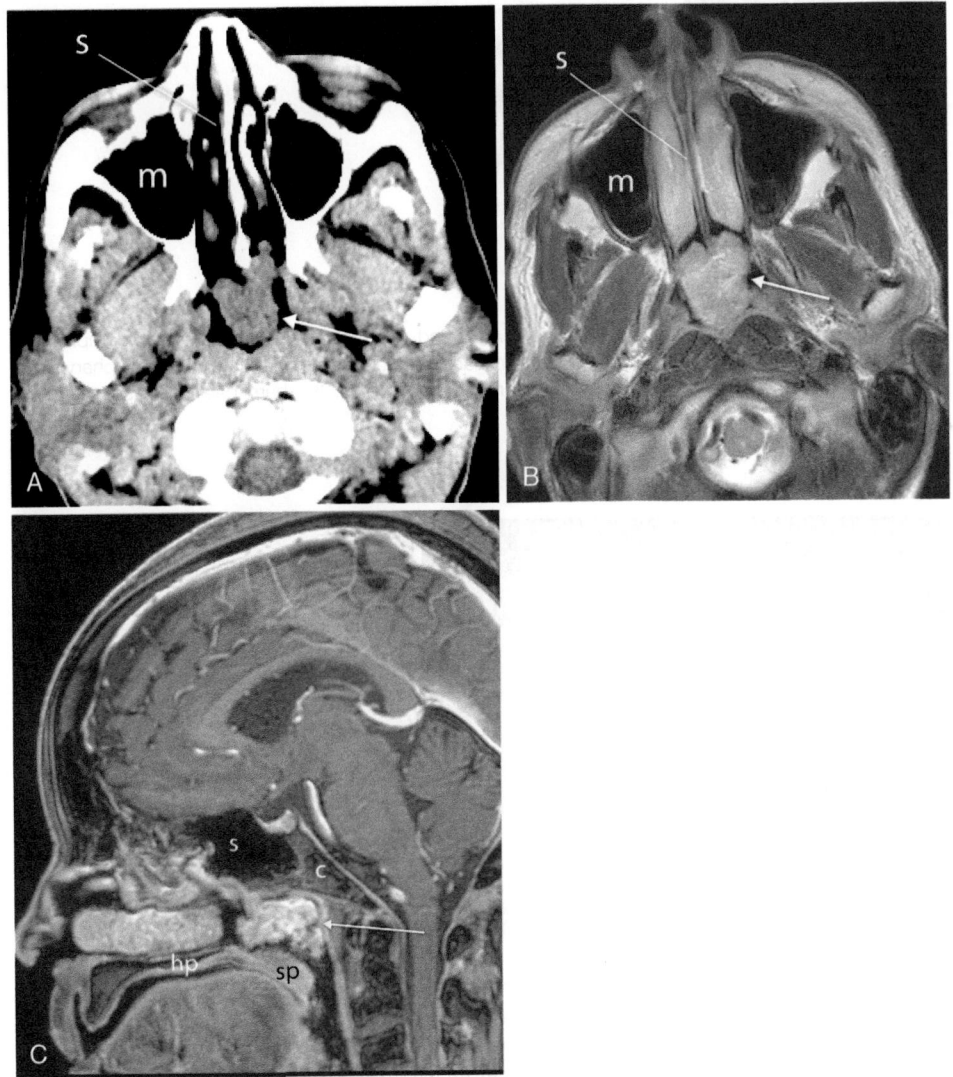

• **Fig. 2.38** Nasopharyngeal polyp. (A) Axial computed tomography (CT), (B) axial T2-weighted magnetic resonance image (MRI), and (C) postcontrast T1-weighted MRI images demonstrating soft tissue polyp within the nasopharynx (*arrows*). *s*, nasal septum; *m*, maxillary sinus; *s*, sphenoid sinus; *c*, Clivus; *hp*, hard palate; *sp*, soft palate.

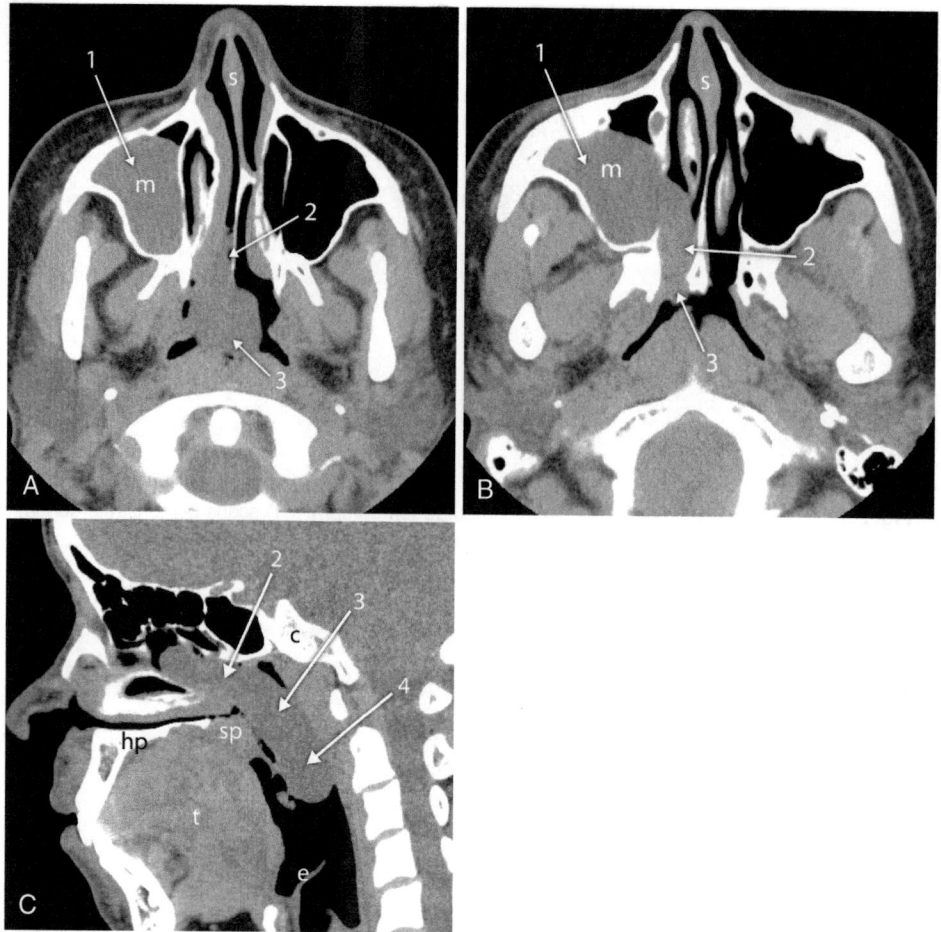

• **Fig. 2.39** Antrochoanal polyposis. (A and B) Axial and (C) sagittal (C) computed tomography (CT) images demonstrate polyps involving the right maxillary sinus (*1*), right nasal cavity (*2*), nasopharynx (*3*), and oropharynx (*4*). *s*, nasal septum; *m*, maxillary sinus; *c*, Clivus; *hp*, hard palate; *sp*, soft palate; *t*, tongue; *e*, epiglottis.

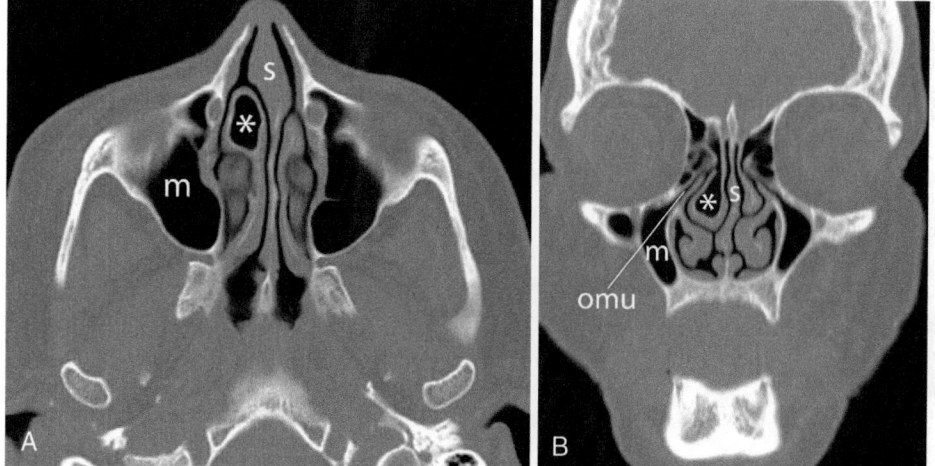

• **Fig. 2.40** Concha bullosa. (A) Axial and (B) coronal computed tomography (CT) scans demonstrate pneumatization (*asterisk*) of the right middle turbinate with slight deviation of the nasal septum (*s*) and anatomic narrowing of the right ostiomeatal unit (*omu*). *m*, Maxillary sinus.

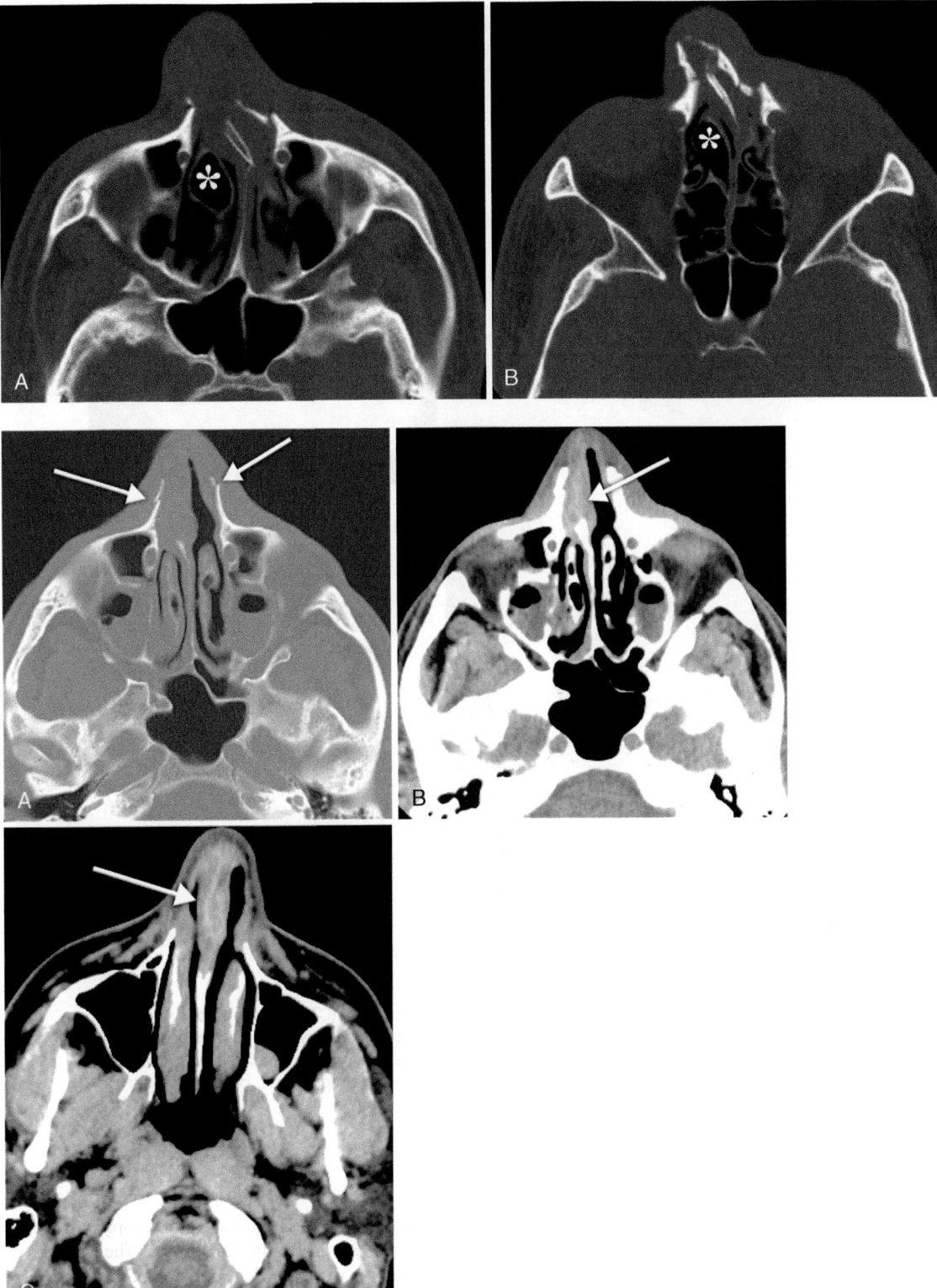

• **Fig. 2.41** Nasal and septal pathology in three patients. Patient 1: (A and B) Axial computed tomography (CT) images demonstrate comminuted fractures of the nasal bones bilaterally as well as a septal fracture. The nasal passages are further compromised by the incidental right concha bullosa (*asterisk*). Patient 2: (C) Axial CT image in bone algorithm shows bilateral anterior maxillary process fractures (*arrows*). (D) Axial CT image in soft tissue algorithm shows thickening and hyperintensity in the anterior nasal septum (*arrow*) compatible with nasal septal hematoma. There is compromise of the right nasal vestibule and pyriform aperture. Patient 3: (E) Axial CT image shows nasal septal hematoma (*arrow*) narrowing the right nasal vestibule in the absence of fracture.

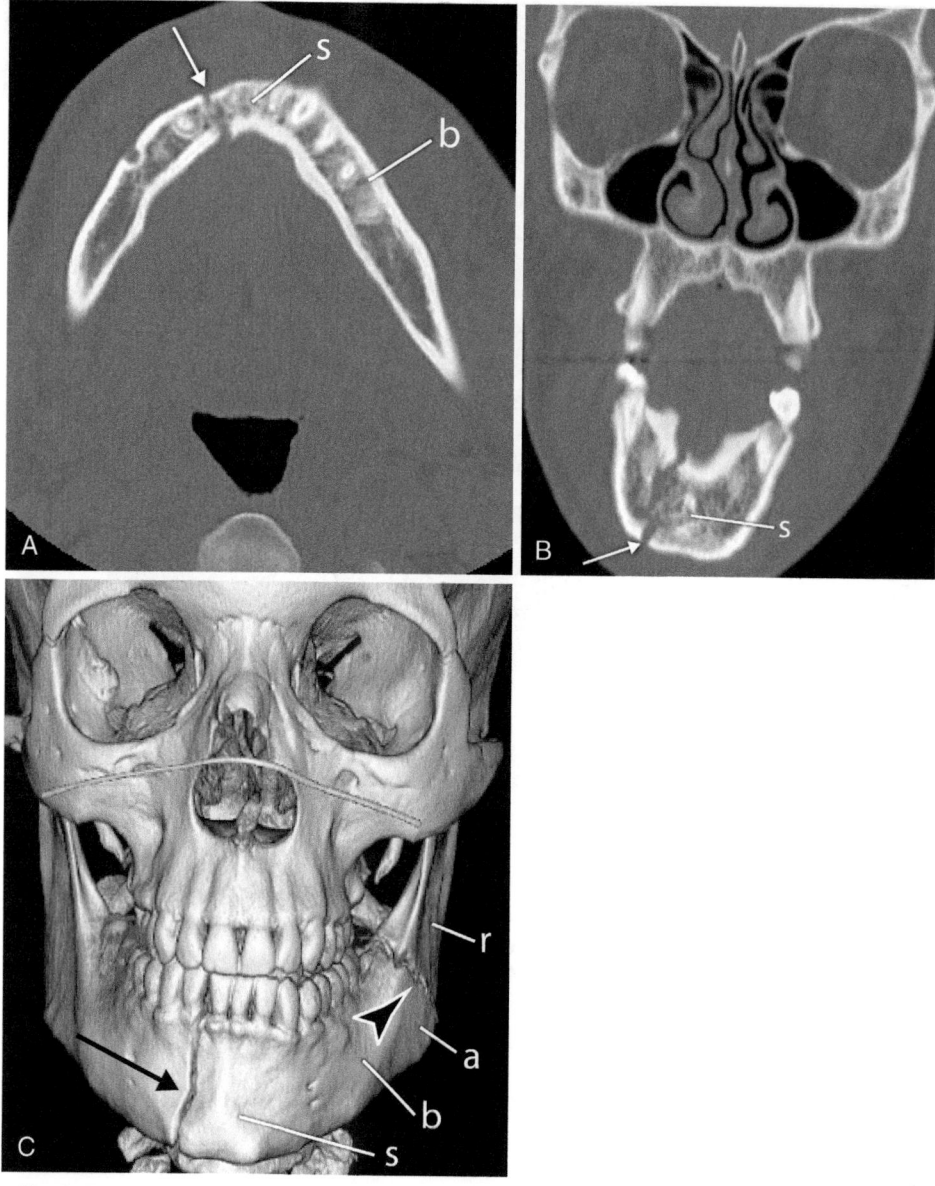

• **Fig. 2.42** Mandibular fracture. (A and B) Axial computed tomography (CT) images demonstrate a fracture of the right parasymphyseal mandible (*arrows*). (C) Fracture is also seen on three-dimensional surface-rendered CT image (*arrow*), which also demonstrates the typical finding of an additional fracture, in this case involving the left mandibular angle (*arrowhead*). *s,* mandibular symphysis; *b,* body of mandible; *a,* Angle of mandible; *r,* mandibular ramus.

anterior displacement of the posterior wall of the maxillary sinus, and erosion of the medial pterygoid plate (Fig. 2.45A–F). Treatment is surgical resection, often with preoperative embolization to decrease the blood supply.

Wegener's granulomatosis, a necrotizing vasculitis, usually affects the upper and lower respiratory tracts and causes a renal glomerulonephritis. It is probably autoimmune in origin. It most often involves the nasal septum first and may arise as a chronic, nonspecific inflammatory process. This process becomes diffuse, and septal ulcerations and perforations occur. Secondary bacterial infection often complicates the clinical and imaging picture (Fig. 2.46A–C).[38] Fibrous dysplasia, an idiopathic bone disorder, is not a tumor but can encroach on the airway and sinuses. Most patients are young at the time of diagnosis. There are monostotic and polyostotic forms. Craniofacial bones are more often involved in the polyostotic form (Fig. 2.47A and B).[38]

Oral Cavity

Development and Structure

The oral cavity, contiguous with the oropharynx, is the primary conduit to the gastrointestinal tract. The development of the mouth, along with the development of the face, is centered on a surface depression, the stomodeum, just below the developing brain. The ectoderm covering the forebrain extends into the stomodeum, where it lies adjacent to the foregut. The junctional zone between the ectoderm and the endoderm is the oropharyngeal membrane, which corresponds to Waldeyer's ring. Dissolution of the oropharyngeal membrane in the fourth gestational week results in establishing patency between the mouth and the foregut.[40] The oral cavity is separated from the oropharynx by the circumvallate papillae, anterior tonsillar pillars, and soft palate. The anterior two-thirds of the tongue (oral tongue), the floor of the

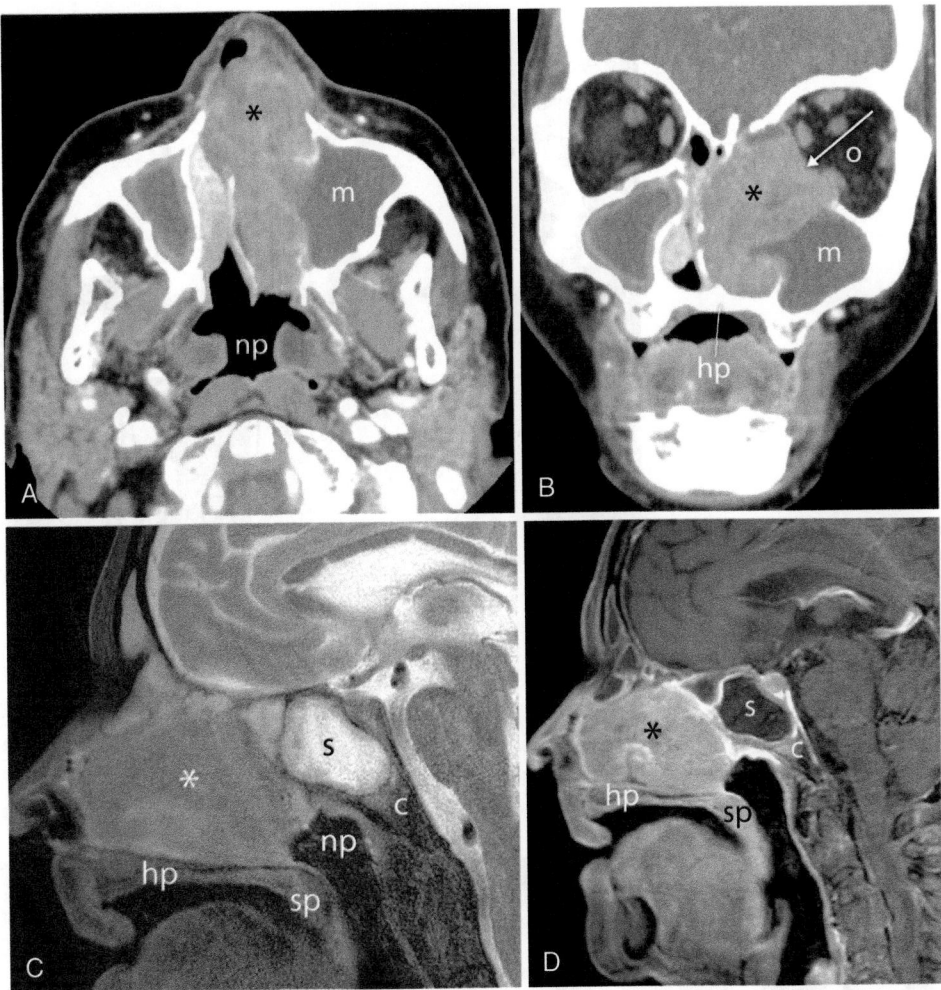

• **Fig. 2.43** Sinonasal lymphoma. (A) Axial and (B) coronal computed tomography (CT), (C) sagittal T2-weighted magnetic resonance imaging (MRI), and (D) sagittal postcontrast T1-weighted MRI images of sinonasal lymphoma (*asterisk*) demonstrating a lesion of the nasal cavity and left maxillary sinus extending into the left extraconal orbit (*arrow* in B). The lesion has intermediate signal on (C) T2-weighted images with enhancement on both CT (A and B) and MRI (D). Inflammatory sinus opacification demonstrated in the sphenoid (*s*) and maxillary (*m*) sinuses is distinguished by (C) high T2-weighted signal, (A an B) low CT attenuation, and (A, B, D) absent enhancement. (B) Bony destruction associated with orbital extension is best seen on CT. *m*, maxillary sinus; *s*, sphenoid sinus; *o*, orbit; *c*, Clivus; *hp*, hard palate; *sp*, soft palate, *np*; nasopharynx.

mouth, the gingivobuccal and buccomasseteric regions, the maxilla, and the mandible are considered oral cavity structures. The anatomic distinction between the oral cavity and the oropharynx has clinical importance. Malignancies in these two regions, especially squamous cell carcinoma, are different in their presentation and prognosis.

Motor innervation of the tongue comes from the hypoglossal nerve (cranial nerve [CN] XII), which courses between the mylohyoid and hyoglossus muscles. The sensory input from the anterior tongue is by the lingual nerve, which is a branch of the trigeminal nerve (CN V). Special sensory taste fibers from the anterior two-thirds of the tongue course with the lingual nerve before forming the chorda tympani nerve, which subsequently joins the facial nerve (CN VII). The special sensory fibers from the posterior one-third of the tongue (tongue base) are supplied by the glossopharyngeal nerve (CN IX). The arterial blood supply to the tongue is from branches of the lingual artery, which itself is

a branch of the external carotid artery. Venous drainage is to the internal jugular vein.[28]

Imaging Anatomy and Pertinent Pathology

CT and MRI are used extensively for evaluation of the oral cavity. The advantages of CT are the speed of data acquisition and the ability to detect calcifications pertinent in the evaluation of inflammatory diseases affecting the salivary glands. For evaluating the extent of tumor infiltration of the soft tissues, MRI is superior to CT but is easily degraded by motion artifacts.

The tongue consists of two symmetrical halves separated by a midline lingual septum. Each half of the tongue is composed of muscular fibers, which are divided into extrinsic and intrinsic muscles. There are four intrinsic tongue muscles: the superior longitudinal muscle, inferior longitudinal muscle, transverse muscle, and vertical muscle. The intrinsic muscles receive motor innervation from the hypoglossal nerve (CN XII) and participate in

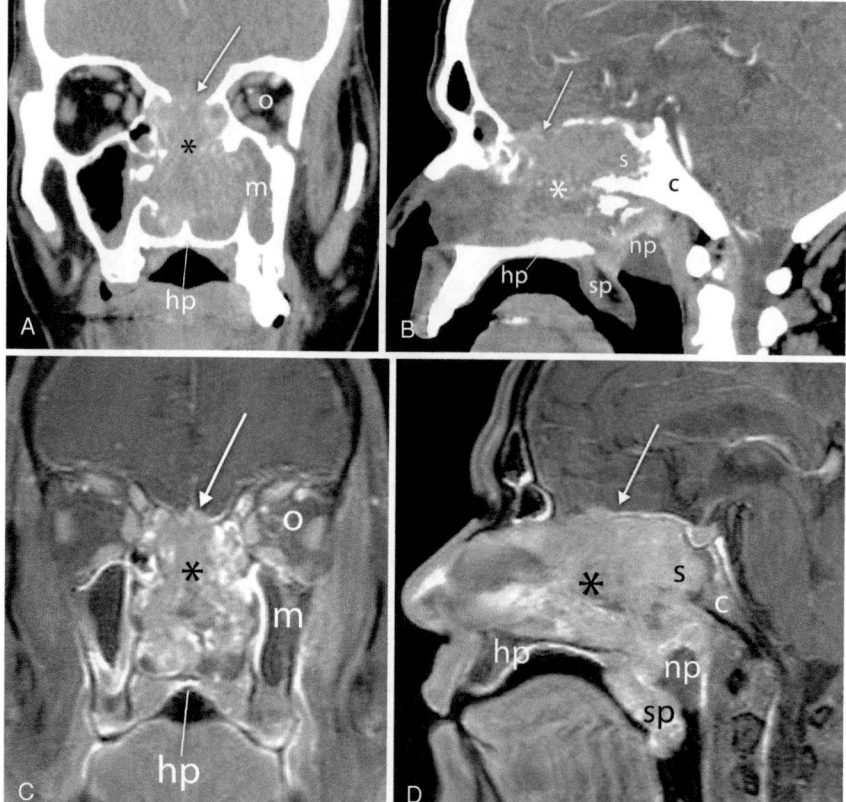

• **Fig. 2.44** Esthesioneuroblastoma. (A) Coronal and (B) sagittal postcontrast computed tomography (CT) images; (C) Coronal and (D) sagittal postcontrast T1-weighted magnetic resonance (MR) images. There is a destructive enhancing mass (*asterisk*) centered in the nasal cavity, ethmoid air cells, and sphenoid sinus. There are nonenhancing obstructive inflammatory changes in the left maxillary sinus. There is mild intracranial extension (*arrows*) with bony destruction of the ethmoid roofs best seen on CT. *m*, maxillary sinus; *s*, sphenoid sinus; *o*, orbit; *c*, Clivus; *hp*, hard palate; *sp*, soft palate, *np*; nasopharynx.

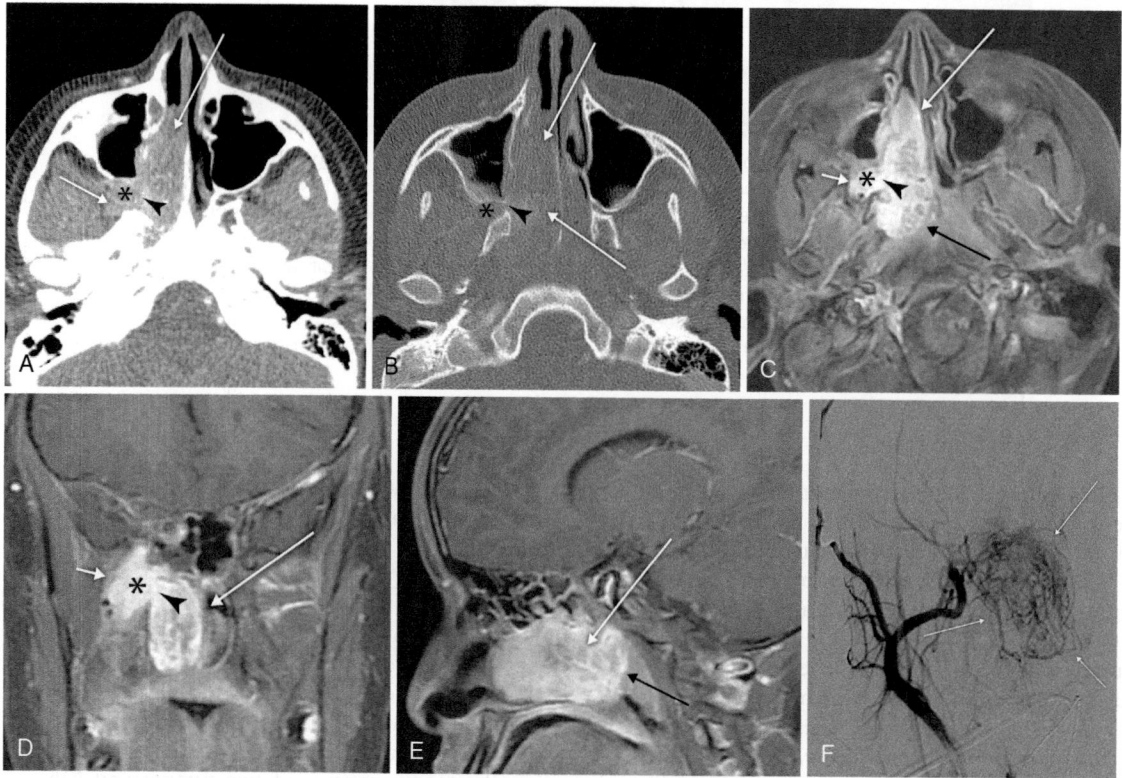

• **Fig. 2.45** Juvenile nasopharyngeal angiofibroma. Axial postcontrast computed tomography (CT) with (A) soft tissue and (B) bone reconstruction algorithm; (C) axial, (D) coronal, and (E) sagittal T1-weighted postcontrast magnetic resonance (MR) images; (F) digital subtraction angiography of right external carotid artery injection. There is a soft-tissue mass involving the right sphenopalatine foramen (*arrowhead A–D*), pterygopalatine fossa (*asterisk A–D*), nasal cavity (*white arrows* in A and B), and nasopharynx (*black arrow* in C and E); lateral extension into the infratemporal fossa (*short white arrow* in A, C, D). There is bony remodeling rather than destruction that is appreciated on bone-algorithm CT images.

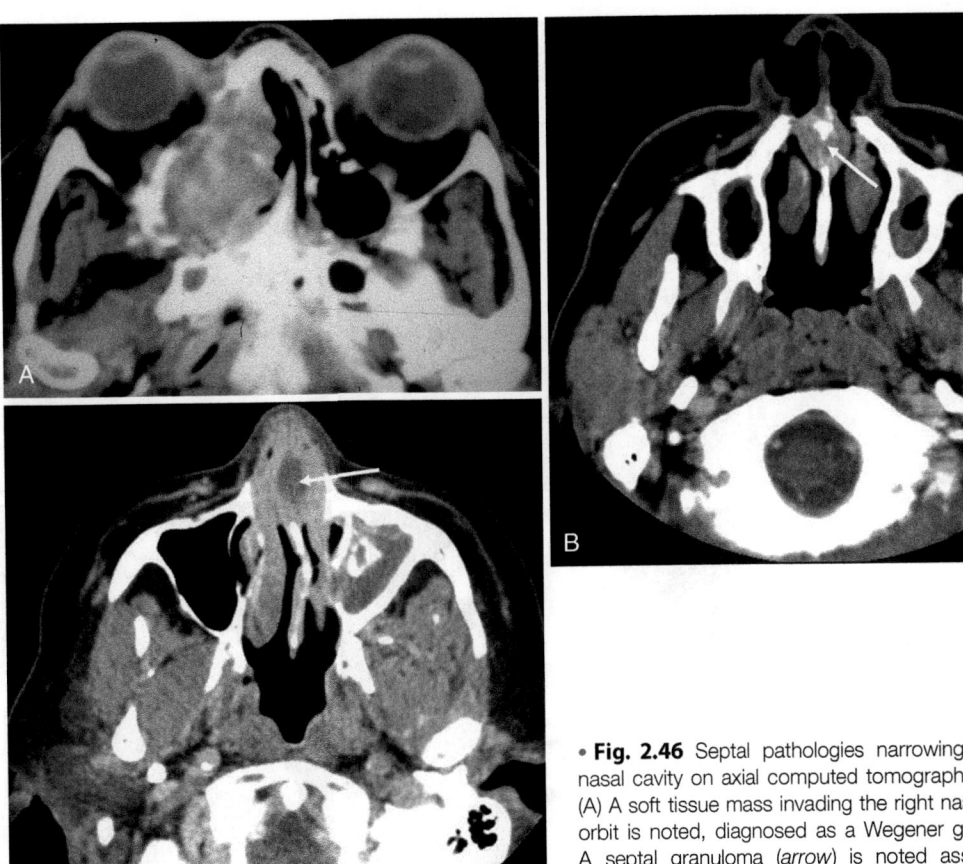

• **Fig. 2.46** Septal pathologies narrowing the anterior nasal cavity on axial computed tomography (CT) scans. (A) A soft tissue mass invading the right nasal cavity and orbit is noted, diagnosed as a Wegener granuloma. (B) A septal granuloma (*arrow*) is noted associated with focal bone destruction. (C) A ring-enhancing lesion of the anterior septum is seen (*arrow*), consistent with a septal abscess.

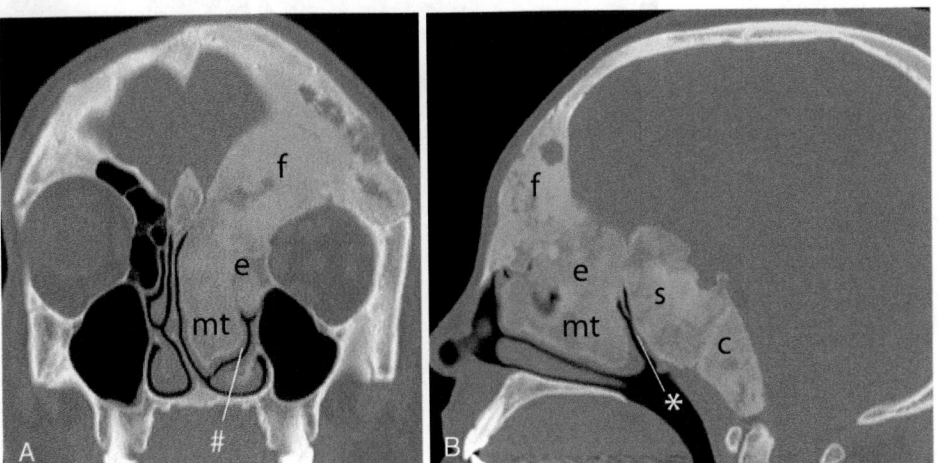

• **Fig. 2.47** Fibrous dysplasia. (A) Coronal and (B) sagittal computed tomography (CT) images demonstrate an expansile bony mass of the anterior and middle skull base with typical "ground glass" appearance. There is involvement of the frontal bone (*f*), ethmoid bone (*e*), middle turbinate (*mt*), sphenoid bone (*s*), and clivus (*c*). There is resultant narrowing of the nasal cavity (*pound sign*) and nasopharynx (*asterisk*).

the enunciation of various consonants. The intrinsic muscles are difficult to distinguish on CT. They are, however, well visualized on MRI, as each muscle bundle is surrounded by high-intensity fibrofatty tissues (Fig. 2.48A–I).[41]

The muscles that originate externally to the tongue but have distal muscle fibers that interdigitate within the substance of the tongue are considered extrinsic muscles of the tongue. The main extrinsic muscles are the genioglossus, hyoglossus, and styloglossus. Sometimes the superior constrictors and the palatoglossus muscle are discussed with the extrinsic muscles of the tongue. The extrinsic muscles attach the tongue to the hyoid, mandible, and styloid process.[41]

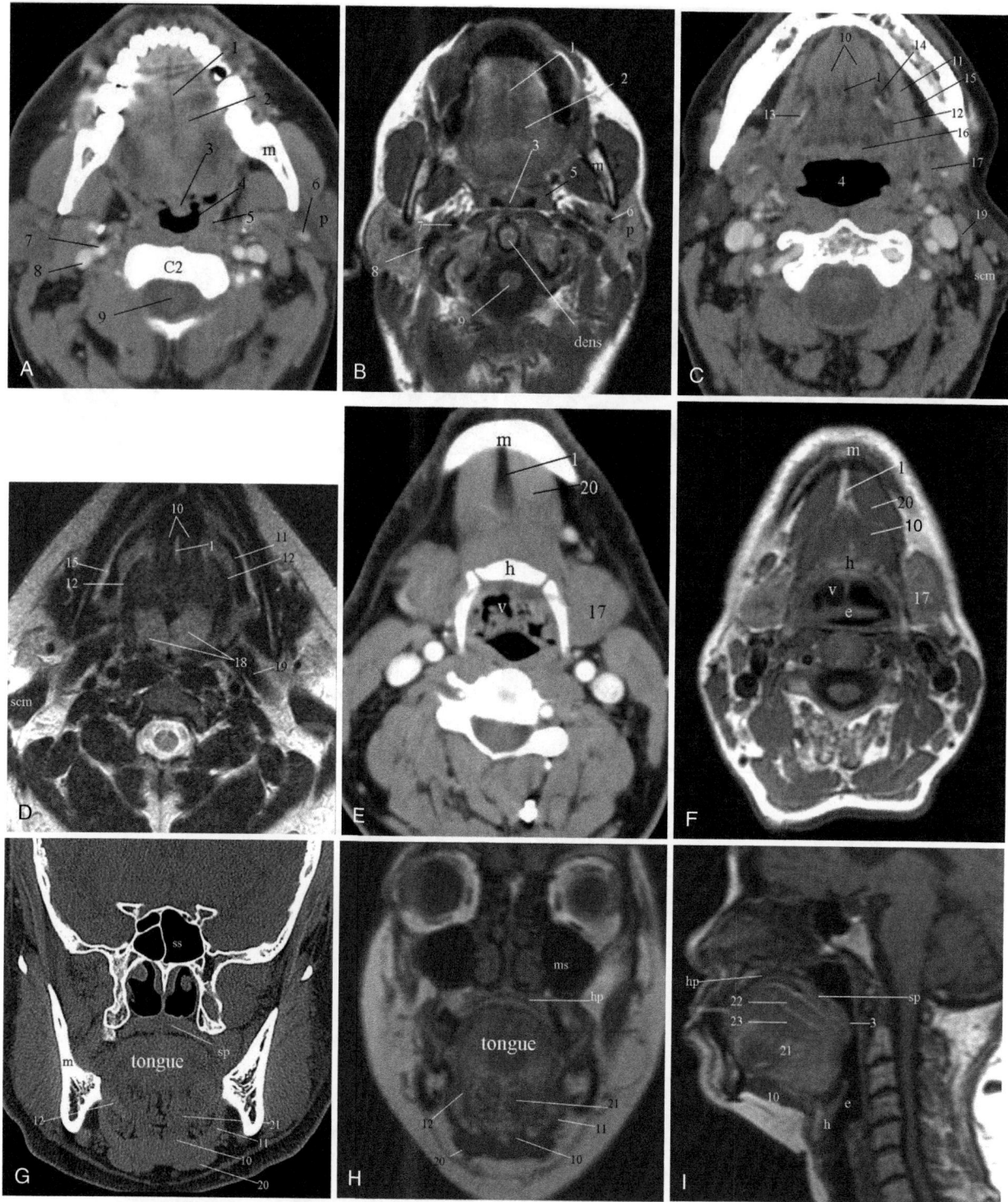

• **Fig. 2.48** Normal anatomy of the oral cavity demonstrated on axial computed tomographic (CT) images (A, C, and E) with corresponding axial magnetic resonance imaging (MRI) scans (B, D, and F), on (G) coronal CT and (H) coronal T1-weighted MRI scans, and on a (I) sagittal T1-weighted MRI image. *1*, Median raphe of tongue (fat is low density on CT and bright on T1-weighted MRI images); *2*, tongue (transverse fibers are seen better on MR imaging); *3*, uvula; *4*, oropharynx; *5*, pharyngeal constrictor muscle; *6*, retromandibular vein; *7*, internal carotid artery; *8*, internal jugular vein; *9*, cervical cord; *10*, paired geniohyoid muscles; *11*, mylohyoid muscle; *12*, hyoglossus muscle; *13*, lingual artery and vein medial to hyoglossus muscle; *14*, Wharton's duct, hypoglossal nerve, and lingual nerve lateral to hyoglossus muscle; *15*, fat in sublingual space; *16*, tongue base; *17*, submandibular gland; *18*, palatine tonsils narrowing oropharynx; *19*, posterior belly of digastric muscle; *20*, paired anterior belly of digastric muscle; *21*, genioglossus muscle; *22*, superior longitudinal muscle; *23*, transverse muscle; *e*, epiglottis; *h*, body of hyoid bone; *hp*, hard palate; *m*, mandible; *ms*, maxillary sinus; *p*, parotid gland; *scm*, sternocleidomastoid muscle; *sp*, soft palate; *ss*, sphenoid sinus; *v*, vallecula.

The floor of the mouth is the tissue layer between the mucosa of the floor of the mouth and the mylohyoid muscle sling. Additional support for the floor is provided by the paired anterior bellies of the digastric muscles and the geniohyoid muscles. The space caudal to the mylohyoid muscle and above the hyoid bone is considered the suprahyoid neck. Through a gap between the free posterior border of the mylohyoid muscle and the hyoglossus muscle, the submandibular gland wraps around the dorsal aspect of the mylohyoid muscle.[41]

Several named spaces and regions in the oral cavity are mentioned in brief because of their anatomic importance with respect to the structures contained within. The sublingual region is below the mucosa of the floor of the mouth, superomedial to the mylohyoid muscle and lateral to the genioglossus-geniohyoid muscles. It is primarily fat filled and is continuous with the submandibular region at the posterior margin of the mylohyoid muscle. The contents of this space include the sublingual gland and ducts, the submandibular gland duct (Wharton's duct), and sometimes a portion of the hilum of the submandibular gland, anterior fibers of the hyoglossus muscle, and the lingual artery and vein. The hyoglossus muscle is an important surgical landmark (see Fig. 2.48C). Lateral to this muscle, one can identify Wharton's duct, the hypoglossal nerve, and the lingual nerve, whereas the lingual artery and vein lie medially. Wharton's duct runs anteriorly from the gland, traveling with the hypoglossal nerve and the lingual (mandibular branch of the trigeminal) nerve. Initially, it lies between the hyoglossus muscle and the mylohyoid muscle. More anteriorly, it lies between the genioglossus and mylohyoid muscles. The duct drains into the floor of the mouth, just lateral to the frenulum of the tongue.[41]

The submandibular space, or fossa, is defined as the space inferior to the mylohyoid muscle, between the mandible and the hyoid bone. At the posterior margin of the mylohyoid muscle, the submandibular space is continuous with the sublingual space and the anterior aspect of the parapharyngeal space. This communication allows the spread of pathology. The submandibular space is primarily fat filled and contains the superficial portion of the submandibular gland and lymph nodes, lymphatic vessels, and blood vessels. The anterior bellies of the digastric muscle lie in the paramedian location in this space. Branches of the facial artery and vein course lateral to the anterior digastric muscle in the fat surrounding the submandibular gland. The artery lies deep to the gland, and the anterior facial vein is superficial.[42] One important anatomic point is that pathology intrinsic to the submandibular gland displaces the facial vein laterally. Other masses lateral to the gland, including nodes, can be identified with the vein interposed between the gland and the mass.[43]

The lips are composed of the orbicularis oris muscle, which is composed of muscle fibers from multiple facial muscles that insert into the lips and additional fibers proper to the lips. The innervation to the lips is from branches of the facial nerve (CN VII). The vestibule of the mouth, or the gingivobuccal region, is the potential space separating the lips and cheeks from the gums and teeth. The parotid gland ducts and mucous gland ducts of the lips and cheek drain into this space, which is contiguous posteriorly with the oral cavity through the space between the last molar tooth and the ramus of the mandible.[42]

Macroglossia

The tongue makes up the bulk of soft tissues in the oral cavity. Enlargement of the tongue, which is defined clinically as protrusion of the tongue beyond the teeth or alveolar ridge in the resting position, compromises the oral airway and makes the insertion of airway devices challenging. Larsson and colleagues defined the appearance of macroglossia on CT imaging as (1) base of the tongue more than 50 mm in the transverse dimension, (2) genioglossus muscle more than 11 mm in the transverse dimension, (3) midline cleft on the tongue surface, and (4) submandibular glands that are normal in size but bulging out of the platysma muscle owing to tongue enlargement.[44] There are congenital and acquired causes of macroglossia. The congenital syndromes in which macroglossia can be seen are trisomy 21, Beckwith-Wiedemann syndrome, hypothyroidism, and mucopolysaccharidoses. The more commonly acquired causes are tumor of the tongue, lymphangioma, hemangioma, acromegaly, and amyloidosis (Figs. 2.49A–C and 2.50A–E). Aggressive floor-of-the-mouth infections (i.e., Ludwig's angina) can also result in enlargement and posterior displacement of the tongue with airway compromise (Fig. 2.51A–D).

Posterior displacement of the tongue or glossoptosis may be observed with macroglossia, micro- or retrognathia, and neuromuscular disorders including unilateral tongue paralysis secondary to hypoglossal nerve (CN XII) denervation. It can also occur in normal patients in a minority of cases. The obvious complication is relative airway obstruction, which, if chronic, results in a myriad of systemic complications.

Micrognathia and Retrognathia

Micrognathia is a term used to describe an abnormally small mandible. *Retrognathia* is defined as abnormal posterior placement of the mandible. These two findings often coexist. Abnormal growth or placement of the mandible can be caused by malformation, deformation, or connective tissue dysplasia.[45] The most familiar syndrome featuring an abnormal mandible is in the Pierre Robin sequence. Other clinical entities include Treacher Collins, Stickler, and DiGeorge syndromes. Thin-section CT with two-dimensional or three-dimensional reformation provides information regarding the size and proportions of the maxilla, nose, mandible, and airway. Micrognathia and retrognathia not only contribute to airway obstruction, these features are also possible indicators of difficult direct laryngoscopy and endotracheal intubation that can lead to life-threatening complications (Figs. 2.52A and B and 2.53A–D).[46,47]

Exostosis

Hyperostosis of the hard palate or mandible is a benign disease that is usually of no clinical significance. Most often these are small exostoses, which may arise from the oral surface of the hard palate (torus palatinus), from the alveolar portion of the maxilla in the molar region, along the lingual surface of the dental arch (torus maxillaris), or along the lingual surface of the mandible (torus mandibularis, Fig. 2.54A–F). Large lesions may restrict tongue motion and distort the airway, leading to speech disturbance.

Tumors

Only 7% of oral cavity lesions are malignant; however, most of these malignant tumors are squamous cell carcinoma. Other neoplasms include minor salivary gland tumors, lymphomas, and sarcomas. Risk factors for squamous cell carcinoma of the oral cavity include a long history of tobacco and alcohol use. Squamous cell carcinoma can arise anywhere in the oral cavity, but it has a predilection for the floor of the mouth, the ventrolateral tongue, the soft palate complex, including the retromolar trigone area and the anterior tonsillar pillar, and base of the tongue (Fig. 2.55A–D). Most lesions are moderately advanced at the time of presentation; 30% to 65% of patients with oral cavity squamous cell carcinoma

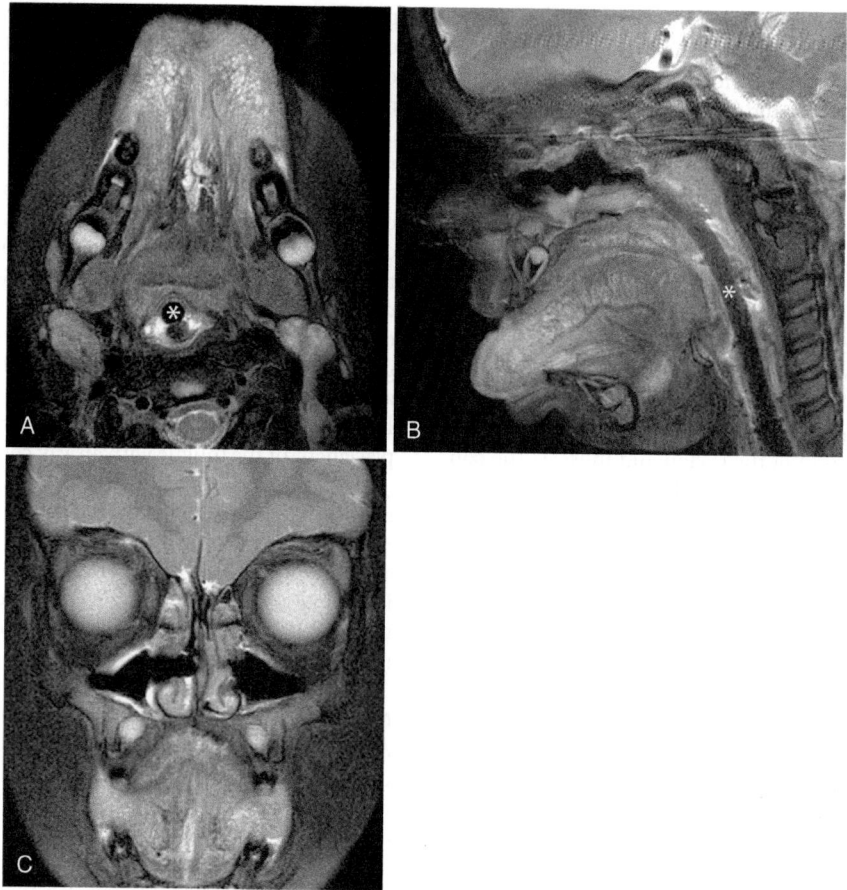

• **Fig. 2.49** Macroglossia. (A) Axial, (B) sagittal, and (C) coronal T2-weighted magnetic resonance (MR) images. There is diffuse enlargement and signal hyperintensity in the tongue with protrusion of the tongue beyond the margin of the oral cavity. There is effacement of the oropharyngeal airway. A nasogastric tube is in place.

have lymph node involvement at the time of diagnosis. The tumors of the oral cavity are usually less aggressive than the squamous cell carcinomas arising from the oropharynx. Both CT and MRI are useful for assessing tumor extent and nodal involvement.[41]

Pharynx

The pharynx is a mucosa-lined tubular structure and is the portion of the aerodigestive tract extending from the skull base to the cervical esophagus. By convention and for ease of discussion, it is divided into three parts: the nasopharynx, oropharynx, and hypopharynx. Anatomically, the nasopharynx is defined as extending from the skull base to the hard palate. The oropharynx extends from the hard palate to the hyoid bone, and the hypopharynx extends from the hyoid bone to the caudal margin of the cricoid cartilage. Below the level of the cricoid cartilage, the cervical esophagus begins. The hypopharynx can be further subdivided into the pyriform sinus region, the posterior wall, the postcricoid region, and the lateral surface of the aryepiglottic folds.[28,42]

The pharyngeal musculature includes the three overlapping constrictor muscles (the superior, middle, and inferior pharyngeal constrictors) and the cricopharyngeus, salpingopharyngeus, stylopharyngeus, palatopharyngeus, tensor veli palatini, and levator veli palatini muscles. Innervation is primarily from the pharyngeal plexus of nerves, to which the vagus (CN X) and glossopharyngeal nerve (CN IX) contribute. The vagus nerve primarily supplies

motor innervation to the constrictors. The mandibular branch of the trigeminal nerve (CN V_3) innervates the tensor veli palatini muscle. Sensory information travels along the glossopharyngeal nerve and the internal laryngeal branch of the superior laryngeal nerve, which arises from the vagus nerve. The arterial supply to the pharynx is from branches of the external carotid artery, including the ascending pharyngeal artery, the tonsillar branches of the facial artery, and the palatine branches of the maxillary artery. Superior and inferior thyroid arteries supply most of the lower pharynx. The primary venous drainage is through the superior and inferior thyroid veins and the pharyngeal veins into the internal jugular veins. The lymphatic drainage is complex and extensive to the jugular, retropharyngeal, posterior cervical, and paratracheal nodes.[28,48]

Imaging studies of the pharynx most commonly include plain film and digital radiographs, barium studies, CT, and MRI. In contrast to CT and MRI, a barium study is a dynamic imaging technique that can demonstrate the sequential contractions of the pharyngeal musculature during deglutition. It can show whether the pharyngeal wall is fixed or pliable and may detect mucosal lesions not apparent on CT or MRI. CT and MRI are most commonly performed with the patient in the supine position and the neck in the neutral position. Intravenous contrast is recommended with CT for evaluation of lymphadenopathy. The inherent differences in signal intensity between tumor, fat, and muscle on MRI often allow accurate delineation of the tumor extent

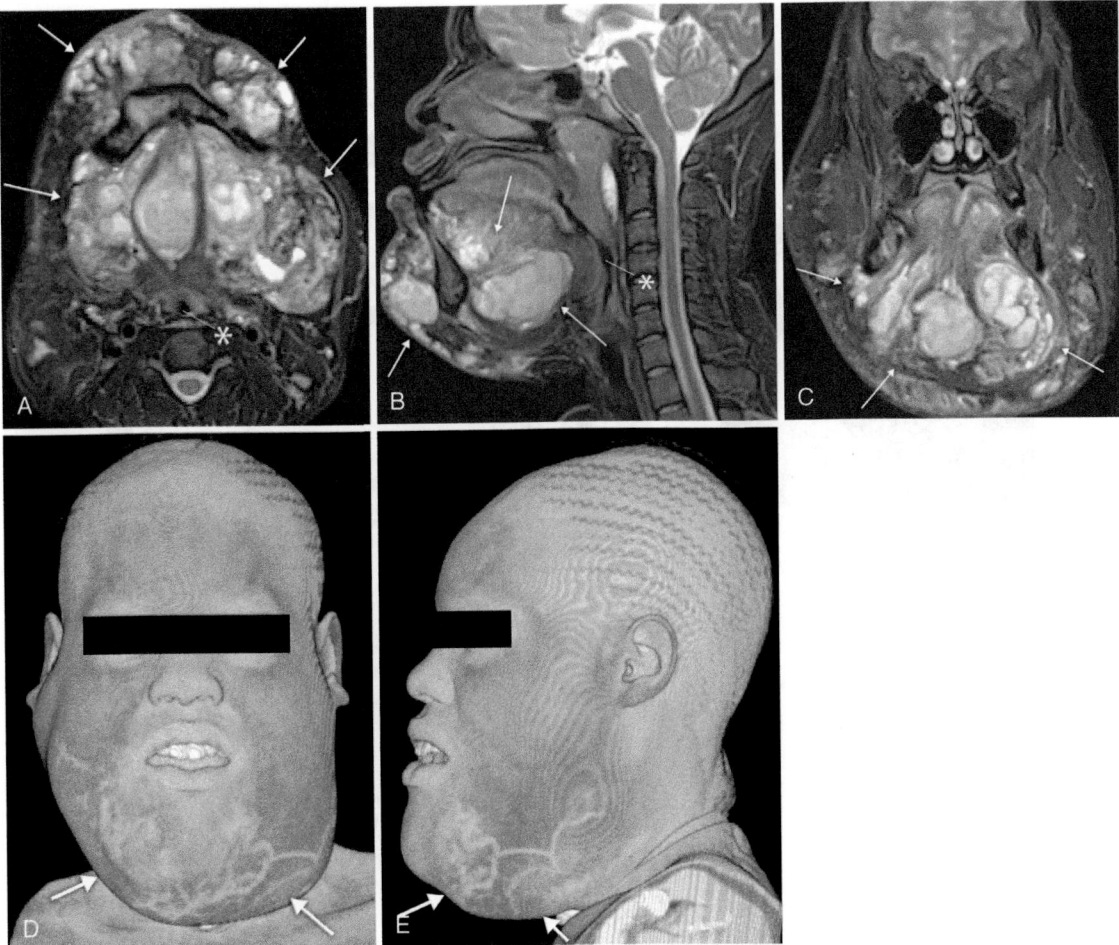

• **Fig. 2.50** Low flow vascular malformation of the oral cavity (formerly referred to as a hemangioma). (A) Axial, (B) sagittal, and (C) coronal T2-weighted magnetic resonance (MR) images demonstrate a lobulated trans-spatial lesion with hyperintense signal (*arrows*) involving the floor of the mouth and submandibular, submental, and buccal spaces. There is effacement of the oropharyngeal airway (*asterisk*). (D) Frontal and (E) lateral three-dimensional surface-rendered computed tomography (CT) images demonstrate clinically apparent contour deformity.

without gadolinium, which is the contrast agent commonly used in clinical practice.[48] Because of the clinical concern for perineural spread of tumor in the head and neck region, however, MRI is usually performed with contrast.

Nasopharynx

The nasopharynx is an air-containing cavity that occupies the uppermost extent of the aerodigestive tract. The roof and posterior wall of the nasopharynx are formed by the sphenoid sinus, clivus, and anterior aspect of the first two cervical vertebrae. The inferior aspect of the nasopharynx is formed by the hard palate, the soft palate, and the ridge of pharyngeal musculature that opposes the soft palate when it is elevated (Passavant's ridge). The lateral nasopharyngeal walls are formed by the margins of the superior constrictor muscle. Anteriorly, the nasopharynx is in direct continuity with the nasal cavity through the posterior choanae. The nasopharynx is in direct communication with the middle ear cavity through the eustachian tubes (Fig. 2.56A–E).[48]

Adenoidal Hypertrophy

The adenoids are lymphatic tissues, located in the upper posterior aspect of the nasopharynx. Prominent adenoids are typical in children;

by the age of 2 to 3 years, the adenoids can fill the entire nasopharynx and extend posteriorly into the posterior choanae. Regression of the lymphoid tissue starts during adolescence and continues into later life. By the age of 30 to 40, adenoidal tissue is minimal, although normal adenoidal tissue may occasionally be seen in adults in their fourth and fifth decades of life.[48] Adenoid tissues appear isodense to muscle on CT imaging (see Fig. 2.56C). On MRI, the adenoids are isointense to muscle on T1-weighted imaging and hyperintense on T2-weighted imaging. If prominent adenoidal tissue is seen in an adult, human immunodeficiency virus should be suspected.[48] Differentiation between lymphomatous involvement and hypertrophy of the adenoids is not possible on imaging, as both are hyperintense on T2-weighted imaging. Enlargement of the adenoids can cause partial obstruction of the nasopharyngeal airway and thus make insertion of a nasogastric tube difficult. Such enlargement may also contribute to the symptom complex of obstructive sleep apnea.

Tornwaldt Cyst

A Tornwaldt cyst is a benign cyst located in the upper nasopharynx and is an occasional incidental finding on MRI (Fig. 2.57A–D). It is usually midline and located between the longus capitis muscles in the posterior nasopharynx. It is a developmental anomaly related to the

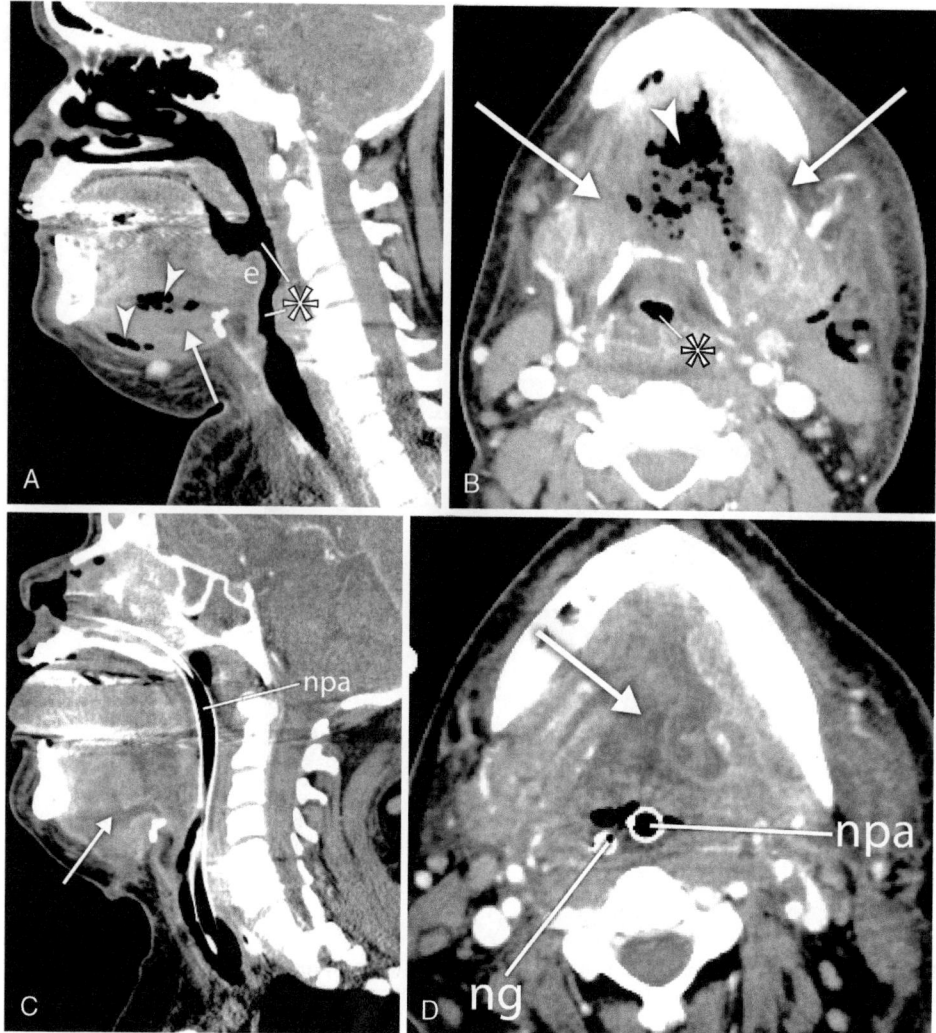

• **Fig. 2.51** Ludwig's angina. (A) Sagittal and (B) axial computed tomography (CT) images with contrast demonstrate fluid collections and edema in the floor of the mouth (*arrows*) compatible with aggressive infection (i.e., Ludwig's angina). Presence of gas (*arrowheads*) indicates infection with gas-forming organisms. There is posterior displacement of the soft tissues with narrowing of the oropharynx, hypopharynx, and supraglottic airway (*asterisk*). Follow-up (C) sagittal and (D) axial CT images demonstrate that the airway has been protected with a nasopharyngeal airway (*npa*). A nasogastric tube is also seen (*ng*). There is persistent edema and residual fluid collections (*arrows*).

ascension of the notochord back into the skull base, pulling a small tag of the developing nasopharyngeal mucosa with it and creating a midline pit or tract that closes over and results in a midline cyst, usually after pharyngitis. These lesions typically have a high signal intensity on T1- and T2-weighted imaging, probably because of the high protein content of the cyst fluid. Tornwaldt cysts can become infected, usually by anaerobic bacteria, and can then empty into the nasopharynx and cause intermittent halitosis. The CT density of the cyst is similar to that of surrounding muscle and lymphoid tissue.[49]

Infection and Abscess

Abscesses in the parapharyngeal and retropharyngeal space may result from tonsillar infection or from iatrogenic or traumatic perforation of the pharynx. Infections may extend from the skull base to the submandibular region and can be difficult to differentiate from a neoplastic process; if large enough, the airway may be compromised. Infection spreading to retropharyngeal nodes, suppurative adenitis, can also obliterate the nasopharyngeal airway (Fig. 2.58A–C).[50,51]

Tumors

Squamous cell carcinoma of the nasopharynx is a relatively rare cancer that accounts for only 0.25% of all malignancies in North America. It has a high rate of incidence in Asia, however, where it is the most common tumor in males, accounting for 18% of cancers in China.[52] Squamous cell carcinoma accounts for 70% or more of the malignancies arising in the nasopharynx, and lymphomas account for approximately 20%. The remaining 10% are a variety of lesions, including adenocarcinoma, adenoid cystic carcinoma, rhabdomyosarcoma, melanoma, extramedullary plasmacytoma, fibrosarcoma, and carcinosarcoma. Risk factors for squamous cell carcinoma in the nasopharynx include the presence of immunoglobulin A antibodies against Epstein-Barr virus, human leukocyte antigen (HLA) (HLA-A2 and HLA-BSin2 serotypes), exposure to nitrosamines or polycyclic hydrocarbons, poor living conditions, and chronic sinonasal infections.[53] The most common presentation is nodal disease. There is no correlation between primary tumor size and the presence of nodal disease. Imaging with

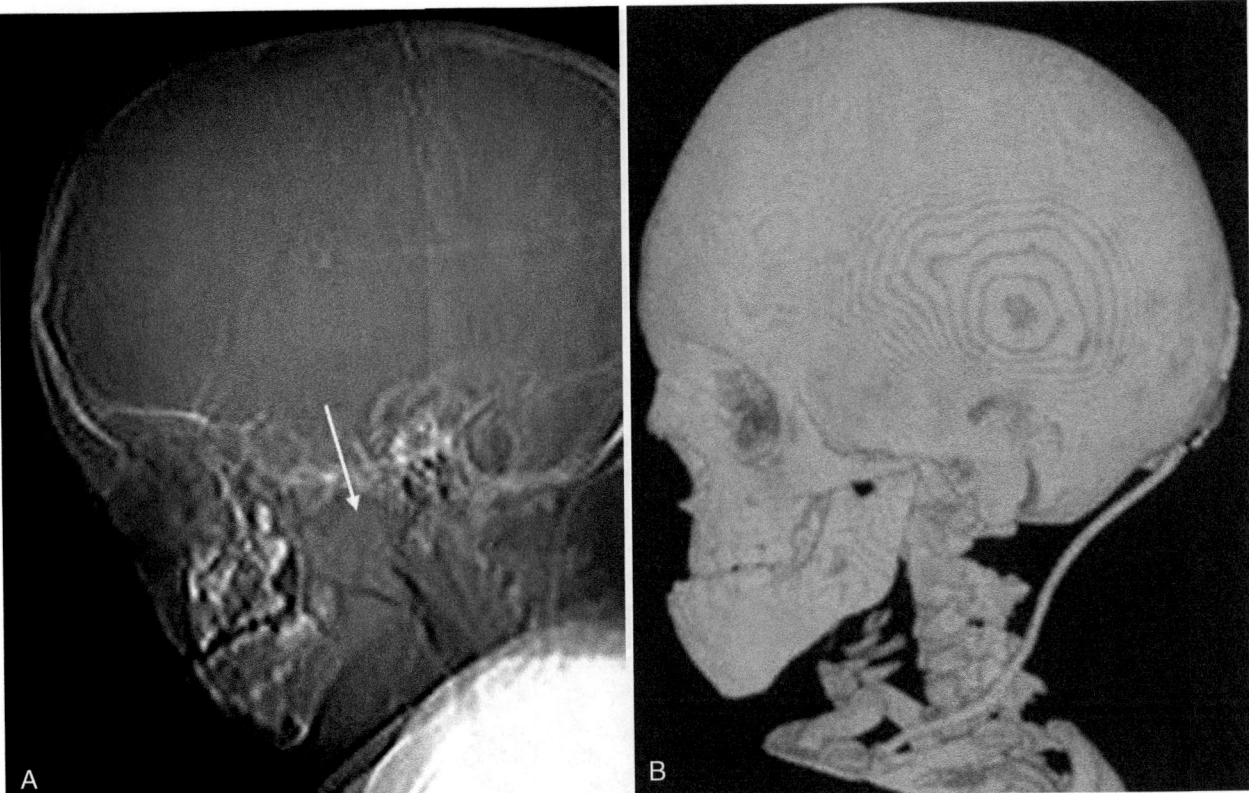

• **Fig. 2.52** Midface regression syndrome in two patients with Jackson-Weiss syndrome demonstrate (A) maxillary regression on computed tomography (CT) scout and (B) three-dimensional surface rendering. Note the presence of a ventriculoperitoneal shunt as hydrocephalus may result from the craniosynostosis associated with this syndrome. The mandible is hypoplastic, and there is soft tissue obscuring the nasopharynx (*arrow*).

CT and MRI is performed to accurately map the extent of the disease, not for histologic diagnosis (Fig. 2.59A–D).

Oropharynx

The oropharynx is the region posterior to the oral cavity that includes the posterior one-third of the tongue (tongue base), the palatine tonsils, the soft palate, and the oropharyngeal mucosa and constrictor muscles. The posterior pharyngeal wall is at the level of the second and third cervical vertebrae. Laterally, there are two mucosa-lined faucial arches; the anterior arch is formed by the mucosa of the palatoglossus muscle, and the posterior arch is formed by the palatopharyngeus muscle. The palatine tonsils are located between the two faucial arches, and the lingual tonsils reside at the base of the tongue. Both sets of lymphoid tissue vary in size and can encroach on the airway; lingual tonsillar hypertrophy is a significant cause of difficult laryngoscopy. The arterial supply to the oropharynx is mainly from the branches of the external carotid artery: the tonsillar branch of the facial artery, the ascending pharyngeal artery, the dorsal lingual arteries, and the internal maxillary and facial arteries. Venous drainage is primarily by the peritonsillar veins, which pierce the constrictor musculature and drain into the common facial vein and the pharyngeal plexus. Lymphatic drainage is mainly to the jugulodigastric chain in the deep upper cervical chain, the retropharyngeal nodes, the parapharyngeal nodes, and sometimes the parotid nodes.

Tonsillar Hypertrophy

During the third and fourth fetal months, lymphoid tissues invade the pharyngeal region of the adenoid tonsils, the palatine region

(palatine tonsils), and the root of the tongue (lingual tonsils).[40] The adenoids are located in the roof of the nasopharynx. As mentioned, enlargement of the palatine and lingual tonsils may compromise the airway (Fig. 2.60A and B).

Tonsillitis and Peritonsillar Abscess

Acute bacterial tonsillitis is most often caused by beta-hemolytic *Streptococcus, Staphylococcus, Pneumococcus,* or *Haemophilus.* It is usually a self-limiting disease; however, uncontrolled infection of the tonsils may result in formation of a peritonsillar abscess or, rarely, in a tonsillar abscess. On CT imaging, the findings of acute or chronic tonsillitis are nonspecific. Focal homogeneous swelling of the palatine tonsils can be present and is difficult to differentiate from tumor. The imaging features of abscess formation are a low-density center and an enhancing rim of soft tissue (Fig. 2.61A–G). Peritonsillar abscess is the accumulation of pus around the tonsils. The infection may extend to the retropharyngeal, parapharyngeal, or submandibular spaces.

Retropharyngeal Abscess

Infection of the retropharyngeal space is usually a result of an infection at a site whose primary drainage is to the retropharyngeal lymph nodes, such as the nose, sinuses, throat, tonsils, oral cavity, and middle ear. The lymph nodes enlarge and undergo suppuration and eventually rupture into the retropharyngeal space, creating an abscess. This can result from a penetrating injury or from cervical spine osteomyelitis or discitis. Before the advent of antibiotics, retropharyngeal infection was potentially life threatening. A retropharyngeal space infection can extend

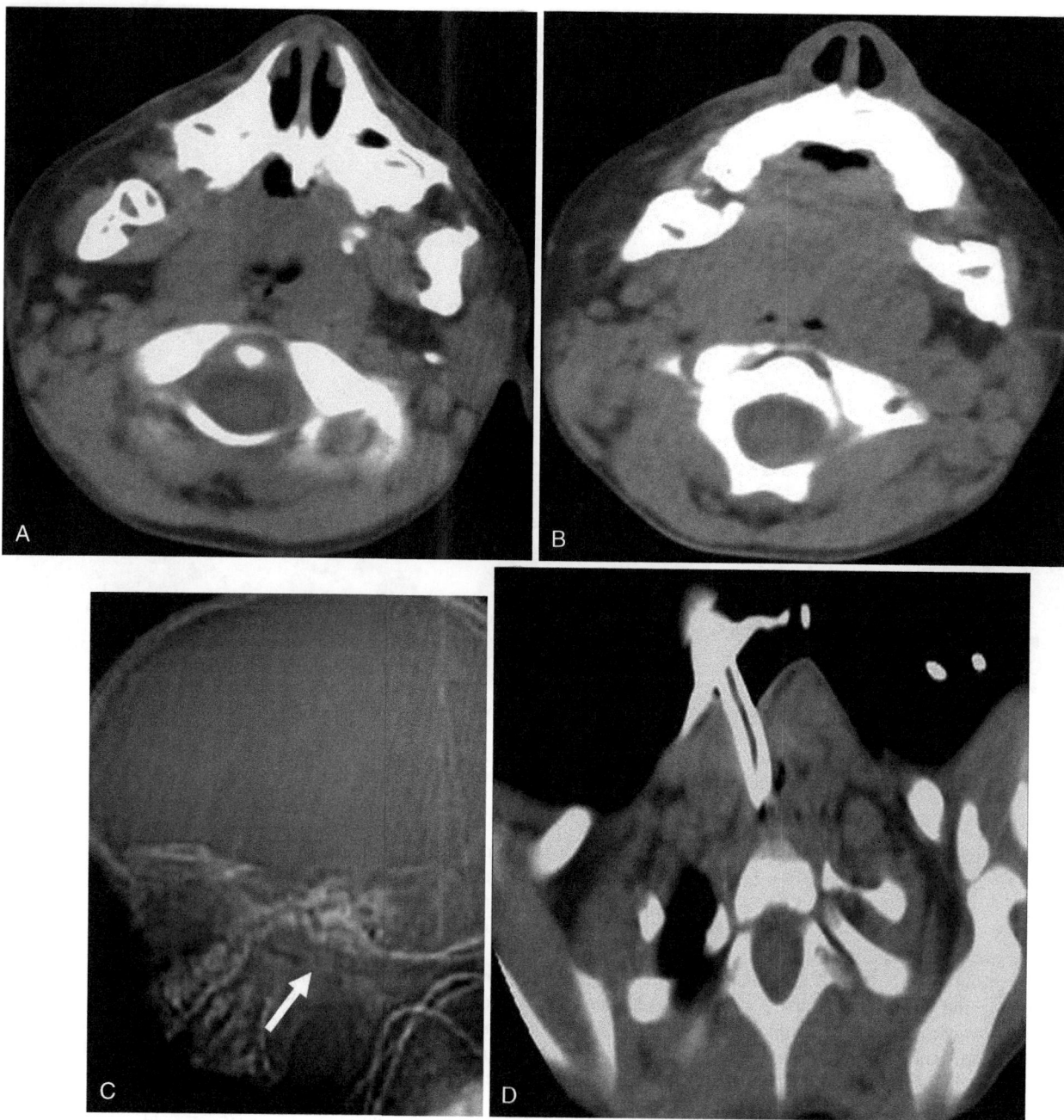

• **Fig. 2.53** Treacher Collins syndrome. Axial computed tomography (CT) scans at the level of the (A) nasopharynx and (B) oropharynx demonstrate near obliteration of the airway by soft tissue, secondary to the facial microsomia. (C) Lateral CT scout view demonstrates marked narrowing (*arrow*) of the airway. Axial CT scan at the thoracic inlet (D) demonstrates the tracheostomy necessitated by this condition.

from the skull base to the carina. On imaging, a retropharyngeal abscess expands the prevertebral space, with enhancement along its margins. Included in the differential diagnosis of a retropharyngeal abscess is tendinitis of the longus colli, which is characterized by inflammation of the tendinous insertion of the longus colli muscle with deposition of calcium hydroxyapatite crystals; an associated effusion may extend from the prevertebral space into the retropharyngeal space and mimic a retropharyngeal abscess. Posttraumatic hematoma may also increase the width of prevertebral space. In addition, cervical spine pathology can extend and enlarge the prevertebral space and cause the airway to deviate anteriorly.

Tortuous Internal or Common Carotid Artery

If the course of either the common carotid artery or the tortuous internal carotid artery is directed medially, bulging of the submucosa of the oropharynx or hypopharynx may result. In this less protected location, the artery is more vulnerable to trauma. Imaging is useful to prevent unnecessary biopsy of this pseudosubmucosal mass (Fig. 2.62A–D).

Tumors

Squamous cell carcinoma is the most common neoplasm of the oropharynx, and its predisposing factors include alcohol and tobacco use. Most recently, epidemiologic and molecular data

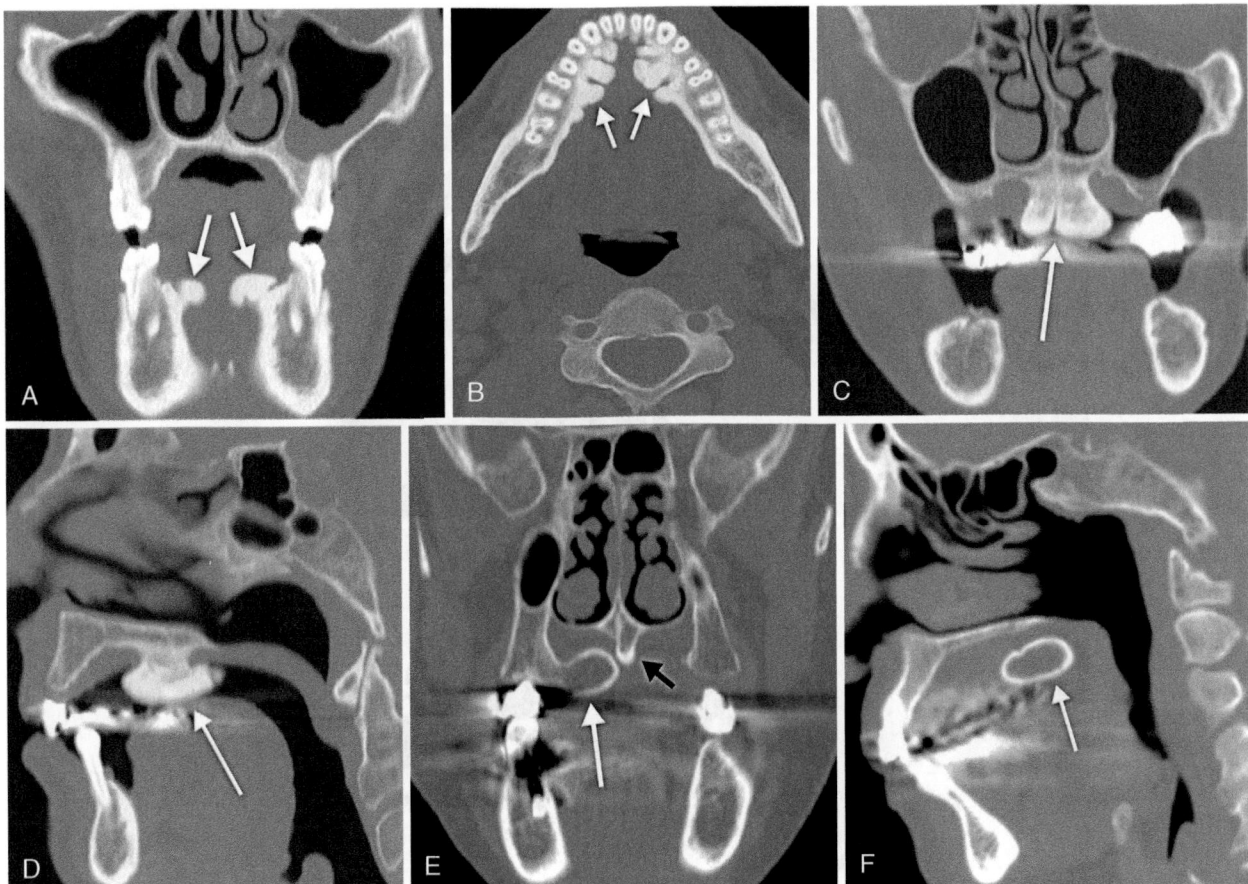

• **Fig. 2.54** Mandibular and maxillary exostoses. (A, B) Torus mandibularis (*arrows*) protruding into the floor of mouth on (A) coronal and (B) axial computed tomography (CT) images. (C, D) Torus palatinus (*arrows*) compromising the oral cavity on (C) coronal and (D) sagittal CT images. (E, F) Right torus maxillarus (*white arrow*) and small torus palatinus (*black arrow*) compromising the oral cavity on (E) coronal and (F) sagittal CT images.

have shown a strong association between human papillomavirus (HPV) exposure or infection, particularly HPV 16, with development of oropharyngeal cancer, especially tonsillar cancer. This comprises a subset of patients with oropharyngeal cancers presenting at a younger age, with distinct molecular and pathologic differences and yet unexplained improved prognosis.[54]

The site of origin determines the spread of the tumor; the most common locations are the anterior and posterior tonsillar pillars, tonsillar fossa, soft palate, and base of the tongue (see Fig. 2.55). Staging of a tumor in the oropharynx is dependent on the size of the tumor and whether it has invaded adjacent structures. Other neoplasms include lymphoma, minor salivary gland tumors, and mesenchymal tumors.

Hypopharynx

The classic boundary of the hypopharynx is defined as the segment of the pharynx extending from the level of the hyoid bone and the valleculae to the cricopharyngeus or the lower level of the cricoid cartilage. The cervical esophagus starts at the caudal end of the cricoid cartilage. The cricopharyngeus muscle acts as the upper esophageal sphincter. It arises from the lower aspect of the inferior constrictor muscle attached to the cricoid. The upper esophageal sphincter is normally closed until a specific volume and pressure in the hypopharynx trigger the relaxation of the cricopharyngeus muscle to allow a bolus of food to pass into the cervical esophagus. The cricopharyngeus muscle then closes

to prevent reflux.[52] The hypopharynx can be divided into four regions: the pyriform sinuses, the posterior wall of the hypopharynx, the postcricoid region, and the lateral surface of the aryepiglottic folds. The pyriform sinus is the anterolateral recess of the hypopharynx. The anterior pyriform sinus mucosa abuts on the posterior paraglottic space. The most caudal portion of each pyriform sinus lies at the level of the true vocal cord. The lateral aspect of the aryepiglottic folds forms the medial wall of the pyriform sinus (Fig. 2.63). This is considered a marginal zone because the aryepiglottic folds are considered part of both the hypopharynx and the supraglottic larynx. Tumors involving the medial surface of the aryepiglottic folds behave like laryngeal tumors. The biologic behavior of tumors arising from the lateral surface of the aryepiglottic folds is similar to that of the more aggressive pharyngeal tumors. The lateral wall of the pyriform sinus is formed by the thyroid membrane and cartilage.[52] The posterior hypopharyngeal wall is continuous with the posterior wall of the oropharynx and begins at the level of the valleculae. It continues caudally as the posterior wall of the cricopharyngeus and the cervical esophagus. The retropharyngeal space lies behind the posterior pharyngeal wall. The anterior wall of the lower hypopharynx is referred to as the postcricoid hypopharynx; the larynx is anterior and the hypopharynx is posterior to this soft tissue boundary. It extends from the level of the arytenoid cartilages to the lower cricoid cartilage. On imaging, the transition from the hypopharynx to the cervical esophagus is denoted by a change in the shape

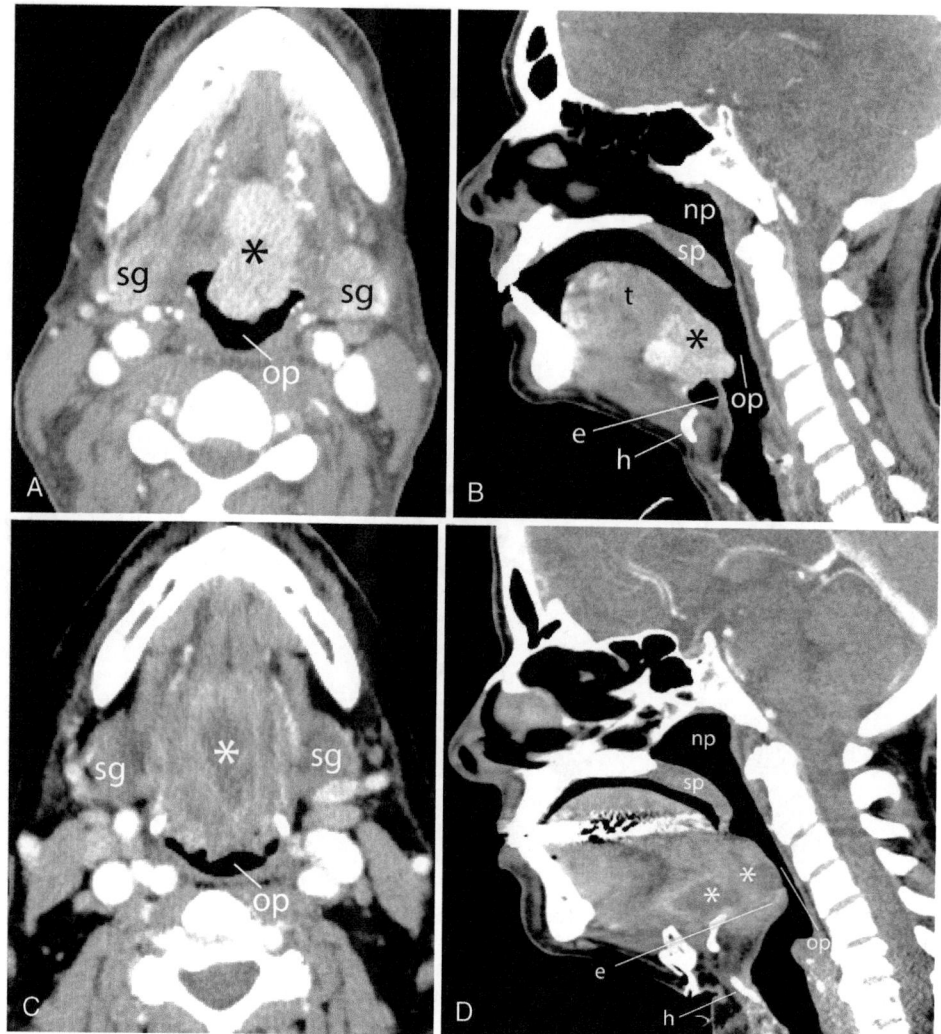

• **Fig. 2.55** Base of tongue lesions in two patients. (A) Axial and (B) sagittal postcontrast computed tomography (CT) images demonstrate a solidly enhancing mass at the tongue base extending into the floor of mouth (*asterisk*). Biopsy confirmed squamous cell carcinoma. (C) Axial and (D) sagittal postcontrast CT images in a different patient demonstrate a peripherally enhancing mass involving the floor of the mouth and the tongue base (*asterisk*), consistent with abscess. There is effacement of the vallecula anterior to the epiglottis and mass effect on the oropharyngeal airway. *sg*, submandibular gland; *op*, oropharynx; *np*, nasopharynx; *sp*, soft palate; *t*, tongue; *h*, hyoid; *e*, Epiglottis.

of the aerodigestive tract, from crescentic or ovoid to round. The arterial supply to the lower pharynx is mainly from the superior and inferior thyroid arteries. Venous drainage is by the superior and inferior thyroid veins and individual pharyngeal veins to the internal jugular vein.

Pharyngitis

In immunocompetent patients, imaging is usually not required for the diagnosis or management of pharyngitis. In AIDS patients, imaging may be helpful to evaluate the extent of disease. Bacterial etiology is not the only concern; opportunistic infection with *Candida* or *Cytomegalovirus* may involve the hypopharynx. These entities do not compromise the airway, but the mucosa is friable and susceptible to injuries from instrumentation.

Pharyngocele

A pharyngocele is a broad-based outpouching of the pharyngeal mucosa of the upper pyriform sinus, which distends with

phonation or during a Valsalva maneuver. These lesions are visible as air-filled structures on CT or as barium-filled areas on a barium swallow test.

Zenker's Diverticulum

Zenker's diverticulum is a diverticulum of the mucosa of the hypopharynx. It is postulated that dyssynergy of the cricopharyngeus muscle plays a role in its formation. The diverticulum usually extends posteriorly and laterally, usually to the left, and may appear as an incidental, air-filled structure in the hypopharynx on CT and MRI. If alerted to the presence of a diverticulum, one should take more caution in the blind advancement of a nasogastric tube, which may take an errant course (Fig. 2.64A–D).

Trauma

Direct trauma or iatrogenic trauma caused by instrumentation, surgery, or a foreign body may result in retropharyngeal hematoma. Patients with hemophilia may be more susceptible to

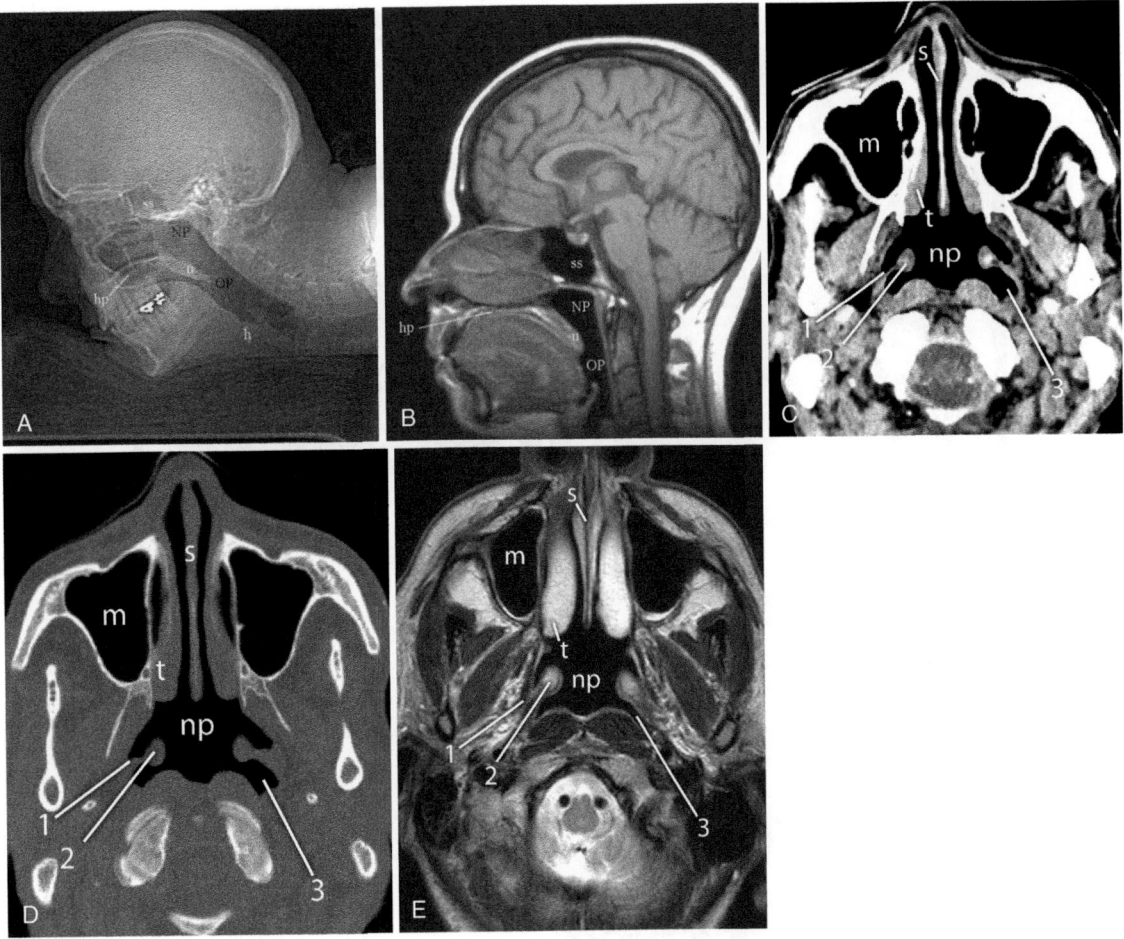

• **Fig. 2.56** Nasopharyngeal anatomy. (A) Computed tomography (CT) scout in prone position. (B) T1-weighted sagittal brain magnetic resonance image (MRI). Axial CT images of a normal nasopharynx in (C) soft tissue and (D) bone reconstruction algorithm. (E) Axial T2-weighted MRI. *1,* Opening of the eustachian tube; *2,* torus tubarius; *3,* fossa of Rosenmüller; *h,* hyoid; *hp,* hard palate; *np,* nasopharynx; *op,* oropharynx; *ss,* sphenoid sinus; *tb,* turbinate, *u,* uvula; *m,* maxillary sinus; *s,* nasal septum.

hematomas with minor trauma. The imaging finding is retropharyngeal or prevertebral soft tissue swelling.

The edema that occurs after radiation therapy may persist for many months or years and is reflective of a radiation-induced obliterative endarteritis. In cases of edema, the pharyngeal and supraglottic mucosa appear swollen, bulging, and hypodense on CT, and the submucosal fat is thickened and streaky. The platysma muscle and skin are also thickened. The result is fibrosis and loss of elasticity of the soft tissues. This increased rigidity of the soft tissues should be considered during laryngoscopy for endotracheal intubation and when selecting the correct size of a laryngeal mask airway.

Tumors and Other Pathology

The hypopharynx is lined by stratified squamous epithelium, and most tumors of the hypopharynx are squamous cell carcinomas (Fig. 2.65A and B). The risk factors for squamous cell carcinoma of the hypopharynx include alcohol abuse, smoking, and previous radiation therapy. Patients with Plummer-Vinson syndrome have a higher incidence of postcricoid carcinoma. Extensive submucosal growth is common and can be appreciated only on imaging. The airway may be effaced and displaced. Most patients have metastases to the cervical nodes at presentation. Between 4% and 15% of patients with squamous cell carcinoma of the hypopharynx have a synchronous or metachronous second primary tumor.[48,55]

Hodgkin lymphoma predominantly affects adolescents and young adults, whereas non-Hodgkin lymphoma is a disease of older patients. In contrast to patients with Hodgkin lymphoma, patients with non-Hodgkin lymphoma present with disease in extranodal sites, such as Waldeyer's ring. The imaging features of extranodal head and neck lymphoma can be difficult to differentiate from those of squamous cell carcinoma. Lymphadenopathy in Hodgkin lymphoma can be quite large without affecting the airways.

Less common primary cancers include minor salivary gland tumors (most often involving the soft palate), rhabdomyosarcomas, granular cell tumors, schwannomas and neurofibromas, hemangiomas, and lipomas.[48,52] Pharyngeal masses can also be the result of amyloidosis or metastatic disease.

Larynx

Structure and Function

The larynx is a conduit to the lungs, provides airway protection against aspiration, and allows vocalization. It has an outer supporting skeleton composed of a series of cartilages, fibrous sheets, muscles, and ligaments, which provide structure and protection for the inner mucosal tube, the endolarynx.

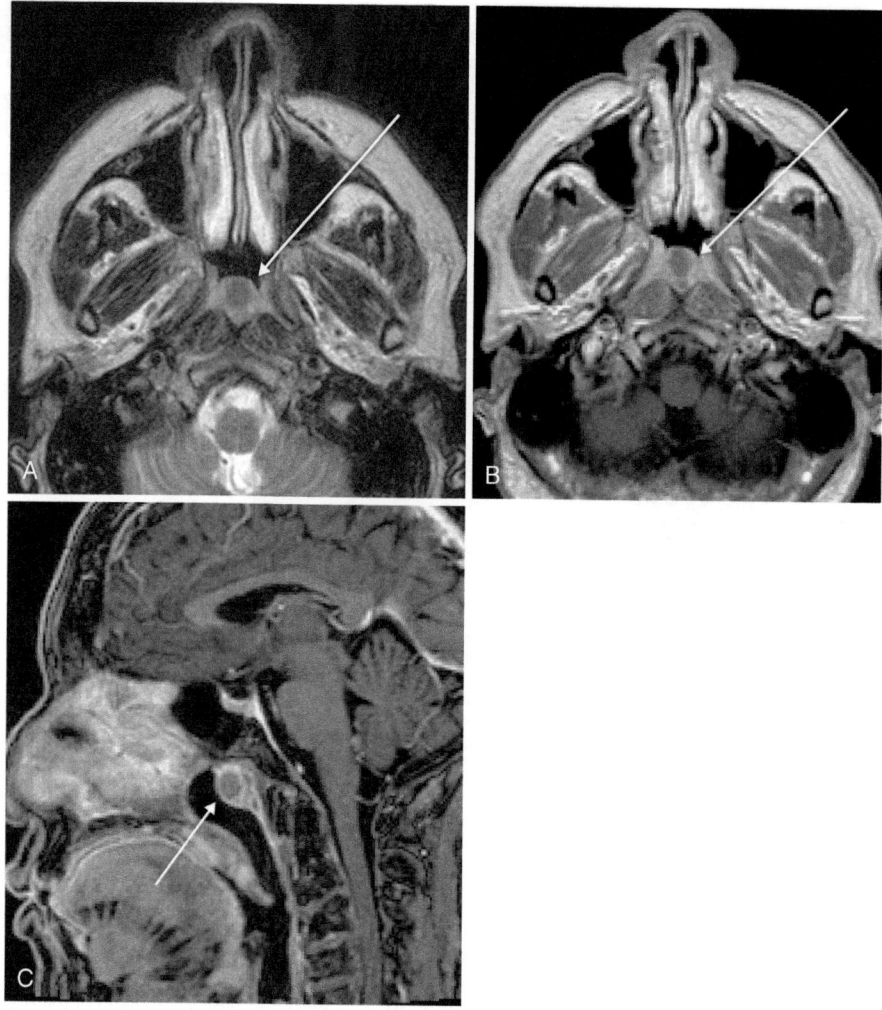

• **Fig. 2.57** Tornwaldt cyst. (A) Axial T2-weighted, (B) axial, and (C) sagittal postcontrast T1-weighted magnetic resonance (MR) images demonstrate a well-defined peripherally enhancing complex cyst (*arrow*) in the midline nasopharynx (*asterisk*) consistent with a Tornwaldt cyst. *s*, Nasal septum.

The thyroid cartilage is the largest cartilage of the larynx. It is made up of two shieldlike laminae that fuse anteriorly to form the laryngeal prominence (Adam's apple). The angle of fusion is usually more acute and more prominent in males. Paired superior and inferior cornua project from the posterior margin of the thyroid cartilage. The superior thyroid cornu is connected to the dorsal tip of the greater cornu of the hyoid bone by the thyrohyoid ligament. The inferior cornu articulates with the lateral facet of the cricoid cartilage to form the cricothyroid joint, where the thyroid cartilage rocks back and forth. Muscles that attach to the external surface of the thyroid cartilage include the sternothyroid and thyrohyoid muscles and the inferior pharyngeal constrictors. The thyrohyoid membrane bridges the gap between the upper surface of the thyroid cartilage and the hyoid bone. Likewise, the cricothyroid membrane spans the distance between the lower margin of the thyroid cartilage and the cricoid cartilage.

The cricoid cartilage, which is shaped like a signet ring with the larger part facing posteriorly, is the base of the larynx. On either side of the cricoid cartilage are facets, which articulate with the inferior horn of the thyroid cartilage. On the upper surface of the cricoid lamina are two paired articular facets, on which are situated the arytenoid cartilages.[28] The arytenoid cartilages are important surgical and imaging landmarks.[28] They are important

in maintaining airway patency and participate in vocalization by altering the opening of the glottis and the tension of the vocal cords. Each cartilage is pyramidal in shape. At the level of the base are two projections: the muscular process situated on the posterolateral margin and the vocal process located anteriorly. The superior process is the apex of the pyramid and is at the level of the false vocal cords. The small corniculate cartilage rests on the superior process. The muscular and vocal processes are at the level of the true vocal cords.

The quadrangular membrane stretches anteriorly from the upper arytenoid and corniculate cartilages to the lateral margin of the epiglottis and contributes to the support of the epiglottis.[56] The superior free margin of this membrane forms the support for the aryepiglottic fold, which stretches from the upper margin of the arytenoids to the lateral margin of the epiglottis. The corniculate and cuneiform cartilages within the aryepiglottic fold help support the edge of each fold. These small, mucosa-covered cartilages are visualized on laryngoscopy as two small protuberances at the posterolateral border of the rima glottidis.

The aryepiglottic folds form the lateral margin of the vestibule of the supraglottic airway. The upper part of the aryepiglottic fold is the aryepiglottic muscle, which functions like a purse string to close the opening of the larynx when swallowing. Lateral to the

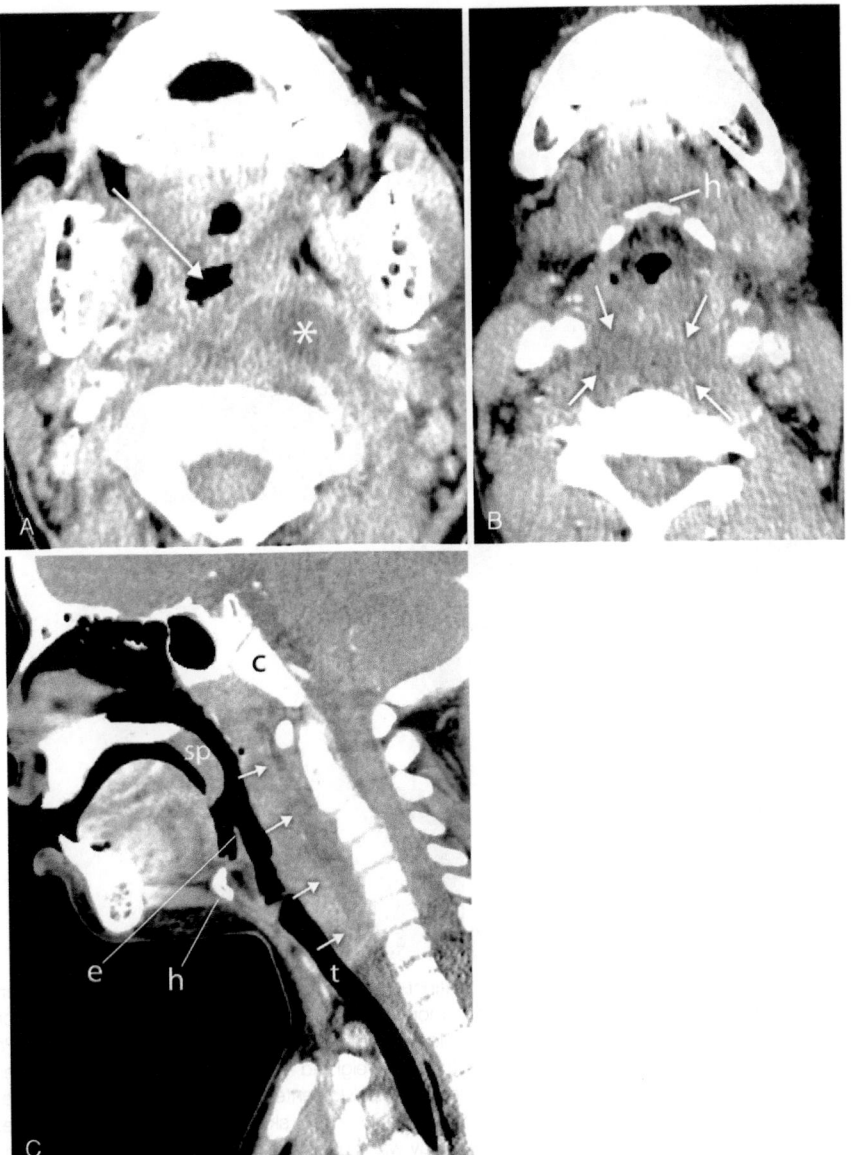

• **Fig. 2.58** Suppurative adenitis. (A) Axial computed tomography (CT) image shows a focal peripherally enhancing collection in the left retropharyngeal space (*asterisk*) with displacement of the oropharyngeal airway (*arrow*). This is a typical location for retropharyngeal lymph nodes, and the appearance is consistent with suppurative adenitis. (B) Axial CT image more inferiorly and (C) midline sagittal CT image show fluid without clear peripheral enhancement more centrally in the retropharyngeal space extending from the skull base toward superior mediastinum (*arrows*) compatible with reactive edema. *c,* Clivus; *sp,* soft palate; *e,* epiglottis; *h,* hyoid; *t,* trachea.

aryepiglottic folds are the pyriform sinuses. The apex, or the most inferior aspect, of the pyriform sinus is at the level of the true vocal cords.

The inferior free margin of the quadrangular membrane forms the ventricular ligament, which extends anteriorly from the superior arytenoid cartilage to the inner lamina of the thyroid cartilage and supports the free edge of the false vocal cords. The false vocal cords are superior to the true vocal cords and are separated by a lateral pouching of the airway, the laryngeal ventricle.[56] The vocal ligaments lie parallel and inferior to the ventricular ligaments; they likewise extend from the vocal process of the arytenoid cartilage to the inner lamina of the thyroid just above the anterior commissure. The vocal ligament provides medial support for the true vocal cords. The space between the left and right vocal cords

is referred to as the rima glottis, through which air passes to allow breathing and vocalization. Extending from the vocal ligament is another fibrous membrane, the conus elasticus, which attaches inferiorly to the upper inner margin of the cricoid cartilage. The conus spans part of the gap between the thyroid and cricoid cartilages.

The muscles of the larynx are categorized as intrinsic and extrinsic muscles. The intrinsic muscles regulate the aperture of the rima glottis: (1) the thyroarytenoid makes up the bulk of the true vocal cord and has a lateral and medial belly, (2) the lateral cricoarytenoids extend from the muscular process of the arytenoid cartilage to the upper lateral cricoid cartilage and function to adduct the cords, (3) the posterior cricoarytenoids extend from the muscular process of the arytenoid cartilage to the posterior

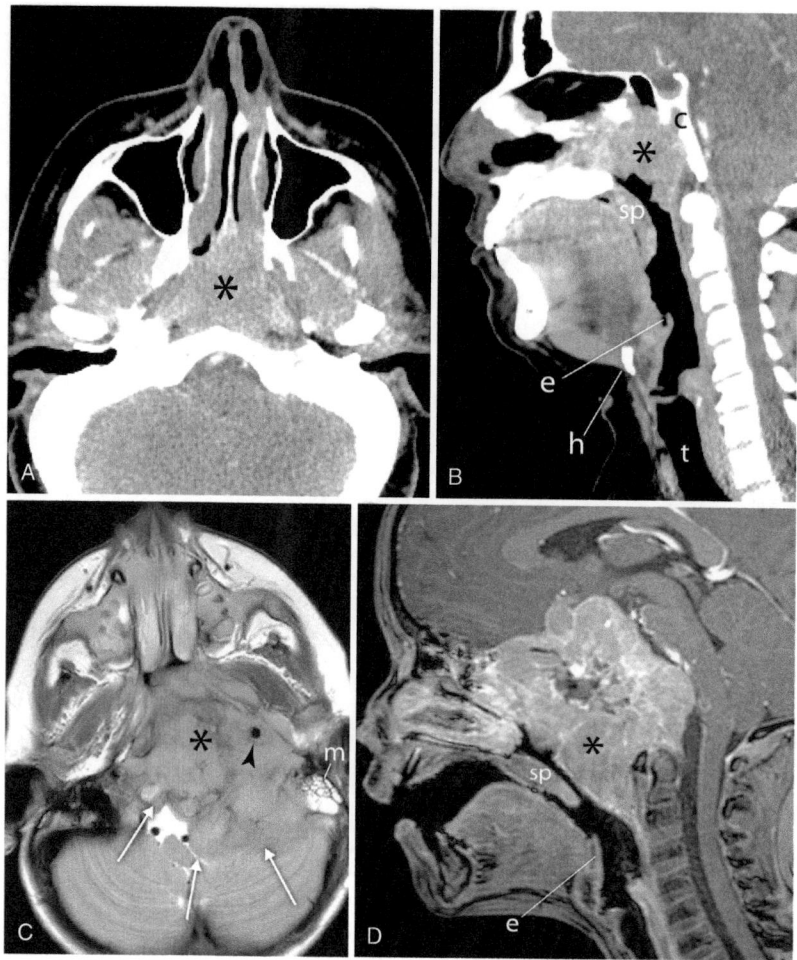

• **Fig. 2.59** Nasopharyngeal neoplasm in two patients. Patient 1: (A) Axial and (B) sagittal postcontrast computed tomography (CT) images in an adult demonstrate enhancing soft tissue effacing the nasopharynx (*asterisk*) with erosive changes of the clivus. Biopsy demonstrated squamous cell carcinoma. Patient 2: (C) Axial T2-weighted and (D) sagittal postcontrast T1-weighted magnetic resonance (MR) images in a child demonstrate a large enhancing soft tissue lesion (*asterisk*) centered on the nasopharynx with extension into the nasal cavity, parapharyngeal space, and invasion of the skull base. There is intracranial extension (*arrows*) with mass effect on the brain. Pathology was consistent with rhabdomyosarcoma. There is encasement of the left internal carotid artery (*arrowhead*). If intracranial extension is not appreciated, an errant nasogastric tube can easily enter the cranium, resulting in brain or vascular injury. *m*, mastoid air cells containing fluid due to eustachian tube dysfunction; *sp*, soft palate; *e*, Epiglottis.

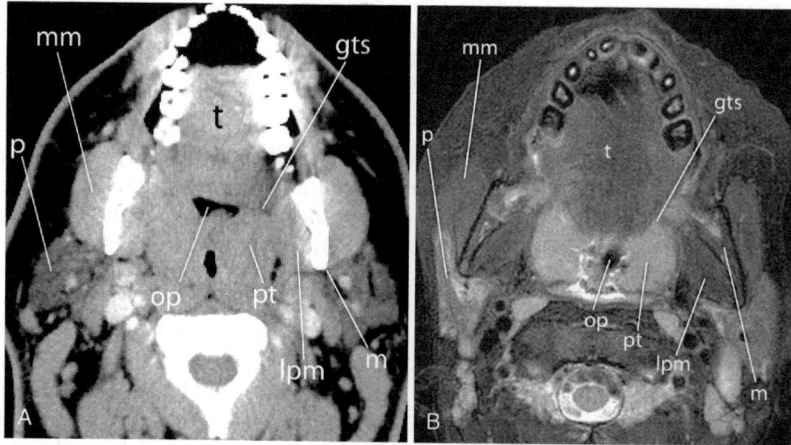

• **Fig. 2.60** Oropharyngeal anatomy. (A) Axial computed tomography (CT) image and (B) axial T2-weighted magnetic resonance (MR) image demonstrate bilateral enlarged palatine tonsils (*pt*) effacing the oropharynx (*op*). *pt*, palatine tonsils; *lt*, lingual tonsils; *o*, oropharynx; *e*, epiglottis; *v*, vallecula; *t*, oral tongue; *bot*, Base of tongue; *gts*, glossotonsillar sulcus; *p*, parotid gland; *m*, mandible; *mm*, masseter muscle; *lpm*, lateral pterygoid muscle.

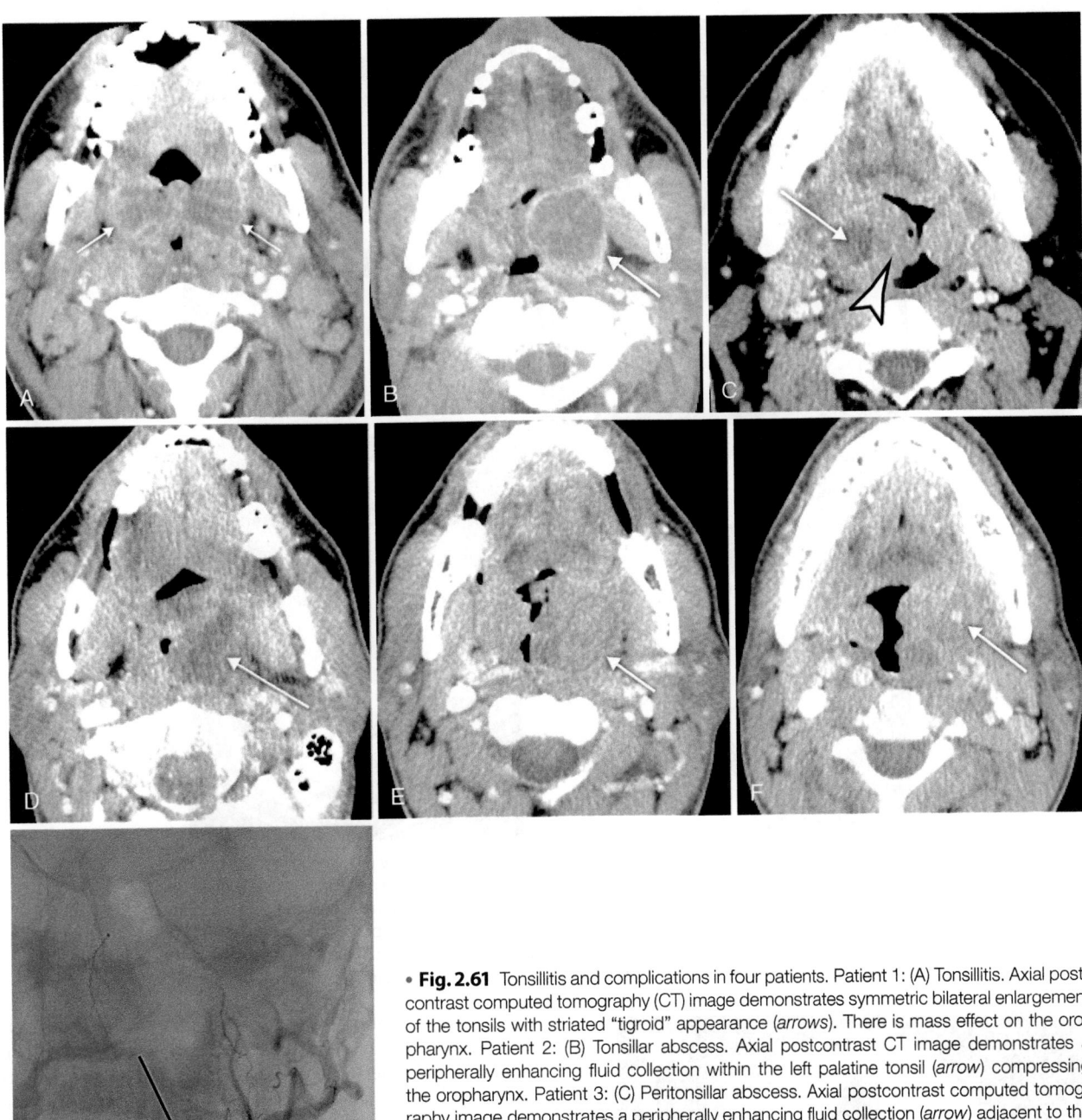

• **Fig. 2.61** Tonsillitis and complications in four patients. Patient 1: (A) Tonsillitis. Axial post-contrast computed tomography (CT) image demonstrates symmetric bilateral enlargement of the tonsils with striated "tigroid" appearance (*arrows*). There is mass effect on the oro-pharynx. Patient 2: (B) Tonsillar abscess. Axial postcontrast CT image demonstrates a peripherally enhancing fluid collection within the left palatine tonsil (*arrow*) compressing the oropharynx. Patient 3: (C) Peritonsillar abscess. Axial postcontrast computed tomography image demonstrates a peripherally enhancing fluid collection (*arrow*) adjacent to the right palatine tonsil (*arrowhead*) compressing the oropharynx. (D–G) Tonsillar abscess with pseudoaneurysm. (D) Axial postcontrast CT image demonstrates a peripherally enhancing fluid collection within the left palatine tonsil compatible with tonsillar abscess (*arrow*). (E) Axial postcontrast CT image on follow-up exam demonstrates increased density within the collection (*arrow*) compatible with hematoma. (F) Axial CT angiography image demonstrates a small collection of arterial enhancement within the hematoma compatible with small pseudoaneurysm (*arrow*). (G) Digital subtraction angiography confirms a small pseudoaneurysm (*arrow*).

surface of the cricoid cartilage and abduct the cords laterally, and (4) the interarytenoid muscle stretches from one arytenoid to the other and functions to adduct the vocal cords.

The extrinsic muscle is the cricothyroid muscle, which extends from the lower thyroid cartilage anteriorly to the upper cricoid carti-lage. The contraction of this muscle pivots the thyroid cartilage for-ward around an axis through the cricothyroid joint, which stretches and tenses the vocal cords, thus affecting pitch in vocalization.[56]

The larynx is innervated primarily by branches of the vagus nerve.[28] The recurrent laryngeal nerve innervates all the intrinsic muscles of the larynx. When vocal cord paralysis is present and nerve damage is suspected, imaging should be tailored to follow the course of the recurrent laryngeal nerve in the neck and upper chest. The vagus nerve, after exiting the jugular foramen, passes vertically down the neck within the carotid sheath, between the internal jugular vein and the internal carotid artery (subsequently

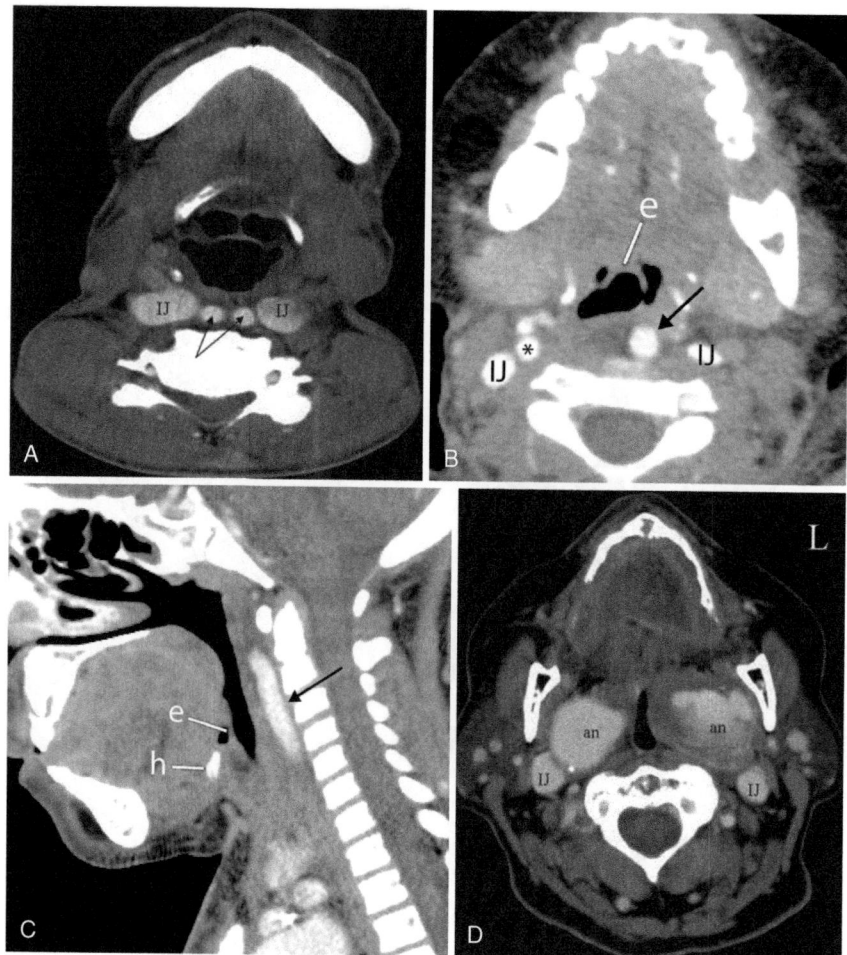

• **Fig. 2.62** Anomalous course of carotids. (A) Axial computed tomography (CT) image with contrast in an adult demonstrates medially deviated retropharyngeal carotids, referred to as "kissing" carotids (*arrows*). (B) Axial and (C) lateral CT with contrast in a child demonstrates a unilateral left retropharyngeal carotid artery (*arrow*). The contralateral right carotid artery is in a normal anatomic position (*asterisk*). (D) Axial CT with contrast shows bilateral carotid aneurysms (*an*) effacing the oropharynx. Note the presence of thrombus in the lumen of the aneurysm on the left. *IJ*, internal jugular vein; *h*, hyoid; *e*, Epiglottis.

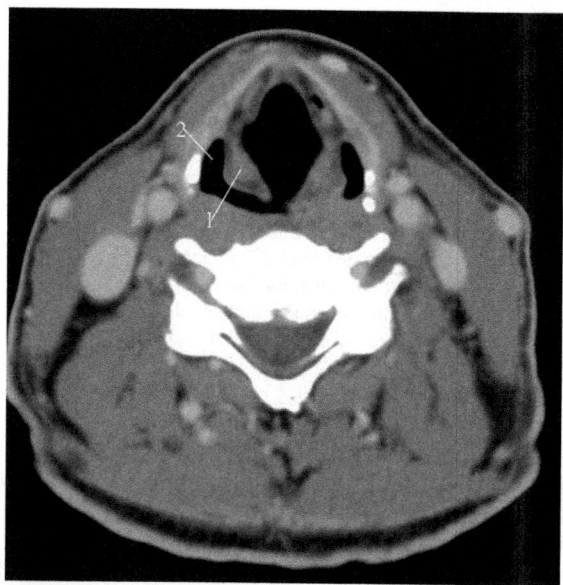

• **Fig. 2.63** Aryepiglottic fold and pyriform sinus. Axial computed tomography (CT) at the level of hypopharynx. *1*, Aryepiglottic fold; *2*, air-containing pyriform sinus.

the common carotid artery) to the root of the neck. In front of the right subclavian artery, the recurrent laryngeal nerve branches from the vagus nerve, loops around the right subclavian artery, and ascends to the side of the trachea behind the common carotid artery, in the tracheoesophageal groove. On the left side, the recurrent laryngeal nerve arises at the level of the aortic arch. It loops around the arch at the point where the ligamentum arteriosum is attached and ascends to the side of the trachea in the tracheoesophageal groove. The recurrent laryngeal nerve enters the larynx behind the cricothyroid joint and innervates all the muscles of the larynx except the cricothyroid muscle, which is an extrinsic muscle of the anterior larynx innervated by the external laryngeal branch of the superior laryngeal nerve, a branch of the vagus nerve in the neck. Sensory input from the laryngeal mucosa is via the internal laryngeal branch of the superior laryngeal nerve, which perforates the posterior lateral portion of the thyrohyoid membrane.[28]

The blood supply to the larynx is from branches of the external carotid artery: the superior and inferior laryngeal arteries. The superior laryngeal artery, a branch of the superior thyroid artery, travels with the internal branch of the superior laryngeal nerve. The inferior laryngeal artery, a branch of the inferior thyroid artery, which itself is a branch of the thyrocervical trunk, accompanies the recurrent laryngeal nerve into the larynx.[28]

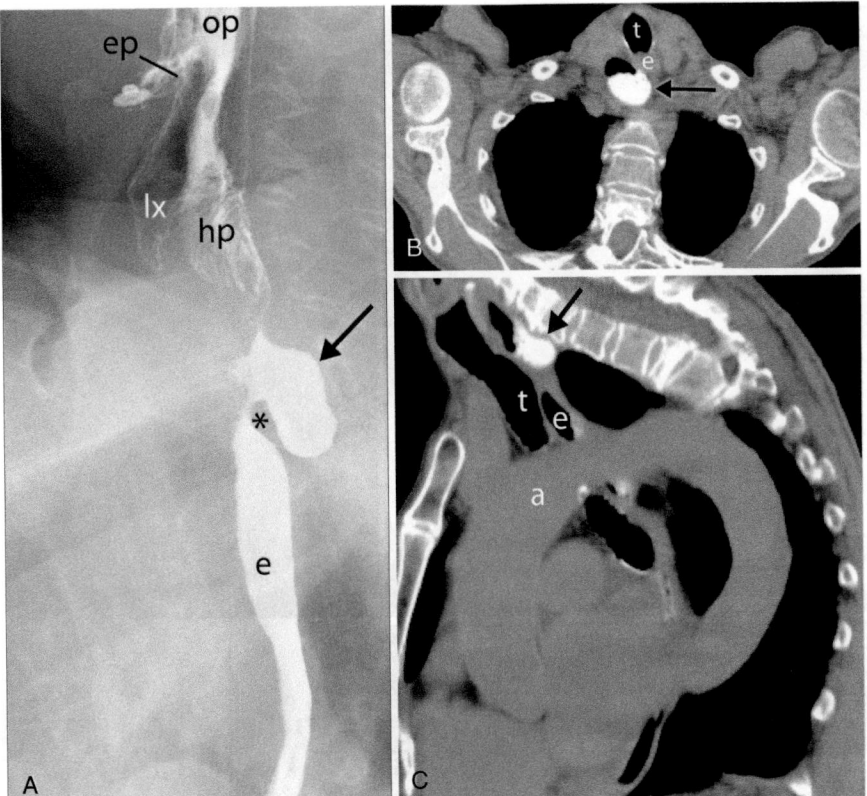

• **Fig. 2.64** Zenker's diverticulum. (A) Right anterior oblique radiograph from a barium esophagram demonstrating a posterior Zenker's diverticulum from the inferior hypopharynx at the pharyngoesophageal junction (*arrow*). Note posterior impression of the cricopharyngeus muscle just superior to diverticulum (*asterisk*). (B) Axial and (C) sagittal computed tomography (CT) images in a different patient demonstrating a posterior Zenker's diverticulum (arrow) in the tracheoesophageal groove containing air and trapped oral contrast from prior esophagram. *op*, oropharynx; *hp*, hypopharynx; *lx*, larynx; *e*, esophagus; *ep*, epiglottis; *t*, trachea; *a*, Aorta.

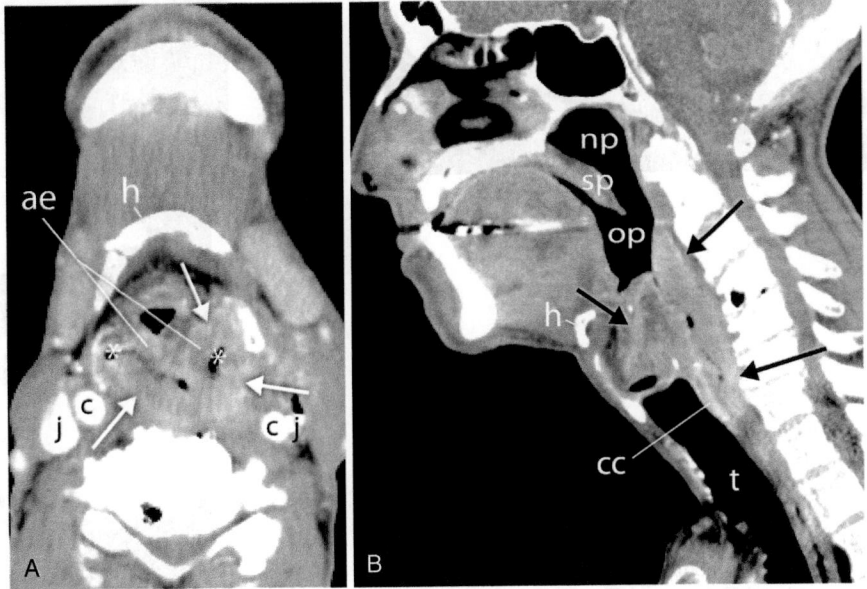

• **Fig. 2.65** Squamous cell carcinoma of the hypopharynx. (A) Axial computed tomography (CT) with contrast demonstrates an enhancing mass (*arrows*) involving bilateral pyriform sinuses and the posterior wall of the hypopharynx with deformity of the airway. There is partial effacement of the pyriform sinuses (*asterisk*). (B) Sagittal CT with contrast demonstrates craniocaudad extent of the mass (*arrows*) from the posterior wall of the oropharynx to the postcricoid hypopharynx. *h*, hyoid; *ae*, Aryepiglottic folds; *np*, nasopharynx; *op* oropharynx; *sp*, soft palate; *cc*, cricoid cartilage; *t*, trachea; *c*, carotid artery; *j*, internal jugular vein.

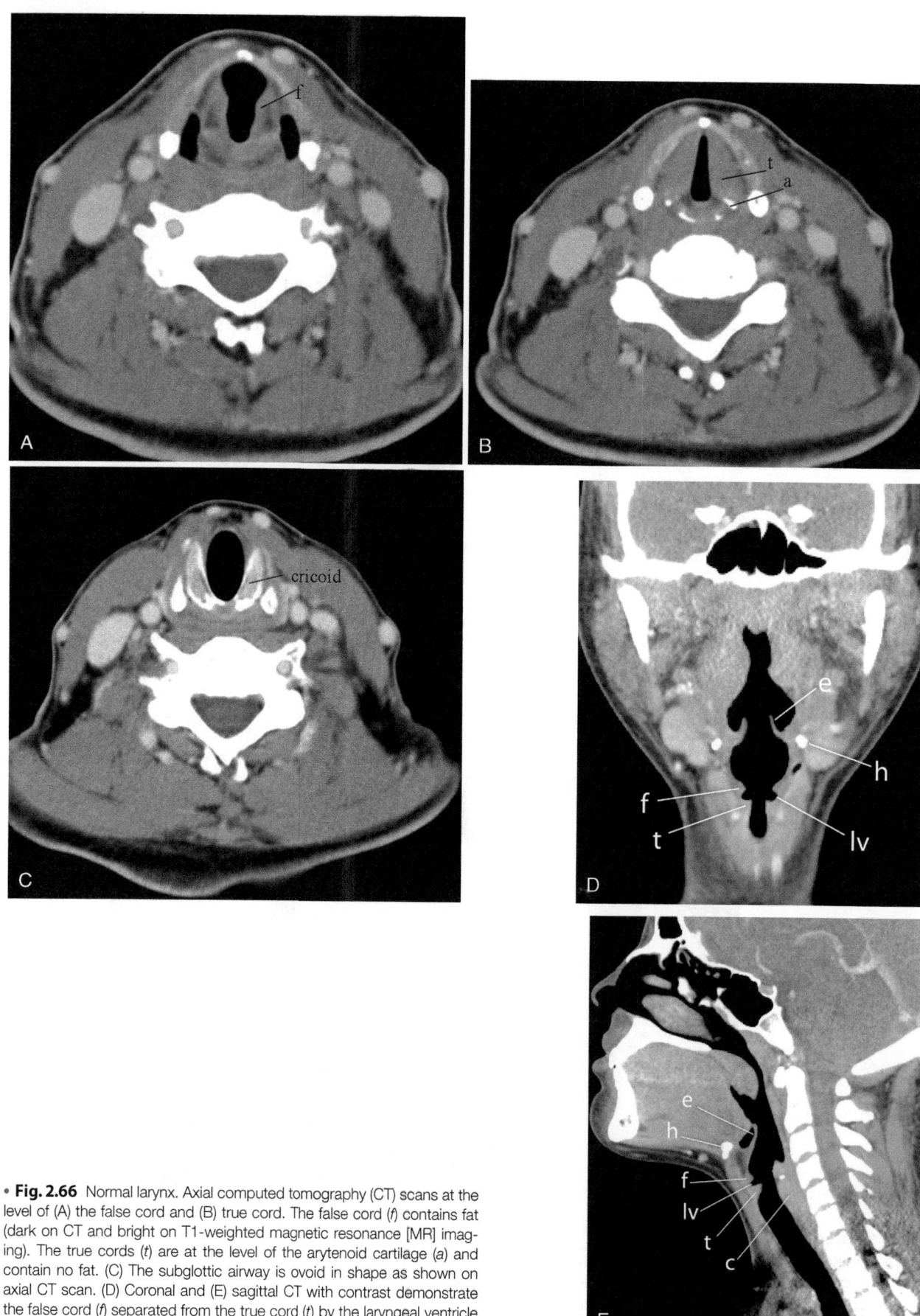

• **Fig. 2.66** Normal larynx. Axial computed tomography (CT) scans at the level of (A) the false cord and (B) true cord. The false cord (*f*) contains fat (dark on CT and bright on T1-weighted magnetic resonance [MR] imaging). The true cords (*t*) are at the level of the arytenoid cartilage (*a*) and contain no fat. (C) The subglottic airway is ovoid in shape as shown on axial CT scan. (D) Coronal and (E) sagittal CT with contrast demonstrate the false cord (*f*) separated from the true cord (*t*) by the laryngeal ventricle (*lv*). *e*, epiglottis; *c*, Cricoid cartilage.

Imaging Anatomy and Pertinent Pathology

Before CT and MRI, examination of the larynx included laryngography and multidirectional tomography. Soft-tissue film of the airway is a good survey study. Barium swallow, which is still in use today, provides dynamic evaluation of the swallowing mechanism.

CT and MRI allow visualization of structures deep to the mucosa (Fig. 2.66A–E); however, breathing and swallowing movements made early CT imaging of the larynx difficult. The faster CT scanning technology available today allows the entire neck to be scanned in a single breath-hold. Helical technology allows reformation of the airway in all three planes. MRI examination of the larynx has been inhibited by motion artifacts intrinsic and extrinsic to the larynx but has a greater ability than CT to separate out various soft tissue planes. Coronal and sagittal reformations from both CT and MRI studies are helpful in evaluating the spaces and mucosal folds. On a sagittal view, one can easily identify the hyoid bone, epiglottis, aryepiglottic folds, and vestibule, which is the space extending from the epiglottis to the level of the false vocal cords. At the level of the thyroid cartilage, a tiny slit of air is seen directed in the anterior-posterior direction. This is the laryngeal ventricle, which separates the false vocal cords from the true vocal cords (see Fig. 2.18). The vocal cords are not static structures, thus the difficulty in imaging. During normal respiration, the vocal cords are abducted, and the airway inlet has a triangular shape. With maximal abduction during deep inspiration, the opening of the glottis adopts more of a diamond shape. The airway opening is narrowed during expiration and phonation. Below the true vocal cords to the cricoid cartilage is the infraglottic cavity. The trachea begins below the level of the cricoid cartilage.

Between the cartilages and the mucosal surface lie the paraglottic and preepiglottic spaces, which contain loose connective tissue, lymphatics, and muscles. Superiorly, the larynx is suspended from the hyoid bone, which is attached to the styloid process at the base of the skull by the stylohyoid ligament. Calcification of the stylohyoid ligament (see Fig. 2.13) has been proposed as a cause of difficult intubation.[25] Muscles attached to the hyoid bone elevate the larynx and move it ventrally, providing the primary protection from aspiration.[56]

Several structures in the endoskeleton of the larynx are worth describing. The epiglottis is a yellow elastic fibrocartilage; the tip defines the cranial margin of the supraglottic larynx. It has a flattened teardrop or leaf shape that tapers to an inferior point called the petiole of the epiglottis, where it is attached to the thyroid cartilage by the thyroepiglottic ligament. The superior and lateral edges are free. Most of the epiglottis extends behind the thyroid cartilage, and the tip may be above the hyoid bone and can sometimes be seen through the oral cavity. It is held in place and stabilized by the hyoepiglottic and thyroepiglottic ligaments. The hyoepiglottic ligament is a tough, fibrous, fanlike ligament extending from the ventral midline of the epiglottis to the dorsal margin of the hyoid cartilage. Immediately above the ligament are the pharyngeal recesses, the valleculae, situated just caudal to the tongue base. The epiglottis helps to guard against aspiration; during swallowing, the aryepiglottic folds pull the sides of the epiglottis down, thereby narrowing the entrance to the larynx.[56]

Congenital Lesions

The respiratory system is formed from an outpouching of the primitive pharynx. The cells on each side of the entrance to the respiratory diverticulum become adherent and form the tracheoesophageal septum, separating the trachea from the primitive foregut. At one point in development, the laryngeal lumen is occluded and later recanalizes. The cartilages arise from the mesenchymal cells on either side of the respiratory tract, which then fuse in the midline to form the thyroid and cricoid cartilages. Congenital lesions are related to delays in the development and maturation of the respiratory system.[34]

Laryngomalacia represents a delay in the development of the laryngeal support system. The structures of the larynx are present but are not mature enough to keep the larynx open. The supraglottic larynx is affected, and the epiglottis may be floppy. As the cartilages mature, the problem resolves.

Webs can be seen at any level of the larynx, but they are usually at the level of the true vocal cords. Subglottic webs are sometimes associated with cricoid abnormalities. Atresia of the larynx results from an incomplete recanalization; there is no air passage to the trachea, which is present. Rarely, incomplete fusion of the tracheoesophageal septum results in a laryngotracheal cleft. A laryngeal cleft can occur in isolation, but often there is an associated tracheal cleft. Stenosis of the larynx or the upper trachea may be caused by a congenital anomaly or by a posttraumatic etiology. Subglottic stenosis is congenital soft-tissue stenosis from the true vocal cords down to the cricoid. This problem is usually outgrown, but sometimes a tracheostomy is needed. The most common cause of stenosis is prolonged intubation. Ingestion of caustic material can also result in strictures of the posterior supraglottic airway. Both plain film radiographic study and CT are good at assessing the extent and length of the stenotic segment.

Trauma

Fracture of the larynx, which usually results from a vehicular accident or blunt trauma to the neck, can involve the thyroid cartilage, cricoid cartilage, or both. Laryngotracheal separation is usually fatal. Dislocation of the arytenoids relative to the cricoid cartilage can be encountered. Malalignment of the thyroid cartilage and cricoid cartilage results in the dislocation of the cricothyroid joint. On imaging, the presence of air in the paraglottic soft tissues is an indication of laryngeal trauma (Fig. 2.67A and B).

Foreign bodies may be the result of trauma but are more commonly attributed to ingestion or aspiration. The pyriform sinus is a common location for a foreign body. If the foreign body enters the larynx, it usually passes through to the trachea or bronchi.

Burn injury to the larynx can result from the inhalation or ingestion of hot material. The supraglottic larynx is most likely to be involved, and generalized edema can occur.

Vocal Cord Paralysis

Vocal cord paralysis may be characterized as either a superior laryngeal nerve deficit, recurrent laryngeal nerve deficit, or total vagus nerve deficit. Imaging should address the entire course of the vagus nerve and the recurrent laryngeal nerve when assessing vocal cord paralysis (Fig. 2.68A–F).

The superior laryngeal nerve, through the external laryngeal branch, innervates only one muscle of the larynx—an extrinsic muscle: the cricothyroid muscle. This muscle extends between the thyroid and cricoid cartilages. As the muscle contracts, the anterior cricoid ring is pulled up toward the lower margin of the thyroid cartilage. This action rotates the upper cricoid lamina (and therefore the arytenoids) posteriorly and puts tension on the true vocal cords. If one side is paralyzed, contraction of one muscle rotates the posterior cricoid to the contralateral paralyzed side.

More commonly, however, vocal cord paralysis is attributed to recurrent laryngeal nerve pathology. All the laryngeal muscles, except for the cricothyroid muscle, are innervated by this nerve.

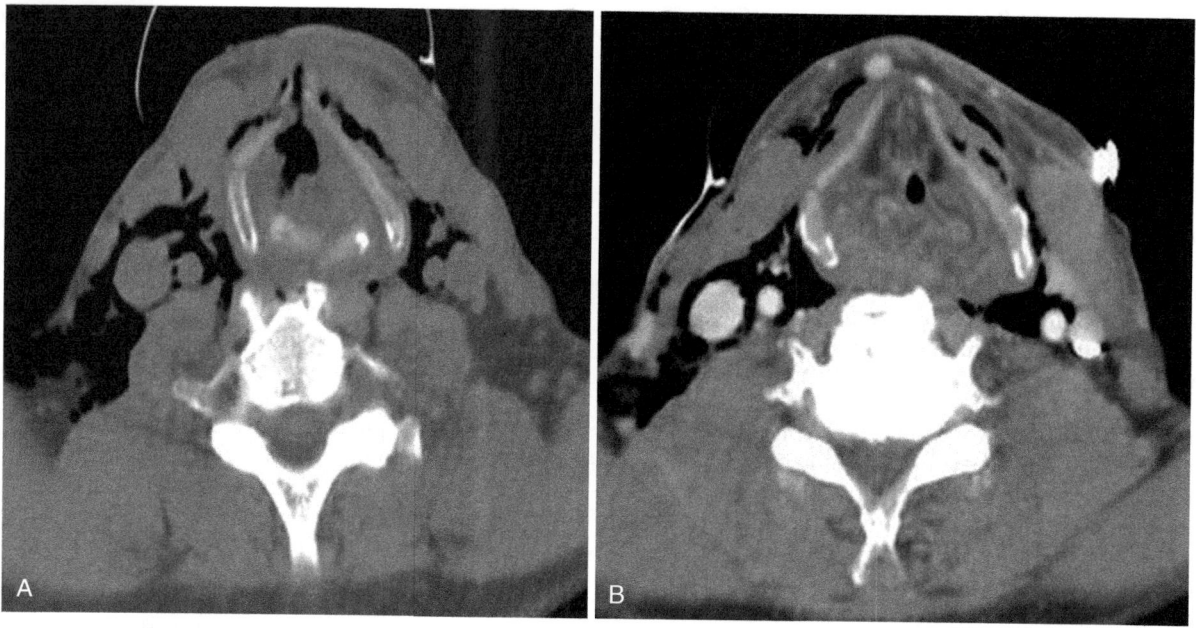

• **Fig. 2.67** Laryngeal fracture. (A) Precontrast and (B) postcontrast axial computed tomography (CT) scans show extensive deep fascial emphysema as well as multiple fractures of the thyroid and cricoid cartilages.

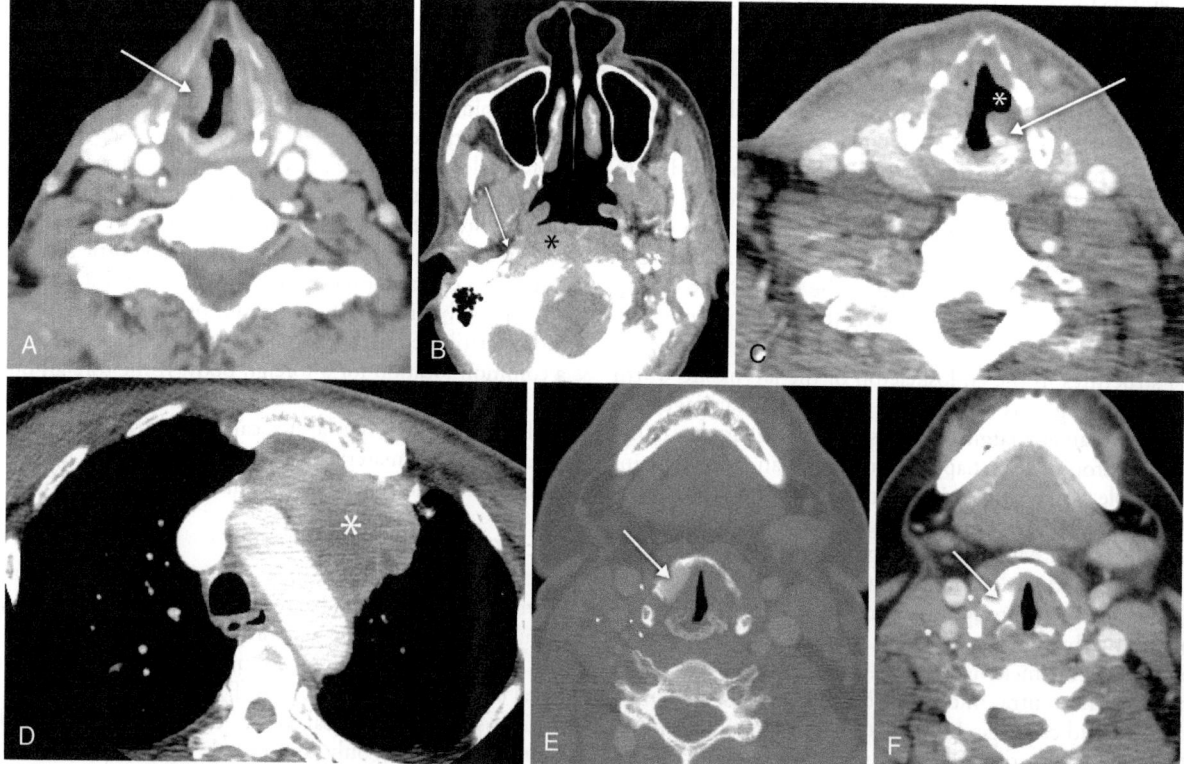

• **Fig. 2.68** Vocal cord paralysis in three patients. Patient 1: (A) Axial computed tomography (CT) scan with contrast demonstrates right vocal cord paralysis that is medially deviated with atrophy. (B) Axial CT scan with contrast demonstrates a skull base mass (*asterisk*) arising from the nasopharynx with involvement of the right carotid space (*arrow*) in the expected location of the right vagus nerve. Patient 2: (C) Axial CT scan with contrast demonstrates left vocal cord paralysis with medial rotation of the left arytenoid cartilage (*arrow*) and asymmetric prominence of the left laryngeal ventricle (*asterisk*). (D) Axial CT scan with contrast demonstrates a mass in the superior mediastinum involving the expected course of the left recurrent laryngeal nerve. Patient 3: Axial CT scan with contrast with (E) bone and (F) soft tissue reconstruction algorithm demonstrates right thyroplasty for treatment of vocal cord paralysis. There is a defect in the right tracheal cartilage with hyperdense implant material at the level of the left true vocal cord (*arrow*). The vocal cord has a normal anatomic position.

Most findings are secondary to atrophy of the thyroarytenoid muscle, the muscle that contributes to the bulk of the true vocal cords. The vocal cords become thinner and more pointed. Compensatory enlargement of the ventricle and the pyriform sinus is seen.[56] In the more acute phase, the paralyzed cord appears flaccid and prolapses medially because of the lack of muscular tone in the thyroarytenoid muscle and demonstrates a lack of movement during breathing maneuvers and phonation.

Tumors and Other Pathology

Most laryngeal tumors are malignant, and squamous cell carcinomas are the most common. These cancers arise on the mucosal surface and can be readily visualized by direct endoscopy. Imaging with CT and MRI is used to define the extent of the disease. Cross-sectional imaging is useful to assess the degree and direction of airway compromise (Fig. 2.69A–C). Other cell types found are adenocarcinoma, verrucous carcinoma, and anaplastic carcinoma. More rare tumors are sarcoma, melanoma, lymphoma, leukemia, plasmacytoma, fibrous histiocytoma, and metastatic disease.

Benign masses encountered in the larynx include vocal cord nodules, juvenile papillomatosis, and other nonepithelial tumors such as hemangiomas, lipomas, leiomyomas, rhabdomyomas, chondromas, neural tumors, paragangliomas, schwannomas, and granular cell tumors.

Mucus-retention cysts can occur along any mucosal surface, but they are most common in the supraglottic larynx. Laryngoceles may be internal, external, or both. The common finding in a supraglottic mass is its connection with the laryngeal ventricle (Fig. 2.70A–E).

Trachea

Development and Structure

The trachea is a tubular structure extending from the cricoid cartilage, at approximately the C6 level, to the carina, usually at the T5 or T6 level. It consists of 16 to 20 C-shaped cartilaginous rings that open posteriorly and are joined by fibroelastic tissue; the trachealis muscle forms the posterior wall of the trachea.

The trachea is approximately 10 to 15 cm in length. The diameter of the tracheal lumen is dependent on the height, age, and gender of the subject but is generally 10 to 25 mm in the coronal imaging plane and from 10 to 27 mm in the sagittal imaging plane in adults.

The innervation of the trachea is from the parasympathetic tracheal branches of the vagus nerve, the recurrent laryngeal nerve, and the sympathetic nerves. The trachea has a segmental blood supply from multiple branches of the inferior thyroidal arteries and bronchial arteries.

Imaging Anatomy and Pertinent Pathology

Radiologic evaluation of the trachea includes radiography of the neck and chest, CT, and MRI. A lateral view of the neck provides a good screening examination for the cervical trachea. CXR allows an initial assessment of the thoracic trachea and mediastinal structures. CT, and especially helical CT, is superior in the evaluation of the tracheal anatomy and pathology because it allows direct visualization of the cross-sectional trachea. With multiplanar reconstruction, the degree and length of stenosis can be fully assessed. Virtual bronchoscopy, which is a three-dimensional reconstruction of helical CT data, allows navigation through the tracheobronchial tree via simulated bronchoscopy. MRI so far has limited use owing to the longer scanning time, intrinsic breathing motion artifacts, and limited resolution.

Early detection of tracheal pathology is unusual because significant compromise of the airway can be present before symptoms manifest. At rest, more than 75% and, with exertion, more than 50% of the luminal diameter must be occluded before symptoms of airway obstruction are manifested.[57] When symptoms are present, a superior mediastinal mass is often found on chest radiograph. Also, the tracheal air column may be deviated or narrowed. Rarely, tracheal enlargement occurs because of tracheomalacia, cystic fibrosis, or Ehlers-Danlos syndrome. Pathology affecting the trachea can largely be classified as extrinsic or intrinsic processes.

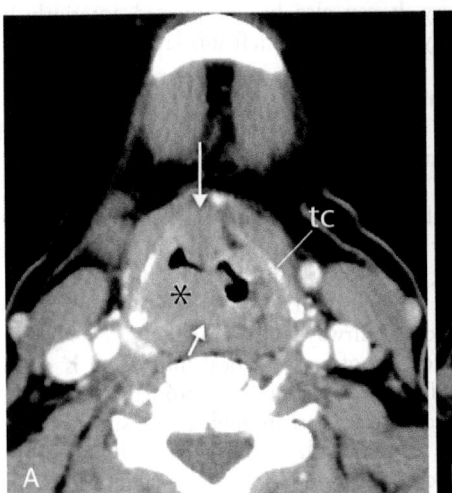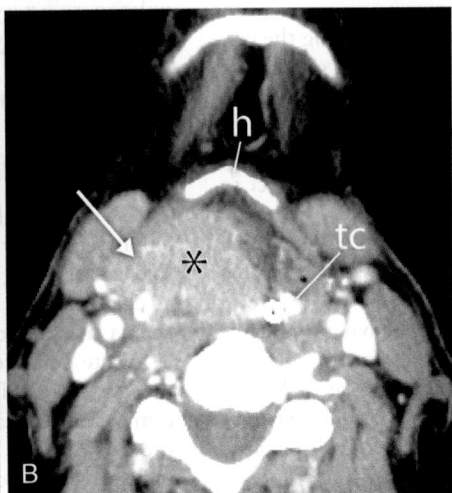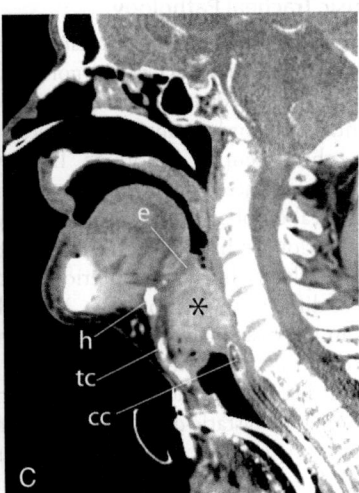

• **Fig. 2.69** Laryngeal carcinoma in two patients. Patient 1: (A) Axial computed tomography (CT) scan with contrast. Squamous cell carcinoma (*asterisk*) involving the right supraglottic larynx extending across the midline anteriorly and posteriorly (*arrows*) to the left with partial effacement of the airway. Patient 2: (B) Axial and (C) sagittal CT scans with contrast. Squamous cell carcinoma of the right supraglottic larynx with complete effacement of the airway. There is extension through the thyrohyoid membrane into the right neck soft tissue (*arrow* in B). Note presence of a nasogastric tube and tracheostomy. *e,* epiglottis; *h,* hyoid; *tc,* tracheal cartilage; *cc,* Cricoid cartilage.

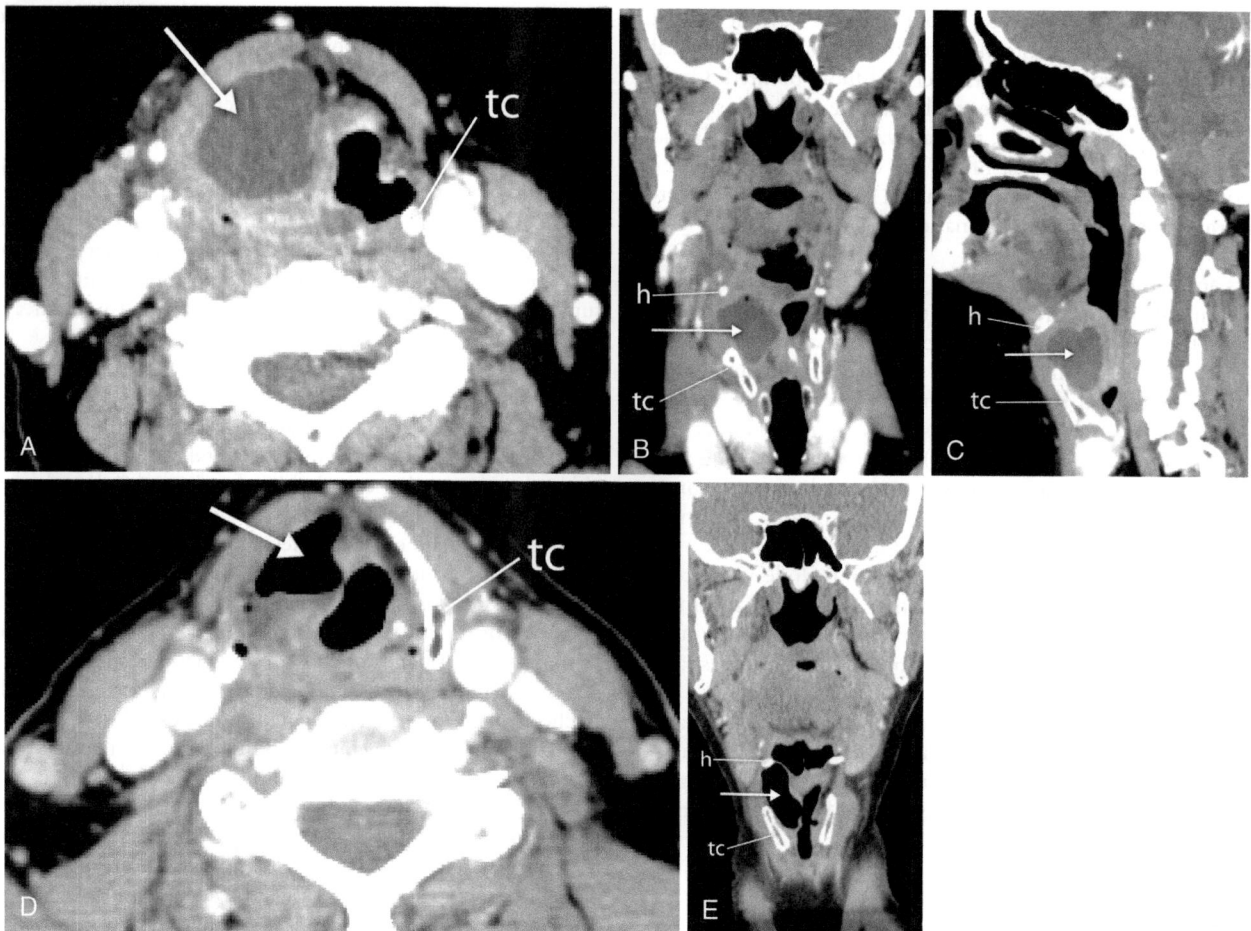

• **Fig. 2.70** Laryngocele. (A) Axial, (B) coronal, and (C) sagittal computed tomography (CT) scans with contrast demonstrate a fluid-filled internal laryngocele on the right (*arrow*) with displacement of the airway. (D) Follow-up axial and (E) coronal CT with contrast after fluid drainage demonstrates that the laryngocele is now air filled with decreased mass effect on the airway. *h*, hyoid; *tc*, thyroid cartilage.

Extrinsic Tracheal Pathology

One of the more common extrinsic pathologies affecting the cervical and substernal trachea is a goiter of the thyroid gland. The trachea is usually displaced laterally, and luminal compression is evident. Vocal cord paralysis, hoarseness, dyspnea, and dysphagia may be the presenting symptoms. These symptoms are all predictable and predicated on the location of the goiter with respect to the trachea, esophagus, and recurrent laryngeal nerve. The lateral and posterior extension of abnormal soft tissue with respect to the larynx displaces the airway anteriorly and laterally and may be a cause of difficult intubation (Fig. 2.71A–D).

As in the case of thyroid goiter, any mass involving or enlarging the thyroid gland can result in airway displacement and compression (Fig. 2.72A and B). Enlarged lymph nodes secondary to lymphoma, metastatic disease, or infection can also cause extrinsic compression anywhere along the aerodigestive tract, including the trachea (Fig. 2.73).

Vascular rings are congenital anomalies of the aorta and great vessels that encircle both the trachea and the esophagus, resulting in airway compression and dysphagia; the most common example is the double aortic arch. Vascular slings are noncircumferential vascular anomalies that may cause airway compromise. The trachea may be compressed posteriorly from a pulmonary artery sling, where the left pulmonary artery arises from the right pulmonary artery. It can also be compressed anteriorly by the innominate artery or an aberrant left subclavian artery.

Intrinsic Tracheal Pathology

Traumatic injury to the trachea is more frequently a result of blunt trauma than of penetrating trauma and is often associated with significant other injuries to the chest, cervical spine, and great vessels. Pneumothorax, pneumomediastinum, and subcutaneous emphysema may be the presenting signs, in addition to endotracheal bleeding and airway compromise. Internal injuries such as chemical and thermal injury to the airway result in mucosal edema and subsequent airway compromise.

A late complication of endotracheal intubation is stenosis at the site of the ETT cuff or tip or at the stoma site of a tracheostomy. Cuff-related trauma is attributable to pressure necrosis from the cuff pressure exceeding the capillary perfusion pressure. The incidence of this complication has decreased significantly with the introduction of the high-volume, low-pressure cuff, which is more pliable and can mold to the contours of the trachea. The blood supply to the anterior cartilages is more susceptible to pressure effects, and anterior tracheal scarring may occur. With increased pressure, the posterior membranous part of the trachea can also become affected, and the scarring becomes more circumferential. This type of injury is related to the position of the cuff and is seen

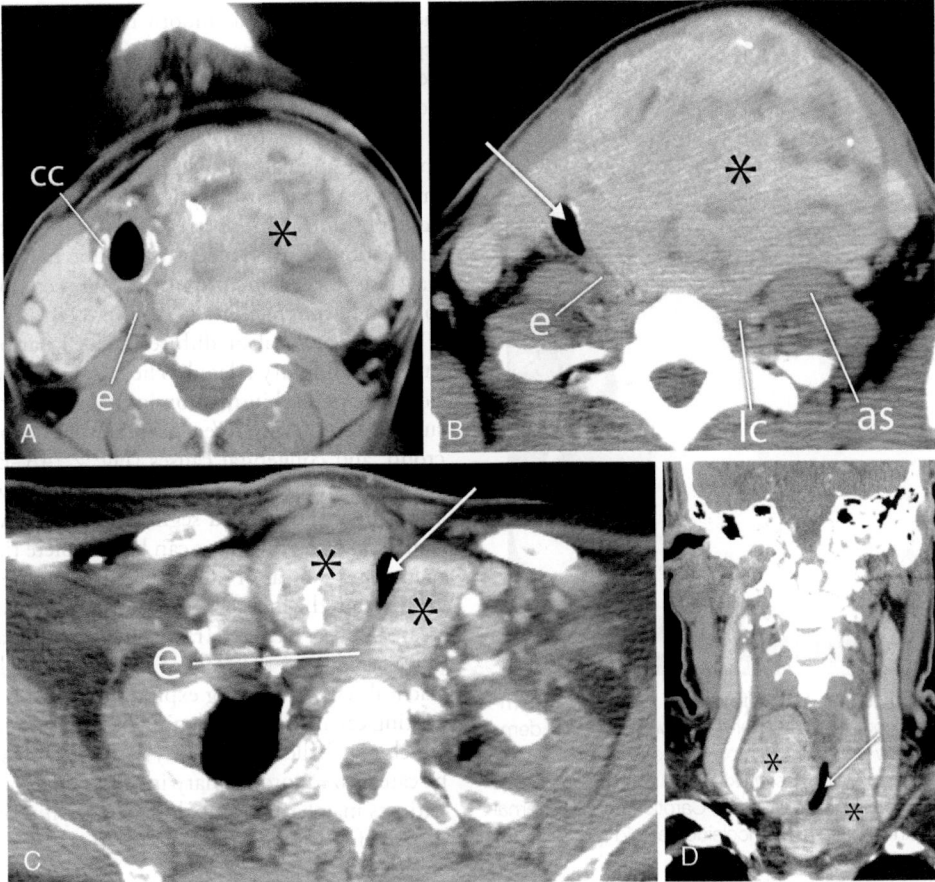

• **Fig. 2.71** Goiter in two patients. Patient 1: (A and B) Axial computed tomography (CT) scans with contrast demonstrate an enlarged heterogenous left thyroid lobe (*asterisk*). (A) At the level of the larynx, the cricoid cartilage (*cc*) is visible with displacement of the airway. (B) More inferiorly, there is displacement and narrowing of the trachea (*arrow*). Patient 2: (C) Axial and (D) coronal CTs with contrast demonstrate enlarged thyroid lobes (*asterisk*) with displacement and narrowing of the trachea (*arrows*). *as,* Anterior scalene muscle; *cc,* cricoid cartilage; *e,* esophagus; *lc,* left carotid.

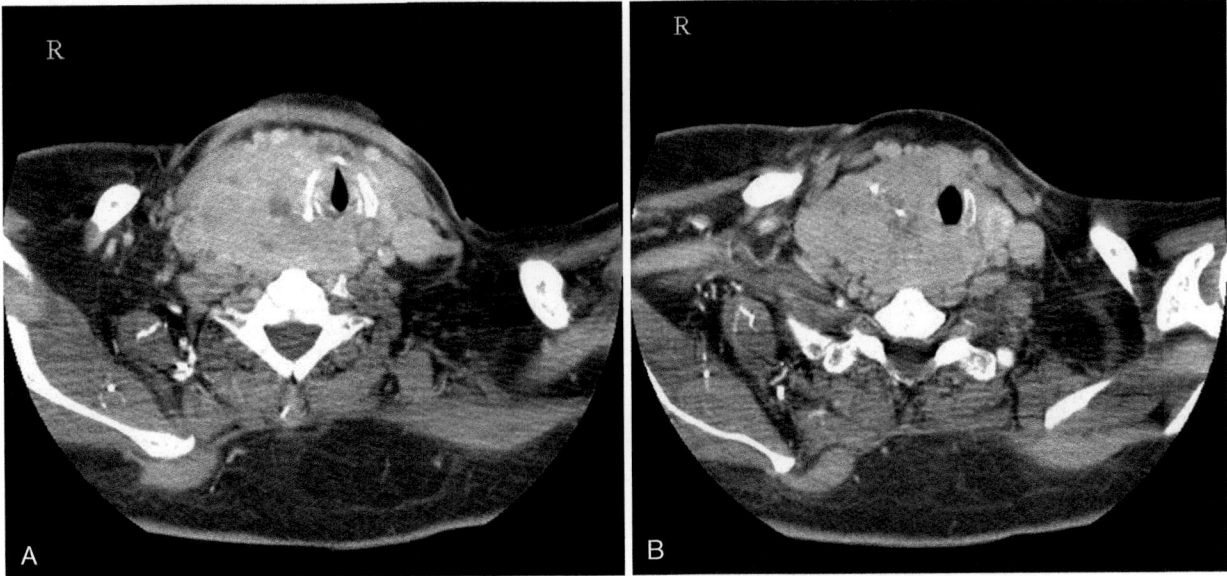

• **Fig. 2.72** Tracheal displacement and effacement. Axial computed tomography (CT) scans of a patient with medullary carcinoma of the thyroid. (A) CT scan demonstrates a right thyroid mass displacing the airway anteriorly and to the contralateral side. (B) The tumor has destroyed the cricoid cartilage on the right and abuts the subglottic airway. R, Right.

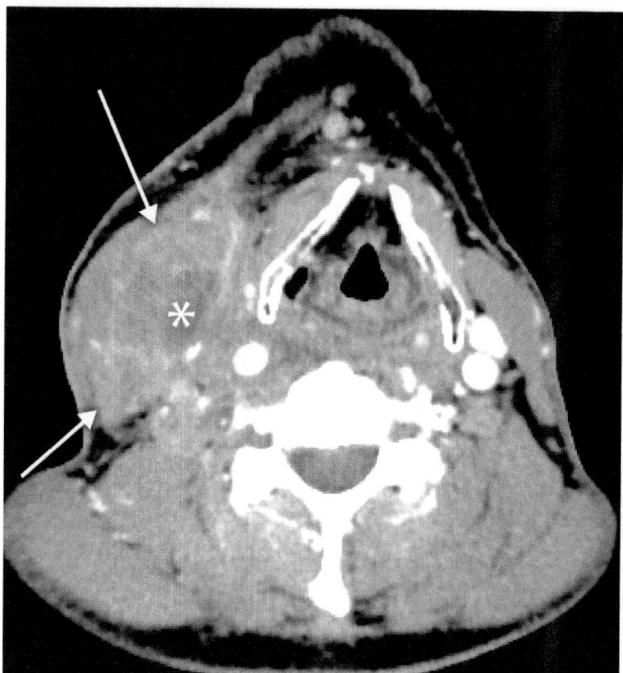

• **Fig. 2.73** *Mycobacterium tuberculosis* infection in an immune-compromised patient. Axial computed tomography (CT) with contrast demonstrates enlarged, irregularly enhancing lymph nodes in the right neck (*arrows*) with areas of central necrosis (*asterisk*). There is displacement of the airway at the level of the supraglottic larynx. *c,* Carotid artery; *ij,* internal jugular vein; *tc.* tracheal cartilage; *scm,* sternocleidomastoid muscle.

radiographically as a smooth tapering over one to two cartilage segments. Symptoms may arise 2 to several weeks after extubation. Less common long-term complications of endotracheal intubation include tracheomalacia and tracheoesophageal fistula.[13,58]

Early tracheostomy complications are usually related to an abnormal angulation of the tube. In contrast to translaryngeal intubation, tracheostomy is not affected by changes in head and neck position because it is not anchored at the nose or mouth. Angulation of the tracheostomy tube may result in increased airway resistance, difficulty in clearing secretions, erosion, and perforation of the trachea.

Causes of focal or diffuse tracheal narrowing, in addition to inhalational injury related to heat, caustic or acid chemicals, radiation therapy, and intubation injury, would include unusual causes such as sarcoidosis, Wegener's granulomatosis, fungal infection, croup, and congenital causes (Fig. 2.74A–E). Congenital stenosis is uncommon and is usually associated with other congenital anomalies. The affected segment has rigid walls with a narrowed lumen, and the cartilages can be complete rings. The stenotic segment can be focal or affect the entire trachea. Symptoms usually arise within the first few weeks or months of age. Most patients are treated conservatively. Tracheomalacia is characterized by abnormal flaccidity of the trachea resulting in collapse of the thoracic tracheal segment during expiration. There is softening of the supporting cartilage and widening of the posterior membranous wall, which may balloon anteriorly into the airway. Tracheomalacia can be categorized into primary intrinsic or secondary extrinsic forms. Patients may have minimal or severe symptoms dependent on the degree of airway obstruction.

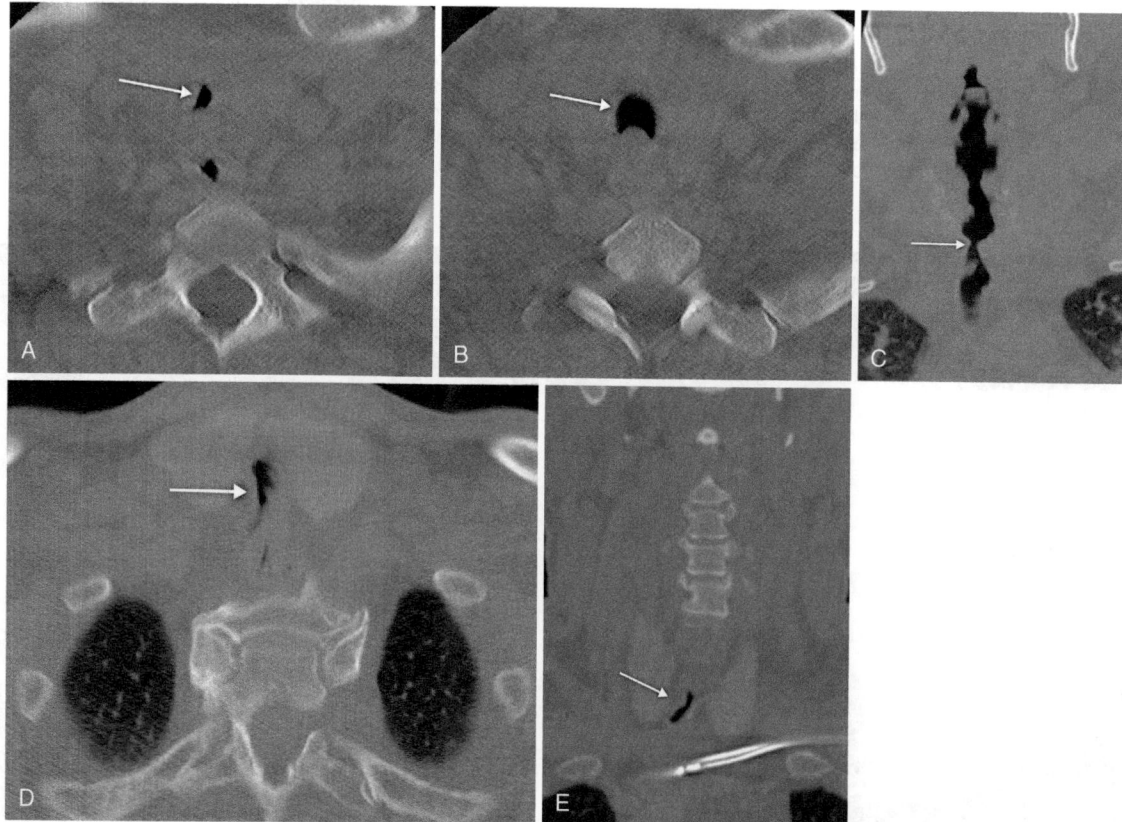

• **Fig. 2.74** Tracheal stenosis in two patients. Patient 1: (A) Axial computed tomography (CT) image in a patient with a history of prolonged intubation demonstrates focal subglottic narrowing of the proximal trachea (*arrow*). (B) Axial CT image just below the stenosis demonstrates normal caliber of the trachea (*arrow*). (C) Focal stenosis is well appreciated on coronal reformatted CT images (*arrow*). Patient 2: (D) Axial and (E) coronal CT images demonstrate another example of focal subglottic narrowing after prolonged intubation.

Tracheoesophageal fistula is a common congenital anomaly, with an incidence of 1 in 3000 to 4000 births. It is often associated with esophageal atresia.[13,58] There are several forms of tracheoesophageal fistula. The most common is a proximal esophageal atresia with a distal tracheoesophageal fistula. This anomaly may be associated with severe neonatal respiratory distress and may require emergent tracheostomy. It is not uncommon to have more than one fistula present, and there may be other associated anomalies affecting the cardiovascular, gastrointestinal, renal, or central nervous systems (Fig. 2.75A and B). Most benign tracheal neoplasms are found in pediatric patients.

Squamous cell papilloma, fibroma, and hemangioma are the most common. In adults, the most common benign tumors are chondroma, papilloma, fibroma, hemangioma, and granular cell myoblastoma. Primary malignant neoplasms of the trachea are rare; laryngeal and bronchial primary tumors are much more common. In adults, however, primary neoplasms of the trachea are more common than benign tumors. The most common malignant tumor is squamous cell carcinoma.[57] The trachea may be secondarily involved by metastatic disease, either from a remote primary tumor or by direct invasion, such as from a thyroid primary (Fig. 2.76A–C).

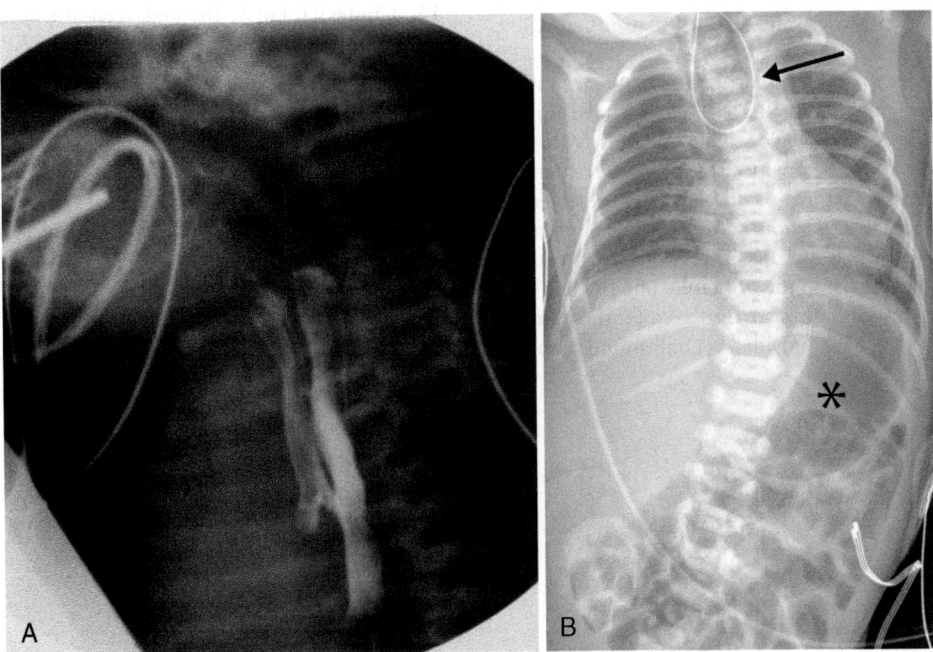

• **Fig. 2.75** Tracheoesophageal fistula (TEF). (A) Oblique radiograph from a swallow study with contrast outlines a classical H-type TEF (Courtesy Dr. Netta Marlyn Blitman, Montefiore Medical Center, Bronx, NY). (B) Posteroanterior radiograph of a different child demonstrates classic findings. A nasogastric tube cannot be passed due to esophageal atresia and is coiled in the midcervical esophagus (*arrow*). However, gas is present in the stomach (*asterisk*) and bowels due to a distal TEF.

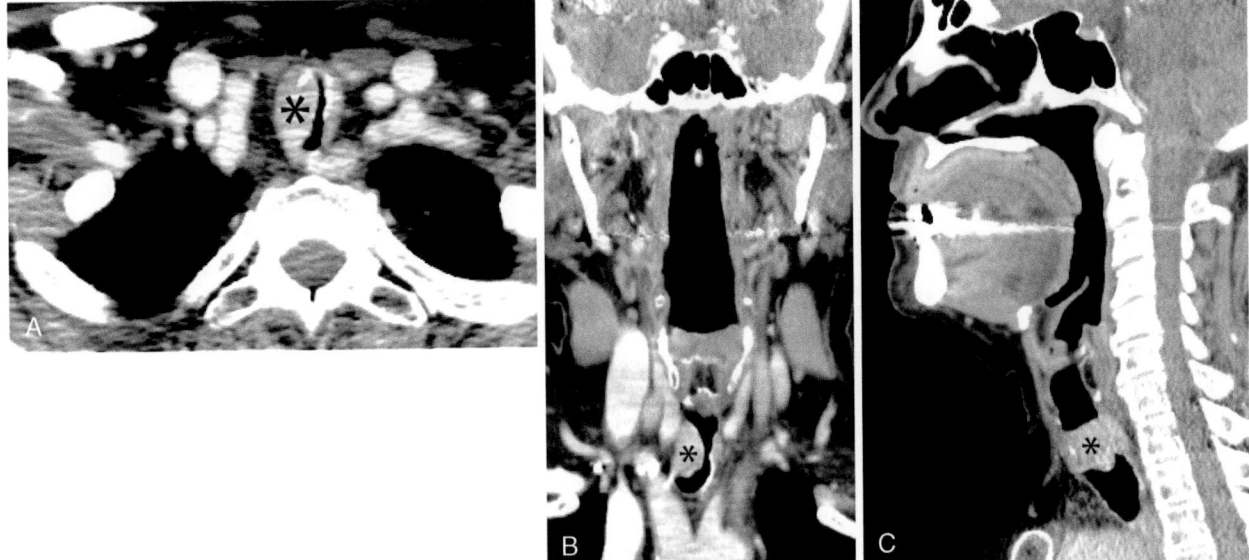

• **Fig. 2.76** Tracheal invasion from thyroid carcinoma. (A) Axial, (B) coronal, and (C) sagittal computed tomography (CT) scans demonstrating a right thyroid mass (*asterisk*) deviating and narrowing the trachea.

Conclusion

Rapid technological advances in the field of radiology allow excellent visualization of airway structures and provide anesthesiologists with essential information to formulate a safe and effective anesthetic plan. The imaging library of each patient is often replete with studies providing gratuitous information of the airway that an anesthesiologist can use in preoperative assessment and anesthetic planning. The airway, in its entirety from the nares to the bronchi, is readily seen on cervical spine and chest radiographs. In addition to cross-sectional images of the upper airway, the scout image or topogram from cross-sectional imaging of the brain, neck, or spine also provides valuable information regarding the airway.

Because radiology is not a part of the curriculum of most anesthesia residency training programs, most anesthesiologists have limited exposure to interpretation of radiologic studies, such as MRI and CT, which are usually a part of the preoperative surgical evaluation. Knowing basic radiographic anatomy of the airway as presented in this chapter allows maximal utilization of the available information to enhance one's anesthetic practice and to improve patient care overall. By updating readers on the principles of MRI and CT and illustrating how airway structures are displayed by these imaging modalities, we hope we have provided a good foundation for gathering clinically useful information from these imaging studies. In addition, we hope that clinicians will incorporate the information from radiologic studies to provide better care to their patients while also considering use of new imaging modalities as powerful research tools for studying the airway.

Selected References

6. Bushberg JT, Boone JM. *Radiography.* 3rd ed. Lippincott Williams & Wilkins; 2012.
9. Hounsfield GN. Computerized transverse axial scanning (tomography): part 1. Description of system. *Br J Radiol.* 1973;46(552):1016-1022.
13. Crosby ET, Lui A. The adult cervical spine: implications for airway management. *Can J Anaesthesia.* 1990;37(1):77-93.
17. Nichol H, Zuck D. Difficult laryngoscopy—the "anterior" larynx and the atlanto-occipital gap. *Br J Anaesthesia.* 1983;55(2):141-144.
20. White A, Kander P. Anatomical factors in difficult direct laryngoscopy. *Br J Anaesthesia.* 1975;47(4):468-474.
33. Bishop MJ, Weymuller EA Jr, Fink BR. Laryngeal effects of prolonged intubation. *Anesth Analg.* 1984;63(3):335-342.
46. Frei FJ, Ummenhofer W. Difficult intubation in paediatrics. *Paediatr Anaesth.* 1996;6(4):251-263.
58. Calder I, Calder J, Crockard H. Difficult direct laryngoscopy in patients with cervical spine disease. *Anaesthesia.* 1995;50(9):756-763.

All references can be found online at eBooks.Health.Elsevier.com.

3

Ultrasonography in Airway Management

MICHAEL SELTZ KRISTENSEN AND WENDY H. TEOH

CHAPTER OUTLINE

KEY POINTS

- Ultrasonography (USG) has many advantages for imaging the airway: It is safe, quick, repeatable, portable, widely available, and gives real-time dynamic images.
- The cricothyroid membrane (CTM) can easily be identified by USG prior to management of a difficult airway, and this technique should be applied if there is uncertainty about the ability to identify it with inspection or palpation methods.
- USG must be used dynamically for maximum benefit and in direct conjunction with airway management (immediately before, during, and after airway interventions).
- Direct observation can be made of whether an endotracheal tube (ETT) is entering the trachea or the esophagus by placing

the ultrasound probe transversely on the neck at the level of the suprasternal notch during intubation; in this way, intubation can be confirmed without the need for ventilation or circulation. Ventilation can be confirmed by observing the lung sliding bilaterally.
- USG should be the first-choice diagnostic approach when a pneumothorax is suspected intraoperatively or during initial trauma evaluation.
- Prandial status can be estimated by determining if the stomach is empty or if it contains fluid or solids and quantifying the amount of gastric fluid.

- Percutaneous dilatational tracheostomy (PDT) can be improved by using USG for identifying the correct tracheal-ring interspace, avoiding blood vessels, and determining the depth from the skin to the tracheal wall.

- Numerous conditions that affect airway management can be diagnosed by preanesthetic USG, but it remains to be determined in which patients the predictive value of such an examination is high enough to recommend USG as a routine approach to airway management planning.

Introduction

Ultrasonography (USG) is becoming an established tool in the hands of physicians[1] for the acute and elective care of patients' airways,[1-3] and its use can now be considered fundamental[4] in management of the difficult airway (DA).[1,5] USG has many potential advantages: It is safe, quick, repeatable, portable, widely available, and gives real-time dynamic images. USG must be used dynamically in direct conjunction with airway procedures for maximum benefit in airway management. For example, if the transducer is placed on the neck, the endotracheal tube (ETT) can be visualized passing into the trachea or the esophagus while it is being placed, whereas the location of the ETT is difficult to visualize if the transducer is placed on the neck of a patient who already has an ETT in place.

The Ultrasound Image and How to Obtain It

Ultrasound refers to sound frequencies beyond 20,000 Hz; frequencies from 2 to 15 MHz are typically used for medical imaging. Ultrasound transducers act as both transmitters and receivers of reflected sound. Tissues exhibit differing acoustic impedance values, and sound reflection occurs at the interfaces between different types of tissues. The impedance difference is greatest at interfaces of soft tissue with bone or air. Some tissues give a strong echo (e.g., fat, bone); these are called *hyperechoic* structures, and they appear white. Other tissues let the ultrasound beam pass easily (e.g., fluid collections, blood in vessels) and, therefore, create only a weak echo; these are *hypoechoic* structures and appear black on the screen. When the ultrasound beam reaches the surface of a bone, a strong echo (i.e., a strong white line) appears, and there is a strong absorption of ultrasound, resulting in depiction of only a limited depth of the bony tissue. Nothing is seen beyond the bone because of acoustic shadowing. Cartilaginous structures, such as the thyroid cartilage, the cricoid cartilage, and the tracheal rings, appear homogeneously hypoechoic (black), but the cartilages tend to calcify with age.[6]

Muscles and connective tissue membranes are hypoechoic but have a more heterogeneous, striated appearance than cartilage. Glandular structures, such as the submandibular and thyroid glands, are homogeneous and are mildly to strongly hyperechoic, in comparison with adjacent soft tissues. Air is a very weak conductor of ultrasound, so when the ultrasound beam reaches a border between tissue and air, a strong reflection (strong white line) appears, and everything on the screen beyond that point represents artifacts, particularly reverberation artifacts, which create multiple parallel white lines on the screen. However, the artifacts that arise from the pleura/lung border often reveal useful information. Visualization of structures, such as the posterior pharynx, posterior commissure, and posterior wall of the trachea, is prevented by intraluminal air.[6]

In B-mode (B = brightness) USG, an array of transducers simultaneously scan a plane through the body that can be viewed as a two-dimensional image on the screen, depicting a "slice" of tissue. In M-mode (M = motion) USG, a rapid sequence of B-mode scans representing one single line through the tissue is obtained. The images follow each other in sequence on the screen, enabling the sonographer to see and measure range of motion as the organ boundaries that produce reflections move relative to the probe. In color Doppler USG, velocity information is presented as a color-coded overlay on top of a B-mode image.

The higher the frequency of the ultrasound wave, the higher the resulting image resolution and the less the penetration in depth.

All modern ultrasound transducers used in airway management have a range of frequencies that can be adjusted during scanning to optimize the image. The linear high-frequency transducer (Fig. 3.1) is the most suitable for imaging superficial airway structures (within 2 to 3 cm from the skin). The curved low-frequency transducer is most suitable for obtaining sagittal and parasagittal views of structures in the submandibular and supraglottic regions,

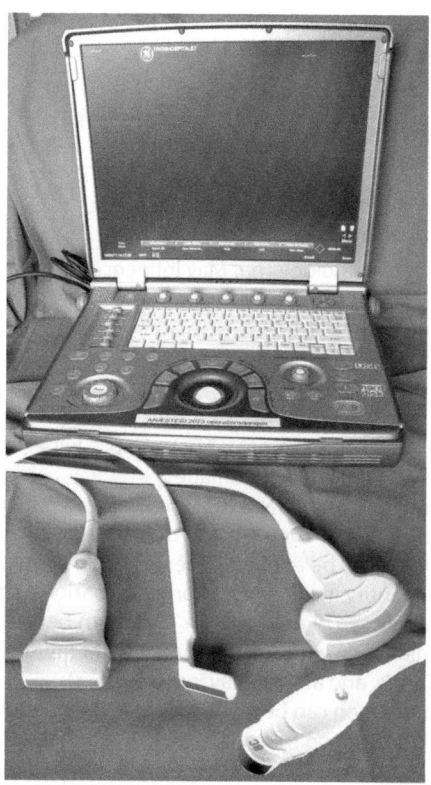

• **Fig. 3.1** Laptop-size ultrasound machine with transducers *(left to right)*: linear 7- to 12-MHz high-frequency transducer; small linear 6- to 10-MHz high-frequency "hockey-stick" transducer; curved, convex 2- to 6-MHz low-frequency transducer; micro convex 4- to 10-MHz transducer *(foreground)*. (From Kristensen MS. Ultrasonography in the management of the airway. *Acta Anaesthesiol Scand*. 2011;55:1155–1173.)

mainly because of its wider field of view. The microconvex transducer gives a wide view of the pleura between two ribs. If only one transducer must be chosen, a linear high-frequency transducer enables the performance of most ultrasound examinations that are relevant to airway management. Portable machines can provide accurate answers to basic questions and are sufficient for airway USG.[7]

Because air does not conduct ultrasound, the probe must be in full contact with the skin or mucosa without any interfacing air.[8] This is achieved by applying judicious amounts of conductive gel between the probe and the skin. Because of the prominence of the thyroid cartilage, it is sometimes a challenge to avoid air under the probe when performing a sagittal midline scan from the hyoid bone to the suprasternal notch in a male patient.

Visualizing the Airway and the Adjacent Structures

With conventional transcutaneous USG, the airway can be visualized from the tip of the chin to the midtrachea, along with the pleural aspect of the most peripheral alveoli and the diaphragm. Additional parts of the airway can be seen with special techniques: The trachea can be seen from the esophagus when performing transesophageal USG, and the tissue surrounding the more distal airway from the midtrachea to the bronchi can be visualized with endoscopic USG via a bronchoscope. These special techniques are not covered in detail in this chapter.

Mouth and Tongue

USG is a simple method for examination of the mouth and its contents. The tongue is composed of an anterior mobile part situated in the oral cavity and a fixed pharyngeal portion. The lingual musculature is divided into the extrinsic muscles, which have a bony insertion and alter the position of the tongue, and intrinsic muscles, whose fibers alter the shape of the tongue.[9] The tongue can be visualized from within the mouth, but the image may be difficult to interpret.[10,11]

The floor of the mouth and the tongue are easily visualized by placing the transducer submentally. If the transducer is placed in the coronal plane, just posterior to the mentum and from there moved posteriorly until the hyoid bone is reached, one can perform a thorough evaluation of all the layers of the floor of the mouth, the muscles of the tongue, and any possible pathologic processes (Fig. 3.2). The scanning image will be flanked by the acoustic shadow of the mandible on each side. The dorsal lingual surface is clearly identified.[12] The width of the tongue base can be measured in a standardized way by locating the two lingual arteries with Doppler ultrasound and measuring the distance between these arteries, where they enter the tongue base at its lower lateral borders.[13] A longitudinal scan of the floor of the mouth and the tongue is obtained if the transducer is placed submentally in the sagittal plane. If a large convex transducer is used, the entire length of the floor of the mouth and the majority of the length of the tongue can be seen in one image (Fig. 3.3). The acoustic shadows from the symphysis of the mandible and from the hyoid bone form the anterior and posterior limits of this image. Detailed imaging of the function of the tongue, including bolus holding, lingual propulsion, lingual-palatal contact, tongue tip and dorsum motion, bolus clearance, and hyoid excursion, can be evaluated in this plane.[12]

When the tongue is in contact with the palate, the palate can be visualized; if there is no contact with the palate, the air at the dorsum of the tongue will make visualization of the palate impossible. An improved image is achievable if water is ingested and retained in the oral cavity. The water eliminates the air-tissue border and allows visualization of most of the oral cavity including the palate (Fig. 3.4), as well as a better differentiation of the hard palate from the soft palate.[9]

The tongue can be visualized in detail with the use of three-dimensional USG.[14] In a child, the major anatomic components of the tongue and mouth are covered by four scanning positions: the midline sagittal, the parasagittal, the anterior coronal, and the posterior coronal planes.[15] In the transverse midline plane just cranial to the hyoid bone, the tongue base and the floor of the mouth are seen. In the transverse (axial) plane in the midline, the lingual tonsils and the vallecula can be imaged. The vallecula is seen just below the hyoid bone, and when the probe is angled caudally, the preglottic and paraglottic spaces and the infrahyoid part of the epiglottis are seen.[16]

Oropharynx

Imaging of a part of the lateral border of the mid-oropharynx can be obtained by placing the transducer vertically with its upper

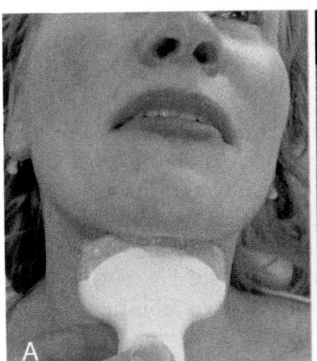
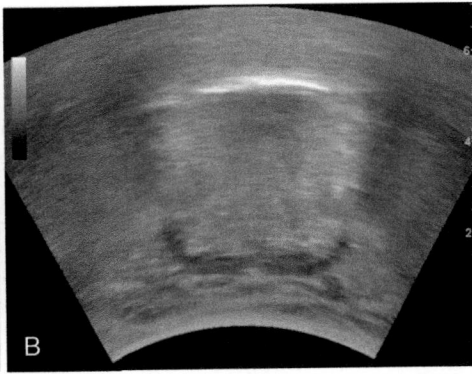
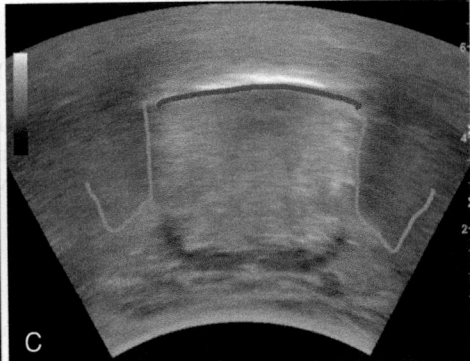

• **Fig. 3.2** Transverse scan of the floor of the mouth and the tongue. (A) Placement of the transducer. (B) The scanning image. (C) The dorsal surface of the tongue is indicated by a *red line*, and shadows arising from the mandible are outlined in *green*. (From Kristensen MS. Ultrasonography in the management of the airway. *Acta Anaesthesiol Scand.* 2011;55:1155–1173.)

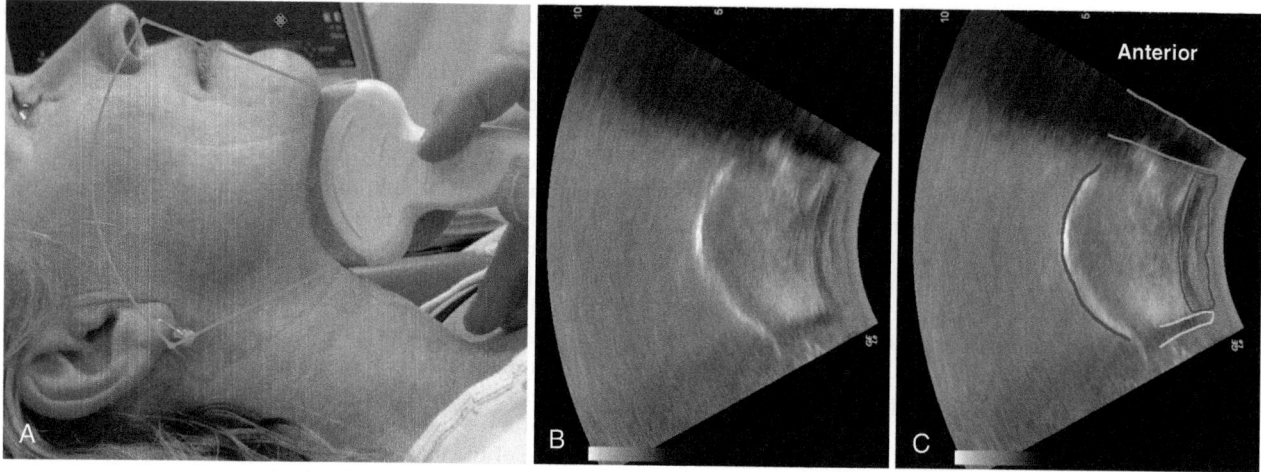

• **Fig. 3.3** Longitudinal scan of the floor of the mouth and the tongue. (A) Placement of the curved low-frequency transducer. The area covered by the scan is outlined in *light blue*. (B) The scanning image. (C) The shadow from the mentum of the mandible is outlined in *green*, the muscles in the floor of the mouth in *purple*, the shadow from the hyoid bone in *yellow*, and the dorsal surface of the tongue in *red*. (From Kristensen MS. Ultrasonography in the management of the airway. *Acta Anaesthesiol Scand.* 2011;55:1155–1173.)

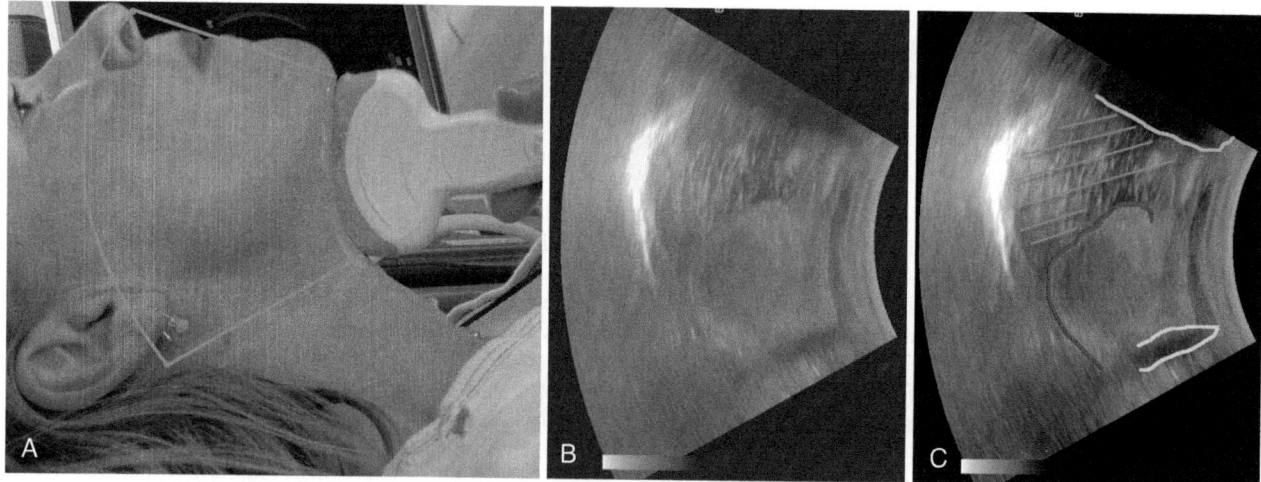

• **Fig. 3.4** The tongue and the mouth are filled with water. Placement of the transducer is the same as in Fig. 3.3. The shadow from the mentum of the mandible is outlined in *green*, the shadow from the hyoid bone in *yellow*, and the dorsal surface of the tongue in *red*. The *blue lines* indicate the water in the mouth. The *thick white line* represents the strong echo from the hard palate. (From Kristensen MS. Ultrasonography in the management of the airway. *Acta Anaesthesiol Scand.* 2011;55:1155–1173.)

edge approximately 1 cm below the external auditory canal.[12] The lateral pharyngeal border and the thickness of the lateral parapharyngeal wall can be determined.[17] The parapharyngeal space can also be visualized via the mouth by placing the probe directly over the mucosal lining of the lateral pharyngeal wall, but this approach is difficult for the patient to tolerate.[18]

Hypopharynx

By performing USG through the thyrohyoid membrane, cricothyroid space, cricothyroid membrane (CTM), thyroidal cartilage lamina, and along the posterior edge of the thyroid lamina, it is possible to locate and classify hypopharyngeal tumors with a success rate as high as that achieved with computed tomography (CT) scanning.[19]

Hyoid Bone

The hyoid bone is a key landmark that separates the upper airway into two scanning areas: the suprahyoid and infrahyoid regions. The hyoid bone is visible on the transverse view as a superficial, hyperechoic, inverted U–shaped, linear structure with posterior acoustic shadowing. On the sagittal and parasagittal views, the hyoid bone is visible in cross-section (see Fig. 3.4) as a narrow, hyperechoic, curved structure that casts an acoustic shadow.[6]

Larynx

Because of the superficial location of the larynx, USG offers images of higher resolution than CT or magnetic resonance imaging (MRI) when a linear high-frequency transducer is used.[16] The different parts of the laryngeal skeleton have different sonographic characteristics.[20] The hyoid bone is calcified early in life, and its bony shadow is an important landmark. The thyroid and cricoid cartilages show variable but progressive calcification throughout life, whereas the epiglottis stays hypoechoic. The true vocal cords overlie muscle that is hypoechoic, whereas the false cords contain hyperechoic fat.

The thyrohyoid membrane runs between the caudal border of the hyoid bone and the cephalad border of the thyroid cartilage and provides a sonographic window through which the epiglottis can be visualized in all subjects when the linear transducer is oriented in the transverse plane (with varying degrees of cephalad or caudad angulation).[6] The midline sagittal scan through the upper larynx from the hyoid bone cranially to the thyroid cartilage distally (Fig. 3.5) reveals the thyrohyoid ligament, the preepiglottic space containing echogenic fat, and, posterior to that, a white line representing the laryngeal surface of the epiglottis.[20] On parasagittal view, the epiglottis appears as a hypoechoic structure with a curvilinear shape; on transverse view, it is shaped like an inverted C. It is bordered anteriorly by the hyperechoic, triangular preepiglottic space and lined posteriorly by a hyperechoic air-mucosa interface.[21] In a convenience sample of 100 subjects, a transverse midline scan cranially to the thyroid cartilage depicted the epiglottis in all subjects and revealed an average epiglottis thickness of 2.39 mm.[22]

In the cricothyroid region, the probe can be angled cranially to assess the vocal cords and the arytenoid cartilages and, thereafter, moved distally to image the cricoid cartilages and the subglottis.[16] With transverse scanning in the paramedian position, the following structures can be visualized (starting cranially and moving distally): faucial tonsils, lateral tongue base, lateral vallecula, strap muscles, laminae of the thyroid cartilage, the lateral cricoid cartilage, and, posteriorly, the piriform sinuses and the cervical esophagus.[16]

The laryngeal cartilage is noncalcified in children, but calcification begins in some individuals before the age of 20 and increases with age. In subjects with noncalcified cartilage, the thyroid cartilage is visible on sagittal and parasagittal views as a linear, hypoechoic structure with a bright air-mucosa interface at its posterior surface. On the transverse view, it has an inverted V shape (Fig. 3.6), within which the true and false vocal cords are visible.[6] By 60 years of age, all individuals show signs of partial calcification, and approximately 40% of the cartilage at the level of the vocal cords is calcified.[22] The calcification is seen as a strong echo with posterior acoustic shadowing. Often the anatomic structures can be visualized despite the calcifications by angling the transducer.

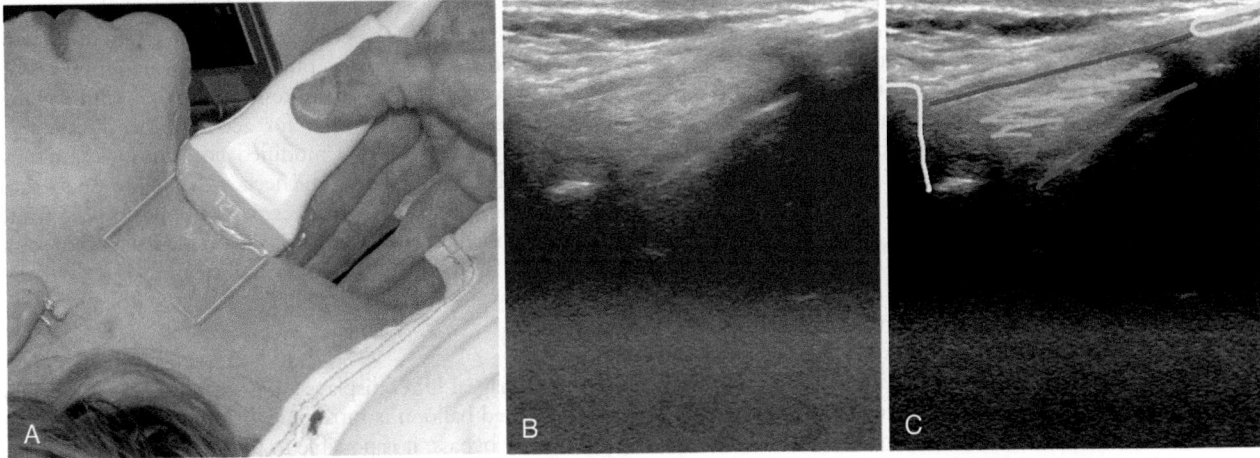

• **Fig. 3.5** Midline sagittal scan from the hyoid bone to the proximal part of the thyroid cartilage. (A) The *light blue outline* shows the area covered by the scan. (B) The scanning image. (C) The shadow from the hyoid bone is marked in *yellow*, the thyrohyoid membrane in *red*, the posterior surface of part of the epiglottis in *blue*, the preepiglottic fat in *orange*, and the thyroid cartilage in *green*. (From Kristensen MS. Ultrasonography in the management of the airway. *Acta Anaesthesiol Scand.* 2011;55:1155–1173.)

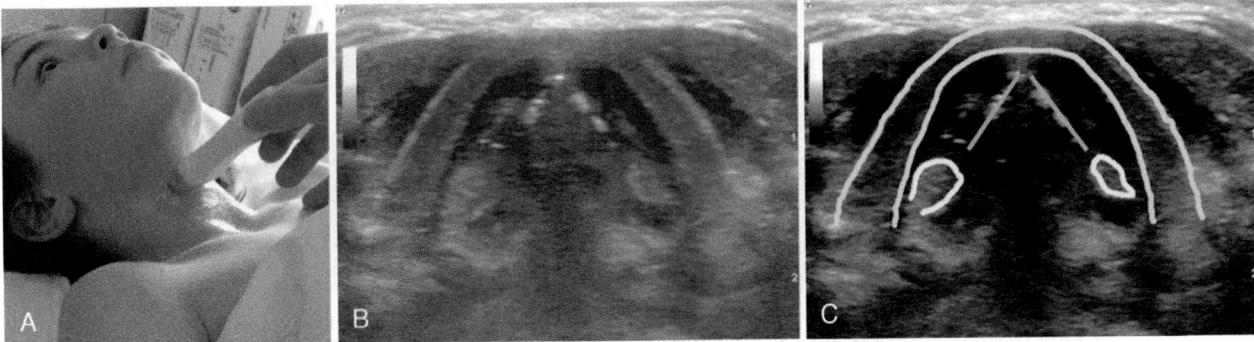

• **Fig. 3.6** Transverse midline scan over the thyroid cartilage in an 8-year-old boy. (A) Placement of the transducer. (B) The scanning image. (C) The thyroid cartilage is marked in *green*, the vocal cords in *orange*, the anterior commissure in *red*, and the arytenoid cartilages in *yellow*. (From Kristensen MS. Ultrasonography in the management of the airway. *Acta Anaesthesiol Scand.* 2011;55:1155–1173.)

In a population of patients who were examined due to suspicion of laryngeal pathology, sufficient visualization of the false cords was obtained in 60% of cases, of the vocal cords in 75%, of the anterior commissure in 64%, and of the arytenoid region in 71%; in 16% of cases, no endolaryngeal structures could be seen.[22]

Vocal Cords

In individuals with noncalcified thyroid cartilages, the false and the true vocal cords can be visualized through the thyroid cartilage.[20] In individuals with a calcified thyroid cartilage, the vocal cords and the arytenoid cartilages can still be seen by combining the scan obtained by placing the transducer just cranial to the superior thyroid notch while angling it caudally, with the scans obtained from the CTM in the midline and on each side with the transducer angled 30 degrees cranially.[16]

The true vocal cords appear as two triangular, hypoechoic structures (the vocalis muscles) outlined medially by the hyperechoic vocal ligaments (see Fig. 3.6). They are observed to oscillate and move toward the midline during phonation.[6] The false vocal cords lie parallel and cephalad to the true cords, are more hyperechoic in appearance, and remain relatively immobile during phonation.

In 24 volunteers with a mean age of 30 years, the thyroid cartilage provided the best window for imaging the vocal cords. In all participants, it was possible to visualize and distinguish the true and false vocal cords by moving the transducer in a cephalic-caudal direction over the thyroid cartilage.[6] In a study of 229 participants ranging in age from 2 months to 81 years, the true and false cords were visible in all female participants; in males, the visibility was 100% for those younger than 18 years and gradually decreased to less than 40% in males 60 years of age and older.[23]

Cricothyroid Membrane and Cricoid Cartilage

The CTM runs between the caudal border of the thyroid cartilage and the cephalad border of the cricoid cartilage. It is clearly seen on sagittal (Fig. 3.7) and parasagittal views as a hyperechoic band linking the hypoechoic thyroid and cricoid cartilages.[6] The cricoid cartilage has a round, hypoechoic appearance on the parasagittal view; on the transverse view, it has an archlike, inverted C-shape appearance with a posterior white lining.

Trachea

The location of the trachea in the midline of the neck makes it a useful reference point for transverse ultrasound imaging. The cricoid cartilage marks the superior limit of the trachea; it is thicker than the tracheal rings below and is seen as a hypoechoic, rounded structure. It serves as a reference point during performance of the sagittal midline scan (see Fig. 3.7). Often, the first six tracheal rings can be imaged when the neck is in mild extension.[18] The trachea is covered by skin, subcutaneous fat, the strap muscles, and, at the level of the second or third tracheal ring, the isthmus of the thyroid gland (see Fig. 3.7). The strap muscles appear hypoechoic and are encased by thin hyperechoic lines from the cervical fascia.[18] A high-riding innominate artery may be identified above the sternal notch as a transverse anechoic structure crossing the trachea.[15] The tracheal rings are hypoechoic, and they resemble a "string of beads" or "string of pearls" in the parasagittal and sagittal plane (see Fig. 3.7). In the transverse view, they resemble an inverted U, or horseshoe, highlighted by a hyperechoic air-mucosa interface with reverberation artifact posteriorly (Fig. 3.8).[6]

Esophagus

The cervical esophagus is most often visible posterolateral to the trachea on the patient's left side at the level of the suprasternal notch (see Fig. 3.8). The concentric muscle layers of the esophagus result in a characteristic "bull's-eye" appearance on USG. The esophagus can be seen to compress and expand with swallowing, and this feature can be used for accurate identification.[18] The patient may be placed in a modified position for examining the esophagus by slightly flexing the neck with a pillow under the head and turning the head 45 degrees to the opposite side while the neck is scanned on either side; this technique makes the esophagus visible also on the right side in 98% of cases.[24]

Lower Trachea and Bronchi

Transesophageal USG displays a part of the lower trachea. When a saline-filled balloon is introduced in the trachea during cardiopulmonary bypass, it is possible to perform USG through the trachea, thus displaying the proximal aortic arch and the innominate

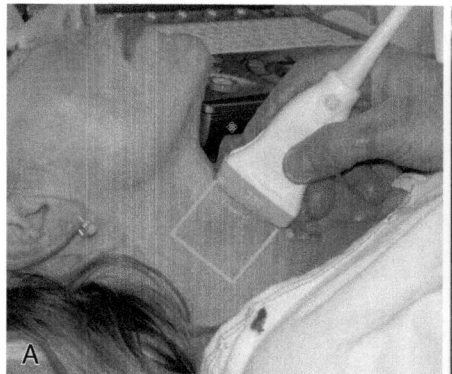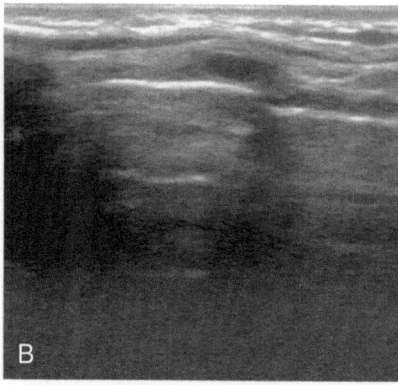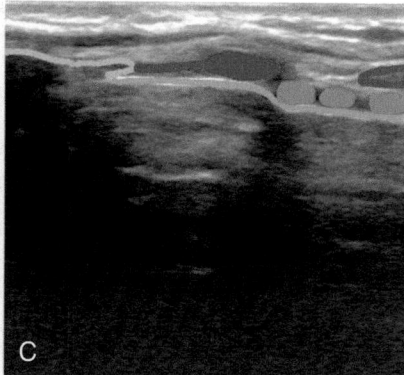

• **Fig. 3.7** Cricothyroid membrane (CTM). (A) The linear high-frequency transducer is placed in the midsagittal plane. The scanning area is marked with *light blue*. (B) The scanning image. (C) The thyroid cartilage is marked in *green*, the cricoid cartilage in *dark blue*, the tracheal rings in *light blue*, the CTM in *red*, the tissue-air border in *orange*, and the isthmus of the thyroid gland in *brown*. Below the *orange line*, only artifacts are seen. (From Kristensen MS. Ultrasonography in the management of the airway. *Acta Anaesthesiol Scand*. 2011;55:1155–1173.)

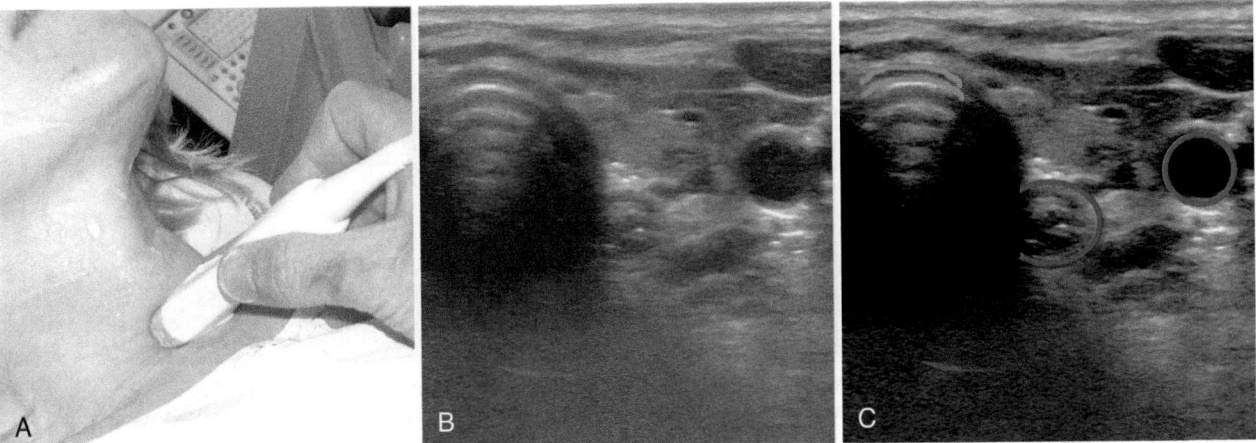

• **Fig. 3.8** Trachea and esophagus. (A) A transverse scan is performed just cranial to the suprasternal notch and to the left side of the patient's trachea. (B) The scanning image. (C) The anterior part of the tracheal cartilage is outlined in *light blue*, the esophagus in *purple*, and the carotid artery in *red*. (From Kristensen MS. Ultrasonography in the management of the airway. *Acta Anaesthesiol Scand.* 2011;55:1155–1173.)

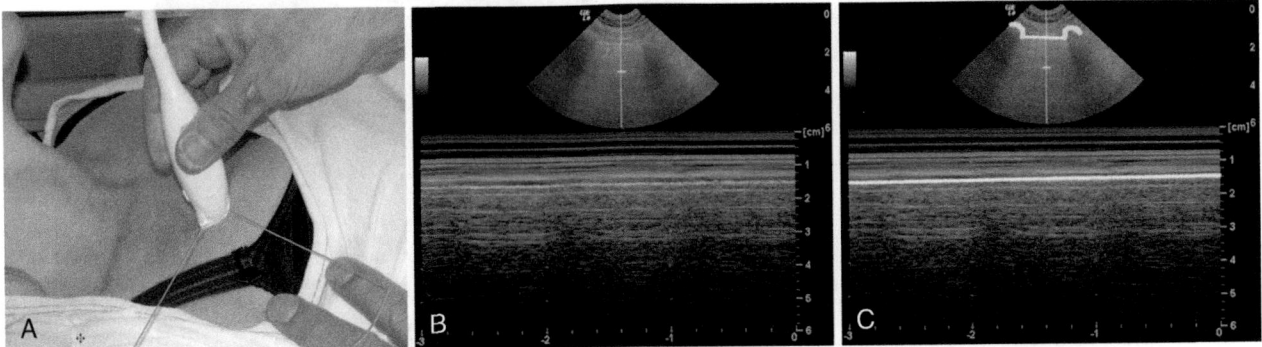

• **Fig. 3.9** Lung sliding. (A) A micro convex probe is placed over an interspace between two ribs during normal ventilation. The light blue line indicates the scanning area. (B) The scanning image, showing B-mode scanning above and M-mode scanning below. (C) The pleural line is marked in *yellow* and the ribs in *orange* (the curved lines at each end of the straight line). Notice that the outline of the ribs and the pleural line forms the image of a flying bat, the "bat sign." In the M-mode image, it is easy to distinguish the non-moving tissue above the pleural line from the artifact caused by respiratory movement of the visceral pleura relative to the parietal pleura. This is called the *seashore sign* or the *sandy beach sign* because the non-moving part resembles waves and the artifact pattern below resembles a sandy beach. (From Kristensen MS. Ultrasonography in the management of the airway. *Acta Anaesthesiol Scand.* 2011;55:1155–1173.)

artery.[25] The bronchial wall and its layers can be visualized from within the airway by passing a flexible ultrasound probe through the working channel of a flexible bronchoscope. This technique, called *endobronchial ultrasound*, reliably distinguishes between airway infiltration and compression by tumor.[26]

Peripheral Lung and Pleura

The ribs are identifiable by their acoustic shadow, and between two ribs a hyperechoic line is visible.[2] This line, called the *pleural line*, represents the interface between the soft tissue of the chest wall and air (Fig. 3.9). In a subject who is either breathing normally or mechanically ventilated, one can identify a to-and-fro movement synchronous with ventilation; this is called *pleural sliding* or *lung sliding*.[27] The movement is striking because the surrounding tissue is motionless.[28] Lung sliding is best seen dynamically, in real time or on video.[29]

Examination of lung sliding should always start by placing the transducer perpendicular to the ribs and in such a way that two rib shadows are identified.[2] The succession of the upper rib, pleural line, and lower rib outlines a characteristic pattern, the "bat sign" (see Fig. 3.9), which must be recognized to correctly identify the pleural line and avoid interpretation errors caused by parietal emphysema. Lung ultrasound examination should, therefore, be considered not feasible if the bat sign is not identified.[28] Lung sliding can be assessed using the time-motion (M) mode, which highlights a clear distinction between a wavelike pattern located above the pleural line and a sandlike pattern below, called the *seashore sign* (see Fig. 3.9).

In breath-holding or apnea, there is no lung sliding, but rather a "lung pulse"—small movements synchronous with the heartbeat (Fig. 3.10).[2] The lung pulse is attributed to the vibrations of the heart that are transmitted through a motionless lung. The lung pulse can also be demonstrated in M-mode scanning. There is a strong echo from the pleural line, and dominant reverberation artifacts of varying strength are seen. They appear as lines parallel to the pleural line and spaced with the same distance as the distance from the skin surface to the pleural line. These "A-lines" are

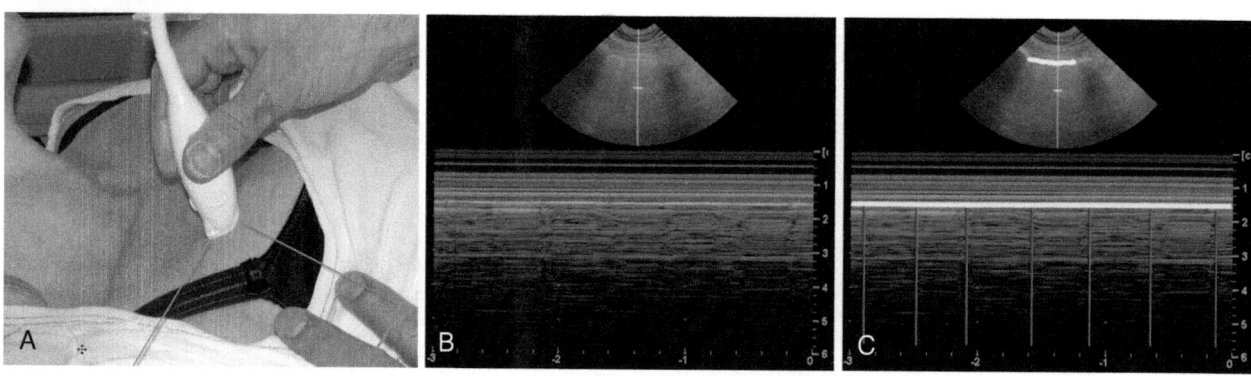

• **Fig. 3.10** Lung pulse. (A) Placement of the transducer. (B) The scanning image, showing B-mode scanning above and M-mode scanning below. In this nonventilated lung, the only movement is that caused by the heartbeat, which creates a subtle movement of the lungs and the pleura. This movement is visualized in the M-mode image synchronous with the heartbeat and is called the *lung pulse*. (C) The pleural line is marked in *yellow* and the superficial outline of the ribs in *orange*. The *red lines* indicate the lung pulse. (From Kristensen MS. Ultrasonography in the management of the airway. *Acta Anaesthesiol Scand.* 2011;55:1155–1173.)

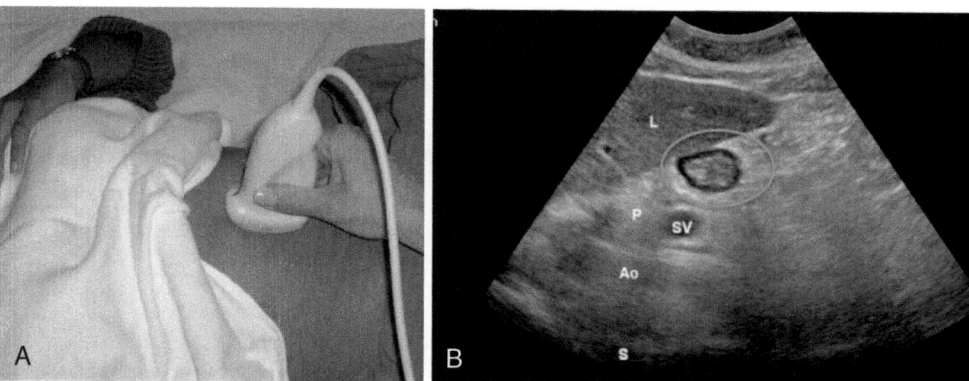

• **Fig. 3.11** Gastric antrum. (A) Sagittal probe orientation in the epigastric area. (B) The antrum (in the *light blue ring*) is located immediately posterior to the left lobe of the liver *(L)*. The pancreas *(P)* is typically hyperechoic and located posterior to the antrum. In this figure, a cross-section of the splenic vein *(SV)* may be seen as it crosses the pancreas from right to left. Posterior to the pancreas, a longitudinal view of the aorta *(Ao)* is seen. The spine *(S)* can also be seen. (Courtesy Anahi Perlas, University of Toronto and Toronto Western Hospital, Toronto, Canada. Figure nested at Rigshospitalet, University Hospital of Copenhagen, http://www.airwaymanagement.dk.)

seen in both the normal and the pathologic lung if the depth of the ultrasound image is sufficiently deep.[30]

The "B-line" is an artifact with seven features: It (1) is a hydrometric comet-tail artifact, (2) arises from the pleural line, (3) is hyperechoic, (4) is well defined, (5) spreads up indefinitely (i.e., spreads to the edge of the screen without fading—up to 17 cm with a probe reaching 17 cm),[28] (6) erases A-lines, and (7) moves with lung sliding when lung sliding is present.[29] Sparse B-lines occur in normal lungs, but the presence of three or more B-lines indicates pathology (e.g., interstitial syndrome).[31] B-lines are also called *ring-down artifacts*.[32]

Diaphragm

The diaphragm and its motion can be imaged by placing a convex transducer in the subxiphoid window in the middle upper abdominal region, just beneath the xiphoid process and the lower margin of the liver. The transducer is tilted 45 degrees cephalad, and bilateral diaphragmatic motion can be seen.[33] The bilateral diaphragm moves toward the abdomen when the lungs are ventilated and toward the chest during the relaxation phase. The liver and spleen movements characterize the overall movement of the corresponding hemidiaphragm during respiration and can be visualized by placing the probe in the longitudinal plane along the right anterior axillary line or the left posterior axillary line, respectively. The movement of the most caudal margin of the liver and spleen with respiration is measured.[34]

Gastric Antrum

The gastric antrum can be visualized by placing a curved, low-frequency probe in a sagittal orientation in the epigastric area. The antrum is usually best visualized in a parasagittal plane just right of the midline, surrounded by the left lobe and caudate lobe of the liver anteriorly and the head or neck of the pancreas posteriorly.[35] The empty antrum appears as a small round or oval structure and may resemble a bull's-eye. When the antrum is empty, only the gastric wall is visible; what appears to be a small amount of gastric content is, in fact, the thickness of all the layers of the gastric wall, which has five distinct sonographic layers (Fig. 3.11). This examination can be performed in the supine patient and in the right lateral decubitus position.[36]

Clinical Applications

Prediction of Difficult Airway Management

USG for screening of patients in order to predict difficulty with airway management has been shown to be useful in smaller series and in subgroups of patients, but its general use for this indication has not yet been fully established. In obese patients, a hyomental distance ratio (i.e., the ratio of the sonographically measured distance between the hyoid bone and the mentum in the fully extended neck position to that in a neutral neck position) of greater than 1.1 predicted a good laryngoscopic view after induction of anesthesia.[37] An inability to visualize the hyoid bone during sublingual USG was shown to be associated with difficult laryngoscopy and had a significantly higher predictive value than the Mallampati score or thyromental distance.[38] In morbidly obese patients, the distance from the skin to the anterior aspect of the trachea correlated with difficult laryngoscopy, but these findings were not reproduced when the end point was laryngoscopy grade without the use of optimal external laryngeal manipulation.[39,40] In recent years, a multitude of small studies have investigated USG-derived parameters including anterior-neck soft-tissue thickness measured at different levels (anterior to the hyoid bone, at the epiglottis, and at the anterior commissure of the vocal cords); hyomental distances measured with the head placed in a neutral, sniffing, or maximally hyperextended position; derived hyomental distance ratios; and tongue thickness, cross-sectional area, width, volume, and thickness-to-oral cavity ratio.[41]

Difficult mask ventilation is significantly correlated with thickness of the base of the tongue >50 mm in both the curarized and the noncurarized patient.[42] Positioning of a ProSeal larlgyneal mask airway (LMA) was verified in three USG planes, and this evaluation was found to be as equally effective as a standard leak test.[43] Most of these measurements have significant predictive values in selected patient groups and skilled hands, but they have not sufficiently proven their superiority over standard clinical measures to be recommended as routine screening procedures.

Evaluation of Pathology That May Influence the Choice of Airway Management Technique

Subglottic hemangiomas, laryngeal stenosis, laryngeal cysts, and respiratory papillomatosis (Fig. 3.12) can all be visualized with USG.[16,44,45] By detecting laryngeal pathology with USG in the patient with stridor,[46,47] a tracheostomy can be chosen instead of a potentially dangerous, or impossible, cricothyrotomy. A pharyngeal pouch (Zenker diverticulum),[48] representing a potential source of regurgitation and aspiration, can be seen on a transverse linear high-frequency scan of the neck; the image in Fig. 3.13 demonstrates one at the posterolateral aspect of the left thyroid lobe.[45] Malignancies and their relationship with the airway can be seen and characterized. Sialolithiasis is a potential contraindication to supraglottic airway placement; salivary stones as small as 2 mm × 3 mm can be recognized as high-level reverberation echoes on USG, accompanied by posterior acoustic shadows or hyperechoic masses.[49]

Fetal airway abnormalities, such as extrinsic obstruction caused by adjacent tumors (e.g., lymphatic malformation, cervical teratoma), can be visualized by prenatal USG (Fig. 3.14). With this information, airway management can be planned, either at birth or as an ex-utero intrapartum treatment (EXIT) procedure. The EXIT procedure can consist of the performance of a cesarean section, followed by tracheal intubation or tracheostomy while the newborn is still attached to the umbilical cord, thus maintaining fetal circulation.

Diagnosis of Obstructive Sleep Apnea

The width of the tongue base measured by USG was found to correlate with the severity of sleep-related breathing disorders,

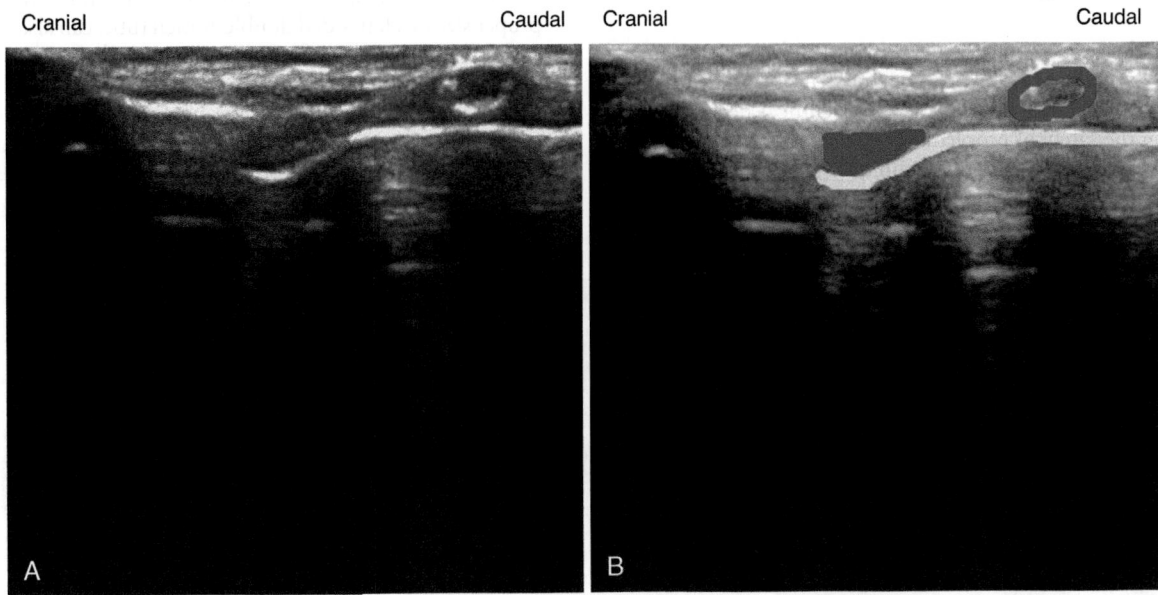

• **Fig. 3.12** Papilloma. Sagittal midline scan of the anterior neck in a patient with a papilloma on the anterior tracheal wall immediately caudal to the anterior commissure. (A) The scanning image. (B) The tissue-air border is marked in *yellow*, the cricoid cartilage in *blue*, and the papilloma in *reddish-brown*. (From Kristensen MS. Ultrasonography in the management of the airway. *Acta Anaesthesiol Scand.* 2011;55:1155–1173.)

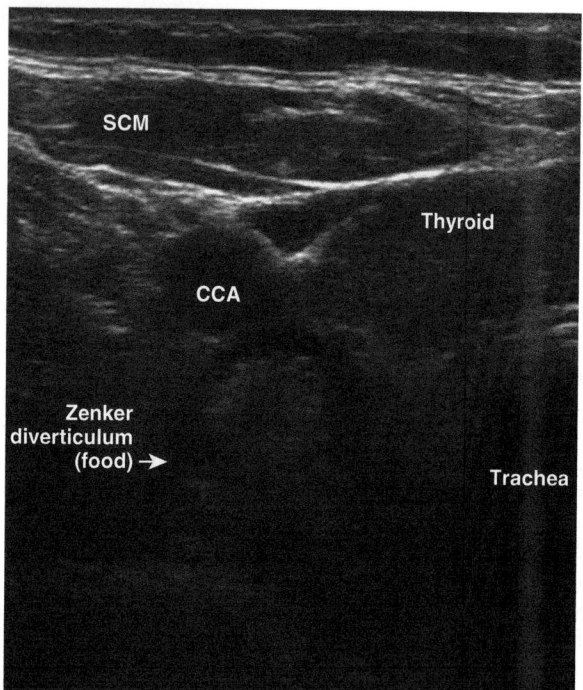

• **Fig. 3.13** Zenker diverticulum is seen laterally to the trachea on a transverse scan of the anterior neck above the suprasternal notch. *CCA*, Common carotid artery; *SCM*, sternocleidomastoid muscle. (Courtesy Peter Cheng, Kaiser Permanente Riverside Medical Center, Riverside, CA.)

A cross-sectional view of the gastric antrum in the epigastric area is obtained with a curved ("abdominal") transducer in the supine and right lateral decubitus positions. The antral findings correlate with those of the entire stomach. First, the type of content is assessed: no content in an empty stomach; hypoechoic, homogeneous content with clear fluids; or heterogeneous and/or hyperechoic content with thick fluids or solids. An empty stomach carries a low risk of aspiration, whereas the presence of solid content represents a high risk.

In the presence of clear fluid content, a volume assessment can help differentiate baseline gastric secretions (Grade 0 or 1 antrum with <1.5 mL/kg) with negligible aspiration risk vs higher-than-baseline volumes that may increase the risk of aspiration (Grade 2 antrum and/or >1.5 mL/kg). If fluid is not visible, this signifies a Grade 0 antrum (empty). If fluid is visible in the antrum in only the right lateral decubitus position, it is referred to as a Grade 1 antrum. If fluid is visible in both supine and right lateral decubitus position, this indicates a Grade 2 antrum. Gastric volume can be quantitatively estimated by measuring the cross-sectional area (CSA) of the gastric antrum:

$$\text{Gastric volume (mL)} = 27 + 14.6 \times \text{Right lateral CSA} \ (\text{cm}^2) - 1.28 \times \text{age (years)}$$

Alternatively, Fig. 3.16 can be used for calculating the volume based on the CSA measurement. Decision-making can be guided by the decision tree depicted in Fig. 3.17.

Prediction of the Appropriate Diameter of an Endotracheal, Endobronchial, or Tracheostomy Tube

In children and young adults, USG is a reliable tool for measuring the diameter of the subglottic upper airway and correlates well with MRI, which is the gold standard.[53,54]

The diameter of the left mainstem bronchus, and thereby the proper size of a left-sided double-lumen tube, can also be estimated with USG. In a series of patients, the outer diameter of the trachea was measured by USG just above the sternoclavicular joint in the transverse plane. The ratio between left mainstem bronchus diameter on CT imaging and outer tracheal diameter measured with USG was found to be 0.68. The sonographic tracheal diameter

including a patient's sensation of choking during the night. The width was measured as the distance between the lingual arteries where they enter the tongue base at its lower lateral borders.[13] The thickness of the lateral pharyngeal wall, as measured with USG, is significantly higher in patients with obstructive sleep apnea than in patients without this condition.[17]

Evaluation of Prandial Status

USG of the gastric antrum makes it possible to determine the volume and nature of stomach contents (empty, fluids, or solids), which can guide risk stratification and clinical decision-making regarding the safety of proceeding with general anesthesia and the choice of airway management technique (Fig. 3.15).[35,36,50–52]

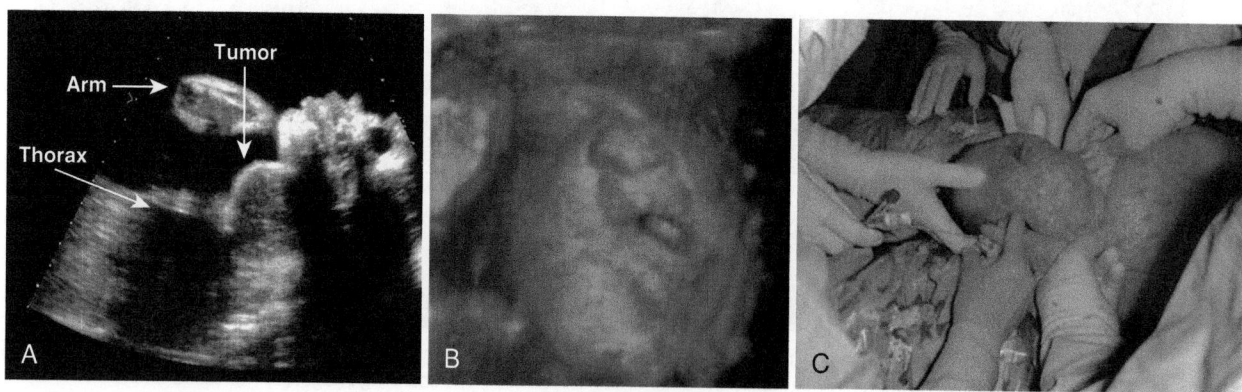

• **Fig. 3.14** (A) A large tumor is seen on the neck of a fetus. (B) Three-dimensional ultrasonographic image. (C) The head is delivered, and the airway is managed while the fetal circulation is still intact. (Courtesy Connie Jørgensen, Rigshospitalet, Copenhagen, Denmark.)

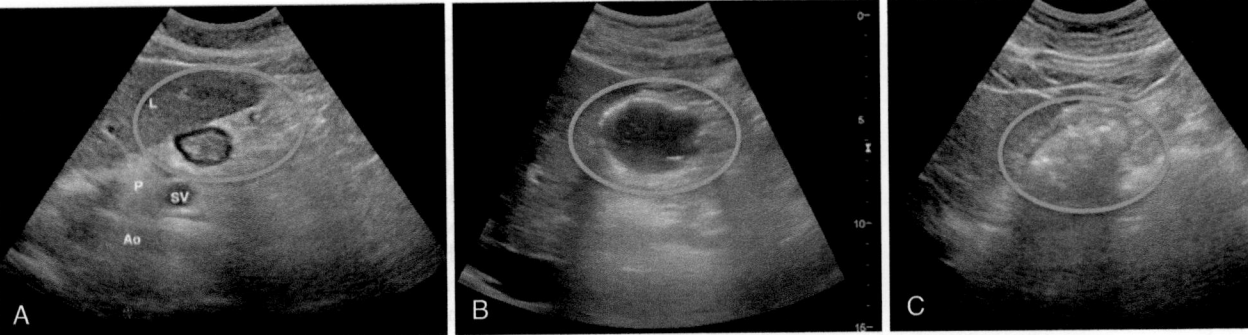

• **Fig. 3.15** Evaluating contents of the gastric antrum *(light blue rings)*. (A) The empty antrum appears as a small round or oval structure that may resemble a bull's-eye target. When the antrum is empty, only the gastric wall is seen; what appears to be a small amount of content is actually the thickness of all the layers of the gastric wall, which has five distinct sonographic layers. The most prominent layer can be clearly seen in this figure as a hypoechoic "ring" that corresponds histologically to the muscularis propria of the stomach. Also seen are the liver *(L)*, the pancreas *(P)*, the splenic vein *(SV)*, and the aorta *(Ao)*. (B) Clear fluid in the stomach (such as water, tea, or normal gastric secretions) can be seen as homogeneous hypoechoic content within the antrum. (C) Solid content in the stomach appears as nonhomogeneous, mostly hyperechoic content. There is usually some amount of air mixed with the solid meal, and this produces multiple "ring down artifacts" that obscure the posterior wall. (Courtesy Anahi Perlas, University of Toronto and Toronto Western Hospital, Toronto, Canada. Figure nested at Rigshospitalet, University Hospital of Copenhagen, www.airwaymanagement.dk.)

Right lat CSA	Age(y)						
	20	30	40	50	60	70	80
2	31	18	5	0	0	0	0
3	45	32	20	7	0	0	0
4	60	47	34	21	9	0	0
5	74	62	49	36	23	10	0
6	89	76	63	51	38	25	12
7	103	91	78	65	52	40	27
8	118	105	93	80	67	54	41
9	133	120	107	94	82	69	56
10	147	135	122	109	96	83	71
11	162	149	136	123	111	98	85
12	177	164	151	138	125	113	100
13	191	178	165	153	140	127	114
14	206	193	180	167	155	142	129
15	220	207	194	182	169	156	143
16	235	222	209	200	184	171	158
17	249	236	224	211	198	185	173
18	164	251	239	226	213	200	187
19	278	266	253	240	227	214	202
20	293	281	268	255	242	229	217
21	307	295	282	269	256	244	231
22	323	310	297	284	271	259	246

• **Fig. 3.16** Table used to determine the volume of gastric contents from antral ultrasound-measured cross-sectional area (CSA). (Reproduced with permission from gastricultrasound.org.)

was then used to select the appropriate-size double-lumen tube; the results were comparable to those obtained using chest radiography as a guide.[55]

In children with tracheostomy, USG measurement of the tracheal width and of the distance from the skin to the trachea can be used to predict the size and shape of a potential replacement tracheostomy tube.[56]

Localization of the Trachea

Obesity, a short thick neck, a neck mass, previous surgery or radiotherapy to the neck, or thoracic pathology resulting in tracheal deviation can make accurate localization of the trachea challenging and cumbersome. Even the addition of chest radiography and techniques of needle aspiration to locate the trachea

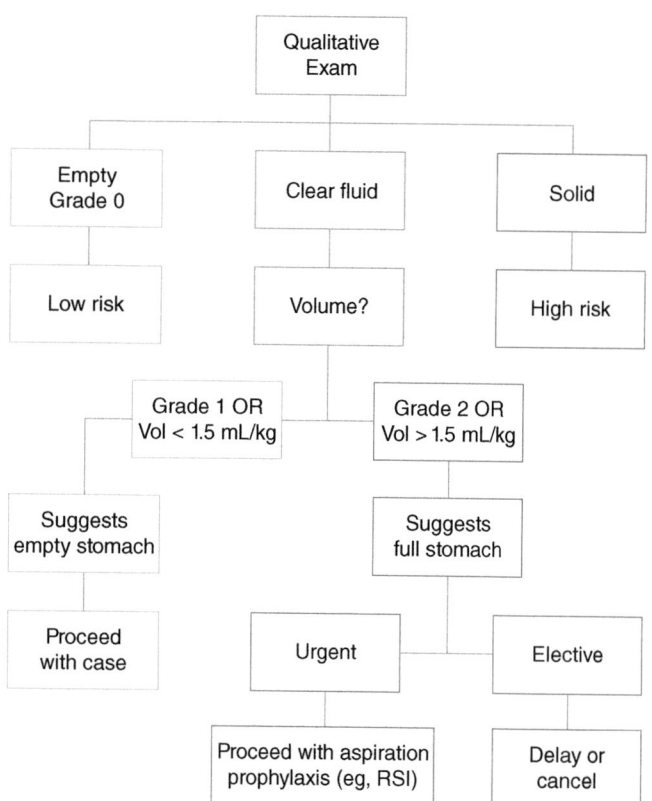

Identification of the Cricothyroid Membrane

The CTM plays a crucial role in airway management, and practitioners must be confident that they can identify it before induction of anesthesia and/or airway management.[59,60] However, it is only correctly identified by anesthesiologists in 0% to 72% of patients by surface landmarks and palpation alone, depending on which population is examined.[61,62] USG allows a reliable, quick, and easily learned method for the identification of the CTM, as preparation for transtracheal cannulation or cricothyrotomy.[5,61,63] Accurate localization of the CTM enables the clinician to approach the difficult airway by placing a transtracheal catheter for infiltration of local anesthesia or emergency transtracheal oxygenation. During awake intubation, it provides the added safety of having localized the CTM in advance should the intubation fail and emergency transcricoid access becomes necessary.

We suggest the following structured, stepwise, "string of pearls" approach for locating the CTM (Fig. 3.19 and Video 3.1):[3,64,65]

1. With the patient's neck extended, the airway practitioner stands on the patient's right side facing the patient.
2. The sternal bone is identified, and the transducer is placed transversely on the patient's neck just cephalad to the suprasternal notch to visualize the trachea, seen as a horseshoe-shaped dark structure with a posterior white line (see Fig. 3.19, first row).
3. The transducer is slid toward the patient's right side (toward the operator), so that the right border of the transducer is positioned midline of the trachea, and the ultrasound image of the tracheal ring is thus truncated in half on the screen (see Fig. 3.19, second row).
4. The right end of the transducer is maintained over the midline of the trachea while the left end is rotated 90 degrees into the sagittal plane, resulting in a longitudinal scan of the midline of the trachea. A number of dark (hypoechoic) rings will be seen anterior to the white hyperechoic line (air-tissue border), akin to a "string of pearls." The dark hypoechoic "pearls" are the anterior parts of the tracheal rings (see Fig. 3.19, third row).
5. The transducer is kept longitudinally in the midline and slid cephalad until the cricoid cartilage comes into view (seen as a larger, more elongated, and anteriorly placed dark "pearl" compared to the other tracheal rings). Further cephalad, the distal part of the thyroid cartilage can be seen as well (see Fig. 3.19,

• **Fig. 3.17** Flowchart for interpreting gastric contents and risk of aspiration. (Reproduced with permission from gastricultrasound.org.)

may be futile.[57] This situation is even more challenging in emergency situations and in cases where awake tracheostomy is chosen because of predicted difficulty with mask ventilation or tracheal intubation, or as an alternative to cricothyrotomy.[47] Under these circumstances, preoperative USG for localization of the trachea (Fig. 3.18) is very useful.[57] This was demonstrated in the case of an obese patient with Ludwig's angina in whom it was not possible to identify the trachea by palpation. A portable ultrasound machine was used, and the trachea was eventually located 2 cm lateral to the midline.[58]

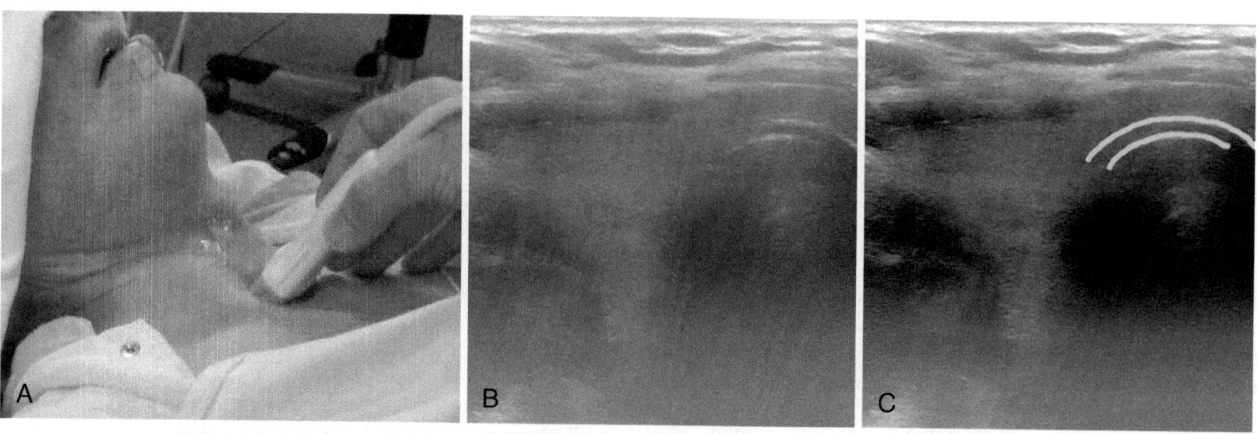

• **Fig. 3.18** Tracheal deviation. (A) The transducer is placed transversely in the midline over the suprasternal notch. (B) The scanning image reveals lateral deviation of the middle part of the trachea. (C) The cartilage of the tracheal ring (*light blue*) is deviated to the patient's left side. (From Kristensen MS. Ultrasonography in the management of the airway. *Acta Anaesthesiol Scand.* 2011;55:1155–1173.)

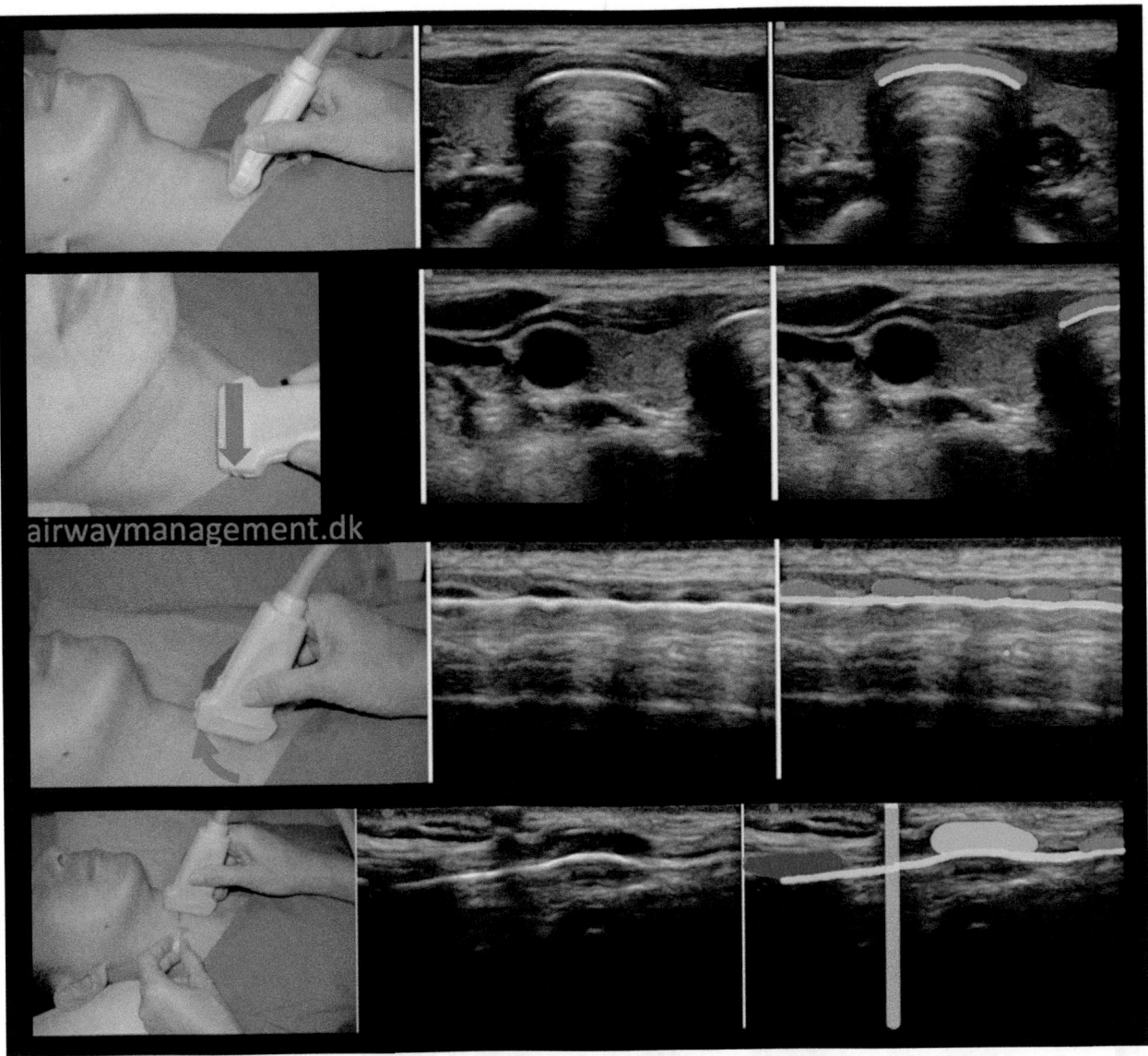

• **Fig. 3.19** The longitudinal "string of pearls" technique for identifying the cricothyroid membrane, the midline of the airway, and the interspaces between tracheal rings. The tracheal rings are marked in *red*, the air-tissue border in *light blue*, the cricoid cartilage in *green*, and the distal end of the thyroid cartilage in *purple*. The shadow created by the needle slid in between the transducer and the skin is shown in *yellow*. (Reproduced with permission from The Scandinavian Airway Management course, www.airwaymanagement.dk.)

fourth row). The longitudinal course of the midline of the airway can be marked with a pen.

6. While still holding the transducer, the other hand is used to slide a needle (as a marker, for its ability to cast a shadow in the ultrasound image) between the transducer and the patient's skin until the needle's shadow is seen midway between the caudal border of the thyroid cartilage and the cephalad border of the cricoid cartilage (see Fig. 3.19, fourth row).

7. The transducer is removed, and the needle marks the center of the CTM in the transverse plane, and this can be marked on the skin with a pen.

This "string of pearls" approach has proven its effectiveness by reducing the rate of failure in identification of the CTM in the morbidly obese female from 63% to 17% when compared with the palpation method,[62] and by significantly reducing the incidence of injury to the larynx following cricothyrotomy in cadavers.[66] Additionally, this approach allows for simultaneous identification of other access points to the airway (e.g., the cricotracheal membrane or the interspace between the second and third tracheal ring to be used for a tracheostomy).[67]

If the neck is too short or cannot be extended for the "string of pearls" approach, one can apply the *TACA technique* (**T**hyroid cartilage, **A**ir line, **C**ricoid cartilage, **A**ir line). See Fig. 3.20 and Video 3.2.[68]

1. With the patient's neck extended, the transducer is placed transversely over the neck, scanning to identify the thyroid cartilage as a hyperechoic, triangular structure (see Fig. 3.20, first row).

2. The transducer is moved caudally until the CTM is identified; this is recognizable as a hyperechoic white line resulting from the echo of the air-tissue border of the mucosal lining on the inside of the CTM, often with parallel white lines (reverberation artefacts) below (see Fig. 3.20, second row).

3. The transducer is moved further caudally until the cricoid cartilage is identified as a black, rotated C-shape with a white lining (see Fig. 3.20, third row).

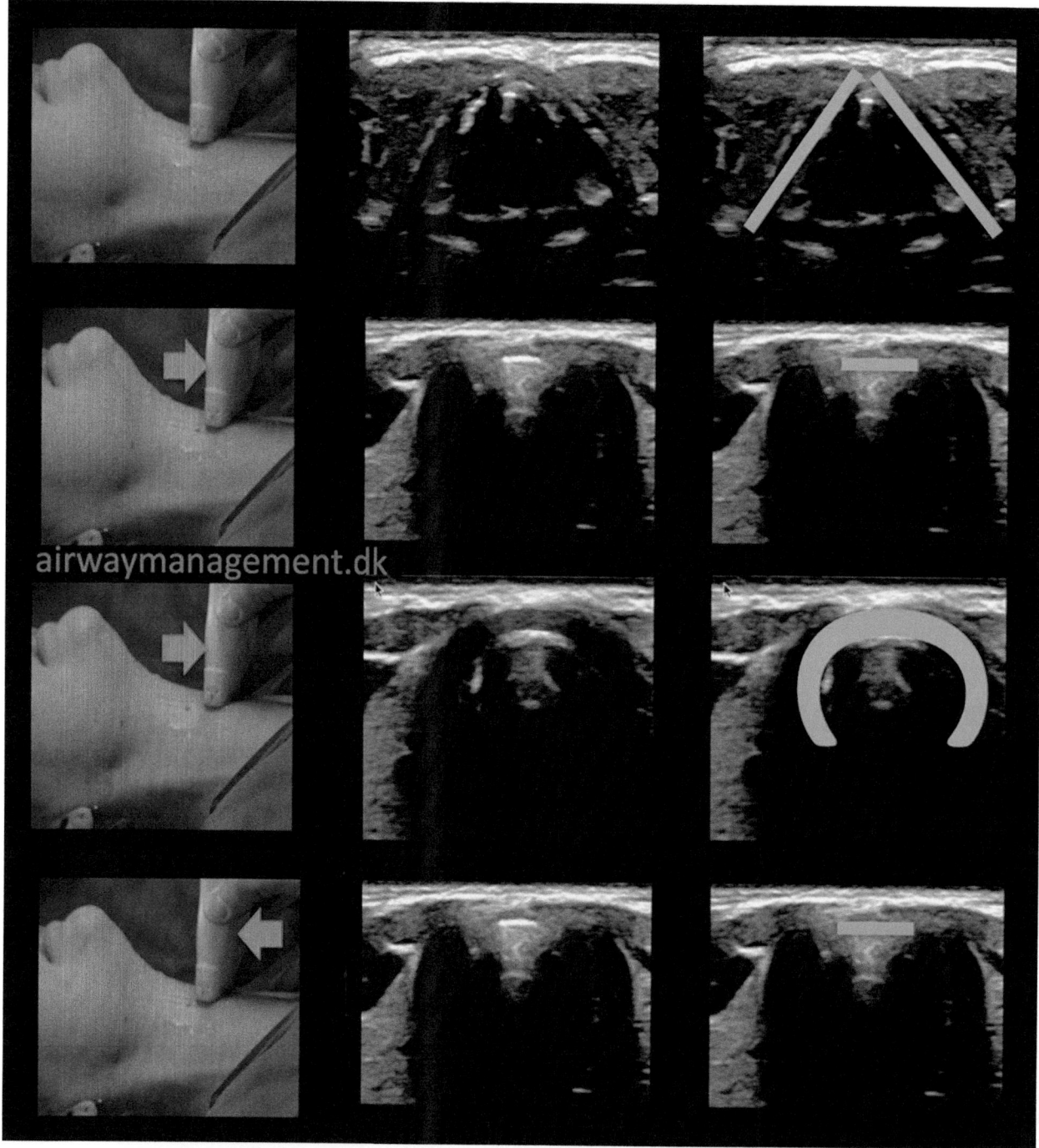

• **Fig. 3.20** The transverse TACA method (Thyroid cartilage, **A**ir line, **C**ricoid cartilage, **A**ir line) for identifying the cricothyroid membrane. (See text for details.) The *blue triangle* represents the thyroid cartilage, the *blue horizontal line* is the "air line," and the cricoid cartilage is seen as a *blue, rotated-C shape*. (Reproduced with permission from The Scandinavian Airwaymanagement course, www.airwaymanagement.dk.)

4. Finally, the transducer is moved back slightly cephalad until the center of the CTM is identified (see Fig. 3.20, fourth row).
5. The center can be marked both transversely and sagittally on the skin with a pen. By identifying the highly characteristic shapes of both the thyroid and the cricoid cartilages, both the cephalad and caudal borders of the cricothyroid membrane can be identified.

The "string of pearls" and TACA techniques can be applied individually or in combination (Video 3.3).[69]

The sum of published data unequivocally documents the superiority of USG for guiding, identification, and marking of the CTM, as well as the severe limitations of palpation methods, especially in the obese and in those with pathology of the neck.[4,70,71] Markings identifying the CTM made in patients with their neck in extension remain accurate if the neck is placed back in the extended position, even after the head and neck are moved and manipulated. This was demonstrated by two studies, which found that markings returned to the correct position in 100% of the combined 34 cases.[72,73] Thus, in patients where visual inspection or palpation methods cannot identify the CTM with certainty, it should be identified with USG and marked with the patient in neck extension. The patient can then be subsequently placed in the desired position for airway management—for example, awake intubation or rapid sequence intubation. In the event that the initial airway management plan fails and emergency invasive airway access is needed, the patient can be quickly placed back in neck extension, and the marking of the center of the CTM will again be in the correct place.[60]

Airway-Related Nerve Blocks

USG has been used to identify and block the superior laryngeal nerve (SLN) as part of the preparation for awake flexible scope intubation (FSI). The greater horn of the hyoid bone and the superior laryngeal artery are identified, and local analgesic is injected between them. In 100 ultrasound examinations of the SLN space (i.e., the space delimited by the hyoid bone, the thyroid cartilage, the preepiglottic space, the thyrohyoid muscle, and the membrane between the hyoid bone and the thyroid cartilage), all components of the space were seen in 81% of cases, and there was a suboptimal, but still useful, depiction of the space in the remaining 19% of cases. The SLN itself was not seen.[74] In a randomized study, the USG-guided SLN block was found to be faster and result in better anesthesia than a landmark palpation technique.[75]

Ultrasound-Guided Intubation

When a sufficient view of the glottic inlet cannot be obtained, it is possible to use USG to assist guiding an ETT into the trachea by (1) scanning at the level of the thyrohyoid membrane, (2) observing the relationship of the ETT to the glottic opening, (3) modifying the trajectory of insertion of the tube to place it through the glottic opening, and (4) confirming tube passage between the vocal cords.[76] In anesthetized patients with neck immobilization, USG-guided intubation had a lower first-pass, but equal overall, success rate when compared with FSI.[77]

Confirmation of Endotracheal Tube Placement

Using USG, confirmation of whether an ETT has entered the trachea or the esophagus can be made directly, in real time, by scanning the anterior neck during the intubation; indirectly, by looking for ventilation at the pleural or the diaphragmatic level; or by a combination of these techniques. Direct confirmation has the advantage that an accidental esophageal intubation is recognized immediately, before ventilation is initiated,[78] and, therefore, before air is forced into the stomach, which results in an increased risk of emesis and aspiration. Confirmation at the pleural level has the advantage of distinguishing, at least to some extent, between tracheal and endobronchial intubation.

Both the direct and the indirect confirmation techniques have an advantage over capnography in that they can be applied in very low cardiac output situations. A recent meta-analysis concluded that USG is a valuable and reliable adjunct for ETT confirmation, including during resuscitation for cardiac arrest.[79] USG is more advantageous than auscultation when performed in noisy environments, such as in helicopters when performing patient retrievals. In a cadaver model in which a 7.5-MHz curved probe was placed longitudinally over the CTM, it was possible for residents given only 5 minutes of training in the technique to correctly identify

esophageal intubation (97% sensitivity) with dynamic examination at the time of intubation. When the examination was performed after the intubation, the sensitivity was very poor.[80]

In a study in children, direct confirmation of ETT placement by scanning via the CTM required multiple views; the USG examination was apparently performed after the intubation, making comparison to other studies difficult, and the feasibility of that approach has been challenged.[81,82] In another pediatric study, when the transducer was placed at the level of the glottis, the vocal cords were always visible. Additionally, passage of the ETT was visible in all children and was characterized by widening of the vocal cords.[83]

Indirect confirmation of ETT placement in 15 patients was performed with the use of a portable, handheld ultrasound machine and routine scanning in the third and fourth intercostal spaces on both sides during the phases of preoxygenation, apnea, bag-mask ventilation, intubation, and positive-pressure ventilation after intubation. ETT placement was confirmed in all cases.[84]

The color power Doppler function has been used as a supplement during observation of lung sliding to detect that a lung was ventilated.[85] The distinction between tracheal and endobronchial intubation can be made by scanning the lung bilaterally. If there is pleural sliding on one side and lung pulse on the other side, the tip of the tube is in the mainstem bronchus on the side on which lung sliding is observed. The ETT is then withdrawn until lung sliding is observed bilaterally, indicating that the tip of the tube is again placed in the trachea.[86] Indirect confirmation of intubation by detection of lung sliding was studied in fresh ventilated cadavers; the tip of the ETT was placed in the esophagus, trachea, or right mainstem bronchus. A high sensitivity (95% to 100%) was found for detection of esophageal versus tracheal or bronchial intubation. The sensitivity for distinguishing a right mainstem bronchus intubation from a tracheal intubation was lower (69% to 78%), most likely because of transmitted movement of the left lung due to expansion of the right lung.[85]

Indirect confirmation of intubation by confirmation of bilateral diaphragmatic movement has been shown to be useful for distinguishing between esophageal and tracheal intubation in a pediatric population.[33] However, when the technique was used to distinguish between endobronchial and tracheal intubation, diaphragmatic ultrasound was not equivalent to chest radiography for determining ETT placement within the airway.[87]

The combination of the direct transverse scan on the neck at the level of the CTM and detection of lung sliding in 30 emergency department patients who required tracheal intubation correctly detected the 3 cases of esophageal intubation, even in the presence of 4 cases of hemopneumothorax.[88]

Filling the ETT cuff with fluid aids in determining the cuff position on USG.[89] On the other hand, use of a metal stylet does not augment visualization of the ETT.[75,90] USG is also useful for confirming the correct position of a double-lumen tube.[55]

The authors recommend the following procedure for USG confirmation of ETT placement (Video 3.4):[91]

1. Perform a transverse scan over the trachea, just above the sternal notch. Note the location and appearance of the esophagus. Proceed with the intubation attempt.
2. If the ETT is visualized passing into the esophagus, remove it without ventilating the patient and make another intubation attempt, possibly using another technique.
3. If the ETT is not seen, or if it is seen in the trachea, ventilate the patient.

4. Move the transducer to an interspace between two ribs bilaterally and look for lung sliding.

5. If there is bilateral lung sliding, it is confirmation that the ETT is in the airway, and very likely in the trachea.

6. If there is lung sliding on one side and lung pulse on the other side, then a mainstem bronchus intubation on the side with the lung sliding is likely, and the tube can be withdrawn gradually until bilateral sliding is present.

7. If there is no lung sliding on either side, but lung pulse is present, there is a small risk that the tube has entered the esophagus.

8. If there is neither lung pulse nor lung sliding, then a pneumothorax should be suspected.

Tracheostomy

Accurate localization of the trachea in the absence of surface landmarks can be very challenging and cumbersome. Preoperative USG for localization of the trachea (see Figs. 3.18 and 3.19) is very suitable for both surgical tracheostomy and percutaneous dilatational tracheostomy (PDT).[57] In children, preoperative USG is of value in verifying the precise tracheostomy position and thereby preventing subglottic damage to the cricoid cartilage and the first tracheal ring, hemorrhage due to abnormally placed or abnormally large blood vessels, and pneumothorax.[92]

USG allows localization of the trachea, visualization of the anterior tracheal wall and pretracheal tissue, including blood vessels, and selection of the optimal intercartilaginous space for the percutaneous dilatational placement of a tracheostomy tube.[93,94] The distance from the skin surface to the tracheal lumen can be measured to predetermine the length of the puncture cannula that is needed to reach the tracheal lumen without perforating the posterior wall.[95] The same distance can be used to determine the optimal length of the tracheostomy cannula.[96]

Ultrasound-guided PDT has been applied in a case in which a bronchoscope-guided technique had been abandoned.[95] Autopsies in three cases of fatal bleeding after PDT revealed that the tracheostomy level was much more caudal than intended and that the innominate vein and the arch of the aorta had been eroded. It is likely that the addition of a USG examination to determine the level for the PDT and to avoid blood vessels could diminish this risk.[97] Ultrasound-guided PDT results in a significantly lower rate of cranial misplacement of the tracheostomy tube compared with "blind" placement.[94] Bronchoscope-guided PDT often results in considerable hypercapnia, whereas Doppler ultrasound–guided PDT does not.[98] The application of USG versus the landmark technique to determine the puncture site significantly improved the first-pass success rate for tracheal puncture in a randomized comparison.[99]

In a prospective series of 72 PDTs, the combination of USG and bronchoscopy was applied. Before the procedures, all subjects had their pretracheal space examined with USG; the findings led to a change in the planned puncture site in 24% of cases and to a change of procedure to surgical tracheostomy in one case in which the ultrasound examination revealed a goiter with extensive subcutaneous vessels.[100] Another approach using real-time ultrasound guidance with visualization of the needle path by means of a linear high-frequency transducer placed transversely over the trachea was more successful and resulted in visualization of the needle path and satisfactory guidewire placement in all of 13 patients.[101]

The addition of USG for PDT reduces the complication rate and facilitates identification of the appropriate tracheostomy tube insertion site.[102] The authors recommend *combining* preprocedural USG with a flexible bronchoscope-guided procedure, when feasible.

Confirmation of Nasogastric Tube Placement

Abdominal USG performed in the intensive care unit (ICU) had a 97% sensitivity for detecting correct gastric placement of a weighted-tip nasogastric tube (NGT). Immediately after insertion of the NGT, the metal stylet was removed and a 2- to 5-MHz convex transducer was used to examine the duodenum in the middle gastric area. If the NGT was not visualized, the probe was oriented toward the left upper abdominal quadrant to visualize the gastric area. If the NGT tip was still not visible, 5 mL saline mixed with air was injected to visualize the hyperechoic "fog" exiting the tip. The tip of the NGT was considered to be correctly located when it was seen surrounded by fluid and echogenic moving formations (related to peristalsis). The tip of the NGT was visualized by USG in 34 of 35 cases. Radiography correctly identified all 35 catheters but lasted on average 180 minutes (range, 113–240 minutes); in contrast, the sonographic examinations lasted 24 minutes on average (range, 11–53 minutes). The authors concluded that bedside USG performed by nonradiologists is a sensitive method for confirming the position of weighted-tip nasogastric feeding tubes, that it is easily taught to ICU physicians, and that conventional radiography can be reserved for cases in which USG is inconclusive.[103] The technique is fast and useful, but the persisting need for radiography in inconclusive cases was confirmed in a review of controlled studies.[104,105]

A Sengstaken-Blakemore tube may be applied for severe esophageal variceal bleeding, but there are considerable complications, including death, from esophageal rupture after inadvertent inflation of the gastric balloon in the esophagus.[106] USG of the stomach can aid in the rapid confirmation of correct placement. If the Blakemore tube is not directly visible, inflation of 50 mL air via the gastric lumen (not the gastric balloon) of the tube should lead to a characteristic jet of echogenic bubbles within the stomach. The gastric balloon is slowly inflated under direct USG guidance and usually appears as a growing echogenic circle within the stomach.[106]

Diagnosis of Pneumothorax

USG is as effective as chest radiography in detecting or excluding pneumothorax.[32] It is even more sensitive in the ICU setting: USG was able to establish the diagnosis in the majority of patients in whom a pneumothorax was invisible on plain radiographs but diagnosed by CT scan.[28] In patients with multiple injuries, USG was faster and had a higher sensitivity and accuracy compared to chest radiography.[107] The value of USG for detecting pneumothorax was recently highlighted in a comprehensive review.[108]

The presence of lung sliding or lung pulse on USG examination indicates that two pleural layers are in close proximity to each other at that specific point under the transducer (i.e., there is no pneumothorax there). If there is free air (pneumothorax) in the part of the pleural cavity underlying the transducer, no lung sliding or lung pulse will be seen, and A-lines (Fig. 3.21) will be more dominant.[30] In M-mode, the "stratosphere sign" will be seen: only parallel lines through all of the depth of the image (see Fig. 3.21). If the transducer is placed right at the border of the pneumothorax, where the visceral pleura intermittently is in contact with the parietal pleura, the "lung point" will be seen; this is a sliding lung

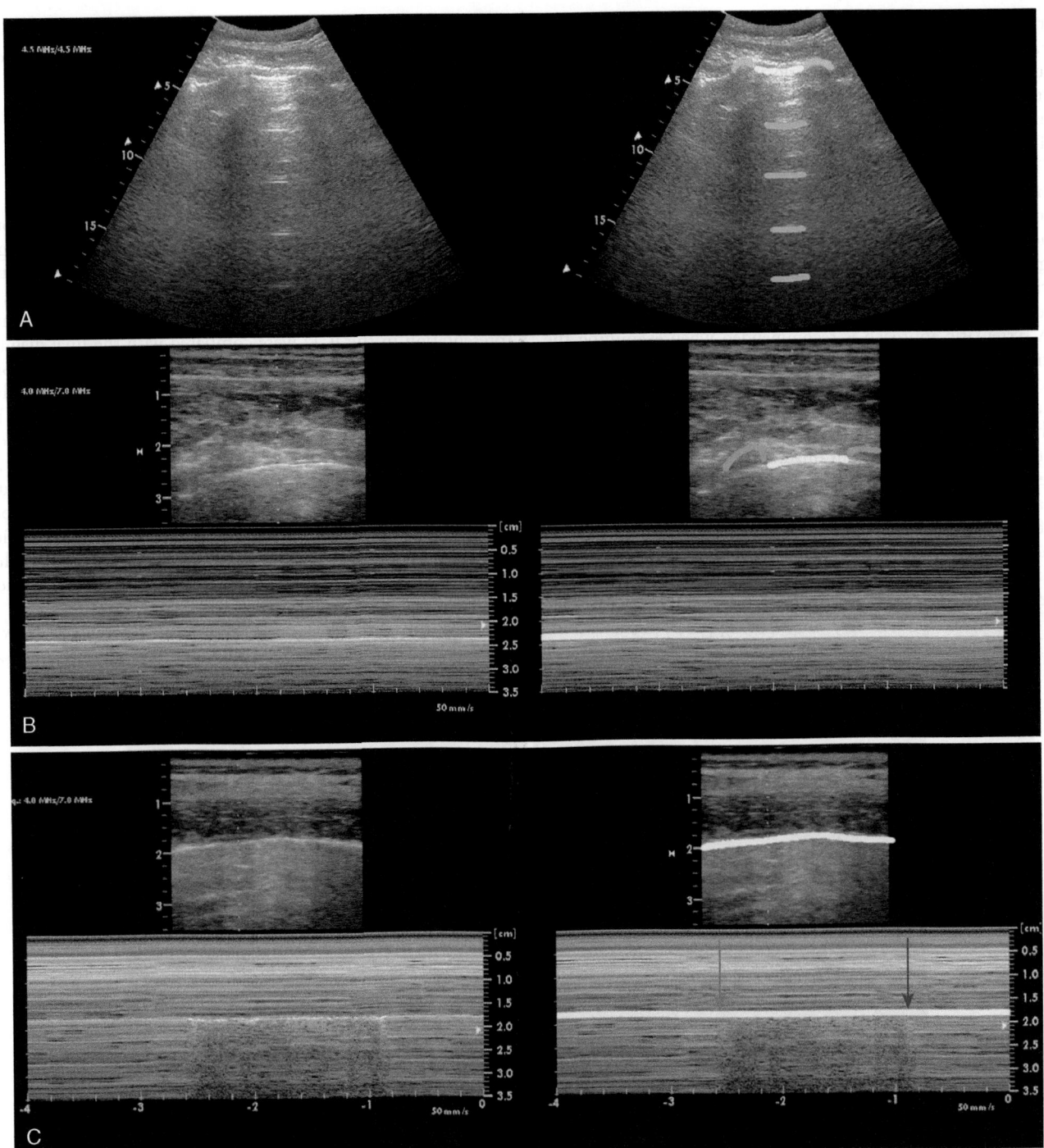

• **Fig. 3.21** Pneumothorax. The scanning images are shown on the *left* and the marked-up images on the *right*. (A) Image obtained with a convex transducer in a rib interspace. The pleural line *(yellow)* represents the surface of the parietal pleura. The ribs *(orange)* create underlying shadows. The "A-lines" *(light blue)* are reverberation artifacts from the pleural line; notice that they are dispersed with the same distance between the A-lines as between the skin surface and the pleural line. (B) Again, the pleural line is marked in *yellow* and the ribs in *orange*. Everything posterior to the pleural line is artifact. There is absence of pleural sliding and absence of lung pulse. The M-mode image consists only of parallel lines, called the *stratosphere sign*. (C) The *green arrow* represents the "lung point," the moment in which the visceral pleura just comes in contact with the parietal pleura at the exact location of the transducer. For the time interval from the *green* to the *blue arrow*, the two pleural layers are in contact with each other and form the "lung sliding" pattern. After the time represented by the *blue arrow*, the two pleural layers are no longer in contact, and the "stratosphere sign" is seen. The lung point can be difficult to see on the static B-mode image, whereas it is easy to recognize with dynamic, real-time, B-mode scanning. (Courtesy Erik Sloth, Aarhus University Hospital, Skejby, Denmark.) (From Kristensen MS. Ultrasonography in the management of the airway. *Acta Anaesthesiol Scand.* 2011;55:1155–1173.)

alternating with A-lines, synchronous with ventilation (Video 3.5). The lung point is pathognomonic for pneumothorax. If a pneumothorax is suspected, the rib interspaces of the thoracic cavity can be systematically "mapped" to confirm or rule out a pneumothorax.

The detection of lung sliding has a negative predictive value of 100%, meaning that when lung sliding is seen, a pneumothorax of the part of the lung beneath the ultrasound probe is ruled out.[28] For diagnosis of occult pneumothorax, the abolition of lung sliding alone had a sensitivity of 100% and a specificity of 78%. Absent lung sliding plus the A-line sign had a sensitivity of 95% and a specificity of 94%. The lung point had a sensitivity of 79% and a specificity of 100%.[30]

A systematic approach is recommended when examining the supine patient for pneumothorax. The anterior chest wall can be divided into quadrants and the probe first placed at the most superior aspect of the thorax with respect to gravity (i.e., the lower part of the anterior chest wall in supine patients). The probe is then positioned on each of the four quadrants of the anterior area, followed by the lateral chest wall between the anterior and posterior axillary lines and the rest of the accessible part of the thorax.[30]

If suspicion for a pneumothorax arises intraoperatively, USG is the fastest way to confirm or rule it out, especially considering that an anterior pneumothorax is often undiagnosed in a supine patient subjected to plain anterior-posterior radiography and that CT, the gold standard, is very difficult to apply in this situation. USG is an obvious first choice for diagnostics if a pneumothorax

is suspected during or after central venous cannulation or nerve blockade, especially if USG is already in use for the procedure itself and, thus, immediately available.

Differentiation Among Different Types of Lung and Pleura Pathology

Seventy percent of the pleural surface is accessible to ultrasound examination,[32] and a wide variety of pulmonary pathological conditions can be investigated with USG (Fig. 3.22).[2] In a study of 260 dyspneic ICU patients with acute respiratory failure, the results of lung USG (performed by a dedicated specialist) on initial presentation in the ICU were compared with the final diagnosis by the ICU team. Three items were assessed: artifacts (horizontal A-lines or vertical B-lines indicating interstitial syndrome); lung sliding; and alveolar consolidation, pleural effusion, or both. Predominant A-lines plus lung sliding indicated asthma or chronic obstructive pulmonary disease (COPD) with 89% sensitivity and 97% specificity. Multiple anterior diffuse B-lines with lung sliding indicated pulmonary edema with 97% sensitivity and 95% specificity (Fig. 3.23). The use of these profiles would have provided correct diagnoses in 90.5% of cases. It was concluded that lung USG can help the clinician make a rapid diagnosis in patients with acute respiratory failure.[31]

USG can detect pleural effusion and differentiate between pleural fluid and pleural thickening, and it is more accurate and

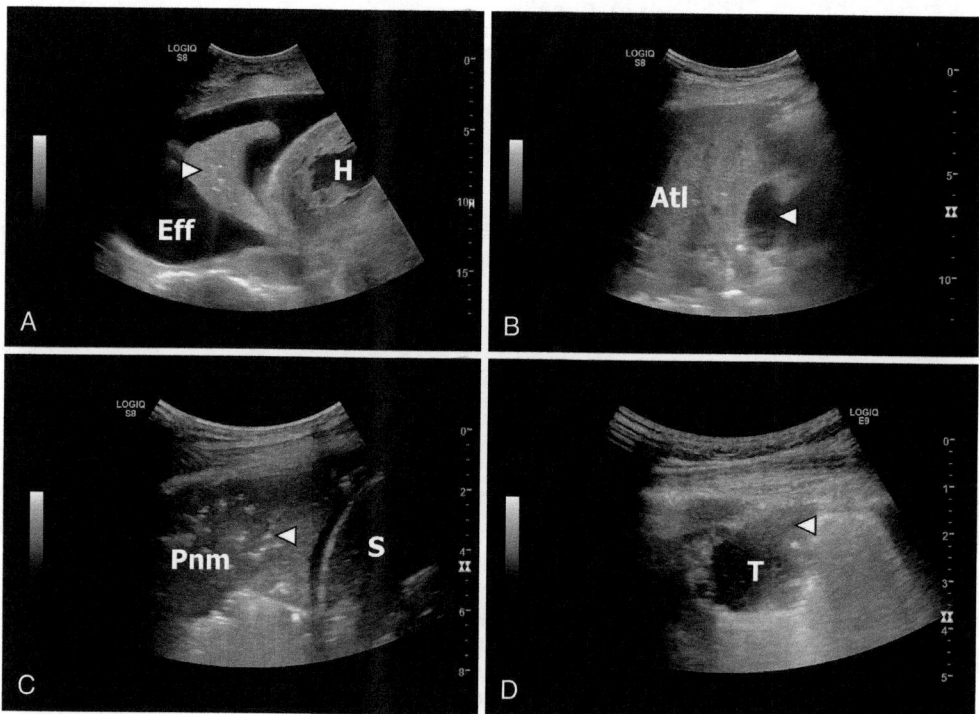

• **Fig. 3.22** Different lung-ultrasound findings. (A) A large, simple, pleural effusion *(Eff)* is present as a hypoechoic area. Underlying compression atelectasis *(arrow)* and the heart *(H)* can also be seen. (B) Complete atelectasis *(Atl)* of the entire right upper lobe. Medially in the image, the superior vena cava can be visualized *(arrow)*. (C) Lobar pneumonia *(Pnm)* of the left lower lobe is present just cranially to the spleen *(S)*. Air bronchograms can be seen as hyperechoic white dots *(arrow)* within the consolidated lung tissue. (D) A lung tumor *(T)* can be seen as a hypoechoic, well-demarcated area just below the pleural line. Invasive growth into the chest wall can be seen *(arrow)*. (Courtesy Christian B. Laursen, Research Unit at the Department of Respiratory Medicine, Odense University Hospital, Odense, Denmark. Figure nested at Rigshospitalet, University Hospital of Copenhagen, http://www.airwaymanagement.dk.)

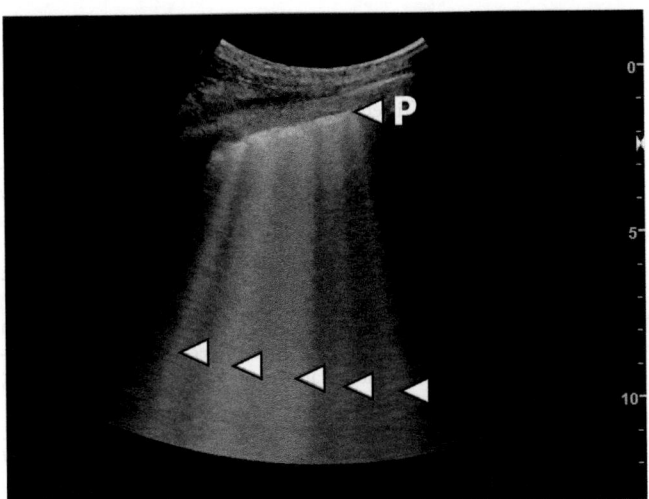

• **Fig. 3.23** Lung ultrasound demonstrating multiple B-lines *(arrows)*, which are seen as vertical reverberation artifacts originating from the pleural line *(P)*. Multiple B-lines, as seen here, indicate the presence of lung interstitial syndrome. (Courtesy Christian B. Laursen, Research Unit at the Department of Respiratory Medicine, Odense University Hospital, Odense, Denmark. Figure nested at Rigshospitalet, University Hospital of Copenhagen, http://www.airwaymanagement.dk.)

preferable to radiographic measurement in the quantification of pleural effusion.[32] Routine use of lung USG in the ICU setting can lead to a reduction of the number of chest radiographs and CT scans performed.[109] A recent review highlights the benefits of thoracic ultrasound.[108]

Prediction of Successful Extubation

In a study of ventilated adult patients, an ultrasound transducer was placed on the CTM with a transverse view of the larynx. The width of the air column was significantly smaller in the group of patients who developed postextubation stridor.[110] However, the number of patients in the stridor group was small (n = 4), and these results need to be evaluated in larger studies.

Intubated patients receiving mechanical ventilation in a medical ICU had their breathing force evaluated by USG. The transducer was placed along the right anterior axillary line and the left posterior axillary line for measurement of liver and spleen displacement in cranio-caudal aspects, respectively. The cutoff value of diaphragmatic displacement for predicting successful extubation was determined to be 1.1 cm. The liver and spleen displacements measured in the study were thought to reflect the "global" functions of the respiratory muscles, and this method provided a good parameter of respiratory muscle endurance and predictor of extubation success.[34] USG of the lungs, heart, and diaphragm is now being used as an integrated tool for planning and execution of successful weaning from mechanical ventilation.[111]

Ultrasonography and the Pediatric Airway

In smaller children, the CTM is very narrow and a tracheal approach to emergency invasive airway access is recommended[112]; USG can be used to identify the trachea before induction of anesthesia.[113] Several other well-established and potential indications for USG in the pediatric population have been described.[113,114]

Special Techniques and Future Aspects

There are a number of miscellaneous applications for USG in airway management. For example, the lateral position of an LMA cuff can be seen on USG if the cuff is filled with fluid; however, the fluid damages the cuff during subsequent autoclaving.[89] Airway obstruction as a result of a prevertebral hematoma after difficult central line insertion may be prevented by using USG for this procedure.[115] Endolaryngeal USG—examination of the larynx from the luminal side—is accomplished using a thin-catheter high-frequency probe with a rotating mirror that spreads the ultrasound ray, producing a 360-degree image rectilinear to the catheter. The larynx and the trachea above the cuff of an ETT are filled with normal saline to obtain sufficient tissue connection and to prevent the retention of air bubbles in the anterior commissure.[116,117] In the near future, 3-D and pocket-size ultrasound devices are likely to move the boundaries for both the quality and the availability of ultrasound imaging of the airway,[118] and automated detection—for example of pleural sliding[119]—is likely to become clinically useful.

Learning Ultrasonography

The following studies provide insight into what (and how little) is required to learn basic airway USG. After 8.5 hours of focused training, comprised of a 2.5-hour didactic course that included essential views of normal and pathologic conditions and three hands-on sessions of 2 hours each, physicians without previous knowledge of USG were able to competently perform basic general USG examinations. The examinations were aimed at diagnosing the presence of pleural effusion, intraabdominal effusion, acute cholecystitis, intrahepatic biliary duct dilation, obstructive uropathy, chronic renal disease, and deep venous thrombosis. In addition, the physicians correctly answered 95% of questions related to a potential therapeutic impact.[7]

The amount of experience needed to make a correct diagnosis with USG is probably task specific. In other words, the basic skill required to detect a pleural effusion may be acquired in minutes but may then improve with experience.[120] A 25-minute instructional session, including both a didactic portion and hands-on practice, was given to critical care paramedics and nurses who were part of a helicopter critical care transport team. The instructional session focused solely on detection of the presence or absence of lung sliding, including secondary techniques such as power Doppler and M-mode USG. The participants' performance was studied on fresh, ventilated cadavers. The presence or absence of lung sliding was correctly identified in 46 of 48 trials, for a sensitivity of 96.9% and a specificity of 93.8%. In a follow-up after 9 months, the presence or absence of lung sliding was correctly identified in all 56 trials, resulting in a sensitivity and specificity of 100%.[121]

As mentioned, residents given only 5 minutes of training were able to correctly identify esophageal intubation with 97% sensitivity when USG was performed dynamically, whereas the sensitivity was very poor when the examination was performed after the intubation.[80]

Conclusion

Important structures relevant to airway management can be identified with the use of USG. These include a large part of the airway and adjacent structures—from the mouth and tongue, to the larynx, to the esophagus and the midtrachea; the pleural layers and their movement; the diaphragm; and the gastric antrum. USG used dynamically, immediately before, during, and after airway interventions, provides real-time images that are highly relevant for several aspects of airway management. Esophageal intubation is detected without the need for ventilation or cardiac output; the CTM is identified before management of a difficult airway; ventilation is seen by observing lung sliding bilaterally, which is also the first choice for ruling out a suspected intraoperative pneumothorax; and PDT is facilitated by identifying the correct tracheal-ring interspace and depth from the skin to the tracheal wall.

Acknowledgments

Acta Anaesthesiologica Scandinavica, the Acta Anaesthesiologica Scandinavica Foundation, and Blackwell Publishing are acknowledged for Figs. 3.1–3.10, 3.12, 3.18, and 3.21, which were first published in Kristensen MS, Ultrasonography in the management of the airway. *Acta Anaesthesiol Scand.* 2011;55:1155–1173.

We also thank Connie Jørgensen, MD, DMSc, Head of the Clinic for Fetal Medicine and Ultrasonography, Rigshospitalet, Copenhagen, Denmark, for illustrations and critical reading of the manuscript; Erik Sloth, MD, PhD, DMSc, Professor in Experimental Ultrasonography, Department of Anaesthesiology and Intensive Care Medicine, Aarhus University Hospital, Skejby, Denmark, for illustrations and videos; Michael Friis-Tvede, MD, Rigshospitalet, Copenhagen, Denmark, for setting up the non-profit home page for academic airway management (www.airwaymanagement.dk) and for incorporating the airway videos; Peter H. Cheng, MD, Director of Regional Anesthesia, Department of Anesthesiology, Kaiser Permanente Riverside Medical Center, Riverside, CA, USA, for illustrations and sparring; Rasmus Hesselfeldt, MD, Rigshospitalet, Copenhagen, Denmark, for help in making the photos and videos; Anahi Perlas, MD, University of Toronto and Toronto Western Hospital, Toronto, Canada, for providing figures and comments; and Christian B. Laursen, MD, PhD, Research Unit at the Department of Respiratory Medicine, Odense University Hospital, Odense, Denmark, for lung ultrasound illustrations and sparring. Peter Van de Putte, MD, PhD, Imelda Hospital, Bonheiden, Belgium, for advice and sharing illustrations from gastricultrasound.org.

Selected References

1. Teoh WH, Kristensen MS. Ultrasonography for airway management. In: Cook T, Kristensen MS, eds. *Core Topics in Airway Management.* Cambridge University Press; 2020:63–71.
2. Kristensen MS, Teoh WH, Graumann O, Laursen CB. Ultrasonography for clinical decision-making and intervention in airway management: from the mouth to the lungs and pleurae. *Insights Imaging.* 2014;5:253–279.
3. Kristensen MS. Ultrasonography in the management of the airway. *Acta Anaesthesiol Scand.* 2011;55:1155–1173.
4. Hung K-C, Chen I-W, Lin C-M, Sun C-K. Comparison between ultrasound-guided and digital palpation techniques for identification of cricothyroid membrane: a meta-analysis. *Br J Anaesth.* 2021;126(1):e9–e11.
29. Rigshospitalet CUH. Ultrasonography in airway management. Rigshospitalet; 2015. Available at https://airwaymanagement.dk/ressources.
31. Lichtenstein DA, Meziere GA. Relevance of lung ultrasound in the diagnosis of acute respiratory failure: the BLUE protocol. *Chest.* 2008;134:117–125.
47. Adi O, Fong CP, Sum KM, Ahmad AH. Usage of airway ultrasound as an assessment and prediction tool of a difficult airway management. *Am J Emerg Med.* 2021;42:263.e1–263.e4.
52. Perlas A, Arzola C, Van de Putte P. Point-of-care gastric ultrasound and aspiration risk assessment: a narrative review. *Can J Anaesth.* 2018;65:437–448.
60. Kristensen MS, Teoh WH. Ultrasound identification of the cricothyroid membrane: the new standard in preparing for front-of-neck airway access. *Br J Anaesth.* 2021;126(1):22–27.
65. Airway Management for Anaesthesiologists. Identification of the Cricothyroid Membrane with Ultrasonography Longitudinal "String of Pearls" Approach. Airwaymanagement.dk. Available at http://airwaymanagement.dk/pearls.
69. Airwaymanagement for Anaesthesiologists. Ultrasound Guided Cricothyrotomy: Confirming with TACA. Airwaymanagement.dk. Available at https://airwaymanagement.dk/ultrasound_needle_cricothyrotomy.
73. Bowness J, Teoh WH, Kristensen MS, et al. A marking of the cricothyroid membrane with extended neck returns to correct position after neck manipulation and repositioning. *Acta Anaesthesiol Scand.* 2020;64(10):1422–1425.

All references can be found online at eBooks.Health.Elsevier.com.

4

Physics of the Airway

D. JOHN DOYLE AND KEVIN F. O'GRADY

CHAPTER OUTLINE

KEY POINTS

- An important formula that quantifies the relationship of pressure, flow, and resistance in laminar flow systems is given by the Hagen-Poiseuille equation. This law states that the fluid flow rate through a horizontal straight tube of uniform bore is proportional to the pressure gradient and the fourth power of the radius and is related inversely to the viscosity of the gas and the length of the tube. This law is valid for laminar flow conditions only.

- When the flow rate exceeds a critical velocity (the flow velocity below which flow is laminar), the flow loses its laminar parabolic velocity profile, becomes disorderly, and is termed *turbulent*. If turbulent flow exists, the relationship between pressure drop and flow is no longer governed by the Hagen-Poiseuille equation. Instead, the pressure gradient required (or the

resistance encountered) during turbulent flow varies as the square of the gas flow rate. In addition, flow becomes inversely related to gas density rather than viscosity (as occurs with laminar flow).

- Clinically, airway-obstructing conditions such as epiglottitis or inhaled foreign bodies are often best modeled as breathing through an orifice. Under such conditions, the approximate flow across the orifice varies inversely with the square root of the gas density, in contrast to laminar flow conditions, in which gas flow varies inversely with gas viscosity. In such conditions, the low density of helium allows it to play a significant clinical role in the management of some forms of airway obstruction.

- Laplace's law predicts that for two alveoli of unequal size but equal surface tension, the smaller alveolus experiences a larger intraalveolar pressure than the larger alveolus, causing the smaller alveolus to collapse. In real life, however, collapse of the smaller alveolus is prevented through the action of pulmonary surfactant, which serves to decrease alveolar surface tension in the smaller alveolus, resulting in equal pressure in both alveoli.

- One of the most important gas laws in physiology is the ideal (or perfect) gas law, PV = nRT (where P = pressure of gas, V = volume of gas, n = number of moles of the gas in volume V, R = gas constant, and T = absolute temperature). This is the equation for ideal gases, which experience no forces of interaction. Real gases, however, experience intermolecular attraction (van der Waals forces), which requires that the pressure-volume gas law be written in a more complex form.
- Most flowmeters measure the drop in pressure that occurs when a gas passes through a known resistance and correlate this pressure drop to flow. When the resistance is an orifice, resistance depends primarily on gas density. Usually, a given flowmeter is calibrated for a particular gas, such as oxygen or air, with conversion tables available to provide flow data for other gases.
- Fick's law of diffusion, applicable to gas flow across lung and placental membranes, states that the rate of diffusion of a gas across a barrier is proportional to the concentration gradient for the gas and inversely proportional to the diffusion distance over which the gas molecules must travel.
- There are five main types of oxygen analyzers: paramagnetic analyzers, fuel cell analyzers, oxygen electrodes, mass spectrometers, and Raman spectrographs. All respond to oxygen partial pressure and not to oxygen concentration.
- The concept of minimum alveolar concentration (MAC) does not apply at higher altitudes and should be replaced by the concept of minimal alveolar partial pressure (MAPP).

The Gas Laws

Ideal Gases

Air is a fluid. Understanding the fundamentals of basic fluid mechanics is essential for grasping the concepts of airway flow. Because air is also a gas, it is important to understand the laws that govern its gaseous behavior. Gases are usually described in terms of pressure, volume, and temperature. Pressure is most often quantified clinically in terms of mm Hg (or torr), volume in mL, and temperature in degrees Celsius. However, calculations often require conversion from one set of units to another and therefore can be quite tedious. We have included a small section at the end of this chapter to simplify these conversions.

Perhaps the most important law governing the state of gas is the ideal gas law, which can be written as follows[1]:

$$PV = nRT \qquad (1)$$

where

P = pressure of gas (pascals or mm Hg)
V = volume of gas (m^3 or cm^3 or mL)
n = number of moles of the gas in volume V
R = gas constant (8.3143 J/mol·K, assuming P in pascals, V in m^3)
T = absolute temperature (in kelvin [K]; 273.16 K = 0°C)

One mole of gas contains 6.023×10^{23} molecules, and this quantity is referred to as *Avogadro's number*. One mole of an ideal gas takes up 22.4138 L at standard temperature and pressure (STP); standard temperature is 273.16 K, and standard pressure is 1 atmosphere (760 mm Hg).[1] Avogadro's law also states that equal volumes of all ideal gases at the same temperature and pressure contain the same number of molecules.

The ideal gas law incorporates the laws of Boyle and Charles.[1] Boyle's law states that, at a constant temperature, the product of pressure and volume (P × V) is equal to a constant. Consequently, P is proportional to 1/V (P ∝ 1/V) at constant T. However, gases do not obey Boyle's law at temperatures approaching their point of liquefaction (i.e., the point at which the gas becomes a liquid).

Boyle's law concerns perfect gases and is not obeyed by real gases over a wide range of pressures (see the following section for a discussion of nonideal gases). However, at infinitely low pressures, all gases obey Boyle's law. Boyle's law does not apply to anesthetic gases and many other gases because of the van der Waals attraction between molecules (i.e., they are nonideal gases).

Charles' law states that, at a constant pressure, volume is proportional to temperature (i.e., V ∝ T at constant P). Gay-Lussac's law states that, at a constant volume, pressure is proportional to temperature (i.e., P ∝ T at constant V).[1] Often, these two laws are shortened for convenience to Charles' law. When a gas obeys both Charles' law and Boyle's law, it is said to be an ideal gas and obeys the ideal gas law.

In clinical situations, gases are typically mixtures of several "pure" gases. Quantifiable properties of mixtures may be determined using Dalton's law of partial pressures. Dalton's law states that the pressure exerted by a mixture of gases is the sum of the pressures exerted by the individual pure gases[1,2]:

$$P_{total} = P_A + P_B + P_C + \cdots + P_N \qquad (2)$$

where P_A, P_B, and P_C are the partial pressures of pure ideal gases.

Nonideal Gases: The van der Waals Effect

Ideal gases have no forces of interaction, but real gases have intermolecular attraction, which requires that the pressure-volume gas law be rewritten as follows[1,2]:

$$\left(P + \frac{a}{V^2}\right) \times (V - b) = nRT \qquad (3)$$

where

P = pressure of gas (pascals or mm Hg)
V = volume of gas (m^3 or cm^3 or mL)
n = number of moles of the gas in volume V
R = gas constant (8.3143 J/mol·K, assuming P in pascals, V in m^3)
T = absolute temperature (K)
a and b = physical constants for a given gas

The values of a and b for a given gas may be found in physical chemistry textbooks and other sources.[1-5] This equation, provided by van der Waals, accounts for intramolecular forces fairly well.

Diffusion of Gases

Clinically, diffusion of gases through a membrane is most applicable to gas flow across lung and placental membranes. The most commonly used relation to govern diffusion is Fick's first law of diffusion, which states that the rate of diffusion of a gas across a barrier is proportional to the concentration gradient for the gas. Fick's law may be expressed mathematically as follows[6]:

$$\text{Flux} = -D\frac{\Delta C}{\Delta X} \tag{4}$$

where

Flux = the number of molecules crossing the membrane each
    second (molecules/cm^2·s)
ΔC = the concentration gradient (molecules/cm^3)
ΔX = the diffusion distance (cm)
D = the diffusion coefficient (cm^2/s)

In general, the value of D is inversely proportional to the gas' molecular weight, as well as intrinsic properties of the membrane.

Because gases partially dissolve when they come into contact with a liquid, Henry's law becomes important in some instances. It states that the mass of a gas dissolved in a given amount of liquid is proportional to the pressure of the gas at constant temperature. As a result, the gas concentration (in solvent) is equal to a constant × P (at constant T).[1]

Pressure, Flow, and Resistance

The laws of fluid mechanics dictate an intricate relationship between pressure, flow, and resistance. Pressure is defined as force per unit area. It is usually measured clinically in mm Hg or cm H$_2$O, but it is most commonly measured scientifically in pascals (Pa), or newtons of force per square meter (1 Pa = 1 N/m^2).

Flow (i.e., the rate of flow) is equal to the change in pressure (pressure drop or pressure difference) divided by the resistance experienced by the fluid. For example, if the flow is 100 mL/s at a pressure difference of 100 mm Hg, the resistance is 100 mm Hg/(100 mL/s), or 1 mm Hg·s/mL. In laminar flow systems only, the resistance is constant, independent of the flow rate.[7,8]

An important formula that quantifies the relationship of pressure, flow, and resistance in laminar flow systems is given by the Hagen-Poiseuille equation. Poiseuille's law states that the fluid flow rate through a horizontal straight tube of uniform bore is proportional to the pressure gradient (ΔP) and the fourth power of the radius (π) and is inversely proportional to the viscosity of the gas (μ, in g/cm·s) and the length of the tube (L, in cm). This law, which is valid for laminar flow only, may be stated as follows[7,8]:

$$\Delta P = \frac{8\mu L}{\pi^4} \times \text{Flow} \tag{5}$$

See the discussion in the section Laminar Flow for further details.

When the flow rate exceeds a critical velocity (the flow velocity below which flow is laminar), the flow loses its laminar parabolic velocity profile, becomes disorderly, and is termed *turbulent* (Fig. 4.1). If turbulent flow exists, the relationship between pressure drop and flow is no longer governed by the Hagen-Poiseuille equation. Instead, the pressure gradient required (or the resistance encountered) during turbulent flow varies as the square of the

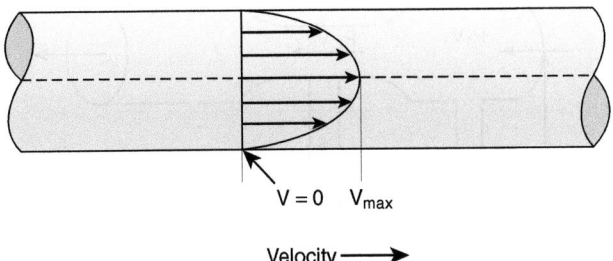

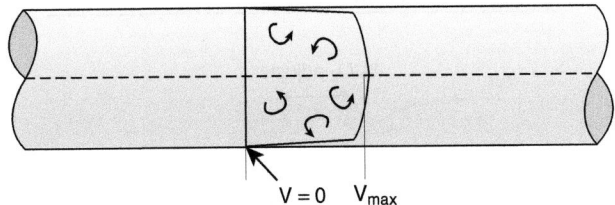

• **Fig. 4.1** Laminar and turbulent flow. *Top,* Laminar flow in a long smooth pipe is characterized by smooth and steady flow with little or no fluctuations. The flow profile is parabolic in nature, with fluid traveling most quickly at the center of the tube and stationary at the edges. *Bottom,* Turbulent flow is characterized by fluctuating and agitated flow. Its flow profile is essentially flat, with all fluid traveling at the same velocity except at tube edges. *V,* Velocity.

flow rate. See the discussion in the section Turbulent Flow for further details.

Viscosity, μ, characterizes the resistance within a fluid to the flow of one layer of molecules over another (shear characteristics).[7] Blood viscosity is influenced primarily by hematocrit, so that at low hematocrit blood flow is easier—that is, blood is more dilute. The critical velocity at which turbulent flow begins depends on the ratio of viscosity (μ) to density (ρ), which is defined as the *kinematic viscosity* (υ)—that is, $\upsilon = \mu/\rho$. (This is illustrated with an example in the section entitled Turbulent Flow.)[7–9] The unit for viscosity is g/cm·s (poise). The typical unit for kinematic viscosity is cm^2/s.

The viscosity of water is 0.01 poise at 25°C and 0.007 poise at 37°C. The viscosity of air is 183 micropoise at 18°C.[10]

Density is defined as mass per unit volume (g/cm^3 or g/mL). The density of water is 1 g/mL. The general relation for the density of a gas is given by the following equation:

$$D = D_0\left(\frac{T_0 P}{T P_0}\right) \tag{6}$$

where D_0 is a known density of the gas at temperature T_0 and pressure P_0, and D is the density of the gas at temperature T and pressure P. For dry air at 18°C and 760 mm Hg (atmospheric pressure), D = 1.213 g/L.[4]

The fall in pressure at points of flow constriction (where the flow velocity is higher) is known as the *Bernoulli effect* (Fig. 4.2).[7,8] This phenomenon is used in devices employing the Venturi principle, such as gas nebulizers, Venturi flowmeters, and some oxygen face masks. The lower pressure related to the Bernoulli effect sucks in (entrains) air to mix with oxygen.

One final consideration that is important in the study of the airway is Laplace's law for a sphere (Fig. 4.3). It states that, for a sphere with one air-liquid interface (e.g., an alveolus), the relation

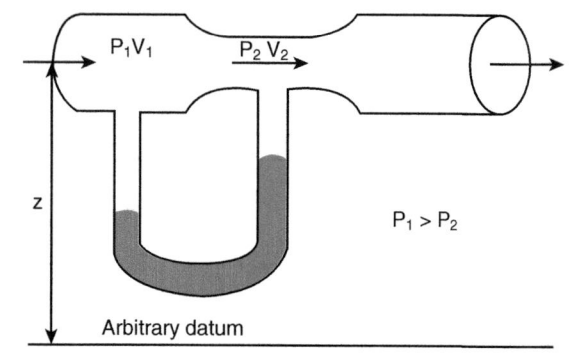

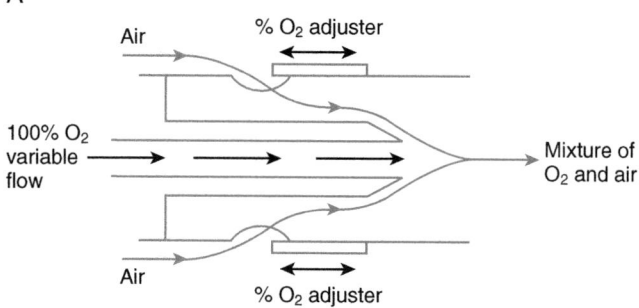

• **Fig. 4.2** Bernoulli effect. (A) Diagram shows fluid flow through a tube with varying diameters. At the point of flow constriction, fluid pressure is less than at the distal end of the tube, as indicated by the height of the manometer fluid column. This effect is described by the Bernoulli equation. In the case of a horizontal pipe, the distance between the centerline of the pipe and an arbitrary datum at two different points will be the same (z). (B) Venturi tube. The lower pressure caused by the Bernoulli effect entrains air to mix with oxygen. *P*, Pressure; *V*, velocity.

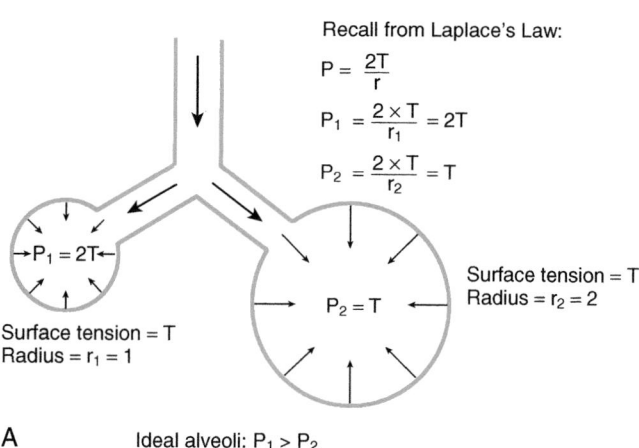

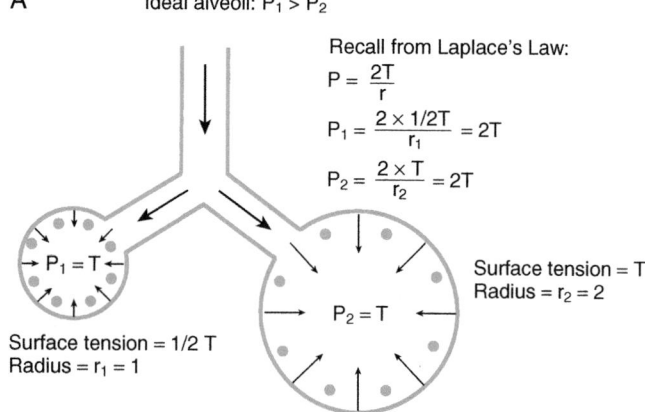

• **Fig. 4.3** Laplace's law for a sphere. (A) Laplace's law dictates that for two alveoli of unequal size but equal surface tension, the smaller alveolus experiences a larger intraalveolar pressure than the larger alveolus. This causes air to pass into the larger alveolus and causes the smaller alveolus to collapse. (B) Collapse of the smaller alveolus is prevented through the action of pulmonary surfactant. Surfactant serves to decrease alveolar surface tension in the smaller alveolus, which results in equal pressure in both alveoli. *P*, Transmural pressure difference; *r*, sphere radius; *T*, surface tension.

between the transmural pressure difference, surface tension, and sphere radius is described by the following equation[11]:

$$P = \frac{2T}{r} \tag{7}$$

where

P = transmural pressure difference (dynes/cm^2; 1 dyne/cm^2 = 0.1 Pa = 0.000751 torr)
T = surface tension (dynes/cm)
r = sphere radius (cm)

The key point in Laplace's law is that the smaller the sphere radius, the higher the transmural pressure. However, real (in vivo) alveoli do not obey Laplace's law because of the action of pulmonary surfactant, which decreases the surface tension disproportionately compared with what is predicted on the basis of physical principles. When pulmonary surfactant is missing from the lungs, the lungs take on the behavior described by Laplace's law.

Example: Transtracheal Jet Ventilation

Transtracheal jet ventilation (TTJV) can be used to oxygenate and ventilate patients in an emergent "cannot intubate, cannot oxygenate" (CICO) scenario.[6] It is a temporizing measure that is used only until an airway can be secured. It is usually employed using equipment commonly available in the operating or emergency room and often using the 50-psi wall oxygen source.[6,12–14]

Analysis

The gas flow through a catheter depends on both the resistance of the catheter–connection hose assembly and the driving pressure applied to it. If the resistance of the assembly is R, the flow (F) from the catheter is F = P$_d$/R, where P$_d$ is the pressure difference between the ends of the catheter-connection assembly. R itself certainly depends on F when the flow becomes turbulent, but the flow relationship still holds. However, P$_d$ is very close to the driving pressure (P) applied to the ventilation catheter, because the lung offers little relative back pressure. (At back pressures greater than 100 cm H$_2$O, the lung is likely to burst, and P is often chosen to be 50 psi, or about 3500 cm H$_2$O.) Therefore, the flow relationship may be simplified to F = P/R.

Next, TTJV is applied through a sequence of "jet pulses," each resulting in a given tidal volume (e.g., 500 mL). Ignoring entrained air effects, the delivered tidal volume is equal to catheter flow × pulse duration. For a catheter flow of 30 L/min, a jet pulse lasting 1 second results in a tidal volume of 30 L/min × $\frac{1}{60}$ min = 0.5 L.

In a TTJV setup consisting of a 14-G angiocatheter connected to a regulated oxygen source by a 4.5-foot polyvinyl chloride

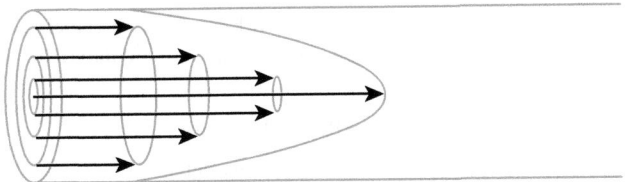

• **Fig. 4.4** Laminar flow. Laminar gas flow through long straight tube of uniform bore has a velocity profile that is parabolic in shape, with the gas traveling most quickly at the center of the tube. Conceptually, it is helpful to view laminar gas flow as a series of concentric cylinders of gas, with the central cylinder moving most rapidly. (From Nunn JF. *Nunn's Applied Respiratory Physiology*. 4th ed. Butterworth-Heinemann; 1993.)

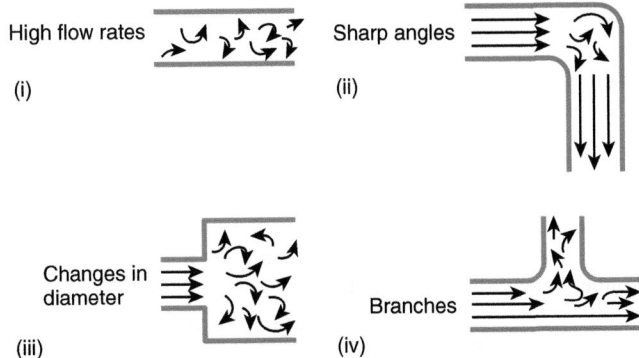

• **Fig. 4.5** Turbulent flow. Four circumstances likely to produce turbulent flow. (From Nunn JF. *Nunn's Applied Respiratory Physiology*. 4th ed. Butterworth-Heinemann; 1993.)

(PVC) tube of $\frac{7}{32}$-inch inner diameter (ID), for oxygen flows between 10 and 60 L/min, the resistance was found to be relatively constant between 0.6 and 0.8 psi/L/min.[15]

Many systems for TTJV choose 50 psi for convenience (50 psi being the oxygen wall outlet pressure), although a regulator is very often used to permit lower pressures. However, 50 psi may not be an optimal pressure choice for TTJV. Using the preceding data, the pressure required for TTJV for a tidal volume of 500 mL can be calculated. Assuming that the setup resistance is 0.7 psi/L/min and the desired flow rate is 30 L/min, the driving pressure should be $0.7 \times 30 = 21$ psi.

Similar analyses can be carried out for other arrangements derived from experiments to obtain resistance data.

Gas Flow

Laminar Flow

In laminar flow, fluid particles flow along smooth paths in layers, or laminas, with one layer gliding smoothly over an adjacent layer.[7] Any tendencies toward instability and turbulence are damped out by viscous shear forces that resist the relative motion of adjacent fluid layers. Under laminar flow conditions through a tube, the flow velocity is greatest at the center of the tube flow and zero at the inner edge of the tube (Fig. 4.4; see also Fig. 4.1). The flow profile has a parabolic shape. Under these conditions in a horizontal tube, the relation between flow, tube, and gas characteristics is given by the Hagen-Poiseuille equation (Eq. 5), restated as follows[7-9]:

$$\dot{V} = \frac{\pi \Delta \mathrm{Pr}^4}{8 \mu L} \tag{8}$$

where

$\dot{V}$ = flow rate (cm³/s)
π = 3.1416
ΔP = pressure gradient (Pa)
r = tube radius (cm)
L = tube length (cm)
μ = gas viscosity (g/cm·s)

Typical units are shown in parentheses. The dot indicates rate of change: V represents volume, and $\dot{V}$ represents the *rate of change of volume*, or *flow rate*. Another way of looking at this concept is that, under conditions of laminar flow through a tube of known radius, the pressure difference across the tube is given by the following proportionality (which is also essentially the same as Eq. 5):

$$\Delta \mathrm{Pressure} \propto \frac{\mathrm{Flow} \times \mathrm{Viscosity} \times \mathrm{Length}}{\mathrm{Radius}^4} \tag{9}$$

The pressure gradient through the airway increases proportionately with flow, viscosity, and tube length but increases exponentially as the tube radius decreases.

The conditions under which flow through a tube is predominantly laminar can be estimated from *critical flow* rates. The critical flow is the flow rate below which flow is predominantly laminar in a given airflow situation.

Laminar Flow Example

Assume a tube of uniform bore that is 1 cm in diameter and 3 m in length. A pressure difference of 5 cm H_2O exists between the ends of the tube, and air is the fluid flowing through the tube. Assuming laminar flow, what flow rate should be expected?

Answer:

The relevant variables are expressed in the centimeter-gram-second (CGS) system of units:

r = 0.5 cm
L = 3000 cm
μ = 183 micropoise = 183×10^{-6} poise = 183×10^{-6} g/cm·s
ΔP = 0.5 cm H_2O = 490 dynes/cm²

Using the Hagen-Poiseuille equation, the laminar flow is determined as follows:

$$\mathrm{Flow} = \frac{\pi \times 490 \times (0.5)^4}{8 \times 183 \times 10^{-6} \times 3000} = 219.06 \, \mathrm{cm}^3/\mathrm{s} \tag{10}$$

Turbulent Flow

Flow in a tube below the critical flow rate remains mostly laminar. However, at flows greater than the critical flow rate, the flow becomes increasingly turbulent. Under turbulent flow conditions, the parabolic flow pattern is lost, and the resistance to flow increases with flow itself. Turbulence may also be created where sharp angles, changes in diameter, and branches are encountered (Fig. 4.5). The flow-pressure drop relationship is given approximately by the following equation[7,8]:

$$V \propto \sqrt{\Delta P} \tag{11}$$

where

V = mean fluid velocity (cm/s)
ΔP = pressure (Pa)

Reynolds Number Calculation Example

The Reynolds number (Re) represents the ratio of inertial forces to viscous forces.[7,8,16] It is useful because it characterizes the flow through a long, straight tube of uniform bore. It is a dimensionless number having the following form:

$$Re = \frac{V \times D \times \rho}{\mu} = \frac{V \times D}{v} = \frac{2 \times \dot{V} \times \rho}{\pi \times r \times \mu} \quad (12)$$

where

Re = Reynolds number
$\dot{V}$ = flow rate (mL/s)
ρ = density (g/mL)
μ = viscosity (poise or g/cm·s)
r = radius (cm)
v = kinematic viscosity (cm²/s) = μ/ρ
D = diameter (cm)
V = mean fluid velocity (cm/s)

Typical units are shown in brackets. For tubes that are long compared with their diameter (i.e., length ÷ diameter >0.06 × Re),[8] the flow is laminar when Re is less than 2000. For shorter tubes, flow is turbulent at Re values as low as 280.

When a tube's radius exceeds its length, it is an orifice; flow through an orifice is always turbulent. Under these conditions, the flow is influenced by the density rather than the viscosity of the fluid.[17] This characteristic explains why a helium-oxygen mixture (heliox) flows better in a narrow edematous glottis: as the following data suggest, helium has a very low density and thus presents less resistance to flow through an orifice.

	Viscosity at 20°C	Density at 20°C
Helium	194.1 micropoise	0.179 g/L
Oxygen	210.8 micropoise	1.429 g/L

How can one predict whether a given gas flow through an endotracheal tube (ETT) is laminar or turbulent? One approach is first to identify the physical conditions. For example, consider the case of an ETT with a 6-mm ID and a length of 27 cm through which 60 L/min of air is passing. In this setting,

L = 27 cm
r = 0.3 cm (size 6.0 ETT)
flow ($\dot{V}$) = 60 L/min = 1000 mL/s
viscosity (μ) = 183 micropoise = 183 × 10⁻⁶ g/cm·s (air at 18°C)
density (ρ) = 1.21 g/L = 0.001213 g/mL (dry air at 18°C)

With this information, one can calculate the Reynolds number:

$$Re = \frac{2 \times 1000 \times 0.001213}{\pi \times 0.3 \times 183 \times 10^{-6}} = 1.41 \times 10^{4} \quad (13)$$

Because this number greatly exceeds 2000, flow is probably quite turbulent.

Critical Velocity

The critical velocity is the point at which the transition from laminar to turbulent flow begins. This point is reached when Re becomes the critical Reynolds number, Re_{crit}. Critical velocity, the flow velocity below which flow is laminar, is calculated by the following equation[8]:

$$V_{crit} = V_{c} = \frac{Re_{crit} \times Viscosity}{Density \times Diameter} \quad (14)$$

where, Re_{crit} = 2000 for circular tubes.

As can be seen from this equation, the critical velocity is proportional to the viscosity of the gas and is related inversely to the density of the gas and the radius of the tube. Viscosity has the dimensions of pascal-second (Pa·s) (equivalent to N·s/m², or kg/m·s).

The critical velocity at which turbulent flow begins depends on the ratio of viscosity to density—that is, μ/ρ. This ratio is known as the *kinematic viscosity*, v, and has typical units of centimeters squared per second (cm²/s). The actual measurement of viscosity of a fluid is carried out with the use of a viscometer, which consists of two rotary cylinders with the test fluid flowing between.

Critical Velocity Calculation Example

Using the same data as in the previous Reynolds number calculation, one can calculate the critical velocity at which laminar flow starts to become turbulent:

$$V_{c} = \frac{2000 \times \left(183 \times 10^{-6} \, poise\right)}{\left(0.001213 \, g/cm^{3}\right) \times \left(2 \times 0.3 \, cm\right)}$$

$$V_{c} = 502.8 \frac{poise}{\left(g/cm^{3}\right) \times cm} = 502.8 \frac{cm}{s} \quad (15)$$

Flow Through an Orifice

Flow through an orifice (defined as flow through a tube whose length is smaller than its radius) is always somewhat turbulent.[17] Clinically, airway-obstructing conditions such as epiglottitis or swallowed obstructions are often best viewed as breathing through an orifice. Under such conditions, the approximate flow across the orifice varies inversely with the square root of the gas density:

$$\dot{V} \propto \frac{1}{\sqrt{Gas \, density}} \quad (16)$$

This is in contrast to laminar flow conditions, in which gas flow varies inversely with gas viscosity. The viscosity values for helium and oxygen are similar, but their densities are very different (Table 4.1). Table 4.2 provides useful data to allow comparison of gas flow rates through an orifice.[18]

TABLE 4.1	Viscosity and Density Differences of Anesthetic Gases	
	Viscosity at 300 K (µPa × s)	Density at 20°C (g/L)
Air	18.6	1.293
Nitrogen	17.9	1.250
Nitrous oxide	15.0	1.965
Helium	20.0	0.178
Oxygen	20.8	1.429

Data from Haynes WM. *CRC Handbook of Chemistry and Physics.* 91st ed. CRC Press; 2010, and Streeter VL, Wylie EB, Bedford KW. *Fluid Mechanics.* 9th ed. McGraw-Hill; 1998.

TABLE 4.2	Gas Flow Rates Through an Orifice			
	%	Density (g/L)	(Density)$^{-1/2}$	Relative Flow
Air	100	1.293	0.881	1.0
Oxygen	100	1.429	0.846	0.96
Helium (He)	100	0.179	2.364	2.68
He-oxygen	20/80	1.178	0.922	1.048
He-oxygen	60/40	0.678	1.215	1.381
He-oxygen	80/20	0.429	1.527	1.73

From Rudow M, Hill AB, Thompson NW, et al. Helium-oxygen mixtures in airway obstruction due to thyroid carcinoma. *Can Anaesth Soc J.* 1986;33:498.

Helium-Oxygen Mixtures

The low density of helium allows it to play a significant clinical role in the management of some forms of airway obstruction.[19–22] For instance, Rudow and colleagues described the use of heliox mixtures in a patient with severe airway obstruction related to a large thyroid mass (see the following section for clinical examples).[18]

The available percentage mixtures of helium and oxygen are typically 80:20 and 70:30. These mixtures are usually administered by a rebreathing face mask to patients who have an increased work of breathing due to airway pathology (e.g., edema) but for whom it is preferable to withhold endotracheal intubation at the time.

Although the use of heliox mixtures in patients with upper airway obstruction has had considerable success, the hope that this approach would also work well for patients with severe asthma has not been borne out. In a systematic review of seven clinical trials involving 392 patients with acute asthma, the authors cautioned, "existing evidence does not provide support for the administration of helium-oxygen mixtures to emergency department patients with moderate-to-severe acute asthma."[23] A similar study noted that "heliox may offer mild-to-moderate benefits in patients with acute asthma within the first hour of use, but its advantages become less apparent beyond 1 hour, as most conventionally treated patients improve to similar levels, with or without it"; however, the authors suggested that its effect "may be more pronounced in more severe cases." They concluded, "There are insufficient data on whether heliox can avert endotracheal intubation, or change intensive care and hospital admission rates and duration, or mortality."[24]

Clinical Vignettes

Rudow and colleagues reported the following clinical illustration of heliox therapy.[18] A 78-year-old woman with both breast cancer and ophthalmic melanoma developed airway obstruction from a thyroid carcinoma that extended into her mediastinum and compressed her trachea. She had a 2-month history of worsening dyspnea, especially when positioned supine. On examination, inspiratory stridor and expiratory stridor were present. The chest radiograph showed a large superior mediastinal mass and pulmonary metastases. A solid mass was identified on a thyroid ultrasound scan. Computed tomography revealed a large mass at the thoracic inlet and extending caudally. Clinically, the patient was exhausted and in respiratory distress.

A 78:22 heliox mixture was administered and provided almost instant relief, with improvements in measured tidal volume and oxygenation. Later, a thyroidectomy was carried out to alleviate the obstruction. For this procedure, topical anesthesia was applied to the airway and awake laryngoscopy and intubation were performed with the patient in the sitting position. After the airway was secured with the use of an armored tube, the patient was given a general anesthetic by intravenous induction. Extubation after the surgery was performed without complication.

Another interesting clinical scenario was published by Khanlou and Eiger.[25] They presented the case of a 69-year-old woman in whom bilateral vocal cord paralysis developed after radiation therapy. Heliox was successfully used for temporary management of the resultant upper airway obstruction until the patient was able to receive a tracheostomy.

A final clinical vignette was reported by Polaner,[26] who used a laryngeal mask airway (LMA) and an 80:20 heliox mixture to administer anesthesia to a 3-year-old boy with asthma and a large anterior mediastinal mass. Clinical management involved an unusual combination of management strategies: The child was kept in the sitting position, spontaneous ventilation with a halothane-in-heliox inhalation induction was used, and airway stimulation was minimized by use of an LMA. However, the author cautioned that cases such as these can readily take a deadly turn, noting that "one must, of course, always be prepared to intervene with either manipulations of patient position in the event of airway compromise (including upright, lateral, and prone) or more aggressive strategies, such as rigid bronchoscopy and even median sternotomy (in the case of intractable cardiovascular collapse), or to allow the patient to awaken if critical airway or cardiovascular compromise becomes evident at any time during the course of the anesthesia."[26]

Pressure Differences

From the analysis of equations governing laminar flow and turbulent flow, the pressure drop along the noncompliant portion of the airway is given approximately by the Rohrer equation[27]:

$$\Delta P = K_1 \dot{V} + K_2 \dot{V}^2 \qquad (17)$$

K_1 and K_2 are known as *Rohrer's constants*, where K_1 is the coefficient of laminar flow and K_2 is the coefficient of turbulent flow. The physical interpretation of this equation is that airway pressure is governed by the sum of two terms:
1. effects proportional to gas flow (laminar flow effects)
2. effects proportional to the square of the gas flow (turbulent flow effects)

It can be seen that the lowest pressure loss across the airway (ΔP) would occur when $\dot{V}$ is small (i.e., with predominantly laminar flow). However, it is known that under conditions of laminar flow, K_1 is largely influenced by viscosity rather than density, and K_2 (the turbulent term) is influenced primarily by density and not viscosity.

Resistance to Gas Flow

When pressure readings are taken at each end of a horizontal tube with a fluid flowing through it, one notices that they are not identical: the pressure at the distal end of the tube is less than the pressure at the proximal end (with fluid flowing from the proximal to the distal end). This pressure loss is attributable to frictional losses incurred by the fluid when in contact with the inside of the tube. This is analogous to heat losses incurred by resistors in an electrical circuit (Fig. 4.6).

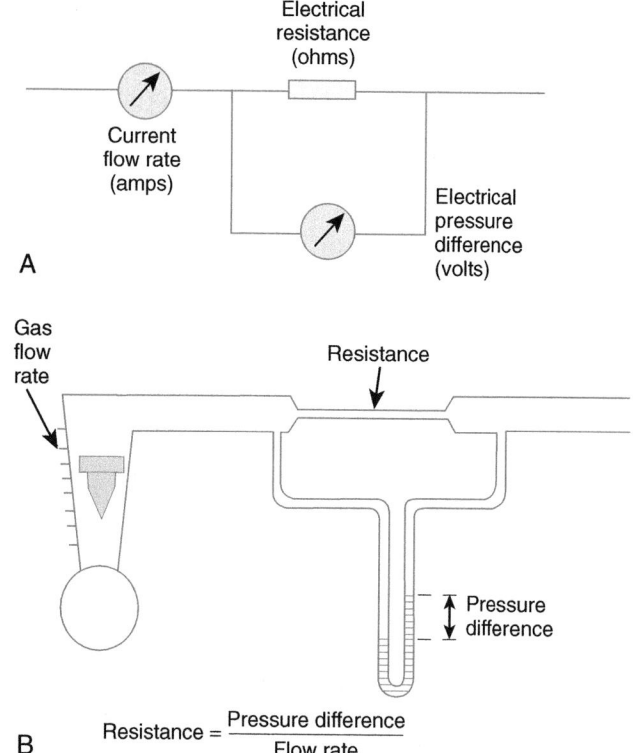

A

B

$$\text{Resistance} = \frac{\text{Pressure difference}}{\text{Flow rate}}$$

• **Fig. 4.6** Analogy between laminar gas flow and flow of electricity through a resistor. (A) Electrical flow rate (current) is measured in amperes; pressure difference (voltage) is measured in volts; resistance is measured in ohms and described by Ohm's law. (B) Gas flow rate is measured as volume/second (e.g., mL/s); pressure difference is measured as force/area (e.g., dynes/cm²); resistance is described by Poiseuille's law. For gases, pressure difference = flow rate × resistance; for electricity, potential difference (voltage) = current × resistance. (From Nunn JF. *Nunn's Applied Respiratory Physiology*. 4th ed. Butterworth-Heinemann; 1993.)

Frictional losses are irreversible—that is, the energy lost cannot be recovered by the fluid and is mostly lost as heat. If the tube is not horizontal, there are additional pressure differences attributable to height differences. The most common relation that describes the flow in a tube is the Bernoulli equation, which is valid for both laminar and turbulent flow[8]:

$$\frac{V_1^2}{2g} + \frac{P_1}{\rho g} + Z_1 = \frac{V_2^2}{2g} + \frac{P_2}{\rho g} + Z_2 + h_f \qquad (18)$$

where

V = velocity (m/s)
g = gravitational constant (9.81 m/s² or 9.81 N/kg)
P = pressure (pascals or N/m²)
ρ = density of fluid (kg/m³)
Z = height from an arbitrary point (datum) (m)
h_f = frictional losses (m)

Typical units are shown in parentheses. Eq. 18 is in units of meters and is termed *meters of head loss*. This is typical of fluid mechanics equations. As mentioned previously, the Bernoulli equation is valid for both laminar and turbulent flow.

Endotracheal Tube Resistance

ETTs, like all tubes, provide resistance to fluid flow (Fig. 4.7). However, ETTs do not add external resistance to the normal airway; rather, they act as a substitute for the normal resistance of the airway from the mouth to the trachea, which accounts for 30% to 40% of normal airway resistance.[28] This is important because, although they can overcome impedance to inspiratory flow during extended periods of artificial respiration, mechanical ventilators do not augment passive exhalation. Resistance to exhalation through a long, small-diameter ETT, which is compounded by turbulence, can seriously constrain ventilation rate and tidal volume.[29,30]

The use of an ETT influences respiration in a number of ways. First, it decreases effective airway diameter and therefore increases the resistance to breathing. Resistance is further increased by the curved nature of the tube; resistance measurements are typically about 3% higher than if the tubes were straight.[31] Also, the passage from the mouth to the larynx is not a smooth curve and may create additional turbulence. Second, studies show that intubated patients experience decreased peak flow rates (inspiratory and expiratory), decreased forced vital capacity, and decreased forced expiratory volume in 1 second (FEV_1).[32] However, the tube may paradoxically increase peak flow rates during forced expiration by preventing dynamic compression of the trachea.[32] Finally, the tube may cause mechanical irritation of the larynx and trachea that may lead to a reflex constriction of the airway distal to the tube.[33]

The combination of tube and connector may cause higher resistance than the tube alone. Moreover, because of turbulence at component connections, the total resistance of a system is not necessarily the sum of the resistances of its component parts, especially if sharp-angled connectors are used (see Fig. 4.5).[25,34] In addition, humidified gases contribute to slightly higher resistances because of the increased density of moist gas, and the resistance of single-lumen tubes is generally lower than that of double-lumen tubes.[35]

The resistance associated with ETTs may be reduced by increasing the tube diameter, decreasing tube length, or decreasing the gas density (hence, the occasional use of heliox mixtures). It has been suggested that the presence of an ETT may double the work of breathing in chronically intubated adults and may lead to respiratory failure in some infants.[31] Therefore it is important to use as large an ETT as is practical in patients who exhibit respiratory dysfunction.

ETT resistance can be measured in the laboratory using differential pressure and flow measurement techniques,[36,37] most commonly by the method of Gaensler and colleagues.[38] Theoretical estimates of resistance under laminar flow conditions can also be obtained by using the Hagen-Poiseuille equation. In vivo measurements of ETT resistance are generally higher than in vitro measurements, perhaps because of secretions, head or neck position, tube deformation, or increased turbulence.[10,39]

Airway resistance may be established from first principles using Poiseuille's law if the gas flow is laminar. If the gas flow is turbulent, resistance is no longer dependent on material properties, and empirical measurements become the only feasible means of characterizing resistance. Intrinsic airway resistance is determined by measuring the transairway pressure—that is, the pressure drop between the airway opening and the alveoli. The following relationship applies[40]:

$$R = \frac{P_{airway} - P_{alveolar}}{\dot{V}} \qquad (19)$$

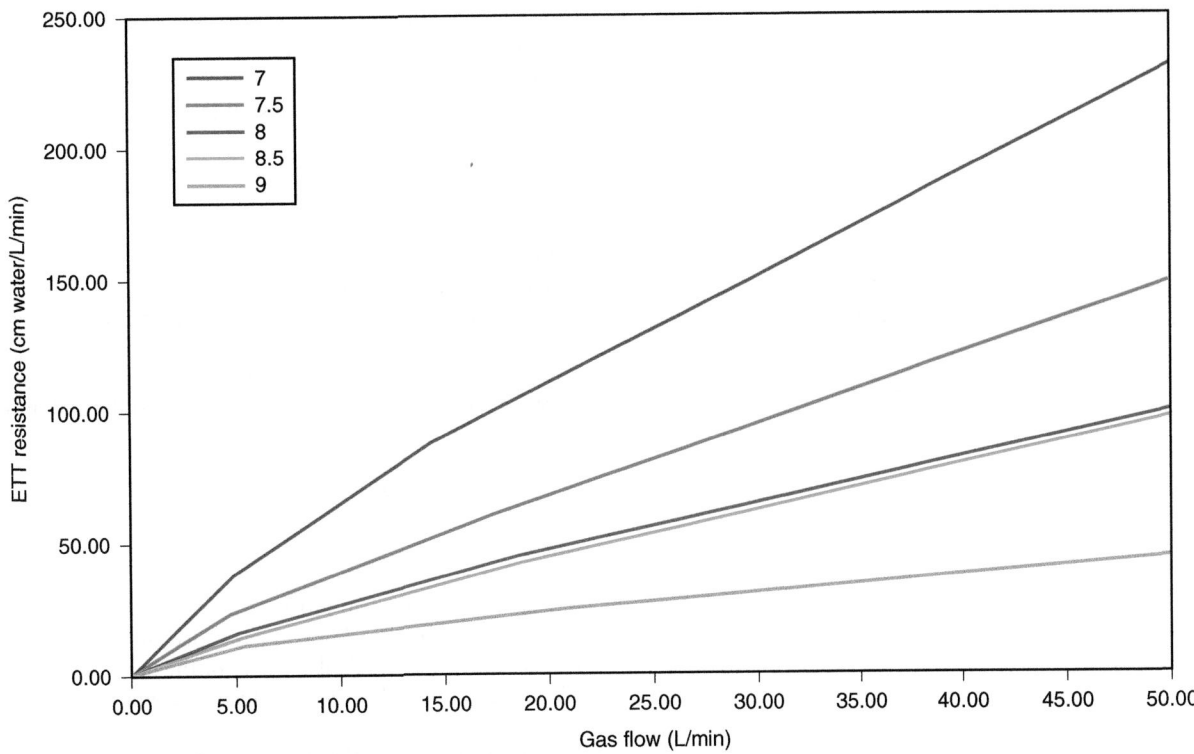

• **Fig. 4.7** Dependence of endotracheal tube (ETT) on flow. The data provided by Hicks in Table 4.3 can be used to show that ETT resistance increases nonlinearly with flow (because of turbulence effects). For pure laminar flow, resistance would be constant, regardless of flow.

where

R = airway resistance (cm $H_2O \cdot s/L$)
P_{airway} = proximal airway pressure (cm H_2O)
$P_{alveolar}$ = alveolar pressure (cm H_2O)
$\dot{V}$ = gas flow rate (L/s)

Typical units used are shown in parentheses.

In clinical practice, airway resistance is most easily determined by using a whole-body plethysmograph. However, this apparatus is unsuitable for critically ill patients. An alternative method of presenting airway resistance was provided by Hicks,[40] who used the following equation and constants:

$$\Delta P = a\,\dot{V}^b \qquad (20)$$

where

ΔP = pressure difference (cm H_2O)
$\dot{V}$ = gas flow (L/min)
a and b = empirical constants

The values for the coefficients a and b depend on tube size and are provided in Table 4.3.

Fig. 4.7 depicts the effects of tube diameter and flow rate on ETT resistance. Notice that resistance is increased as a result of increasing turbulence caused by decreasing ETT diameter and increasing flow rate.

Clinically, the issue of ETT resistance is perhaps most important in pediatrics and during T-piece trials. In a laboratory study, Manczur and colleagues sought to determine the resistances of ETTs commonly used in neonatal and pediatric intensive care

TABLE 4.3	Coefficients for Airway Resistance Computations	
Tube	a	b
7.0	9.78	1.81
7.5	7.73	1.75
8.0	5.90	1.72
8.5	4.61	1.78
9.0	3.90	1.63

From Hicks GH: Monitoring respiratory mechanics. *Probl Respir Care.* 1989;2:191.

units.[41] They examined straight tubes with IDs of 2.5 to 6 mm and shouldered (Cole) tubes with ratios of ID to outer diameter ranging from 2.5:4 mm to 3.5:5 mm. Predictably, they found that resistance increased as ETT diameter decreased. The resistances of the 6-mm ID ETTs were 3.1 and 4.6 cm $H_2O \cdot s/L$ at flows of 5 and 10 L/min, respectively, and the resistances of the 2.5-mm ID ETT were 81.2 and 139.4 cm $H_2O \cdot s/L$, respectively. The authors reported that shortening an ETT to a length appropriate for the patient (e.g., shortening a 4.0-mm ID ETT from 20.7 to 11.3 cm) reduced resistance on average by 22%. They also noted that the resistance of a Cole tube was "about 50% lower than that of a straight tube with an ID corresponding to the narrow part of the shouldered tube."

Using an acoustic reflection research method, Straus and colleagues sought to study the influence of ETT resistance during T-piece trials by comparing the work of breathing in 14 successfully

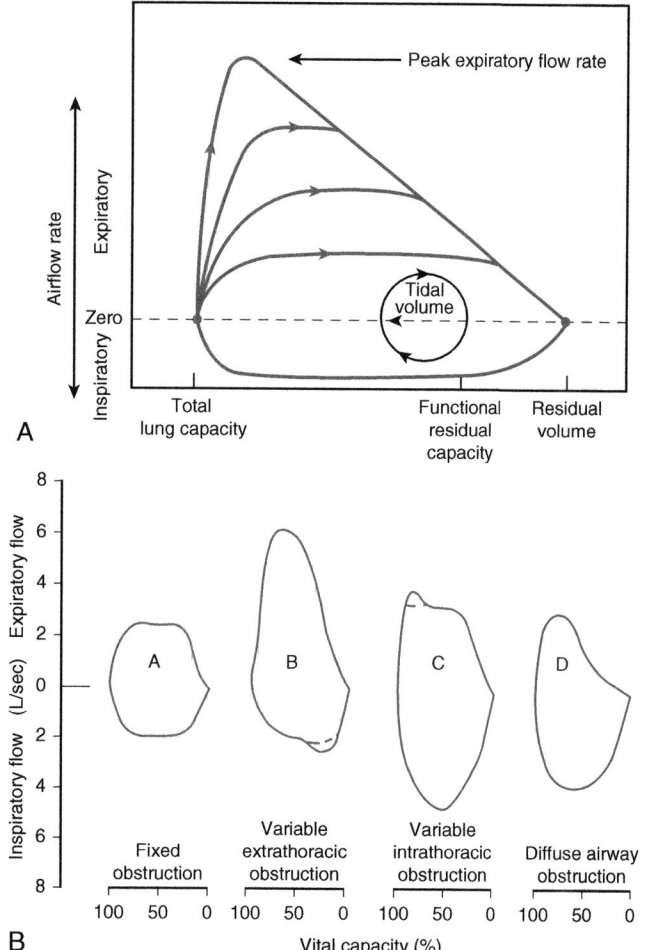

B

| | 100 | 50 | 0 | 100 | 50 | 0 | 100 | 50 | 0 | 100 | 50 | 0 |

Vital capacity (%)

• **Fig. 4.8** Flow-volume curves. (A) A flow-volume curve consists of a plot of gas flow against lung volume. Four loops are shown, corresponding to four different levels of expiratory effort. Peak expiratory flow is effort dependent, but toward the end of expiration the curves converge (as flow is limited by dynamic airway collapse). From a diagnostic viewpoint, the expiratory portion of the loop is of more value than the inspiratory portion. (B) Maximum inspiratory and expiratory flow-volume curves (flow-volume loops) in four types of airway obstruction. (A, From Nunn JF. *Nunn's Applied Respiratory Physiology*. 4th ed. Butterworth-Heinemann; 1993. B, From Gal TJ. *Anesthesia*. 2nd ed. Churchill Livingstone; 1986.)

extubated patients at the end of a 2-hour trial and after extubation.[42] They found that the work of breathing was identical in both groups and there was no significant difference between the beginning and the end of the T-piece trial. The work caused by the ETT amounted to about 11.0% of the total work of breathing, and the supralaryngeal airway resistance was significantly smaller than the ETT resistance. The authors concluded that "a 2-hour trial of spontaneous breathing through an ETT well mimics the work of breathing performed after extubation, in patients who pass a weaning trial and do not require reintubation."

Work of Breathing

Breathing comprises a two-part cycle: inspiration and expiration. During normal breathing, inspiration is an active, energy-consuming process, and expiration is ordinarily a passive process in which the diaphragm and intercostal muscles relax (Figs. 4.8

and 4.9). However, expiration becomes an active process during forced expiration, such as during exercise or during expiration against a resistance load. Several studies have examined the work of breathing in various clinical settings.[43–48]

Considering only normal breathing, the work of breathing is given by the following formulas:

work = force × distance
force = pressure × area
distance = volume ÷ area
work = (pressure × area) × (volume/area) = pressure × volume

Because the air pressure in the lung varies with lung volume and pressure measurements are obtained distal to the end of the ETT, work may be expressed as follows[49]:

$$\text{WORK}_{\text{INSPIRATION}} = \int_{\text{FRC}}^{\text{FRC+TV}} P\,dV \tag{21}$$

where

P = airway pressure (cm H_2O)
dV = (infinitesimal) volume of gas added to the lung (mL)
FRC = functional residual capacity of the lungs (mL)
TV = tidal volume breathed in during respiration (mL)

When the pressure varies as a function of time, Eq. 21 may be integrated in the following manner:

$$\text{Let } dV = \frac{dV}{dt} \times dt = \dot{V}dt \tag{22}$$

Changing the limits of integration yields the following:

$$\text{WORK}_{\text{INSPIRATION}} = \int_{t_1}^{t_2} P(t)\,\dot{V}(t)\,dt \tag{23}$$

where

t_1 = time at the beginning of inspiration (s)
t_2 = time at the end of inspiration (s)
P = pressure measured at a point of interest in the airway (e.g., at the tip of the ETT or at the carina) (cm H_2O)
$\dot{V}$ = flow (mL/s)

The preceding equation is cumbersome to integrate quickly. However, it is sometimes reasonable to assume that the pressure during inspiration remains fairly constant. Under these circumstances, integration of the original work equation during constant-pressure inspiration yields the following approximation:

$$\text{WORK}_{\text{INSPIRATION}} = P_{\text{AVE}} \times TV \tag{24}$$

where

P_{AVE} = mean airway pressure during inspiration (cm H_2O)
TV = tidal volume of inspiration (mL)

During anesthesia, an ETT is often inserted, and additional energy is required to overcome the friction effects of the ETT. The added work of breathing presented by an ETT is given by the following equation:

$$\text{WORK}_{\text{ETT}} = \int_{\text{FRC}}^{\text{FRC+TV}} \Delta P\,dV \tag{25}$$

where ΔP is the pressure drop across the tube.

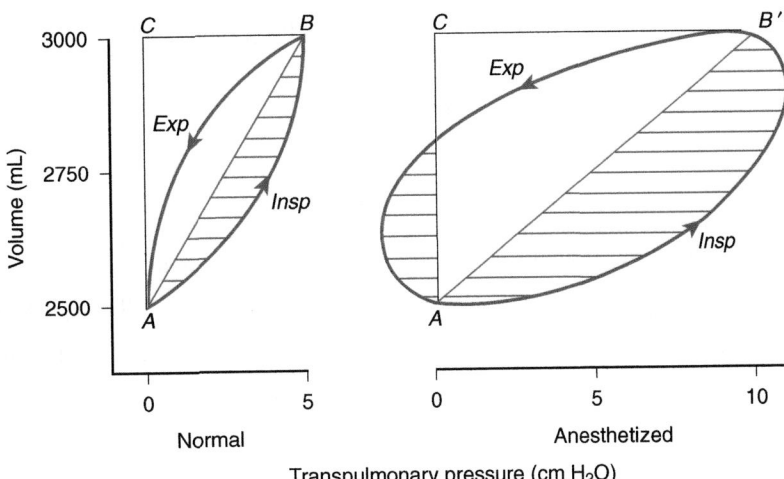

• **Fig. 4.9** Work of breathing. Lung volume is plotted against transpulmonary pressure in a pressure-volume diagram for an awake *(Normal)* patient and an anesthetized *(Anesthetized)* patient. The total area within the oval and triangles has the dimensions of pressure multiplied by volume and represents the total work of breathing. The hatched area to the right of lines *AB* and *AB'* represents the active inspiratory work necessary to overcome resistance to airflow during inspiration *(Insp)*. The hatched area to the left of the triangle *AB'C* represents the active expiratory work necessary to overcome resistance to airflow during expiration *(Exp)* in the anesthetized subject. Expiration is passive in the normal subject because sufficient potential energy is stored during inspiration to produce expiratory airflow. The fraction of total inspiratory work necessary to overcome elastic resistance is shown by triangles *ABC* and *AB'C*. The anesthetized patient has decreased compliance and increased elastic resistance work (triangle *AB'C*) compared with the normal patient's compliance and elastic resistance work (triangle *ABC*). The anesthetized patient shown has increased airway resistance to both inspiratory and expiratory work. (From Benumof JL. *Anesthesia.* 2nd ed. Churchill Livingstone; 1986.)

Often, the pressure gradient ΔP is relatively constant during inspiration, and therefore:

$$WORK_{ETT} = \Delta P \int_{FRC}^{FRC+TV} dV = \Delta P \times \Delta V \quad (26)$$

where

ΔP = pressure drop across ETT during inspiration (mm Hg)
ΔV = volume added to lungs = tidal volume (mL)

The total work done, measured in joules (kg·m²/s²), is as follows:

$$WORK_{TOTAL} = WORK_{ETT} + WORK_{INSPIRATION} \quad (27)$$

Pulmonary Biomechanics

Respiratory Mechanics Equation

Approximately 3% of the body's total energy is required to maintain normal respiratory function.[11] Energy is required to overcome three main forces: (1) the elastic resistance of the lungs, which restores the lungs to their original size after inflation; (2) the force required to move the rib cage, diaphragm, and appropriate visceral contents; and (3) the dissipative resistance of the airway and any breathing apparatus.[50] The respiratory system is commonly modeled as the frictional airway (R_L) that is in series with the lung compliance (C_L). Such a model is analogous to a resistor and capacitor in series that form a resistive-capacitive (R_C) circuit (Fig. 4.10).

A transmural (P_{TM}) pressure gradient exists between the airway at the mouth (i.e., at atmospheric pressure) and the pressure inside the pleural cavity. This pressure gradient is responsible

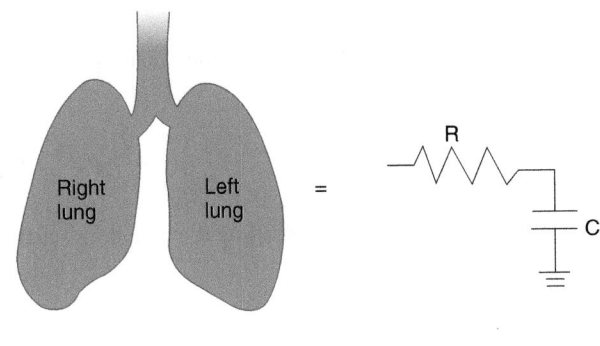

R = Resistance = $\dfrac{\text{Pressure change}}{\text{Flow rate}}$

C = Compliance = $\dfrac{\text{Volume change}}{\text{Pressure change}}$

• **Fig. 4.10** Resistance-compliance (RC) model of the lungs. Resistance of lungs to airflow and natural ability to resist stretch (compliance) enable lungs to be modeled as an electrical circuit. A resistor of resistance *R* placed in series with a capacitor of capacitance *C* is a simple and convenient analogy on which to base pulmonary biomechanics.

for the lungs "hugging" the thoracic cavity as the chest enlarges during inspiration. The presence of an external breathing apparatus causes a further pressure loss (P_{EXT}). The total pressure drop between the atmosphere and the pleural cavity is given by the respiratory mechanics equation and may be modeled as follows[50]:

$$P_{TOTAL} = P_{EXT} + P_{TM} = R_{EXT}\, \dot{V} + \frac{V}{C_L} + R_L\, \dot{V} \quad (28)$$

$$P_{EXT} = R_{EXT} \dot{V} \tag{29}$$

$$P_{TM} = \frac{V}{C_L} + R_L \dot{V} \tag{30}$$

where

P_{TOTAL} = pressure drop between atmosphere and pleural cavity
P_{EXT} = pressure drop across external breathing apparatus
P_{TM} = transmural pressure gradient
R_{EXT} = external apparatus resistance (e.g., an ETT)
$\dot{V}$ = dV/dt = gas flow rate into the lungs
C_L = lung compliance
R_L = airway resistance
V = volume of gas above the FRC in the lungs

Thus, the pressure required to inflate the lungs depends on both lung compliance and gas flow rate. The time required to inflate the lungs is measured in terms of a pulmonary time constant. This time constant (t) is simply the product $R_L \times C_L$. However, determination of the time constant is not a trivial matter, and attention is now turned to that determination.

Pulmonary Time Constant

Using the previous formula (Eq. 29) in the case that no external resistance exists, one can show that, during passive expiration, the volume in the lungs in excess of FRC takes on the following form[51]:

$$V = V_0 e^{-t/\tau} \tag{31}$$

where V_0 is the volume taken in during inspiration and $\tau = R_L C_L$ is the time constant for the lungs.

Flow from the lungs is obtained by differentiating this equation with respect to time:

$$\dot{V} = \frac{dV}{dt} = V_0 \frac{d\left(e^{-t/\tau}\right)}{dt} = V_0 e^{-t/\tau}\left(-\frac{1}{\tau}\right) = -\frac{V_0}{\tau}e^{-t/\tau} \tag{32}$$

Tau (τ) may now be estimated by dividing the preceding equation by the first one:

$$\frac{\dot{V}}{V} = \frac{V_0 e^{-t/\tau}\left(-\dfrac{1}{\tau}\right)}{V_0 e^{-t/\tau}} = -\frac{1}{\tau} \tag{33}$$

Therefore, τ can be estimated as the negative of the reciprocal of the average slope of the plot of flow ($\dot{V}$) against volume (V) during expiration. Another means of estimating τ is by taking the natural logarithm of the volume equation $V = V_0 e^{-t/\tau}$.

The value of τ can also be estimated as the negative reciprocal of the average slope of the natural logarithm of the lung volume plotted against time.

$$\ln V = \ln\left(V_0\right) = \frac{t}{\tau} = \frac{d\left(\ln V\right)}{dt} = -\frac{1}{\tau} \tag{34}$$

Determination of Rohrer's Constants

A more complete approach to modeling the pressure-flow relationship of the respiratory system assumes that a single time constant τ may be inadequate to describe pulmonary biomechanics in some situations. The classical form of the equation,[27]

$$\frac{V}{\dot{V}} = -\tau = C_L \times R_L \tag{35}$$

can be changed to a more elaborate form of:

$$\frac{V}{\dot{V}} = -C_L\left(K_1 + K_2 \dot{V}\right) \tag{36}$$

where K_1 and K_2 are known as Rohrer's constants and $(K_1 + K_2)$ is a form of R_L.

In this situation, the resistance of the pulmonary system is not assumed to be constant; rather, it is assumed to be flow dependent:

$$R = K_1 + K_2 \dot{V} \tag{37}$$

When this equation is expressed in the following form,

$$\frac{V}{C_L \dot{V}} = -(K_1 + K_2 \dot{V}) \tag{38}$$

K_1 and K_2 may be determined as the intercept and slope, respectively, of a plot of $V/C_L\dot{V}$ against $\dot{V}$.

Compliance

Pulmonary compliance measurements reflect the elastic properties of the lungs and thorax and are influenced by factors such as degree of muscular tension, degree of interstitial lung water, degree of pulmonary fibrosis, degree of lung inflation, and alveolar surface tension.[52] Total respiratory system compliance is given by the following calculation[40]:

$$C = \frac{\Delta V}{\Delta P} \tag{39}$$

where

ΔV = change in lung volume
ΔP = change in airway pressure

This total compliance may be related to lung compliance and thoracic (chest wall) compliance by the following relation:

$$\frac{1}{C_T} = \frac{1}{C_L} + \frac{1}{C_{Th}} \tag{40}$$

where

C_T = total compliance (e.g., 100 mL/cm H_2O)
C_L = lung compliance (e.g., 200 mL/cm H_2O)
C_{Th} = thoracic compliance (e.g., 200 mL/cm H_2O)

The values shown in parentheses are some typical normal adult values that can be used for modeling purposes.[40] *Elastance*, the reciprocal of compliance, offers notational advantage over compliance in some physiologic problems. However, its use has not been popular in clinical practice.

Compliance may be estimated using τ, the pulmonary time constant. If a linear resistance of known value (ΔR) is added to the patient's airway, the time constant will change to τ' as follows[27]:

$$\tau' = \left(R_L + \Delta R\right) \times C_L = \tau + \left(C_L + \Delta R\right) = \tau + \Delta \tau \tag{41}$$

Therefore, if ΔR is known and τ and τ' are determined experimentally, one can solve for C_L and then for R_L:

$$C_L = \frac{\tau' - \tau}{\Delta R} = \frac{\Delta \tau}{\Delta R} \qquad R_L = \tau \times \frac{\Delta R}{\Delta \tau} = \frac{\tau \times \Delta R}{\tau' - \tau} \tag{42}$$

Advanced Formulation of the Respiratory Mechanics Equation

An alternative to the elementary respiratory mechanics equation may be used to describe the physical behavior of the lungs. The original formulation of this advanced respiratory mechanics equation was carried out by Rohrer during World War I, but the first completely correct formulation was devised by Gaensler and colleagues and has the following form[38]:

$$P = \frac{V}{C} + K_1\dot{V} + K_2\dot{V}^2 \qquad (43)$$

where

P = airway pressure
V = lung volume
$\dot{V}$ = gas flow rate into (out of) lung
C = compliance of the pulmonary system
K_1 and K_2 = empirical Rohrer's constants

This equation is more advanced than the elementary respiratory mechanics equation because it is able to account for flow losses attributable to turbulence. Because turbulent flow conditions are most likely to exist during anesthesia, the $\dot{V}^2$ term is very important in accurately quantifying the pressure losses of respiration. In addition, the advanced equation combines the resistance losses into the constants K_1 and K_2, which require only empirical determination.

Anesthesia at Moderate Altitude

The parameters that govern the administration of anesthesia are altered slightly when the elevation above sea level is increased. Generally, a change in the atmospheric (or barometric) pressure is responsible for these differences. This section briefly examines the consequences of a moderate change in altitude.

The approximate alveolar gas equation is a useful tool in quantifying the differences that occur at higher elevations[53]:

$$PAO_2 = PIO_2 - \frac{PaCO_2}{R} \quad PIO_2 = (P_B - 47) \times FIO_2 \qquad (44)$$

where

PAO_2 = alveolar oxygen tension
PIO_2 = inspired oxygen tension partial pressure
$PaCO_2$ = arterial carbon dioxide tension
R = 0.8 → gas exchange coefficient (CO_2 produced/O_2 consumed)
P_B = barometric pressure (760 mm Hg at sea level)
47 = water vapor pressure at 37°C
FIO_2 = fraction of inspired oxygen = 0.21 at all altitudes (room air)

All tensions are in mm Hg (torr).

Altered Partial Pressure of Gases

The effect of altitude is very apparent on the partial pressure of administered gases. The partial pressure of oxygen is given by $PIO_2 = (P_B - PH_2O) \times 0.21$. At 1524 m (5000 ft) above sea level, PIO_2 is reduced to 128 mm Hg from 158 mm Hg at sea level, so that the maximum PaO_2 is about 83 mm Hg (assuming $PaCO_2 = 36$).[54] At 3048 m (10,000 ft), PIO_2 is 111 mm Hg, and the maximum PaO_2 is 65 mm Hg.[54] In order to counteract the effects of the hypoxia, ventilation is increased, so that at 5000 ft, $PaCO_2 = 36$ mm Hg and at 3048 m, $PaCO_2 = 34$ mm Hg on average.[54] The effectiveness of nitrous oxide (N_2O) decreases with altitude because of an absolute reduction of its partial pressure (tension).

Oxygen Analyzers

There are five main types of oxygen analyzers: paramagnetic analyzers, fuel cell analyzers, oxygen electrodes, mass spectrometers, and Raman spectrographs. All respond to oxygen partial pressure (not concentration) so that the output changes with barometric pressure. At 1524 m, an analyzer set to measure 21% O_2 at sea level reads 17.4%. If these devices were to calculate the amount of oxygen in terms of partial pressure, the scale readings would reflect the true state of oxygen availability, but clinical practice dictates that a percentage scale be used anyway.

Carbon Dioxide Analyzers and Vapor Analyzers

Absorption of infrared radiation by gas is the usual analytic method used to determine the amount of CO_2 in a gas mixture, although other methods (e.g., Raman spectrographs) also work well. This type of method measures partial pressures, not percentages. To operate accurately, these machines must either be calibrated using known CO_2 concentrations at the correct barometric pressure or have the scale converted to read partial pressures.

Similar arguments apply to modern vapor analyzers, all of which respond to partial pressures, not concentrations, despite the fact that the output of these devices, by clinical custom, is usually calculated in percentages.

Vapors and Vaporizers

Practically speaking, the saturated vapor pressure of a volatile agent depends only on its temperature. At a given temperature, the concentration of a given mass of vapor increases as barometric pressure decreases, but its partial pressure remains unchanged. Similarly, the output of calibrated vaporizers is altered with changes in barometric pressure. Only the concentration of the vapor changes; the partial pressure remains the same, as does the patient's response at a given setting as compared with sea level. This assumes that the vaporizer characteristics do not change with altered density and viscosity of the carrier gases.

Flowmeters

Most flowmeters measure the drop in pressure that occurs when a gas passes through a resistance and correlate this pressure drop with flow. The pressure drop depends on gas density and viscosity. If the resistance is an orifice, resistance depends primarily on gas density. For laminar flow through a tube, viscosity determines resistance (Hagen-Poiseuille equation). Some flowmeters employ a floating ball or bobbin supported by the stream of gas in a tapered tube. The float is fluted so that it remains in the center of the flow. At low flow, the device depends primarily on laminar flow, and as the float moves up the tube, the resistance behaves progressively more like an orifice.

The density of a gas changes, of course, with barometric pressure, but the viscosity changes little, being primarily dependent on temperature. Gas flow through an orifice is inversely proportional to the square root of gas density: As the density falls, flow increases

Name	Symbol	GMW
Hydrogen	H	1.00797
Helium	He	4.0026
Nitrogen (molecular)	N_2	28.0134
Oxygen (molecular)	O_2	31.9988
Neon	Ne	20.183
Argon	Ar	39.948
Xenon	Xe	131.30
Halothane	$CF_3CClBrH$	197
Isoflurane	$CF_2H\text{-}O\text{-}CHClCF_3$	184.5
Enflurane	$CF_2H\text{-}O\text{-}CF_2CFHCl$	184.5
Nitrous oxide	N_2O	44.013

TABLE 4.4 Gram Molecular Weight (GMW) for Some Common and Anesthetic Gases

TABLE 4.5 Minimum Alveolar Concentration (MAC) at Various Altitude Levels and Comparative Values for Minimal Alveolar Partial Pressure (MAPP)

Agent	Sea Level	5000 ft	10,000 ft	(kPa)	(mm Hg)
	MAC (%)			MAPP	
Nitrous oxide	105.0	126.5	152.2	106.1	798.0
Ethyl ether	1.92	2.31	2.78	1.94	14.6
Halothane	0.75	0.90	1.09	0.76	5.7
Enflurane	1.68	2.02	2.43	1.70	12.8
Isoflurane	1.2	1.45	1.73	1.22	9.1

MAPP, MAC × 0.01 × 760 mm Hg.
Adapted from James MFM, White JF. Anesthetic considerations at moderate altitude. *Anesth Analg.* 1984;63:1097.

(orifice size being constant). Therefore, at high altitude the actual flowmeter flow is greater than that indicated by the float position:

$$\text{Actual flow} = \text{Nominal flow} \times \sqrt{\frac{760 \text{ mm Hg}}{P_B}} \quad (45)$$

Flowmeter Calibration

The calibration of standard flowmeters, such as the Thorpe tube, depends on gas properties. Usually, a particular flowmeter is calibrated for a particular gas, such as oxygen or air. The factor used to convert nominal flow measurements to actual flow measurements is given by the following equation[53]:

$$k = \frac{\sqrt{GMW_A}}{\sqrt{GMW_B}} \quad (46)$$

where

A = the gas for which the flowmeter was originally designed
B = the gas actually used
GMW = the gram molecular weight of the gas in question
A list of common anesthetic gases and their respective GMWs is presented in Table 4.4.

Example Calculation 1

Determine the actual flow rate of a 70:30 heliox mixture if it is passed through an oxygen flowmeter that reads 10 L/min.
Answer:

$$GMWO_2 = 32 \text{ g/mol} \quad (47)$$

$$GMW_{heliox} = 0.3(32) + 0.7(4) = 12.4 \text{ g/mol} \quad (48)$$

The actual flow rate of heliox is given by the following equation:

$$\text{Actual flow rate} = 10 \times \frac{\sqrt{GMWO_2}}{\sqrt{GMW_{helix}}} \quad (49)$$

$$= 10 \times \frac{\sqrt{32}}{12.4} = 16.1 \text{ L/min}$$

Example Calculation 2

Determine the appropriate multiplier if oxygen is passed through an airflow meter.
Answer:

$$\text{Multiplier} = \frac{\sqrt{GMW_{AIR}}}{\sqrt{GMWO_2}} = \frac{\sqrt{0.2(32) + 0.79(28)}}{\sqrt{32}} = .95 \quad (50)$$

Anesthetic Implications

At 10,000 ft a 30% O_2 mixture has the same partial pressure as a 20% O_2 mixture at sea level.[54] In addition, the reduction in partial pressure of N_2O that occurs seriously impairs the effectiveness of the agent, and its administration may be of no benefit. The concept of minimum alveolar concentration (MAC) does not apply at higher altitudes and should be replaced by the concept of minimal alveolar partial pressure (MAPP) (Table 4.5). The use of this concept would eliminate many of the problems identified earlier.

Estimation of Gas Rates

Estimation of Carbon Dioxide Production Rate

The carbon dioxide production rate ($\dot{V}CO_2$) of a patient may be estimated in the following manner. The CO_2 production rate can be described as the product of the amount of CO_2 produced per breath and the number of breaths per minute (BPM), with typical units of mL/min. Therefore, $\dot{V}CO_2$ may be expressed as follows:

$$VCO_2 = CO_2 \text{ produced per breath} \times BPM \quad (51)$$

$$VCO_2 = VCO_2 \times BPM \quad (52)$$

The amount of CO_2 produced per breath is calculated as follows:

$$VCO_2 = \int_{t=0}^{t=t_{end} \text{ expiration}} CCO_2(t) \times Q(t) \times \gamma dt \quad (53)$$

where

$CCO_2(t)$ = capnogram signal (mm Hg)
$Q(t)$ = gas flow rate signal (mL/min)

γ = scaling factor to switch dimensions from mm Hg to concentration % = 100% ÷ 760 mm Hg = 0.1312

Estimation of Oxygen Consumption Rate

The oxygen consumption rate may be estimated similarly to $\dot{V}_{CO_2}$. The oxygen consumption rate can be expressed as the product of oxygen consumed per breath and the number of breaths per minute. Mathematically, this may be written as follows:

$$\dot{V}O_2 = O_2 \text{ consumed per breath} \times \text{number of breaths per minute} \quad (54)$$

$$\dot{V}O_2 = \dot{V}O_2 \times BPM \quad (55)$$

The amount of O_2 consumed per breath can now be expressed as follows:

$$\dot{V}O_2 = \int_{t=0}^{t=t_{end} \text{ expiration}} (PIO_2 - CO_2) \times Q(t) \times \gamma dt \quad (56)$$

where

PIO_2 = inspiratory oxygen pressure = $(P_B - 47) \times FIO_2$ (mm Hg)
CO_2 = oxygen signal (mm Hg)
$Q(t)$ = gas flow rate signal (mL/min)
γ = scaling factor = 0.1312

Interpretation of Carbon Dioxide Production and Oxygen Consumption Rates

The rates $\dot{V}O_2$ and $\dot{V}CO_2$ are linked by the respiratory exchange coefficient RQ (RQ = $\dot{V}CO_2$ / $\dot{V}O_2$), which is governed largely by diet; some diets produce less CO_2 than others and have a smaller RQ. Typically, RQ = 0.8. $\dot{V}O_2$ and $\dot{V}CO_2$ both go up with increases in metabolism, which may be related to factors such as fever, sepsis, light anesthesia, shivering, malignant hyperthermia, and thyroid storm. Decreases in $\dot{V}CO_2$ and $\dot{V}O_2$ may also have many causes (e.g., hypothermia, deep anesthesia, hypothyroidism).

Ventilation via Narrow-Bore Catheters

Earlier, this chapter discussed the physics behind TTJV, where oxygen is injected percutaneously under high pressure (e.g., 20 psi) via a narrow-bore, high-resistance cannula. This is ordinarily done in order to oxygenate a patient in whom establishing a conventional airway has failed and the situation is emergent. Unfortunately, this technique of ventilation comes with a special concern—expiration of the injected gas in this setting must take place via the nose and/or mouth since passive expiration via the transtracheal catheter is not possible (because of its very high resistance). Consequently, in situations where complete airway obstruction exists and no gas egress pathway exists, repeated injections of oxygen will only lead to patient harm, as the resulting pressure buildup will result in barotrauma in the form of a pneumothorax, subcutaneous emphysema, hemodynamic deterioration, or even complete cardiac arrest.

Instead of passive compliance-dependent expiration via a narrow-bore catheter (which takes place far too slowly because of its high resistance), envision a system that uses active expiration—that is, a system that aids expiration by actively sucking gas through the catheter. This is the novel scheme devised by Dr. Dietmar Enk,

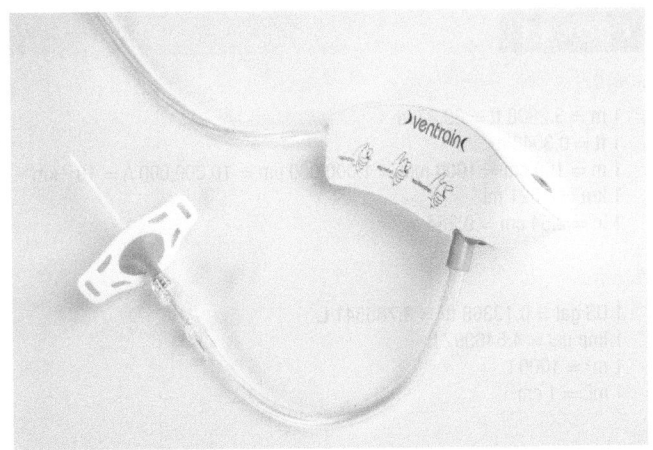

• **Fig. 4.11** The Ventrain ventilation system (Ventinova Medical, Eindhoven, The Netherlands) hooked up to a 75-mm-long transtracheal ventilation catheter (Cricath) utilizing an inner diameter of only 2 mm. Unlike with conventional TTJV catheters, both inspiration and expiration take place through the catheter. (Courtesy Ventinova Medical, Eindhoven, The Netherlands.)

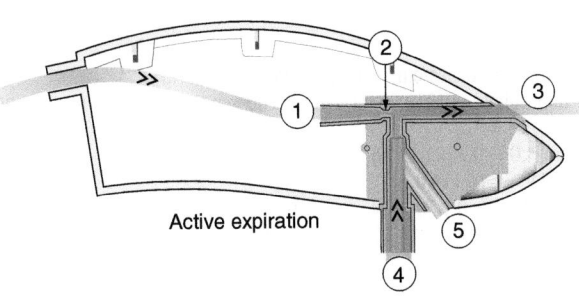

Active expiration

• **Fig. 4.12** Schematic diagram of the Ventrain ventilation system. Active expiration (i.e., expiration assisted by suction) is achieved via an arrangement striking a balance between the Bernoulli effect and jet entrainment. Oxygen flows via the inlet (1) through a very narrow nozzle (2) and exhaust pipe (3) to the outside. The flow entrains gas from the side port (4), which is connected to a catheter, to achieve active expiration. Insufflation occurs by closing the exhaust pipe (3). The bypass control (5) functions as an on/off switch. (Adapted from Ventinova Medical, Eindhoven, The Netherlands.)

who has developed an apparatus that uses fluidic technology for exactly such a purpose. Figs. 4.11 and 4.12 illustrate the design of the system. The Ventrain (Ventinova Medical, Eindhoven, The Netherlands) is a manually operated, flow-controlled ejector ventilator. The driving oxygen flow, manually set according to clinical needs, allows one to easily estimate the oxygen volume insufflated per second (e.g., flow of 12 L/min = 200 mL/s). As the gas encounters a very narrow nozzle, high gas pressure proximal to the jet nozzle is converted into a region of high gas velocity distal to the jet nozzle that results in subatmospheric pressure (via Bernoulli's principle); that subatmospheric pressure effectively assists expiration by suction, the same way lift is generated on an aircraft wing.

Note that the physics of the Ventrain system differs from that of classical TTJV in several important ways. First, the insufflation pressures are much lower (less than 3 psi compared to 20 psi or more for TTJV). Second, the gas flow, usually set to approximately 15 L/min in adult patients (in children, a lower flow is

• BOX 4.1   Selected Dimensional Equivalents

Length

1 m = 3.2808 ft = 39.37 in
1 ft = 0.3048 m
1 m = 100 cm = 1000 mm = 1,000,000 µm = 10,000,000 Å = 10^{-3} km
1 km = 0.621 mi
1 in = 2.54 cm = 0.254 m

Volume

1 US gal = 0.13368 ft^3 = 3.785541 L
1 Imp gal = 4.546092 L
1 m^3 = 1000 L
1 mL = 1 cm^3

Mass

1 kg = 1000 g = 2.2046 lb_m = 0.068521 slugs
1 lb_m = 0.453592 kg
1 slug = 1 $lb_f \cdot s^2/ft$ = 32.174 lb_m

Force

1 lb_f = 4.448222 N = 4.448 × 10^5 dynes
1 N = 1 kg·m/s^2 = 10,000 dynes = 10,000 g·cm/s^2

Pressure

1 N/m^2 = 10 dynes/cm^2 = 1 Pa = 0.007501 mm Hg
1 atmosphere = 1013.25 millibars = 760 mm Hg = 101,325 Pa = 14.696 lb/in^2
1 cm H_2O = 0.735 mm Hg
1 lb/in^2 = 51.71 mm Hg
1 dyne/cm^2 = 0.1 Pa = 145.04 × 10^{-7} lb/in^2
1 bar = 10^5 N/m^2 = 14.504 lb/in^2 = 106 dynes/cm^2

Viscosity

1 kg/(m·s) = 1 N × s/m^2 = 0.6729 lb_m/(ft·s) = 10 poise

Energy

1 joule (J) = 1 kg·m^2/s^2
1 Btu = 778.16 ft·lb_f = 1055.056 J = 252 cal = 1.055 × 10^{10} ergs
1 cal = 4.1868 J

Power

1 watt (W) = 1 kg·m^2/s^3 = 1 J/s
1 hp = 550 ft·lb_f/s = 745.699 W

advisable), is known and can readily be adjusted, whereas the gas flow in the case of TTJV is neither directly known nor directly adjustable. Finally, when a cuffed catheter is used with the Ventrain there is no air entrainment effect to consider, whereas compared to classic jet ventilation the much lower insufflation pressure associated with the Ventrain system reduces the air entrainment effect to remarkably lower levels when uncuffed catheters are used.

In addition to the use of the Ventrain device during emergency transtracheal ventilation, other possible uses include transoral/translaryngeal ventilation in otolaryngologic cases requiring very narrow catheters (e.g., where a regular microlaryngeal tube [MLT] may be too large). In addition, the Ventrain may be used as an

alternative to transoral/translaryngeal (subglottic) jet ventilation using, for instance, the Hunsaker MonJet Catheter (Medtronic Xomed, Jacksonville, FL, USA) in conjunction with a Monsoon jet ventilator (Acutronic Medical Systems, Hirzel, Switzerland). For additional information, the interested reader is referred to references.[55–63]

Transnasal Humidified Rapid-Insufflation Ventilatory Exchange (THRIVE)

High-flow nasal oxygen therapy provides a means to deliver humidified and heated oxygen at rates that may exceed 100 L/min.[64,65] Primarily used to greatly extend apnea time in adult patients undergoing airway procedures under general anesthesia, THRIVE supports apneic oxygenation (oxygenation in the absence of spontaneous respiration or mechanical ventilation). In addition, the technique may well be helpful at CO_2 elimination.[66] For additional information, the interested reader is referred to references.[64–69]

Selected Dimensional Equivalents

Discussions regarding physics in anesthesia may be confusing because of the variety of units used in the clinical literature. The list in Box 4.1 is a compilation of units and equivalents that one is likely to encounter.

Conclusion

An understanding of a number of basic principles of physics can be very helpful in clinical airway management. This is especially true for the physics of fluid flow, such as the relationships between pressure, flow, and resistance under laminar and turbulent flow conditions.

In addition to the application of basic physics principles to airway situations, the application of mathematical methods and physiologic modeling can sometimes be enormously helpful in obtaining insights into complex physiologic systems related to the airway, such as the determination of arterial blood oxygenation under various conditions. In many cases, such modeling can produce results that would be extremely difficult to obtain by recourse to pure experimentation alone.

Selected References

11. Sherwood L. Human Physiology: From Cells to Systems. 9th ed. Nelson; 2015.
20. Kemper KJ, Ritz RH, Benson MS, Bishop MS. Helium-oxygen mixture in the treatment of postextubation stridor in pediatric trauma patients. *Crit Care Med*. 1991;19:356–359.
23. Rodrigo GJ, Rodrigo C, Pollack CV, Rowe B. Use of helium-oxygen mixtures in the treatment of acute asthma: a systematic review. *Chest*. 2003;123:891–896.
25. Khanlou H, Eiger G. Safety and efficacy of heliox as a treatment for upper airway obstruction due to radiation-induced laryngeal dysfunction. *Heart Lung*. 2001;30:146–147.
26. Polaner DM. The use of heliox and the laryngeal mask airway in a child with an anterior mediastinal mass. *Anesth Analg*. 1996;82:208–210.

42. Straus C, Louis B, Isabey D, et al. Contribution of the endotracheal tube and the upper airway to breathing workload. *Am J Respir Crit Care Med.* 1998;157:23–30.

49. Bolder PM, Healy TE, Bolder AR, et al. The extra work of breathing through adult endotracheal tubes. *Anesth Analg.* 1986;65:853–859.

50. Davis PD, Kenny GNC. Basic Physics and Measurement in Anaesthesia. 5th ed. Elsevier Health Science; 2003.

54. James MF, White JF. Anesthetic considerations at moderate altitude. *Anesth Analg.* 1984;63:1097–1105.

60. Paxian M, Preussler NP, Reinz T, Schlueter A, Gottschall R. Transtracheal ventilation with a novel ejector-based device (Ventrain) in open, partly obstructed, or totally closed upper airways in pigs. *Br J Anaesth.* 2015;115(2):308–316.

All references can be found online at eBooks.Health.Elsevier.com.

5

Physiology of the Airway

WILLIAM C. WILSON AND JONATHAN L. BENUMOF

CHAPTER OUTLINE

KEY POINTS

- The ventilated gas that participates in gas exchange is referred to as *alveolar ventilation* ($\dot{V}A$). The volume of gas that is wasted is referred to as *dead space* (VD). The aggregate total of dead space is referred to as the *physiologic dead space* ($VD_{physiologic}$) and is divided into two subcomponents. The volume of gas that ventilates the conducting airways is called the *anatomic dead space* ($VD_{anatomic}$), and the volume of gas that ventilates nonperfused alveoli is the *alveolar dead space* ($VD_{alveolar}$).
- Ventilation/perfusion ($\dot{V}A/\dot{Q}$) relationships are important in pulmonary gas exchange. At the top of the lung there is relatively high $\dot{V}A/\dot{Q}$, whereas at the bottom, there is relatively low $\dot{V}A/\dot{Q}$.

However, most of the perfusion and most of the ventilation occur at the base, and perfusion is well matched throughout the lung in normal, young, healthy individuals. Alveolar ventilation without perfusion results in alveolar dead space, and alveolar perfusion without ventilation results in a right-to-left transpulmonary shunt.

- The functional residual capacity (FRC) is the amount of gas in the lungs at end-expiration during normal tidal breathing. The FRC is also equal to the sum of the expiratory reserve volume and the residual volume. The FRC has important clinical significance because it represents the major reservoir of oxygen in the body and is directly related to the time until desaturation after apnea. The FRC is also inversely proportional to the degree of low-$\dot{V}A/\dot{Q}$ alveoli and shunt. For example, morbidly obese patients have low FRCs, tend to desaturate quickly, and have many more atelectatic alveoli and shunt units than normal, age-matched patients.

- Lung compliance (CL, volume/pressure) is the inverse of elastance. CL is bimodal: It is low at low lung volumes, highest at normal lung volumes (normal FRC), and low at very high lung volumes. The formula for compliance is analogous to the mathematical formula used to calculate capacitance in electronics.
- Factors that affect airway resistance include lung volume, bronchial smooth muscle tone, and the density/viscosity of the inhaled gas.
- Pulmonary vessels constrict in response to hypoxia, hypercarbia, and acidosis, whereas systemic vessels dilate when exposed to these factors.
- Increased oxygen affinity shifts the oxygen-hemoglobin (oxy-Hb) dissociation curve to the left (i.e., it increases the affinity of Hb for oxygen, thus reducing P_{50}, the oxygen concentration at which Hb is 50% saturated), whereas decreased oxygen affinity shifts the oxy-Hb curve to the right (i.e., it decreases Hb affinity for oxygen and thus increases P_{50}). The four primary processes that shift the oxy-Hb curve to the right are increased hydrogen ion (H^+) concentration, increased partial pressure of carbon dioxide (PCO_2), increased 2,3-diphosphoglycerate (2,3-DPG), and increased temperature.
- The Bohr effect refers to the effect of PCO_2 and H^+ ions on the oxy-Hb curve (i.e., increasing the propensity for oxygen to offload from Hb).
- The Haldane effect describes the shift in the CO_2 dissociation curve caused by oxygenation of Hb. Low PO_2 shifts the CO_2 dissociation curve to the left so that the blood can pick up more CO_2 (e.g., in capillaries of rapidly metabolizing tissues). Highly oxygenated Hb (as occurs in the lungs) reduces the affinity of Hb for CO_2, shifting the CO_2 dissociation curve to the right and thereby increasing CO_2 removal.
- CO_2 is transported in the blood primarily in three different forms: physically dissolved in blood, bound to amino groups of proteins (e.g., Hb) as carbamate compounds, and as bicarbonate ions.

Introduction

Anesthesiologists, nurse anesthetists, emergency medicine physicians, and other healthcare professionals responsible for airway management require an extensive knowledge of respiratory physiology to provide optimal patient care. Mastery of the normal respiratory physiologic processes is a prerequisite to understanding the mechanisms of impaired gas exchange that occur during anesthesia, during surgery, and with disease. This chapter is divided into two major sections. The first section reviews the normal (nonanesthetized) condition with emphasis on the distribution of perfusion and ventilation (both gravity and nongravity determined), compliance, resistance, work of breathing (WOB), transport of respiratory gases, pulmonary reflexes, and special functions of the lung. In the second section, these processes and concepts are discussed in relation to the common mechanisms of impaired gas exchange that occur during anesthesia, during surgery, and with disease.

Normal Respiratory Physiology (Nonanesthetized)

Atmospheric air is a mixture of oxygen (O_2, 20.95%), nitrogen (N_2, 78.09%), argon (Ar, 0.93%), carbon dioxide (CO_2, 0.03%), and water vapor (0% to 2%). For practical purposes, we typically assume air is 21% O_2 and 79% N_2 and ignore the contributions from CO_2 and Ar. Under physiologic conditions, inhaled gas becomes fully saturated with water at the alveolar level, constituting about 6% of the alveolar gas. Accordingly, at sea level (760 mm Hg), and at normal core body temperature (37°C), the water vapor pressure of gas in the lung is 47 mm Hg. During airway management, augmenting the fraction of inspired oxygen (FIO_2) provides a measure of safety in the event of a cannot intubate/cannot oxygenate situation. Following intubation, during mechanical ventilation, the FIO_2 should be decreased to as low as practicable to maintain a safe oxygen saturation (SpO_2) of ≥92%. Prolonged duration at excessively high FIO_2 levels (particularly >0.6) in adults can lead to oxygen toxicity. Neonates can suffer manifestations of oxygen toxicity even at much lower levels of FIO_2 (discussed in greater detail later in this chapter).

Gravity-Determined Distribution of Perfusion and Ventilation

For cells to utilize the oxygen in the atmosphere, it must be transported to the tissues and cells. The first step is inspiration, the transfer of atmospheric air (including oxygen) to the alveoli, where it is brought in close proximity to the pulmonary capillary blood to allow efficient gas exchange (oxygen crosses the alveolar-capillary membrane and enters the capillary blood, whereas CO_2 exits the capillary blood and enters the alveolar space), followed by movement of alveolar air back to the environment (expiration), where CO_2 is eliminated. Ventilation (inspiration and expiration) is closely coupled with perfusion of the alveoli. The interaction of ventilation and perfusion ultimately determines the gas exchange in the lungs. There are gravitational and nongravitational determinants of both perfusion and ventilation, and the elements controlling these factors will be described next, beginning with perfusion.

Distribution of Pulmonary Perfusion

Contraction of the right ventricle imparts kinetic energy manifested as the ejection of blood into the main pulmonary artery, with subsequent flow into the right and left pulmonary arteries and the subsequent branches. As this energy is dissipated in climbing a vertical hydrostatic gradient, the absolute pressure in the pulmonary artery (Ppa) decreases by 1 cm H_2O per centimeter of vertical distance up the lung (Fig. 5.1). At some height above the heart, Ppa becomes zero (i.e., equal to atmospheric pressure), and still higher in the lung Ppa becomes relatively negative (lower than atmospheric pressure).[1] In this region the alveolar pressure (PA) exceeds Ppa and pulmonary venous pressure (Ppv), which is relatively negative at this vertical height. Because the pressure outside the vessels is greater than the pressure inside, the vessels in this region of the lung are collapsed, and no blood flow occurs; this has been described by John West as *zone 1* (PA > Ppa > Ppv).[1] Because there is no blood flow through zone 1 capillaries, gas exchange

The four zones of the lung

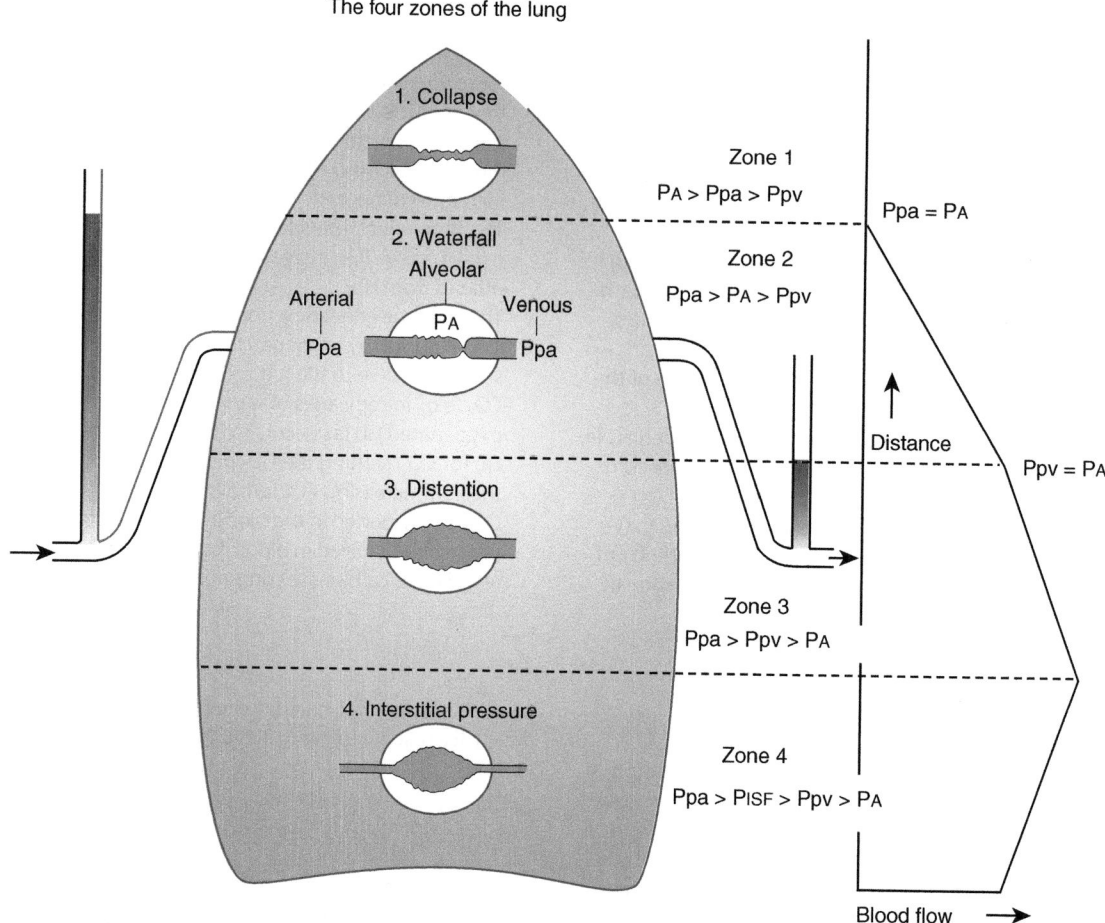

• **Fig. 5.1** Schematic diagram showing the distribution of blood flow in the upright lung. In zone 1, alveolar pressure *(PA)* exceeds pulmonary artery pressure *(Ppa)*, and no flow occurs because the intraalveolar vessels are collapsed by the compressing alveolar pressure. In zone 2, Ppa exceeds PA, but PA exceeds pulmonary venous pressure *(Ppv)*. Flow in zone 2 is determined by the Ppa – PA difference (Ppa – PA) and has been likened to an upstream river flowing over a dam. Because Ppa increases down zone 2 whereas PA (at end-expiration) remains constant, perfusion pressure increases, and flow steadily increases down the zone. In zone 3, Ppv exceeds PA, and flow is determined by the Ppa – Ppv difference (Ppa – Ppv), which is constant down this portion of the lung. However, transmural pressure across the wall of the vessel increases down this zone, so the caliber of the vessels increases (resistance decreases), and therefore flow increases. Finally, in zone 4, pulmonary interstitial pressure *(PISF)* becomes positive and exceeds both Ppv and PA. Consequently, flow in zone 4 is determined by the Ppa – PISF difference (Ppa – PISF). (Modified from West JB. *Ventilation/Blood Flow and Gas Exchange.* 4th ed. Blackwell Scientific; 1970.)

does not occur, and the region functions as alveolar dead space, or wasted ventilation. Little or no zone 1 exists in the lung under normal conditions,[2] but the amount of zone 1 lung can be greatly increased if Ppa is reduced, as in hypovolemic shock, or if PA is increased, as in the application of excessively large tidal volumes (VT) or levels of positive end-expiratory pressure (PEEP) during positive-pressure ventilation.

Further down the lung, absolute Ppa becomes positive, and blood flow begins when Ppa exceeds PA *(zone 2,* Ppa > PA > Ppv). At this vertical level in the lung, PA exceeds Ppv, and blood flow is determined by the mean Ppa – PA difference rather than by the more conventional Ppa – Ppv difference (see later discussion).[3] In zone 2, the relationship between blood flow and alveolar pressure has physical characteristics similar to a waterfall flowing over a dam. The height of the upstream river (before reaching the dam) is equivalent to Ppa, and the height of the dam is equivalent to PA. The rate of water flow over the dam is proportional to only

the difference between the height of the upstream river and the dam (Ppa – PA), and it does not matter how far below the dam the downstream riverbed (Ppv) is. This phenomenon has various names, including the waterfall, Starling resistor, weir (dam made by beavers), and sluice effect. Because mean Ppa increases down this region of the lung, but mean PA is relatively constant, the mean driving pressure (Ppa – PA) increases linearly; therefore, mean blood flow increases linearly as one descends down this portion of the lung. Respiration and pulmonary blood flow, however, are cyclic phenomena. Therefore, absolute instantaneous Ppa, Ppv, and PA are changing continuously, and the relationships among Ppa, Ppv, and PA are dynamically determined by the phase lags between the cardiac and respiratory cycles. Consequently, a specific point in zone 2 may actually be in either a zone 1 or a zone 3 condition at a given moment, depending on where the patient is in respect to respiratory systole and diastole, as well as cardiac systole and diastole.

Still lower in the lung is a vertical level at which Ppv becomes positive and also exceeds PA. In this region, blood flow is governed by the pulmonary arteriovenous pressure difference, Ppa – Ppv (*zone 3*, Ppa > Ppv > PA), for here both of these vascular pressures exceed PA, and the capillary systems are thus permanently open and blood flow is continuous. In descending zone 3, gravity causes both absolute Ppa and Ppv to increase at the same rate, so the perfusion pressure (Ppa – Ppv) is unchanged. However, the pressure outside the vessels—namely, pleural pressure (Ppl)—increases less than Ppa and Ppv. Therefore, the transmural distending pressures (Ppa – Ppl and Ppv – Ppl) increase down zone 3, the vessel radii increase, vascular resistance decreases, and blood flow consequently increases further.

Finally, whenever pulmonary vascular pressures (Ppa) are extremely high—as they are in a severely volume-overloaded patient, in an extremely dependent lung (far below the vertical level of the left atrium), and in patients with pulmonary embolism or mitral stenosis—fluid can transude out of the pulmonary vessels and into the pulmonary interstitial compartment. In addition, pulmonary interstitial edema can be caused by extremely negative Ppl and perivascular hydrostatic pressure, such as may occur in a spontaneously breathing patient with an obstructed airway due to obstructive sleep apnea (OSA), laryngospasm, upper airway masses (e.g., tumors, hematoma, abscess, edema), strangulation, infectious processes (e.g., epiglottitis, pharyngitis, croup), or vocal cord paralysis; with rapid reexpansion of the lung; or with the application of very negative Ppl during thoracentesis.[4,5] Transudated pulmonary interstitial fluid can alter the distribution of pulmonary blood flow by exerting pressure on pulmonary capillaries.

When the flow of fluid into the interstitial space is excessive and the fluid cannot be cleared adequately by the lymphatics, it accumulates in the interstitial connective tissue compartment around the vessels and airways and forms peribronchial and periarteriolar edema fluid cuffs. The transuded pulmonary interstitial fluid fills the pulmonary interstitial space and may eliminate the normally present negative and radially expanding interstitial tension on the extraalveolar pulmonary vessels. Expansion of the pulmonary interstitial space by fluid causes pulmonary interstitial pressure (PISF) to become positive and to exceed Ppv (*zone 4*, Ppa > PISF > Ppv > PA).[6,7] In addition, the vascular resistance of extraalveolar vessels may be increased at a very low lung volume (i.e., residual volume); at such volumes, the tethering action of the pulmonary tissue on the vessels is also lost, and as a result PISF increases positively (see later discussion of lung volume).[8,9] Consequently, zone 4 blood flow is governed by the arteriointerstitial pressure difference (Ppa – PISF), which is less than the Ppa – Ppv difference, and therefore zone 4 blood flow is less than zone 3 blood flow. In summary, zone 4 is a region of the lung from which a large amount of fluid has transuded into the pulmonary interstitial compartment or is possibly at a very low lung volume. Both circumstances produce positive interstitial pressure, which causes compression of extraalveolar vessels, increased extraalveolar vascular resistance, and decreased regional blood flow.

It should be evident that as Ppa and Ppv increase, three important changes take place in the pulmonary circulation—namely, recruitment or opening of previously unperfused vessels, distention or widening of previously perfused vessels, and transudation of fluid from very distended vessels.[10,11] Thus, as mean Ppa increases, zone 1 arteries may become zone 2 arteries, and as mean Ppv increases, zone 2 veins may become zone 3 veins. The increase in both mean Ppa and Ppv distends zone 3 vessels according to their compliance and decreases the resistance to flow through

them. Zone 3 vessels may become so distended that they leak fluid and become converted to zone 4 vessels. In general, pulmonary capillary recruitment is the principal change as Ppa and Ppv increase from low to moderate levels; distention is the principal change as Ppa and Ppv increase from moderate to high levels; and transudation is the principal change when Ppa and Ppv increase from high to very high levels.

Distribution of Ventilation

Gravity also causes differences in vertical Ppl, which in turn causes differences in regional alveolar volume, compliance, and ventilation. The vertical gradient of Ppl can best be understood by imagining the lung as a plastic bag filled with semifluid contents; in other words, it is a viscoelastic structure. Without the presence of a supporting chest wall, the effect of gravity on the contents of the bag would cause the bag to bulge outward at the bottom and inward at the top (i.e., it would assume a globular shape). Inside the supporting chest wall, the lung cannot assume a globular shape. However, gravity still exerts a force on the lung to assume a globular shape; this force creates relatively more negative pressure at the top of the pleural space (where the lung pulls away from the chest wall) and relatively more positive pressure at the bottom of the lung (where the lung is compressed against the chest wall) (Fig. 5.2). The density of the lung determines the magnitude of this pressure gradient. Because the lung has about one-fourth the density of water, the gradient of Ppl (in cm H_2O) is about one-fourth the height of the upright lung (30 cm). Thus, Ppl increases positively by 30/4 = 7.5 cm H_2O from the top to the bottom of the lung.[12]

Because PA is the same throughout the lung, the Ppl gradient causes regional differences in transpulmonary distending pressure (PA – Ppl). Ppl is most positive in the dependent basilar lung regions, so alveoli in these regions are more compressed and are, therefore, considerably smaller than the superior, relatively

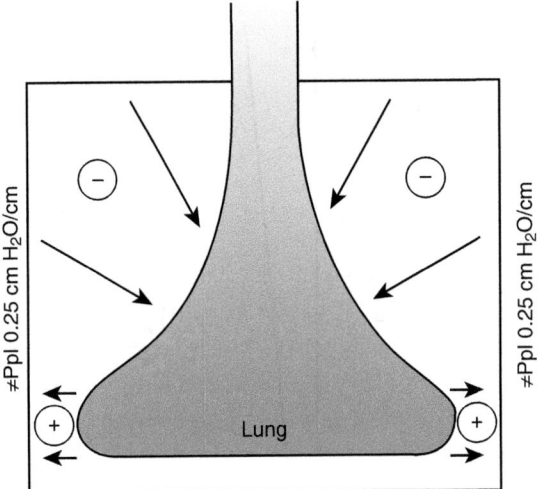

Chest wall

• **Fig. 5.2** Schematic diagram of the lung within the chest wall showing the tendency of the lung to assume a globular shape because of gravity and the lung's viscoelastic nature. The tendency of the top of the lung to collapse inward creates a relatively negative pressure at the apex of the lung, and the tendency of the bottom of the lung to spread outward creates a relatively positive pressure at the base of the lung. Therefore, alveoli at the top of the lung tend to be held open and are larger at end-expiration, whereas those at the bottom tend to be smaller and compressed at end-expiration. Pleural pressure increases by 0.25 cm H_2O per centimeter of lung dependence.

noncompressed apical alveoli (the volume difference is approximately fourfold).[13] If regional differences in alveolar volume are translated to a pressure-volume (compliance) curve for normal lung (Fig. 5.3), the dependent small alveoli are on the midportion, and the nondependent large alveoli are on the upper portion of the S-shaped compliance curve. Because the different regional slopes of the composite curve are equal to the different regional lung compliance values, dependent alveoli are relatively compliant (steep slope), and nondependent alveoli are relatively noncompliant (flat slope). Therefore, most of the VT is preferentially distributed to dependent alveoli that expand more per unit of pressure change than the nondependent alveoli.

Ventilation/Perfusion Ratio

Blood flow and ventilation (both shown on the left vertical axis of Fig. 5.4) increase linearly with distance down the normal upright lung.[14] The ventilation/perfusion ratio ($\dot{V}A/\dot{Q}$, right vertical axis of Fig. 5.4) describes the amount of ventilation relative to perfusion in any given lung region. Because blood flow increases from a very low value and more rapidly than ventilation does with distance down the lung, $\dot{V}A/\dot{Q}$, which is very high at the top of the lung, decreases rapidly at first and then more slowly toward the bottom of the lung, where $\dot{V}A/\dot{Q}$ is low ($\dot{V}A/\dot{Q} < 1$).

Fig. 5.5 shows the calculated ventilation ($\dot{V}A$) and blood flow ($\dot{Q}$), the $\dot{V}A/\dot{Q}$ ratio, and the alveolar partial pressures of oxygen (PAO_2) and carbon dioxide ($PACO_2$) for horizontal slices from the top (7% of lung volume), middle (11% of lung volume), and bottom (13% of lung volume) of the lung.[15] PAO_2 increases by more

than 40 mm Hg, from 89 mm Hg at the base to 132 mm Hg at the apex, whereas $PACO_2$ decreases by 14 mm Hg, from 42 mm Hg at the bottom to 28 mm Hg at the top. Therefore, in keeping with the regional $\dot{V}A/\dot{Q}$ ratio, the bottom of the lung is relatively hypoxic and hypercapnic compared with the top of the lung.

$\dot{V}A/\dot{Q}$ inequalities have different effects on arterial CO_2 tension ($PaCO_2$) than on arterial oxygen tension (PaO_2). Blood passing through underventilated alveoli tends to retain its CO_2 and does not take up enough oxygen; blood traversing overventilated alveoli gives off an excessive amount of CO_2 but cannot take up a proportionately increased amount of oxygen because of the flatness of the oxygen-hemoglobin (oxy-Hb) dissociation curve in this region (see Fig. 5.25). A lung with uneven $\dot{V}A/\dot{Q}$ relationships can eliminate CO_2 from the overventilated alveoli to compensate for the underventilated alveoli. As a result, with uneven $\dot{V}A/\dot{Q}$ relationships, $PACO_2$-to-$PaCO_2$ gradients are small; whereas, PAO_2-to-PaO_2 gradients are usually large.

In 1974, Wagner and colleagues described a method of determining the continuous distribution of $\dot{V}A/\dot{Q}$ ratios within the lung based on the pattern of elimination of a series of intravenously infused inert gases.[16] Gases of differing solubility are dissolved in physiologic saline solution and infused into a peripheral vein until a steady state is achieved (20 minutes). Toward the end of the infusion period, samples of arterial and mixed expired gas are collected, and total ventilation and total cardiac output ($\dot{Q}T$) are measured. For each gas, the ratio of arterial to mixed venous concentration (retention) and the ratio of expired to mixed venous concentration (excretion) are calculated, and retention-solubility

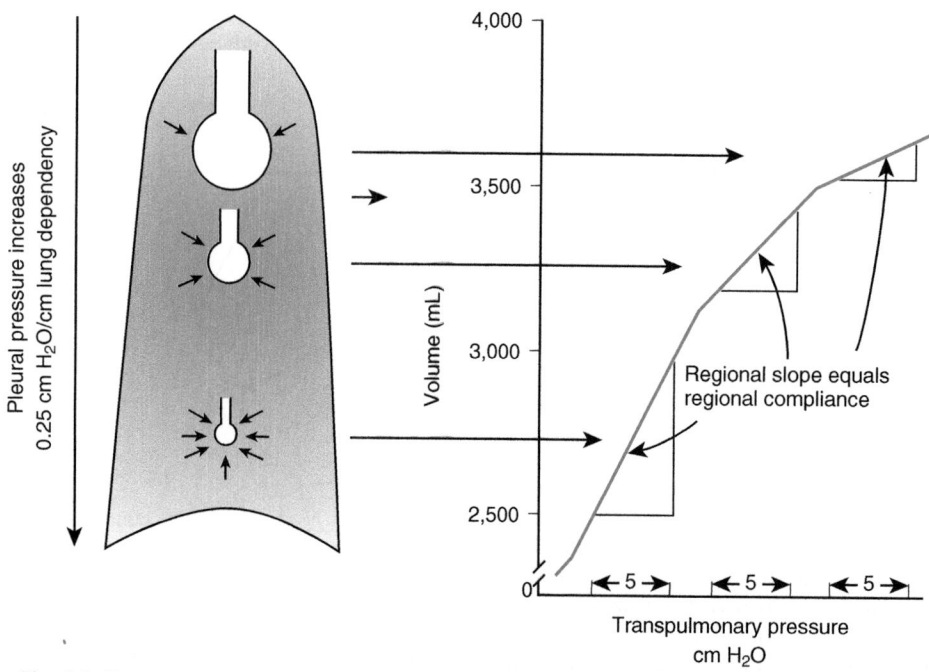

• **Fig. 5.3** Pleural pressure increases by 0.25 cm H_2O every centimeter down the lung. This increase in pleural pressure causes a fourfold decrease in alveolar volume from the top of the lung to the bottom. The caliber of the air passages also decreases as lung volume decreases. When regional alveolar volume is translated to a regional transpulmonary pressure–alveolar volume curve, small alveoli are seen to be on a steep portion of the curve (large slope), and large alveoli are on a flat portion of the curve (relatively small slope). Because the regional slope equals regional compliance, the dependent small alveoli normally receive the largest share of the tidal volume. Over the normal tidal volume range, the pressure-volume relationship is linear: Lung volume increases by 500 mL, from 2500 mL (normal functional residual capacity) to 3000 mL. The lung volume values in this diagram are derived from the upright position.

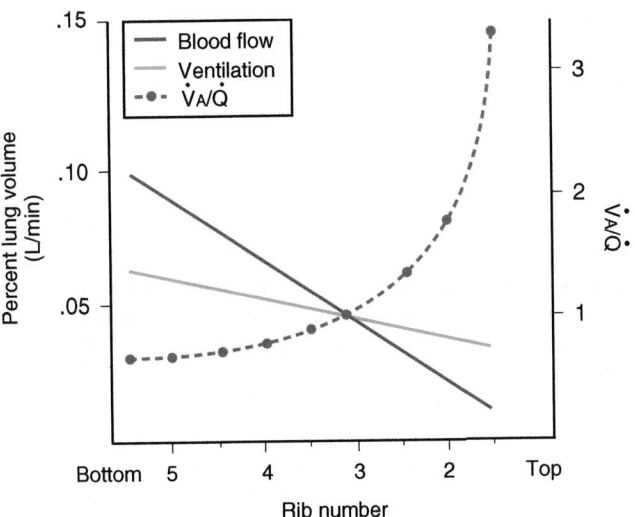

• **Fig. 5.4** Distribution of ventilation and blood flow (left vertical axis) and the ventilation/perfusion ratio ($\dot{V}_A/\dot{Q}$), right vertical axis) in normal upright lung. Both blood flow and ventilation are expressed in liters per minute per percentage of alveolar volume and have been drawn as smoothed-out linear functions of vertical height. The *closed circles* mark the $\dot{V}_A/\dot{Q}$ ratios of horizontal lung slices (three of which are shown in Fig. 5.5). A cardiac output of 6 L/min and a total minute ventilation of 5.1 L/min were assumed. (Modified from West JB. *Ventilation/Blood Flow and Gas Exchange.* 4th ed. Blackwell Scientific; 1970.)

and excretion-solubility curves are drawn. The retention- and excretion-solubility curves can be regarded as fingerprints of the particular distribution of $\dot{V}_A/\dot{Q}$ ratios that give rise to them.

Fig. 5.6 shows the types of distributions found in young, healthy subjects breathing air in the semirecumbent position.[17] The distributions of both ventilation and blood flow are relatively narrow. The upper and lower 9% limits shown (vertical interrupted lines) correspond to $\dot{V}_A/\dot{Q}$ ratios of 0.3 and 2.1, respectively. Note that these young, healthy subjects had no blood flow perfusion areas with very low $\dot{V}_A/\dot{Q}$ ratios, nor did they have any blood flow to unventilated or shunted areas ($\dot{V}_A/\dot{Q} = 0$) or unperfused areas ($\dot{V}_A/\dot{Q} = 8$). Fig. 5.6 also shows P_{AO_2} and P_{ACO_2} in respiratory units with different $\dot{V}_A/\dot{Q}$ ratios. Within the 95% range of $\dot{V}_A/\dot{Q}$ ratios (i.e., 0.3 to 2.1), P_{AO_2} ranges from 60 to 123 mm Hg, whereas the corresponding P_{ACO_2} range is 44 to 33 mm Hg.

Nongravitational Determinants of Blood Flow Distribution

Passive Processes

Cardiac Output

The pulmonary vascular bed is a high-flow, low-pressure system under normal health conditions. As total pulmonary blood flow (cardiac output [$\dot{Q}_T$]) increases, pulmonary vascular pressures

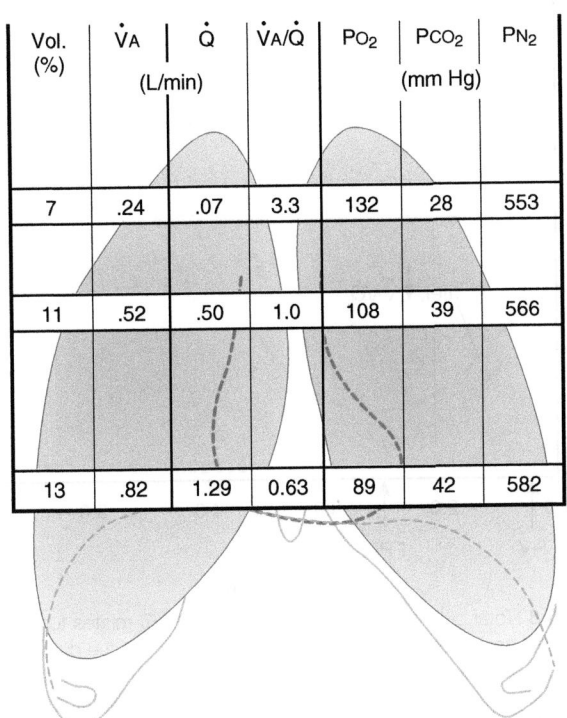

Vol. (%)	$\dot{V}_A$	$\dot{Q}$	$\dot{V}_A/\dot{Q}$	P_{O_2}	P_{CO_2}	P_{N_2}
	(L/min)			(mm Hg)		
7	.24	.07	3.3	132	28	553
11	.52	.50	1.0	108	39	566
13	.82	1.29	0.63	89	42	582

• **Fig. 5.5** Ventilation/perfusion ratio ($\dot{V}_A/\dot{Q}$) and the regional composition of alveolar gas. Values for regional flow ($\dot{Q}$), ventilation ($\dot{V}_A$), partial pressure of oxygen (P_{O_2}), and partial pressure of carbon dioxide (P_{CO_2}) were derived from Fig. 5.4. Partial pressure of nitrogen (P_{N_2}) represents what remains from total gas pressure (760 mm Hg including water vapor, which equals 47 mm Hg). The percentage volumes (*Vol.*) of the three lung slices are also shown. When compared with the top of the lung, the bottom of the lung has a low $\dot{V}_A/\dot{Q}$ ratio and is relatively hypoxic and hypercapnic. (From West JB. Regional differences in gas exchange in the lung of erect man. *J Appl Physiol.* 1962;17:893.)

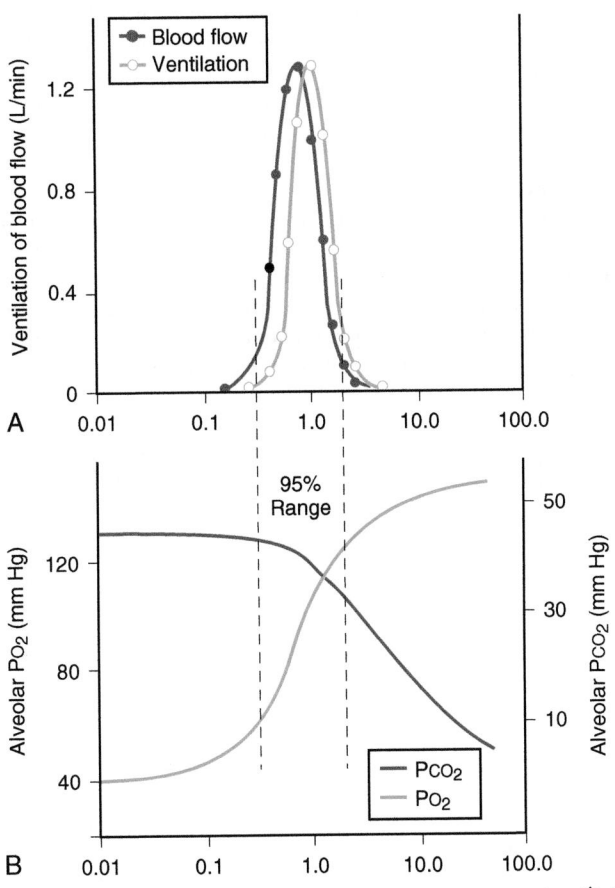

• **Fig. 5.6** (A) Average distribution of ventilation/perfusion ratios ($\dot{V}_A/\dot{Q}$) in normal, young, semirecumbent subjects. The 95% range (between *dashed lines*) is 0.3 to 2.1. (B) Corresponding variations in partial pressures of oxygen (P_{O_2}) and carbon dioxide (P_{CO_2}) in alveolar gas. (From West JB. Blood flow to the lung and gas exchange. *Anesthesiology.* 1974;41:124.)

increase minimally.[18] However, increases in $\dot{Q}T$ distend open vessels and recruit previously closed vessels. Accordingly, pulmonary vascular resistance (PVR) drops because the normal pulmonary vasculature is quite distensible (and partly because of the addition of previously unused vessels to the pulmonary circulation). As a result of the distensibility of the normal pulmonary circulation, an increase in Ppa increases the radius of the pulmonary vessels, which causes PVR to decrease (Fig. 5.7). Conversely, the opposite effect occurs within the pulmonary vessels during a decrease in $\dot{Q}T$. As $\dot{Q}T$ decreases, pulmonary vascular pressures decrease, the radii of the pulmonary vessels are reduced, and PVR consequently increases. In contrast to the normal situation, the pulmonary vessels of patients with significant pulmonary arterial hypertension (PAH) are less distensible, acting more like rigid pipes. In this setting, Ppa will increase sharply with any increase in $\dot{Q}T$ because PVR in these stiff vessels does not decrease significantly due to minimal expansion of their radii.

Understanding the relationships among Ppa, PVR, and $\dot{Q}T$ during passive events is a prerequisite to recognition of active vasomotion in the pulmonary circulation (see section "Lung Volume"). Active vasoconstriction occurs whenever $\dot{Q}T$ decreases and Ppa either remains constant or increases. Increased Ppa and PVR have been found to be "a universal feature of acute respiratory failure."[19]

Active pulmonary vasoconstriction can increase Ppa and Ppv, contributing to the formation of pulmonary edema, and in that way it has a role in the pathophysiology of adult respiratory distress syndrome (ARDS). Active vasodilation occurs whenever $\dot{Q}T$ increases and Ppa either remains constant or decreases. When deliberate hypotension is achieved with sodium nitroprusside or nitroglycerine infusions, $\dot{Q}T$ often remains constant or increases, but Ppa decreases, and therefore so does PVR.

Lung Volume

Lung volume and PVR have an asymmetric, U-shaped relationship because of the varying effect of lung volume on small intraalveolar and large extraalveolar vessels, which in both cases is minimal at functional residual capacity (FRC). FRC is defined as the volume of gas in the lungs at end-expiration during normal tidal breathing. Ideally, this means that the patient is inspiring a normal VT, with

minimal or no muscle activity or pressure difference between the alveoli and atmosphere at end-expiration. Total PVR is increased when lung volume is either increased or decreased from FRC (Fig. 5.8).[20–22] The increase in total PVR above FRC results from alveolar compression of small intraalveolar vessels, which results in an increase in small-vessel PVR (i.e., creation of zone 1 or zone 2).[23] As a relatively small counterbalancing effect to the compression of small vessels, the large extraalveolar vessels can be expanded by the increased tethering of interstitial connective tissue that occurs at high lung volumes (and, with spontaneous ventilation only, the negativity of perivascular pressure at high lung volumes). The increase in total PVR with lung volumes below FRC results from an increase in the PVR of large extraalveolar vessels (passive effect). The increase in large-vessel PVR is partly due to mechanical tortuosity or kinking of these vessels (passive effect). In addition, small or grossly atelectatic lungs become hypoxic, and it has been shown that the increased large-vessel PVR in these lungs is also caused by an active vasoconstrictive mechanism known as hypoxic pulmonary vasoconstriction (HPV).[24] The effect of HPV (discussed in greater detail in the section "Alveolar Gases") is significant whether the chest is open or closed and whether ventilation is by positive pressure or spontaneous.[25]

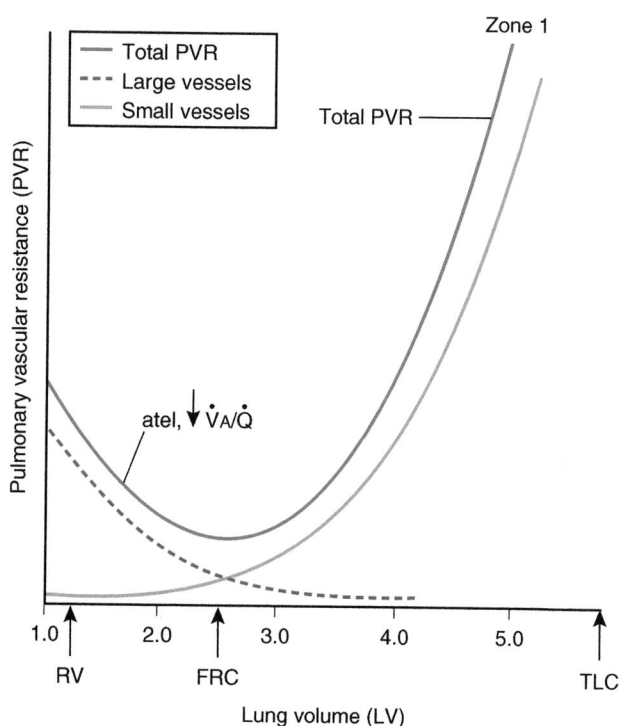

• **Fig. 5.8** Total pulmonary vascular resistance *(PVR)* relates to lung volume as an asymmetric, U-shaped curve. The trough of the curve occurs when lung volume equals functional residual capacity *(FRC)*. Total PVR is the sum of the resistance in small vessels (increased by increasing lung volume *[LV]*) and the resistance in large vessels (increased by decreasing LV). The end point for increasing LV toward total lung capacity *(TLC)* is the creation of zone 1 conditions, and the end point for decreasing LV toward residual volume *(RV)* is the creation of low ventilation/perfusion *(V̇A/Q̇)* and atelectatic *(atel)* areas that demonstrate hypoxic pulmonary vasoconstriction. (Data from Bhavani-Shankar K, Hart NS, Mushlin PS. Negative pressure induced airway and pulmonary injury. *Can J Anaesth.* 1997;44:78; Berggren SM. The oxygen deficit of arterial blood caused by nonventilating parts of the lung. *Acta Physiol Scand Suppl.* 1942;4:11; and Benumof JL. One lung ventilation: which lung should be PEEPed? *Anesthesiology.* 1982;56:161.)

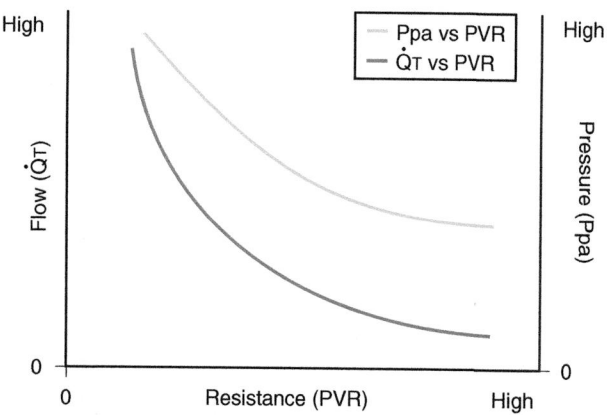

• **Fig. 5.7** Passive changes in pulmonary vascular resistance *(PVR)* as a function of pulmonary artery pressure *(Ppa)* and pulmonary blood flow *(Q̇T)*: PVR = Ppa/Q̇T. As Q̇T increases, Ppa also increases, but to a lesser extent, and PVR decreases. As Q̇T decreases, Ppa also decreases, but to a lesser extent, and PVR increases. (Modified from Fishman AP. Dynamics of the pulmonary circulation. In: Hamilton WF, ed. *Handbook of Physiology.* Section 2: Circulation, Vol. 2. Williams & Wilkins; 1963:1667.)

TABLE 5.1	Local Tissue (Autocrine/Paracrine) Molecules Involved in Active Control of Pulmonary Vascular Tone			
Molecule	Subtype	Site of Origin	Site of Action	Response
Nitric oxide	NO	Endothelium	Sm. muscle	Vasodilation
Endothelin	ET-1	Endothelium	Sm. muscle (ET_A receptor) Endothelium (ET_B receptor)	Vasoconstriction Vasodilation
Prostaglandin	PGI_2	Endothelium	Endothelium	Vasodilation
Prostaglandin	PGF_{2a}	Endothelium	Sm. muscle	Vasoconstriction
Thromboxane	TXA_2	Endothelium	Sm. muscle	Vasoconstriction
Leukotriene	LTB_4–LTE_4	Endothelium	Sm. muscle	Vasoconstriction

ET_A receptor, ET-1 receptor located on the smooth muscle cell membrane; *ET_B receptor*, ET-1 receptor located on the endothelial cell membrane; *Sm. muscle*, pulmonary arteriole smooth muscle cell.

Active Processes and Pulmonary Vascular Tone

Four major categories of active processes affect the pulmonary vascular tone of normal patients: (1) local tissue (endothelial- and smooth muscle–derived) autocrine or paracrine products, which act on smooth muscle (Table 5.1); (2) alveolar gas concentrations (chiefly hypoxia), which also act on smooth muscle; (3) neural influences; and (4) humoral (or hormonal) effects of circulating products within the pulmonary capillary bed. The neural and humoral effects work by means of either receptor-mediated mechanisms involving the autocrine/paracrine molecules listed in Table 5.1 or related mechanisms ultimately affecting the smooth muscle cell.[26] These four interrelated systems, each affecting pulmonary vascular tone, are briefly reviewed in sequence.

Tissue (Endothelial- and Smooth Muscle–Derived) Products

The pulmonary vascular endothelium synthesizes, metabolizes, and converts numerous vasoactive substances and plays a central role in the regulation of PVR. However, the main effecter site of pulmonary vascular tone is the pulmonary vascular smooth muscle cell, which both senses and produces a multitude of pulmonary vasoactive compounds.[27] The autocrine/paracrine molecules listed in Table 5.1 are all actively involved in the regulation of pulmonary vascular tone during various conditions. Numerous additional compounds bind to receptors on the endothelial or smooth muscle cell membranes and modulate the levels (and effects) of these vasoactive molecules.

Nitric oxide (NO) is the predominant endogenous vasodilatory compound. Its discovery by Palmer and colleagues more than 45 years ago ended the long search for the so-called endothelium-derived relaxant factor (EDRF).[28] Since then, a massive amount of laboratory and clinical research has demonstrated the ubiquitous nature of NO and its predominant role in vasodilation of both pulmonary and systemic blood vessels.[29] In the pulmonary endothelial cell, L-arginine is converted to L-citrulline by means of nitric oxide synthase (NOS) to produce the small, yet highly reactive NO molecule.[30] Because of its small size, NO can diffuse freely across membranes into the smooth muscle cell, where it binds to the heme moiety of guanylate cyclase (which converts guanosine triphosphate to cyclic guanosine monophosphate [cGMP]).[31] cGMP activates protein kinase G, which dephosphorylates the myosin light chains of pulmonary vascular smooth muscle cells and thereby causes vasodilation.[31] NOS exists in two forms: constitutive (cNOS) and inducible (iNOS). cNOS is permanently expressed in certain cells, including pulmonary vascular endothelial cells, and produces short bursts of NO in response to changing levels of calcium, calmodulin, and shear stress. The cNOS enzyme is also stimulated by linked membrane-based receptors that bind numerous molecules in the blood (e.g., acetylcholine and bradykinin).[31] In contrast, iNOS is produced only when triggered by inflammatory mediators and cytokines and, when stimulated, produces large quantities of NO for an extended duration.[31] It is well known that NO is constitutively produced in normal lungs and contributes to the maintenance of low PVR.[32,33]

Endothelin-1 (ET-1) is a pulmonary vasoconstrictor and mitogen.[34] The endothelins are 21-amino-acid peptides that are produced by a variety of cells. ET-1 is the only family member produced in pulmonary endothelial cells, and it is also produced in vascular smooth muscle cells.[34] ET-1 exerts its major vascular effects through activation of two distinct G protein-coupled receptors (ET_A and ET_B). ET_A receptors are found in the medial smooth muscle layers of the pulmonary (and systemic) blood vessels and in atrial and ventricular myocardium.[34] When stimulated, ET_A receptors induce vasoconstriction and cellular proliferation by increasing intracellular calcium.[35] ET_B receptors are localized on endothelial cells and some smooth muscle cells.[36] Activation of ET_B receptors stimulates the release of NO and prostacyclin, thereby promoting pulmonary vasodilation and inhibiting apoptosis.[30] Bosentan, a competitive ET_A and ET_B antagonist, has produced modest improvement in the treatment of PAH.[37] Selective ET_A receptor antagonists (e.g., sitaxsentan and ambrisentan) may have additional benefits in improving PAH.[38] However, all of these ET-1 receptor antagonists are associated with an increased risk of liver toxicity; sitaxsentan was removed from the market in 2010 for this reason.[39] In summary, it appears that there is a normal balance between NO and ET-1, with a slight predominance toward NO production and vasodilation in health.

Similarly, various eicosanoids are elaborated by the pulmonary vascular endothelium, with a balance toward the vasodilatory compounds in health. Prostaglandin I_2 (PGI_2), now called epoprostenol (previously known as prostacyclin), causes vasodilation and is continuously elaborated in small amounts in healthy endothelium. In contrast, thromboxane A_2 and leukotriene B_4 are expressed under pathologic conditions and are involved in the pathophysiology of PAH associated with sepsis and reperfusion injury.[26]

Epoprostenol has been used successfully to decrease PVR in patients with chronic PAH when infused or inhaled.[40,41] Synthetic PGI_2 (iloprost) is a commonly used inhaled eicosanoid for reduction of PVR in patients with PAH.[41] Although many patients with chronic PAH are unresponsive to an acute vasodilator challenge with short-acting agents such as epoprostenol, adenosine, or

NO,[42] long-term administration of epoprostenol has been shown to decrease PVR in these patients.[43] Furthermore, some patients with previously severe PAH have been weaned from epoprostenol after long-term administration, with dramatically decreased PVR and improved exercise tolerance.[42] The vascular remodeling required to provide such a dramatic reduction in PVR is probably the result of mechanisms besides simple local vasodilation, as predicted by Fishman in an editorial in 1998.[44] One such mechanism that appears to be important is the increased clearance of ET-1 with long-term epoprostenol administration.[45]

Alveolar Gases

Hypoxia-induced pulmonary vasoconstriction constitutes a fundamental difference between pulmonary vessels and all systemic blood vessels (which vasodilate in the presence of hypoxia). Alveolar hypoxia of in vivo and in vitro whole lung, unilateral lung, lobe, or lobule of lung results in localized pulmonary vasoconstriction. This phenomenon is widely referred to as HPV and was first described more than 70 years ago by Von Euler and Liljestrand.[46] The HPV response is present in all mammalian species and serves as an adaptive mechanism for diverting blood flow from poorly ventilated to better ventilated regions of the lung and thereby improving $\dot{V}_A/\dot{Q}$ ratios.[47] The HPV response is also critical for fetal development because it minimizes perfusion of the unventilated lung.

The HPV response occurs primarily in pulmonary arterioles of about 200 μm internal diameter (ID) in humans (60 to 700 μm ID in other species).[48] These vessels are advantageously situated anatomically in close relation to small bronchioles and alveoli, which permits rapid and direct detection of alveolar hypoxia. Indeed, blood may actually become oxygenated in small pulmonary arteries because of the ability of oxygen to diffuse directly across the small distance between the contiguous air spaces and vessels.[49] This direct access that gas in the airways has to small arteries makes possible a rapid and localized vascular response to changes in gas composition.

The oxygen tension at the HPV stimulus site (P_{SO_2}) is a function of both P_{AO_2} and mixed venous oxygen pressure ($P\bar{v}_{O_2}$).[50] The P_{SO_2}-HPV response curve is sigmoidal, with a 50% response when P_{AO_2}, $P\bar{v}_{O_2}$, and P_{SO_2} are approximately 30 mm Hg. Usually, P_{AO_2} has a much greater effect than $P\bar{v}_{O_2}$ does because oxygen uptake is from the alveolar space to the blood in the small pulmonary arteries.[50]

Numerous theories have been developed to explain the mechanism of HPV.[46,51–53] Many vasoactive substances have been proposed as mediators of HPV, including leukotrienes, prostaglandins, catecholamines, serotonin, histamine, angiotensin, bradykinin, and ET-1, but none has been identified as the primary mediator. In 1992, Xuan proposed that NO has a pivotal role in modulating PVR.[54] NO is involved, but not precisely in the way that Xuan first proposed. There are multiple sites of oxygen sensing with variable contributions from the NO, ET-1, and eicosanoid systems (previously described). In vivo, HPV is currently thought to result from the synergistic action of molecules produced in both endothelial cells and smooth muscle cells.[55] However, HPV can proceed in the absence of intact endothelium, suggesting that the primary oxygen sensor is in the smooth muscle cell and that endothelium-derived molecules modulate only the primary HPV response.

The precise mechanism(s) of HPV continue to be studied. However, abundant data support the smooth muscle mitochondrial electron transport chain as the HPV sensor (Fig. 5.9).[56] In addition, reactive oxygen species (including H_2O_2 and superoxide) are

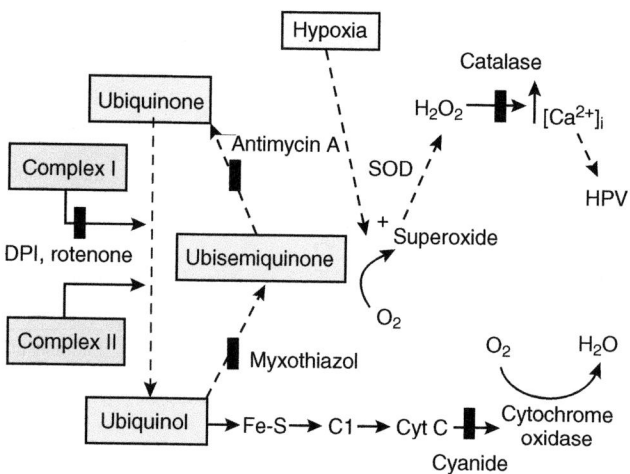

• **Fig. 5.9** Schematic model of the mitochondrial oxygen-sensing and effector mechanism responsible for hypoxic pulmonary vasoconstriction *(HPV)*. In this model, reactive oxygen species (ROS) are released from electron transport chain complex III and act as second messengers in the hypoxia-induced calcium *(Ca²⁺)* increase and resultant HPV. The *solid arrows* represent electron transfer steps; *solid bars* show sites of electron chain inhibition. Normal mitochondrial electron transport involves the movement of reducing equivalents generated in the Krebs cycle through complex I or II and then through complex III (ubiquinone) and complex IV (cytochrome oxidase). The Q cycle converts the dual electron transfer in complex I and II into a single electron transfer step used in complex IV. The ubisemiquinone (a free radical) created in this process can generate superoxide, which in the presence of superoxide dismutase *(SOD)* produces H_2O_2, the probable mediator of the hypoxia-induced increase in Ca²⁺ and HPV. This process is amplified during hypoxia. Diphenyleneiodonium *(DPI)*, rotenone, and myxothiazol are inhibitors of the proximal portion of the electron transport chain; cyanide is an inhibitor of cytochrome oxidase. (From Waypa GB, Marks JD, Mack MM, et al. Mitochondrial reactive oxygen species trigger calcium increases during hypoxia in pulmonary artery myocytes. *Circ Res.* 2002;91:719.)

released from complex III of the electron transport chain and probably serve as second messengers to increase calcium in pulmonary artery smooth muscle cells during acute hypoxia.[57] Alternative (less likely) mechanisms are also being investigated. One alternative hypothesis suggests that smooth muscle microsomal reduced nicotinamide adenine dinucleotide phosphate (NADPH) oxidoreductase or sarcolemmal NADPH oxidase is the sensing mechanism.[57] Although the precise oxygen sensing and signal transduction mechanisms remain under investigation,[57] it is now clear that the mitochondria of the pulmonary artery smooth muscle cells are the focus of these effects.[58] Indeed, a recent study by Zhou and colleagues demonstrated that transplantation of mitochondria from femoral arterial smooth muscle cells into the pulmonary artery smooth muscle cells attenuates the HPV response.[58]

In summary, HPV results from a direct action of alveolar hypoxia on pulmonary smooth muscle cells, sensed by the mitochondrial electron transport chain, with reactive oxygen species (probably H_2O_2 or superoxide) serving as second messengers to increase calcium and smooth muscle vasoconstriction. The endothelium-derived products serve to both potentiate (ET-1) and attenuate (NO, PGI_2) to achieve the HPV response. Additional mechanisms (humoral and neurogenic influences) modulate baseline pulmonary vascular tone and affect the magnitude of the HPV response.

Elevated P_{ACO_2} has a pulmonary vasoconstrictor effect. Both respiratory acidosis and metabolic acidosis augment HPV, whereas respiratory and metabolic alkalosis cause pulmonary vasodilation and serve to reduce HPV.

The clinical effects of HPV in humans can be classified under three basic mechanisms. First, life at high altitude or whole-lung respiration of a low FIO_2 increases Ppa. This is true for newcomers to high altitude, for the acclimatized, and for natives.[53] The vasoconstriction is considerable; in healthy people breathing 10% oxygen, Ppa doubles, whereas pulmonary wedge pressure remains constant.[59] The increased Ppa increases perfusion of the apices of the lung (through recruitment of previously unused vessels), which results in gas exchange in a region of lung not normally used (i.e., zone 1). Therefore, with a low FIO_2, PaO_2 is greater and the alveolar-arterial oxygen tension difference and the ratio between dead space and tidal volume (V_D/V_T) are less than would be expected or predicted on the basis of a normal (sea level) distribution of ventilation and blood flow. High-altitude PAH is an important component in the development of mountain sickness subacutely (hours to days) and cor pulmonale chronically (weeks to years).[60] There is now good evidence that in both patients with chronic obstructive pulmonary disease (COPD) and those with OSA, nocturnal episodes of arterial oxygen desaturation (caused by episodic hypoventilation) are accompanied by elevations in Ppa that can eventually lead to sustained PAH and cor pulmonale.[61]

Second, hypoventilation (low $\dot{V}A/\dot{Q}$ ratio), atelectasis, or nitrogen ventilation of any region of the lung usually causes a diversion of blood flow away from the hypoxic to the nonhypoxic lung (40% to 50% in one lung, 50% to 60% in one lobe, 60% to 70% in one lobule) (Fig. 5.10).[62] The regional vasoconstriction and blood flow diversion are important in minimizing transpulmonary shunting and normalizing regional $\dot{V}A/\dot{Q}$ ratios during unilateral lung disease, one-lung ventilation (see Chapter 26), inadvertent intubation of a mainstem bronchus, and lobar collapse.

Third, in patients who have COPD, asthma, pneumonia, or mitral stenosis without bronchospasm, administration of pulmonary vasodilator drugs such as isoproterenol, nitroprusside, or nitroglycerin inhibits

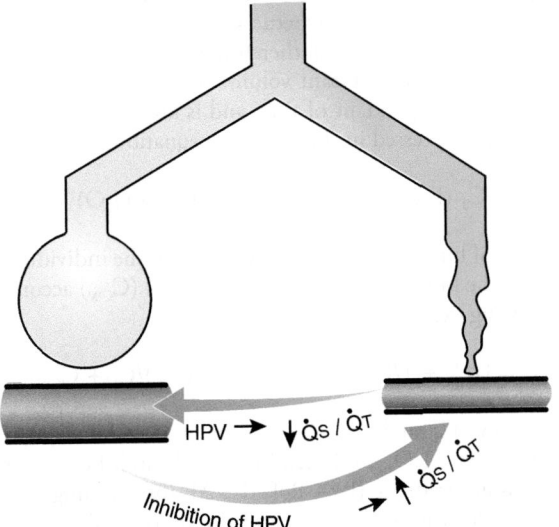

• **Fig. 5.10** Schematic drawing of regional hypoxic pulmonary vasoconstriction *(HPV)*; one-lung ventilation is a common clinical example of regional HPV. HPV in the hypoxic atelectatic lung causes redistribution of blood flow away from the hypoxic lung to the normoxic lung, thereby diminishing the amount of shunt flow *(Qs/QT)* that can occur through the hypoxic lung. Inhibition of hypoxic lung HPV causes an increase in the amount of shunt flow through the hypoxic lung, thereby decreasing the alveolar oxygen tension (PAO$_2$).

HPV and causes a decrease in PaO_2 and PVR and an increase in right-to-left transpulmonary shunt.[63] The mechanism for these changes is thought to be deleterious inhibition of preexisting and, in some conditions, geographically widespread HPV without concomitant bronchodilation.[63] In accordance with the latter two lines of evidence (one-lung or regional hypoxia and vasodilator drug effects on generalized or whole-lung disease), HPV can divert blood flow away from hypoxic regions of the lung, thereby serving as an autoregulatory mechanism that protects PaO_2 by favorably adjusting regional $\dot{V}A/\dot{Q}$ ratios. Factors that inhibit regional HPV are extensively discussed by other authors,[64,65] and further explained in this chapter (In Section Inhibition of Hypoxic Pulmonary Vasoconstriction (pp. 151–152)).

Neural Influences on Pulmonary Vascular Tone

The three systems used to innervate the pulmonary circulation are the same ones that innervate the airways: the sympathetic, parasympathetic, and nonadrenergic, noncholinergic (NANC) systems.[26] Sympathetic (adrenergic) fibers originate from the first five thoracic nerves and enter the pulmonary vessels as branches from the cervical ganglia, as well as from a plexus of nerves arising from the trachea and mainstem bronchi. These nerves act mainly on pulmonary arteries down to a diameter of 60 µm.[26] Sympathetic fibers cause pulmonary vasoconstriction through α_1-receptors. However, the pulmonary arteries also contain vasodilatory α_2-receptors and β_2-receptors. The α_1-adrenergic response predominates during sympathetic stimulation, such as occurs with pain, fear, and anxiety.[26] The parasympathetic (cholinergic) nerve fibers originate from the vagus nerve and cause pulmonary vasodilation through a NO-dependent process.[26] Binding of acetylcholine to the muscarinic (M_3) receptor on the endothelial cell increases intracellular calcium and stimulates cNOS.[26] NANC nerves cause pulmonary vasodilation through NO-mediated systems by using vasoactive intestinal peptide as the neurotransmitter. The functional significance of this system is still under investigation.[26]

Humoral Influences on Pulmonary Vascular Tone

Numerous molecules are released into the circulation that either affect pulmonary vascular tone (by binding to pulmonary endothelial receptors) or are altered by the pulmonary endothelium and subsequently become activated or inactivated (Table 5.2). The basic effects that various circulating factors have on pulmonary vascular tone are increasingly understood, and it is unlikely that these compounds significantly modulate pulmonary vascular tone under normal circumstances. However, they can have marked effects during disease (e.g., ARDS or sepsis).

Endogenous catecholamines (epinephrine and norepinephrine) bind to both α_1- (vasoconstrictor) and β_2- (vasodilator) receptors on the pulmonary endothelium, but when elaborated in high concentration, they have a predominant α_1- (vasoconstrictive) effect. The same is true for exogenously administered catecholamines. Other amines (e.g., histamine and serotonin) are elaborated systemically or locally after various challenges and have variable effects on PVR. Histamine can be released from mast cells, basophils, and elsewhere. When histamine binds directly to H_1-receptors on endothelium, NO-mediated vasodilation occurs. In contrast, stimulation of H_1-receptors on the smooth muscle membrane results in vasoconstriction, whereas direct stimulation of H_2-receptors on smooth muscle cell membranes causes vasodilation. Serotonin (5-hydroxytryptamine) is a potent vasoconstrictor that can be elaborated from activated platelets (e.g., after pulmonary embolism) and can contribute to acute severe PAH.[66]

Numerous peptides circulate and cause either pulmonary vasodilation (e.g., substance P, bradykinin, and vasopressin [a systemic

TABLE 5.2	Action of Pulmonary Endothelium on Compounds Passing Through the Pulmonary Circulation		
Molecule Type	**Activated**	**Unchanged**	**Inactivated**
Amines		Dopamine Epinephrine Histamine	5-Hydroxytryptamine Norepinephrine
Peptides	Angiotensin I	Angiotensin II Oxytocin Vasopressin	Bradykinin Atrial natriuretic peptide Endothelins
Eicosanoids	Arachidonic acid	PGI_2 PGA_2	PGD_2 PGE_1, PGE_2 PGF_{2a} Leukotrienes
Purine derivatives			Adenosine ATP, ADP, AMP

ADP, Adenosine diphosphate; *AMP,* adenosine monophosphate; *ATP,* adenosine triphosphate; *PG,* prostaglandin.

Modified from Lumb AB. Non-respiratory functions of the lung. In: Lumb AB, ed. *Nunn's Applied Respiratory Physiology.* 5th ed. Butterworths; 2000:309.

vasoconstrictor]) or vasoconstriction (e.g., neurokinin A and angiotensin). These peptides only produce clinically detectable effects on PVR in high concentrations, such as with exogenous administration or in disease.

Two other classes of molecules must be mentioned for completeness: eicosanoids (whose vasoactive effects were previously discussed) and purine nucleosides (which are similarly highly vasoactive).[26] Adenosine is a pulmonary vasodilator in normal subjects, whereas adenosine triphosphate (ATP) has a variable effect, depending on the baseline pulmonary vascular tone.[67]

Alternative (Nonalveolar) Pathways of Blood Flow Through the Lung

Blood can also traverse the lung from the right to the left side of the heart without being fully oxygenated or oxygenated at all. For example, blood flow through poorly ventilated alveoli (regions of low $\dot{V}_A/\dot{Q}$ with an $FIO_2 < 0.3$) have a right-to-left shunt effect on oxygenation, and blood flow through nonventilated alveoli (in atelectatic or consolidated regions, $\dot{V}_A/\dot{Q} = 0$) does not contribute to gas exchange at any FIO_2 values; both are sources of right-to-left transpulmonary shunting. Low-$\dot{V}_A/\dot{Q}$ and atelectatic lung units occur in conditions in which the FRC is less than the closing capacity (CC) of the lung (see section "Lung Volume, Functional Residual Capacity, and Closing Capacity").

In addition, several right-to-left blood flow pathways traverse the lungs and heart without passing by or involving alveoli at all. The bronchial and pleural circulations originate from systemic arteries and empty directly into the left side of the heart without being oxygenated; these circulations constitute the 1% to 3% true right-to-left shunt normally present. With chronic bronchitis, and in cases of severe chronic thromboembolic pulmonary hypertension (CTEPH), the bronchial circulation can markedly increase, carrying as much as 10% of the cardiac output, and with pleuritis the pleural circulation can increase to carry 5% of the cardiac output. Consequently, as much as a 10% or 15% obligatory right-to-left shunt can be present under pathologic conditions.

Intrapulmonary arteriovenous anastomoses are normally closed, but in the presence of acute PAH, such as may be caused by a pulmonary embolus, they may open and result in a direct increase in right-to-left shunting. A patent foramen ovale (PFO) is present in 20% to 30% of individuals, but it usually remains functionally closed because left atrial pressure normally exceeds right atrial pressure. When a PFO is present, any condition that causes right atrial pressure to be greater than left atrial pressure can produce a right-to-left shunt, with resultant hypoxemia and possible paradoxical embolization. Such conditions include PAH, the use of high levels of PEEP, pulmonary embolization, COPD, pulmonary valvular stenosis, congestive heart failure, and postpneumonectomy states.[68] Even such common events as mechanical ventilation and reaction to the presence of an endotracheal tube (ETT) during the excitement phase of emergence from anesthesia have caused right-to-left shunting across a PFO and severe arterial desaturation (with the potential for paradoxical embolization).[69,70] Transesophageal echocardiography (TEE) has been demonstrated to be a sensitive modality for diagnosing a PFO in anesthetized patients with elevated right atrial pressure.[71]

Esophageal to mediastinal to bronchial to pulmonary vein pathways of right-to-left shunt have been described and may explain, in part, the hypoxemia associated with portal hypertension and cirrhosis. Thebesian vessels nourish the left ventricular myocardium and originate and empty into the left side of the heart. There are no known conditions that selectively increase thebesian blood flow.

Nongravitational Determinants of Pulmonary Compliance, Resistance, Lung Volume, Ventilation, and Work of Breathing

Pulmonary Compliance

For air to flow into the lungs, a pressure gradient (ΔP) must be developed to overcome the elastic resistance of the lungs and chest wall to expansion. These structures are arranged concentrically, and their elastic resistance is therefore additive. The relationship between ΔP and the resultant volume increase (ΔV) of the lungs and thorax is independent of time and is known as total compliance (C_T), as expressed in the following equation:

$$C_T \ (\text{L/cm } H_2O) = \Delta V \ (\text{L})/\Delta P \ (\text{cm } H_2O) \tag{1}$$

The C_T of lung plus chest wall is related to the individual compliance of the lungs (C_L) and of the chest wall (C_{CW}) according to the following expression:

$$1/C_T = 1/C_L + 1/C_{CW} \ [\text{or } C_T = (C_L)(C_{CW})/C_L + C_{CW}] \tag{2}$$

Normally, C_L and C_{CW} each equal 0.2 L/cm H_2O; hence $C_T = 0.1$ L/cm H_2O. To determine C_L, ΔV and the transpulmonary pressure gradient ($P_A - P_{pl}$, the ΔP for the lung) must be known; to determine C_{CW}, ΔV and the transmural pressure gradient ($P_{pl} - P_{ambient}$, the ΔP for the chest wall) must be known; and to determine C_T, ΔV and the transthoracic pressure gradient ($P_A - P_{ambient}$, the ΔP for the lung and chest wall together) must be known. In clinical practice, only C_T is measured, which can be done dynamically or statically, depending on whether a peak or a plateau inspiratory ΔP (respectively) is used for the C_T calculation.

During a positive- or negative-pressure inspiration of sufficient duration, transthoracic ΔP first increases to a peak value and then decreases to a lower plateau value. The peak transthoracic pressure value is the pressure required to overcome both elastic and airway resistance (see section "Airway Resistance"). Transthoracic pressure decreases to a plateau value after the peak value because, with time, gas is redistributed from stiff alveoli (which expand only slightly and therefore have only a short inspiratory period) into more compliant alveoli (which expand a great deal and therefore have a long inspiratory period). Because the gas is redistributed into more compliant alveoli, less pressure is required to contain the same volume of gas, which explains why the pressure decreases. In practical terms, dynamic compliance is the volume change divided by the peak inspiratory transthoracic pressure, and static compliance is the volume change divided by the plateau inspiratory transthoracic pressure. Therefore, static C_T is usually greater than dynamic C_D, because the former calculation uses a smaller denominator (lower pressure) than the latter. If the patient is receiving PEEP, that pressure must first be subtracted from the peak or plateau pressure before thoracic compliance is calculated (i.e., compliance is equal to the volume delivered divided by the peak or plateau pressure—PEEP).

Alveolar pressure deserves special comment. The alveoli are lined with a layer of liquid. When a curved surface (a sphere or cylinder, such as the alveoli, bronchioles, and bronchi) is lined with liquid, a surface tension is created that tends to make the surface area that is exposed to the atmosphere as small as possible. Simply stated, water molecules crowd much closer together on the surface of a curved layer of water than elsewhere in the fluid. As the alveolar size decreases, the degree of curvature and the retractive surface tension will increase.

According to the Laplace expression, shown in Eq. 3, the pressure in an alveolus (P, in dynes/cm²) is higher than ambient pressure by an amount that depends on the surface tension of the lining liquid (T, in dynes/cm) and the radius of curvature of the alveolus (R, in cm). This relationship is expressed in the following equation:

$$P = 2T/R \qquad (3)$$

Although surface tension contributes to the elastic resistance and retractive forces of the lung, two difficulties must be resolved. First, the pressure inside a small alveolus should be higher than that inside a large alveolus, a conclusion that stems directly from the Laplace equation (R in the denominator). From this reasoning, one would expect a progressive discharge of each small alveolus into a larger one until eventually only one gigantic alveolus would be left (Fig. 5.11A). The second problem concerns the relationship between lung volume and transpulmonary ΔP (P_A – P_{pl}). Theoretically the retractive forces of the lung should increase as lung volume decreases. If this were true, lung volume would decrease in a vicious circle, with an increasingly progressive tendency to collapse as lung volume diminishes.

These two problems are resolved by the fact that the surface tension of the fluid lining the alveoli is variable and decreases as its surface area is reduced. The substance responsible for the reduction (and variability) in alveolar surface tension is secreted by the intraalveolar type II pneumocyte; it is a lipoprotein called *surfactant*, which floats as a 50-Å-thick film on the surface of the fluid lining the alveoli. When the surface film is reduced in area and the

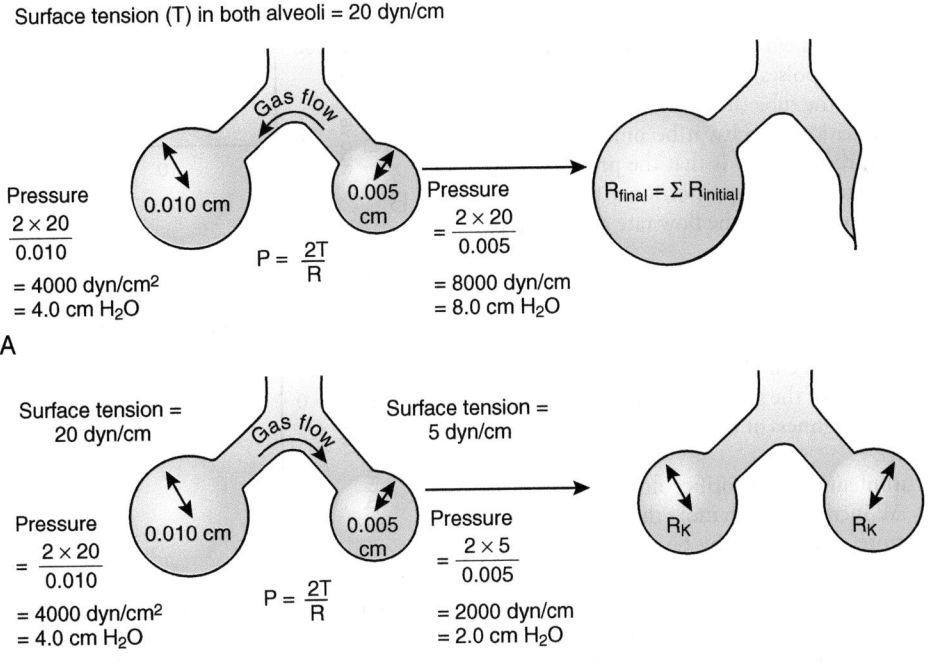

• **Fig. 5.11** Relationship between surface tension *(T)*, alveolar radius *(R)*, and alveolar transmural pressure *(P)*. The left side of each diagram shows the starting condition; the right side shows the expected result in alveolar size (using the Laplace equation to calculate the starting pressure). In (A) the surface tension in the fluid lining both the large and the small alveolus is the same (no surfactant). Accordingly, the direction of gas flow is from the higher-pressure small alveolus to the lower-pressure large alveolus, which results in one large alveolus ($R_{final} = \Sigma R_{initial}$). (B) Shows the expected changes in surface tension when surfactant lines the alveolus (less tension in the smaller alveolus). The direction of gas flow is from the larger to the smaller alveolus until the two are of equal size and are volume stable *(R_K)*. *K*, Constant; *ΣR*, sum of all individual radii.

concentration of surfactant at the surface is increased, the surface-reducing pressure is increased and counteracts the surface tension of the fluid lining the alveoli.

The surface tension of alveolar fluid can reach levels that are well below the normal range for body fluids such as water and plasma. When an alveolus decreases in size, the surface tension of the lining fluid falls to an extent greater than the corresponding reduction in radius; as a result, the transmural pressure gradient (equal to 2T/R) diminishes. This explains why small alveoli do not discharge their contents into large alveoli (see Fig. 5.11B) and why the elastic recoil of small alveoli is less than that of large alveoli.

Airway Resistance

For air to flow into the lungs, a ΔP must also be developed to overcome the nonelastic airway resistance (R_{AW}) of the lungs to airflow. The R_{AW} describes the relationship between ΔP and the rate of airflow ($\dot{V}$).

$$R(cm\,H_2O \cdot s/L) = \frac{\Delta P(cm\,H_2O)}{\Delta \dot{V}(L/s)} \quad (4)$$

The ΔP along the airway depends on the caliber of the airway and the rate and pattern of airflow. There are three main patterns of airflow. Laminar flow occurs when the gas passes down parallel-sided tubes at less than a certain critical velocity. With laminar flow, the pressure drop down the tube is proportional to the flow rate and may be calculated from the equation derived by Poiseuille:

$$\Delta P = \dot{V} \times 8\,L \times \mu/\pi r^4 \quad (5)$$

where ΔP is the pressure drop (in cm H_2O), $\dot{V}$ is the volume flow rate (in mL/s), μ is viscosity (in poises), L is the length of the tube (in cm), and r is the radius of the tube (in cm).

When flow exceeds the critical velocity, it becomes turbulent. The significant feature of turbulent flow is that the pressure drop along the airway is no longer directly proportional to the flow rate but is proportional to the square of the flow rate according to Eq. 6 for turbulent flow:

$$\Delta P = \dot{V}^2 \rho f\,L/4\pi^2 r^5 \quad (6)$$

where ΔP is the pressure drop (in cm H_2O), $\dot{V}$ is the volume flow rate (in mL/s), ρ is the density of the gas (or liquid), f is a friction factor that depends on the roughness of the tube wall, and r is the radius of the tube (in cm).[72]

With increases in turbulent flow (or orifice flow, as described in the next paragraph), ΔP increases much more than $\dot{V}$ and therefore R_{AW} also increases more, as predicted by Eq. 4.

Orifice flow occurs at severe constrictions such as a nearly closed larynx, subglottic stenosis or stricture, or a kinked ETT. In these situations, the pressure drop is also proportional to the square of the flow rate, but density replaces viscosity as the important factor in the numerator. This explains why a low-density gas such as helium diminishes the resistance to flow (by threefold in comparison to air) in the setting of severe upper airway obstruction.

Because the total cross-sectional area of the airways increases as branching occurs, the velocity of airflow decreases in the distal airways; laminar flow is therefore chiefly confined to the airways below the main bronchi. Orifice flow occurs at the larynx, and flow in the trachea is turbulent during most of the respiratory cycle. By examining the components that constitute each of the

preceding airway pressure equations, one can see that many factors can affect the pressure drop down the airways during ventilation. However, variations in diameter of the smaller bronchi and bronchioles are particularly critical, because bronchoconstriction may convert laminar flow to turbulent flow and the pressure drop along the airways can become much more closely related to the flow rate.

Different Regional Lung Time Constants

Thus far, the compliance and airway resistance properties of the chest have been discussed separately. In the following analysis, pressure at the mouth is assumed to increase suddenly to a fixed positive value (Fig. 5.12) that overcomes both elastic and airway resistance and to be maintained at this value during inflation of the lungs.[73] The ΔP required to overcome nonelastic airway resistance is the difference between the fixed mouth pressure and the instantaneous height of the dashed line in Fig. 5.12 and is proportional to the flow rate during most of the respiratory cycle.

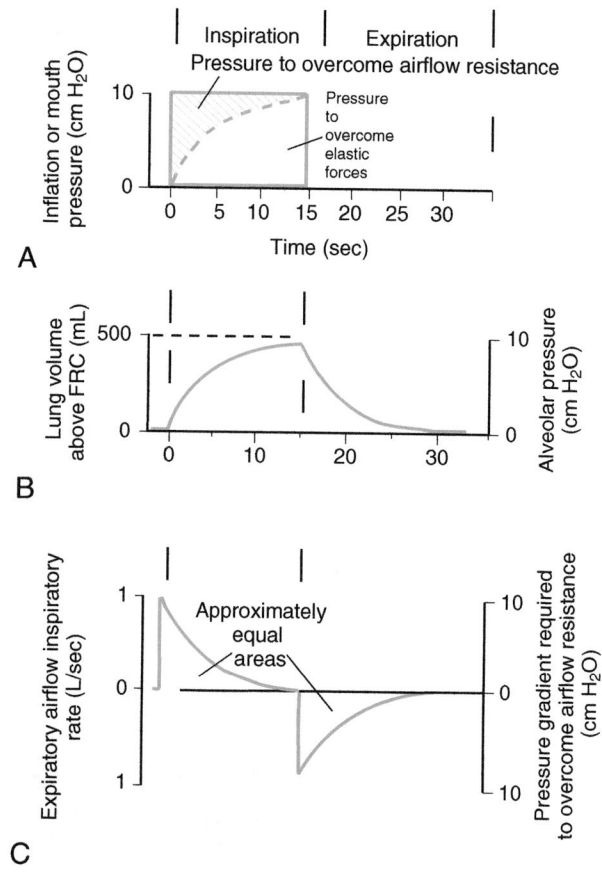

• **Fig. 5.12** Artificial ventilation by intermittent application of constant pressure (square wave) followed by passive expiration. The pressure required to overcome airway resistance (*hatched lines* in A) and the airflow rate (in C) from Eq. 4 in the text are proportional to one another and decrease exponentially (assuming that resistance to airflow is constant). The pressures required to overcome the elastic forces (*height of the dashed line* in A and lung volume in B) are proportional to one another and increase exponentially. Values shown are typical for an anesthetized supine paralyzed patient: total dynamic compliance, 50 mL/cm H_2O; pulmonary resistance, 3 cm H_2O/L/s; apparatus resistance, 7 cm H_2O/L/s; total resistance, 10 cm H_2O/L/s; time constant, 0.5 s. *FRC*, functional residual capacity. (From Lumb AB. Artificial ventilation. In: Lumb AB, ed. *Nunn's Applied Respiratory Physiology.* 5th ed. Butterworths; 2000:590.)

The ΔP required to overcome nonelastic airway resistance is maximal initially but then decreases exponentially (see Fig. 5.12A, *hatched lines*). The rate of filling therefore also declines in an approximately exponential manner. The remainder of the pressure gradient overcomes the elastic resistance (the instantaneous height of the *dashed line* in Fig. 5.12A) and is proportional to the change in lung volume. The ΔP required to overcome elastic resistance is minimal initially but then increases exponentially, as does lung volume. Alveolar filling ceases (lung volume remains constant) when the pressure resulting from the retractive elastic forces balances the applied (mouth) pressure (see Fig. 5.12A, *dashed line*).

Because only a finite time is available for alveolar filling and because alveolar filling occurs in an exponential manner, the degree of filling depends on the duration of the inspiration. The rapidity of change in an exponential curve can be described by its time constant τ, which is the time required to complete 63% of an exponentially changing function if the total time allowed for the function change is unlimited ($2\tau = 87\%$, $3\tau = 95\%$, and $4\tau = 98\%$). For lung inflation, $\tau = C_T \times R$; normally, $C_T = 0.1$ L/cm H_2O, $R = 2.0$ cm H_2O/L/s, $\tau = 0.2$ s, and $3\tau = 0.6$ s.

When this equation is applied to individual alveolar units, the time taken to fill such a unit clearly increases as airway resistance increases. The time required to fill an alveolar unit also increases as compliance increases, because a greater volume of air is transferred into a more compliant alveolus before the retractive force equals the applied pressure. The compliance of individual alveoli differs from top to bottom of the lung, and the resistance of individual airways varies widely depending on their length and caliber. Therefore, various time constants for inflation exist throughout the lung.

Pathways of Collateral Ventilation

Collateral ventilation is another nongravitational determinant of the distribution of ventilation. Four pathways of collateral ventilation are known. First, interalveolar communications (pores of Kohn) exist in most species; their number ranges from 8 to 50 per alveolus, and they may increase with age and with the development of obstructive lung disease. Their precise role has not been defined, but they probably function to prevent hypoxia in neighboring but obstructed lung units. Second, distal bronchiole-to-alveolus communications are known to exist (channels of Lambert); their function in vivo is speculative but may be similar to that of the pores of Kohn. Third, respiratory bronchiole-to-terminal bronchiole connections have been found in adjacent lung segments (channels of Martin) in healthy dogs and in humans with lung disease. Fourth, interlobar connections exist; the functional characteristics of interlobar collateral ventilation through these connections have been described in dogs,[74] and they have been observed in humans as well.[75]

Work of Breathing

The pressure-volume characteristics of the lung also determine the WOB. Because

$$\text{Work} = \text{Force} \times \text{Distance}$$
$$\text{Force} = \text{Pressure} \times \text{Area} \quad (7)$$
$$\text{Distance} = \text{Volume/Area}$$

work is defined by the equation

$$\text{Work} = (\text{Pressure} \times \text{Area})(\text{Volume/Area}) = \quad (8)$$
$$\text{Pressure} \times \text{Volume}$$

and ventilatory work may be analyzed by plotting pressure against volume.[76] In the presence of increased airway resistance or decreased C_L, increased transpulmonary pressure is required to achieve a given V_T with a consequent increase in the WOB. The metabolic cost of the WOB at rest constitutes only 1% to 3% of the total oxygen consumption in healthy subjects, but it is increased considerably (up to 50%) in patients with severe lung disease.

Two different pressure-volume diagrams are shown in Fig. 5.13. During normal inspiration, transpulmonary pressure increases from 0 to 5 cm H_2O while 500 mL of air is drawn into the lung. Potential energy is stored by the lung during inspiration and is expended during expiration; consequently, the entire expiratory cycle is passive. The hatched area plus the triangular area ABC represents pressure multiplied by volume and is the WOB during one breath. Line AB is the lower section of the pressure-volume curve of Fig. 5.13. The triangular area ABC is the work required to overcome elastic forces (C_T), whereas the hatched area is the work required to overcome airflow or frictional resistance (R). The second graph applies to an anesthetized patient with diffuse obstructive airway disease resulting from the accumulation of mucous secretions. There is a marked increase in both the elastic (triangle AB'C) and the airway (hatched area) resistive components of respiratory work. During expiration, only 250 mL of air leaves the lungs during the passive phase when intrathoracic pressure reaches the equilibrium value of 0 cm H_2O. Active effort-producing work is required to force out the remaining 250 mL of air, and intrathoracic pressure becomes positive.

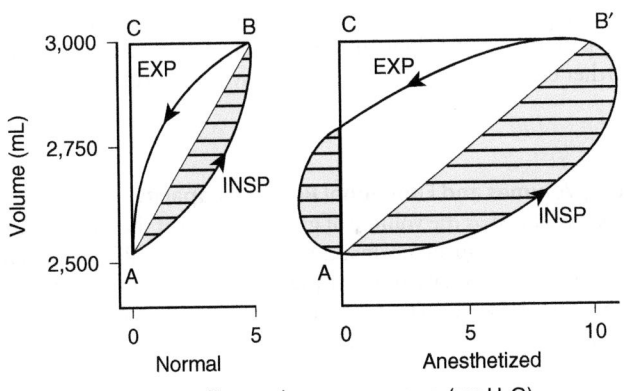

• **Fig. 5.13** Lung volume plotted against transpulmonary pressure in a pressure-volume diagram for a healthy awake patient *(Normal)* and an anesthetized patient. The lung compliance of the awake patient (slope of line AB = 100 mL/cm H_2O) equals that shown for the small dependent alveoli in Fig. 5.3. The lung compliance of the anesthetized patient (slope of line AB' = 50 mL/cm H_2O) equals that shown for the medium midlung alveoli in Fig. 5.3 and for the anesthetized patient in Fig. 5.12. The total area within the oval and triangles has the dimensions of pressure multiplied by volume and represents the total work of breathing. The hatched areas to the right of lines AB and AB' represent the active inspiratory work necessary to overcome resistance to airflow during inspiration *(INSP)*. The hatched area to the left of the triangle AB'C represents the active expiratory work necessary to overcome resistance to airflow during expiration *(EXP)*. Expiration is passive in the healthy subject because sufficient potential energy is stored during inspiration to produce expiratory airflow. The fraction of total inspiratory work necessary to overcome elastic resistance is shown by the triangles ABC and AB'C. The anesthetized patient has decreased compliance and increased elastic resistance work (triangle AB'C) compared with the healthy patient's compliance and elastic resistance work (triangle ABC). The anesthetized patient represented in this figure has increased airway resistance to both inspiratory and expiratory work.

The full WOB over time must include the ventilatory frequency. The following equation depicts the variables included in the WOB equation:

$$WOB = \dot{V}_E \times \frac{R_{AW}}{C_L} \qquad (9)$$

Evaluating each component in the WOB equation, $\dot{V}_E$ is the minute ventilation (RR × V_T) required to achieve a normal $Paco_2$. When patients have increased CO_2 production (as occurs with fever), the $\dot{V}_E$, and hence the WOB, will need to be higher. When the dead space (either alveolar or anatomic) is increased, the $\dot{V}_E$ will need to increase to achieve a normal $Paco_2$. Similarly, when airway resistance (R_{AW}) is increased or compliance (C_L) is decreased, there will be a corresponding increase in the WOB.

Furthermore, for any constant minute volume, the work done against elastic resistance is increased when breathing is deep and slow. On the other hand, the work done against airflow resistance is increased when breathing is rapid and shallow. If the two components are summed and the total work is plotted against respiratory frequency, there is an optimal respiratory frequency at which the total WOB is minimal (Fig. 5.14).[77] In patients with diseased lungs in which elastic resistance is high (e.g., pulmonary fibrosis, pulmonary edema, or in infants), the optimal frequency is increased, and rapid, shallow breaths are favored. Like other muscles, respiratory muscles can become fatigued, especially with rapid, shallow breathing.[78] When airway resistance is high (e.g., in asthma or COPD), the optimal frequency is decreased, and slow, deep breaths are favored. Although the optimal frequency is slow (allowing a prolonged expiratory phase), a rapid, shallow breathing pattern also develops in these patients when fatigued, which further exacerbates their primary (airway resistance) problem.[78]

Lung Volumes, Functional Residual Capacity, and Closing Capacity

Lung Volumes and Functional Residual Capacity

FRC is defined as the volume of gas in the lung at the end of a normal expiration during normal tidal breathing. At FRC, there is no airflow and PA equals ambient pressure. Under these conditions, expansive chest wall elastic forces are exactly balanced by retractive lung tissue elastic forces (Fig. 5.15).[79]

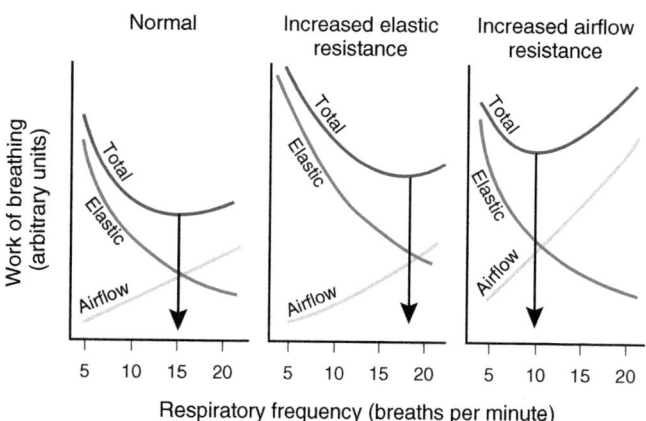

• **Fig. 5.14** The diagrams show the work done against elastic and airflow resistance, both separately and summed to indicate the total work of breathing at different respiratory frequencies. The total work of breathing has a minimal value at approximately 15 breaths/min under normal circumstances. For the same minute volume, minimal work is performed at higher frequencies with stiff (less compliant) lungs and at lower frequencies when airflow resistance is increased. (Modified from Lumb AB. Pulmonary ventilation: mechanisms and the work of breathing. In: Lumb AB, ed. *Nunn's Applied Respiratory Physiology*. 5th ed. Butterworths; 2000:128.)

The FRC includes the *expiratory reserve volume* (the additional gas beyond the tidal volume that can be forcibly exhaled) along with the *residual volume*. Therefore, FRC equals residual volume plus expiratory reserve volume (Fig. 5.16). With regard to the other lung volumes shown in Fig. 5.16, V_T, vital capacity, inspiratory capacity, inspiratory reserve volume, and expiratory reserve volume can be measured by simple spirometry. Total lung capacity (TLC), FRC, and residual volume contain a fraction (residual volume) that cannot be measured by simple spirometry. However, if one of these three volumes is measured, the others can easily be derived, because the other lung volumes, which relate these three volumes to one another, can be measured by simple spirometry.

Residual volume, FRC, and TLC can be measured by any of three techniques: (1) nitrogen washout, (2) inert gas dilution (e.g., helium wash-in), and (3) total-body plethysmography. The first

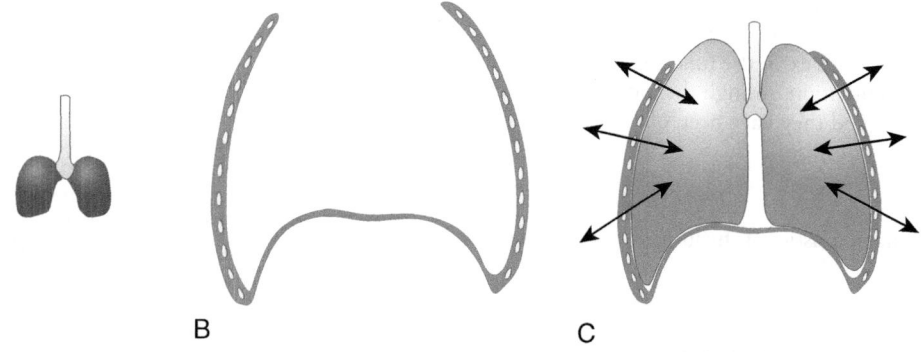

• **Fig. 5.15** (A) The resting state of normal lungs when they are removed from the chest cavity—that is, elastic recoil causes total collapse. (B) The resting state of a normal chest wall and diaphragm when the thoracic apex is open to the atmosphere and the thoracic contents are removed. (C) The lung volume that exists at the end of expiration is the functional residual capacity (FRC). At FRC, the elastic forces of the lung and chest walls are equal and in opposite directions. The pleural surfaces link these two opposing forces. (Modified from Shapiro BA, Harrison RA, Trout CA. The mechanics of ventilation. In: Shapiro BA, Harrison RA, Trout CA, eds. *Clinical Application of Respiratory Care*. 3rd ed. Year Book; 1985:57.)

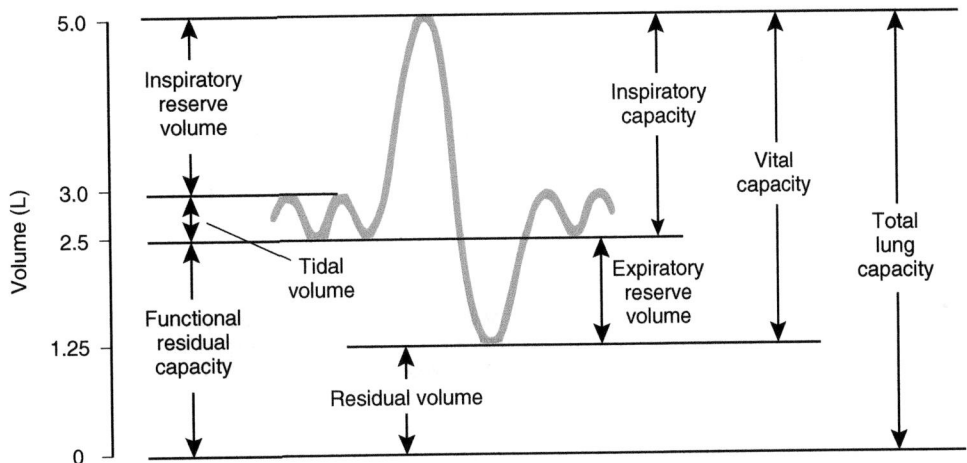

• **Fig. 5.16** The dynamic lung volumes that can be measured by simple spirometry are tidal volume, inspiratory reserve volume, expiratory reserve volume, inspiratory capacity, and vital capacity. The static lung volumes are residual volume, functional residual capacity, and total lung capacity. Static lung volumes cannot be measured by simple spirometry and require separate methods of measurement (e.g., inert gas dilution, nitrogen washout, or total-body plethysmography).

method, the nitrogen washout technique, is based on measuring expired nitrogen concentrations before and after the patient breathes pure oxygen for several minutes; the difference is the total quantity of nitrogen eliminated. If, for example, 2 L of N_2 is eliminated and the initial alveolar N_2 concentration was 80%, the initial volume of the lung was 2.5 L. The second method, the inert gas dilution technique, uses the wash-in of an inert tracer gas such as helium. If 50 mL of helium is introduced into the lungs and, after equilibration, the helium concentration is found to be 1%, the volume of the lung is 5 L. The third method, the total-body plethysmography technique, uses Boyle's law ($P_1V_1 = P_2V_2$, where P_1 = initial pressure, V_1 = initial volume). The subject is confined within a gas-tight box (plethysmograph) so that changes in the volume of the body during respiration may be readily determined as a change in pressure within the sealed box. Although each technique has technical limitations, all are based on sound physical and physiologic principles and provide accurate results in normal patients. Disparity between FRC as measured in the body plethysmograph and as determined by the helium dilution method is often used as a way of detecting large, nonventilating, air-trapped blebs.[80]

Airway Closure and Closing Capacity

As discussed (see section "Distribution of Ventilation"), Ppl increases when proceeding from the top to the bottom of the lung and determines regional alveolar size, compliance, and ventilation. Of even greater importance to the clinician is the recognition that these gradients in Ppl may lead to airway closure and collapse of alveoli.

Patient with Normal Lungs. Fig. 5.17A illustrates the normal resting end-expiratory (FRC) position of the lung–chest wall combination. The distending transpulmonary ΔP and the intrathoracic air passage transmural ΔP are 5 cm H_2O, and the airways remain patent. During the middle of a normal inspiration (see Fig. 5.17B), there is an increase in transmural ΔP (to 6.8 cm H_2O) that encourages distention of the intrathoracic air passages. During the middle of a normal expiration (see Fig. 5.17C), expiration is passive; PA is attributable only to the elastic recoil of the lung (2 cm H_2O), and there is a decrease (to 5.2 cm H_2O) but still a favorable (distending) intraluminal transmural ΔP. During the

middle of a severe forced expiration (see Fig. 5.17D), Ppl increases far higher than atmospheric pressure and is communicated to the alveoli, which have a pressure that is still higher because of the elastic recoil of the alveolar septa (an additional 2 cm H_2O).

At high gas flow rates, the pressure drop down the air passage is increased, and there is a point at which intraluminal pressure equals either the surrounding parenchymal pressure or Ppl; that point is termed the *equal pressure point* (EPP). If the EPP occurs in small noncartilaginous air passages (distal to the 11th generation, the airways have no cartilage and are called *bronchioles*), they may be held open at that point by the tethering effect of the elastic recoil of the immediately adjacent or surrounding lung parenchyma. If the EPP occurs in large cartilaginous air passages (proximal to the 11th generation, the airways have cartilage and are called *bronchi*), they may be held open at that point by their cartilage. Downstream of the EPP (in either small or large airways), transmural ΔP is reversed (–6 cm H_2O), and airway closure occurs. Thus, the patency of airways distal to the 11th generation is a function of lung volume, and the patency of airways proximal to the 11th generation is a function of intrathoracic (pleural) pressure. In bronchi, the posterior membranous sheath appears to give first by invaginating into the lumen.[81] If lung volume were abnormally decreased (e.g., because of splinting) and expiration were still forced, the caliber of the airways would be relatively reduced at all times, which would cause the EPP and point of collapse to move progressively from larger to smaller air passages (closer to the alveolus).

In adults with normal lungs, airway closure can still occur even if expiration is not forced, provided that residual volume is approached closely enough. Even in patients with normal lungs, as lung volume decreases toward residual volume during expiration, small airways (0.5 to 0.9 mm in diameter) show a progressive tendency to close, whereas larger airways remain patent.[82,83] Airway closure occurs first in the dependent lung regions (as directly observed by computed tomography) because the distending transpulmonary pressure is less and the volume change during expiration is greater.[32] Airway closure is most likely to occur in the dependent regions of the lung whether the patient is in the supine or the lateral decubitus position and whether ventilation is spontaneous or positive-pressure ventilation.[32,84,85]

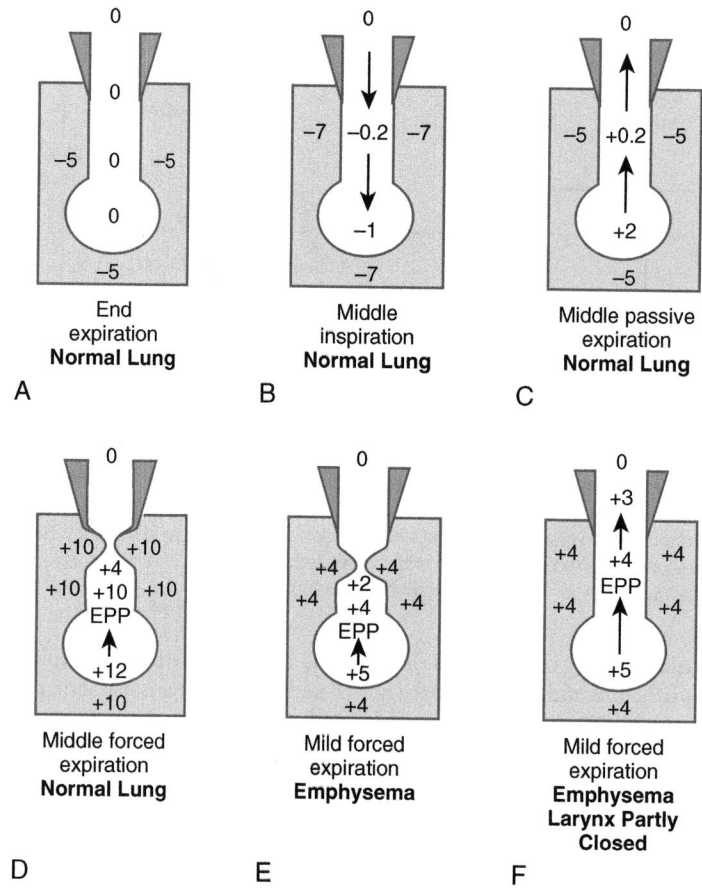

• **Fig. 5.17** Pressure gradients across the airways. The airways consist of a thin-walled intrathoracic portion (near the alveoli) and a more rigid (cartilaginous) intrathoracic and extrathoracic portion. During expiration, the pressure from elastic recoil is assumed to be +2 cm H_2O in normal lungs (A–D) and +1 cm H_2O in abnormal lungs (E, F). The total pressure inside the alveolus is pleural pressure plus elastic recoil. The arrows indicate the direction of airflow. *EPP,* Equal pressure point. See text for explanation. (Modified from Benumof JL. *Anesthesia for Thoracic Surgery.* 2nd ed. Saunders; 1995:Chapter 8.)

Patients With Abnormal Lungs. In patients with emphysema, bronchitis, asthma, or interstitial pulmonary edema, airway closure occurs with milder active expiration, lower gas flow rates, and higher lung volumes and occurs closer to the alveolus. In all four conditions, the increased airway resistance causes a larger decrease in pressure from the alveoli to the larger bronchi, thereby creating the potential for negative intrathoracic transmural ΔP and narrowed and collapsed airways. In addition, the structural integrity of the conducting airways may be diminished because of inflammation and scarring; therefore, these airways may close more readily for any given lung volume or transluminal ΔP.

In emphysema, the elastic recoil of the lung is reduced (to 1 cm H_2O in Fig. 5.17E), the air passages are poorly supported by the lung parenchyma, the point of airway resistance is close to the alveolus, and transmural ΔP can become negative quickly. Therefore during only a mild forced expiration in an emphysematous patient, the EPP and the point of collapse are near the alveolus (see Fig. 5.17E). The use of pursed-lip or grunting expiration (the equivalents of partly closing the larynx during expiration), PEEP, or continuous positive airway pressure in an emphysematous patient restores a favorable (distending) intrathoracic transmural air ΔP (see Fig. 5.17F). In bronchitis, the airways are structurally weakened and may close when only a small negative transmural ΔP is present (as with mild forced expiration). In asthma, the

midsize airways are narrowed by bronchospasm and, if expiration is forced, they are further narrowed by a negative transmural ΔP. Finally, with pulmonary interstitial edema, perialveolar interstitial edema compresses the alveoli and acutely decreases FRC; the peribronchial edema fluid cuffs (within the connective tissue sheaths around the larger arteries and bronchi) compress the bronchi and acutely increase closing volume (CV).[86–88]

Measurement of Closing Capacity. CC is a sensitive test of early small-airways disease and is performed by having the patient exhale to residual volume (Fig. 5.18).[89] As inspiration from residual volume toward TLC begins, a bolus of tracer gas (e.g., xenon 133 or helium) is injected into the inspired gas. During the initial part of this inspiration from residual volume, the first gases to enter the alveolus are the dead space (VD) gas and the tracer bolus. The tracer gas enters only alveoli that are already open (presumably the apices of the lung) and does not enter alveoli that are already closed (presumably the bases of the lung). As the inspiration continues, the apical alveoli complete filling and the basilar alveoli begin to open and fill, but with gas that does not contain any tracer gas.

A differential tracer gas concentration is thus established, with the gas in the apices having a higher tracer concentration than that in the bases (see Fig. 5.18). As the subject exhales and the diaphragm ascends, a point is reached at which the small airways just

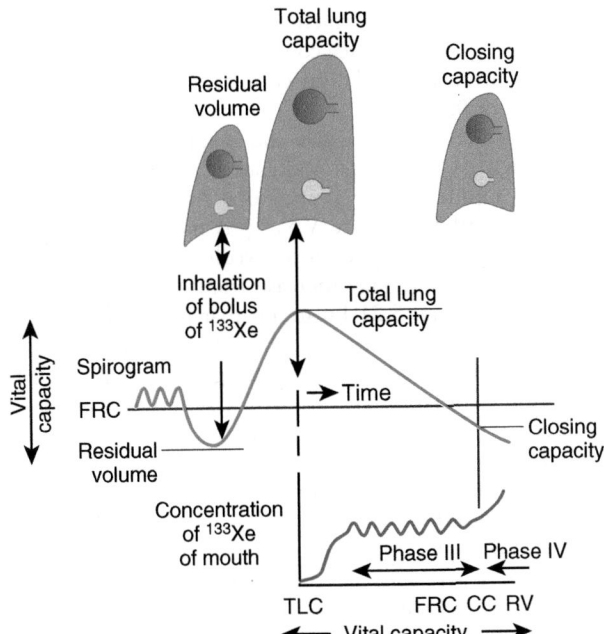

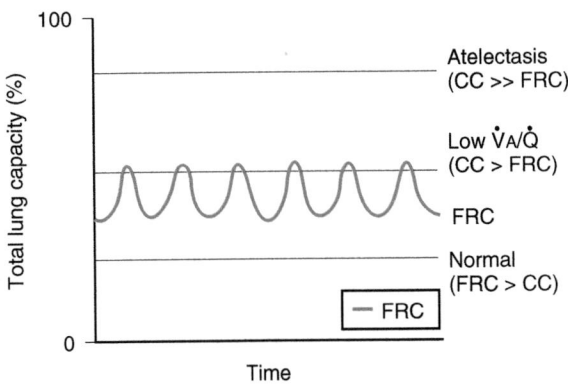

• **Fig. 5.18** Measurement of closing capacity *(CC)* with the use of a tracer gas such as xenon-133 *(^{133}Xe)*. The bolus of tracer gas is inhaled near residual volume *(RV)* and, because of airway closure in the dependent lung, is distributed only to nondependent alveoli whose air passages are still open. During expiration, the concentration of tracer gas becomes constant after the dead space is washed out. This plateau *(Phase III)* gives way to a rising concentration of tracer gas *(Phase IV)*, when there is once again closure of the dependent airways because the only contribution made to expired gas is by the nondependent alveoli with a high ^{133}Xe concentration. *FRC,* Functional residual capacity; *TLC,* total lung capacity. (Modified from Lumb AB. Respiratory system resistance: Measurement of closing capacity. In: Lumb AB, ed. *Nunn's Applied Respiratory Physiology.* 5th ed. Butterworths; 2000:79.)

• **Fig. 5.19** Relationship between functional residual capacity *(FRC)* and closing capacity *(CC)*. FRC is the amount of gas in the lungs at end-expiration during normal tidal breathing, shown by the level of each trough of the sine wave tidal volume. CC is the amount of gas that must be in the lungs to keep the small conducting airways open. This figure shows three different CCs, as indicated by the three different straight lines. See the text for an explanation of why the three different FRC-CC relationships depicted result in normal or low ventilation/perfusion *($\dot{V}$A/$\dot{Q}$)* relationships or atelectasis. (From Benumof JL. *Anesthesia for Thoracic Surgery.* 2nd ed. Saunders; 1995:Chapter 8.)

above the diaphragm start to close and thereby limit airflow from these areas. The airflow now comes more from the upper lung fields, where the alveolar gas has a much higher tracer concentration, which results in a sudden increase in the tracer gas concentration toward the end of expiration (Phase IV of Fig. 5.18).

CV is the difference between the onset of phase IV and residual volume; because it represents part of a vital capacity maneuver, it is expressed as a percentage of vital lung capacity. CV plus residual volume is known as CC and is expressed as a percentage of TLC. Smoking, obesity, aging, and the supine position increase CC.[90] In healthy individuals at a mean age of 44 years, CC = FRC in the supine position, and at a mean age of 66 years, CC = FRC in the upright position.[91]

Relationship Between Functional Residual Capacity and Closing Capacity. The relationship between FRC and CC is far more important than consideration of FRC or CC alone, because it is this relationship that determines whether a given respiratory unit is normal or atelectatic or has a low $\dot{V}$A/$\dot{Q}$ ratio. The relationship between FRC and CC is as follows. When the volume of the lung at which some airways close is greater than the entire VT, lung volume never increases enough during tidal inspiration to open any of these airways. As a result, these airways stay closed during the entire tidal respiration. Airways that are closed all the time are equivalent to atelectasis (Fig. 5.19). If the CV of some airways lies within VT, as lung volume increases during inspiration, some previously closed airways open for a short time until lung

volume recedes once again below the CV of these airways. Because these opening and closing airways are open for a shorter time than normal airways are, they have less chance or time to participate in gas exchange, a circumstance equivalent to a low-$\dot{V}$A/$\dot{Q}$ region. If the CC of the lung is below the whole of tidal respiration, no airways are closed at any time during tidal respiration; this is a normal circumstance. Anything that decreases FRC relative to CC or increases CC relative to FRC converts normal areas to low-$\dot{V}$A/$\dot{Q}$ and atelectatic areas,[83] which causes hypoxemia.

Mechanical intermittent positive-pressure breathing (IPPB) may be efficacious because it can take a previously spontaneously breathing patient with a low-$\dot{V}$A/$\dot{Q}$ relationship, in which CC is greater than FRC but still within VT (Fig. 5.20, spontaneous ventilation), and increase the amount of inspiratory time that some previously closed (at end-expiration) airways spend in fresh gas exchange,

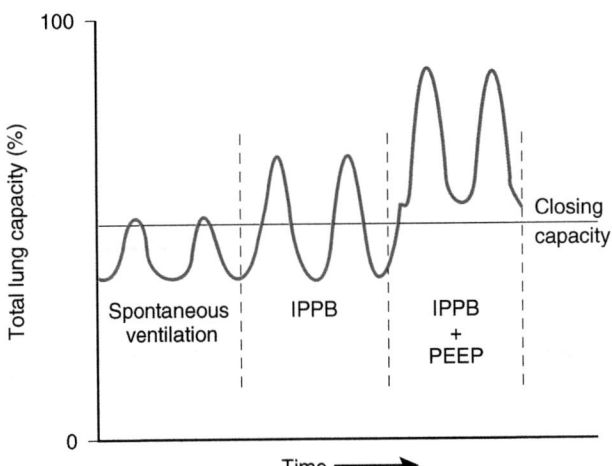

• **Fig. 5.20** Relationship of functional residual capacity (FRC) to closing capacity (CC) during spontaneous ventilation, intermittent positive-pressure breathing *(IPPB)*, and IPPB with positive end-expiratory pressure *(IPPB + PEEP)*. See the text for an explanation of the effect of the two ventilatory maneuvers (IPPB and PEEP) on the relationship of FRC to CC.

thereby increasing $\dot{V}_A/\dot{Q}$ (see Fig. 5.20, IPPB). However, if PEEP is added to IPPB, PEEP increases FRC to a lung volume equal to or greater than CC, thereby restoring a normal FRC-to-CC relationship so that no airways are closed at any time during the tidal respiration (see Fig. 5.20, IPPB + PEEP). Indeed, anesthesia-induced atelectasis (quantified by computed tomography) in the dependent regions of patients' lungs may persist with IPPB alone but is fully reversed with IPPB plus PEEP (5 to 10 cm H_2O).[32]

Oxygen and Carbon Dioxide Transport

Alveolar and Dead Space Ventilation and Alveolar Gas Tensions

In normal lungs, approximately two-thirds of each breath reach perfused alveoli to take part in gas exchange. This constitutes the effective or alveolar ventilation ($\dot{V}_A$). The remaining third of each breath takes no part in gas exchange and is therefore termed the V_D. The relationship is as follows: alveolar ventilation ($\dot{V}_A$) = frequency (f) × (V_T – V_D). The physiologic (or total) dead space ($V_{D_{physiologic}}$) may be further divided into two components: a volume of gas that ventilates the conducting airways, the anatomic dead space ($V_{D_{anatomic}}$), and a volume of gas that ventilates unperfused alveoli, the alveolar dead space ($V_{D_{alveolar}}$). Clinical examples of $V_{D_{alveolar}}$ ventilation include zone 1, pulmonary embolus, and destroyed alveolar septa; such ventilation does not participate in gas exchange. Fig. 5.21 shows a two-compartment model of the lung in which the anatomic and

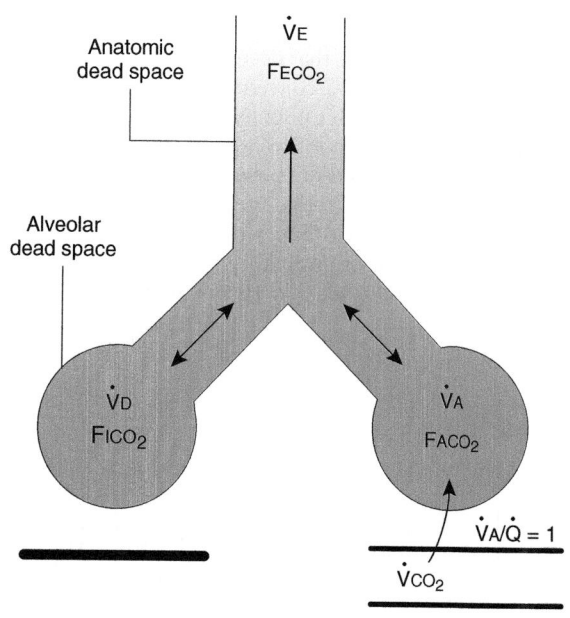

$\dot{V}_D$ = Total dead space ventilation
    = Anatomic + alveolar dead space ventilation

• **Fig. 5.21** Two-compartment model of the lung in which the anatomic and alveolar dead space compartments have been combined into the total (physiologic) dead space ventilation ($\dot{V}_D$). $FACO_2$ = alveolar CO_2 fraction; $FECO_2$ = mixed expired CO_2 fraction; $FICO_2$ = inspired CO_2 fraction; $\dot{V}_A$ = alveolar ventilation; $\dot{V}CO_2$ = carbon dioxide production; $\dot{V}E$ = expired minute ventilation. $\dot{V}_A/\dot{Q} = 1$ means that ventilation and perfusion are equal in liters per minute. Normally, the amount of CO_2 eliminated at the airway ($\dot{V}E × FECO_2$) equals the amount of CO_2 removed by alveolar ventilation ($\dot{V}_A × FACO_2$) because there is no CO_2 elimination from alveolar dead space ($FICO_2 = 0$).

alveolar dead space compartments have been combined into the total (physiologic) dead space compartment; the other compartment is the alveolar ventilation compartment, whose idealized $\dot{V}_A/\dot{Q}$ ratio is 1.0.

$V_{D_{anatomic}}$ varies with lung size and is approximately 2 mL/kg of body weight (150 mL in a 70-kg adult). In a normal, healthy adult lying supine, $V_{D_{anatomic}}$ and total V_D are approximately equal to each other, because $V_{D_{alveolar}}$ is normally minimal. In the erect posture, the uppermost alveoli may not be perfused (zone 1), and $V_{D_{alveolar}}$ may increase from a negligible amount to 60 to 80 mL. Fig. 5.21 illustrates that in a steady state, the volume of CO_2 entering the alveoli ($\dot{V}CO_2$) is equal to the volume of CO_2 eliminated in the expired gas, ($\dot{V}E$)($FECO_2$), where $\dot{V}E$ = minute ventilation and $FECO_2$ = fraction of expired CO_2. Thus $\dot{V}CO_2 = (\dot{V}E)(FECO_2)$. However, the expired gas volume consists of alveolar gas, ($\dot{V}_A$)($FACO_2$), and V_D gas, ($\dot{V}_D$)($FICO_2$), where $FACO_2$ and $FICO_2$ are the alveolar and inspired fractions of CO_2, respectively. Thus $\dot{V}CO_2 = (\dot{V}_A)(FACO_2) + (\dot{V}_D)(FICO_2)$. Setting the first equation equal to the second equation and using the relationship $\dot{V}E = \dot{V}_A + \dot{V}_D$, subsequent algebraic manipulation (including setting $PACO_2$ equal to $PaCO_2$) results in the modified Bohr equation:

$$V_D/V_T = (PaCO_2 - PECO_2)/PaCO_2 \qquad (10)$$

The CO_2 tension in expired gas, $PECO_2$, may be obtained by measuring expired CO_2 in a large (Douglas) bag or, more commonly, by using end-tidal CO_2 tension ($PETCO_2$) as a surrogate. In severe lung disease, physiologic V_D/V_T ratio provides a useful expression of the inefficiency of ventilation. In a healthy adult, this ratio is usually less than 30%—that is, ventilation is more than 70% efficient. In a patient with COPD, V_D/V_T may increase to 60% to 70%. Under these conditions, ventilation is obviously grossly inefficient. Fig. 5.22 shows the relationship between $\dot{V}E$ and $PaCO_2$ for several V_D/V_T values. As $\dot{V}E$ decreases, $PaCO_2$ increases for all V_D/V_T values. As V_D/V_T increases, a given decrease in $\dot{V}E$ causes a much greater increase in $PaCO_2$. If $PaCO_2$ is to remain constant while V_D/V_T increases, $\dot{V}E$ must increase more.

The alveolar concentration of a gas is equal to the difference between the inspired concentration and the ratio of the output (or uptake) of the gas to $\dot{V}_A$. Thus, for gas X during dry conditions, $P_{AX} = (P_{dry\ atm})(F_{IX}) ± \dot{V}_X$ (output or uptake)/$\dot{V}_A$, where P_{AX} = alveolar partial pressure of gas X, F_{IX} = inspired concentration of gas X, $P_{dry\ atm}$ = dry atmospheric pressure = $P_{wet\ atm}$ – P_{H_2O} = 760 – 47 = 713 mm Hg, $\dot{V}_X$ = output or uptake of gas X, and $\dot{V}_A$ = alveolar ventilation.

For CO_2, $PACO_2$ = 713 ($FICO_2 + \dot{V}CO_2/\dot{V}_A$). Because $FICO_2 = 0$ and using standard conversion factors:

$$PACO_2 = 713*(\dot{V}CO_2[mL/min\ STPD]/\dot{V}_A \\ [L/min/BTPS]*0.863) \qquad (11)$$

where BTPS = body temperature and pressure, saturated (i.e., 37°C, P_{H_2O} = 47 mm Hg), and STPD = standard temperature and pressure, dry. For example, 36 mm Hg = (713) * (200/4000).

For oxygen,

$$PAO_2 = 713*(FIO_2 - \dot{V}O_2\ [mL/min]/\dot{V}_A\ [mL/min]) \qquad (12)$$

where $\dot{V}O_2$ = oxygen consumption by the body. For example, 100 mm Hg = (713) * (0.21 – 225/3200).

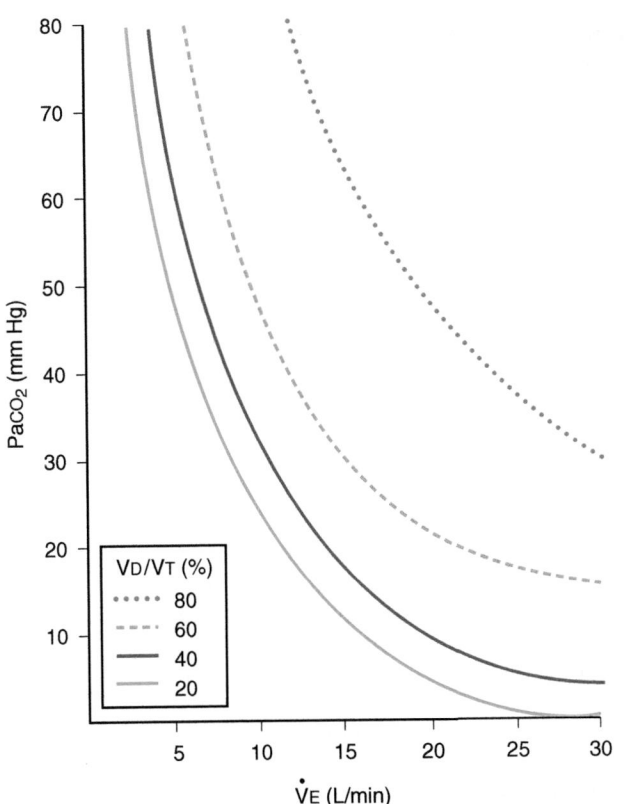

• **Fig. 5.22** Relationship between minute ventilation *(V̇E, L/min)* and arterial partial pressure of carbon dioxide *(PaCO₂)* for a family of ratios of total dead space to tidal volume *(VD/VT)*. These curves are hyperbolic and rise steeply at low V̇E values. See Eq. 10 in the text.

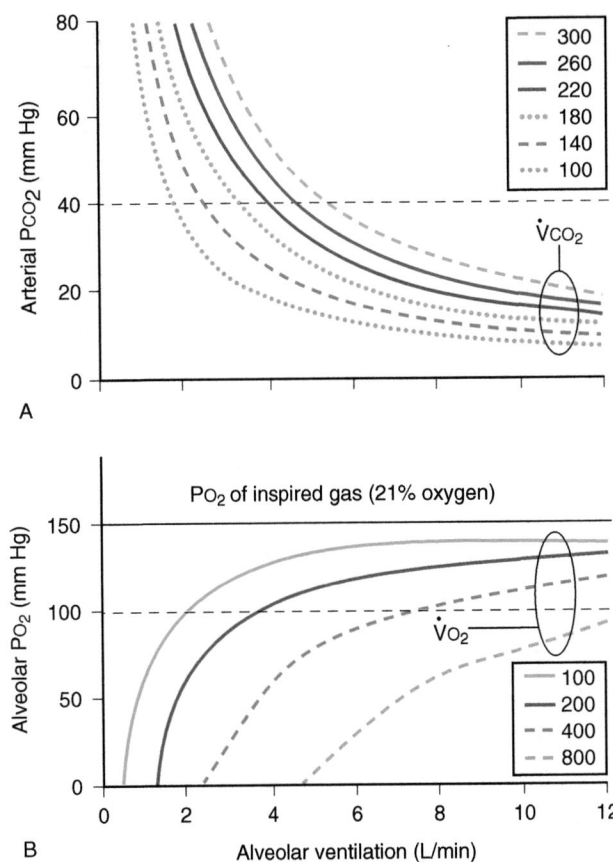

• **Fig. 5.23** (A) The relationship between alveolar ventilation and arterial carbon dioxide tension (PaCO₂) for a group of different CO₂ production values (V̇CO₂). (B) The relationship between alveolar ventilation and alveolar oxygen tension (PAO₂) for a group of different oxygen consumption values (V̇O₂). Values are derived from Eqs. 10 and 11 in the text, and the curves are hyperbolic. As alveolar ventilation increases, PAO₂ and PaCO₂ approach inspired concentrations. Decreases in alveolar ventilation to less than 4 L/min are accompanied by precipitous decreases in PAO₂ and increases in PaCO₂.

Fig. 5.23 shows the hyperbolic relationships expressed in Eqs. 10 and 11 between PaCO₂ and V̇A (see Fig. 5.22), and between PAO₂ and V̇A for different levels of V̇CO₂ and V̇O₂, respectively. PaCO₂ is substituted for PACO₂ because PACO₂-to-PaCO₂ gradients are small (as opposed to PAO₂-to-PaO₂ gradients, which can be large). Note that as V̇A increases, the second term on the right side of Eqs. 11 and 12 approaches zero and the composition of the alveolar gas approaches that of the inspired gas. In addition, Figs. 5.22–5.24 show that, because anesthesia is usually administered with an oxygen-enriched gas mixture, hypercapnia is a more common result of hypoventilation than hypoxemia is. Another perspective on these relationships is the very important observation that all patients who are hypoventilating should receive low-dose supplemental oxygen to protect from hypoxemia that would otherwise occur.

Oxygen Transport

Overview

The principal function of the heart and lungs is supporting oxygen delivery to and CO₂ removal from the tissues in accordance with metabolic requirements while maintaining arterial blood oxygen and CO₂ partial pressures within a narrow physiologic range. The respiratory and cardiovascular systems are linked in series to accomplish this function over a wide range of metabolic requirements, which can increase 30-fold from rest to heavy exercise. The functional links in the oxygen transport chain are as follows: (1) ventilation and distribution of ventilation with respect to perfusion, (2) diffusion of oxygen into blood, (3) chemical reaction of oxygen with hemoglobin (Hb), (4) total cardiac output of arterial blood, and (5) distribution of blood to tissues and release of oxygen (Table 5.3). The system is seldom stressed except at exercise, and the earliest symptoms of cardiac or respiratory diseases are often seen only during exercise.

The maximum functional capacity of each link can be determined independently. Table 5.3 lists these measured functional capacities for healthy, young people. Because theoretical maximal oxygen transport at the ventilatory step or at the diffusion and chemical reaction step (approximately 6 L/min in healthy humans at sea level) exceeds the oxygen transportable by the maximum cardiac output and distribution steps, the limit to oxygen transport is the cardiovascular system. Respiratory diseases would not be expected to limit maximum oxygen transport until functional capacities are reduced by 40% to 50%.

Oxygen-Hemoglobin Dissociation Curve

As a red blood cell (RBC) passes by the alveolus, oxygen diffuses into plasma and increases PaO₂. As PaO₂ increases, oxygen diffuses into the RBC and combines with Hb. Each Hb molecule consists of four heme molecules attached to a globin molecule. Each heme molecule consists of glycine, α-ketoglutaric acid, and iron in the ferrous (Fe²⁺) form. Each ferrous ion has the capacity

TABLE 5.3	Functional Capacities and Potential Maximum Oxygen Transport of Each Link in the Oxygen Transport Chain in Normal Humans[a] at Sea Level		
Link in Chain	**Functional Capacity in Normal Humans**		**Theoretical Maximum Oxygen Transport Capacity**
Ventilation	200 L/min (MVV)		$0.030 \times MVV = 6.0$ L O_2/min
Diffusion and chemical reaction			$DL_{O_2} = 6.1$ L O_2/min
Cardiac output	20 L/min		
O_2 extraction	75%		$0.16 \times$ Cardiac output $= 3.2$ L O_2/min
($Ca_{O_2} - C\bar{v}_{O_2}$ difference)	(16 mL O_2/100 mL or 0.16)		

$Ca_{O_2} - C\bar{v}_{O_2}$, Arteriovenous oxygen content difference; DL_{O_2}, diffusing capacity of lung for oxygen; MVV, maximum voluntary ventilation.

[a]Hemoglobin = 15 g/dL; physiologic dead space in percentage of tidal volume = 0.25; partial alveolar pressure of oxygen >110 mm Hg.

From Cassidy SS. Heart-lung interactions in health and disease. *Am J Med Sci.* 1987;30:451–461.

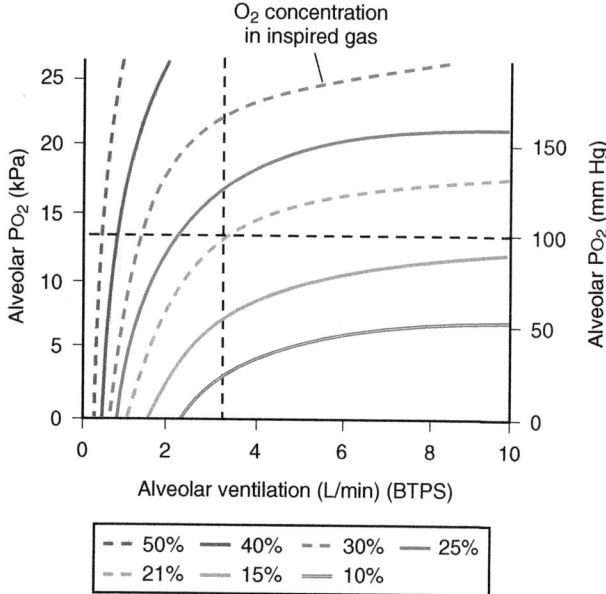

• **Fig. 5.24** For any given oxygen concentration in inspired gas, the relationship between alveolar ventilation and alveolar oxygen tension (PA_{O_2}) is hyperbolic. As the inspired oxygen concentration is increased, the amount that alveolar ventilation must decrease to produce hypoxemia is greatly increased. *BTPS,* Body temperature, ambient pressure, saturated. (From Lumb AB. Respiratory system resistance: measurement of closing capacity. In: Lumb AB, ed. *Nunn's Applied Respiratory Physiology.* 5th ed. Butterworths; 2000:79.)

to bind with one oxygen molecule in a loose, reversible combination. As the ferrous ions bind to oxygen, the Hb molecule becomes saturated.

The oxy-Hb dissociation curve relates the saturation of Hb (rightmost vertical axis in Fig. 5.25) to PA_{O_2}. Hb is fully saturated (100%) by a P_{O_2} of approximately 700 mm Hg. The saturation at normal arterial pressure (point *a* on upper, flat part of the oxy-Hb curve in Fig. 5.25) is 95% to 98%, achieved by a Pa_{O_2} of about 90 to 100 mm Hg. When P_{O_2} is less than 60 mm Hg (90% saturation), saturation falls steeply, and the amount of Hb uncombined with oxygen increases greatly for a given decrease in P_{O_2}. Mixed venous blood has a P_{O_2} ($P\bar{v}_{O_2}$) of about 40 mm Hg and is approximately 75% saturated, as indicated by the middle of the three points ($\bar{v}$) on the oxy-Hb curve in Fig. 5.25.

The oxy-Hb curve can also relate the oxygen content (C_{O_2}) (vol%, or mL of O_2 per dL of blood; see Fig. 5.25) to P_{O_2}. Oxygen is carried both in solution in plasma (0.003 mL of O_2/mm Hg P_{O_2} per dL) and combined with Hb (1.39 mL of O_2/g of Hb), to the extent (percentage) that Hb is saturated. Therefore:

$$C_{O_2} = (1.39)(Hb)(\text{percent saturation}) + 0.003(P_{O_2}) \quad (13)$$

For a patient with an Hb content of 15 g/dL, a Pa_{O_2} of 100 mm Hg, and a $P\bar{v}_{O_2}$ of 40 mm Hg, the arterial oxygen content (Ca_{O_2}) = (1.39)(15)(1) + (0.003)(100) = 20.9 + 0.3 = 21.2 mL/dL; the mixed venous oxygen content ($C\bar{v}_{O_2}$) = (1.39)(15)(0.75) + (0.003)(40) = 15.6 + 0.1 = 15.7 mL/dL. Therefore, the normal arteriovenous oxygen content difference is approximately 5.5 mL/dL of blood.

Note that Eq. 13 uses the constant 1.39, which means that 1 g of Hb can carry 1.39 mL of oxygen. Controversy exists over the magnitude of this number. Originally, 1.34 had been used,[92] but with determination of the molecular weight of Hb (64,458), the theoretical value of 1.39 became popular.[93] After extensive human studies, Gregory observed in 1974 that the applicable value was 1.31 mL O_2/g of Hb in human adults.[94] The lower clinically measured C_{O_2} value, compared to the theoretical 1.39, is probably due to the small amount of methemoglobin and carboxyhemoglobin normally present in blood.

The oxy-Hb curve can also relate oxygen transport (L/min) to the peripheral tissues (see Fig. 5.25) to P_{O_2}. The term *oxygen transport* is synonymous with the term *oxygen delivery.* This value is obtained by multiplying the oxygen content by $\dot{Q}_T$ (O_2 transport $= \dot{Q}_T \times Ca_{O_2}$). To perform this calculation, the content unit of mL/dL must be converted to mL/L by multiplying by 10; subsequent multiplication of mL/L against $\dot{Q}_T$ in L/min yields mL/min. Thus, if $\dot{Q}_T$ = 5 L/min and Ca_{O_2} = 20 mL of O_2/dL, the arterial point corresponds to 1000 mL O_2/min going to the periphery, and the venous point corresponds to 750 mL O_2/min returning to the lungs, with $\dot{V}_{O_2}$ = 250 mL/min.

The oxy-Hb curve can also relate the oxygen available to the tissues (leftmost vertical axis in Fig. 5.25) as a function of P_{O_2}. Of the 1000 mL/min of oxygen normally going to the periphery, 200 mL/min of oxygen cannot be extracted because it would lower P_{O_2} below the level at which organs such as the brain can survive (*f* *dashed line* in Fig. 5.25); the oxygen available to tissues is therefore 800 mL/min. This amount is approximately three to four times the normal resting $\dot{V}_{O_2}$. When $\dot{Q}_T$ = 5 L/min and

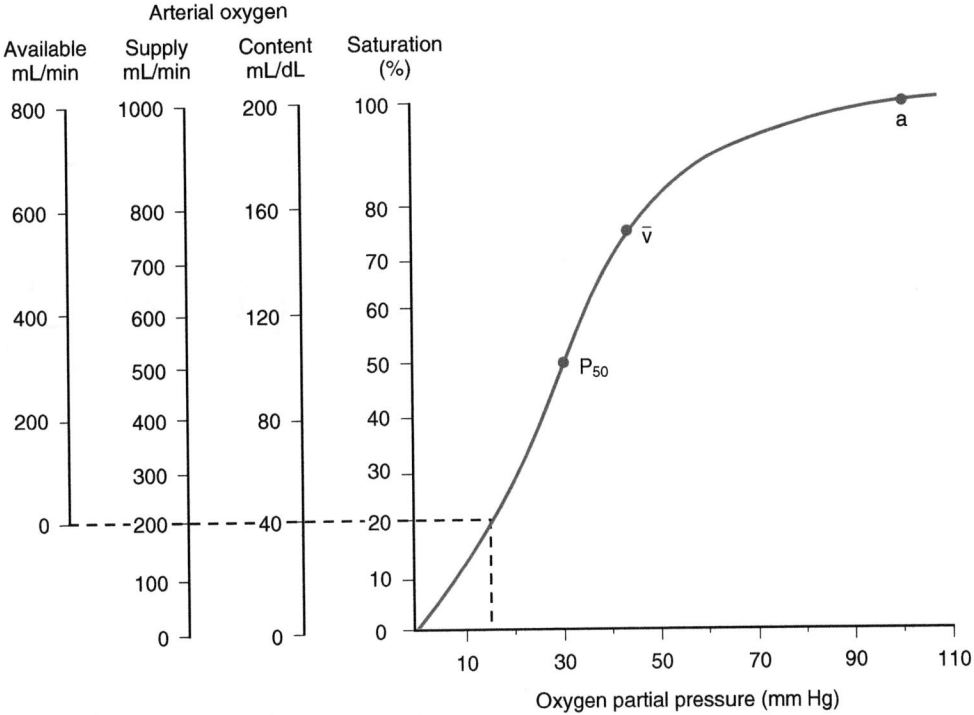

Arterial oxygen

• **Fig. 5.25** Oxygen-hemoglobin dissociation curve. Four different ordinates are shown as a function of oxygen partial pressure (horizontal axis). In order from right to left, they are arterial oxygen saturation (%), arterial oxygen content (mL of O_2/dL of blood), oxygen supply to peripheral tissues (mL/min), and oxygen available to peripheral tissues (mL/min), which is oxygen supply minus the approximately 200 mL/min that cannot be extracted below a partial pressure of 20 mm Hg. Three points are shown on the curve: *a*, normal arterial partial pressure; *v̄*, normal mixed venous partial pressure; and P_{50}, the partial pressure (27 mm Hg) at which hemoglobin is 50% saturated.

arterial saturation is less than 40%, the total flow of oxygen to the periphery is reduced to 400 mL/min; the available oxygen is then 200 mL/min, and oxygen supply just equals oxygen demand. Consequently, with low arterial saturation, tissue demand can be met only by an increase in $\dot{Q}_T$ or, in the longer term, by an increase in Hb concentration.

The affinity of Hb for oxygen is best described by the P_{O_2} level at which Hb is 50% saturated (P_{50}) on the oxy-Hb curve. The normal adult P_{50} is 26.7 mm Hg (see Fig. 5.25). The effect of a change in P_{O_2} on Hb saturation is related to both P_{50} and the portion of the oxy-Hb curve at which the change occurs.[95] In the region of normal P_{aO_2} (75 to 100 mm Hg), the curve is relatively horizontal, and shifts of the curve have little effect on saturation. In the region of mixed venous P_{O_2}, where the curve is relatively steep, a shift of the curve leads to a much greater difference in saturation. A P_{50} lower than 27 mm Hg describes a left-shifted oxy-Hb curve, which means that at any given P_{O_2}, Hb has a higher affinity for oxygen and is therefore more saturated than normal. This lower P_{50} may require higher-than-normal tissue perfusion to produce the normal amount of oxygen unloading. Causes of a left-shifted oxy-Hb curve are alkalosis (metabolic and respiratory—the Bohr effect), hypothermia, abnormal fetal Hb, carboxyhemoglobin, methemoglobin, and decreased RBC 2,3-diphosphoglycerate (2,3-DPG) content. The last condition may occur with the transfusion of old acid citrate-dextrose-stored blood; storage of blood in citrate-phosphate-dextrose minimizes changes in 2,3-DPG with time.[95] A P_{50} higher than 27 mm Hg describes a right-shifted oxy-Hb curve, which means that at any given P_{O_2}, Hb has a low affinity for oxygen and is less saturated than normal. This higher P_{50} may allow a lower

tissue perfusion than normal to produce the normal amount of oxygen unloading. Causes of a right-shifted oxy-Hb curve are acidosis (metabolic and respiratory—the Bohr effect), hyperthermia, abnormal Hb, increased RBC 2,3-DPG content, and inhaled anesthetics (see later discussion).[95] Abnormalities in acid-base balance result in alteration of 2,3-DPG metabolism to shift the oxy-Hb curve to its normal position. This compensatory change in 2,3-DPG requires between 24 and 48 hours. Therefore, with acute acid-base abnormalities, oxygen affinity and the position of the oxy-Hb curve change. However, with more prolonged acid-base changes, the reciprocal changes in 2,3-DPG levels shift the oxy-Hb curve and oxygen affinity back toward normal.[95]

Many inhaled anesthetics have been shown to shift the oxy-Hb dissociation curve to the right.[96] Isoflurane shifts P_{50} to the right by 2.6 ± 0.07 mm Hg at a vapor pressure of approximately 1 MAC (minimum alveolar concentration) (1.25%).[97] On the other hand, high-dose fentanyl, morphine, and meperidine do not alter the position of the curve.

Effect of $\dot{Q}_S/\dot{Q}_T$ on Alveolar Oxygen Tension

P_{aO_2} is directly related to F_{IO_2} in normal patients. P_{aO_2} and F_{IO_2} also correspond to P_{aO_2} when there is little to no right-to-left transpulmonary shunt ($\dot{Q}_S/\dot{Q}_T$). Fig. 5.26 shows the relationship between F_{IO_2} and P_{aO_2} for various amounts of right-to-left transpulmonary shunt; the calculations assume a constant and normal $\dot{Q}_T$ and P_{aCO_2}. With no $\dot{Q}_S/\dot{Q}_T$, a linear increase in F_{IO_2} results in a linear increase in P_{aO_2} (solid straight line). As the shunt is increased, the lines relating F_{IO_2} to P_{aO_2} become progressively flatter.[98] With a shunt of 50% of $\dot{Q}_T$, an increase in F_{IO_2} results in

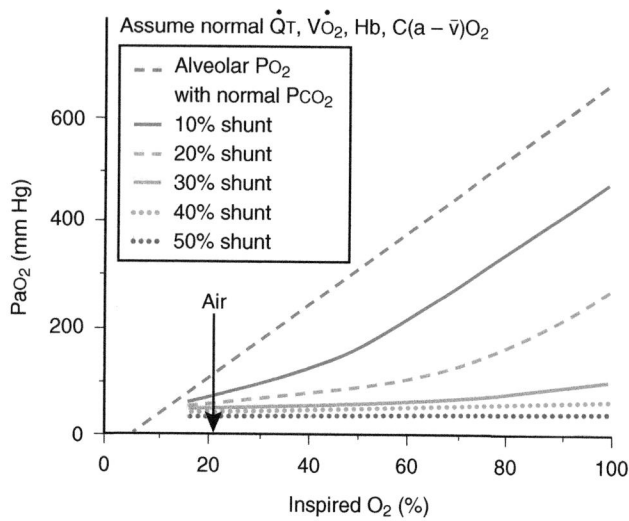

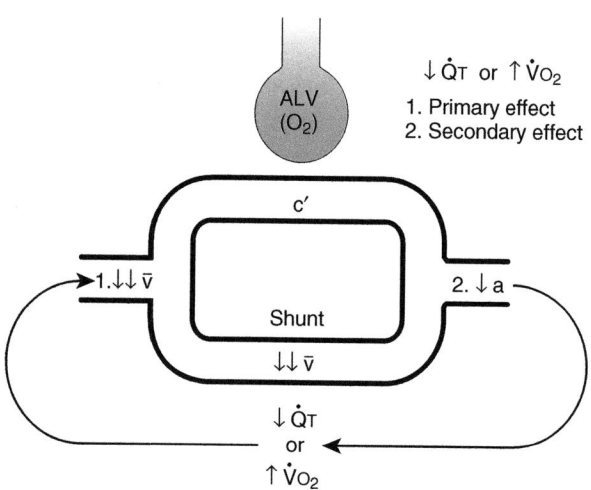

• **Fig. 5.26** Effect of changes in inspired oxygen concentration on arterial oxygen tension (PaO_2) for various right-to-left transpulmonary shunts. Cardiac output ($\dot{Q}_T$), hemoglobin (Hb), oxygen consumption ($\dot{V}O_2$), and arteriovenous oxygen content differences $C(a - \bar{v})O_2$ are assumed to be normal. PCO_2, Partial pressure of carbon dioxide; PO_2, Partial pressure of oxygen.

• **Fig. 5.27** Effect of a decrease in cardiac output ($\dot{Q}_T$) or an increase in oxygen consumption ($\dot{V}O_2$) on mixed venous and arterial oxygen content. Mixed venous blood ($\bar{v}$) either perfuses ventilated alveolar capillaries (ALV) and becomes oxygenated end-pulmonary capillary blood (c') or perfuses whatever true shunt pathways exist and remains the same in composition (i.e., desaturated). These two pathways must ultimately join together to form mixed arterial (a) blood. If $\dot{Q}_T$ decreases or $\dot{V}O_2$ increases, or both, the tissues must extract more oxygen per unit volume of blood than under normal conditions. Thus the primary effect of a decrease in $\dot{Q}_T$ or an increase in $\dot{V}O_2$ is a decrease in mixed venous oxygen content. The mixed venous blood with a decreased oxygen content must flow through the shunt pathway as before (which may remain constant in size) and lower the arterial content of oxygen. Thus, the secondary effect of a decrease in $\dot{Q}_T$ or an increase in $\dot{V}O_2$ is a decrease in arterial oxygen content.

almost no increase in PaO_2. The solution to the problem of hypoxemia secondary to a large shunt is not to increase FIO_2 but rather to reduce the shunt (e.g., with PEEP, patient positioning, suctioning, flexible bronchoscopy, diuretics, or antibiotics).

Effect of $\dot{Q}_T$ and $\dot{V}O_2$ on Arterial Oxygen Content

In addition to an increased $\dot{Q}s/\dot{Q}_T$, CaO_2 is decreased by decreased $\dot{Q}_T$ (for a constant $\dot{V}O_2$) and by increased $\dot{V}O_2$ (for a constant $\dot{Q}_T$). In either case, along with a constant right-to-left shunt, the tissues must extract more oxygen from blood per unit blood volume, and therefore $C\bar{v}O_2$ must primarily decrease (Fig. 5.27). When blood with lower $C\bar{v}O_2$ passes through whatever shunt exists in the lung and remains unchanged in its $\dot{V}O_2$, it must inevitably mix with oxygenated end-pulmonary capillary blood (c' flow) and secondarily decrease CaO_2. The amount of oxygen flowing per minute through any lung unit, as depicted in Fig. 5.27, is a product of blood flow times the oxygen content of that blood—thus $\dot{Q}_T \times CaO_2 = \dot{Q}c' \times Cc'O_2 + \dot{Q}s \times C\bar{v}O_2$. With $\dot{Q}c' = \dot{Q}_T - \dot{Q}s$ and further algebraic manipulation,[99]

$$\dot{Q}s/\dot{Q}_T = Cc'O_2 - CaO_2/Cc'O_2 - C\bar{v}O_2 \qquad (14)$$

The larger the intrapulmonary shunt, the greater the decrease in CaO_2, because more venous blood with lower $C\bar{v}O_2$ can admix with end-pulmonary capillary blood (c') (see Fig. 5.37, later in the chapter)[100,101] Therefore, the alveolar-arterial oxygen difference $P(A - a)O_2$ is a function both of the size of the $\dot{Q}s/\dot{Q}_T$ and of what is flowing through the $\dot{Q}s/\dot{Q}_T$—namely, $C\bar{v}O_2$—and $C\bar{v}O_2$ is a primary function of $\dot{Q}_T$ and $\dot{V}O_2$. Fig. 5.28 shows the equivalent circuit of the pulmonary circulation in a patient with a 50% shunt, a normal $C\bar{v}O_2$ of 15 mL/dL, and a moderately low CaO_2 of 17.5 mL/dL. Decreasing $\dot{Q}_T$ or increasing $\dot{V}O_2$, or both, causes a larger primary decrease in $C\bar{v}O_2$ to 10 mL/dL and a smaller but still significant secondary decrease in CaO_2 to 15 mL/dL; the ratio of change in $C\bar{v}O_2$ to change in CaO_2 in this example of 50% $\dot{Q}s/\dot{Q}_T$ is 2:1.

If a decrease in $\dot{Q}_T$ or an increase in $\dot{V}O_2$ is accompanied by a decrease in $\dot{Q}s/\dot{Q}_T$, there may be no change in PaO_2 (i.e., a

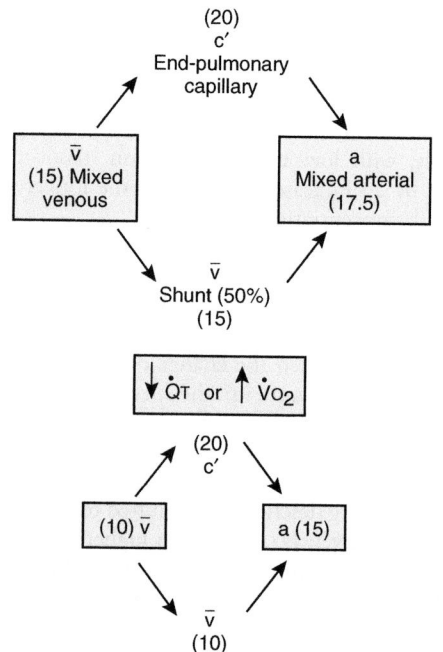

• **Fig. 5.28** The equivalent circuit of the pulmonary circulation in a patient with a 50% right-to-left shunt. Oxygen content is in mL/dL of blood. In this example, a decrease in cardiac output ($\dot{Q}_T$) or an increase in oxygen consumption ($\dot{V}O_2$) can cause a decrease in mixed venous oxygen content, from 15 to 10 mL/dL, which in turn causes a decrease in the arterial content of oxygen, from 17.5 to 15.0 mL/dL). In this 50% shunt example, the decrease in mixed venous oxygen content was twice the decrease in arterial oxygen content: a, Arterial blood; c', end-pulmonary capillary blood; $\bar{v}$, mixed venous blood.

TABLE 5.4	Relationship Between Cardiac Output ($\dot{Q}_T$), Shunt ($\dot{Q}_S/\dot{Q}_T$), and Venous ($P\bar{v}O_2$) and Arterial (PaO_2) Oxygenation

Changes	Clinical Situation
If $\dot{Q}_T \downarrow \rightarrow \downarrow P\bar{v}O_2$ and $\dot{Q}_S/\dot{Q}_T = 0 \rightarrow PaO_2 \downarrow$	Decreased cardiac output, stable shunt
If $\dot{Q}_T \downarrow \rightarrow \downarrow P\bar{v}O_2$ and $\dot{Q}_S/\dot{Q}_T \downarrow \rightarrow PaO_2 =$ no Δ	Application of PEEP in ARDS
If $\dot{Q}_T \downarrow \rightarrow \downarrow P\bar{v}O_2$ and $\dot{Q}_S/\dot{Q}_T \uparrow \rightarrow PaO_2 \downarrow\downarrow$	Shock combined with ARDS or atelectasis

$\downarrow$, decrease; $\uparrow$, increase; *ARDS*, acute respiratory distress syndrome; *no Δ*, no change; *PEEP*, positive end-expiratory pressure.

decreasing effect on PaO_2 is offset by an increasing effect on PaO_2) (Table 5.4). These changes sometimes occur in diffuse lung disease. However, if a decrease in $\dot{Q}_T$ or an increase in $\dot{V}O_2$ is accompanied by an increase in $\dot{Q}_S/\dot{Q}_T$, PaO_2 may be greatly decreased (i.e., a decreasing effect on PaO_2 is compounded by another decreasing effect on PaO_2). These changes sometimes occur in regional ARDS and atelectasis.[102]

Fick Principle

The Fick principle allows calculation of $\dot{V}O_2$ and states that the amount of oxygen consumed by the body ($\dot{V}O_2$) is equal to the amount of oxygen leaving the lungs ($\dot{Q}_T$)(CaO_2) minus the amount of oxygen returning to the lungs ($\dot{Q}_T$)($C\bar{v}O_2$):

$$\dot{V}O_2 = (\dot{Q}_T)(CaO_2) - (\dot{Q}_T)(C\bar{v}O_2) = \dot{Q}_T(CaO_2 - C\bar{v}O_2) \quad (15)$$

Condensing the content symbols yields the usual expression of the Fick equation:

$$\dot{V}O_2 = (\dot{Q}_T)[C(a - \bar{v})O_2] \quad (16)$$

This equation states that oxygen consumption is equal to $\dot{Q}_T$ times the arteriovenous oxygen content difference [$C(a - \bar{v})O_2$]. Normally, (5 L/min)(5.5 mL/dL) = 0.27 L/min (see "Oxygen-Hemoglobin Dissociation Curve").

Similarly, the amount of oxygen consumed by the body ($\dot{V}O_2$) is equal to the amount of oxygen brought into the lungs by ventilation ($\dot{V}_I$)(FiO_2) minus the amount of oxygen leaving the lungs by ventilation ($\dot{V}_E$)(FeO_2), where $\dot{V}_E$ is expired minute ventilation and FeO_2 is the mixed expired oxygen fraction: $\dot{V}O_2 = (\dot{V}_I)(FiO_2) - (\dot{V}_E)(FeO_2)$. Because the difference between $\dot{V}_I$ and $\dot{V}_E$ is due to the difference between $\dot{V}O_2$ (normally 250 mL/min) and $\dot{V}CO_2$ (normally 200 mL/min) and is only 50 mL/min (see later discussion), $\dot{V}_I$ essentially equals $\dot{V}_E$.

$$\dot{V}O_2 = \dot{V}_E(FiO_2) - \dot{V}_E(FeO_2) = \dot{V}_E(FiO_2 - FeO_2) \quad (17)$$

Normally, $\dot{V}O_2 = 5.0$ L/min (0.21 – 0.16) = 0.25 L/min. In determining $\dot{V}O_2$ in this way, $\dot{V}_E$ can be measured with a spirometer, FiO_2 can be measured with an oxygen analyzer or from known fresh gas flows, and FeO_2 can be measured by collecting expired gas in a bag for a few minutes. A sample of the mixed expired gas is used to measure PeO_2. To convert PeO_2 to FeO_2, one simply divides PeO_2 by dry atmospheric pressure: $PeO_2/713 = FeO_2$.

In addition, the Fick equation is useful in understanding the impact of changes in $\dot{Q}_T$ on PaO_2 and $P\bar{v}O_2$. If $\dot{V}O_2$ remains constant (K) and $\dot{Q}_T$ decreases ($\downarrow$), the arteriovenous oxygen content difference has to increase ($\uparrow$):

$$\dot{V}O_2 = K = (\downarrow)\dot{Q}_T \times (\uparrow)C(a - \bar{v})O_2 \quad (18)$$

The $C(a - \bar{v})O_2$ difference increases because a decrease in $\dot{Q}_T$ causes a much larger and primary decrease in $C\bar{v}O_2$ versus a smaller and secondary decrease in CaO_2, as follows[101]:

$$(\uparrow)C(a - \bar{v})O_2 = C(\downarrow a - \downarrow\downarrow \bar{v})O_2 \quad (19)$$

Thus $C\bar{v}O_2$ and $P\bar{v}O_2$ are much more sensitive indicators of $\dot{Q}_T$ because they change more with changes in $\dot{Q}_T$ than CaO_2 (or PaO_2) does (see Figs. 5.27 and 5.28 as well as and 5.37, later in the chapter).

Carbon Dioxide Transport

The amount of CO_2 circulating in the body is a function of both CO_2 elimination and CO_2 production. Elimination of CO_2 depends on pulmonary blood flow and alveolar ventilation. Production of CO_2 ($\dot{V}CO_2$) parallels oxygen consumption ($\dot{V}O_2$) according to the respiratory quotient (RQ):

$$RQ = \frac{\dot{V}CO_2}{\dot{V}O_2} \quad (20)$$

Under normal resting conditions, RQ is 0.8—that is, only 80% as much CO_2 is produced as oxygen is consumed. However, this value changes as the nature of the metabolic substrate changes. If only carbohydrate is used, the RQ is 1.0. Conversely, with the sole use of fat, more oxygen combines with hydrogen to produce water, and the RQ value drops to 0.7. CO_2 is transported from mitochondria to the alveoli in several forms. In plasma, CO_2 exists in physical solution, hydrated to carbonic acid (H_2CO_3), and as bicarbonate (HCO_3^-). In the RBC, CO_2 combines with Hb as carbaminohemoglobin (Hb-CO_2). The approximate values of H_2CO_3 ($H_2O + CO_2$), HCO_3^-, and Hb-CO_2 relative to the total CO_2 transported are 7%, 80%, and 13%, respectively.

In plasma, CO_2 exists both in physical solution and as H_2CO_3:

$$H_2O + CO_2 \rightarrow H_2CO_3 \quad (21)$$

The CO_2 in solution can be related to the partial pressure of CO_2 (PcO_2) by the use of the Henry law.[103]

$$PcO_2 \times a = [CO_2] \text{ in solution} \quad (22)$$

where a is the solubility coefficient of CO_2 in plasma (0.03 mmol/L/mm Hg at 37°C).

However, the major fraction of CO_2 produced passes into the RBC. As in plasma, CO_2 combines with water in the RBC to produce H_2CO_3. However, unlike the slow reaction in plasma, in which the equilibrium point lies toward the left, the reaction in an RBC is catalyzed by the enzyme carbonic anhydrase. This zinc-containing enzyme moves the reaction to the right at a rate 1000 times faster than in plasma. Furthermore, almost 99.9% of the H_2CO_3 dissociates to HCO_3^- and hydrogen ions (H^+):

$$H_2O + CO_2 \xrightarrow[\substack{H_2CO_3 \rightarrow H^+ + HCO_3^-}]{\text{carbonic anhydrase}} H_2CO_3 \quad (23)$$

The H^+ produced from H_2CO_3 in the production of HCO_3^- is buffered by Hb ($H^+ + Hb \rightleftharpoons HHb$). The HCO_3^- produced passes out of the RBC into plasma to perform its function as a buffer. To maintain electrical neutrality within the RBC, chloride ion (Cl⁻) moves in as HCO_3^- moves out (Cl⁻ shift).

Finally, CO_2 can combine with Hb in the erythrocyte to produce Hb-CO_2. Again, as in HCO_3^- release, an H^+ ion is formed in the reaction of CO_2 and Hb. This H^+ ion is also buffered by Hb.

Bohr and Haldane Effects

Just as the percent saturation of Hb with oxygen is related to Po_2 (described by the oxy-Hb curve), so the total CO_2 in blood is related to Pco_2. In addition, Hb has variable affinity for CO_2; it binds more avidly in the reduced state than as oxy-Hb.[95] The Bohr effect describes the effect of Pco_2 and H^+ ions on the oxy-Hb curve. Hypercapnia and acidosis both shift the curve to the right (reducing the oxygen-binding affinity of Hb), and hypocapnia and alkalosis both shift the curve to the left. Conversely, the Haldane effect describes the shift in the CO_2 dissociation curve caused by oxygenation of Hb. Low Po_2 shifts the CO_2 dissociation curve to the left so that the blood can pick up more CO_2 (as occurs in capillaries of rapidly metabolizing tissues). Conversely, oxygenation of Hb (as occurs in the lungs) reduces the affinity of Hb for CO_2, and the CO_2 dissociation curve is shifted to the right, thereby increasing CO_2 removal.

Pulmonary Microcirculation, Interstitial Space, and Pulmonary Edema

The ultrastructural appearance of an alveolar septum is depicted schematically in Fig. 5.29.[104] Capillary blood is separated from alveolar gas by a series of anatomic layers: capillary endothelium, endothelial basement membrane, interstitial space, epithelial basement membrane, and alveolar epithelium (of the type I pneumocyte).

On one side of the alveolar septum (the thick, upper, fluid- and gas-exchanging side), the epithelial and endothelial basement membranes are separated by a space of variable thickness containing connective tissue fibrils, elastic fibers, fibroblasts, and macrophages. This connective tissue is the backbone of the lung parenchyma; it forms a continuum with the connective tissue sheaths around the conducting airways and blood vessels. Thus, the pericapillary, perialveolar

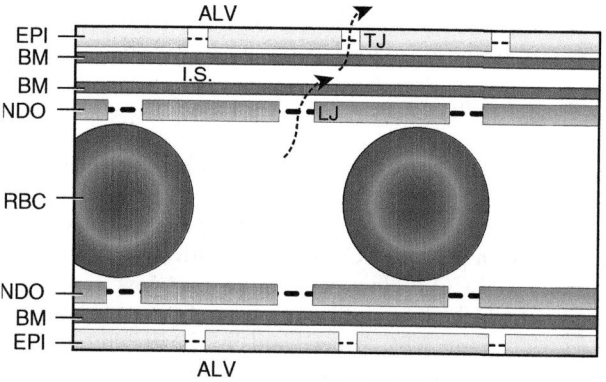

• **Fig. 5.29** Schematic summary of the ultrastructure of an alveolar septum. On the upper side of the capillary, the endothelial (*ENDO*) and epithelial (*EPI*) basement membranes (*BM*) are separated by an interstitial space (*I.S.*), whereas the lower side contains only fused ENDO and EPI BM. The *dashed arrows* indicate a potential pathway for fluid to move from the intravascular space to the I.S. through loose junctions (*LJ*) in the endothelium and from the I.S. to the alveolar space (*ALV*) through tight junctions (*TJ*) in the epithelium. *RBC*, Red blood cell. (From Fishman AP. Pulmonary edema: the water-exchanging function of the lung. *Circulation.* 1972;46:390.)

interstitial space is continuous with the interstitial tissue space that surrounds terminal bronchioles and vessels, and both spaces constitute the connective tissue space of the lung. There are no lymphatics in the interstitial space of the alveolar septum. Instead, lymphatic capillaries first appear in the interstitial space surrounding terminal bronchioles, small arteries, and veins.[105]

The opposite side of the alveolar septum (the thin, lower, solely gas-exchanging side) contains only fused epithelial and endothelial basement membranes. The interstitial space is greatly restricted on this side because of fusion of the basement membranes. Interstitial fluid cannot separate the endothelial and epithelial cells from one another. As a result, the space and distance barrier to fluid movement from the capillary to the alveolar compartment is reduced; it is composed of only the two cell linings with their associated basement membranes.[106]

Between the individual endothelial and epithelial cells are holes or junctions that provide a potential pathway for fluid to move from the intravascular space to the interstitial space and finally from the interstitial space to the alveolar space (see Fig. 5.29). The junctions between endothelial cells are relatively large and are therefore termed *loose*; the junctions between epithelial cells are relatively small and are therefore termed *tight*. Pulmonary capillary permeability is a direct function of, and is essentially equivalent to, the size of the holes in the endothelial and epithelial linings.

To understand how pulmonary interstitial fluid is formed, stored, and cleared, it is necessary first to develop the concepts that (1) the pulmonary interstitial space is a continuous space between the periarteriolar and peribronchial connective tissue sheath and the space between the endothelial and epithelial basement membranes in the alveolar septum and (2) the space has a progressively negative distal-to-proximal ΔP.

The concepts of a continuous connective tissue sheath–alveolar septum interstitial space and a negative interstitial space ΔP are prerequisite to understanding interstitial fluid kinetics. After entering the lung parenchyma, both the bronchi and the arteries run within a connective tissue sheath that is formed by an invagination of the pleura at the hilum and ends at the level of the bronchioles (Fig. 5.30A). This results in a potential perivascular space between the arteries and the connective tissue sheath and a potential peribronchial space between the bronchi and the connective tissue sheath. The negative pressure in the pulmonary tissues surrounding the perivascular connective tissue sheath exerts a radial outward traction force on the sheath. This radial traction creates negative pressure within the sheath that is transmitted to the bronchi and arteries and tends to hold them open and increase their diameters.[106] The alveolar septum interstitial space is the space between the capillaries and alveoli (or, more precisely, the space between the endothelial and epithelial basement membranes) and is continuous with the interstitial tissue space that surrounds the larger arteries and bronchi. Studies indicate that the alveolar interstitial pressure is also uniquely negative but not as much so as the negative interstitial space pressure around the larger arteries and bronchi.[107]

The forces governing net transcapillary–interstitial space fluid movement are as follows: The net transcapillary flow of fluid (F) out of pulmonary capillaries (across the endothelium and into the interstitial space) is equal to the difference between pulmonary capillary hydrostatic pressure (P_{inside}) and interstitial fluid hydrostatic pressure ($P_{outside}$) and the difference between capillary colloid oncotic pressure (π_{inside}) and interstitial colloid oncotic pressure ($\pi_{outside}$). These four forces produce a steady-state fluid flow (F) during a constant capillary permeability (K) as predicted by the Starling equation:

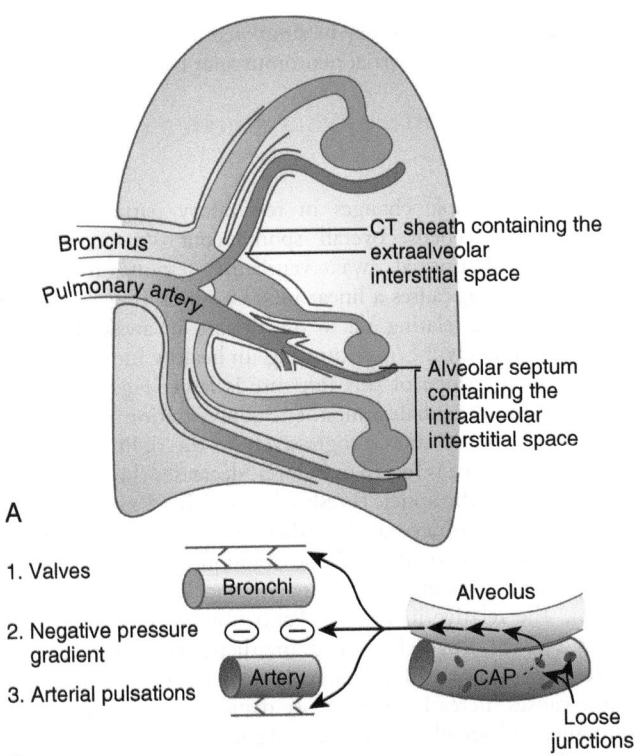

1. Valves

2. Negative pressure gradient

3. Arterial pulsations

B

• **Fig. 5.30** (A) Schematic diagram of the concept of a continuous connective tissue sheath–alveolar septum interstitial space. The entry of the mainstem bronchi and pulmonary artery into the lung parenchyma invaginates the pleura at the hilum and forms a surrounding connective tissue sheath. The connective tissue sheath ends at the level of the bronchioles. The space between the pulmonary arteries and bronchi and the interstitial space is continuous with the alveolar septum interstitial space. The alveolar septum interstitial space is contained within the endothelial basement membrane of the capillaries and the epithelial basement membrane of the alveoli. (B) Schematic diagram showing how interstitial fluid moves from the alveolar septum interstitial space (no lymphatics) to the connective tissue interstitial space (lymphatic capillaries first appear). The mechanisms are the presence of one-way valves in the lymphatics, a negative pressure gradient (sump), and the massaging action of arterial pulsations. *CAP,* Capillary; *CT,* connective tissue. (Modified from Benumof JL. *Anesthesia for Thoracic Surgery.* 2nd ed. Saunders; 1995:Chapter 8.)

$$F = K[(P_{inside} - P_{outside}) - (\pi_{inside} - \pi_{outside})] \qquad (24)$$

K is a capillary filtration coefficient expressed in mL/min/mm Hg/100 g. The filtration coefficient is the product of the effective capillary surface area in a given mass of tissue and the permeability per unit surface area of the capillary wall to filter the fluid. Under normal circumstances and at a vertical height in the lung that is at the junction of zones 2 and 3, intravascular colloid oncotic pressure ($\approx$ 26 mm Hg) acts to keep water in the capillary lumen; working against this force, pulmonary capillary hydrostatic pressure ($\approx$ 10 mm Hg) acts to force water across the loose endothelial junctions into the interstitial space. If these were the only operative forces, the interstitial space and, consequently, the alveolar surfaces would be constantly dry and there would be no lymph flow. In fact, alveolar surfaces are moist, and lymphatic flow from the interstitial compartment is constant ($\approx$ 500 mL/day). This can be explained in part by $\pi_{outside}$ ($\approx$ 8 mm Hg) and in part by negative $P_{outside}$ (−8 mm Hg).

Negative (subatmospheric) interstitial space pressure would promote, by suction, a slow loss of fluid across the endothelial holes.[108] Indeed, extremely negative pleural (and perivascular hydrostatic) pressure, such as may occur in a vigorously spontaneously breathing patient with an obstructed airway, can cause pulmonary interstitial edema, so-called *negative pressure pulmonary edema* (Box 5.1).[109] Relative to the vertical level of the junction of zones 2 and 3, as lung height decreases (lung dependence), absolute P_{inside} increases, and fluid has a propensity to transudate; as lung height increases (lung nondependence), absolute P_{inside} decreases, and fluid has a propensity to be reabsorbed. However, fluid transudation induced by an increase in P_{inside} is limited by a concomitant dilution of proteins in the interstitial space and therefore a decrease in $\pi_{outside}$.[110] Any change in the size of the endothelial junctions, even if the foregoing four forces remain constant, changes the magnitude and perhaps even the direction of fluid movement. Increased size of endothelial junctions (increased permeability) promotes transudation, whereas decreased size of endothelial junctions (decreased permeability) promotes reabsorption.

No lymphatics are present in the interstitial space of the alveolar septum. The lymphatic circulation starts as blind-ended lymphatic capillaries, first appearing in the interstitial space sheath surrounding terminal bronchioles and small arteries and ends at the subclavian veins. Interstitial fluid is normally removed from the alveolar interstitial space into the lymphatics by a sump (pressure gradient) mechanism, which is caused by the presence of more negative pressure surrounding the larger arteries and bronchi.[3,111] The sump mechanism is aided by the presence of valves in the lymph vessels. In addition, because the lymphatics run in the same sheath as the pulmonary arteries, they are exposed to the massaging action of arterial pulsations. The differential negative pressure, the lymphatic valves, and the arterial pulsations all help propel the lymph proximally toward the hilum through the lymph nodes (pulmonary to bronchopulmonary to tracheobronchial to paratracheal to scalene and cervical nodes) to the central venous circulation (see Fig. 5.30B). An increase in central venous pressure, which is the backpressure for lymph to flow out of the lung, would decrease lung lymph flow and perhaps promote pulmonary interstitial edema.

If the rate of entry of fluid into the pulmonary interstitial space exceeds the capability of the pulmonary interstitial space to clear the fluid, the pulmonary interstitial space fills with fluid. The fluid, now under an increased and positive driving force (P_{ISF}), crosses the relatively impermeable epithelial wall holes, and the alveolar space fills. Intraalveolar edema fluid also causes alveolar

---

• **BOX 5.1** **Causes of Extremely Negative Pulmonary Interstitial Fluid Pressure ($P_{outside}$) in Pulmonary Edema**

Vigorous spontaneous inhalation efforts against an obstructed (or partially obstructed) airway
    Laryngospasm
    Upper airway mass (e.g., tumor, hematoma, abscess, or foreign body)
    Upper airway stricture (e.g., from chronic scarring or from infection, inflammation, or edema)
    Vocal cord paralysis
    Strangulation
Rapid reexpansion of lung
Vigorous pleural suctioning (thoracentesis, chest tube)

collapse and atelectasis, thereby promoting further accumulation of fluid and worsening right-to-left transpulmonary shunt.

Respiratory Function During Anesthesia

Arterial oxygenation is impaired in most patients during anesthesia with either spontaneous or controlled ventilation.[112–117] In otherwise normal patients, it is generally accepted that the impairment in arterial oxygenation during anesthesia is more severe in the elderly,[118,119] the obese,[120] and smokers.[121] In various studies of healthy, young to middle-aged patients under general anesthesia, venous admixture (shunt) has been found to average 10%, and the scatter in $\dot{V}_A/\dot{Q}$ ratios is small to moderate.[119,122] In patients with a more marked deterioration in preoperative pulmonary function, general anesthesia causes considerable widening of the $\dot{V}_A/\dot{Q}$ distribution and large increases in both low-$\dot{V}_A/\dot{Q}$ (0.005 < $\dot{V}_A/\dot{Q}$ < 0.1) (underventilated) regions and shunting.[118,121,123] The magnitude of shunting correlates closely with the degree of atelectasis.[118,123]

In addition to these generalizations concerning respiratory function during anesthesia, the effect of a given anesthetic on respiratory function depends on the depth of general anesthesia, the patient's preoperative respiratory condition, and the presence of special intraoperative anesthetic and surgical conditions.

Anesthetic Depth and Respiratory Pattern

A patient's respiratory pattern is altered by the induction and deepening of anesthesia. When the depth of inhalational anesthesia is inadequate, the respiratory pattern may vary from excessive hyperventilation and vocalization to breath-holding. As anesthetic depth proceeds to "light" general anesthesia, irregular respiration progresses to a more regular pattern that is associated with a larger than normal V_T. However, during light but deepening anesthesia, the approach to a more regular respiratory pattern may be interrupted by a pause at the end of inspiration (a "hitch" in inspiration), followed by a relatively prolonged and active expiratory phase in which the patient seems to exhale forcefully rather than passively. As general inhalational anesthesia deepens to moderate levels, the respiratory rate becomes faster and more regular but shallower. The respiratory pattern is a sine wave losing both the inspiratory hitch and lengthened expiratory pause. There is little or no inspiratory or expiratory pause, and the inspiratory and expiratory periods become equivalent. Intercostal muscle activity is still present, and there is normal movement of the thoracic cage with lifting of the chest during inspiration.

The respiratory rate is generally slower and the V_T larger with opioid-based anesthetic techniques in combination with nitrous oxide or propofol infusion than with anesthesia involving halogenated agents. During deep anesthesia with halogenated agents, increasing respiratory depression is manifested by increasingly rapid and shallow breathing (panting). On the other hand, with deep opioid–nitrous oxide anesthesia, respirations become slower but typically remain deep. In the case of very deep anesthesia with all inhaled drugs, respirations often become jerky or gasping in character and irregular in pattern. This situation results from loss of the active intercostal muscle contribution to inspiration. As a result, a rocking boat movement occurs in which there is out-of-phase depression of the chest wall during inspiration, flaring of the lower chest margins, and billowing of the abdomen. The reason for this type of movement is that inspiration becomes dependent solely on diaphragmatic effort. Independent of anesthetic depth,

similar chest movements may be simulated by upper or lower airway obstruction or by partial neuromuscular blockade.

Anesthetic Depth and Spontaneous Minute Ventilation

Despite the variable changes in respiratory pattern and rate as anesthesia deepens, overall spontaneous $\dot{V}_E$ progressively decreases. In the normal, awake ventilatory response to CO_2, an increasing P_{ETCO_2} causes a linear increase in $\dot{V}_E$ (Fig. 5.31). The slope of the line relating $\dot{V}_E$ to the P_{ETCO_2} in awake individuals is approximately 2 L/min/mm Hg. In healthy individuals, the variation in the slope of this response is large. Fig. 5.31 shows that increasing the inhaled anesthetic concentration displaces the ventilation/response curve progressively to the right (i.e., at any P_{ETCO_2}, ventilation is less than before), decreases the slope of the curve, and shifts the apneic threshold to a higher P_{ETCO_2}.[124] Similar alterations are observed with other halogenated anesthetics, as well as with opioid-based anesthetic techniques.[125] Figs. 5.22–5.24 show that decreases in $\dot{V}_E$ cause increases in $PaCO_2$ and decreases in PaO_2. The relative increase in $PaCO_2$ caused by depression of $\dot{V}_E$ (<1.24 MAC) by halogenated anesthetics is desflurane = isoflurane > sevoflurane > halothane. At higher concentrations, desflurane causes increasing ventilatory depression, even more than isoflurane, and sevoflurane causes a degree of ventilatory depression similar to isoflurane.

Preexisting Respiratory Dysfunction

Anesthesiologists frequently care for patients with acute chest injuries and disease (e.g., pulmonary infection or atelectasis) or systemic diseases (e.g., sepsis, cardiac failure, or renal failure) who require emergency operations. In addition, many patients are heavy smokers

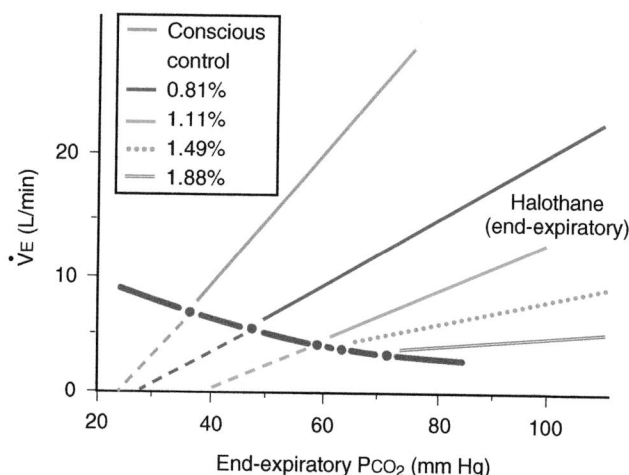

• **Fig. 5.31** In conscious controls, increasing end-expiratory concentration of carbon dioxide (PCO_2, horizontal axis) increases pulmonary minute volume ($\dot{V}_E$, vertical axis). The *dashed line* is an extrapolation of the CO_2 response curve to zero ventilation and represents the apneic threshold. Increases in end-expiratory anesthetic (halothane) concentration progressively diminish the slope of the CO_2 response curve and shift the apneic threshold to a higher PCO_2. The heavy line interrupted by dots shows the decrease in minute ventilation and the increase in PCO_2 that occur with increasing depth of anesthesia. (Modified from Munson ES, Larson CP Jr, Babad AA, et al. The effects of halothane, fluroxene and cyclopropane on ventilation: A comparative study in man. *Anesthesiology.* 1966;27:716.)

or have hyperreactive airways, whereas others have emphysematous and bronchitic problems or obesity with susceptibility to decreases in FRC during anesthesia.[126]

The nature and magnitude of these preexisting respiratory conditions determine, in part, the effect of a given standard anesthetic on respiratory function. For example, in Fig. 5.32, the FRC-CC relationship is depicted for normal, obese, bronchitic, and emphysematous patients. In a healthy patient, FRC exceeds CC by approximately 1 L. In the latter three respiratory conditions, CC is 0.5 to 1 L less than FRC. If anesthesia causes a 1-L decrease in FRC in a healthy patient, there is no change in the qualitative relationship between FRC and CC. In patients with special respiratory conditions, however, a 1-L decrease in FRC causes CC to exceed FRC and changes the previous marginally normal FRC-CC relationship to either a grossly low $\dot{V}A/\dot{Q}$ or an atelectatic FRC-CC relationship. Similarly, patients with chronic bronchitis, who have copious airway secretions, may suffer more than other patients from an anesthetic-induced decrease in mucus

flow velocity. Finally, if an anesthetic inhibits HPV, shunting can increase more in patients with preexisting HPV than in those without preexisting HPV. Thus, the effect of a standard anesthetic can be expected to produce varying degrees of respiratory change in patients who have different degrees of preexisting pulmonary dysfunction.

Special Intraoperative Conditions

Some special intraoperative conditions (e.g., surgical position, massive blood loss, surgical retraction on the lung) can cause impaired gas exchange. For example, some surgical positions (e.g., lithotomy, jackknife, or kidney rest positions) and surgical exposure requirements may decrease $\dot{Q}T$, cause hypoventilation in a spontaneously breathing patient, and/or reduce FRC. The type and severity of preexisting respiratory dysfunction, as well as the number and severity of special intraoperative conditions that can embarrass respiratory function, magnify the respiratory depressant effects of any anesthetic.

Mechanisms of Hypoxemia During Anesthesia

Equipment Malfunction

Mechanical Failure of Anesthesia Apparatus to Deliver Oxygen to the Patient

Hypoxemia resulting from mechanical failure of the oxygen supply system or the anesthesia machine is a recognized hazard of anesthesia. Disconnection of the patient from the oxygen supply system (usually at the juncture of the ETT and the elbow connector) is by far the most common cause of mechanical failure to deliver oxygen to the patient. Other reported causes of failure of the oxygen supply during anesthesia include the following: an empty or depleted oxygen cylinder, substitution of a nonoxygen cylinder at the oxygen yoke because of absence or failure of the pin index, an erroneously filled oxygen cylinder, insufficient opening of the oxygen cylinder (which hinders free flow of gas as pressure decreases), failure of gas pressure in a piped oxygen system, faulty locking of the piped oxygen system to the anesthesia machine, inadvertent switching of the Schrader adapters on piped lines, crossing of piped lines during construction, failure of a reducing valve or gas manifold, inadvertent disturbance of the setting of the oxygen flowmeter, use of the fine oxygen flowmeter instead of the coarse flowmeter, fractured or sticking flowmeters, transposition of rotameter tubes, erroneous filling of a liquid oxygen reservoir with nitrogen, and disconnection of the fresh gas line from machine to in-line hosing.[127–131] Monitoring of the inspired oxygen concentration with an in-line F_{IO_2} analyzer and monitoring of airway pressure should detect most of these causes of failure to deliver oxygen to the patient.[127–131]

Improper Endotracheal Tube Position

Esophageal intubation results in almost no ventilation. Aside from disconnection, almost all other mechanical problems with ETTs (e.g., kinking, blockage of secretions, herniated or ruptured cuffs) cause an increase in airway resistance that may result in hypoventilation. Intubation of a mainstem bronchus results in absence of ventilation of the contralateral lung; although potentially minimized by HPV, some perfusion to the contralateral lung always remains, causing an increase in shunting and a decrease in Pa_{O_2}. An ETT previously well positioned in the trachea may enter a bronchus after the patient or the patient's head is turned or moved into a new position.[132] Flexion of the head causes the tube to

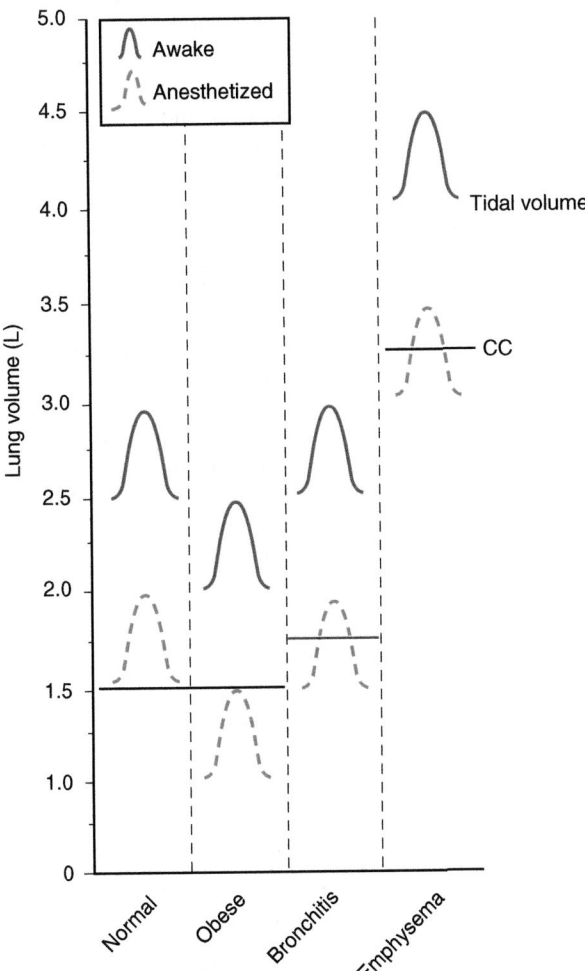

• **Fig. 5.32** The lung volume (vertical axis) at which a tidal volume is breathed decreases by 1 L from the awake state to the anesthetized state. Functional residual capacity (FRC), which is the volume of gas existing in the lung at the end of a tidal breath, therefore also decreases (by 1 L) from the awake to the anesthetized state. In healthy, obese, bronchitic, and emphysematous patients, the awake FRC considerably exceeds the closing capacity (CC, horizontal lines), but the anesthetized state causes FRC to be less than CC. In healthy patients, anesthesia causes FRC to equal CC.

migrate deeper (caudad) into the trachea, whereas extension of the head causes cephalad (outward) migration of the ETT.[132] A high incidence of mainstem bronchial intubation after the institution of a 30-degree Trendelenburg position has been reported.[133] Cephalad shift of the carina and mediastinum during the Trendelenburg position can cause a previously "fixed" ETT to migrate into a mainstem bronchus. Mainstem bronchial intubation can obstruct the ipsilateral upper lobe in addition to the contralateral lung.[134,135] Rarely, the right upper bronchus or one of its segmental bronchi branches from the lateral wall of the trachea (above the carina) and may be occluded by a properly positioned ETT.

Hypoventilation

Patients under general anesthesia may have a reduced spontaneous V_T for two reasons. First, increased WOB can occur during general anesthesia as a result of increased airway resistance and decreased C_L. Airway resistance can be increased because of reduced FRC, tracheal intubation, the presence of the external breathing apparatus and circuitry, and possible airway obstruction in patients whose tracheas are not intubated.[136–138] C_L is reduced as a result of some (or all) of the factors that can decrease FRC.[89] Second, patients may have a decreased drive to breathe spontaneously during general anesthesia (i.e., decreased chemical regulation of breathing) (see Fig. 5.31).

Decreased V_T may cause hypoxemia in two ways.[117] First, shallow breathing can promote atelectasis and cause a decrease in FRC (see section "Ventilation Pattern [Rapid Shallow Breathing]").[40,139] Second, decreased $\dot{V}_E$ decreases the overall $\dot{V}_A/\dot{Q}$ ratio of the lung, which decreases Pa_{O_2} (see Figs. 5.23 and 5.24).[117] This is likely to occur with spontaneous ventilation during moderate to deep levels of anesthesia, in which the chemical regulation of breathing is significantly altered.

Hyperventilation

Hypocapnic alkalosis (hyperventilation) can occasionally be associated with a decreased Pa_{O_2} due to several indirect mechanisms: decreased $\dot{Q}_T$ and increased $\dot{V}_{O_2}$[140,141] (see "Decreased Cardiac Output and Increased Oxygen Consumption"),[99,101,140,141] a left-shifted oxy-Hb curve (see "Oxygen-Hemoglobin Dissociation Curve"), decreased HPV (see "Inhibition of Hypoxic Pulmonary Vasoconstriction"),[142] and increased airway resistance and decreased compliance (see "Increased Airway Resistance").[143] Although these theoretical causes of hypoxemia exist, they are seldom a major factor in the clinical realm.

Decrease in Functional Residual Capacity

The effect of decreased FRC on hypoxemia is very significant clinically. Induction of general anesthesia is consistently accompanied by a pronounced 15% to 20% decrease in FRC,[32,83,144] which usually causes a decrease in C_L.[89] The maximum decrease in FRC appears to occur within the first few minutes of anesthesia,[32,145] and in the absence of any other complicating factor, FRC does not seem to decrease progressively during anesthesia. During anesthesia, the reduction in FRC is of the same order of magnitude whether ventilation is spontaneous or controlled. Conversely, in awake patients, FRC is only slightly reduced during controlled ventilation.[146] In obese patients, the reduction in FRC is far more pronounced than in normal patients, and the FRC decreases exponentially as the body mass index (BMI) increases.[147] The reduction in FRC continues into the postoperative period.[148] For individual patients, the reduction in FRC correlates well with the increase in the alveolar-arterial P_{O_2} gradient during anesthesia

with spontaneous breathing,[149] during anesthesia with artificial ventilation,[146] and in the postoperative period.[148] The reduced FRC can be restored to normal or above normal by the application of PEEP.[82,150] The following discussion considers the most common causes of reduced FRC.

Supine Position

Anesthesia and surgery are usually performed with the patient in the supine position. With a change from the upright to the supine position, FRC decreases by 0.5 to 1.0 L because of a 4-cm cephalad displacement of the diaphragm by the abdominal viscera (Fig. 5.33).[32,83,144] Pulmonary vascular congestion can also contribute to the decrease in FRC in the supine position, particularly in patients with symptoms of orthopnea preoperatively.

Induction of General Anesthesia: Change in Thoracic Cage Muscle Tone

At the end of a normal (awake) expiration, there is slight tension in the inspiratory muscles and no tension in the expiratory muscles. Therefore, at the end of a normal expiration, there is a force tending to maintain lung volume and no force decreasing lung volume. After induction of general anesthesia, there is a loss of inspiratory tone and an appearance of end-expiratory tone in the abdominal expiratory muscles at the end of expiration. The end-expiratory tone in the abdominal expiratory muscles increases intraabdominal pressure, forces the diaphragm cephalad, and decreases FRC (see Fig. 5.33).[145,151] Thus after the induction of general anesthesia, there is loss of the force tending to maintain lung volume and gain of the force tending to decrease lung volume. Indeed, neuroleptanesthesia with droperidol and fentanyl may increase tone in expiratory muscles to such an extent that the reduction in FRC with neuroleptanesthesia without neuromuscular blockade is greater than when combined with neuromuscular blockade induced by succinylcholine.[151,152]

In emphysema, expiration can be accompanied by pursing of the lips or grunting (i.e., with a partially closed larynx). An emphysematous patient exhales in either of these ways because both these maneuvers cause an expiratory retardation that produces PEEP in the intrathoracic air passage and decreases the possibility of airway closure and a decrease in FRC (see Fig. 5.17F).

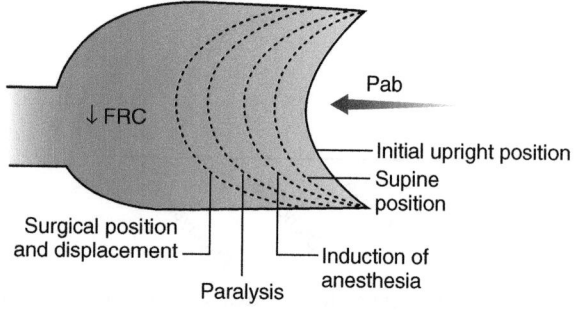

Progressive Cephalad Displacement of the Diaphragm

↓FRC

Pab

Initial upright position
Supine position
Surgical position and displacement
Induction of anesthesia
Paralysis

• **Fig. 5.33** Anesthesia and surgery may cause a progressive cephalad displacement of the diaphragm. The sequence of events involves assumption of the supine position, induction of anesthesia, establishment of paralysis, assumption of several surgical positions, and displacement by retractors and packs. Cephalad displacement of the diaphragm results in decreased functional residual capacity (↓ FRC). *Pab,* Pressure of abdominal contents. (Modified from Benumof JL. *Anesthesia for Thoracic Surgery.* 2nd ed. Saunders; 1995:Chapter 8.)

Tracheal intubation bypasses the lips and glottis and can abolish the normally present pursed-lip or grunting expiration in a patient with COPD and, in that way, contributes to airway closure and loss of FRC in some spontaneously breathing patients.

Neuromuscular Blockade

In an upright subject, FRC and the position of the diaphragm are determined by the balance between lung elastic recoil pulling the diaphragm cephalad and the weight of the abdominal contents pulling it caudad.[153] There is no transdiaphragmatic pressure gradient.

The situation is more complex in the supine position. The diaphragm separates two compartments of markedly different hydrostatic gradients. On the thoracic side, pressure increases by approximately 0.25 cm H_2O/cm of lung height,[38,154] and on the abdominal side, it increases by 1.0 cm H_2O/cm of abdominal height.[153] Therefore, in horizontal postures, progressively higher transdiaphragmatic pressure must be generated toward dependent parts of the diaphragm to keep the abdominal contents out of the thorax. In an unparalyzed patient, this tension is developed either by passive stretch and changes in shape of the diaphragm (causing an increased contractile force) or by neurally mediated active tension. With neuromuscular blockade, neither of these two mechanisms can operate, and a shift of the diaphragm to a more cephalad position occurs (see Fig. 5.33).[155] The latter position expresses the true balance of forces on the diaphragm, unmodified by any passive or active muscle activity.

During general anesthesia, the cephalad shift in the FRC position of the diaphragm because of expiratory muscle tone is equal to the shift observed during neuromuscular blockade (awake or anesthetized patients).[145,156] The equal shift suggests that the pressure on the diaphragm caused by an increase in expiratory muscle tone during general anesthesia is equal to the pressure on the diaphragm caused by the weight of the abdominal contents during neuromuscular blockade. The magnitude of these changes in FRC related to neuromuscular blockade also depends on body habitus.

Light or Inadequate Anesthesia and Active Expiration

Induction of general anesthesia can result in increased expiratory muscle tone,[151] but the increased expiratory muscle tone is not coordinated and does not contribute to the expired volume of gas. In contrast, spontaneous ventilation during light general anesthesia usually results in a coordinated and moderately forceful active expiration and larger expired volumes. Excessively inadequate anesthesia (relative to a given stimulus) results in very forceful active expiration, which can produce expired volumes of gas equal to an awake expiratory vital capacity.

As during an awake expiratory vital capacity maneuver, forced expiration during anesthesia raises intrathoracic and alveolar pressure considerably above atmospheric pressure (see Fig. 5.17). This increase in pressure results in rapid outflow of gas, and because part of the expiratory resistance lies in the smaller air passages, a drop in pressure occurs between the alveoli and the main bronchi. Under these circumstances, intrathoracic pressure rises considerably above the pressure within the main bronchi. Collapse occurs if this reversed pressure gradient is sufficiently high to overcome the tethering effect of the surrounding parenchyma on the small intrathoracic bronchioles or the structural rigidity of cartilage in the large extrathoracic bronchi. Such collapse occurs in a normal subject during a maximal forced expiration and is responsible for the associated wheeze in both awake and anesthetized patients.[157]

In an anesthetized patient with neuromuscular blockade, the use of a subatmospheric expiratory pressure phase is analogous to a forced expiration in a conscious subject; the negative phase may set up the same adverse ΔP, which can cause airway closure, gas trapping, and a decrease in FRC. An excessively rapidly descending bellows of a ventilator during expiration has caused subatmospheric expiratory pressure and resulted in wheezing.[158]

Increased Airway Resistance

The overall reduction in all components of lung volume during anesthesia results in reduced airway caliber, which increases airway resistance and any tendency toward airway collapse (Fig. 5.34). The relationship between airway resistance and lung volume is well established (Fig. 5.35). The decreases in FRC caused by the supine position (≈ 0.8 L) and induction of anesthesia (≈ 0.4 L) are

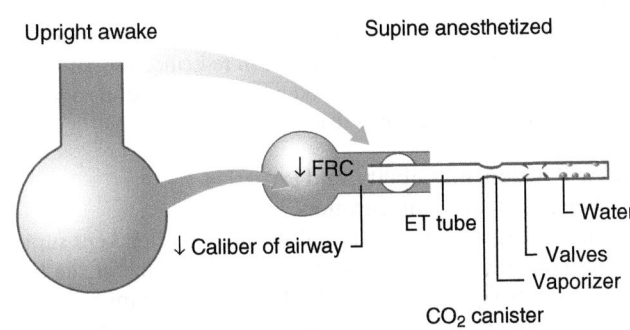

• **Fig. 5.34** An anesthetized patient in the supine position has increased airway resistance as a result of decreased functional residual capacity (FRC), decreased caliber of the airways, tracheal intubation, and connection of the endotracheal tube (ET tube) to the external breathing apparatus and circuitry. ↓, decreased. (Modified from Benumof JL. *Anesthesia for Thoracic Surgery*. 2nd ed. Saunders; 1995:Chapter 8.)

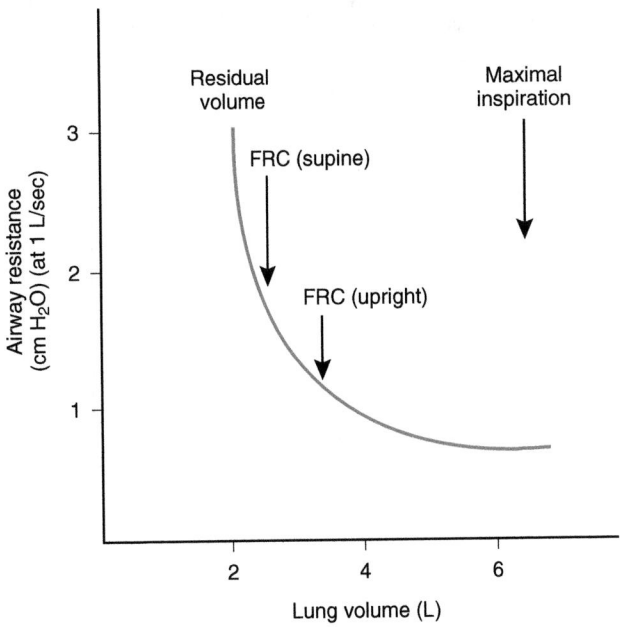

• **Fig. 5.35** Airway resistance is an increasing hyperbolic function of decreasing lung volume. Functional residual capacity (FRC) decreases with a change from the upright to the supine position. (Modified from Lumb AB. Respiratory system resistance. In: Lumb AB, ed. *Nunn's Applied Respiratory Physiology*. 5th ed. Butterworths; 2000:67.)

often sufficient to explain the increased resistance seen in a healthy anesthetized patient.[137]

In addition to this expected overall increase in airway resistance in anesthetized patients, there are several potential sites of focally increased airway resistance, including the ETT (if present), the upper and lower airway passages, and the external anesthesia apparatus. Tracheal intubation reduces the size of the airway at the level of the trachea, usually by 30% to 50% (see Fig. 5.34). Pharyngeal obstruction, a normal feature of unconsciousness, is common; a minor degree of this type of obstruction occurs in snoring. Laryngospasm and obstructed ETTs (e.g., secretions, kinking) are not uncommon and can be life-threatening.

The respiratory apparatus often causes resistance that is considerably higher than the resistance in the normal human respiratory tract (see Fig. 5.34).[89] When certain resistors, such as those shown in Fig. 5.34, are joined in a series to form an anesthetic gas circuit, their effects are generally additive and produce larger resistance (as with resistance in a series in an electrical circuit). The increase in resistance associated with commonly used breathing circuits and ETTs can impose an additional WOB that is two to three times that of normal.[136]

Supine Position, Immobility, and Excessive Intravenous Fluid Administration

Patients undergoing anesthesia and surgery are often kept supine and immobile for long periods. In these cases, some of the lung can be continually dependent and below the left atrium and therefore in a zone 3 or 4 condition. Being in a dependent position, the lung is predisposed to both atelectasis and fluid accumulation. Coupled with excessive fluid administration, conditions sufficient to promote transudation of fluid into the lung are present and result in pulmonary edema and decreased FRC.

When dogs were placed in a lateral decubitus position and anesthetized for several hours (Fig. 5.36), expansion of the extracellular space with fluid caused the P_{O_2} of blood draining the dependent lung to decrease precipitously to mixed venous levels (no oxygen uptake).[159] Blood draining the nondependent lung maintained its P_{O_2} for a period but declined after 5 hours in the presence of

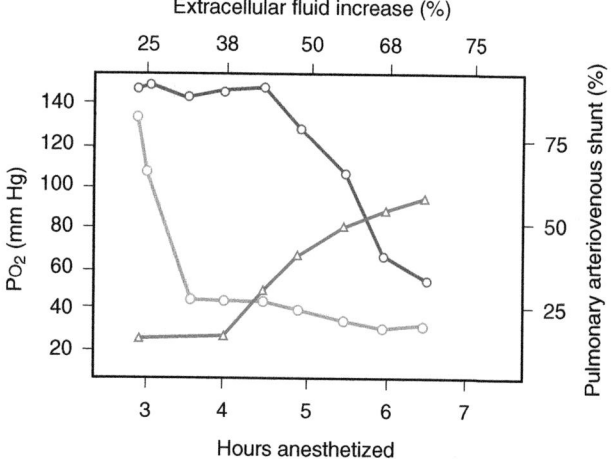

• **Fig. 5.36** Dogs anesthetized with pentobarbital were placed in a lateral decubitus position and subjected to progressive extracellular fluid expansion. They had a marked decrease in the partial pressure of oxygen *(Po₂)* of blood draining the dependent lung *(yellow line)* and a smaller, much slower decrease in the Po₂ of blood draining the nondependent lung *(purple line)*. The pulmonary arteriovenous shunt rose progressively *(blue line)*. (From Ray JF, Yost L, Moallem S, et al. Immobility, hypoxemia, and pulmonary arteriovenous shunting. *Arch Surg.* 1974;109:537.)

the extracellular fluid expansion. Transpulmonary shunting progressively increased. If the animals were turned every hour (and received the same fluid challenge), only the dependent lung, at the end of each hour period, suffered a decrease in oxygenation. If the animals were turned every half-hour and received the same fluid challenge, neither lung suffered a decrease in oxygenation.

In patients who undergo surgery in the lateral decubitus position (e.g., pulmonary resection), in which they have or will have a restricted pulmonary vascular bed and receive excessive intravenous fluids, the risk of the dependent lung's becoming edematous is increased. These considerations also explain, in part, the beneficial effect of a continuously rotating (side-to-side) bed on the incidence of pulmonary complications in critically ill patients.[160]

High Inspired Oxygen Concentration and Absorption Atelectasis

General anesthesia is usually administered with an increased F_{IO_2}. In patients who have areas of moderately low $\dot{V}_A/\dot{Q}$ ratios (0.1 to 0.01), administration of F_{IO_2} greater than 0.3 adds enough oxygen into the alveolar space in these areas to eliminate the shuntlike effect that they create, and total measured right-to-left shunting decreases. However, when patients with a significant amount of blood flow perfusing lung units with very low $\dot{V}_A/\dot{Q}$ ratios (0.01 to 0.0001) have a change in F_{IO_2} from room air to 1.0, the very low $\dot{V}_A/\dot{Q}$ units virtually disappear, and a moderately large right-to-left shunt appears.[16,17,161] In these studies, the increase in shunting was equal to the amount of blood flow previously perfusing the areas with low $\dot{V}_A/\dot{Q}$ ratios during the breathing of air. Thus, the effect of breathing oxygen was to convert units that had low $\dot{V}_A/\dot{Q}$ ratios into shunt units. The pathologic basis for these data is the conversion of low $\dot{V}_A/\dot{Q}$ units into atelectatic units. The cause of the atelectatic shunting during oxygen breathing is presumably a large increase in oxygen uptake by lung units with low $\dot{V}_A/\dot{Q}$ ratios.[161,162] A unit that has a low $\dot{V}_A/\dot{Q}$ ratio during breathing of air will have a low P_{AO_2}. When an enriched oxygen mixture is inspired, P_{AO_2} rises, and the rate at which oxygen moves from alveolar gas to capillary blood increases greatly. The oxygen flux can increase so much that the net flow of gas into blood exceeds the inspired flow of gas, and the lung unit becomes progressively smaller. Collapse is most likely to occur if F_{IO_2} is high, the $\dot{V}_A/\dot{Q}$ ratio is low, the time of exposure of the unit with low $\dot{V}_A/\dot{Q}$ to high F_{IO_2} is long, and $C\bar{v}_{O_2}$ is low. Given the right $\dot{V}_A/\dot{Q}$ ratio and time of administration, an F_{IO_2} as low as 50% can produce absorption atelectasis.[161,162] This phenomenon is of considerable significance in the clinical situation for two reasons. First, enriched oxygen mixtures are often used therapeutically, and it is important to know whether this therapy is causing atelectasis. Second, the amount of shunt is often estimated during breathing of 100% oxygen, and if this maneuver results in additional shunt, the measurement is hard to interpret.

Surgical Position

In the supine position, the abdominal contents force the diaphragm cephalad and reduce FRC.[83,145,151,156] The Trendelenburg position allows the abdominal contents to push the diaphragm further cephalad so that the diaphragm must not only ventilate the lungs but also lift the abdominal contents out of the thorax. The result is a predisposition to decreased FRC and atelectasis.[163] The decrease in FRC related to Trendelenburg position is exacerbated in obese patients.[147] Increased pulmonary blood volume and gravitational force on the mediastinal structures are additional factors that may decrease pulmonary compliance and

FRC. In the steep Trendelenburg position, most of the lung can be below the left atrium and therefore in a zone 3 or 4 condition. In this condition, the lung may be susceptible to the development of pulmonary interstitial edema. Thus, patients with elevated Ppa, such as those with mitral stenosis, do not tolerate the Trendelenburg position well.[164]

In the lateral decubitus position, the dependent lung experiences a moderate decrease in FRC and is predisposed to atelectasis, whereas the nondependent lung may have increased FRC. The overall result is usually a slight to moderate increase in total-lung FRC.[165] The kidney and lithotomy positions also cause small decreases in FRC above that caused by the supine position. The prone position may increase FRC moderately.[165]

Ventilation Pattern (Rapid Shallow Breathing)

Rapid shallow breathing is often a feature of deep levels of general anesthesia. Monotonous shallow breathing can cause a decrease in FRC, promote atelectasis, and decrease compliance.[40,139,166] These changes with rapid shallow breathing are probably due to progressive increases in surface tension.[166] Initially, these changes can cause hypoxemia with normocapnia and may be prevented or reversed by periodic large mechanical inspirations, recruitment breaths, PEEP, or a combination of these techniques.[166–168]

Decreased Removal of Secretions (Decreased Mucociliary Flow)

Tracheobronchial mucous glands and goblet cells produce mucus, which is swept by cilia up to the larynx, where it is swallowed or expectorated. This process clears inhaled organisms and particles from the lungs. The secreted mucus consists of a surface gel layer lying on top of a more liquid sol layer in which the cilia beat. The tips of the cilia propel the gel layer toward the larynx (upward) during the forward stroke. As the mucus streams upward and the total cross-sectional area of the airways diminishes, absorption takes place from the sol layer to maintain a constant depth of 5 μm.[169]

Poor systemic hydration and low inspired humidity reduce mucociliary flow by increasing the viscosity of secretions and slowing the ciliary beat.[170–172] Mucociliary flow varies directly with body or mucosal temperature (low inspired temperature) over a range of 32°C to 42°C.[173,174] High F_{IO_2} decreases mucociliary flow.[175] Inflation of an ETT cuff suppresses tracheal mucus velocity,[176] an effect that occurs within 1 hour, and apparently it does not matter whether a low- or high-compliance cuff is used. Passage of an uncuffed tube through the vocal cords and keeping it in situ for several hours does not affect tracheal mucus velocity.[176]

The mechanism for suppression of mucociliary clearance by the ETT cuff is speculative. In the report of Sackner and colleagues,[176] mucus velocity was decreased in the distal portion of the trachea, but the cuff was inflated in the proximal portion. Therefore, the phenomenon cannot be attributed solely to damming of mucus at the cuff site. One possibility is that the ETT cuff causes a critical increase in the thickness of the layer of mucus proceeding distally from the cuff. Another possibility is that mechanical distention of the trachea by the ETT cuff initiates a neurogenic reflex arc that alters mucous secretions or the frequency of ciliary beating.

Other investigators showed that when all the foregoing factors were controlled, halothane reversibly and progressively decreased but did not stop mucus flow over an inspired concentration of 1 to 3 MAC.[177] The halothane-induced depression of mucociliary clearance was probably due to depression of the ciliary beat, an effect that caused slow clearance of mucus from the distal and peripheral airways. In support of this hypothesis is the finding that cilia are morphologically similar throughout the animal kingdom. Inhaled anesthetics in clinical doses, including halothane, have been found to cause reversible depression of the ciliary beat of protozoa.[115]

Decreased Cardiac Output and Increased Oxygen Consumption

Decreased $\dot{Q}_T$ in the presence of constant oxygen consumption ($\dot{V}_{O_2}$), increased $\dot{V}_{O_2}$ in the presence of a constant $\dot{Q}_T$, and decreased $\dot{Q}_T$ concomitant with increased $\dot{V}_{O_2}$ must all result in lower $C\bar{v}_{O_2}$. Venous blood with lowered $C\bar{v}_{O_2}$ then flows through whichever shunt pathways exist, mixes with the oxygenated end-pulmonary capillary blood, and lowers Ca_{O_2} (see Figs. 5.27 and 5.28). Fig. 5.37 shows these relationships quantitatively for several different transpulmonary shunts.[100,101] The larger the transpulmonary shunt, the greater the decrease in Ca_{O_2}, because more venous blood with lower $C\bar{v}_{O_2}$ can admix with end-pulmonary capillary blood. Decreased $\dot{Q}_T$ may occur with myocardial failure and hypovolemia; the specific causes of these two conditions are beyond the scope of this chapter. Increased $\dot{V}_{O_2}$ may occur with excessive stimulation of the sympathetic nervous system, hyperthermia, or shivering and can further contribute to impaired oxygenation of arterial blood.[178]

Inhibition of Hypoxic Pulmonary Vasoconstriction

Decreased regional Pa_{O_2} causes regional pulmonary vasoconstriction, which diverts blood flow away from hypoxic regions of the lung to better-ventilated, normoxic regions. The diversion of blood flow minimizes venous admixture from the underventilated or nonventilated lung regions. Inhibition of regional HPV could impair arterial oxygenation by permitting increased venous admixture from hypoxic or atelectatic areas of the lung (see Fig. 5.9).

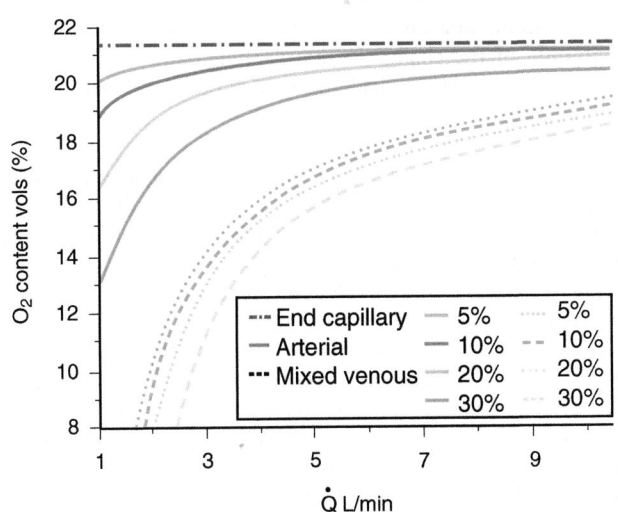

• **Fig. 5.37** Effects of changes in cardiac output $(\dot{Q})$ on the oxygen content of end-pulmonary capillary, arterial (*solid lines*), and mixed venous (*dashed lines*) blood for various transpulmonary right-to-left shunts. The magnitudes of the shunts are indicated by the percentages; the oxygen content of end-capillary blood is unaffected by the degree of shunting. Note that a given decrease in $\dot{Q}$ results in a greater decrease in the arterial content of oxygen with larger shunts. (From Kelman GF, Nunn JF, Prys-Roberts C, et al. The influence of the cardiac output on arterial oxygenation: a theoretical study. *Br J Anaesth*. 1967;39:450.)

Because the pulmonary circulation is poorly endowed with smooth muscle, any condition that increases the pressure against which the vessels must constrict (i.e., Ppa) decreases HPV. Numerous clinical conditions can increase Ppa and therefore decrease HPV. Mitral stenosis,[179] volume overload,[179] low (but greater than room air) FIO_2 in nondiseased lung,[74] a progressive increase in the amount of diseased lung,[74] thromboembolism,[74] hypothermia,[180] and vasoactive drugs can all increase Ppa.[64] Direct vasodilating drugs (e.g., isoproterenol, nitroglycerin, or nitroprusside),[64,59] inhaled anesthetics,[65] and hypocapnia can directly decrease HPV.[64,142] Selective application of PEEP to only the nondiseased lung can selectively increase PVR in the nondiseased lung and may divert blood flow back into the diseased lung.[181]

Neuromuscular Blockade

In the supine position, the weight of the abdominal contents pressing against the diaphragm is greatest in the dependent or posterior part of the diaphragm and least in the nondependent or anterior part of the diaphragm. In an awake patient breathing spontaneously, active tension in the diaphragm can overcome the weight of the abdominal contents, and the diaphragm moves least in the anterior portion and most in the posterior portion (because the posterior of the diaphragm is stretched higher into the chest, it has the smallest radius of curvature and therefore contracts most effectively). This circumstance is beneficial because the greatest amount of ventilation occurs in areas with the most perfusion (posteriorly or dependently), and the least amount occurs in areas with the least perfusion (anteriorly or nondependently). During neuromuscular blockade and positive-pressure ventilation, the passive diaphragm is displaced by the positive pressure preferentially in the anterior, nondependent portion (where there is the least resistance to diaphragmatic movement) and is displaced minimally in the posterior, dependent portion (where there is the most resistance to diaphragmatic movement). This circumstance is detrimental to gas exchange because the greatest amount of ventilation now occurs in areas with the least perfusion, and the least amount occurs in areas with the most perfusion.[156] However, the magnitude of the change in the diaphragmatic motion pattern with neuromuscular blockade varies with body position.[156,182]

Right-to-Left Interatrial Shunting

Acute arterial hypoxemia from a transient right-to-left shunt through a PFO has been described, particularly during emergence from anesthesia.[70] However, unless a real-time technique of imaging the cardiac chambers is used (e.g., transesophageal echocardiography with color flow Doppler imaging),[71] it is difficult to document an acute and transient right-to-left intracardiac shunt as a cause of arterial hypoxemia. Nonetheless, right-to-left shunting through a PFO has been described in virtually every conceivable clinical situation that afterloads the right side of the heart and increases right atrial pressure. When right-to-left shunting through a PFO occurs because of transiently increased PAH, administration of inhaled NO can decrease PVR and functionally close the PFO.[183]

Involvement of Mechanisms of Hypoxemia in Specific Diseases

In any given pulmonary disease, many of the previously listed mechanisms of hypoxemia can be involved.[117] Pulmonary embolism with air, fat, or thrombi (Fig. 5.38) and the evolution of ARDS (Fig. 5.39) are used to illustrate this point. A significant pulmonary embolus can cause severe increases in Ppa, and these

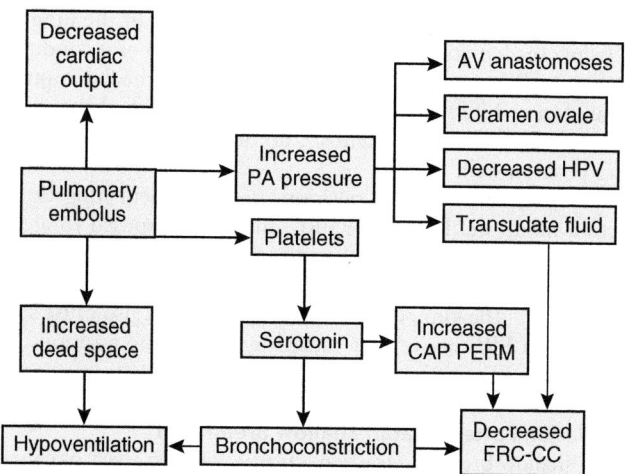

• **Fig. 5.38** Mechanisms of hypoxemia during pulmonary embolism. See the text for an explanation of the pathophysiologic flow diagram. *AV,* Arteriovenous; *CAP PERM,* Capillary permeability; *CC,* closing capacity; *FRC,* functional residual capacity; *HPV,* hypoxic pulmonary vasoconstriction; *PA,* pulmonary artery. (Modified from Benumof JL. *Anesthesia for Thoracic Surgery.* 2nd ed. Saunders; 1995:Chapter 8.)

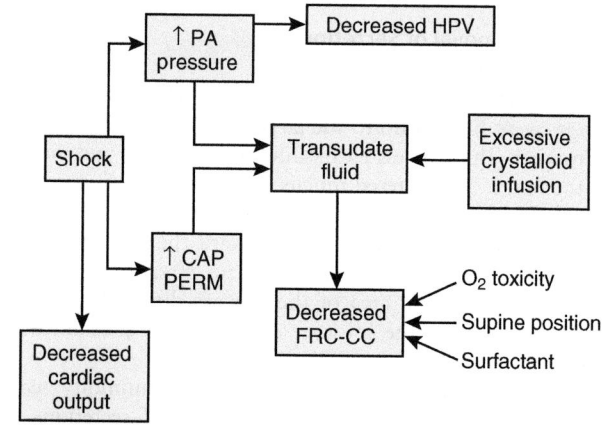

• **Fig. 5.39** Mechanisms of hypoxemia during adult respiratory distress syndrome. See the text for an explanation of the pathophysiologic flow diagram. *CAP PERM,* Capillary permeability; *CC,* closing capacity; *FRC,* functional residual capacity; *HPV,* hypoxic pulmonary vasoconstriction; *PA,* pulmonary artery. (Modified from Benumof JL. *Anesthesia for Thoracic Surgery.* 2nd ed. Saunders; 1995:Chapter 8.)

increases can result in right-to-left shunting through opened arteriovenous anastomoses and the foramen ovale (patent in 20% of patients), pulmonary edema in nonembolized regions of the lung, and inhibition of HPV. The embolus can also cause hypoventilation through increased dead space ventilation. If the embolus contains platelets, serotonin can be released, and such release can cause hypoventilation and pulmonary edema from bronchoconstriction and increased pulmonary capillary permeability, respectively. Finally, the pulmonary embolus can increase PVR (by platelet-induced serotonin release,[4] among other mechanisms) and decrease cardiac output.

After major hypotension, shock, sepsis, aspiration, massive transfusion, or other conditions, noncardiogenic pulmonary edema can occur, leading to acute respiratory failure or ARDS.[184] The syndrome can evolve during and after anesthesia and has the hallmark characteristics of decreased FRC and compliance and hypoxemia. After shock or trauma, plasma levels of serotonin, histamine, kinins, cytokines, lysozymes, reactive oxygen species, fibrin degradation products, products of complement metabolism, and fatty acids all increase. Increased levels of activated complement and cytokines stimulate neutrophils into chemotaxis in patients with inflammatory pathologies, such as trauma or pancreatitis; activated neutrophils can damage endothelial cells. These factors, along with pulmonary contusion (if it occurs during trauma), can individually or collectively increase pulmonary capillary permeability. Afterward, acidosis, increased circulating catecholamines and sympathetic nervous system activity, leukotriene and prostaglandin release, microembolism (with serotonin release), and alveolar hypoxia can occur and may individually or collectively (particularly after resuscitation) cause a moderate increase in Ppa. After shock, the normal compensatory response to hypovolemia is movement of a protein-free fluid from the interstitial space into the vascular space to restore vascular volume. Dilution of vascular proteins by protein-free interstitial fluid can cause decreased capillary colloid oncotic pressure. Increased pulmonary capillary permeability and Ppa along with decreased capillary colloid oncotic pressure results in fluid transudation and pulmonary edema. In addition, decreased $\dot{Q}_T$, inhibition of HPV, immobility, the supine position, excessive fluid administration, lung injury from high tidal volumes and peak pulmonary pressures, and an excessively high F_{IO_2} can all contribute to the development of ARDS.

Mechanisms of Hypercapnia and Hypocapnia During Anesthesia

Hypoventilation, increased dead space ventilation, increased CO_2 production, and an exhausted or malfunctioning CO_2 absorber can all cause hypercapnia (Fig. 5.40).

Hypoventilation

Patients spontaneously hypoventilate during anesthesia because it is more difficult to breathe (abnormal surgical position, increased airway resistance, decreased compliance) and because they are less willing to breathe (decreased respiratory drive due to anesthetics). Hypoventilation results in hypercapnia (see Figs. 5.22 and 5.23).

Increased Dead Space Ventilation

A decrease in Ppa, as during deliberate hypotension,[185] can cause an increase in zone 1 and alveolar dead space ventilation. An increase in airway pressure (as with PEEP) can also cause an increase in zone 1 and alveolar dead space ventilation. Pulmonary embolism, thrombosis, and vascular obliteration (e.g., kinking, clamping, or blocking of the pulmonary artery during surgery) can increase the amount of lung that is ventilated but unperfused. Vascular obliteration can also increase dead space ventilation; this occurs naturally with age (V_D/V_T % = 33 + age/3). Rapid, short inspirations can be distributed preferentially to noncompliant (short time constant for inflation) and badly perfused alveoli, whereas slow inspiration allows time for distribution to more compliant (long time constant for inflation) and better perfused alveoli. Thus rapid, short inspirations may have a dead space ventilation effect.

The anesthesia apparatus increases total dead space ratio (V_D/V_T) for two reasons. First, the apparatus simply increases the anatomic dead space. Inclusion of normal apparatus dead space increases the V_D/V_T ratio from 33% to about 46% in intubated patients and to about 64% in patients breathing through a mask.[186] Second, anesthesia circuits cause rebreathing of expired gases, which is equivalent to dead space ventilation. The rebreathing classification by Mapleson during spontaneous ventilation with

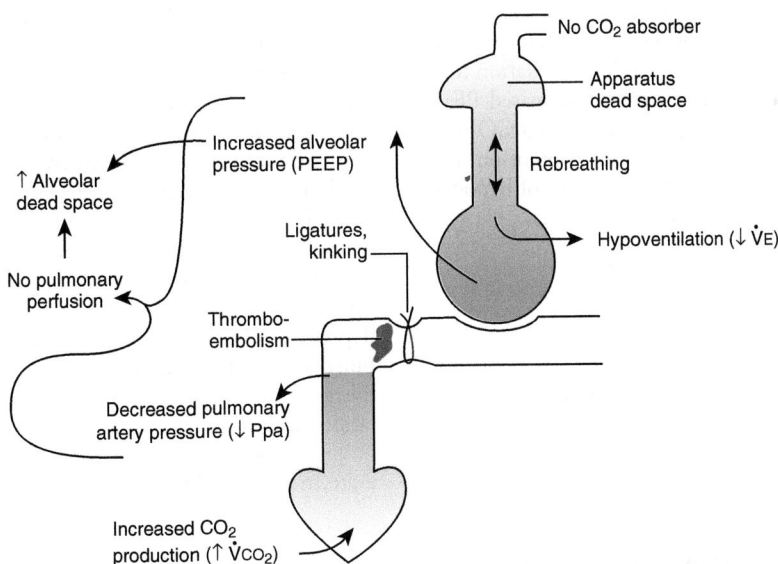

• **Fig. 5.40** Schematic diagram of the causes of hypercapnia during anesthesia. An increase in carbon dioxide (CO_2) production ($\dot{V}CO_2$) increases the arterial partial pressure of CO_2 ($PaCO_2$) with a constant minute ventilation ($\dot{V}E$). Several events can increase alveolar dead space: a decrease in pulmonary artery pressure (Ppa), the application of positive end-expiratory pressure ($PEEP$), thromboembolism, and mechanical interference with pulmonary arterial flow (ligatures and kinking of vessels). Most commonly in trauma, surgery, and critical care, hypovolemia due to hemorrhage or third spacing leads to increased alveolar dead space and consequently to increased $PaCO_2$. A decrease in $\dot{V}E$ causes an increase in $PaCO_2$ with a constant $\dot{V}CO_2$. It is possible for some anesthesia systems to cause rebreathing of CO_2. Finally, the anesthesia apparatus may increase the anatomic dead space, and depletion or malfunction of the CO_2 absorber in the presence of low fresh gas flow can increase $PaCO_2$. ↑, increase; ↓, decrease. (Modified from Benumof JL. *Anesthesia for Thoracic Surgery.* 2nd ed. Philadelphia: Saunders; 1995:Chapter 8.)

Mapleson circuits in order of increasing rebreathing is A (Magill), D, C, and B. The order of increasing rebreathing (decreasing clinical merit) during controlled ventilation is D, B, C, and A. There is no rebreathing in system E (Ayre T-piece) if the patient's respiratory diastole is long enough to permit washout with a given fresh gas flow (a common event) or if the fresh gas flow is greater than the peak inspiratory flow rate (an uncommon event).

The effects of an increase in dead space can usually be counteracted by a corresponding increase in the respiratory $\dot{V}E$. If, for example, the $\dot{V}E$ is 10 L/min and the V_D/V_T ratio is 30%, alveolar ventilation is 7 L/min. If a pulmonary embolism occurred and resulted in an increase in the V_D/V_T ratio to 50%, $\dot{V}E$ would need to be increased to 14 L/min to maintain an alveolar ventilation of 7 L/min (14 L/min × 0.5).

Increased Carbon Dioxide Production

All causes of increased oxygen consumption also increase CO_2 production; these causes include hyperthermia, shivering, catecholamine release (light anesthesia), hypertension, thyroid storm, and malignant hyperthermia. If $\dot{V}E$, total dead space, and $\dot{V}A/\dot{Q}$ relationships are constant, an increase in CO_2 production results in hypercapnia.

Malfunction or Exhaustion of a Carbon Dioxide Absorber

Many factors, such as patients' ventilatory responsiveness to CO_2 accumulation, fresh gas flow, circle system design, and CO_2 production, determine whether hypercapnia results from malfunction or depletion of a circle CO_2 absorber. However, high fresh gas flows (≥5 L/min) minimize the problem with almost all systems for almost all patients.

Hypocapnia

The mechanisms of hypocapnia are the reverse of those that produce hypercapnia. Thus, all other factors being equal, hyperventilation (spontaneous or controlled), decreased V_D ventilation (e.g., change from a mask airway to an ETT airway, decreased PEEP, increased Ppa, or decreased rebreathing), and decreased CO_2 production (e.g., hypothermia, deep anesthesia, or hypotension) lead to hypocapnia. By far the most common mechanism of hypocapnia is iatrogenic hyperventilation by mechanical means.

Physiologic Effects of Abnormalities in Respiratory Gases

Hypoxia

The end products of aerobic metabolism (oxidative phosphorylation) are CO_2 and water, both of which are easily diffusible and lost from the body. The essential feature of hypoxia is the cessation of oxidative phosphorylation when mitochondrial Po_2 falls below

a critical level. Anaerobic pathways, which produce energy (ATP) inefficiently, are then used. The main anaerobic metabolites are H^+ and lactate ions, which are not easily excreted. They accumulate in the circulation, where they can be quantified in terms of the base deficit and the lactate-pyruvate ratio.

Because the various organs have different blood flow and oxygen consumption rates, the manifestations and clinical diagnosis of hypoxia are usually related to symptoms arising from the most vulnerable organ. This organ is usually the brain in an awake patient and the heart in an anesthetized patient (see later discussion), but in special circumstances it may be the spinal cord (e.g., aortic surgery), kidney (e.g., acute tubular necrosis), liver (e.g., hepatitis), or limb (e.g., claudication, gangrene).

The cardiovascular response to hypoxemia is a product of both reflex (neural and humoral) and direct effects (Table 5.5).[187-189] The reflex effects occur first and are excitatory and vasoconstrictive. The neural reflex effects result from aortic and carotid chemoreceptor, baroreceptor, and central cerebral stimulation, and the humoral reflex effects result from catecholamine and renin-angiotensin release. The direct local vascular effects of hypoxia are inhibitory and vasodilatory and occur late. The net response to hypoxia in a subject depends on the severity of the hypoxia, which determines the magnitude and balance between the inhibitory and excitatory components; the balance may vary according to the type and depth of anesthesia and the degree of preexisting cardiovascular disease.

Mild arterial hypoxemia (arterial saturation less than normal but still 80% or higher) causes generalized activation of the sympathetic nervous system and release of catecholamines. Consequently, the heart rate, stroke volume, $\dot{Q}T$, and myocardial contractility—as measured by a shortened preejection period (PEP), left ventricular ejection time (LVET), and a decreased PEP/LVET ratio—are increased (Fig. 5.41).[190] Changes in systemic vascular resistance (SVR) are usually slight. However, in patients under anesthesia treated with β-blockers, hypoxia (and hypercapnia when present) may cause circulating catecholamines to have only an α-receptor effect, the heart to be unstimulated (or even depressed by a local hypoxic effect), and SVR to increase. Consequently, $\dot{Q}T$ may be decreased in these patients. With moderate hypoxemia (arterial oxygen saturation 60% to 80%), local vasodilation begins to predominate and SVR and blood pressure decrease, but the heart rate may continue to be increased because of a systemic hypotension-induced stimulation of baroreceptors. Finally, with severe hypoxemia (arterial saturation <60%), local depressant effects dominate and blood pressure falls rapidly; the pulse slows, shock develops, and the heart develops malignant dysrhythmias, including ventricular tachycardia, ventricular fibrillation, and ultimately asystole.

Significant preexisting hypotension converts a mild or moderate hypoxemic hemodynamic profile into a moderate or severe

TABLE 5.5	**Cardiovascular Response to Hypoxemia**					
Hemodynamic Variable Oxygen Saturation (%)	Heart Rate	Systemic Blood Pressure	Stroke Volume	Cardiac Output	SVR	Predominant Response
>80	↑	↑	↑	↑	No change	Reflex, excitatory
60–80	↑ Baroreceptor	↓	No change	No change	↓	Local, depressant > reflex, excitatory
<60	↓	↓	↓	↓	↓	Local, depressant

↑, increase; ↓, decrease; *SVR,* systemic vascular resistance.

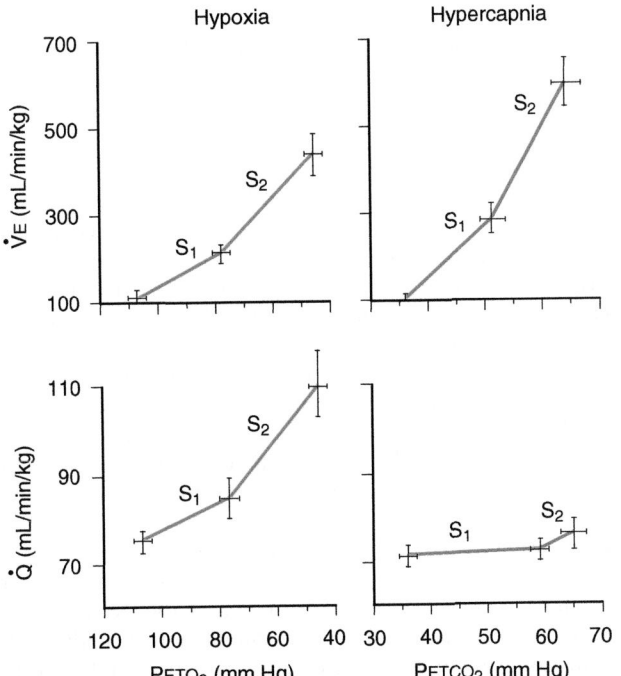

• Fig. 5.41 Changes in minute ventilation circulation of healthy awake humans during progressive isocapnic hypoxia and hyperoxic hypercapnia. $PETCO_2$, End-tidal PCO_2; $PETO_2$, End-tidal PO_2; $\dot{Q}$ cardiac output; S_1, slope during the first phase of slowly increasing ventilation and/or circulation; S_2, slope during the second phase of sharply increasing ventilation and/or circulation; $\dot{V}E$, expired minute ventilation. (From Serebrovskaya TV. Comparison of respiratory and circulatory human responses to progressive hypoxia and hypercapnia. *Respiration.* 1992;59:35.)

hypoxemic hemodynamic profile. Similarly, in well-anesthetized or sedated patients, early sympathetic nervous system reactivity to hypoxemia may be reduced and the effects of hypoxemia may be expressed only as bradycardia with severe hypotension and, ultimately, circulatory collapse.[191]

Hypoxemia-induced cardiac dysrhythmias can be caused by multiple interrelated mechanisms that all cause a decrease in the myocardial oxygen supply-demand ratio, which in turn increases myocardial irritability. First, arterial hypoxemia can directly decrease the myocardial oxygen supply. Second, early tachycardia may result in increased myocardial oxygen consumption, and decreased diastolic filling time may lead to decreased myocardial oxygen supply. Third, early increased systemic blood pressure can cause an increased afterload on the left ventricle, which increases left ventricular oxygen demand. Fourth, late systemic hypotension can decrease myocardial oxygen supply because of decreased diastolic perfusion pressure. Fifth, coronary blood flow reserve can be exhausted by a late, maximally increased coronary blood flow because of maximal coronary vasodilation.[192] The level of hypoxemia that causes cardiac dysrhythmias cannot be predicted with certainty because the myocardial oxygen supply-demand relationship in a given patient is not known (i.e., the degree of coronary artery atherosclerosis may not be known). However, if a myocardial area (or areas) becomes hypoxic or ischemic, or both, unifocal or multifocal premature ventricular contractions, ventricular tachycardia, and ventricular fibrillation can occur.

The cardiovascular response to hypoxia includes several other important effects. Ventilation is stimulated regardless of the reason for the hypoxia (see Fig. 5.41). The pulmonary distribution

of blood flow is more homogeneous because of increased Ppa. Chronic hypoxia causes an increased Hb concentration and a right shift of the oxy-Hb curve (because of either an increase in 2,3-DPG or acidosis), which tends to raise tissue PO_2.

Hyperoxia (Oxygen Toxicity)

The dangers associated with inspiration of excessive oxygen are multiple. Exposure to high oxygen tension clearly causes pulmonary damage in healthy individuals.[193,194] A dose-time toxicity curve for humans is available from several studies.[193–195] Because the lungs of normal human volunteers cannot be directly examined to determine the rate of onset and the course of toxicity, indirect measures such as onset of symptoms have been used to construct dose-time toxicity curves. Examination of the curve indicates that 100% oxygen should not be administered for more than 12 hours, 80% oxygen for more than 24 hours, and 60% oxygen for more than 36 hours.[193–195] No measurable changes in pulmonary function or blood-gas exchange occur in humans during exposure to less than 50% oxygen, even for long periods.[195] Nevertheless, it is important to note that, in the clinical setting, these dose-time toxicity relationships are often obscured because of the complex multivariable nature of the clinical setting.[196]

The dominant symptom of oxygen toxicity in human volunteers is substernal discomfort, which begins as mild irritation in the area of the carina and may be accompanied by occasional coughing.[197] As exposure continues, the pain becomes more intense, and the urge to cough and to breathe deeply also becomes more intense. These symptoms progress to severe dyspnea, paroxysmal coughing, and decreased vital capacity when the FIO_2 has been 1.0 for longer than 12 hours. If excessive oxygen is discontinued at this point, recovery of mechanical lung function usually occurs within 12 to 24 hours, but more than 24 hours may be required in some individuals.[195] As toxicity progresses, results of other pulmonary function studies such as compliance and blood gases show deterioration. In animals, the lesion progresses pathologically from tracheobronchitis (exposure for 12 hours to a few days), to involvement of the alveolar septa with pulmonary interstitial edema (exposure for a few days to 1 week), to pulmonary fibrosis of the edema (exposure for >1 week).[198]

Excessive oxygen administration can lead to ventilatory depression in patients who, by reason of drugs or disease, have been ventilating in response to a hypoxic drive. Ventilatory depression that results from removal of a hypoxic drive through increasing the inspired oxygen concentration causes hypercapnia but does not necessarily produce hypoxia (because of the increased FIO_2). The role of this phenomenon in the development of hypercapnic respiratory failure in patients with COPD administered a high FIO_2 is likely not as significant as the contribution of increased CO_2 unloading due to the Haldane effect (see section "Bohr and Haldane Effects") and the contribution of impaired HPV in poorly ventilated areas of the lung (see section "Active Processes and Pulmonary Vascular Tone").

Absorption atelectasis was described earlier (see section "High Inspired Oxygen Concentration and Absorption Atelectasis"). Retrolental fibroplasia, an abnormal proliferation of the immature retinal vasculature of an infant born prematurely, can occur after exposure to hyperoxia. Extremely premature infants (i.e., those <1.0 kg in birth weight and <28 weeks of gestation) are most susceptible to retrolental fibroplasia. The risk of retrolental fibroplasia exists whenever the FIO_2 causes PaO_2 to be greater than 80 mm Hg for longer than 3 hours in an infant whose gestational age plus chronological age combined is less than 44 weeks. If the ductus arteriosus is patent, arterial blood samples should be drawn from the right radial artery and pulse oximetry should be monitored on the right hand; umbilical, left-upper extremity, or lower extremity Pao_2 is lower than the Pao_2 to which the eyes are exposed because of ductal shunting of unoxygenated blood.

The mode of action of oxygen toxicity in tissues is complex, but interference with metabolism seems to be widespread. Most importantly, many enzymes, particularly those with sulfhydryl groups, are inactivated by oxygen-derived free radicals.[196] Neutrophil recruitment and release of mediators of inflammation occur next and greatly accelerate the extent of endothelial and epithelial damage and impairment of the surfactant systems.[196] The most acute toxic effect of oxygen in humans is a convulsive effect, which occurs during exposure to pressures more than 2 atmospheres (atm) absolute.

High inspired oxygen concentrations can be of use therapeutically. Clearance of gas loculi in the body may be greatly accelerated by the inhalation of 100% oxygen. Inhalation of 100% oxygen creates a large nitrogen gradient from the gas space to the perfusing blood. As a result, nitrogen leaves the gas space, and the space diminishes in size. Administration of oxygen to remove gas from extraanatomic spaces has been used clinically—for example, to ease intestinal gas pressure in patients with intestinal obstruction, to decrease the size of an air embolus, and to aid in the absorption of pneumocephalus, pneumothorax, or pneumoperitoneum.

Hypercapnia

The effects of CO_2 on the cardiovascular system are as complex as those of hypoxia. Like hypoxemia, hypercapnia appears to cause direct depression of both cardiac muscle and vascular smooth muscle, but at the same time it causes reflex stimulation of the sympathoadrenal system, which compensates to a greater or lesser extent for the primary cardiovascular depression (see Fig. 5.41).[189,192] With moderate to severe hypercapnia, a hyperkinetic circulation results with increased $\dot{Q}_T$ and increased systemic blood pressure.[190] Even in patients under inhalational anesthesia, plasma catecholamine levels increase in response to increased CO_2 levels in much the same way as in conscious subjects. Thus hypercapnia, like hypoxemia, may cause increased myocardial oxygen demand (tachycardia, early hypertension) and decreased myocardial oxygen supply (tachycardia, late hypotension).

Table 5.6 summarizes the interaction of anesthesia with hypercapnia in humans; increased $\dot{Q}_T$ and decreased SVR should be emphasized.[199,200] The increase in $\dot{Q}_T$ is most marked during anesthesia with drugs that enhance sympathetic activity and least marked with nitrous oxide. The decrease in SVR is most marked during anesthesia and hypercapnia. Hypercapnia is a potent pulmonary vasoconstrictor even after the inhalation of 3% isoflurane for 5 minutes.[199]

Dysrhythmias have been reported in unanesthetized humans during acute hypercapnia, but they have seldom been of serious importance. A high $Paco_2$ level is, however, more dangerous during general anesthesia. With halothane anesthesia, dysrhythmias frequently occur above a $Paco_2$ arrhythmic threshold that is often constant for a particular patient. Furthermore, halogenated anesthetics have been shown to prolong the QT interval in humans, thereby increasing the risk for torsades de pointes, which in turn is notorious for decompensating into ventricular fibrillation.[201]

The maximum stimulatory respiratory effect is attained by a $Paco_2$ of about 100 mm Hg. At a higher $Paco_2$, stimulation is reduced, and at extremely high levels, CO_2 narcosis depresses brain function and respiratory drive until ventilation ceases altogether. Anesthetics and other depressant drugs displace the Pco_2 ventilation/response curve to the right and reduce its slope.[202] With deep anesthesia, the response curve can be flat or even sloping downward, and CO_2 then acts as a respiratory depressant. In patients with ventilatory failure, CO_2 narcosis occurs when $Paco_2$ rises to greater than 90 to 120 mm Hg. A 30% CO_2 concentration is sufficient for the production of anesthesia, and this concentration causes total but reversible flattening of the electroencephalogram.[203] Hypercapnia causes bronchodilation in both healthy persons and patients with lung disease.[204] Apart from the effect on ventilation, CO_2 exerts two other important effects that influence oxygenation of the blood.[117] First, if the concentration of nitrogen (or other inert gas) remains constant, the concentration of CO_2 in alveolar gas can increase only at the expense of oxygen, which must be displaced. Thus, Pao_2 and Pao_2 may decrease. Second, hypercapnia shifts the oxy-Hb curve to the right, thereby facilitating tissue oxygenation.[95]

Chronic hypercapnia results in increased reabsorption of bicarbonate by the kidneys, which further raises the plasma bicarbonate level and constitutes a secondary or compensatory metabolic alkalosis. The decrease in renal reabsorption of bicarbonate in patients with chronic hypocapnia results in a further fall in plasma bicarbonate and produces a secondary or compensatory metabolic acidosis. In each case, arterial pH returns toward the normal value, but the bicarbonate ion concentration departs even further from normal.

Hypercapnia is accompanied by leakage of potassium from cells into plasma. Much of the potassium comes from the liver, probably from glucose release and mobilization, which occurs in response to the rise in plasma catecholamine levels.[205] Because the plasma potassium level takes an appreciable amount of time to return to normal, repeated bouts of hypercapnia at short intervals result in a stepwise rise in plasma potassium. Finally, hypercapnia can predispose the patient to other complications in the operating room—for example, the oculocardiac reflex is far more common during hypercapnia than during eucapnia.[206]

TABLE 5.6 **Cardiovascular Responses to Hypercapnia ($Paco_2$ = 60–83 mm Hg) During Isoflurane Anesthesia (1 MAC) and Nitrous Oxide[a]**

Anesthesia	Heart Rate	Contractility	Cardiac Output	Systemic Vascular Resistance
Conscious	↑↑	↑↑	↑↑↑	↓
Nitrous oxide	0	↑	↑↑	↓↓
Isoflurane	↑↑	↑↑↑	↑↑↑	↓

[a]The increase in the partial arterial pressure of carbon dioxide ($Paco_2$) in conscious subjects was 11.5 mm Hg from a normal level of 38 mm Hg.

↑, <10% increase; ↑↑, 10–25% increase; ↑↑↑, >25% increase; 0, no change; ↓, <10% decrease; ↓↓, 10–25% decrease; MAC, Minimum alveolar concentration for adequate anesthesia in 50% of subjects.

Hypocapnia

In this section, hypocapnia is considered to be produced by iatrogenic hyperventilation. Hypocapnia can cause a decrease in $\dot{Q}_T$ by three separate mechanisms. First, if it is present, an increase in intrathoracic pressure decreases $\dot{Q}_T$. Second, hypocapnia is associated with withdrawal of sympathetic nervous system activity, and such withdrawal can decrease the inotropic state of the heart. Third, hypocapnia can increase pH, and the increased pH can decrease ionized calcium, which can, in turn, decrease the inotropic state of the heart. Hypocapnia with alkalosis also shifts the oxy-Hb curve to the left, which increases Hb affinity for oxygen and thus impairs oxygen unloading at the tissue level. The decrease in peripheral flow and the impaired ability to unload oxygen to the tissues are compounded by an increase in whole-body oxygen consumption because of increased pH-mediated uncoupling of oxidation from phosphorylation.[207] A $Paco_2$ of 20 mm Hg increases tissue oxygen consumption by 30%. Consequently, hypocapnia may simultaneously increase tissue oxygen demand and decrease tissue oxygen supply. To have the same amount of oxygen delivery to the tissues, $\dot{Q}_T$ or tissue perfusion must increase at a time when it may not be possible for it to do so. The cerebral effects of hypocapnia may be related to a state of cerebral acidosis and hypoxia because hypocapnia can cause a selective reduction in cerebral blood flow and shifts the oxy-Hb curve to the left.[208] Hypocapnia can cause $\dot{V}_A/\dot{Q}$ abnormalities by inhibiting HPV or by causing bronchoconstriction and decreased C_L. Finally, hypocapnia promotes apnea.

Conclusion

The primary purpose of the respiratory system is to facilitate gas exchange of oxygen and CO_2 in the alveoli. At the alveoli, oxygen combines with Hb and is transported throughout the body by the circulatory system, while at the same time, CO_2 that has been transported from the tissues is removed to be exhaled via the alveoli. These respiratory functions are achieved by coordinated action of the upper and lower airways, alveoli, pulmonary blood flow, respiratory muscles, and metabolic sensors, along with medullary- and neural-based control centers.

The lungs also serve several very important nonpulmonary metabolic and humoral functions, as described in this chapter.

Ventilation is the process of bringing in oxygen-rich air through the airways to the alveoli (inspiration), where gas exchange occurs; then, during expiration, the oxygen-depleted air (along with CO_2 produced in tissues) is returned to the external environment. The process of ventilation is tightly regulated by neural and nonneural mechanisms.

Perfusion relates to the quantity of blood flowing by the alveoli. Pulmonary perfusion is generally equal to cardiac output unless shunts occur. Ventilation is closely coupled with perfusion of the alveoli. The interaction between ventilation and perfusion ($\dot{V}_A/\dot{Q}$) ultimately determines gas exchange in the lungs.

The transport of oxygen requires reversible binding of oxygen to Hb, which is then unloaded at the tissues. The oxygen flows through its concentration gradient to the extracellular space and cells. Intracellular concentrations of oxygen vary within the cell, with the mitochondrial Po_2 being very low compared to arterial and even mixed venous blood values. Furthermore, interaction of the circulatory system with the respiratory system adds another level of fine-tuning and complexity to the process of perfusion, ventilation, and ventilation/perfusion interaction.

Cardiac and respiratory functions are closely integrated with numerous feedback mechanisms designed to match ventilation with perfusion. The lungs and the heart are the only organs that receive the full pulmonary blood flow ($\dot{Q}_T$). Accordingly, the lungs are anatomically well situated to perform many secondary (nonpulmonary) functions. The list of nonpulmonary functions continues to grow and includes filtering of metabolic products, conversion of important enzymes, and immune protection.

Pulmonary and nonpulmonary functions adapt to the constantly changing needs of the body. Understanding the basic physiologic mechanisms involved in pulmonary and nonpulmonary functions of the lungs is the key to appreciating the pathophysiology of respiratory disorders and the rational management of respiratory function during resuscitation, perioperative management, and critical care.

Selected References

1. West JB, Dollery CT, Naimark A. Distribution of blood flow in isolated lung: relation to vascular and alveolar pressures. *J Appl Physiol*. 1961;19:713.
17. West JB. Blood flow to the lung and gas exchange. *Anesthesiology*. 1974;41:124.
24. Benumof JL. Mechanism of decreased blood flow to the atelectatic lung. *J Appl Physiol*. 1978;46:1047.
40. Bendixen HH, Bullwinkel B, Hedley-Whyte J, et al. Atelectasis and shunting during spontaneous ventilation in anesthetized patients. *Anesthesiology*. 1964;25:297.
65. Lumb AB, Slinger P. Hypoxic pulmonary vasoconstriction: physiology and anesthetic implications. *Anesthesiology*. 2015;122(4):932–946.
112. Hedenstierna G. Gas exchange during anaesthesia. *Br J Anaesth*. 1990;64:507.
117. Wilson WC, Shapiro B. Perioperative hypoxia: the clinical spectrum and current oxygen monitoring methodology. *Anesthesiol Clin North Am* 2001;19:769.
147. Pelosi P, Croci M, Ravagnan I, et al. The effects of body mass on lung volumes, respiratory mechanics, and gas exchange during general anesthesia. *Anesth Analg*. 1998;87:654.
156. Froese AB, Bryan CA. Effects of anesthesia and paralysis on diaphragmatic mechanics in man. *Anesthesiology*. 1974;41:242.

All references can be found online at eBooks.Health.Elsevier.com.

6

Airway Pharmacology

SRIKANTH SRIDHAR AND NAVEEN VANGA

CHAPTER OUTLINE

KEY POINTS

- The selection of pharmacologic agents should consider the effects on airway patency, airway reflexes, and airway reactivity.
- Delivery of inhalational drugs should be optimized to prevent inefficient administration, and dedicated devices may be necessary to increase the amount of drug that reaches the target site.
- Topical local anesthetics can be safely administered in the upper airway with a low potential for toxicity. The upper limit of dose is unclear, but doses of lidocaine up to 9 mg/kg have been shown to be safe.
- Sedative/hypnotic agents used in anesthesia generally reduce the patency of the upper airway, and caution must be exercised with their use. The loss of patency is related to loss of coordination of the upper airway musculature from decreased arousal. These agents also generally have bronchodilating effects.
- The use of neuromuscular blocking drugs increases the chance of successful airway management during anesthesia. These

agents can be safely administered during induction of general anesthesia, as all aspects of airway management will be facilitated with their use.
- Patients with asthma should have a targeted preoperative evaluation discussing the current pharmacologic therapy they are receiving, and consideration should be given to adequacy of the therapy and optimization of symptoms. Inhaled glucocorticoids are a mainstay of treatment and should be initiated and continued perioperatively.
- The risk of perioperative bronchospasm should be considered in patients with reactive airway disease and other risk factors, and it should be adequately prepared for in all phases of the perioperative period.
- Intraoperative bronchospasm can become an anesthetic emergency, and a structured approach to its management will lead to the highest likelihood of a successful outcome.

Introduction

The modern practice of medicine is heavily influenced by the development and use of pharmacologic agents to achieve a therapeutic effect. This influence spreads to every corner of medical practice and, therefore, has a large impact on the discussion and practice of airway management. In this chapter, we will examine the various aspects of pharmacology that are relevant to the physiology, function, and maintenance of the normal airway. The concept of airway pharmacology can be approached from various perspectives. First, drugs can be viewed as having a direct or indirect effect on the airway. Second, drugs can be classified based on therapeutic intent—that is, whether they are administered with the primary intent to affect airway function or whether they are administered for another reason and have a secondary effect on airway function. Third, drugs can be classified based on their site of action in the airway, namely the upper airway (superior to the glottis) or the lower airway (inferior to the glottis). Finally, drugs can be conceptualized based on their observed effect on the airway—for example, bronchodilation or loss of airway patency.

This chapter will encompass these perspectives when they are relevant to a particular drug or class of drugs. The discussion will begin with a review of some overarching themes regarding pharmacology and normal airway function and physiology. It will continue with a review of common classes of agents used in the perioperative period that have an effect on airway management and function, and it will consider a clinically relevant model of airway disease (i.e., asthma) as well as common drugs with therapeutic effects on the airway. This chapter is not intended to be a comprehensive scientific review of the literature surrounding specific pharmacologic agents with effects on the airway. Indeed, such a review would require an independent textbook. The intent of this chapter is to present information regarding clinical concerns relevant to airway management that would be most useful in daily practice. For those readers desiring a more granular examination of the pharmacologic concepts addressed, a selection of references has been provided for further review.

General Pharmacologic Concepts and Clinical Considerations

There are several general concepts that warrant review at the outset—specifically, some basic pharmacologic concepts and some basic concepts regarding the airway and its clinical significance.

Pharmacologic Concepts

When selecting a pharmacologic agent, there are several considerations. A therapeutic effect must ideally be achieved for the desired time frame and with the intended degree. A drug's potential side effects, interaction with other agents, metabolism, and cost must be weighed against its potential benefit. Each of these concepts will be discussed with each drug class in the rest of this chapter, but the basic elements of each will be described here.

Pharmacodynamics

Pharmacodynamics refers to the properties of a drug at the site of action and its resulting effects, including the intensity of therapeutic and adverse effects. It describes a drug or drug class on the basis of mechanism of action, such as receptor binding or enzymatic action, and the subsequent effect of that action. The effect of a drug can be described on a molecular level, such as in the example of a G protein–coupled receptor creating a cascade of intracellular events or a sodium channel closing and altering resting ion conductance across the cell membrane. Alternatively, the effect can be described on a systemic basis, or by the therapeutic change effected by the drug's action. Examples of this include a change in airway resistance with dilation of a respiratory bronchiole or numbing of the airway resulting from loss of sensory input with blockade of nerve conduction. Analysis of a drug's effect based on the amount of drug given, or a dose-response relationship, is also under the scope of pharmacodynamics. Finally, description of drug action compared with other drugs also falls under the umbrella of pharmacodynamics. For example, classifying drugs as agonists, antagonists, or partial agonists at a receptor site is a pharmacodynamic concept.

Pharmacokinetics

Pharmacokinetics includes the absorption, distribution, metabolism, and excretion properties of a drug in relation to the body. Essentially, it describes where a drug goes when it is administered, or the volume of distribution. Drug delivery falls within these considerations, as does drug elimination from the body—clearance. A more granular view of pharmacokinetics would describe the complex processes of drug distribution and redistribution within the body, as well as the factors that govern how a drug molecule reaches its site of action and how that drug is removed from its site of action to terminate the effect. Drug distribution and redistribution require an intricate knowledge of how much drug is present in various sites in the body at a given time after administration, and, in fact, several complex mathematical models attempt to describe this idea in a very discrete manner. Finally, the physical aspects and molecular structure of a drug often play into its pharmacokinetics because this is one of the primary determinants of a drug's ability to travel in the body. For example, a drug's ability to cross a lipid membrane may be very important in determining its onset of action or the concentration in the blood required to initiate an effect.

Adverse Reactions, Side Effects, and Toxicity

With any administration of a drug, there are side effects, adverse reactions, and toxicity that must be taken into consideration. The first concept to introduce is that of local and systemic effects of drugs. For example, agents directly involved in airway management may have systemic considerations; conversely, systemic treatments may have effects on the airway. In fact, a drug administered with an intended effect may actually act in a completely remote area of the body to create that effect. This leads into the concept of side effects of drugs, which describes effects that a drug may have secondary to its intended therapeutic use. An example of this would be with sympathomimetic agents, which may be given with the intent of airway smooth muscle relaxation but have a separate effect of increased heart rate and blood pressure. This side effect of a drug may or may not be considered also to be an adverse reaction of the drug, which is an unintended effect with the potential to create harm or injury to a patient. Another example of an adverse reaction is a drug allergy; however, the two are not equivalent terms.

One way to describe a drug's ability to create harm or adverse effects is the concept of toxicity. This describes the extent to which a drug can cause harm and is often related to the amount of drug in the body. Many drugs have an established toxicity level based on observation after clinical use. For example, lidocaine has the ability to create toxic effects at or above serum concentrations of 5 to 6 µg/mL. This introduces the concept of a therapeutic range of a drug, which is a conceptualization of the amount of drug that will create and maximize the intended therapeutic effect with minimal toxic side effects. Some drugs have a therapeutic range below a toxic concentration range, but some drugs create therapeutic effects at similar concentrations that create toxic effects. A situation in which administration of a drug simultaneously results in benefit and harm creates a dilemma for the practitioner in the drug prescribing process and requires special consideration. Unfortunately, this is frequently the case when managing the airway and in the perioperative period or with critically ill patients.

Routes of Drug Administration to the Airway

One special pharmacokinetic consideration when thinking about the airway is the route of delivery of a drug. The choice of route of delivery is based primarily on the available routes for a particular drug or class of drugs, but other factors also influence this decision. Some available methods of delivery for drugs that affect the airway are inhalation, topical application, and oral and parenteral routes.

Inhalation delivery is particularly useful for drugs with an effect on the airway. This route tends to provide optimal delivery of the drug to the lungs and airways (especially useful if these are the target tissues) but requires a dedicated device for administration, which may not always be available.[1] First, the device must be able to convert a drug into an aerosol form that is available for inhalation. For drugs that are in liquid or powder form, this would require the use of an actuator to agitate the drug and create the aerosol. For drugs that are supplied in gas or vapor form, this is not necessary. The size of particles that comprise the aerosol can be very consequential. Optimal particle size is between 0.5 and 5 µm.[2] Smaller particles are inhaled and immediately exhaled before they can take effect, and larger particles tend to deposit in more proximal tissues such as the nasal passage and oropharynx rather than reaching the lungs for absorption. Second, an ideal delivery device would assist in driving the drug away from the site of aerosol formation. Various inhalation devices accomplish this differently. For example, many inhaler devices use a propellant gas to carry the aerosol particles and aid delivery to the airway. Inhalation of aerosols has the detriment of requiring a great deal of patient education and cooperation for successful use, but it is one of the most widely used forms of drug delivery to the airway.

An alternate form of inhalation delivery is nebulization. This is an option available for liquid medications and involves driving a gas (usually oxygen or air) through the liquid to draw it into droplets that are carried by the flowing gas for inhalation.[3] This is, unfortunately, a very inefficient mechanism for drug delivery because of the loss of a large portion of drug externally as a mist and deposition of the drug droplets into proximal tissues. It is, however, a very frequently used modality because it requires far less patient cooperation, allows for delivery of oxygen to patients who require it (as many conceivably do when presenting with airway pathology), and is relatively easy to use interchangeably in patients with or without airway instrumentation in place.

Topical administration is more typically used for delivering drug to the upper airway and can be in the form of liquids, creams, gels, or powders. The anatomic difficulty of topically applying a drug to the lower airway limits its use in this regard. An example of topical administration of a drug in airway management is the practice of directly applying local anesthetic to the oropharynx and palate in preparation for awake intubation.

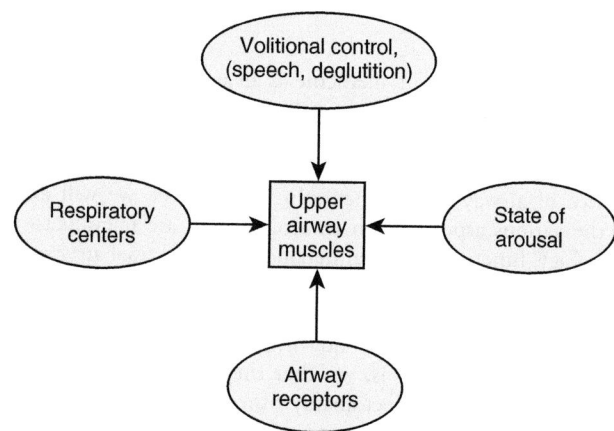

• **Fig. 6.1** A schematic representation of some of the factors that influence the activity of muscles in the upper airway.

Oral administration of drugs that affect the airway is used infrequently but is most often used when inhalation delivery is problematic or impossible. Additionally, this route can be used when the need for an airway is urgent and action or delivery of the drug by other routes would be inefficient.

Parenteral administration is most frequently used in emergency situations for drugs that are intended to affect the airway, but the effect of parenteral drugs used for sedation and anesthesia and their effects on the airway are readily seen on a daily basis. The secondary airway effects of these drug types will be discussed later in the chapter.

Anatomy and Physiology of the Airway

Airway anatomy has already been covered in great detail in Chapter 1, and airway physiology has been covered extensively in Chapter 5; however, a brief review of key elements that are relevant to the administration and effect of drugs that are frequently used with airway effect is warranted. Particularly with the upper airway, a number of factors at play have a very clinically significant result in the caliber of the airway (Fig. 6.1).

Anatomy

Anatomic considerations include age, body habitus, and posture. As individuals age, the cartilaginous structures of the airway continue to grow and increase in rigidity. Obesity, particularly in the cervical region, can restrict range of movement as well as decrease the volume of the upper airway. In the supine position, the effect of gravity is such that the tissue will tend to collapse on the airway, potentially creating a partial or complete obstruction. Similarly, the lower airway can be affected with changes in lung volumes and functional residual capacity.

The upper airway is most susceptible to anatomic change and loss of patency because of the complex muscle arrangements that coordinate function, such as passage of air, swallowing, and speech.[4,5] Activation of these muscles prevents collapse of the space with the negative pressure of inspiration. This concept will present itself in various forms when various drug classes are considered with their effects on neuromuscular function and upper airway patency.

Neuromuscular Function

The upper airway is primarily comprised of skeletal muscles that are innervated by motor neurons. This is not to say that the muscles are always and completely under voluntary control. In fact, the complex relationships between muscles for contraction and relaxation to maintain patency of the airway are controlled by the respiratory centers and, to some extent, by the arousal centers and reticular activating system. A phasic contraction and relaxation in the oropharynx[6] and the glottic musculature[7–10] is related to and controlled by the central respiratory control centers. Additionally, reflex arcs exist in response to mechanical and chemical stimuli that create coordinated contractions of the upper airway musculature to protect the airway.[11]

The lower airway is primarily comprised of smooth muscle that is involuntary and under autonomic control. It also, however, has reflex activity that serves to protect the airway in the presence of noxious stimuli[12,13] and to prevent the aspiration of unwanted material into the lungs.

Hypoxia and hypercarbia serve to increase the respiratory drive, triggering the upper airway muscles, diaphragm, and accessory muscles of the lung to increase airway patency and function.

Autonomic Nervous System

Airway dynamics are controlled by the surrounding musculature, which provides either dilating or constricting effects. The autonomic nervous system is the principal regulator of airway tone. Environmental stressors, such as exercise, increase sympathetic nervous activity, which dilates the upper and lower airways.

The lower airway is where the autonomic system has the greatest influence. Adrenergic receptors are present in the lower airway; however, no sympathetic nerves actually innervate the smooth muscle fibers of the airway—rather, they are influenced by the sympathetic nervous system when there is an increase in circulating epinephrine. The resulting phenomenon is one of autonomic control by primarily vagal output (Fig. 6.2). The effect of parasympathetic activity is of muscarinic activation, which leads to bronchoconstriction, increase in mucus production and secretion, and pulmonary vasodilation.

Another influence on lower airway musculature and function is a nonadrenergic, noncholinergic (NANC) system that may be mediated by nitric oxide (NO) and by-products as well as vasoactive intestinal peptide (VIP).[14–16] This system is rather complex, but it is increasingly implicated in the development of airway inflammatory disease, cytokine release, and pathologic structural change in the airway.

Voluntary Regulation of Airway Patency

Upper airway patency is somewhat dependent on arousal,[17] with the reticular activating system playing a role in the contraction of musculature and maintenance of patency. Sleep tends to have a countereffect by typically increasing airway resistance,[18] whereas general anesthesia blunts the response of the sympathetic nervous system to external stimuli such as pain.

Voluntary activities that involve coordination of muscular activity include speech and swallowing. The use of the term *voluntary* is not to indicate that the muscles of the oropharynx are under voluntary control individually but that the central processing and output of that coordinated activity is under voluntary control. Indeed, it is rather easy to voluntarily swallow, but it is rather difficult to voluntarily contract one's stylopharyngeus muscle. An exception to this rule in the upper airway is the tongue; its movements are largely under voluntary control to facilitate speech and swallowing. It does, however, undertake centrally controlled muscular contraction in coordination with the remainder of the pharyngeal apparatus.

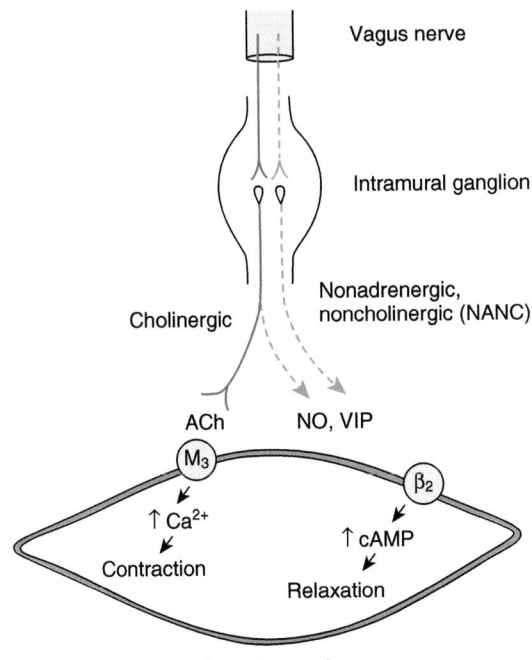

• **Fig. 6.2** Some of the systems that control lower airway smooth muscle tone. Note that β2-receptors on airway smooth muscle are not innervated. It is unclear if the nonadrenergic, noncholinergic system (depicted by *dashed lines*) uses independent neural pathways or if its mediators nitric oxide (*NO*) and vasoactive intestinal peptide (*VIP*) are cotransmitters released with acetylcholine (*ACh*) from postganglionic nerves. *cAMP*, Cyclic adenosine monophosphate.

Disease Affecting the Airway

Various pathologies, such as malignancy, genetic conditions, neuromuscular disease, infection, asthma, chronic obstructive pulmonary disease (COPD), restrictive lung disease, obesity, and obstructive sleep apnea (OSA), can affect the airway in a number of ways. Airway sensitivity, resistance, patency, and anatomy can be affected and must be considered when selecting a pharmacologic agent in the setting of these problems.

Clinical Issues Regarding the Airway

The functional aspects of the airway that are clinically significant from a pharmacology perspective are those that are modifiable by an administered drug. Throughout the remainder of this chapter, drug action will be discussed in the context of modulation of airway patency, protection, reactivity, and resistance. These are the primary modifiable qualities of the airway that are commonly encountered by the clinician and should be considered when choosing a therapeutic regimen for a patient needing airway management.

Airway Patency

Patency of the upper airway is of great concern and is the most modifiable airway parameter affected by pharmacologic agents. Centrally or locally effective agents may affect upper airway patency, and the changes involve both motor output and sensory feedback. As with all agents, the effects may be directly initiated or indirectly caused by action at another site.

Upper airway patency may also be diminished by physical factors, such as malignancy, mass, or inflammation. These types of

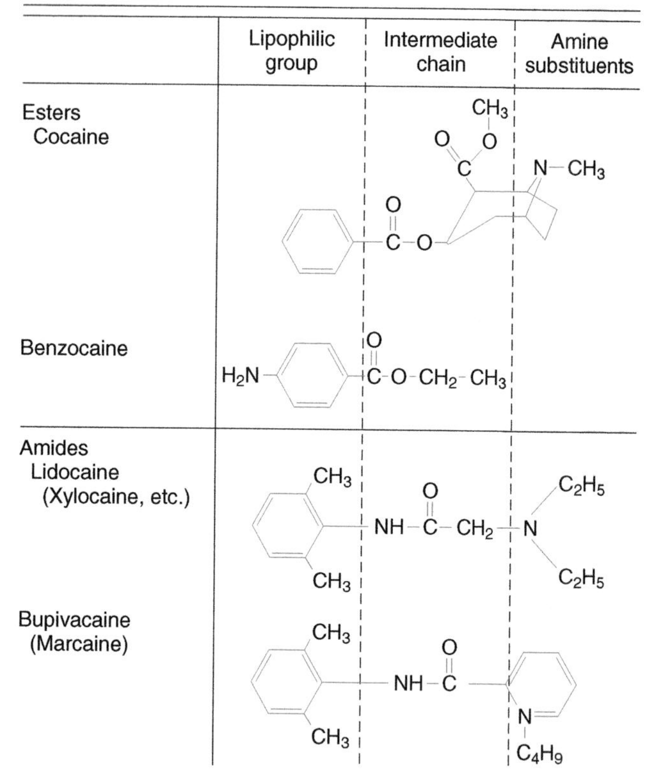

	Lipophilic group	Intermediate chain	Amine substituents
Esters Cocaine			
Benzocaine			
Amides Lidocaine (Xylocaine, etc.)			
Bupivacaine (Marcaine)			

• **Fig. 6.3** Chemical structure of some of the local anesthetics used for topical airway anesthesia.

obstructions may not be amenable to pharmacologic treatment, but they undoubtedly affect a drug regimen that may be used during airway management.

Airway Protection

Protection of the airway was described earlier in the chapter and is associated with arousal and reflex pathways. Upper airway reflexes play a role in airway protection and are diminished in a state of hypnosis. Lower airway reflexes prevent aspiration of particulate matter or liquids into the lungs that would impede oxygen delivery and gas exchange. The loss of these reflexes can be dangerous to a patient, and potentially life-threatening complications may ensue. As a result, protection of the airway must be a serious concern when it is pharmacologically eliminated from normal functionality.

The pharyngeal reflex (gag reflex) plays a vital role in airway management because there are scenarios where its preservation or its suppression is required. As a reflex arc mediated afferently by the glossopharyngeal nerve and efferently by the vagus nerve, the principal function of the pharyngeal reflex is to prevent aspiration. Pharmacologic agents can directly or indirectly suppress this reflex, facilitating airway instrumentation in a sedated or even awake patient. Inadvertent suppression of the reflex must also be carefully considered, as an unprotected airway can lead to aspiration of gastric contents.

Airway Reactivity and Resistance

Upper airway resistance is almost entirely related to patency and was discussed earlier in the chapter. Lower airway resistance and reactivity are closely related phenomena. Increases in resistance and reactivity may be markers of irritability of the airway, and caution should be taken with instrumentation and manipulation. Reactivity and resistance can be adversely affected by disease

processes, such as infection and inflammation; noxious external stimuli, such as aspirated gastric contents; and pharmacologic agents, such as some volatile anesthetics. Airway reactivity will be discussed in much further detail at the end of this chapter.

Anesthetic Drugs and Effect on the Airway

Almost all pharmacologic agents used for sedation and general anesthesia have an effect on the airway. Those effects may be directly on the structures of the airway, or they may be mediated by indirect action. In some instances, there are both direct and indirect effects that combine to create an overall observed effect. This section will address various classes of these anesthetic drugs and review their effects on the airway.

Local Anesthetics

Local anesthetics are some of the most used drugs with effects on the airway. They are a very appropriate example of a drug being used specifically for an airway effect when used for preparation for awake tracheal intubation or when used intravenously to blunt afferent sensory input from the airway during airway instrumentation or manipulation. Generally, the effect of local anesthetics on the airway is that of blockade of afferent nervous input for reflex activity (i.e., protective reflexes in the upper airway or response to noxious stimuli in the lower airway). Additionally, the upper airway undergoes a loss of muscle tone and subsequent loss of patency.[19,20] In higher doses, local anesthetics may directly irritate airway mucous membranes, which may limit the use of some agents as a result of this counterproductive effect.

Local anesthetics bind to transmembrane sodium channels in neurons and block their function to prevent initiation and propagation of action potentials.[21,22] They are weak bases and are comprised of a lipophilic chemical group that is connected to an ionizable group consisting of an ester or an amide chain (Fig. 6.3). The ionizable group allows the drug to be present in the body in two forms that exist in equilibrium: an ionized form that is present in the plasma and a nonionized form that is more lipophilic and able to diffuse across membranes. Local anesthetics formulated with an amide chain are metabolized in the liver, and those with an ester linkage are hydrolyzed in the plasma. After conversion, all are excreted in the urine. The onset of action of these drugs is dependent upon diffusion of the drug to the target site, which, in turn, is dependent upon the availability of nonionized drug to do so. Physiologic states that reduce the amount of nonionized drug in equilibrium will affect the action of local anesthetics, but this effect is variable for different agents with different dissociation constants based on individual chemical structure.

Local anesthetics are widely available and exist in multiple formulations and concentrations. They can be administered topically to the upper airway with the use of gels or liquids; the use of atomizing devices or special instruments to instill the drug more distally in the airway allows for more effective and targeted delivery onto the mucous membranes. Local anesthetics may also be delivered via the inhalational route, with the most common method being nebulization of a liquid drug for passage into the lower airways. Finally, parenteral delivery is available, with the options of direct administration into the bloodstream or, alternatively, targeted injection into the soft tissues surrounding sensory nerves to allow diffusion directly to the nerve for effect. An example of the latter includes the use of local anesthetics for nerve blocks in the head and neck in preparation for awake tracheal intubation.

Toxicity attributed to local anesthetics is exceedingly rare when administered for airway management purposes. Lidocaine is the most commonly used and extensively studied agent, so it will be used as an example here. A generally accepted serum level of toxicity for lidocaine ranges from 5 to 6 μg/mL, and the maximum dose is commonly cited as 4.5 mg/kg; however, most studies have failed to demonstrate serum levels approaching toxicity with clinically relevant doses or even with large doses used in the airway. In fact, one study has demonstrated no patients with a toxic level even after administration of 9 mg/kg of lidocaine.[23] The exception to this seems to be with gargling of the drug, where 6 mg/kg may have been associated with a near toxic serum level.[24] Some case reports have implicated local anesthetics in adverse effects, so caution and close monitoring are recommended when large doses of lidocaine are required for topical anesthesia, and generally using the least amount that is effective is considered best practice in this regard. Strategies to minimize the need for local anesthetic use in topical airway anesthesia are discussed in the chapter dedicated to preparation for awake intubation (Chapter 13).

Intravenous (IV) administration of lidocaine has long been used as a modality to reduce airway reactivity and allow a patient to "tolerate" an endotracheal tube (ETT) and the stimulus it creates by blunting airway reflexes and preventing bronchoconstriction. The result is mixed, and the evidence for this practice is equivocal. IV dosing of lidocaine has indeed been shown to blunt reflex bronchoconstriction and relax airway smooth muscle,[25] but there are also reports of lidocaine possibly causing bronchoconstriction and having the opposite of the intended effect.[26] IV use for this purpose persists in the anesthesia community, so exercising caution and close monitoring are the most prudent choice, as with any other pharmacologic agent given for a therapeutic purpose.

Adverse reactions from toxic levels of local anesthetics include central nervous system effects, such as tinnitus and even convulsions, or cardiovascular effects, such as conduction abnormalities and even cardiovascular collapse. Some local anesthetic agents (particularly esters) may be associated with allergic reactions, but these types of reactions are rare. Benzocaine, in particular, has been associated with methemoglobinemia, but the dose required to reach a clinically significant problem with oxygen delivery is unclear. Finally, swallowing significant amounts of local anesthetics, such as might occur in preparation for intubation, can lead to significant nausea and vomiting and complicate management of the airway.

Adrenergic Drugs

Adrenergic drugs that affect the airway generally fall under the category of sympathomimetics. These drugs will be discussed more extensively later in the section regarding management of reactive airway disease, as that is the primary use for β-adrenergic drugs with respect to the lower airway. α-adrenergic activity, however, can also be relevant in the management of upper airway problems. Topical administration of sympathomimetics can be used to alter mucosal blood flow by their α-receptor effects causing vasoconstriction of small vessels. The most commonly used drug is epinephrine given in a nebulized form, which can be useful for postextubation croup or other clinical scenarios where there is a potential for upper airway bleeding. Phenylephrine and oxymetazoline are other commonly used drugs that are applied topically, cause vasoconstriction in the mucous membranes, and are potentially helpful when instrumentation of the airway is planned. This is particularly applicable when instrumenting the nasal passages because the chances of traumatic instrumentation

are high, and the ability to stop bleeding in that area is relatively low. Additionally, epinephrine is frequently added to local anesthetic formulations in an effort to prevent systemic spread by creating reduced blood flow to the applied area, leading to increased duration of action and reduced systemic absorption and toxicity.[27]

Care must be taken when using vasoactive adrenergic drugs in the airway, as there is a significant potential for systemic absorption and effect. Generally, the effects seen are cardiovascular in nature and include tachycardia or bradycardia, hypertension, dysrhythmia, tremor, and anxiety.

Volatile Anesthetics

The effects of volatile general anesthetic agents can be seen in both the upper and lower airways and in the form of both direct and indirect effects. In the upper airway, the effects are primarily indirect. The loss of coordinated muscle function in the pharynx leads to potential airway collapse. As indicated earlier, central suppression of arousal and respiratory control centers creates difficulty in maintaining a patent upper airway. This dynamic collapse is most often observed in spontaneous ventilation, because it is actually ameliorated in positive-pressure ventilation settings; this is similar to the phenomenon seen with neuromuscular blockade, which will be discussed later in the chapter. There is also a differential effect on the airway musculature in response to loss of central control. For example, the muscles controlled by the hypoglossal nerve seem to be more sensitive than other nerves to the loss of tone,[28] resulting in an initial posterior displacement of the tongue and soft palate creating airway collapse. This is indicative of the primary need for muscle coordination to maintain patency of the upper airway rather than simply muscle tone.

The effects of volatile agents on the lower airway have been well studied. Direct effects on the smooth muscle of the bronchial tree demonstrate a reduction in resting muscle tone as well as a reduction in the ability of the musculature to create bronchoconstriction.[29-35] These effects are thought to be mediated by intracellular actions of the volatile agents that reduce extracellular calcium influx, intrinsic calcium release to contractile components in the cell, and calcium sensitivity, as well as by intracellular blockade of the G-protein second messengers employed by cell membrane receptors to create muscle contraction in response to a stimulus, such as cholinergic input from the vagus nerve.[36] Additionally, volatile agents exert an indirect effect in that they are able to suppress the reflex neural pathways that contribute and lead to bronchoconstriction. The direct and indirect effects on the lower airway smooth muscle can be important in different situations. For example, bronchoconstriction in response to a noxious stimulus that is reflex mediated would respond more readily to the indirect effects of volatile anesthetics; however, constriction in response to locally mediated inflammation or tissue damage might respond more readily to the direct, cell-mediated effects of the drugs.

Volatile agents may also cause undesirable effects in the airway. Some halogenated agents can be irritating to the airway tissues and create bronchoconstriction independent of other stimuli. Isoflurane and desflurane have been implicated as being more irritating than halothane.[37] Desflurane may be the worst offender; isoflurane creates a net relaxation of bronchial smooth muscle despite its irritant effects, but desflurane has been shown to possibly increase overall airway resistance despite its anesthetic effects.[38] The stimulation of airway receptors possibly contributes to the tachycardia and hypertension that accompany high concentrations of desflurane administration.[39] Evidently, the irritant effects may be manageable and modulated because opioids given concomitantly have been shown to decrease them.[40] Sevoflurane demonstrates less airway irritation than the other available volatile anesthetics,[41] and as a result it is frequently used as the preferred agent for inhalational induction of general anesthesia. Other detrimental effects of volatile anesthetics include decreased mucociliary function and the inability to effectively clear secretions from the lower airway by either direct or indirect mechanisms.[42–45] The potential harmful sequelae from this would be evident in postoperative pulmonary complications after anesthesia, which are potentially catastrophic to patients; however, the clinical significance of the contribution of volatile agents to any particular pulmonary complication is unclear.

Intravenous Anesthetics

The effect of IV anesthetic agents on the upper airway is very similar to the effect of volatile anesthetics. The comparison is an apt one; both types of agents create their effects by loss of reticular activating system input to motor neurons of the upper airway. Again, the loss of coordination of the pharyngeal musculature rather than specific muscle dysfunction produces a dynamic airway collapse with spontaneous ventilation. In the case of IV agents, there is variable differential resistance to the effects of the anesthetic; as a result, it seems that airway collapse may be more resultant from posterior displacement of the soft palate and epiglottis rather than the tongue (Fig. 6.4).[46] The effects of IV anesthetics on the upper airway are comparable to the effects of sleep.

IV agents affect the lower airway indirectly by suppression of reflex neural pathway bronchoconstriction, in much the same way as the indirect effects of volatile agents. Barbiturates have this effect, but they also have been reported to create bronchoconstriction as well. The variable effects of different barbiturates are well described and range from direct constriction to histamine-mediated constriction to thromboxane-mediated increases in airway resistance.[47,48] The likelihood, however, is that none of these mechanisms creates a clinically significant effect on airway resistance.[49,50] Propofol is another anesthetic agent that strongly blunts neurally mediated airway reflexes; in addition, there seems to be some direct bronchodilatory effect with this drug.[51–54] Airway reactivity in patients who may be prone to bronchospasm seems to be blunted with propofol as compared with barbiturates.[55]

Ketamine is an interesting IV anesthetic drug in that its function as a sympathomimetic drug creates bronchodilation that may be more significant than that seen with other IV agents.[56] It has been used in the treatment of status asthmaticus successfully, so there is evidence for a clinically significant benefit. Ketamine also depresses neural reflex pathways like the other IV anesthetics, but it does not have the same differential effect on upper airway musculature that many other drugs have.[57] The effect of this may be one of possible preservation of upper airway patency and muscular coordination.

Benzodiazepines

Benzodiazepines seem not to have a significant impact on the function of the airway. They have the same general effects on the upper airway that other hypnotic drugs have, in that they have the ability to reduce the patency of the upper airway indirectly by decreasing arousal and muscle tone. There are γ-aminobutyric acid receptors in airway nerves that may contribute to the attenuation of reflex bronchoconstriction,[58] but the importance of this is unclear. There may also be some central action that reduces resting

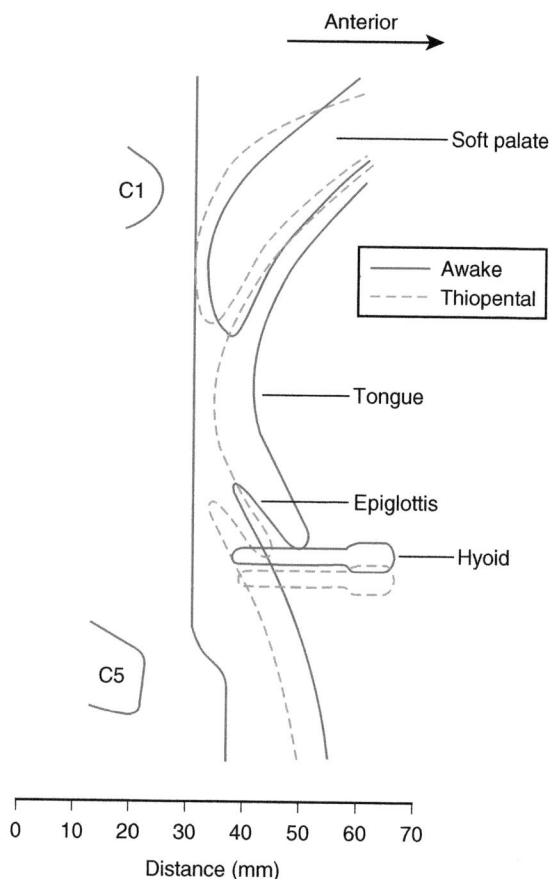

• **Fig. 6.4** Effects of thiopental anesthesia on airway dimensions. Notice that the primary site of obstruction is at the level of the soft palate. (Modified from Nandi PR, Charlesworth CH, Taylor SJ, et al. Effect of GA on the pharynx. *Br J Anaesth.* 1991;66:157.)

smooth muscle tone; but again, the clinical significance is questionable. At the very least, we can confidently state that benzodiazepines do not have a detrimental effect on lower airway smooth muscle tone and have an expected effect on the patency of the upper airway that is comparable with other IV hypnotic agents.

Opioids

Opioids have numerous effects on the airway.[59] First and foremost, upper airway tone and patency may be reduced to a similar degree as with hypnotic agents if sufficient opioids are administered to induce somnolence in a patient. Some opioids (e.g., morphine and meperidine) are implicated in causing histamine release, which may cause bronchoconstriction in susceptible patients. The clinical relevance of this is controversial because opioids have inversely been shown to decrease reflex bronchoconstriction and attenuate vagally mediated bronchial tone.[60] Contradictory evidence has also been presented that demonstrates that fentanyl and morphine may actually increase tracheal tone,[61] but this does not seem to be clinically relevant.

When opioid medications are combined with hypnotic agents, attenuation of airway reflexes is increased beyond what is seen with either agent alone.[62] This indicates a variable mechanism that can be initiated and increased with the use of multiple agents; this is a potentially clinically significant finding for conducting an anesthetic or for simply managing the airway in patients who may be prone to airway reactivity. Such strategies will be discussed at the end of this chapter when looking specifically at patients at risk for bronchospasm. Other effects of opioids on the lower airway are of questionable significance.

Another effect of opioids is that of muscle rigidity with administration of large doses in a short period of time, especially with the phenylpiperidine class of opioids (i.e., fentanyl, sufentanil, etc.). This can lead to difficulty with mask ventilation, which is commonly attributed to "chest wall rigidity." Studies in intubated patients and patients with tracheostomies, however, have shown that decreases in pulmonary compliance as a result of chest wall rigidity are not sufficient to explain an inability to mask ventilate after a large dose of opioid,[63] and examination of the vocal cords during induction with opioids has shown that vocal cord closure is the primary cause of difficult ventilation after opioid-induced anesthesia.[64] Treatment with small doses of neuromuscular blocking drugs (NMBDs), naloxone, or topical lidocaine (laryngotracheal anesthesia) can be effective in relaxing the vocal cords to allow for mask ventilation and/or intubation.[64] The ability of opioids to significantly blunt airway reflexes, in combination with the pharmacokinetic profile of ultrashort-acting opioids such as remifentanil, allows the practitioner to have more options when managing the airway. Intubation can be reliably performed without neuromuscular blockade using high doses of remifentanil; because of remifentanil's short duration of action, this technique adequately blunts the hemodynamic effects of laryngoscopy while allowing a fast recovery.[65,66] Another technique allows patients to be emerged from hypnotic anesthesia under the influence of deep remifentanil analgesia and able to tolerate an ETT while awake; this may possibly reduce the need to rely on deep extubation for patients who have reactive airways and allows for rapid emergence and extubation from anesthesia without the detrimental hemodynamic effects that may be seen from activation of airway reflexes. Finally, short-acting drugs like remifentanil have, in many instances, replaced other sedative agents for procedures that require some level of sedation but not general anesthesia. Caution must be exercised, however, because of the potential for upper airway collapse and apnea with increasing doses of opioids.

Neuromuscular Blocking Drugs

NMBDs are frequently used during airway management to prevent patient movement and facilitate intubation by removing the motor reflex response to airway manipulation. These agents only work at nicotinic acetylcholine (ACh) receptors, meaning that they only cause neuromuscular blockade in the skeletal muscle fibers of the upper airway but not in the smooth muscle fibers of the lower airway. Similar to inhalational and intravenous anesthetic agents, NMBDs create differential effects in the various skeletal muscles of the airway. The diaphragm and laryngeal muscles are most resistant to their effects (and are among the most resistant in the body),[67] meaning that a higher serum level of drug is required to completely block their function than is required for other muscles in the upper airway or in the body. This differential blockade carries a great deal of clinical importance. First, when establishing intubating conditions with the use of these agents, a sufficient dose must be given to abolish the motor control of the larynx; the consequence of insufficient block may be reflex activation of the laryngeal muscles and, possibly, laryngospasm. Second, differential blockade may be manifested to the detriment of the patient during the recovery from neuromuscular blockade and extubation of the trachea. Assessment of spontaneous ventilation

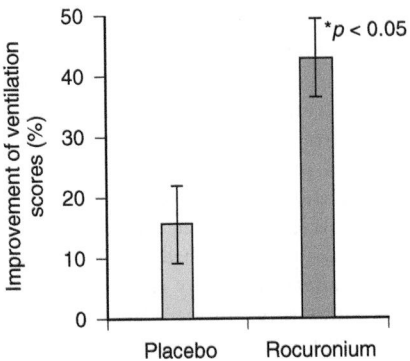

• **Fig. 6.5** Efficacy of face-mask ventilation in anesthetized patients with or without neuromuscular blockade. (From Szabo TA, Reves JG, Spinale FG, et al. Neuromuscular blockade facilitates mask ventilation. *Anesthesiology.* 2008;109:A184.)

before extubation without confirmation of complete recovery from neuromuscular blockade may be insufficient to determine successful ventilation after removal of the artificial airway. The reason is that adequate spontaneous ventilation can be achieved with only recovery of the diaphragm, but when an artificial airway is removed and the upper airway musculature is weak, there is a high likelihood of airway collapse and an inability to ventilate. Monitoring of neuromuscular blockade in the least resistant muscles, such as those innervated by peripheral motor nerves, is recommended to prevent such a circumstance from occurring.

Patency of the upper airway is an important factor modulated by NMBDs, and the effect is essentially the same as that seen with other anesthetic agents. Essentially, the loss of muscle tone and neural control leads to flaccid paralysis and increased airway collapsibility. Again, when a low level of drug is introduced and there is differential blockade, the loss of coordination of the pharyngeal apparatus becomes paramount and creates a tendency toward collapse with the negative inspiratory forces created by the diaphragm. NMBDs are somewhat different, however, in that a sufficiently high dose will create flaccid paralysis in all the musculature equally. Although the effects of this are obvious in spontaneously ventilating patients (apnea), there is some debate regarding the effects of NMBDs when positive-pressure mask ventilation is performed. Dogmatic views of airway management in the past have mandated the avoidance of neuromuscular blockade without confirmation of the ability to mask ventilate a patient; the fear of a possible situation where neither mask ventilation nor intubation is possible was the driving force behind this principle. In fact, however, more recent evidence has demonstrated an improved ability to manage the upper airway in the presence of rocuronium-induced blockade (Fig. 6.5).[68] The mechanism for this is postulated to be primarily attributable to relaxation of the laryngeal musculature, preventing vocal cord closure that would interfere with mask ventilation. Emerging thought processes in management of the airway advocate early use of neuromuscular blockade in a difficult airway situation in an attempt to facilitate maneuvers that would rescue it, such as mask ventilation, supraglottic airway placement, tracheal intubation, and surgical airway.[69,70] If the airway is, in fact, easier to manage with the effects of NMBDs, then it may be conceptualized that the upper airway has "increased patency" compared with an upper airway without neuromuscular blockade. It should be noted that the "increased patency" is dependent on active positive-pressure ventilation, and there would be airway collapse without that.

There are various effects of NMBDs on the lower airway. Some agents, such as tubocurarine or atracurium, cause histamine release and the associated potential for bronchoconstriction.[71] Others, such as pancuronium and rapacuronium, have been shown to create secondary muscarinic antagonism and possible increased airway resistance because of preganglionic parasympathetic M_2-receptor blockade.[72] Succinylcholine may have the effect of increasing tracheal tone by occupying muscarinic receptors and creating a surrogate for vagal activity. Additionally, succinylcholine has been shown to increase airway reactivity to ACh and possibly causes bronchospasm by this mechanism.[73] The clinical significance of any of these effects is unclear, and the potential for bronchospasm does not prevent succinylcholine from being widely used when indicated for rapid sequence induction or for any other purposes to create depolarizing neuromuscular blockade. The other agents mentioned previously are no longer widely used in the United States, and the newer agents that are commonly used do not have the complex side effect pharmacology that confounds their usage.

Reversal Agents for Neuromuscular Blocking Drugs

The use of neostigmine or other anticholinesterase medications for reversal of nondepolarizing NMBDs may potentially lead to increases in lower airway resistance. This potential effect is countered by coadministration with an anticholinergic drug, such as glycopyrrolate, and no change in airway smooth muscle tone is usually noted.[74] Inadequate reversal of neuromuscular blockade is more problematic, however, with pulmonary complications creating the bulk of morbidity and mortality.[75]

The modified γ-cyclodextrin sugammadex provides an alternative reversal agent for the aminosteroid NMBDs rocuronium and vecuronium.[76] Sugammadex binds aminosteroids within minutes and is rapidly cleared through the kidneys as an unmodified drug complex. It is contraindicated in patients with severe renal disease. The dosage is largely dependent on patient weight and the depth of neuromuscular block and is ineffective in the setting of non-aminosteroid NMBDs, such as cisatracurium or succinylcholine.

Cyclodextrins are ringlike structures composed of sugar units with a hydrophobic interior and a hydrophilic exterior. As rocuronium has a steroidlike structure, it binds to sugammadex with 1:1 stoichiometry and with high affinity as it becomes encapsulated within the hydrophobic core of the modified γ-cyclodextrin. This reverses muscle paralysis by reducing the plasma levels of free rocuronium.

Pharmacokinetic competitive binding analysis with other drugs has found that interference of sugammadex binding of NMBDs is unlikely; however, encapsulation of etonogestrel, a progestin used in contraception, is possible, and it is recommended that nonhormonal means of contraception should be used for up to 1 week after administration.[77] Despite this, the administration of 4 mg/kg of sugammadex to humans has shown no clinical effects to serum progesterone or related steroid hormones.[78] Potential adverse effects, while rare, include hypersensitivity (particularly at higher doses) and cardiac arrhythmias (e.g., bradycardia).[79]

Airway Pharmacology for Reactive Airway Disease

Overview

Pharmacology with respect to the airway also involves primary airway pathology and drugs that are used to treat such pathology.

The best example of this is in the group of conditions referred to as "reactive airway disease," which includes asthma and some forms of COPD. Patients with these conditions exhibit a heightened tendency toward bronchoconstriction and airway irritability and, in fact, may be at higher risk for complications in the perioperative period or the time surrounding airway instrumentation.[50,80] This section will use the pathology and treatment of asthma as a model for discussing some of the commonly used drugs that directly impact the airway and, later on, as a model for the prevention and treatment of perioperative bronchospasm, as the pharmacology surrounding both conditions is very similar.

Pathology

Asthma is one of the most prevalent diseases in the United States, with over 10 million cases, and in the rest of the world, with over 300 million cases. It is also a large driver of healthcare costs and hospital visits and is a potentially fatal disease, with hundreds of thousands of deaths each year.[81] The cause for its development in any one patient is unclear, and like many other systemic diseases, it is likely caused by a combination of factors. Nevertheless, there are common traits among many of the patients who suffer with asthma, and one of the most common traits is a tendency toward atopy, or a tendency to create antibody-mediated reactions toward one or many triggering allergens. Many patients also have a strong family history of asthma, indicating a genetic predisposition toward its development. Environmental and other controllable factors often play a role in either the development and/or exacerbation of asthma, such as obesity and exposure to tobacco smoke or dust mites.

Several features related to the airway are typical of the patient with asthma, and the four key features that seem to play the largest roles are (1) inflammation of the lower airway, (2) airway hyperresponsiveness, (3) loss of patency of the lower airways, and (4) remodeling of the airway structure over the long term. The inflammatory response is likely the most important and most insidious of the four. Hundreds of mediators are implicated in creating an inflammatory response in the airway, and that response may be attributable to any number of triggers in a particular patient. The humoral immune responses of atopic individuals are amplified, so the inflammation is triggered even more swiftly in these individuals. The same mediators that govern the inflammatory response also create in airway smooth muscles an overreaction to noxious stimuli, leading to the hallmark of airway hyperresponsiveness commonly seen in asthmatics. These patients will often have clinically significant bronchoconstriction that is more severe than what is seen in a normal subject. This hyperreactivity leads directly to the possibility of decreased airway patency as a result of constriction of bronchial smooth muscle, manifested by some of the previously discussed reflex pathways that mediate the airway response to an unwanted stimulus. Another reason for loss of airway patency is the remodeling of the structural elements of the airway that is seen in asthma patients. Although smooth muscle contractions are primarily responsible for acute asthma symptoms, remodeling is at least partially responsible for the natural history of the disease over the lifetime of the patient. Fig. 6.6 illustrates some of the cell types that lead to such structural changes.

Treatment of Asthma

The clinical management of asthma involves controlling all the processes detailed previously with regard to the disease process. Each patient must be evaluated as to the extent of the disease and the types of symptoms that are experienced. For example,

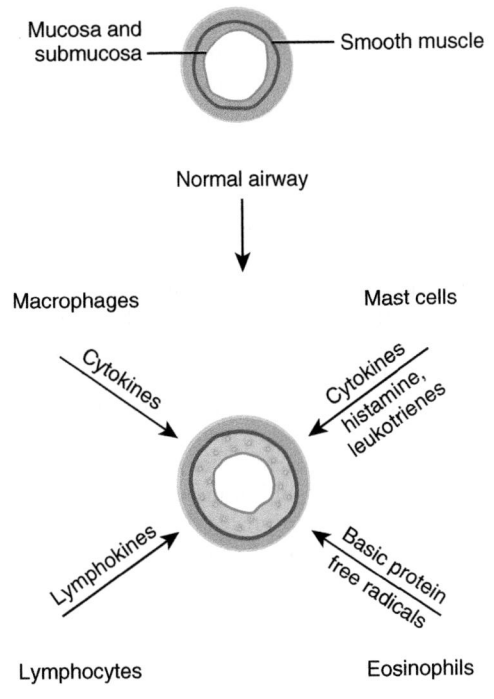

• **Fig. 6.6** Changes in the cross-sectional anatomy of normal and asthmatic airways, with some of the factors influencing the physical changes in the lower airways. Note the thickening of the smooth muscle and submucosa, associated with infiltration of inflammatory cells.

TABLE 6.1	Stepwise Approach to Asthma Management in Adults	
Asthma Treatment Step	**Drug Therapy**	
1. Mild intermittent asthma	SABA as needed	
2. Persistent mild asthma	IGC + as needed SABA or as needed SABA/IGC combination	
3. Add-on controller therapy	LABA with IGC (LM and/or LAMA)	
4. Therapy for persistent poor control	Increase IGC/LABA and add LAMA (or LM, consider biologic therapy)	
5. Therapy with continual or frequent systemic GC	Increase IGC/LABA/LAMA (add alternative agents/biologics)	

BA, β-Agonist; *GC*, glucocorticoid; *IGC*, inhaled glucocorticoid; *LABA*, long-acting β-agonist; *LAMA*, long-acting muscarinic antagonist; *LM*, leukotriene modifier; *SABA*, short-acting β-agonist.
For drugs listed in parentheses, consider addition of one or more agents.

some patients may only experience episodic wheezing and airway reactivity that may only require symptomatic treatment, whereas others may experience a more severe course involving continuous inflammation that requires continuous pharmacologic therapy with multiple agents. The primary goals of therapy are to reduce the severity of symptoms experienced by the patient and to reduce the risk of severe complications of the disease, such as hospitalization as a result of acute attacks and morbidity related to poor pulmonary status. The treatment for asthma varies with the presentation of the disease, and four distinct clinical states can be observed: episodic presentation, persistent asthma, exacerbation of chronic symptoms, and severe acute asthma. The last category includes the most worrisome and immediately life-threatening entity, status asthmaticus, which is often found to be resistant to commonly used pharmacologic agents and may require mechanical ventilation. Several medical societies in various countries have set forth guidelines and updates on the development of new strategies to manage asthma, and they attempt to educate healthcare providers in the best strategies to manage patients with this complex disease.[82–84] These guidelines are publicly available and are intended to educate both practitioners and patients about the disease process and provide information on therapies and coping strategies. Table 6.1 outlines a stepwise approach to organize pharmacologic therapy in asthma patients.

Drug Treatments for Asthma

The mainstay for asthma treatment is pharmacologic therapy, and multiple different classes of agents are used. A helpful approach to conceptualizing each drug is to categorize it as a reliever or a controller. In other words, some drugs (usually those with a rapid onset and short duration of action) are most useful in relieving acute symptoms of asthma during episodic presentation or exacerbation. Other drugs are more useful over the long term for controlling persistent symptoms, preventing acute exacerbations, reducing inflammatory processes, and, hopefully, inhibiting airway remodeling. Finding the best combination of drugs that will maximize both patient compliance and disease management is a complex and dynamic goal.

Beta-adrenergic Agonists

Adrenergic agents have been discussed previously with respect to the upper airway, but the primary use of these drugs is in the lower airway to modulate airway smooth muscle tone. To this end, β-adrenergic agonists are used because of the presence of a large number of β_2-adrenergic receptors in the lower airway. The action of these drugs is to bind to the receptor and initiate an intracellular G protein–coupled response that increases intracellular cyclic adenosine monophosphate (cAMP) and subsequently decreases the intracellular availability of calcium ions to participate in the contraction of smooth muscle.[85] Thus, the effect is more related to prevention of smooth muscle contraction rather than active relaxation of the muscle; however, the clinical effect is the same because of the fact that airway smooth muscle is controlled by a baseline vagal tone. Although the primary, and most useful, effect of β-agonists is in modulating airway resistance, there are secondary actions as well. There is evidence that they help modulate the actions of other neurotransmitters such as ACh and prevent degranulation of mast cells, and it is possible that they reduce inflammation, alter bronchial blood flow by modulating vascular tone, stimulate mucociliary action, and change the composition of mucous secretions in the airway.

β-agonist drugs can be classified as short acting or long acting with respect to their utility for treatment of asthma. They can additionally be classified based on the specificity of their interactions with β-receptors: Some are mixed β_1- and β_2-agonists, some are β_1-selective agonists, and others are β_2-selective agonists. Selective β_1-agonists will not be discussed because the predominant adrenergic receptor present in the airway is the β_2-receptor.

The differentiation between the selectivity of the various agents is important in predicting their effects and side effects. The most commonly prescribed drug for the treatment of asthma is albuterol, a short-acting, β_2-selective drug. It can be administered as an aerosolized suspension by metered dose inhaler or by nebulizer and has a duration of action of 4 to 6 hours.[86,87] Terbutaline is another selective β_2-agonist that is less commonly used in the treatment of asthma. It has a similar duration of action to albuterol and is essentially equivalent when inhaled[88]; however, it is the only selective agent that can be also be administered parenterally (IV or subcutaneously [SQ]) and consequently has clinical utility in patients who are unable to receive the drug directly in the airway. The most commonly used long-acting β-agonists are salmeterol and formoterol, and these drugs have a duration of action as long as 12 hours.[89] They are frequently administered in conjunction with glucocorticoids via inhalation and are useful for long-term control of asthma symptoms and prevention of exacerbation. Finally, nonselective agents are available, such as epinephrine and isoproterenol. Generally, their use is avoided on a routine basis because of the high risk of cardiovascular side effects with nonselective adrenergic receptor stimulation; however, they may be useful in emergency situations. Epinephrine, in particular, can be administered SQ or IV and has been shown to be greatly effective as a first-line emergency drug for severe bronchoconstrictive attacks.

As discussed, β-agonists have potential cardiovascular side effects, including tachycardia, hypertension, hypotension, and dysrhythmia. Other side effects include tremor and anxiety. An additional consideration with regard to the treatment of asthma with β-agonists is the evidence suggesting that using these agents as monotherapy results in an increase in asthma-related mortality; this phenomenon has been termed the "asthma paradox."[90] A number of explanations are proposed for this finding,[91–95] some of which postulate that long-term β-agonism may lead to enhanced airway reactivity by an unknown mechanism. Another theory suggests that continuous β-receptor-driven bronchodilation may mask underlying inflammatory symptoms that then go untreated; the result is continual airway inflammation with remodeling and thickening of the airway wall that eventually can no longer be compensated for.[96] Regardless of the mechanism, current recommendations are to avoid sole therapy with β-agonist drugs in treating chronic asthma for fear of increased mortality.

Glucocorticoids

Glucocorticoids are the most effective and one of the most widely used drug types in the treatment of asthma. Glucocorticoids can be administered via various routes including topical, oral, and IV; however, most effective and useful for this discussion is the inhaled route. Inhaled glucocorticoids have become a mainstay in the treatment of asthma and other pulmonary disorders; they are formulated such that they can be aerosolized and administered by metered dose inhalers, much like β-agonists. Unlike β-agonists, however, they are not useful for acute control of asthma exacerbations but rather are used in chronic therapy for long-term control of persistent disease.

Glucocorticoids exert their actions primarily by a single mechanism; they enter the cytoplasm of a target cell to bind cytoplasmic steroid receptors and subsequently enter the nucleus of the cell to alter DNA activity and change gene expression by either activating or repressing transcription. The downstream effect of this is an alteration in normal cellular function at multiple levels, but the observed effect is the result of changes in the amount and types of enzymes, receptors, cytokines, adhesion molecules, and so on produced by the cell and expressed on the cell membrane, functioning within the cell, or released by the cell into the surrounding environment.[97,98] In the case of glucocorticoids in relation to

asthma, there is a clear reduction in inflammatory cell recruitment, survival, and activity.[99,100] Another beneficial effect seen with glucocorticoid treatment is a reduction in lung hyperperfusion that is seen in asthmatic patients; this results in a reduction in the washout by the pulmonary circulation of asthma-related drugs from the effect site in the lungs, leading to an increase in the duration of action and a decrease in clearance of partner drugs.[101] Finally, glucocorticoids have an important synergistic interaction with β-agonists resulting in a potentiation of their actions.[102,103] In terms of pharmacokinetics, glucocorticoids have a relatively large volume of distribution in the body and are cleared by the hepatic cytochrome P450 system, so they are subject to drug interactions and physiologic states that alter liver enzyme activity.

The adverse effects of systemic glucocorticoid therapy present a problematic concern in the treatment of asthma. Although low-dose therapy with inhaled agents does not typically carry a large risk, some systemic absorption is nonetheless possible. In patients with severe disease, high-dose inhaled therapy or oral therapy may be necessary, with a real risk of systemic side effects, including osteoporosis, osteonecrosis, systemic hypertension, diabetes mellitus, obesity, skin thinning, myopathy, cataracts, and glaucoma.[83] A common concern with chronic, systemic steroid therapy is suppression of the hypothalamic-pituitary-adrenal axis and possible acute adrenal crisis if therapy is interrupted or discontinued; this is not as likely with low-dose inhaled therapy. A particular problem seen with inhaled glucocorticoids is the development of oral candidiasis,[104] so patients receiving chronic therapy should be monitored.

Inhaled glucocorticoids are either administered individually or combined with long-acting β-agonists for concurrent therapy. Examples of commonly available agents are beclomethasone, budesonide, fluticasone, flunisolide, and mometasone. Oral and parenteral therapy are also available in a variety of agents, some of which are used in a daily prescription, whereas others are more commonly used for higher-dose "pulse" treatment in patients who have experienced an exacerbation or life-threatening event. Examples include prednisone, prednisolone, methylprednisone, methylprednisolone, betamethasone, dexamethasone, and hydrocortisone.

Methylxanthines

Methylxanthines represent a class of drug that has been commonly used in asthma therapy for several decades. The most often used agents are theophylline and aminophylline; other naturally occurring compounds such as caffeine and theobromine may also have therapeutic value. These drugs are typically classified as phosphodiesterase inhibitors, but they have a multitude of additional actions that seem to be unrelated to phosphodiesterase inhibition.[105,106] They cause an increase in intracellular cAMP levels that should create a similar bronchodilating effect as β-agonists, but the plasma levels required to achieve this effect are not achieved at standard therapeutic doses. They also increase mucociliary clearance, increase ventilatory drive and diaphragm function, and perhaps have some degree of antiinflammatory action. Individually, these effects seem to fail the test of clinical significance, but the overall picture observed with these drugs is a reduction in symptomatic burden in chronic asthma sufferers. Additionally, IV loading of aminophylline is useful in the treatment of acute asthma exacerbation. This class of drug has fallen off the mainstay of asthma treatment and is generally used as an adjuvant therapy in poorly controlled patients or those who tolerate traditional medications poorly.

Methylxanthines are metabolized in the liver and have clearance rates that are highly variable. Smokers and patients with low cardiac output are especially prone to prolonged clearance times, and these agents should be used with caution in these populations. Regular monitoring of theophylline levels is recommended in patients who are undergoing therapy as a result of the potential for adverse side effects. The most common problems encountered are central nervous system stimulation, tremor, insomnia, convulsions, and cardiovascular toxicity with atrial and ventricular dysrhythmias. Nausea and vomiting are also commonly seen during treatment with methylxanthines.

Leukotriene Modifiers

Leukotrienes, one of the end products of arachidonic acid metabolism, are inflammatory mediators involved in the body's general inflammatory response, particularly in the airway. They cause bronchoconstriction, increase blood flow, support inflammatory processes, and also create localized edema, glandular secretion, and cell recruitment for inflammation.[107–109] Modulation of this activity was thought to be a potential new avenue for asthma treatment, and, indeed, antagonist agents were developed and entered clinical practice as the most recent advancement in asthma therapy. This class of drug can be separated into leukotriene antagonists, which bind to transmembrane receptors and competitively inhibit leukotriene action, and 5-lipoxygenase inhibitors, which prevent the production of leukotrienes and reduce their availability in the body to create undesirable effects. There is only one 5-lipoxygenase inhibitor on the market: zileuton. Available leukotriene antagonists include the drugs montelukast, pranlukast, and zafirlukast.

Leukotriene modifiers are used as controlling medications and are not useful in the event of an acute asthma attack. As monotherapy, they are less effective than other available agents for asthma control, but they are frequently added to a patient's regimen in an attempt to reduce the dose of steroid necessary and are effective in that regard.[110] They are orally administered and are most frequently administered in several doses each day, so patient compliance can be an issue. Toxicity is rare, but there is potential for elevation of liver enzymes that may require monitoring, particularly with zileuton. Additional side effects include abdominal discomfort, muscle weakness, and pain.

Anticholinergic Agents

The contribution of parasympathetic activity to resting bronchial smooth muscle tone in the airway and the potential for increased muscarinic activity to create an effective reduction in lower airway patency have been previously discussed. Of the three types of muscarinic receptors whose activity may be modulated by anticholinergic drugs, the M_3-receptor is the most important in that it is present on the surface of airway smooth muscle cells. M_1-receptors are ganglionic receptors that facilitate parasympathetic transmission, so blockade of these receptors is also beneficial to asthma control. M_2-receptors, however, are ganglionic receptors that block ACh release in the ganglion, so blockade of these would actually increase parasympathetic transmission and would be detrimental to treatment. Thus, the ideal treatment with anticholinergic agents would be one with local effect that avoids ganglionic effects altogether; this is accomplished via inhalational administration. Available anticholinergic agents for inhalational administration are ipratropium, which has an onset of 15 to 30 minutes and a duration of action of 3 to 5 hours, and tiotropium, which has a slower onset and a longer duration of action as long as 1 week.

Other available drugs are parenteral anticholinergics that are well known for other purposes, such as atropine and glycopyrrolate. This is a far less used approach because of the high incidence of side effects that can occur from systemic administration, such as increased heart rate, blurry vision, dry mouth, and confusion.

The utility of anticholinergic therapy is highly dependent on the individual and the baseline contribution of parasympathetic activity to bronchial tone. Anticholinergics do not have antiinflammatory action and, thus, are unlikely to alter the overall progression of disease. They can, however, be effective in acute management or in long-term management of bronchoconstrictive symptoms. In fact, the combination of ipratropium and β-agonists has been shown to be superior to monotherapy with β-agonists, and ipratropium has also shown effectiveness in patients with bronchoconstriction related to β-blocker overdose.[111–113] Tiotropium has become a common drug used in the treatment of COPD, and we have seen a resurgence of long-acting muscarinic antagonist medications in the treatment of persistent asthma. Several new agents on the market include combination therapy with a steroid, long-acting β-agonist, and long-acting muscarinic antagonist as a single inhalational therapy.

Chromoglycates

Cromolyn sodium and nedocromil comprise the group of drugs called *chromoglycates*. These are plant-derived agents that are somewhat useful in prevention of asthma symptoms and bronchospasm. Their efficacy is moderate, and the proposed mechanism of action is the prevention of mast cell degranulation and the downstream inflammatory effects that occur as a result. The exact mechanism of the prevention of release of inflammatory substances from mast cells is somewhat unclear, but some usefulness for these drugs is seen in immunoglobulin-mediated, antigen-induced asthma. They are also frequently used as pretreatment in patients with exercise-induced asthma before exertion. Note that chromoglycates are not effective after bronchospasm has occurred; they must be administered before the event as a controller and preventer, hence the efficacy in patients who have known and discrete inciting factors for asthma attacks. Response to these drugs is quite variable, and therapeutic trials in individual patients will help determine a benefit from these agents.

Chromoglycates are administered via the inhalational route by metered dose inhalers and are poorly absorbed into the systemic circulation. Cromolyn is also available for nebulization. The formulations are somewhat irritating to the oropharyngeal mucosa but, otherwise, significant toxicity or side effects are rare. Anaphylaxis is reported but also very rare. The drugs are excreted in urine and bile without being metabolized significantly.

Alternative Agents and Future Directions

Several other agents exist that are infrequently used in patients who are refractory to traditional therapy or require additional therapy to minimize the use of steroids or other agents because of adverse effects. That discussion is beyond the scope of this chapter, and these agents can be reviewed in detail in the review articles listed in the Selected References section at the end of this chapter.

Current avenues of research are attempting to uncover new classes of drugs that might have some action in the airway;[114] most are exploring different ways to modulate the inflammatory response and remodeling that occur with asthma because these are the features that are currently the most difficult to effectively control in patients with very severe disease. Newer biologic agents currently in use target the humoral immune response of asthma patients (anti-IgE) and cytokines produced from chronic airway inflammation (anti-IL5/4/13). These treatments are reserved for patients with severe persistent disease or those with a clear allergic component precipitating asthma symptoms. Finally, nonpharmacologic treatments are also under development, such as radiofrequency treatment of the airway to reduce smooth muscle mass. Long-term outcomes for these therapies are still under investigation.

Perioperative Approach to the Patient With a Reactive Airway

The perioperative period presents an opportunity to examine the management of asthma and the ramifications of managing the airway of an asthmatic in an acute setting. One of the most potentially dangerous consequences that can arise in the patient with reactive airway disease perioperatively is a severe broncho-constrictive process that is commonly referred to as *bronchospasm*. The result of bronchospasm in a patient is a potential inability to ventilate and oxygenate, often resulting in desaturation events and hypercarbia; the event can be so severe as to be life threatening.

The keys to preventing such a disastrous outcome include identifying those patients who may be at increased risk for these events, assessing if the patient's condition is optimized to minimize the risk of such an event occurring, developing a prevention plan for the perioperative period that involves appropriate pharmacologic agents and an optimal anesthetic plan, and developing an action plan for the treatment of bronchospasm if it were to occur in the period involving the management of the airway or during an operation. The preceding sections of this chapter have set forth a strong foundation for understanding the pharmacologic concepts and agents that are available for modulating this perioperative risk, so the remaining task is to understand how to select the proper agents and identify the correct actions to prevent an undesirable outcome with a patient.

Proactive Management—Prevention of Bronchospasm

The first step in prevention of bronchospasm is identification of those at increased risk for the event. Generally, people with a diagnosis of asthma or COPD are considered to be particularly at risk given that a component of their disease is airway hyperreactivity. Those patients with poor control over their disease are at highest risk; those with well-controlled and mild disease may not necessarily face an increased risk of perioperative events. Additionally, those who are currently or have recently suffered from respiratory illness are noted to be at heightened risk for bronchospasm as well; this becomes particularly important in the pediatric population given a seasonal propensity for upper and lower respiratory infections. There is debate regarding the appropriate optimization and necessary timing surrounding a respiratory infection and scheduling of an elective surgery; that discussion is beyond the scope of this chapter. Smokers and patients suffering from gastroesophageal reflux disease are also potentially at heightened risk for bronchospasm. Patients who have previously experienced bronchospasm around the time of surgery have an independent risk factor, and such a history should be elicited in the preoperative evaluation whenever possible. Finally, the location of surgery may pose an additional risk; those patients having surgery on the airway or in major body cavities (abdomen or thorax) seem to have a higher incidence of events.

The next consideration is proper optimization of a patient's medical status before undergoing an operation to minimize, as much as possible, his or her individual risk for bronchospasm. This involves ensuring medication compliance if a patient is currently being treated for a disease involving the airway; patients often show poor compliance and a lack of control of the disease resulting from that. Smoking cessation for as long as possible is a key factor in reducing risk of bronchospasm[115]; ideally, 2 months of smoking cessation would be achieved before undergoing an elective procedure. Adequate control of reflux disease is important as well, as there is an association between patients with reactive airway disease and acid reflux symptoms. Whenever possible, medications used for treatment of these conditions should be continued through the day of surgery and restarted in the perioperative period as soon as possible. Delaying elective surgery until control of active symptoms is achieved would be the most prudent option in preventing a potentially dangerous event from occurring[116]; it is inadvisable to place a patient at risk for such an event for the sake of expediency.

Prevention of bronchospasm before and during a procedure involves action at several steps along the way (Box 6.1). Preoperatively, one should ensure that airway inflammation is at the minimum level possible with adequate glucocorticoid administration. This may involve placing an at-risk patient on a 5-day "pulse" before the operation, and appropriate consideration should be given to the requirement of additional steroids perioperatively for those patients who have been on them chronically and have potential suppression of the hypothalamic axis and poor adrenal output. Next, still in the preoperative phase, adequate anxiolysis should be established because asthma may be exacerbated by emotional stress. This may be achieved with benzodiazepines or with other agents, such as the α_2-adrenergic agonists, clonidine, or dexmedetomidine. The latter agents may even provide some measure of bronchodilation. Third, the use of bronchodilators in the form of β-agonists and anticholinergics is indicated around the time of airway manipulation to attenuate the reflex bronchoconstriction that is bound to occur with such action.

The selection of an appropriate anesthetic plan is critical. Regional anesthesia may be a good option in that manipulation of the airway can be entirely avoided; however, evidence supporting this notion as a protective action is lacking. If general anesthesia is required, it may be beneficial to opt for a volatile anesthetic-based technique given that these agents are potent bronchodilators and will help attenuate any airway irritation or reactivity that is encountered during the course of a procedure. Choice of agent

---

• BOX 6.1 Prevention of Perioperative Bronchospasm

Optimization of baseline pharmacologic therapy and symptoms, continue medications up to day of surgery
Appropriate and adequate glucocorticoid preparation, if appropriate
Adequate preoperative anxiolysis and analgesia
Use of inhaled β-agonists (± anticholinergics) before airway instrumentation
Individually tailored anesthetic plan to provide bronchodilation with volatile agents when appropriate
Utilization of regional anesthesia and avoidance of airway instrumentation if possible
Topical or regional anesthesia of the airway before manipulation if indicated
Balanced anesthetic administration with use of intravenous lidocaine, propofol, opioids, and ketamine as indicated

is key because, as has been discussed, agents such as desflurane may have an increased airway irritant quality compared with other choices and may be better avoided. Additionally, nitrous oxide and opioid-based anesthetics seem to increase bronchospastic events and may not be the optimal choice of anesthetic technique.

When a patient with reactive airway disease requires an awake intubation, adequate preparation of the airway is critical with respect to topical local anesthetics or upper airway nerve blocks, as these techniques can help to blunt airway reflexes to noxious stimuli and prevent adverse events (see Chapter 13). Finally, a balanced anesthetic plan involving adequate analgesia with opioids or other drugs (e.g., propofol, ketamine, intravenous lidocaine), which have beneficial profiles with respect to bronchospasm, is beneficial. Intratracheal lidocaine may not be desirable during the time of airway manipulation because of the possibility of airway irritation. Extubation may be carried out under a deep level of anesthesia if deemed appropriate, but concerns regarding airway patency should take precedence in that decision.

Reactive Management—Treatment of Bronchospasm

The incidence of intraoperative bronchospasm is anywhere from 1.7% to 16%,[117] so it is a phenomenon that is encountered rather frequently during the provision of anesthetic care or management of the airway. Inciting events may include anaphylaxis, preexisting asthma or COPD, or simply the act of intubation when instrumenting the airway. These events are also commonly seen during the induction and emergence events perioperatively when the anesthetic level may be inadequate to suppress the airway's protective reflexes. It occurs in graded severity, but critical intraoperative bronchospasm is an anesthetic emergency. Following is a brief discussion of the management plan for intraoperative bronchospasm and some of the pharmacologic agents that can be employed in its management (Box 6.2).

The first step is to recognize the event as bronchospasm so that appropriate interventions can be performed; this requires a high level of vigilance during patient care. An examination of the patient may reveal wheezing, prolonged expiration, or loss of breath sounds in severe cases. Increased airway pressures are seen during mechanical ventilation, and capnography may show an upsloping curve indicative of an obstructive airway process. A differential diagnosis should be considered, and included in that should be the possibility of pneumothorax, mechanical

---

• **BOX 6.2** Management of Intraoperative Bronchospasm

Establish resources to be available before starting care of an at-risk patient.
Quickly recognize the problem and establish a differential diagnosis for evaluation.
Deepen level of anesthesia with volatile agent if possible.
Consider the use of intravenous hypnotic agents to deepen the anesthetic level if needed (propofol, lidocaine, ketamine).
Rapidly utilize inhaled β-agonists and consider the use of intravenous agents such as epinephrine in emergent or deteriorating situations.
Recognize the need for early use of corticosteroids and administer intravenously if needed for prevention of subsequent attacks.
Adjust ventilatory parameters to avoid excessive airway pressures and allow for adequate time for prolonged exhalation.

---

obstruction, aspiration, and pulmonary edema. These should be quickly ruled out as indicated by the situation, and attention should be given to the appropriate treatment immediately. The first treatment action should be to increase the anesthetic depth in a way that promotes bronchodilation. Adding or increasing volatile anesthetics may accomplish this, but delivery of these drugs may be difficult in severe bronchospasm. Intravenous agents such as propofol, ketamine, or lidocaine may alternatively be used. Inhaled bronchodilators (i.e., β-agonists) should be administered as soon as possible because they provide an additive benefit to that provided by volatile anesthetics; higher doses may be necessary as a result of deposition of the drug in the breathing equipment and reduced efficiency of delivery in acute bronchospasm.

In the event that all of the above interventions fail, intravenous bronchodilators may be necessary to overcome the severe bronchospasm. Epinephrine is the drug of choice and has proven to be beneficial when other drugs fail. Care should be taken to avoid undesirable cardiovascular side effects, but the urgency of treatment may supersede concerns about side effects. Glucocorticoids should also be considered for severe cases (both intravenous and inhalational), but the onset of action is slower and the benefit conferred will be for subsequent events. Other agents that may prove helpful include magnesium sulfate and nitrates. Methylxanthines do not seem to be helpful in acute treatment and only increase the risk of dysrhythmia.

Recovery from an acute bronchospastic event may not be straightforward. Up to 20% of patients will experience a postoperative deterioration in pulmonary status, so planning is necessary for additional care and appropriate monitoring.[118,119] Hospital admission may be necessary, and in some cases admission to the intensive care unit may be appropriate. In unexpected cases, anaphylaxis testing should be performed to identify possible inciting allergens and aid in prevention of future attacks.

Conclusion

Airway pharmacology is an important topic in the discussion of airway management. This chapter reviewed the general concepts related to pharmacology and physiology with regard to the airway and looked at the specific processes in the airway that are affected by pharmacologic agents. The effects of anesthetic drugs on the function and patency of the airway were discussed, highlighting the significant risk for airway compromise with the use of these drugs. The pharmacologic treatment of asthma was used as a model for illustrating the effects of various drugs that are intended to act in the airway. Finally, the pathophysiology of bronchospasm was reviewed with a focus on the use of pharmacologic agents to prevent and treat intraoperative bronchospasm. A sound understanding of the available drugs that act on the airway and the benefits and pitfalls associated with these drugs are critical to a thorough understanding of airway management.

Selected References

46. Nandi PR, Charlesworth CH, Taylor SJ, et al. Effect of general anaesthesia on the pharynx. *Br J Anaesth.* 1991;66:157–162.
56. Sih K, Campbell SG, Tallon JM, et al. Ketamine in adult emergency medicine: controversies and recent advances. *Ann Pharmacother.* 2011;45(12):1525–1534.
59. Ehsan Z, Mahmoud M, Shott SR, et al. The effects of anesthesia and opioids on the upper airway: a systematic review. *Laryngoscope.* 2016;126(1):270–284.

65. Durmus M, Ender G, Kadir BA, et al. Remifentanil with thiopental for tracheal intubation without muscle relaxants. *Anesth Analg.* 2003;96:1336–1339.

69. Calder I. Could "safe practice" be compromising safe practice? Should anaesthetists have to demonstrate that face mask ventilation is possible before giving a neuromuscular blocker? *Anaesthesia.* 2008;63:113–115.

80. Pinto Pereira LM, Orrett FA, Balbirsingh M. Physiological perspectives of therapy in bronchial hyperreactivity. *Can J Anaesth.* 1996;43:700–713.

83. Bateman ED, Hurd SS, Barnes PJ, et al. Global strategy for asthma management and prevention: GINA executive summary. *Eur Respir J.* 2008;31:143–178.

92. Page CP. Beta agonists and the asthma paradox. *J Asthma.* 1993;30:155–164.

116. Pera T, Penn RB. Bronchoprotection and bronchorelaxation in asthma: new targets, and new ways to target the old ones. *Pharmacol Ther.* 2016;164:82–96.

119. Woods BD, Sladen RN. Perioperative considerations for the patient with asthma and bronchospasm. *Br J Anaesth.* 2009;103:i57–i65.

All references can be found online at eBooks.Health.Elsevier.com.

7

Physiologic and Pathophysiologic Responses to Intubation

CHRISTOPHER ROSS

CHAPTER OUTLINE

KEY POINTS

- Laryngoscopy can variably induce bradycardia (via the vagal nerve) or hypertension (HTN) and tachycardia (mediated by the cardioaccelerator nerves and sympathetic chain ganglia). The former is most common in infants and children, whereas the latter is typical for adolescents and adults.

- Laryngoscopy and intubation result in stimulation of the central nervous system and may increase cerebral blood flow (CBF), which may result in elevated intracranial pressure (ICP). The exact ramifications of this short-term increase during intubation remain unclear. Sustained elevations in ICP can lead to brain herniation.

- Ischemic electrocardiographic changes lasting less than 10 minutes during airway manipulation have not been shown to correlate with postoperative myocardial infarction. Electrocardiographic changes that are more prolonged should be treated carefully as potential myocardial ischemia.

- Succinylcholine is associated with bradycardia in children, particularly when doses are repeated. The clinical relevance of this, however, may be negligible. In adults it appears to be a cardiovascular stimulant.

- Succinylcholine may directly elevate CBF and ICP, an effect that can be blunted by pretreatment with a nondepolarizing agent and adequate induction of anesthesia with intravenous agents. The administration of defasciculating doses of a nondepolarizing neuromuscular blocking drug (NMBD) to blunt elevations in ICP during intubation has not been shown to be effective.

- The application of cricoid pressure can result in a greater heart rate (HR) and blood pressure (BP) response to tracheal intubation than when it is not used; this should be considered when evaluating the risk-benefit ratio of this procedure in individual patients. This is especially true in pediatric patients for whom the evidence recommends against cricoid pressure.

- Fentanyl provides a graded response in blunting hemodynamic responses to intubation, with 2 µg/kg IV given several minutes before induction only partially preventing HTN and tachycardia during rapid sequence intubation (RSI).
- Fentanyl and propofol require several minutes, to achieve effect-site equilibrium after IV bolus administration. Therefore, the commonly observed practice of administering a 50 to 100 µg bolus of fentanyl simultaneously with administration of other induction medications would not be expected to have an adequate effect based on inadequate dose and inappropriate timing of administration.

- When given in a bolus of 1.5 mg/kg IV, lidocaine adds approximately 0.3 MAC (minimum alvaolar concentration) of anesthetic potency, but it is not reliable at blunting the cardiovascular or airway response to laryngoscopy or intubation.
- For surgeries lasting longer than 2 hours, cough and throat complaints may be decreased by inflating the cuff of the endotracheal tube (ETT) with a buffered solution containing 40 mg of lidocaine. This can be accomplished by using a 10-mL syringe containing 5 mL 1% lidocaine, 1 mL 8.4% $NaHCO_3$ solution, and 4 to 5 mL of sterile diluent and inflating the cuff until no leak is present.

Introduction

Airway management involves a myriad of manipulations to the airway and associated anatomic structures that vary from simple to complex. Airway assessment, laryngoscopy, tracheal intubation, and other airway manipulations (e.g., placement of a supraglottic airway [SGA]) are stimuli that have the potential to induce profound changes in cardiovascular and respiratory function. Although these responses may be of short duration and of little consequence in healthy individuals, serious complications can occur in the critically ill and in patients with underlying comorbidities, including hypertension (HTN),[1] coronary artery disease,[2] reactive airways,[3] and intracranial neuropathology.[4]

Cardiovascular Responses During Airway Manipulation

Cardiovascular Reflexes

The cardiovascular responses to airway manipulation are initiated by sensory receptors responding to tissue irritation in the supraglottic region and in the trachea.[5] Located in close proximity to the airway mucosa, these sensory receptors consist of mechanoreceptors with small-diameter myelinated fibers, slowly adapting stretch receptors with large-diameter myelinated fibers, and polymodal endings of nonmyelinated nerve fibers.[6,7] The superficial location of these receptors and their nerves makes topical local anesthesia of the airway an effective means of blunting cardiovascular responses to airway interventions.[8] The glossopharyngeal and vagal afferent nerves transmit these impulses to the brainstem, leading to widespread autonomic activation through the sympathetic and parasympathetic nervous systems.[9] Bradycardia, often elicited in infants and small children during laryngoscopy or intubation, is the autonomic equivalent of the laryngospasm response. Although seen only rarely in adults, this reflex results from an increase in vagal tone at the sinoatrial node and is essentially a monosynaptic response to a noxious stimulus in the airway.[10]

In adults and adolescents, the more common response to airway manipulation is HTN and tachycardia mediated by the cardioaccelerator nerves and sympathetic chain ganglia. This response includes widespread release of norepinephrine from adrenergic nerve terminals and secretion of epinephrine from the adrenal medulla.[11] Notably, patients with pheochromocytoma or other catecholamine-secreting tumors may have a markedly exaggerated sympathetic response with airway manipulation.[12] A component of the hypertensive response to tracheal intubation also

results from activation of the renin-angiotensin system, including release of renin from the renal juxtaglomerular apparatus via direct stimulation by β-adrenergic nerves.[1]

In addition to activation of the autonomic nervous system, laryngoscopy and tracheal intubation result in stimulation of the central nervous system, as evidenced by increases in electroencephalographic (EEG) activity, cerebral metabolic rate of oxygen consumption ($CMRo_2$), and cerebral blood flow (CBF).[13] In patients with compromised intracranial compliance due to head injury, increases in CBF may result in elevated intracranial pressure (ICP), which, if prolonged, may result in herniation of brain contents and severe neurologic compromise.[14] Tachycardia and HTN associated with tracheal intubation have not been shown to be the cause of severe complications of head injury in isolation.

The effects of tracheal intubation on the pulmonary vasculature are poorly understood as they are often coupled with changes in airway reactivity associated with intubation. Acute bronchospasm or mainstem bronchial intubation results in a marked maldistribution of perfusion to poorly ventilated lung units, increasing transpulmonary shunting, which subsequently reduces systemic arterial oxygen tension and leads to an increase in pulmonary vascular resistance triggered by hypoxic pulmonary vasoconstriction.[15] In addition, impaired venous return to the left side of the heart from the pulmonary circulation as a result of positive end-expiratory pressure (PEEP) after tracheal intubation causes a reduction in cardiac output (CO). The impact of these changes can be profound in patients who have compromised myocardial function or depleted intravascular volume.[16,17]

Intubation in the Presence of Cardiovascular Disease

Perioperative myocardial ischemia often occurs in patients with preexisting cardiac risk factors, such as advanced age, smoking history, HTN, obesity, hypercholesterolemia, diabetes mellitus, or a family history of coronary artery disease. However, it has also been reported in young, healthy patients without notable risk factors during emergence from general anesthesia.[18]

Myocardial ischemia results from an imbalance between myocardial oxygen supply and demand. In the presence of stable oxygen content in the blood, myocardial oxygen supply is determined almost entirely by coronary blood flow and distribution, because oxygen extraction at the cellular level is near maximum even under resting conditions.

The chief components of myocardial oxygen demand are heart rate (HR) and myocardial wall tension. Of the two, increases in HR are of greatest concern, because cardiac inotropy (contractility) subserves cardiac chronotropy (rate). Not only does tachycardia increase myocardial oxygen consumption per minute at a constant wall tension, but elevations in rate effectively reduce the diastolic period. This reduces the time for full diastolic relaxation and leads to an increase in resting wall tension, impairing subendocardial blood flow and thereby reducing myocardial oxygen supply. It follows, then, that neuroendocrine responses to airway manipulation resulting in tachycardia and HTN may result in a variety of complications in patients with underlying cardiac disease, particularly myocardial ischemia. This explains the ischemic electrocardiographic ST-segment depression and increased pulmonary artery diastolic blood pressure (BP) sometimes observed when intubation is performed in patients with arteriosclerosis; patients who experience greater increases in BP and HR during intubation exhibit a higher rate of ischemic electrocardiography (ECG) changes.[19] Occasionally, these episodes foreshadow the occurrence of a perioperative myocardial infarction. Short, transient ischemic episodes (<10 minutes) evidenced by electrocardiographic ST-segment depression, such as those associated with brief airway manipulation, have not been shown to correlate with postoperative myocardial infarction. In contrast, ST-segment changes of a single duration lasting longer than 20 minutes or cumulative durations lasting longer than 1 hour do seem to be an important factor associated with adverse perioperative cardiac outcomes.[20,21]

Patients with aneurysmal disease of the cerebral and aortic circulation may also be at increased risk of complications related to a sudden increase in BP during airway instrumentation. Laplace's law defines the transmural wall tension of a blood vessel (the determinant of its likelihood of rupture) as the product of the pressure inside the vessel and its radius divided by the wall thickness. The presence of a thin-walled vascular aneurysm (higher transmural wall tension at baseline) combined with a sudden increase in intraluminal pressure can lead to rupture of the affected vessel and abrupt deterioration in the patient's status. Leaking or ruptured aortic aneurysms are partially tamponaded by intraabdominal pressure but can suddenly expand into the retroperitoneal space during abrupt or sustained arterial HTN. This results in significant blood loss and additional technical challenges during surgical resection of the lesion and/or placement of a vascular prosthesis. Similarly, sudden increases in BP and contractility can result in propagation of false lumens in patients with aortic dissection.[22]

Implications for Patients With Neurovascular Disease

Intracranial aneurysms and arteriovenous malformations (AVMs) may present with a "sentinel" hemorrhage that could serve as a warning for further neurologic risk. During subsequent periods of elevated arterial BP, these lesions can rebleed, which may result in sudden and permanent neurologic injury.[23] Many neurosurgeons and interventional neuroradiologists attempt to stabilize cerebral aneurysms and AVMs soon after hospitalization in an effort to minimize the risk of rebleeding, necessitating anesthesia and airway manipulation at a time when the clot tamponading the aneurysm or AVM is particularly delicate. A small increase in arterial transmural pressure during tracheal intubation can increase the shearing forces on the vessel and could cause rerupture.[24] It is important, therefore, to pay meticulous attention to attenuating these responses during the course of anesthetic induction and tracheal intubation.

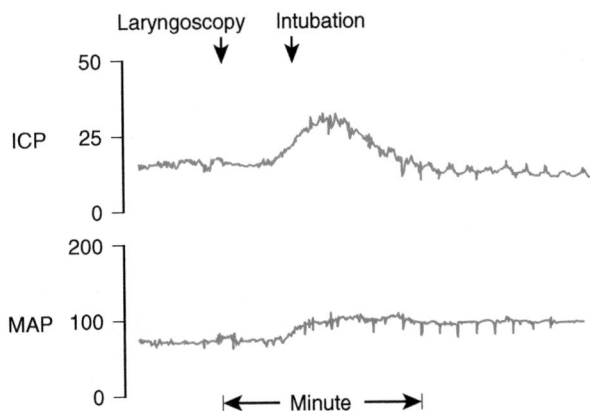

• **Fig. 7.1** Increases in systemic mean arterial pressure (MAP) and intracranial pressure (ICP) in response to tracheal intubation in a patient with a small brain tumor. Notice the minimal response to rigid laryngoscopy. There is a sustained increase in MAP but only a transient increase in ICP, which returns to normal as cerebrovascular autoregulation becomes operative. (From Bedford RF. Circulatory responses to tracheal intubation. *Probl Anesth.* 1988;2:201.)

Intubation in Patients With Neuropathologic Disorders

Reflex responses to tracheal intubation causing intracranial HTN are also potential hazards to patients with compromised intracranial compliance resulting from neuropathologic processes such as intracranial mass lesions, brain edema, or acute hydrocephalus. Uncontrolled coughing can result in a marked increase in intrathoracic and intraabdominal pressure that, in turn, increases cerebrospinal fluid pressure and may compromise cerebral perfusion. In patients with impaired cerebral autoregulation (e.g., brain trauma, cerebrovascular accidents, or neoplasms), the normal tendency for CBF to remain constant over the mean BP range of 70 to 150 mm Hg is impaired. When tracheal intubation causes an increase in arterial BP in these patients, there is a marked increase in CBF and cerebral blood volume, which in turn can cause dangerous increases in ICP.[25] This effect is magnified by the fact that noxious stimuli, such as airway manipulation, also result in increased CBF, which summates with the cardiovascular response, occasionally causing profound increases in ICP (Fig. 7.1).

The presence of a spinal cord injury may attenuate or enhance the hemodynamic response to intubation, depending on the spinal cord level and the chronicity of the injury. Patients with a high-level injury leading to quadriplegia (injury above C7) tend not to have the typical increase in BP but do exhibit an increase in HR in response to tracheal intubation. In contrast, patients with acute paraplegia (injury below T5) often have an exaggerated hypertensive response that tends to normalize over time.[26] Furthermore, patients with traumatic brain injury can show a severe hypertensive response to laryngoscopy and intubation that can worsen cerebral edema and place them at risk for secondary injury.[27]

Neuromuscular Blocking Drugs and Cardiovascular Responses

Neuromuscular blocking drugs (NMBDs) are often administered to optimize conditions for intubation. Accordingly, it is appropriate to consider the cardiovascular and cerebrovascular responses to the administration of these agents. Indeed, the hypertensive-tachycardic response to tracheal intubation was not identified until NMBDs were introduced into clinical practice. Before that time, intubation was performed only with the patient under such deep levels of anesthesia that relatively little cardiovascular response was generated.[28]

The depressor effects of benzylisoquinolinium relaxants (atracurium and mivacurium) are mediated by histamine release.[29] This effect could be viewed as a potential antagonist to the pressor response to laryngoscopy and tracheal intubation. In the case of patients at risk for intracranial HTN, however, histamine-induced cerebral vasodilation may produce increases in ICP, even as the BP falls.[30] By contrast, pancuronium, rocuronium, and, to a lesser extent, vecuronium may initiate a hyperdynamic cardiovascular state that can potentiate the cardiovascular responses seen after tracheal intubation in anesthetized patients.[31]

Succinylcholine is associated with bradycardia as a result of muscarinic stimulation, particularly when doses are repeated and, more commonly, in children. Studies of this phenomenon demonstrate that treatment with atropine had no effect on patient outcomes so routine administration for "reflex" treatment is not advised.[7]

In adults, succinylcholine is typically a cardiovascular stimulant.[32] This phenomenon is often associated with activation of the EEG, and patients with brain tumors may sustain marked increases in ICP after succinylcholine administration if intracranial compliance is compromised and cerebrovascular autoregulation is impaired.[33] This has been demonstrated to be a result of increased CBF related primarily to succinylcholine-induced increases in afferent muscle spindle activity at the time of fasciculation and secondarily to an elevated arterial carbon dioxide tension from fasciculation-induced carbon dioxide production.[34] The evidence to substantiate the clinical relevance of these findings is lacking, however. While it has been reported that succinylcholine administered to patients with brain tumors may elevate ICP by a mean of 5 to 12 mm Hg, cerebral perfusion pressure does not change significantly, and a negative effect on neurologic outcome has not been established.[35] Classical teaching that this phenomenon can be prevented by pretreatment with defasciculating doses of nondepolarizing NMBDs has not been demonstrated in the literature.[36] Furthermore, when adequate ventilation is maintained, succinylcholine administered to intubated patients being treated for intracranial HTN of various causes had no effect on ICP, cerebral perfusion pressure, or CBF.[37] As a result, succinylcholine is still considered a first-line agent for rapid sequence induction and intubation (RSI) in patients with acute head injury.[38]

Cardiopulmonary Consequences of Positive-Pressure Ventilation

The transition from spontaneous, negative-pressure ventilation to positive-pressure ventilation (PPV) at the time of intubation and subsequent mechanical ventilation significantly alters hemodynamics via compression of mediastinal structures by the lungs as positive inspiratory pressures cause an increase in mean intrathoracic pressure. Elevated intrathoracic pressure diminishes the gradient driving venous blood from the periphery to the right atrium, reducing the flow of blood through the right heart and pulmonary circulation, ultimately impairing left ventricular preload. This can lead to decreased CO, especially in preload-dependent states such as hypovolemia, atrial arrythmias, tachycardias, ventricular diastolic failure, and decreased ventricular afterload.[39] As CO drops, mean arterial blood pressure (MAP) falls with especially

exaggerated hypotension observed in patients unable to compensate due to intravascular volume depletion or a significant vasodilatory response from anesthetic induction agents.[40] One common clinical scenario is a patient who responds to intubation with a brisk increase in BP and then suddenly develops acute hypotension as PPV is instituted. In such a situation, volume expansion, positional changes, and judicious use of α-adrenergic agents such as phenylephrine may be needed.[41]

Whereas preexisting impaired cardiac function may worsen in the setting of PPV, some patients see improvement in cardiac function, depending on the variable impacts of decreased preload and decreased afterload. PPV, particularly PEEP or continuous positive airway pressure (CPAP), diminishes the transmural wall tension of the left heart by raising juxtacardiac pressures, leading to decreased left ventricular afterload and potentially improved left ventricular performance.

It should also be noted that both hypoxemia and hypercapnia lead to a stress-induced catecholamine response that may mask other potential causes of hypotension. This becomes readily apparent after intubation in critically ill patients when the stress is relieved and the underlying hemodynamics are unmasked. Prophylactic volume expansion and the immediate availability of vasoactive infusions decrease the risk of severe hemodynamic collapse in this situation.[42]

Prevention of Cardiovascular Responses

Minimizing Stimulation of Airway Sensory Receptors

As a general rule, cardiovascular responses to airway maneuvers can be minimized by limiting airway sensory receptor stimulation, including manipulation of the larynx itself. Application of cricoid pressure results in a significantly greater HR and BP response to tracheal intubation than does gentle palpation of the cricoid area.[43] This underrecognized effect of cricoid pressure should be considered when estimating the risk-benefit ratio of this procedure in individual patients.

Laryngoscopy is a moderately stimulating procedure, and the use of a straight blade (e.g., a Miller blade) with elevation of the vagally innervated posterior aspect of the epiglottis results in significantly higher arterial BP than does the use of a curved blade (e.g., a Macintosh blade).[44] Video-assisted laryngoscopy (VAL), which does not require approximation of the anatomical axes for adequate visualization of the glottis and subsequent intubation, has the potential to minimize the pressor response to airway manipulation, but this has be countered with the fact that VAL may take longer than direct laryngoscopy (DL). Manikin studies have demonstrated that VAL requires less force to displace oropharyngeal tissues than DL with a Macintosh blade.[45,46] Channel-based videolaryngoscopes also have been shown to attenuate the hemodynamic responses of tracheal intubation compared to a Macintosh laryngoscope.[47]

However, some studies show no difference between VAL and DL with respect to increases in HR and BP.[48,49] One possible explanation for the lack of hemodynamic advantage to less stimulating intubation devices is that the act of tracheal intubation is far more hemodynamically stimulating than laryngoscopy itself. For example, the use of a lighted intubation stylet fails to prevent hemodynamic stimulation once an ETT is advanced past the vocal cords. This has also been demonstrated with VAL.[50,51]

Insertion of a laryngeal mask airway (LMA) after induction of general anesthesia with thiopental or propofol and fentanyl has been shown to cause a lower cardiovascular and endocrine response than laryngoscopy or tracheal intubation.[52,53] The LMA has the advantage of avoiding the vagally mediated infraglottic stimulation entailed by the use of a laryngoscope, thus requiring lighter levels of general anesthesia. Furthermore, because neuromuscular blockade is not required for airway control, spontaneous ventilation and avoidance of the adverse hemodynamic consequences of PPV are possible. In contrast, tracheal intubation via an intubating LMA results in a hemodynamic and endocrine response similar to that of DL and intubation after propofol induction.[54] Therefore, if tracheal intubation is necessary, there may not be a hemodynamic advantage to instrumenting the airway with the intubating LMA or other less stimulating devices. Notably, placement of a Combitube (Kendall-Sheridan Catheter Corp., Argyle, NY) was found to cause significantly greater elevations in BP and catecholamine release when compared with tracheal intubation or LMA placement as there is gross stimulation of multiple airway structures as well as the esophagus.[55]

Whichever technique is used to manage the airway, it must be emphasized that the hypertensive-tachycardic response to intubation may be a manifestation of insufficient anesthesia, which is often caused by a failure to maintain an appropriate level of anesthetic during intubation. Insofar as the pressor response can also be influenced by prolonged intubation time, rapid first-attempt success is also of particular importance, with multiple attempts being associated with increased risk of hemodynamic complications including bradycardia and cardiac arrest.[56]

Topical and Regional Anesthesia

Topical anesthesia applied to the upper airway is effective in blunting hemodynamic responses to tracheal intubation,[57] but it has almost invariably proven to be less effective than systemic administration of lidocaine. During general anesthesia, DL and instillation of lidocaine solution initiate the same adverse reflexes caused by placement of an ETT (Fig. 7.2).[58] Furthermore, a laryngotracheal spray of lidocaine solution may, in itself, produce profound cardiovascular stimulation in adults, and in children it may produce the same sort of bradycardic response associated with tracheal intubation.[59] If topical lidocaine is administered to the upper airway, there should be an intervening period of at least 2 minutes to allow initiation of anesthetic effect before airway instrumentation begins.[60]

Excellent topical anesthesia of the airway obtained before awake flexible scope intubation (FSI) results in less cardiovascular stimulation after this procedure than after intubation with DL.[61] Later studies performed with patients under general anesthesia demonstrated no difference between the two modes of intubation with regard to hemodynamic impact, probably because the more profound stimulus resulting from placement of the ETT below the level of the glottis had been suppressed by local anesthetic topicalization in the patients undergoing awake intubation.[62,63] This further supports the concept that intubation of the trachea with the ETT predominates over laryngoscopy as the major noxious driver of the hemodynamic response to intubation.

Increasing the concentration of lidocaine used, and thus the total dose, also does not appear to provide any increased benefit, although it may improve intubating conditions during awake FSI.[64,65] Although both 2% and 4% lidocaine administered through a flexible intubation scope (FIS) by a "spray-as-you-go"

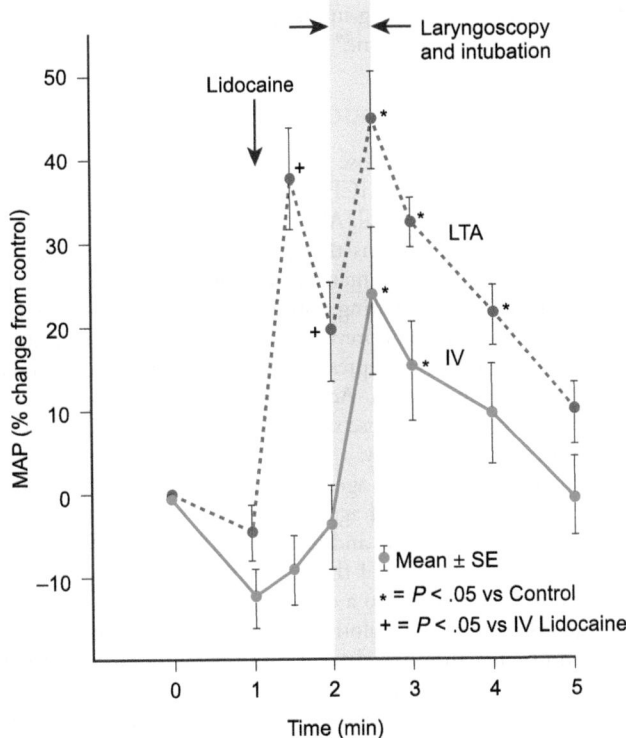

• **Fig. 7.2** Mean arterial pressure (MAP) response to tracheal intubation after either intravenous (IV) or intratracheal (LTA) lidocaine instillation. (From Hamill JF, Bedford RF, Weaver DC, Colohan AR. Lidocaine before tracheal intubation: IV or laryngotracheal? *Anesthesiology.* 1981;55:578.)

technique provided similar intubating conditions and hemodynamic profiles, the former resulted in a smaller overall dose, lower plasma levels, and therefore a reduced risk of toxicity.[64] Lower concentrations of lidocaine (1%) provided even lower plasma levels and similar hemodynamics but appeared to provide less optimal intubating conditions than atomized 2% lidocaine when used for topical anesthesia before airway manipulation.[65] Lidocaine has been compared in both spray and viscous form for procedural topical airway anesthesia and the spray form has been demonstrated to result in a higher procedural completion rate, greater ease of intubation, and greater patient and proceduralist satisfaction and is currently recommended.[66]

In contrast to topical anesthesia of the airway, which appears to provide inconsistent benefit, regional blocks of airway sensory nerves have been shown to prevent hemodynamic responses to intubation. The superior laryngeal nerve (SLN) innervates the superior surface of the larynx, and the glossopharyngeal nerve innervates the oropharynx. Injecting local anesthetic at each cornu of the hyoid bone can block the SLN. Blockade of the glossopharyngeal nerve is performed at the tonsillar pillars or palatoglossal fold.[67,68] The inferior surfaces of the larynx and trachea are innervated by the recurrent laryngeal nerve and the vagus, which cannot be directly blocked, and require topical anesthesia (see Chapter 13).

Instillation of lidocaine via an ETT can be effective in preventing alterations in cerebrovascular hemodynamics after tracheal intubation in patients with severe head injury. A dose of 1.7 mg/kg of lidocaine at body temperature instilled slowly (1 mL/s) through a fine tube advanced to the end of the ETT, but not in contact with the tracheal mucosa, was reported to effectively prevent tracheal suctioning-induced ICP increase and cerebral perfusion pressure reduction.[69]

Inhalational Anesthetics

Defining the anesthetic dose required to effectively block (or blunt) hemodynamic and ICP responses to tracheal intubation has remained an elusive goal. Airway management maneuvers are relatively brief interventions that produce short-lived responses during a dynamic airway management period, with drug concentrations rapidly fluctuating both in plasma and at effect sites. Agents that are capable of preventing responses may also produce profound cardiovascular depression before and after the stimulation of tracheal intubation. Accordingly, there are relatively few well-controlled dose-response studies, and those that are available have limited practical utility.

Inhalational anesthetic agents can have profound hemodynamic effects. Halogenated agents including sevoflurane, desflurane, isoflurane, enflurane, and halothane all decrease MAP with increasing concentrations of the anesthetic gas in a dose-dependent manner. This is due to a decrease in systemic vascular resistance (SVR), except for halothane, which directly depresses the myocardium and therefore decreases CO without affecting SVR. Sevoflurane has demonstrated less hemodynamic impact than desflurane and isoflurane. Nitrous oxide does not affect MAP and has a good hemodynamic safety profile, making it useful for sedation for minor procedures. CO is reduced as the concentration of inhaled agent increases. This is usually compensated for with an increased HR. In healthy adults this has no clinical ramifications, but in those with underlying cardiovascular disease or the elderly, this could be harmful.[70]

Tracheal intubation using these agents in doses in the range of the minimum alveolar concentration (1 MAC) results in marked cardiovascular stimulation during anesthesia with nitrous oxide (N_2O) supplemented with either halothane or morphine.[71] It should not be surprising that 1 MAC is insufficient, because it is known that approximately 1.5 to 1.6 MAC is needed to block the adrenergic and cardiovascular responses to a simple surgical skin incision (MAC-BAR).[72] The dose of anesthetic required to prevent coughing during tracheal intubation in 50% of patients with sevoflurane may be as high as 4.5% expired in adults (2 MAC),[73] although the dose in children was found to be approximately 2.7% expired (1.3 MAC).[74]

Accordingly, the dose of volatile anesthetic required to block the cardiovascular response to tracheal intubation in adults can result in profound cardiovascular depression before tracheal intubation, limiting its usefulness.[75,76] From a cerebrovascular viewpoint, this approach is highly impractical, because high doses of volatile anesthetics cause cerebral vasodilation and marked increases in ICP in patients with compromised intracranial compliance. Furthermore, the arterial hypotension and reduced cerebral perfusion pressure before intubation would be unacceptable for patients with cerebrovascular disease or brain injury.[76]

Intravenous Agents

Propofol, barbiturates, and benzodiazepines are all associated with profound hypotension at doses that suppress the hemodynamic and ICP responses to intubation.[77,78] In the case of etomidate, the effective dose for blocking the cardiovascular response to intubation can be identified by a burst-suppression pattern on the cortical surface EEG, indicating fairly deep cerebral depression.[79]

Because etomidate supports BP at such deep levels of anesthesia, it is probably the only contemporary agent that, by itself, can achieve suppression of cardiovascular responses without first producing undue arterial hypotension and compromise of coronary and cerebral perfusion. Because it is clinically impractical to achieve sufficient anesthetic depth to prevent a hyperdynamic response to intubation solely with an intravenous (IV) or inhalational agent (etomidate excepted), a wide variety of anesthetic drug combinations, adjuvants, or both have been used in attempts to potentiate anesthetic effects while minimizing hemodynamic depression.[80]

Opioids are the adjuvant agents most commonly co-administered with IV or inhalational agents to facilitate induction of anesthesia and subsequent airway manipulation by reducing the hemodynamic responses.[81] Their use in this capacity stems from the historical strategy of using a N_2O-narcotic anesthetic in patients with marginal cardiac reserve. With greater potency and a more rapid onset, fentanyl (and its derivatives) has become the preferred opioid to suppress the hemodynamic response to intubation. Fentanyl may not achieve its peak central nervous system effect until 10 minutes after bolus IV injection.[82] Fentanyl appears to blunt the hemodynamic responses in a dose-dependent manner: 2 µg/kg IV given several minutes before induction only partially prevented HTN and tachycardia during an RSI with thiopental and succinylcholine, whereas 6 µg/kg was considerably more effective.[83] Higher doses of fentanyl, such as greater than 5 µg/kg, have been demonstrated to be effective in blunting both HR and BP responses following laryngoscopy and intubation.[84] Interestingly, in patients intubated using postinduction FSI, pretreatment with fentanyl reduced the sympathetic response to intubation compared with patients not given opioid, but it did not reduce the response in patients undergoing DL, which suggests that fentanyl attenuates the response to the passage of the ETT into the trachea more than stimulus of DL.[81] In doses that prevent a hemodynamic response to intubation, however, fentanyl is not a short-acting agent, and the risk of prolonged postoperative respiratory depression must be weighed against the advantages of perioperative cardiovascular stability. With this risk in mind, it has been observed that pretreatment with 2 µg/kg IV fentanyl given 10 minutes before intubation during an infusion of propofol prevented a significant increase in HR or BP compared with awake preanesthetic values.[85] Similar results were observed when intubation was performed after administration of 2 µg/kg IV fentanyl and propofol bolus doses of 2.0 to 3.5 mg/kg.[82]

Fentanyl and propofol require 6.4 and 2.9 minutes, respectively, to achieve effect-site equilibrium after IV bolus administration. Therefore, the common practice of administering a bolus of fentanyl simultaneously with other induction medications would not be expected to have the desired effect of blunting the hemodynamic response to intubation due to inadequate accumulation of the drug at the effect site at the time of intubation. Rather, a peak effect occurring well after intubation may provide a more plausible explanation for hypotension observed during the quiescent period between tracheal intubation and surgical incision. It is strongly recommended that laryngoscopy and intubation be timed to coincide with the peak effect of these agents.

Opioids with shorter onset and offset times have some advantages over fentanyl for modulating circulatory responses to intubation. Alfentanil has a smaller steady-state distribution volume and shorter terminal elimination half-life than fentanyl.[86] A preinduction bolus dose of 15–45 µg/kg of alfentanil effectively suppresses the hemodynamic and catecholamine response to tracheal intubation.[87]

Remifentanil has been found to be highly effective in preventing hemodynamic responses to intubation, albeit with the cost of dose-dependent bradycardia and/or hypotension before and after airway manipulation.[88] Many studies have used vagolytic agents to avoid bradycardia, at the risk of an elevated HR response after intubation. Remifentanil's half-time for equilibration between blood and effect site is 1.3 minutes,[89] and it has a brief half-life of 3 to 5 minutes due to hydrolysis by tissue and blood esterases.[90] Typical remifentanil infusion rates used for blunting hemodynamic responses are 0.25 to 1.0 μg/kg/min in association with cautious propofol administration and nondepolarizing neuromuscular blockade.[91] For RSI with thiopental and succinylcholine, the optimal dose of remifentanil appears to be 1.0 μg/kg administered over 30 seconds, with laryngoscopy performed 1 minute after induction. A bolus dose of 1.25 μg/kg was associated with unsatisfactory bradycardia, whereas 0.5 μg/kg resulted in excessive cardiovascular stimulation.[92] This dosing recommendation is supported by another report that found remifentanil 1 μg/kg given over 30 seconds, followed by thiopental 5 mg/kg and rocuronium 1 mg/kg 100 seconds later, was more effective than lidocaine and esmolol in attenuating the hemodynamic response to RSI.[93] Care should be taken with these agents in elderly patients who may be particularly sensitive to hypotension induced by alfentanil or remifentanil.[94]

IV dexmedetomidine acts as a sedative/hypnotic and catecholamine suppressor via activation of central, presynaptic α_2-adrenergic receptors that reduce central sympathetic outflow and subsequent activation of the peripheral sympathetic nervous symptom. These properties have led to investigations into its ability to suppress the hemodynamic response to intubation and potentially reduce perioperative ischemic events.[95] An IV bolus dose of 1 μg/kg of dexmedetomidine over 10 minutes followed by a continuous infusion at 0.7 μg/kg/h administered 15 minutes prior to anesthetic induction blunts the cardiovascular response to tracheal intubation while minimizing the decrease in BP associated with anesthetic induction.[96] A meta-analysis of 23 randomized trials evaluating the perioperative use of α_2-adrenergic agonists—including dexmedetomidine and clonidine—on mortality and cardiovascular complications in surgical patients demonstrated reductions in mortality and cardiovascular events in vascular and cardiac surgery patients.[97]

IV lidocaine blunts hemodynamic and cerebrovascular responses to intubation.[98] When given as a bolus of 1.5 mg/kg IV, it adds approximately 0.3 MAC of anesthetic potency.[98] Significant reductions in hemodynamic response to tracheal intubation have been noted when lidocaine (3 mg/kg) was used as an adjunct to high-dose fentanyl anesthesia,[99] as well as during other light anesthetic techniques, such as thiopental-N_2O-oxygen.[100] However, smaller doses of lidocaine (1.5 mg/kg) have not been consistently reported to be effective in reducing the hemodynamic response to laryngoscopy and tracheal intubation in adults and children.[101,102] The general anesthetic properties of lidocaine tend to reduce CMR_{O_2} and CBF, thus lowering ICP in patients with compromised intracranial compliance. Theoretically, these properties of lidocaine might be exploited to mitigate rises in ICP during airway manipulation in those patients with acute intracranial pathology or compromised intracranial compliance.[103,104] However, a general statement can be made that there is no high-quality evidence that pretreatment of a patient with lidocaine will prevent or reduce a rise in ICP caused by laryngoscopy and tracheal intubation.[105]

With regard to the patient at risk for intracranial HTN, it is important that agents used to control cardiovascular responses to intubation also have a minimal adverse impact on ICP. Agents that act as cerebral vasodilators, such as volatile anesthetics, nitroglycerin, nitroprusside, or hydralazine, are generally avoided if there is a serious risk of intracranial HTN.

Nonanesthetic Adjuvant Agents

A final means for modifying the cardiovascular responses to tracheal intubation is prophylactic administration of vasoactive substances that directly affect the cardiovascular system. There have been several studies advocating the use of various vasodilators and adrenergic blocking agents as pretreatment before tracheal intubation, including diltiazem, verapamil, and nicardipine[106,107]; hydralazine[108]; nitroprusside[109]; nitroglycerin[110]; labetalol[111]; esmolol[112]; and clonidine.[113] Virtually all of these agents appear to be somewhat effective when compared with placebo, particularly when used in high doses. Currently, the optimal use of any of these agents is undefined, although their use as adjuncts to RSI is reasonable, taking into account evidence-based dosing recommendations for the situation.

Airway Effects of Tracheal Intubation

Upper Airway Reflexes

Because the upper airway reflexes protect the respiratory gas exchange surface from noxious substances, it is appropriate that the nose, mouth, pharynx, larynx, trachea, and carina have an abundance of sensory nerve endings and brisk motor responses. Anesthesiologists are especially familiar with the glottic closure reflex (laryngospasm), which is invariably encountered early in their training. The sneeze, cough, and swallow reflexes are equally important upper airway reflexes.

Afferent pathways for laryngospasm and the cardiovascular responses to tracheal intubation are initiated by the glossopharyngeal nerve when stimulation occurs superior to the anterior surface of the epiglottis and by the vagus nerve when stimulation occurs from the level of the posterior epiglottis down into the lower airway. Because the laryngeal closure reflex is mediated by vagal efferents to the glottis, it is virtually a monosynaptic response, occurring primarily when a patient is lightly anesthetized as vagally innervated sensory endings in the upper airway are stimulated and conscious respiratory efforts cannot override the reflex.

Dead Space

Patients with severe chronic lung disease may find it easier to breathe after intubation or a tracheostomy. The improvement is most likely due to reduced dead space. The normal extrathoracic anatomic dead space, based on cadaveric measurements, is between 70 and 75 mL.[114] The exact volume of the ETT is easily calculated as that of a cylinder using the formula $V = \pi r^2 l$, where r is the radius of the tube and l is the length. For example, an ETT that has an 8-mm inner diameter (ID) and a length of 25 cm has a volume of 12.6 mL. Intubation should therefore result in a reduction in dead space of approximately 60 mL, assuming no additional circuitry. Tracheostomy tubes are shorter than oral ETTs and have an even smaller dead space, although the difference as a proportion of tidal volume (V_T) is negligible.

In normal individuals, the reduction in dead space with intubation or insertion of a tracheostomy tube is negligible relative to a normal V_T, so there is little benefit. In a patient with severe restrictive lung disease, such as in end-stage kyphoscoliosis, however, V_T may be as low as 100 mL, and intubation can confer a major benefit. Similarly, patients with emphysema who are switched from mouth breathing to tracheostomy demonstrate a reduction in required minute ventilation and a decrease in total body oxygen consumption, presumably due to a decreased work of breathing (WOB).[115] Most likely, the decreased volume required more than compensates for the slight increase in resistance.

Upper Airway Resistance

Anesthesiologists are aware that adequate ventilation can be maintained with an ETT as small as 6 mm ID in place in most healthy, anesthetized patients. However, intensivists caring for a patient with respiratory failure often insist that an ETT has a minimum ID of 8 mm. These tube sizes are appropriate for the clinical situations described. The high resistance of the 6-mm ETT is inconsequential for the low minute ventilation required under general anesthesia, but the high flow rates required for a patient with respiratory failure may render the resistance of a small ETT prohibitive.

The relatively small caliber of an ETT creates a mechanical burden for a spontaneously breathing patient in the form of a fixed upper airway resistance. Gas flows whenever there is a pressure difference across the ETT, whether it is caused by subatmospheric pressure generated during spontaneous breathing or by positive pressure generated from a mechanical ventilator. The apparent resistance of an ETT is influenced by the shape of the tube and by two types of friction: the friction among gas molecules and the friction between gas molecules and the tube wall. Irregular surfaces created by secretions or by ridges from wire reinforcement may create greater friction and resistance. ETTs and tracheostomies have a higher resistance than the normal upper respiratory tract.[116,117]

The relationship between pressure difference and flow rate depends on the nature of the flow: laminar, turbulent, or a mixture of the two. In an ETT, turbulent flow predominates. During turbulent flow, the measured resistance is not a constant but varies with the flow rate, becoming markedly higher at high flow rates. Instead of the laminar flow relationship of pressure being directly proportional to flow, the pressure required to move the gas through an ETT with turbulent flow is proportional to the square of the flow. The relationship can therefore be described by a parabolic curve, as in Fig. 7.3. The apparent resistance of a tube is proportional to the fourth power of the radius during laminar flow (Poiseuille's law) but to the fifth power during turbulent flow. Assuming turbulent flow, the estimated relative resistance of a 6-mm ETT versus an 8-mm ETT is 4^5, or 4.2 times as great as depicted in Fig. 7.3. The slope of the pressure-flow graph is the apparent resistance. The parabolic shape of the graphs demonstrates the primarily turbulent nature of the flow through an ETT.

Although the resistance of the ETT may be severalfold greater than the resistance of the normal human upper airway, this is of relatively little consequence at low minute ventilation with low flow rates. With a typical peak inspiratory flow of 25 to 30 L/min, approximately 0.5 cm H_2O pressure must be generated to overcome the resistance of the upper respiratory tract. This represents about 10% of the total WOB. Even a doubling or tripling of that resistance by placement of an ETT does not result in a clinically worrisome increase in the total WOB.[118]

Theoretically, the patient's native airway should have less resistance than any size of ETT. However, a patient who has been intubated for an extended period may not have a normal upper

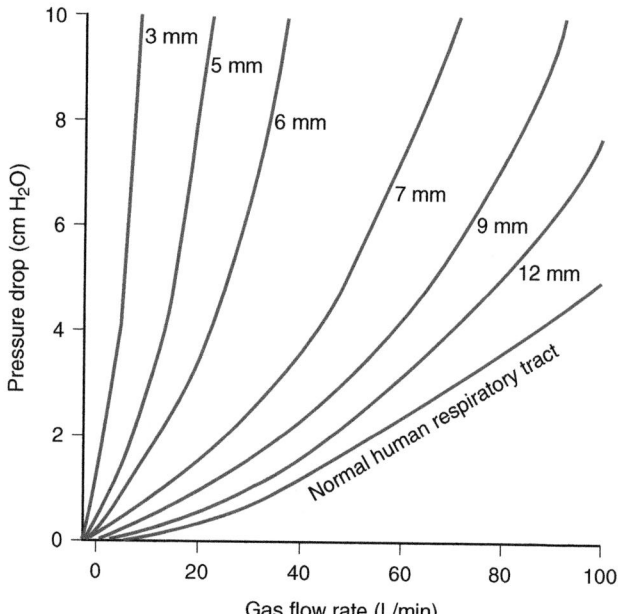

• **Fig. 7.3** Pressure drop across endotracheal tubes of various sizes at flow rates ranging from 0 to 100 L/min. Note the wide disparity between 6- and 7-mm tubes as flow rate increases to the range typically seen in patients with respiratory failure. (Modified from Nunn JF. *Modified Respiratory Physiology.* Butterworths; 1987.)

airway. Indeed, some evidence suggests that WOB may actually increase after extubation, perhaps due to high upper airway resistance.[119] Therefore if the patient is close to successful weaning, a reasonable approach may be to attempt extubation rather than to change ETTs, recognizing that the need for reintubation is a possibility. Alternatively, pressure support ventilation can be used to compensate for the added WOB through the smaller tube until extubation is warranted.[120]

Tracheostomy tubes have lower resistance than ETTs of comparable diameters because they are shorter. However, there is little, if any, difference in the WOB imposed by fresh tracheostomy tubes and ETTs of comparable ID.[121] On the other hand, tracheostomy does appear to decrease the WOB in patients who have undergone prolonged intubation and mechanical ventilation. This paradox may be explained by a reduction in the ID of an ETT over time, perhaps as a result of accumulated secretions or conformational changes.[122] This size reduction may explain the observation that patients being weaned from mechanical ventilation are sometimes more rapidly weaned after a tracheostomy is performed,[123] although it may also reflect the increased comfort of clinicians in discontinuing ventilatory support after the airway is secured.

Lower Airway Resistance

Bronchospasm after induction of anesthesia is a relatively uncommon but well-recognized event and is likely related to a reflex response to tracheal intubation. Several studies provide some evidence regarding the frequency of bronchospasm. One study noted that bronchospasm accounted for 5.3% of fatal or near-fatal periinduction complications.[124] The largest study found 246 cases of bronchospasm to have occurred out of a total of 136,929 anesthesia inductions, for an incidence of 1.7 per 1000.[125] However, the exact incidence undoubtedly depends substantially on the prevalence of disease in the patient population.

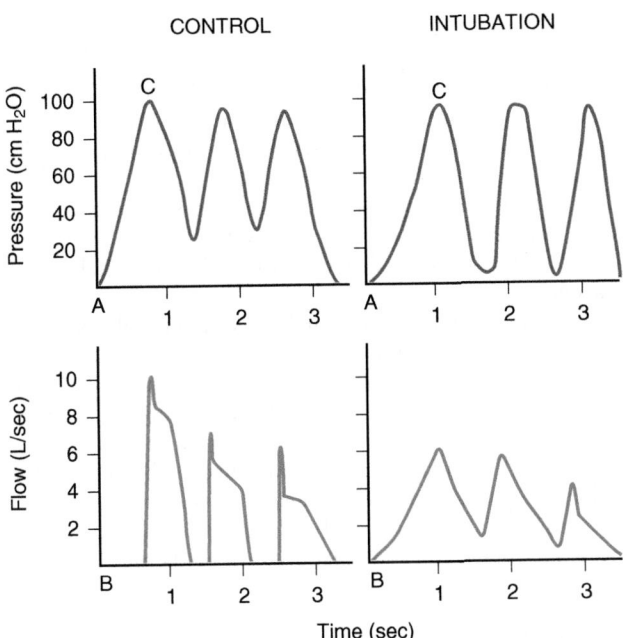

CONTROL   INTUBATION

• **Fig. 7.4** Pressure and flow curves (labeled *A* and *B*, respectively) generated during a burst of three successive coughs *(C)* by a volunteer before (control) and after tracheal intubation. Notice that the flows and pressures generated are only modestly diminished after intubation. (From Gal TJ. How does tracheal intubation alter respiratory mechanics? *Probl Anesth.* 1988;2:191.)

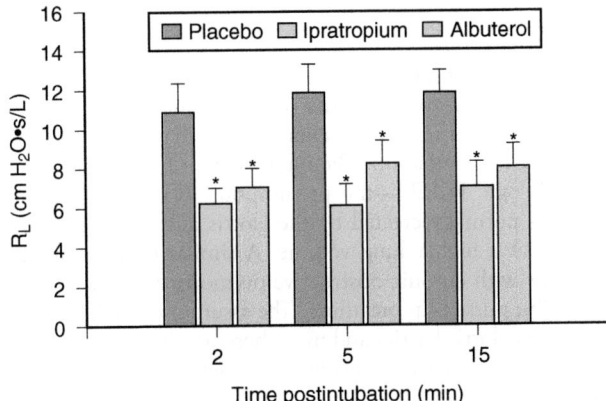

• **Fig. 7.5** Lung resistance (R_L) at 2, 5, and 15 minutes after intubation in patients pretreated with either a placebo, the anticholinergic drug ipratropium bromide, or the β-adrenergic agonist albuterol. Both drugs markedly diminished lung resistance for longer than 15 minutes after tracheal intubation under thiopental-narcotic anesthesia. (From Kil HK, Rooke GA, Ryan-Dykes MA, et al. Effect of prophylactic bronchodilator treatment on lung resistance after tracheal intubation. *Anesthesiology.* 1994;81(1):43–48.)

The incidence of postintubation bronchospasm may be decreasing because of the increasing use of propofol as an induction agent (propofol being more effective than thiopental at preventing this complication). However, ventilation problems combined with hypoxia due to acute bronchospasm still represent important sentinel anesthesia events.[126]

Whereas the incidence of overt clinical bronchospasm is low, a subclinical reflex-driven increase in airway resistance may occur much more often. Receptors in the larynx and upper trachea may cause large airway constriction distal to the ETT, which in turn may extend to the smaller peripheral airways (Fig. 7.4).[127]

Bronchoconstriction also occurs after tracheal intubation of normal subjects who have received thiopental/narcotic anesthesia. In a series of patients pretreated before anesthesia with either a β-adrenergic agonist (albuterol) or an inhaled anticholinergic agent (ipratropium bromide), measured airway resistance after intubation was markedly lower compared with placebo treatment (Fig. 7.5).[128] On the other hand, premedication with albuterol in school-age children did not reduce the incidence of perioperative respiratory events.[129]

Increases in airway resistance may result from changes in intrinsic smooth muscle tone, airway edema, or intraluminal secretions. Rapid changes in airway caliber after airway instrumentation are thought to result largely from parasympathetic nervous system activation of airway smooth muscle. Cholinergic innervation predominates in the larger central airways, with efferent nerves arising in the vagal nuclei of the brainstem and synapsing with ganglia in the airway walls. Postganglionic parasympathetic nerves release acetylcholine, activating muscarinic receptors on airway smooth muscle that lead to smooth muscle constriction. Such responses can be blocked via muscarinic blockade, using either systemic or inhaled anticholinergic agents.[130]

Tracheal intubation also may induce bronchospasm by causing coughing. A cough reduces lung volume, which in turn markedly increases bronchoconstriction in response to a stimulus. In the patient with a known reactive airway, prevention of coughing at the time of tracheal intubation by use of either a deep level of anesthetic or neuromuscular blockade may help to minimize the likelihood of bronchospasm.[131]

Endotracheal Tube Resistance and Exhalation

In normal patients, exhalation is usually completed well before the next inhalation begins, even when breathing at moderately elevated minute ventilation. By contrast, patients with obstructive lung disease may not complete full exhalation before the start of the next inhalation. In other words, inhalation begins before exhalation to functional residual capacity (FRC), resulting in the sequential accumulation of retained gases in the alveoli. This phenomenon is called auto-PEEP or dynamic hyperinflation, and it is associated with air trapping, elevated intrathoracic pressure, and hemodynamic compromise.[132]

Auto-PEEP most commonly occurs in patients with obstructive lung disease and high minute ventilation, but it also may occur rarely in patients with relatively normal airways who are ventilated at a very high minute ventilation. This has been observed in patients with burns or sepsis who may require a minute ventilation of as much as 30 to 40 L/min. Under these circumstances, the resistance of the ETT may limit expiratory flow such that full exhalation does not occur. This has been demonstrated experimentally, with the magnitude of the auto-PEEP correlating directly with the resistance of the ETT.[133] Among patients under anesthesia, major resistance to exhalation caused by the ETT is of no consequence in routine cases and is only rarely seen in critically ill patients. However, low levels of auto-PEEP due to tube resistance probably occur frequently in patients with high minute ventilation and during single-lung ventilation via a double-lumen ETT.[123]

Functional Residual Capacity

The effect of tracheal intubation on FRC has been a subject of considerable controversy. Intensivists are familiar with instances of patients recovering from respiratory failure where oxygenation improved after extubation. The improvement has been attributed to "physiologic PEEP"—the presumption that a small positive pressure is normally created by the glottis and that this leads to breathing at a higher lung volume. A similar effect is observed in patients with chronic obstructive pulmonary disease (COPD) who exhibit pursed-lip breathing. The assumption is that an ETT removes the glottic barrier and may, therefore, lower lung volume. However, the existence of positive intratracheal pressure has never been documented.[127-134]

By contrast, different conclusions were reached in a series of patients who were studied just before and after extubation following recovery from respiratory failure. In this situation, both FRC and arterial oxygen tension (Pao_2) were found to increase after extubation, supporting the concept that the presence of an ETT decreases FRC.[135]

Cough

Although it is widely recognized that cough efficiency is reduced whenever an ETT is in place, it is a common observation that a disconnected ETT is likely to produce a plug of sputum whenever the patient is stimulated to cough. Studies have demonstrated that a cough performed with an ETT in place leads to peak airway flow that is reduced but still adequate to enable secretion clearance. Large airway collapse is important for producing maximum force against secretions. Because an ETT prevents collapse of the trachea by acting as a stent, maximum efficiency of expectoration cannot be achieved, explaining why removing secretions from the trachea through an ETT often requires the use of a suction catheter.[127]

Humidification of Gases

Under normal circumstances, the upper airway warms, humidifies, and filters 7000 to 10,000 L of inspired air daily, adding up to 1 L of moisture to the gases. When the upper airway is bypassed by intubation, the gas must be warmed and humidified in the trachea if it is not adequately humidified before inhalation. In an anesthetized patient breathing dry gases, up to 10% of the average metabolic rate may be required to perform these tasks.[136] Delivery of cool, dry gases may also have a significant effect on mucociliary transport, a critical defense mechanism of the respiratory tract. Inhalation of unconditioned gas rapidly leads to abnormal mucosal ciliary motion, with subsequent thickening and encrustation of tracheal secretions. These changes occur as early as 30 minutes after intubation and, theoretically, may lead to an increase in postoperative complications. Accordingly, assurance of adequate gas conditioning should be standard for all but very brief tracheal intubations.[137]

Control and Treatment of the Respiratory Responses to Airway Instrumentation

Preventing Upper Airway Responses

Cough and laryngospasm in response to intubation appear to be sound protective reflexes. Under most circumstances, the body needs to prevent further intrusion by a foreign body and tries to expel it from the airway. However, these responses can be troublesome during induction of anesthesia or at the time of extubation. Cough can lead to bronchospasm as lung volume is reduced, and it can also result in desaturation as the lung volume drops to residual volume. Laryngospasm may result in life-threatening abnormalities of blood gases. Consequently, anesthesiologists routinely try to prevent these responses with the use of medications delivered topically, via inhalation, or intravenously.

Inhibition of upper airway reflexes can certainly be accomplished by performing tracheal intubation after the administration of NMBDs. If circumstances preclude the use of NMBDs, laryngeal and tracheal reflexes are difficult to inhibit by deep levels of general anesthesia alone.[138] The clinician must then give consideration to how best to prevent discomfort, gagging, coughing, and laryngospasm during tracheal intubation: avoidance of tracheal intubation, use of regional and topical anesthesia, very deep general anesthesia, or a combination of all modalities.

Minimizing Airway Stimulation

Although placement of an SGA is likely to be less noxious than DL and tracheal intubation, it remains a highly stimulating procedure that can lead to gagging, laryngospasm, and coughing.[139] Instrumentation of the upper airway by any technique will illicit protective reflexes that must be obtunded with local or general anesthesia (or both).

Regional and Topical Anesthesia

The mucosal surfaces of the mouth and nose are easily anesthetized with topical anesthetic sprays or gels. Lidocaine is equally effective as cocaine and less toxic; it can be combined with a vasoconstrictor to give equivalent intubating conditions. Administration of an antisialagogue 30 to 60 minutes before application of topical anesthetic results in better anesthesia and intubating conditions by minimizing dilution of the applied anesthetic.[140-142]

The supraglottic larynx derives its sensory innervation from the SLN, a branch of the vagus, and intubation can be facilitated by blocking it bilaterally. The nerve block relies on the consistent relationship of the SLN to the lateral horns of the hyoid bone. When combined with topical anesthesia of the nose or mouth and adequate anesthesia of the infraglottic larynx, this nerve block provides excellent intubating conditions, and most patients are able to accept an ETT without cough, gag, or laryngospasm. Equal success in blunting upper airway reflexes can be achieved by careful spraying of the larynx with topical anesthesia. Topical anesthesia spares the patient the need for two injections.[143]

The infraglottic larynx derives sensory innervation from the recurrent laryngeal nerves, which run along the posterolateral surfaces of the trachea. Again, topical anesthesia rather than nerve block is the method of choice for obtunding reflexes. Injection of several milliliters of 4% lidocaine into the trachea via the cricothyroid membrane routinely results in excellent blockade of sensation.

The efficacy of topical and nerve block anesthesia at suppressing airway reflexes during intubation is evident. Several studies have documented that topical anesthesia applied preoperatively (for brief cases) or intraoperatively can suppress cough and laryngospasm at the time of extubation.[144] The incidence of coughing, stridor, or laryngospasm at the time of extubation can be reduced by application of topical lidocaine at the time of intubation.[145,146]

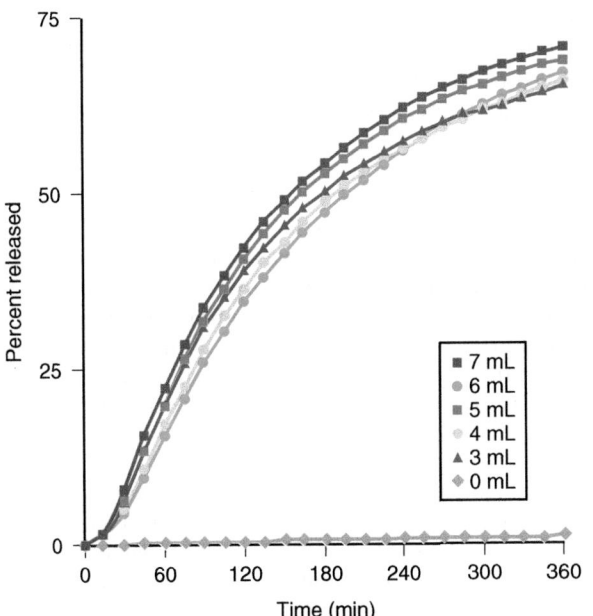

• **Fig. 7.6** Percentage of lidocaine released in vitro as a function of time from an endotracheal tube (ETT) cuff filled with 2 mL of 2% lidocaine (40 mg) with 8.4% sodium bicarbonate solution added to equal 0, 3, 4, 5, 6, or 7 mL. (From Estebe JP, Dollo G, Le Corre P, et al. Alkalinization of intracuff lidocaine improves ETT-induced emergence phenomena. *Anesth Analg.* 2002;94:227–230.)

The use of an aqueous lidocaine-bicarbonate mixture rather than air to inflate the cuff of the ETT after intubation has also been reported to be effective in diminishing emergence phenomena. Inflating the ETT cuff with 40 mg of lidocaine (2 mL of 2% solution) and then adding 3 to 7 mL of 8.4% sodium bicarbonate until no cuff leak was present resulted in significant reductions in coughing, restlessness, and BP during emergence. In addition, postoperative complaints of sore throat, postoperative dysphonia, and hoarseness after extubation were all reduced when compared with cuff inflation with air[147,148] (Fig. 7.6). Because standard NaHCO$_3$ is a basic solution with a calculated pH of 7.8 (range 7 to 8.5), the addition of more than 2 mL of bicarbonate to the 2 mL of 2% lidocaine (calculated pH 6, range 5 to 7) already injected into the ETT cuff results in a basic solution; this leads to concern about tracheal mucosal burn injury in the event of a cuff rupture. However, a direct comparison between solutions of 2 mL of 2% lidocaine with 8.4% versus 1.4% bicarbonate reported similar efficacy in reducing postoperative sore throat complaints and the occurrence of various emergence phenomena.[148] Therefore in clinical practice, a favorable risk-benefit balance can be achieved by using the following combination in a 10-mL syringe: 5 mL 1% lidocaine, 1 mL 8.4% NaHCO$_3$ solution, and 4 mL of sterile diluent. As a potentially simpler alternative, benzydamine hydrochloride (1.5 mg/mL) sprayed on the outside of the ETT cuff prior to intubation also reduces postoperative sore throat.[149]

Intravenous Agents

Given a high enough dose, virtually all agents used as IV anesthetics will suppress the cough response to intubation. However, different agents appear to vary in their ability to inhibit upper airway reflexes when judged on the basis of equal potency in depressing consciousness and in depressing the cardiovascular system. Propofol/narcotic anesthesia may be adequate for intubating the trachea in some patients even without the use of NMBDs.[150] On the other hand, ketamine clinically appears to enhance laryngeal reflexes at doses that provide adequate anesthesia for surgery.[151]

IV lidocaine is frequently used to prevent cough and laryngospasm at the time of intubation or extubation. Although the studies are not uniform in documenting efficacy, the preponderance of evidence supports the use of lidocaine.[152,153] The maximal efficacy of IV lidocaine occurs 1 to 3 minutes after injection and requires a dose of 1.5 mg/kg or more. This corresponds to a plasma level in excess of 4 μg/mL.[154]

The ability of IV lidocaine to suppress cough appears to be related to factors beyond induction of general anesthesia, because cough suppression occurs at levels routinely seen in awake patients being treated with the drug. A comparison of the antitussive effects of lidocaine compared with meperidine and thiopental demonstrated that severe respiratory depression occurs with the latter drugs in achieving the same antitussive efficacy that can be achieved with lidocaine with virtually no respiratory depression.[154] Further evidence showing reduction of coughing and sore throat has been discussed previously in this chapter.

Preventing Bronchoconstriction

Bronchoconstriction is a frequent consequence of tracheal intubation. In healthy subjects, it appears to be of a moderate degree, but the exaggerated response seen in patients with hyperactive airways can be life-threatening. Even though the incidence of severe bronchospasm only accounts for 2% of adverse events in the American Society of Anesthesiologists Closed Claims Project, over 90% of these claims involved severe brain injury or death.[155] Prevention or treatment of this response can be achieved with the use of topical anesthetics, inhaled bronchodilators, or IV agents. Inhaled anesthetic agents also inhibit the response through direct absorption by smooth muscle or inhibition of reflexes.

Bronchospasm after intubation is likely cholinergically mediated. Afferent parasympathetic fibers travel to bronchial smooth muscle and then produce bronchoconstriction by stimulating M$_3$ cholinergic receptors on bronchial smooth muscle. In addition, stimulation of M$_3$ cholinergic receptors on airway smooth muscle potentiates bronchospasm by inhibiting β-adrenergic–mediated smooth muscle relaxation.[156] The ability to prophylactically treat with bronchodilators is controversial and has not been shown to be effective. Patients who have existing bronchoconstriction should be aggressively treated with usual protocols.

Minimizing Airway Stimulation

Avoidance of tracheal intubation is the most logical first step in terms of limiting airway irritation and bronchoconstriction. If general anesthesia is required, an SGA may be preferable to tracheal intubation in terms of provocation of bronchospasm, but, as alluded to previously, an SGA will not prevent coughing in the absence of neuromuscular blockade.[139] However, SGAs do appear to result in reduced lower airway resistance when compared with tracheal intubation after induction of general anesthesia. This difference is assumed to result from induction of reversible bronchospasm by the ETT. In addition, use of an SGA results in fewer pulmonary complications and improved pulmonary function when compared with tracheal intubation in infants born prematurely with bronchopulmonary dysplasia and in adults without lung disease.[157,158] If tracheal intubation is absolutely required, minimizing the time instrumenting the airway must be a priority.

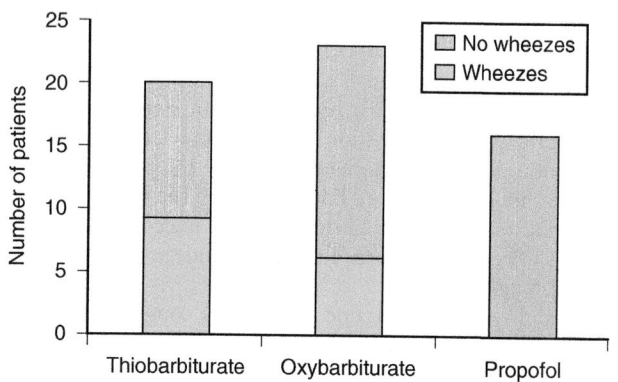

• **Fig. 7.7** Incidence of wheezing after tracheal intubation in asthmatics when induction was performed with either an oxybarbiturate (methohexital), a thiobarbiturate (thiopental or thiamylal), or propofol ($P < 0.05$ for either thiobarbiturate or oxybarbiturate versus propofol). (From Pizow R, Brown RH, Weiss YS, et al. Wheezing during induction of general anesthesia in patients with and without asthma: a randomized, blinded trial. *Anesthesiology.* 1995;81:1111.)

Topical Anesthesia

Studies have demonstrated a doubling of lower airway resistance after tracheal intubation of awake volunteers under topical anesthesia.[159] The bronchoconstrictor response must indeed be a powerful one if local anesthesia sufficient to permit awake intubation was not sufficient to prevent the reflex bronchoconstriction. A study of awake fiberoptic intubation in asthmatics demonstrated a marked decrease in forced expiratory volume in 1 minute (FEV_1) after intubation. This decrease was somewhat mitigated by topical lidocaine, although lidocaine was not as effective as albuterol in preventing bronchoconstriction.[160]

Intravenous Agents

A variety of drugs have been studied for their bronchodilating properties. Although IV β_2-agonists clearly produce bronchodilation, there is no benefit to parenteral administration of these agents compared with inhalational administration. Among anesthetic induction agents, considerable experimental evidence suggests that ketamine has both direct and indirect relaxant effects on airway smooth muscle through non–β-receptor mechanisms.[161,162] However, the clinical data supporting the use of ketamine for prevention or treatment of bronchospasm are largely anecdotal, or unimpressive in more rigorous trials. This may relate to a lack of evaluation of a range of doses of ketamine and a reluctance to routinely use ketamine at high doses because of its side effects, including dysphoria, emergence reactions, and sympathetic stimulation.[163]

Propofol, midazolam, and etomidate all relax airway smooth muscle in vitro, although generally at higher effect-site concentrations than would be used clinically.[164,165] In contrast, barbiturates may have direct bronchoconstricting effects.[166] Propofol may also have indirect effects on airway constriction, perhaps through inhibition of vagal tone.[167] Clinically, propofol has been shown to be superior to the barbiturates and to etomidate in reducing wheezing and airway resistance in both asthmatic and nonasthmatic subjects.[168,169] When asthmatics were induced with either thiopental, methohexital, or propofol at equipotent doses, none of the patients given propofol wheezed after tracheal intubation, whereas both of the barbiturates resulted in a significant incidence of wheezing (Fig. 7.7).[168]

It has been shown that in patients with bronchial hyperreactivity, IV lidocaine reduces the bronchoconstrictor response

to histamine challenge and has an additive effect with albuterol in reducing this response.[168] However, a double-blind, placebo-controlled trial of IV lidocaine (1.5 mg/kg) or inhaled albuterol in asthmatics found that albuterol, but not lidocaine, prevented postintubation bronchoconstriction.[170] Although lidocaine may inhibit reflex-induced bronchospasm, it may also cause contraction of bronchial smooth muscle in the absence of reflex mechanisms. A published best-evidence review also failed to find support for the use of IV lidocaine during intubation in patients with status asthmaticus.[171] In summary, the evidence in support of IV lidocaine to prevent postintubation bronchospasm when used without the concomitant administration of an inhaled β-agonist is scant, and there is a potential risk of worsening airway resistance; therefore its use for this indication cannot be endorsed.

Inhaled Agents

All of the volatile anesthetics have direct and perhaps indirect relaxant effects on airway smooth muscle in experimental models.[172–174] Although these agents have differences in potency in vitro, the clinical importance of these differences remains unclear. In adult patients, sevoflurane is more effective than isoflurane, desflurane, or halothane in reducing airway resistance after tracheal intubation[175–177] but does not prevent an increase in airway resistance after intubation of asthmatic children.[178] However, given the available data, sevoflurane is probably the volatile agent of choice, and desflurane should be avoided in high-risk patients (Fig. 7.8).

There are no prospective, controlled studies comparing deep inhalational anesthesia to IV induction with bronchoprotective agents such as ketamine or propofol in high-risk patients. Achieving a deep plane of anesthesia with a bronchoprotective agent before intubation is likely the most important point in preventing severe bronchospasm in high-risk patients, rather than the choice of IV versus inhalational induction techniques.

Pretreatment of patients with inhaled β_2-adrenergic agonists or an inhaled anticholinergic markedly reduced lung resistance following tracheal intubation and should be used routinely in patients known to have bronchospasm.[128,179] Additionally, in bronchospastic patients with severely impaired ventilation, a liquid bolus of albuterol via the ETT may have utility as a rescue agent when albuterol via metered dose inhaler is ineffective.[180]

Choice of Neuromuscular Blocking Drug

The choice of NMBDs can influence bronchial tone after tracheal intubation. Of the NMBDs currently in use, rocuronium is most frequently associated with anaphylaxis.[181] Several case reports have emerged of providers successfully using the reversal agent sugammadex to block an immunologic response to rocuronium via chemical encapsulation.[182]

Conclusion

Airway manipulations of any kind can result in complex reflex-mediated changes in cardiopulmonary physiology. The type and depth of anesthesia provided must be individualized for the type of airway being used and the clinical situation for which it is required. Additionally, clinicians should be prepared to treat profound alterations in HR, BP, airway resistance, and ICP occurring during or immediately following airway manipulation. Although these responses may be of short duration and of little consequence in healthy individuals, serious complications can occur in patients with underlying cardiovascular, respiratory, or intracranial pathology.

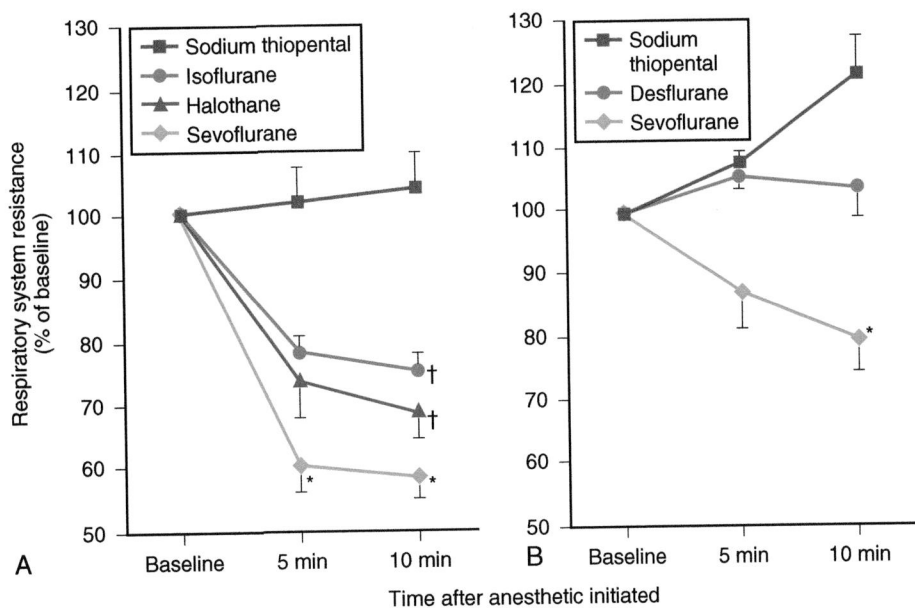

• **Fig. 7.8** Respiratory system resistance (percent of baseline) during maintenance anesthesia. (A) Isoflurane, halothane, and sevoflurane are compared with thiopental 0.25 mg/kg/min plus 50% nitrous oxide. * $P < 0.05$ versus isoflurane, halothane, and thiopental. †$P < 0.05$ versus thiopental. (B) Desflurane and sevoflurane are compared with thiopental 0.25 mg/kg/min. *$P < 0.05$ versus desflurane and thiopental. (A, Modified from Rooke GA, Choi JH, Bishop MJ. The effect of isoflurane, halothane, sevoflurane, and thiopental/nitrous oxide on respiratory system resistance after tracheal intubation. *Anesthesiology.* 1997;86:1294; B, From Goff MJ, Arain SR, Ficke DJ, et al. Absence of bronchodilation during desflurane anesthesia: a comparison to sevoflurane and thiopental. *Anesthesiology.* 2000;93:404.)

Selected References

4. Kramer N, Lebowitz D, Walsh M, Ganti L. Rapid sequence intubation in traumatic brain-injured adults. *Cureus.* 2018;10(4):e2530. doi:10.7759/cureus.2530.

17. Alviar CL, Rico-Mesa JS, Morrow DA, et al. Positive pressure ventilation in cardiogenic shock: review of the evidence and practical advice for patients with mechanical circulatory support. *Can J Cardiol.* 2020;36(2):300–312. doi:10.1016/j.cjca.2019.11.038.

27. Perkins ZB, Wittenberg MD, Nevin D, Lockey DJ, O'Brien B. The relationship between head injury severity and hemodynamic response to tracheal intubation. *J Trauma Acute Care Surg.* 2013;74(4):1074–1080. doi:10.1097/TA.0b013e3182827305.

38. Bucher J, Koyfman A. Intubation of the Neurologically Injured Patient. *J Emerg Med.* 2015;49(6):920–927. doi:10.1016/j.jemermed.2015.06.078.

51. Buhari FS, Selvaraj V. Randomized controlled study comparing the hemodynamic response to laryngoscopy and endotracheal intubation with McCoy, Macintosh, and C-MAC laryngoscopes in adult patients. *J Anaesthesiol Clin Pharmacol.* 2016;32(4):505–509. doi:10.4103/0970-9185.194766.

70. Eis S, Kramer J. Anesthesia Inhalation Agents Cardiovascular Effects. In: *StatPearls* [Internet]. StatPearls Publishing; 2020. Accessed January 11, 2021. http://www.ncbi.nlm.nih.gov/books/NBK541090.

88. Grape S, Kirkham KR, Frauenknecht J, Albrecht E. Intra-operative analgesia with remifentanil vs. dexmedetomidine: a systematic review and meta-analysis with trial sequential analysis. *Anaesthesia.* 2019;74(6):793–800. doi:10.1111/anae.14657.

154. Yang SS, Wang N-N, Postonogova T, et al. Intravenous lidocaine to prevent postoperative airway complications in adults: a systematic review and meta-analysis. *Br J Anaesth.* 2020;124(3):314–323. doi:10.1016/j.bja.2019.11.033.

175. Ehsan Z, Mahmoud M, Shott SR, Amin RS, Ishman SL. The effects of anesthesia and opioids on the upper airway: A systematic review. *The Laryngoscope.* 2016;126(1):270–284. doi:10.1002/lary.25399.

181. Harper NJN, Cook TM, Garcez T, et al. Anaesthesia, surgery, and life-threatening allergic reactions: epidemiology and clinical features of perioperative anaphylaxis in the 6th National Audit Project (NAP6). *Br J Anaesth.* 2018;121(1):159–171. doi:10.1016/j.bja.2018.04.014.

All references can be found online at eBooks.Health.Elsevier.com.

PART 2

The Difficult Airway: Definition, Assessment, Planning, and Algorithms

8

Definition and Incidence of the Difficult Airway

P. ALLAN KLOCK JR.

CHAPTER OUTLINE

KEY POINTS

- The inability to manage a difficult airway (DA) is responsible for a large proportion of deaths and morbidity directly attributable to anesthesia.
- While it is important to have common definitions for common problems, the literature continues to report variable nomenclature related to DA management. It is important to have an understanding of the incidence of significant airway problems for the specialty to make advances in this area.
- Difficult mask ventilation (DMV) has been reported at a rate of 1 to 2 per 100 anesthetics, and impossible mask ventilation (IMV) can be expected at a rate of 1 to 2 times per 1000 anesthetics.
- Most studies report the failure rate for supraglottic airway (SGA) devices at approximately 2% for the classical laryngeal mask airway (CLMA) and flexible LMA (FLMA) and 1% for the intubating LMA (ILMA), unique LMA (ULMA), and ProSeal LMA (PLMA). A 2015 study showed difficulty in 0.5% of SGA uses and failure of the device 0.2% of the time.

- Fewer data exist regarding failure for video-assisted laryngoscopy (VAL) than for direct laryngoscopy (DL), but the incidence of failed intubation with these devices ranges from 0.4% to 2.6% in patients with a normal airway and 2.4% to 3.6% for patients with a DA.
- When difficult laryngoscopy is defined as a Cormack-Lehane (CL) grade 2 or 3 view requiring multiple attempts or blades, the reported incidence varies from 1% to 18% of surgical cases, but the majority of these patients are successfully intubated.
- Unsuccessful intubation with DL occurs at a rate of 5 to 35 per 10,000 anesthetics, and the cannot intubate/cannot oxygenate (CICO) scenario occurs at a rate of 0.01 to 2 patients per 10,000 anesthetics.
- Large multicenter studies will be required to refine our understanding of the incidence of serious airway problems.

Introduction

The fundamental responsibility of an anesthesiologist is to ensure adequate gas exchange for the patient. Failure to maintain oxygenation for more than a few minutes could result in catastrophic anoxic injury. Data from closed claims of respiratory-related malpractice in 1990 reported brain damage or death in over 85% of patients.[1] In the closed claims data from 2006, subsequent improvements in airway management techniques and monitoring standards reduced the number of intubation-related claims,[2] but

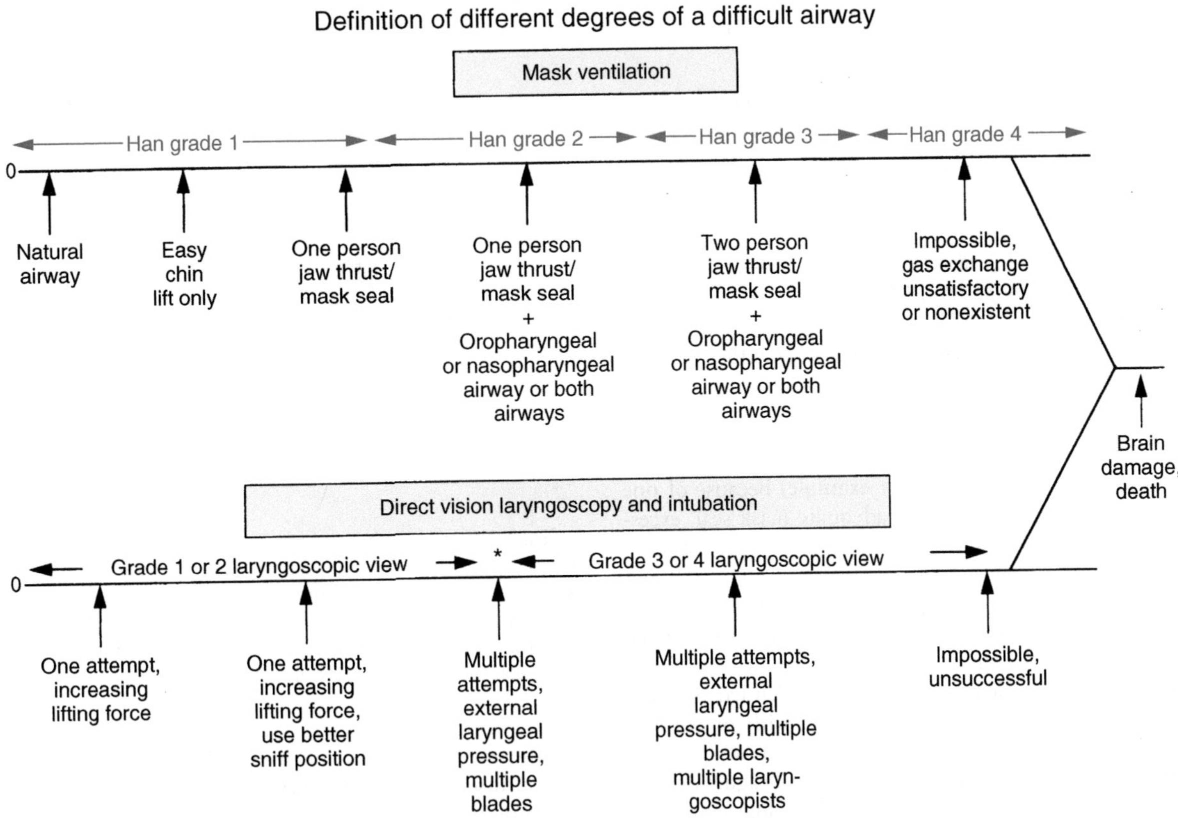

Definition of different degrees of a difficult airway

• **Fig. 8.1** Conceptualization of the difficult airway. Difficult intubation (DI) is one or more of the following: difficult laryngoscopy, difficult video-assisted laryngoscopy, or difficult flexible scope visualization. The widespread use of supraglottic airways (SGAs) has elevated them to immediate rescue devices in cannot intubate/cannot oxygenate situations. The triad of difficult mask ventilation, difficult SGA placement, and DI increases the risk of hypoxic brain injury and death.

difficulties with airway management during emergence remain among the leading causes of serious perioperative problems.[3] It has been estimated that the inability to successfully manage a difficult airway (DA) is responsible for as many as 30% of deaths and the majority of cardiac arrests directly attributable to anesthesia.[4]

In general, greater degrees of difficulty in maintaining airway patency are more likely to engender greater risk of brain damage or death. Before discussing the specific management of a DA, we must (1) define the DA, (2) classify the degrees of difficulty in maintaining a patent airway, and (3) determine the incidence of each class or type of DA. In this discussion, it is assumed that a reasonably well-trained anesthesia provider always attempts to maintain airway patency.

Definition and Classification of the Difficult Airway

There are three common ways of maintaining airway patency and gas exchange. First, mask ventilation (MV) delivers inspired gas via a mask that is sealed to the patient's face, while the natural airway from the face to the vocal cords is kept patent with or without external jaw thrust maneuvers or internal upper airway devices. Second, inspired gas can be delivered via a supraglottic airway (SGA), such as a laryngeal mask airway (LMA). Third, with tracheal intubation, inspired gases are delivered via a tube that traverses the vocal cords, providing continuity from the respiratory circuit to the trachea. Maintenance of airway patency via a surgically inserted device is not discussed in this chapter.

The term *difficult airway* spans a spectrum of clinical situations (Fig. 8.1) from difficulty or inability to ventilate the patient with a face mask or SGA to difficulty or inability to intubate the trachea. The combined "cannot intubate/cannot oxygenate" (CICO) scenario carries the highest risk of brain damage or death. To better describe the layers of difficulty, we have chosen several categories: difficult mask ventilation (DMV) or impossible mask ventilation (IMV); difficult placement of or ventilation via an SGA; difficult laryngoscopy; and difficult intubation (DI) using a direct laryngoscope, videolaryngoscope (VL), or flexible intubation scope (FIS), such as a flexible bronchoscope.

Difficult or Impossible Face-Mask Ventilation

Causes of Difficult Mask Ventilation

There are two main causes of inadequate MV. One cause is an inability to establish an adequate seal between the face and the mask, causing a leak of respiratory gas. The second cause is inadequate patency of the airway at the level of the nasopharynx, oropharynx, hypopharynx, larynx, or trachea. These manifest as either an inability to generate adequate airway pressure to drive gas into the lungs or an inability to move gas into the lungs despite an adequate driving pressure.

Definition of Difficult Mask Ventilation

The American Society of Anesthesiologists (ASA) *Practice Guidelines for Management of the Difficult Airway* define DMV as the inability "to provide adequate ventilation (as confirmed by

TABLE 8.1	Han Mask Ventilation Scale and Incidence of Difficult Mask Ventilation	
Grade	Description	Incidence, *n* (%)
1	Ventilated by mask	37,857 (71.3)
2	Ventilated by mask with oral airway/adjuvant, with or without muscle relaxant	13,966 (26.3)
3	Difficult ventilation (inadequate, unstable, or requiring two providers) with or without muscle relaxant	1,141 (2.2)
4	Unable to mask ventilate with or without muscle relaxant	77 (0.15)

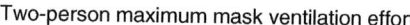

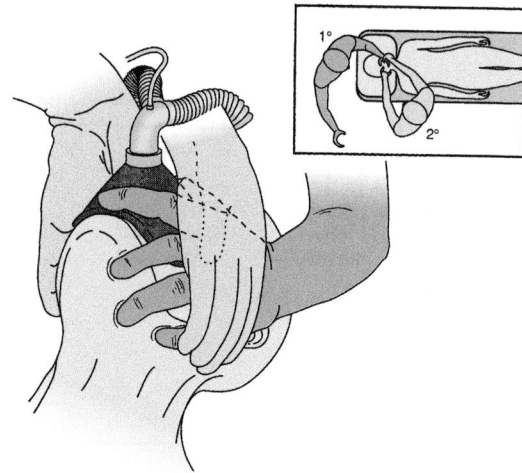

• **Fig. 8.2** Optimal two-person mask ventilation effort. The primary practitioner stands at the head of the patient and uses left and right hands in the standard classical fashion. The secondary (assisting) person stands facing the primary practitioner at the level of the patient's shoulder and uses the right hand to help achieve left-sided jaw thrust and mask seal while the left hand achieves right-sided jaw thrust and mask seal.

end-tidal carbon dioxide detection, for example) because of one or more of the following problems: inadequate mask seal, excessive gas leak, or excessive resistance to the ingress or egress of gas."[5]

The most commonly cited MV scale in contemporary literature was described by Han and colleagues in 2004 (Table 8.1).[6] In this scale, the progressive grades of difficulty are (1) ventilated by mask; (2) ventilated by mask with oral airway or other adjuvant, with or without muscle relaxant; (3) DMV defined as "inadequate, unstable, or requiring two providers," with or without muscle relaxant; and (4) IMV with an inability to mask ventilate, with or without muscle relaxant. Langeron and colleagues defined DMV as "the inability of an unassisted anesthesiologist to maintain oxygen saturation >92%, as measured by pulse oximetry, or to prevent or reverse signs of inadequate ventilation during positive-pressure MV under general anesthesia."[7] In that study, MV was considered difficult if one or more of six criteria were present:
• inability of the unassisted anesthesiologist to maintain oxygen saturation >92% using 100% oxygen and positive-pressure MV;
• significant gas flow leak by the face mask;
• need to increase gas flow to >15 L/min and to use the oxygen flush valve more than twice;
• no perceptible chest movement;
• need to perform a two-handed MV technique; or
• change of operator required.

El-Ganzouri and colleagues defined DMV as the "inability to obtain chest excursion sufficient to maintain a clinically acceptable capnogram waveform despite optimal head and neck positioning and use of muscle paralysis, use of an oral airway, and optimal application of a face mask by anesthesia personnel."[8]

Incidence of Difficult Mask Ventilation

Two studies by Kheterpal and colleagues on DMV and IMV represent the largest investigations to date on the topic. The incidence of DMV was 1.4% in 22,660 patients and 2.2% in a subsequent study of 50,000 patients.[9,10] The incidence of IMV ranged from 0.15% to 0.16% in these two large studies.[9,10] Langeron and colleagues reported a 5% incidence of DMV with 1 of 1502 patients impossible to ventilate with a face mask (0.07%).[7] Thomsen and colleagues reported a DMV or IMV (Han grade 3 or 4) incidence of 0.07% in 658,104 anesthetic records.[11] Other large prospective studies show an incidence ranging from 0.07% to 1.4%, although this was not always the primary outcome being assessed.[8,12,13] In summary, DMV can be expected between 1 and 2 times per 100 anesthetics, and IMV can be expected between 1 and 2 times per 1000 anesthetics.

Techniques for improving airway patency include the head-tilt, jaw-thrust, and chin-lift maneuvers, as well as insertion of oral or nasal airways. If mask seal is poor, the practitioner may choose a different face mask, use a two-handed or two-person technique, insert bolsters between the alveolar ridge and the cheeks, or employ other methods to improve the interface between the face and the mask. When two providers are needed, ideally the primary practitioner stands at the patient's head and initiates jaw thrust with the left hand at the angle of the left mandible and left-sided mask seal, while the right hand compresses the reservoir bag. The standard position for the primary practitioner is shown in Fig. 8.2. The secondary (assisting) person stands at the patient's side, at the level of the patient's shoulder, facing the primary practitioner. The right hand of the secondary practitioner should cover the left hand of the primary practitioner and contribute to left-sided jaw thrust and mask seal, and the left hand of the secondary person initiates right-sided jaw thrust and mask seal. In this way, all four hands are doing something important without interfering with one another, and there is almost no redundant effort. With this positioning, the secondary person can watch the monitors continuously, manipulate the larynx externally, and hand equipment to the primary practitioner.

Difficulty With Supraglottic Airways

SGAs have become a mainstay of airway management. They have a role in routine airway management and are an essential part of all difficult airway algorithms (DAAs). Most studies of SGAs describe first-attempt and overall success rates. Difficulties with the devices include failure of insertion, failure to form a clear passage to the trachea from obstruction or laryngospasm, and failure to form an effective seal in the airway.[14,15]

Most of the studies examining difficulties with SGAs focus on LMAs (Teleflex, Inc., Morrisville, NC). Among these, the failure rate is 1% for the LMA Unique (ULMA), intubating LMA (LMA Fastrach; ILMA), and the LMA ProSeal (PLMA), and it is 2% for the LMA Classic (CLMA) and LMA Flexible (FLMA).[14,15]

Definition of Difficult Placement

The ASA *Practice Guidelines for Management of the Difficult Airway* define difficult supraglottic airway ventilation as the inability

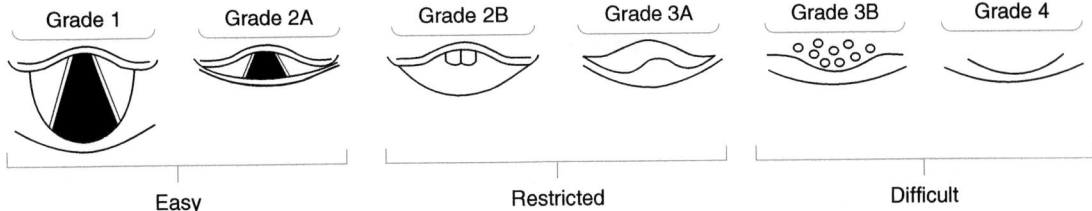

• **Fig. 8.3** Grading of laryngoscopic view. (Top) Cormack-Lehane grading system. Grade 1 is visualization of the entire laryngeal aperture; grade 2A is partial visualization of the vocal cords; grade 2B is visualization of only the posterior commissure of the vocal cords or arytenoid cartilages; grade 3A is visualization of only the epiglottis (epiglottis can be lifted); grade 3B is visualization of only the epiglottis (epiglottis cannot be lifted off the posterior pharynx); and grade 4 is visualization of only the soft palate. (Bottom) Cook grading system. *Easy*, the laryngeal inlet is visible; *Restricted*, the posterior glottic structures are visible and the epiglottis can be lifted; *Difficult*, the epiglottis cannot be lifted, or no laryngeal structures are visible. (Adapted from Cook TM. A new practical classification of laryngeal view. *Anaesthesia.* 2000;55:274–279.)

"to provide adequate ventilation because of one or more of the following problems: difficult SGA placement, SGA placement requiring multiple attempts, inadequate SGA seal, excessive gas leak, or excessive resistance to the ingress or egress of gas."[5]

Success rates after one, two, or three attempts are a quantifiable way to characterize the difficulty of placement of an SGA. Other methods include time taken for successful placement, Likert-based difficulty scales (very easy, easy, or difficult), and secondary measures, such as evidence of trauma during insertion.

Incidence of Success

The CLMA has reported success rates ranging from 95.3% to 99.8%.[13,16,17] A large observational study of the ULMA found a 1.1% failure rate. In this study, failure was defined as the need for tracheal intubation because of hypoxia, hypercarbia, or obstruction.[15]

For the PLMA, first-attempt success rates range from 76% to 100% (mean, 87.3%), and overall success rates range from 90% to 100% (mean, 98.4%).[18] A study published in 2015 reported a retrospective chart review of over 14,000 anesthetics using various SGAs, including the CLMA, PLMA, LMA Supreme (SLMA), and ILMA, as well as the i-gel (Intersurgical Ltd, Wokingham, Berkshire, UK). Difficult ventilation, defined as excessive leak, poor seal, or excessive resistance to ingress of gas, was reported in 0.5% of patients, and failure of the device was reported in 0.2%.[19]

One of the important rescue functions of the SGA is as a conduit for the FIS, previously referred to as a *flexible bronchoscope*. An inability to visualize the vocal cords using a trans-SGA FIS technique is a significant impediment to successful tracheal intubation. The incidence of difficult laryngeal visualization ranges from 0% to 26% with the PLMA.[18] Although it is possible that success rates may differ with other SGAs, the inherent variability in success is an important point. Early recognition of unsuccessful placement and institution of alternate airway plans are essential to prevent morbidity from failure of an SGA.

Difficult Direct Laryngoscopy

Laryngeal Visualization

The appearance of the laryngeal inlet on direct laryngoscopy (DL) is most often described by the Cormack-Lehane (CL) grade of laryngeal view (Fig. 8.3).[20] DL is most commonly defined as presence of a grade 3 or 4 view on laryngoscopy.[21] Several maneuvers improve the laryngeal view on laryngoscopy, but in general, poorer laryngeal views progressively contribute to greater difficulty in achieving successful tracheal intubation.[20,22] An alternative system for classifying glottic exposure was proposed by Cook

in 2000.[23] This system uses an "easy," "restricted," and "difficult" ordinal scale. During easy DL, part or all of the vocal cords are visible (CL grade 2A or 1). During restricted DL, only the arytenoids are visible, or the epiglottis is visible and can be lifted (CL grade 2B or 3A). With difficult DL, the epiglottis adheres to the posterior pharynx (i.e., it cannot be lifted) or no laryngeal structures are seen (CL grade 3B or 4). The advantage of the Cook system is that it correlates better than the CL classification with the time required for intubation and the need for adjuncts. The ASA *Practice Guidelines for Management of the Difficult Airway* define difficult laryngoscopy as the inability "to visualize any portion of the vocal cords after multiple attempts at laryngoscopy."[5]

As the laryngeal view worsens, increasing anterior lifting force with the laryngoscope blade, reinstituting optimal sniffing position, making multiple attempts, manipulating the larynx externally (see Chapter 20), or opting for alternative devices or a more experienced laryngoscopist may be required to achieve intubation. A learning curve exists for management of a DA, and a poor laryngeal view observed by an inexperienced laryngoscopist may easily be improved by a more experienced or skillful individual with, perhaps, a different blade. Although a CL grade 3 or 4 laryngoscopic view may be overcome by the occasional successful "blind" intubation, these views more commonly render intubation impossible. Therefore, early recognition of a DA and immediate availability of skilled help and advanced equipment for airway management are essential components of DA management.

Incidence of Difficult Laryngeal Visualization

The incidence of difficult laryngoscopy or intubation in the general surgical population varies greatly depending on the laryngeal view, the individual study population, and the definition used. A grade 2 or 3 laryngoscopic view requiring multiple attempts and/or blades (and presumably external laryngeal manipulation) is relatively common and is found in 1% to 18% of cases. Grade 3 laryngeal views resulting in a successful intubation occur at a rate of 1% to 4%. Intubation is unsuccessful in 5 to 35 patients per 10,000, and the CICO scenario occurs in 0.01 to 2 patients per 10,000 (Table 8.2).

For studies of difficult laryngoscopy to be reliable and for the laryngoscopic grading system to be helpful, the reported grades must describe the best view that was obtained, which depends on the best possible performance of laryngoscopy. The components of best performance of laryngoscopy consist of proper sniffing position, complete muscle relaxation, firm forward traction on the laryngoscope, and, if necessary, optimal external laryngeal manipulation (OELM). The application of OELM may reduce the incidence of a grade 3 view from 9% to between 5.4% and 1.3%.[13] When the laryngeal view is insufficient, the practitioner,

TABLE 8.2   Incidence of Various Levels of Difficult Intubation

Degree of Difficulty With Intubation	RANGE OF INCIDENCE		References
	Per 10,000	%	
Tracheal intubation successful but multiple attempts and/or blades may be required; probable grade 2 or 3	100–1800	1–18	13,20
Tracheal intubation successful but multiple attempts and/or blades and/or laryngoscopists required; grade 3	100–400	1–4	13,22
Tracheal intubation not successful; grade 3 or 4	5–35	0.05–0.35	13,20,22
Cannot ventilate by mask, cannot intubate; transtracheal jet ventilation, tracheostomy, brain damage, or death	0.01–2.0	0.0001–0.02	13,25,28,32,34

while performing laryngoscopy with the left hand, should quickly apply external pressure over the laryngeal cartilages with the right hand. In a matter of seconds, the vector and force of pressure that afford the best laryngeal view can be determined (i.e., OELM). Having found the position that gives the best view, the laryngoscopist should ask the assistant to carefully press on the same spot. OELM by the assistant must be directed by the laryngoscopist, even if the assistant is fully trained. The best performance of laryngoscopy avoids awkward high-arm postures, positioning the laryngoscope blade over the middle of the tongue, gripping the laryngoscope at the junction of the handle and blade with rotation about a horizontal axis, choosing the wrong blade size or shape, and placing the blade incorrectly. Theoretically, if the components of best performance of laryngoscopy are used and the pitfalls avoided, all laryngoscopists (novice and expert) should have close to the same laryngoscopic view.

Difficult Intubation During Direct Laryngoscopy

Unlike DMV and difficult laryngoscopy, there is no uniformly accepted method of classifying DI. The Intubation Difficulty Score (IDS) validated by Adnet and colleagues describes a spectrum of intubation difficulty.[24] The assessment variables for the IDS are number of additional attempts, number of additional operators, number of alternative intubation techniques used, CL laryngeal view (minus one), need for excessive lifting force, need for laryngeal pressure, and vocal cord adduction. Each variable carries 1 point, and DI is defined as an IDS score >5, indicating moderate to major difficulty, with a score of infinity (∞) being assigned to an impossible intubation. Kheterpal and colleagues defined DI as CL grade 3 or 4, or intubation requiring more than three attempts by anesthesia attending staff to secure the airway with an endotracheal tube (ETT).[10]

Incidence of Difficult Intubation

The incidence of DI ranges from 1% to 18% in various studies of elective surgical cases. The true incidence is probably 5% to 8% in most practice settings. A study of emergent tracheal intubations in a university hospital showed a 10.3% incidence of DI.[25] The incidence of failed tracheal intubation ranges from 0.05% to 0.35%; the low and high ends of this range are associated with elective surgical and obstetric patients, respectively. The incidence of failed intubation is approximately 8 times higher in the obstetrical population than in others, with a 13-fold increase in the risk of death.[26]

Combined Difficult Mask Ventilation and Difficult Intubation

In one study from the Multicenter Perioperative Outcomes Group, the incidence of combined DMV and DI was 0.40%.[27] Patients whose lungs were impossible to ventilate via mask had a risk for DI of 25%, significantly higher than that for the overall population. One in three patients with combined IMV and DI required an alternative intubation technique to secure the airway, with 10% of such patients requiring a surgical airway. Similarly, one of the significant findings in another study was that DMV conferred a 4-fold greater risk for DI and 12-fold greater risk of an impossible intubation.[8] A more recent report of 658,104 Danish anesthetics reported DA management in 4898 patients for a rate of 0.74%. Of the 975 patients with DMV or IMV, 516 (53% of DMV patients and 0.08% of cohort) were difficult or impossible to intubate.[11]

Impossible Mask Ventilation and Intubation

The incidence of CICO has been estimated to range from 0.01 to 2 per 10,000 patients.[26–29] In a cohort of 53,041 patients, Kheterpal and colleagues reported 77 cases of IMV (14.5 per 10,0000); of these, 66 patients were ultimately intubated using conventional DL, leaving 11 patients (2.07 per 10,000) impossible to mask ventilate and intubate with conventional DL.[10] The Danish study cited above had the subjective "cannot intubate, cannot mask ventilate" box selected in 455 records, resulting in a prevalence of 6.9 per 10,000 anesthetics, but many of these patients were ventilated with an SGA and there were likely fewer DL attempts compared to earlier studies.[11] Despite recent advances in airway devices and techniques, most busy hospitals encounter several such events every year, making it imperative to ensure that DA recognition and management remain central tenets of anesthesiology education and training.

Variability in Incidence of Difficult Laryngoscopy and Difficult Intubation

Difficult laryngoscopy (a grade 3 or 4 CL laryngeal view) is synonymous with DI in the majority of patients.[20] However, tracheal intubation and laryngoscopy have slightly differing skill requirements, which may contribute to variability in the occurrence of difficult laryngoscopy and DI. In one prospective study examining respiratory complications in 1005 patients undergoing tracheal intubation, three patients had grade 4 laryngeal views. One patient was easy to intubate, one was "moderately difficult" to intubate, and one was "difficult" to intubate.[12] In the same study among 68 patients with a grade 3 laryngoscopic view, 13 (19%) were easy to intubate, 50 (74%) were moderately difficult to intubate, and 5 (7%) were difficult to intubate. A number of scenarios can explain some of the discordance between difficult laryngoscopy and DI. First, some patients with a grade 3 view have a trachea that can be intubated on the first or second attempt if the distal end of the endotracheal tube is appropriately curved by a malleable stylet (hockey-stick shape) or if a small

TABLE 8.3	Overall Videolaryngoscope Intubation Success Rate			
Device	**Intubations (n)**	**Patients (N)**	**Success Rate (%)**	**References**
Storz C-Mac (Karl Storz SE and Co. KG, Tuttlingen, Germany)	1395	1400	99.6	42–46
GlideScope (Verathon Inc., Bothell, WA)	3164	3250	97.4	37,44,45,47–56
McGrath (Medtronic, Minneapolis, MN)	432	440	98.2	44,45,57–59
Pentax AWS (Nihon Kohden, Tokyo, Japan)	1663	1669	99.6	39,52,54,55,60–67

curved introducer is used (e.g., a gum elastic bougie). Second, grade 3 laryngoscopic views have been variously described as seeing all of the epiglottis or as seeing just the tip of the epiglottis.[30] These different classes of a grade 3 view may respond differently to adjustments, such as OELM, and therefore may differ initially and subsequently with respect to difficulty of tracheal intubation. Third, when using a curved blade placed in the vallecula, a grade 3 view caused by a long, floppy epiglottis may convert to a grade 1 or 2 view if either a curved or straight blade is placed posterior to the epiglottis and used to lift the epiglottis anteriorly.[31] Fourth, the epiglottis may be fixed or mobile, depending on anatomy or pathologic changes such as inflammation or fibrosis. Finally, certain pathologic conditions, such as a laryngeal web, laryngeal tumor, or tracheal stenosis, may disassociate ease of laryngoscopy from difficulty of tracheal intubation.

Complications of Difficult Laryngoscopy and Difficult Intubation

Anesthesia in a patient with a DA can lead to direct airway trauma and morbidity from hypoxia and hypercarbia. The incidence of brain damage, cardiac arrest, and death related to airway disasters appears to be decreasing.[3,28,32] Directly mediated laryngovagal reflexes (airway spasm, apnea, bradycardia, arrhythmia, or hypotension) and laryngospinal reflexes (coughing, vomiting, or bucking) are the sources of some morbidity. In the Fourth National Audit Project (NAP4) of the United Kingdom, aspiration was the most common cause of death from adverse airway events.[33] In general, DA management is more likely to be associated with use of physical force during laryngoscopy and more attempts to secure the airway; together these increase the incidence of complications. Repeated laryngoscopy attempts often convert a can ventilate–cannot intubate situation to the dreaded CICO scenario.[33,34]

Difficult Video-Assisted Laryngoscopy

Video-assisted laryngoscopy (VAL) has been increasingly used in both difficult and routine airway management. In general, VAL provides a better laryngoscopic view than DL. It is important to note, however, that an improved CL laryngoscopic grade does not always guarantee successful intubation of the trachea.[35] Many VLs use a highly angulated blade with a camera positioned to allow the user to "see around the corner" of the tongue. While DL creates a straight line between the operator's eye and the vocal cords, allowing straightforward intubation, highly curved VLs maintain the natural curvature of the airway, necessitating special techniques to pass a tube into the trachea.

An excellent review of VAL in adult airway management published in 2010 pools data from 27 studies in adult patients (Tables 8.3 and 8.4).[35] The operators using the devices were different, and criteria for successful intubation and the definition of a DA were inconsistently applied from study to study, so direct comparisons cannot be made between the devices listed. Nevertheless, the intubation success rate was found to be 97.1% to 99.6% overall and 95.8% to 100% in patients with a predicted DA. A 2012 review by Healy and colleagues analyzes the available VAL data more rigorously and provides a summary of strength of evidence for individual devices, but the overall success rates do not differ significantly from the earlier study.[36]

There are fewer data examining the role of VAL in managing patients with a DA. One study of over 2000 patients found that intubation with the GlideScope (Verathon Inc., Bothell, WA) was successful in 96% of patients with predicted DI. When applied to patients with failed DL, the GlideScope-aided intubation was successful in 94% of patients.[37] Another randomized controlled trial of 300 patients with risk factors for DI showed that the Storz C-Mac (Karl Storz SE and Co. KG, Tuttlingen, Germany) had a first-pass success rate of 93%, whereas DL had an 84% success rate.[38] Other smaller studies of patients with predicted DI showed rates of successful intubation ranging from 95.8% to 100% with VAL.

Difficult Flexible Scope Intubation

Definition of Difficult Flexible Scope Intubation

Flexible scope intubation (FSI) skills are now considered essential for all practicing anesthesia providers. Although FSIs have enhanced patient safety, especially when difficulty with airway management is anticipated, they are by no means fail-safe. A difficult or impossible FSI can be described broadly as inadequate laryngeal visualization with or without difficulty in advancing an ETT. The ease of laryngeal exposure was defined by Ovassapian as *not difficult*, *moderately difficult* (needing some manipulation of the scope in all directions), and *difficult* (needing extensive manipulation of the scope in all directions with or without change in position).[39]

Incidence of Difficult or Failed Flexible Scope Intubation

Inadequate laryngeal visualization is a result of several factors acting individually or in tandem: inexperienced operators, presence of blood or secretions, inadequate topical anesthesia (for awake FSI), distorted airway anatomy, and equipment failure. Factors that typically have little impact on DL, such as the presence of a large, floppy epiglottis, or small amounts of pharyngeal blood, could pose significant hurdles to successful FSI. The incidence of difficult laryngeal visualization has been reported to be 6.7% during orotracheal and 4.4% during nasotracheal awake FSI. The lower incidence of difficult laryngeal visualization using the orotracheal approach under general anesthesia (4.4%) likely reflects differences in the types of

TABLE 8.4	Videolaryngoscope Intubation Success Rate in Patients with a Predicted Difficult Airway			
Device	Intubations (*n*)	Patients (*N*)	Success Rate (%)	References
Storz C-Mac (Karl Storz SE and Co. KG, Tuttlingen, Germany)	405	415	97.6	30,38,44,46,57,68
GlideScope (Verathon Inc., Bothell, WA)	1490	1546	96.4	37,44,47,49,51,53
McGrath (Medtronic, Minneapolis, MN)	133	138	96.4	44,57,68,69

patients who are chosen for awake FSI (e.g., those with distorted upper airway anatomy or a severely compromised airway). The incidence of difficult FSI using an orotracheal approach was 29.1% in awake and 24.1% in anesthetized patients. In contrast, the incidence during nasotracheal intubation was markedly lower at 6.0% in awake and 11.0% in anesthetized patients, reflecting important technical differences between the two approaches. FSI fails in 1.4% to 2.1% of awake and anesthetized patients, respectively, with the primary cause equally distributed between difficulty with laryngeal visualization and inability to advance the ETT.[40]

Other Considerations

The rates of different types of DA management will change over time. Surgical patients will continue to become older, and the prevalence of morbid obesity will likely increase, leading to greater difficulties with MV and intubation using DL. Increased use of awake airway management, improved adherence to airway management algorithms, and access to SGAs and VLs should reduce the rates of failed intubations and inadequate ventilation.

It is expected that as these technologies are increasingly adopted as first-line techniques, clinicians' skill with MV and DL will diminish. Similar trends in medicine have been observed as the use of ultrasound has reduced clinical skills using surface anatomy for regional anesthesia and central venous access. One large prospective study showed a fourfold reduction in the rate of failed tracheal intubation in 16 hospitals comparing epochs of 2002 to 2009 and 2010 to 2015.[41] The reader should remember this because many of the success rates for ventilation and tracheal intubation will change over time as new technologies are adopted and skills with older technologies fade.

Conclusion

Inability to adequately ventilate or oxygenate patients remains an important cause of anesthesia-related morbidity and mortality. It is incumbent upon the anesthesia provider to ensure adequate gas exchange and oxygenation for his or her patient. DMV has been reported at a rate of 1 to 2 per 100 anesthetics, and IMV can be expected at a rate of 1 to 2 per 1000 anesthetics. Most studies report the failure rate for SGAs to be approximately 2% for the CLMA and FLMA and 1% for the ILMA, ULMA, and PLMA. A 2015 study demonstrated difficulty in 0.5% of SGA uses and failure of the device 0.2% of the time. Difficult laryngoscopy occurs at a rate of 1% to 18% of surgical cases, but the majority of these patients are successfully intubated. Unsuccessful intubation with DL occurs at a rate of 5 to 35 per 10,000 anesthetics, and the CICO scenario occurs at a rate of 0.01 to 2 patients per 10,000 anesthetics. Fewer data exist regarding failure of video and optical laryngoscopy than for DL, but the incidence of failed intubation

with these devices ranges from 0.4% to 2.6% in patients with a normal airway and 2.4% to 3.6% for patients with a DA.

Because the incidence of serious airway problems occurs at a low rate, large populations must be examined to improve our understanding of the causes and incidence of these events. Our understanding of management of the DA will improve as we collect data from multicenter trials. If electronic medical and anesthesia records use common language and definitions, data can be pooled from multiple institutions, providing the resources for effective analysis of the serious problem of DA management. This will become increasingly important as advances in technology and techniques reduce the incidence of the DA.

Selected References

1. Caplan RA, Posner KL, Ward RJ, Cheney FW. Adverse respiratory events in anesthesia: a closed claims analysis. *Anesthesiology.* 1990;72:828–833.
2. Joffe, AM, Aziz MF, Posner KL, Duggan LV, Mincer SL, Domino KB. Management of difficult tracheal intubation: a closed claims analysis. *Anesthesiology* 2019;131(4): 818–829.
3. Cheney FW, Posner KL, Lee LA, Caplan RA, Domino KB. Trends in anesthesia-related death and brain damage: a closed claims analysis. *Anesthesiology.* 2006;105:1081–1086.
7. Langeron O, Masso E, Huraux C, et al. Prediction of difficult mask ventilation. *Anesthesiology.* 2000;92:1229–1236.
8. el-Ganzouri AR, McCarthy RJ, Tuman KJ, Tanck EN, Ivankovich AD. Preoperative airway assessment: predictive value of a multivariate risk index. *Anesth Analg.* 1996;82:1197–1204.
10. Kheterpal S, Martin L, Shanks AM, Tremper KK. Prediction and outcomes of impossible mask ventilation: a review of 50,000 anesthetics. *Anesthesiology.* 2009;110:891–897.
11. Thomsen, JLD, Nørskov AK, Rosenstock CV. Supraglottic airway devices in difficult airway management: a retrospective cohort study of 658,104 general anaesthetics registered in the Danish Anaesthesia Database. *Anaesthesia.* 2019;74(2): 151–157.
15. Ramachandran SK, Mathis MR, Tremper KK, et al. Predictors and clinical outcomes from failed Laryngeal Mask Airway Unique: a study of 15,795 patients. *Anesthesiology.* 2012;116:1217–1226.
20. Cormack RS, Lehane J. Difficult tracheal intubation in obstetrics. *Anaesthesia.* 1984;39:1105–1111.
33. Cook TM, Woodall N, Frerk C. Fourth National Audit Project. Major complications of airway management in the UK: results of the Fourth National Audit Project of the Royal College of Anaesthetists and the Difficult Airway Society. Part 1: anaesthesia. *Br J Anaesth.* 2011;106:617–631.
36. Healy DW, Maties O, Hovord D, et al. A systematic review of the role of videolaryngoscopy in successful orotracheal intubation. *BMC Anesthesiol.* 2012;12:32.
41. Schroeder RA, Pollard R, Dhakal I, et al. Temporal trends in difficult and failed tracheal intubation in a regional community anesthetic practice. *Anesthesiology.* 2018;128(3): 502–510.

All references can be found online at eBooks.Health.Elsevier.com.

9

Airway Assessment and Prediction of the Difficult Airway

P. ALLAN KLOCK JR.

CHAPTER OUTLINE

KEY POINTS

- Poor airway assessment may contribute to poor patient outcomes.
- An airway history and physical examination should be performed in all patients undergoing airway management. Relevant diagnostic studies should be reviewed.
- No single test reliably predicts difficult mask ventilation (DMV), difficulty with a supraglottic airway (SGA), difficult laryngoscopy, or difficult intubation (DI).
- A greater number of airway abnormalities imply increasing difficulty.
- Proposed predictors of impossible face-mask ventilation include neck radiation changes, beard, male gender, obstructive sleep apnea (OSA), and modified Mallampati class of III or IV.

- Proposed predictors of SGA airway failure include male sex, high BMI, poor dentition, and surgical table rotation.
- Some factors that predict a DI include a history of a difficult airway (DA), interincisor distance <3 cm, failed temporomandibular joint (TMJ) translation, small mandibular space, limited cervical spine mobility, temporomandibular distance translation <6 cm, modified Mallampati class of III or IV, and a short, thick neck.
- Because most DAs are not expected, clinicians should develop a comprehensive airway strategy rather than a single airway plan for every patient even if the airway assessment is normal.

Introduction

An airway evaluation, including history, physical examination, and other diagnostic tests, should be performed for all patients who are undergoing anesthesia or have a need for airway management.[1] When the 2013 American Society of Anesthesiologists (ASA) Guidelines for Management of the Difficult Airway (DA) were developed, 100% of consultants and ASA members agreed that a preanesthetic examination should include an airway assessment.[2] The Fourth National Audit Project (NAP4) of the United Kingdom, one of the largest population-based studies of complications of airway management, concluded that lack of airway assessment was correlated with poor planning and patient morbidity and mortality.[3]

An assessment of the airway focuses on medical history and physical features that impact the patient's risk for difficult mask ventilation (DMV), difficult intubation (DI), supraglottic airway (SGA) failure, challenging surgical airway, increased risk for aspiration of gastric contents, or poor tolerance of apnea. Variations or abnormalities are found by reviewing records, taking an anesthetic- and airway-focused history, examining the patient, and reviewing relevant laboratory and radiologic studies.

Patient History

History of a Difficult Airway

A history of a DA is a strong predictor of future airway problems.[4,5] The inverse is not necessarily true; a history of problem-free airway management suggests straightforward airway management but does not guarantee it. Factors such as weight, age, dental issues, or pathology may have altered the airway after previous procedures. If a patient reports a history of DMV or DI, additional investigation is warranted. If possible, medical records from those procedures should be obtained. Questions are then asked regarding the nature and context of the event. Noting the year an event occurred may be helpful, especially if newer airway devices were not available at the time. History of severe sore throat, trauma to the airway, unanticipated postoperative intubation, or reintubation also may indicate that providers experienced difficulty. Disease processes such as obstructive sleep apnea (OSA) or respiratory illness may have influenced extubation.

Medical Conditions

Diabetes

The incidence of DI in patients with long-standing diabetes is 21% to 41%.[6-9] Nonenzymatic glycosylation of collagen may lead to limited joint mobility.[10] Poor glycemic control in long-standing disease increases the likelihood of developing joint problems.[11] If the atlanto-occipital joint or laryngeal joints become involved, then neck extension and laryngeal mobility may become limited, making laryngoscopy or intubation difficult. Collagen glycosylation starts in the fourth and fifth interphalangeal joints, preventing the patient from approximating the palms and fingers of the hands; therefore, limited phalangeal extension may be used as a predictor of DA management caused by neck and larynx stiffness. The prayer sign and palm print test have been suggested as tests of phalangeal joint immobility.[7] For the prayer sign, the patient is asked to place his hands in the prayer position with the palms approximated as much as possible; the ability of the

interphalangeal joints to oppose one another so that the fingers lie flat against each other can be assessed.[7] Difficulty with intubation is considered more likely in patients with less ability to oppose the joints successfully. To perform the palm print test, the patient's hand is painted with black ink and pressed against a piece of paper. The fraction of the palm print present in ink is deemed inversely proportional to intubation difficulty. Several studies of the predictive value of these tests found sensitivity ranged from 13% to 75%, and specificity from 69% to 96%.[8,12-14] Although these individual tests have poor predictive value, the palm print test or prayer sign may give additional information about difficulty of intubation in patients with diabetes.[8]

Rheumatoid Arthritis

Rheumatoid arthritis (RA) is a chronic autoimmune disorder that affects joints throughout the body. It can cause immobility or hypermobility of the joints of the jaw, larynx, and neck. The temporomandibular joint (TMJ), cricoarytenoid joint, cricothyroid joint, atlantoaxial joint, and cervical spine may be involved.[15,16]

Some manifestations of the disease are laryngeal nodules, mucosal edema, and swelling of the arytenoids or surrounding tissue. Dysphonia, dysphagia, sore throat, and poor exercise tolerance can occur. Cricoarytenoid arthritis can cause voice changes, hoarseness, pain on swallowing, dyspnea, stridor, and tenderness over the larynx.[15] If the vocal cords move poorly as a result of arytenoid edema,[17] the larynx may be more difficult to identify during laryngoscopy.[18] Swelling may be so severe that the glottis is obscured. Not only can arthritis influence airway management, but instrumenting the airway can also exacerbate the condition. Worsening of laryngeal symptoms after tracheal intubation or SGA placement in patients with RA has been reported.[19] Postextubation stridor in patients may indicate aggravation of the arthritis.[20] The patient with RA should be asked about symptoms, length of diagnosis, and steroid use. Cervical spine disease is correlated with duration of arthritis, significant peripheral joint erosion, long-standing steroid use, older age, and neck symptoms.[16,20] Depending on symptoms, surgical plan, or other factors, additional diagnostic work-up such as radiographs, laryngoscopy, or even pulmonary function tests (PFTs) may be warranted.

Ankylosing Spondylitis

Ankylosing spondylitis is a seronegative spondyloarthropathy affecting the bony insertion points of ligaments. The disease can lead to fusion and rigidity of joints including the spine, the TMJ, and, in some cases, the cricoarytenoid joint. The disease is progressive, leading to spinal immobility and the characteristic "bamboo spine" on radiograph. Osteoporosis also develops, causing bones to be more fragile.[21] Preoperative evaluation is guided by the severity of the disease and procedure to be performed. Disease duration can indicate severity.[22] Cervical fractures and spinal nerve root compression can occur. During the airway assessment, any related neurologic deficits should be documented. Atlantoaxial subluxation occurs in 21% of patients with the condition.[22] Care with airway instrumentation is of utmost importance in these patients, as the lower cervical spine can fracture with improper neck extension. Neurologic injury, including quadriplegia after cervical spine injury during intubation, has been reported.[21,23]

Temporomandibular Disorders

Temporomandibular disorders can arise from joint problems (articular) or nonarticular causes. Articular disorders can be associated with RA, ankylosing spondylitis, gout, infectious arthritis, or osteoarthritis. Nonarticular causes include fibromyalgia, muscle spasm, and acute muscle sprain.[24] Patients with muscle disorders, disc condyle disorders, joint inflammation, or hypermobility will likely display normal mouth opening after the induction of general anesthesia.[25] Synovitis of the TMJ leads to reduced mandibular motion, causing a reduced oral aperture. Severe forms of juvenile RA (Still's disease) can involve the TMJ, leading to poor mandibular development (micrognathia).

TMJ disease or dysfunction should be noted in the patient's medical history. Patients with TMJ disease may be more difficult to intubate, and many experience worsening of symptoms postoperatively.[26] The patient should be asked about any clicking or grinding with mandibular movement, periauricular pain, pain that radiates to the head or neck, pain with chewing, restricted movement, and joint hypermobility.[25] The presence of symptoms should prompt the practitioner to discuss the possibility that symptoms may worsen postoperatively. Patients with or without preexisting signs and symptoms may develop TMJ dysfunction or dislocation even after uneventful laryngoscopy and intubation.[26–28] Absence of symptoms or a diagnosis does not preclude disease or provide immunity to postoperative symptoms.

Bleeding Risk

Bleeding in the airway during instrumentation can obscure the view of the glottis. Bleeding can be especially problematic during flexible scope intubation (FSI) or video-assisted laryngoscopy (VAL). The patient with an inherited or acquired clotting factor deficiency may develop severe epistaxis with nasal intubation, and some consider nasal intubation to be contraindicated in these patients. Patients taking anticoagulants that have been discontinued pose only a relative contraindication to nasal intubation.[29] Nasal intubation is not contraindicated in patients taking antiplatelet medication. Patients with severe coagulation abnormalities may be at risk of developing a tongue hematoma, which can cause partial or complete airway obstruction that may not manifest until the airway device is removed.

Cardiopulmonary Illness

Although time to oxyhemoglobin desaturation after preoxygenation is not a predictor of DA management, it is an important consideration when developing an airway management strategy. The longer the time available to secure the airway, the greater the likelihood of successful intubation. Patients with a reduced functional residual capacity (FRC), decreased diffusion of oxygen across the lung parenchyma, or increased oxygen consumption tolerate less apneic time before desaturation begins. Restrictive lung disease, advanced pregnancy, and morbid obesity are common causes of reduced FRC.

Airway manipulation in patients with obstructive airway disease such as asthma or chronic obstructive pulmonary dysfunction (COPD) may lead to severe bronchospasm, hypoxia, and even death.[30] The National Asthma Education and Prevention Program (NAEPP) Expert Panel Report[31] and the GOLD Guidelines[32] provide stepwise approaches to the assessment and treatment of patients with asthma and COPD, respectively. Clinicians can refer to these guidelines when optimizing the medical status of patients preoperatively.[33] Cardiac illness should also be assessed. The patient with severe cardiac disease may not be able to withstand a long apneic period or the sympathetic responses to intubation and extubation.

Congenital Abnormalities

Developmental abnormalities of the first and second pharyngeal arches can lead to craniofacial abnormalities, including cleft lip, cleft palate, and micrognathia. Specific syndromes include Treacher-Collins syndrome, Pierre Robin syndrome, and Goldenhar syndrome.[34] In some severe cases of micrognathia, airway obstruction can occur even during normal wakefulness. Macroglossia, an abnormally large tongue, can also lead to difficulty with airway management. Macroglossia is associated with Down syndrome and the mucopolysaccharidoses. It is not important to remember each syndrome and its accompanying features. Rather, practitioners should educate themselves on the syndrome preoperatively and, if appropriate, refer the patient to a tertiary center for care.

Masses of the Head, Neck, and Airway

Any anatomic abnormality relating to the nose, face, mouth, pharynx, or larynx should be thoroughly investigated. Changes may be caused by pathology or treatments including surgery, radiation therapy, and chemotherapy. A history of voice changes indicates laryngeal pathology. Difficulty swallowing or inspiring deeply may indicate airway narrowing caused by an intrinsic or extrinsic mass. Radiation therapy to the head and neck can cause inflammation and fibrosis. These may lead to difficult or impossible face-mask ventilation and direct laryngoscopy (DL).[35] Patients with vocal cord paralysis may be at increased risk for aspiration.

Many supraglottic and glottic tumors or other pathologies are hidden from view during routine physical examination and remain undiagnosed before induction of anesthesia. Mask ventilation and intubation may be difficult in such cases. Masses can reside at the base of the tongue or occupy space in the vallecula, preventing optimal placement of Macintosh blades and interfering with displacement of the epiglottis by Miller blades.[36] Pharyngeal problems that can complicate laryngoscopy include acute lingual tonsillitis,[37] lingual tonsillar abscesses, lingual thyroids,[38] and thyroglossal cysts.[39,40] In the case of lingual tonsillar hypertrophy, enlarged lymphoid tissue pushes the epiglottis posteriorly, preventing visualization of the glottis and obstructing mask ventilation.[41] Ovassapian and colleagues analyzed 33 cases of unanticipated DI. Postoperative fiberoptic pharyngoscopy revealed lingual tonsil hypertrophy in all of these patients.[42]

Infections of the face and neck, such as epiglottitis or acute cellulitis of the submandibular space (Ludwig's angina), distort the patient's airway anatomy and can progress rapidly to a life-threatening airway obstruction.

Patients may be unable to swallow oral secretions and may be most comfortable sitting up, leaning forward to expectorate their oral secretions. Their airway may become obstructed in the supine position. Awake tracheostomy or FSI, possibly in the seated position, may be considered appropriate in these patients.

Various types of imaging can diagnose supraglottic and glottic tumors; however, relatively few patients benefit from such studies. Diagnostic studies should be pursued if the results will impact management.

Burns

Thermal injury to the head or neck complicates airway management in several ways. One retrospective study showed that burn patients with inhalational injury had three times the mortality of those without inhalational injury.[43] Airway burns are to be suspected when the victim was trapped in a closed space with the fire, suffered loss of consciousness, or if another victim died at the scene.[44] Thermal damage to the upper airway may cause massive soft tissue swelling within 2 to 24 hours.

Respiratory distress, stridor, hoarseness, blistering of the oropharynx, singed nasal hairs, and carbonaceous material in the mouth, nares, or pharynx are clinical signs of inhalational injury.[44] The risk of airway compromise and DI in patients with inhalational injury is significant. Elective prophylactic intubation is often indicated for such patients. If intubation is not deemed necessary, regular reassessments should be performed. A scoring system based on mucosal injury as assessed with nasal endoscopy has been suggested.[45]

For burn survivors, chronic airway problems are frequent. Inelastic scars over the face and neck limit mobility of the TMJ and cervical spine. These changes can result in a small mouth opening and an inability to achieve the sniffing position. Scar release under local anesthesia may restore mobility to the joints and improve intubating conditions. See Chapter 35 for more detailed discussion.

Acromegaly

Acromegaly results from excess growth hormone produced by a pituitary tumor. The incidence of difficult laryngoscopy and DI in acromegaly is four to five times higher than that in the general population.[46] Typical acromegalic features are characterized by a large nose and tongue, thick mandible, full lips, elevated nasolabial folds, and prominent frontal sinuses. Patients with acromegaly appear to experience overgrowth of mucosa and soft tissues of the pharynx, larynx, and vocal cords.[47,48] Many experience central apnea or OSA.[49,50] Early in the disease process, joint spaces may be widened; later, arthritis develops, which may limit range of motion at the TMJ or cricoarytenoid joints, leading to a small mouth opening or limited vocal cord abduction, respectively. Overgrowth of tissues can produce vocal cord abnormalities resulting in hoarseness or recurrent laryngeal nerve paralysis.

The clinical features of acromegaly predispose to DMV, difficult laryngoscopy, and DI. In one study of acromegalic patients, the incidence of difficult laryngoscopy was 26% and of DI was 10%.[51] The tongue and/or epiglottis may be enlarged, leading to airway obstruction and difficult laryngoscopy and intubation. A large or long mandible increases the distance between teeth and vocal cords, necessitating a longer laryngoscope blade. Thickened vocal cords and subglottic narrowing may require smaller tracheal tubes than would otherwise be selected. Nasal turbinate enlargement may obstruct the nasal airway and prevent the passage of a tube. Dyspnea on exertion, stridor, or hoarseness may suggest laryngeal abnormalities that can complicate intubation.

Obesity

Body mass index (BMI), an estimate of body fat, is used to classify obesity. BMI is calculated by dividing body weight in kilograms by body surface area in meters squared. A BMI of 18.5 to 24.9 kg/m² is normal, 25 to 29.9 kg/m² is overweight, between 30 and 39.9 kg/m² is obese, and greater than 40 kg/m² indicates morbid obesity.[52] Several studies indicate that airway difficulty occurs more often in obese than in lean patients.[3,53–55] Although morbid obesity alone does not appear to be a strong independent predictor of a DI,[56–60] obesity creates anatomic or physiologic changes that make airway management more difficult. Face-mask ventilation and laryngoscopy may be complicated by large cheeks, a short immobile neck, a large tongue, and pharyngeal adipose deposits. Adipose tissue may be deposited in the lateral pharyngeal walls, protruding into the airway. During periods of negative airway

• BOX 9.1   STOP-BANG Questionnaire

1. Snoring: Do you snore loudly (louder than talking or loud enough to be heard through closed doors)?
2. Tired: Do you often feel tired, fatigued, or sleepy during daytime?
3. Observed: Has anyone observed you stop breathing during your sleep?
4. Blood Pressure: Do you have or are you being treated for high blood pressure?
5. BMI: BMI more than 35 kg/m²?
6. Age: Age over 50 years old?
7. Neck circumference: Neck circumference greater than 40 cm?
8. Gender: Gender male?

Scoring

High risk of OSA: answering yes to three or more items
Low risk of OSA: answering yes to less than three items

From Chung F, Yegneswaran B, Liao P, et al. STOP questionnaire: a tool to screen patients for obstructive sleep apnea. *Anesthesiology.* 2008;108:812–821.

pressure, such as during inspiration, the tissue is drawn further into the airway, predisposing to OSA and its side effects (see Chapter 40). Increasing BMI corresponds to decreasing FRC and less tolerance to apneic periods.[61] Adipose tissue of the neck and upper back can decrease cervical flexion and atlanto-occipital extension. Measuring neck circumference (NC) during assessment may aid in determining risk. An NC greater than 43 cm (16.9 in) or a ratio of NC to thyromental distance (TMD) greater than 5 predicts DI.[53,62]

Obstructive Sleep Apnea

A diagnosis of OSA is suggested by a history of heavy snoring, daytime somnolence, impaired memory, inability to concentrate, and frequent accidents. Associated findings include hypoxemia, polycythemia, systemic hypertension, pulmonary hypertension, and hypercarbia. Risk factors for OSA are male gender, middle age or older, obesity, increased NC, evening alcohol consumption, and drug-induced sleep. Definitive diagnosis is made by polysomnography. Treatment frequently centers on the application of continuous positive airway pressure (CPAP) during sleep, but not all patients tolerate the mask. Alternative therapies include oral appliances and nocturnal administration of oxygen. Surgical options also exist, such as uvulopalatopharyngoplasty, genioglossus advancement, maxillomandibular advancement, and tracheostomy.

Most patients with sleep apnea are not diagnosed before surgery.[63] Polysomnography in every at-risk patient is not a viable option. Among many screening tools that exist, the STOP-BANG questionnaire (Box 9.1) is easy to use and has a high sensitivity and positive predictive value (PPV).[64]

OSA is a predictor of a difficult or even impossible mask ventilation.[35] There are conflicting data regarding OSA as a predictor of DI.[65,66] OSA is associated with an increase of postoperative complications including postoperative desaturation.[67,68] A complete discussion of preoperative assessment of sleep apnea can be found in Chapter 40.

Pregnancy

Airway management is one of the most important factors contributing to maternal mortality.[69,70] Airway difficulties pose a risk of pulmonary aspiration and hypoxic cardiopulmonary arrest. A comprehensive airway strategy should be developed for all pregnant patients because the risk of unanticipated DI is very high. Rocke and colleagues reported some degree of difficulty during intubation in almost 8% of full-term pregnant patients undergoing cesarean section.[57] One study of 239 consecutive patients who received general anesthesia for cesarean section found 14 patients (6%) were difficult to intubate. Only 3 of the 14 (21%) patients had any risk factors suggesting a possible DI.[71] A registry study from the UK enrolled pregnant patients having general anesthesia for obstetric and nonobstetric surgery from May 2017 to August 2018. DI was reported in 163 of 3117 anesthetics (5.2%), and failed intubation was reported in 0.32%. Surprisingly, VAL was used in only 1.9% of the anesthetics.[72]

Mallampati classification increases during labor; therefore, the airway of any pregnant patient should be assessed when developing an airway strategy and immediately before taking the patient to the operating room.[73] For more detailed information regarding airway management in the obstetric patient, see Chapter 37.

Aspiration Risk

Assessment of aspiration risk is an important part of the preoperative evaluation. For patients at high risk, rapid sequence induction or awake intubation may be necessary. The incidence of aspiration in elective surgery is about 1 in 2000 to 3000 anesthetics.[74] Although aspiration is rare, aspiration of gastric contents was the most common cause of death from airway events in the NAP4 study.[3] Many of the aspiration events may have been prevented with better patient assessment or planning.[3] Some predisposing risk factors for aspiration are nonfasting status, gastrointestinal obstruction, gastroesophageal reflux disease, emergent surgery, delayed gastric emptying due to diabetes or use of opioids, pregnancy, hiatal hernia, previous gastrointestinal surgery, and obesity. A full discussion of aspiration risk and prevention can be found in Chapter 14.

Psychosocial Context

Although a patient's desires and mental health should not dictate airway management strategy, they should be considered on a case-by-case basis. The presence and severity of anxiety should be ascertained, especially if awake intubation is being considered. When caring for singers, actors, or patients for whom voice quality is important, the risks and benefits of specific airway techniques, such as using an SGA or smaller endotracheal tube (ETT), should be discussed.[75]

Physical Examination

Oral Aperture

Mouth opening determines the space available for placing and manipulating laryngoscopes and airway devices.[76] Mouth opening depends on the TMJ, which has both a hingelike movement and a gliding motion known as *translation*. In the hingelike movement, the mandible pivots on the maxilla. The more the mandible swings away from the maxilla, the bigger the mouth opening. The adequacy of mouth opening is assessed by measuring the interincisor distance. An interincisor distance of 3 cm is sufficient space for DL, absent other complicating factors. The aperture can be measured with a small ruler or by inserting fingers (corresponding to 3 cm) into the patient's mouth to estimate the aperture.

Factors that interfere with mouth opening include masseter muscle spasm, TMJ dysfunction, and integumentary conditions, including burn scar contractures and progressive systemic sclerosis. Patients with mandibular or facial fractures can experience masseter muscle spasm or pain when opening the mouth; induction of anesthesia and administration of muscle relaxants may allow the mouth to be opened in these patients. Mechanical problems at the TMJ itself may remain unaltered by induction of anesthesia. Occasionally, patients with adequate mouth opening when awake have an inadequate opening after anesthesia induction[77]; the problem can often be relieved by pulling the mandible forward. A mouth opening that was sufficient for a previous anesthetic may not be adequate after TMJ surgery or temporal neurosurgical procedures.[78]

Investigations of the predictive value of oral aperture did not produce favorable results. In a 2005 meta-analysis, the area under the receiver operating characteristic (ROC) curve for oral aperture alone was 0.72.[79] Patients with very small oral openings were likely excluded from the studies analyzed. Small interincisor distance as a single factor does not cause most DA situations, but small mouth opening by itself may make laryngoscopy difficult or impossible. Common sense dictates that if a device cannot fit into the patient's mouth, other options must be considered.

Dentition

Missing, loose, or damaged teeth and dental appliances should be documented as part of the airway assessment. It is helpful to use systematic notation. The Universal Numbering System is commonly used in the United States. Each permanent tooth is assigned a number from 1 to 32, and each primary (baby) tooth is assigned a letter A–T. Children typically lose their primary teeth between the ages of 6 and 12 years (Fig. 9.1).

Instrumentation of the airway places the teeth at risk for damage. Teeth may be dislodged or broken, leading to pain, inability to chew, and costly repair. Broken teeth can fall into the bronchial tree and cause obstruction or lead to abscess. Loose teeth that can be extracted easily with digital pressure should probably be removed before laryngoscopy. Patients with poor dentition may be more at risk than others for tooth damage or dislodgment. In these patients, extra efforts should be made to avoid placing pressure on maxillary incisors. This may result in the laryngoscope being manipulated into less than ideal positions for visualization of the larynx and glottis. In some cases, use of a flexible intubation scope may prevent tooth damage. Poor dentition can also lead to problems with placement of oral airways and SGAs. In one study, poor dentition (missing or broken teeth, dentures) was one of four independent factors for SGA failure.[80]

Prominent maxillary incisors complicate laryngoscopy because they protrude into the mouth and block the line of sight to the larynx. On the other hand, edentulous patients tend to be easy to intubate because the airway practitioner can adjust the line of sight to an advantageous angle.

Tongue

The tongue occupies space in the mouth and oropharynx, and its base lies close to the glottic aperture. Visualization of the larynx with a rigid laryngoscope requires displacing the tongue base anteriorly and sometimes laterally, pushing it into the submental space. As a result, a line of sight to the glottis is created. The new position of the tongue is within the mandibular space—the area between the two rami of the mandible. When the tongue is too large to fit in the mandibular space, visualization of the larynx is sometimes inadequate. A large tongue, a small mandible, or a combination thereof can influence the ability to obtain an adequate laryngeal view during DL.

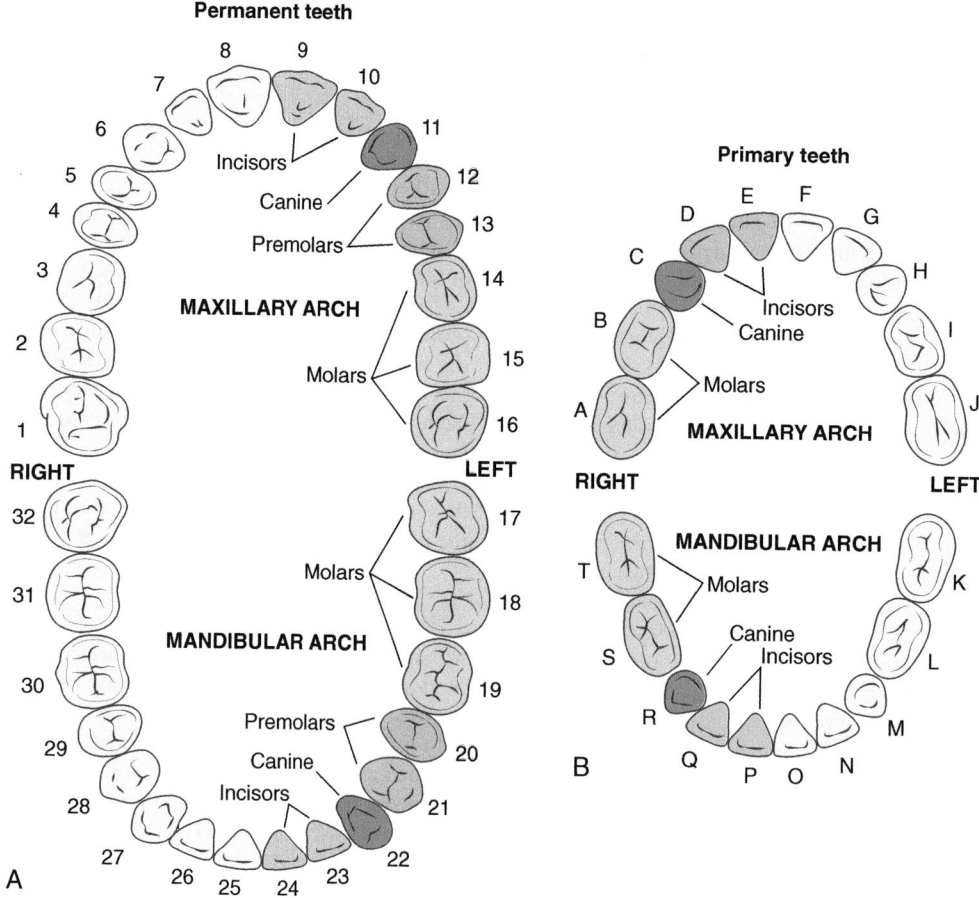

• **Fig. 9.1** Dental Nomenclature: Universal Numbering System: (A) Permanent teeth are numbered sequentially from 1 to 32, starting from the patient's rear right upper tooth. (B) Primary teeth are noted alphabetically from A through T, starting from the patient's rear right upper tooth.

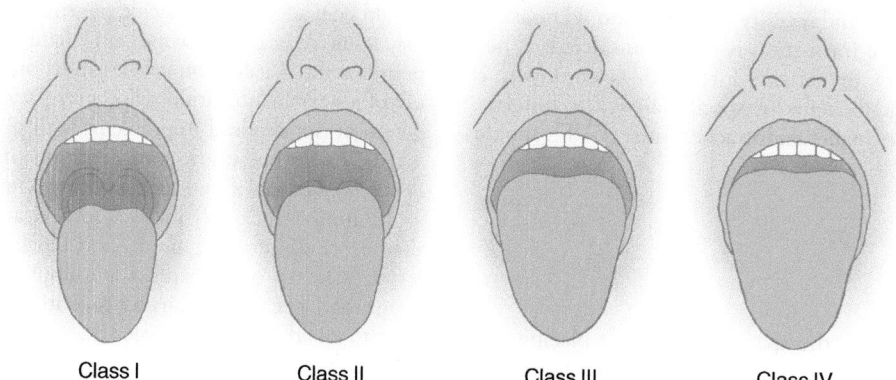

• **Fig. 9.2** Modified Mallampati classification system. The oropharynx is divided into four classes based on the structures visualized: *Class I*, soft palate, fauces, uvula, pillars; *Class II*, soft palate, fauces, uvula; *Class III*, soft palate, base of uvula; *Class IV*, soft palate not visible. (Modified from Samsoon GL, Young JR. Difficult tracheal intubation: a retrospective study. *Anaesthesia*. 1987;42:487–490.)

Mallampati Classification

To recognize the implications of tongue size for successful airway management, Mallampati and colleagues devised a classification system to predict difficult laryngoscopy.[81] Mallampati reasoned that a large tongue could be identified on visual inspection of the open mouth. Samsoon and Young modified the original system in 1987, increasing categorization into four groups instead of the original three (Fig. 9.2).[82] The Samsoon and Young classification is commonly referred to as the *modified Mallampati classification* and is ubiquitous in clinical practice. In a patient with a normal-size tongue, oropharyngeal structures can be visualized. As the tongue size increases, some structures become hidden from view.

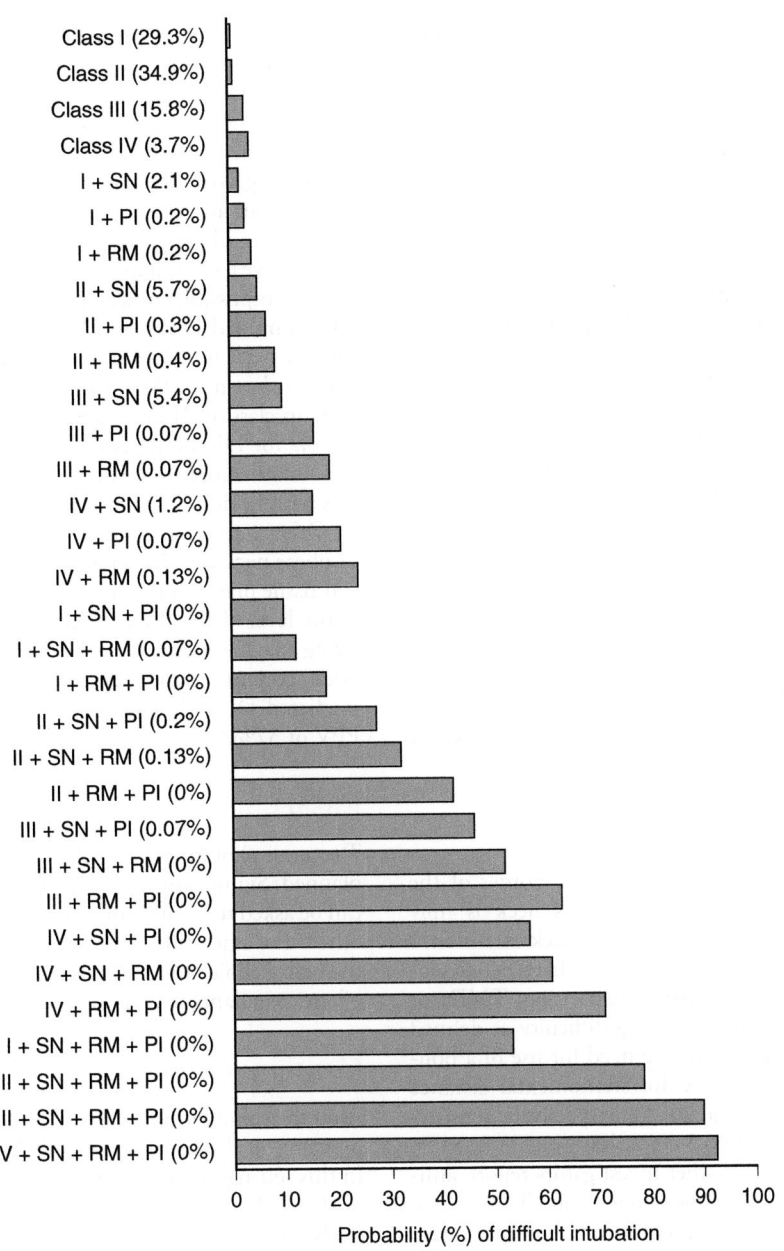

• **Fig. 9.3** Probability of difficult intubation. Roman numerals *I–IV* refer to the modified Mallampati class. *PI*, Protruding incisors; *RM*, receding mandible; *SN*, short neck. (From Rocke DA, Murray WB, Rout CC, Gouws E. Relative risk analysis of factors associated with difficult intubation in obstetric anesthesia. *Anesthesiology.* 1992;77:67.)

Determination of a patient's modified Mallampati class is straightforward. The patient is seated in the neutral upright position. If the patient is supine, the Mallampati class may appear higher, but sensitivity and specificity in either position are similar. Performing the test with the patient in both sitting and supine positions may better reveal the anatomy of the patient.[83,84] The mouth is opened as wide as possible, and the tongue is protruded as far as possible. Phonation is discouraged because it raises the soft palate, allowing visualization of additional structures.[85] The observer looks for specific anatomic landmarks: the fauces, tonsillar pillars, uvula, and soft palate.

Airway assessment is often performed to determine if DL will be difficult. In 1984, Cormack and Lehane described a grading system for comparing laryngoscopic views.[86] Cormack-Lehane (CL) grade 1 views show the entire glottic opening; grade 2 views show the posterior laryngeal aperture but not the anterior portion; grade 3 views are of the epiglottis but not part of the larynx; and grade 4 views are of the soft palate but not the epiglottis. Initial investigations suggested a positive correlation between modified Mallampati classification and CL laryngoscopic grades (i.e., a higher modified Mallampati classification predicts a higher laryngoscopic grade for any given patient).[81,82] In 1992, however, Rocke and colleagues examined several classic predictors of DI. They found that none, including the Mallampati classification, was reliable as a predictive test (Fig. 9.3).[57] Despite the fact that the Mallampati classification in isolation has limited utility, it should be measured as part of a comprehensive airway assessment. A modified Mallampati class of III or IV has been shown to be associated with DMV and difficult laryngoscopy.[35,87]

Thyromental Distance

A small mandible correlates with DI. The size of the mandible can be estimated by measuring the TMD. The patient's head is extended at the atlanto-occipital joint, the mentum of the mandible and the thyroid cartilage are identified, and the distance between the thyroid cartilage and the mentum is measured using a gauge, ruler, or the observer's fingers. A TMD <6 cm correlates with intubation difficulty.[88] Three finger breadths is commonly cited as corresponding to 6 cm. The mean width of the middle three fingers is 5.38 cm for women and 5.91 cm for men;[89] practitioners should calibrate the width of their fingers with a ruler. The predictive value of the TMD increases as the TMD gets smaller.[79] The positive likelihood ratio for DI as defined by a CL grade 3 or higher was 4.1 when a threshold of TMD 6 cm or less was used.[90] Investigators have also studied the value of combining the TMD with another test for airway prediction. TMD combined with Mallampati classification showed good accuracy (an area under the ROC curve of 0.84). When the TMD was combined with NC in obese patients, an NC/TMD ratio of 5.0 or more had a higher sensitivity and negative predictive value (NPV) than other common bedside tests and indices (an area under the ROC curve of 0.86).[53]

Sternomental Distance

Sternomental distance, measured from the upper border of the manubrium to the mentum while the patient's neck is fully extended with the mouth closed, is a measure of neck extension.[91] A sternomental distance <12.5 cm was shown to have better sensitivity and specificity than Mallampati classification, TMD, or mandibular protrusion in predicting airway difficulty as defined by a Cormack-Lehane 3 or 4 view or the need for use of a bougie.[91] Sensitivity, specificity, and PPV for sternomental distance 12.5 cm or less were 82%, 89%, and 26.9%, respectively; sensitivity, specificity, and PPV for TMD 6.5 cm or less were 65%, 81%, and 8.9%, respectively. Although other investigators report similarly poor predictive value of both sternomental and TMD alone for laryngoscopic view,[92] they are important for a comprehensive assessment of airway anatomy.

Neck Anatomy and Mobility

Neck mobility is important for the oral, pharyngeal, and tracheal axes to align. When they do, there is a direct line of sight to the glottis during DL. Airway management can be difficult in patients with limited neck range of motion from immobility or functional limitation (i.e., pain with movement). To achieve the sniffing position, the lower cervical spine must flex and the atlantoaxial joint and upper cervical spine must extend.[93] Both flexion and extension of the neck should be assessed with the patient seated in a neutral position. Flexion is measured when the patient places the chin on the chest. It is important to assess the contour of the neck to determine how much the cervical vertebrae are able to flex. Flexion of the atlanto-occipital joint is not helpful during DL. Extension of the atlanto-occipital joint is measured when the patient extends the neck backward with the mouth open. The angle between the occlusal surface of the upper teeth or jaw and a horizontal line parallel to the ground is estimated. A goniometer may be used

for more accuracy. Normal atlanto-occipital extension measures 35 degrees; limitation of extension is an indication of potential difficulty with DL.[94] If neck movement elicits pain, tingling, or numbness of the neck or arms, then a neutral position of the neck should be maintained during intubation; this precaution can make DL more challenging. Inability to flex or extend the neck predicts a DI.[95]

Mashour and colleagues studied the relationship between neck mobility and laryngoscopy, and intubation.[96] In patients younger than 60 years, limitation of neck mobility was associated with DMV, impossible mask ventilation, difficult laryngoscopy, DI, and combined DMV and DI. In patients aged 60 years or older, limited neck mobility was associated with difficult laryngoscopy and DI, but not DMV. In patient aged 48 years or older, a Mallampati class of III or IV and TMD <6 cm were independent predictors for DI among patients with limited neck mobility. There was no difference in the incidence of a DA, whether the limitation was with flexion or extension.

Other neck features may impact airway management. A thick or obese neck can decrease neck flexion and extension, and excess soft tissue may complicate jaw thrust maneuvers. Quantifying NC at the level of the thyroid cartilage with use of a tape measure or string may be useful in predicting airway difficulty. One study of obese patients found that an NC greater than 43 cm (16.9 in) predicted DI with a sensitivity of 92%, specificity of 84%, and PPV of 37%.[62]

Nasal Characteristics

The nose should be examined, especially if nasal intubation is planned. Significant septal deviation should be noted. The patient can be asked to occlude one nostril and breathe deeply through the other. The side with less obstructed breathing may be larger and the better choice for tube placement. Bleeding disorders or the use of anticoagulants is a relative contraindication to nasal intubation.

Mandibular Protrusion

After the submandibular space is filled with the tongue, additional pressure on the laryngoscope blade lifts the mandible anteriorly. In this setting, mandibular displacement depends on the mobility of the TMJ. The ability to translate the mandible in the TMJ is easily assessed. The patient is asked to place the mandibular incisors (bottom teeth) in front of the maxillary incisors (upper teeth). If the patient is unable to perform this simple task, the TMJ may not glide, predicting DI.[97]

The upper lip bite test (ULBT) has been proposed as a modification of the TMJ displacement test.[98] It is performed by asking the patient to place the mandibular incisors as high on the upper lip as possible, similar to biting the upper lip. Contact of the mandibular teeth above or on the vermilion border is thought to predict adequate laryngoscopic views, whereas inability to touch the vermilion border is thought to predict poor laryngoscopic views (Fig. 9.4). The predictive ability of this maneuver has been confirmed.[91,97] A specificity of 91.7% and area under the ROC curve of 91% were greater for the ULBT than any other bedside diagnostic test.[91] Similarly high specificity and accuracy are found in the upper lip *catch* test in edentulous patients.[99]

Facial Features

Abnormal appearance or dissymmetry of the face with or without a diagnosis of a specific syndrome should heighten the practitioner's

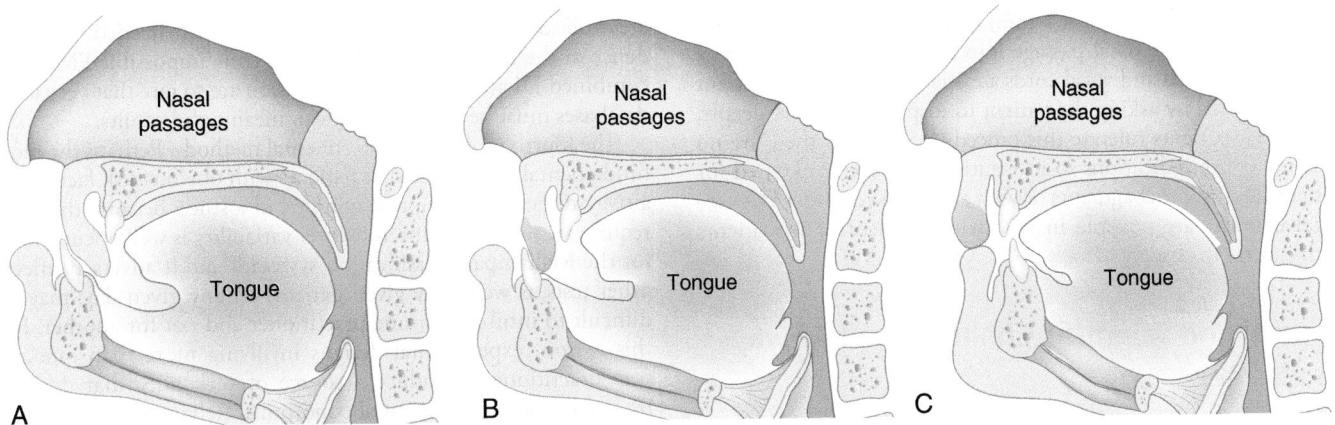

• **Fig. 9.4** Cross-section view of the upper lip bite test. (A) Class I: lower incisors biting the upper lip, mucosa of lip entirely invisible. (B) Class II: lower incisors half-biting the upper lip, mucosa partially visible. (C) Class III: lower incisors unable to bite the upper lip, mucosa of lip fully visible. (Modified from Khan ZH, Kashfi A, Ebrahimkhani E. A comparison of the upper lip bite test [a simple new technique] with modified Mallampati classification in predicting difficulty in endotracheal intubation: a prospective blinded study. *Anesth Analg*. 2003;96:595–599.)

attention to airway assessment. History of facial trauma, surgical changes, or distortive disease processes must be considered. Many congenital syndromes are associated with airway abnormalities; additional information can be gained from textbooks devoted to the anesthetic management of patients with uncommon diseases and dysmorphisms.

A beard can impede mask ventilation by preventing an adequate seal.[35,100] If there is a concern, the patient can be requested to shave. If he refuses on personal or religious grounds, the beard may be covered with occlusive dressing, plastic wrap, gel, or gauze.[100,101]

Diagnostic Studies

All preoperative patient assessments should include pertinent laboratory tests and consultations necessary for the delivery of anesthesia care.[102] Radiographs and other imaging techniques are too expensive and inconvenient to serve as routine screening tests for a DA; however, using specialized imaging can be helpful if a known or suspected DA exists. Computed tomography (CT), magnetic resonance imaging (MRI), or ultrasound may be helpful for patients with a goiter, tumors that may compress the airway, and anterior or lateral displacement of the cervical larynx and trachea. Particularly worrisome findings include tumors in the upper or lower airway, extrinsic masses that cause a narrowing of the airway, and lesions that displace the larynx anteriorly or laterally. Imaging may help evaluate for the presence of chondromalacia when extrinsic compression of the airway is long standing. Flexion-extension radiographs of the cervical spine may be useful in patients with RA or Down syndrome because of possible atlantoaxial instability.

Ultrasound has been advocated as a safe, real-time, dynamic tool to aid in airway assessment. In obese patients, it may show whether pretracheal fat will interfere with intubation.[103] Other potential clinical applications include evaluating head and neck pathology, aiding in the diagnosis of sleep apnea, predicting the appropriate diameter of an ETT, evaluating prandial status, localizing the trachea and cricothyroid membrane, and guiding the placement of airway-related nerve blocks. Measuring the width of the air column at the level of the thyroid with ultrasonography has been suggested as a test to evaluate the risk of postextubation

stridor, although its predictive value remains to be determined (see Chapter 3).[104,105]

An endoscopic airway examination is a common procedure performed by otolaryngologists to assess the nasopharynx, larynx, and glottis. Tumor staging or dynamic function of the vocal cords and larynx can be determined. Anesthesiologists may find a preoperative endoscopic airway examination (PEAE) useful in certain patients. With this bedside test, head and neck disease, abnormalities of the base of the tongue, and tumors or abscesses that distort normal anatomy can be examined. Electronic medical records may allow the anesthesia provider to view still or video images from an endoscopic airway exam performed in the clinic setting; in this case, another endoscopy is usually unnecessary. In the patient with stridor or breathing difficulty, an endoscopic examination may guide airway management. PEAE may also influence the decision of whether to intubate after induction of general anesthesia or perform an awake intubation. Rosenblatt and colleagues performed PEAEs on 138 patients. Forty-four patients had an initial plan of awake intubation; after a PEAE, only 16 were felt to need an awake intubation. There were 94 patients for whom intubation after induction of anesthesia was planned; 8 of these patients had the plan changed to an awake technique after the PEAE.[106]

A PEAE can be performed in the preoperative holding area or during a preoperative clinic visit. The patient is placed in a semirecumbent position. A nasal vasoconstrictor such as oxymetazoline is sprayed in the naris; this shrinks the nasal mucosa, increasing the diameter of the nasal passage and decreasing bleeding risk. Topical anesthesia can be accomplished with various local anesthetic solutions including 2% or 4% lidocaine with or without epinephrine or a 3:1 mix of 4% lidocaine and 1% phenylephrine. The selection of local anesthetic depends on availability and patient comorbidities. The maximum dose of topical lidocaine in the airway is debated; many practitioners limit the dose to 5 mg/kg to reduce the risk of local anesthetic toxicity, while some guidelines suggest a maximum dose of 9 mg/kg. Local anesthetics can be sprayed into the naris with an atomizer or with a syringe attached to an angiocatheter. Alternatively, pledgets or cotton-tipped swabs are soaked in the solution and advanced into the naris. Lidocaine 5% ointment can be placed on swabs or on a small nasal trumpet and gently and gradually inserted into the naris. After topicalization, a small flexible scope (3.7–4.1 mm) is inserted into the naris and guided through the nasal passage into the posterior nasopharynx until the epiglottis and vocal cords are seen. Vocal cord movement can be assessed by asking the patient to inspire and expire deeply. In general, patients tolerate this procedure well, and there are no absolute contraindications to it. Caution, however, is advised for patients taking anticoagulants or with a bleeding disorder.[106] Vasovagal episodes are possible in an anxious patient or in patients with cardiac disease.

Clinical and Scientific Challenges of Airway Assessment

Despite decades of work and hundreds of studies on the topic, there is no single practical tool that can reliably predict which patients will have a DA and which will not. It is helpful to understand how predictive tests are created. To establish a predictive test requires three steps: the outcome must be defined, patients with the outcome must be found, and the test must be correctly validated. To predict airway difficulties, there are obstacles at each step.[107]

One problem is nomenclature. According to the 2013 ASA Practice Guidelines, a DA is defined as "the clinical situation in which a conventionally trained anesthesiologist experiences difficulty with face mask ventilation of the upper airway, difficulty with tracheal intubation, or both."[2] The guidelines further define difficult mask and SGA ventilation, SGA placement, laryngoscopy, and intubation.

Although helpful, these definitions do not resolve all issues. Studies published before publication of these definitions may have used alternate definitions. The definitions themselves lack the precision required for scientific investigation. For example, some practitioners may perform a single laryngoscopy and, based on the view obtained, elect to forgo further attempts at laryngoscopy in favor of another technique. This situation does not meet the formal definition of a DI, although it would have if a second attempt at intubation had been made. *Failed intubation* may be an easier term to understand. A failed intubation exists when the airway practitioner gives up, deciding that conventional intubation will not be successful. The end point is clear and occurs with an incidence of 1 in 100 for patients in the emergency room,[108] 1 in 250 obstetric patients,[109] and up to 3 in 1000 among the general surgical population.[82,110] With the advent of the videolaryngoscope, practitioners may be using it as a first choice in many patients. This will confound further study of the incidence of difficult conventional laryngoscopy.

The second problem is identifying features that predict DI. Characteristics have been described in patients who have proven difficult to intubate; however, information is lacking about the characteristics in patients who are easy to intubate. Although large databases are becoming available, the normal values for many prediction criteria remain unknown.[111] A better method is to apply multivariate analysis to populations of patients in a prospective manner. In this way, a single factor can be compared in difficult and easy intubations. Various scoring systems have been introduced, such as the Wilson score and Intubating Difficulty Score.[95,112] These rating systems combine multiple predictors into a formula, but to date none has clinical utility. They are either statistically unsatisfactory or too onerous for clinical application.

The third problem is validating the tests. Validation tests performed on the same population of patients identified by the tests

are misleading. Different sample populations are needed. The incidence of the most serious problems of truly impossible FMV and combined DI and impossible ventilation are so rare that very large databases must be analyzed to glean meaningful results.

The fourth problem is experimental methods. Perhaps the most fundamental problem is that patients with obvious risk factors for airway difficulty will not be enrolled in a study because they will require an awake FSI. Interobserver variability is well documented for the Mallampati classification system,[84] and it adversely affects other tests as well. Any given patient, on any given day, may be difficult to intubate for one practitioner and not for another. For this reason, experimental designs involving more than one airway practitioner introduce a source of variability that detracts from control of experimental conditions. Relying on a single airway practitioner obviates this problem but limits the number of patients who can be enrolled into a single study.

Another source of experimental error is observer variation. Just as airway practitioners differ, so do observers.[113,114] Observations performed by different experimenters are subject to variability and introduce another source of error in data. The best way to prevent this problem is to have all observations performed by a single experimenter. This also limits the number of patients enrolled in a single study and does not mimic the clinical environment.

Sensitivity, PPV, and NPV are statistical measures used to characterize the usefulness of a particular predictor or test. Sensitivity is the proportion of patients with a DA who are correctly identified as such. For example, consider a sample in which five patients are difficult to intubate. If a predictor correctly identifies all five patients, its sensitivity is 100%. If the predictor correctly identifies only two of the five patients, the sensitivity is 2/5, or 40%.

PPV is the probability that patients identified by a test as being difficult to intubate are, in fact, difficult to intubate. If the test predicts that five patients will be difficult to intubate and all five of those patients experience a DI, the PPV of the test is 100%. If the test predicts that 10 patients will be difficult to intubate but only 5 of them are, in fact, difficult to intubate, its predictive value is 5/10, or 50%. Similarly, NPV is the probability that patients identified as not being difficult to intubate are, in fact, not difficult. Unfortunately, studies calculating the sensitivity, PPV, and NPV for classic DA predictors have led to unfavorable results.[13,107] A Cochrane review of bedside tests to predict DA management published in 2019 showed sensitivities ranging from 17% to 67% and specificities ranging from 87% to 95% (Table 9.1).[115]

Classic prediction criteria essentially consider surface anatomy. They screen for some factors associated with intubation but fail to evaluate others. Moreover, some potential problems are not revealed by examination of surface anatomy. Glottic and supraglottic abnormalities, such as lingual tonsil hypertrophy or epiglottic prolapse into the glottic opening, cannot be diagnosed by standard physical examinations for predicting intubation difficulty.[5,116,117] Pathophysiologic factors, such as mobile TMJ discs or disc fragments, may cause severe limitation of mouth opening after induction of anesthesia when none existed before.[116] Precise measurements of atlantoaxial motion sometimes fail to predict a DI.[118] Supraglottic, glottic, or subglottic pathology may be unrecognized by standard tests but complicate intubation nonetheless.[119] As of this writing, no single factor reliably predicts intubation difficulty. As the number of traits found in a patient increases, so does the likelihood of difficulty.[1,95,114,120,121]

Consequently, using scoring systems that synthesize multiple factors may improve predictive ability. However, patients' anatomies are highly variable, and some may not fit well into these

TABLE 9.1   Statistical Characteristics of Bedside Tests for Predicting Difficult Airways

Test	Number of Subjects (studies)	Sensitivity	Specificity	Positive Predictive Value	Negative Predictive Value
Difficult Direct Laryngoscopy (Prevalence: 10%)					
Mallampati test	2165 (6)	0.40	0.89	0.29	0.93
Modified Mallampati test	232,939 (80)	0.53	0.80	0.23	0.94
Wilson risk score	5862 (5)	0.51	0.95	0.53	0.95
Thyromental distance	33,189 (42)	0.37	0.89	0.27	0.93
Sternomental distance	12,211 (16)	0.33	0.92	0.31	0.92
Mouth opening test	22,179 (24)	0.22	0.94	0.29	0.91
Upper lip bite test	19,609 (27)	0.67	0.92	0.48	0.96
Difficult Intubation (Prevalence: 11%)					
Modified Mallampati test	191,849 (24)	0.51	0.87	0.33	0.93
Thyromental distance	5089 (10)	0.24	0.90	0.23	0.90
Mouth opening test	6091 (9)	0.27	0.93	0.32	0.91
Difficult Intubation (Prevalence: 11%)					
Modified Mallampati test	56,323 (6)	0.17	0.90	0.17	0.90

Modified from Roth D, Pace NL, Lee A, et al. Airway physical examination tests for detection of difficult airway management in apparently normal adult patients. *Cochrane Database Syst Rev.* 2018;5:CD008874.

models. Likewise, it may not be practical to assess multiple patient characteristics for all patients and analyze them in a cumbersome algorithm.

Conclusion

How does the practitioner interpret the information that has been gathered about a patient's history, physical examination, and diagnostic studies? It would be beneficial to have rules, scoring systems, or tests that provide a high NPV and a high PPV for a DA. Unfortunately, despite attempts at finding single predictors of difficulty or creating elaborate scoring systems, airway assessment tools that influence clinical practice remain elusive.[121,122]

Perhaps the most important reason for that elusiveness is that difficulty with airway management is caused by a variety of anatomic or pathologic factors. For example, a patient with ankylosing spondylitis may have a normal oral aperture and Mallampati class but be difficult to intubate because of neck immobility. Another patient may have normal neck range of motion but have TMJ dysfunction that limits mouth opening, preventing DL. No single test can detect all causes of difficulty with intubation or ventilation. Elaborate multifactorial scoring systems have failed to gain popular use because they may overlook some obvious cases and still miss cases with no discernable risk factors.

Practitioners should base their assessment on information gathered from the patient's history, physical examination, and diagnostic studies. The airway management strategy should be based on the assessment, the clinical context, and the risks and benefits of the possible options for management. The strategy should consider criteria that correlate with DMV (Box 9.2), difficulty with an SGA (Box 9.3), DI (Table 9.2), and, especially, combined DMV and DI (Box 9.4).[123]

• BOX 9.2   Risk Factors for Difficult and Impossible Mask Ventilation

Predictors of Difficult Mask Ventilation

Obesity
Beard
Edentulousness
History of snoring
History of obstructive sleep apnea
Age older than 55 years
Large tongue
Poor translation
Poor atlanto-occipital extension
Pharyngeal pathology
Lingual tonsil hypertrophy
Lingual tonsil abscess

Predictors of Impossible Mask Ventilation

Neck radiation changes
Beard
Male gender
Sleep apnea
Mallampati Class III or IV

Modified from Kheterpal S, Han R, Tremper KK, et al. Incidence and predictors of difficult and impossible mask ventilation. *Anesthesiology.* 2006;105:885–891; and Langeron O, Masso E, Huraux C, et al. Prediction of difficult mask ventilation. *Anesthesiology.* 2000;92:1229–1236.

Despite our best efforts, some causes of DI or DA management are not detectable with conventional screening. In fact, most patients with a DA will have a normal history and physical examination.[87,122] This may lead the clinician to wonder if it is worthwhile to perform an airway assessment. Because the consequences of a combined DI and DMV are so grave, the ASA and every other organization that has published guidelines on this matter recommend an airway assessment before formulating an anesthetic plan. The NAP4 study found that many patients injured by airway management had risk factors that were overlooked or disregarded, and one of the key conclusions of the study was that poor assessment led to poor outcomes.[3] Many patients will have obvious signs on examination, and some patients will report a history of prior airway difficulty. These patients deserve a special airway management strategy.

Continued research should focus on formulating tests that are painless, quick, and simple to apply and require little or no equipment. Optimally, the tests should be objective, reliable, and reproducible with little interexaminer variation. High degrees of sensitivity and NPV are crucial.

The lack of sensitivity of our assessment tools requires that airway management be approached with a strategy rather than a single plan. In other words, it is possible that a patient with a normal airway assessment may be difficult to intubate and/or ventilate. For that reason, the practitioner should be able to rapidly execute a strategy that includes plans for mask ventilation, SGA ventilation, and tracheal intubation for every patient.

TABLE 9.2	Generally Accepted Predictors of Difficult Intubation	
Criterion	**Suggestion of Difficult Intubation**
History of difficult intubation	Positive history
Length of upper incisors	Relatively long
Interincisor distance	Less than two finger breadths (<3 cm)
Overbite	Maxillary incisors override mandibular incisors
Temporomandibular joint translation	Inability to extend mandibular incisors anterior to maxillary incisors
Mandibular space	Small, indurated, encroached upon by mass
Cervical vertebral range of motion	Cannot touch chin to chest or cannot extend neck
Thyromental distance	Less than three finger breadths (<6 cm)
Modified Mallampati classification	Class III or IV—relatively large tongue: uvula not visible
Neck	Short, thick

From Apfelbaum JL, Hagberg CA, Caplan RA, et al. American Society of Anesthesiologists Task Force on Management of the Difficult Airway. Practice guidelines for management of the difficult airway: an updated report by the American Society of Anesthesiologists Task Force on Management of the Difficult Airway. *Anesthesiology.* 2013;118:251–270.

Selected References

2. Apfelbaum JL, Hagberg CA, Caplan RA, et al. American Society of Anesthesiologists Task Force on Management of the Difficult Airway. Practice guidelines for management of the difficult airway: an updated report by the American Society of Anesthesiologists Task Force on Management of the Difficult Airway. *Anesthesiology.* 2013;118:251–270.

3. Cook TM, Woodall N, Frerk C, Fourth National Audit Project. Major complications of airway management in the UK: results of the Fourth National Audit Project of the Royal College of Anaesthetists and the Difficult Airway Society. Part 1: anaesthesia. *Br J Anaesth.* 2011;106:617–631.

5. el Ganzouri AR, McCarthy RJ, Tuman KI, et al. Preoperative airway assessment: predictive value of a multivariate risk index. *Anesth Analg.* 1996;82:1197–1204.

35. Kheterpal S, Martin L, Shanks AM, et al. Prediction and outcomes of impossible mask ventilation: a review of 50,000 anesthetics. *Anesthesiology.* 2009;110:891–897.

79. Shiga T, Wajima Z, Inou T, et al. Predicting difficult intubation in apparently normal patients: a meta-analysis of bedside screening test performance. *Anesthesiology.* 2005;103:429–437.

80. Ramachandran SK, Mathis MR, Tremper KK, et al. Predictors and clinical outcomes from failed Laryngeal Mask Airway Unique: a study of 15,795 patients. *Anesthesiology.* 2012;116:1217–1226.

87. Langeron O, Masso E, Huraux C, et al. Prediction of difficult mask ventilation. *Anesthesiology.* 2000;92:1229–1236.

92. Khan ZH, Mohammadi M, Rasouli MR, et al. The diagnostic value of the upper lip bite test combined with sternomental distance, and interincisor distance for prediction of easy laryngoscopy and intubation: a prospective study. *Anesth Analg.* 2009;109:822–824.

106. Rosenblatt W, Ianus AI, Sukhupragarn W, et al. Preoperative endoscopic airway examination (PEAE) provides superior airway information and may reduce the use of unnecessary awake intubation. *Anesth Analg.* 2011;112:602–607.

110. Rose DK, Cohen MM. The airway: problems and predictions in 18,500 patients. *Can J Anaesth.* 1994;41:372–383.

115. Roth D, Pace NL, Lee A, et al. Airway physical examination tests for detection of difficult airway management in apparently normal adult patients. *Cochrane Database of Systematic Reviews.* 2018;5. CD008874. doi:10.1002/14651858.CD008874.pub2.

122. Norskov AK, Rosenstock CV, Wetterslev J, et al. Diagnostic accuracy of anaesthesiologists' prediction of difficult airway management in daily clinical practice: a cohort study of 188 064 patients registered in the Danish Anaesthesia Database. *Anaesthesia.* 2015;70:272–281.

123. Kheterpal S, Healy D, Aziz MF, et al. Incidence, predictors, and outcome of difficult mask ventilation combined with difficult laryngoscopy: a report from the multicenter perioperative outcomes group. *Anesthesiology.* 2013;119(6):1360–1369.

All references can be found online at eBooks.Health.Elsevier.com.

10

Development of an Airway Management Plan

WILLIAM H. ROSENBLATT

"I have no intention of following the algorithm down to a surgical airway … can't we just do a spinal?"

ANONYMOUS RESIDENT

CHAPTER OUTLINE

KEY POINTS

- Decision bias can be reduced by considering each aspect of airway management separately.
- The utility of any airway device is dependent on prior experience and availability; two different practitioners may justifiably come to widely opposing management decisions.
- The Cormack and Lehane (CL) laryngeal view score has not been validated as indicating the ease or difficulty of tracheal intubation.
- The vast majority of difficult airways (DAs) are not predicted.

- The degree of lingual tonsil hyperplasia and its effect on ease of laryngoscopy may vary with seasonal allergies and patient conditions.
- A prior history of no difficulty with ventilation or intubation is an indicator, but not a guarantee, of ease of management east.
- Airway evaluation indices have poor sensitivity and specificity.
- Preoperative endoscopic airway evaluation (PEAE) provides improved information about the invisible airway.
- An examination of neck surface landmarks should be part of the routine airway evaluation in every patient.

Introduction

A multitude of algorithms, techniques, and opinions focused on management of both the routine and difficult airway (DA) patient can be found in the anesthetic literature. Airway management practitioners study the mechanics of airway evaluation and history taking and can apply devices and procedures once a course of action is chosen. Less distinctly described are the "hows" and "whys" of arriving at this plan. Perhaps this lack of attention occurs because too many algorithms, techniques, opinions, and devices exist, and because the availability of tools and our experience with them vary greatly among practitioners.[1]

The patient with an anticipated DA is often, therefore, an enigma. The large database of the Danish Society of Anesthesiology highlights the gap between the anesthesiologist's prediction and outcome of a DA.[2,3] In this collection of nearly 200,000 anesthetic cases, 93% and 94% of difficult intubation (DI) and difficult mask ventilation (DMV) cases, respectively, were unanticipated, whereas predictions of difficulty were correct only 25% of the time.

Similarly, confounding the issue is the condition of the patient and the experience of the operator.[1] For example, a patient presenting for elective abdominal surgery in the operating room may be easy to manage (in terms of his or her airway) with a videolaryngoscope (VL). That same patient presenting emergently a week later with ileus, hypoxemia, and a depressed level of consciousness to a junior physician in a community-based emergency department where a standard direct laryngoscope is the device of choice must be treated differently and may result in a different outcome.[4]

Indeed, making decisions regarding one's ability to intubate the trachea or ventilate via face mask or supraglottic airway (SGA) and what other risks the patient faces (e.g., pulmonary aspiration of gastric contents, tolerance of oxyhemoglobin desaturation) must be individualized not only to the patient but also to the practitioner, context, and time.[3]

Decision-Making

Decision-making can be flawed.[5] A variety of cognitive models have been described, and all are influenced by biases that result in a preference for including or excluding evidentiary factors in the process of making a decision and formulating a plan. In airway management, several biases can affect the course of the clinician's cognitive processes. *Confirmation bias* is the act of seeking information that confirms ones predetermined opinion. *Fixation bias* or "tunnel vision" causes the clinician to focus on a single aspect of the patient to the detriment of other (possibly more important) pieces of information. *Visceral bias* is the VIP phenomena—someone "important" or to whom the operator has an attachment is treated out of the norm. *Retrospective bias* refers to applying a prior positive or negative outcome as proof for or against a correct decision. *Omission bias* may be one of the strongest in the field of airway management: inaction out of fear of causing harm or damaging one's reputation, especially in the presence of an "authority." The Fourth National Audit Project (NAP4) of the Royal College of Anaesthetists and the Difficult Airway Society (DAS) demonstrated these phenomena in instances where clinicians seemingly avoided awake intubation in favor of inappropriately using SGAs or regional anesthetics or ignored physical examination findings and historic evidence suggestive of a DA because of skill and confidence-related issues.[6]

A component-by-component approach to the airway management decision-making process can encourage the isolation of biases and empower the clinician to arrive at a rational plan. Although the derived plan may be outside the operator's comfort level or rejected by another invested clinician (e.g., the surgeon), knowledge that a logical, step-by-step approach was employed should fortify the conclusion. In some cases, this may lead to the seeking of help from skilled personnel, delaying of procedures, or a change in the care plan.[7] For example, in the case of a patient with COVID-19 infection who requires tracheal intubation for intensive care, advice might be given to the primary care team that airway management is too hazardous and non-invasive repiratory support might be sought.

Evaluation of the Airway

The value of a history of difficulty with airway management is limited, unless there is clear and extensive documentation.[8] For example, a history of difficult or failed tracheal intubation by direct laryngoscopy (DL) is a strong predictor (6- and 22-fold, respectively) of difficulty on a future presentation[9,10]; yet, multiple studies have demonstrated a 94% to 95% rate of rescue of failed DL by video-assisted laryngoscopy (VAL).[11] The number of available techniques and devices is vast, and the range of experience with a particular device will vary greatly between practitioners. Documentation of the success of laryngoscopy for the purpose of communication most often relies on the Cormack and Lehane (CL) grading scale, which was not developed for VAL, flexible intubation scopes (FISs), or other modern devices.[12] The CL grade has not been validated as an indicator of the ease

or difficulty of intubation with DL, but much of the literature assumes that the ability to see the glottis correlates with ease of tracheal intubation.[13] For example, Rose and Cohen, in a prospective study of 18,500 tracheal intubations, described that poor visualization of the glottic structures was associated with a higher rate of DI by DL.[14] Cook, modifying the original CL grading system to more practically describe the findings of a full or partial laryngeal view, a visible and mobile or immobile epiglottis, or no view, was able to correlate CL grade to time to intubation as well as the need for airway adjuncts.[15] Contrary to this, Adnet and colleagues noted that in a study of 331 patients the majority of patients with poor CL grades on DL were intubated on first attempt, and 4 patients with complete views of the larynx were difficult to intubate.[16] Aziz and colleagues noted that 35% of intubation failures during use of the GlideScope VL (Verathon Inc., Bothell, WA) were associated with complete views of laryngeal structures[11]; similarly, Cooper and colleagues found the rate to be 54%.[17] Because the incidence of an adequate view of the larynx during VAL is high (99.78% in one study), an adequate laryngeal view is likely irrelevant to the success or failure of intubation—other factors influencing tracheal tube delivery being more important.[18]

Invisible and asymptomatic changes in the airway's anatomy can have profound effects on the ability to manipulate the airway with any one device.[19] Findings such as lingual tonsil hyperplasia may vary with time, season, allergies, or other factors.[20] Therefore, any history of difficulty with airway management should raise the suspicion that more than routine procedures may be required and should be prepared for. Alternatively, a previous history of a DA does not destine the patient to special procedures and concerns in all future events.

Should a history of difficulty be elicited from the patient or medical record, an effort should be made to determine not only the nature of the encounter, but also how each facet of management (e.g., intubation, mask ventilation [MV], SGA ventilation) was performed and affected. Critical information includes the experience of the airway manager, the device(s) used, and contextual issues.[21] This information guides the practitioner's decision on the individual components of airway management.

The Need to Control the Airway

Although it is one of the most common procedures of the anesthesia practitioner, controlling the airway entails risk to the patient. Not only are intrinsic respiratory drives and reflexes obtunded, but difficulty in airway control via face mask, SGA, or tracheal intubation may ensue or complications in successful management may be encountered even after uneventful management. In the American Society of Anesthesiologists (ASA) Closed Claims Database, 80% of laryngeal trauma claims were associated with cases of routine airway management and no suspicion of injury.[22] The risks and benefits of airway control should always be considered and balanced. A common example of this balance is the preference for regional anesthesia in obstetric anesthesia; a 10-fold increase in airway-related maternal morbidity and mortality is well documented and is in great part responsible for this practice.[23] Patient and surgeon preference, as well as the operator's skill level, must be considered in this decision, with the latter taking priority. The guidelines of the ASA Task Force for Management of the DA caution similarly and recommend that there be a preformulated strategy for managing the airway, as well as dedicated equipment available, when regional anesthesia is selected for any procedure.[24]

This same recommendation is made in the airway management guidelines of other international expert organizations.[25,26]

Laryngoscopy and Intubation

Definitive airway management has traditionally been understood to mean tracheal intubation by some means (e.g., by DL, VAL, or flexible scope intubation [FSI]). Although it may be argued that face mask or SGA ventilation may constitute as secure an airway as tracheal intubation, this discussion will assume the traditional meaning. This is not to say that all decisions regarding airway management should result in a plan for tracheal intubation; rather, by assuming tracheal intubation as the default plan, the safety of a plan can be incrementally evaluated when the default plan (i.e., tracheal intubation) appears impossible or difficult. Several factors are considered in the assessment of the ease of tracheal intubation: airway evaluation indexes, practitioner experience, and device availability.

Airway Evaluation Indices

A variety of airway evaluation indices have been developed and have subsequently undergone validation studies by independent researchers. Roth and colleagues found that clinical bedside predictors of difficult DL have poor sensitivity and modest specificity.[27] El-Ganzouri and colleagues, by weighing these predictors in a multivariate index, achieved an improved positive predictive value for poor laryngeal view as compared with the use of the Mallampati class alone.[28]

Overall, and despite the use of these indices, the ability of practitioners to reliably predict the difficulty of tracheal intubation has been shown to be poor.[2] Data extracted from the Danish Anesthesia Database, a national clinical quality assurance database, indicated that 75% to 93% of DI events were unanticipated based on historical findings and physical examination. Of those patients who were anticipated to be difficult to intubate, only 25% proved to be.

Occasionally, studies have examined the relative effect of one anatomic finding on the predictive performance of other measures. For example, Ayoub and colleagues found that when patients were segregated by thyromental space (greater or less than 4 cm) the predictive value of the Mallampati score improved.[29] Calder and colleagues demonstrated that maximal interincisor gap was dependent on the ability of the patient to extend the head on the neck.[30] As shown by Brodsky and colleagues, the Samsoon and Young classification of the oropharyngeal view experienced higher sensitivity for predicting difficult DL in patients with a BMI greater than 35.[31] In his editorial, Yentis goes further in explaining the lack of utility of these measures.[32]

In a Special Article in *Anaesthesia*, Greenland reviewed the unique problem of the patient who may have anatomic distortion or a space-occupying lesion of the "middle column" of the airway—the pharynx behind the tongue, the hypopharynx, and the glottis.[33] This would include the patient presenting with or after previous therapy for an upper airway cancer. These areas are invisible during routine preoperative assessment. The otolaryngologist bringing the patient to the operating room may have performed an upper airway endoscopy during the preoperative assessment. Although the results of this examination may be available to the practitioner managing the airway, this evaluation differs from the assessment needed by the airway manager, and performing a preoperative endoscopic airway evaluation (PEAE) can be used to make

decisions regarding the ability to rapidly intubate, ventilate via face mask, or use an SGA.[34] PEAE is discussed in detail in Chapter 9.

Practitioner Experience

Confounding the interpretation of airway predictors and indices is the operator's tolerance for an error in judgment. Unless any test is 100% sensitive (i.e., all patients who are difficult to intubate are detected by this test), there will remain some number of patients who will not be detected and will therefore be at risk of facing a failed intubation. Likewise, if a test is not 100% specific (i.e., all patients who are straightforward to intubate are excluded), some number of patients will be managed with unnecessary procedures, with the potential for wasting time and resources, and possibly causing the patient stress, discomfort, and morbidity. As Yentis notes, many of the indices used in the evaluation for difficult laryngoscopy and intubation are evaluated on a continuous scale (e.g., centimeters of interincisor gap, degrees of head extension at the occiput).[32] Altering the point along the scale at which the test is considered positive or negative will affect sensitivity and specificity. Changing that point might depend on other measures (as discussed) or on the operator's recent or cumulative experience. Sakles and colleagues reported the improvement in VAL and intubation success with anesthesiology trainees over a 7-year period.[35] Whereas first-year trainees demonstrated a 74.4% intubation success rate with a GlideScope, the same trainees achieved a 90% success rate in their third year of training. A less sophisticated, albeit fascinating, result from the same data set demonstrated that the entire department (trainees and attending anesthesiologists) experienced increased overall intubation success with the GlideScope over the same period.[36] Availability of the device, the introduction of faculty more accustomed to VAL, and other factors resulted in institutional improvement.

Device Availability

A large number and variety of devices that aid in tracheal intubation have been introduced over the last half-century, and each has seen its proponents and detractors. Studies, case reports, and opinion articles have attempted to link particular devices and pathology.[37,38] Despite the literature endorsing or decrying any particular device, the practitioner's experience with the intubation aid must be weighed, as previously illustrated.[17,35,36] Likewise, a device encouraged in the literature for a specific clinical situation might not be available at any one institution or at the time of a particular patient's presentation.

Summary

The practitioner's interpretation of standard indices for ease of laryngoscopy/intubation, as mitigated by the device being considered, the experience of the operator (both cumulative and recent), the practitioner's tolerance for error, and the availability of a particular intubation tool may result in vastly different interpretations of similar clinical situations. When fully confident that induction of anesthesia, with or without the use of muscle relaxants, and the application of the chosen (and available) technique of laryngoscopy will result in rapid tracheal intubation, the operator can proceed without further considerations. Failure of laryngoscopy/intubation can occur, and a number of expert groups have provided algorithms for this eventuality.[24,39–43] See Box 10.1 for integration into a preoperative plan.

Ventilation

Face mask and SGA ventilation have been the subjects of far fewer investigations than tracheal intubation.[44] The incidence of difficult ventilation via face mask or SGA has been described as 0.5% to 5%; failed ventilation by face mask or SGA occurs at a rate of 0.07% to 0.2%.[45,46] Independent factors that inform the practitioner's expectation that face mask and SGA ventilation may be difficult are listed in Box 10.2. Skill with SGAs increases rapidly with experience.[47] Technical errors probably account for most failures of SGAs in patients with normal anatomy (Archie Brain MD, Michael Frass MD, and Muhammad Nasir MD, personal communications). Judging the feasibility of using a face mask or SGA must be based on the practitioner's personal experience and the availability of devices with which the practitioner is familiar. As discussed, PEAE may be helpful in determining the risks associated with face mask or SGA ventilation. See Box 10.1 for integration into a preoperative plan.

Risk of Aspiration of Gastric Contents

Pulmonary aspiration of gastric contents is a rare but serious complication of sedation and anesthetic induction, with an incidence between 0.025% and 0.2%, depending on the risk factors in specific populations[48]; aspiration has a mortality of 5%.[48] A significant risk factor is the presence of gastric contents, and expert groups have recommended fasting guidelines for elective and urgent surgical patients.[43] A variety of factors may affect the degree of risk, including obesity, metabolic disease, pregnancy, advanced age, reduced level of consciousness, ileus or bowel obstruction, history of reflux or hiatal hernia, pain and pain therapy, advanced liver or renal dysfunction, critical illness, increasing ASA status, and proper use of pharmacologic agents such as proton pump inhibitors or prokinetic agents.[48,49]

For patients who are evaluated to have a low risk for difficult tracheal intubation, yet a significant risk for aspiration, a rapid sequence induction is often chosen. Although rapid sequence induction and intubation are considered the standard practice for patients who are at risk of gastric contents aspiration, this technique is contraindicated for patients whose airway may be difficult to manage (because of the prolonged duration of the airway being unprotected). Likewise, face mask and SGA ventilation, two techniques not designed to protect the airway from aspiration, are not considered safe techniques in patients at high risk.[6]

Assessing which patients are at risk of pulmonary aspiration of gastric contents and the degree to which this should guide the management of the airway is multifactorial.[48] Based on the clinical situation, the physiologic status of the patient, and the risk of DA management, the clinician must make a carefully considered decision as to the relative degree of risk. See Box 10.1 for integration into a preoperative plan.

Tolerance of Apnea

Errors in judgment may result in periods of apnea during the process of airway management. The inability to intubate or oxygenate by face mask or SGA may occur despite a thorough evaluation.

TABLE 10.1	Time to Significant Oxyhemoglobin Desaturation in Apneic Patients Without an Established Airway Following Preoxygenation[50-54]	
Neonate		2.5 min
1-year-old		3.5 min
Child		4 min
Teen		5.5 min
Healthy adult		8.6 ± 1 min
Healthy adult smoker		6.8 ± 0.9 min
Healthy adult (not preoxygenated)		0.5–1.5 min
Obese adult		3–3.5 min
Pregnant (term) adult		2–3 min
Adult (critically ill)[a]		1–4 min

[a]Includes significant cardiac and/or pulmonary disease, sepsis, other oxygen-deficit process.

Thorough preoxygenation and continuous nasal oxygen have been shown to prolong the safe apneic period. Some populations of patients will be at higher risk of oxyhemoglobin desaturation than others. Table 10.1 summarizes the literature on patient conditions and the time to desaturation to under 90% oxyhemoglobin saturation as measured by pulse oximetry. See Box 10.1 for integration into a preoperative plan.

Emergency Invasive Airway Access

In the recommendations and guidelines published by expert groups, airway access through the neck and into the larynx or trachea is the advised salvage method when a "cannot intubate/cannot oxygenate" (CICO) situation develops.[24,25,39,40,43] Because errors may occur in the assessment of one or more components of the airway management process, the potential to salvage the patient with emergency invasive airway access should always be considered. Groups such as the ASA Task Force on Management of the DA counsel the practitioner to evaluate the patient for "difficult surgical airway" before initiating airway management. When a patient's anatomy is not conducive to rapid invasive access (e.g., obesity, prior neck surgery, or radiation), planning invasive rescue may not be practical.

Unfortunately the feasibility of relying on emergency invasive airway access for airway salvage has been questioned.[6] The NAP4 study found that failure of emergency invasive airway access was common in the hands of the anesthesia provider. Failure to learn and practice emergency invasive airway techniques, lack of familiarity with the anatomic structures, and a hesitancy to do invasive procedures were considered as major contributing factors by the NAP4 authors.

Integration: The Airway Approach Algorithm

Previously presented are six components to be contemplated before initiating airway management. The order in which these components are considered can provide clear management choices. A decision-tree approach to preoperative assessment that integrates these components, the Airway Approach Algorithm (AAA), has been described (Fig. 10.1).[55] The end goal of this decision tree is the choice between managing the patient's airway after the induction of anesthesia and awake airway management, as recommended by expert guidelines,

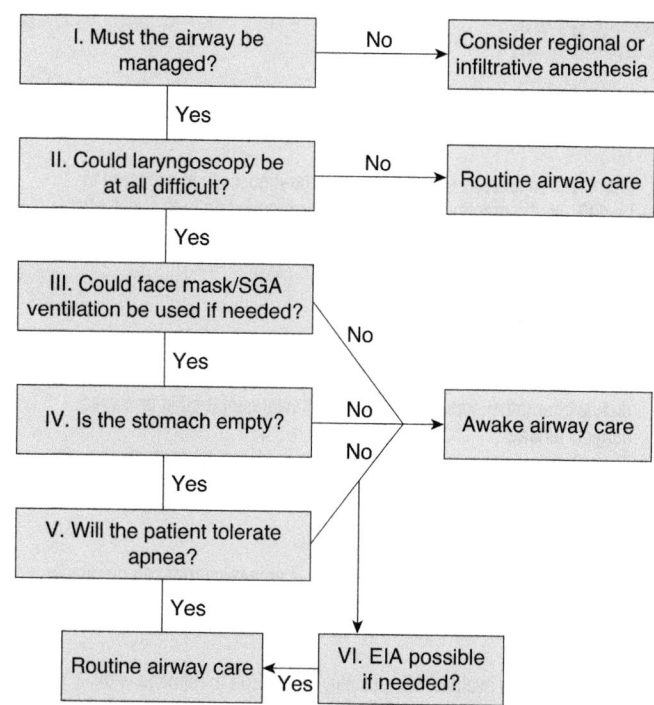

• **Fig. 10.1** The Airway Approach Algorithm is a decision-tree approach to integration of segregated airway management decisions. *EIA*, Emergency invasive airway *SGA*, supraglottic airway. (Modified from Rosenblatt, WH. The Airway Approach Algorithm: a decision tree for organizing preoperative airway information. *J Clin Anes.* 2004;16:312–316.)

such as those of the ASA, the Canadian Airway Focus Group, and others.[24,40,43] The AAA decision tree is organized in a single trunk; branch points from this trunk lead to a clinical pathway.

The entry point into the AAA is the decision to pursue airway management (Fig. 10.1, I.). If airway management is not required, the operator is encouraged to consider the decision tree in preparation for failed nongeneral anesthesia care. If airway control is planned, the airway manager considers the potential for difficult laryngoscopy and intubation (Fig. 10.1, II.). If, after a thorough evaluation and consideration of the earlier discussion, laryngoscopy and intubation are expected to be straightforward, no further evaluation is required. The prototypical patient is the one in which rapid sequence induction is planned—there is no intent to ventilate the patient by face mask or SGA. Indeed, airway management might fail as a result of unforeseen reasons, and the algorithms and discussions of many expert groups provide strategies.[24,25,39,40,43]

If, for any reason, it is suspected that laryngoscopy and intubation may be difficult, the practitioner proceeds to question III of the AAA: "Could face mask/SGA ventilation be used if needed?" If, after considering the preceding discussion, doubts remain regarding the rescue potential of ventilation, the practitioner has determined the patient to be at risk for intubation failure and ventilation failure. As this conclusion is arrived at in the preoperative setting, the practitioner has the opportunity to avoid a potential CICO situation by choosing to manage the patient with an alternative approach, including awake intubation, awake elective invasive airway, or an alternative anesthetic technique (e.g., regional anesthesia).

Should face mask/SGA ventilation be judged as straightforward despite concerns regarding laryngoscopy and intubation, the operator now considers the risk for aspiration of gastric contents (Fig. 10.1, IV.). As discussed, face mask/SGA ventilation is considered to be contraindicated in the elective situation when there is an aspiration risk. If the practitioner judges that there is a risk for aspiration, a conclusion of possible failed intubation and contraindicated ventilation is reached, and an alternative approach including awake intubation or awake surgical airway is chosen.

If the operator decides that there is no aspiration threat, the risk of an error in judgment is considered (Fig. 10.1, V.). As discussed, the evaluation of ease of laryngoscopy and intubation and face mask/SGA ventilation is multifactorial and inexact. Should a judgment error have occurred, a CICO scenario may occur after the induction of anesthesia. The clinician must weigh the risk to the patient in this scenario. If the patient is considered at high risk for oxyhemoglobin desaturation, an alternative, awake approach is chosen. Alternatively, if the patient is judged to be able to tolerate apnea while corrective actions (including a surgical airway) are taken, the practitioner progresses to induction of anesthesia and airway care.

Conclusion

The DA is an enigma. Although common usage of the term frequently refers to the patient whose difficulty is only discovered after the induction of anesthesia, preoperative assessment is designed to identify these patients before a precarious situation is encountered. Likewise, difficulty may concern laryngoscopy and intubation, MV, SGA ventilation, aspiration risk, the difficulty of performing a rapid surgical airway if needed, or combinations of these techniques. Lastly, a variety of biases and judgment errors can affect outcomes. A careful component-by-component consideration of each facet of airway management and a coherent approach to their integration into an airway plan can both provide safe care and remove doubt from airway decision-making.

Selected References

2. Nørskov AK, Rosenstock CV, Wetterslev J, et al. Diagnostic accuracy of anaesthesiologists' prediction of difficult airway management in daily clinical practice: a cohort study of 188 064 patients registered in the Danish Anaesthesia Database. *Anaesthesia.* 2015;70:272–281.
12. Angadi SP, Frerk C. Video laryngoscopy and Cormack and Lehane grading. *Anaesthesia.* 2011;66:628–629.
19. Ovassapian A, Glassenberg R, Randel GI, et al. The unexpected difficult airway and lingual tonsil hyperplasia: a case series and a review of the literature. *Anesthesiology.* 2002;97:124–132.
21. Cooper RM. Preparation for and management of "failed" laryngoscopy and/or intubation. *Anesthesiology.* 2019;130(5):833–849.
32. Yentis SM. Predicting difficult intubation—worthwhile exercise or pointless ritual? *Anaesthesia.* 2002;57(2):105–109.
33. Greenland KB. A proposed model for direct laryngoscopy and tracheal intubation. *Anaesthesia.* 2008;63:156–161.
34. Rosenblatt W, Andreea I, Sukhupragarn W, et al. Preoperative endoscopic airway examination (PEAE) provides superior airway information and may reduce the use of unnecessary awake intubation. *Anesth Analg.* 2011;112:602–607.
40. Law JA, Broemling N, Cooper RM, et al. The difficult airway with recommendations for management—Part 1—difficult tracheal intubation encountered in an unconscious/induced patient. *Can J Anaesth.* 2013;60:1089–1118.
46. Kheterpal S, Han R, Tremper K, et al. Incidence and predictors of difficult and impossible mask ventilation. *Anesthesiology.* 2006;105:885–891.
55. Rosenblatt WH. The Airway Approach Algorithm: a decision tree for organizing preoperative airway information. *J Clin Anesth.* 2004;16:312–316.

All references can be found online at eBooks.Health.Elsevier.com.

11

Algorithms for Management of the Difficult Airway

THOMAS HEIDEGGER AND CARIN A. HAGBERG

CHAPTER OUTLINE

KEY POINTS

- Adherence to the principles of an airway management algorithm and widespread adoption of such a structured plan should result in a reduction of respiratory catastrophes and a decrease in perioperative morbidity and mortality.
- Airway evaluation should consider any characteristics of the patient that could lead to difficulty in the performance of (1) face mask or supraglottic airway (SGA) ventilation, (2) direct or video-assisted laryngoscopy (VAL), (3) intubation, (4) invasive airway access, or (5) extubation.
- In the anesthetized patient whose trachea has proved to be difficult to intubate, it is necessary to try to maintain oxygenation by mask ventilation between and during intubation attempts, whenever possible. The use of transnasal humified rapid insufflation ventilator exchange (THRIVE) should be considered when available.
- Repeated attempts at difficult intubation (perseveration) can result in serious soft tissue injury and rapidly deteriorate into a cannot intubate/cannot oxygenate (CICO) situation that requires a cricothyrotomy as a potentially lifesaving procedure.

- SGA devices are not helpful if there is complete airway obstruction located above, at, or below the glottic opening.
- A well-selected number of alternative airway devices and techniques should be available and routinely practiced.
- Extubation of the patient with a DA should be carefully assessed and performed, and the anesthesiologist should develop a strategy for safe extubation of these patients.
- The presence and nature of the airway difficulty should be documented in the medical record.
- Further research should address aspects such as adherence to national and local guidelines in emergency situations, the detailed experience with new and already established airway devices, and the specific role and limitations of new devices as they reach clinical practice.
- As difficult airway (DA) guidelines and algorithms will continue to be modified, airway practitioners must keep abreast of new advances in both techniques and theory related to DA management.

Introduction

The difficult airway (DA) remains one of the most relevant and challenging clinical situations faced by anesthesiologists due to the occurrence of major adverse consequences if airway patency is not established, such as brain injury and death.[1] There is strong evidence that successful airway management in the perioperative environment depends on specific strategies. Suggested strategies from various subfields of medicine are now being linked to form more comprehensive treatment plans or algorithms. Many national anesthesiology societies have developed guidelines for management of the DA that are based on expert opinion and scientific evidence. Algorithms have been developed to assimilate these guidelines in a stepwise fashion to facilitate management of the DA and reduce the likelihood of adverse outcomes. Additionally, efforts are currently underway to develop a universal airway management guideline that can be applied across clinical disciplines, patient types, geographic regions, and contexts of care.

There has been tremendous growth in the literature on management of the DA in anesthesia practice. In order for DA guidelines to reflect the most current evidence, they should be reviewed regularly for their content and continued relevance. Some of the most significant changes in DA guidelines over the past two decades have been the incorporation of new airway devices or techniques. As the practice of airway management becomes more advanced, anesthesiologists must become both knowledgeable and proficient in the use of various airway devices and techniques in both the nonemergent and emergent setting. Nonetheless, there are also nontechnical factors involved when an anesthesiologist is confronted with an unexpected DA in either setting. Anesthesiology as a specialty must address the impact of environmental, technical, and psychological factors on the practitioner's performance. A better understanding of the human factors involved in a DA crisis is crucial to ensure patient safety, and further research into their role in the cause of airway complications is needed.

Usefulness of Airway Algorithms

The effectiveness of guidelines for airway management in daily practice is not straightforward, as indicated in several outcome studies.[2–4] One of the largest outcome studies in airway management is the Fourth National Audit Project of the Royal College of Anaesthetists and the Difficult Airway Society (NAP4),[5] which analyzed 2.9 million anesthetics in the United Kingdom. Major complications occurred in 1:22,000 anesthetics leading to an airway-related mortality rate of 1:180,000 cases. However, as the number of cases may have been underreported, the true incidence of severe events might actually have been 4 times higher (~1:5,500).[6] From a more pessimistic point of view, the estimated number of critical airway incidents (near-misses) that do not lead to actual harm, such as failed intubation with mild or moderate hypoxic episodes, is considerably more common than 1:5,500.

The original Difficult Airway Society (DAS) guidelines[7] were in effect during the time period the NAP4 survey was conducted. Thus, the actual positive impact of the airway guidelines may be questioned. On the other hand, results from the implementation of the guidelines from the American Society of Anesthesiologists (ASA) Practice Guidelines for the Management of the DA[8] and from institutional guidelines suggest that routine application of an algorithmic approach to failed intubation was associated with much higher success rates once implemented.[9–13] Unfortunately, results of the newest analysis of the Closed Claims Project in the United States with regard to difficult tracheal intubation have yielded worrisome figures as well.[14] Compared to the period from 1993 to 1999, the latest figures from the years 2000 to 2012 show that the incidence of brain damage or death at induction was 5.5 times greater in the latter time period.

When considering the sobering results of the NAP4 study and the recent Closed Claims analysis, perhaps it is the nonobligatory use or the flexibility when using algorithms or guidelines in daily practice that is problematic. In fact, the practitioner may deviate from a predefined plan according to the actual clinical situation. This is very different from civil aviation, where "following the rules" is considered paramount in terms of safety.[15] "The big difference is not so much the safety toolkit, which is similar for most industries," as Amalberti and colleagues stated, "but in an industry's willingness to abandon historical and cultural precedents and beliefs that are linked to performance and autonomy, in a constant drive toward a culture of safety."[16] From this point of view, it is conceivable that the nonobligatory nature to use airway algorithms/guidelines may be partly responsible for the disappointing result of NAP4. Thus, perhaps following such algorithms should be compulsory and considered standard of care, such as the use of basic monitoring (electrocardiography [ECG], pulse oximetry, capnography) when providing general anesthesia, regional anesthesia, or monitored anesthesia care.[17]

The use of algorithms for patient care may be problematic for practitioners because of complexity and information overload, which makes it very difficult to distinguish between relevant and irrelevant information.[18] To aid compliance in adhering to algorithms, flowcharts have been developed and successfully used by a range of practitioners. The classic flowcharts of this nature are the resuscitation algorithms that provide evidence-based guidance during cardiopulmonary resuscitation worldwide, such as the American Heart Association Life Support guidelines.[19] Additionally, cognitive aids are increasingly being used during emergencies and have been demonstrated to improve anesthesia decision making in the DA setting.[20,21]

Further consideration regarding the effectiveness of algorithms should include the quality of the evidence. Just because a guideline or an algorithm claims to be evidence based does not necessarily mean that it provides correct recommendations.[22] On the other hand, if there is a requirement for only strong evidence to manage a DA, a decision may not be made at all. It is sometimes necessary, especially in the area of airway management, to sacrifice internal validity to achieve generalizability.[23] In other words, even though randomized controlled trials provide high-quality evidence, these studies may have only limited relevance in clinical practice. A key question regarding the usefulness of airway algorithm guidelines is whether or not they actually reflect best clinical practice since they are primarily based on experience and expert opinion rather than strong evidence.[24]

Nonetheless, airway guidelines do help guide clinicians and allow the community to improve standards, ensure that certain equipment is available, and ensure that training for the skills and processes required to follow such guidelines are in place.[25] The pros and cons regarding the usefulness of algorithms and guidelines are shown in Table 11.1.

Definition of Terms and Degree of Obligation

In the practice of anesthesiology, guidelines and standards have long been used. For instance, many anesthesia societies have implemented mandatory protocols for perioperative monitoring.[17,26–28]

TABLE 11.1 Usefulness of Algorithms—Pros and Cons

Pro Arguments	Con Arguments
Quality assurance (through activities that are proven to be effective); use in "high-risk" technology; support for rare but critical events[63,64]	"Cookbook" medicine; prevents innovation[26]; "what is best for patients overall may be inappropriate for individuals"[15]
Information and involvement of patients in decision-making by using guidelines[65]	Questionable health effect and questionable sustained effect on long-term behavior[66]
"Use of standards makes sense"[15]	Far away from practice[67]; risk for overruling[68]
Routine application of institutional guidelines is associated with higher success rates[9]	Questionable effect on outcome because of a lack of obligation[68]
Simple and logical algorithms increase survival[19]	Noncompliance due to information overload and high complexity[18]
Opportunity to improve standards and availability of equipment[25]	Questionable value because guidelines are built on expert opinion and group consensus rather than on hard evidence, and because they are outdated due to a limited lifespan (new evidence, new technologies)[9,69]

In airway management, numerous flowcharts, guidelines, and algorithms have been developed over time. Theoretically, there are differences between algorithms, guidelines, recommendations, standards, protocols, and so on, but in practice it is difficult to differentiate these terms. Table 11.2 contrasts the definitions and the degrees of obligation of the different terms. The main difference relates to the degree of obligation of the practitioner, which means that standards—such as the use of ECG, pulse oximetry, or capnography for monitoring purposes—are obligatory, whereas all others (algorithms, guidelines, protocols, etc) are, strictly speaking, voluntary.[29,30] Nonetheless, in the courtroom when there is an airway mishap, these terms are often used interchangeably.

National Anesthesia Society Guidelines

Many national anesthesia societies have published their own guidelines for management of the DA, including the ASA,[8] the DAS of the United Kingdom,[31] the Canadian Airway Focus Group (CAFG),[32,33] the Italian Society for Anesthesia Analgesia Resuscitation and Intensive Care Medicine (SIAARTI),[34] the French Society of Anesthesia and Intensive Care (SFAR),[35] the German Society of Anesthesiology and Intensive Care Medicine (DGAI),[36] the Chinese Society of Anesthesiology,[37] the Japanese Society of

Anesthesiologists,[38] and the All India Difficult Airway Association (AIDAA).[39]

Similar to the ASA's DA guidelines, the CAFG, SIAARTI, and AIDAA guideline methodologies include a systematic review of the literature with classification of the level of evidence. Guidelines published by the other national societies include literature reviews but do not aggregate and classify evidence in a systematic fashion.[40] The DGAI's guidelines grade the organization's statements into "strongly recommend," "recommend," and "unclear recommendation." With the exception of the DAS and the AIDAA guidelines, which only focus on the management of *unanticipated* difficult intubation, all other national guidelines also include recommendations for management of the *anticipated* DA.

All national societies regard awake flexible scope intubation (FSI) as the technique of choice to manage the *anticipated* DA, and all societies have incorporated cricothyrotomy for management of a "cannot intubate/cannot oxygenate" (CICO) scenario.[41]

Thus, training and subsequently retaining skills with these techniques remain crucial. This has been impressively confirmed by the recent Closed Claims analysis of the United States.[14] One of the modifications is the addition of video-assisted laryngoscopy (VAL). However, there is still debate as to whether VAL should be a routine, first-line technique or whether it should be reserved

TABLE 11.2 Definition of Terms and Degree of Obligation[60,70]

Terms	Definition	Degree of Obligation
Standards	Generally accepted principles for patient management; exceptions are rare and failure to follow is often difficult to justify	Mandatory
Strategy	A well-planned series of steps for achieving a goal	Voluntary
Guidelines	Systematically developed statements to assist the practitioner in specific clinical circumstances; incorporates the best scientific evidence with expert opinion	Voluntary
Practice policies	Describe present recommendations issued to influence practitioners in reaching decisions about interventions	Voluntary
Recommendations	Suitable and useful strategies; not as strict as standards and guidelines	Voluntary
Options	Different possibilities are available; neutral assessment	Voluntary
Protocols/Algorithms	Stepwise procedures or decision trees to guide the practitioner through the diagnosis and treatment of various clinical problems	Voluntary

for those patients who are predicted or found to be difficult to intubate.[42,43] Even though there is a range in the various guidelines for the number of intubation attempts, most algorithms strictly limit the number of intubation attempts to a maximum of three attempts. Many guidelines place increased emphasis on communication (e.g., declaration of failure), situational awareness, strategy, and planning, rather than on tools and devices, which is regarded as an important step toward the improvement of safety.[25,44,45]

American Society of Anesthesiologists' Practice Guidelines for Management of the Difficult Airway

The ASA Task Force on Management of the DA developed the original ASA Difficult Airway Algorithm (DAA) over a 2-year period. The task force included both academic and private anesthesiologists and a statistical methodologist. This algorithm was introduced by the ASA as a practice guideline in 1993.[46] In 2003, the ASA Task Force presented a revised algorithm that essentially retained the same concept but recommended a wider range of airway management techniques than was previously included, based on more recent scientific evidence and the advent of new technology. In 2013, this revised algorithm was further modified, taking into account additional updated evidence obtained from scientific literature and technology since the last revision and findings from new surveys of expert consultants as well as randomly selected ASA members.[8,47]

The ASA DA guidelines were most recently revised and published in 2022 (Fig. 11.1).[48] Their intended use has now broadened to all airway management and anesthetic care delivered in inpatient (e.g., perioperative, nonoperating room, emergency department, and critical care settings) and ambulatory settings (e.g., ambulatory surgery centers, office-based surgery, and procedure centers performing invasive airway procedures) and applies to anesthesiologists and all other practitioners who perform anesthesia care or airway management. As in the past, the guidelines are intended for all patients with either an anticipated or unanticipated DA, including but not limited to obstetric, intensive care, and critically ill patients. Of note, the 2022 ASA DA guidelines include separate DA algorithms for adult and pediatric patients, and each algorithm is accompanied by an infographic that can be utilized in real time or for educational purposes.

The 2022 ASA DA guidelines for adult patients differ from the 2013 DA guidelines in the following significant ways:
1. Developed by an international task force of anesthesiologists representing several anesthesiology, airway, and other medical organizations;
2. Broadens the intended use of the guidelines to all individuals who perform anesthesia care or airway management, both anesthesiologists and non-anesthesiologists;
3. Provides considerations for the development of a difficult airway management strategy, including considerations for awake airway management and assessments to predict risk of aspiration;
4. Provides guidance for entering the awake intubation vs. airway management after the induction of anesthesia pathways based on assessment particular to the airway practitioner, context, and resources;
5. Provides recommendations for managing failure in the awake intubation pathway;
6. Broadens its descriptions of the difficult airway to include inadequate ventilation, difficult or failed tracheal intubation,

extubation of the difficult airway, and difficult or failed invasive airway;
7. Recommends optimization of oxygenation before initiating and throughout difficult airway management, including the extubation process;
8. Specifies limiting initial attempts at intubation, limiting intubation attempts if ventilation is adequate but intubation is unsuccessful, and limiting attempts at placing an SGA in a "cannot intubate, cannot ventilate" scenario;
9. Explicitly mentions awake intubation techniques, such as flexible bronchoscopy or combination techniques;
10. Provides an opinion-based recommendation to limit attempts at laryngoscopy and intubation or SGA attempts to three, with one additional attempt by a clinician with a high skill set;
11. Broadens noninvasive and invasive alternatives for difficult airway management to include the use of combination techniques, rigid bronchoscopy, and extracorporeal membrane oxygenation;
12. Provides updated recommendations for the contents of a portable storage unit, as well as recommendations for airway management items in all anesthetizing locations;
13. Provides more robust recommendations for precautions during extubation of the difficult airway and additional recommendations for follow-up care;
14. Includes consideration of human factors (including environmental factors, team behaviors, and individual performance) as part of airway preparation, management, and post-event airway care;
15. Provides new algorithms and infographics for adult and pediatric difficult airway management.

Difficult Airway Society Guidelines for Management of Unanticipated Difficult Intubation in Adults

Unlike the ASA DA guidelines, which address both the anticipated and the unanticipated DA, the DAS guidelines focus on the unanticipated DA, an unpredictable problem. The new 2015 DAS guidelines[31] differ from the original 2014 DAS DA guidelines in that they are more concise and more pragmatic, with considerable emphasis placed on preparedness and accountability of the practitioner, by optimizing conditions and minimizing patient morbidity in a DA situation (Figs. 11.2–11.4). Training of physicians with alternative airway devices and techniques, including emergency invasive airway access, is considered not only essential but expected.[49]

After an unsuccessful initial intubation attempt, restoration of ventilation is the priority, by either noninvasive (e.g., SGA) or invasive intervention, or by awakening the patient. Repeated attempts at intubation should not delay noninvasive airway ventilation or emergency invasive airway access. The new guidelines favor the use of second-generation SGAs in this situation, because they have specifically designed features to reduce the risk of aspiration and provide a better airway seal. Similar to recommendations by other national societies, the new guidelines incorporate the use of VAL for management of the DA. Although all anesthesia society guidelines incorporate the performance of a cricothyrotomy for management of the CICO situation, the new DAS guidelines no longer recommend the cannula technique, due to the findings from the NAP4 study that this technique was inferior to the surgical technique.[5] The new guidelines recommend consideration of

ASA DIFFICULT AIRWAY ALGORITHM: ADULT PATIENTS

Pre-Intubation: Before attempting intubation, choose between either an awake or post-induction airway strategy. Choice of strategy and technique should be made by the clinician managing the airway.[1]

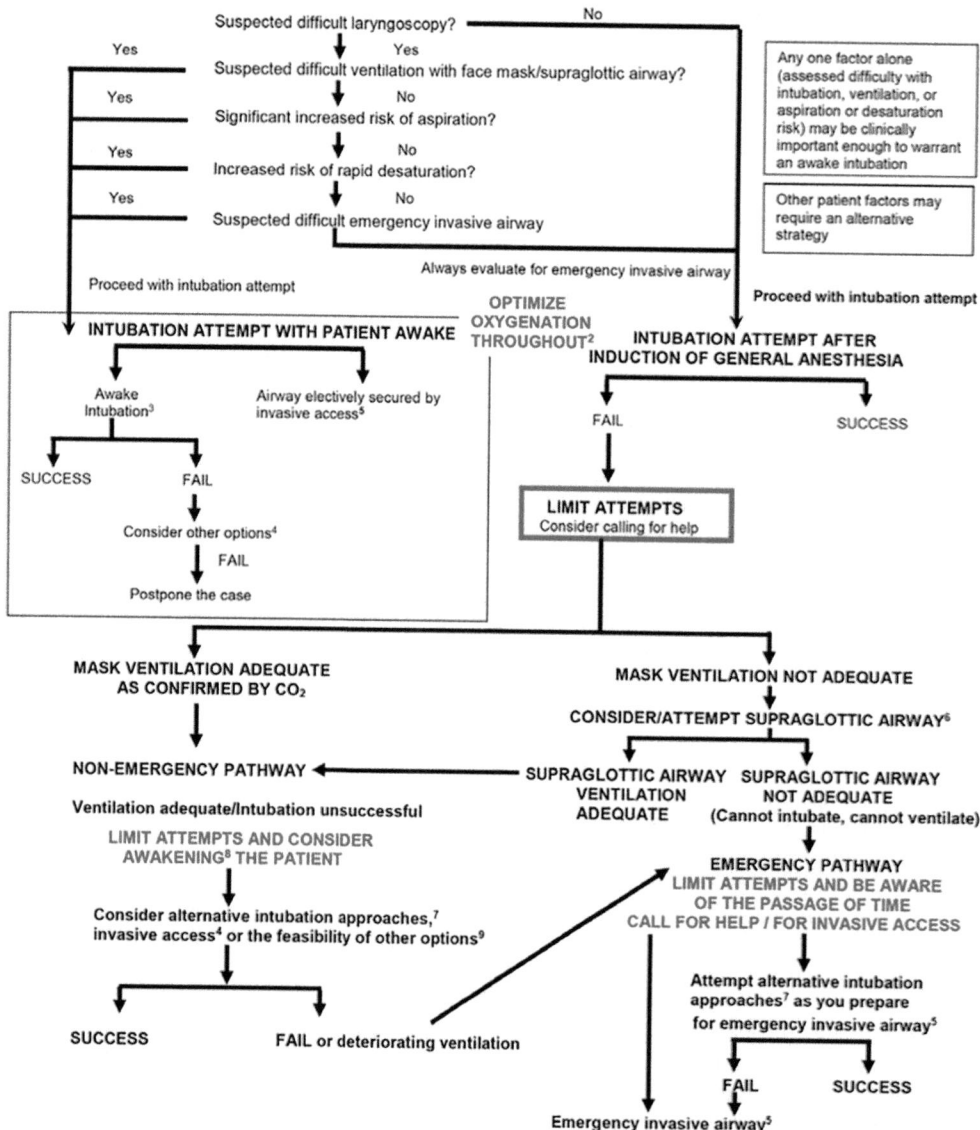

Difficult airway algorithm: Adult patients. [1]The airway manager's choice of airway strategy and techniques should be based on their previous experience; available resources, including equipment, availability and competency of help; and the context in which airway management will occur. [2]Low- or high-flow nasal cannula, head elevated position throughout procedure. Noninvasive ventilation during preoxygenation. [3]Awake intubation techniques include flexible bronchoscope, videolaryngoscopy, direct laryngoscopy, combined techniques, and retrograde wire-aided intubation. [4]Other options include, but are not limited to, alternative awake technique, awake elective invasive airway, alternative anesthetic techniques, induction of anesthesia (if unstable or cannot be postponed) with preparations for emergency invasive airway, and postponing the case without attempting the above options. [5]Invasive airway techniques include surgical cricothyrotomy, needle cricothyrotomy with a pressure-regulated device, large-bore cannula cricothyrotomy, or surgical tracheostomy. Elective invasive airway techniques include the above and retrograde wire–guided intubation and percutaneous tracheostomy. Also consider rigid bronchoscopy and ECMO. [6]Consideration of size, design, positioning, and first *versus* second generation supraglottic airways may improve the ability to ventilate. [7]Alternative difficult intubation approaches include but are not limited to video-assisted laryngoscopy, alternative laryngoscope blades, combined techniques, intubating supraglottic airway (with or without flexible bronchoscopic guidance), flexible bronchoscopy, introducer, and lighted stylet or lightwand. Adjuncts that may be employed during intubation attempts include tracheal tube introducers, rigid stylets, intubating stylets, or tube changers and external laryngeal manipulation. [8]Includes postponing the case or postponing the intubation and returning with appropriate resources (*e.g.*, personnel, equipment, patient preparation, awake intubation). [9]Other options include, but are not limited to, proceeding with procedure utilizing face mask or supraglottic airway ventilation. Pursuit of these options usually implies that ventilation will not be problematic.

• **Fig. 11.1** 2022 American Society of Anesthesiologists Practice Guidelines for Management of the Difficult Airway *ECMO*, extracorporeal membrane oxygenation. (From Apfelbaum JL, Hagberg CA, Connis RT, et al. 2022 American Society of Anesthesiologists Practice Guidelines for Management of the Difficult Airway. *Anesthesiology.* 2022;136:31–81.)

DAS Difficult Intubation Guidelines – Overview

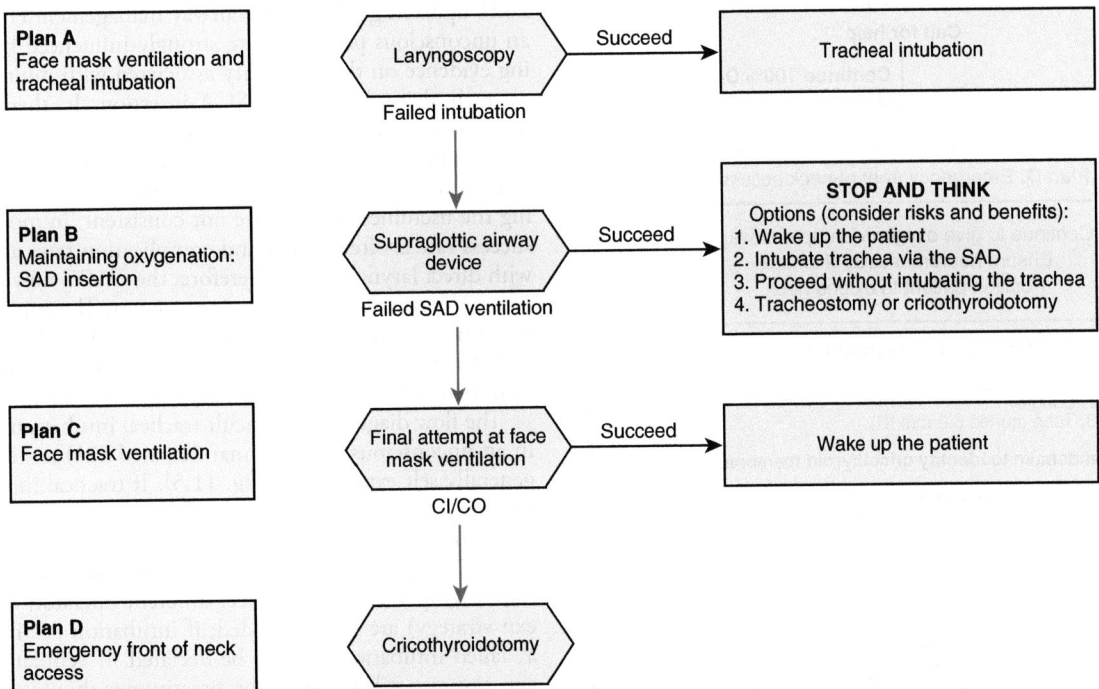

• **Fig. 11.2** Overview of Difficult Airway Society Guidelines. *DAS,* Difficult Airway Society; *CI/CO,* cannot intubate/cannot oxygenate; *SAD,* supraglottic airway device. (From Frerk C, Mitchell VS, McNarry AF, et al. Difficult Airway Society 2015 guidelines for management of unanticipated difficult intubation in adults. *Br J Anaesth.* 2015;115(6):827–848.)

Management of Unanticipated Difficult Tracheal Intubation in Adults

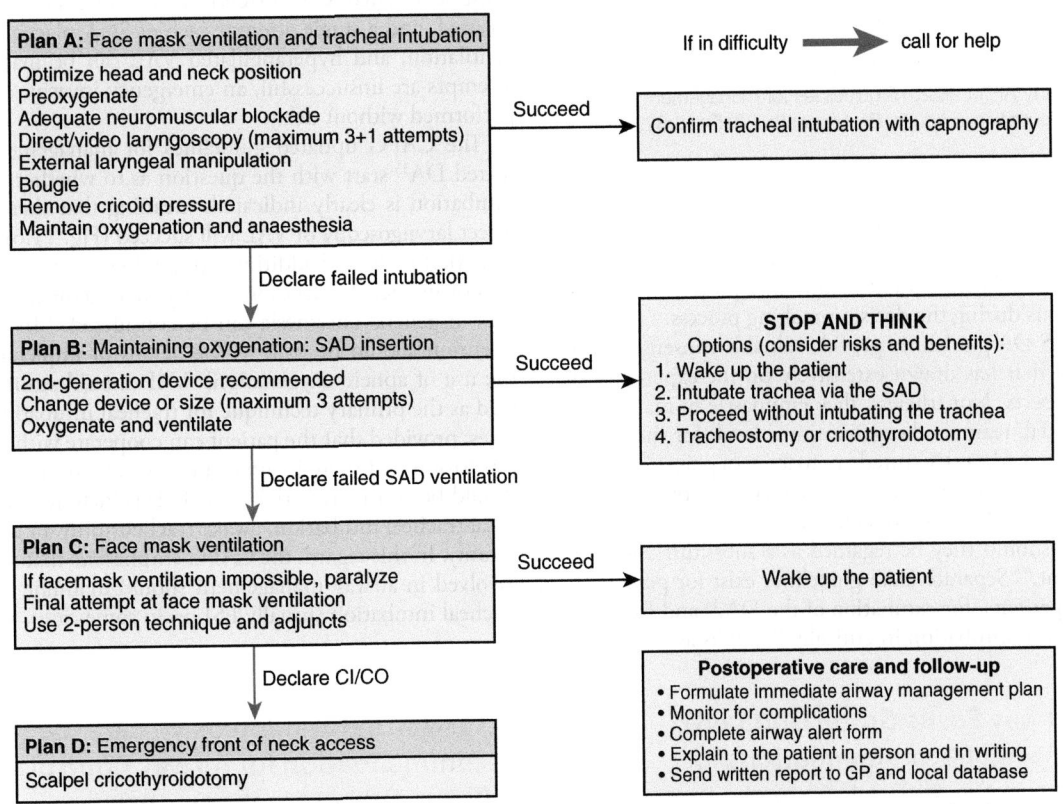

• **Fig. 11.3** Difficult Airway Society Guidelines for management of unanticipated difficult intubation in adults. *CI/CO,* Cannot intubate/cannot oxygenate; *SAD,* supraglottic airway device. (From Frerk C, Mitchell VS, McNarry AF, et al. Difficult Airway Society 2015 guidelines for management of unanticipated difficult intubation in adults. *Br J Anaesth.* 2015;115(6):827–848.)

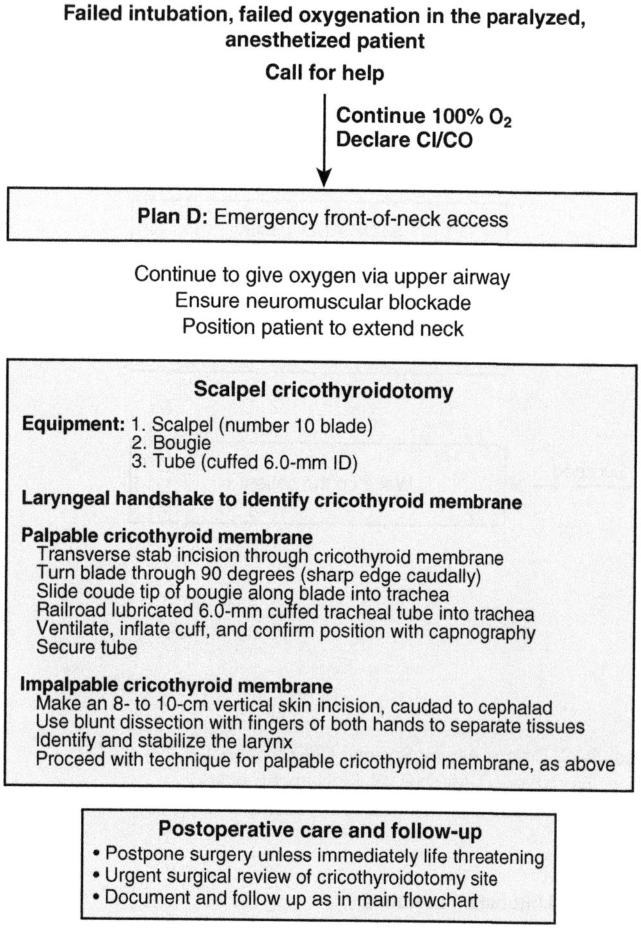

**Failed intubation, failed oxygenation in the paralyzed,
anesthetized patient**

Call for help

Continue 100% O_2
Declare CI/CO

↓

Plan D: Emergency front-of-neck access

Continue to give oxygen via upper airway
Ensure neuromuscular blockade
Position patient to extend neck

Scalpel cricothyroidotomy

Equipment: 1. Scalpel (number 10 blade)
2. Bougie
3. Tube (cuffed 6.0-mm ID)

Laryngeal handshake to identify cricothyroid membrane

Palpable cricothyroid membrane
Transverse stab incision through cricothyroid membrane
Turn blade through 90 degrees (sharp edge caudally)
Slide coude tip of bougie along blade into trachea
Railroad lubricated 6.0-mm cuffed tracheal tube into trachea
Ventilate, inflate cuff, and confirm position with capnography
Secure tube

Impalpable cricothyroid membrane
Make an 8- to 10-cm vertical skin incision, caudad to cephalad
Use blunt dissection with fingers of both hands to separate tissues
Identify and stabilize the larynx
Proceed with technique for palpable cricothyroid membrane, as above

Postoperative care and follow-up
• Postpone surgery unless immediately life threatening
• Urgent surgical review of cricothyroidotomy site
• Document and follow up as in main flowchart

• **Fig. 11.4** Difficult Airway Society Guidelines for failed intubation, failed oxygenation in the paralyzed, anaesthetized patient: technique for scalpel cricothyrotomy. CI/CO, Cannot intubate/cannot oxygenate. (From Frerk C, Mitchell VS, McNarry AF, et al. 2015 guidelines for management of unanticipated difficult intubation in adults. *Br J Anaesth.* 2015;115:827–848.)

the technique of nasal oxygen during efforts securing a tube (NO DESAT)[50] and transnasal humidified rapid-insufflation ventilatory exchange (THRIVE)[51] to relieve the time pressure of falling oxygen saturations during the decision-making process.

The new DAS DA guidelines provide valuable consensus from an expert panel that has drawn extensively on the experience of international experts. Nonetheless, they emphasize human factor issues at individual, team, and organizational levels for their optimization. They provide a structured approach to a potentially life-threatening clinical situation and consider current practice and recent developments. They do not constitute a minimum standard of practice, nor should they be regarded as a substitute for good clinical judgment.[49] Separate DAS guidelines exist for pediatric[52] and obstetric[53] patients, for extubation of the DA,[54] and for management of tracheal intubation in critically ill adults as well.[55]

Canadian Airway Focus Group Updated Consensus-Based Recommendations for Management of the Difficult Airway

The CAFG initially published recommendations for the unanticipated DA in 1998; their updated recommendations also including

management of the anticipated DA were published in 2013. Their 2021 updated guidelines for airway management encountered in an unconscious patient[32] were strongly influenced by the emerging evidence on the morbidity associated with multiple attempts at tracheal intubation and SGA insertion. It, therefore, underscores the need to optimize for success on the first attempt and to limit further attempts to a maximum of three before stopping to consider "exit strategy" options. Even though findings regarding the usefulness of VAL are not consistent, in most studies the success rate is often higher and complication rates are lower than with direct laryngoscopy. Therefore, the CAFG now recommends use of VAL on the first intubation attempt. The guidelines further recommend that SGA insertion attempts should also be limited and that neuromuscular blockade should be ensured in case of a cannot ventilate/cannot oxygenate (CVCO) situation.

The flow diagram for difficult tracheal intubation encountered in an unconscious patient (unanticipated DA) is still simple and generally self-explanatory (Fig. 11.5). If tracheal intubation (one attempt) is unsuccessful (left path of the algorithm), the next decision is whether ventilation and oxygenation by face mask or SGA are possible or not. If yes, up to two additional intubation attempts (different device, different operator, or proceed to exit strategy) are recommended; if intubation is still impossible, a "failed intubation" should be declared. If ventilation and oxygenation are still possible, the practitioner should pause to consider an "exit strategy," such as awakening the patient (if feasible), temporary SGA placement, an additional intubation attempt, or, in rare circumstances, a surgical airway could be chosen. If ventilation and oxygenation cannot be ensured, a CVCO situation must be declared and a "call for help" is mandatory (right path of the algorithm). Preparing for emergency invasive airway access must be initiated. Concurrently, neuromuscular blockade must be ensured, and a single attempt each at SGA placement, face-mask ventilation, and hyperangulated VAL can be made. If all these attempts are unsuccessful, an emergency invasive airway must be performed without delay.

The CAFG updated guidelines for management of the predicted DA[33] start with the question as to whether awake tracheal intubation is clearly indicated, meaning that there is no chance direct laryngoscopy or VAL will succeed (Fig. 11.6). If the answer is no (left path) and additional physiological and contextual issues do not impact the decision, airway management after the induction of general anesthesia can be considered.[56] In this case, close attention should be paid to the details of implementation (e.g., the use of apneic oxygenation). VAL should strongly be considered as the primary technique for tracheal intubation. In all other cases, provided that the patient can cooperate with awake tracheal intubation and there is sufficient time, awake tracheal intubation should be considered (right path). This includes an awake oral or nasal tracheal intubation, awake tracheostomy, or awake cricothyrotomy. In this regard, the CAFG emphasizes that all practitioners involved in airway management should maintain skills in awake tracheal intubation (usually FSI or, in some cases, VAL).

Italian Society of Anesthesia Analgesia Resuscitation and Intensive Care Medicine's Recommendation for Airway Control and Difficult Airway Management

The original SIAARTI DA guidelines published in 1998 were updated in 2013.[34] The recommendation for management of the

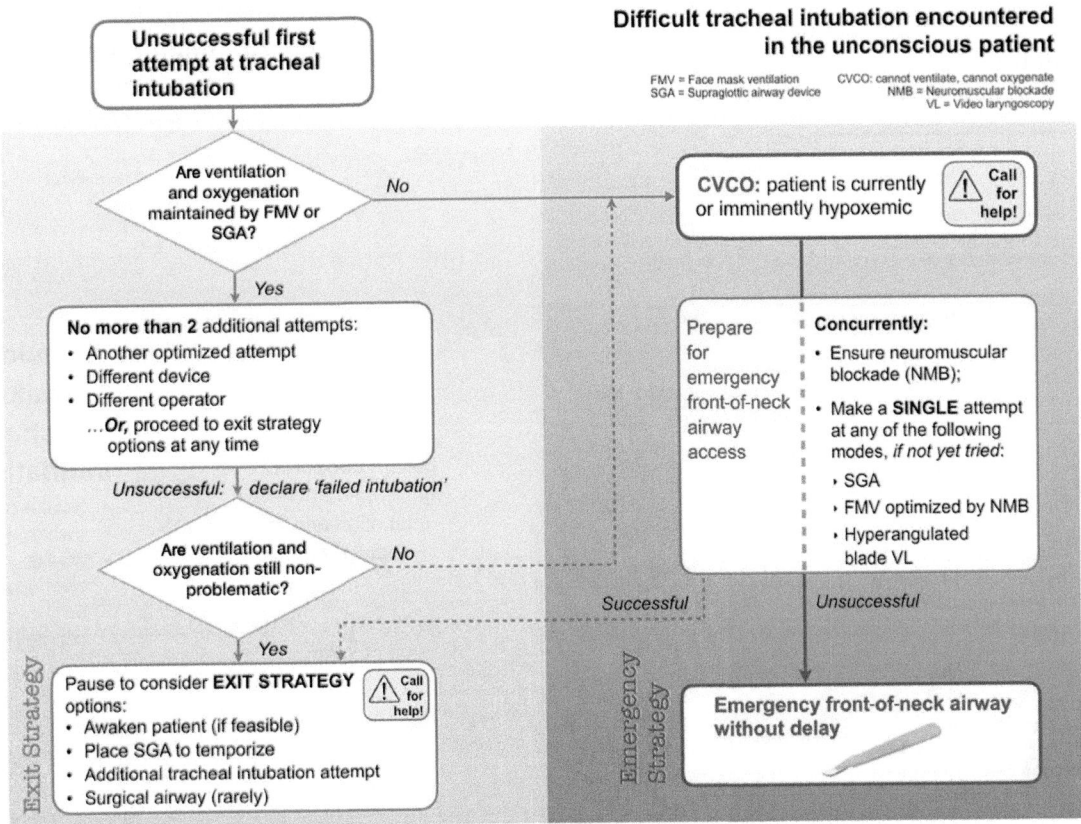

Difficult tracheal intubation encountered in the unconscious patient

FMV = Face mask ventilation CVCO: cannot ventilate, cannot oxygenate
SGA = Supraglottic airway device NMB = Neuromuscular blockade
VL = Video laryngoscopy

Unsuccessful first attempt at tracheal intubation

Are ventilation and oxygenation maintained by FMV or SGA? — No →

Yes ↓

No more than 2 additional attempts:
• Another optimized attempt
• Different device
• Different operator
...*Or*, proceed to exit strategy options at any time

Unsuccessful: ↓ declare 'failed intubation'

Are ventilation and oxygenation still non-problematic? — No →

Yes ↓

Pause to consider **EXIT STRATEGY** options: ⚠ Call for help!
• Awaken patient (if feasible)
• Place SGA to temporize
• Additional tracheal intubation attempt
• Surgical airway (rarely)

Exit Strategy

CVCO: patient is currently or imminently hypoxemic ⚠ Call for help!

Prepare for emergency front-of-neck airway access

Concurrently:
• Ensure neuromuscular blockade (NMB);
• Make a **SINGLE** attempt at any of the following modes, *if not yet tried*:
 ‣ SGA
 ‣ FMV optimized by NMB
 ‣ Hyperangulated blade VL

Successful | *Unsuccessful*

Emergency front-of-neck airway without delay

Emergency Strategy

• **Fig. 11.5** Canadian Airway Focus Group flow diagram for difficult tracheal intubation encountered in the unconscious patient. *CVCO,* Cannot ventilate, cannot oxygenate; *FMV,* face-mask ventilation; *NMB,* neuromuscular blockade; *SGA,* supraglottic airway; *VL,* video laryngoscopy. (From Law JA, Duggan LV, Asselin M, et al. Canadian Airway Focus Group updated consensus-based recommendations for management of the difficult airway: part 1. Difficult airway management encountered in an unconscious patient. *Can J Anaesth.* 2021;68(9):1373–1404.)

DA is divided into "unpredicted difficulty" and "predicted difficulty." The flow diagram for the unpredicted DA starts with a "call for help" and the question of whether face-mask ventilation is possible or not. If not, rapid tracheal access is recommended. If face-mask ventilation is possible, up to four laryngoscopy attempts with alternative devices are allowed. The flow diagram for management of the predicted DA is divided into a "borderline" (ventilation likely possible, low aspiration risk, and availability and competency in alternative devices) and "severe" pathway. In case of a "severe" DA, awake FSI is recommended; otherwise, airway management after induction of general anesthesia is preferred.

French Society of Anesthesiology and Resuscitation's Guidelines on Difficult Intubation and Extubation in Adult Anesthesia

The most recent SFAR guidelines on difficult intubation and extubation in adult anesthesia are updated from the 2006 guidelines.[35] The panel provided 13 statements on difficult intubation (both unexpected and expected) and extubation with various levels of agreement. Five of these statements have a high level of agreement (grade 1+): (1) preventing arterial oxygen desaturation during tracheal intubation or SGA insertion maneuvers because of the risk of morbidity and mortality; (2) to definitively prevent arterial desaturation during tracheal intubation or insertion of an SGA,

a preoxygenation procedure (3 minutes/8 deep inspirations), including for the management of emergencies, is recommended; (3) during scheduled surgery, VAL should be used as an initial strategy for patients in whom mask ventilation is possible and who present at least two criteria for difficult intubation; (4) maintaining a deep level of anesthesia using rapidly reversible agents in order to optimize conditions of mask ventilation and intubation; and (5) using decision trees and algorithms to optimize the management of DA control. All the recommendations are summarized in six algorithms including two algorithms for extubation.

German Society of Anaesthesiology and Intensive Care Medicine's Guidelines on Airway Management

The DGAI updated its original 2004 DA guidelines in 2015.[36] The recommendations are divided into "strongly recommend," "recommend," and "open recommendation." Flowcharts address the anticipated and unanticipated DA. The flowchart for the anticipated DA recommends maintenance of spontaneous ventilation; FSI has the highest priority in this setting.

The flowchart management of the unanticipated DA starts with the rather unclear term *failed airway protection*, which is—didactically—probably more confusing than helpful. In the case of unexpected difficult/impossible mask ventilation, the administration of

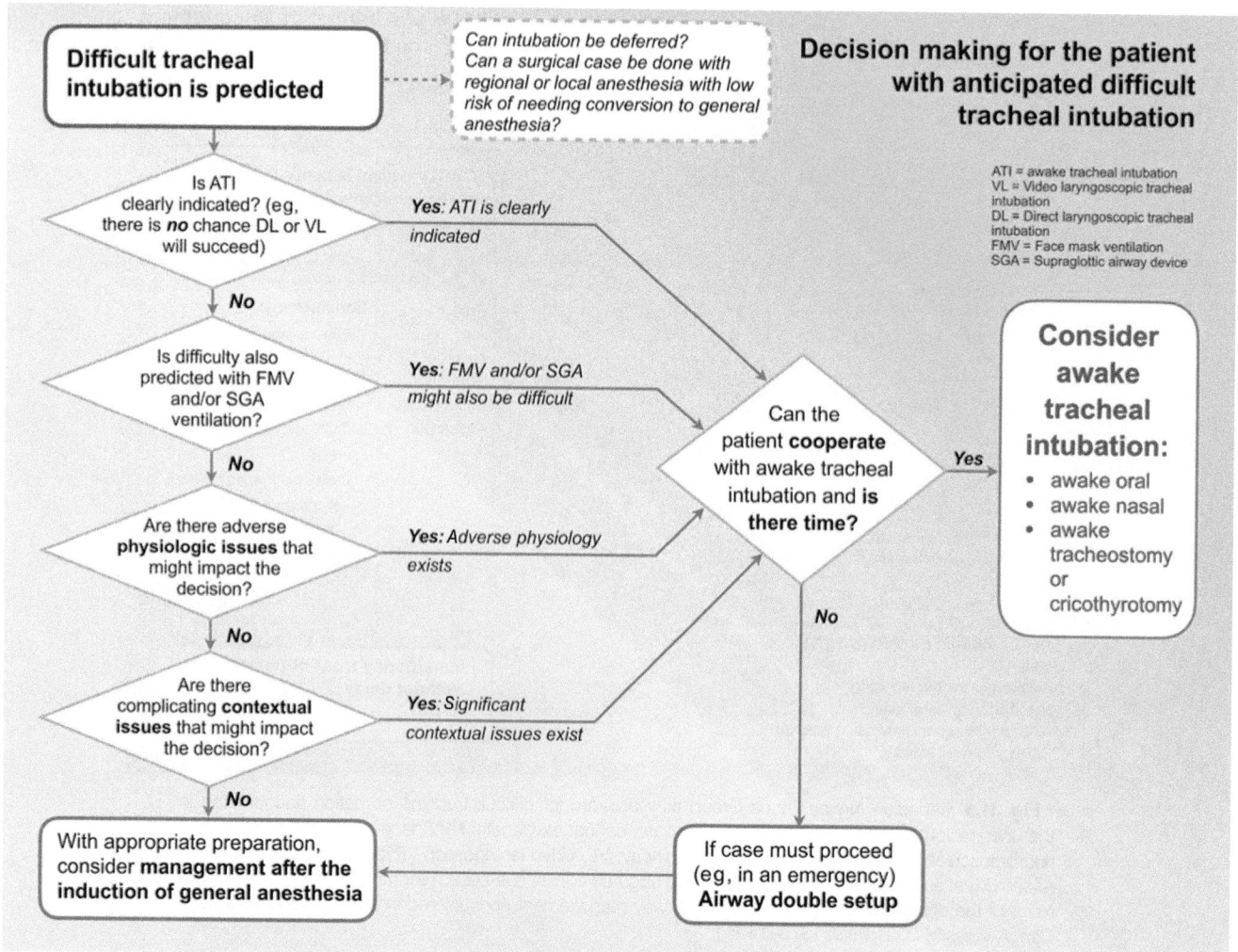

• **Fig. 11.6** Canadian Airway Focus Group flow diagram for anticipated difficult tracheal intubation. *ATI*, Awake tracheal intubation; *DL*, direct laryngoscopy; *FMV*, face-mask ventilation; *SGA*, supraglottic airway; *VL*, video laryngoscopy. (From Law JA, Duggan LV, Asselin M, et al. Canadian Airway Focus Group updated consensus-based recommendations for management of the difficult airway: part 2. Planning and implementing safe management of the patient with an anticipated difficult airway. *Can J Anaesth.* 2021;68(9):1405–1436.)

neuromuscular blocking agents, the use of an SGA or direct/indirect laryngoscopy, return to spontaneous ventilation, or the use of alternative techniques, such as FSI, should be considered. The urgent "call for help" is crucial from the beginning. In case of a CICO situation, a translaryngeal or transtracheal access technique is recommended. If mask ventilation is possible, various options to secure the airway, such as optimized direct laryngoscopy (up to two attempts), VAL, SGA, FSI, and awakening the patient should be considered.

Chinese Society of Anesthesiology's Guidelines for Management of the Difficult Airway

The 2013 Chinese DA guidelines[37] are similar to the ASA DA guidelines with the philosophy to prepare, evaluate, and execute airway procedures in a stepwise fashion to ensure safer and more effective results. Eight steps are used in a flowchart fashion, including preoxygenation, type of DA (anticipated versus unanticipated), anesthetic induction, mask ventilation grading, laryngoscopic view grading, approach to airway, judgment, and final disposition. These guidelines differentiate anticipated and unanticipated DAs. Those pertaining to management of an anticipated DA are divided into an "identified" DA, for which

an awake intubation is recommended, and "suspected" DA, in which the preservation of spontaneous ventilation should be considered. Further steps in management of an unanticipated DA depend on the difficulty/grading of mask ventilation, and in the case of an "emergency airway" (grade 4, decreasing saturation), invasive airway access (cricothyrotomy) is recommended.

Japanese Society of Anesthesiologists' Airway Management Guidelines

In 2014, the Japanese DA guidelines[38] were developed. They divide airway management into three different areas using traffic signal zones, depending on the degree of patient risk and ability to achieve successful ventilation: green for a safe condition, yellow for a semiemergency condition, and red for a critical emergency condition. The Japanese guidelines do not use the severity of hypoxemia but, rather, the adequacy of ventilation via capnogram waveform as criteria for progressing through the different zones. The guidelines are considered for general airway management and not necessarily DA management. Specific airway devices are not mentioned. However, skills with alternative techniques, such as

SGA, VAL, FSI, and surgical techniques, are regarded as fundamental rescue airway skills and should be used when necessary. In patients at risk for difficult face-mask ventilation or aspiration, awake tracheal intubation should be considered.

All India Difficult Airway Association Guidelines for the Management of Unanticipated Difficult Tracheal Intubation in Adults

The AIDAA guidelines[39] developed in 2016 provide a structured, stepwise approach for management of the unanticipated DA in adults (Fig. 11.7). Optimum preoxygenation and nasal insufflation of 15 L/min of oxygen during apnea in all patients is recommended, calling for help if the initial attempt at intubation is unsuccessful and using THRIVE when available. Further recommended are no more than three attempts at tracheal intubation and two attempts at SGA insertion if intubation fails, provided oxygen saturation remains ≥95%. If SGA insertion fails, one final attempt at mask ventilation should be tried after ensuring neuromuscular blockade using the optimal technique for mask ventilation. In case of "complete ventilation failure" (cannot intubate/cannot ventilate using SGA and FMV), an emergency cricothyrotomy (surgical or cannula technique) should be performed.

Project for Universal Management of Airways Guidelines

The Project for Universal Management of Airways (PUMA) was initiated following some very passionate conversations at the 2015 World Airway Management meeting in Dublin about the need for a universal airway management guideline. This guideline is not intended to compete with any existing national guidelines but, rather, to serve as airway management principles that could apply across medical specialties and geographic boundaries that reflect the current consensus of all the major published international airway guidelines.

A recent review article by Edelman and colleagues identified 38 published airway management algorithms in the last 20 years, 14 of which were published by national or international airway societies.[57] They concluded that universal endorsement of a single airway algorithm that can be adequately adapted to a range of clinical scenarios could be most effective in further improving DA management. The frequency of algorithm publication has increased recently, yet adherence and implementation outcome data remain limited. Their results highlight the lack of a single algorithm that is universally endorsed, recognized, and applicable to all DA management situations. There remains a lack of published evidence as to whether the implementation of airway algorithms results in modification of clinical practice or a change in patient outcomes.

The PUMA guideline emphasizes the predominance of recommendations that are common across *all* guidelines. The specific requirements of particular circumstances are accounted for via a limited number of context-specific caveats and exceptions. The result is a single "universal" guideline that can be applied to every episode of airway management, routine or challenging, and independent of context (including geography, provider, location, patient, indication, urgency, and complexity). The PUMA guideline can also be applied independently of the intended airway device, addressing a significant gap in other guidelines, which almost exclusively address the situation in which the planned airway is an endotracheal tube (ETT). The PUMA guideline provides the practitioner with a consistent framework with which to approach every case rather than having to invoke a novel approach for each patient type or situation. Although the current guidelines are excellent, they often have limitations that are specific for certain patient categories, such as for adults,[39] pediatric patients,[58] obstetric patients,[52] and critically ill patients.[55] While algorithms have been developed across the spectrum of disciplines, the overwhelming majority of algorithms developed by the major airway societies have been mostly anesthesiology based, incorporating concepts like "cancel surgery" that potentially make them difficult for other disciplines to use.

The PUMA task force was developed in 2016 by the formulation of a 14-member working group, composed of 11 anesthesiologists (3 of whom are intensivists) and 3 emergency medicine physicians, all considered to be experts and opinion leaders in airway management and guideline development. Although members of the working group were spread across four continents, they met on average every 2 weeks via videoconference, as well as in person at different scientific meetings over a 4-year period from 2017 to 2021. The process for developing the PUMA principles conforms with the criteria specified in the Appraisal of Guidelines Research and Evaluation checklist.[59] The first step was to review the 24 "existing guidelines" to develop a universal guideline for airway management that reflects the current consensus of all the major published international airway guidelines. From this review, statements of common principles consistent with all guidelines were generated. Emphasis was placed on similarities rather than differences. Not every statement is relevant to all airway management contexts, but no statement conflicts with the management principles of a particular context. As such, all statements are applicable to any of the contexts to which they are relevant.

Additionally, a 60-plus-member working group (from 17 countries) was formed to provide expertise from other countries and disciplines—paramedics, airway assistants, human factors experts, head and neck surgeons, and so on—and tasked with reviewing any statements in which consensus could not be reached among the working group or where an existing consensus could not be identified in the literature. Statements were also generated for areas about which existing guidelines were silent or had novel ideas. These statements were put to the working group as online surveys. Statements were rated on the Likert scale and free text comments included. Any disputed statements were reviewed at biweekly (on average) videoconferences. Extensive literature review using keywords was determined by each reviewer, as well as generated from the expert consensus statements.

Five documents are in the process of production, including *Universal Principles for Airway Evaluation, Risk Evaluation, Airway Strategy* (including methods to extend safe apnea time, determining the first-line approach to airway management, rapid sequence intubation [RSI], and extubation), *Airway Rescue* (what traditional DA guidelines address), and *Communication of Airway Outcomes*, including what the issues were during the airway episode and what should be communicated to the next person. The PUMA guideline is really a set of comprehensive recommendations for airway management that will be an iterative, freely accessible, and updated virtual document.

After publication of all five documents, a training program will follow. There will be an accompanying web-based educational resource for translation of the PUMA guidelines into clinical practice. Additionally, there will be PUMA workshops at both online and in-person conferences. Future iterations of the PUMA

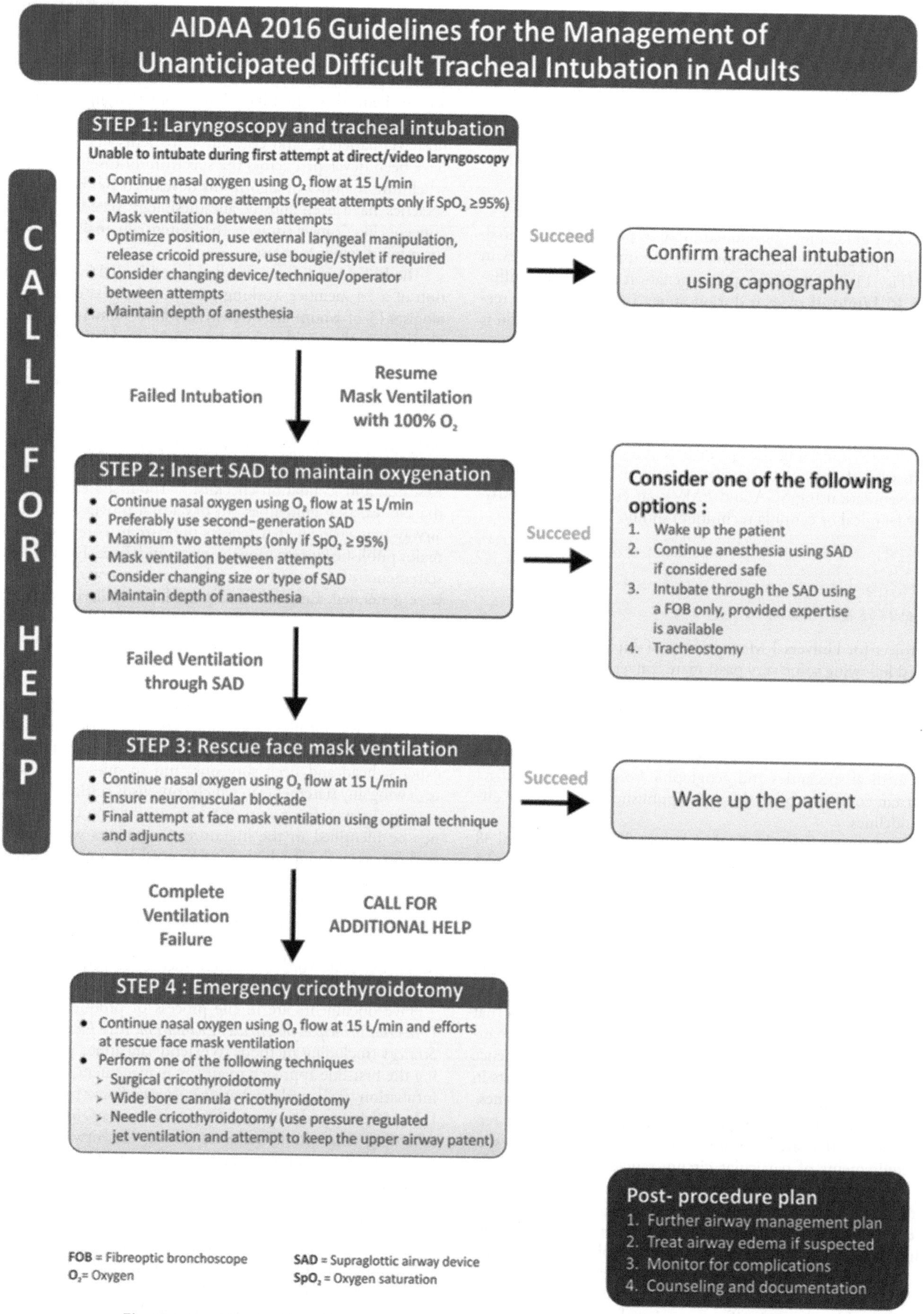

AIDAA 2016 Guidelines for the Management of Unanticipated Difficult Tracheal Intubation in Adults

CALL FOR HELP

STEP 1: Laryngoscopy and tracheal intubation

Unable to intubate during first attempt at direct/video laryngoscopy

- Continue nasal oxygen using O_2 flow at 15 L/min
- Maximum two more attempts (repeat attempts only if SpO_2 ≥95%)
- Mask ventilation between attempts
- Optimize position, use external laryngeal manipulation, release cricoid pressure, use bougie/stylet if required
- Consider changing device/technique/operator between attempts
- Maintain depth of anesthesia

Succeed → **Confirm tracheal intubation using capnography**

Failed Intubation — Resume Mask Ventilation with 100% O_2

STEP 2: Insert SAD to maintain oxygenation

- Continue nasal oxygen using O_2 flow at 15 L/min
- Preferably use second–generation SAD
- Maximum two attempts (only if SpO_2 ≥95%)
- Mask ventilation between attempts
- Consider changing size or type of SAD
- Maintain depth of anaesthesia

Succeed → **Consider one of the following options :**
1. Wake up the patient
2. Continue anesthesia using SAD if considered safe
3. Intubate through the SAD using a FOB only, provided expertise is available
4. Tracheostomy

Failed Ventilation through SAD

STEP 3: Rescue face mask ventilation

- Continue nasal oxygen using O_2 flow at 15 L/min
- Ensure neuromuscular blockade
- Final attempt at face mask ventilation using optimal technique and adjuncts

Succeed → **Wake up the patient**

Complete Ventilation Failure

CALL FOR ADDITIONAL HELP

STEP 4 : Emergency cricothyroidotomy

- Continue nasal oxygen using O_2 flow at 15 L/min and efforts at rescue face mask ventilation
- Perform one of the following techniques
  - Surgical cricothyroidotomy
  - Wide bore cannula cricothyroidotomy
  - Needle cricothyroidotomy (use pressure regulated jet ventilation and attempt to keep the upper airway patent)

Post- procedure plan
1. Further airway management plan
2. Treat airway edema if suspected
3. Monitor for complications
4. Counseling and documentation

FOB = Fibreoptic bronchoscope   SAD = Supraglottic airway device
O_2= Oxygen SpO_2 = Oxygen saturation

• **Fig. 11.7** The All India Diffcult Airway Association 2016 algorithm for the management of unanticipated difficult tracheal intubation in adults. (From Myatra SN, Shah A, Kundra P, et al. All India Difficult Airway Association 2016 guidelines for the management of unanticipated difficult tracheal intubation in adults. *Indian J Anaesth.* 2016;60:885–898.)

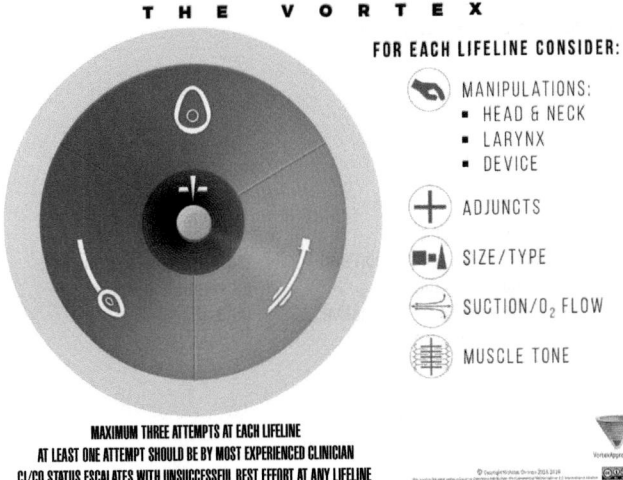

• **Fig. 11.8** The Vortex Implementation Tool. (Modified from Chrimes N. *The Vortex Approach to Airway Management*, 2nd ed. Simpact; 2016. Available from http://www.VortexApproach.org)

guidelines may involve formal representation from the national professional airway groups that have produced the existing guidelines. Lastly, a PUMA app is being developed, which will allow the practitioner to easily apply the PUMA guidelines in real time on a case-by-case basis. Additional information on the project is available at https://www.UniveralAirway.org.

Vortex Approach to Airway Management

The Vortex cognitive aid categorizes itself as a "high acuity implementation tool" and has been specifically designed for real-time use during an evolving airway emergency.[49,50] Instead of an algorithm, the design of the Vortex employs a simple, low-content graphic that uses the visual metaphor of spiraling into a funnel to enhance team situational awareness of concepts relating to DA management—a process referred to as "conceptual imprinting" (Fig. 11.8). Rather than advocating a specific sequence of airway management techniques, the Vortex provides visual cues reminding clinical teams to implement general strategies to restore airway patency that target recognized failings in emergency airway management. This includes prompts to ensure that best efforts at face-mask ventilation, SGA, and intubation are all attempted and that, if these are unsuccessful, progression to "CICO rescue" (emergency invasive airway) occurs. A distinctive feature of the Vortex is the concept of the "Green Zone," which provides a prompt for clinicians to stop and consider their options whenever airway patency has been restored. This represents an attempt to address the process of repeated airway instrumentation often seen in adverse airway events, which can potentially convert a "can oxygenate" scenario into a "cannot oxygenate" scenario.

The design of the Vortex provides it with the flexibility to be applied to any circumstances in which airway management takes place. This makes the Vortex unique in providing a common tool that can be used not only in anesthesiology but across all specialties engaged in airway management. Although the Vortex Approach does include more detailed foundation materials that allow it to be used as a stand-alone tool, because the strategies for its use are largely consistent with the basic principles of all national anesthesia society guidelines, it can be used in conjunction with any of them. As such, this approach does not represent an alternative to national airway guidelines but rather provides a complementary tool with the potential to facilitate implementation of these guidelines during an airway emergency (see Chapter 12).

Difficult Airway Scenarios: Comparison of National Societies

A comparison between algorithms for management of the DA can be based primarily on different clinical scenarios.[60,61] A logical and process-oriented classification is as follows: "anticipated DA," "unexpected difficult mask ventilation," "unexpected difficult SGA ventilation," "unexpected difficult intubation," and "CICO." Interestingly, many guidelines do not explicitly consider management of the unexpected difficult mask ventilation or unexpected difficult SGA ventilation, even though difficulty with either may be faced by the practitioner after induction of general anesthesia. Difficult intubation can be divided into three categories: (1) difficult laryngoscopy but easy intubation, (2) easy laryngoscopy but difficult intubation, and (3) difficult laryngoscopy and difficult intubation. National anesthesia society algorithms, however, do not differentiate these situations. Table 11.3 compares the recommendations from the various national anesthesia societies concerning these clinical scenarios.

Extubation of the Patient With a Difficult Airway

Extubation of the patient with a DA should be carefully assessed and performed. Although the ASA DA guidelines do not include an algorithm specific to extubation, recommendations pertaining to extubation have been in place since their first iteration in 1993.[46] The clinician should develop a strategy for safe extubation of these patients, depending on the type of surgery, the condition of the patient, and the skills and preferences of the clinician. Additional considerations include the following:

- Awake extubation versus extubation before return of consciousness
- Clinical symptoms with the potential to impair ventilation (e.g., altered mental status, abnormal gas exchange, airway edema, inability to clear secretions, inadequate return of neuromuscular function)
- Airway management plan if the patient is not able to maintain adequate ventilation
- Short-term use of an airway exchange catheter (AEC), which can be used to facilitate reintubation

The ideal method of extubation of a patient with a DA is gradual, step by step, and reversible at any time. Extubation over an AEC closely approximates this ideal.[62] The equipment that should be immediately available for the extubation of a DA includes the same equipment necessary for intubation of the DA.

The 2022 ASA DA guidelines provide more robust recommendations for extubation of the DA:

- Have a preformulated strategy for extubation and subsequent airway management. This strategy will depend, in part, on the surgery/procedure, other perioperative circumstances, the condition of the patient, and the skills and preferences of the clinician.
- Assess patient readiness for extubation.
- Ensure that a skilled individual is present to assist with extubation, when feasible.

TABLE 11.3 **Comparison Between National Anesthesia Society Guidelines Recommendations for Different Clinical Scenarios**

Algorithm	CLINICAL SCENARIO			
	Anticipated Difficult Airway	Unexpected Difficult Mask Ventilation or Difficult SGA Ventilation	Unexpected Difficult Intubation	Cannot Intubate/Cannot Oxygenate
United States: ASA (2013)	Awake intubation: noninvasive (e.g., FSI) vs invasive access (surgical or percutaneous cricothyrotomy)	Algorithm begins with unexpected difficult intubation; no specific recommendation for unexpected difficult mask ventilation or SGA ventilation	Consider returning to spontaneous ventilation and awakening patient If FMV adequate → alternative approaches to intubation (e.g., VAL) If FMV inadequate, attempt → SGA ventilation and proceed down emergency pathway	Invasive airway access (surgical or percutaneous, jet ventilation, retrograde intubation)
UK: DAS (2015)	No recommendation	Optimize airway position, chin lift and jaw thrust maneuver, oral or nasopharyngeal airway, improve inadequate anesthesia and neuromuscular blockade	DL or VAL (maximum 3+1 attempts) → Declare failed intubation 2nd-generation SGA (maximum 3 attempts) → Declare failed SGA ventilation Revert to FMV, paralyze → Declare CICO → Emergency invasive airway access	Scalpel cricothyrotomy
Canada: CAFG (2021)	If difficulty is not predicted with FMV and/or SGA, and there are no physiological or contextual issues that impact the decision, airway management after the induction of general anesthesia might be considered. In all other cases, awake tracheal intubation should be considered	Algorithm starts with unexpected difficult intubation; no specific recommendation for unexpected difficult FMV or SGA ventilation In case of ventilation and oxygenation by FMV or SGA cannot be maintained → declaration of CVCO and call for help	No more than 2 further intubation attempts (another optimized attempt, different device, different operator) or proceed to exit strategy (call for help) → Awaken patient (if feasible), place SGA to temporize, additional tracheal intubation attempt, or surgical airway (rarely)	Prepare for emergency invasive airway access and concurrently ensure neuromuscular blockade, make a single attempt at SGA, FMV, and/or hyperangulated VAL If unsuccessful → emergency invasive airway (surgical cricothyrotomy)
Italy: SIAARTI (2005)	Borderline cases: general anesthesia and laryngoscopy (DL vs VAL) Severe cases: in cooperative patients, awake intubation under local anesthesia (FSI, retrograde intubation); in uncooperative patients, FSI under general anesthesia	Algorithm begins with unexpected difficult intubation; no specific recommendation for unexpected difficult FMV or SGA ventilation	If FMV possible, a second intubation attempt followed by two further intubation attempts with alternative devices If FMV impossible, call for help and rapid tracheal access	Tracheal puncture, cricothyrotomy
France: SFAR (2018)	Call for help from the beginning. Apneic technique → DL or VAL (maximum of 2 attempts); in case of failure → Intubating LMA Spontaneous ventilation technique→ FSI; in case of failure →awakening patient or awake tracheostomy	Intubating laryngeal mask If ventilation/intubation fails → oxygenation algorithm (transtracheal oxygen)	If FMV is effective → DL or VAL (maximum of 2 attempts); in case of failure → Intubating LMA If FMV is ineffective → Intubating LMA; if failure → oxygenation algorithm (transtracheal oxygen)	Cricothyrotomy or tracheostomy
Germany: DGAI (2015)	Maintenance of spontaneous ventilation, awake technique: FSI first choice, intubation via SGA, indirect laryngoscopy, transtracheal oxygenation	Call for help SGA Direct/indirect laryngoscopy, spontaneous ventilation, VAL Transtracheal access	Optimized laryngoscopy (maximum 2 intubation attempts) VAL SGA Rigid or flexible scope intubation Awakening patient	Translaryngeal or transtracheal access

TABLE 11.3 Comparison Between National Anesthesia Society Guidelines Recommendations for Different Clinical Scenarios—cont'd

Algorithm	CLINICAL SCENARIO			
	Anticipated Difficult Airway	Unexpected Difficult Mask Ventilation or Difficult SGA Ventilation	Unexpected Difficult Intubation	Cannot Intubate/ Cannot Oxygenate
China: Chinese Society of Anesthesiologists (2013)	Awake intubation or intubation under preservation of spontaneous ventilation	Call for help; SGA, one more intubation attempt, TTJV, cricothyrotomy	Nonemergency noninvasive airway access (VAL or other options; eg, awakening patient) vs emergency airway (invasive airway access)	Invasive airway access (cricothyrotomy)
Japan: Japanese Society of Anesthesiologists (2014)	Awake (flexible) intubation	One best intubation attempt; consider restoring consciousness and spontaneous breathing If failed → cricothyroid membrane identification (cricothyrotomy or tracheostomy	Not more than two attempts for each provider and for each airway device SGA Consider awakening patient	Cricothyrotomy (puncture kit or surgical)
India: AIDAA (2016)	No recommendation	Algorithm begins with unexpected difficult intubation with DL or VAL Continuous apneic oxygenation via nasal cannula throughout	Step 1: Not more than two attempts; consider changing device, technique, or operator Step 2: SGA to maintain oxygenation Step 3: Ensure neuromuscular blockade; final attempt at FMV using optimal technique	Cricothyrotomy Surgical technique Wide-bore cannula or needle technique

CICO, Cannot intubate/cannot oxygenate; *CVCO*, cannot ventilate/cannot oxygenate; *DL*, direct laryngoscopy; *FMV*, face-mask ventilation; *FSI*, flexible scope intubation; *LMA*, laryngeal mask airway; *SGA*, supraglottic airway; *TTJV*, transtracheal jet ventilation; *VAL*, video-assisted laryngoscopy.

- Select an appropriate time and location for extubation, when possible.
- Assess the relative clinical merits and feasibility of the short-term use of an AEC and/or SGA that can serve as a guide for expedited reintubation. The use of AECs should be minimized with pediatric patients.
- Before attempting extubation, evaluate the risks and benefits of elective surgical tracheostomy.
- Evaluate the risks and benefits of awake extubation versus extubation before the return to consciousness.
- When feasible, use supplemental oxygen throughout the extubation process.
- Assess the clinical factors that may produce an adverse impact on ventilation after the patient has been extubated.

The DAS,[54] the DGAI,[36] and the SFAR[35] have developed separate guidelines for extubation of the DA, which stratify low-risk to high-risk patients. A step-by-step process is elucidated in the DAS guidelines (see also Chapter 47):
- *Step 1.* Develop a plan for extubation in which an airway assessment is performed and general risk factors are acknowledged.
- *Step 2.* Prepare for extubation by optimizing the patient and any risk factors and categorizing the patient as either low or high risk. At-risk patients include those in which the ability to oxygenate is uncertain, reintubation is potentially difficult, and/or general risk factors, such as specific surgical requirements or medical conditions, are present.

- *Step 3.* Perform the extubation using the "low risk" or "at risk" algorithm.
- *Step 4.* Determine postextubation care (recovery room, step-down unit or intensive care setting).

Follow-Up Care of the Patient With a Difficult Airway

The ASA DA guidelines[8] also suggest that follow-up care should be performed on any patient with a DA. The presence and nature of the airway difficulty should be documented in the medical record. The intent of this documentation is to guide and facilitate the delivery of future care. Aspects of documentation that may prove helpful include the following:
- Description of the airway difficulties, which should distinguish between difficulties with mask ventilation and those with tracheal intubation.
- Description of the airway management techniques used, which should indicate the beneficial or detrimental role of each technique in management of the DA.
- Information given to the patient (or responsible person) concerning the airway difficulty that was encountered. The intent of this communication is to assist the patient (or responsible person) in guiding and facilitating the delivery of future care. The information conveyed may include, for instance, the presence of a DA, the apparent reasons for the difficulty, and implications for future care.

Additional recommendations for follow-up care in the 2022 ASA DA guidelines include:

- Use postextubation steroids and/or racemic epinephrine, when appropriate.
- Instruct the patient to register with an emergency notification service (such as MedicAlert), when appropriate and feasible (see Chapter 50).

Finally, the anesthesiologist should evaluate and observe the patient for potential complications of DA management, such as airway edema, bleeding, tracheal or esophageal perforation, pneumothorax, and aspiration.

Conclusion

Specific strategies for DA management can be linked together to form more comprehensive treatment plans or algorithms. However, there is not enough data to support the selection of a particular strategy made in these various algorithms. Rather, trust is placed in experts' recommendations, based on the best available published evidence and consensus of the involved task forces, which has led to widespread dissemination and integration of DA guidelines in daily practice.[9] As the practice of airway management becomes more advanced, practitioners must become both knowledgeable and proficient in the use of various airway devices and techniques. Although no airway algorithm can be practiced in its entirety on a regular basis, these alternative devices and techniques must be incorporated into routine practice so that the confidence and skill required for their successful use in the emergent setting can be developed. The regular use of only a well-selected number of devices is a prerequisite to acquire and maintain the appropriate expertise. Many adverse airway events occur as a result of the lack of anticipation, strategy (human factors and ergonomics), training, or adequate equipment for DA management. Further research should address adherence to national and local guidelines in emergency situations, the detailed experience with new and already established airway devices, and the specific role and limitations of new devices as they reach clinical practice.[49] Appropriate follow-up and communication should be performed so that future caretakers will not unwittingly reproduce the same experience and risk. Finally, lifelong training by airway practitioners is necessary, as there will be further updates of DA guidelines

in the future, which will require successful assimilation into their clinical practice.

Selected References

5. Cook TM, Woodhall N, Frerk C, on Behalf of the Fourth National Audit Project. Major complications of airway management in the UK: results of the Fourth National Audit Project of the Royal College of Anaesthetists and the Difficult Airway Society. Part 1: anaesthesia. *Br J Anaesth.* 2011;106:617–631.

6. O'Sullivan E, Laffey J, Pandit JJ. A rude awakening after our fourth 'NAP': lessons for airway management. *Anaesthesia.* 2011;66:331-334.

8. Apfelbaum JL, Hagberg CA, Caplan RA, et al. Practice guidelines for management of the difficult airway: an updated report by the American Society of Anesthesiologists Task Force on Management of the Difficult Airway. *Anesthesiology.* 2013;118:291–307.

9. Crosby ET. An evidence-based approach to airway management: is there a role for clinical practice guidelines? *Anaesthesia.* 2011;66(2):112–118.

11. Heidegger T, Gerig HJ, Ulrich B, et al. Validation of a simple algorithm for tracheal intubation: daily practice is the key to success in emergencies – an analysis of 13,248 intubations. *Anesth Analg.* 2001:92:517-522.

15. Woolf SH, Grol R, Hutchinson A, et al. Clinical guidelines. Potential benefits, limitations, and harms of clinical guidelines. *BMJ.* 1999;318:527–530.

31. Frerk C, Mitchell VS, McNarry AF, et al. Difficult Airway Society 2015 guidelines for management of unanticipated difficult intubation in adults. *Br J Anaesth.* 2015;115:827–848.

32. Law JA, Duggan LV, Asselin M, et al. Canadian Airway Focus Group updated consensus-based recommendations for management of the difficult airway: part 1. Difficult airway management encountered in an unconscious patient. *Can J Anesth.* 2021;68(9):1373–1404. https://link.springer.com/article/10.1007/s12630-021-02007-0.

33. Law JA, Duggan LV, Asselin M, et al. Canadian Airway Focus Group updated consensus-based recommendations for management of the difficult airway: part 2. Planning and implementing safe management of the patient with an anticipated difficult airway. *Can J Anesth.* 2021;68(9):1405–1436.

47. Normand K, Hagberg CA. Understanding the ASA Difficult Airway Algorithm. In: Doyle DJ, Abdelmalak B, eds. *Clinical Airway Management: An Illustrated Case-Based Approach.* Cambridge University Press; 2017.

All references can be found online at eBooks.Health.Elsevier.com.

12
Human Factors in Airway Management

STUART D. MARSHALL AND NICHOLAS CHRIMES

CHAPTER OUTLINE

KEY POINTS

- Airway management occurs within the broad and complex sociotechnical system of healthcare delivery.
- Aspects of design, training, and team functioning can be modified to improve safety.
- Airway management is now a "team sport," and interventions to improve safety should focus on team performance rather than individuals' skills alone.

- Explicit communication involving the use of cognitive aids and other checklists should be used in all nonroutine airway management episodes.
- Improvements and safety should be addressed at a systems level with lessons from successes and failures distributed as widely as possible.

Introduction

Until relatively recently, the primary emphasis of efforts to improve success at airway management has been on the technical performance of the relevant procedural skills.[1] In addition to requiring technical skill, however, airway management tasks often must be performed under time pressure with little margin for error while under threat of serious patient morbidity or mortality as outcomes.[2] The varied circumstances of airway management in terms of patient variability, environmental differences, and team-related

considerations mean that every airway management episode will be unique. These contextual factors can not only compromise the motor skills required for technical performance but may also impair cognitive performance, resulting in poor decision-making.[3,4] In recognition of this, attempts have been made to create standardized or "normative" processes for airway management, put into place to ensure that efficient completion of tasks with the widest possible margin of safety for the patient. Difficult airway algorithms, beginning with the first published failed intubation drill in 1976, are one example of this.[5] Nonetheless, effective airway management, particularly in an emergency setting, requires much more than a clinician having the skills to perform a nominated task and a defined trigger for initiating them.[6] Recognition that a trigger for performing an intervention has arisen depends on the relevant cues being evident, detected, correctly interpreted, and their implications understood. This, in turn, can be affected by factors such as the design and settings of monitors, the perception and attention of team members, and their experience and knowledge. When an individual other than the one responsible for undertaking the intervention recognizes a trigger, social factors, such as assertiveness and language, influence the effectiveness with which that information is communicated to the airway practitioner.[7] Even once a trigger is recognized, the ability to access equipment in a timely manner will depend on use of language, how and where the equipment is stored and labeled, and the familiarity of supporting staff with these factors. The social aspect of airway management, and indeed of all other areas of healthcare provision, is commonly overlooked in theoretical descriptions of clinical care, but it is of vital importance in the practical performance of tasks. Airway management requires social interaction not only to coordinate the required physical tasks, but also for assessment, understanding, and trust of other team members' skills. Airway management thus takes place within a complex sociotechnical system. Multiple interactions must occur between a minimum of two but often among several health professionals, as well as the patient, the equipment, and both a physical and an organizational environment.[8]

The scientific field of human factors, or ergonomics, seeks to optimize the components and processes of complex systems to improve their efficiency and safety.[9] Its focus is often misunderstood as being restricted only to nontechnical or teamwork skills such as leadership or communication.[10] In addition to examining the interactions between clinicians, however, the field of human factors also addresses the interactions of clinicians with all the other elements in a system. A further misconception is that the science of human factors seeks to target the human element as the weakest link in the system. Although some human behavior can predispose to error, the adaptability of humans has the potential to greatly improve the ability of a system to operate safely under widely varying conditions. A well-designed system will both augment the ability of humans to enhance safe and effective performance and minimize the human vulnerabilities that contribute to errors. The field of human factors is multidisciplinary, bringing together diverse groups, such as engineers, architects, psychologists, and anthropometrists, to explore how clinicians behave and

work in particular situations. The ultimate aim is to adapt the processes and equipment to support humans more effectively, with the consequence of providing safer and more efficient care. Put simply, human factors science is directed at making it easy for the team to "get it right."

Over the past decade, there has been an increasing recognition of the significant contribution of human factors to the safety and effectiveness of airway management. In 2011, the Fourth National Audit Project of the Royal College of Anesthetists (RCoA) and the Difficult Airway Society (DAS) in the United Kingdom (NAP4) initially estimated that 40% of major airway complications involved human factors contributions.[11] However, when a random subset of cases was examined in detail, all were found to have elements of failure at a human factors level related to task, planning, or communication with a median of 4.5 failures per case.[6] The initial difference between these studies derives from appreciation of the scope of human factors beyond nontechnical skills. Human factors, in fact, contribute to the occurrence or severity of nearly all adverse airway events.

In order to conceptualize all the components in airway management and the complex interactions among them, a model, such as the extended Systems Engineering Initiative for Patient Safety (SEIPS 3.0), can be helpful (Figure 12.1).[12] The work system described in the SEIPS 3.0 model is typical of many other sociotechnical systems with interactions of people and technology, and it places the humans ("care team") at the center of the work system. Careful attention to all aspects of the design of the work system can guard against failure of one component, such as the clinician managing an airway under time pressure. We will take each of these components and processes from the SEIPS 3.0 framework, in turn, to explain how human factors, or cognitive engineering, can improve safety and efficiency even in the face of extreme physiological compromise.

Components of Airway Management

Each of the components of the airway management sociotechnical system is interdependent. For example, the availability or introduction of new technology can affect how tasks are performed, who performs those tasks, decisions about when to perform them, and how the physical organization of the room can be optimized. When video-assisted laryngoscopy (VAL) was first introduced into clinical practice, clinicians quickly realized that it altered the optimal layout for equipment and that this may vary further, depending on

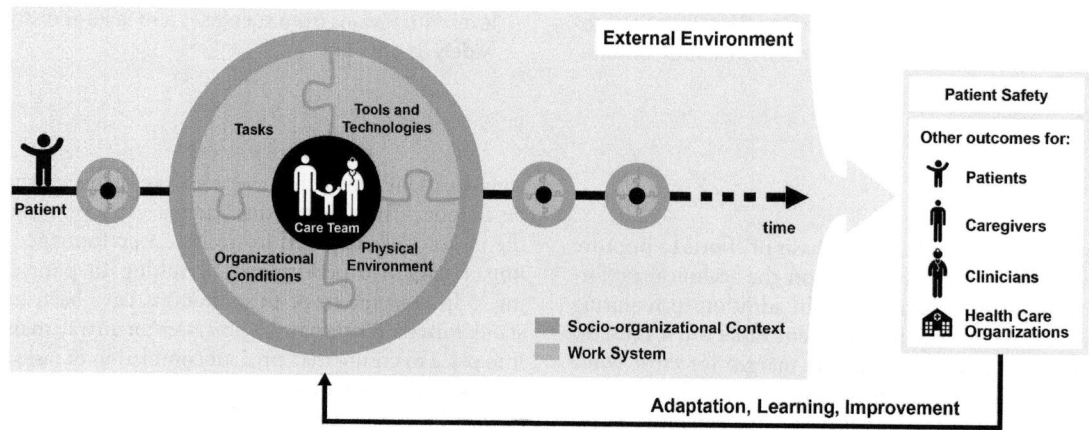

• **Fig. 12.1** SEIPS 3.0 model: sociotechnical systems approach to patient safety.

where the display is located with different devices (i.e., a freestanding screen vs one attached to the laryngoscope handle). Furthermore, the ability of the assistant to see the screen augmented the contribution they were able to make to airway interventions (e.g., by providing improved external laryngeal manipulation). Consequently, this changed the teamwork dynamic between the assistant and the airway operator. As such, additional or modified training was required to account for the equipment, the different roles, and the different setups required when using a videolaryngoscope (VL). Thus, if the equipment to manage an airway changes, so must the task and the training for that task change with the new equipment. This is just one example of the domino effects of changing one element in an airway management system. Notwithstanding this, for clarity the following sections will address the components of airway management as if they were separate, but this underlying complexity must always be kept in mind.

Physical Environment

The physical characteristics of the environment in which airway management is performed greatly influence other components of airway management. Light, noise, and physical space are just a few of the potential factors that might adversely affect the completion of airway management tasks.

Any clinician who has performed an intubation in a prehospital setting knows that ambient light can be a complicating factor. Glare on screens or the impaired ability to see the airway structures due to the contrast and light adaptation of the eyes may hamper the ability to perform intubation.

Noise can make communications between airway team members difficult, impeding the coordination of tasks.[13] As with lighting issues, noise is also a more commonly encountered problem in prehospital settings but can be an issue within healthcare facilities, in areas such as imaging rooms or other places where equipment without adequate sound shielding is used.[14] Most often though, noise distraction results from other individuals talking during airway management procedures. Such noise tends to escalate during an airway crisis, further impeding clear communication when it becomes most crucial. Several solutions have been devised to minimize this. One technique borrowed from aviation is the "sterile cockpit" or "below-ten-thousand" rule.[15] In commercial aviation, the usual procedure is to avoid all nonessential communication not directly relating to the task at hand when the aircraft is climbing or descending below 10,000 feet. These periods correlate with times of high workload, namely taking off and landing when distraction could be dangerous. Similarly, in medicine, the act of airway management could also be seen as a period of high workload or activity, when minimizing noise and distraction might theoretically improve communication and coordination. Attempts to enact the "sterile cockpit" principle have had mixed success, perhaps because of the awkward association with aviation and the terminology used. Alternative terms for the same strategy, such as *critical period* or *focus,* may have more success in the future.

The effect of the physical arrangement of the workspace on the ability to perform airway management is frequently underacknowledged. In the United Kingdom, it is common to anesthetize the patient in a separate anesthetic room adjacent to the operating room (OR). As noted, while this might minimize noise and distraction, it can also introduce additional complications such as the need to transfer an anesthetized patient into another room after an airway device has been inserted. Distractions from maintaining oxygen and anesthetic agent delivery during such times may

occur, which might conceivably negate other potential advantages.[16] Furthermore, equipment might not be easily available in the anesthetic room and surgical assistance might be slower and impeded by the limited space outside of the OR.

Airway management often occurs in environments, such as the emergency department or the intensive care unit (ICU), that might not be primarily designed for this purpose. As such, access for providers and to equipment for the patient's airway may be impeded— a phenomenon that may become compounded during a crisis as more staff and equipment are called upon to assist.[17] Orienting monitors so that they are easily visible to the airway team may also become challenging in such environments. Increasingly, elective anesthesia is being conducted in locations, such as diagnostic imaging or cardiology rooms, where confined spaces are combined with bulky scanning equipment that also aggravates these issues.

With the combination of factors previously noted, it is not surprising that airway management in areas of the hospital outside of the OR is associated with higher risks of complications, such as death and hypoxic brain injury. Some estimates suggest these complications are up to 60 times more likely to occur in the ICU.[18] The reasons for this are multifactorial, including patient factors and those related to training and equipment. However, it is easy to appreciate that airway management in environments that may be remote from additional advanced equipment and clinicians with advanced skills might be performed less favorably than it would in an area where expertise and equipment are concentrated. Many attempts have been made to address this, specifically the creation of difficult airway response teams (DARTs). These teams are similar in structure to cardiac arrest teams with preallocated roles and responsibilities and equipment that is taken to the location of the airway event.[19] There is currently limited evidence of their effectiveness, but anecdotally they appear to improve outcomes of patients with complex airways in clinical areas outside of the OR.

Tools and Technologies

It is evident how the availability of different equipment might affect how airway management is performed. It may not be perceived as cost-effective to purchase expensive, specialized equipment (e.g., flexible intubation scopes; FISs) for environments where they are rarely used. However, inability to access required equipment derives not only from an absolute deficit, where the facility simply does not possess the equipment. Proximity, signage, presentation, and staff familiarity with storage locations may influence the ability to retrieve equipment within the required timeframe during an airway emergency. This once again illustrates the interdependence between different system components (organizational, physical, and individuals) in ultimately determining the availability of equipment. Equipment may also become unavailable due to damage, maintenance, or cleaning. This has become a greater issue with the increased use of more expensive and technologically advanced airway equipment, which may be purchased in smaller numbers and may be more vulnerable to damage. The increasing availability of disposable FISs and VL blades has somewhat mitigated these issues, but this solution comes at an environmental cost. Equipment deficits might also apply to more basic equipment, such as supraglottic airways (SGAs) through a simple failure to restock local stores. This may have implications beyond the lack of availability simply preventing immediate use of a device. In a study of 16 critical airway events, Schnittker and colleagues discovered that merely not having the equipment visible led to clinicians failing to consider that equipment as a potential option for rescue in five cases.[20] Similarly, when equipment was available and its location was known, it helped prompt actions that enabled critical decisions. This demonstrates that clinicians may fail to request a device not present at the bedside, even though it could be retrieved from a remote location. Furthermore, equipment that is present may not be requested simply because a cluttered layout results in it not being readily visible. Decision-making is therefore not merely a product of training of the clinicians undertaking airway management but is also influenced by the context, environment, and prompts from equipment visibility. Historically, the difficult airway cart has typically been stocked with a multitude of specialized airway devices in an attempt to satisfy the needs of all clinicians and circumstances. More recently, however, a more restrained, strategic, and standardized approach to selecting equipment for the difficult airway cart has been advocated. The intent is to reduce clutter, improving visibility and simplifying decision-making in an emergency. Several researchers have also investigated the design of the difficult airway cart to ensure that it aligns with the decisions and prompts needed during an emergency. Typically, the drawers or compartments of a difficult airway cart correspond to specific equipment. Chrimes and colleagues described the "next generation airway trolley" as having a layout that aligns with the functions and decisions made during an airway emergency (Figure 12.2).[21] The ideal cart uses the same key elements as in the associated cognitive aid training and is standardized across all clinical locations. An alternative to this functionally based approach may be used in pediatric settings where equipment is grouped according to the size of the child. The equipment for routine airway management should be similarly organized such that performance in an emergency is familiar to reduce the stress and cognitive load of clinicians. A simple arrangement of the work-surface using a "kit dump" approach can be used. In this way, the key equipment that is required is presented in a clear and ordered manner and the omission of any item is immediately obvious.[22] Ideally, the arrangement of the equipment on the surface aligns with the processes that are to be followed or are grouped in a logical manner. Work to determine how these surfaces should be arranged has already been undertaken using a codesign process based on simulation and feedback from clinical staff.[23]

There are, of course, additional processes underpinning availability and usability of equipment for airway management that must be in place to ensure that the equipment is ready and serviceable when required. As noted, regulation of devices is needed to make sure devices are durable and fit for purpose. Furthermore, organizational arrangements must be made to safeguard the purchasing and upkeep of airway management equipment. An individual should be assigned this role in every organization.

Tasks

To a large extent, the tasks that must be performed during airway management are already predetermined with little scope for redesign. However, there are situations where revisiting the allocation of tasks within roles can be beneficial and a small amount of additional training might improve overall outcomes. For example, the role of the airway assistant in tracheal intubation has traditionally been limited to handing equipment to the practitioner performing the intubation. This arrangement developed because, until recently, the assistant was unable to visualize what the practitioner was seeing. The customary way to circumvent this was for the practitioner to verbalize what they were doing and seeing, and indeed this remains good practice. However, with the advent of

VAL, there is an opportunity for the assistant to be more engaged and active in the process. With shared vision on the VL screen, the assistant is able to share the awareness of the practitioner and actively assist by external manipulation of the larynx toward the location of the tube. Furthermore, the experienced assistant can also make targeted suggestions and help guide decision-making under stress beyond vague suggestions such as "Would a bougie help?" as is commonly the case when visualization is otherwise limited. This is a good example of shared cognition. Rather than accepting that all of the perception, decision-making and monitoring of the situation must be performed by each individual, and relying solely on the leader who is often the operator, these functions can be assisted by other team members. As we will see later, sharing the cognitive load by using effective communication and cognitive aids can help prevent task fixation.

To establish other methods of performing tasks, human factors practitioners (ergonomists) commonly undertake task analyses. These task analyses take different forms, depending on the task and the purpose of the analysis. Hierarchical task analyses examine the detailed nature of the tasks required to reach the management goals. These analyses are useful for understanding physical tasks, such as intubation and the ordering and distribution of the tasks. Other forms of analyses might be more appropriate where information exchange and decision-making are central. Cognitive task analyses examine what information is required to make a particular decision and where that information is obtained. Task analyses can be useful when redesigning equipment and monitors and can guide how processes can be made safer and more efficient and where there may be gaps in training.

The appropriateness of task allocation may vary according to the situation. In a routine elective anesthetic setting, it would not be uncommon for the airway practitioner to also function in a leadership role, but as an airway crisis unfolds, assuming the dual role of leader and technician may become infeasible. A common problem in airway management in emergency situations is the loss of situational awareness.[24] Loss of situational awareness, or "fixation error," occurs when the team has failed to recognize the true nature of the situation and that solutions other than the solutions immediately available are required. As noted earlier, this might lead to repeated attempts at intubation or SGA placement beyond the number deemed reasonable by published guidelines. One of the roles that can be assigned to prevent this is that of a leader who does not get involved in performing other physical tasks but whose job it is to have an overall view of the situation.[25] This can be problematic, as the leader in a difficult airway scenario is usually the most experienced in airway management, but in an airway emergency this person will usually be allocated to the airway practitioner role. Reframing the leadership role and renaming the person tasked with the overall view as the "coordinator" might remove this perception. This may allow a more junior member of the team or a nonmedical professional to adopt the role.

Team Members

The final component of the airway management work system are the people involved in performing the work—those centrally placed in the model. Health professionals must have specific characteristics to ensure that they can perform the work required of them during airway management episodes. Apart from the necessary professional qualifications and certifications, they must have undertaken specific training related to their roles. The training required can be described in terms of technical and nontechnical skills.

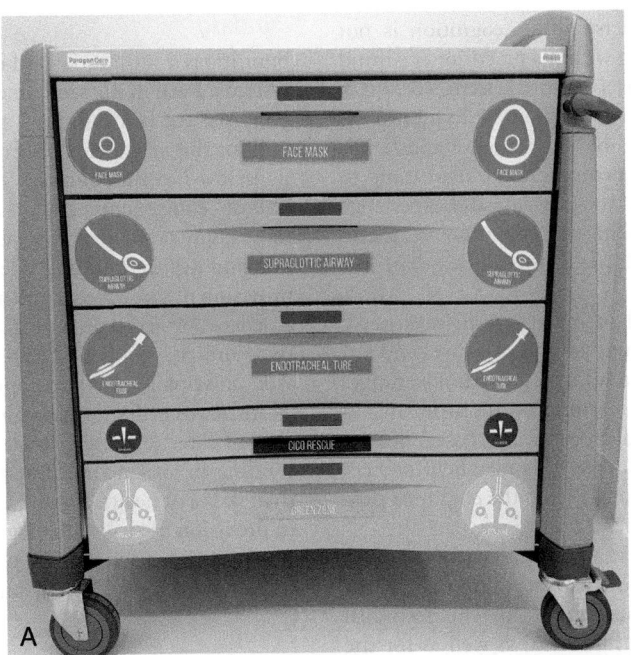

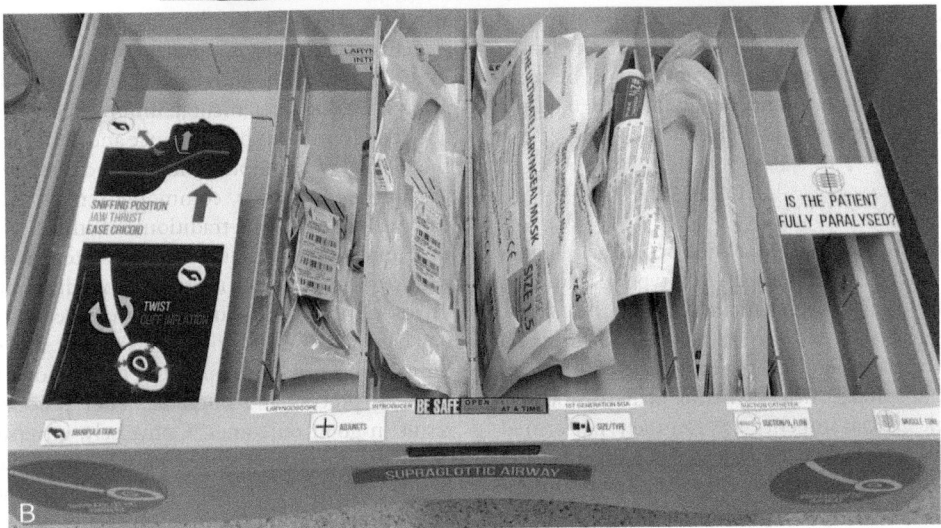

• **Fig. 12.2** (A) The Vortex Airway Rescue Cart is a dedicated emergency airway cart that uses a Vortex-based layout and icons. (B) In addition to prompting for the use of specific equipment, visual cues are used to prompt nonequipment-based interventions.

Technical skills include the physical actions required to perform an airway management task, such as the hand-eye coordination of laryngoscopy or flexible scope techniques. These tasks are easy to learn and best managed with a mastery approach to learning, where not just competency is achieved, but there is deliberate repetition with focused feedback on performance.[26] In this way, the ability to manage novel situations under pressure is developed rather than a lower level of performance. Ideally, practice is spaced over time to enhance retention and includes situations with varying levels of complexity and difficulty in order to train to respond to different and adverse circumstances. Lack of confidence in specialized techniques may lead clinicians to find excuses to avoid performing them in favor of less safe practices, even when the former are clearly indicated. In several adverse airway events identified in NAP4, lack of confidence while performing awake tracheal intubation was thought to be a contributory factor in the decision to induce apnea and unconsciousness despite identification of a clearly difficult airway.[11]

The cognitive skills required for airway management are commonly underappreciated. Even seemingly simple tasks, such as bag-mask ventilation, are complex cognitive tasks requiring detection of cues, processing of meaning of these cues, and adaptation.[27] Observations of the visual scanning patterns of experienced clinicians performing infant bag-mask ventilation compared to novices are instructive. They demonstrated that experts rely on clinical cues in comparison to novices who rely on vital signs such as pulse oximetry that lag behind the immediate clinical picture of poor ventilation.

Decision-making is a key task of airway management teams. Teams must collectively gather information, evaluate potential options with their potential advantages and disadvantages, and plan for each technique. This planning often occurs in a time-pressured situation where information may be uncertain, and the situation evolves rapidly. Furthermore, teams must devise a strategy of how to move from one airway management technique to another, recognizing when one method has failed and must be abandoned, as well as how to and who should activate the next attempt. Contrary to common understanding, cognition is not dependent solely on what is occurring within a practitioner's mind but is an emergent property of the overall work system. As noted, cognition is affected by the positioning of equipment to prompt its use, suggestions offered by team members, availability and familiarity with cognitive aids such as mnemonics and algorithms to prompt a standardized approach, and the expertise and experience of individual clinicians. Decision-making and cognition are, therefore, an intangible amalgam of multiple factors rather than just knowledge and training.

Health professionals experienced in managing airways make decisions primarily by pattern matching to previous cases and situations, rather than by weighing the advantages and disadvantages of every potential approach. When teaching decision-making in airway management, emphasis should be on case-based discussions and the decision-making of experts. This may help novices develop decision-making skills vicariously from the cognitive processes of more experienced practitioners.

It also should not be forgotten that at the center of the airway management work system are the patients. Including the patient in decision-making is technically important for the technical purposes of keeping them calm and informed, as well as for the ethical and legal responsibilities related to consent. Truly informed consent is perhaps impossible in health care, and especially in airway management where procedures and decisions might be complex and difficult for a layperson to understand and weigh all the options. Nevertheless, explanation and inclusion are vital.

Organizational Conditions

Planning at the level of the healthcare service occurs at a higher level of management above the clinician is. The types of patients, staffing, rosters, and funding arrangements in each healthcare facility, such as clinics and hospitals, may have profound effects on the practice of airway management. There may be stark differences in the function of the hospital—such as whether pediatric, obstetric, or head and neck cancer surgeries are routinely performed there—which will invariably affect the way that the organization manages highly specialized activities. The organization also might play a significant role in ensuring that professionals in training are exposed to high-complexity cases and perhaps research to advance knowledge in subspecialty areas. In contrast, a more generalist facility may require distributed expertise and capability across a diverse range of clinical areas. The internal structure of the organization must be matched to these requirements.

Purpose

Depending on the clinical needs, emergency departments, ICUs, and ORs will schedule staff to specific activities. The scheduling must consider the skill mix and number of clinicians and ensure that staff are adequately rested, as clinical emergencies requiring airway assistance can occur day or night. It is self-evident that schedules and fatigue management systems which do not adequately account for the basic human requirements of the clinical staff will lead to impaired individuals who are less able to make effective decisions and perform clinical tasks to a high standard.[28] Appropriate scheduling includes ensuring adequate breaks (and access to food and drink) during shifts, appropriate rest intervals between shifts, and judicious scheduling of overnight shifts. Despite the widespread availability of scheduling and fatigue management resources for clinical departments, it is still unfortunately common to have extended shift hours and patterns that contribute to both acute and cumulative sleep debt.

Funding

Funding is a substantial and ongoing problem in many healthcare systems. Even in high-income countries, the availability of VLs for every patient is still limited and thus a barrier to providing a core tool for the management of difficult airways.

In low-income countries, resources are extremely limited. Reuse of basic equipment such as latex gloves remains commonplace in these countries where the average daily income is less than $3 per day, and health spending is less than $50 per person per year. The provision of safe surgery and anesthesia in these countries has been aided by projects such as Lifebox, the Global Oximetry Initiative, and the Global Capnography Project. These charities provide pulse oximeters and capnography equipment to low-income countries in order to maintain minimum global standards for safe patient care. Although donations account for over 30% of health funding in low-income countries, these charities still provide less than 0.2% of health funding globally.[29] Clearly, there is a disparity in provision of airway management between the richest and poorest countries, where the poorest third of the world's population has access to only 3.5% of surgery performed worldwide.

Culture

It is now well-established across many industries that the safety of patients (or workers/customers) and the safety culture of an organization are highly correlated.[30] High-reliability organizations are always seeking incremental improvements in safety by learning about their previous performance and aiming to be better. This takes the form of two complementary mindsets: learning from failure and learning from success, commonly termed *Safety I* and *Safety II*.[31] Safety II differs from traditional methods of larger-scale learning that concentrates on failures in the system and seeks to rectify them with regulations, more restriction, or education to change behavior. Thankfully, in the field of airway management the incidence of serious harm or death is now very low, but this makes it increasingly difficult to learn from failures. Furthermore, there is a disconnect between process and outcome. Poor process frequently will still result in good outcomes. Conversely, adverse outcomes may still occur despite best practice. As such, outcomes cannot necessarily be attributed to "good" or "bad" actions by the clinicians involved. By focusing only on the poor outcomes, the capacities of the individuals and the organization to learn are restricted. A true learning culture seeks to identify circumstances that successfully prevent or mitigate adverse events, even when the outcome is favorable. In the realm of safety science, the ability of a system to minimize or avoid adverse outcomes in the face of threats to patient safety is termed *resilience*. This term is starkly different when applied to individuals and their ability to cope with circumstances that are suboptimal.

The hierarchy within an organization is one aspect of safety culture directly affecting airway management. When individuals are able to speak up about events that they deem unsafe, they can avert clinical disasters. In many examples of death and injury from airway management, an inexperienced or junior member of staff speaking up may have prevented harm. For instance, merely pointing out that no end-tidal carbon dioxide tracing is present, that the oxygen saturations are not recovering, or that repeated attempts at tracheal intubation are against current guidelines and unlikely to be successful may lead an airway operator to attempt an alternative strategy, such as use of an SGA. A successful culture within an organization or clinical workgroup actively encourages questioning of senior members of the team.

Culture is developed over time by the actions of individuals performing the clinical work and by the managers who incentivize or reprimand specific behaviors that these individuals exhibit. Changing the culture of an organization is always difficult but can be accomplished over time by being consistent with regular education and reinforcement in the workplace. Such change requires a top-down approach. Leaders at the management and clinical levels should set an expectation for team members to speak up for the safety of patients or when they are uncomfortable with situations. Episodes of speaking up should be positively acknowledged and even rewarded to encourage this behavior.

External Environment

In terms of hierarchy, the external environment oversees the regulatory environment in which the health system and organization operate. The regulation and certification of the health professionals working within the healthcare system, the healthcare facility, and the equipment used are all required and relevant parts of developing a safe and effective system for provision of airway care.

The direct effects of the external environment on airway management became clear during the COVID-19 pandemic. Some areas of the world saw government policy and actions driving increased numbers of infections while simultaneously limiting supplies of personal protective equipment (PPE)[32]. Clinicians who genuinely feared for their safety were compelled to adapt their techniques for airway management to address this lack of PPE by developing barriers intended to protect them from infectious aerosols generated during airway interventions. Acrylic "aerosol boxes" and plastic sheets created into makeshift tents around patients' heads were disseminated and used widely.[33] Approval of such devices by the Therapeutic and Goods Administration (a component of the external environment) through an emergency process condoned their use and implied that they were safe, which greatly increased their popularity. Subsequently, several studies have suggested not only that the level of protection provided by the boxes is much less than first expected but that they might actually increase the risk to the team managing the airway, with increased exposure and the risk of damage to their PPE[34]. Furthermore, by impeding the performance of airway interventions, the risk to the patient is amplified. This failure of regulation arguably led to a detrimental change in the practice of airway management for many patients with COVID-19 during the pandemic. This is a clear illustration of how the external environment can influence the conduct of a clinical process and, consequently, how safe that process is.

Processes of Airway Management

The processes of airway management and how providers, equipment, and environment interact should be conducted in a way that ensures maximal efficiency and safety for the patient. Earlier versions of the SEIPS model included explicit reference to the processes that emerge from the components of the system, but these can be difficult to distinguish from the components themselves.[8] Coordination of actions among healthcare providers requires a mutual understanding of the order of these actions. A well-coordinated team has a clear understanding of the clinical problems, the overarching goal, and how it will be achieved. This understanding requires a clear division of roles, an understanding of how each person's role fits into the whole procedure, and what will happen if certain obstacles or events are encountered. This understanding is collectively known as the "mental model" of the team.

A shared mental model of a problem and how it will be addressed is important to allow the team members to prepare themselves for their role and anticipate others' needs. Furthermore,

with a clear plan and expectation of how events will proceed, it is obvious to all team members if the airway practitioner or others become fixated on a particular solution. With a shared strategy comes implicit permission to challenge actions and reestablish situational awareness.

Explicit Protocols and Plans

Protocols are systems of suggested actions that help guide an airway management team under specific circumstances to progress through steps rapidly and comprehensively. Adherence to protocols allows for efficiently and robustly creating a shared mental model of a problem and the actions required. An example is an RSI protocol for a specified situation such as prehospital care, where the context and actions are well-defined. However, despite protocols being designed by experts for these generic circumstances, they commonly do not anticipate the specific problem faced by the practitioner. There will always be variations in the context, patient characteristics, pathology, and comorbidities that have not been foreseen by the expert group. Inevitably, modifications to the protocol must be made to suit the exact circumstances faced by the practitioner.

Tailoring the actions of a protocol to a specific clinical context means that the appropriate care can be delivered without the unnecessary or impractical steps of the protocol being included. A series of actions can be planned that are more efficient and context specific. For example, if a patient with limited mouth opening is being managed and the practitioner believes that an SGA cannot be inserted, this might reasonably be removed from the list of prospective options. The more specific the protocols, however, the greater the number of protocols that a clinical team must be familiar with and able to recall, which can increase cognitive load.

Other airway protocols relate to specific emergencies, such as the unanticipated difficult intubation. These protocols are designed as series of predetermined actions to be trained for and practiced so that performing them is as automatic as possible in case of a rare emergency.

Thus, these are the three levels of planned behaviors:
- Strategies for individual patients (comprised of a coordinated combination of plans)
- Protocols for specific (nonemergency) circumstances
- Emergency protocols

All three types of preplanned actions must be clearly understood in detail by the airway management team. Which protocols and plans are followed may or may not be explicitly communicated among the team members at the time of the event. However, the team should be able to justify any deviation from the initial plan, such as when a piece of equipment malfunctions unexpectedly or the clinical picture changes.

Communication of Plans and Protocols

There are two methods by which members of an airway team can know the order of tasks related to an airway management event. First, they might learn a specific order of actions by rote, such as by memorizing the sequence of an already defined protocol. Second, the team might have the progression of tasks laid out in the form of a checklist, flowchart, or other graphical representation that is readily at hand. Both approaches have advantages and disadvantages depending on the circumstances.

Rote learning and repeated simulation of events leads to the development of high levels of familiarity with normative processes and protocols and relatively automatic action. This can be particularly useful in situations that require urgent and standardized actions under time pressure, such as when performing an emergency invasive airway access technique. However, where there are nuances or ambiguities that must be addressed, automatic completion of a series of tasks might lead to an inadvertent outcome. For instance, an algorithm learned by rote might suggest a procedure on a patient in a situation where the pathology might render it dangerous or inadvisable. It is feasible that a practitioner working on an automatic, preprogrammed series of actions might perform the procedure anyway, which might put the patient at risk. Examples might include application of high-flow nasal oxygen in the presence of a basal skull fracture or a rapid sequence intubation for a patient with an anterior mediastinal mass.

The alternative method of ensuring that the correct order of tasks is performed is to have a checklist, algorithm, or descriptive flowchart at the point of care. These reminders of a course of action are termed *cognitive aids* and may take a variety of forms, including mnemonics that are remembered for the actual sequence of events.[35]

Cognitive Aids

Cognitive aids provide prompts for action by putting the information needed for clinicians to perform their work where the work takes place.[36] The most common forms of cognitive aids in airway management are flowcharts from sources such as difficult airway algorithms from the American Society of Anesthesiologists or the Difficult Airway Society, which consist of branched decision trees that depend on responses during the event.

To be useful, the manner of presentation of cognitive aids must take into account the nature and context of the work. For instance, a cognitive aid that requires interaction with a touch screen will be useless if the clinician is using both hands in a manual task. Similarly, a cognitive aid that provides auditory prompts will be impractical in a noisy environment where such prompts would be inaudible.[37]

The design of cognitive aids for clinical emergencies, such as airway emergencies, has recently been investigated in substantial detail. Branched algorithms, as have traditionally been presented, have been found to be more difficult to follow during such time-pressured situations.[38] Where possible, information should be

presented in a concise, linear format that is easier for teams to follow during stressful events. Linear cognitive aids also appear to contribute to improved team communication and overall team performance in contrast to more complex designs.

The Vortex approach is a linear cognitive aid for management of the unanticipated difficult airway that involves the recollection of a simple visual image (Figure 12.3).[39] The visual representation of a funnel divided in three reminds the clinician that there are three techniques for managing the airway from above the larynx. The central area at the lower point of the cone represents the requirement for emergency invasive airway access if the other options fail. The graphic prompts the airway management team to consider the options available to manage the event and, to some extent, the order of the actions. Additional graphic elements visually convey danger, safety, and urgency according to context, promoting team situational awareness and facilitating development of a shared mental model for ongoing management. In addition to the Vortex image, icons represent methods for optimizing each of the supraglottic airway management techniques as a linear list of actions. The Vortex approach makes extensive use of images rather than words, prompting nonverbal recognition, which has been demonstrated to be more effective in situations such as road safety.[40]

Research into the effectiveness of teams using cognitive aids has identified a benefit to having a specified reader of the cognitive aid to assist the leader in decision-making by prompting with the required actions.[41] In this situation, the reader becomes a default co-leader, helping to recall complex procedural information while the team leader may be dealing with coordination of the broader team's activities.[42]

Benefiting from a cognitive aid requires the team to be previously trained in its use. It is unrealistic to expect that reaching for an unfamiliar tool for the first time in an emergency will improve performance. It may, in fact, impair performance by adding to cognitive load.

Deviation From Protocols and Resilience

Protocols and algorithms can never encompass all the potential situations that an airway management team may face. There are as many anatomic variations of the airway as there are humans. Coupled with the potential physiological, pathological, and contextual variations, the combinations of clinical presentations for airway management are infinite. Of course, the vast majority of airway management events will be routine and will not require variation from standard pathways. However, deviation from standard protocols will occasionally be needed, not because individuals wish to violate the standardized norms that are judged as safe but, rather, to create additional safety.

There are many case reports of extraordinary actions that prevent harm to patients in extraordinary circumstances.[43,44] These isolated reports remind us that there is still room for lateral thinking beyond the published algorithms and protocols. Reviewing these innovations occasionally leads to further research and wider incorporation of ideas. One example in airway management is the implementation of apneic oxygenation techniques during laryngoscopy on three patients, as described by Levitan, after rediscovery of a number of papers from over half a century earlier.[45] The incorporation of new and innovative techniques used in difficult circumstances is another demonstration of Safety II: an ability to learn from extraordinary successes and to integrate them into new clinical guidelines.

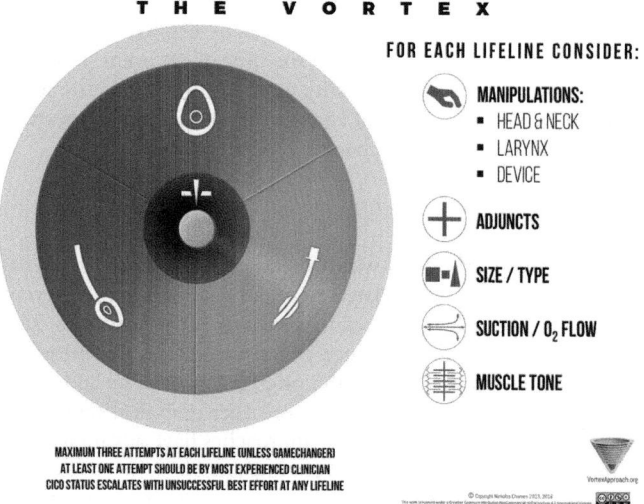

MAXIMUM THREE ATTEMPTS AT EACH LIFELINE (UNLESS GAMECHANGER)
AT LEAST ONE ATTEMPT SHOULD BE BY MOST EXPERIENCED CLINICIAN
CICO STATUS ESCALATES WITH UNSUCCESSFUL BEST EFFORT AT ANY LIFELINE

• **Fig. 12.3** The Vortex approach cognitive aid.

Implicit and Explicit Coordination

As noted, team members who are following role-learned protocols and procedures may not require much or any communication to coordinate their activities. Individuals who work together frequently can identify other clinicians' progress and adapt or assist to create an efficient work activity without verbal clarification.[46] Such activity is termed *implicit coordination* and in airway management is regularly seen in anesthetic teams performing RSI. Commonly performed interventions, such as RSI, often follow a defined normative process where an expected set of events is enacted in a particular order. Experienced practitioners who work together frequently might not need to discuss these expectations. Consequently, an airway operator well-versed in the process may not need to communicate their own or the assistant's steps, dependencies, or actions. Without any talking, the endotracheal tube (ETT) stylet may be removed, the tracheal cuff inflated, and the airway circuit connected.

Implicit coordination may lead to efficient and rapid completion of a predetermined order of tasks in experienced practitioners. Occasionally, however, events do not go according to plan, there is some deviation or difficulty, and discussion is needed. Similarly, individuals with less experience might need guidance or coaching that also will require communication. This *explicit coordination* requires clear unambiguous messaging.

Communication

Clinical communication is commonly imprecise and of a social nature, even during clinical emergencies. For communication to be effective, the content and structure must be unequivocal and directed toward the appropriate team members.[47] Where there is doubt about the requests or the accuracy of information being conveyed, team members must be empowered to speak up and question what is being stated. This ability to speak up has previously been mentioned as part of the culture of the team environment but deserves comment again as a vital part of communication.

Closed Loop Communication

There are many ways within a team environment to foster open communication and speaking up. The most commonly referenced method is the use of closed loop communication, which involves the repeating back (or read-back) of vital information. The model commonly given is that of aviation where, as part of the standard phraseology of the International Civil Aviation Organization (ICAO), read-back is required for specifics such as actions and clearances.[48] Using this technique, it becomes clear that the recipient of the information has both heard and understood the instruction given. A further, longer feedback loop can also be used after the instruction has been carried out to let the leader know that the item is completed and perhaps also that the team member is available for a further task. The use of names is also particularly helpful when assigning tasks to ensure that the correct individual is assigned the correct role.

Callouts or Situation Reports

Another method of inviting open communication and suggestions is to regularly give a summary of the progress made. This updates other team members as to the current state and is particularly useful if some team members have been preoccupied with other tasks. By providing a summary and requesting input, team members can suggest other courses of action that may not have been obvious to the team leader. These callouts or situation reports are typically undertaken every 5 or 10 minutes and also can be performed when there is a significant change in the patient's condition.

Critical Language

The term *critical language* refers to the precise terminology needed to avoid ambiguity. Chrimes and Cook suggest that terms used in airway management should be "precisely defined, consistently used, memorable, easy to articulate, and readily understood by all team members" to prevent any confusion.[49]

In particular, several words and phrases in airway management are imprecise and potentially dangerous. For example, does the term *oxygenation* refer to the process of providing oxygen to the alveoli or to a state of having sufficient oxygen for cellular processes? Arguably the most critical communication in any airway crisis—declaring a need to perform an emergency invasive airway access—is associated with a multitude of ill-defined phrases and words that might delay prompt action. Whichever term is chosen, it should be clear, unambiguous, and stimulate immediate action.

Alarms and Alerts

Automated alarms are important tools for maintaining awareness of the state of the patient. Despite their importance, these alarms are commonly missed among the noise of a time-critical event, and announcement of an alarm by a member of the team may be helpful. For example, the duration of a period of oxygen desaturation may be helpful for a team member to announce in order to prompt others to ensure that prolonged attempts at instrumentation of the airway are not undertaken.

Other alerts that convey patient status include the pitch of the pulse oximeter tone. This provides an auditory representation of critical information that can be perceived by the whole team and stimulate appropriate action. Variable tone oximetry provides a key safety measure despite the lack of standardization and methods that manufacturers use to represent changes in oxygen levels.[50]

Role Allocation

Allocation of roles on an airway management team should be carefully considered, particularly before embarking on complex airway management events, and requires matching of the clinician skill set to the specific tasks required of the role. Shared leadership is an emerging concept in healthcare action teams that appears to have promise in improving team effectiveness in clinical scenarios. A co-leader can identify deficits in the leader's plan and make suggestions or assist with assigning roles to other team members.

Another important aspect of role allocation is ensuring that a designated clinician is available to perform an emergency invasive airway access should it be required. Evidence is emerging to suggest that designating one person removes some of the cognitive burden of the decision to perform this procedure. It also makes logical sense to have an additional operator if the original clinician that cared for the patient lacks confidence in performing the rescue after having failed to secure an airway using upper airway approaches. Furthermore, in situations where clinicians from multiple specialties are present, those clinicians with the greatest expertise in securing the airway noninvasively may be different from those most expert at performing an emergency invasive airway.

Practical Design Methods for Airway Management

The final section of this chapter brings together the theoretical threads of human factors redesign, discussed in previous sections, into practical suggestions that may be implemented in a healthcare organization. These will be considered in terms of organizational preparedness, precase planning, management of airway events, and review of outcomes.

Organizational Preparedness

The cornerstones of organizational preparedness are standardization and codesign of processes. Wherever possible, equipment, processes, and education should be designed with the input of the clinicians who will be involved in the clinical events. Ideally, airway emergencies occurring in different areas of the organization should have the same equipment, processes, and education such that staff from one area could seamlessly manage patients in another area with little additional anxiety.

Risk Assessment

A regular review of relevant guidelines should be undertaken from a delegated lead in each department, and any changes should be communicated to the clinicians in the department. Similarly, an understanding of the types of patients and areas where airway events could occur should be assessed. Where appropriate, a DART should be considered to ensure that the appropriate skills are immediately available at all times.

Equipment

An individual in each organization should be tasked with the purchase and maintenance of airway equipment. The design of difficult airway carts should be considered when assembling the equipment to ensure that vital equipment is readily at hand, particularly in emergencies. The design should reflect the processes and education that will be followed and should involve clinicians at all stages of the design.

Similarly, new clinical spaces also should be designed with airway management in mind. Most architects specializing in healthcare facilities are aware of the basic standards related to clinical buildings, but they must also consider the position of power and gas pipeline outlets for vital emergency equipment. Lighting, ventilation, and noise are also key considerations. The configuration of negative pressure rooms, filtration, and the number of air exchanges became of great interest during the COVID-19 pandemic. Attention to the design of future spaces in case of new pandemics should now be considered.

Education

The case mix within an organization will, to some extent, determine the core skills required of clinicians. These proficiencies should include cognitive skills, such as the ability to determine if alveolar ventilation is adequate. Training programs for junior staff should include basic technical and cognitive skills that provide a foundation for the advanced techniques required for their roles.

Skills maintenance may be problematic for senior staff members due to the specifics of scheduling and subsequently limited access for certain procedures. This is particularly true for less frequently performed procedures, such as awake intubation. To some extent, simulation and continuing education can address these issues by supporting a well-managed continuing professional development and credentialing program. However, access to suitable candidates for some procedures might always be limited, and consideration should be given to limiting the number of staff undertaking certain advanced techniques. Some infrequently performed procedures, such as emergency invasive airway access, must be considered core skills for all airway practitioners due to the unpredictable and time-critical nature of their performance. Training for these procedures must include both the technical skills and nontechnical (teamwork) skills to ensure safe and efficient action when needed.

Simulation

Rehearsal of rare events in a simulation setting is valuable to ensure that all members of the team are prepared for airway emergencies. Ideally, training should take place where providers will be expected to perform so that familiarity with procedures and location of equipment can be ingrained. Where possible, the use of actual monitors and cognitive aids should be employed in real time with a whole team, reflecting the old military adage of "Train as you fight, fight as you train," to improve the performance of the team should the event occur. Simulating actual events that occurred in the clinical setting can provide important insights into how situations might be better managed. In situ simulation in the actual clinical setting allows for deeper insights into the design, processes, and education that might create a more resilient organizational response.

Pre-Case Planning

The preparation of clinicians faced with an anticipated difficult airway is covered extensively within this book. However, some general points may help to improve management of the actual event.

Pre-Brief

A meeting prior to the commencement of a case might identify problems that individual clinicians have not themselves considered. Discussion of these helps to form a shared mental model. This will help in the preparation of equipment, assigning roles, and creating expectations of how the case will proceed.

At the end of the pre-brief, a specified series of plans for the patient should be clear to all team members. Writing these plans on a whiteboard or display visible to the team during the case acts as a cognitive aid for this event. Importantly, specific criteria also should be identified for when one method has failed and another should be commenced. Predefining these points ensures that team members do not persist with failing techniques and do not become fixated. Furthermore, it allows other team members to step in and prevent multiple failed attempts at, for example, laryngoscopy. By the addition of these decision points, the airway plan becomes a strategy with clear end points and triggers for progression.

Simulation has been mentioned previously as a method for education, and simulating cases before they are managed is becoming an increasingly common method of preparation for teams. Such rehearsals have been undertaken for rare, complex cases such as the EXIT procedure where the airway (or extracorporeal oxygenation) of a fetus is established before delivery by cesarean.[51] The widening availability of 3D-printed training airways and virtual reality technologies that mirror pathological abnormalities may make these simulations more commonplace in the future.[52]

Equipment

After an airway strategy has been discussed, the equipment for each plan within the strategy should be prepared. If multiple methods have been considered, it might not be possible to have all of the equipment in the room because of spatial constraints. Assigning individuals to remove used equipment and bring prepared equipment to the operator might be a consideration when assigning tasks.

Checklists and Algorithms

The availability of cognitive aids is particularly useful in areas where airway management is not a routine event. Undertaking a checklist at these times commonly uncovers omissions in preparation that were not immediately evident to the team. Frequently overlooked equipment includes specific monitors, such as the capnography monitor, in clinical areas where they are not routinely used. Preoxygenation and optimal positioning of patients prior to intubation are also commonly missed without reference to a checklist. As with other cognitive aids, the value of a checklist is dependent not only on its content but also on its presentation and the manner with which the checklist is implemented. Using a challenge-response format to work through the checklist as a confirmation of actions performed rather than as a prompt to perform them provides a mechanism for clinicians to prepare for airway management in the individualized manner to which they are accustomed, all while maintaining a standardized mechanism to ensure that items are not overlooked. The importance of checklists, particularly when nonroutine or high-stakes situations for airway management arise or when unfamiliar team members are brought together, has been highlighted by the COVID-19 pandemic.

Role Allocation

The team leader must ensure that all roles are allocated including, if necessary, who will perform emergency invasive airway access if required. Dividing the team into subteams may assist in some instances—for example, for preparation of equipment for different approaches. This may help in the preparation of complex equipment, such as for flexible scope techniques.

Specific roles that must be allocated prior to any complex airway management episode include, but are not limited to, a leader (or coordinator), an airway operator for each technique, an airway assistant for each technique, and a reader of the relevant cognitive aid.

During Airway Management

Teamwork aspects such as communication and coordination techniques that have been practiced in training and simulation should be implemented in the real clinical situation.

Team Structure

Omissions and miscommunications commonly occur when information is not fed back centrally to the team leader or coordinator. Any important observations should be announced to the leader that might affect the planned actions. Similarly, observation of team members' performance and either helping or feeding back to the leader that help is needed are expectations of all team members.

Communication

The default method of coordination must be explicit, with ongoing verbalization of the strategy and actions undertaken by the leader and the team members. Use of names and closed loop communication should be the norm in all situations and is essential in emergency situations. During airway management, there should be no communication or noise unrelated to the clinical circumstances to prevent distraction. A written strategy on a whiteboard or large computer screen should be referred to by the leader and the reader of any cognitive aid, such that new team members and team members who have been distracted can immediately identify how the team is progressing with its strategy.

Situation Reports or Callouts

Intermittently, the team leader or cognitive aid reader should recap the clinical situation and progress using a structured callout. This will ensure that all team members are aware of the progress and problems identified and will invite input. Team members must feel able to speak up and highlight any concerns they have, and callouts assist in their ability to do that.[53]

Following Airway Management

Similar to a planned simulation education event, team debriefing after real clinical cases can be used to help understand what the strengths of the team were (to reinforce these behaviors) and what may be areas for improvement. These debriefs may take place immediately (hot debriefs) to capture any immediate thoughts and as way to support team members should the outcome have been suboptimal. Learning may be limited from these hot debriefs, however, because of a lack of reflection and overriding emotion. A delayed debrief might be more appropriate but may be hampered by the ability to assemble all members of the team due to the practicalities of scheduling.

Review of multiple cases in a structured education session or audit session is also helpful for institutional learning. Aggregation of data from multiple cases might suggest areas where education or system redesign might have the most effect in improving management.

Conclusion

Human factors engineering principles include the redesign of the components and processes of airway management to make it safer and more efficient. This involves understanding how the different technical, social, and cognitive aspects of airway management interact. In the absence of detailed system analyses, simple universal methods of planning, team organization, communication, and coordination can be implemented. These include prebriefing; the use of checklists and algorithms; clear, structured communication; and methods to learn from each clinical event.

Selected References

1. Marshall SD, Chrimes N. Time for a breath of fresh air: Rethinking training in airway management. Editorial. *Anaesthesia.* 2016;71(11):1259–1264.
6. Flin R, Fioratou E, Frerk C, Trotter C, Cook TM. Human factors in the development of complications of airway management: preliminary evaluation of an interview tool. *Anaesthesia.* 2013;68:817–825.
8. Holden RJ, Carayon P, Gurses AP, et al. SEIPS 2.0: a human factors framework for studying and improving the work of healthcare professionals and patients. *Ergonomics.* 2013;56(11):1669–1686. doi:10.1080/00140139.2013.838643

10. Russ AL, Fairbanks RJ, Karsh B-T, Militello LG, Saleem JJ, Wears RL. The science of human factors: separating fact from fiction. *BMJ Qual Saf.* 2013;22(10):802–808.

17. Petrosoniak A, Hicks C, Barratt L, et al. Design Thinking-Informed Simulation: An innovative framework to test, evaluate, and modify new clinical infrastructure. *Simul HC.* 2020;15(3):205–213.

20. Schnittker R, Marshall SD, Horberry T, Young K. Human factors enablers and barriers for successful airway management - an in-depth interview study. *Anaesthesia.* 2018;73(8):980–989.

21. Chrimes N, Bradley WPL, Gatward JJ, Weatherall AD. Human factors and the 'next generation' airway trolley. *Anaesthesia.* 2019;74(4):427–433.

23. Schnittker R, Marshall SD, Horberry T, Young K. The codesign process of a decision support tool for airway management. *Advances in Intelligent Systems and Computing* (AISC). 2019;818:111–120.

27. Mumma JM, Durso FT, Dyes M, Dela Cruz R, Fox VP, Hoey M. Bag valve mask ventilation as a perceptual-cognitive skill. *Hum Factors.* 2018;60:212–221.

31. Schnittker R, Marshall SD. Safe anaesthetic care: Further improvements require a focus on resilience. *Br J Anaesth.* 2015;115(5):643–645. doi:10.1093/bja/aev153.

33. Turner MC, Duggan LV, Glezerson BA, Marshall SD. Thinking outside the (acrylic) box: a framework for the local use of custom-made medical devices. *Anaesthesia.* 2020;75(12):1566–1569. doi:10.1111/anae.15152.

39. Chrimes N. The Vortex: a universal 'high-acuity implementation tool' for emergency airway management. *Br J Anaesth.* 2016;117(suppl_1):i20-i27. doi:10.1093/bja/aew175.

All references can be found online at eBooks.Health.Elsevier.com.

PART 3

Preintubation-Ventilation Procedures

13

Preparation of the Patient for Awake Intubation

PAUL POTNURU AND CARLOS A. ARTIME

CHAPTER OUTLINE

KEY POINTS

- When faced with a difficult airway (DA), awake intubation is the gold standard for airway management.
- There are no absolute contraindications to awake intubation other than patient refusal, or a patient who is unable to cooperate (e.g., a child, a patient with an intellectual disability, or an intoxicated, combative patient).
- Preparation begins with a careful history and physical examination and a detailed discussion of the procedure with the patient.
- The goals of premedication are to alleviate anxiety, provide a clear and dry airway, protect against the risk of aspiration, and enable adequate topicalization.
- The nasal mucosa and nasopharynx are highly vascular. When a patient requires nasotracheal intubation, adequate vasoconstriction is essential because bleeding can make visualization of the larynx extremely difficult.

- Sedation may be accomplished with benzodiazepines, opioids, or intravenous hypnotics, either alone or in combination; these agents must be titrated carefully to maintain cooperation and adequate spontaneous ventilation.
- Adequate topicalization of the airway with local anesthetics is the key to a successful awake intubation. When using local anesthetics, the practitioner must be familiar with the speed of onset, duration of action, optimal concentration, maximum recommended dosage, and signs and symptoms of toxicity.
- If airway topicalization is insufficient, airway nerve blocks may be employed to supplement airway anesthesia.
- Many choices are involved when preparing for awake intubation. Safety should be the primary consideration.

Introduction

The American Society of Anesthesiologists (ASA) Practice Guidelines for Management of the Difficult Airway (ASA DA Guidelines), together with the airway management guidelines of several other international anesthesiology societies, advocate for the consideration of airway management before induction of general anesthesia (awake intubation) as a primary strategy for management of the predicted difficult airway (DA).[1–4] Although awake fiberoptic or flexible scope intubation (FSI) has traditionally been the technique of choice for awake intubation, awake video-assisted laryngoscopy (VAL) has gained acceptance.[5]

Regardless of the intubation technique, however, awake tracheal intubation is considered the gold standard for management of the DA for the following reasons:[6,7]

- Spontaneous ventilation is maintained.
- Patency of the airway is maintained by upper pharyngeal muscle tone.
- The larynx does not move to a more anterior position, as it does after induction of anesthesia, resulting in an easier intubation.

Awake intubation can also be used for the patient with cervical spine pathology to allow for neurologic monitoring during and after the intubation procedure. An awake patient is also able to monitor his or her own neurologic symptoms to guard against further neurologic injury. In the unstable cervical spine, care must be taken to ensure that the topicalization and intubation do not result in coughing because this could result in further injury.

Another indication for awake intubation is the patient at high risk for pulmonary aspiration, particularly when the airway assessment predicts difficulty with airway management. With careful topicalization and the avoidance or judicious use of sedation, the patient can protect his or her own airway from aspiration during the intubation process.

A summary of the general indications for awake intubation is presented in Box 13.1. There are no absolute contraindications to awake intubation other than patient refusal, or a patient who is unable to cooperate (e.g., a child, a patient with an intellectual disability, or an intoxicated, combative patient).[7] Although allergy to local anesthetics has been cited as a contraindication to awake intubation, awake intubation without the use of local anesthetics has been reported utilizing sedation with remifentanil or dexmedetomidine (see later discussion).

Preoperative Preparations

Chart Review

Whenever possible, previous anesthetic records should be examined, especially those involving airway management.[1,8] Information regarding ease of mask ventilation, effective ventilation using a supraglottic airway device (SGA), and previously successful intubation techniques are particularly valuable. One should be alert for evidence of reactions to local anesthetics or respiratory depression with minimal doses of sedatives. All available anesthetic records should be reviewed, if possible; although the most recent intubation may have been routine, prior intubations may have been difficult. One should also note the surgical procedures involved—previous intubations may have been routine; however, the operation subsequently performed may have rendered the airway difficult.

When reviewing the chart, one should focus on four important features:

1. Degree of difficulty of tracheal intubation (the difficulty encountered and the method used)
2. Positioning of the patient during laryngoscopy (e.g., sniffing position, use of a ramp)
3. Equipment used (even if the intubation was performed routinely in one attempt, a videolaryngoscope [VL] or a flexible intubation scope [FIS] may have been used, potentially masking a DA)
4. Whether the technique that was used is a familiar one (one should not attempt to learn a new technique on a DA)

For patients with head and neck pathology having otorhinolaryngologic surgery, the ear, nose, and throat (ENT) surgeon's notes should be reviewed in detail, with specific attention to characterizations of the patient's airway, as well as any findings from nasopharyngeal laryngoscopy performed earlier. Imaging of the airway (e.g., computed tomography), if performed, should also be examined before formalizing an airway management plan.

The Patient Interview

After the medical records have been reviewed, a careful patient history should be obtained with particular attention to symptoms that may indicate airway obstruction, such as stridor or paroxysmal nocturnal dyspnea.[9] The preoperative interview should also address the possibility of events having occurred since the last anesthetic that may impact ease of intubation, such as weight gain, airway radiation, facial cosmetic surgery, or worsening temporomandibular joint disorder or rheumatoid arthritis.

Once the anesthesia practitioner has made the decision that awake intubation is necessary, communication with the patient and psychological preparation are of the utmost importance to maximize the odds for a successful awake intubation.[7] In a careful, unhurried manner, the anesthesiologist should describe to the patient conventional intubation contrasted with awake intubation and focus on the fact that, although the former is easier and less time consuming, the latter is safer in light of the patient's own anatomy or condition. The anesthesiologist should present himself or herself as a knowledgeable, caring physician who is willing to

---

• BOX 13.1   Indications for Awake Intubation

1. Previous history of difficult intubation
2. Anticipated difficult airway (DA) based on physical examination:
   Small mouth opening
   Receding mandible/micrognathia
   Macroglossia
   Short, muscular neck
   Limited range of motion of the neck (rheumatoid arthritis, ankylosing spondylitis, prior cervical fusion)
   Congenital airway anomalies
   Morbid obesity
   Pathology involving the airway (tracheomalacia)
   Airway masses (malignancy of the tongue, tonsils, or larynx; large goiter; mediastinal mass)
   Upper airway obstruction
3. Unstable cervical spine
4. Trauma to the face or upper airway
5. Anticipated difficult mask ventilation
6. Severe risk of aspiration
7. Severe hemodynamic instability
8. Respiratory failure

From Kopman AF, Wollman SB, Ross K, et al. Awake endotracheal intubation: a review of 267 cases. *Anesth Analg.* 1975;54:323–327; Thomas JL. Awake intubation: indications, techniques and a review of 25 patients. *Anaesthesia.* 1969;24:28–35; Bailenson G, Turbin J, Berman R. Awake intubation: indications and technique. *Anesth Prog.* 1967;14:272–278.

take extra measures to ensure the patient's safety and comfort. Recommendations should be presented to the patient with conviction, and if the patient is skeptical about proceeding as such, assistance from the surgeon may be enlisted. Because the patient has an established relationship with their surgeon, the surgeon's reinforcement of the anesthesiologist's opinion may be quite helpful. If this and subsequent discussion with the patient are unsuccessful, the anesthesiologist should document these efforts in the chart.

Complications of awake intubation should also be presented, including local anesthetic toxicity, airway trauma, epistaxis, discomfort, coughing or gagging, and failure to secure the airway.[10,11] The possibility of recall of the intubation procedure should be discussed; the incidence of recall after awake intubation varies depending on the different sedative agents used and their dosage. Recall rates as low as 0% and as high as 90% have been reported; however, higher rates of recall do not seem to be associated with patient dissatisfaction.[12–14]

Staff

According to the ASA DA Guidelines, there should be "at least one additional individual who is immediately available to serve as an assistant in difficult airway management."[1] Whenever possible, it is preferable to have a second member of the anesthesia care team who can assist in the monitoring, ventilation, and pharmacotherapy of the patient and can provide an extra set of hands during the intubation procedure. For patients in extremis and those who refuse awake intubation, a surgeon trained in performing a surgical airway should be available with a tracheostomy/cricothyrotomy tray, ready to perform an emergency surgical airway, if necessary.

Monitors

During awake intubation, the routine use of electrocardiography (ECG), pulse oximetry, noninvasive blood pressure monitoring, and capnography is required as part of standard, basic intraoperative monitoring. Depending on the patient's cardiovascular history and hemodynamic status, invasive hemodynamic monitoring may be necessary before awake intubation. Specific indications include hemodynamic instability, severe ischemic or valvular heart disease, and a patient for whom hypertension and tachycardia are potentially dangerous (e.g., the patient with aortic dissection or intracerebral aneurysm).

Supplemental Oxygen

The ASA DA Guidelines encourage the clinician to actively pursue opportunities to administer supplemental oxygen throughout the process of DA management, whenever possible.[1] Arterial hypoxemia has been well documented during bronchoscopy and is associated with increased cardiac strain and dysrhythmias.[15] In addition, sedation administered to supplement topicalization for awake intubation may result in unintended respiratory depression or apnea. Preoxygenation and supplemental oxygen delivery during the awake intubation procedure (including sedation, topicalization, intubation, and extubation) can prevent the onset of hypoxemia.

Traditional preoxygenation (≥3 minutes of tidal volume ventilation) or fast-track preoxygenation (i.e., four vital-capacity breaths in 30 seconds) is effective in delaying arterial desaturation during subsequent apnea.[1] Supplemental oxygen has been shown to delay circulatory arrest resulting from local anesthetic toxicity in animals.[16]

Oxygen delivery by nasal cannula can easily be administered during orotracheal intubation, regardless of the intubation technique. During nasotracheal intubation, the nasal cannula can be placed over the mouth. Transnasal humidified rapid-insufflation ventilatory exchange (THRIVE) via high-flow nasal cannula is associated with decreased incidence of desaturation during awake intubation and is considered the technique of choice when available (see Chapter 15).[4,17,18] In a patient in extremis, transtracheal jet ventilation (TTJV) can be used to administer oxygen while a definitive airway is established.[7,19,20]

Airway Equipment

The ASA DA Guidelines recommend the ready availability of a portable storage unit that contains specialized equipment for DA management.[1] The concept of preassembled carts for emergency situations is not new; examples include crash carts for cardiac arrest and malignant hyperthermia carts. Suggested contents of this portable unit are listed in Box 13.2.

Many techniques can be used to secure the airway in the awake patient. Direct laryngoscopy (DL), VAL, intubating laryngeal mask airways (ILMAs), FSI, rigid fiberoptic laryngoscopy, retrograde intubation, lighted stylets, and blind nasal intubations have all been used successfully to perform awake intubation.[6,10,21,22] No matter which technique is selected, all of the necessary equipment should be prepared ahead of time and readily available, when needed. The practitioner should also have several backup modalities in mind with the required equipment available, in case the initial technique used is ineffective.

Premedication and Sedation

Before awake intubation, premedication is commonly employed to alleviate anxiety, provide a clear and dry airway, protect against the risk of aspiration, and enable adequate topicalization of the airway. The pharmacologic agents most commonly used in preparation for awake intubation include antisialagogues, mucosal vasoconstrictors, aspiration prophylaxis agents, and sedatives/hypnotics.

• BOX 13.2 **Suggested Contents of the Portable Unit for Difficult Airway Management**

1. Rigid laryngoscope blades of alternative designs and sizes from those routinely used; may include a rigid fiberoptic laryngoscope
2. Videolaryngoscopes (with both Macintosh-shaped blades and highly curved or distally angulated blades)
3. Endotracheal tubes (ETTs) of assorted sizes and styles, such as the Parker Flex-Tip tube (Parker Medical, Highlands Ranch, CO)
4. ETT guides, such as semirigid stylets, ventilating tube changers, light wands, and forceps designed to manipulate the distal portion of the ETT
5. Supraglottic airways of assorted sizes and styles, such as the intubating laryngeal mask airway
6. FSI equipment
7. Equipment suitable for emergency surgical airway access (e.g., cricothyrotomy)
8. An exhaled CO_2 detector

The items listed represent suggestions. The contents of the portable storage unit should be customized to meet the specific needs, preferences, and skills of the practitioner and the healthcare facility.

Modified from Apfelbaum JL, Hagberg CA, Caplan RA, et al. Practice guidelines for management of the difficult airway: an updated report by the American Society of Anesthesiologists Task Force on Management of the Difficult Airway. *Anesthesiology.* 2013;118(2):251–270.

Antisialagogues

One of the goals of premedication for awake intubation is drying of the airway. Secretions can obscure the view of the glottis, especially when an FIS or VL is being used to intubate. In addition, secretions can prevent local anesthetics from reaching intended areas, resulting in failed sensory blockade, or they can wash away and dilute local anesthetics, diminishing their potency and duration of action.

The medications most often used for their antisialagogic properties are the anticholinergics, which inhibit salivary and bronchial secretions by way of their antimuscarinic effects.[23] They should be administered as early as possible for maximal effect (preferably at least 30 minutes in advance) because they do not eliminate existing secretions but rather prevent new secretion formation. The anticholinergics most often used in clinical practice are glycopyrrolate, scopolamine, and atropine. A summary of their pharmacologic properties is presented in Table 13.1.

Glycopyrrolate

Glycopyrrolate (0.2 to 0.4 mg intravenous [IV] or intramuscular [IM]) is the anticholinergic of choice for most clinical circumstances because of its marked antisialagogic effect and rapid onset after IV dosing of 1 to 2 minutes; the onset after IM dosing is 20 to 30 minutes. It has a moderate vagolytic effect, which lasts 2 to 4 hours; its antisialagogic effect lasts longer. Glycopyrrolate is devoid of central nervous system (CNS) effects because its quaternary amine structure prevents passage through the blood-brain barrier.

Scopolamine

Scopolamine (0.4 mg IV or IM) has an onset of 5 to 10 minutes after IV dosing and 30 to 60 minutes after IM. The duration of action is about 2 hours after IV dosing and 4 to 6 hours after IM dosing. In addition to being a very effective antisialagogue, scopolamine has very potent CNS effects, with sedative and amnestic properties. In some patients, however, this may lead to restlessness, delirium, and prolonged emergence following short procedures. Because it is the least vagolytic of the anticholinergics in clinical use, it may be the drug of choice for patients in whom tachycardia is contraindicated. Scopolamine for injection was discontinued by the sole manufacturer in the United States in 2015 with no plans for reintroduction.

Atropine

Atropine (0.4 to 0.6 mg IV or IM) has a rapid onset after IV administration of 1 minute; the onset after IM dosing is 15 to 20 minutes. Atropine produces only a mild antisialagogic effect but causes significant tachycardia because of its potent vagolytic effects. As such, it is not an ideal drug for use in drying the airway. As a tertiary amine, it easily crosses the blood-brain barrier and causes mild sedation. It may occasionally cause delirium, especially in elderly patients.

Nasal Mucosal Vasoconstrictors

The nasal mucosa and nasopharynx are highly vascular. When a patient requires nasotracheal intubation, adequate vasoconstriction is essential for preventing epistaxis. Blood in the nasal passage can make visualization of the larynx extremely difficult, especially during FSI. Nasal mucosal vasoconstrictors should be applied 15 minutes before nasal intubation. One commonly used agent is 4% cocaine, which has vasoconstrictive as well as local anesthetic effects (see later discussion). Alternatively, a mixture of lidocaine 3% and phenylephrine 0.25% can be made by combining lidocaine 4% and phenylephrine 1% in a 3:1 ratio.[24] This combination has anesthetic and vasoconstrictive properties similar to those of cocaine and can be used as a substitute. This mixture can be either sprayed intranasally or applied with cotton-tipped applicators. Commercially available nasal decongestants containing either oxymetazoline 0.05% (Afrin) or phenylephrine 0.5% (Neo-Synephrine) may also be applied to nasal mucosa.[25] The usual dose is two sprays in each nostril.

Aspiration Prophylaxis

Routine prophylaxis against aspiration pneumonitis is not recommended for healthy patients who are appropriately fasted. However, it may be beneficial in patients with risk factors for aspiration, such as a full stomach, symptomatic gastroesophageal reflux disease, gastrointestinal motility disorders, morbid obesity, diabetic gastroparesis, or pregnancy.[26] In these patients, nonparticulate antacids, histamine (H_2)-receptor antagonists, and metoclopramide may be used alone or in combination.

Antacids

Preoperative administration of a nonparticulate antacid, such as sodium citrate, provides effective buffering of gastric acid pH.[27] Total gastric volume is increased, but this effect is offset by an increase in the pH of gastric fluid so that, if aspiration occurs, morbidity and mortality are significantly lower.[28] One disadvantage of sodium citrate is the potential to cause emesis because of its unpleasant taste.[29] The use of particulate antacids, such as magnesium trisilicate, is not recommended for prophylaxis.[26]

Histamine Receptor Antagonists

H_2-receptor antagonists selectively and competitively inhibit secretion of hydrogen ion (H^+) by gastric parietal cells and also decrease the secretion of gastric fluid. With IV administration of cimetidine 300 mg, famotidine 20 mg, or ranitidine 50 mg, peak effects are achieved within 30 to 60 minutes, increasing gastric pH and decreasing gastric volume.[30,31] Of the three, ranitidine is probably the drug of choice because it has fewer adverse effects, greater efficacy, and a longer duration of action.[32,33]

Proton Pump Inhibitors

Proton pump inhibitors (PPIs), such as pantoprazole, lansoprazole, and omeprazole, have not been shown to be as effective as H_2-receptor antagonists at increasing gastric pH and decreasing gastric volume preoperatively, particularly when administered

TABLE 13.1	Pharmacologic Characteristics of Anticholinergic Drugs		
Drug	Tachycardia	Antisialagogue Effect	Sedation
Glycopyrrolate	++	++	0
Scopolamine	+	+++	+++
Atropine	+++	+	+

0, No effect; +, minimal effect; ++, moderate effect; +++, marked effect.
Modified from Stoelting RK, Flood P, Rathmell JP, Shafer S. *Stoelting's Handbook of Pharmacology and Physiology in Anesthetic Practice.* 3rd ed. Wolters Kluwer Health; 2015:144.

TABLE 13.2	Sedative Drugs for Awake Airway Management		
Drug	Class	Sedative Dose	Notes
Midazolam	Benzodiazepine	1–2 mg IV, repeated prn (0.025–0.1 mg/kg)	Frequently used in combination with fentanyl
Fentanyl	Opioid	25–200 µg IV (0.5–2 µg/kg)	Usually used in combination with other agents (e.g., midazolam, propofol)
Alfentanil	Opioid	500–1500 µg IV (10–30 µg/kg)	Faster onset, shorter duration than fentanyl
Remifentanil	Opioid	Bolus 0.5 µg/kg IV followed by an infusion of 0.1 µg/kg/min	Infusion can subsequently be titrated by 0.025 µg/kg/min to 0.05 µg/kg/min in 5-minute intervals to achieve adequate sedation
Propofol	Hypnotic	0.25 mg/kg IV, in intermittent boluses or Continuous IV infusion of 25–75 µg/kg/min, titrated to effect	Can also be used in combination with remifentanil (decrease dose of both drugs)
Ketamine	Hypnotic	0.2–0.8 mg/kg IV	Pretreat with antisialagogue Consider administration of midazolam to attenuate undesirable psychological effects
Dexmedetomidine	Alpha-2 agonist	Bolus 1 µg/kg IV over 10 minutes, followed by an infusion of 0.2–0.7 µg/kg/h	Reduce dose in the elderly and in patients with depressed cardiac function

From Artime CA, Hagberg CA. Airway management in the adult. In: Gropper MA, Miller RD, eds. *Miller's Anesthesia*. 9th ed. Elsevier; 2020:1373–1412.

orally.[34,35] PPIs may have a role in aspiration prophylaxis for the patient on chronic H_2-receptor antagonist therapy.[36]

Metoclopramide

Metoclopramide is a cholinergic agent and dopamine (D_2)-receptor antagonist that stimulates motility of the upper gastrointestinal tract and increases lower esophageal sphincter tone. The net effect is accelerated gastric emptying with minimal effect on gastric pH.[26] The standard adult dose is 10 mg IV. Onset after IV administration is rapid, within 1 to 3 minutes, and its effects may persist for up to 2 hours.[37] Metoclopramide can precipitate extrapyramidal symptoms and should be avoided in patients with Parkinson disease.[38]

Sedatives/Hypnotics

Depending on the clinical circumstance, IV sedation may be useful in allowing the patient to tolerate awake intubation by providing anxiolysis, amnesia, and analgesia. Benzodiazepines, opioids, hypnotics, α_2-agonists, and neuroleptics can be used alone or in combination. These agents should be carefully titrated to effect, because oversedation can render a patient uncooperative and make awake intubation more difficult.[7] Spontaneous respiration with adequate oxygenation and ventilation should always be maintained. Extreme caution should be taken in the presence of critical airway obstruction, because awake muscle tone is sometimes necessary in these patients to maintain airway patency.[39] In these situations, sedation should be used sparingly or avoided altogether. Avoidance of oversedation is also important in the patient with a full stomach, because an awake patient can protect his or her own airway if regurgitation should occur.[7] See Table 13.2 for a summary of sedative regimens for awake intubation.

Benzodiazepines

Benzodiazepines, via their action at the γ-aminobutyric acid (GABA)–benzodiazepine receptor complex, have hypnotic,

sedative, anxiolytic, and amnestic properties.[40] They have also been shown to depress upper airway reflex sensitivity,[41] a property that is desirable for awake intubation. Benzodiazepines are frequently used to achieve sedation for awake intubation in combination with opioids,[42] and they are used for their amnestic and anxiolytic effects when other sedatives (e.g., dexmedetomidine, ketamine, remifentanil) are chosen as the primary agent.[43,44] Three benzodiazepine receptor agonists are commonly used in anesthesia practice: midazolam, diazepam, and lorazepam.[40]

Midazolam

Because of its more rapid onset and relatively short duration, midazolam is the most commonly used agent. Sedation with midazolam is achieved with doses of 0.5 to 1 mg IV repeated until the desired level of sedation is achieved. The IM dose is 0.07 to 0.1 mg/kg. Onset is rapid, with peak effect usually achieved within 2 to 3 minutes of IV administration. The duration of action is 20 to 30 minutes, with termination of effect resulting primarily from redistribution. Although recovery is rapid, the elimination half-life is 1.7 to 3.6 hours, with increases noted in patients with cirrhosis, congestive heart failure, renal failure, or morbid obesity, as well as in the elderly. It is extensively metabolized by the liver and renally eliminated as glucuronide conjugates.[40,45]

Diazepam and Lorazepam

Diazepam has a slightly slower onset and longer duration of action than midazolam and has been shown to be a less potent amnestic.[40,45,46] It can cause pain on IV injection and has the added risk of thrombophlebitis.[47] Lorazepam possesses more profound sedating and amnestic properties; however, it is less suitable for sedation during awake intubation because these effects are slower in onset and longer lasting than with either midazolam or diazepam.[40]

Precautions

Care must be used when using benzodiazepines in combination with other sedative drugs. The pharmacologic effects of benzodiazepines are augmented synergistically by other medications used for sedation, including opioids and α_2-agonists.[48] Propofol has been shown to increase the plasma concentration of midazolam by decreasing distribution and clearance.[49] Systemic absorption of local anesthetics used for airway topicalization may also lead to potentiation of the sedative/hypnotic effects of midazolam.[50]

The primary adverse effect of oversedation with benzodiazepines is respiratory depression, which may lead to hypoxemia or apnea.[40] Flumazenil, a specific benzodiazepine antagonist, may be used to reverse the sedative and respiratory effects of benzodiazepines if a patient becomes too heavily sedated. It is given in incremental IV doses of 0.2 mg, repeated as needed to a maximum dose of 3 mg. It has a rapid onset, with peak effect occurring in 1 to 3 minutes. Because it has a half-life of 0.7 to 1.8 hours, resedation can be a problem if flumazenil is being used to reverse high doses or longer-acting benzodiazepines, and patients should be monitored carefully in those circumstances. Although flumazenil may precipitate withdrawal symptoms in benzodiazepine-dependent patients, it is generally safe and devoid of major side effects when used for the reversal of the clinical effects of benzodiazepines administered in anesthesia practice.[40,51,52]

Opioids

Opioids, by way of their agonist effect on opioid receptors in the brain and spinal cord, provide analgesia, depress airway reflexes, and prevent hyperventilation associated with pain or anxiety. These properties make them a useful addition to the sedative regimen for awake intubation. Although any opioid could theoretically be used for this purpose, fentanyl, alfentanil, and remifentanil are particularly useful because of their rapid onset, relatively short duration of action, and ease of titration.[8]

Fentanyl

Fentanyl is widely used in anesthesia practice and, prior to the introduction of remifentanil, was the most commonly used opioid for awake intubation.[53] The sedative dose ranges from 0.5 to 2 µg/kg IV. Onset is rapid, within 2 to 3 minutes. The relatively short duration of action of a single bolus dose (30 to 45 minutes) is as a result of redistribution of fentanyl to a large peripheral compartment rather than rapid elimination; thus, the duration of action after cessation of a prolonged infusion is markedly longer as a result of redistribution to the central compartment from the peripheral compartment.[54]

Sufentanil

Sufentanil is 7 to 10 times more potent than fentanyl and has a similar pharmacokinetic profile after a single bolus dose. The primary difference is a significantly faster recovery after prolonged infusion compared with fentanyl.[55] Adequate sedation with sufentanil can be achieved in adult patients with 5 to 20 µg IV in divided doses; alternatively, a loading dose of 0.2 µg/kg followed by an infusion rate of 0.1 µg/kg/h has been shown to be an effective regimen in combination with midazolam.[56] When using target-controlled infusion (TCI), an effect-site concentration of 0.2–0.3 ng/mL provides satisfactory sedation for awake intubation.[57]

Alfentanil

Compared with fentanyl and sufentanil, alfentanil has an even quicker onset (1.5 to 2 minutes). It is approximately 1/70 as potent as fentanyl; however, because of rapid plasma to effect-site equilibration, comparatively smaller doses are needed to achieve a similar peak effect. Because smaller doses are needed relative to its potency, recovery from a single bolus of alfentanil is faster than with the other agents of this class, potentially making alfentanil the drug of choice when a transient peak effect after a single bolus is desired, as in awake intubation.[55] Sedative doses range from 10 to 30 µg/kg IV, administered in 3–5 µg/kg aliquots.[8] In one study, alfentanil 20 µg/kg IV significantly improved intubating conditions and attenuated the hemodynamic effects of awake nasal FSI in patients premedicated with oral diazepam. Moderate respiratory depression was noted without overt apnea or hypoxia.[58]

Remifentanil

Remifentanil is an ultrashort-acting opioid that is unique compared with the other short-acting agents in that it is rapidly metabolized by nonspecific plasma and tissue esterases, resulting in a context-sensitive half-time of 3 minutes that is independent of infusion duration.[59] Its potency approximates that of fentanyl.[60] Several studies have shown the effectiveness and safety of remifentanil sedation for awake intubation as a single agent in combination with topical anesthesia,[43,44,61] in combination with midazolam or propofol,[12,62–64] and as a sole agent with no premedication or topicalization.[65]

Remifentanil is usually administered as a weight-based infusion. Several different remifentanil dosing strategies have been described in the literature for awake intubation, with infusion rates ranging between 0.06 and 0.5 µg/kg/min, with or without an initial bolus of 0.5 to 1.5 µg/kg.[61,62,66] Studies using remifentanil TCI for awake intubation have demonstrated that the mean effect-site concentration of remifentanil needed for awake intubation is 2 to 3 ng/mL[12,44,63,64]; higher effect-site concentrations in the 6 to 8 ng/mL range were necessary when using remifentanil as a sole agent without topicalization.[65] The dosing strategy described by Atkins and Mirza,[67] a bolus of 0.5 µg/kg followed by an infusion of 0.1 µg/kg/min, rapidly achieves an effect-site concentration of 2 to 2.5 ng/mL according to the Minto pharmacokinetic model.[68] The infusion can subsequently be titrated by 0.025 to 0.05 µg/kg/min in 5-minute intervals to achieve adequate sedation.

Precautions

The most serious adverse effect of opioids is respiratory depression leading to overt apnea. Opioids reduce the stimulatory effect of carbon dioxide (CO_2) on ventilation while increasing the apneic threshold and the resting end-tidal CO_2. Factors that increase susceptibility to opioid-induced respiratory depression include old age, obstructive sleep apnea, and concomitant administration of CNS depressants.[69]

Naloxone, an opioid antagonist, can be used to restore spontaneous ventilation in patients after an opioid overdose. Onset after IV administration is rapid, within 1 to 2 minutes, and the duration of action is 30 to 60 minutes. Naloxone should be administered in 0.04 to 0.08 µg IV boluses every 2 to 3 minutes. Doses of 1 to 2 µg/kg will restore adequate spontaneous ventilation in most cases, while preserving adequate analgesia. Potential complications of naloxone administration are reversal of analgesia, tachycardia, hypertension, and, in severe cases, pulmonary edema or myocardial ischemia. Because of the relatively short duration of action of naloxone, one should carefully monitor for recurrence of respiratory depression, especially when it is used to reverse longer-acting opioids such as morphine or hydromorphone. In those situations, an IM dose of 2 times the required IV dose or a continuous IV infusion (2.5 to 5 µg/kg/h) should be considered.[69]

Chest wall rigidity leading to ineffectual bag-mask ventilation is commonly cited as a potential adverse effect of opioids, particularly fentanyl, sufentanil, alfentanil, and remifentanil. Opioids do have the potential to cause muscle rigidity, but clinically significant rigidity usually occurs only after an opioid dose sufficient to cause apnea, just as or after the patient loses consciousness.[69] Studies in intubated patients and patients with tracheostomies have shown that decreases in pulmonary compliance as a result of chest wall rigidity are not sufficient to explain an inability to maintain bag-mask ventilation after a large dose of opioid,[70,71] and flexible scope examination of the vocal cords during induction with sufentanil has shown that vocal cord closure is the primary cause of difficult ventilation after opioid-induced anesthesia.[72] Careful titration to prevent overdose is perhaps the best way to prevent rigidity-associated difficult ventilation. Should it occur, treatment with naloxone or neuromuscular blocking agents is effective.[73,74]

Intravenous Anesthetics

Propofol

Propofol (2,6-diisopropylphenol) is the most frequently used IV anesthetic today.[39] Its primary effect is hypnosis, which is primarily mediated by interaction with GABA receptors. Propofol has a rapid onset of approximately 90 seconds, with rapid recovery (4 to 5 minutes after an induction dose) as a result of both elimination and redistribution. It attenuates airway responses in induction doses via an unclear mechanism and provides a smooth induction with few excitatory effects. Although it is frequently used as an induction agent in doses of 1.5 to 2.5 mg/kg IV, intermittent doses of approximately 0.25 mg/kg IV or a continuous IV infusion of 25 to 75 µg/kg/min provide an easily titratable level of sedation with rapid recovery.

The use of propofol in awake intubation is well described both as a single agent and in combination with remifentanil.[12,75–77] TCI studies have shown that the effective plasma concentration of propofol to facilitate awake intubation is 1 to 2 µg/mL.[10,62,71] Care should be taken if the patient has a critical airway, because propofol causes reduction of tidal volumes and an increase in respiratory frequency at sedative doses. At sufficiently elevated plasma concentrations, propofol can lead to apnea. Other common adverse effects are a decrease in arterial blood pressure and pain on injection. An additional benefit of propofol is its antiemetic properties.

Dexmedetomidine

Dexmedetomidine is a centrally acting, highly selective α_2-adrenoreceptor agonist with several properties that make it well suited for use in awake intubation. It has sedative, analgesic, anxiolytic, antitussive, and antisialagogic effects while causing minimal respiratory impairment, even at high doses. Compared with clonidine, it is 8 to 10 times more specific for the α_2- versus the α_1-adrenergic receptor and has a shorter half-life (2 to 3 hours). Dexmedetomidine sedation provides unique conditions in which the patient is asleep but is easily arousable and cooperative when stimulated. It is approved for continuous IV sedation in intubated and mechanically ventilated patients and for sedation in nonintubated patients undergoing surgical or other procedures.[78,79]

There are several studies of dexmedetomidine sedation in awake FSI,[80] including a phase IIIb Food and Drug Administration (FDA) study specifically for this indication.[81] Dosing for awake intubation is a 1 to 1.5 µg/kg load over 10 minutes, usually followed by a continuous infusion of 0.2 to 0.7 µg/kg/h.[80,82] Some patients may require higher maintenance doses.[83] A reduced loading dose of 0.5 µg/kg and a reduction in the maintenance infusion should be considered in elderly patients (age >65 years) and in those with hepatic or renal impairment.[84] For awake intubation, dexmedetomidine is usually combined with airway topicalization, although its successful use as a sole agent without local anesthetics has been reported.[85] Although lowering of bispectral index scores (BIS) and partial amnesia have been reported with its use,[86,87] dexmedetomidine is not a reliable amnestic and is frequently combined with midazolam to decrease the incidence of recall.[88]

Dexmedetomidine can cause adverse hemodynamic effects including bradycardia, hypotension, and hypertension. During the loading dose, hypertension and bradycardia can occur as a result of stimulation of peripheral postsynaptic α_{2B}-adrenergic receptors resulting in vasoconstriction. Central α_{2A}-mediated sympatholysis eventually leads to bradycardia, hypotension, and decreased cardiac output.[89] The bradycardic effect can be mitigated by pretreatment with an anticholinergic (e.g., glycopyrrolate) or by combining the dexmedetomidine with ketamine for its cardiostimulatory properties.[14,90] Caution should be used in patients with depressed systolic function.[84]

Ketamine

Ketamine is a phencyclidine derivative and N-methyl-D-aspartate (NMDA) antagonist that produces dissociative anesthesia, which manifests clinically as a cataleptic state with eyes open and many reflexes intact, including the corneal, cough, and swallow reflexes.[40] Ketamine-induced anesthesia is associated with amnesia, nystagmus, and the potential for hallucinations and other undesirable psychological reactions. Benzodiazepines are commonly administered to attenuate or treat these reactions; dexmedetomidine has also been shown to reduce the incidence and severity of ketamine-induced delirium.[91,92] Ketamine has an opioid-sparing effect and produces analgesia that extends well into the postoperative period, because plasma levels required for analgesia are considerably lower than those required for loss of consciousness. Usual doses for sedation range from 0.2 to 0.8 mg/kg IV, with peak plasma levels occurring after less than 1 minute and a duration of hypnosis of 5 to 10 minutes. At these doses, minute ventilation, tidal volume, functional residual capacity (FRC), and the minute ventilation response to CO_2 are maintained. Although airway reflexes and upper airway skeletal muscle tone are preserved, airway protection remains necessary in patients who are at risk for aspiration.

Ketamine increases blood pressure, heart rate, cardiac output, and myocardial oxygen consumption via a centrally mediated stimulation of the sympathetic nervous system. Ketamine is a direct myocardial depressant, however, and in patients with depleted catecholamine stores (e.g., the patient in shock or after repeated administrations), it may cause hypotension.[93] Its successful use in awake intubation has been described in combination with benzodiazepines, and it has been shown to provide better sedation and hemodynamic stability when used in combination with dexmedetomidine compared with dexmedetomidine alone.[6,14] Patients receiving ketamine sedation should always be pretreated with an antisialagogue because ketamine causes increased airway secretions that can lead to upper airway obstruction or make FSI or VAL difficult.

Droperidol

Droperidol, a butyrophenone, is a neuroleptic medication occasionally used in anesthesia practice for its sedative and antiemetic properties.[40] Its mechanism of action is antagonism of dopamine receptors in the CNS; it also interferes with GABA-, norepinephrine-, serotonin-, and acetylcholine-mediated neuronal activity.

In combination with fentanyl, it produces a state of hypnosis, analgesia, and immobility classically referred to as *neuroleptanalgesia*. In combination with a hypnotic or nitrous oxide, droperidol and fentanyl produce general anesthesia (*neuroleptanesthesia*), not unlike the dissociative state produced by ketamine. In this state, patients may experience extreme fear and apprehension despite appearing outwardly calm; droperidol is also a poor amnestic. For this reason, benzodiazepines should be administered for anxiolysis and amnesia. Neuroleptanalgesia has been used for awake intubation with favorable results.[6,94-96]

Doses of droperidol for neuroleptanalgesia range from 2.5 to 5 mg IV; the antiemetic dose is 0.625 to 1.25 mg. Onset is in 20 minutes, with a half-life of about 2 hours. Side effects include mild hypotension as a result of peripheral α-adrenergic blockade, dysphoria, and extrapyramidal symptoms. Droperidol can also cause QT prolongation, especially in larger doses. This has led to an FDA "black box" warning concerning the risk for potentially fatal torsades de pointes. Therefore, droperidol should not be administered to patients with a prolonged QT interval (>440 milliseconds for males, >450 milliseconds for females), and ECG monitoring should be performed during treatment and for 2 to 3 hours after treatment with neuroleptic doses.[97]

Topicalization

Topicalization of the airway with local anesthetics should, in most cases, be the primary anesthetic for awake intubation; many times, it is all that is needed.[4,7] When using local anesthetics, the practitioner must be familiar with the speed of onset, duration of action, optimal concentration, signs and symptoms of toxicity, and maximum recommended dosage of the drug chosen. The rate and amount of topical local anesthetic absorption vary depending on the site of application, the concentration and total dose of local anesthetic applied, the hemodynamic status of the patient, and individual patient variation. Local anesthetic absorption is more rapid from the alveoli than from the tracheobronchial tree, and more rapid from the tracheobronchial tree than from the pharynx. The most commonly used agents for topical anesthesia of the airway are lidocaine and cocaine.

Although awake intubation with airway topicalization is considered the safest method of airway management for the patient with a DA, it is not without risk.[98] Local anesthetic systemic toxicity (LAST), ranging from mild symptoms to major neurologic and cardiovascular toxicity, is a real concern[99,100]; death attributed to lidocaine toxicity of a healthy volunteer undergoing bronchoscopy has occurred.[101] In addition, total airway obstruction during topical anesthesia in a nonsedated patient with a critical airway has been reported. This was postulated to have been caused by dynamic airway obstruction related to loss of upper airway tone as a result of topicalization.[102] Early symptoms of local anesthetic toxicity include euphoria, dizziness, tinnitus, confusion, and a metallic taste in the mouth. Signs of severe local anesthetic systemic toxicity include seizures, respiratory failure, loss of consciousness, and circulatory collapse.[103] LAST can have a variable presentation of signs and symptoms with regard to timing of onset and order of presentation after local anesthetic administration.[104] Early treatment with 20% intravenous lipid emulsion is a cornerstone of successful LAST management.[105] An initial bolus of 100 mL should be administered over 2 to 3 minutes for patients over 70 kg or 1.5 mL/kg if the weight is less than 70 kg. Additional boluses can be administered if the patient remains unstable and an infusion should be started after the initial dose. Use of

cognitive aids (e.g., checklists) and guideline-driven management of LAST is strongly recommended.[104]

Lidocaine

Lidocaine, an amide local anesthetic, is the most commonly used agent for airway topicalization.[106,107] It is available in various concentrations (1% to 10%) and in preparations including aqueous and viscous solutions, ointments, and jellies. For infiltration and minor nerve blocks, 1% to 2% lidocaine is commonly used; for topical anesthesia, the concentration used is 2% to 10%.[108] Lidocaine is an excellent choice for airway anesthesia because of its reasonably rapid onset of 2 to 5 minutes and its high therapeutic index. Its duration of action is 30 to 60 minutes after topical application or infiltration; addition of epinephrine extends the duration to 2 to 3 hours when used for infiltration. It is hepatically metabolized with a half-life of 90 minutes; caution should be exercised in patients with hepatic failure.

The maximum recommended dosage for infiltration of lidocaine without epinephrine is 5 mg/kg of lean body mass.[107] For topicalization of the airway, the maximum dose is less well established. The British Thoracic Society recommends using the lowest dose of lidocaine possible, noting that while doses of 15.4 mg/kg may be used without serious adverse events, doses higher than 9.6 mg/kg can be associated with subjective symptoms of lidocaine toxicity (e.g., dizziness, euphoria).[109] Studies using total doses as high as 9.3 mg/kg failed to demonstrate signs or symptoms of lidocaine toxicity.[110-113] Other studies using higher doses reported an increased incidence of signs and symptoms of lidocaine toxicity.[114] Common to these studies, however, is significant variability among patients with regard to absorption depending on patient factors, mode of delivery, and timing of administration. Some authors, therefore, recommend using the lower limit of 5 mg/kg[107] and encourage the use of 2% lidocaine for airway topicalization.[115] DAS guidelines for airway topicalization advise a maximum lidocaine dose of 9 mg/kg.[4]

Cocaine

Cocaine, a naturally occurring ester anesthetic, is used primarily for anesthesia of the nasal mucosa when the nasal route is planned for awake intubation. It has a vasoconstrictor property that makes it particularly useful for this application, because the nose is highly vascularized and bleeding can make FSI or VAL impossible. It is available commercially as a 4% (40 mg/mL) solution and can be applied to the nasal mucosa using cotton pledgets or cotton-tipped swabs. The maximum recommended dosage for intranasal application is 1.5 to 3 mg/kg. Systemic absorption from a soaked cotton pledget placed in the nose is approximately 40%.[116] After topical application of cocaine to the nasal mucosa, peak plasma levels are achieved in 30 to 45 minutes, and the drug persists in the plasma for 5 to 6 hours.[117]

Cocaine is primarily metabolized by plasma pseudocholinesterase; it also undergoes slow hepatic metabolism and is excreted unchanged by the kidney. The signs and symptoms of cocaine toxicity include tachycardia, cardiac dysrhythmia, hypertension, and fever. Severe complications include convulsions, respiratory failure, coronary spasm, cardiac arrest, stroke, and death. It should not be administered to patients with uncontrolled hypertension, coronary artery disease, hyperthyroidism, pseudocholinesterase deficiency, or preeclampsia and in those patients taking monoamine oxidase inhibitors.

The use of cocaine for topicalization and vasoconstriction is no longer advised[4,109] because of the higher risk of cardiovascular toxicity compared to the combination of lidocaine and phenylephrine, which is equally as effective.[118]

Other Local Anesthetics

Benzocaine is a water-insoluble ester-type local anesthetic agent that is mainly useful for topical application. The onset of action is rapid (<1 minute), and the effective duration is 5 to 10 minutes. Benzocaine is most commonly available as a 20% aerosol spray that is easily applied to the oropharyngeal mucosa. The limiting factor in benzocaine use is the potential development of clinically significant methemoglobinemia. In some patients, this can occur with as little as 1 to 2 seconds of spraying.[119] The risk increases by almost 20-fold when benzocaine exposure is repeated within 1 week. Although most patients tolerate benzocaine airway topicalization without any adverse effects, it is not possible to identify in advance those patients who are at risk for significant methemoglobinemia. Some have advocated for the cessation of benzocaine use for airway anesthesia.[120] Symptoms of early methemoglobinemia toxicity can be seen with methemoglobin levels of 5% and include cyanosis, tachycardia, and tachypnea. As levels increase to 20% to 30%, patients may develop chest pain, ischemic changes on ECG, hypotension, altered mental status, syncope, or coma. The most severe cases have led to neurologic hypoxic injury, myocardial infarction, and death. Should symptomatic methemoglobin occur, treatment is with methylene blue 1 to 2 mg/kg IV given over 5 minutes.[121] Because recent shortages of methylene blue have been reported, benzocaine should only be used if methylene blue is confirmed to be clinically available. When methylene blue is unavailable or contraindicated (e.g., glucose-6-dehydrogenase deficiency), ascorbic acid (vitamin C) 10 g IV can be used to treat severe or symptomatic methemoglobinemia.[122,123]

Tetracaine is an amide local anesthetic agent with a longer duration of action than lidocaine or cocaine. It is available as 0.5% to 1% solutions for local use. It is metabolized through hydrolysis by plasma cholinesterase. Severe toxic reactions after tetracaine overdose include convulsions, respiratory arrest, and circulatory collapse. Fatalities have been reported with the topical application of 100 mg of tetracaine to anesthetize mucous membranes.[124] These issues have limited its use as a primary local anesthetic for airway topicalization, although its safe use in a large cohort has been reported.[125]

Cetacaine is a topical application spray containing 14% benzocaine, 2% tetracaine, and 2% butyl aminobenzoate (a local anesthetic similar to benzocaine). Like 20% benzocaine spray, this combination produces rapid airway anesthesia, but with a prolonged duration of action compared with benzocaine alone. The risk of methemoglobinemia is still a consideration, and cases of severe toxicity have been reported.[126]

Eutectic mixture of local anesthetics (EMLA) cream contains 2.5% lidocaine and 2.5% prilocaine and is a topical anesthetic for use on intact skin. Although the manufacturer does not recommend its use on mucosal surfaces because of faster systemic absorption, it has been employed safely as a topical anesthetic for awake intubation. A case series of 20 adult patients who underwent awake FSI using 4 g of EMLA applied over the upper airway found that peak plasma concentrations of lidocaine or prilocaine[127] did not reach toxic levels, and methemoglobin levels did not exceed normal values (1.5%).

Application Techniques

Local anesthetic may be directly applied to the airway mucosa by several different methods. As long as the total dose of local anesthetic administered falls under the maximum dosage guidelines, these techniques can be used in combination to achieve adequate topical airway anesthesia. It is helpful to differentiate the airway into three distinct areas: the nasal cavity and nasopharynx; the oral cavity and oropharynx; and the larynx, trachea, and hypopharynx. The basis for this distinction involves the innervation of these different areas and is explained in more detail later in this chapter.

Direct Application

The mucosa of the airway can be topicalized by the direct application of local anesthetic. Nasal anesthesia can be achieved by placing cotton pledgets or cotton-tipped swabs soaked in lidocaine 4% with epinephrine 1:200,000, or a 3:1 mixture of lidocaine 4% and phenylephrine 1% in the nares. The benefits of this technique are that initial topicalization of the nasal cavity is achieved, the angle of endotracheal tube (ETT) insertion can be predicted, and patency of the nasal cavity is assessed. The pledgets or swabs can then be followed by placement of a nasopharyngeal airway (nasal trumpet) coated in 2% to 5% lidocaine ointment, viscous solution, or jelly; a 32-French nasopharyngeal airway predicts easy passage of a 7.0-mm internal diameter (ID) ETT.

Topicalization of the oral cavity is not necessary for awake intubation per se. The gag reflex and the posterior oropharynx, however, do require anesthesia, particularly if the airway management technique chosen will be stimulating these areas (e.g., awake VAL). A 2% to 4% aqueous or viscous solution of lidocaine can be used to "swish, gargle, and spit." This technique adequately anesthetizes the oral and pharyngeal mucosa, although the larynx and trachea may require additional topicalization.

Laryngeal anesthesia can be achieved via the aspiration of local anesthetic. Several methods are available to achieve this. A "lidocaine lollipop" can be made by placing lidocaine 5% ointment or lidocaine 2% to 4% jelly on the end of a tongue depressor.[106] This is then placed lidocaine-side-down onto the posterior tongue. The patient is encouraged not to swallow, but rather to allow the lidocaine to "melt" and run down the base of the tongue and pool above the glottis, where it is then aspirated. The "toothpaste method" is a similar concept that involves placing a line of lidocaine 5% ointment down the middle of the tongue.[128] The patient is instructed to place the tongue against the roof of the mouth and is encouraged not to swallow. Aspiration of an aqueous solution of lidocaine can also be achieved by slowly trickling 10 to 12 mL of lidocaine 2% onto the back of the tongue, while the tongue is held by the operator between two pieces of gauze. This prevents the patient from swallowing and results in aspiration of the lidocaine, resulting in adequate laryngotracheal anesthesia.[129]

Atomizers

Atomization is another common method of local anesthetic application to the airway. Disposable plastic atomizers are available for this purpose (Fig. 13.1). The atomizer reservoir is filled with 2 to 4% lidocaine, and tubing is connected from the atomizer to a regulated oxygen source with a flow rate of 8 to 10 L/min. The phalange is depressed, and the spray of local anesthetic solution is directed toward the soft palate and posterior pharynx to topicalize the mucosa. Any residual anesthetic agent in the oropharynx should be suctioned out to reduce absorption from the

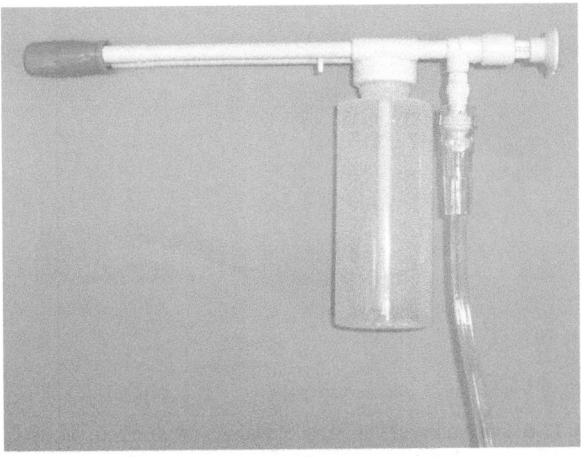

• **Fig. 13.1** Typical disposable atomizer.

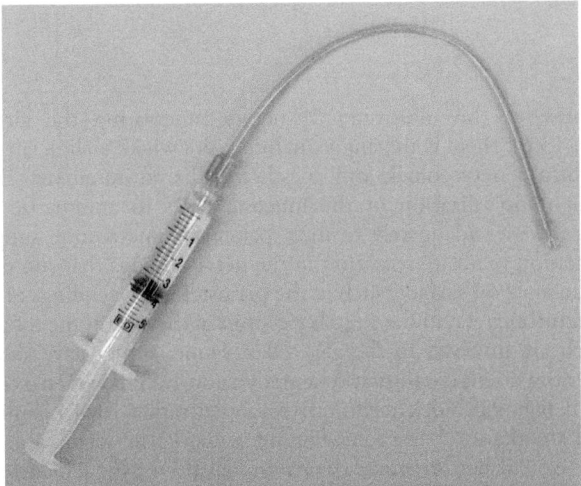

• **Fig. 13.2** MADjic Mucosal Atomization Device. (Courtesy Teleflex, Research Triangle Park, NC.)

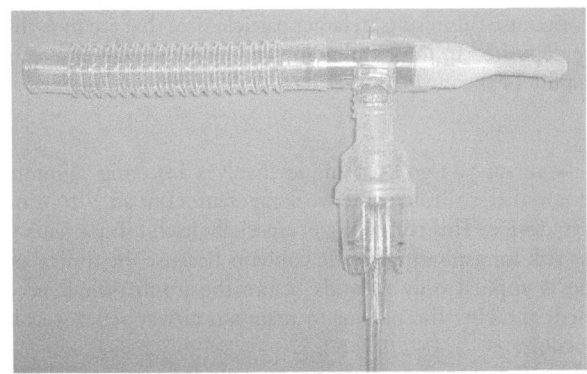

• **Fig. 13.3** Typical mouthpiece-type nebulizer.

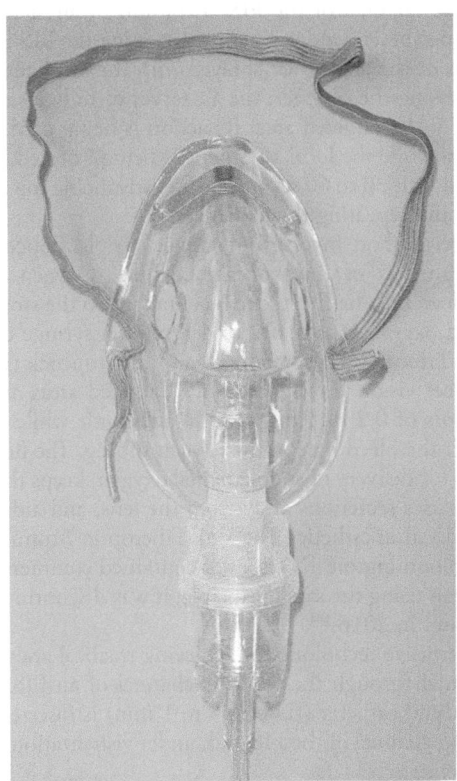

• **Fig. 13.4** Typical face-mask-type nebulizer.

gastrointestinal tract. A disadvantage with this method is the difficulty in controlling the exact amount of local anesthetic administered.

Alternatively, the MADjic Mucosal Atomization Device (Teleflex Medical, Morrisville, NC) is an inexpensive, disposable, latex-free device that, when attached to a Luer-fitted syringe containing local anesthetic, can be used to dispense a fine mist to the oropharyngeal or nasal mucosa (Fig. 13.2). The tubing is malleable, allowing for delivery of local anesthetic to deeper pharyngeal structures and the glottis. Because a syringe is used, a known amount of local anesthetic can be administered. The primary disadvantage of this device is that smaller particle sizes are not achieved, limiting the amount of local anesthetic that reaches the trachea.

Nebulizers

Nebulizers may also be used to apply local anesthetic to the airway. The advantages of this technique include ease of application and safety. A standard mouthpiece-type nebulizer (Fig. 13.3) can topicalize the oropharynx and trachea. If nasal cavity anesthesia is needed, a face-mask–type nebulizer (Fig. 13.4) can be used; the patient is instructed to breathe in through the nose. Because it is associated with less coughing and gagging, nebulization is especially advantageous for patients with increased intracranial pressure (ICP), open eye injury, or severe coronary artery disease.[130] A study comparing the administration of lidocaine using two different modalities (nebulizer-atomizer combination and atomizer alone) in patients undergoing bronchoscopy found that the nebulizer-atomizer combination was more efficacious, resulting in a reduction of the dose required to anesthetize the upper airway.[131] A typical dose of lidocaine used in a standard nebulizer is 4 mL of 4% lidocaine; this results in a total dose of 160 mg of lidocaine, which is well within the safe dosage range.[109] Studies using 6 mg/kg of 10% lidocaine showed that peak plasma concentrations are much lower than would be expected if all the lidocaine had been absorbed—evidence that some of the local anesthetic is lost during exhalation.[132] When nebulizing local anesthetics for airway topicalization, lower oxygen flow rates (2 to 4 L/min) should be used, because this results in larger particle sizes that are more likely to be deposited in the oropharynx and upper airway, where anesthesia for awake intubation is needed.[133]

Spray-as-You-Go

The "spray-as-you-go" technique involves injecting aliquots of local anesthetic through the working channel of an FIS or other airway device. This technique is especially useful in patients who are at risk for aspirating gastric contents because the topical anesthetic is applied only seconds before the intubation is accomplished, allowing the patient to maintain airway reflexes as long as possible.

The most common method is to draw 0.5 to 1 mL of 2% to 4% lidocaine into a 5- or 10-mL syringe. The plunger is then pulled back so that when the syringe is inverted and inserted into the working channel of the FIS, a column of air sits on top of the local anesthetic. Under visualization using the FIS image, targeted areas of the airway are sprayed with the local anesthetic by fully depressing the plunger; the air serves to fully eject the local anesthetic at the targeted area. If suction is being used, it should be clamped while the local anesthetic is being injected. The clinician should wait 30 to 60 seconds before advancing toward deeper structures and repeating the maneuver.[106]

Another method involves attaching a triple stopcock to the proximal portion of the working channel. Oxygen tubing in which a bleed hole has been cut is connected to the stopcock and a regulated oxygen source at 2 to 4 L/min. A syringe containing 2% to 4% lidocaine is also connected to the stopcock (Fig. 13.5). Under direct vision through the FIS, targeted areas are sprayed with aliquots of 0.2 to 1 mL of local anesthetic while a finger is placed over the bleed hole in the oxygen tubing. The flow of oxygen allows for delivery of supplemental oxygen, keeps the FIS lens clean, disperses secretions away from the lens, and aids in nebulizing the local anesthetic. The Enk Fiberoptic Atomizer (Cook Medical, Bloomington, IN) is a self-contained commercial device that operates using the same principle; it was discontinued by the manufacturer in 2016.[134]

A noninvasive technique for achieving tracheal anesthesia can be performed through the working channel of an FIS. A multiorifice epidural catheter (ID of 0.5 to 1 mm) is inserted through the working channel of the FIS and, under visualization, is guided

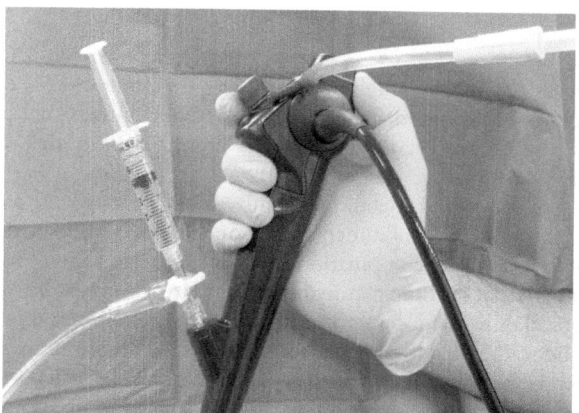

• **Fig. 13.5** "Spray-as-you-go" technique. An oxygen hose and a triple stopcock are attached to the suction port of a flexible bronchoscope with syringe attached containing local anesthetic.

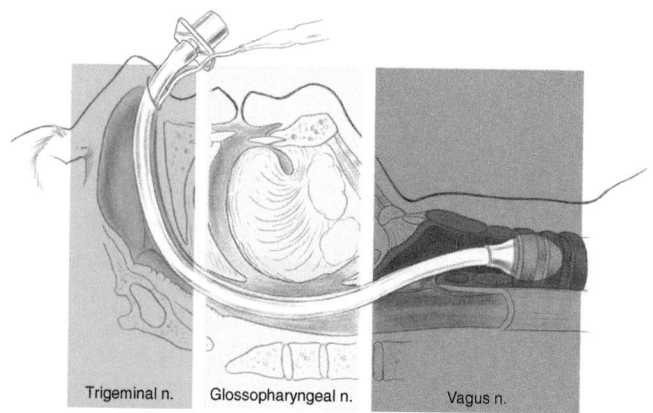

Trigeminal n.   Glossopharyngeal n.   Vagus n.

• **Fig. 13.6** Innervation of the upper airway. *n.,* nerve. (From Brown D, ed. *Atlas of Regional Anesthesia.* 2nd ed. Saunders; 1999.)

into the trachea, where 1 to 2 mL of 2% to 4% lidocaine is administered.[135]

Nerve Blocks

Because of the multitude of nerves innervating the airway (Fig. 13.6), there is no single anatomic site where a clinician can perform a nerve block and anesthetize the entire airway. Even though topicalization of the mucosa serves to anesthetize the entire airway adequately in most patients, some require supplementation to ablate sensation in the nerve endings that run deep to the mucosal surface, such as the periosteal nerve endings of the nasal turbinates and the stretch receptors at the base of the tongue, which are involved in the gag reflex. Some studies have shown superior patient comfort and hemodynamic stability when a combined regional block technique was used rather than nebulized local anesthetic.[136] The following nerve blocks are remarkable for their ease of performance, their minimal risk to the patient, and their speed of onset. Nerve blocks are applied to the nasal cavity and nasopharynx, the oropharynx, the larynx, and the trachea and vocal cords.

Nasal Cavity and Nasopharynx

Anatomy

Most of the sensory innervation of the nasal cavity is derived from two sources: the sphenopalatine ganglion and the anterior ethmoidal nerve. The sphenopalatine ganglion (also referred to as the *pterygopalatine, nasal,* or *Meckel's ganglion*) is a parasympathetic ganglion that is in the pterygopalatine fossa (Fig. 13.7A), posterior to the middle turbinate. Its sensory root is derived from sphenopalatine branches of the maxillary nerve, cranial nerve (CN) V_2. As they pass through the sphenopalatine ganglion, these sensory branches form the greater and lesser palatine nerves, which provide sensory innervation to the nasal cavity, as well as the roof of the mouth, soft palate, and tonsils. The anterior ethmoidal nerve (see Fig. 13.7B) is one of the sensory branches of the ciliary ganglion, which is located within the orbital cavity and inaccessible to nerve blocks. It provides sensory innervation to the anterior portion of the nasal cavity.[137]

Sphenopalatine Nerve Block
Nasal Approach

The most common approach to the sphenopalatine block is noninvasive and takes advantage of the ganglion's shallow position

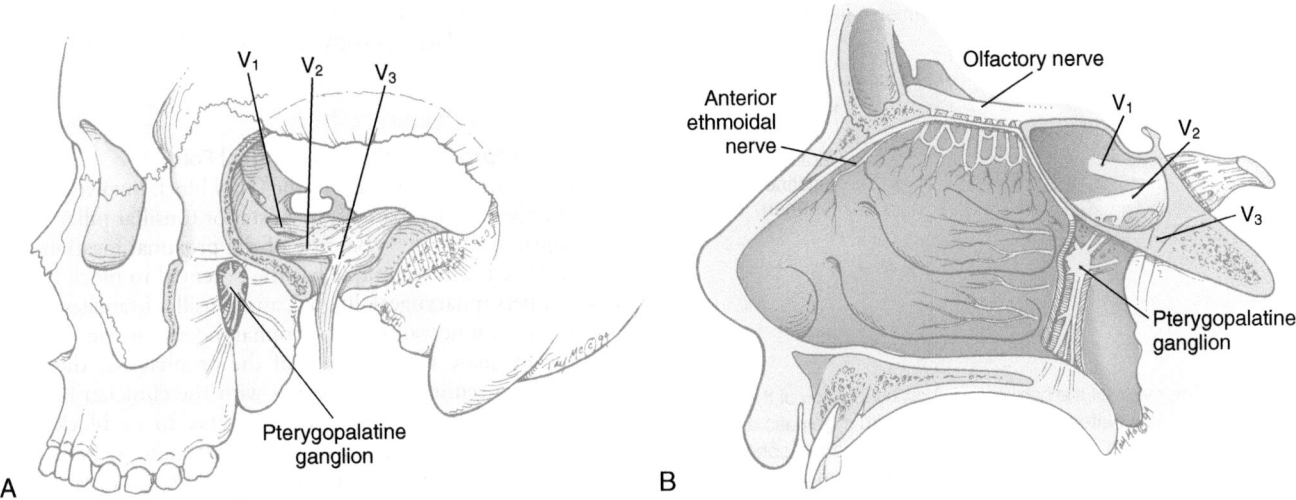

• **Fig. 13.7** (A) Left lateral view of the skull with temporal bone removed depicting the trigeminal ganglion with the three branches (V_1 to V_3) of the trigeminal nerve. V_2 is the major contributor to the sphenopalatine (pterygopalatine) ganglion, shown as it sits in the pterygopalatine fossa. (B) Left lateral view of the right nasal cavity depicting the anterior ethmoidal nerve, olfactory nerve, and trigeminal nerve (V_1 to V_3). The pterygopalatine ganglion lies just beneath the mucosal surface on the caudad surface of the sphenoid sinus and forms the roof of the pterygopalatine fossa. (From Difficult Airway: Teaching Aids. Irvine, University of California, Department of Anesthesia.)

beneath the nasal mucosa. This block anesthetizes the greater and lesser palatine nerves, as well as the nasociliary and nasopalatine nerves, which also contribute to the sensory innervation of the nasal cavity. In addition to providing anesthesia to the nasal cavity, it also blocks sensation from the roof of the mouth, soft palate, and tonsils, making it useful even when a transoral intubation is planned. The block should be performed bilaterally.

A long cotton-tipped swab soaked in either 4% lidocaine with epinephrine 1:200,000 or 3% lidocaine/0.25% phenylephrine is

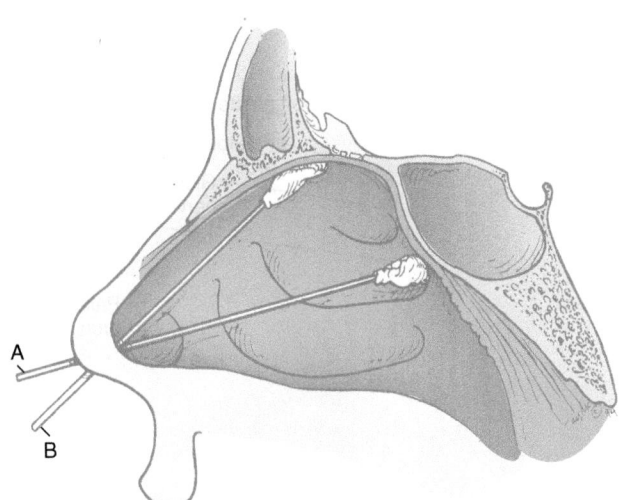

• **Fig. 13.8** Left lateral view of the right nasal cavity, showing long cotton-tipped swabs soaked in local anesthetic. (A) Swab angled at 45 degrees to the hard palate with cotton swab over the mucosal surface overlying the sphenopalatine ganglion. (B) Swab placed parallel to the dorsal surface of the nose, blocking the anterior ethmoidal nerve. (From Difficult Airway: Teaching Aids. Irvine, University of California, Department of Anesthesia.)

applied to the mucosal surface overlying the ganglion (Fig. 13.8A). The swab is passed along the upper border of the middle turbinate at an angle of approximately 45 degrees to the hard palate and directed posteriorly until the upper posterior wall of the nasopharynx (sphenoid bone) is reached. The swab is then left in place for approximately 5 minutes. Alternatively, cotton pledgets soaked in a local anesthetic solution may be used and applied to the nasal cavity in the same manner using bayonet forceps.[138,139]

Oral Approach

An oral approach to the sphenopalatine ganglion block has been described. It is rarely used for airway anesthesia, however, because of its technical difficulty and higher risk of complications; it is included here for completeness. With the patient in the supine position, the clinician stands facing the patient on the contralateral side of the nerve to be blocked. Using the nondominant index finger, the clinician identifies the greater palatine foramen. It is located on either side of the roof of the mouth between the second and third maxillary molars, approximately 1 cm medial to the palatogingival margin, and it can usually be palpated as a small depression near the posterior edge of the hard palate. In approximately 15% of the population, the foramen is closed and inaccessible. A 25-gauge spinal needle, bent 2 to 3 cm proximal to the tip to an angle of 120 degrees, is inserted through the foramen in a superior and slightly posterior direction to a depth of 2 to 3 cm. An aspiration test is performed to ascertain that the sphenopalatine artery has not been cannulated, and 1 to 2 mL of 2% lidocaine with epinephrine 1:100,000 is injected. (Fig. 13.9). The epinephrine is used as a vasoconstrictor for the sphenopalatine artery, which runs parallel to the nerves, to decrease the incidence of epistaxis. The injection of the local anesthetic should be performed in a slow, continuous fashion (preventing acute increases in pressure within the fossa) to decrease sympathetic stimulation. Complications include bleeding, infection, nerve trauma,

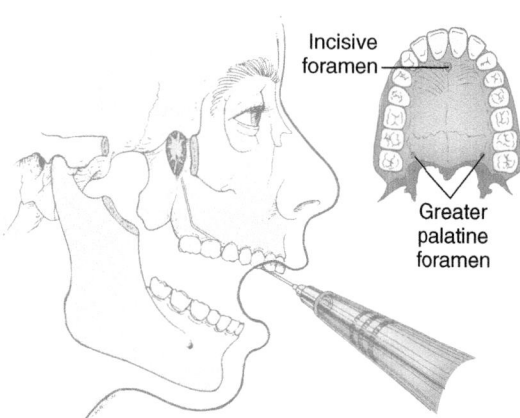

• **Fig. 13.9** Inferior view of the hard palate showing location of the greater palatine foramen. Right lateral view of the head with zygomatic arch and coronoid process of the mandible removed to expose the sphenopalatine ganglion, with angulated spinal needle in place. (From Difficult Airway: Teaching Aids. Irvine, University of California, Department of Anesthesia.)

intravascular injection of local anesthetic, and hypertension. Pain on insertion of the needle can be prevented by application of 2% viscous lidocaine with a cotton-tipped applicator for 1 to 2 minutes before the block is applied.[138,140]

Anterior Ethmoidal Nerve Block

The anterior third of the nasal cavity can usually be sufficiently anesthetized by either topical or inhalational local anesthetic; however, selective blockade of the anterior ethmoidal nerve can also be performed. A long cotton-tipped swab, soaked in either 4% cocaine or 4% lidocaine with epinephrine 1:200,000, is inserted parallel to the dorsal surface of the nose until it meets the anterior surface of the cribriform plate (see Fig. 13.8B). The applicator is held in position for 5 minutes.[140]

Oropharynx

Anatomy

The somatic and visceral afferent sensory fibers of the oropharynx are supplied by a plexus derived from the vagus (CN X), facial (CN VII), and glossopharyngeal (CN IX) nerves. The glossopharyngeal nerve (GPN) emerges from the skull through the jugular foramen and passes anteriorly between the internal jugular and carotid vessels, traveling along the lateral wall of the pharynx. It supplies sensory innervation to the posterior third of the tongue via the lingual branch and to the valleculae, the anterior surface of the epiglottis, the posterior and lateral walls of the pharynx, and the tonsillar pillars. Its only motor innervation in the pharynx is to the stylopharyngeus muscle, one of the muscles of deglutition.[137]

In most patients, topicalization of the mucosa of the oropharynx is sufficient to allow instrumentation of the airway. In some, however, the gag reflex is so pronounced that topicalization alone may be insufficient for awake intubation. The afferent limb of the gag reflex arises from stimulation of deep pressure receptors found in the posterior third of the tongue, which cannot be reached by the diffusion of local anesthetics through the mucosa. Various measures can minimize this problem: instructing the patient to breathe in a nonstop panting fashion, avoiding pressure on the base of the tongue by performing a nasal FSI, administering

opioids, or performing blockade of the GPN. The GPN block is easy to perform and is highly effective in abolishing the gag reflex and decreasing the hemodynamic response to laryngoscopy, including awake laryngoscopy. Several different approaches have been described.

Glossopharyngeal Nerve Block

Posterior Approach (Palatopharyngeal Fold)

The classic intraoral approach to the GPN block involves injecting local anesthetic at the base of the posterior tonsillar pillar (palatopharyngeal fold).[106,141,142] Because of the proximal location of the nerve targeted, this technique has the potential to block both the sensory fibers (pharyngeal, lingual, and tonsillar branches) and the motor branch innervating the stylopharyngeus muscle.

After adequate topicalization of the oropharynx, the patient is placed in a semireclined position with the clinician facing the patient on the ipsilateral side of the nerve to be blocked. The patient's mouth is opened wide. With a tongue depressor held in the nondominant hand, the tongue is displaced caudad and medially, exposing the soft palate, uvula, palatoglossal arch, tonsillar bed, and palatopharyngeal arch (Fig. 13.10). This maneuver stretches both the palatopharyngeal arch and the palatoglossal arch, making them more accessible. A size 3 Macintosh laryngoscope blade may also be useful for retraction, because it provides additional light.[143] The dominant hand holds a 23-gauge tonsillar needle attached to a syringe. Alternatively, a 22-gauge, 9-cm spinal needle with the distal 1 cm of the needle bent at a 90-degree angle may be used. The needle is inserted submucosally into the caudad portion of the posterior tonsillar pillar. After an attempt to aspirate blood, 5 mL of 0.5% to 1% lidocaine is slowly injected. If blood is aspirated or the patient complains of headache during injection, the needle should be removed and repositioned. The procedure is repeated on the contralateral side.

Because of the proximity of the GPN at this location to the internal carotid artery, care must be taken to avoid intraarterial injection, which could result in headache or seizure. Hypopharyngeal swelling and mucosal bleeding may occur. Tachycardia may

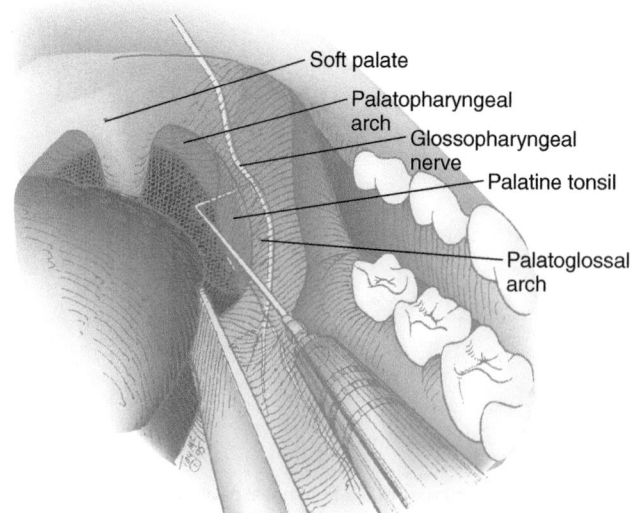

• **Fig. 13.10** Left glossopharyngeal nerve block, posterior approach. A 25-gauge spinal needle bent at a right angle (or a tonsillar needle) is placed behind the midportion of the palatopharyngeal fold. (From Difficult Airway: Teaching Aids. Irvine, University of California, Department of Anesthesia.)

also result from blockade of the afferent nerve fibers of the GPN that arise from the carotid sinus.[144]

Anterior Approach (Palatoglossal Fold)

The lingual branch of the GPN provides sensory innervation to the posterior third of the tongue and is the afferent limb of the gag reflex. The anterior approach, which isolates this branch as it passes medially to the base of the anterior tonsillar pillar, is easier and is better tolerated by the patient because it requires less exposure.[7,145,146]

The patient is placed in the sitting position with the clinician facing the patient on the contralateral side of the nerve to be blocked. The patient's mouth is opened wide with the tongue protruded. With the nondominant hand, the clinician uses a tongue blade or a Macintosh size 3 laryngoscope blade to displace the tongue medially, forming a gutter or trough along the floor of the mouth between the tongue and the teeth. The gutter ends in a cul-de-sac formed by the base of the palatoglossal arch (also known as the *anterior tonsillar pillar*), which is a U- or J-shaped structure that starts at the soft palate and runs along the lateral aspect of the pharynx. A 25-gauge spinal needle is inserted 0.25 to 0.5 cm deep at the base of the palatoglossal arch, just lateral to the base of the tongue, and an aspiration test is performed (Fig. 13.11). If air is aspirated, the needle has been advanced too deeply (i.e., the tip has advanced all the way through the palatoglossal arch) and should be withdrawn until no air can be aspirated; if blood is aspirated, the needle should be redirected more medially. Next, 2 mL of 1% to 2% lidocaine is injected, and the procedure is repeated on the contralateral side. The same procedure can be performed noninvasively with cotton-tipped swabs soaked in 4% lidocaine; the swab is held in place for 5 minutes (see Video 13.1).

Although this block is targeted at the lingual branch of the GPN, studies using methylene blue dye have shown that, in some cases, retrograde submucosal tracking of local anesthetic occurs, blocking more proximal branches of the GPN (i.e., pharyngeal and tonsillar branches). Serious complications are rare for this approach, although one study reported that 91% of patients undergoing this procedure experienced oropharyngeal discomfort for at least 24 hours after the procedure.[147]

External Approach (Peristyloid)

The external approach is most useful when the patient's mouth opening is insufficient to allow adequate visualization to perform one of the intraoral blocks.[106,142] The patient is placed supine with the head in a neutral position. The styloid process is located by identifying the midpoint of the line between the mastoid process and the angle of the jaw. A skin wheal with local anesthetic is made at this location, and a 22-gauge spinal needle is advanced perpendicularly to the skin until the styloid process is contacted. Depending on the patient's habitus, this should occur at a depth of 1 to 2 cm. The needle is then redirected posteriorly, and as soon as contact is lost with the styloid process, 5 to 7 mL of 0.5% to 1% lidocaine is injected after a negative aspiration for blood (Fig. 13.12). The procedure is then repeated on the opposite side. Similar precautions should be taken for the peristyloid approach as for the posterior approach because of the proximity of the GPN at this anatomic location to both the internal carotid artery and the internal jugular vein.

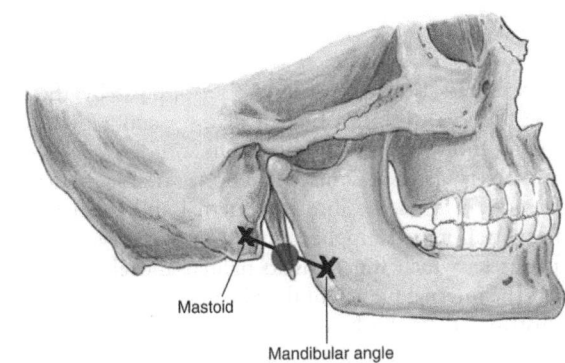

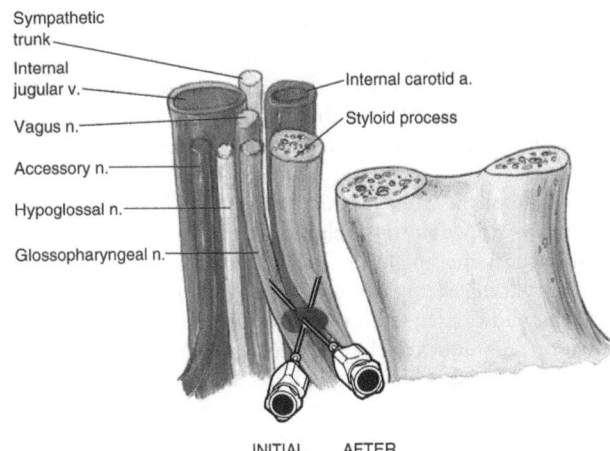

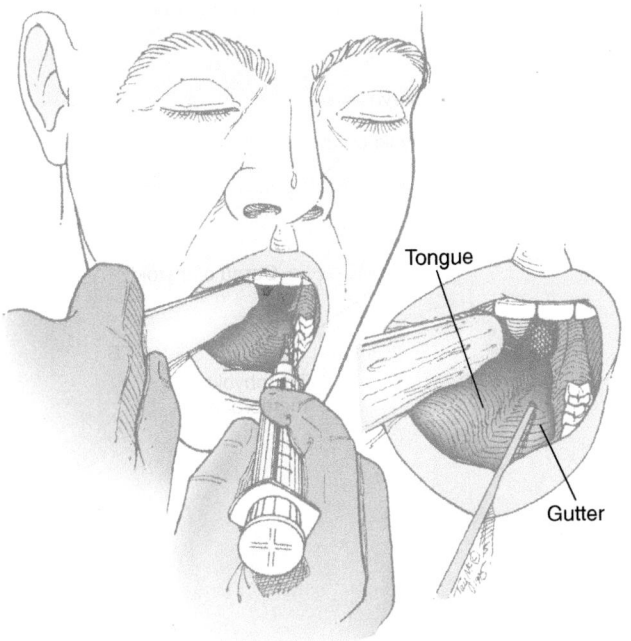

• **Fig. 13.11** Left glossopharyngeal nerve block, anterior approach. The tongue is displaced medially, forming a gutter (glossogingival groove), which ends distally in a cul-de-sac. A 25-gauge spinal needle is placed at the base of the palatoglossal fold. (From Difficult Airway: Teaching Aids. Irvine, University of California, Department of Anesthesia.)

• **Fig. 13.12** Glossopharyngeal nerve block, peristyloid approach. A 22-gauge spinal needle is inserted to contact the styloid process. It is then redirected posteriorly, putting the tip of the needle near the glossopharyngeal nerve. *a.,* Artery; *n.,* nerve; *v.,* vein. (From Brown D, ed. *Atlas of Regional Anesthesia.* 2nd ed. Saunders; 1999.)

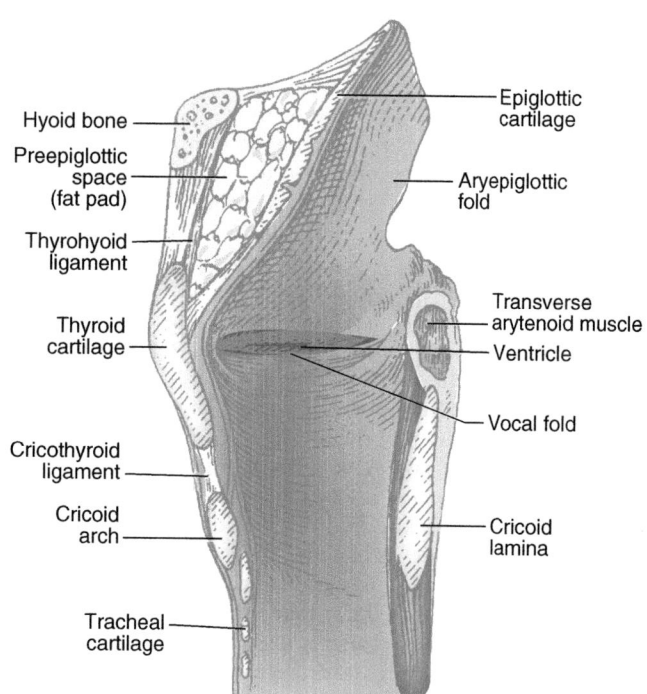

Hyoid bone
Preepiglottic space (fat pad)
Thyrohyoid ligament
Thyroid cartilage
Cricothyroid ligament
Cricoid arch
Tracheal cartilage

Epiglottic cartilage
Aryepiglottic fold
Transverse arytenoid muscle
Ventricle
Vocal fold
Cricoid lamina

• **Fig. 13.13** Midsagittal view of the larynx showing the preepiglottic space containing fat pad and thyrohyoid ligament.

Larynx

Anatomy

Sensory innervation of the larynx is supplied by the superior laryngeal nerve (SLN), a branch of the vagus nerve. The SLN originates from the ganglion nodosum and descends deep to the carotid artery. It then courses anteriorly, and at the level of the hyoid bone it branches into the external and internal branches. The external branch supplies motor innervation to the cricothyroid muscle, which functions to tighten and elongate the vocal cords. The internal branch of the SLN contains sensory fibers that are distributed to the base of the tongue, valleculae, epiglottis, aryepiglottic folds, arytenoids, and glottis down to the level of the vocal cords. It passes medially between the greater horn of the hyoid bone and the superior horn of the thyroid cartilage and pierces the thyrohyoid membrane along with the superior laryngeal artery and vein. The nerve then lies in the paraglottic space, a closed space bounded by the thyrohyoid membrane laterally and the laryngeal mucosa medially, where it ramifies (Figs. 13.13 and 13.14).

Blockade of the SLN produces dense anesthesia of the hypopharynx and upper glottis, including the valleculae and the laryngeal surface of the epiglottis. When performed in combination with oropharyngeal topical anesthesia, with or without a GPN block, this allows adequate airway anesthesia for a variety of awake intubation techniques, including direct laryngoscopy. In the external approach, local anesthetic is injected into the paraglottic or preepiglottic space, targeting the nerve soon after it pierces the thyrohyoid ligament. The internal approach targets the nerve as it courses submucosally in the region of the pyriform recess.

Superior Laryngeal Nerve Block

External Approach

In the external approach, the patient is placed in the supine position, head slightly extended, with the clinician standing on the

side to be blocked. The two main anatomic structures that are useful to identify are the hyoid bone and the superior horn of the thyroid cartilage. The hyoid bone lies above the thyroid cartilage. It is identified by deep palpation; this can be uncomfortable to the patient and is difficult in patients who have a short or thick neck. Because it does not articulate with any other bones, the hyoid is freely movable, which helps in its identification. The greater horn of the hyoid is the most lateral aspect of the bone that can be palpated. One side can be made more prominent by displacing the contralateral side toward the side being blocked. The superior lateral horn of the thyroid cartilage can be identified by palpating the superior thyroid notch, the "Adam's apple," and tracing the upper edge of the thyroid cartilage laterally until the most lateral aspect is identified. Three techniques using different landmarks have been described (see Fig. 13.14).[106,141,148–150] Using 1% to 2% lidocaine, satisfactory sensory blockade is achieved within 5 minutes, with a success rate of 92% to 100%.[148]

Greater Horn of the Hyoid. After identifying the greater horn of the hyoid, the clinician uses the nondominant index finger to depress the carotid artery laterally and posteriorly. With the dominant hand, a 25-gauge needle is "walked off" the horn of the hyoid bone (see Fig. 13.14A) in an anterior-inferior direction, aiming toward the middle of the thyrohyoid membrane. A slight resistance is felt as the needle is advanced through the membrane, usually at a depth of 1 to 2 cm (2 to 3 mm deep to the hyoid bone). The needle at this point has entered the preepiglottic space. Aspiration through the needle should be attempted. If air is aspirated, the needle has gone too deep and may have entered the pharynx; it should be withdrawn until no air can be aspirated. If

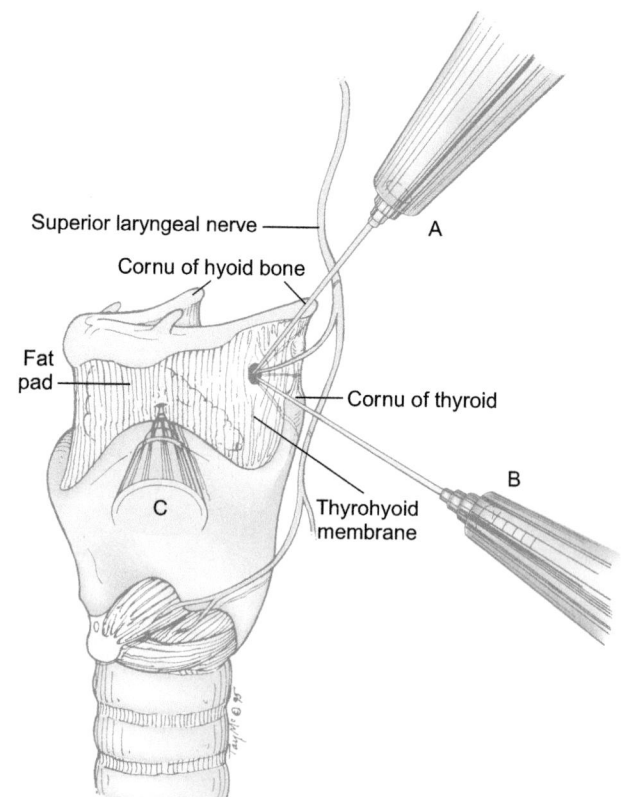

Superior laryngeal nerve
Cornu of hyoid bone
Fat pad
Cornu of thyroid
Thyrohyoid membrane
A
B
C

• **Fig. 13.14** Superior laryngeal nerve block, external approach using as a landmark (A) the greater horn of the hyoid bone, (B) the superior horn of the thyroid cartilage, or (C) the thyroid notch. (From Difficult Airway Teaching Aids. Irvine, University of California, Department of Anesthesia.)

blood is aspirated, the needle has cannulated the superior laryngeal artery or vein or the carotid artery; the needle should be directed more anteriorly. After satisfactory needle placement is achieved, 2 to 3 mL of local anesthetic is injected as the needle is withdrawn. The block is repeated on the opposite side.

Superior Horn of the Thyroid. A similar technique to the one previously described uses the superior lateral horn of the thyroid as the landmark. The benefit of this technique is that, in many patients, this structure is easier and less painful to palpation than the hyoid bone. A 25-gauge needle is walked off the horn of the thyroid cartilage (see Fig. 13.14B) in a superior-anterior direction, aiming toward the lower third of the thyroid membrane. The same precautions as before are taken, and 2 to 3 mL local anesthetic solution is injected as the needle is withdrawn. The block is repeated on the opposite side.

Thyroid Notch. The easiest landmark to identify in many patients, especially in the morbidly obese, is the superior thyroid notch (Adam's apple), the most medial and superficial aspect of the thyroid cartilage. The thyroid notch is palpated, and the upper border of the thyroid cartilage is traced laterally for approximately 2 cm (see Fig. 13.14C). With a 25-gauge needle, the thyrohyoid ligament is pierced just above the thyroid cartilage at this location, and the needle is advanced in a posterior and cephalad direction to a depth of 1 to 2 cm from the skin. The tip of the needle is then in the preepiglottic space, which normally contains the terminal branches of the internal branch of the SLN imbedded in a fat pad (see Fig. 13.13). After an aspiration test, 2 to 3 mL of local anesthetic is injected into the preepiglottic space, and the needle is withdrawn. The block is repeated on the opposite side. An added benefit of this approach is the decreased likelihood of blocking the motor branch of the SLN.

Ultrasound-Guided Technique. The use of ultrasonography to facilitate SLN blockade may be beneficial when the patient's anatomy is difficult to ascertain as a result of obesity, malignancy, or abscess. The technique that has been most used clinically involves sonographic visualization of the hyoid bone and SLN.[151,152] A potentially simpler technique involving identification of the thyrohyoid membrane without visualization of the SLN has been studied in cadavers.[153] A prospective, randomized study of this latter technique in 40 patients demonstrated improved quality of anesthesia and slightly shorter time to intubation with the ultrasound-guided technique compared to a landmark-guided one.[154] One primary difference of these ultrasound-guided techniques compared with the anatomically guided techniques is that the local anesthetic is injected anterior to the thyrohyoid membrane, targeting the SLN before it pierces the thyrohyoid membrane.

When performing an SLN block, care should be taken to avoid insertion of the needle into the thyroid cartilage, to preclude the possibility of injecting the local anesthetic at the level of the vocal cords, which could cause laryngeal edema and airway obstruction. The carotid artery should be identified and displaced posteriorly to minimize the risk of intravascular injection; even small amounts (0.25 to 0.5 mL) of local anesthetic injected into the carotid artery can induce seizures.[155]

Hypotension and bradycardia have also been associated with SLN blockade. A number of possible causes of this reaction have been postulated, including (1) vasovagal reaction related to painful stimulation; (2) digital pressure on the carotid sinus; (3) excessive manipulation of the larynx, causing vasovagal reaction; (4) large doses of or accidental intravascular administration of local anesthetic drugs; and (5) direct neural stimulation of the branch of the vagus nerve by the needle.[156] It is recommended that anticholinergics be administered before the block is performed.

Complications of the external approach also include hematoma and pharyngeal puncture, resulting in the aspiration of air. The needle should be withdrawn until no more air is aspirated before local anesthetic is injected. Contraindications to the external approach include local infection, local tumor growth, and coagulopathy. Although not universally accepted, some have advocated avoidance of SLN anesthesia in patients who are at high risk for aspiration.[157,158]

Internal Approach

A noninvasive SLN block can be performed by applying local anesthetic to the pyriform recess. At this anatomic location, the internal branch of the SLN lies submucosally, and blockade is possible by diffusion of concentrated local anesthetic.[159] After adequate topicalization of the oropharynx, the patient is placed in the sitting position with the clinician standing on the contralateral side of the nerve to be blocked. The patient's mouth is opened widely with the tongue protruded. The tongue is grasped with the nondominant hand using a gauze pad and gently pulled anteriorly, or it is depressed with a tongue blade. With the dominant hand, a Krause forceps holding a sponge soaked in 4% lidocaine is advanced over the lateral posterior curvature of the tongue along the downward continuation of the tonsillar fossa (Fig. 13.15). The tip of the forceps is advanced until it cannot be advanced any farther (Fig. 13.16); at that point, the handle of the forceps should be in a horizontal position and the tip should be resting in the pyriform recess. The position of the tip of the forceps may be checked by palpating the neck lateral to the posterior-superior aspect of the thyroid cartilage. The forceps are kept in this position for 5 minutes or longer, and then the process is repeated on the opposite side. This approach requires a considerable length of time and is limited to those patients who can open their mouths sufficiently wide.

Trachea and Vocal Cords

Anatomy

The sensory innervation of the trachea, inferior larynx, and vocal cords is supplied by the recurrent (inferior) laryngeal nerves, which are branches of the vagus nerve. The right recurrent laryngeal nerve (RLN) originates at the level of the right subclavian artery; the left originates at the level of the aortic arch, distal to the ligamentum

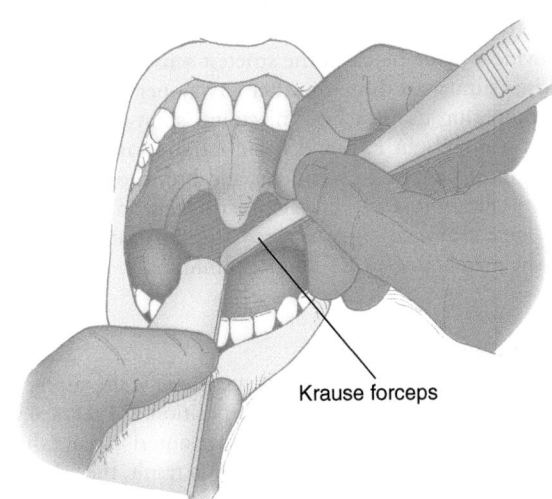

• **Fig. 13.15** Superior laryngeal nerve block, internal approach. A Krause forceps is advanced over the tongue toward the pyriform sinus. (From Difficult Airway: Teaching Aids. Irvine, University of California, Department of Anesthesia.)

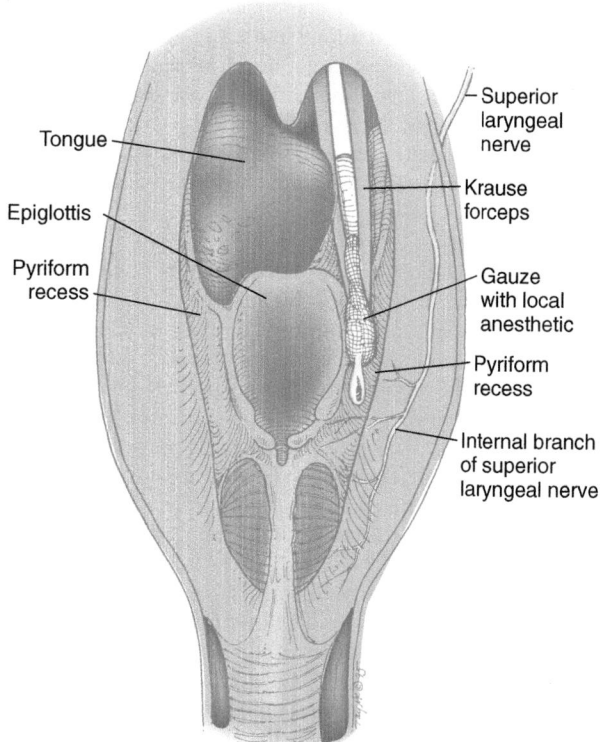

Tongue

Epiglottis

Pyriform
recess

Superior
laryngeal
nerve

Krause
forceps

Gauze
with local
anesthetic

Pyriform
recess

Internal branch
of superior
laryngeal nerve

• **Fig. 13.16** Superior laryngeal nerve block, internal approach. Posterior view of the larynx showing tip of Krause forceps at the level of the pyriform sinus. (From Difficult Airway: Teaching Aids. Irvine, University of California, Department of Anesthesia.)

arteriosum. Both ascend along the tracheoesophageal groove to supply sensory innervation to the tracheobronchial tree up to and including the vocal cords, as well as supplying motor nerve fibers to the intrinsic muscles of the larynx (except the cricothyroid muscle). Because the sensory and motor fibers run together, nerve blocks cannot be performed because they would result in bilateral vocal cord paralysis and complete airway obstruction.

The alternative is topicalization of the tracheal mucosa. In addition to the use of a nebulizer, atomizer, or "spray-as-you-go" technique, topicalization of the trachea may be achieved by transtracheal (translaryngeal) injection. Although this technique does not provide a nerve block in the strictest sense, it is invasive and bears risks similar to those of other airway nerve blocks. In one study comparing transtracheal injection, "spray-as-you-go" topicalization through an FSI, and nebulization, transtracheal injection was most preferred by patients and bronchoscopists.[160] Tracheal topicalization is also of particular benefit in cases in which a neurologic examination is required after intubation, because it makes the presence of an ETT more comfortable.

Transtracheal (Translaryngeal) Anesthesia
Positioning and Landmarks
The ideal position for transtracheal anesthesia is the supine position with the neck in extension. In this position, the cervical vertebrae push the trachea and cricoid cartilage anteriorly and displace the strap muscles of the neck laterally. As a result, the cricoid cartilage and the structures above and below it are easier to palpate. The thyroid cartilage is palpated at midline and followed caudally until a depression and a firm ring of tissue are identified. These are the cricothyroid groove and the cricoid cartilage, respectively. Overlying the cricoid groove is the cricothyroid membrane.

Technique
The clinician should stand at the side of the patient with the dominant hand closest to the patient. The patient is asked not to talk, swallow, or cough until instructed. The midline of the cricothyroid membrane is identified as the needle insertion site. The index and middle finger of the nondominant hand can be used to mark this spot and stabilize the trachea (Fig. 13.17). Using a tuberculin syringe or a 25-gauge needle, the clinician raises a small skin wheal. A 20-gauge angiocatheter attached to a 5- to 10-mL syringe containing 3 to 5 mL saline is used. The needle is advanced through the skin perpendicularly or slightly caudally while aspirating. When air is freely aspirated, the sheath of the angiocatheter is advanced slightly, the needle is removed, and a syringe containing 3 to 5 mL of 2% to 4% lidocaine is carefully attached to the catheter sheath that has been left in place. Aspiration of air is reconfirmed, the patient is warned to expect vigorous coughing, and the local anesthetic is injected rapidly during inspiration (Fig. 13.18). The sheath of the angiocatheter may be left in place until the intubation is complete in case more local anesthetic is needed and to decrease the likelihood of subcutaneous emphysema. Coughing helps to nebulize the local anesthetic so that the inferior and superior surfaces of the vocal cords can be anesthetized along with the tracheobronchial tree and inferior larynx. Anesthesia of the epiglottis, valleculae, tongue, and posterior pharyngeal wall are possible but unreliable. The success of transtracheal anesthesia has been found to be as high as 95% and is attributed to both topicalization of the airway and systemic absorption (see Video 13.2).[106,140]

This technique may also be performed using a standard 20- or 22-gauge needle. This may, however, increase the risk of airway injury from the sharp metal bevel as the patient coughs. If this technique is used, care should be taken to remove the needle immediately after injection of the local anesthetic. This technique has also been described using a 25-gauge needle, but this is not recommended because it introduces the risk of needle breakage as a result of movement of the cricoid cartilage cephalad when the patient coughs.[161] The use of ultrasonography to identify the cricothyroid membrane is more reliable than palpation alone, and may be particularly useful in patients with anatomic landmarks that are difficult to identify.[162]

To avoid laryngeal trauma and to ensure adequate spread of local anesthetic below the vocal cords, the tip of the needle should never be aimed in a cephalad direction. Because this procedure eliminates the patient's ability to protect the airway from aspiration, it should not be performed in patients who are at high risk for aspiration. Coughing elicited by this block may result in increased heart rate, mean arterial blood pressure, ICP, and intraocular pressure. Therefore, it is contraindicated in patients with elevated ICP or open globe, and care should be taken in patients with significant cardiac disease. It is also relatively contraindicated in patients with cervical instability, although its routine use in these patients has been described without complications.[163] Transtracheal injection should be avoided in patients with local tumor or large goiter.

Potential complications are similar to those described for retrograde intubation (see Chapter 21). They include subcutaneous and intratracheal bleeding, infection, subcutaneous emphysema,[164] pneumomediastinum, pneumothorax, vocal cord trauma, and esophageal perforation. These complications are rare, as was illustrated by a review of 17,500 cases of transtracheal puncture that showed an incidence of complications of less than 0.01%.[158]

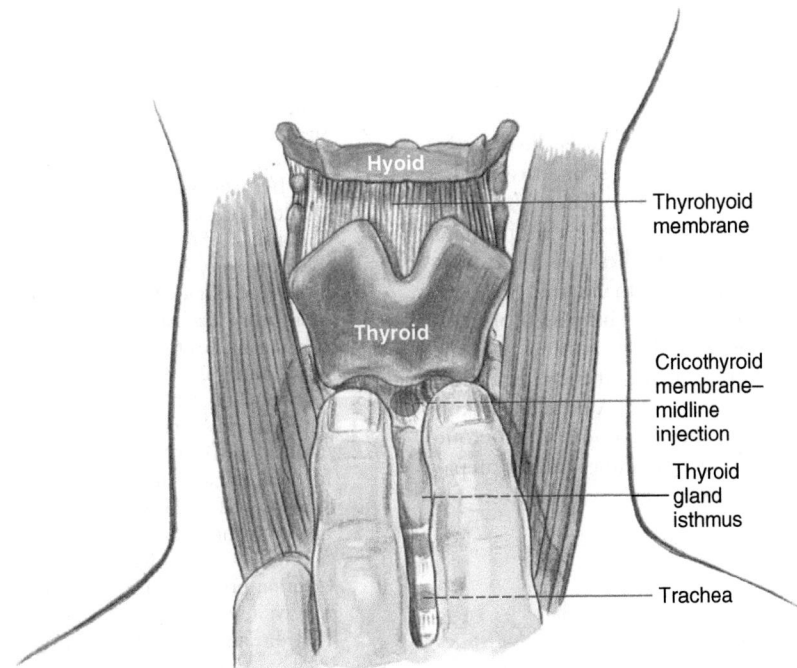

• **Fig. 13.17** Transtracheal anesthesia, anatomic landmarks. (From Brown D, ed. *Atlas of Regional Anesthesia*. 2nd ed. Saunders; 1999.)

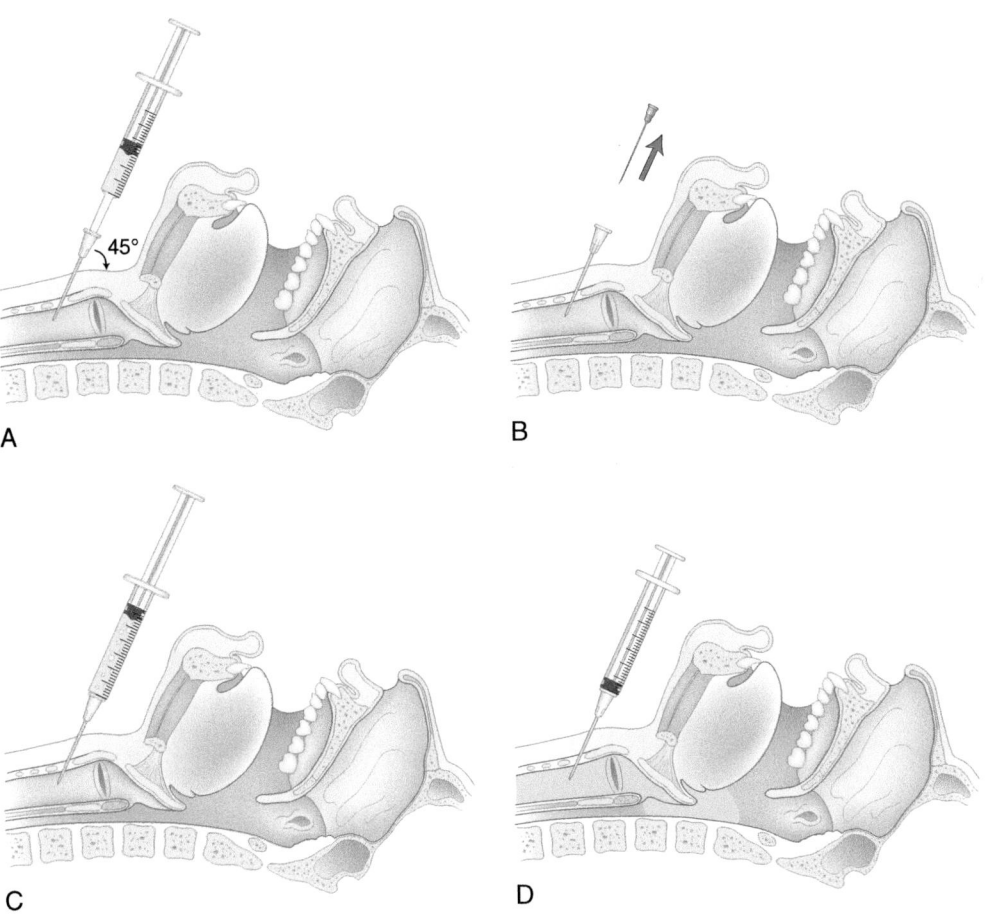

• **Fig. 13.18** Transtracheal anesthesia (midsagittal view of the head and neck). (A) The angiocatheter is inserted at the cricothyroid membrane, aimed caudally. An aspiration test is performed to verify the position of the tip of the needle in the tracheal lumen. (B) The needle is removed from the angiocatheter. (C) With the syringe containing local anesthetic attached, the aspiration test is repeated. (D) Local anesthetic is injected, resulting in coughing and nebulization of the local anesthetic *(shaded area)*. (From The Retrograde Cookbook. Irvine, University of California, Department of Anesthesia.)

Conclusion

Once the decision to perform an awake intubation has been made, the clinician has many choices to make regarding the mode of preparation and the technique to be used. Regardless of the indication for awake intubation, these clinical situations involve greater risk than a standard anesthetic technique. Safety should be the primary concern. Sedation should generally be a supplement to, rather than a substitute for, topical anesthesia of the airway. As long as the patient is awake, cooperative, maintaining the airway, and spontaneously ventilating, no bridges have been burned. The clinician should be comfortable with the techniques used for topicalization and intubation—during management of a critical airway is not the time to learn a new technique. A detailed backup plan should be in place in the event that the primary technique planned is unsuccessful. With the proper planning, patient preparation, and technique, awake intubation is an invaluable tool for management of the DA.

Selected References

1. Apfelbaum JL, Hagberg CA, Caplan RA, et al. Practice guidelines for management of the difficult airway: an updated report by the American Society of Anesthesiologists Task Force on Management of the Difficult Airway. *Anesthesiology.* 2013;118(2):251–270.

4. Ahmad I, El-Boghdadly K, Bhagrath R, et al. Difficult Airway Society guidelines for awake tracheal intubation (ATI) in adults. *Anaesthesia.* 2020;75(4):509–528.

7. Benumof JL. Management of the difficult adult airway. With special emphasis on awake tracheal intubation. *Anesthesiology.* 1991;75(6):1087–1110.

10. Law JA, Morris IR, Brousseau PA, de la Ronde S, Milne AD. The incidence, success rate, and complications of awake tracheal intubation in 1,554 patients over 12 years: an historical cohort study. *Can J Anaesth.* 2015;62(7):736–744.

17. Patel A, Nouraei SA. Transnasal Humidified Rapid-Insufflation Ventilatory Exchange (THRIVE): a physiological method of increasing apnoea time in patients with difficult airways. *Anaesthesia.* 2015;70(3):323–329.

53. Johnston KD, Rai MR. Conscious sedation for awake fibreoptic intubation: a review of the literature. *Can J Anaesth.* 2013;60(6):584–599.

67. Atkins JH, Mirza N. Anesthetic considerations and surgical caveats for awake airway surgery. *Anesthesiol Clin.* 2010;28(3):555–575.

106. Simmons ST, Schleich AR. Airway regional anesthesia for awake fiberoptic intubation. *Reg Anesth Pain Med.* 2002;27(2):180–192.

108. Cabrini L, Baiardo Redaelli M, Ball L, et al. Awake Fiberoptic intubation protocols in the operating room for anticipated difficult airway: a systematic review and meta-analysis of randomized controlled trials. *Anesth Analg.* 2019;128(5):971–980.

140. Hagberg CA. Airway blocks. In: Chelly JE, ed. *Peripheral Nerve Blocks: A Color Atlas.* Wolters Kluwer Health/Lippincott Williams & Wilkins; 2009.

All references can be found online at eBooks.Health.Elsevier.com.

14

Aspiration Prevention and Prophylaxis: Preoperative Considerations for the Full Stomach Patient

MARKO ZDRAVKOVIC AND OLIVIER LANGERON

CHAPTER OUTLINE

KEY POINTS

- The incidence of pulmonary aspiration in the general surgical population is low, but it is slightly increased among obstetric, pediatric, and trauma patients. It remains the leading cause of death related to airway management.
- Regurgitation and aspiration can result from "light" anesthesia, coughing, or gagging in the patient whose airway is not protected with a cuffed endotracheal tube (ETT).
- Patients manifesting no evidence of respiratory impairment for 2 hours after a known or suspected aspiration episode are highly unlikely to become significantly symptomatic later.
- Preoperative ultrasonography of the gastric antrum may be used to screen patients at risk for perioperative pulmonary aspiration of regurgitated gastric contents.
- Both pain and opioids significantly delay gastric emptying.
- Aspiration of particulate antacids can induce a severe granulomatous pneumonitis.

- Ingestion of clear liquids 2 to 3 hours before anesthetic induction does not appear to increase the risk of gastric content aspiration in patients with no gastrointestinal pathology.
- Cricoid pressure can compromise ventilation by either face mask or supraglottic airway and can interfere with direct laryngoscopy, thus requiring discontinuation in certain circumstances.
- Routine preoperative use of gastrointestinal stimulants, H_2-receptor antagonists, and proton pump inhibitors is not recommended in patients with no increased risk of pulmonary aspiration.
- Meticulous attention to airway management during induction, through emergence, and after extubation is crucial for patients at risk for pulmonary aspiration. Approximately 50% of all cases of perioperative aspiration occur at times other than anesthetic induction.

Introduction

Pulmonary aspiration is a rare event. Yet, it is still about 10 times more common as an airway management complication than is the failure to oxygenate. Prevention of pulmonary aspiration is thus one of the basic goals of anesthetic care. In this chapter we will provide a thorough review of risk factors for pulmonary aspiration, preventive techniques, medical prophylaxis, and management strategies. The need for conscious adherence to deliberate practice principles and to development and maintenance of expertise in airway management as a key for the anesthesia provider to minimize the risk of pulmonary aspiration is highlighted.

Perioperative Aspiration

Perioperative pulmonary aspiration of regurgitated gastric contents is conceptually defined as the presence of gastric or bilious secretions or particulate matter in the tracheobronchial tree. In research and clinical practice, the method of diagnosis differs substantially: from visual confirmation (either direct visual or bronchoscopic confirmation), biochemical analysis of tracheal aspirate (pepsin A or pH), or postoperative imaging that demonstrates lung infiltrates not previously identified on a preoperative chest radiograph. The pulmonary aspiration of gastric contents has generated a body of research and recrimination that might seem disproportionate to its reported incidence. Yet, it remains one of the leading causes of mortality and morbidity related to the management of the airways.[1]

Most cases of pulmonary aspiration occur during induction of anesthesia and initial airway management (50%) or during and after emergence from anesthesia.[2-5] The basic tenet of a safe anesthesia management plan for reducing the incidence of pulmonary aspiration of gastric contents is preoperative fasting, which, in the past, led to prolonged rituals that have been more recently challenged, at least with respect to fluids. Crucial to pulmonary aspiration prevention is identifying those at risk and applying appropriate airway management techniques that may reduce the risk of pulmonary aspiration.

Incidence

The overall incidence of perioperative pulmonary aspiration is between 1 and 5 per 10,000 anesthetics.[1-5] A multicenter, prospective study of almost 200,000 surgeries performed in France found the overall incidence of clinically apparent aspiration to be 1.4 per 10,000 anesthetics.[2] Warner and colleagues retrospectively reviewed more than 215,000 general anesthetics and found an incidence of aspiration of 3.1 per 10,000 cases.[3] Olsson and colleagues examined the records of more than 175,000 anesthetics administered at one hospital over more than 13 years and reported an incidence of aspiration of 4.7 per 10,000.[4] In their 1999 review of 133 Australian cases, Kluger and Short reported that the incidence of passive regurgitation was three times that of active vomiting and that a majority of aspiration episodes accompanied anesthetics delivered by face mask or supraglottic airway (SGA).[5] Among those who aspirated, 38% developed radiographic infiltrates, more often in the right lung than in the left. The authors also noted that a recurring theme in many incidents was inadequate depth of anesthesia leading to coughing/straining and subsequent regurgitation/vomiting.[5]

Aspiration of gastric contents was the primary adverse event in 17% of major complications as reported in the Fourth National Audit Project (NAP4) of the Royal College of Anaesthetists and the Difficult Airway Society, which examined records for major complications among 2.9 million general anesthetics and airway management procedures across the United Kingdom.[1] The audit revealed 184 serious airway-related complications that led to unanticipated admission to or prolonged stay in the intensive care unit, emergency invasive airway access, brain damage, and/or death. The report showed that pulmonary aspiration remains a serious issue and was responsible for 50% of anesthesia-related deaths related to airway management.[1]

Several authors have observed that only 50% or less of episodes of perioperative aspiration occur during anesthetic induction and intubation, perhaps because concern is less heightened at other times.[1-7] These potentially catastrophic events also take place before induction (when the unguarded patient may be excessively sedated), during anesthesia maintenance, and during or after emergence and extubation. Interestingly, the incidence of pulmonary aspiration rises to 50 per 10,000 anesthetics for patients who are managed with rapid sequence induction and intubation (RSI) and to 280 per 10,000 when RSI is performed outside the operating room.[8,9]

Consequences

When aspiration does occur, the subsequent clinical course can range from benign to fatal. Olsson and colleagues reported that 18% of patients who aspirated perioperatively required mechanical ventilatory support and 5% died; all those who died had a poor preoperative physical status.[4] Warner and colleagues reported that 64% of patients did not exhibit coughing, wheezing, radiographic abnormalities, or a 10% decrease in arterial oxygen saturation from preoperative room air values during the first 2 hours after aspiration.[3] Such patients, who remained asymptomatic for 2 hours, developed no respiratory sequelae. Of the patients who did manifest signs or symptoms of pulmonary aspiration within 2 hours after the event, 54% required mechanical ventilatory support for 6 hours or longer, and 25% were ventilated for more than 24 hours. Approximately 50% of those ventilated for 24 hours or longer died, generating an overall mortality rate of up to 5% of all aspiration events.[3]

Mortality rates resulting from perioperative pulmonary aspiration have ranged from less than 5% to more than 80% in other reports.[3,10,11] In the aforementioned studies of Warner and Olsson, there were no deaths in healthy patients undergoing elective surgery.[3,4] In a review of more than 85,000 Scandinavian anesthetics, only 3 of 25 patients who aspirated developed serious morbidity, 2 of whom endured a prolonged course of illness but all of whom survived.[12] In general, most healthy patients who aspirate only gastric fluid can expect to survive without residual respiratory impairment, as long as aspiration is promptly recognized and adequately managed.

Risk Factors

Demographic

Published surveys have associated some patient characteristics or circumstances with an increased incidence of aspiration. Warner and colleagues noted that the relative risk of aspiration was more than four times higher for emergency surgeries compared with elective surgeries.[3] A higher American Society of Anesthesiologists (ASA) physical status classification also was associated with a higher risk of aspiration. The incidence of aspiration increased from 1.1 per 10,000 elective anesthetics in ASA class I patients to 29.2 per 10,000 emergency anesthetics in ASA class IV and V patients. Age, gender, pregnancy, concurrent administration of opioids, obesity, experience of anesthesia provider, and types of surgical procedure—contrary to conventional wisdom—were not

Regurgitation or vomiting
Hypotension
Opioids
Increased intragastric volume and pressure
Decreased lower esophageal barrier pressure
Incompetent laryngeal protective reflexes
Neurologic disease
Neuromuscular disease
Central nervous system depressants
Advanced age or debility

Increased gastric filling
Air insufflation during mask ventilation
Increased gastric acid production
Gastrin
Histamine$_2$ (H$_2$) receptor stimulation
Recent ethanol ingestion
Recent hypoglycemic episode
Decreased gastric emptying
Intestinal obstruction
Diabetic gastroparesis
Opioids
Anticholinergics
Sympathetic stimulation (pain and anxiety)

independent risk factors for pulmonary aspiration.[3] In Warner's study, the most common predisposing condition in all patients was gastrointestinal obstruction.[3] In a retrospective review of pediatric cases, aspiration occurred significantly more often in patients with greater severity of underlying illness (Box 14.1).[13]

Olsson and colleagues found that children and the elderly were more likely than patients of intermediate ages to aspirate perioperatively.[4] Statistically, the risk of aspiration was more than three times higher in emergency surgeries than in elective operations. The incidence of aspiration was increased more than sixfold when surgery was performed at night rather than during daylight hours. More recent studies of both adult and pediatric cases have confirmed an impressive increase in the incidence of perioperative aspiration in emergency situations.[1,8,9,12]

Pulmonary aspiration has been demonstrated to occur more frequently after difficulty with airway management.[2] In Olsson's study, 15 of 83 aspirations occurred in patients with no known risk factors; of these, 10 were associated with airway difficulty, suggesting that unanticipated difficult airway may be an important risk factor for pulmonary aspiration.[4]

Although regional techniques are often favored for patients at increased risk for aspiration, elderly patients, in particular, have been reported to vomit and aspirate during spinal anesthesia. Hypotension resulting from neuraxial sympathectomy can induce nausea and vomiting, and supplemental analgesics and sedatives given during lengthy operations can significantly obtund protective airway reflexes.[4,14,15]

Barrier Pressure

Patients who are likely to have gastric contents of increased volume or acidity, elevated intragastric pressure, or decreased tone of the lower esophageal sphincter (LES) traditionally are considered to be at increased risk for perioperative pulmonary aspiration (Boxes 14.1 and 14.2).[11,16] The LES forms a boundary between the stomach and the esophagus, creating a sling around the abdominal esophagus to prevent reflux of gastric contents into the esophagus. Intragastric pressure is normally less than 7 mm Hg; the difference between LES pressure and gastric pressure is the *barrier pressure*, which is typically 15 to 25 mm Hg in conscious individuals. An incompetent LES reduces barrier pressure, increasing the risk of regurgitation of gastric contents, such as in patients with gastroesophageal reflux disease (GERD). Likewise, elevated intragastric pressure, such as when the stomach is distended postprandially, reduces barrier pressure and increases the risk of regurgitation.[17] Gastric distention with increased intragastric pressure causes reflex relaxation of the LES with resultant reflux.

Anesthetic agents relax the LES, reduce barrier pressure, and predispose the patient to regurgitation.[18] Cricoid pressure (CP)

application and laryngoscopy during anesthesia also decrease LES tone.[19] Drugs that lower LES tone include anticholinergics, benzodiazepines, dopamine, sodium nitroprusside, thiopental, tricyclic antidepressants, β-adrenergic stimulants, opioids, and propofol.[20] Inhalational anesthetic agents can reduce the LES pressure below the intragastric pressure, depending on the degree of relaxation.[18] Recent ethanol ingestion or hypoglycemic episodes stimulate gastric acid secretion, whereas tobacco inhalation temporarily lowers LES tone. LES tone also has been found to be reduced by gastric fluid acidity, caffeine, chocolate, and fatty foods.[11] Drugs that increase LES pressure include antiemetics, cholinergic drugs, succinylcholine (also increases the intragastric pressure), pancuronium, metoclopramide, neostigmine, metoprolol, α-adrenergic stimulants, and antacids.[18]

Surgical outpatients traditionally have been thought to have increased gastric volume and reduced gastric pH, possibly because of preoperative anxiety. Clinical studies, however, have not consistently confirmed this expectation and have failed to confirm an increased risk of pulmonary aspiration in the outpatient, with no correlation between anxiety or outpatient status and gastric residual.[2] Furthermore, Hardy and colleagues contradicted several conventional notions by finding that neither gastric volume nor pH correlated with preoperative anxiety, body mass index (BMI), ethanol or tobacco intake, or history of GERD.[16]

Obesity

Obese patients traditionally have been thought to pose a relatively high risk for aspiration because of increased gastric volume and acidity, increased intragastric pressure, and a higher incidence of GERD[20]; however, this assumption has been challenged. In 1998, Harter and colleagues studied 232 fasted, nondiabetic surgical patients who had received no relevant preoperative medication; they found that obese patients had a lower incidence of elevated gastric volume and acidity compared with nonobese patients.[20] Grading obesity by BMI, they also found no association between degree of obesity and gastric fluid volume or pH.[20] Verdich and colleagues reported that obese and lean patients did not differ in rate of gastric emptying during the first 3 hours after a test meal.[21] LES pressure also has been shown not to differ significantly between obese and nonobese patients.[20]

On the other hand, the difficulties with airway management that arise from obesity, along with the association between airway difficulty and aspiration, appear to increase the risk of aspiration in obese patients regardless of their gastrointestinal motility.

Clinical studies on the incidence of difficult intubation in the obese have been contradictory.[22–25] In a review of the topic, it has been reported that obese patients develop oxygen desaturation faster than the nonobese, and the safe apneic period is reduced from more than 5 minutes to less than 2 to 3 minutes in the preoxygenated state.[7] In addition, because obese patients are at a high risk for difficult mask ventilation,[26] gastric insufflation may occur as a result of increased airway pressures during mask ventilation. Thus, the risk of regurgitation in an obese patient may be increased because of intragastric pressure increases. Nevertheless, morbidity in obese patients occurs more often from hypoxemia related to decreased functional residual capacity during difficult or failed intubation than from aspiration.[7] With the increased frequency of bariatric procedures, clinicians should recognize that patients who have previously undergone bariatric surgery are at particular risk for aspiration because of their gastric dysfunction.[27]

Systemic Diseases

Patients with connective tissue, neurologic, metabolic, or neuromuscular disease may be at risk for esophageal dysfunction or laryngeal incompetence. Progressive systemic sclerosis and myotonic dystrophy have been specifically mentioned in case reports.[28–30] Gastric emptying time in patients with Parkinson disease was shown to be delayed compared with control volunteers and was even slower in patients treated with levodopa.[31] Advanced age may be associated with attenuated cough or gag reflexes.

Long-standing diabetes mellitus is well known to delay gastric emptying and also may compromise LES function.[32] Several authors have reported a high incidence of gastroparesis and prolonged mean gastric emptying times, at least for solid foods, in diabetic patients compared with control subjects.[33–36] Impairment of gastric motility was usually found to correlate with findings of autonomic neuropathy but not with peripheral neuropathy or with indices of glycemic stability.

Pregnancy

Pregnancy imposes a constellation of potential risk factors for regurgitation of gastric contents. The enlarging uterus increases intragastric pressure by compressing the stomach, physically delays gastric emptying by pushing the pylorus cephalad and posteriorly, and promotes gastroesophageal reflux by altering the angle of the gastroesophageal junction. Progesterone decreases LES tone, and excess gastrin produced by the placenta promotes gastric acid secretion.[32,37,38] The alterations in anatomy that are typical of late pregnancy can interfere with laryngoscopy and tracheal intubation. It has been observed that the incidence of Mallampati classes III and IV increases during labor compared with the prelabor period.[39] Laryngeal and upper airway edema are also common in the parturient and can be exaggerated by preeclampsia.[40]

Studies of gastric emptying in pregnancy have produced somewhat inconsistent results. Wong and colleagues found that water was readily cleared from the stomachs of nonobese, nonlaboring parturients at term.[41] Other recent studies of gastric emptying in nonlaboring term women also suggest that gastric emptying is not delayed during pregnancy.[41] Chiloiro and colleagues found that gastric emptying time did not become slower with the progress of gestation but that total orocecal transit time did.[42]

A more common clinical concern is the parturient in labor. Laboring patients who consumed a light solid meal had significantly greater gastric volumes than those allowed only water.[43] Although pain, in any circumstance, is thought to delay gastric emptying, Porter and colleagues suggest that pain does not appear

to be the sole cause of gastric slowing in late labor because there was a similar delay in women in late labor who had received either epidural local anesthetic alone or no analgesia.[44]

Pain and Analgesics

Pain and its treatment are risk factors for aspiration, notably in patients presenting with trauma. Crighton and colleagues found that circulating catecholamines have an inhibitory effect on gastric emptying, and noradrenaline release in response to painful stimuli may cause inhibition of gastric tone and emptying.[45] Trauma patients, especially those in acute pain who are scheduled for emergency surgery, have decreased gastrointestinal motility and increased gastrointestinal secretion despite fasting preoperatively. The incidence of pulmonary aspiration increases markedly after trauma because of recent ingestion of food, depressed consciousness, diminished or absent airway reflexes, or gastric stasis induced by increased levels of catecholamines. Patients with spinal cord or brain injuries also have been shown to manifest delayed gastric emptying of both liquid and solid contents.[46,47]

Administration of opioids to alleviate pain may further impair gastrointestinal function. Opioid receptors can be found throughout the gastrointestinal tract; human and animal studies suggest that there are central and peripheral mechanisms by which these drugs delay gastric emptying.[48] Even modest intravenous doses of morphine demonstrably prolong gastric transit times in clinical studies.[45,49–51]

Neuraxial opioids also can prolong gastric emptying. In parturients, the administration of fentanyl 25 μg intrathecally delayed gastric emptying in labor compared with both extradural fentanyl 50 μg with bupivacaine and extradural bupivacaine alone.[52] On the other hand, the addition of fentanyl (2 or 2.5 μg/mL) to dilute bupivacaine for epidural infusion during labor was not found to affect gastric motility.[44,53]

Pathophysiology

When gastric contents enter the lungs, the resultant pulmonary pathology depends on the nature of the material aspirated (Box 14.3). Food particles small enough to enter the distal airways induce a foreign body reaction of inflammation and eventual granuloma formation. The aspiration of particulate antacids produces the same adverse response.[40,54] Acid aspiration induces an inflammatory response that begins within minutes and progresses over 24 to 36 hours.[54,55] In 1940, Irons and Apfelbach described the characteristic microscopic changes as intense engorgement of the alveolar capillaries, edema, hemorrhage into the alveolar spaces, and extensive desquamation of the lining of the bronchial tree.[56] Other authors also have described hemorrhagic pulmonary edema, intense inflammation, and derangement of the pulmonary epithelium.[55,57] The membranous epithelial cells that produce surfactant are damaged or destroyed by the acid and replaced by

• BOX 14.3 Pathophysiology of Aspiration

Particulate aspiration → Airway obstruction →
Granulomatous inflammation → Acid aspiration →
Neutrophilic inflammation → Hemorrhagic pulmonary edema →
Destruction of airway epithelium → Loss of type I alveolar cells →
Loss of surfactant → Alveolar instability and collapse →
Disruption of alveolar-capillary membrane → Plasma leakage from pulmonary capillaries → Noncardiogenic pulmonary edema → Hypovolemia

granular epithelial cells.[15] As surfactant production fails, lung units progressively collapse. Fibrin and plasma leak from the capillaries into the pulmonary interstitium and alveoli, producing noncardiogenic pulmonary edema often referred to as adult respiratory distress syndrome.[15,55,58,59] With effective supportive care, the acute inflammation can diminish, and epithelial regeneration can begin within 72 hours.

The clinical features of aspiration pneumonitis have been well described for more than 70 years. Even earlier, in 1887, Becker referred to bronchopneumonia as a postoperative complication related to the inhalation of gastric contents.[56] Hall, in 1940, published the first description of gastric fluid inhalation in obstetric patients. He distinguished between the aspiration of solid material, which could quickly kill by suffocation, and the aspiration syndrome produced by gastric fluid, for which he coined the term *chemical pneumonitis.*[60] Mendelson, in 1946, described the clinical features of 66 cases of peripartum aspiration observed from 1932 to 1945.[61] Solid food produced airway obstruction, which was quickly fatal in two instances. Otherwise, wheezing, rales, rhonchi, tachypnea, and tachycardia were prominent.[61] Subsequent reports have not found wheezing to be as universal a manifestation, occurring in about one-third of aspirations. When present, wheezing is thought to result from bronchial mucosal edema and from a reflex response to acidic airway irritation.[11,55,62]

Refractory hypoxemia can ensue almost immediately as bronchospasm, airway edema, airway obstruction, and alveolar collapse or flooding increase the effective intrapulmonary shunt fraction (Box 14.4). The awake patient may experience intense dyspnea and may cough up pink, frothy sputum characteristic of pulmonary edema.[11,38,55] More modest aspirations may not become clinically evident for several hours.[38,63,64]

Hemodynamic derangements also can demand therapeutic attention. As the alveolar-capillary membrane loses its integrity, plasma leaks out of the pulmonary vasculature. With increasing volumes of fluid leaking into the lung, the loss of circulating volume can produce hemoconcentration, hypotension, tachycardia, and even shock.[11,38] Pulmonary vasospasm also may contribute to right ventricular dysfunction.[11]

Radiographic evidence of pulmonary aspiration may become evident immediately, if aspiration is massive, or after a delay of several hours. There is no pattern on the chest radiograph that is specific for aspiration. The distribution of infiltrates depends on the volume of material inhaled and the patient's position at the time of the event. As a result of bronchial anatomy, aspiration occurring in the supine patient affects the right lower lobe most commonly and the left upper lobe least often.[11,38] In most cases, infiltrates are seen in dependent parts of the lungs, predominating in the lower lobes (Fig. 14.1). If pulmonary aspiration is not complicated by secondary events, improvement in symptoms can be anticipated within 24 hours, although the radiographic picture may continue to worsen for another day.[38]

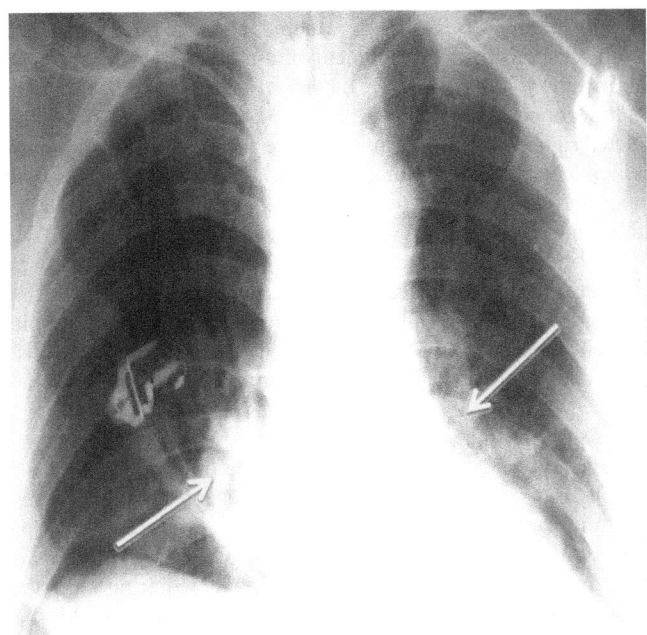

• **Fig. 14.1** Chest x-ray performed after tracheal intubation. Pulmonary infiltrates are seen in the dependent parts of the lungs *(arrows).*

Determinants of Morbidity

pH and Volume of Aspirate

In his 1946 report, Mendelson set out to determine the relationship between gastric fluid acidity and pulmonary morbidity.[61] When liquid containing hydrochloric acid (HCl) was instilled into rabbits' tracheas, the animals developed a syndrome similar in many respects to that observed in humans following liquid aspiration[61]: cyanosis, dyspnea, and pink, frothy sputum. On the other hand, when neutral liquid was instilled into the trachea, the rabbits endured a brief symptomatic period; within a few hours, however, they were apparently back to normal and able to carry on rabbit activities uninhibited.[61] Since Mendelson's report, numerous attempts have been made to define the "critical" volume and pH of gastric contents required to inflict significant damage on the lungs. Such neatly defined threshold values may not be realistic clinically. Nonetheless, almost all researchers in the field of aspiration pneumonitis have made some use of critical values to define the success or failure of drug therapies in the modification of gastric contents.

In 1952, Teabeaut injected HCl solutions of different volumes and acidities into rabbits' tracheas.[65] He found that solutions with a pH higher than 2.4 caused a relatively benign tissue response similar to that induced by the intratracheal injection of water.[65] As the pH of the injectate was reduced from 2.4 to 1.5, a progressively more severe tissue reaction was elicited. At pH 1.5, the damage was maximal and equal to that found at lower pH values.[65] From this study stemmed the popular concept of the pH value of 2.5 as a threshold for chemical pneumonitis.

The determination of a critical volume of gastric contents required to produce severe aspiration pneumonitis has been even more contentious than that of a critical pH. In dogs, pulmonary injury became independent of pH as the volume of aspirate was increased from 0.5 to 4.0 mL/kg.[11] Gastric fluid instillation into the right mainstem bronchus of a single monkey long ago led to the acceptance of 0.4 mL/kg as the volume of gastric fluid that places a subject at risk for development of aspiration pneumonitis.[66-68] Clearly, the volume of aspirate that is considered hazardous depends on how much morbidity or pathology must be produced to be considered significant. Arguments also have been made concerning the experimental instillation of gastric fluid into one lung versus both lungs and the reliability of gastric fluid volume measurements. In addition, even if a critical volume for aspiration pneumonitis could be reliably determined, it cannot be known how much fluid must be present in the stomach to deposit this critical volume into the lung or lungs.[66] The ASA Task Force on Preoperative Fasting, despite extensive scrutiny of the existing data, has been unable to establish a link between residual gastric volume and pulmonary aspiration.[69]

Particulate Matter

Volume and acidity are not, of course, the only determinants of injuries and sequelae when gastric contents enter the lungs. Gastric fluid containing particulate antacids can produce severe aspiration pneumonitis, even at near-neutral pH, with symptoms of wheezing, pulmonary edema, and hypoxemia requiring mechanical ventilatory support.[70] Animal studies have confirmed that nonparticulate gastric acid and particulate antacid solutions have similar potentials for pulmonary injury if aspirated.[63] Although blood and digestive enzymes do not appear to induce chemical pneumonitis, feculent gastric contents with a high bacterial density readily produce pneumonitis and death in animals (acidic gastric contents are normally sterile). Another study demonstrated that the mucus present in the gastric fluid of dogs with intestinal obstruction produced diffuse small airway obstruction and pulmonary injury when aspirated.[11]

Prevention of Aspiration

The clinical challenges of perioperative pulmonary aspiration are prevention, prophylaxis, and treatment. Ideally, gastric contents can be physically prevented from entering the lungs in the first place. Should prevention fail, pharmacologic prophylaxis may modify the volume and character of gastric contents so that they inflict minimal damage on the lungs. Least desirably, aspiration pneumonitis can require intensive medical treatment and ventilatory support.

The nonpharmacologic means of keeping gastric contents out of the lungs are preoperative fasting, gastric decompression, and optimal airway management.

Preoperative Fasting

The most common means of keeping gastric contents out of the lungs is to minimize the volume of such contents through preoperative fasting. However, both the utility and the necessity of adhering to traditional NPO (Latin: *nil per os*, or "nothing by mouth") regimens for clear liquids have been challenged. As noted by Sethi and colleagues, the stomach can never be completely empty even after a midnight fast because it continues to secrete gastric juices.[71] The issue has been studied in both pediatric and adult surgical patients and has become particularly contentious in obstetric anesthesia.

Pediatric Patients

Conventional preoperative fasting can impose physical and emotional discomfort on children and their parents and may be difficult to enforce reliably in outpatients. Dehydration in infants and hypoglycemia in neonates also may result from prolonged fasting

times.[2,10] The normal stomach can empty 80% of a clear liquid load within 1 hour after ingestion. The stomach continues to secrete and reabsorb fluid throughout the fasting period, whereas ingested clear liquids are completely passed into the duodenum within 2.25 hours.[72] Several researchers have, therefore, sought to demonstrate that children may safely be allowed to drink clear liquids until just 2 to 3 hours before elective surgery.

It has been shown that healthy infants can drink limited volumes of clear liquids 3 to 4 hours before surgery with no effect on gastric content volumes.[73] Splinter and colleagues found that healthy infants could drink clear liquids freely until 2 hours before anesthetic induction without altering gastric fluid volume or pH.[74] (Gastric fluid pH was quite variable, and mean pH was less than 2.5 in all groups of patients studied, regardless of the duration of fasting.) In a study of 97 healthy infants undergoing elective surgery, gastric fluid volume was not increased when the fasting time for formula was reduced from 8 hours to either 6 or 4 hours.[75] When gastric contents of children subjected to conventional preoperative fasting (mean fasting time of 13.5 hours) were compared with those of children permitted clear liquids until 2 hours before anesthetic induction (mean fasting time of 2.6 hours), the gastric fluid volumes actually tended to be somewhat smaller in the children allowed to drink clear liquids up to 2 hours preoperatively.[76] Furthermore, almost all children in both groups had gastric content pH values of 2.5 or less.[76] Several other studies all concluded that permitting children to drink nonparticulate fluids 2 to 3 hours before surgery had either no effect or a small beneficial influence on the quantity and acidity of their gastric contents.[77-80] Ingestion of clear liquids alone therefore appears to pose no demonstrable hazard if taken no later than 2 hours before anesthesia by children without gastrointestinal pathology. On the other hand, milk or formula intake on the morning of surgery (4 to 6 hours before induction) was associated with the presence of curds in many of the gastric aspirates. This was considered to represent an unacceptable risk of particulate aspiration. The authors therefore concurred with previous recommendations that infants not be allowed milk or formula on the morning of surgery.[74]

The ASA's Practice Guidelines for Preoperative Fasting and the Use of Pharmacologic Agents to Reduce the Risk of Pulmonary Aspiration were updated in 2017. The ASA Committee on Standards and Practice Parameters supports in healthy patients undergoing elective procedures a fasting period of 2 hours after the ingestion of clear liquids (infants and children) and, for neonates and infants, 4 hours after breast milk and 6 hours after infant formula (i.e., unchanged recommendations from those published in 2011).[69]

Adult Patients

In adult surgical patients as well, considerable evidence has demonstrated that clear liquid intake within 2 to 3 hours of anesthetic induction does not increase the risk of aspiration. Note that these studies typically involved healthy, nonpregnant, nonobese patients who were free of known gastrointestinal pathology, were not receiving opioids or other medications known to interfere with gastric emptying, and were undergoing elective surgery. The results of such studies cannot, therefore, be reliably applied to any other groups of patients.[81-84] With adults, as with children, the basic arguments favoring relaxed fasting regimens for clear liquids involve their normally rapid gastric clearance. More than 90% of a 750-mL bolus of isotonic saline was found to pass from the normal stomach within 30 minutes.[85] After 2 hours of fasting, the fluid in the stomach primarily represents the acid secreted by the stomach itself. Exogenous clear liquids tend to dilute endogenous gastric acid and may even accelerate gastric emptying.[76,83] Solids, lipids, and hyperosmotic liquids are thought to delay gastric emptying, and their intake would therefore be considered ill-advised before anesthetic induction. In addition, the particulate elements of a light breakfast do not completely exit after 4 hours.[86]

Reflecting a consensus of clinical comfort, the aforementioned ASA Task Force recommends a fasting period of 2 hours after the ingestion of clear liquids, a 6-hour preoperative fast following a "light meal," and a fast of 8 hours or longer for a meal that included fried or fatty foods or meat.[69] Both the amount and types of food ingested should be considered when evaluating the fasting status.[69]

Pregnant Patients

As preoperative fasting standards became more relaxed, strenuous debate arose over the necessity of adhering to conventional fasting regimens for patients in labor. On the one hand, anesthesiologists have long recognized that advanced gestation increases the risk of gastric content aspiration. However, proponents of liberalizing oral intake for parturients cited the infrequency of aspiration pneumonitis in modern practice, the futility of fasting in ensuring an empty stomach, and the detrimental effects of fasting on maternal and fetal well-being. An ultrasound study in which almost two-thirds of patients in labor had solid food in the stomach, regardless of how long they had fasted, contributed to the arguments against conventional fasting guidelines.[2]

It has been suggested that administration of narcotics, not labor itself, appears to be the major factor in delaying stomach emptying.[87] Evidence suggests that pregnancy by itself does not delay gastric emptying, including in obese term pregnant patients, who also have been found to have normal gastric emptying.[88] Nevertheless, these findings apply only to patients who are not in labor.[88]

The Report on Confidential Enquiries into Maternal Deaths in England and Wales 1982–1984 found that 7 of 19 anesthesia-associated maternal deaths resulted from aspiration of gastric contents into the lungs.[89] In a study comparing obstetric and nonobstetric anesthesia malpractice claims, it was reported that complications attributable to aspiration were significantly more common among the obstetric cases (4%) than in nonobstetric cases (1%), and the standard of care was judged to have been met in 46% of obstetric cases and in 39% of nonobstetric cases.[90]

The pregnant patient with a difficult airway cannot always be avoided, nor can general anesthesia for cesarean section, no matter how aggressively regional anesthesia is promoted. Regardless of gastric fluid volume or acidity, the presence of solid food imparts the immediate hazard of asphyxiation. Therefore, current recommendations are that pregnant patients should undergo a fasting period of 6 to 8 hours before elective cesarean delivery, and solid foods should be avoided in actively laboring patients. Finally, there is insufficient evidence to suggest changes in the risk of aspiration in the first 24 hours of the postpartum period, when operative procedures are common; therefore, similar precautions should be emphasized.[91]

Role of Preoperative Ultrasonography

Ultrasonography (USG) has been proposed as a useful, noninvasive, bedside tool to determine gastric content and volume in the perioperative period.[92] In a prospective observational study, 183 patients undergoing scheduled surgery were consecutively included, allowing 180 measurements of antral cross-sectional area.[92] A significant positive relationship between antral cross-sectional area and aspirated fluid volume was found with a cutoff value of antral area of

340 mm^2 for the diagnosis of "risk stomach," defined by an aspirated fluid volume of gastric contents greater than 0.8 mL/kg and/or the presence of solid particles. Area under the receiver operating characteristic curve for the diagnosis of risk stomach was 90% with a sensitivity of 91% and a specificity of 71%. The authors concluded that ultrasonographic measurement of antral cross-sectional area could be an important help for the anesthesiologist in minimizing the risk of pulmonary aspiration of gastric contents during general anesthesia.[92] Another prospective trial performed an ultrasonographic qualitative and quantitative analysis of the gastric antrum in 200 fasted patients undergoing elective surgery by assigning a grade to each patient on a 3-point grading scale.[93] Eighty-six patients were categorized as grade 0, suggesting an empty antrum (0 mL); 107 patients as grade 1, suggesting minimal fluid volume (16 ± 36 mL) detected only in the right lateral decubitus position; and 7 patients as grade 2, suggesting a distended gastric antrum with fluid 180 ± 83 mL visible in supine and right lateral decubitus positions.[93] Results of this study of elective surgical patients indicate that preoperative USG may be used to help identify patients who are at higher risk of pulmonary aspiration.

Because certain patient populations (e.g., trauma patients and patients with advanced diabetes) are known to be at high risk for pulmonary aspiration and the associated morbidity and mortality, it seems prudent to use USG as a screening tool preoperatively for these patients. Furthermore, a recent study demonstrated that the decision to perform the appropriate induction technique (RSI vs standard) for nonelective pediatric surgery could be improved from 49% (based on clinical assessment alone) to 85% with the use of point-of-care gastric USG.[94] These findings support the routine use of point-of-care gastric USG before all nonelective surgeries to optimize the airway management approach.

Preinduction Gastric Emptying

When a patient who is at increased risk for aspiration presents for surgery, the stomach can be emptied, at least in part, by an orogastric or nasogastric tube (NGT). Some patients, of course, already have such tube placed for gastric decompression, particularly if intestinal obstruction has been diagnosed. In such cases, the anesthesiologist must decide whether or not to remove the gastric tube before induction. If gastric decompression has not been attempted, the anesthesiologist may wish to do so while the patient's protective airway reflexes remain intact. There are some controversies as to whether an NGT should be inserted and then removed before induction of anesthesia or left in situ during a RSI. It has long been argued that the presence of a gastric tube interferes with the function of the LES and promotes gastroesophageal reflux.[11,91] In addition, the presence of a foreign body in the pharynx also could interfere with laryngoscopy. In one study, when attempts were made to provoke gastroesophageal reflux with a device that elevated abdominal pressure in a stepwise fashion to 100 mm Hg, gastroesophageal reflux was not detected at any level of abdominal pressure regardless of the presence or size of an NGT in normal subjects.[95] Salem and colleagues had previously demonstrated that CP is effective in sealing the esophagus around an esophageal tube against an intraesophageal pressure up to 100 cm H_2O.[96] They also advocated the utility of an NGT as a "blow-off valve" for increased intragastric pressure during induction.[96] In addition, Vanner and Asai advised that an NGT already inserted should be suctioned and left in place for anesthetic induction because its presence does not reduce the efficacy of CP.[97] On the other hand, others contested the recommendation that a NGT should be left in situ during a RSI as this is not supported by the evidence.[98] None of these discussions addressed the decision concerning which patients should have NGTs placed before entering the operating room. Gastric decompression during surgery also may reduce the risk of regurgitation and aspiration during surgery, extubation, and the early postoperative period.

Several authors have studied the thoroughness of gastric emptying attainable by gastric tube suctioning, usually in the context of comparing different methods for estimating gastric residual volume. Ong and colleagues reported as early as 1978 that the volume of fluid obtained by orogastric suctioning correlated poorly with the gastric residual volume calculated by a dilution method, with the volume aspirated being frequently much less than the volume calculated.[99] They concluded that suctioning through a gastric tube will not empty the stomach completely; consequently, mechanical decompression of the stomach before induction may therefore be of limited reliability and thus provide a false sense of security.[99] On the other hand, only 0 to 13 mL of residual gastric volume was found following aspiration through an 18-French Salem sump tube in 24 patients.[100] The authors concluded that the volume of aspirated gastric fluid is a very good estimate of the volume present in the stomach at the time of induction and that gastric tube suctioning also could be suitable to empty the stomach of its liquid contents before anesthesia.[100]

It can be argued that any reduction in intragastric volume and pressure before anesthetic induction is desirable and therefore should be attempted. On the other hand, particulate matter is impossible to evacuate through the lumen of an ordinary nasogastric tube. There is currently no consensus to dictate preinduction placement of an NGT in any set of patients without intestinal obstruction. In any case, gastric decompression in no way substitutes for proper perioperative management of the airway.

Although an NGT helps to reduce intragastric volume and pressure, it does not guarantee that the stomach is completely empty. Preoperative NGT insertion and stomach decompression are recommended only in patients with a distended stomach (e.g., bowel obstruction) or achalasia.[101] A recent global survey of over 10,000 anesthesia providers revealed that this is performed by 60% to 80% of practitioners in patients with intestinal obstruction, with increasing frequency in lower-income countries.[102] Furthermore, over 350 respondents reported that their key lesson from having experienced aspiration was to address gastric decompression before anesthesia, which includes placing an NGT if not already present, applying suction through it, administering a small amount of saline to unblock a potentially obstructed tube, and changing the patient position on the operating table to facilitate gastric emptying.[102] There is insufficient evidence to make a recommendation on whether or not an NGT should be removed after suctioning or left in place.

Awake Tracheal Intubation

For the patient whose stomach is assumed to be full, the anesthesiologist must first decide whether to secure the airway before or after anesthetic induction. Awake intubation, with topical anesthesia of the airway, can always be considered. Securing the airway with the patient awake avoids many of the pitfalls of RSI in patients with a full stomach and a difficult airway including the loss of protective airway reflexes, failure of CP to prevent pulmonary aspiration, and failed tracheal intubation leading to hypoxia, brain death, and cardiovascular collapse. However, patients can still aspirate during the process of awake tracheal intubation.[102,103]

A full-stomach patient with an anticipated difficult airway (i.e., difficult intubation) warrants an awake tracheal intubation; on the other hand, a patient with predicted difficult mask ventilation can be safely managed with an RSI if intubation is predicted to be straightforward. No single feature on physical examination accurately predicts a difficult intubation, but a variety of simple diagnostic tests have been suggested to identify patients with difficult airways. Successful accomplishment of awake intubation in patients at risk for pulmonary aspiration depends on several factors, including adequate psychological preparation, use of an IV antisialagogue to dry oropharyngeal secretions, judicious IV sedation, topicalization, and expertise of the practitioner performing the intubation.[103] The drawback of using anticholinergic drugs in patients with a full stomach is that they can reduce LES tone and barrier pressure, creating a potentially increased risk for pulmonary aspiration. The goal of sedation in this scenario is to provide comfort for the patient and tolerance of the procedure while maintaining patient responsiveness to commands and the ability to protect his or her own airway. It should be emphasized that sedation should not be used as a substitute for inadequate airway topicalization.[103] Recent Difficult Airway Society guidelines for awake tracheal intubation in adults recommend breaking down this procedure into sedation, topicalization, oxygenation, and performance to improve clinical practice.[103] While topicalization of the lower airway (i.e., below the vocal cords) in an awake patient at risk for pulmonary aspiration is controversial, there exists a lack of quality evidence in support of any particular approach. One option is to delay the laryngeal and infraglottic topicalization until just before tracheal intubation, using a "spray-as-you-go" technique (see Chapter 13).

Rapid Sequence Induction and Cricoid Pressure

If anesthetic induction is to precede tracheal intubation, the standard protective maneuver for 5 decades has been RSI with CP. The technique of RSI of anesthesia to protect the airway from pulmonary aspiration of gastric contents has evolved since the introduction of succinylcholine in 1951 and the first description of CP by Sellick in 1961.[104] The primary objective of RSI is to minimize the time interval between loss of protective airway reflexes and tracheal intubation. The traditional components of this technique include preoxygenation and denitrogenation of the lungs, rapid administration of anesthetic induction and neuromuscular blocking agents with brief onset times, application of CP, avoidance of manual ventilation by mask, and (ideally) tracheal intubation immediately after loss of consciousness and onset of neuromuscular blockade. Abstention from positive-pressure ventilation (PPV) during RSI is based on the idea that the resulting gastric insufflation will increase the likelihood of regurgitation and aspiration of gastric contents before tracheal intubation and may prolong the time from loss of consciousness to intubation. Of course, if the patient becomes hypoxemic, manual ventilation becomes mandatory.

Propofol has replaced thiopental as the most popular induction agent for RSI in hemodynamically stable patients[105,106]; other IV induction agents include ketamine and etomidate. Opioids are used more than 80% of the time, and succinylcholine remains the muscle relaxant of choice for use in RSI, although the use of high-dose rocuronium is becoming more common.[105,106]

As opined by El-Orbany and Connolly, RSI has achieved a status close to being a standard of care for induction of general anesthesia in patients with a full stomach.[107] Despite the widespread use of the technique, however, there is still no agreement on how it should best be performed.[107] The practice of RSI has generated contention regarding almost all aspects of the technique. Thus, the huge variability in practice shown in the survey of over 10,000 anesthesiologists from 141 countries might not come as a surprise.[102] The authors of this survey aimed to explore RSI practice variation with respect to departmental standards, patient factors, socioeconomic factors, training, and supervision. They showed that the level of training of respondents and the existence of national or local guidelines influenced preferences less than the national income of the country of respondents and patient factors. For example, for a hypothetical patient with intestinal obstruction, there was a preference for the head-up or head-down position, nasogastric tube insertion, and CP application, as compared with a patient without intestinal obstruction requiring RSI.[102] Also, with decreasing national income of the respondent's location, the preference for supine position, CP, and NGT insertion increased.[102] What was specifically pointed out is the evident lack of deliberate practice—that is, a consistent practice of the three technical aspects of RSI (patient positioning, CP, and NGT use) in order to develop/maintain the expert-level performance.[102,108]

The utility of CP has been challenged on many fronts. Initially described by Sellick in 1961, the maneuver consists of occlusion of the upper end of the esophagus/hypopharynx by posterior pressure on the cricoid cartilage against the bodies of the cervical vertebrae.[104,109] Pressure is maintained until intubation and inflation of the cuff of the ETT are completed.[104] Sellick originally suggested that CP should be applied "lightly" initially and then with firm pressure as soon as consciousness is lost. Traditional teaching of the required force has been 44 N (4.4 kg),[110] while a reasonable recommendation to apply 10 N (1 kg) to the cricoid cartilage when the patient is awake and to increase the force to 30 N (3 kg) once the patient has lost consciousness has been more recently proposed.[111]

In Sellick's original report of 26 high-risk cases, 23 patients neither vomited nor regurgitated at any time around induction, and in the other 3 cases the release of CP after intubation was followed immediately by reflux into the pharynx of gastric or esophageal contents, suggesting (but not proving) that in these three cases CP had been effective.[104]

Two of the principal arguments against the use of CP for RSI stem from studies demonstrating that the application of CP worsens the laryngeal view[112,113] and leads to reduction in lower and upper esophageal sphincter tone,[19,114] decreasing barrier pressure and potentially increasing the risk of regurgitation. Interestingly, however, the largest randomized controlled trial to date with 3472 patients showed that RSI with CP prolonged the median time to intubation by only 4 seconds, which may not be clinically relevant.[8,113] The results of other studies examining the impact of CP on laryngoscopic view have been contradictory. The authors of one study reported that the effect of CP on laryngoscopy is variable.[115] In some subjects, the view may improve, whereas in others the view deteriorates; however, in a subset of individuals, a force close to that currently recommended (30 N) may cause a complete loss of the glottic view.[115] Other authors have contended that CP interferes with intubation using a lighted stylet or flexible intubation scope techniques.[116,117] On the other hand, in a randomized study of 700 adult surgical patients, Turgeon and colleagues concluded that CP applied by trained personnel does not increase the rate of failed intubation.[118] Given the current level of evidence, the take-home message for daily practice is to release CP if it is difficult to obtain a sufficient view of the laryngeal inlet.

Other authors have noted the inconsistency with which CP is applied. Great variability in the application of CP was reported in an observational study, identifying 10 different techniques in 32

observations; in addition, misapplication does occur with possible patient harm.[119] In a study of simulated CP, the target pressures could be sustained with a flexed arm for a mean of only 3.7 to 6.4 minutes and with an extended arm for 7.6 to 10.8 minutes.[120] Regular training has been shown to be required to more reliably apply CP, and correct site recognition of the cricoid cartilage is improved with the use of USG.[121,122]

A rising chorus of skepticism concerning the efficacy of CP has been sounded.[8,113,123] Not only are there reports of lethal aspiration occurring despite the application of CP and potential significant complications,[5,124] but there also is no quality evidence that CP, in fact, prevents pulmonary aspiration.[112] Specifically addressing medicolegal arguments, Jackson contended that there is no scientific validation for the commonly held belief that improper application of CP might explain any failures to prevent aspiration.[125]

Current national guidelines reflect the opposing views on the utility of CP. While its use is recommended in the guidelines of the Difficult Airway Society from the United Kingdom, guidelines from Germany and Scandinavia no longer recommend its routine use.[112] Current global practice on CP use during RSI seems to be split as well: it would be used in 50% for a hypothetical patient without intestinal obstruction who undergoes RSI, but in 71% for a hypothetical patient with intestinal obstruction.[102]

Cook emphasized that the risks of CP should balance the benefits and suggested that properly applied CP does not worsen the view at laryngoscopy nor significantly interfere with mask ventilation.[126] Therefore, to ensure that CP is properly applied, those applying it should be adequately trained in the technique.[1,121,122] It has been reported that the required force is equal to the force necessary to depress a capped air-filled 50-mL syringe from 50 to 32 mL; training assistants using this model improves the reliability of the force applied and the CP technique.[127]

In summary, anyone performing RSI should be adequately trained by following the deliberate practice principles. While many aspects of the optimal RSI technique remain controversial, it is clear that the target has remained the same for over 50 years: to insert a cuffed endotracheal tube swiftly. The patient should be adequately oxygenated, fully paralyzed, and CP should not be slavishly pursued to the detriment of gas exchange and airway securement and should be released to potentially improve a poor laryngeal view. The application of CP should not be confused with displacement of the larynx by backward, upward, and rightward pressure on the thyroid cartilage, also known as the BURP maneuver.[128] This maneuver has been shown to improve visualization of the glottis and serves as an important adjunct in the management of difficult direct laryngoscopy—one might need to release CP during RSI and attempt the BURP maneuver to improve the laryngeal view.

Tracheal Extubation

Tracheal extubation is typically the last step of airway management. It is a step, however, with high risk for serious, and potentially fatal, respiratory complications. It has been reported that the incidence of respiratory complications immediately or shortly after tracheal extubation was significantly higher than that during induction of anesthesia.[129] More recently, the UK report identified pulmonary aspiration as a leading cause of airway-related anesthetic deaths, most cases having identifiable risk factors.[1] In this audit, events at emergence and in recovery accounted for 29% of cases and were all related with airway obstruction; although aspiration of gastric contents was not listed as the primary event in any of the adverse events at extubation, the authors could not state that aspiration was not a contributory factor in at least some of the episodes.[1] Nevertheless, when an awake intubation or RSI is indicated to prevent pulmonary aspiration, an awake tracheal extubation is recommended to prevent airway complications and to enhance patient safety during emergence from general anesthesia, at extubation, and in the postanesthesia care unit.[130] The patient should be awake, conscious, and appropriately responding to commands before extubation. In a survey of tracheal extubation of adult surgical patients who were still deeply anesthetized, most respondents who otherwise used the technique considered the risk of pulmonary aspiration a contraindication to deep tracheal extubation.[131]

The Difficult Airway Society has developed guidelines for the safe management of tracheal extubation in adult perioperative practice.[132] A strategic, stepwise approach to extubation was promoted. The guidelines discuss the problems arising during extubation and recovery, in particular pulmonary aspiration, emphasizing the importance of planning and preparation, including practical techniques for use in clinical practice and recommendations for postextubation care.

Medical Prophylaxis of Aspiration

Gastroesophageal Motility

Although preparation of the patient (i.e., a rational fasting strategy and perhaps gastric suctioning) and expedient airway management are the twin pillars of aspiration prevention, pharmacologic prophylaxis has been promoted as an adjunct to patient safety. Because gastric contents must first pass through the esophagus before entering the pharynx and trachea, the LES is a focus of attention. The LES consists of functionally (although not anatomically) specialized smooth muscle, of about 2 to 4 cm in length, just proximal to the stomach. The sphincteric muscle maintains closure of the distal esophagus through a mechanism of tonic contraction.[133] Normally, a cholinergic reflex loop acts to increase LES pressure when intragastric or intraabdominal pressure rises.[4] As previously described, the pressure gradient between the LES and the stomach, referred to as the barrier pressure, is responsible for preventing gastroesophageal reflux (Boxes 14.5 and 14.6).[14,134,135]

LES function is modulated by neurohumoral influences. Cholinergic stimulation increases LES tone, whereas dopaminergic and adrenergic stimuli reduce it.[14,30,134] β-Adrenergic agonists and theophylline reduce LES pressure and promote gastroesophageal reflux, often with symptomatic heartburn in awake patients. β-Adrenergic blockade, on the other hand, elevates LES pressure.[136] Anticholinergics attenuate LES tone and impair the efficacy of

---

• BOX 14.5   Factors That Decrease Lower Esophageal Barrier Pressure

Gastric fluid components
Increased gastric acidity
Lipids
Hyperosmolar fluid
Progesterone
Pharmacologic agents
Dopaminergic agonists
β-Adrenergic agonists
Theophylline and caffeine
Anticholinergics
Opioids

• BOX 14.6   Factors That Increase Lower Esophageal Barrier Pressure

Dopaminergic antagonists
Metoclopramide
β-Adrenergic antagonists
Gastrointestinal cholinergic agonists

---

medications given to increase LES barrier pressure.[2,32,63,137,138] Although prochlorperazine raises LES pressure (presumably by an antidopaminergic effect), promethazine lowers LES pressure because of its anticholinergic properties.[14] Among the wide variety of other drugs that may reduce LES tone are benzodiazepines, opioids, barbiturates, dopamine, tricyclic antidepressants, calcium channel blockers, nitroglycerin, and nitroprusside.[2,32] Although succinylcholine-induced fasciculations can elevate intraabdominal pressure, LES tone concurrently rises, and the barrier pressure is maintained or increased.[2,14] Apart from pharmacologic influences, the barrier pressure may be reduced after insertion of an LMA during anesthesia with spontaneous ventilation.[135]

In many cases, agents that increase LES contractility also promote forward passage of gastric contents, and the factors that attenuate LES tone also retard gastric emptying. This correlation compounds pharmacologic opportunities for either protection or potential harm. Opioids and anticholinergics inhibit gastrointestinal motility, increasing the volume of gastric contents available for vomiting or regurgitation.[138,139] Although pain and anxiety delay gastric emptying through sympathetic stimulation, the administration of an opioid for analgesia can further delay the emptying of gastric contents into the duodenum.[32,134]

Metoclopramide

Gastric prokinetic drugs are available to promote gastric emptying while simultaneously enhancing LES barrier pressure. Metoclopramide is the prototypical agent in this category. The mechanisms of action proposed for metoclopramide include central antidopaminergic activity and prolactin stimulation, peripheral blockade of dopamine receptors, and stimulation of cholinergic function in the upper gastrointestinal tract. Although metoclopramide retains its prokinetic effect in vagotomized subjects, atropine has been shown to interfere with its effects.[133,140] Metoclopramide both raises LES contractility and barrier pressure and accelerates gastric emptying. The latter effect is achieved by intensifying gastric longitudinal muscle contraction while relaxing the pyloric sphincter and increasing the coordination of gastrointestinal peristalsis. Metoclopramide has no effect on gastric acid secretion.[63,133]

Metoclopramide has been extensively investigated as a chemoprophylactic agent for aspiration pneumonitis in children and in adults. Several original studies of patients given metoclopramide, in a dose of 10 or 20 mg either orally or IV, demonstrated the drug's utility in reducing gastric residual volume.[63,141,142] It was found that 10 mg of metoclopramide, in combination with a nonparticulate antacid or an H_2-receptor antagonist, provides the most effective control of gastric volume and pH.[63] Administered orally, metoclopramide has an onset of action that varies from 30 to 60 minutes, with a duration of action of 2 to 3 hours.[63] It has been demonstrated that either a 10- or 20-mg IV dose of metoclopramide can reliably empty the stomach within 10 to 20 minutes.[133] Metoclopramide also was found to reduce the volume of gastric contents in pediatric trauma patients.[143]

Other researchers have found metoclopramide to be less uniformly effective, especially in the context of opioid coadministration or the recent ingestion of a solid meal.[137] Christensen and colleagues demonstrated no influence of metoclopramide 0.1 mg/kg on the gastric pH or volume of healthy pediatric patients.[144] As a perioperative antiemetic, metoclopramide was shown to be inconsistently useful.[137] Side effects attributed to metoclopramide have included somnolence, dizziness, and faintness. These problems may surface more frequently in elderly or severely ill patients.[13,133] Extrapyramidal reactions are a more serious problem but reportedly occur in only 1% of subjects.[133] A case report was published of a patient with traumatic brain injury in whom metoclopramide 10 mg IV repeatedly induced a severe rise in intracranial pressure as a result of increased cerebral blood flow.[145]

Metoclopramide also has been investigated in obstetric anesthesia. The drug has been shown to increase LES tone in pregnant women and therefore may be a useful prophylactic agent before cesarean section.[137,140] However, studies of gastric emptying in parturients have provided less consistent results. Metoclopramide was shown to accelerate gastric emptying in patients undergoing scheduled or urgent cesarean section.[140,142] On the other hand, in a study 58 healthy, fasting parturients, metoclopramide 10 mg IV had no significant effect on mean gastric volume, gastric pH, or the proportion of patients with a gastric content volume exceeding 25 mL.[140] The study authors suggested that the drug might be more useful in the emergency setting for patients with active labor, recent food intake, pain, and anxiety. Maternal metoclopramide administration does produce detectable and variable neonatal blood levels of the drug but without reported effects on Apgar scores or neurobehavioral test results.[140,146]

Erythromycin

Erythromycin is a macrolide antibiotic that has been in common use for more than 60 years. Administered IV, it has been shown to improve gastric motility in patients with diabetic gastroparesis. Enteral feedings with erythromycin also pass more quickly through the stomach than control feedings. This action is thought to arise from the stimulation of motilin receptors in gastric smooth muscle.[147] IV erythromycin increases gastric emptying in a dose-response manner but is associated with nausea and stomach cramping at the highest dose (3 mg/kg).[148] In a double-blind crossover study, erythromycin 250 mg IV significantly improved gastric emptying for solids, but not liquids, in volunteers subjected to a standardized acute painful stimulus, which can alter gastric emptying.[149] The authors concluded that erythromycin was effective as a prokinetic drug for solids in acute painful situations.[149] Another prospective, double-blind, placebo-controlled clinical trial in patients undergoing emergency surgery under general anesthesia found that patients who received erythromycin 3 mg/kg IV were more likely to have gastric contents of less than 40 mL with no solid matter than patients who received placebo; this beneficial effect was seen only in the non-trauma population.[150] However, patients who received erythromycin experienced higher rates of nausea and stomach cramping.[150]

Reduction of Gastric Acid Content

Chemoprophylaxis of aspiration pneumonitis also can include the inhibition of gastric acid secretion or the neutralization of HCl already in the stomach. The former should eventually increase the pH and reduce the volume of gastric contents but has no effect on acidic fluid already in place. The latter should elevate gastric fluid pH but also may increase gastric fluid volume. The aspiration of particulate antacids can pose hazards equivalent to those of gastric acid inhalation, as previously described. Studies have demonstrated severe pulmonary pathology in rabbits resulting from aspiration of a commercial particulate antacid[151]; therefore, oral antacid prophylaxis should include only soluble, nonparticulate agents.

Neutralization of Gastric Acid

The clear antacid solutions most studied are sodium citrate (0.3 molar solution) and Bicitra, a combination of sodium citrate and citric acid. The pH of sodium citrate solutions typically exceeds 7.0, whereas that of Bicitra is 4.3.[151] When fasted, non-obese surgical outpatients were given Bicitra 15 or 30 mL orally, only 32% or 16%, respectively, had a gastric content pH of 2.5 or less, whereas 88% of the patients in the matched control group had such a low pH.[141]

Sodium citrate has been evaluated as a sole prophylactic agent in a variety of surgical settings, with inconsistent results. In one study, sodium citrate 30 mL, taken shortly before elective surgery, resulted in gastric fluid pH values greater than 3.5 in 95% of patients.[152] In other reports, however, sodium citrate failed to alter gastric fluid pH in surgical patients. In a 0.3 molar solution, 30 mL may be more consistently effective than 15 mL, but it may still not have prolonged effects in patients with rapid gastric emptying.[14,153,154] Antacid prophylaxis may therefore be adequate at the induction of anesthesia but inadequate at the time of awakening. Larger volumes of sodium citrate can induce nausea and vomiting or diarrhea.[141]

Inhibition of Gastric Acid Secretion

H$_2$-Receptor Blockade

Gastric acid production is strongly modulated by the action of histamine (H$_2$) receptors. H$_2$-receptor blockade inhibits both basal acid secretion and acid secretion stimulated by the presence of gastrin or food. Both H$_2$-antagonists and anticholinergic agents block the neural stimulation of gastric acid secretion.[133] However, the anticholinergic effect is overridden by the inhibition of gastrointestinal motility so that gastric volume is not reduced and gastric pH is elevated only inconsistently.[63] Although H$_2$-antagonists do not delay gastric emptying, their inhibition of acid secretion tends to correlate inconsistently with both the timing and the magnitude of maximal drug concentration in the plasma.[91] Various H$_2$-antagonists have been evaluated in both surgical and obstetric settings, with different doses and routes of administration, and with and without other prophylactic medications, to produce an expansive volume of findings.

Cimetidine. Given before elective surgery, a variety of cimetidine regimens can ensure that most patients have gastric fluid volume or pH values, or both, in the safe range, as defined by the investigators. These usually effective regimens include cimetidine 300 mg orally at bedtime followed by 300 mg orally or intramuscularly (IM) on the morning of surgery; cimetidine 300 to 600 mg orally given 1.5 to 2 hours preoperatively; and cimetidine 200 mg IV given 1 hour before surgery. In one study, cimetidine most reliably produced gastric content safety when combined with preoperative metoclopramide.[2] The reliability of oral cimetidine is generally improved if the drug is administered both the night before and on the morning of anesthesia.[11]

A gastric fluid pH of 2.5 or lower has been found in 5% to 35% of patients treated with single 300-mg doses of cimetidine given orally, IM, or IV in different studies. Significant elevation of gastric pH requires 30 to 60 minutes to become evident after the IV administration of cimetidine and 60 to 90 minutes after IM or oral dosing. Effective inhibition of gastric acid secretion persists for 4 to 6 hours.[64,137]

Cimetidine chemoprophylaxis also has been evaluated in obstetric anesthesia. In a study of 100 patients undergoing emergency cesarean section, cimetidine 200 mg IM was administered as soon as surgical delivery was decided upon, followed by oral intake of a 0.3-molar solution of sodium citrate 30 mL just before induction.[154] None of these patients had a gastric fluid pH lower than 2.7, and only 1 of 100 had a gastric fluid pH lower than 3.0.[154] Cimetidine administered in this fashion would most likely reduce gastric acidity by the time of extubation, whereas sodium citrate would be required to neutralize the acid already present.

Although cimetidine has a well-established record of safety when administered for perioperative aspiration prophylaxis, there are potential and observed side effects. The rapid IV infusion of large doses (e.g., 400 to 600 mg) has reportedly induced both hypotension and dangerous ventricular dysrhythmias.[134,137] It is advised that IV cimetidine be infused over at least a 10-minute period.[154] Other side effects sporadically associated with cimetidine include confusion, dizziness, headaches, and diarrhea, although these have not been reported to occur with single-dose preoperative administration.[133,134,147] Cimetidine competitively inhibits the hepatic mixed-function oxidase system (cytochrome P450 enzyme) and also reduces hepatic perfusion.[134,136,137] As a result, cimetidine may elevate the blood concentrations of other drugs that are cleared by the liver, including warfarin, propranolol, diazepam, theophylline, phenytoin, meperidine, bupivacaine, and lidocaine. Clinically, this seems to be a greater concern with long-term use than with one-dose or two-dose administration.[133,137]

Ranitidine. After cimetidine, ranitidine emerged as the next option for H_2-receptor blockade. Ranitidine is considered to exert little or no inhibition on hepatic enzymes, has a longer duration of action (6 to 8 hours), and has an efficacy greater than or equal to that of cimetidine. Effective onset times for the two drugs appear to be similar.[2,63,137,155] Smith and colleagues reported that ranitidine 50 mg, given IV over 2 minutes to 20 critically ill patients, led to variable, transient reductions in mean arterial pressure and systemic vascular resistance.[156] These hemodynamic effects occurred less frequently and were of lesser degree and duration than those resulting from cimetidine 200 mg, similarly administered. Previous sporadic case reports associated significant bradycardia with the IV administration of either cimetidine or ranitidine.

In a study of adult surgical outpatients, ranitidine 150 mg orally, administered 2.5 hours before anesthetic induction, significantly decreased gastric residual volume and significantly increased gastric fluid pH compared with placebo.[85] In no patient was there the conventional (but arbitrary) at-risk combination of gastric pH lower than 2.5 and gastric volume greater than 25 mL.[85] McAllister and colleagues treated adult patients with a single oral dose of ranitidine 300 mg administered 2 hours before surgery and found both a significant increase in mean gastric fluid pH and a significant decrease in mean gastric fluid volume compared with placebo treatment.[157] Noting the occasional patient with gastric fluid pH lower than 2.5, the authors cautioned that it is unsafe to assume that H_2-antagonists will always eliminate the risk of acid aspiration pneumonitis.[157] Single-dose IV administration of ranitidine, 40 to 100 mg, also has been found to reliably generate gastric fluid pH values greater than 2.5 in adults, manifesting a greater efficacy than that of cimetidine 300 mg IV.[2]

Sandhar and colleagues evaluated the efficacy of a single oral dose of ranitidine, 2 mg/kg, given 2 to 3 hours before surgery to patients ages 1 to 14 years.[72] Although ranitidine significantly reduced both the volume and the acidity of gastric contents compared with placebo, 6 of 44 children receiving ranitidine did have gastric fluid pH values of 2.5 or lower.[72] These findings confirmed those of a similar study by Goudsouzian and Young,[158] although other authors have not demonstrated such a consistent reduction in gastric fluid volume.[2,85]

Papadimitriou and colleagues compared ranitidine 150 mg IV with cimetidine 400 mg IV and placebo given 1 hour before anesthetic induction to emergency surgical patients.[159] Ranitidine and cimetidine caused similar reductions in gastric volume and acidity; only the reductions in acidity were statistically significant. Although the mean pH values in the cimetidine and ranitidine groups were similar, only ranitidine consistently produced safe gastric pH values (all of which were 5.0 or higher).[159] In morbidly obese surgical patients, ranitidine was found to be superior to cimetidine in elevating gastric fluid pH.[160]

The effect of oral ranitidine (150 mg, given 2 to 3 hours before the scheduled time of surgery) with or without oral metoclopramide (10 mg, given 1 hour before surgery) and/or sodium citrate (30 mL on call to the operating room) on gastric fluid volume and pH was measured in 196 elective surgical inpatients.[161] Although no combination guaranteed a safe combination of fluid volume and pH, a single oral dose of ranitidine was statistically as effective as triple prophylaxis.[161] In pediatric patients, two separate studies showed that oral ranitidine (either 2 mg/kg or 75 mg) effectively elevated gastric fluid pH with no appreciable effect on gastric volume.[80,162] In a study of the IV administration of these drugs 15 minutes before anesthetic induction, it was concluded that prophylactic ranitidine 50 mg IV and metoclopramide 10 mg IV may be an easy and useful method to decrease the volume while increasing the pH of gastric contents.[163]

Ranitidine also has been evaluated for prophylactic use in obstetric anesthesia. A recent study published in the *Cochrane Database of Systematic Reviews* concluded that, although the quality of the evidence was poor, the evidence suggests that the combination of antacids plus H_2-antagonists is superior to antacids alone in increasing gastric pH in women before cesarean section.[164] When a single agent is used, antacids alone are superior to H_2-antagonists.[164]

Other H_2-Receptor Blockers. A voluminous body of evidence documents the general safety and efficacy of preoperative cimetidine and ranitidine in ameliorating the acidity and volume of gastric contents. Newer agents, such as famotidine (20 mg orally or IV) and nizatidine, also have been evaluated, with generally favorable results.[160,165] For example, nizatidine 300 mg orally was uniformly effective in maintaining gastric content pH above 2.5 and volume below 25 mL when given 2 hours before surgery.[165]

Based on the presumably high ratio of benefit to risk, H_2-blocking agents have been recommended for surgical patients who have an increased likelihood of aspirating gastric contents.[2] However, given the infrequency of perioperative aspiration pneumonitis, proof of the actual clinical benefit of this practice has yet to be established. In a review by Warner and colleagues of more than 215,000 general anesthetics in adults, 35 patients with acknowledged risk factors did aspirate perioperatively.[3] Of these 35, 17 had been given prophylactic medication. In this small sample, aspiration prophylaxis produced no discernible difference in the incidence of pulmonary complications.[3] In general, the routine preoperative use of H_2-antagonists is not considered either essential or cost-effective because it has yet to be proven that prophylaxis against acid aspiration changes morbidity or mortality in healthy patients having elective surgery.[2]

Proton Pump Inhibition. Proton pump inhibitors (PPIs) constitute a newer class of agents for the suppression of gastric acid production. Acetylcholine, histamine, and gastrin all stimulate HCl secretion by the gastric parietal cell. Although these agonists stimulate different populations of receptors, their mechanisms of action all eventually result in the formation of cyclic adenosine monophosphate (cAMP). cAMP activates the proton pump, hydrogen potassium adenosine triphosphatase (H^+/K^+-ATPase), which exchanges intraluminal potassium ions for intracellular hydrogen ions. Hydrogen ions are thereby secreted from the parietal cell into gastric fluids.[72,157] Omeprazole, the prototypical PPI, is actually a pro-drug that is absorbed in the small intestine and is activated in the highly acidic milieu of the gastric parietal cell. Activated omeprazole then remains in the parietal cell for up to 48 hours, inhibiting the proton pump in a prolonged manner.[146,166–168] Inhibition of gastric acid secretion can be nearly complete, with no discernible side effects. A single dose of omeprazole, 20 to 40 mg, reduces gastric acidity for up to 48 hours. On the other hand, PPIs are characterized by variable first-pass metabolism with resulting inconsistencies in the plasma concentration after any given oral dose. As is the case with H_2-antagonists, there is also an unpredictable relationship between peak plasma concentration and peak inhibition of gastric acid production.[91]

Omeprazole has been evaluated as a preoperative agent for the chemoprophylaxis of aspiration pneumonitis. When omeprazole 40 mg was administered orally to healthy patients either the evening before or 2 hours before elective surgery, mean gastric fluid pH was significantly higher and gastric fluid volume lower with omeprazole treatment than with placebo.[166] Yet, 6 of 30 patients receiving omeprazole had gastric fluid pH values lower than 2.5 at the time of induction.

Omeprazole also has been evaluated in obstetric anesthesia and found to be effective at reducing gastric volume and increasing gastric pH parturients presenting for elective cesarean delivery.[146] Administration of omeprazole 40 mg orally the night before surgery with an additional 40 mg dose the morning of surgery was found to be more effective than a single dose of 80 mg on the morning of surgery. Coadministration of metoclopramide 20 mg IM was shown to improve the beneficial effect of omeprazole in both dosing regimens.

In other studies, PPIs have been found most effective when given in two doses: one on the night before and one on the morning of surgery.[91] Given the dwindling proportion of patients hospitalized before elective surgery, however, two-dose regimens for chemoprophylaxis would seem somewhat impractical. Furthermore, it was reported that a single preoperative oral dose of ranitidine was more effective in reducing gastric acid content than two-dose regimens of rabeprazole or lansoprazole.[169] On the other hand, Pisegna and colleagues found that pantoprazole 40 mg IV decreased gastric acid output and volume and increased pH within 1 hour of dosing. Effects were sustained for up to 12 hours following single-dose administration.[170]

Management of Pulmonary Aspiration

When a fully conscious person aspirates foreign substances into the tracheobronchial tree, a brief but effective bout of coughing can clear the aspirate. Patients with observed pulmonary aspiration under sedation should have the mouth and pharynx suctioned immediately so that the patency of the upper airway is restored. Suctioning solid or liquid material allows recovery of the aspirated material so that it is not reaspirated and stimulates coughing to further expel the aspirate (provided the cough reflex is preserved). Turning the patient's head to the side and placing the patient in the Trendelenburg position can help promote the flow of gastric contents out of the mouth and avoid further pulmonary aspiration.

After an aspiration event, patients who are obtunded or whose clinical status has deteriorated should be tracheally intubated. A suction catheter should be advanced into the trachea to clear the airways prior to initiation of PPV.[171] It is essential, though, not to make prolonged efforts at suctioning the trachea at the expense of adequate oxygenation and ventilation.[171] Bronchoscopy also can be performed to clear the obstructing material from the lower airways, but it remains debated whether it should be routinely performed or reserved for patients who have aspirated sufficient solid material to cause significant airway obstruction and/or for those who aspirated particulate material that needs to be lavaged.[171,172] One might anticipate the need for additional equipment to be able to grab, hold, and remove foreign material from the airways if it cannot be suctioned. Chemical damage to the mucosa of the tracheobronchial tree occurs within seconds, but bronchial secretions neutralize the aspirated acid within minutes.[173] Attempts to neutralize the acid aspirate with saline or bicarbonate lavage have proved to be futile and may increase the damage.[174]

The treatment of pulmonary aspiration of gastric contents is aimed at restoring pulmonary function to normal as soon as possible. If the patient is awake and able to maintain a reasonable arterial oxygen tension (Pa_{O_2}), a conservative approach is to provide supplemental oxygen through a nasal cannula or a face mask. The inspired oxygen concentration (Fi_{O_2}) can be increased to maintain the Pa_{O_2} at approximately 60 to 70 mm Hg. This may suffice in a patient with a mild condition, but more aggressive therapy is indicated if aspiration is more severe. Severe bronchospasm may be treated by the inhalation of a β-adrenergic bronchodilator.[174,175]

When severe pulmonary aspiration is suspected, early ventilatory support is the mainstay of treatment. Early continuous positive airway pressure (CPAP) is indicated in awake and alert patients who do not respond to oxygen supplementation. CPAP up to 12 to 14 mm Hg can be administered through a tight-fitting mask. If higher levels are required, mechanical ventilation should be considered. The level of CPAP can be reduced as the patient improves, but it should not be completely withdrawn before the alveoli can maintain stability. A high Fi_{O_2} level can be used initially but should be decreased as soon as possible.[176]

If the patient is obtunded, an ETT should be placed and mechanical ventilation initiated. Positive end-expiratory pressure (PEEP) should be applied, and the Fi_{O_2} should be decreased as soon as possible while adequate oxygenation is maintained. PEEP is commonly used to improve functional residual capacity and prevent atelectasis resulting from poor ventilatory efforts.[175] It also improves the ventilation-perfusion ratio and allows the use of less toxic levels of oxygen to be administered, giving the lungs a chance to recover.[173] Caution should be exercised when using PEEP because high levels can worsen pulmonary damage by causing increased transudation of fluid through injured capillary beds.[177] Cereda and colleagues investigated the effect of PEEP in patients with acute lung injury and found that a PEEP of at least 15 cm H_2O was needed to prevent a decay in respiratory system compliance.[178]

Despite these measures, if hypoxemia persists along with bilateral lung infiltrates and poor lung compliance, management should be like that for acute respiratory distress syndrome (ARDS). A large, multicenter, randomized trial sponsored by the

National Institutes of Health compared ventilation with lower versus traditional tidal volumes in patients with ARDS.[179] Smaller tidal volumes (6 mL/kg predicted body weight) and hypoventilation with permissive hypercapnia were associated with a 10% reduction in mortality, along with a shorter period using mechanical ventilation. The lower tidal volume ventilation approach protected the lungs from excessive stretch, improving several important clinical indicators of outcome in patients with ARDS.[179] An alveolar recruitment maneuver using a CPAP of 40 cm H_2O for 40 seconds improved oxygenation in patients with early ARDS who did not have impairment of the chest wall.[180] A recruitment maneuver with a smaller tidal volume was associated with a survival rate of 62%, compared with a rate of 29% when using conventional ventilation without the recruitment maneuver.[181]

Use of prophylactic antibiotics is not recommended.[182] Antibiotics alter the normal flora of the respiratory tract, which predisposes the susceptible patient to secondary infection with resistant organisms. In mice, it was demonstrated that acid aspiration–induced epithelial injury led to subsequent bacterial infection.[183] Approximately 20% to 30% of patients who manifest initial gastric content aspiration eventually develop a secondary infection.[182] Antibiotics should be reserved for patients who show signs of clinical infection and for patients who have aspirated grossly contaminated material into their lungs.[171]

Wolfe and colleagues found that pneumonia resulting from gram-negative bacteria was more common after pulmonary aspiration among patients treated with corticosteroids than those who were not treated.[184] Corticosteroids interfered with the healing of granulomatous lesions in rabbit models.[185] The consensus appears to be that corticosteroids play no role in the treatment of aspiration pneumonitis.[171,186]

In the most severe cases of lung injury, extracorporeal membrane oxygenation therapy and/or lung transplantation may need to be considered.[171]

Conclusion

It is clearly best to prevent gastric contents of any volume or pH from entering the trachea. Although this ideal may not always be attainable by even the most skillful of clinicians, its likelihood would appear to be favored by optimal preparation of patients and a carefully executed, well-designed plan for anesthetic induction and airway management, including tracheal extubation. There is a growing body of evidence for the preoperative use of point-of-care gastric USG for assessing gastric contents and better identifying patients with the highest risk of aspiration of gastric contents. The role of awake intubation and preinduction gastric emptying in high-risk cases is influenced by patients' characteristics and practitioners' experience and confidence. RSI is a well-accepted induction technique to reduce the incidence of pulmonary aspiration. CP is a variably practiced maneuver in conjunction with RSI, with differing recommendations from different national societies. It should be recognized that laryngoscopic view may be adversely affected by CP and that airway management and effective ventilation may mandate its modification or discontinuation.

An impressive array of pharmacologic agents now can be employed to promote antegrade gastric emptying, inhibit gastroesophageal reflux, and reduce the acidity of gastric fluids. These drugs have an established record of safety and offer the reasonable expectation of rendering gastric fluid less threatening to the lungs.

However, because of the low incidence of clinically significant perioperative aspiration, it may not be possible to demonstrate statistically that the use of these agents actually improves patient outcomes. In reference to gastric prokinetic drugs, antacids, and inhibitors of acid secretion, the ASA Task Force concluded that the routine preoperative use of such medications in patients who have no apparent increased risk for pulmonary aspiration is not recommended.[69] Chemoprophylaxis is only an adjunct to and not a substitute for otherwise sound clinical practice. It is, of course, less desirable to have aspirated and survived than never to have aspirated at all.

Acknowledgments

The authors would like to acknowledge Drs. Romain Deransy, Ashutosh Wali and Uma Munnur for their work on this chapter in previous editions.

Selected References

1. Cook TM, Woodall N, Frerk C, for the National Audit Project. Major complications of airway management in the UK. Results of the Fourth National Audit Project of the Royal College of Anaesthetists and the Difficult Airway Society. Part 1: Anesthesia. *Br J Anaesth.* 2011;106:617–631.

3. Warner MA, Warner ME, Weber JG. Clinical significance of pulmonary aspiration during the perioperative period. *Anesthesiology.* 1993;78:56–62.

8. Birenbaum A, Hajage D, Roche S, et al. Effect of cricoid pressure compared with a sham procedure in the rapid sequence induction of anesthesia. The IRIS randomized clinical trial. *JAMA Surg.* 2019;154:9–17.

69. Practice Guidelines for Preoperative Fasting and the Use of Pharmacologic Agents to Reduce the Risk of Pulmonary Aspiration: Application to Healthy Patients Undergoing Elective Procedures: An Updated Report by the American Society of Anesthesiologists Task Force on Preoperative Fasting and the Use of Pharmacologic Agents to Reduce the Risk of Pulmonary Aspiration. *Anesthesiology.* 2017;126:376–393.

101. Salem MR, Khorasani A, Saatee S, Crystal GJ, El-Orbany M. Gastric tubes and airway management in patients at risk of aspiration: history, current concepts, and proposal of an algorithm. *Anesth Analg.* 2014;118:569–579.

102. Zdravkovic M, Berger-Estilita J, Sorbello M, Hagberg CA. An international survey about rapid sequence intubation of 10,003 anaesthetists and 16 airway experts. *Anaesthesia.* 2020;75(3):313–322.

108. Hastings RH, Rickard TC. Deliberate practice for achieving and maintaining expertise in anesthesiology. *Anesth Analg.* 2015;120:449–559.

109. Rice MJ, Mancuso AA, Gibbs C, Morey TE, Gravenstein N, Deitte LA. Cricoid pressure results in compression of the post-cricoid hypopharynx: the esophageal position is irrelevant. *Anesth Analg.* 2009;109:1546–1552.

112. Salem MR, Khorasani A, Zeidan A, Crystal GJ. Cricoid pressure controversies: narrative review. *Anesthesiology.* 2017;126:738–752.

132. Difficult Airway Society Extubation Guidelines Group, Popat M, Mitchell V, et al. Difficult Airway Society Guidelines for the management of tracheal extubation. *Anaesthesia.* 2012;67:318–340.

164. Paranjothy S, Griffiths JD, Broughton KH, et al. Interventions at caesarean section for reducing the risk of aspiration pneumonitis (review). *Cochrane Database Syst Rev.* 2010;(1):CD004943.

171. Gaba DM, Fish KJ, Howard SK, Burden A. Crisis Management in Anesthesiology. 2nd ed. Elsevier/Saunders; 2015:181–184.

All references can be found online at eBooks.Health.Elsevier.com.

15

Perioxygenation

FIONA ROBERTS, ELIZABETH C. BEHRINGER, AND ANIL PATEL

CHAPTER OUTLINE

KEY POINTS

- The mainstay technique for increasing the apneic window is through preoxygenation with spontaneous face-mask ventilation and 100% oxygen.
- More recently, there has been increased emphasis on *perioxygenation*, which also involves providing oxygenation during the apneic period.
- Preoxygenation denitrogenates the lungs and creates an alveolar oxygen reservoir. The size of this reservoir can be increased by reducing dependent atelectasis through head-up patient positioning and raising mean airway pressure. Ultimately, however, the size of the oxygen reservoir is fixed at the end of preoxygenation, and, once apnea begins, it does not get replenished.
- Preoxygenation techniques include tidal volume breathing of oxygen by face mask for 3 to 5 minutes, deep breathing

techniques by face mask up to 2 minutes, continuous positive airway pressure (CPAP), and noninvasive positive-pressure ventilation (NIPPV), or bi-level positive airway pressure (BiPAP).
- Apneic oxygenation describes the physiologic phenomenon in which, provided that a patent air passageway exists between the lungs and the exterior (nasopharyngeal and oropharyngeal airspace), the difference between the alveolar rates of oxygen removal from the lungs and carbon dioxide excretion into the lungs generates a negative pressure gradient of up to 20 cm H_2O that drives oxygen into the lungs from the nasopharyngeal and oropharyngeal reservoirs. Techniques of apneic oxygenation serve to prolong the duration of apnea without desaturation.

- Techniques that prolong apnea time include low-flow nasal oxygen at flows less than 15 L/min (NO DESAT), pharyngeal oxygen insufflation, and high-flow humidified nasal oxygen at 30 to 70 L/min (THRIVE).

- Head-up positioning is especially useful in that it both improves other efforts at preoxygenation and aids in prolonging the duration of apnea without desaturation.

Introduction

During induction of anesthesia, maintenance of arterial oxyhemoglobin saturation levels is critical in an apneic patient until airway control has been achieved, with desaturation leading to dysrhythmias, hemodynamic decompensation, hypoxic brain injury, and ultimately death.[1,2] These saturation levels are maintained via the process of "perioxygenation" (Fig. 15.1).[3] The term *perioxygenation* includes both preoxygenation and apneic oxygenation. Preoxygenation ends when apnea starts due to induction of anesthesia and neuromuscular blockade; thereafter, apneic oxygenation (and ventilation) occur.[3] Perioxygenation has become a universally accepted strategy designed to increase oxygen reserves and thereby delay the onset of arterial oxyhemoglobin desaturation during periods of hypoventilation and apnea.

Apnea time is defined as the length of time from cessation of breathing or ventilation until the onset of significant arterial desaturation (typically, an arterial oxyhemoglobin saturation [Sao_2] <90%). The primary method for increasing apnea time during airway management is through preoxygenation with spontaneous face-mask ventilation and 100% oxygen before induction of anesthesia. Preoxygenation denitrogenates the lungs and creates an alveolar oxygen reservoir. The size of this reservoir can be increased by reducing dependent atelectasis through head-up patient positioning and by raising mean airway pressure; ultimately, however, the size of the oxygen reservoir is fixed at the end of preoxygenation, and, once apnea begins, it does not get replenished unless ventilation resumes or other strategies are employed.

Apneic oxygenation describes the physiologic phenomenon in which, provided that a patent air passageway exists between the lungs and the atmosphere (i.e., the nasopharyngeal and oropharyngeal airspace), the difference between the alveolar rates of oxygen removal from the lungs and carbon dioxide (CO_2) excretion into the lungs generates a negative pressure gradient of up to 20 cm H_2O that drives oxygen into the lungs from the nasopharyngeal and oropharyngeal reservoir.[4,5–11] A continuous flow of nasal oxygen therefore allows maintenance of oxygenation without spontaneous or administered ventilation and increases the apnea time beyond that of standard face-mask preoxygenation. Three techniques use this concept: nasal oxygen during efforts securing an ETT (NO DESAT),[12] pharyngeal oxygen insufflation,[13] and transnasal humidified rapid-insufflation ventilatory exchange (THRIVE).[14]

The first version of the American Society of Anesthesiologists (ASA) Practice Guidelines for Management of the Difficult Airway did not mention preoxygenation. In the updated 2003 report, the topic of "face mask preoxygenation before initiating management of the difficult airway" was added.[15] Routine preoxygenation has become a new minimum standard of care, not only during induction of anesthesia but also during emergence from anesthesia and tracheal extubation.[16–19]

Physiologic Considerations

The principles important to understanding the physiology of perioxygenation include body oxygen stores, the physiology of apnea, and the concept of apneic oxygenation.

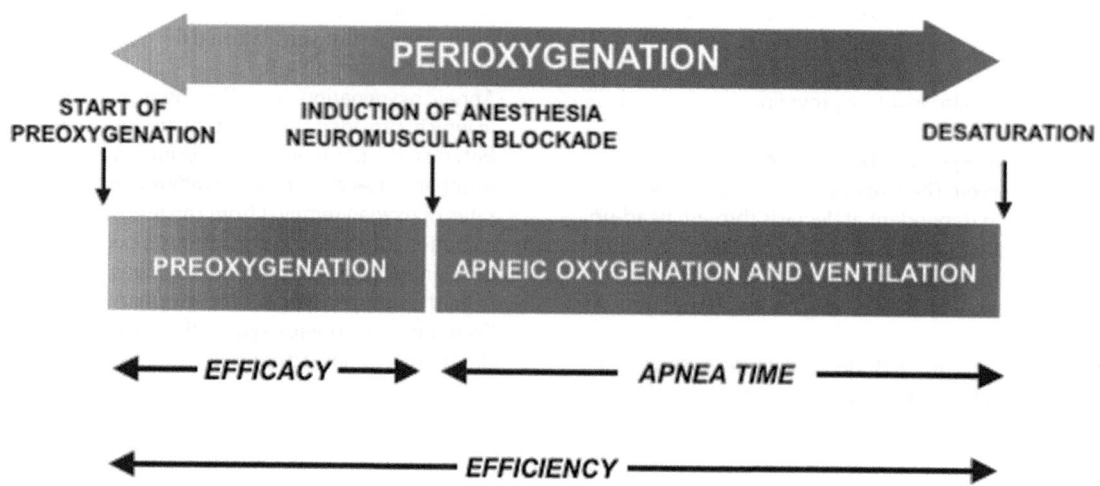

- **Fig. 15.1** Perioxygenation. (Modified from Patel A, El-Boghdadly K. Apnoeic oxygenation and ventilation: Go with the flow. *Anaesthesia.* 2020;75:1002–1005.)

Body Oxygen Stores

Oxygen is carried in the blood in two forms: the greater portion is in reversible chemical combination with hemoglobin (Hb), and the smaller part is dissolved in plasma.[20] The ability to carry large amounts of oxygen in Hb is important, because without it the amount carried in the plasma would be so small that cardiac output would need to be increased 20 times or more to yield adequate oxygen delivery.[20] The amount of chemically bound oxygen is directly related to the concentration of Hb and how saturated the Hb is with oxygen. Arterial oxygen content (CaO_2) can be calculated from the following equation:

where

   1.36 = estimated mass volume of oxygen that can be bound by
      1 g of normal Hb
   SaO_2 = arterial oxyhemoglobin saturation (when fully saturated, SaO_2 = 100%)
   PaO_2 = arterial partial pressure of oxygen
   0.003 = solubility coefficient of oxygen in human plasma

The CaO_2 with a Hb concentration of 15 g/dL and 100% SaO_2 is approximately 20 mL of oxygen per 100 dL of blood. In addition, approximately 0.3 mL of oxygen/100 dL blood is in physical solution at a normal physiologic PaO_2; this amount of dissolved oxygen normally accounts for only 1.5% of the total oxygen content, but its contribution increases when PaO_2 is increased (dissolved oxygen is linearly related to PaO_2). The venous oxygen content (C_vO_2) can be calculated with the same formula using mixed venous oxygen tension (P_vO_2) and mixed venous oxyhemoglobin saturation (S_vO_2).

The pattern of uptake and release of oxygen by Hb is demonstrated by the oxyhemoglobin dissociation curve, which is a plot of Hb saturation as a function of partial pressure of oxygen (PO_2). The sigmoid shape of the curve reflects the fact that the four binding sites on a given Hb molecule interact with each other.[20] When the first site has bound a molecule of oxygen, the binding of the next site is facilitated, and so forth. The result is a curve that is steep up to a PO_2 of 60 mm Hg and shallower thereafter, approaching 100% saturation asymptotically. At a PO_2 of 100 mm Hg (the normal arterial value), 97% of the hemes have bound oxygen; at 40 mm Hg (a typical value for PvO_2 in a resting person), the saturation declines to about 75%. The shape of the oxyhemoglobin dissociation curve has important physiologic implications. The flatness of the curve above a PO_2 of 80 mm Hg ensures a relatively constant SaO_2 despite wide variations in alveolar oxygen pressure. The steep portion of the curve between 20 and 60 mm Hg permits unloading of oxygen from Hb at relatively high PO_2 values, which favors the delivery of large amounts of oxygen into the tissues by diffusion.

The oxygen-binding properties of Hb are influenced by several factors, including pH, partial pressure of carbon dioxide (PCO_2), and temperature.[20] These factors cause shifts of the oxyhemoglobin dissociation curve to the right or left without changing the slope of the curve. For example, an increase in temperature or a decrease in pH, such as may occur in active tissues, decreases the affinity of Hb for oxygen and shifts the oxyhemoglobin dissociation curve to the right. As a result, a higher PO_2 is required to achieve a given saturation, facilitating the unloading of oxygen at the tissue. To quantify the extent of a shift of the oxyhemoglobin dissociation curve, the P_{50} is used—that is, the PO_2 required for 50% saturation. The P_{50} of normal adult Hb at 37°C and normal pH and PCO_2 is 26 to 27 mm Hg.

Despite its great importance, oxygen is a very difficult gas to store in a biologic system. In subjects breathing air, oxygen stores

Storage Site (mL)	Room Air (mL)	100% O_2
In the lungs (FRC)	450	3000
In the blood	850	950
Dissolved in tissue fluids	50	100
In combination with myoglobin	200	200
Total	1550	4250

TABLE 15.1 Body Oxygen Stores During Room Air and 100% Oxygen Breathing

FRC, Functional residual capacity; O_2, oxygen.
From Nunn JF, ed. *Nunn's Applied Respiratory Physiology*. 4th ed. Butterworth-Heinemann; 1993:288.

are small (Table 15.1).[20,21] The relatively steep oxyhemoglobin dissociation curve and the small oxygen stores imply that factors affecting PaO_2 produce their full effects very quickly. This contrasts with CO_2, for which the large size of the stores buffers the body against rapid changes. Therefore, in a subject breathing air, a pulse oximeter probably gives an earlier indication of hypoventilation than does CO_2 measurement. In contrast, in a subject breathing a high fraction of inspired oxygen (FIO_2), CO_2 measurement gives an earlier indication of hypoventilation.[20]

The amounts of body oxygen in the various storage sites of a person breathing air are increased with breathing an FIO_2 of 100% (Fig. 15.2; see also Table 15.1).[20,21] The largest increase in oxygen stores occurs in the functional residual capacity (FRC). Storage of oxygen in the tissue is rather difficult to assess, but assuming that Henry's law applies and that the partition coefficient for gases approximates the gas-water coefficients, breathing oxygen for 3 minutes significantly increases tissue oxygen stores.[21]

Physiology of Apnea

During apnea in the paralyzed patient there is no diaphragmatic movement or lung expansion, and the total body oxygen consumption ($\dot{V}O_2$) remains fairly constant at about 230 mL/min.

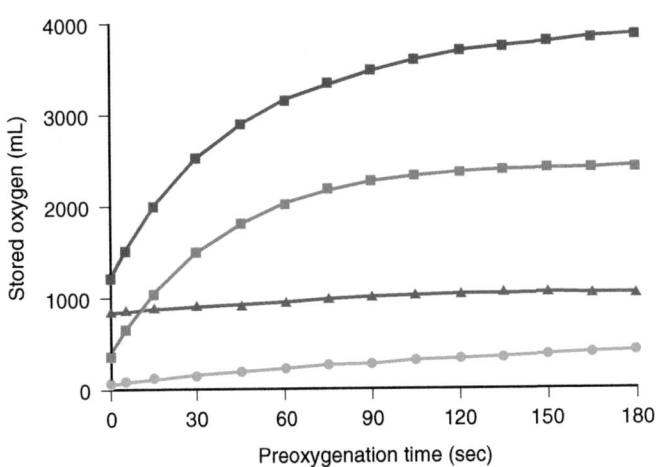

• **Fig. 15.2** Variation in volume of oxygen stored in the functional residual capacity *(blue)*, the blood *(red)*, the tissue *(turquoise)*, and the whole body *(purple)* with duration of preoxygenation. (From Campbell IT, Beatty PCW. Monitoring preoxygenation. *Br J Anaesth.* 1994;72:3–4.)

Consequently, Pao_2 decreases rapidly because of the depletion of the diminishing oxygen stores in the lungs. If the airway becomes obstructed, oxygen removal will generate a substantial and immediate negative pressure, contributing to a further decrease of Pao_2. Although the Pao_2 falls in direct relation to the alveolar oxygen concentration (Pao_2), Sao_2 remains 90% or more as long as Hb can be reoxygenated in the lungs.[8,11,22,23] Sao_2 begins to decrease only after lung oxygen stores are depleted and the Pao_2 is lower than 60 mm Hg. It is for this reason that oximetry is not the best physiologic means, compared with Pao_2, for predicting the onset of hypoxemia. However, because it detects decreases in Sao_2 before other clinical signs, oximetry is an invaluable clinical monitor that adds to the safety of anesthetic management.[23] Critical oxyhemoglobin desaturation may be defined as Sao_2 80% or less; for patients with Sao_2 80% or less, the range in the rate of decrease is 20% to 40% per minute during apnea.

Apneic Oxygenation

The physiologic nomenclature for describing apneic oxygenation has changed several times since the phenomenon was discovered by Volhard in 1908.[4] It has been described as "diffusion respiration" by Draper and Whitehead,[24] as "aventilatory mass flow" by Bartlett and colleagues,[5] and as "apneic oxygenation" by Frumin and colleagues.[8] What all of these studies describe is oxygenation using only the difference in the rates of excretion of CO_2 and absorption of oxygen as the driver of gaseous flow.

Mechanism

Preoxygenation followed by oxygen insufflation during subsequent apnea maintains Sao_2 by apneic oxygenation.[8,11] In the apneic adult, $\dot{V}o_2$ averages 230 mL/min, whereas the output of CO_2 to the alveoli is limited to about 20 mL/min, and the remaining CO_2 production (approximately 90%) is buffered within the body tissues. The difference in gas solubility between oxygen and CO_2 and the affinity of oxygen for Hb accounts for the difference in movement of oxygen and CO_2 across the alveolar membrane.

Lung gas volume initially decreases because of the net negative gas exchange rate of 210 mL/min. Therefore, a pressure gradient is created between the upper airway and the alveoli, and if the airway is patent, this results in a mass movement of oxygen down the trachea into the alveoli, prolonging apnea time. Conversely, CO_2 is not exhaled because of this mass movement of oxygen down the trachea, and the alveolar CO_2 concentration ($Paco_2$) shows an initial rise of about 8 to 16 mm Hg during the first minute and a subsequent fairly linear rise of about 3 mm Hg/min.[10]

Fraioli and colleagues emphasized the importance of the ratio of FRC to body weight during apneic oxygenation and demonstrated that patients with a low FRC/body weight ratio could not tolerate apnea for more than 4 minutes, whereas those with a high FRC/body weight ratio (>53.3 ± 7 mL/kg) maintained Pao_2 at 90% of the control value for 15 minutes or longer.[11] Some studies demonstrated that with a patent airway and an Fio_2 of 1.0, Sao_2 can be maintained at greater than 90% for up to 100 minutes with apneic oxygenation.[8,11]

The success of apneic oxygenation depends on airway patency to allow oxygen to move into the apneic lungs. In the presence of airway obstruction, not only does lung gas volume decrease rapidly, but intrathoracic pressure also decreases at a rate that is dependent on $\dot{V}o_2$ and thoracic compliance, subsequently leading to a marked decrease in Pao_2. When airway obstruction is relieved, rapid flow of oxygen into the lungs occurs, and with high Fio_2, rapid reoxygenation resumes.[23]

Apneic oxygenation can be achieved by preoxygenation followed by insufflation of oxygen through a nasopharyngeal or oropharyngeal cannula or through a needle inserted in the cricothyroid or cricotracheal membrane. This provides at least 10 minutes of adequate oxygenation in healthy apneic patients whose airways are unobstructed and therefore has many practical applications.[13] In patients who are difficult to intubate or ventilate, pharyngeal oxygen insufflation (or tracheal insufflation, in cases of upper airway obstruction) may allow additional time for laryngoscopy and endotracheal intubation.[7,13,25] This can be advantageous in patients who have decreased oxygen reserves, such as children, pregnant women, obese patients, and patients with acute respiratory distress syndrome (ARDS).[25] The combination of preoxygenation and apneic oxygenation can be used during bronchoscopy and can provide an otolaryngologist adequate time for glottic surgery unimpeded by the presence of an endotracheal tube (ETT) or by a patient's respiratory movements.[6]

The relationship between the ambient oxygen fraction and the time to development of dangerous hypoxemia (apnea time) has been investigated in a computational modeling analysis by McNamara and Hardman.[26] As the ambient oxygen fraction increases, the onset of hypoxia is delayed irrespective of shunt fraction, and the increase in time to desaturation is very much greater with very high ambient oxygen fractions (Fig. 15.3).[26] Increasing the ambient oxygen fraction from 0.9 to 1.0 more than doubles the time to desaturation compared with increasing the ambient oxygen fraction from 0.21 to 0.9.[26] This effect was maintained over a wide range of shunt fractions (1% to 30% of cardiac output) during apnea. These findings have significant implications for anesthetic practice, where assurance of effective apneic oxygenation involves ensuring the patency of the airway and the provision of 100% oxygen. Failure to provide 100% oxygen to the apneic patient's open airway greatly hastens the development of hypoxemia.[26]

Effect on Clearance of Carbon Dioxide

Apneic oxygenation provides very little, if any, CO_2 clearance. Although apneic oxygenation can largely meet physiologic oxygen demands for an increased period, it does not prevent a rapid and eventually fatal rise in CO_2 concentration. In Frumin's experiments, apneic oxygenation was carried out in 8 human subjects for periods between 15 and 55 minutes; in 2 out of 8 human subjects,

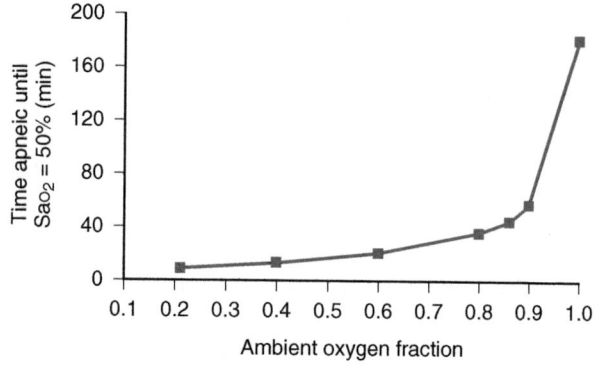

• **Fig. 15.3** The time (duration of apnea) required to reach 50% Sao_2 with an open airway exposed to various ambient O_2 fractions. (From McNamara MJ, Hardman JG. Hypoxaemia during open-airway apnoea: a computational modelling analysis. *Anaesthesia*. 2005;60:741–746.)

the trial was prematurely terminated because of the development of ventricular arrhythmias associated with respiratory acidosis.[8] In an apneic oxygenation study in 12 dogs, 1 died, likely from CO_2 toxicity.[6] There were also suggestions of patient death and altered cerebral function in early studies of apneic oxygenation.[27,28] Joels and Samueloff demonstrated that apneic oxygenation caused a progressive respiratory acidosis that rapidly overwhelmed the blood's buffering mechanisms and progressed into a mixed acidosis that proves fatal.[29] Death is principally caused by the limited tolerance of the myocardial contractile and conductive mechanisms to acidosis.[30,31] Joels and Samueloff's experiments placed the upper limit of the 95% confidence interval for occurrence of death attributed to acidosis at a pH of 6.9.[29]

Efficacy and Efficiency of Preoxygenation

Studies of preoxygenation have focused on measurements of indices reflecting its efficacy and efficiency.[32] Measurements of alveolar oxygen,[33-35] alveolar nitrogen,[36] or Pa_{O_2} reflect the efficacy of preoxygenation, whereas the drop in Sa_{O_2} during apnea is indicative of its efficiency.[32,36-39] Sa_{O_2} is misleading as a guide to alveolar denitrogenation. An oxygen saturation as measured by pulse oximetry (Sp_{O_2}) of 100% is not a reason to cease preoxygenation and may occur well before the lungs are adequately denitrogenated. Conversely, failure of Sp_{O_2} to increase substantially during denitrogenation does not necessarily indicate failure of preoxygenation or lack of its value; patients with substantial pulmonary shunting may achieve excellent pulmonary oxygen reservoirs while remaining hypoxemic.[40]

Efficacy of Preoxygenation

Preoxygenation increases alveolar oxygen concentration and decreases alveolar nitrogen in a parallel fashion (Fig. 15.4); it is the washout of nitrogen from the lungs that is the key to achieving preoxygenation.[36,41] Historically, preoxygenation and denitrogenation have been used interchangeably, although a change in focus from preoxygenation to denitrogenation has been suggested.[36] With normal lung function, oxygen wash-in and nitrogen wash-out are exponential functions; therefore the rate of preoxygenation (or denitrogenation) is governed by the time constant (τ) of the exponential curves. This constant is the same for both the wash-in and wash-out curves and is proportional to the ratio of alveolar ventilation ($\dot{V}_A$) to FRC. Because the oxygen flow used for $\dot{V}_A$ is delivered via an anesthesia circuit, preoxygenation occurs in two sequential stages according to the time constant, which is the time necessary for a given flow through a container to equal the volume of the container. These are the two stages:

1. Wash-out of the anesthesia circuit by oxygen flow
2. Wash-out of the FRC by alveolar ventilation

After 1 τ, the oxygen concentration of the FRC will be increased by approximately 63% of its original value; after 2 τ, to 86%; after 3 τ, to 95%; and after 4 τ, to about 98% of its original value.

To hasten denitrogenation, it is advisable to wash out (flush) the anesthesia circuit with a high oxygen flow before applying the face mask to the patient. During preoxygenation, an oxygen flow rate that eliminates rebreathing should be used.

In summary, three steps should be followed to enhance preoxygenation: (1) the anesthesia circuit is flushed by a high oxygen flow, (2) a nonleaking face mask is used to avoid air entrainment, and (3) an oxygen flow of 5 L/min is used for tidal volume breathing (TVB), and a flow of 10 L/min is used for deep breathing.

The end points of maximal alveolar preoxygenation or denitrogenation have been defined as an end-tidal oxygen concentration (EtO_2) of approximately 90% and an end-tidal nitrogen concentration (EtN_2) of 5%.[18,38] In an adult with a normal FRC and $\dot{V}_{O_2}$, an EtO_2 of 90% or more means that the lungs contain more than 2000 mL of oxygen (8 to 10 times the $\dot{V}_{O_2}$).[23] Because of the obligatory presence of CO_2 and water vapor in the alveolar gas, an EtO_2 greater than 97% cannot be easily achieved. Factors affecting the efficacy of preoxygenation include Fi_{O_2}, duration of breathing, and the $\dot{V}_A$/FRC ratio (Box 15.1).

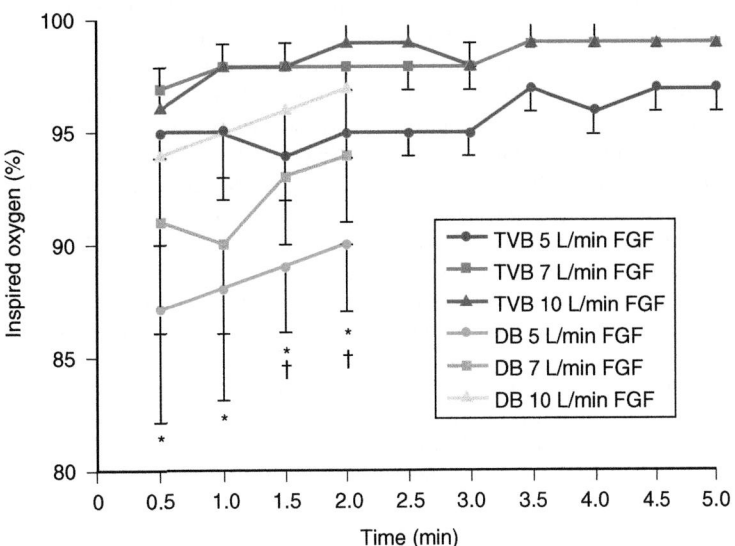

• **Fig. 15.4** Comparison of tidal volume breathing (TVB) and deep breathing (DB) preoxygenation techniques on inspired oxygen using 5, 7, and 10 L/min fresh gas flow (FGF). *Significant difference ($p < 0.05$) between 5, 7, and 10 L/min FGF; †significant difference ($p < 0.05$) from deep breaths at 0.5 and 1 minute. (From Nimmagadda U, Chiravuri SD, Salem MR, et al. Preoxygenation with tidal volume and deep breathing techniques: The impact of duration of breathing and fresh gas flow. *Anesth Analg.* 2001;92:1337–1341.)

Fraction of Inspired Oxygen

The main reasons for failure to achieve an F_{IO_2} close to 1.0 are a leak under the face mask,[32,42-45] rebreathing of exhaled gases, and the use of systems incapable of delivering a high oxygen concentration, such as resuscitation bags.[41] Even the presence of minor leaks may not be fully compensated for by increasing the fresh gas flow (FGF) or by increasing the duration of preoxygenation. Bearded patients, edentulous patients, patients with sunken cheeks, the presence of nasogastric tubes, use of a wrong face mask size, improper use of head straps, and use of systems allowing air entrainment under the face mask are all common factors causing leaks between the mask and the patient's face that result in a lower F_{IO_2}. Clinical endpoints indicative of a sealed system include movement of the reservoir bag with inhalation and exhalation, the presence of a normal capnogram and end-tidal CO_2 ($EtCO_2$), and measurements of inspired and $EtCO_2$ values.[32]

Although anesthetic circuits can deliver 100% oxygen, the F_{IO_2} is influenced by the type of breathing, the level of FGF, and the duration of breathing.[46] In a study that compared preoxygenation techniques using a semiclosed circle absorber with varying FGFs in the same subjects, it was found that with TVB, inspired oxygen concentration was 95% with FGF of 5 L/min, increasing to 98% with FGFs of 7 and 10 L/min. However, with deep breathing, the inspired oxygen concentration was only 88% at 5 L/min, 91% at 7 L/min, and 95% at 10 L/min FGF (see Fig. 15.4).[46] These findings imply that increasing the FGF from 5 to 10 L/min has little impact on increasing F_{IO_2} during TVB but has a noticeable effect during deep breathing.[43] Because of the breathing characteristics of the circle system, the minute ventilation during deep breathing may exceed the FGF, resulting in rebreathing of exhaled gases (N_2) and consequently decreasing the F_{IO_2}; in contrast, during TVB, rebreathing of exhaled gases is negligible, and increasing the FGF from 5 to 10 L/min has only a slight effect on F_{IO_2}.[46,47]

Duration of Breathing, Functional Residual Capacity, and Alveolar Ventilation

Sufficient time is needed to accomplish maximal preoxygenation. With an F_{IO_2} close to 1.0, most healthy adult patients can reach the target level of EtO_2 90% or more (or EtN_2 ≤5%) within 3 to 5 minutes of TVB. The half-time for exponential change in fraction

of alveolar oxygen concentration (Fa_{O_2}) with an immediate change in F_{IO_2} for a nonrebreathing system is described by the equation:

$$F_{AO_2} = 0.693 \times \frac{V_{FRC}}{\dot{V}_A}$$

where V_{FRC} = volume of functional residual capacity.

With a V_{FRC} of 2.5 L, the half-times are 26 seconds when $\dot{V}_A = 4$ L/min and 13 seconds when $\dot{V}_A = 8$ L/min.[32] Therefore most of the oxygen that can be stored in the lungs may be brought in by hyperventilation with an F_{IO_2} of 1.0 for a shorter period of time than that needed with TVB.[32] This is the basis for the deep breathing techniques, which have been introduced as an alternative to TVB.[32,39]

Changes in $\dot{V}_A$ and FRC can have a marked effect on the rate of rise in EtO_2 (and decrease in EtN_2) during preoxygenation. In pregnant women, because of an increased $\dot{V}_A$ and decreased FRC, EtO_2 rises faster than in nonpregnant women.[42,48,49] Similarly, preoxygenation can be accomplished faster in infants and children than in adults.[50]

Efficiency of Preoxygenation

Preoxygenation can markedly delay arterial oxyhemoglobin desaturation during apnea. In healthy individuals breathing room air, desaturation to 70% can occur within 1 minute, whereas with adequate preoxygenation, desaturation occurs after 5 minutes. The delay in desaturation during apnea depends on the efficacy of preoxygenation, the capacity for oxygen loading, and $\dot{V}_{O_2}$ (see Box 15.1). Patients with a decreased capacity for oxygen loading (decreased FRC, Pa_{O_2}, Ca_{O_2}, or cardiac output) or with increased $\dot{V}_{O_2}$, or both, desaturate much faster during apnea than healthy patients do.[51-54] The main difference in the rate of apnea-induced oxyhemoglobin desaturation after different preoxygenation techniques is observed between Sa_{O_2} levels of 100% and 99%.[23,32,50,51] This range represents the flat portion of the oxyhemoglobin dissociation curve. When oxygen reserves are depleted, rapid desaturation occurs regardless of the technique of preoxygenation and is like that observed in patients breathing air.

Farmery and Roe developed a computer model describing the rate of oxyhemoglobin desaturation during apnea.[52] This model was found to agree reasonably well with actual data from patients whose weight and degree of preoxygenation were reliably known (Fig. 15.5).[51,52] Because it would be dangerous to obtain data on time to marked oxyhemoglobin desaturation in humans, this model is uniquely useful for analysis of oxyhemoglobin desaturation below 90%.[51,52] As the pre-apnea Fa_{O_2} is progressively decreased from 0.87 to 0.8, 0.7, 0.6, 0.5, 0.4, 0.3, and 0.13 (Fa_{O_2} at room air) in a healthy 70-kg patient, the apnea time to 60% Sa_{O_2} is progressively decreased from 9.9 to 9.31, 8.38, 7.30, 6.37, 5.40, 4.40, 3.55, and 2.8 minutes, respectively.[51,52] Fig. 15.5 shows that for a healthy 70-kg adult, a moderately ill 70-kg adult, a healthy 10-kg child, and an obese 127-kg adult, 80% Sa_{O_2} is reached after 8.7, 5.5, 3.7, and 3.1 minutes, respectively, whereas 60% Sa_{O_2} is reached at 9.9, 6.2, 4.23, and 3.8 minutes, respectively.[32,51]

Techniques for Preoxygenation and Prolongation of Apnea Time

Various techniques and regimens have been described to ensure (1) adequate preoxygenation to optimize the oxygen reservoir before induction of anesthesia and (2) techniques to prolong the duration

Time to hemoglobin desaturation with initial F$_{AO_2}$ = 0.87

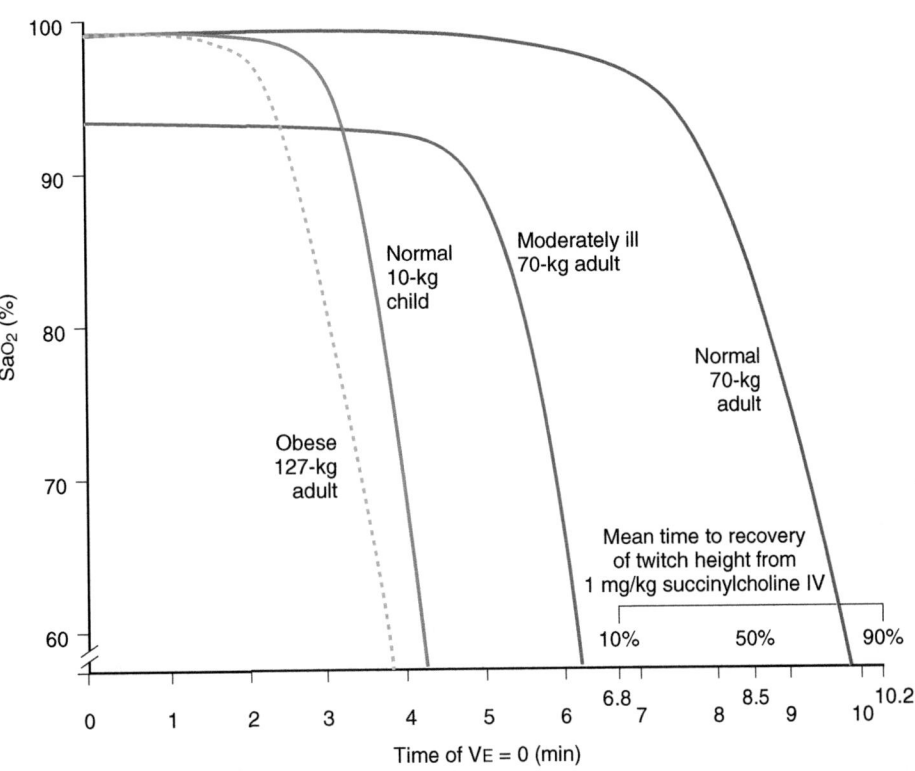

• **Fig. 15.5** Arterial oxyhemoglobin saturation (Sao$_2$) versus time of apnea in an obese adult, a 10-kg child (low functional residual capacity [FRC] and high oxygen consumption [V̇o$_2$]), and a moderately ill adult, compared with a healthy adult. F$_{AO_2}$, Fractional alveolar oxygen concentration; V$_E$, expired volume. (From Benumof JL, Dagg R, Benumof R. Critical hemoglobin desaturation will occur before return to unparalyzed state from 1 mg/kg succinylcholine. *Anesthesiology.* 1997;87:979–982.)

of apnea after the induction of anesthesia and administration of muscle relaxants. Regardless of the technique used, preoxygenation and prolongation of the apnea time after induction of anesthesia have become an integral component of the rapid sequence induction and intubation (RSI) technique and are particularly important if manual ventilation is not desirable following the induction of anesthesia, if difficulty with ventilation or endotracheal intubation is anticipated, and in patients with oxygen transport limitations. Because the "cannot intubate, cannot oxygenate" (CICO) situation is largely unpredictable, the desirability of maximal preoxygenation is theoretically present for all patients.[32]

Techniques for Preoxygenation

Several methods of preoxygenation are described in the scientific literature. Traditional techniques include TVB, deep breathing, and positive airway pressure (Box 15.2). THRIVE can also be used for preoxygenation (see later discussion).

Tidal Volume Breathing

The classic maneuver of TVB with 100% oxygen remains an effective technique for preoxygenation. Maximally effective preoxygenation using this technique requires 3 to 5 minutes at an F$_{IO_2}$ close to 1.0. Various anesthetic breathing circuits (circle absorber,[38,47] Mapleson A,[55–57] Mapleson D,[56–59] and nonrebreathing systems) and FGFs ranging from 5 to 35 L/min have been used successfully.[42,45,56,57,59] The circle absorber system (the

---

• BOX 15.2   Techniques for Preoxygenation

Tidal Volume Breathing

Traditional tidal volume breathing (3 to 5 minutes)
One vital capacity breath followed by tidal volume breathing

Deep Breathing

Single vital capacity breath
Four deep breaths (4 inspiratory capacity breaths)
Eight deep breaths (8 inspiratory capacity breaths)
Extended deep breathing (12 to 16 inspiratory capacity breaths)
One vital capacity breath followed by deep breathing

Preoxygenation and an Additional Maneuver

Preoxygenation and continuous positive airway pressure (CPAP)
Preoxygenation and oxygen insufflation
Preoxygenation and bi-level positive airway pressure (BiPAP)

THRIVE

Tidal volume breathing with mouth closed for 3 minutes

---

system most commonly used in the operating room [OR]) with an FGF as low as 5 L/min is as effective as other TVB methods.[41] Increasing the FGF from 5 to 10 L/min has little effect on enhancing preoxygenation during TVB in normal subjects (Fig. 15.6).[41]

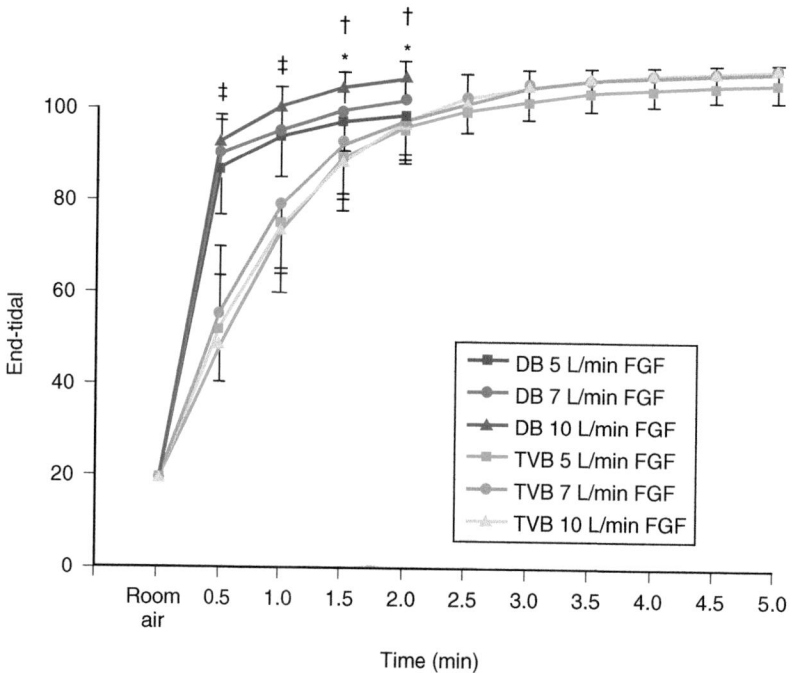

• **Fig. 15.6** Comparison of tidal volume breathing (TVB) and deep breathing (DB) preoxygenation techniques on end-tidal oxygen using 5, 7, and 10 L/min fresh gas flow (FGF). *Significant difference ($p < 0.05$) from DB at 5 and 7 L/min FGF; †Significant difference ($p < 0.05$) from DB at 0.5 and 1.0 minute; ‡Significant difference ($p < 0.05$) from TVB. (From Nimmagadda U, Chiravuri SD, Salem MR, et al. Preoxygenation with tidal volume and deep breathing techniques: the impact of duration of breathing and fresh gas flow. *Anesth Analg.* 2001;92:1337–1341.)

Deep Breathing Techniques

Based on the assumption that alveolar denitrogenation can be achieved rapidly by deep breathing, Gold and colleagues introduced a deep breathing method of preoxygenation consisting of 4 deep breaths (DBs) over 30 seconds (4 DB/30 seconds).[38] They showed that the Pao$_2$ after 4 DB/30 seconds was no different from the Pao$_2$ after TVB for 3 minutes. Although a few studies corroborated their findings,[60,61] other investigations showed that 3 minutes of TVB provided better preoxygenation (Fig. 15.7) and longer protection against hypoxemia during apnea than the 4 DB/30 seconds method did, particularly in pregnant women, patients with morbid obesity, and elderly patients.[42,47,58,59]

The primary reason why the 4 DB/30 seconds method is inferior to TVB is that ventilation during deep breathing is much greater than the oxygen inflow rate, resulting in rebreathing of exhaled nitrogen and a decreased FiO$_2$. Nimmagadda and colleagues confirmed that 4 DB/30 seconds provided suboptimal preoxygenation in volunteers; no subject achieved an EtO$_2$ value of 90% or better.[46] Another possible reason why patients preoxygenated with 4 DB/30 seconds desaturate more quickly is that the tissue and venous compartments need longer than 30 seconds to fill with oxygen.[21,32] These compartments likely have the capability of storing additional oxygen above that contained while breathing room air.[32,46] Such stored oxygen increases exponentially. It is possible that the 4 DB/30 seconds technique leads to rapid arterial oxygenation without substantial increase in the tissue oxygen stores and hence results in more rapid desaturation during subsequent apnea than would a longer period of preoxygenation with TVB.[32] Because the 4 DB/30 seconds technique yields submaximal preoxygenation, it should be reserved for emergency situations when time is limited.[46]

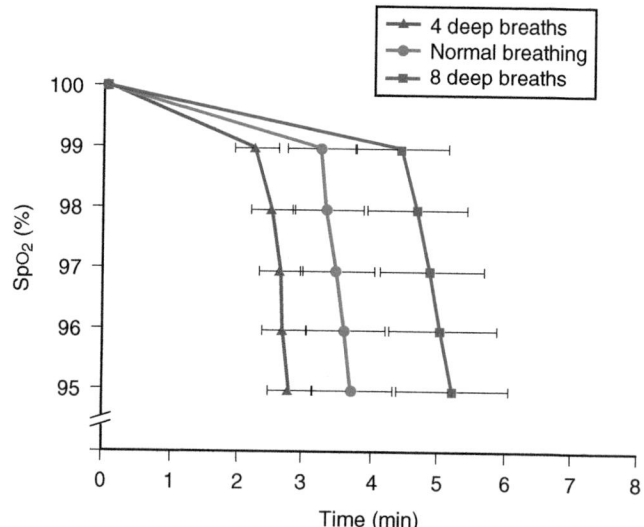

• **Fig. 15.7** Mean times to reach percentage decrease in hemoglobin saturation during apnea after three different preoxygenation techniques (4 deep breaths, normal breathing, 8 deep breaths). Spo$_2$, Oxygen saturation from pulse oximetry. (From Baraka AS, Taha SK, Aouad MT, et al. Preoxygenation: comparison of maximal breathing and tidal volume breathing techniques. *Anesthesiology.* 1999;91:612–616.)

To optimize the deep breathing method of preoxygenation, investigators have focused on (1) extending the duration of deep breathing to 1, 1.5, and 2 minutes (to allow 8, 12, and 16 DBs, respectively) and (2) using high FGF (≥ 10 L/min).[42,43] These maneuvers result in maximal preoxygenation (evidenced by higher EtO$_2$, Pao$_2$, and lower EtN$_2$) and improved efficiency (delayed onset of oxyhemoglobin desaturation during apnea) compared with the original 4 DB/30 seconds method.[37,46] One investigation suggested that preoxygenation using 8 DBs over 1 minute with an FGF of 10 L/min is associated with slower oxyhemoglobin desaturation than that using 4 DB/30 seconds or TVB for 3 minutes (see Fig. 15.6).[37] Several explanations were given for this finding, including leftward shift of the oxyhemoglobin dissociation curve secondary to hyperventilation-induced reduction in $Paco_2$ (Fig. 15.8) and the occurrence of several extra DBs during anesthetic induction.[32,62]

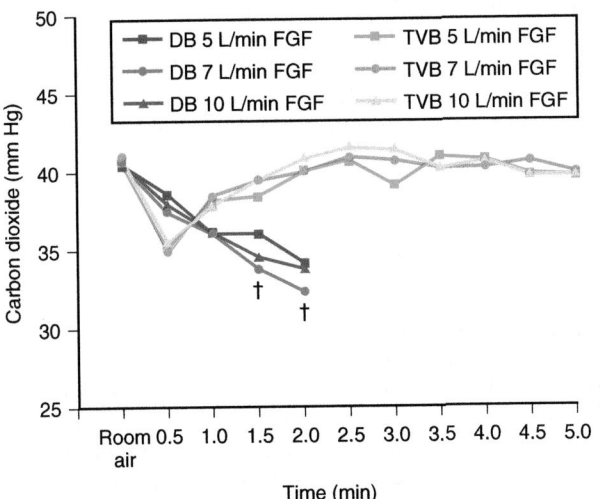

• **Fig. 15.8** Effect of the deep breathing technique on end-tidal carbon dioxide tension using 5, 7, and 10 L/min fresh gas flow (FGF). *DB,* Deep breathing; *TVB,* tidal volume breathing. †Significant difference ($p < 0.05$) from deep breaths at 0.5 and 1.0 minute. (From Nimmagadda U, Chiravuri SD, Salem MR, et al. Preoxygenation with tidal volume and deep breathing techniques: the impact of duration of breathing and fresh gas flow. *Anesth Analg.* 2001;92:1337–1341.)

The use of maximal exhalation before any preoxygenation maneuver has been suggested.[25,63] In a healthy subject with an FRC of 3 L, forced exhalation to the residual volume decreases the lung volume to approximately 1.5 L. This 50% reduction in the FRC leads to a 50% reduction in the time constant of the oxygen wash-in (nitrogen wash-out) curve.[64] The influence of prior maximal exhalation on preoxygenation using TVB or deep breathing has been studied.[65] TVB after maximal exhalation resulted in a more rapid rise in EtO_2 during the first minute than did TVB without prior maximal exhalation; however, the time required to reach maximal preoxygenation ($EtO_2 \geq 90\%$) was the same (Fig. 15.9).[66] During preoxygenation with deep breathing, the time courses for denitrogenation with and without prior maximal exhalation were identical. Apparently, the decrease in FRC resulting from maximal exhalation is minor in comparison with the level of $\dot{V}A$ associated with deep breathing. Regardless of whether prior maximal exhalation was used, deep breathing for 1.5 minutes was still required to reach an EtO_2 of 90% or more. As a result, prior maximal exhalation confers little or no additional practical benefit to preoxygenation.[65]

It has been demonstrated that preoxygenation using a single vital capacity breath (SVCB) technique can, within 30 seconds, result in a Pao_2 comparable to that achieved by TVB for 3 minutes.[66] This technique involves a triphasic process. The first phase consists of forced exhalation to the residual volume, which minimizes lung nitrogen content and the subsequent dilution of incoming oxygen. The second phase is deep inspiration to expand the lungs to their total capacity, with a consequent maximal increase in Pao_2. The third phase consists of holding the breath in full inspiration, which may allow gas movement from more-compliant alveoli to less-compliant alveoli because the time constants of filling between alveoli are not uniform.[66] The SVCB technique can provide adequate preoxygenation, especially when it is used for rapid induction of inhalational anesthesia.[66]

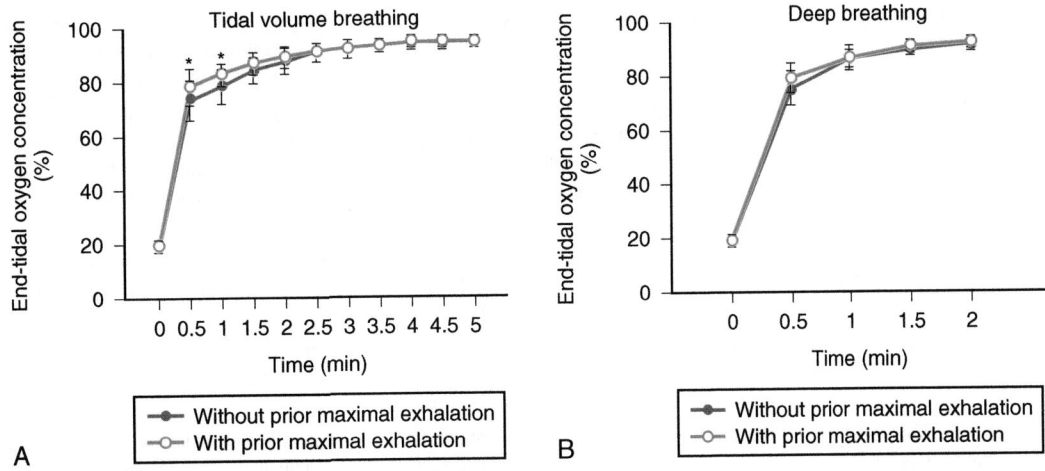

• **Fig. 15.9** (A) Comparison of end-tidal oxygen concentration values (mean ± SD) over 5-minute periods during simulated preoxygenation using tidal volume breathing (TVB) technique after maximal exhalation (*blue* O) versus TVB without prior maximal exhalation (*purple* •). *Statistically significant difference ($p < 0.05$) between techniques (TVB with or without prior maximal exhalation) at that time period. (B) Comparison of end-tidal oxygen concentration values (mean ± SD) over 2-minute periods during simulated preoxygenation using deep breathing technique after maximal exhalation (*blue* O) versus deep breathing without prior maximal exhalation (*purple* •). *SD,* Standard deviation. (From Nimmagadda U, Salem MR, Joseph NJ, Miko I. Efficacy of preoxygenation using tidal volume and deep breathing techniques with and without prior maximal exhalation. *Can J Anesth.* 2007;54:448–452.)

Head-Up Positioning

The supine position is not optimal for maximizing preoxygenation. The supine state hinders a patient's ability to take DBs, leading to dependent atelectasis and decreased FRC. As a result, the time to desaturation following the onset of apnea is shortened.[1] The back-up/head-elevated (BUHE) position improves the efficacy of preoxygenation and prolongs apnea time when compared with the supine position in both normal and obese patients.[67–70] In patients who are immobilized (e.g., those with potential spinal cord injury), reverse Trendelenburg position with the head 30 degrees higher than the foot improves preoxygenation.[1,69]

The BUHE position has benefits beyond those of improving the efficacy of preoxygenation. Khandelwal and colleagues found that placing patients in the BUHE position during emergency tracheal intubation in the ward and the intensive care unit (ICU) was associated with reduced odds of airway-related complications including hypoxemia.[71]

Noninvasive Positive-Pressure Ventilation

Obese, pregnant, or critically ill patients are at risk for reduced efficacy of traditional preoxygenation methods because their pathophysiologic state results in reduced FRC, increased risk of atelectasis, and right to left shunt. Recent studies have recommended maximizing preoxygenation in obese and/or critically ill patients by combining breathing 100% oxygen with noninvasive positive-pressure ventilation (NIPPV) with positive end-expiratory pressure (PEEP) in the reverse Trendelenburg position.[1,72,73] NIPPV and PEEP serve to increase mean airway pressure, thereby recruiting alveoli that contribute to increased right-to-left shunt in vulnerable patient populations. Weingart and Levitan detailed several studies that supported preoxygenation techniques that increase mean airway pressure (Table 15.2).[1]

Baillard and colleagues conducted a randomized, prospective study in two medical/surgical intensive care units (ICUs) in France.[75] Preoxygenation was performed before RSI in two study groups: the control group was preoxygenated with 3 minutes of TVB using a nonrebreather bag-valve mask, whereas the study group received NIPPV via an ICU ventilator through a face mask. The study groups were matched for age, disease severity, diagnosis, and SaO_2 before preoxygenation. SaO_2 was higher in the NIPPV group at the end of preoxygenation, at time of intubation, and 5 minutes after intubation. SaO_2 dropped below 80% in 46% of patients in the control group compared with 7% of patients in the NIPPV group. The incidence of regurgitation and new infiltrate on postprocedure chest radiograph did not vary between study groups and occurred in 3 and 4 cases, respectively. The authors concluded that preoxygenation using NIPPV is more effective for intubation of hypoxemic patients than the standard method of TVB.

Techniques for Prolongation of Apnea Time

Nasal Oxygen During Efforts Securing a Tube

Nasal oxygen during efforts securing a tube (NO DESAT) is a technique originally described by Levitan as a simple, accessible method to extend the apneic period during RSI in the emergency department (ED).[1,12] Nasal cannulae are placed on a patient under either a face mask or bag-valve mask device during initial preoxygenation. Once anesthesia is induced with ensuing apnea, the nasal cannula flow rate is increased to a maximum of 15 L/min. At this flow rate, nearly 100% FiO_2 is provided, facilitating apneic oxygenation. This technique is dependent upon the maintenance of airway patency throughout airway management, either by jaw thrust or laryngoscopy itself.

TABLE 15.2 Evidence for Increased Mean Airway Pressure as a Preoxygenation Technique

Study	Patients	Intervention	Comparator	Outcome
Delay et al.[74]	RCT of 28 obese operative patients	Noninvasive ventilation	Spontaneous ventilation at zero pressure	The patients in the NIPPV group achieved faster and more complete denitrogenation than the standard group, as measured by an exhaled oxygen level >90%.
Futier et al.[77]	RCT of 66 obese operative patients	Two treatment groups: noninvasive ventilation or noninvasive ventilation with posttracheal intubation recruitment maneuver	Spontaneous ventilation at zero pressure	At the end of preoxygenation, PaO_2 was higher in the NIPPV and NIPPV + RM groups compared with the spontaneous ventilation group and remained higher after intubation and the onset of mechanical ventilation.
Cressey et al.[76]	RCT of 20 morbidly obese women undergoing bariatric surgery	CPAP preoxygenation	Spontaneous ventilation at zero pressure	Showed a 40-s increase in time to desaturation using NIPPV. Nonsignificant primary outcome.
Gander et al.[78]	RCT of 30 morbidly obese operative patients	CPAP preoxygenation	Spontaneous ventilation at zero pressure	The time until reaching a saturation of 90% after apnea was expected by a minute in the CPAP group.
Herriger et al.[80]	RCT of 40 ASA PS I–II operative patients	CPAP preoxygenation	Spontaneous ventilation at zero pressure	Application of positive airway pressure during induction of anesthesia in adults prolongs the nonhypoxic apnea duration by >2 min.
Antonelli et al.[84]	RCT of 26 hypoxemic ICU patients requiring bronchoscopy	Noninvasive ventilation	Spontaneous ventilation at zero pressure	The PaO_2/FiO_2 ratio improved in the NIPPV group and worsened in the high-FiO_2-alone group.

ASA PS, American Society of Anesthesiologists Physical Status; *CPAP*, continuous positive airway pressure; *FiO_2* fraction of inspired oxygen; *NIPPV*, noninvasive positive pressure ventilation; *PaO_2* arterial partial pressure of oxygen; *RCT*, randomized, controlled trial; *RM*, recruitment maneuver.
From Weingart SD, Levitan RM. Preoxygenation and prevention of desaturation during emergency airway management. *Ann Emerg Med.* 2012;59(3):165–175.

Bhagwan described a small case series of RSIs in infants with pyloric stenosis using NO DESAT. The author commented that this was an easy and helpful technique. Desaturation and bradycardic events were infrequent. There were no reported cases of poor mask seal with the nasal cannula in place. Neither nosebleeds nor pneumothorax was noted in this series.[79]

Semler and colleagues published a randomized trial of apneic oxygenation during endotracheal intubation in 150 critically ill ICU patients.[81] The goal of the study was to determine if apneic oxygenation increased the lowest arterial oxygen saturation experienced by patients undergoing endotracheal intubation in the ICU by comparing the NO DESAT technique during laryngoscopy with no supplemental oxygen during the apneic period of laryngoscopy. The median lowest arterial oxygen saturation was 92% with apneic oxygenation versus 90% with the usual care group. There was no difference between study groups in the incidence of oxygen saturation below 90%. The authors concluded that use of the NO DESAT technique is not supported for routine use in critically ill adults. Further investigation is warranted to fully assess this simple and accessible method of apneic oxygenation in a wider variety of patients.

Pharyngeal Oxygen Insufflation

The technique of pharyngeal oxygen insufflation during the apneic period was first described by Teller and colleagues in 1988.[13] Twelve healthy patients scheduled for elective surgery breathed oxygen for 3 minutes from a circle system at an F_{IO_2} of 1; they were then instructed to hyperventilate until their $EtCO_2$ reached approximately 25 mm Hg, ensuring that, after 10 minutes of apnea, arterial CO_2 tension would not exceed 100 mm Hg. Following induction of anesthesia and neuromuscular blockade with succinylcholine, an 8-French catheter was inserted into the oropharyngeal airspace via the nose. Study patients were randomized to either 3 L/min of oxygen via the 8-French catheter or no oxygen. Anesthesia was maintained with a succinylcholine infusion and additional doses of thiopental, fentanyl, and midazolam. Apnea continued until either an Sao_2 of 92% was reached or 10 minutes of time elapsed. The Sao_2 of patients in the pharyngeal insufflation group never fell below 97%, and all patients in the group achieved the 10-minute predetermined apnea time. Patients who did not receive pharyngeal insufflation only achieved 6.8 minutes of apnea time with a minimum Sao_2 of 91%. The authors concluded that preoxygenation followed by pharyngeal oxygen insufflation provided 10 minutes of safe apnea time in healthy patients in whom the airway was unobstructed and the trachea was not intubated.

Baraka and colleagues studied supplementation of preoxygenation with nasopharyngeal oxygen insufflation (5 L/min) in 34 morbidly obese patients undergoing either gastric band or gastric bypass surgery.[19] Half of the patients received nasopharyngeal oxygen insufflation following preoxygenation, whereas the control group received preoxygenation alone. The time from the onset of apnea until Sao_2 of 95% was reached was compared between study groups with a cut-off time of 4 minutes. In the control group, Sao_2 fell from 100% to 95% in 147 ± 27 seconds during the apneic period; the time to desaturation was inversely correlated to body mass index (BMI). In the pharyngeal insufflation group, Sao_2 was maintained in 16 of 17 patients at 100% for the entire 4-minute study period. The authors concluded that nasopharyngeal oxygenation following preoxygenation in morbidly obese patients delayed the onset of oxyhemoglobin desaturation during subsequent apnea.

Heard and colleagues investigated the influence of buccal oxygenation using a preformed 3.5-mm internal diameter (ID) tracheal tube cut short so that its distal end was positioned in the buccal space.[82] Forty morbidly obese patients with a BMI of 30 to 40 kg/m^2 were randomly assigned to standard care (no buccal oxygenation) or buccal oxygenation at 10 L/min. After induction of general anesthesia, laryngoscopy was maintained during the study period until the Spo_2 dropped below 95% or 750 seconds (12.5 minutes) elapsed. Recipients of buccal oxygenation were less likely to develop an Spo_2 less than 95% during the apneic period, and the authors concluded that clinically important prolongation of safe apnea times could be achieved by delivering buccal oxygen to obese patients on induction of anesthesia.

Pharyngeal oxygen insufflation has also been studied in an experimental model of acute lung injury,[83] following preoxygenation using the four-deep-breath technique,[85] via a modified Macintosh laryngoscopy blade,[86] and during Airtraq laryngoscopy in infants and small children.[87]

THRIVE

THRIVE was first described in 2015 by Patel and Nouraei and involved the administration of high-flow (30 to 70 L/min) warmed, humidified oxygen to adult patients with difficult airways (DAs) using Optiflow, a commercial transnasal humidified oxygen delivery system (Fig. 15.10; Fisher & Paykel Healthcare, Auckland, New Zealand).[14] In healthy, awake volunteers, THRIVE for 3 minutes at 60 L/min has been shown to be as effective at preoxygenation as 3 minutes of face mask TVB with 10 L/min of oxygen.[14] THRIVE extends the safe apnea time before desaturation and reduces the accumulation of CO_2 as compared to conventional measures of apneic oxygenation using low-flow oxygen delivery devices.[88] Since its introduction, it has become a vital asset to anesthesia practice worldwide and has been included in several updated airway guidelines.[16] The beneficial effects of THRIVE have now been demonstrated in many studies and are reproducible across several patient groups including adults, pediatrics,

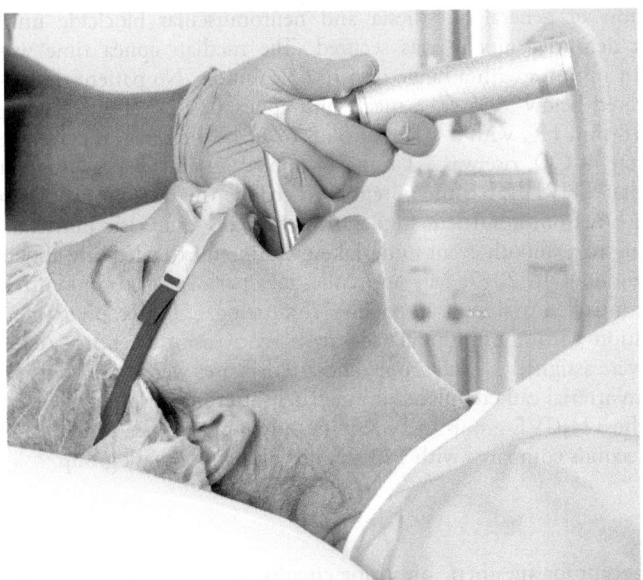

• **Fig. 15.10** Optiflow being used to provide THRIVE (transnasal humidified rapid-insufflation ventilatory exchange) during direct laryngoscopy to prolong apnea time. (Image courtesy Fisher & Paykel Healthcare, Auckland, NZ.)

obese patients, and the critically ill.[89,90] By utilizing the concept of perioxygenation, THRIVE increases the margin of safety while a definitive airway is secured, thus facilitating safer training during DA management and allowing the provision of a "tubeless" anesthesia technique if required.[90]

Despite the widespread use of THRIVE, the exact underlying physiological mechanisms have not been completely elucidated. It is now known that THRIVE provides only minimal positive airway pressure (as opposed to high-flow nasal oxygen [HFNO]), and thus that is not a significant mechanism of action. Cardiac oscillations have been postulated as a potential mechanism for increased CO_2 clearance; however, oscillations occur with all forms of oxygen delivery systems (e.g., low-flow systems) and thus cannot be the sole contributor. Physical airway models suggest that enhanced CO_2 clearance with THRIVE arises from interactions between entrained, turbulent supraglottic flow vortices generated by HFNO (turbulence proportional to flow rate), as well as cardiogenic oscillations.[91] This interaction creates a mechanism enhancing CO_2 removal from carina to pharynx, while also providing a means of increasing oxygen delivery from pharynx to carina—an "active" oxygenation component.[91] Apneic ventilation further increases P_{AO_2} as a result of its reciprocal reduction in the arterial partial pressure (Pa_{CO_2}) as explained by the alveolar gas equation:

$$P_{AO_2} = (F_{IO_2} \times [P_{atm} - P_{H_2O}]) - (Pa_{CO_2}/R)$$

where

P_{atm} = atmospheric pressure

P_{H_2O} = partial pressure of water

R = gas exchange ratio (ratio of CO_2 production to oxygen consumption)

Results from computational modeling in adults support these findings.[92]

In 2015, Patel and Nouraei described 25 adult patients undergoing general anesthesia for hypopharyngeal or laryngotracheal surgery in whom the presence of a DA was known and whose body mass index (BMI) or underlying cardiorespiratory disease made rapid oxygen desaturation at induction of anesthesia likely.[14] THRIVE was administered from preoxygenation through induction of general anesthesia and neuromuscular blockade until a definitive airway was secured. The median apnea time was 14 minutes with a range of 5 to 65 minutes. No patient desaturated below 90%. The mean post-apnea CO_2 level was 58.5 ± 18 mm Hg, with a range of 36.8 to 114.8 mm Hg; the average rate of CO_2 rise was 1.1 mm Hg/min. Patel and Nouraei suggest that THRIVE has the potential to change the nature of securing a DA from a hurried, stop-start, potentially traumatic undertaking to a smooth event undertaken within an extended safe apneic window. In 2017, Mir and colleagues performed a randomized controlled trial with 40 patients comparing THRIVE preoxygenation with conventional face-mask ventilation. Twenty patients were assigned to each group, and arterial gases were sampled using an arterial catheter placed immediately after induction. Patients in the THRIVE group had a significantly longer apnea time of 248 seconds compared with 123 seconds in the face mask group.[93]

Oxygen Delivery Systems

Except for anesthetic breathing circuits, virtually all oxygen delivery systems are nonrebreathing. In nonrebreathing circuits, the inspiratory gas is not made up in any part by the exhaled tidal volume (V_t), and the only CO_2 inhaled is that in any entrained room air. To avoid rebreathing, exhaled gases must be sequestered by one-way valves, and inspired gases must be presented in sufficient volume and flow to satisfy the high peak-flow rates and minute ventilation demonstrated in critically ill patients. Inspiratory entrainment of room air or the use of inspiratory reservoirs (including the anatomic dead space of the nasopharynx, oropharynx, and non–gas-exchanging portion of the bronchial tree) and one-way valves typifies nonrebreathing systems and defines them as two groups.[94–96] Low-flow systems depend on inspiration of room air to meet inspiratory flow and volume demands. High-flow systems attempt to provide the entire inspiratory demand. High-flow systems use reservoirs or very high flow rates to meet the large peak inspiratory flow demands and the exaggerated minute volumes found in many critically ill patients.

Low-Flow Oxygen Systems

A low-flow, variable-performance system depends on room air entrainment to meet the patient's peak inspiratory and minute ventilatory demands that are not met by the inspiratory gas flow or oxygen reservoir alone. Low-flow devices include the nasal cannula, simple face mask, partial rebreathing mask, nonrebreathing mask, and tracheostomy collar. Low-flow systems are characterized by the ability to deliver high and low values of F_{IO_2}. The F_{IO_2} becomes unpredictable and inconsistent when these devices are used for patients with abnormal or changing ventilatory patterns.[95] Low-flow systems produce F_{IO_2} values of 21% to 80%. The F_{IO_2} may vary with the size of the oxygen reservoir, oxygen flow, and the patient's ventilatory pattern (e.g., V_t, peak inspiratory flow, respiratory rate, minute ventilation). With a normal ventilation pattern, these devices can deliver a relatively predictable and consistent F_{IO_2} level.

Low-flow systems do not mean low F_{IO_2} values. With changes in V_t, respiratory rate, oxygen reservoir size, and so on, the F_{IO_2} can vary dramatically at comparable oxygen flow rates. The following examples are theoretical mathematical estimates of an F_{IO_2} produced by a low-flow system (e.g., nasal cannula) in two clinical conditions.

The example for estimation of F_{IO_2} from a low-flow system is based on the standard normal patient and ventilatory pattern. Several assumptions are used for the F_{IO_2} calculation. The anatomic reservoir for a nasal cannula consists of nose, nasopharynx, and oropharynx, and it is about one-third of the entire normal anatomic dead space, including the trachea. For example, 150 mL ÷ 3 = 50 mL; assume a nasal cannula oxygen flow rate of 6 L/min (100 mL/s), V_t of 500 mL, respiratory rate of 20 breaths/min, inspiratory (I) time of 1 second, and expiratory (E) time of 2 seconds. If the terminal 0.5 second of the 2-second expiratory time has negligible gas flow, the anatomic reservoir (50 mL) completely fills with 100% oxygen, assuming an oxygen flow rate of 100 mL/s. Using the preceding normal variables, the F_{IO_2} is calculated for a patient with a 500-mL and a 250-mL V_t (Tables 15.3 and 15.4).

The preceding 50% variability in F_{IO_2} at 6 L/min of oxygen flow clearly demonstrates the effects of a variable ventilatory pattern. In general, the larger the V_t or faster the respiratory rate, the lower the F_{IO_2}. The smaller the V_t or lower the respiratory rate, the higher the F_{IO_2}.

Low-flow oxygen devices are the most commonly employed oxygen delivery systems because of simplicity, ease of use, familiarity, economics, availability, and acceptance by patients. In most clinical situations (see sections "High-Flow Oxygen Systems" and "High-Flow Devices"), these systems should be initially employed.

TABLE 15.3 Example 1: If V_T Is Decreased to 500 mL

Cannula	6 L/min	V_T 500 mL
Mechanical reservoir	None	I/E ratio = 1:2
Anatomic reservoir	50 mL	Rate = 20 breaths/min
100% oxygen provided/sec	100 mL	Inspiratory time = 1 second
Volume inspired oxygen		
Anatomic reservoir	50 mL	
Flow/second	100 mL	
Inspired room air (0.20 × 350 mL)	70 mL	
Oxygen inspired	220 mL	

$$F_{IO_2} = 200\ mL\ O_2 \div 500\ mL\ O_2 = 0.44$$

F_{IO_2}, Fraction of inspired oxygen; *I/E ratio*, inspiration/expiration ratio; V_T, tidal volume.

TABLE 15.4 Example 2: If V_T Is Decreased to 250 mL

Volume Inspired Oxygen	
Anatomic reservoir	50 mL
Flow/sec	100 mL
Inspired room air (0.20 × 100 mL)	20 mL
Oxygen inspired	170 mL

$$F_{IO_2} = 170\ mL\ O_2 \div 250\ mL\ O_2 = 0.68$$

F_{IO_2}, Fraction of inspired oxygen; V_T, tidal volume.

Oxygen Delivery Devices

Low-Flow Devices

Nasal Cannulas

Because of their simplicity and the ease with which patients tolerate them, nasal cannulas are the most frequently used oxygen delivery devices. The nasal cannula consists of two prongs, one inserted into each naris, delivering 100% oxygen. To be effective, the nasal passages must be patent, but the patient need not breathe through the nose. The flow rate settings range from 0.25 to 6 L/min. The nasopharynx serves as the oxygen reservoir (Fig. 15.11). Gases should be humidified to prevent mucosal drying if the oxygen flow exceeds 4 L/min. For each 1 L/min increase in flow, the F_{IO_2} is assumed to increase by 4% (Table 15.5).

An F_{IO_2} of 0.24 to 0.44 can be delivered predictably if the patient breathes at a normal minute ventilation rate with a normal respiratory pattern. Increasing flows to more than 6 L/min does not significantly increase the F_{IO_2} above 0.44 and is often poorly tolerated by the patient.

The components of a nasal cannula are nasal cannula prongs, delivery tubing, and an adjustable, restraining headband. Additional equipment includes an oxygen flowmeter to provide controlled gas delivery from a wall outlet; a humidification system increases patients' comfort at higher flows (≥4 L/min).

Procedurally, the initiation of oxygen therapy should be preceded by a review of the chart and documentation of the oxygen concentration and device ordered. If a humidifier (typically prefilled, single use, and disposable) is used, it should be filled to the appropriate level with sterile water and connected to the flowmeter. The nasal prongs should be secured in the patient's nares and the cannula secured around the patient's head by a restraining strap.

Avoidance of undue cutaneous pressure is essential. Gauze may be needed to pad pressure points around the cheeks and ears during prolonged use. The flowmeter should be adjusted to the prescribed liter flow to attain the desired F_{IO_2} (see Table 15.5).

High-Flow Oxygen Systems

High-flow, fixed-performance systems are nonrebreathing systems that provide the entire inspiratory atmosphere needed to meet the peak inspiratory flow and minute ventilatory demands of the patient. The flow rate and reservoir are essential to meet the patient's peak inspiratory flow. Flows of 30 to 40 L/min (or three to four times the measured minute volume) are often necessary. High-flow devices include aerosol masks and T-pieces that are powered by air-entrainment nebulizers or air-oxygen blenders and Venturi masks (see section "Oxygen Delivery Devices"). Regardless of the patient's respiratory pattern, high-flow systems are expected to deliver predictable, consistent, and measurable high and low F_{IO_2} values. High-flow systems also can control the humidity and temperature of the delivered gases. The primary limitations of these systems are cost, bulkiness, and patients' tolerance.

There are two primary indications for high-flow oxygen devices:

1. Patients who require a consistent, predictable, minimal F_{IO_2} to reverse hypoxemia but prevent respiratory compromise because of excessive oxygen delivery (see section "Complications of Perioxygenation"); and
2. The patient with increased minute ventilation and abnormal respiratory pattern who needs predictable and consistent high F_{IO_2} values.

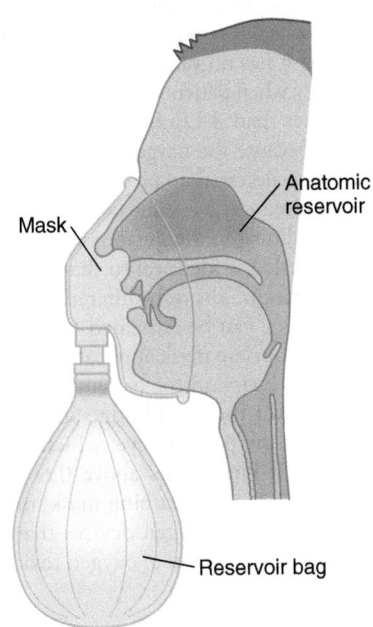

• **Fig. 15.11** The three reservoirs of low-flow oxygen therapy. (From Vender JS, Clemency MV. O_2 delivery systems, inhalation therapy, and respiratory care. In Benumof JL, ed. *Clinical Procedures in Anesthesia and Intensive Care*. Lippincott; 1992:63–87.)

TABLE 15.5	Approximate F_{IO_2} Delivered by Nasal Cannula	
Flow Rate (L/min)	Approximate F_{IO_2}[a]
1	0.24
2	0.28
3	0.32
4	0.36
5	0.40
6	0.44

F_{IO_2}, Fraction of inspired oxygen.
[a]Based on normal ventilatory patterns.

TABLE 15.6	Approximate F_{IO_2} Delivered by Simple Face Mask	
Flow Rate (L/min)	F_{IO_2}[a]
5–6	0.4
6–7	0.5
7–8	0.6

F_{IO_2}, Fraction of inspired oxygen.
[a]Based on normal ventilatory patterns.

Although nasal cannulas are simple and safe to use, several potential hazards and complications exist. Oxygen supports combustion, and any type of oxygen therapy is a fire hazard. Nasal trauma from prolonged use of or pressure from the nasal prongs can cause tissue damage. With poorly humidified, high gas flows, the airway mucosal surface can become dehydrated. This mucosal dehydration can result in mucosal irritation, epistaxis, laryngitis, ear tenderness, substernal chest pain, and bronchospasm.[94,96,97] Because this is a low-flow system, the F_{IO_2} can be inaccurate and inconsistent, leading to the potential for underoxygenation or overoxygenation. Overoxygenation may induce respiratory distress in patients with severe COPD by reversing protective hypoxic pulmonary vasoconstriction, depressing ventilation, and minimizing the Haldane effect (see section "Complications of Perioxygenation"). Underoxygenation potentiates any problems associated with hypoxemia.

Simple Face Mask

To provide a higher F_{IO_2} than that provided by nasal cannula with low-flow systems, the size of the oxygen reservoir must increase (see Fig. 15.11). A simple face mask consists of a mask with two side ports. The mask serves as an additional oxygen reservoir of 100 to 200 mL. The side ports allow room air entrainment and egress of exhaled gases. The mask has no valves. An F_{IO_2} of 0.40 to 0.60 can be achieved predictably when patients exhibit normal respiratory patterns. Gas flows greater than 8 L/min do not significantly increase the F_{IO_2} above 0.60 because the oxygen reservoir is filled. A minimum flow of 5 L/min is necessary to prevent CO_2 accumulation and rebreathing. The delivered oxygen value depends on the ventilatory pattern of the patient, similar to the situation with nasal cannulas.

The equipment needed is identical to that used for nasal cannula oxygen administration. The only difference is the use of a face mask. The predicted F_{IO_2} can be estimated from the oxygen flow rate (Table 15.6). Appropriate mask application is needed with all masks to maximize the F_{IO_2} and the patient's comfort. The mask should be positioned over the nasal bridge and the face, restricting oxygen escape into the patient's eye, which can cause ocular drying and irritation. If F_{IO_2} values above 0.60 are required, a partial rebreathing mask, nonrebreathing mask, or high-flow system should be employed. All oxygen devices that deliver higher values of F_{IO_2} increase the potential of oxygen toxicity (see section "Complications of Perixoygenation").

Partial Rebreathing Mask

To deliver an F_{IO_2} level of more than 60% with a low-flow system, the oxygen reservoir system must be increased (see Fig. 15.11).[96] A partial rebreathing mask adds a reservoir bag with a capacity

of 600 mL to 1000 mL. Side ports allow entrainment of room air and the egress of exhaled gases. The distinctive feature of this mask is that the first 33% of the patient's exhaled volume fills the reservoir bag. This volume is derived from the anatomic dead space and contains little CO_2. During inspiration, the bag should not completely collapse. A deflated reservoir bag results in a decreased F_{IO_2} because of entrained room air. With the next breath, the first exhaled gas (which is in the reservoir bag) and fresh gas are inhaled—accounting for the name *partial rebreather*. Fresh gas flows should be greater than 8 L/min, and the reservoir bag must remain inflated during the entire ventilatory cycle to ensure the highest F_{IO_2} and adequate CO_2 evacuation. An F_{IO_2} of 0.60 to 0.80 or more can be delivered with this device if the mask is applied appropriately and the ventilatory pattern is normal (Table 15.7). This mask's rebreathing capacity allows oxygen conservation and may be useful during transportation, when oxygen supply may be limited. Complications with partial rebreathing oxygen delivery systems are similar to those with other mask devices with low-flow systems.

Nonrebreathing Mask

A nonrebreathing mask (Fig. 15.12) is similar to a partial rebreathing mask but adds three unidirectional valves. One valve is located on each side of the mask to permit the venting of exhaled gases and to prevent room air entrainment. The third unidirectional valve is situated between the mask and the reservoir bag and prevents exhaled gases from entering the bag.

The bag must be inflated throughout the ventilatory cycle to ensure the highest F_{IO_2} and adequate CO_2 evacuation. Typically, the F_{IO_2} level is 0.80 to 0.90. Fresh gas flow is usually 15 L/min (range, 10 to 15 L/min). If room air is not entrained, an F_{IO_2} value approaching 1.0 can be achieved. If fresh gas flows or reservoir volume do not meet ventilatory needs, many masks have a spring-loaded tension valve that permits room air entrainment if

TABLE 15.7	Approximate F_{IO_2} Delivered by Mask With Reservoir Bag	
Flow Rate (L/min)	F_{IO_2}[a]
6	0.6
7	0.7
8	0.8
9	0.8+
10	0.8+

F_{IO_2}, Fraction of inspired oxygen.
[a]Based on normal ventilatory patterns.

Nonrebreathing oxygen mask

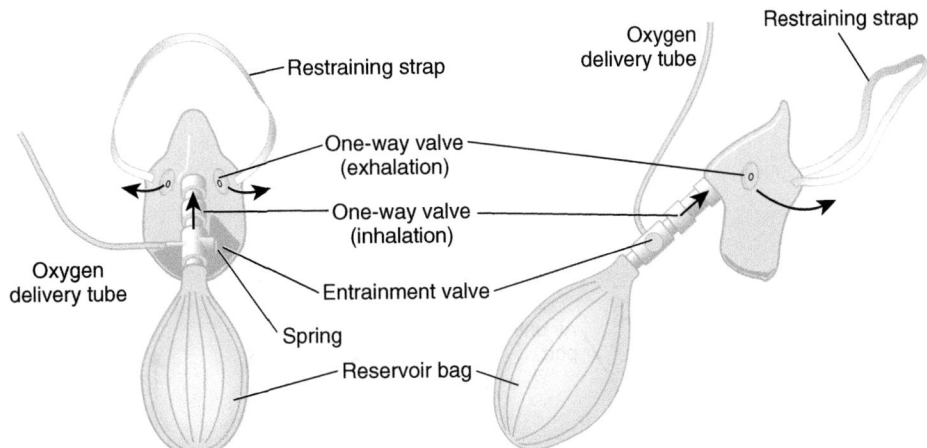

• **Fig. 15.12** A nonrebreathing oxygen mask. In addition to the exhalation valve, the mask has a one-way inhalation valve. (From Vender JS, Clemency MV. Oxygen delivery systems, inhalation therapy, and respiratory care. In Benumof JL, ed. *Clinical Procedures in Anesthesia and Intensive Care*. Lippincott; 1992.)

the reservoir is evacuated. This spring valve is often called a *safety valve*. The spring valve tension should be checked periodically. If such a valve is not present, one of the unidirectional valves on the mask should be removed to allow room air entrainment if needed to meet ventilatory demands. This may be required to meet the increased inspiratory drive of critically ill patients. If the total ventilatory needs are met without room air entrainment, the rebreathing mask performs like a high-flow system. The operational application of a nonrebreathing mask is similar to that of other mask devices. To optimize the system, the mask should fit snugly (without excessive pressure) to avoid air entrainment around the mask, which would dilute the delivered gas and lower the F_{IO_2}. If the mask fit is appropriate, the reservoir bag responds to the patient's inspiratory efforts.

Tracheostomy Collars

Tracheostomy collars are used primarily to deliver humidity to patients with artificial airways. Oxygen may be delivered with these devices, but as with other low-flow delivery systems, the F_{IO_2} is unpredictable, inconsistent, and dependent on ventilatory pattern because of the limited reservoir volume. The consistency of delivered F_{IO_2} by tracheostomy also depends on the patient's breathing entirely through the tracheostomy. Cuff deflation or tube fenestration allows entrainment of air through the upper airways, and this may alter the concentration of delivered oxygen.

High-Flow Devices

Venturi Masks

High-flow systems have flow rates and reservoirs large enough to provide the total inspired gases reliably. Most high-flow systems use gas entrainment at some point in the circuit to provide the flow and F_{IO_2} needs. Venturi masks entrain air by the Bernoulli principle and constant pressure-jet mixing.[98] This physical phenomenon is based on a rapid velocity of gas (e.g., oxygen) moving through a restricted orifice. This action produces viscous shearing forces that create a decreased pressure gradient (subatmospheric) downstream relative to the surrounding gases. The pressure gradient causes room air to be entrained until the pressures are equalized. Fig. 15.13 illustrates the Venturi principle.

Venturi principle

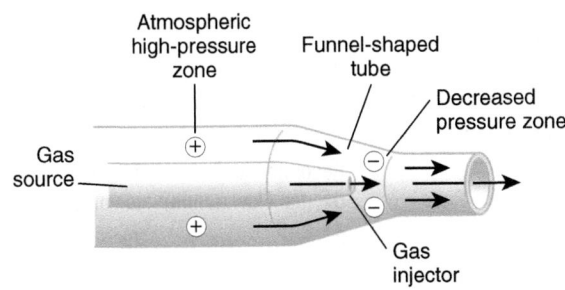

• **Fig. 15.13** Application of the Venturi principle. (From Vender JS, Clemency MV. Oxygen delivery systems, inhalation therapy, and respiratory care. In Benumof JL, ed. Clinical Procedures in *Anesthesia and Intensive Care*. Lippincott; 1992.)

Altering the gas orifice or entrainment port size causes the F_{IO_2} value to vary. The oxygen flow rate determines the total volume of gas provided by the device. It provides predictable and reliable F_{IO_2} values of 0.24 to 0.50 that are independent of the patient's respiratory pattern. These masks come in two varieties:

1. A fixed F_{IO_2} model, which requires specific inspiratory attachments that are color coded and have labeled jets that produce a known F_{IO_2} with a given flow.
2. A variable F_{IO_2} model (Fig. 15.14), which has a graded adjustment of the air entrainment port that can be set to allow variation in delivered F_{IO_2}.

To use any air entrainment device properly to control the F_{IO_2}, the standard air-oxygen entrainment ratios and minimum recommended flows for a given F_{IO_2} level must be used (Table 15.8). The minimum total flow requirement should result from entrained room air added to the fresh oxygen flow and should equal three to four times the minute ventilation. This minimal flow is required to meet the patient's peak inspiratory flow demands. As the desired F_{IO_2} increases, the air-oxygen entrainment ratio decreases with a net reduction in total gas flow. The higher the desired F_{IO_2}, the greater the probability of the patient's needs exceeding the total flow capabilities of the device.

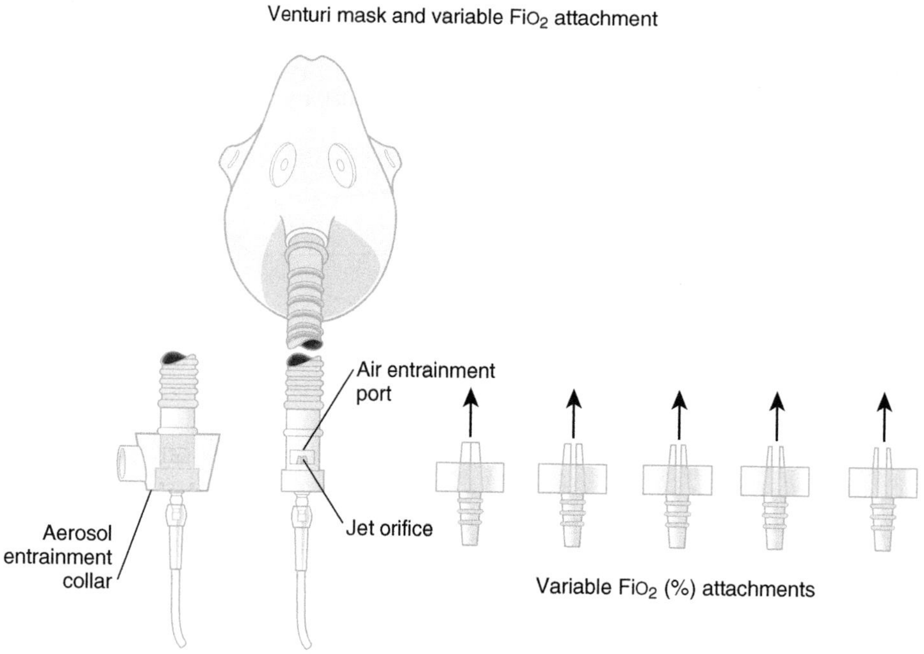

Venturi mask and variable FiO₂ attachment

Air entrainment
port

Aerosol
entrainment
collar

Jet orifice

Variable FiO₂ (%) attachments

• **Fig. 15.14** Graded air entrainment by the Ventimask provides specific F_{IO_2} levels through the jet orifices. (From Vender JS, Clemency MV. Oxygen delivery systems, inhalation therapy, and respiratory care. In Benumof JL, ed. *Clinical Procedures in Anesthesia and Intensive Care*. Lippincott; 1992.)

TABLE 15.8	Approximate Air Entrainment Ratio and Gas Flow (F_{IO_2})		
F_{IO_2} (%)	Ratio	Recommended Oxygen Flow (L/min)	Total Gas Flow to Port (L/min)[a]
24	25.3:1	3	79
26	14.8:1	3	47
28	10.3:1	6	68
30	7.8:1	6	53
35	4.6:1	9	50
40	3.2:1	12	50
50	1.7:1	15	41

F_{IO_2}, Fraction of inspired oxygen.
[a]Varies with manufacturer.

Venturi masks are often useful when treating patients with COPD who may develop worsening respiratory distress and dead space ventilation with supplemental increases in oxygen fraction.[99,100] The Venturi mask's ability to deliver a high flow with no particulate H_2O makes it beneficial in treating asthmatics, in whom bronchospasm may be precipitated or exacerbated by aerosolized H_2O administration.

Several specific concerns regarding the application of a Venturi mask must be recognized to provide appropriate function. Obstructions distal to the jet orifice can produce back pressure and an effect referred to as *Venturi stall*. When this occurs, room air entrainment is compromised, causing a decreased total gas flow and an increased F_{IO_2}. Occlusion or alteration of the exhalation ports can also produce this situation. Aerosol devices should not be used with these devices. Water droplets can occlude the oxygen injector. If humidity is needed, a vapor-type humidity adapter collar should be used.

High-Flow Nasal Oxygen

HFNO systems have been developed that can provide humidified gas flows up to 50 L/min while achieving 72% to 100% F_{IO_2}.[101] Consistent delivery of humidification is also maintained at 72% to 99.9% relative humidity using specialized nasal cannulas,[102] larger tubing, high-flow humidifiers, and oxygen blenders. HFNO can generate moderate levels of continuous positive airway pressure (CPAP) in nasal-breathing and mouth-breathing patients[103–105] and reduce anatomic dead space by washing out room air from the upper airway.[104,106] It does not require a face mask, unlike most other high-flow systems, and this affords patients the opportunity to verbally communicate and eat in a normal manner.

In observational studies of hypoxemic patients, the use of HFNO was associated with lower rates of intubation in comparison to noninvasive ventilation (NIV) and standard oxygen therapy.[104,107] Although the use of HFNO in patients with hypoxemic respiratory failure did not reduce rates of intubation in a randomized controlled trial,[106] it did improve mortality and ventilator-free days in comparison to NIV and standard oxygen therapy. Additionally, HFNO has shown some benefit in reducing $Paco_2$ similar to NIV in patients with stable hypercapnic COPD.[108] In a randomized controlled trial of intubated ICU patients, application of HFNO after extubation was associated with better oxygenation and lower reintubation rates in comparison with the Venturi mask.[109] Use of HFNO was found to be noninferior to noninvasive bi-level positive airway pressure (BiPAP) use in a randomized trial of cardiothoracic surgery patients.[110] Several types of HFNO systems are available for adults: the High Flow Adult Cannula (Salter Labs, Lake Forest, IL), the Optiflo (Fisher & Paykel Healthcare, Auckland, New Zealand), and Precision Flow (Vapotherm, Exeter, NH). All achieve high relative humidity and high F_{IO_2} values. The High Flow Adult Cannula and Precision Flow resemble a regular nasal cannula at the patient interface. The High Flow Adult Cannula includes larger three-channel tubing that is colored green and can provide flow rates up to 15 L/min, whereas the Precision Flow includes a circuit comprised of a nasal cannula delivery tube, disposable water path, and vapor transfer cartridge, providing flow rates up to 40 L/min.

Aerosol Masks and T-Pieces With Nebulizers or Air-Oxygen Blenders

Large-volume nebulizers and wide-bore tubing are optimal for delivering F_{IO_2} levels greater than 0.40 with a high-flow system. Aerosol masks, in conjunction with air entrainment nebulizers or air-oxygen blenders, deliver consistent and predictable F_{IO_2} levels, regardless of the patient's ventilatory pattern. A T-piece is used in place of an aerosol mask for patients with an artificial airway.

Air entrainment nebulizers can deliver F_{IO_2} of 0.35 to 1.00 and produce an aerosol. The maximum gas flow through the nebulizer is 14 to 16 L/min. As with the Venturi masks, less room air is entrained with higher F_{IO_2} values. As a result, total flow at high F_{IO_2} values is decreased. To meet ventilatory demands, two nebulizers may feed a single mask to increase the total flow, and a short length of corrugated tubing may be added to the aerosol mask side ports to increase the reservoir capacity (Fig. 15.15). If the aerosol mist exiting the mask side ports disappears during inspiration, room air is probably being entrained, and flow should be increased.

Circuit resistance can increase as a result of water accumulation or kinking of the aerosol tubing. The increased pressure at the Venturi device decreases room air entrainment, increases the F_{IO_2} level, and decreases total gas flow. If a predictable F_{IO_2} level of more than 0.40 is desired, an air-oxygen blender should be used. Air-oxygen blenders can deliver consistent and accurate F_{IO_2} values from 0.21 to 1.0 and flows of up to 100 L/min with humidification. The higher flows tend to produce excessive noise through the large-bore tubing. Air-oxygen blenders are recommended for patients with increased minute ventilation who require a high F_{IO_2} level and in whom bronchospasm may be precipitated or worsened by a nebulized H_2O aerosol. With an artificial airway,

a 15- to 20-inch reservoir tube should be added to the Briggs T-piece (Hudson RCI, Temecula, CA) to prevent the potential of entraining air into the system.

Humidifiers

Humidity is the water vapor in a gas. When air is 100% saturated at 37°C, it contains 43.8 mg of H_2O/L. The amount of water vapor contained in a volume of gas depends on the temperature and water availability. The vapor pressure exerted by the water vapor is equal to 47 mm Hg. Alveolar gases are 100% saturated at 37°C. When the inspired atmosphere contains less than 43.8 mg of H_2O/L or has a vapor pressure of less than 47 mm Hg, a gradient exists between the respiratory mucosa and the inhaled gas. This gradient causes water to leave the mucosa and to humidify the inhaled gas.

Room air that has a relative humidity of 50% at 21°C has a relative humidity of 21% at 37°C. Under normal conditions, the lungs contribute about 250 mL of H_2O per day to maximally saturate inspired air.[96]

The administration of dry oxygen lowers the water content of the inspired air. The upper respiratory tract filters, humidifies, and warms inspired gases. Nasal breathing is more efficient than oral breathing for conditioning inspired gases. The use of an artificial airway bypasses the nasopharynx and oropharynx, where a significant amount of warming and humidification of inspired gases are accomplished. As a result, oxygen administration and the use of artificial airways increase the demand on the lungs to humidify the inspired gases.

The increased demand ultimately leads to mucosal drying, inspissated secretions, and decreased mucociliary clearance, which can eventually result in bacterial infections, mucous plugging, atelectasis, and pneumonia. To prevent these complications, a humidifier or nebulizer should be used to increase the water content of the inspired gases.

Indications for humidity therapy include high-flow therapeutic gas delivery to nonintubated patients, delivery of gases through

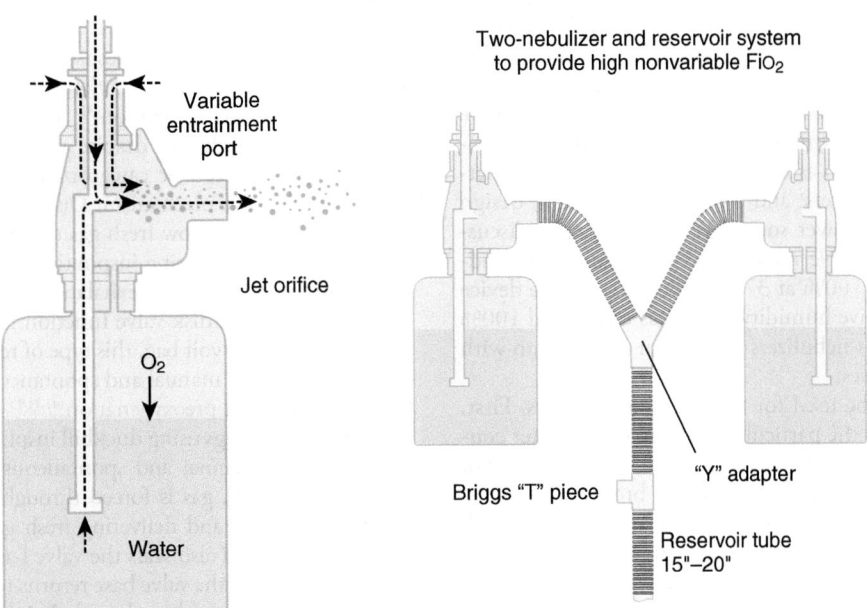

• **Fig. 15.15** Single-unit and double (tandem)-unit mechanical aerosol systems. (From Vender JS, Clemency MV. Oxygen delivery systems, inhalation therapy, and respiratory care. In Benumof JL, ed. *Clinical Procedures in Anesthesia and Intensive Care.* Lippincott; 1992.)

artificial airways, and reduction of airway resistance in asthma. Low flows (1 to 4 L/min) usually do not need humidification except in specific individuals, but all oxygen delivered to infants should be humidified.

A humidifier increases the heated or unheated water vapor in a gas. This can be accomplished by passing gas over heated water (heated pass over humidifier); by fractionating gas into tiny bubbles as gas passes through water (bubble diffusion or jet humidifiers); by allowing gas to pass through a chamber that contains a heated, water-saturated wick (heated wick humidifier); and by vaporizing water and selectively allowing the vapor to mix with the inspired gases (vapor-phase humidifier). Other variations of humidification systems exist but are beyond the scope of this chapter.[111]

Bubble humidifiers can be used with nasal cannulas, simple face masks, partial and nonrebreathing masks, and air-oxygen blenders. They increase the relative humidity of gas from 0% to 70% at 25°C, which is approximately equal to 34% at 37°C.[112,113] Large-volume bubble-through humidifiers are available for use with ventilator circuits or high-gas-flow delivery systems.

A heated humidifier may be used when delivering dry gases to patients with ETTs because it allows delivery of gases with an increased water content and relative humidity exceeding 65% at 37°C. When heated humidifiers are used, proximal airway temperature should be monitored to ensure a gas temperature that allows maximum moisture-carrying capacity but prevents mucosal burns.

Heat and moisture exchangers (HMEs) are simple, small humidifier systems designed to be attached to an artificial airway. The HMEs are often referred to as an *artificial nose*. The efficiency of these devices is quite variable, depending on the HME design, V_t, and atmospheric conditions. HMEs are typically used for short-term ventilatory support and for humidification during anesthesia. Several contraindications include use in neonatal and small pediatric patients; copious secretions; significant spontaneous breathing, in which the patient's V_t exceeds the HME specifications; and large-volume losses through a bronchopleural fistula or leakage around the ETT.[111]

A nebulizer increases the water content of the inspired gas by generating aerosols (small droplets of particulate water) that become incorporated into the delivered gas stream and then evaporate into the inspired gas as it is warmed in the respiratory tract. There are two basic kinds of nebulizers: pneumatic and electric. Pneumatic nebulizers operate from a pressured gas source and are jet or hydrodynamic. Electric nebulizers are powered by an electrical source and are referred to as *ultrasonic*. There are several varieties of both types of nebulizers, and they depend more on design differences than on the power source. A more in-depth discussion of nebulizers is available elsewhere.[96] The resultant humidity ranges from 50% to 100% at 37°C, depending on the device used. If heated, the relative humidity of the gas can exceed 100% at 37°C. Air entrainment nebulizers are used in conjunction with aerosol masks and T-pieces.

Aerosol therapy can be used for three general purposes. First, aerosol therapy increases the particulate and molecular water content of the inspired gases. The aerosol increases the water content of desiccated and retained secretions, enhancing bronchial hygiene. This does not alleviate the need for systemic hydration. Second, delivery of medications is a primary indication for aerosol therapy. For example, β_2-agonists, corticosteroids, anticholinergics, and antiviral-antibacterial agents may be delivered to patients' airways by aerosol therapy. Third, aerosol therapy can be employed for sputum induction. The success of aerosol therapy depends on appropriate application and proper technique of administration.

The aerosol generated by the nebulizer can precipitate bronchospasm of hyperactive airways.[94,96] Prophylactic bronchodilator therapy should be employed before or during the aerosol treatment. Fluid accumulation and overload have been reported. These problems are more common in treating pediatric patients and with continuous ultrasonic nebulizers rather than intermittent or jet therapy. Dry secretions are hydrophilic and can swell because of the absorbed water content. If secretions swell, they can obstruct airways. Mobilization of secretions limits this problem. Aerosol therapy for drug delivery has been reported to precipitate the same side effects as systemic drug delivery. Therapeutic aerosols have been implicated in nosocomial infections.[114] Cross-contamination between patients must be avoided.

Manual Resuscitation Bags

Manual resuscitation bags are used primarily for resuscitation and manual ventilation of ventilator-dependent patients. These bags can deliver an FIO_2 of more than 0.90 and V_t values up to 800 mL when oxygen flows to the bag are 10 to 15 mL/min. Factors that promote the highest FIO_2 level include the use of an oxygen reservoir, connection to an oxygen source, and slow rates of ventilation that allow the bag to refill completely. Positive end-expiratory pressure (PEEP) valves should be used for patients who require more than 5 cm H_2O of PEEP. The clinician should be aware of different capabilities among various resuscitation bags in the delivery of maximum FIO_2.[115–117]

Breathing Systems for Preoxygenation

The design of the breathing system used for preoxygenation can have significant impact on the efficacy of denitrogenation. The degree of rebreathing during spontaneous respiration is less with the Mapleson A system than with the Mapleson D system.[56] Therefore when using the Mapleson A or the circle system for preoxygenation by TVB, an oxygen flow of 5 L/min can adequately preoxygenate the patient within 3 minutes, whereas an oxygen flow of 10 L/min is required to achieve a similar EtO_2 with the Mapleson D system.[56,57] In contrast, when deep breathing is used, an oxygen flow of 10 L/min is required irrespective of the anesthesia circuit.[57]

In the critical care setting, resuscitation bags are commonly used for preoxygenation. However, their effectiveness differs markedly during spontaneous respiration.[41] Some, because of their design, cannot deliver a high FIO_2 despite an FGF of 15 L/min or greater. Resuscitation bags can be categorized into two groups depending on the type of valve mechanism. Disk-type valve systems use single or multiple disks to allow fresh gas to flow to the patient (and seal the exhalation port) during inspiration. The disk returns to its former position and opens the exhalation port during exhalation (Fig. 15.16). Because the disk valve function is not dependent on compression of the reservoir bag, this type of resuscitation bag functions equally well during manual and spontaneous ventilation and therefore can be used for preoxygenation.[41,118]

Resuscitation bags using duckbill inspiratory valves function differently during manual and spontaneous ventilation.[41,118] During manual ventilation, gas is forced through the valve base, opening the duckbill valve, and delivering fresh gas to the patient's lungs. The force generated also seals the valve base to the exhalation port. During exhalation, the valve base returns to its former position, and exhaled gases are vented to the exhalation port (Fig. 15.17). Mills and colleagues found that duckbill-type resuscitation bags, without one-way exhalation valves to prevent air entrainment, showed variability in delivered oxygen concentration during spontaneous

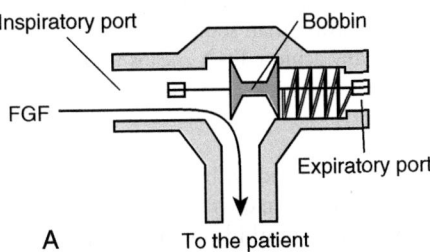

Inspiratory phase

Inspiratory port — Bobbin

FGF

Expiratory port

A   To the patient

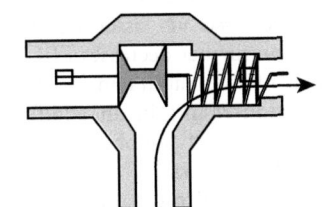

Expiratory phase

B

• **Fig. 15.16** Diagram of a typical disk valve in a disk-type resuscitation bag. (A) During inhalation, the piston seals the exhalation port and allows fresh gas to flow to the patient. (B) During exhalation, the fresh gas port is sealed by the piston while gas is allowed to flow to the exhalation port. *FGF,* Fresh gas flow. (From Moyle JTB, Davey A, eds. *Ward's Anaesthetic Equipment.* Saunders; 1998:190.)

respiration.[118] These findings were confirmed by Nimmagadda and colleagues, who showed that some duckbill resuscitation bags cannot deliver a high F_{IO_2} during spontaneous ventilation even if a high FGF is used.[41] In the absence of a one-way valve on the exhalation port, generation of sufficient negative pressure to open the duckbill valve becomes impossible. During inspiration, the unsealed valve base allows room air to enter through the exhalation port and mix with oxygen from a partially open duckbill valve (see Fig. 15.17). With the addition of a one-way valve on the exhalation port, duckbill-type resuscitation bags can reliably deliver an F_{IO_2} of 0.9 or more with an FGF of 15 L/min. This valve seals the exhalation port during inspiration and allows the patient to generate sufficient negative pressure to open the duckbill valve, permitting oxygen to flow without dilution (see Fig. 15.17).[41]

The inability of a resuscitation bag to deliver a high F_{IO_2} may have serious consequences during RSI in the critical care setting or during transport of the spontaneously breathing critically ill patient.[41] Clinicians should ascertain that the resuscitation bags used for preoxygenation in their institutions can deliver a high F_{IO_2} during spontaneous ventilation.[41]

Special Situations

Investigations have highlighted risk factors for the rapid development of hypoxemia during apnea. These factors are additive and include a reduced FRC, inadequate denitrogenation, hypoventilation before

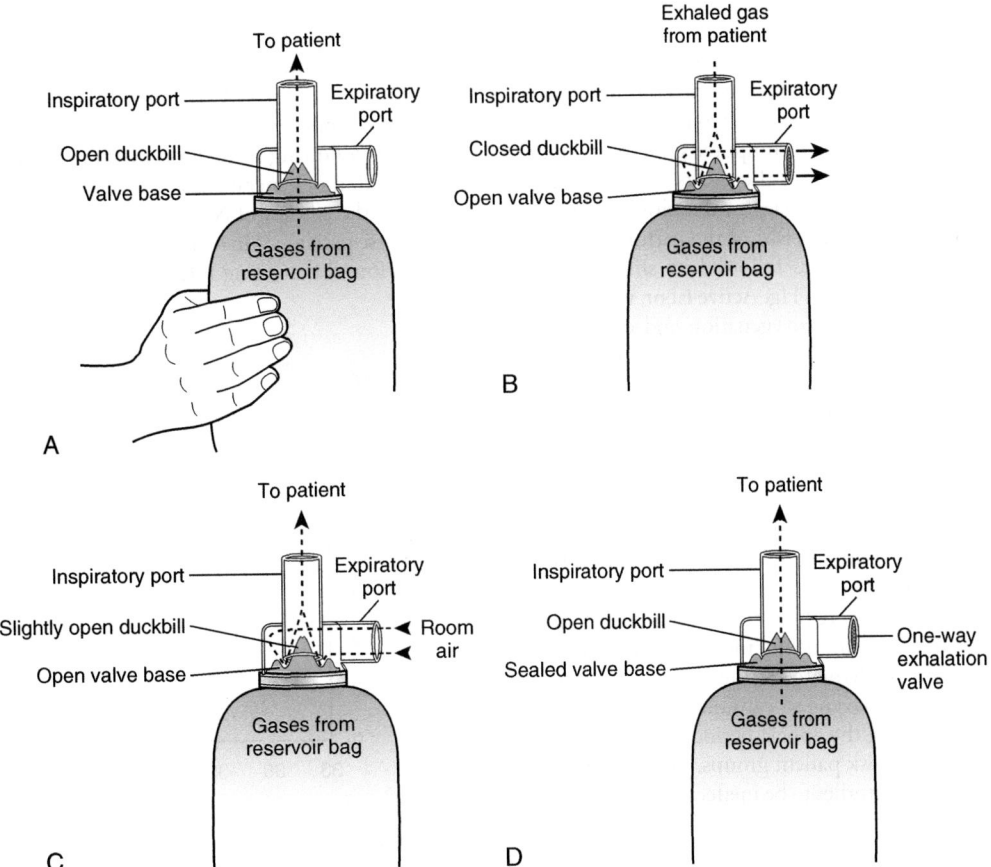

• **Fig. 15.17** Schematic diagrams of (A) a duckbill-type resuscitation bag during inspiration by manual ventilation, (B) exhalation by manual or spontaneous ventilation, (C) spontaneous inspiration without a one-way exhalation valve, and (D) spontaneous inspiration with a one-way exhalation valve. (From Nimmagadda U, Salem MR, Joseph NJ, et al. Efficacy of preoxygenation with tidal volume breathing: comparison of breathing systems. *Anesthesiology.* 2000;93:693–698.)

apnea, increased $\dot{V}o_2$, and airway obstruction.[34,113] Patients with a combination of these risk factors should be considered as high risk for hypoxemia during apnea.

Pregnancy

Maximal preoxygenation can be achieved faster in pregnant than in nonpregnant women because of increased $\dot{V}A$ and decreased FRC.[49,60,119] However, during apnea, pregnant women become hypoxemic more rapidly because of the limited oxygen stores in their smaller FRC and increased $\dot{V}o_2$.[19] From the fifth month of pregnancy, FRC decreases to 80% of that in the nonpregnant state, whereas $\dot{V}o_2$ increases by 30% to 40%. Hypoxemia after induction of the pregnant patient is further compounded by pregnancy-associated airway changes that can result in delay in securing the airway.[23]

In pregnant women, preoxygenation can be accomplished by TVB for 2 to 3 minutes or by deep breathing for 1 minute or longer before anesthetic induction. A combination of both techniques may also be used. Because of the increased $\dot{V}A$ during pregnancy, an oxygen flow of 10 L/min or higher is necessary (using a circle system) during TVB or deep breathing.[119] However, the 4 DB/30 seconds technique should be used only in emergency situations when time is limited.

The influence of preoxygenation on apnea time in the supine position versus the 45-degree head-up position has been investigated.[47] The average time for Spo_2 to reach 95% was shorter in pregnant than in nonpregnant patients (173 vs 243 seconds) in the supine position.[47] Use of the head-up position resulted in an increase in apnea time in nonpregnant patients but had no effect in pregnant patients. The reason for this finding is unclear; the head-up position has been shown to increase FRC in pregnant women.[120]

Using the Nottingham physiology computer simulation model, McClelland and colleagues investigated the effects of labor, obesity, sepsis, preeclampsia, maternal hemorrhage, and multiple pregnancy on preoxygenation and apnea during RSI of the parturient.[121] Preoxygenation with 100% oxygen was followed by simulated RSI when EtN2 reached less than 7.5 mm Hg. Active labor, morbid obesity, and sepsis accelerated both preoxygenation and desaturation during apnea. A subject with a BMI of 50 kg/m² in active labor had the most rapid desaturation during the apneic period.[121]

The Obstetric Anaesthetists' Association and Difficult Airway Society (DAS) guidelines for the management of difficult and failed tracheal intubation in obstetrics were published in 2015 and included specific recommendations for preoxygenation in pregnant patients [122,123]: head-up positioning should be considered as it increases FRC in pregnant patients; a fresh gas flow rate of 10 L/min or more is required for effective denitrogenation, and a tight mask-to-face seal is essential to reduce air entrainment[119]; clinical research and computational modeling indicate that a 2-minute period of preoxygenation is adequate for the pregnant woman at term[34,119]; and nasal or nasopharyngeal cannula administration of oxygen should be used during the apneic period.

As opposed to other high-risk patient groups, the use of HFNO has been shown in numerous studies to be ineffective as a method of preoxygenation in term pregnant women.[123,124] Tan and colleagues studied 73 term parturients who all underwent a 3-minute preoxygenation protocol with HFNO. Only 60% of patients reached the target of EtO2 >90%, demonstrating the HFNO protocol to be ineffective.[123] Similarly, Shippam and colleagues performed a randomized physiologic study comparing HFNO preoxygenation to standard 15 L/min face mask preoxygenation in pregnant patients.

Twenty patients in each group underwent both 3 minutes of TVB and 30 seconds of TVB followed by eight vital capacity breaths. HFNO performed worse than standard face mask preoxygenation, and it did not reliably achieve EtO2 means >90%.[124]

Morbid Obesity

Morbid obesity is associated with a more rapid decrease in Spo_2 during apnea after induction of anesthesia.[43,68,76,125] This is particularly hazardous because morbid obesity complicated by obstructive sleep apnea may be associated with an increased risk of difficult intubation (DI) and difficult mask ventilation (DMV). The more rapid Hb desaturation in the patient with morbid obesity is attributed to increased $\dot{V}o_2$ associated with a decreased FRC. The supine position further decreases FRC because of the cephalad displacement of the diaphragm by the abdominal contents. Anesthetic induction results in an additional reduction of the FRC; whereas the FRC of nonobese patients decreases by 20% after induction of anesthesia, it decreases by 50% in morbidly obese patients. The V_T of the patient with morbid obesity may fall within the closing capacity, resulting in atelectasis and a subsequent increase in intrapulmonary shunting.

In the patient with morbid obesity, the time required for Spo_2 to fall to 90% during apnea after preoxygenation with TVB for 3 minutes is significantly reduced compared with the time in nonobese patients.[126,127] In one study, the time to desaturation to an Spo_2 of 90% after preoxygenation was 6 minutes for patients of normal weight but 2.7 minutes for those with morbid obesity.[125] A significant negative correlation between BMI and time to oxyhemoglobin desaturation has been described (Fig. 15.18).[127]

CPAP of 10 cm H_2O at an Fio_2 for 5 minutes increases the duration of apnea without desaturation and reduces the amount of atelectasis following intubation in morbidly obese patients during the induction of general anesthesia.[78,128] Delay and colleagues demonstrated the efficacy of NIPPV to enhance preoxygenation of morbidly obese patients.[74] In a randomized, controlled clinical study, the authors found that using NIPPV with pressure support ventilation

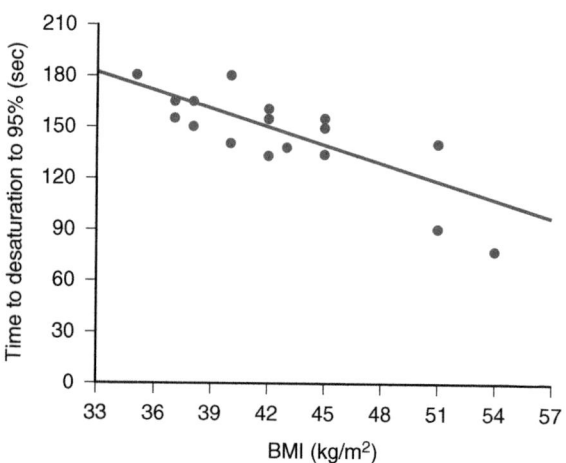

• **Fig. 15.18** Correlation between time required for desaturation to 95% in seconds and body mass index (BMI) in kg/m² during apnea after preoxygenation in morbidly obese patients. The time to desaturation is inversely related to the body mass index: $R^2 = 0.66$ ($p < 0.05$). (From Baraka AS, Taha SK, Siddik SM, et al. Supplementation of pre-oxygenation in morbidly obese patients using nasopharyngeal O_2 insufflation. *Anaesthesia.* 2007;62:769–773.)

(PSV) of 8 cm H_2O and PEEP of 6 cm H_2O for 5 minutes was safe, effective, and efficient in a group of morbidly obese patients. In this study, 95% of patients achieved EtO_2 of 90% compared with only 50% of study patients receiving oxygen alone.

Shah and colleagues have published a comprehensive review of preoxygenation and intraoperative ventilation strategies in obese patients.[129] Several of the techniques described in this chapter—including head-up positioning, NIPPV, and apneic oxygenation—have all been described to enhance oxygenation in morbidly obese patients. The authors concluded the following based on the strength of existing scientific literature: Head-up positioning enhances preoxygenation in obese patients[68]; CPAP enhances preoxygenation in obese patients[78]; and apneic oxygenation increases the duration of safe apnea in obese patients.[127]

In the critically ill, morbidly obese patient with respiratory failure, traditional preoxygenation with or without subsequent nasopharyngeal oxygen insufflation may not prevent rapid desaturation during apnea. This can be attributed to atelectasis and decreased FRC with marked intrapulmonary shunting. In this situation, the use of BiPAP can improve alveolar recruitment with a consequent decrease in intrapulmonary shunting.[130] BiPAP preoxygenation can achieve a notable increase in SaO_2 associated with less hypercarbia compared with the traditional technique of preoxygenation.[129]

HFNO has also been shown to be an effective method of preoxygenation in the morbidly obese. Wong and colleagues performed a randomized controlled trial on 40 patients undergoing general anesthesia. HFNO, compared to classic face mask preoxygenation, provided a longer safe apnea time by 40% (77.7 seconds vs 185.5 seconds in the HFNO group) and a higher minimum SpO_2 (91% vs 88%) in morbidly obese patients during anesthesia induction.[131]

Pediatric Patients

Because of their smaller FRC and increased metabolic requirements, children are at increased risk for developing faster oxyhemoglobin desaturation than adults whenever there is an interruption of their oxygen delivery.[50,132–136] The younger the child, the faster the onset of hypoxemia.[132–137] With a satisfactory mask fit, the efficacy of preoxygenation depends on the age and the duration and type of breathing.[50,133,137] Studies in children have demonstrated that maximal preoxygenation can be reached faster than in adults. With TVB, an EtO_2 of 90% or greater is reached within 60 to 100 seconds in almost all children.[50,133,137] Among those in the first year of life, it is reached in 36 seconds (range: 20 to 60 seconds); between 3 and 5 years of age, it is reached in 50 seconds (range: 30 to 90 seconds); and in those older than 5 years, it is reached in 68 seconds (range: 30 to 100 seconds).[133] Deep breathing in children results in faster preoxygenation than TVB and also faster preoxygenation than deep breathing in adults (Fig. 15.19).[137] Optimal preoxygenation can be accomplished in children with the use of deep breathing for 30 seconds.[137]

Several factors affect the onset of apnea-induced oxyhemoglobin desaturation after preoxygenation in children. These include the efficacy of preoxygenation, the child's age (or weight), the presence of disease, and the composition of gases in the lungs. Some studies have examined the time required for SpO_2 to decrease from 100% to 95% (Fig. 15.20)[136]; others have targeted a level as low as 90%.[132,136,138] In a comparison of three groups of children who breathed 100% oxygen at TVB for 1, 2, and 3 minutes before apnea, the times needed for SpO_2 to decrease from 100% to 98%,

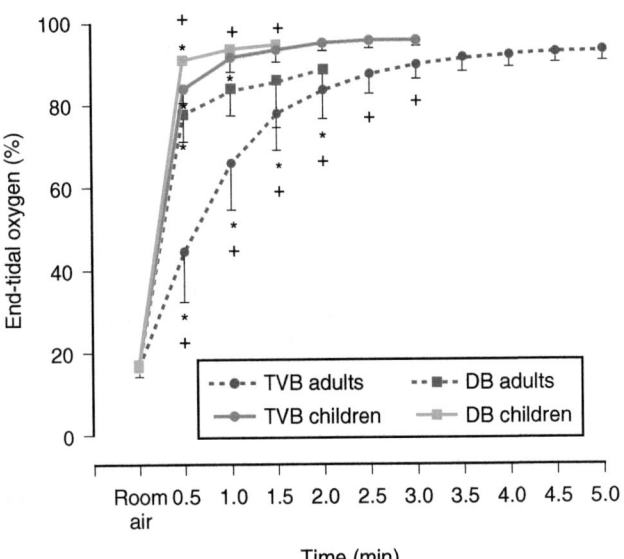

• **Fig. 15.19** Comparison of the effects of tidal volume breathing (TVB) and deep breathing (DB) preoxygenation techniques on end-tidal oxygen in adults and children. *Significant difference from all other time periods; +Significant difference ($p < 0.01$) between adults and children. (From Salem MR, Joseph NJ, Villa EM, et al. Preoxygenation in children: comparison of tidal volume and deep breathing techniques [abstract]. *Anesthesiology.* 2001;97:A1247.)

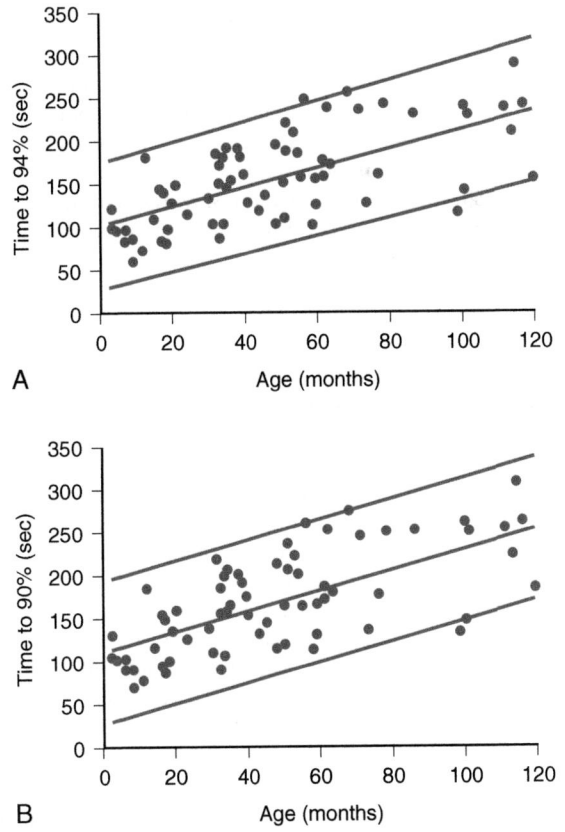

• **Fig. 15.20** Relationship between desaturation times to 94% (A) and to 90% (B) versus age with a prediction interval of 95 ($p < 0.001$). (From Dupeyrat A, Dubreuil M, Ecoffey C. Preoxygenation in children [letter]. *Anesth Analg.* 1994;79:1027.)

95%, and 90% were shorter in those who had breathed oxygen for 1 minute.[138] On the basis of these findings, 2 minutes of preoxygenation with TVB in children seems to provide maximum benefit and allows at least 2 minutes of safe apnea.[138] In a 1-month-old infant, the rate of decline in PaO_2 during apnea is three times more rapid than in an adult.[139] The times for SpO_2 to decrease from 100% to 95% and to 90% are shorter in younger children than in older children. Most infants reach an SpO_2 of 90% in 70 to 90 seconds (see Fig. 15.20).[136] This duration is shortened in the presence of upper respiratory infection.[136] The benefit of preoxygenation is greater in the older child than in the infant.[139] In an 8-year-old patient, the time after the onset of apnea to 90% SaO_2 is 28 seconds without preoxygenation but slightly longer than 5 minutes with preoxygenation.[139]

Although the time for desaturation is mainly dependent on the oxygen content of the lungs at the start of apnea, other gas components may play a role. If 60% nitrous oxide (N_2O) in oxygen is used, the time for SpO_2 to decrease to 95% is shortened to approximately one-third, but it is still longer than the apnea time after breathing an air-oxygen mixture with the same oxygen concentration.[132] This can be explained by the second-gas effect. Compared with nitrogen, in the case of air-oxygen breathing, N_2O continues to dissolve into the blood and is carried away from the lungs, resulting in an increase in the PaO_2 and hence delaying the onset of desaturation.[132]

It should be emphasized that the apnea-desaturation studies were performed in healthy children with a patent airway. The presence of cardiac or respiratory disease or airway obstruction could lead to faster desaturation during apnea.[132]

Premature infants are usually given a low FIO_2 using an air-oxygen mixture because of fear of retinopathy. Oxyhemoglobin desaturation occurs very quickly in these infants even after a short period of apnea. Transiently increasing the FIO_2, limiting apnea to very short periods, and close monitoring are important considerations.[140] The respiratory rate in preterm infants is 30 to 60 breaths/min. Rapid respirations tend to maintain the FRC by not allowing time for complete exhalation; slow respirations or apnea results in marked decrease of FRC and fast desaturation after apnea in preterm infants.[140]

Critically Ill Patients

Critically ill patients undergoing advanced airway management are prone to significant oxygen desaturation and hypoxemia, potentially leading to catastrophic complications such as cardiac arrest, arrhythmias, anoxic brain injury, and death. Patients suffering from a variety of conditions, such as sepsis, pneumonia, pulmonary edema, ARDS, and trauma, are at risk.[2,141] Those patients with a known or suspected DA are especially vulnerable for complications during advanced airway management in the ICU.[142]

Maximizing preoxygenation is therefore crucial in the critically ill patient population. To understand its application in the critically ill, remember the purpose of preoxygenation, which is to maintain Hb saturation despite continued oxygen consumption during the apneic period.[141] Preoxygenation denitrogenates alveoli so that the FRC serves as an oxygen reservoir. Clinical conditions that negatively impact FRC will have a negative impact on the efficacy of preoxygenation. In contrast with healthy patients, preoxygenation in critically ill patients must involve more than simple measures of denitrogenation. A variety of patient and pathophysiologic factors lead to this. Increased oxygen consumption leads to rapid Hb desaturation and resulting reduction in the

duration of apnea. In critically ill patients, as the alveolar-arterial (A-a) gradient increases, the oxygen reservoir stored in FRC is less efficient in saturating Hb with oxygen.[141] As the A-a gradient increases, because of a variety of disease processes, preoxygenation must involve improving CaO_2 and delivery in addition to denitrogenation.[141] In ARDS, lung injury leads to an increased shunt fraction (i.e., fewer alveoli are able to participate in gas exchange); increasing shunt fraction also limits the ability to saturate Hb with oxygen despite maximal denitrogenation.

Mosier and colleagues published a cogent summary of preoxygenation and apneic oxygenation during intubation of the critically ill.[141] They suggested that preoxygenation should be defined as the initiation of denitrogenation to the initiation of mechanical ventilation and thus includes the apneic period (i.e., the modern concept of perioxygenation). Denitrogenation should begin with maximum exhalation followed by high-flow oxygen administration with a tight-fitting mask for at least 3 minutes. In the presence of a mask leak, a nasal cannula should be added; in patients with a high A-a gradient, preoxygenation with NIPPV should be performed for at least 3 minutes for alveolar recruitment. Promising pilot data suggest that HFNO may be useful as well. The efficacy of apneic oxygenation depends on denitrogenation adequacy, the A-a gradient, and the degree of shunt. Apneic oxygenation performed with HFNO capable of 40 to 60 L/min may be effective, and, if not available, a standard nasal cannula at 15 L/min may be added after adequate denitrogenation. NIPPV by nasal mask can provide similar oxygen flows and the addition of PEEP when the mouth is closed.

Mort studied the efficacy of preoxygenation with 100% oxygen and a tight-fitting bag-valve mask assembly in critically ill patients requiring emergency intubation in a tertiary-care ICU.[143,144] This nonrandomized clinical study included critically ill patients who were failing noninvasive respiratory support techniques and required urgent endotracheal intubation and mechanical ventilatory support. Using this technique in his study population, the PaO_2 only increased by a mean of 37 mm Hg after 4 minutes of preoxygenation with 100% oxygen. Over one-third of study patients had negligible changes in their baseline PaO_2 (baseline PaO_2 was 67 ± 19.6 mm Hg [range: 43–88 mm Hg]).[143] In a subsequent study, Mort studied the efficacy of prolonging the preoxygenation period from 4 to 6 to 8 minutes in a group of critically ill patients suffering from cardiopulmonary deterioration.[144] Interestingly, after 8 minutes, one-quarter of patients experienced deterioration in the PaO_2 achieved after 4 minutes of tight-fitting bag-valve mask ventilation with 100% oxygen. Most important, nearly 50% of the study patients desaturated during the intubation procedure. Mort's studies suggest that this traditional method of preoxygenation is marginally useful in critically ill patients and must be combined with other techniques to prevent desaturation during endotracheal intubation.

Baillard and colleagues studied the use of NIPPV as a preoxygenation technique before intubation in hypoxemic patients.[75] The incidence of severe hypoxemia, defined as an SpO_2 less than 80%, within 30 minutes of intubation was 7% in the NIPPV group compared with 42% in the oxygen-only group. NIPPV study patients received PSV of 5 to 15 cm H_2O, PEEP of 5 to 10 cm H_2O, and FIO_2 of 100% for 3 to 5 minutes in the semi-sitting position.

Doyle and colleagues published a prospective, observational study where THRIVE was introduced in the ICU, OR, and ED during emergency intubation of patients at high risk of peri-intubation hypoxemia, including patients intubated in the ICU or ED, patients with a high metabolic rate, acute respiratory disease, anticipated DA, BMI greater than 30, chronic respiratory disease, or patients with pathology known to decrease FRC.[145] The THRIVE protocol consisted of 3 minutes of preoxygenation using HFNO at 60 L/min with 100% oxygen before induction of general anesthesia. The authors reported no complications associated with this technique and concluded that preoxygenation and apneic oxygenation using THRIVE were associated with a low incidence of desaturation during emergency intubation of patients at high risk of hypoxia.

In 2018, the DAS published specific guidelines for the management of tracheal intubation in the critically ill that detail a comprehensive strategy to optimize oxygenation, airway management, and intubation in the critically ill. They include guidance on "optimizing preoxygenation" by aiming for an EtO_2 >85% and urge consideration of NIPPV or HFNO.[16]

COVID-19

Severe acute respiratory syndrome coronavirus 2 (SARS-CoV-2), which causes coronavirus disease 2019 (COVID-19), led to a worldwide pandemic and brought safe airway management back to the forefront of anesthesia practice. Airway management of patients with COVID-19 hypoxemic respiratory failure is challenging for multiple reasons: (1) the severity of hypoxemia and the resultant physiologic difficulty, (2) the risk of aerosol generation and cross-contamination, and (3) the volume of patients presenting with the illness and the limited nature of resources.

The DAS, the Association of Anaesthetists the Intensive Care Society, the Faculty of Intensive Care Medicine, and the Royal College of Anaesthetists produced consensus guidelines for managing the airway in COVID-19. They aimed to provide guidance to make airway management in these patients "safe, accurate, and swift."[146] Likewise, the Society of Airway Management published a consensus statement on management of the airway in patients with COVID-19.[147] Both guidelines stress the importance of effective preoxygenation with a tight-fitting face mask and advocate for an RSI to minimize the need for face-mask ventilation. Less definitive is the recommendation for apneic oxygenation during intubation attempts; it can be considered but is not routinely recommended, particularly in patients who are not hypoxemic prior to induction.[146]

International guidelines published in the *British Journal of Anaesthesia* in January 2021 produced consensus opinions on some of the main controversies surrounding airway management in COVID-19.[148] These included the use of personal protective equipment (PPE), early vs late intubation, and the use of HFNO. The expert consensus on PPE is to use the highest level of protection available, particularly when performing aerosol-generating procedures (e.g., intubation, tracheostomy, extubation). Mask fit testing and supervised donning and doffing of PPE are considered crucial steps in the avoidance of cross-infection of healthcare workers. The expert consensus on early vs late intubation was that the appropriate decision may depend on the individual patient's pathophysiology and clinical picture. Further evidence is required before a definitive statement can be made.[148]

COVID-19 has also generated the question of whether virus-laden aerosols are generated during HFNO therapy in infected patients, thereby posing a risk to healthcare workers. As a result of limitations in the availability of ICU support during significant waves of the pandemic, HFNO was widely used in patients with respiratory failure in lieu of intubation despite initial skepticism.

This resulted in numerous clinical and laboratory-based studies assessing HFNO and the potential risk of aerosol generation. To date, there is no convincing evidence to support the hypothesis that HFNO increases the risk of transmission of COVID-19 to healthcare workers wearing appropriate PPE,[149] and—crucially—it does not appear to result in increased aerosol generation when compared to other modes of oxygen delivery.

Complications of Perioxygenation

Complications related to oxygen delivery can be subdivided into those related to the oxygen delivery systems themselves (see sections in this chapter that discuss individual devices) and the pathophysiologic complications related to oxygen therapy. Pathophysiologic complications related to oxygen therapy can lead to serious consequences—primarily hypoventilation, absorption atelectasis, and oxygen toxicity.

Oxygen therapy must be used appropriately in patients with severe COPD because of the risk of developing respiratory distress. Conventional teaching of hypoxic drive theory and excessive oxygen delivery have not been consistently supported in the literature.[150] Disturbances in ventilation/perfusion ($\dot{V}/\dot{Q}$) matching develop in patients with COPD, and through hypoxic pulmonary vasoconstriction, perfusion is redistributed to areas of higher oxygen tension. In the presence of low oxygen tension, pulmonary arterioles constrict, resulting in increased vascular resistance. This results in shunting of blood flow to areas of higher oxygen tension. Increasing mixed venous or alveolar oxygen tension can reverse this shunting and worsen $\dot{V}/\dot{Q}$ matching.[151]

In addition to regional ventilation disturbances, patients with severe COPD typically have a chronically elevated $Paco_2$, a normal pH, and a Pao_2 level that usually is less than 60 mm Hg. Patients may become desensitized to ventilatory stimulation from changes in $Paco_2$ because their increased baseline $Paco_2$ is compensated for with an increased bicarbonate ion concentration in arterial blood and cerebrospinal fluid. Instead, chemoreceptors in the aortic and carotid bodies stimulate ventilation. They are sensitive to Pao_2 values less than 60 mm Hg. When worsening hypoxemia is treated with supplemental oxygen, the goal is to raise the Pao_2 to the patient's chronic level. Although many patients will demonstrate an initial decrease in respiratory rate with hyperoxia, minute ventilation soon normalizes.[151] By means of the Haldane effect, deoxygenated Hb binds to and reduces dissolved CO_2. By displacing CO_2 from Hb, the elevated oxygen concentration reverses the compensatory mechanism of the Haldane effect.[152]

Absorption atelectasis occurs when high alveolar oxygen concentrations cause alveolar collapse. Nitrogen, already at equilibrium, remains within the alveoli and "splints" alveoli open. When high Fio_2 values are administered, nitrogen is washed out of the alveoli, which are then filled primarily with oxygen. In areas of the lungs with reduced $\dot{V}/\dot{Q}$ ratios, oxygen is absorbed into the blood faster than ventilation can replace it. The affected alveoli become smaller and smaller and eventually collapse with increased surface tension. Progressively higher fractions of inspired oxygen greater than 0.8 lead to absorption atelectasis in healthy individuals. Fio_2 values of 0.5 or greater may precipitate this phenomenon in patients with decreased $\dot{V}/\dot{Q}$ ratios.

Oxygen toxicity, the third pathophysiologic complication of oxygen therapy, becomes clinically important after 8 to 12 hours of exposure to a high Fio_2 level.[153] Oxygen toxicity probably results from direct exposure of the alveoli to a high Fio_2 level. Healthy lungs appear to tolerate Fio_2 values of less than 0.6. In damaged lungs, Fio_2 values greater than 0.50 can result in a toxic alveolar oxygen concentration. Because most oxygen therapy is delivered at 1 atm barometric pressure, the FIO_2 and the duration of exposure become the determining factors in the development of most clinically significant oxygen toxicity.

The mechanism of oxygen toxicity is related to the significantly higher production of oxygen free radicals, including superoxide anions (O_2^-), hydroxyl radicals (OH^-), hydrogen peroxide (H_2O_2), and singlet oxygen. These free radicals affect cell function by inactivating protein sulfhydryl enzymes, disrupting DNA synthesis, and disrupting cell membrane integrity by lipid peroxidation. Vitamin E, superoxide dismutase, and sulfhydryl compounds promote normal, protective free radical scavenging within the lung. During periods of lung tissue hyperoxia, these protective mechanisms are overwhelmed, and toxicity results.[153]

The classic clinical manifestations of oxygen toxicity include cough, substernal chest pain, dyspnea, rales, pulmonary edema, progressive arterial hypoxemia, bilateral pulmonary infiltrates, decreasing lung compliance, and atelectasis. These signs and symptoms are nonspecific, and oxygen toxicity is frequently difficult to distinguish from severe underlying pulmonary disease. Often, only subtle progression of arterial hypoxemia heralds the onset of pulmonary oxygen toxicity.

Classic oxygen toxicity in animal models occurs in two distinct phases. The early or exudative phase, observed during the first 24 to 48 hours, is characterized by capillary endothelial thinning and vacuolization,[154] destruction of type I pneumocytes, and development of interstitial and intraalveolar hemorrhage and edema. The late or proliferative phase, which begins after 72 hours, is characterized by reabsorption of early infiltrates, hyperplasia, proliferation of type II pneumocytes, and increased collagen synthesis. When oxygen toxicity progresses to the proliferative stage, permanent lung damage may result from scarring, fibrosis, and proliferation of type II pneumocytes.[154]

The best treatment for oxygen toxicity is preventing it from occurring altogether. Oxygen therapy should be directed at improving oxygenation with the minimum FIO_2 needed to obtain an arterial oxygenation (SaO_2) of more than 90%. Inhalation treatments and raised expiratory airway pressure may be useful adjuncts in improving pulmonary toilet, decreasing $\dot{V}/\dot{Q}$ mismatch, and improving arterial oxygenation. These therapies may be used to maintain adequate oxygenation at an FIO_2 of 0.50 or less.

In a review of the risks associated with preoxygenation, Nimmagadda and colleagues include delayed diagnosis of esophageal intubation and cardiovascular responses in addition to the previously discussed issues of absorption atelectasis and creation of oxygen free radicals.[155] Because preoxygenation prolongs the onset of hypoxemia, the detection of inadvertent intubation of the esophagus could be delayed. This risk factor emphasizes the importance of the use of end-tidal CO_2 detection following intubation.[155]

Animal studies have demonstrated a vasoconstrictor response to hyperoxia affecting the peripheral vascular supply to the kidney, gastrointestinal tract, and extremities. Again, the relatively brief period of preoxygenation makes this an unlikely clinical consideration. Human studies have demonstrated that hyperoxia causes a modest decrease in heart rate, a parallel decrease in cardiac output, an increase in systemic vascular resistance and arterial blood pressure, as well as decreases in coronary and cerebral blood flow because of vasoconstriction. However, the clinical manifestations of this are mild and variable; therefore, there is little justification for limiting preoxygenation, even in patients with susceptible disease states.[155]

Conclusion

Perioxygenation is the cornerstone of the safe and uncomplicated conduct of advanced airway management in a variety of clinical situations. It encompasses both preoxygenation and apneic oxygenation, with the goal of prolonging the safe apnea time.[3] An increasing amount of information is available on techniques that can be used to optimize perioxygenation. These include head-up patient positioning, nasal oxygen during efforts securing a tube (NO DESAT), pharyngeal oxygen insufflation, transnasal humidified rapid-insufflation ventilatory exchange (THRIVE), and noninvasive positive-pressure ventilation (NIPPV). Clinicians involved in advanced airway management are urged to understand the applicability of these techniques and incorporate many of them into their routine clinical practice. These techniques are especially critical in those patients at risk for desaturation during advanced airway management.

Selected References

1. Weingart SD, Levitan RM. Preoxygenation and prevention of desaturation during emergency airway management. *Ann Emerg Med.* 2012;59(3):165–175.
3. Patel A, El-Boghdadly K. Apnoeic oxygenation and ventilation: Go with the flow. Anaesthesia 2020, 75, 1002–1005.12. Levitan R. NO DESAT! (Nasal oxygen during efforts securing a tube). Emergency Physicians Monthly. 2010.
14. Mir F, Patel A, Iqbal R, Cecconi M. A randomised controlled trial comparing transnasal humidified rapid insufflation ventilatory exchange (THRIVE) pre-oxygenation with facemask pre-oxygenation in patients undergoing rapid sequence induction of anaesthesia. *Anaesthesia.* 2017;72(4):439–443.
16. Higgs A, McGrath BA, Goddard C, et al. Guidelines for the management of tracheal intubation in critically ill adults. *Br J Anaesth.* 2018;120:323–352.
35. Bhatia PK, Bhandari SC, Tulsiani KL, Kumar Y. End-tidal oxygraphy and safe duration of apnoea in young adults and elderly patients. *Anaesthesia.* 1997;52(2):175–178.
41. Nimmagadda U, Salem MR, Joseph NJ, et al. Efficacy of preoxygenation with tidal volume breathing. Comparison of breathing systems. *Anesthesiology.* 2000;93(3):693–698.
46. Nimmagadda U, Chiravuri SD, Salem MR, et al. Preoxygenation with tidal volume and deep breathing techniques: the impact of duration of breathing and fresh gas flow. *Anesth Analg.* 2001;92(5):1337–1341.
73. Tanoubi I, Drolet P, Donati F. Optimizing preoxygenation in adults. *Can J Anaesth.* 2009;56(6):449–466.
124. Shippam W, Preston R, Douglas J, et al. High-flow nasal oxygen vs. standard flow-rate facemask pre-oxygenation in pregnant patients: a randomised physiological study. *Anaesthesia.* 2019;74(4):450–456.
141. Mosier JM, Hypes CD, Sakles JC. Understanding preoxygenation and apneic oxygenation during intubation in the critically ill. *Intensive Care Med.* 2017;43(2):226–228.
155. Nimmagadda U, Salem MR, Crystal GJ. Preoxygenation: physiologic basis, benefits, and potential risks. *Anesth Analg.* 2017;124(2):507–517.

All references can be found online at eBooks.Health.Elsevier.com.

16

Techniques to Induce General Anesthesia

JOSHUA B. KNIGHT, KATHRYN K. WALKER, SHAWN T. BEAMAN, AND JOSEPH J. QUINLAN

CHAPTER OUTLINE

Introduction

Standard Intravenous Induction With Neuromuscular Blockade

Intravenous Induction Without Neuromuscular Blockade

Rapid Sequence Induction and Intubation

Inhalational Induction

Conclusion

KEY POINTS

- Neuromuscular blockade has been shown to improve the ability to face-mask ventilate and perform laryngoscopy.
- A ketamine induction is likely to preserve spontaneous ventilation; however, apnea has been reported, and airway obstruction is always possible.
- Succinylcholine, despite its side effects, is still recommended as the neuromuscular blocking drug of choice for rapid sequence induction and intubation (RSI) over rocuronium because of the advantages of its quick offset. However, the recent wider availability of sugammadex may change this recommendation.
- Although cricoid pressure (CP) may be important in reducing the risk of aspiration during airway management, it has been

shown to result in greater difficulty with face-mask ventilation and to impair laryngoscopy, laryngeal mask airway (LMA) insertion, ventilation via an LMA, and intubation via an LMA.
- Inhalational induction can be performed using either vital capacity "single breath" or conventional breathing techniques.
- Pediatric patients experience a more rapid induction of anesthesia than adults with inhalational anesthetics because of a higher alveolar ventilation to functional residual capacity ratio.
- Spontaneous ventilation may be maintained with inhalational induction, but recovery from airway obstruction is highly variable and may require a prolonged period of time.

Introduction

Airway management usually requires some form of anesthesia to blunt airway reflexes, attenuate the hemodynamic response to airway instrumentation, and provide patient comfort. When clinically indicated, an "awake" technique, utilizing local anesthesia of the airway with or without sedation, can be used to meet these goals (see Chapter 12). In emergency settings where the patient is obtunded or comatose, such as during acute respiratory or cardiac arrest, anesthesia may not be required at all. Most commonly, however, airway management is performed after induction of general anesthesia.[1]

Induction of general anesthesia is often achieved with anesthetic agents that produce airway obstruction and some degree of central apnea as a side effect; the addition of neuromuscular blocking drugs (NMBDs) to an intravenous (IV) induction guarantees apnea. Although it is not within the scope of this chapter, induction of general anesthesia should only be performed after careful consideration and prediction of the ability to manage the

patient's airway once apnea ensues (see Chapter 13). This chapter reviews common strategies to induce general anesthesia and their implications on airway management. Techniques that ablate spontaneous ventilation are discussed first, followed by techniques that are more likely to preserve spontaneous ventilation.

Standard Intravenous Induction With Neuromuscular Blockade

The most common technique for induction of general anesthesia is an IV induction, which includes the administration of a rapidly acting IV anesthetic, followed by an NMBD. Muscle relaxation achieved by the administration of NMBDs improves intubating conditions by facilitating laryngoscopy, preventing reflex laryngeal closure, and preventing coughing postintubation.[1]

The use or avoidance of and the timing of administration of NMBDs during airway management are important topics. Although use of such medications should be considered with caution given the resulting guarantee of apnea, the literature demonstrates widespread use and efficacy in airway management, including in cases that prove to be difficult. In a study examining difficult mask ventilation (DMV), 77 out of 53,041 patients were found to have impossible mask ventilation. Nevertheless, all but 4 of the 77 patients had received NMBDs at some point during airway management.[2] In subsequent retrospective work, the authors found that neuromuscular blockade improved the ability to face-mask ventilate patients and that the incidence of DMV, as well as DMV combined with difficult laryngoscopy, was higher in patients who did not receive NMBDs.[3] At least three prospective trials have determined that NMBDs improve face-mask ventilation and/or improve expired tidal volumes.[4–6] The report and findings of the Fourth National Audit Project (NAP4) of the Royal College of Anaesthetists, which reviewed the incidence of major complications of airway management during anesthesia in the United Kingdom, made two recommendations regarding neuromuscular blockade. First, when face-mask ventilation or ventilation via a laryngeal mask airway (LMA) is complicated by hypoxia, neuromuscular blockade should be entertained early to treat laryngospasm. Second, the report recommends the use of neuromuscular blockade before a failed airway intervention proceeds to a surgical airway.[7]

The clinical introduction of sugammadex and its ability to rapidly reverse the effects of rocuronium and vecuronium has important implications for airway management.[8–11] At a dose of 16 mg/kg, sugammadex reverses rapid sequence induction and intubation (RSI) doses of rocuronium of 1.2 mg/kg within 3 minutes of administration.[12] This outweighs the clinical benefit of succinylcholine's rapid offset, as trials have demonstrated significantly faster recovery from previously stated doses of rocuronium relative to 1 mg/kg of succinylcholine.[13] However, it should be appreciated that the recognition of the need to reverse an NMBD and subsequent reversal treatment will take longer than 3 minutes. Although bradycardia is an uncommon side effect of sugammadex, it has been demonstrated to be less prevalent than in patients receiving traditional reversal with neostigmine, particularly in children.[14] The most concerning adverse reactions involving sugammadex are hypersensitivity and anaphylaxis, which have been shown to be rare and dose dependent, thus far.[15]

Intravenous Induction Without Neuromuscular Blockade

Despite the value of neuromuscular blockade in facilitating airway management, the use of neuromuscular blockade may be undesirable in certain clinical circumstances. A classic scenario includes a desired short duration of neuromuscular blockade coupled with the necessity to avoid succinylcholine because of a concern for a predisposition to hyperkalemia, malignant hyperthermia, or myalgia. As already discussed, the availability of sugammadex potentially allows the use of nondepolarizing NMBDs, even in the setting of a short operative procedure. Nonetheless, coupling an induction agent, such as propofol with high-dose remifentanil, has been shown to provide acceptable intubating conditions in the absence of NMBDs in both adults and children.[16–18] Doses of remifentanil between 1 and 5 mcg/kg have been described; higher doses provide better and more reliable intubating conditions but also produce a greater degree of bradycardia and hypotension.[16] Disadvantages of this technique include a potentially higher incidence of difficult intubation and an increased risk for laryngeal morbidity.[19] This technique also introduces the risk of

opioid-induced muscle rigidity, resulting in difficulty with mask ventilation. While this difficulty is commonly attributed to chest wall rigidity, studies have shown that decreases in pulmonary compliance as a result of chest wall rigidity are not sufficient to explain an inability to mask ventilate after a large dose of opioid. Rather, vocal cord closure is the primary cause of difficult ventilation after opioid-induced anesthesia.[1,20] Treatment with small doses of NMBDs or topical lidocaine (laryngotracheal anesthesia) can be effective in relaxing the vocal cords to allow for mask ventilation and/or intubation.[1,20,21]

An alternative approach to the induction of general anesthesia to facilitate endotracheal intubation without NMBDs is to simply use high-dose propofol. This approach is commonly taken when utilizing supraglottic airways; however, higher doses are necessary when tracheal intubation is undertaken.[1] Naturally, greater reductions in systemic vascular resistance result from increasing doses of propofol.[1]

An alternative IV induction approach maintains spontaneous ventilation. Ketamine is the only known IV medication capable of inducing general anesthesia without the risk of profound respiratory depression. In sedative doses, protective airway reflexes are maintained.[22] When administered as a single induction agent, spontaneous ventilation is maintained, and central apnea is exceedingly rare.[23] The classic clinical indication for IV induction with ketamine is cardiac tamponade. Preservation of spontaneous ventilation protects systemic venous return and, thereby, safeguards against hemodynamic collapse caused by further compression of an already compromised right ventricle. Cases of apnea have, however, been reported, and airway obstruction is possible.[24] Ketamine acts as a potent sympathomimetic and can cause tachycardia and hypertension, especially in induction doses. These side effects may, in certain clinical situations, be undesirable, especially in patients who are already hypertensive or tachycardic or have flow-limiting coronary artery lesions. There is some evidence that ketamine in isolation acts as a direct myocardial depressant and can produce hypotension or decreased myocardial function in patients who are in extremis or catecholamine depleted.[25–27] Airway management may also be affected by the excessive salivation that can result after an induction dose of ketamine and is often treated effectively with an antisialagogue premedication, such as glycopyrrolate.[28]

Rapid Sequence Induction and Intubation

Rapid sequence induction and intubation (RSI) is the long-standing method of inducing general anesthesia and intubating the trachea when it is suspected that the patient has an increased risk of pulmonary aspiration of gastric contents. The goal of an RSI is to shorten, as much as possible, the time between the loss of airway reflexes and placement of a cuffed endotracheal tube (ETT), thereby minimizing the time a patient is at risk for aspiration. Exactly how an RSI is achieved has varying effects on the medical decision-making regarding the patient's airway management. Nevertheless, inherent in the technique is the rapid administration of an induction agent and a muscle relaxant which mandate a high degree of confidence that intubation can be reasonably achieved once paralysis and the resultant apnea ensue.

Stept and Safar initially described RSI in 1970.[29] The key components of the technique include cricoid pressure (CP), administration of a predetermined IV dose of anesthetic immediately followed by a rapid-acting muscle relaxant, and avoidance of positive-pressure ventilation (PPV). The medications first employed were sodium thiopental and succinylcholine.[22] Significant deviation from the initially described method is commonly practiced.[30-32] Variation has been found to exist in the medications employed, the use and timing of CP, as well as the use of PPV in RSI. In a UK survey of consultant anesthetists and trainees published in 2016, the most common induction agent employed during RSI was propofol, followed by thiopental, etomidate, and ketamine.[32] Although individual patient hemodynamic conditions most frequently determine the choice of induction agent, studies have been performed attempting to delineate the quality of intubating conditions using various induction agents during RSI. No difference in intubating conditions was found between thiopental and etomidate as the induction agent for RSI when using high-dose rocuronium as the muscle relaxant.[33] Propofol was found to produce better intubating conditions compared to thiopental during RSI, also with high-dose rocuronium in both groups.[34] Etomidate is commonly used for RSI in hemodynamically compromised patients. Intubating conditions have been found to be similar with etomidate or ketamine together with succinylcholine.[35] However, a randomized multicenter study demonstrated that etomidate administration leads to adrenal insufficiency, which may be particularly detrimental in septic patients.[35,36]

Beyond the selection of the induction agent used for RSI, perhaps greater variation exists regarding the choice of muscle relaxant employed. Stept and Safar originally advocated for succinylcholine as the drug of choice because of its rapid onset time; however, clinically viable alternatives were not available at the time of their work. Controversy still exists regarding the optimal muscle relaxant in RSI. A randomized trial of high-dose rocuronium versus succinylcholine in RSI with propofol concluded that rocuronium 1 mg/kg provided intubating conditions clinically equivalent to succinylcholine 1 mg/kg.[37] Conversely, it has also been demonstrated that the choice of induction agent only affects intubating conditions when rocuronium is used as the muscle relaxant in RSI and that, regardless of induction agent, succinylcholine produces better intubating conditions.[38] The choice of succinylcholine versus rocuronium in RSI remains an important issue because succinylcholine can significantly increase plasma potassium concentration and can trigger malignant hyperthermia. It also affords a rapid offset time relative to rocuronium, although with the increasing availability of sugammadex this difference may not be as clinically relevant in many anesthetizing locations. Although rocuronium does not trigger malignant hyperthermia or raise potassium levels, without high-dose sugammadex on hand it does not offer a clinically meaningful chance of return to spontaneous ventilation, especially not in the doses used for RSI. In 2015, a Cochrane Review was published on the topic that added 13 studies to the 37 included in a prior 2008 review, which resulted in 4151 participants being included in the meta-analysis.[31] The review concluded that there was no statistical difference in intubating conditions between succinylcholine and rocuronium 1.2 mg/kg for RSI. Studies using multiple induction agents were included. However, the summary recommendation of the review was that, despite the potential negative side effects, succinylcholine is clinically superior because of its shorter duration of action.[31] Given new data by Lee and colleagues regarding faster recovery with sugammadex as described previously, these recommendations may be changed in future reviews.[13]

The use of CP during RSI, as classically described, is also a subject of debate. Sellick published a description of the maneuver as a means for preventing aspiration before the initial description of RSI. His original cadaver study demonstrated that the maneuver prevents gastric reflux and pulmonary aspiration.[39] The proposed mechanism was that applying backward pressure to the cricoid cartilage compressed the esophagus against the underlying vertebral body, occluding the esophagus. Since his initial description, and the incorporation of the maneuver into RSI, as described by Stept and Safar, CP has become universally adopted. Several studies have demonstrated the effectiveness of CP in preventing aspiration in cadavers and human subjects. Nonetheless, despite its wide use, there is no randomized controlled trial evidence supporting its effectiveness.[40]

Unfortunately, many reports of pulmonary aspiration can be found in the anesthesia, emergency medicine, and obstetric literature, despite the application of CP.[38] This may be attributed in part to the reduction of lower esophageal sphincter (LES) tone caused by the application of CP, which has been demonstrated in awake volunteers (see Chapter 14). A large body of evidence has also debated the intrinsic failure of the technique because of anatomic variation as well as inappropriate application and/or inability by providers to properly identify landmarks.[41,42] Magnetic resonance imaging (MRI) studies have demonstrated that the esophagus often lies lateral to the larynx and that CP often displaces it laterally.[43]

Perhaps even more concerning is the evidence that the application of CP may make routine airway management maneuvers less successful. A series of studies show that the application of CP negatively impacts face-mask ventilation.[41] Reduced tidal volumes, increased peak inspiratory pressures, and a total inability to ventilate were described. Asai has published a series of studies demonstrating that CP impedes placement of an LMA, may inhibit ventilation via an LMA, and impedes flexible scope intubation (FSI) via an LMA.[44-46] Further work has demonstrated that CP leads to difficulty with FSI without using an LMA as a conduit and that CP prevents placement of a laryngeal tube.[47-49] A body of data also suggests that CP or bimanual manipulation degrades the direct laryngoscopic view of the glottis.[41,50] A randomized study investigating the ability to insert a bougie into the trachea while CP is applied also found that CP degraded the laryngoscopic view of the glottis.[51] The most recent Difficult Airway Society guidelines for management of unanticipated difficult intubation in adults, published in 2015, reaffirms that CP should be removed if intubation is difficult during an RSI.[52] Perhaps most compelling is a large randomized double-blind trial demonstrating noninferiority of a sham application of CP to actual CP in prevention of aspiration in operative locations.[53]

Given the available evidence, the authors of this chapter routinely use CP when indicated to reduce the risk of pulmonary aspiration. It is also common to reduce or remove the CP if tracheal intubation proves to be difficult. The most recent survey of RSI practice in the United States revealed a significant variation from the classical description of RSI with respect to PPV.[54] The survey reports that 71% of respondents, all of whom practiced in academic medical centers, used PPV via a face mask before securing the airway during RSI.[54] The authors refer to the technique of preoxygenation and CP accompanied by PPV after the induction of general anesthesia, as modified RSI.[54,55]

Inhalational Induction

Inhalational induction is commonly used for patients without IV access, particularly pediatric patients who are often unwilling to tolerate IV catheter placement. Another common indication for inhalational induction is when spontaneous ventilation is preferred, such as in the patient with an anterior mediastinal mass. This section of the chapter focuses on inhalational agents, induction techniques, patient selection, inhalational induction as an approach to the known difficult airway (DA), and important differences in the pediatric population.

Volatile anesthetics used most commonly during induction include sevoflurane and nitrous oxide (N_2O). Isoflurane and desflurane are not amenable to mask induction because of their noxious smell and airway-irritating properties, which can cause a higher incidence of cough, breath holding, and laryngospasm.[56,57] Historically, halothane was developed in the 1950s and used extensively for inhalational inductions because of its sweet smell and lack of airway irritation. Sevoflurane became popular in the 1990s as an induction agent and has widely replaced halothane in the developed world because of its more favorable cardiac safety profile.[58] N_2O has been widely used since its discovery in the 1700s. It is odorless and not irritating to the airways. N_2O can be used alone for procedural sedation and has been used extensively for dental procedures. The minimum alveolar concentration of N_2O is not deliverable without a hyperbaric chamber, and thus it cannot be used as the sole agent for general anesthesia. However, it is frequently used as an adjuvant to the more potent volatile agents.[59]

There are several options for inducing general anesthesia using inhalation of volatile agents. If the patient is cooperative, a vital capacity rapid induction or "single breath" induction technique can be performed. A vital capacity breath is a maximal inspiration starting from residual volume. The circuit must first be primed with a high concentration of volatile anesthetic. The patient is instructed first to exhale completely and then take as deep a breath as possible. Sevoflurane 8%, both with and without 66% N_2O, has been shown to produce more rapid induction than 5% halothane with 66% N_2O.[60]

Noncooperative patients may be induced using more gradual techniques during which a normal breathing pattern is maintained. A volatile agent may be incrementally increased every few breaths, or a high concentration of volatile agent may be applied from the start. Either of these techniques may use a volatile agent by itself or combined with N_2O. A study compared incremental sevoflurane with a high initial concentration of sevoflurane in children and found that immediate use of a high concentration of sevoflurane produced a more rapid induction.[61]

The addition of N_2O to a volatile agent during inhalational induction is controversial. High concentrations of N_2O during induction will lead to an increase in the alveolar concentration of other volatile agents, or the "second gas effect."[62] However, it is difficult to show a difference in the speed of induction with or without N_2O.[63,64] N_2O may be used as premedication to sedate a patient before the initiation of a volatile agent, particularly in pediatric patients who may accept a mask with a pleasant scent by using scented oil or lip balm, along with the odorless N_2O. Once the patient is sedated, a volatile agent may then be added. The smell of a volatile agent, even the less-noxious sevoflurane, can sometimes be intolerable.

Inhalational induction is faster in the pediatric patient than the adult patient because of several factors related to differences in ventilation, cardiac output, and the solubility of agents in both tissue and blood.[65] Infants have a higher ratio of alveolar ventilation to functional residual capacity (5:1 in infants compared with 1.5:1 in adults), which allows for a faster rise in the alveolar concentration of volatile agent. Infants have a higher cardiac index, which allows for delivery of the agent to the brain faster than in adults who have a greater proportion of other tissue types such as fat and muscle. When using an inhalational technique to induce general anesthesia in larger pediatric or adult patients, it is prudent to

remain aware of the extended time it may take to reach Guedel Stage III, as compared with an infant.

Maintenance of spontaneous ventilation is possible using either "single breath" or conventional breathing induction of anesthesia, in both pediatric and adult patients. One study of adult patients using a modified vital capacity technique (specifically exhalation to residual volume, then three maximum capacity breaths followed by assisted ventilation) demonstrated that it was possible to insert an oral airway, an LMA, and an ETT without significant complications.[63] Airway obstruction during induction of anesthesia is very common and may occur at multiple levels of the upper airway. Careful attention during mask induction must be paid to the development of airway obstruction. Insertion of an airway device, such as an oropharyngeal airway or supraglottic airway device, during Guedel Stage II anesthesia can cause laryngospasm, rendering ventilation impossible. If partial obstruction is present, it is prudent to first apply continuous positive airway pressure (CPAP) and positive end-expiratory pressure (PEEP) until IV access is obtained so that an additional route to deliver medications is established before insertion of an airway device.

In the patient with a known DA, inhalational induction may be possible and even preferred, depending on the clinical situation. Inhalational induction may be especially helpful in the pediatric population or in an adult who is unwilling or unable to cooperate with awake intubation. Several groups have reported success with inhalational induction in patients with known or suspected DA.[66–69] One technique that allows continued ventilation during an intubation attempt is to place a nasopharyngeal airway and connect the anesthesia circuit to it via an ETT adaptor. The volatile agent is then continuously administered with the patient breathing spontaneously while an intubation attempt is made.

Some have argued that if the airway becomes obstructed and ventilation becomes difficult or impossible during an inhalational induction, the volatile agent will quickly redistribute, the patient will awaken, and the obstruction will be relieved. This hypothesis was tested in healthy volunteers with simulated airway obstruction with both sevoflurane and halothane.[70] In this study, halothane allowed for a more rapid awakening, which was thought to be because of halothane's greater solubility. Another group came to the opposite conclusion, demonstrating more rapid redistribution of sevoflurane, following simulated airway obstruction.[23] A recent study used the Gas Man computer simulation program (Med Man Simulations, Inc., Boston, MA) to examine recovery from sevoflurane and halothane while varying multiple parameters, including minimum alveolar concentration (MAC) levels before obstruction, cardiac output, functional residual capacity, and vessel-rich group perfusion.[71] This study showed that recovery was possible but varied significantly depending on the parameters adjusted and the agent used. Recovery occurred within 35 to 749 seconds with sevoflurane and within 13 to 222 seconds with halothane. The variability highlights the dynamic circumstances inherent in the practice of anesthesia.

Conclusion

Induction for airway management remains one of the most clinically crucial periods of anesthesia and critical care. A wide range of patient physiology, comorbidities, and anatomy must be assimilated into a crucial moment that is not static but quite dynamic. Choices of airway devices, anesthetic agents, neuromuscular blockade, and patient ventilation can have profound impacts on patient care and outcomes. Further advances in the science of airway managementwill be helpful in keeping our patients as safe as possible during induction of general anesthesia for airway management.

Selected References

1. Hagberg C, Artime C. Airway management in the adult. In: Miller RD, Cohen NH, Eriksson LI, et al., eds. Miller's Anesthesia. 8th ed. Elsevier; 2015.

2. Kheterpal S, Martin L, Shanks AM, et al. Prediction and outcomes of impossible mask ventilation: a review of 50,000 anesthetics. *Anesthesiology.* 2009;110:891–897.

3. Kheterpal S, Healy D, Aziz MF, et al. Incidence, predictors, and outcome of difficult mask ventilation combined with difficult laryngoscopy: a report from the multicenter perioperative outcomes group. *Anesthesiolgy.* 2013;119:1360–1369.

7. Report and Findings of the 4th National Audit Project of the Royal College of Anaesthetists. Available at: https://www.nationalaudit-projects.org.uk/downloads/NAP4%20Full%20Report.pdf.

13. Lee C, Jahr JS, Candiotti KA, et al. Reversal of profound neuromuscular block by sugammadex administered three minutes after rocuronium: a comparison with spontaneous recovery from succinylcholine. *Anesthesiology.* 2009;110(5):1020–1025

29. Stept WJ, Safar P. Rapid induction/intubation for prevention of gastric-content aspiration. *Anesth Analg.* 1970;49:633–636.

30. El-Orbany M, Connolly LA. Rapid sequence induction and intubation: current controversy. *Anesth Analg.* 2010;110:1318–1325.

31. Tran DTT, Newton EK, Mount VAH, et al. Rocuronium versus succinylcholine for rapid sequence induction intubation. *Cochrane Database Syst Rev.* 2015;CD002788.

32. Sajayan A, Wicker J, Ungureanu N, et al. Current practice of rapid sequence induction of anaesthesia in the UK - a national survey. *Br J Anaesth.* 2016;117(suppl 1):i69–i74.

41. Ellis DY, Harris T, Zideman D. Cricoid pressure in emergency department rapid sequence tracheal intubations: a risk-benefit analysis. *Ann Emerg Med.* 2007;50:653–665.

50. Levitan RM, Kinkle WC, Levin JL, et al. Laryngeal view during laryngoscopy, comparing cricoid pressure, backward-upward-rightward-pressure and bimanual laryngoscopy. *Ann Emerg Med.* 2006;47:548–555.

54. Ehrenfeld JM, Cassedy EA, Forves VE, et al. Modified rapid sequence induction and intubation; a survey of United States current practice. *Anesth Analg.* 2012;115:95–101.

69. Kandasamy R, Sivalingam P. Use of sevoflurane in difficult airways. *Acta Anaesthesiol Scand.* 2000;44:627–629.

71. Kuo AS, Vijjeswarapu MA, Philip JH. Incomplete spontaneous recovery from airway obstruction during inhaled anesthesia induction: a computational simulation. *Anesth Analg.* 2016;122:698–705.

All references can be found online at eBooks.Health.Elsevier.com.

PART 4

The Airway Techniques

17

History of Airway Management

CHRISTINE M. BALL AND DAVID J. WILKINSON

"Everything has been said before, but since nobody listens, we have to keep going back and beginning all over again."

Andre Gidé, Le traité du Narcisse: Theorie du symbole, 1891

CHAPTER OUTLINE

KEY POINTS

- The early evolution of airway management techniques and equipment for anesthesia was largely driven by surgical need, the requirement for airway protection, and the treatment of infectious diseases, such as polio and diphtheria.
- The concept of a "difficult airway" was appreciated by the first practitioners of anesthesia with London-based anesthesiologist Joseph Clover (1825-1882) carrying his homemade difficult airway equipment with him to every case.
- Although many historical techniques, such as cricothyrotomy, tracheotomy and insufflation have been abandoned for the routine management of the airway, all still have a place in the management of a difficult airway.
- Basic airway management remains as important a skill today as it was in 1846.
- The laryngeal mask airway (LMA), which has revolutionized airway management over the past 25 years, was based on a concept briefly explored in the 1930s. Great developments are often built on ideas from the past; it is important to have knowledge of history.

- Coordinated airway planning with consensus guidelines and difficult intubation trolleys is a modern phenomenon, largely driven by the rapid development of equipment.
- Modern technological developments are now generally focused on the management of the "difficult airway." The vast array of

- devices currently available commercially necessitates regular, coordinated reappraisals of consensus guidelines.
- The Macintosh laryngoscope blade remains the most important laryngoscope blade invented, with its usefulness now further enhanced by video technology.

Introduction

Accidents, drowning and neonatal asphyxia led to the development of simple airway techniques long before the discovery of anesthesia. But the advent of anesthesia soon tested the limits of these techniques. As surgeons gained confidence with unconscious patients, they embarked on more adventurous operations, requiring deeper planes of anesthesia and often encroaching on the shared airway. Improved airway management techniques and equipment evolved out of necessity, testing the inventiveness and imagination of early anesthesiologists. Later pharmacological developments, like the discovery of muscle relaxants, also had an influence on airway management. Today we have a bewildering array of techniques and devices for managing the airway requiring special interest groups, societies, and algorithms to help the airway practitioner plan their approach to various problems. It is worth reflecting on the historical journey, the way that many of these techniques have developed, to assist with the process and to guide future developments.

Before Anesthesia

A Patent Airway

A patent airway was essential for life until the introduction of the cardiopulmonary bypass machine in the early 1950s. Despite the limited freedom provided by this innovation, a patent airway remains a fundamental requirement of anesthesia practice. Prior to the discovery of anesthesia, loss of a patent airway was usually associated with accidents, such as head injury drowning, or infections such as diphtheria; the exception was neonates who were frequently born apneic, requiring either simple stimulation or more complex airway relief. While definitive proof is difficult to obtain, extensive review of historical literature suggests that attempts to initiate neonatal respiration were more commonplace than any endeavors to resuscitate drowned, comatose, or diphtheric patients until the middle of the 18th century. Future translations of Chinese, Arabic, and Indian texts may result in modification of these views.

Early Anatomical and Physiological Experiments

Andreas Vesalius (1514–1564) performed a tracheostomy on a sheep and reported that ventilation with bellows preserved the life of the animal.[1] This advancement established the importance of understanding anatomy in the airway management of a living creature. In the 17th century, Robert Hooke (1635–1703) repeated the experiment with a dog.[2] In a further experiment some years later, he opened the thorax of a dog and pierced several small holes in the surface of the lungs. He then kept the dog alive with fully inflated lungs, providing a constant air supply equal to that leaking through the holes.[3] He concluded that a supply of fresh air was required to sustain life, not motion of the lungs. It was Richard Lower (1631–1691) who made the crucial step in physiological understanding by observing that blue blood entering the lungs had turned red by the

time it returned to the left side of the heart. He suggested this was as a result of the absorption of air used to inflate the lungs during his experiments.[4] Further experimentation by John Mayow (1643–1679) confirmed Lower's findings.[5] There is no evidence that any of these experiments had an impact on medical practice at the time, but they established an understanding of physiological principles that would become important in subsequent airway management.

Resuscitation

Neonatal Resuscitation

The practice of stimulating a neonate to induce respiration appears to have been commonplace from very early times. Positive-pressure ventilation seems to have been less popular, but in 1754 Benjamin Pugh (1715–1796) described the use of an air-pipe, which he would introduce into the mouth of a child during a breech delivery. This would ensure that respiration could take place even if delivery of the head were delayed (Fig. 17.1). *"The air-pipe, as big as a swan's quill in the inside, ten inches long, is made of a small common wire, turned very close (in the manner wire springs are made) will turn any*

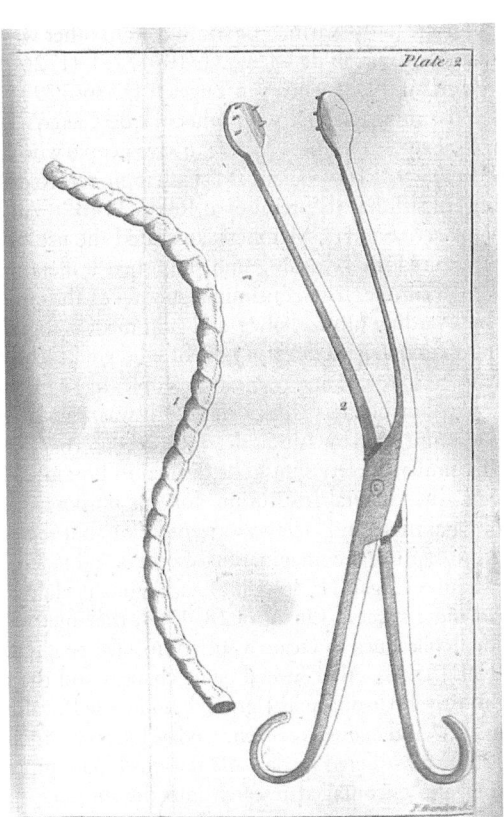

• **Fig. 17.1** Benjamin Pugh's air pipe. (From Pugh, B. *A Treatise of Midwifery.* J. Buckland; 1754.

way; and covered with soft leather, one end is introduced with the palm of the hand and between the fingers that are in the child's mouth as far as the larynx, the other end external."[6] He used this device frequently and said he had made the tube because *"I found many children were lost in this way for want of air."* Pugh also describes mouth-to-mouth ventilation as a normal practice if the onset of natural respiration was delayed after delivery: *"If the child does not breathe immediately upon delivery, which sometimes it will not, . . . wipe its mouth, and press your mouth to the child's, at the same time pinching the nose with the thumb and finger, to prevent the air escaping; inflate the lungs, rubbing it before the fire, by which method I have saved many."*[6]

A New Approach in Adults

During the 18th century, a change occurred in the approach to those who had died as a result of drowning or other accidents. Since life was associated with movement, it was believed that excitatory stimulation of the dead body to restore movement might also restore life. It was some time before establishing an open airway and attempting to restart respiration became regular practice. Dr. John Wilkinson (1746–1819) wrote *Tutamen Nauticum* or *The seaman's preservation from shipwreck, diseases, and other calamities incident to mariners* in 1759. The second edition in 1764 had an extensive section on restoring life to drowned sailors. *"A wholesome strong person ought to blow warm air into his lungs . . . which may be effectuated by a pipe, funnel, faucet, reed, can, hollow stick, quill or the like tube introduced into the mouth. This air blown forcibly, the nostrils being stopped at this time, will make its way into the lungs. . . By this introduced air, the lungs are dilated, and, if any life remains, the circulation immediately recommences."*[7] This contributed to a change in approach across most of Europe—a growing understanding that drowned individuals could be resuscitated if the airway and ventilation could be restored, the lungs inflated with air, and the body warmed or stimulated in other ways.

In Amsterdam, Jacob de Clercq (1710–1777), (1726–1777), a rich merchant, and Cornelius van Engelen (1726–1793), a Mennonite Baptist minister, met with others in de Clercq's house on October 26, 1767, to found a society to save people who appeared to have drowned.[8] The society, Maatschappij tot Redding van Drenkelingen, still has its premises at Rokin 114B in Amsterdam and remains active today. Members advocated the use of mouth-to-mouth expired air breathing and published leaflets that soon spread across Europe. The continuing success of the process was ensured by awarding bronze, silver, and gold medals, together with a payment of up to 6 gold ducats (3.5G of solid gold each), to those who attempted to rescue and resuscitate people. In 1773, they published an account of their work. This work was translated in the UK in the same year by Alexander Johnson (1716–1790), who suggested a similar society should be formed in London.[9] Johnson established "The General Institution" for this purpose, suggesting the use of nasal tubes and bellows for ventilation, but the organization failed to capture the imagination of others and faded away.

Drs. Thomas Cogan (1736–1808) and William Hawes (1736–1818) had more success. On April 18, 1774, they met with some like-minded colleagues to create a society to save people drowned in the River Thames. After several name changes and the eventual granting of Royal patronage, the group became the Royal Humane Society in 1787; it remains in existence today. Like the Dutch society, the English society offered medals and rewards for attempted resuscitation but also encouraged research into the subject. A series of essays resulted, as well as special tubes that were developed for passing blindly into the trachea, allowing ventilation of the lungs with bellows. One of the first to suggest this was James Curry (d. 1819),

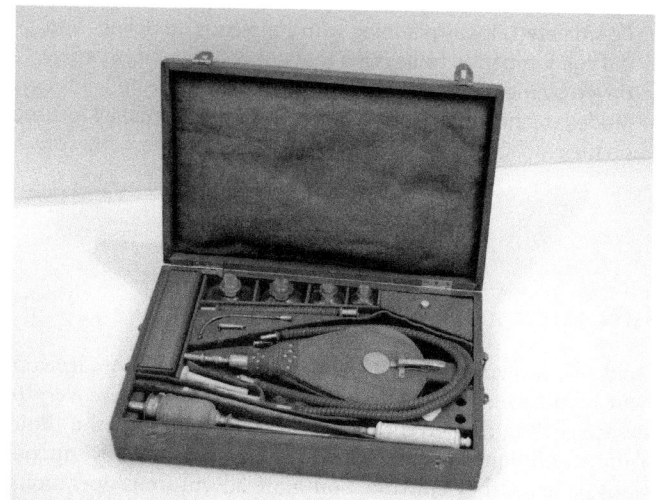

• **Fig. 17.2** Resuscitation set of Royal Humane Society on permanent loan to Association of Anaesthetists, London, showing curved metal tube for blind laryngeal intubation. (Photograph reproduced with the kind permission of The Association of Anaesthetists.)

who subsequently moved from Northampton south to London. The Royal Humane Society adopted his ideas, offering sets of apparatus, including the tubes for intubation, to those who wished to try the technique (Fig. 17.2). Curry noted that, if oral placement of the "cannula" into the trachea was not possible, the only subsequent treatment available was bronchotomy. *"The operation consists of making a longitudinal incision, of about an inch in length, through the skin, so as to lay bare that portion of the wind-pipe immediately below the protuberance which appears in the fore part of the neck; a transverse opening is then made between the rings of the wind-pipe, just large enough to admit the tip of the silver cannula, through which the air must be blown and the lungs inflated. It is scarcely necessary to add that this cannot be done properly but by a medical person."*[10]

Intubation of the larynx and direct lung ventilation ceased fairly abruptly after the publication of research on the forcible ventilation of animals by Jean Jacques Joseph Leroy D'Etiolles (1798–1860).[11] He demonstrated that administering high pressures and large volumes to the lungs with bellows via tubes could result in lung rupture, with the resulting pneumothorax preventing successful resuscitation. He presented this work to the French Academy, who proceeded to ban the use of tracheal tubes and bellows. The Royal Humane Society rapidly followed suit, but there is evidence that this form of resuscitation continued in London hospitals for at least another 20 years.[12]

The only field of medicine in which intubation of the larynx continued unabated was in neonatal resuscitation. In 1807, François Chaussier (1746–1828), Professor of Obstetrics in Paris, described an intubation cannula with a small sponge at the distal end to provide a seal at the larynx, along with a detailed description of mouth-to-mouth expired air ventilation of neonates.[13] He also had previously advocated the use of oxygen therapy in apneic neonates.[14]

Introduction of Anesthesia

Airway Obstruction

Simple Airway Management

Initially, unconsciousness resulting from the inhalation of ether vapor was not associated with airway problems. In the 1840s, light anesthesia allowing patients to move or even talk during procedures meant that respiratory obstruction was relatively rare. As practitioners began to administer deeper anesthesia, reports emerged of "stertorian breathing" and even cyanosis; the latter sign interpreted to be breath holding at a light plane of anesthesia.[15] Most operations were performed with the patient sitting upright in a chair so the airway remained clear, with the jaw, tongue, and soft tissues falling forward to allow relatively unhindered respiration. When more extensive surgery was undertaken, patients were placed supine or only slightly head up; in this position the airway obstructed as consciousness was lost. This problem became more apparent when chloroform anesthesia was administered.

The standard treatment of this respiratory obstruction was described by Jacob Heiberg (1843–1888), a Norwegian general surgeon: "[T]here are several circumstances which may occur during the administration of chloroform, and cause anxiety to the operator and his assistants. These cases are chiefly associated with incomplete, rattling respiration, pale livid color of the face, feeble pulse[,] etc. It is especially the imperfect respiration which causes anxiety and gives the impression that the entrance to the trachea is, as it were, closed by a valve. As a remedy for this evil, which is, so to say, of daily occurrence in every surgical infirmary, a special treatment has been methodized. A peculiar gag is applied, with a screw which forces the teeth apart, and the tongue is then drawn out with forceps or with pointed hooks"[16] (Fig. 17.3).

This technique was effective and popular, but it was also brutal. Joseph Clover, then the leading anesthetist in England, did not recommend it; he found that merely raising the chin from the sternum, "to give effect to the muscles between the chin and hyoid bone," was enough to relieve the airway obstruction.[17] Heiberg also abandoned tongue forceps, highlighting broken teeth and lacerated tongues as a common outcome. His treatment, developed over two and a half years, was both simple and effective: "This consists in drawing forward the under-jaw in toto." He had tried this technique on over a thousand consecutive chloroform cases and had not needed any other manipulation or alteration in the anesthesia. His technique went like this: "Standing preferably behind the reclining patient, the operator places both his thumbs on the symphysis of the lower jaw, presses the second joint of the bent forefingers behind the posterior margin of the rami ascendentes of the under-jaw, and thus holding the whole bone fast between the two hands, draws it forcibly upwards. . . . the head of the jaw slips forward over the tuberculum with an appreciable jerk,

the whole under-jaw slides forward. . . . When the experiment is successful, a deep complete respiration will immediately take place, and will be continued as long as the jaw is kept 'luxated' forward."[16] Earlier, Friedrich von Esmarch (1823–1908) had described a similar technique in his handbook for battlefield surgery.[18,19] He did not claim to have invented it, saying he had been shown the technique by an unknown British surgeon.[20] Toward the end of the century, when anesthesia textbooks, such as those of Sir Frederic Hewitt (1857–1916) and James Gwathmey (1862–1944), appeared, they contained descriptions and illustrations of this simple airway management technique.[21,22]

Oral Airways

In the early 20th century, airway management was augmented by the introduction of a simple straight oral airway.[23] Sir Frederic Hewitt was one of the great innovators of his era in anesthesia. He described respiratory obstruction under anesthesia as "auto-asphyxia" and recognized it was more common in patients who were "thick-set" or in whom the surgical operating position—for example, steep head down—caused the tongue to naturally fall backward across the airway. His airway was constructed with "a circular metal ring, with an internal diameter of half an inch, and a deep groove in its outer circumference to allow the ring being held firmly by the teeth." The initial airway was a straight 0.5-inch diameter rubber tube, 3.25 inches long, attached to the metal ring with the distal opening beveled and directly opposite the laryngeal opening when correctly inserted. After a few years this straight tube was altered to a curved one, which more appropriately reflected the anatomical structures in the mouth and pharynx (Fig. 17.4). Oral airways subsequently became very popular, and a large variety were developed, each with a specific name and shape. Construction materials also varied, with rubber, metal, and plastic all finding a place. The first metal airway was a flattened version of Hewitt's, designed by Karl Connell (1878–1941) (Fig. 17.5).[24] Other metal airways were created by Mona Dew Roberts (1878–1936), a Liverpool anesthetist,[25] and Ralph Waters (1883–1979) (Fig. 17.6). Ralph Waters did not describe this airway in the literature. The device, which had a side tube for insufflation of gases, appears in the Foregger Catalogue of 1930, where it is listed as "Waters' insufflation or suction airway."[26] However, correspondence in the University of Wisconsin Archives dates the airway to August 1928 or even earlier.[27] The ubiquitous Guedel airway, still in common use, was described by Arthur Guedel (1883–1956) in 1933.[28]

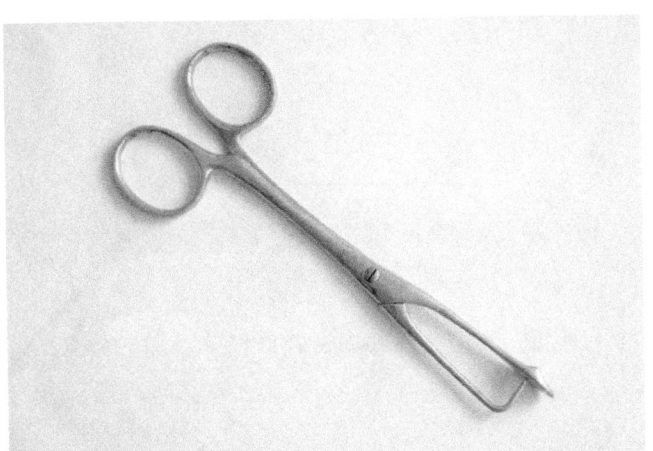

• **Fig. 17.3** Tongue forceps. (Courtesy Geoffrey Kaye Museum of Anaesthetic History, Melbourne, Victoria, Australia.)

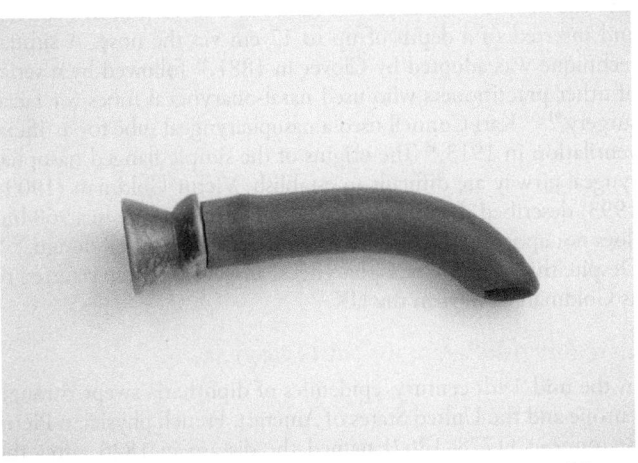

• **Fig. 17.4** Hewitt's airway. (Courtesy Geoffrey Kaye Museum of Anaesthetic History, Melbourne, Victoria, Australia.)

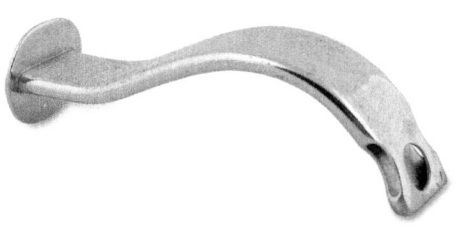

• **Fig. 17.5** Connell airway. (Courtesy Wood Library-Museum, Schaumburg, IL, USA.)

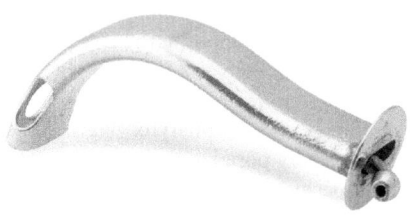

• **Fig. 17.6** Waters airway. (Courtesy Wood Library-Museum, Schaumburg, IL, USA.)

Nasal Airways

In 1859 in Paris, Gustave Fauré (1843–1924) utilized a technique developed by Joseph François Malgaigne (1806–1865) for ether in 1847, giving chloroform anesthesia via a rubber tube passed into the nostril.[29,30] The rubber tube was 8 to 13 mm in diameter and inserted to a depth of up to 17 cm via the nose. A similar technique was adopted by Clover in 1881,[31] followed by a series of other practitioners who used nasal-pharyngeal tubes for facial surgery.[32–35] Karl Connell used a nasopharyngeal tube for artificial ventilation in 1913.[36] The origins of the simple flanged nasopharyngeal airway are difficult to establish; Victor Goldman (1903–1993) described the soft plastic version of this airway in 1968 but does not appear to have been responsible for the initial design.[37,38] Despite this, modern nasopharyngeal airways are often referred to as Goldman airways in the UK.[39]

Infection: A Different Airway Challenge

In the mid-19th century, epidemics of diphtheria swept through Europe and the United States of America. French physician Pierre Bretonneau (1778–1862) named the disease in 1826, after the "leather-like" membrane that gradually obstructs the larynx of the afflicted child.[40] Bretonneau was also the first to distinguish

this disease from scarlet fever and reportedly the first to successfully treat the disease with tracheostomy.[41] However, there were isolated prior reports of tracheostomy used to treat membranous croup, a disease that was almost certainly diphtheria.[42] Initially tracheostomy provided the only hope of recovering the airway: a surgical procedure that carried a very high morbidity in a moribund hypoxic child. Physicians in several countries (Johann Dieffenbach [1792–1847] in Berlin, Germany, in 1839; Jean François Reybard [1795–1863] in Lyon, France in 1855; and Josef Weinlechner [1829–1906] in Vienna, Austria in 1866)[43] tried to introduce some form of catheter into the larynx to overcome diphtheric obstruction. They were rarely successful, and their techniques were impossible for others to duplicate. In 1858, Eugène Bouchut (1818–1891) presented seven cases of laryngeal intubation to the Academy of Science in Paris.[44] He placed short metal tubes into the larynx, leaving them in place for a couple of days, but the tubes were anatomically inaccurate, causing severe pain and often hemorrhage. The Academy was influenced by Armand Trousseau (1801–1867), who had refined and advocated the use of tracheostomy for diphtheria and opposed to this practice, so Bouchut's experiments eventually ceased.[42] Nearly 30 years later Joseph P. O'Dwyer (1841–1898), appalled by the pediatric mortality from diphtheria in New York and apparently unaware of Bouchut's work, worked in the hospital mortuary dissecting the necks of diphtheric children to perfect an anatomically accurate laryngeal tube. His first cases of successful treatment were presented in 1885.[45] He continued to develop and perfect this apparatus over the following decades (Fig. 17.7). Later he created a series of tubes for the treatment of syphilitic tracheal stenosis,[46] as well as a 'tube' to attach to the bellows ventilator developed by George Fell (1849–1918) for the resuscitation of opium overdoses. Fell's original apparatus was connected to a face mask or directly to the trachea by a tracheostomy.[47] The Fell-O'Dwyer apparatus, an elegant combination of an adult O'Dwyer tube and the Fell bellows, proved to be very successful.[48]

Intubation for Anesthesia

The Trendelenburg Cone

In 1871, Friederich Trendelenburg (1844–1924) described a cone and cuffed metal cannula for the delivery of anesthesia via

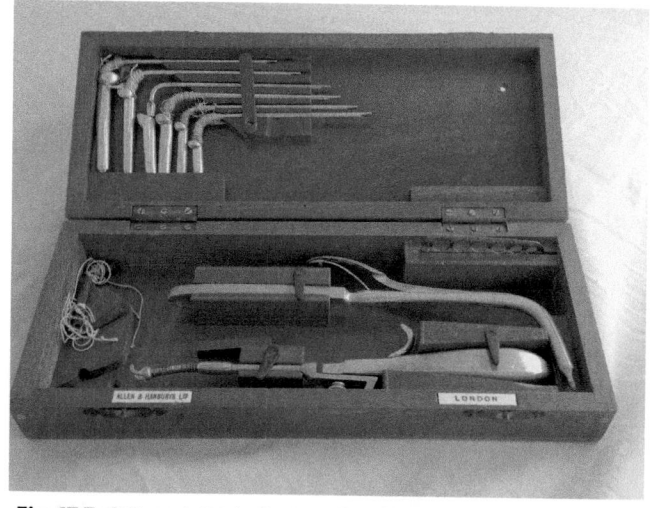

• **Fig. 17.7** O'Dwyer's intubation set. (Courtesy Geoffrey Kaye Museum of Anaesthetic History, Melbourne, Victoria, Australia.)

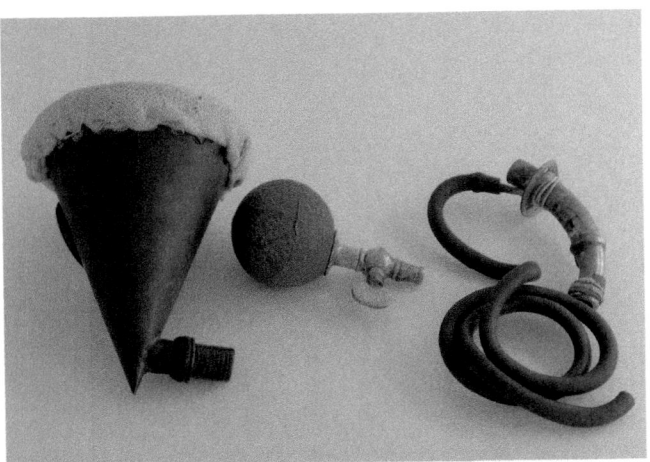

• **Fig. 17.8** Trendelenburg cone and cannula. The cuff on the cannula has perished. (Courtesy Geoffrey Kaye Museum of Anaesthetic History, Melbourne, Victoria, Australia.)

a tracheotomy (Fig. 17.8).[49] His objective was to overcome the problem of blood contaminating the airway during oral surgery. Although effective, it was a disfiguring and unpopular technique that was never widely adopted. Karl Maydl (1853–1903), working in Prague, connected a glass Trendelenburg Cone to an O'Dwyer laryngeal tube, packing the pharynx with gauze to protect the airway during anesthesia delivery.[50] Viktor Eisenmenger (1864–1932) had a similar idea, but he connected a hard rubber tube with a tracheal cuff to the Trendelenburg Cone.[51] Both inserted their tubes with the aid of an oral mirror. These techniques partly overcame the issues faced by oral surgeons, but the thoracic cavity remained a problem. Once surgeons opened the chest in a spontaneously breathing patient, respiration was no longer possible, as the lung collapsed. This made all but the shortest operations in the chest impossible. In Paris, Eugene Doyen (1859–1916) created a special introducer to insert a laryngeal tube. Once inserted, the tube was connected via rubber tubing to hand bellows, which could both blow and aspirate air.[52] The soft tubing connectors were easily obstructed by the patient's teeth, but it was a preliminary attempt to maintain lung volumes during thoracic surgery. By attaching a Trendelenburg Cone to the Fell-O'Dwyer apparatus, Rudolph Matas (1860–1957) created a more effective system of ventilation and anesthesia for thoracic surgery.[53]

Early Experience With Intubation for Anesthesia

William Macewen (1848–1924) experimented with tracheal tubes for airway management, developing a series of 18- to 20-gauge rubber and gum elastic catheters.[54] Using cadavers and himself, he developed a technique of blind intubation using a finger passed over the back of the tongue. He first tried the technique on a patient requiring excision of a pharyngeal tumor in early 1878.[55] He practiced inserting the tube with the patient several times before actually performing the surgical procedure. After the success of this procedure, he used the tubes on two other occasions for patients with airway obstruction, one with inhalational burns and the other with a prolonged ulceration of the larynx. These cases were remarkably successful, leading him to attempt a second anesthetic. Unfortunately, this fourth patient died after the patient himself removed the tube.[56] Macewen did not report any more cases of intubation for anesthesia but continued to use the tubes for the treatment of diphtheria in a similar way to Joseph O'Dwyer.[57]

Franz Kuhn (1866–1929) a head and neck surgeon working in Kassel, Germany, became intent on finding a way to secure the

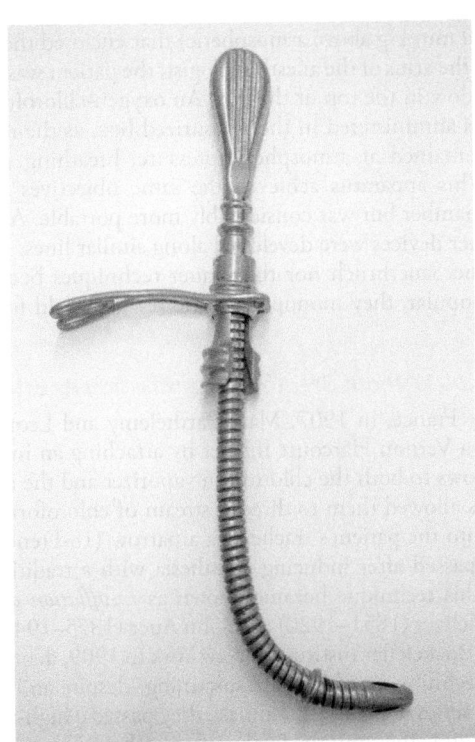

• **Fig. 17.9** Kuhn tube with stylet. (Courtesy Geoffrey Kaye Museum of Anaesthetic History, Melbourne, Victoria, Australia.)

airway after the sudden death of a patient from a pharyngeal hemorrhage.[58,59] By 1902, he had designed a flexible, oral metallic tube with a flange to prevent it being inserted too far and a stylet for introduction (Fig. 17.9). The epiglottis and arytenoid cartilages were palpated with one hand, as the tube was introduced into the trachea with the other; anesthesia was then maintained with a Trendelenburg Cone attached to the tube, and the pharynx was packed with oiled gauze. An added refinement was the connection of a monoaural stethoscope to the side of the cone, thus permitting the anesthesiologist to listen to respiration and heart sounds. Kuhn continued to modify and develop his tubes and also reported a nasotracheal version.[60] He invented two positive-pressure circuits for use with these tubes, but neither progressed beyond the experimental stage, presumably because of their excessive dead space and the high resistance in the small-diameter breathing tube.[13] The Kuhn tube was the forerunner of the modern tracheal tube. It was used in the UK on occasions for oral surgery but was never widely adopted.[61]

Surgical Requirements

Pressure Chambers

The need to operate in the thorax drove many developments in anesthesia and airway management toward the end of the 19th century and into the next. Ferdinand Sauerbruch (1871–1955) felt that positive-pressure insufflation was unphysiologic. In 1904, he developed a pressure chamber that surrounded the whole patient, except for the head. The pressure was then reduced in the chamber to 10 mm Hg below atmospheric pressure. The patient continued to breathe spontaneously, but the lung remained inflated when the chest was opened. The entire surgical team worked inside the negative pressure chamber while the anesthesiologist remained outside at the patient's head.[62]

The concept was reversed by Ludolf Brauer (1865–1951), a colleague of Sauerbruch. His apparatus consisted of a pressurized box (at 10 mm Hg above atmospheric) that enclosed the patient's head and the arms of the anesthesiologist; the patient was observed via a window in the top of the box. An oxygen-chloroform anesthetic was administered in the pressurized box, as the rest of the patient remained at atmospheric pressure, breathing spontaneously.[63] This apparatus achieved the same objectives as Sauerbruch's chamber but was considerably more portable. As a result, many other devices were developed along similar lines. Although neither the Sauerbruch nor the Brauer techniques became universally popular, they monopolized the research field for around 20 years.[13]

Respiration Without Breathing: Insufflation Anesthesia

In Nancy, France, in 1907, Marc Barthélemy and Leon Dufour modified a Vernon Harcourt Inhaler by attaching an insufflating hand bellows to both the chloroform vaporizer and the air bypass inlet. This allowed them to direct a stream of chloroform and air directly into the patient's trachea via a narrow (18-French gauge) catheter, passed after inducing anesthesia with a traditional face mask.[64] This technique became known as *insufflation anesthesia*. Samuel Meltzer (1851–1920) and John Auer (1875–1948), working at the Rockefeller Institute in New York in 1909, demonstrated that the technique could be life sustaining, despite an open thorax.[65] In a series of paralyzed animals, they passed a high-flow mixture of air and ether into the trachea via a catheter inserted close to the bifurcation. Using foot bellows to generate the flow, they were able to achieve pressures of 15 to 20 mm Hg. Effectively duplicating Robert Hooke's experiment some 250 years previously, they described it as respiration without respiratory movement.

The surgeon Charles A. Elsberg (1871–1948) was the first to test this technique in humans in 1910, thereby demonstrating its effectiveness for anesthesia for thoracic surgery.[66] The following year, Frederic J Cotton (1869–1938) and Walter Boothby (1880–1953) established that anesthesia could be maintained with nitrous oxide/oxygen insufflation and subsequently promoted the technique extensively.[67,68] Insufflation anesthesia was popularized in the UK by the Liverpool surgeon Robert E. Kelly (1879–1944)[69] and adopted by Frederick Silk (1858–1943) in London.[70] Rubens Wade (1880–1940), who took over from Silk at the military hospital at Aldershot, worked with plastic surgeon Harold Gillies (1882–1960) there and then at Queens Hospital, Sidcup.[71] Also providing anesthesia there was John C. Clayton, who was probably one of the first to routinely use nasal insufflation catheters to allow the surgeon free access to the mouth. He would attach the catheter to a funnel and, by holding the funnel to his ear, position the catheter *"somewhere just above the epiglottis where breathing is comfortable."*[72] In Gillies's seminal work on plastic surgery of the face, Wade advocated the use of the nasopharyngeal tube, recommending loosely packing the pharynx around the tube and using a special right-angled metal connector at the level of the ala to prevent the tube kinking. Referring to Silk's influence, he stated that for large operations around the mouth *"intratracheal administration in some form has been adopted as routine."*[73] Wade also recommended an apparatus designed by Francis Shipway (1876–1968): an insufflation device that provided warmed ether, chloroform, or a mixture of the two.[74] He particularly favored this apparatus when the patient needed to be operated on when lying flat, insufflating through a metal tube attached to a Hewitt's airway. The Shipway apparatus was designed to assist with temperature maintenance during long cases, the only oral surgery cases not performed in the sitting position (Fig. 17.10).[75] Shipway also believed that warmed ether was less irritating, resulting in less mucous production and calmer respiration.[76]

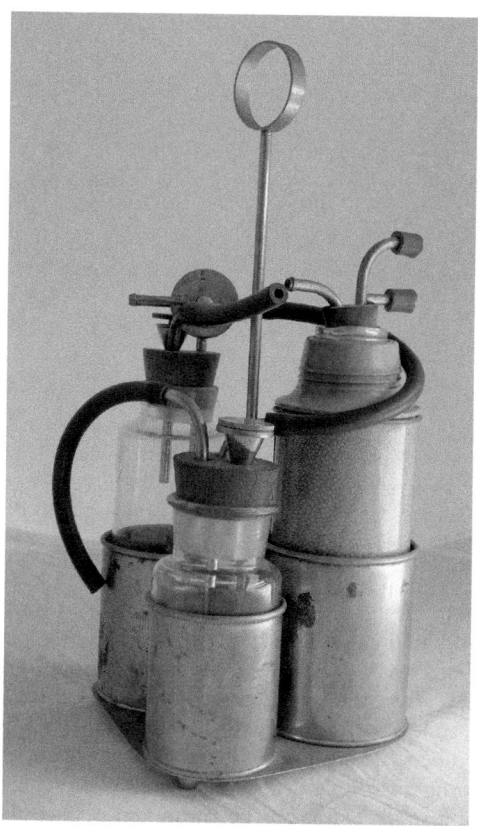

• **Fig. 17.10** Shipway insufflation apparatus for delivery of warmed ether. (Courtesy Geoffrey Kaye Museum of Anaesthetic History, Melbourne, Victoria, Australia.)

Wide-Bore Tracheal Tubes

At the end of World War I, Rubens Wade left Queen's Hospital, Sidcup, to return to St. Bartholomew's Hospital. His place was taken by Ivan Magill (1888–1986), who was soon joined by Stanley Rowbotham (1890–1979). Over 60,000 British soldiers suffered head and eye injuries during the war, often from simply peering over the edge of the trench.[77] Queen's Hospital was the treatment center for these devastating, complex facial injuries, presenting the anesthesiologists and surgeons with an extraordinary array of problems. Building on the experience of his predecessors Wade, Silk, and Clayton, Magill applied his inventive skills to find new solutions to airway management. Insufflation anesthesia provided a clear airway but also exposed the surgeon to a constant spray of blood and ether. Magill inserted a second insufflation tube, packing the pharynx around both tubes so the exhaled air was directed away from the surgical field.[78] He placed both catheters under direct vision using a laryngoscope he also devised—a modification of the Jackson laryngoscope.[79] Initially Magill manipulated the catheters with a metal rod inserted through the eye of the catheter, developing his well-known forceps in 1920 (Fig. 17.11).[80]

Faced with a particularly complex patient, Magill resorted to placing a wide-bore piece of tubing *"after the manner of Kahn[1] [sic]"* through the patient's nose.[78] Using a large endotracheal tube allowed spontaneous ventilation, rather than insufflation, and soon became a preferred technique. Working with Rowbotham on all these concepts, Magill perfected oral intubation with a similar tracheal tube,

---

[1]He was referring to the work of Franz Kuhn, acknowledging his invention of the wide-bore tracheal tube.

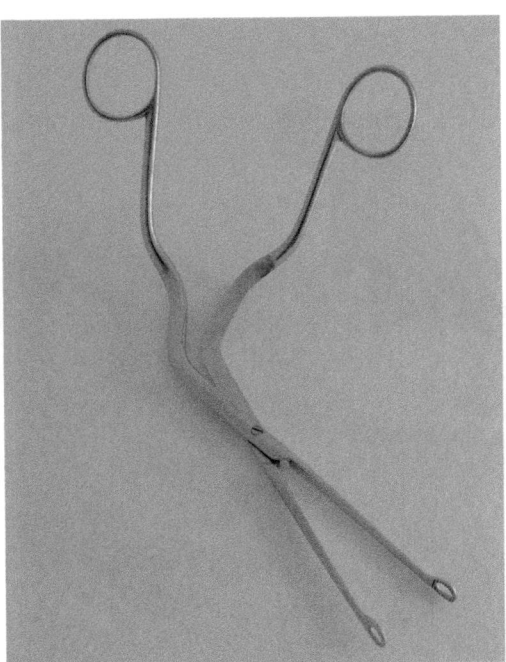

• **Fig. 17.11** Magill forceps. (Courtesy Geoffrey Kaye Museum of Anaesthetic History, Melbourne, Victoria, Australia.)

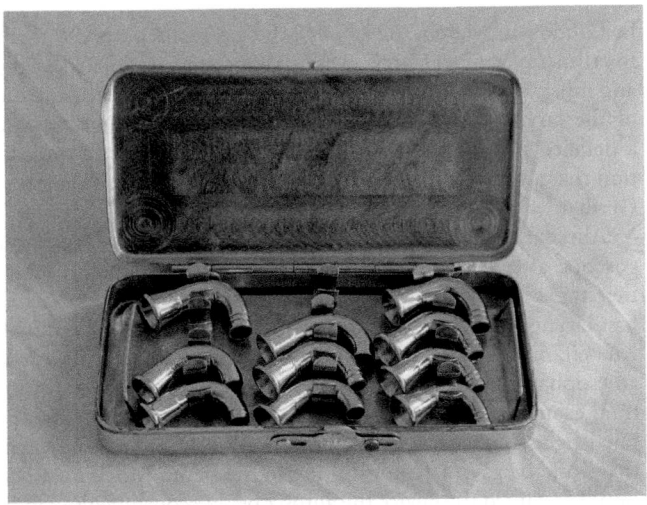

• **Fig. 17.12** Set of Magill metal nasal tube connectors. (Courtesy Geoffrey Kaye Museum of Anaesthetic History, Melbourne, Victoria, Australia.)

developing special connectors to prevent kinking of the tubes as they exited the nose or mouth (Fig. 17.12).[81] Magill's development of blind nasal intubation under relatively deep ether anesthesia became a source of amazement to the many visitors who came to watch him work at Sidcup. His manual dexterity was legendary, and he would often divert the visitor's attention at the exact moment that he placed the tube so that they missed the little twist and push he gave the tube as it approached the larynx [personal communication, Ivan Magill (DJW)]. This technique was recorded in a 1944 film that is available to watch at https://www.youtube.com/watch?v=PRi5MA1cJeY. An interview with Sir Ivan Magill is also available for viewing at https://wellcomelibrary.org/item/b16734178#?c=0&m=0&s=0&cv=0.

Improvements to Tracheal Tubes

Due to the work of Magill and Rowbotham, wide-bore tracheal tubes quickly spread internationally, resulting in subtle changes by

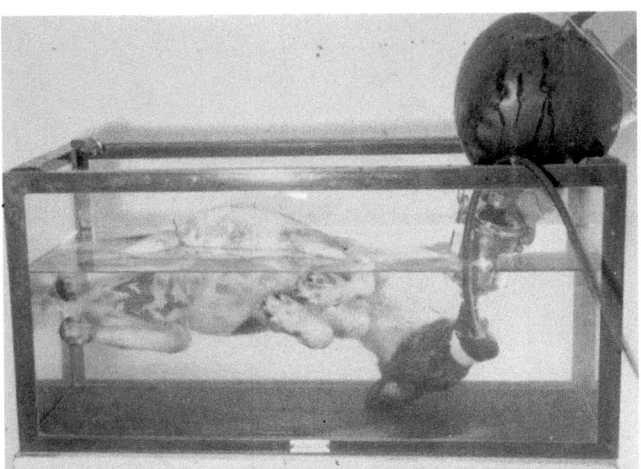

• **Fig. 17.13** Dunked dog experiment. (Courtesy Wood Library-Museum, Schaumburg, IL, USA.)

other practitioners. The most noteworthy of these was the addition of an inflatable cuff by Arthur E. Guedel (1883–1956) and Ralph M. Waters (1883–1979) in the late 1920s. The efficacy of the tracheal cuff was dramatically displayed in the "dunked dog" demonstration. An intubated anesthetized dog immersed underwater in an aquarium was wheeled onto a lecture theater stage. After an hour, the dog awoke and was extubated with no ill effects (Fig. 17.13).[82] The dog lived for a while with the Guedel family, eventually moving to live with the Waters family; sadly he went missing after two years: *"I think someone stole him."*[83] Red rubber tubes made for nasal and oral placement continued to evolve and their quality improved steadily. The next improvement was the addition of a pilot balloon by Christopher L. Hewer (1896–1986) to guide the degree of cuff distention and to minimize cuff perforation.[84] A lateral opening, the so-called "Murphy eye," was added following the work of Frank Murphy (1900–1972) in Detroit.[85]

In 1940, a London-based dentist born in Poland, Sydney Leader (1898–1964), began experimenting with plastic for medical and dental uses. He formed the company Portland Plastics (as his flat was located on Great Portland Street, London), later renamed Portex, which manufactured dental tubing from polyvinyl chloride (PVC). He was invited to Basingstoke General Hospital in 1943 by the anesthesiologist Harry L. Thornton (1906–1987) to investigate the possibility of making PVC tracheal tubes.[86] Thornton was subsequently deployed to France and Belgium, where he found these tubes to be very satisfactory, even though they became discolored by regular boiling (Fig. 17.14).[87] Thornton and his military colleagues were supplied with coiled lengths of tubing that they cut to length, creating a bevel with scissors and, if necessary, smoothing the tip with a hot spatula before polishing the tube with a chloroform-soaked cloth.[88] Subsequently, PVC tubes, in a variety of sizes, were made available to civilian anesthesiologists by Portex and were found to be satisfactory for both adults and children.[89,90] Bernard Branstater (1929–2020), at the American University Hospital in Beirut, was the first to report successful long-term intubation of infants and children with PVC tubes.[91] Integrated cuffs were added by 1958,[92] followed by radio-opaque markers and pilot tube inflation lines within the annulus, enhancements that were impossible with rubber tubes.[93] In the late 1960s, as prolonged intubation became more common, concerns developed about mucosal damage due to pressure and the leaching of toxic substances used in the manufacture of PVC.[94] Low-pressure

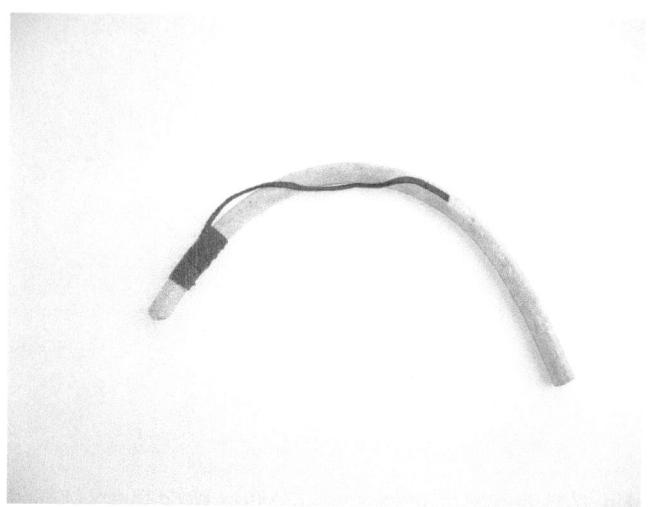

• **Fig. 17.14** An example of an early plastic tube with a removable cuff. (Courtesy Geoffrey Kaye Museum of Anaesthetic History, Melbourne, Victoria, Australia.)

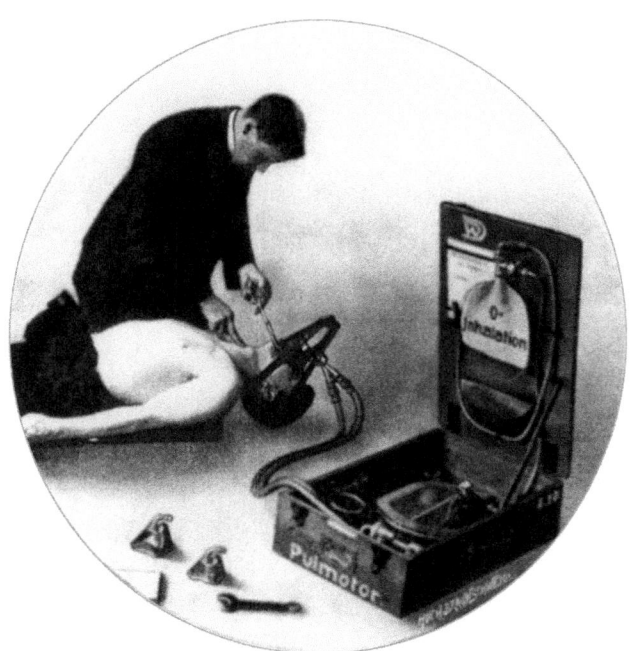

• **Fig. 17.15** "Rothscher Handgriff" during mechanical face mask ventilation with "Pulmotor," 1912. (Courtesy Dräger Archives, Lubeck, Germany.)

cuffs were developed, initially for tracheostomy tubes,[95] and by 1975 the importance of maintaining the cuff pressure lower than the mucosal capillary pressure was evident.[96]

In 1968, animal experiments established that PVC could cause toxic reactions.[97] Concerns about toxicity and the lack of compatibility between various device connections led to the development of standards by the American Society for Testing and Materials (ASTM) and the American National Standards Institute (ANSI).[98] Initially these issues were addressed by the Z-79 committee, with compliant, appropriately tested PVC tubes permitted to be marked "Z79-IT." Standards for tracheal tubes are currently managed by the Airways and Related Equipment Committee, ISO/TC 121/SC 2.[99] Subsequently, in 1968 concerns about toxic substances released by sterilization led to the first calls for single-use PVC tubes.[100]

Airway Protection: Cricoid Pressure

Cricoid pressure was first suggested by the anatomist/surgeon John Hunter (1728–1793) and his contemporary Alexander Monro secundis (1733–1817), as a means of preventing aspiration during resuscitation from drowning accidents.[101,102] James Curry also drew attention to it in his treatise on resuscitation from drowning.[10] The technique was revived by Professor Otto Roth (1863–1944), surgeon and advisor to the Dräger company in Lubeck, Germany, who strongly recommended the use of cricoid pressure in resuscitation. Subsequently, cricoid pressure, or "Handgriff nach Otto Roth," became an important part of the training manuals accompanying the Dräger Pulmotor, an internationally used resuscitation device in the early part of the twentieth century (Fig. 17.15).[103] In Britain in 1961, Brian Sellick (1918–1966) introduced into anesthesia the use of cricoid pressure with cuffed tracheal tubes.[104] It has been standard practice for rapid sequence inductions since then, although its effectiveness is often debated.[105,106]

Visualizing the Larynx

Early Laryngoscope Development

Using the sun as a light source, then medical student Benjamin Guy Babington (1794–1866) created a "glottiscope" to visualize the larynx, presenting it to a meeting of the Hunterian Society

in London in March 1829.[107] He did no further work with this instrument. Manuel García (1805–1906), the great Spanish singer and music teacher, was the first to describe the functional anatomy of the larynx. Using sunlight and a dental mirror, he prepared a detailed paper for the Royal Society of London,[108] a presentation that awarded him an honorary medical degree in Königsberg, Germany, in 1862.[109]

Alfred Kirstein (1863–1922) designed the first direct laryngoscope after learning that a colleague had accidentally entered the trachea while performing esophagoscopy;[110,111] this was the first laryngoscope that did not require the use of mirrors. Initially Kirstein modified a headlamp to provide direct illumination down an esophagoscope; later he added a Casper lamp, derived for urethral examination, on to the esophagoscope, creating an incorporated light source. In 1895, just over 3 weeks after commencing this work, he gave a demonstration to the Berlin Medical Association. He named the device the autoscope. He continued to modify the autoscope, replacing the esophagoscope with a blade not dissimilar to modern laryngoscopes, describing the ideal position for use as the "sniffing" position, which is still used today.[112] Kirstein suggested that his autoscope could be useful for the removal of foreign bodies but was reluctant to pass it through the vocal cords into the trachea due to the visible pulsations of the aorta.[111,113] It was Gustav Killian (1860–1921), inspired by Kirstein's presentation, who developed the art of bronchoscopy for removal of foreign bodies. He developed the first suspension laryngoscope, allowing the surgeon to work freely with both hands.[114,115]

The American surgeon Chevalier Jackson (1865–1958) worked independently in Pittsburgh, Pennsylvania, but he did meet with Killian in 1907.[113] He developed endoscopic instruments for the esophagus, larynx, and trachea, becoming a world leader in endoscopic foreign body retrieval.[116,117] His U-shaped laryngoscope, designed to be held in the left hand, became popular with otolaryngologists (Fig. 17.16). It was also adopted by anesthesiologists following his publication of its use for the introduction of insufflation catheters.[118,119] Like Kirstein, Jackson realized the importance

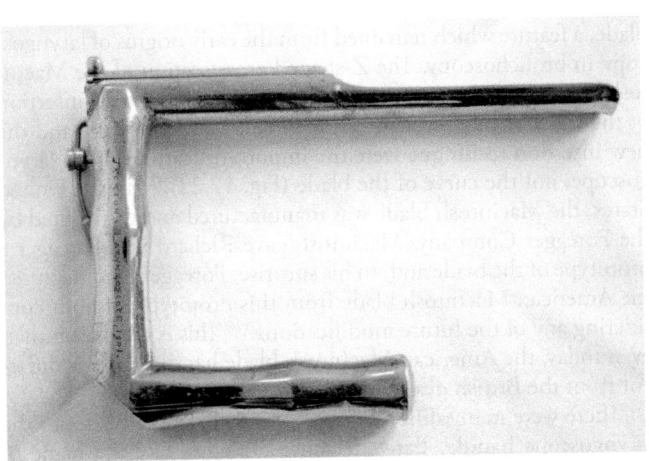

• **Fig. 17.16** Chevalier Jackson laryngoscope. (Courtesy Geoffrey Kaye Museum of Anaesthetic History, Melbourne, Victoria, Australia.)

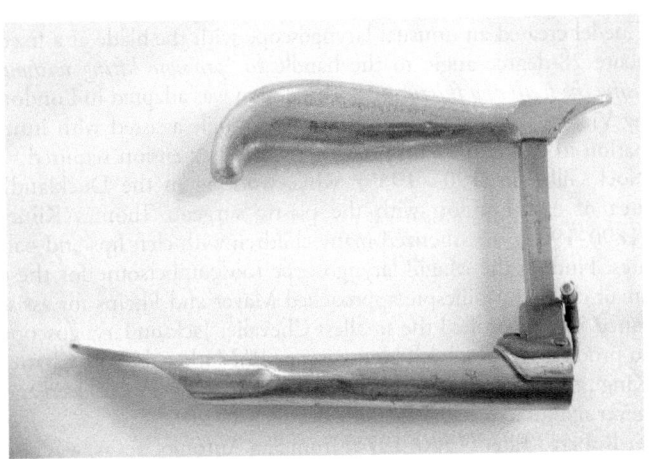

• **Fig. 17.17** Magill laryngoscope. (Courtesy Geoffrey Kaye Museum of Anaesthetic History, Melbourne, Victoria, Australia.)

of a good light source and incorporated it into the distal portion of the laryngoscope handle. Not everyone found it easy to use. Harris Peyton Mosher (1867–1954) from Boston complained of difficulty visualizing the upper end of the esophagus with the Jackson laryngoscope, leading him to devise his own speculum, best used with the patient's head in the lateral position.[120] Rubens Wade (1880–1940) used Mosher's speculum at Aldershot and Sidcup to assist with airway management for Gillies's plastic surgery.[73]

Laryngoscopes for Anesthesia

Henry H. Janeway (1873–1921) was the first to design a laryngoscope specifically for the placement of insufflation tubes for anesthesia.[121] His complex device incorporated a telescopic prism with an eyepiece above a long curved speculum. The catheter was passed through the speculum, guided by the curve of the lumen and kept in place by a central notch. Eventually, he shortened the lumen, allowing direct vision and dispensing with the need for the prism. The laryngoscope had two dry cell batteries in the handle with a push button to activate the light. Janeway used this device extensively, but it was never widely adopted by others.

When Ivan Magill developed his double insufflation catheter technique, he devised his own laryngoscope to assist with the passage of the catheters.[79] He found this laryngoscope equally useful when he wanted to insert a single, wide-bore tracheal tube.[78] Bearing many similarities to Jackson's laryngoscope, Magill's laryngoscope was initially powered by an external power source; later designs incorporated batteries in the handle (Fig. 17.17). In New York, Paluel Flagg (1886–1970), aware of Magill's work with single lumen, wide-bore tracheal tubes, worked closely with Chevalier Jackson to develop an anesthetic technique using a single tracheal tube.[122] His cooperation with Jackson may explain why his tubes were so different to those of Magill; the distal end of the chrome-plated tubes was straight and rigid, and the proximal part was a tight spiral of wire with a removable rubber coating (Fig. 17.18). The tubes, introduced over a stylet, bore a resemblance to bronchoscopes. Flagg used Jackson's laryngoscope before eventually designing his own (Fig. 17.19).[123] The blade was long and straight, with a slight curve at the end, designed to lift the epiglottis after establishing deep ether anesthesia; it retained the cross-sectional C-shape favored by bronchoscopists.[124–126] The laryngoscope was made with detachable blades in several sizes; both the blades and the lamp could be sterilized by boiling, but in practice Flagg used either alcohol or ether.

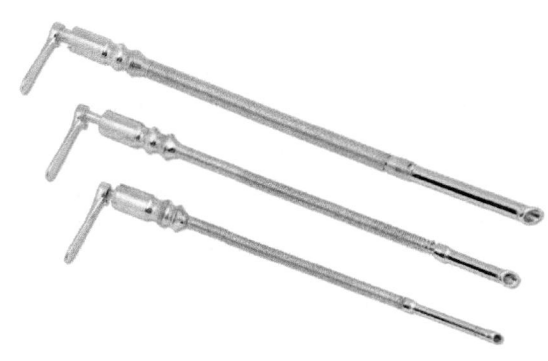

• **Fig. 17.18** Flagg endotracheal tube. (Courtesy Wood Library-Museum, Schaumburg, IL, USA.)

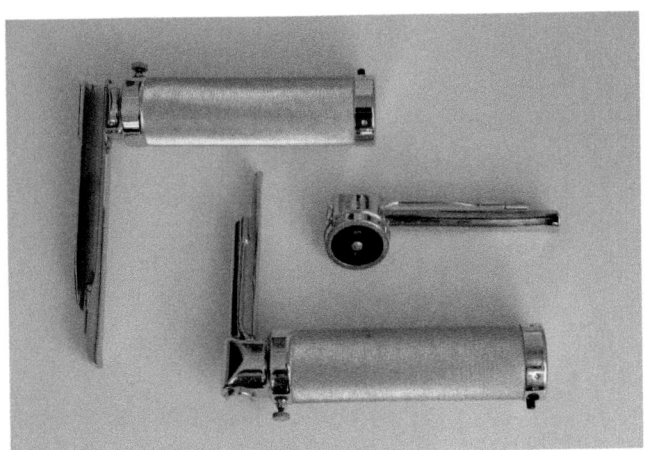

• **Fig. 17.19** Flagg laryngoscope with detachable blades. (Courtesy Geoffrey Kaye Museum of Anaesthetic History, Melbourne, Victoria, Australia.)

In the early 1930s, John Lundy (1894–1973) described a laryngoscope made by the Welch Allyn Company to his specifications.[127] Shortly thereafter, almost every anesthesiologist of note was requesting modifications from the manufacturers. Arthur

Guedel created an unusual laryngoscope with the blade at a fixed acute 28-degree angle to the handle to *"promote lifting without using the teeth as a fulcrum."*[128] This design was adapted in London by Victor Goldman, who felt the acute angle assisted with intubation in children by minimizing the head extension required.[129] Noel Gillespie (1904–1955), while working in the Dockland's area of east London with the plastic surgeon Thomas Kilner (1890–1964), anesthetized many children with cleft lips and palates. Finding the Magill laryngoscope too cumbersome for these small children, Gillespie approached Mayer and Phelps for assistance. They modified the smallest Chevalier Jackson laryngoscope to produce the Shadwell laryngoscope.[130] Marketed by A. Charles King Ltd., this laryngoscope was made specifically for children and never manufactured in an adult size (Fig. 17.20).

Robert Miller (1906–1976) from San Antonio, Texas, was also concerned with damaging teeth. Feeling that the available laryngoscopes were too thick at the base of the blade, he approached Welch Allyn to find a solution. The result was the long, narrow Miller blade. Released in 1941, it was designed to pass beyond the epiglottis and was particularly useful when mouth opening was limited (Fig. 17.21).[131] The most successful of the straight blades, it has been through several modifications but remains available today in a range of sizes.[132] The biggest revolution in laryngoscope design was initiated by a serendipitous observation. Robert Macintosh (1897–1989) was assisting with the insertion of a Boyle-Davis Gag for a tonsillectomy when he saw the vocal cords clearly displayed.[133] Realizing the potential of this observation, he summoned the department technician, Richard Salt, and by noon Salt had soldered a Davis blade onto a laryngoscope handle. Crucial to the success of this modification was the realization that the blade did not have to be passed over the epiglottis but could be inserted into the vallecula. Macintosh described the new technique along with his curved laryngoscope blade in 1943.[134] The curved Macintosh blade became the most popular blade around the world; its enduring legacy is most clearly demonstrated by the transition of the design into modern video laryngoscopy. The Macintosh blade also marked the end of the C-shaped cross-sectional laryngoscope blade, a feature which remained from the early origins of laryngoscopy in bronchoscopy. The Z-shaped cross-section of the Macintosh blade allows better visualization of the larynx during insertion of the tracheal tube; Macintosh believed that this feature and the new insertion technique were the important features of his laryngoscope, not the curve of the blade (Fig. 17.22).[135] In the United States, the Macintosh blade was manufactured and distributed by the Foregger Company. Macintosh gave Richard von Foregger a prototype of the blade and, to his surprise, Foregger manufactured the American Macintosh blade from this prototype without considering any of the future modifications.[136] This is the reason that, even today, the American Macintosh blade has dimensions different from the British design.

There were many different ways of attaching the blades to the laryngoscope handle. Early detachable blades, like the blade of the Flagg laryngoscope (see Fig. 17.19), screwed into the handle. Both Medical & Industrial Equipment Ltd and the Longworth Company used hinged fittings, the Longworth consisting of a removable hinge-pin and spring clip (see Fig. 17.21). Welch

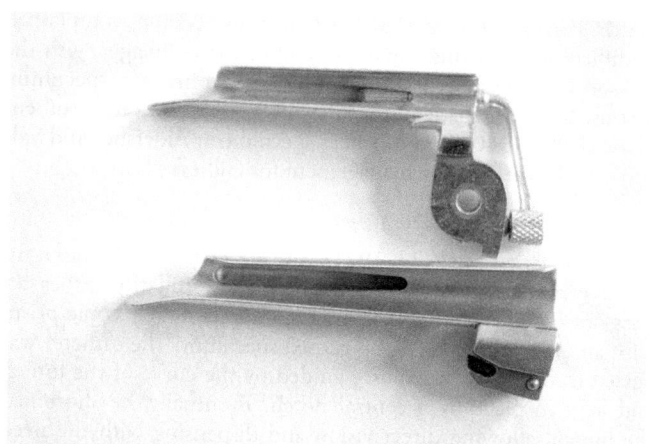

• **Fig. 17.21** Miller blades. The top demonstrates an earlier removable hinge-pin attachment; the lower demonstrates a modern hinged connection. (Courtesy Geoffrey Kaye Museum of Anaesthetic History, Melbourne, Victoria, Australia.)

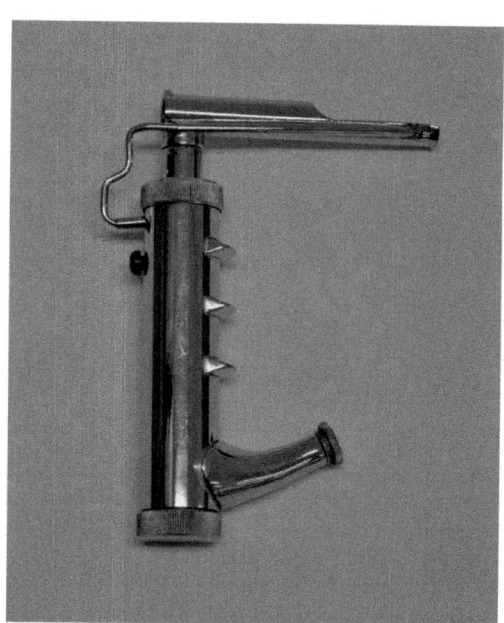

• **Fig. 17.20** Shadwell infant laryngoscope. (Courtesy Harry Daly Museum, Australian Society of Anaesthetists, North Sydney, NSW, Australia.)

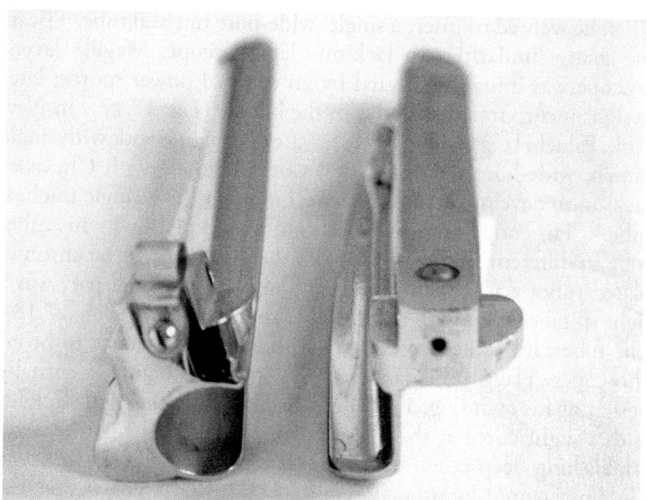

• **Fig. 17.22** Left: C-shaped cross-section of an early Miller blade. Right: Z-shaped cross-section of a Macintosh blade. (Courtesy Geoffrey Kaye Museum of Anaesthetic History, Melbourne, Victoria, Australia.)

Allyn designed the hook-on fitting that was eventually adopted by all the companies; Welch Allyn only patented this fitting in the United States.[137]

Further Development of Pharyngeal Airways

Cuffed Pharyngeal Airways

Closed-circuit anesthesia attracted a lot of attention in the 1930s. William B. Primrose (1892–1977) from Glasgow was attempting to perfect a closed system anesthesia delivery when he designed his pharyngeal airway in 1934.[138] The pharyngeal tube, which had a cuff at the distal end, was positioned close to the laryngeal opening before the cuff was inflated. This was probably the first example of a cuffed pharyngeal airway. The following year in London, Francis Shipway described a bulbous pharyngeal airway with an inflatable cuff designed to protect the trachea from contamination from blood or pus during nasal operations.[139] A year later, the Foregger catalogue presented a "Lessinger Airway cuff" that was almost identical. Beverley Leech (1898–1960) from Regina, Canada, described a "pharyngeal bulb gasway" in 1937; it had a solid rubber cuff, which was not inflatable (Fig. 17.23).[140] Like the Primrose airway, it was intended to provide an airway seal during cyclopropane anesthesia, allowing closed-circuit anesthesia without resorting to tracheal intubation. The bulb sealed with the soft tissues of the pharyngeal wall posteriorly and with the tongue anteriorly. The cuffed pharyngeal airway was a short-lived invention; airway protection with a cuffed tracheal tube became universally accepted and the cuffed pharyngeal airway was largely forgotten.

Development of the Laryngeal Mask Airway

After decades without development, the concept of a cuffed pharyngeal airway was re-explored by Archie Brain (1942–), once again looking for a way to seal the airway without resorting to a tracheal tube.[141] Brain, working in east London, noticed that the inflatable cuff of the Goldman Dental Facemask he was using had a shape very similar to the area surrounding the larynx. Working with cadaveric molds, he developed his first prototype laryngeal mask airway (LMA) in 1981, attaching the cuff of a Goldman mask to the proximal part of a 10-mm plastic tracheal tube with acrylic adhesive. By the time the first clinical trial was reported in 1983, the black rubber prototypes had been used on over a thousand cases, proving very successful (Fig. 17.24).[142] Believing that silicone would be a better material for the LMA, Brain

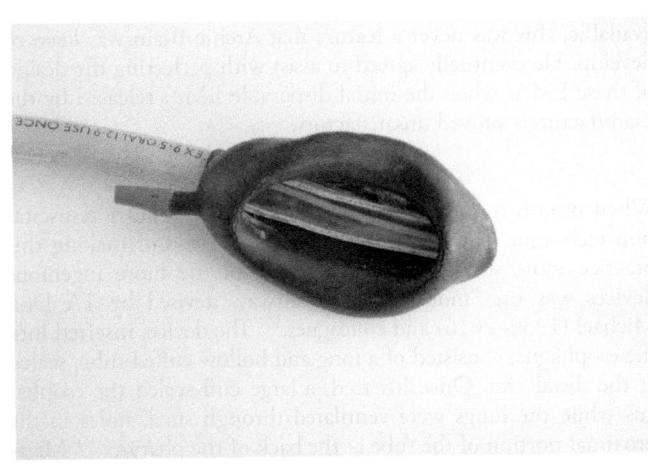

• **Fig. 17.24** Prototype laryngeal mask airway. (Courtesy Geoffrey Kaye Museum of Anaesthetic History, Melbourne, Victoria, Australia.)

approached the Dunlop Rubber Company for assistance. After many modifications and improvements, Brain was able to provide Dr. John Nunn at Northwick Park Hospital with two new silicone LMA devices for the first independent trial.[143] The first commercially available LMA, the LMA Classic, became available in Britain in 1988. The new device was an instant success, and within three years of its introduction, it had been used on over two million patients.[144] It was particularly fortunate that the timing of the introduction of the LMA coincided with the release of propofol as an induction agent. The airway relaxation created by an induction dose of propofol creates ideal conditions for the insertion of a laryngeal mask. Whereas an induction dose of thiopentone, previously the most commonly used intravenous anesthetic agent, maintains these reflexes, making LMA insertion difficult.

Refinements of the Laryngeal Mask Airway

Archie Brain had already been working on a solution to the problem of the kinking of LMAs by the time they were reported.[145,146] With the aid of some wire reinforcing, the LMA tube was strengthened to produce the flexible LMA, with the first clinical trial of this device reported in 1990.[147]

Classic LMAs were intermittently used to assist with intubation, but they had many deficiencies when used in this way. A few individuals experimented with a split LMA,[148] but it was evident that a complete redesign was required. The first clinical trial of the prototype intubating LMA was conducted at the Royal Berkshire Hospital in 1995 with fairly disappointing results.[149] After further design work, the Intubating LMA was released in 1997 with a single epiglottic lifting bar.[150,151] It was accompanied by a specially designed cuffed silicone tracheal tube.

Archie Brain was very aware that the LMA Classic did not provide protection against aspiration of gastric contents, leading him to state that it "was not therefore regarded by the inventor as the ultimate form of the device."[152] In 1995, he described a prototype with a second mask to isolate the upper end of the esophagus, concluding that it needed further improvement.[152] Various modifications were produced, which were all rather stiff and bulky, but clinical testing proved them to be effective in preventing aspiration.[153] After a series of improvements, the LMA ProSeal was available for clinical testing in 1999.[144] Since then, further refinements have resulted in the LMA Supreme, which combines the desirable features of the LMA ProSeal and the Intubating LMA. It should be noted that, although there are now single-use LMAs

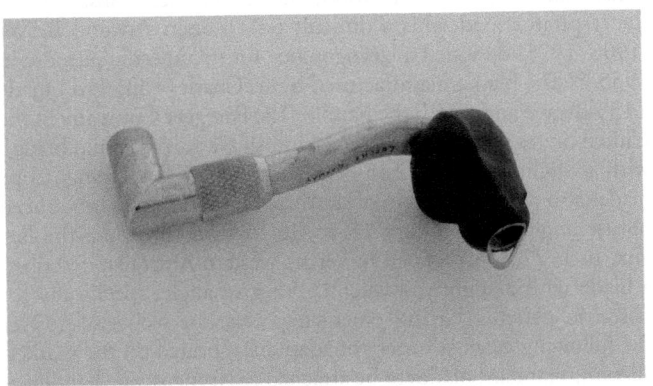

• **Fig. 17.23** Leech pharyngeal bulb "gasway." (Courtesy Geoffrey Kaye Museum of Anaesthetic History, Melbourne, Victoria, Australia.)

available, this was never a feature that Archie Brain was keen to develop. He eventually agreed to assist with perfecting the design of these LMAs when the initial disposable LMAs released by the manufacturers proved unsatisfactory.

Other Supraglottic Airway Devices

When mouth-to-mouth respiration became a popular resuscitation technique in the 1960s, many sought ways of making this practice more socially acceptable. One of the more ingenious devices was the "mouth-to-lung" airway, devised by TA Don Michael (1932–2016) and colleagues.[154] The device, inserted into the esophagus, consisted of a long and hollow cuffed tube, sealed at the distal end. Once inserted, a large cuff sealed the esophagus while the lungs were ventilated through small holes in the proximal portion of the tube at the back of the pharynx.[154] Many modifications were made to this device, which was widely used by emergency services. It was not without controversy, with Smith and colleagues reporting an 18% failure rate with the device.[155]

The principal problem with Don Michael's airway was that no ventilation was possible if it entered the trachea. The Esophageal Tracheal Combitube (ETC) was specifically intended to overcome this problem, allowing ventilation regardless of whether it entered the trachea or the esophagus.[156] It has two lumens, one of which is open at the distal end to allow ventilation if inserted in the trachea. If the tube travels into the esophagus, ventilation will then continue via the pharyngeal holes, as in the original version. The ETC was designed principally as a rescue and resuscitation aid for emergency workers and was never intended for anesthesia. It is now part of a bewildering array of constantly changing, supraglottic airways (SGAs) on the market, many of which are unfamiliar to anesthesiologists.[157] Nevertheless, the availability of an SGA rescue device, in addition to the LMA, is part of difficult airway guidelines around the world.[158]

Difficult Airway Management

Recognition and Early Approaches

Bougies and Stylets

The work of Magill and Rowbotham popularized the use of tracheal tubes, but it was soon apparent that it was not always easy to pass the tube through the laryngeal opening. Some tubes came with in-built stylets to stiffen them, but improvization was often required. Emery Rovenstine (1895–1960) wrote to Robert Macintosh (1897–1989) in 1939 suggesting that a knitting needle could be used for this purpose.[159] Metal and plastic knitting needles became popular as introducers but, as they were hazardous, a variety of copper and brass stylets were subsequently devised, usually with blunt ends and often a sliding stop to limit the depth to which they were inserted (Fig. 17.25).[160,161] In 1948, Robert Minnitt (1889–1974) and John Gillies (1895–1976) suggested that a semi-rigid gum-elastic catheter, normally used for urethral dilation, could be used as an aid to intubation. The following year, Robert Macintosh provided detailed instructions for its use for this purpose.[162]

In 1957, Macintosh and Harry Richards described a vinyl-coated introducer with a light at the distal tip.[163] The technique of tracheal transillumination was described 2 years later when the first successful blind intubation with a lighted introducer was reported by Hideo Yamamura and his colleagues.[164] In the early 1970s Paul Venn, working as the anesthetic advisor to Eschmann Bros. & Walsh Ltd., developed a new introducer colloquially known as

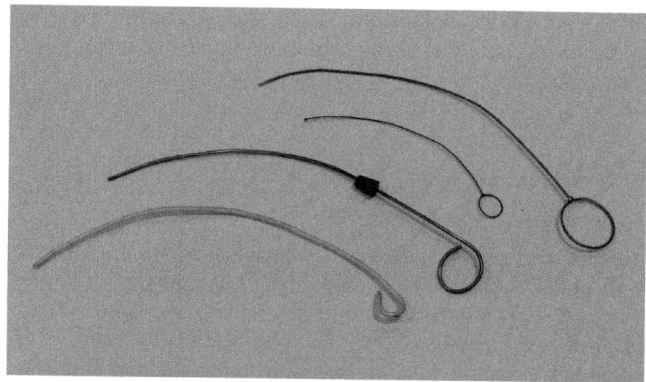

• **Fig. 17.25** A selection of early stylets with a modern example at the bottom of the picture. (Courtesy Geoffrey Kaye Museum of Anaesthetic History, Melbourne, Victoria, Australia.)

the *gum elastic catheter* or *bougie* (after the catheter originally used by Macintosh).[165] The 60-cm-long Eschmann introducer was not made of gum elastic and had three unique features: a woven polyester core with a coat of resin, a distal 40-degree coudé (French for "elbow bend"), and a much greater length than other introducers. These introducers became extremely popular in the United Kingdom during the 1980s but were seldom used in the United States; subsequent studies demonstrated their effectiveness, and they were eventually incorporated into the American Society of Anesthesiologists (ASA) guidelines.[166,167] In the 1990s, single-use equipment became increasingly popular, and the Eschmann introducer was replaced by the disposable Portex Venn Tracheal Introducer.

Laryngoscopes for Difficult Intubations

Tracheal intubation had obvious benefits, but it was soon evident there were hazards associated with the procedure.[168] Many practitioners incorporated tracheal tubes into their practice without skill or experience, commonly performing blind nasal intubations. Among the reports of morbidity associated with tracheal tubes, it was also noted that *"Death has been known to follow copious and persistent pharyngeal hemorrhage caused by attempts at blind intubation."*[168] The introduction of muscle relaxants in the 1940s further increased the need for a controlled airway, and as the polio epidemic spread around the world in the 1950s, intubation became necessary in increasingly complex situations.

Polio patients, managed in negative-pressure ventilators, still occasionally required intubation, and the physical constraints of the respirator made this a difficult task. Robert Atwood Beaver (1906–1975) designed a laryngoscope for this specific purpose in 1955.[169] The blade, manufactured by A. Charles King Ltd., made a 155-degree angle with the handle. The Foregger Company in the United States sold a modified Macintosh blade, the "polio blade," with a slightly smaller 135-degree angle.[92] These laryngoscope blades also proved useful in obstetric patients, but the pronounced obtuse angle made it difficult to lift upward to expose the larynx. In 1977, John Kessell in Perth, Western Australia, described a blade with a slightly smaller 110-degree angle, specifically for obstetric patients having emergency cesarean sections.[170] Over the following years, a variety of adapters appeared on the market, allowing standard blades to be attached to laryngoscope handles at different angles. The vast number of available adapters led Dhara and Cheong to describe an adjustable multiple-angle adapter in

1991. The adapter provided incremental angles from 5 to 180 degrees, allowing for many different scenarios.[171]

In 1956, Ephraim Siker (1926–2013) described some of the anatomic problems that contribute to a difficult intubation: a recessed mandible, protruding upper incisors, and a large tongue. Patients with these anatomical features are more likely to have a high anterior larynx, which Siker found he could view more easily by placing a mirror in an angled laryngoscope blade. To prevent fogging of the mirror, the mirror attachment was encased in copper, making the larynx potentially easier to see, but the reverse image made the blade difficult to use without practice.[172] Henry Janeway had used prisms in the earliest anesthetic laryngoscope,[121] but it was the nurse anesthetist John Huffman who suggested the prism as a potential aid to difficult intubations.[173,174] Initially he added a prism to a Macintosh blade but found this crowded the pharynx, making intubation difficult despite an improved view of the larynx (Fig. 17.26). He therefore designed his own laryngoscope to accommodate the prism, and a later model with two prisms. Further variations by others followed. Christopher P. Bellhouse, combining the concepts developed by Siker and Huffman, designed an angled blade with an associated prism in 1988.[175] Three years later, Jay Choi described a multi-angled blade intended to overcome the need for mirrors or prisms.[176]

Another novel approach was that devised by Eamon P. McCoy and Rajinder K. Mirakhur in Belfast in 1993. They modified a standard Macintosh blade, removing the tip and reattaching it with a hinged mechanism. Once inserted in the vallecula, the hinged tip was elevated via a spring-loaded lever, lifting the hyoepiglottic ligament and exposing the larynx.[177] One of the aims of this laryngoscope was to provide a fulcrum point inside the pharynx, decreasing the risk to the patient's teeth.

Many other laryngoscope blades have been invented over the past 30 years; some have survived, whereas others have faded into obscurity as modern technological advances have come to dominate the field of airway management.

Transtracheal Ventilation

Transtracheal ventilation as a means of sustaining life was first demonstrated in Robert Hooke's experiments of 1667. In 1877, Joseph Clover successfully resuscitated an anesthetized patient with complete airway obstruction using a cricothyrotomy.[178] Eighty years later, there was a resurgence of interest in this technique, as a means of resuscitation in the patient with complete airway obstruction, particularly in relation to anesthesia. Porter Reed and his colleagues reported a series of experiments with dogs,[179] and a series of case reports followed in the 1970s, with suggestions for simple ways of adapting available equipment in an emergency.[180,181] The use of simple equipment gained widespread acceptance in 1989 with the publication of Jon Benumof's review of transtracheal ventilation: *"There is widespread agreement in the literature that percutaneous transtracheal jet ventilation (TTJV) using a large IV catheter inserted through the cricothyroid membrane is a simple, relatively safe, extremely effective treatment of choice for the desperate cannot ventilate/cannot intubate situation."*[182] Equipment for emergency transtracheal jet ventilation is now an important part of many difficult airway guidelines.[158]

Airway Classification

Ronald Cormack and John Lehane from Northwick Park Hospital in north London noted that anesthetic obstetric deaths in the United Kingdom had remained constant at around 14 deaths a year for over a decade; the majority of these were due to failed intubation.[183] Believing that this was unacceptable, they devised a classification of the airway according to the view of the larynx. The now familiar classification identifies Grade 3 as a view of the epiglottis only and Grade 4 as being unable to see even the epiglottis. Assuming that Grade 4 was very uncommon, usually predictable, and often associated with known airway pathology, they postulated that most of the airway-related deaths in obstetrics were related to unexpected Grade 3 laryngeal views. They proposed that a Grade 3 view should be simulated for trainees who could then practice various drills to effectively intubate someone with a Grade 3 larynx. The drill they recommended was the Macintosh method, not invented by Macintosh but named after him due to the use of the Oxford tube.[184] The method was simple: Using the epiglottis as a guide, an introducer was inserted in the midline, maintaining an anterior position. Once the introducer was in place, an Oxford tube was placed over an introducer and inserted blindly into the trachea. Interestingly, at no point in this oft-cited article do the authors mention using this classification to inform the patient or future anesthesiologists of potential difficulty. The article is principally in support of a training exercise, but its legacy is an invaluable warning system. The modification of this classification was proposed in 1998, allowing subclassification of Grade 2 laryngeal views, providing more information to subsequent anesthesiologists.[185] However, the Cormack-Lehane classification, as the authors acknowledged, is not predictive. A predictive system came later with the work of Seshagiri Rao Mallampati from Boston.

In 1983 Mallampati hypothesized that examining the patient's throat with the mouth fully open and the tongue protruded provided clues to the difficulty of subsequent intubation.[186] A subsequent study established the predictability of this test. The initial scaling system included three classes; the modified Mallampati scoring system has four classes and is widely used.[187] Subsequent analysis has suggested it is best used as one tool in the total assessment of the airway.[188]

Technological Advances

Flexible Intubation Scopes
The first flexible endoscope was constructed by gastroenterologist, Basil Hirschowitz (1925–2013) in the mid-1950s, when physicists were finally able to perfect optically insulated fibers.[189,190] The original fiberscope, created to visualize the upper gastrointestinal tract, was 1 meter long with a central group of image-carrying

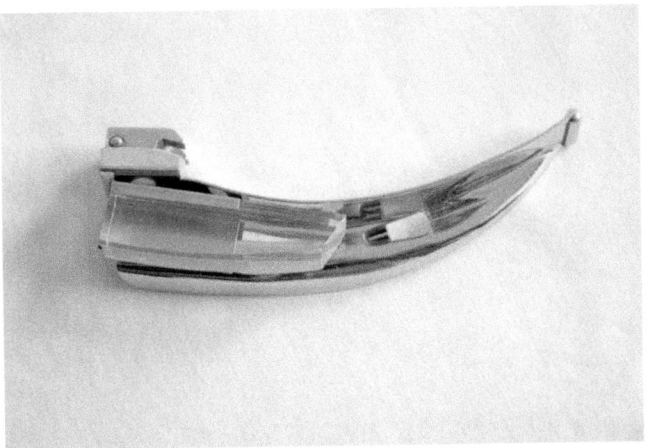

• **Fig. 17.26** Huffman prism in a Macintosh blade. (Courtesy Geoffrey Kaye Museum of Anaesthetic History, Melbourne, Victoria, Australia.)

fibers surrounded by transmitting fibers carrying light from an external source. By the 1960s, similar fiberscopes were being commercially manufactured for a range of procedures, with the first flexible bronchoscope commissioned in 1967 by Shigeto Ikeda (1925–2001). He reported 184 diagnostic bronchoscopies in 1968, concluding 3 years later that flexible fiberoptic broncshoscopy was an effective aid to the diagnosis of lung cancer.[191,192]

Before the first flexible bronchoscope appeared on the market, Peter Murphy, a senior anesthesia trainee at the National Hospital, Queen Square, London, chanced upon an article in the Lancet describing a flexible choledochoscope for looking into the common bile duct during cholecystectomy.[193] Realizing the potential of this instrument for difficult intubations, he made inquiries of American Cystoscope Makers Inc (ACMI). which to his surprise sent him one to test with a request to inform the company of his progress. Given that the instrument was expensive and delicate, it is a testament to both Murphy and ACMI that this work could proceed. Murphy quickly established that the instrument was extremely useful in the management of the airway, reporting some of his findings in a letter to the editor of Anaesthesia.[194] By the early 1970s, there were many reports of airway management with both flexible bronchoscopes and purpose built flexible fiberoptic laryngoscopes.[195–198] Opinions were mixed; seen by some as a new era in airway management, others felt the cost would be prohibitive in many settings.[195,199] Because distal camera chip technology has largely replaced fiberoptic bundles in the flexible laryngoscopes on the market today, the term flexible fiberoptic laryngoscope has been replaced with flexible intubation scopes (FIS), and the procedure in which these instruments are used is now referred to as flexible scope intubation (FSI). Today, FSI is viewed as a basic skill requirement for anesthesiologists, with awake flexible scope intubations reported in observational studies to be successful in 88% to 100% of difficult intubations (Category B3-B evidence).[200]

Intubating Stylets

Although aids to FSI were developed rapidly in the 1970s, no equipment was small enough for children. In 1977, Down Bros. and Mayer and Phelps Ltd. constructed a very fine fiberoptic bundle for Charles A. Foster, at St. Thomas' Hospital in London.[201] Foster used this to perform a blind nasal intubation with laryngeal transillumination on a child whose mouth would not open. The bundle fitted easily down a 4-mm tracheal tube and connected to a standard fiberoptic light source. The following year, M. Ducrow used an existing surgical light, the Flexi-lum, to achieve the same result in an adult.[202] This light was a single-use surgical device, not intended for this purpose but subsequently widely used for this technique until a dislodged light globe complicated a difficult intubation.[203] A number of commercial devices were then developed for performing blind intubation with transillumination. The technique has proved to be effective and useful in a variety of scenarios, including in remote and austere environments.[204] Lighted stylets are recognized as a useful tool in a difficult intubation, listed under "Strategies for Intubation and Ventilation" in the current American Society of Anesthesiologists (ASA) Practice Guidelines.[200]

In 1979, Ronald Katz and George Berci described a "rigid, straight optical instrument that permits us 'to see through' the endotracheal tube."[205] This was essentially a fiberoptic telescope that allowed a 60-degree view of the larynx but could only operate in a straight line. Most commonly used with a regular laryngoscope to displace the tongue from view, it was felt by the authors to be most useful as a teaching aid. They described using it in difficult intubations as a method of visualizing the larynx, while passing the tracheal tube over a separate curved stylet.

Indirect Laryngoscopes

Fiberoptic technology also allowed a reappraisal of indirect laryngoscopy. Roger Bullard filed several patents in the late 1970s relating to the first indirect rigid fiberoptic laryngoscope,[206–208] with the first clinical report appearing in 1979 (Fig. 17.27).[209] Optical fibers were used to transmit an image from the distal end of the blade to an eyepiece, allowing the laryngoscope to be used with minimal mouth opening and a neutral head position.[210] Working ports were added for integrated intubating forceps and additional oxygen or suction as required. Subsequent modifications to the Bullard laryngoscope included a conventional laryngoscope handle and a video camera attachment. Other indirect fiberoptic laryngoscopes, such as the Wu-Scope[211] and the Upsher Scope,[212] appeared on the market in the 1990s, but video technology soon made these redundant.

Videos in Laryngoscopy

Fiberoptic technology allowed anesthesiologists to see around tight bends, but like all early endoscopists, they were required to look through a small eyepiece at the end of the endoscope. Early attempts at projecting the image onto a screen required heavy external cameras. In the early 1980s, Welch Allyn was able to take advantage of the new charge-coupled devices (CCD) on the market and incorporate video technology within an endoscope.[213] Their prototype video endoscope for colonoscopy was the beginning of a revolutionary change in endoscopic technology.[214,215] A rash of patents were lodged, but the microprocessor technology crucial to these developments was freely available, and all the leading companies began to harness this technology. New camera chips, built-in display monitors and single-use sheaths are among the many developments on this rapidly changing scene. Despite this, many fiberoptic intubations are still conducted via a single eyepiece.

Video Laryngoscopes

The application of modern technology to the humble laryngoscope has seen a revolution in laryngoscope design in the past 20 years. Video laryngoscopes were created by adding a miniature

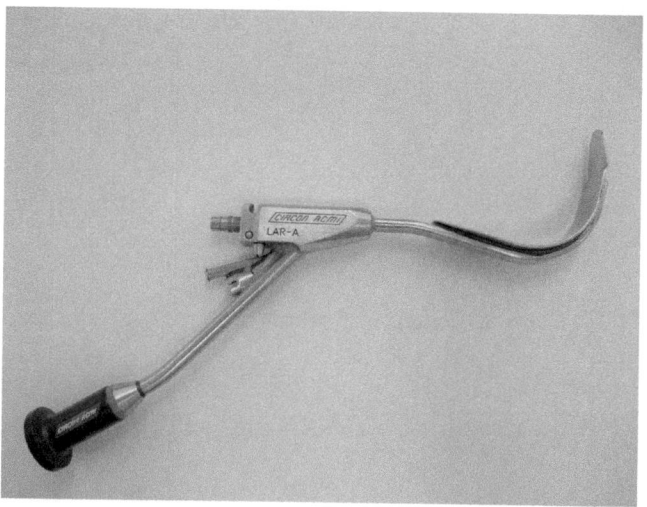

• **Fig. 17.27** The Bullard laryngoscope. (Courtesy Wood Library-Museum, Schaumburg, IL, USA.)

video camera or fiberoptic bundle to the blade of a standard laryngoscope. The captured image is transmitted to a monitor, either mounted on the handle or on a separate screen, giving an enhanced view of the larynx and the passage of the tracheal tube.

In 1988, Peter Bumm, an ear, nose, and throat surgeon, patented a way of achieving a similar view by inserting a fiberoptic bronchoscope next to a conventional laryngoscope. This method then became part of the patent filed by Dr. Wilfried Ilias, describing *"a laryngoscope within a laryngoscope which is connected with a laryngoscope."*[216] Karl Storz, an endoscope manufacturer, working with the surgeon George Berci and anesthesiologist Marshal Kaplan, developed this patent to produce a video laryngoscope with limited views in 1999. The technology was improved over the next 12 months to project a larger image onto the screen (Fig. 17.28).

The Video Macintosh Intubating Laryngoscope System incorporated the camera into the handle of a standard Macintosh laryngoscope, allowing visualization of the larynx both directly and on the portable screen. Kaplan and his colleagues reported only one failed intubation in the first series of 235 patients, attributing the success to their adaptation of existing familiar equipment.[217] Subsequently, the camera has been incorporated into the blade of the laryngoscope (CMAC, Storz, Tuttlingen, Germany). Although there is evidence a projected image is better than a direct view,[218] many manufacturers have now added this combined functionality to their products.

Swiss anesthesiologist Markus Weiss created a channel inside the blade of a plastic Macintosh laryngoscope, using this to guide a fine endoscope to the end of the blade.[219] This was another adaptation of Bumm's technique, which was demonstrated to be useful in children requiring intubation with manual inline stabilization.[220] These were the first publications using video technology with conventional laryngoscopes. Jon Berall lodged the first US patent for a video laryngoscope in 1997, aiming to provide a light, portable laryngoscope with a screen on the handle.[221] This laryngoscope was released to the market in 2005 (Coopdech, Daiken, Osaka, Japan).

In 2001, a single-piece, plastic videolaryngoscope (Glidescope, Saturn Biomedical, Indianapolis, IN, USA) was developed by the Canadian surgeon John Pacey. Successful intubation with this video laryngoscope requires a stylet in the tracheal tube and a slight change of technique from direct laryngoscopy.[222]

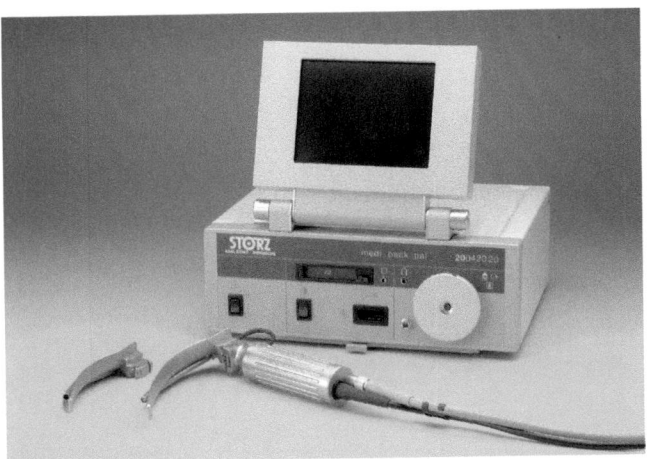

• **Fig. 17.28** Early video laryngoscope (2001 MVM Medipack) with fibers and no camera chip, developed by the surgeon George Berci, MD. (Image courtesy of Karl Storz & Co. KG, Tuttlingen, Germany.)

Video laryngoscopes have been integrated into anesthesia practice with startling rapidity; whether they ultimately come to completely replace the standard laryngoscope remains to be seen.[223] Video-assisted laryngoscopy is discussed further in Chapter 23.

Airway Planning

Difficult Airway Trolley

The first person to realize that equipment for the management of a difficult airway should be readily available for every anesthetic was Joseph Clover. Clover practiced anesthesia in London from 1858 until his death in 1882, carrying an emergency laryngotomy trochar and cannula with him throughout his career. He only used it on one occasion, but the case report clearly documents that the procedure, carried out with the assistance of the surgeon, saved the patient's life. He cautioned: *"I should regret if this record were to lead anyone to open the larynx without sufficient necessity. I have never used the cannula before, although it has been my companion at some thousands of anaesthetic cases."*[178]

A century later, a plethora of airway management devices were available, but there was little consistency surrounding the management of a difficult airway. Toward the end of the 1980s, anesthesia departments in a number of countries began to construct their own difficult intubation sets, generally assembling equipment in their respective facilities. Initially there was little formal reporting of this trend; it developed gradually in individual departments and spread by word of mouth. In 1990, James Diaz described a "Difficult intubation kit" that could be *assembled quickly from vascular catheters and sheaths commonly available in surgical facilities.*[224] The kit, which was accompanied by a set of guidelines for its use, allowed for *"continuous oxygen administration throughout all phases of its application in difficult upper airway management."* The same year, in a letter to the editor, Philip Larson of Stanford University Hospital described a difficult intubation cart containing *"all the equipment and supplies necessary to accomplish a difficult tracheal intubation."*[225] The cart had been in use for 2 years, with a comprehensive list of contents. Along with a fiberoptic laryngoscope, various sizes of Macintosh and Miller laryngoscope blades were recommended, along with a Siker mirror, an illuminated stylet, a cricothyrotomy set with a transtracheal jet ventilation system, and an optional tracheostomy set. As equipment for difficult intubations has evolved, so too has the difficult intubation trolley. Although every institution will have its own preferred equipment, current ASA guidelines recommend *"at least one portable storage unit that contains specialized equipment for difficult airway management should be readily available."*[200]

Difficult Airway Algorithms

By the 1990s, a complex array of equipment and options were available for managing the difficult airway but with no single coordinated approach. The ASA Taskforce on the Management of the Difficult Airway produced the first set of national guidelines in 1993.[226] These have been updated every 10 years, with the latest iteration released in 2013 and the most recent update currently being drafted.[200] Many other countries released their own guidelines over the next 10 years along similar lines.[158] In the UK, the Difficult Airway Society was founded in 1995 after discussions among Ray Towey, Adrian Pearce (both from London), and Ralph Vaughan (from Cardiff), primarily to teach fiberoptic intubation skills to anaesthesiologists.[227] In 2004 they questioned the ASA guidelines, suggesting that the flow diagrams in the document allowed for too much choice.[228] Fundamental to the UK guidelines was the development of three simple algorithms for specific situations: unanticipated difficult tracheal intubation in routine induction of anesthesia, unanticipated difficult tracheal intubation during a rapid sequence induction, and the "can't intubate, can't ventilate" scenario. The Difficult Airway Society upgraded its difficult intubation guidelines in 2015 and have since provided other guidelines for specific scenarios, such as airway management in the critically ill patient.[229,230]

Checklists for Airway Management

Checklists have been essential to the airline industry for decades. They have gained more traction in the medical world since the introduction of the World Health Organization (WHO) Surgical Safety Checklist in 2009.[231,232] This checklist has been widely adopted across surgical services throughout the world and has increased debate about the value of checklists in other areas of medicine, such as airway management. Checklists for intubation have since been adopted by many prehospital services and in hospital areas outside the operating room. In 2011, the Royal College of Anaesthetists in the UK conducted a national audit of airway complications (NAP4).[233] The auditors found a high incidence of complications in emergency department and intensive care settings, which they attributed to teams with limited experience working in unfamiliar places. Despite limited evidence, one of their recommendations was the use of checklists in these situations. A 2016 review of the use of airway management checklists also acknowledged the dearth of evidence but concluded that airway checklists have been increasingly adopted. *"Use of checklists is intuitive and likely to be of benefit, providing regular educational update and review within a robust governance structure."*[234]

In late 2019, the emergence of severe acute respiratory syndrome coronavirus 2 (SARS-Co-V-2) focused attention on the need to protect staff involved in the airway management of patients with airborne infectious diseases. As well as mandating specific personal protective equipment, many institutions and anesthesiology departments instituted checklists and other cognitive aids for intubation and extubation to standardize management and ensure the safety of their staff.[235,236]

Pictorial flow charts, algorithms, guidelines, and other cognitive aids are all essential to modern anesthesia practice, but success in the management of the airway ultimately depends on the preparedness and skill of the individual, appropriate assistance, and knowledge of the available equipment.

Conclusion

The maintenance of a patent airway has been a fundamental requirement of safe anesthesia since the first ether anesthetics in the 1840s. The specialty of anesthesia has always attracted physicians with inquiring minds who can envisage ways of incorporating new technology into their practice. As advances in engineering have resulted in new compounds and technology, these have been rapidly assimilated into anesthesia, particularly in the area of airway management. Small steplike changes have been interspersed with huge paradigm shifts, such as the current explosion of video technology. Although it is interesting to speculate about the future of such technology, an understanding of anesthesia's historical heritage suggests we should constantly reappraise old techniques in the light of modern technology. History provides a different and hopefully useful perspective on the techniques that are fundamental to our daily practice.

Selected References

10. Curry J. Popular Observations on Apparent Death from Drowning, Suffocation, etc. T Dicey and Co.; 1792.
16. Heiberg J. A new expedient in administering chloroform. *Medical Surgical Gazette.* 1874;1:36.
23. Hewitt F. An artificial "air-way" for use during anaesthetisation. *Lancet.* 1908;1:490–491.
45. O'Dwyer J. Intubation of the larynx. *New York Medical Journal.* 1885;421:145–147.
78. Magill I. Endotracheal anaesthesia. *Proc R Soc Med.* 1928;22: 83–89.
86. Thornton H. Vinyl-"Portex" tubing. *Br Med J.* 1944;2:14.
100. Rendell-Baker L. Hazards of prolonged intubation and tracheotomy equipment. *JAMA.* 1968;204:624–625.
141. Brain AIJ. The development of the larngeal mask - a brief history of the invention, early clinical studies and experimental work from which the laryngeal mask evolved. *European Journal of Anaesthesiology.* 1991;(suppl 4):5–17.
178. Clover JT. Laryngotomy in chloroform asphyxia. *BMJ.* 1877;1: 132–133.
193. Calder I. Classic Paper. Murphy P. A fibre-optic endoscope used for nasal intubation. *Anesthesia.* 1967;22:489–491. *Anaesthesia.* 2010;65:1133–1136.

All references can be found online at eBooks.Health.Elsevier.com.

18

Noninvasive Management of the Airway

JAMES DUCANTO, ADRIAN MATIOC, AND RICHARD E. GALGON

CHAPTER OUTLINE

KEY POINTS

- The most important upper airway (UA) soft tissue obstruction site is the soft palate.
- The one-handed face-mask ventilation (FMV) technique airway maneuver is the chin-lift/head extension (CL/HE) maneuver applied in the sagittal plane (on the occipito-atlanto-axial joint). The two-handed airway maneuver is the jaw thrust applied in the transverse plane (on the temporomandibular joints).
- The chin elevation (by head extension or mandibular advancement) can be estimated by the increase of the chin–sternum (UA stretching) and chin–cervical spine (UA enlargement) distance.
- The objective marker for the CL/HE is the head extension angle (optimal = 42 degrees), and for the mandibular advancement, the distance achieved between the mandibular and maxillary incisors (optimal = 16.2 ± 3.2 mm).
- The objective markers for the outcome of an FMV attempt are the tidal volume, airway pressure, and end-tidal CO_2.

- An unexpected difficult mask ventilation (DMV), just like an unexpected difficult intubation attempt, should be quickly diagnosed using objective markers. Oxygen desaturation is a late sign of FMV failure.
- The most efficient airway technique is the triple airway maneuver that combines a simultaneous CL/HE with a jaw thrust and an open mouth.
- The traditional escalating FMV approach (from simple to complex techniques) deters the operator from tailoring an optimal first response to the predictors of an expected DMV producing extended periods of apnea.
- The oropharyngeal airway is an underused device. It should be used with the first attempt in the expected DMV in obese, obstructive sleep apnea, edentulous, and fixed cervical spine patients and early in an unexpected DMV attempt.

Overview

Introduction

Core airway management skills common to all prehospital, emergency medicine, critical care, and anesthesiology providers begin with the recognition of airway patency, as well as the familiarity with the tools and techniques to maintain oxygenation and ventilation before invasive airway management. Too frequently, many caregivers believe that definitive airway management necessitates intubation of the trachea. Noninvasive management of the airway, of which face-mask ventilation (FMV) represents the most time-critical procedure in patients with acute respiratory failure, is an essential skill for providers tasked with caring for critically ill patients. Establishing and maintaining a patent airway has been the cornerstone of resuscitation and life support since the technique of cardiopulmonary resuscitation was introduced in 1961 by Safar and colleagues.[1] Despite the relative deemphasis on airway management in current American Heart Association (AHA) Resuscitation guidelines[2] (often misinterpreted by professionals and laypeople), airway management with noninvasive methods and tools represents a vital component of preserving and restoring life to critically ill patients. This chapter will specifically discuss simple tools and methods to achieve airway patency as well as the use of the FMV for passive, assisted, and active ventilatory support. Additionally, we will discuss the functional anatomy of the upper airway (UA) and its contribution to airway patency and obstruction.

The Enduring Importance of Face Mask Ventilation

FMV and the management of the nonintubated UA are central to the concept of continuous patient oxygenation. The face mask (FM) is the oldest airway management device in continuous use since 1847, when British physician John Snow introduced it for the administration of inhalational anesthesia. The bag-valve-mask (BVM) device (otherwise known as the Air-Shields-Manual-Breathing Unit [AMBU]) is a ubiquitous ventilation system used across prehospital and hospital environments that retains its relevance even in the era of advanced airway management devices.[3,4] Although FMV is apparently intuitive to perform and master with BVM or anesthesia circle systems, the technique has proven difficult to learn, retain, and apply in critical situations by inexperienced providers.[5] FMV represents an essential backup skill to failed attempts at supraglottic airway (SGA) or endotracheal tube (ETT) placement (and thus is portrayed as such in all of the guidelines for difficult airway management). In the critically ill patient its effective use prior to tracheal intubation can reduce the incidence of severe hypoxemia.[6] Therefore competency in this procedure must be reinforced in caregivers whenever possible.

A recent innovation to simplify FMV for novice, as well as experienced, rescuers is the use of automatic resuscitation management systems (ARMS), which are flow-controlled oxygen-powered resuscitators to simplify mask ventilation. These devices allow the use of both hands to ensure adequate mask seal, including proper airway maneuvers, such as head-tilt and jaw thrust, and use a flow-controlled system that prevents overpressurization of the airway in the presence of airway obstruction. A study of 104 prehospital providers tasked with FMV in anesthetized patients using standard BMV systems compared with an oxygen-powered automated resuscitator unit (Oxylator FR-300) demonstrated reduced gastric insufflation and improved tidal volume (TV) per respiratory cycle.[7] This study suggests that the use of ARMS devices can simplify and improve the quality of ventilation via FM in novice healthcare providers and that more investigation in simplifying FMV is indicated in this area. An example of the use of an ARMS unit with capnography monitoring is provided in the video supplement to this chapter (Video 18.1).

It is important to state that the plethora of invasive airway management devices in use today (such as SGAs) has been said to have "cannibalized the experience of younger anesthetists" with the FMV technique, leading to inconsistent and suboptimal practice.[8] Current and future emphasis on acquiring and maintaining prowess in the FMV technique should be a goal of training programs in anesthesiology, emergency medicine, and critical care as well as prehospital providers.

Functional Anatomy and Its Role in Upper Airway Obstruction

Upper Airway Functional Anatomy

Noninvasive airway management seeks to maintain UA patency with minimal equipment and interventions. We shall now review the pertinent anatomy and physiology of the UA, as it applies to providing clinically effective maneuvers to relieve obstruction to ventilation. The UA extends from the anterior nares or lips to the larynx and includes two cavities (nasal and oral), which subdivide the pharynx. The adult pharynx is a 12- to 15-cm-long convoluted and collapsible muscular tube that is subdivided into functional compartments: nasopharynx, velopharynx (retropalatal), oropharynx (retroglossal), and laryngopharynx (retroepiglottic) (Fig. 18.1). The cervical spine defines the solid posterior wall of the UA, while soft expandable (and collapsible) tissues form the

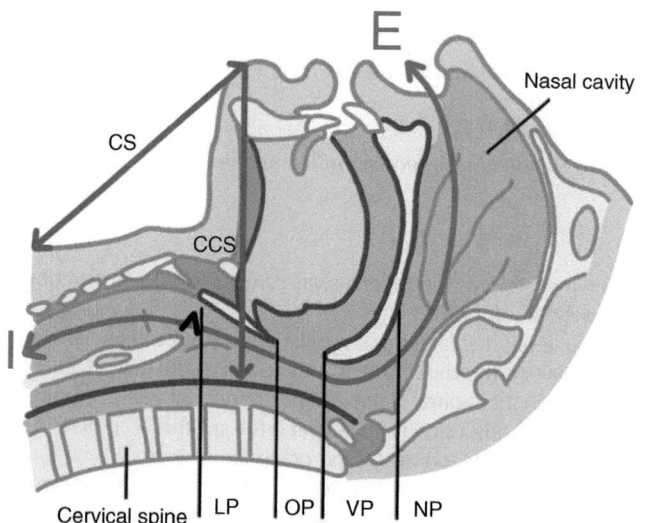

• **Fig. 18.1** The upper airway pharyngeal compartments: the nasopharynx *(NP)*, velopharynx *(VP)*, oropharynx *(OP)*, and laryngopharynx *(LP)*. The anatomic sites of UA soft tissue collapse in an unconscious patient are the soft palate, the most important being the tongue and epiglottis. The generic markers of chin elevation (by head extension or mandibular advancement) are the increase of the chin–sternum *(CS)* and chin–cervical spine *(CCS)* distance. The nasal ventilation route (with the mouth closed)—*red line*—cumulates all the potential obstruction sites: nasal cavities, *NP, VP, OP, LP,* and the glottis in expiration *(E)* and inspiration *(I)*.

anterior and lateral pharyngeal wall. The pharynx supports deglutition, phonation, and respiration. The UA is a dynamic structure defined by the interaction between soft tissues (muscle, mucosa, lymphatic structure) and enclosing solid structures (bones posteriorly as the cervical spine and cartilages anteriorly and inferiorly as the thyroid cartilages). In a supine unconscious patient the soft tissues collapse posteriorly and medially, generating UA obstruction. To relieve the UA obstruction in such a case, the provider applies airway maneuvers by manipulating two solid structures (the cervical spine and the mandible) to stretch the anterior neck structures, thus mobilizing and tensing the collapsed soft tissue structures.

Upper Airway Collapsibility and Obstruction

Patency in the UA is maintained by the balance between the inward narrowing forces (negative airway pressure during inspiration and the effect of gravity) and the outward dilating forces (pharyngeal dilator muscles). Pharyngeal dilator muscles are dependent on efferent neural control to maintain UA patency. When neural control of the pharyngeal dilator muscles is impaired or abolished by sedatives, intoxicants, anesthetics, REM sleep, or neuromuscular disease, the UA collapses, and airway obstruction ensues.[9] Failure of UA patency leading to upper airway obstruction (UAO) can occur at several anatomic sites from the nasal cavities to the larynx and is highly dependent upon the anatomic and physiologic state of the patient.

The nasal ventilation route (with the mouth closed) has five possible obstruction sites: the nasal cavities and nasopharynx, soft palate, base of the tongue, epiglottis, and glottis (glottic closure with the extreme of laryngospasm) (see Fig. 18.1). Ventilation via the oral route (with the mouth open) has three sites of potential obstruction: the base of the tongue, the epiglottis, and the glottis. Of these potential airway obstruction sites, two respond consistently to externally applied airway maneuvers (the base of the tongue and the epiglottis). The following is a summary of the potential sites of UAO and the effects of sedative medications.

Nasopharyngeal obstruction can occur because of physical deformities, such as septal deviation and nasal foreign bodies (as seen in children) and physiologic derangements, such as allergic rhinitis or epistaxis. Preprocedure assessment of nasal patency can be evaluated clinically by requesting the patient to breathe alternatively through one nostril while gently blocking the other with a fingertip. The assessment of airflow in this manner will allow the clinician to predict the degree of airway obstruction as a result of restriction of nasal airflow and will also help identify the laterality of the appropriate nare for nasopharyngeal airway (NPA) placement, should that become necessary.

Safar radiographically confirmed the role of the tongue in UAO in the unconscious patient in his seminal work on exhaled air-rescue (mouth-to-mouth) breathing. He also correlated neck flexion with epiglottis downfolding and soft palate obstruction.[10] A more recent assessment of the tongue's contribution to UAO during anesthetic induction using ultrasound scanning of the hypopharynx did not indicate that the tongue is the major cause of airway obstruction.[11] The soft palate is considered a primary site of UAO in unconscious or anesthetized patients, because it is the most compliant structure in normal and in obstructive sleep apnea (OSA) subjects.[12–14] Boidin demonstrated in anesthetized, nonparalyzed patients using flexible bronchoscopy that the epiglottis has a more important contribution to UAO than the tongue, as it closes the flow of gas to the larynx when resting against the posterior pharynx.[15]

Drug-induced UAO generated by propofol,[16] sufentanil,[17] isoflurane,[18] sevoflurane,[19] and dexmedetomidine[20] is difficult to compare, because there is no reliable pharmacodynamic indicator of the depth of unconsciousness. Ketamine preserves the hypopharyngeal size, whereas the neuromuscular agents generate profound relaxation of skeletal muscle activity (including the upper esophageal sphincter). In sedated patients reduction of UA patency occurs to a greater extent at the level of the soft palate and the epiglottis than at the level of the tongue. Dexmedetomidine, compared with propofol, may produce less UAO in light to moderately sedated patients but not in patients under deep sedation.[21–25] Ketamine may preserve UA patency better than either propofol or dexmedetomidine.[26]

Partial UAO is insidious in onset, leading to hypoxemia, hypercapnia, and respiratory acidosis. Clinical signs are noisy breathing (inspiratory stridor), use of accessory muscles, tachycardia, tachypnea, paradoxical chest, abdominal movement ("see-sawing"), agitation, reduced consciousness level, and cyanosis as a late sign. Complete UAO with the absence of airway noises is a critical event and, if left untreated, leads rapidly to hypoxia and cardiac arrest.

The site of airway obstruction may change during the respiratory cycle. In a sedated/anesthetized patient inspiratory efforts tend to cause pharyngeal collapse because of negative inspiratory pressure on the tissues of the pharynx, tongue, and epiglottis.[27] In the unconscious patient inspiratory obstruction can be generated by any of the collapsible sites.

Expiratory UAO is less well known and understood. In a sample of paralyzed patients the incidence of expiratory UAO with the mouth closed was 34%. The obstruction site was the velopharynx, where the soft palate acts as a one-way valve blocking the nasal egress of gas.[28] Expiratory UAO should be suspected in all cases of ineffective FMV that cannot be corrected by routine airway maneuvers. Positive pressure ventilation in the context of an inadequate airway maneuver may forcefully open the airway during inspiration followed by collapse as a result of low airway pressure in expiration. The "poof sign" raises clinical suspicion for expiratory UAO: forced egress of gas through a closed mouth indicating forced diversion from the nasal route.[29] Other clinical signs of expiratory UAO are subtle: chest rise but not fall (breath stacking) and lack of substantial end-tidal CO_2 ($EtCO_2$) waveform. Insertion of an oral or nasal airway will bypass the soft palate obstruction in inspiration and expiration.

Specific cases of UAO can be related to gender, age, and body habitus factors. Male predisposition to pharyngeal collapse is attributed to an increase in the length of the vulnerable pharyngeal airway, as well as an increased soft palate size.[30] Mechanisms that may predispose to pharyngeal collapse in elderly patients are the decrease in negative pressure reflex, increase in the deposition of parapharyngeal fat, increased pharyngeal airway length in older women, and "acquired" retrognathia.[31] Also, rhinitis in the elderly is a common but often neglected source of nasal obstruction. OSA in obese patients is a risk factor for UAO because of excess adipose tissue deposition in the anterior and especially lateral parapharyngeal walls, narrowing the UA and increasing the wall compliance and the extraluminal pressure. The anatomic imbalance between increased soft tissue volume within a limited craniofacial bony enclosure defines the severity of the OSA and airway obstruction.[32] OSA in nonobese patients is related to a caudal positioning of the hyoid bone. The tongue in these patients may be enlarged and expanded anteroposteriorly, as well as caudally, conditions that may result in an increased pharyngeal length and an increased distance from the mandibular plane to the hyoid.[33] Other pathologic conditions related to UAO are tonsillar hyperplasia; oral, maxillary, pharyngeal, or laryngeal tumors; airway edema after prolonged UA manipulation; laryngeal spasm; external compression by large neck masses and neck hematoma; and UA trauma.

Airway Maneuvers Applied to Bony Structures

Deliberate manipulation of a patient's head to achieve craniocervical extension at the occipito-atlanto-axial joint is the airway maneuver that defines both the chin-lift/head extension maneuver (CL/HE) and the extent of mouth opening. Patients with poor craniocervical extension (because of advanced age, trauma, cervical spine disease) may demonstrate a restricted CL/HE and mouth opening, conditions that can complicate both invasive and noninvasive airway management. A short thyromental distance acts as a surrogate for inadequate head extension.[34,35] The temporomandibular joints (TMJs) are synovial articulations between the mandible and the temporal bones and allow both rotational and translational mandibular movement. Two types of movements occur naturally in the TMJ, namely, rotational (the movement that occurs when the mouth opens and closes around a fixed axis within the TMJ) and translational (the mandible advances anteriorly by the sliding motion of the condyles in the TMJ). Mandibular advancement or jaw thrust can be initiated only after translational movement has occurred.[27] The cervical spine and the occipito-atlanto-axial joint are positioned in the sagittal plane, whereas the TMJs and the mandible are positioned in the transverse plane. These are the planes where optimal airway maneuvers should be implemented on the specific joints.

Understanding Anatomic Links Between Soft Tissues of the Airway and the Mobile Solid Structures

Understanding the direct anatomic links between the obstructing soft tissues and the mobile solid structures is essential to understanding the mechanism of action of airway maneuvers (Fig. 18.2). The tongue (genioglossus) has direct links with the mandible. The epiglottis is a mobile cartilaginous structure connected to the thyroid by the thyroepiglottic ligament (which acts as a hinge) and to the hyoid bone by the hyoepiglottic ligament (which acts as a lever). The epiglottic maneuverability is therefore hyoid dependent. The hyoid bone provides attachment to the muscles of the floor of the mouth, the tongue, the larynx, the epiglottis, and the pharynx. The hyoid is the central point of a muscular hammock that connects suprahyoid (mandible, tongue) and infrahyoid (larynx, styloid, sternum, clavicles) structures. The stretching of this muscular hammock along with the deep cervical fascia and platysma by the use of airway maneuvers will displace anteriorly the tongue-hyoid-thyroid-epiglottis complex and stiffen and dilate the pharyngeal airway. The soft palate connects only to bordering soft tissues (palatoglossus, palatopharyngeus, and tensor palati) without direct structural connection to mobile solid structures. As a result of their direct connections to bony structures, the tongue and the epiglottis respond consistently to external airway maneuvers, which can be externally manipulated, whereas the soft palate does not because it lacks direct connections to structures. Relief of an obstructed UA is achieved through manipulation of the bony structures to elevate the chin of the supine patient and effectively enlarge the solid space occupied by the soft tissues (see Fig. 18.1).

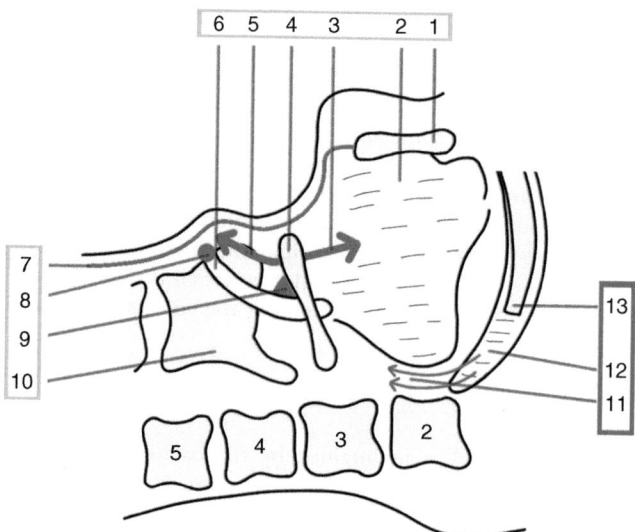

• **Fig. 18.2** Upper airway soft and solid tissue connections essential for the relief of the airway obstruction by airway maneuvers: *1*, mandible; *2*, tongue (genioglossus, hyoglossus); *3*, suprahyoid muscles (digastric, stylohyoid, geniohyoid, mylohyoid); *4*, hyoid bone; *5*, infrahyoid muscles (sternohyoid, sternothyroid, thyrohyoid, omohyoid); *6*, epiglottis; *7*, platysma; superficial and middle cervical fascia; *8*, thyroepiglottic ligament (works as a hinge); *9*, hyoepiglottic ligament (works as a lever); *10*, thyroid; *11*, palatoglossus, palatopharyngeus; tensor veli palate; *12*, soft palate; *13*, hard palate. *Green boxes:* direct soft–solid tissue connections with consistent response to airway maneuvers. *Red box:* indirect soft–solid tissue connections with inconsistent response to airway maneuvers (bypassed by the use of oropharyngeal airway and nasopharyngeal airway).

Cause of Airway Obstruction Unrelated to Soft Tissue Collapse

Airway obstruction unrelated to soft tissue collapse is generated by laryngospasm and glottic closure, often in response to a noxious stimulus at the level of the larynx and is accomplished by the contraction of the external laryngeal muscles. Resolution of laryngospasm (with attendant glottis closure) can occur spontaneously with time and with gentle positive pressure applied through mask ventilation if appropriate (stable vital signs with adequate oxygenation maintained per pulse oximetry monitoring) or through the administration of medications (neuromuscular relaxant medication such as succinylcholine or rocuronium, or hypnotic medications at the discretion of the clinician). Posterior to the larynx, the upper esophageal sphincter is located at the lower end of the pharynx and has two major functions: to prevent air from entering into the esophagus during breathing and to prevent the reflux of esophageal contents into the pharynx.

Techniques and Devices Used to Secure Airway Patency

Validated Airway Maneuvers

The validated airway maneuvers are two-handed techniques, described by Elam and colleagues for an expiratory air ventilation applied in resuscitation (i.e., mouth-to-mouth resuscitation) without a BVM system.[36] UA soft tissue structures are anteriorly displaced with the elevation of the chin, and the anterior neck

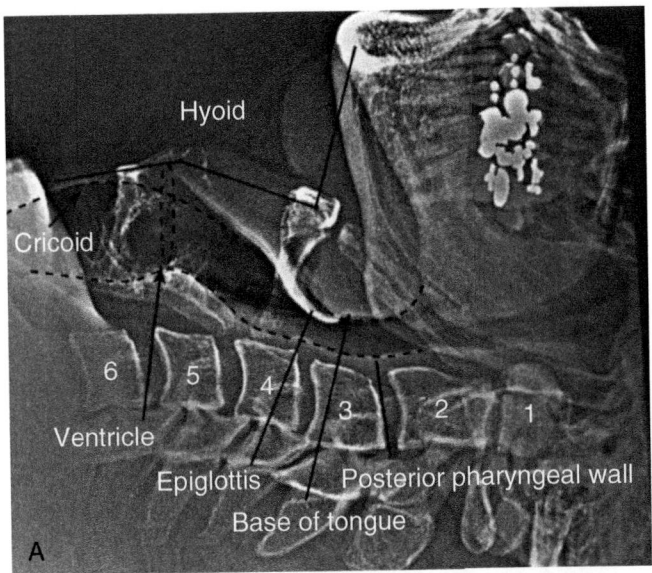

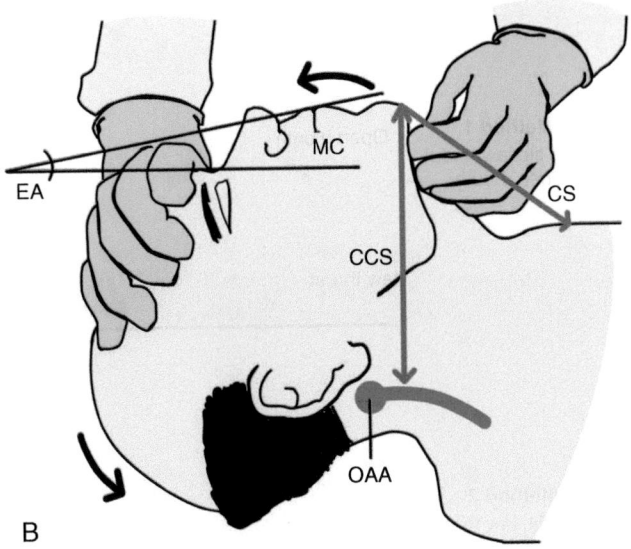

• **Fig. 18.3** (A) Lateral xenogram of the head and neck shows the extended position (head extension) in an awake and supine patient. The mentum is superior to the hyoid bone, the base of the tongue and the epiglottis are farther from the posterior pharyngeal wall, and the thyroid and cricoid cartilages are at the C4–C5 level. The hyoid bone has been raised and elevated from C3–C4 to C2–C3. (B) The validated chin lift/head extension (CL/HE) is a two-handed technique applied in the sagittal plane with one hand on the chin and the other on the forehead/occiput to extend the head on the cervical spine at the occipito-atlanto-axial *(OAA)* joint, stretching the anterior neck structures. The objective marker of a CL/HE is the extension angle *(EA)* and the increase in the chin–sternum *(CS)* and chin–cervical spine *(CCS)* distance. Maximal EA corresponding to a maximal extension is 42 degrees in both men and women. *MC,* Mouth closed.

structures are stretched, producing tension in these tissues that support airway patency in patients with a relaxed UA tone.[37,38]

The CL/HE maneuver engages the occipito-atlanto-axial joint and the cervical spine. The hands are positioned in the sagittal plane: one hand is placed underneath the mentum and elevates the chin, while simultaneously, the second hand generates downward pressure on the forehead. The CL/HE maneuver is performed with the mouth closed. In healthy awake supine patients maximal head extension is 42 degrees. This angle can be estimated during an FMV attempt as the angle between a horizontal line (longitudinal axis of the operating room bed) and the longitudinal axis of the FM at the cushion level. It may be used as an objective marker for a CL/HE attempt (Fig. 18.3).[39] Older patients often have restricted cervical spine movement with suboptimal head extension due to age-related pathologic changes.

The jaw thrust engages the mandibular rami to subluxate the TMJs. The hands are in the transverse plane positioned on the ascending rami of the mandible and forcefully advancing the mandible, placing the mandibular incisors anterior to the maxillary incisors with the mouth open (Fig. 18.4). The mandible is readily retracted into the TMJ once the bilateral maneuver is concluded. The jaw thrust maneuver is initiated and maintained with two hands.[40] In normal adults under propofol anesthesia, maximum mandibular advancement is required to restore the pharyngeal airway to its preanesthetic size. This corresponds to 16.2 ± 3.2 mm mandibular incisor advancement anterior to the maxillary incisors.[41] The distance between the mandibular and maxillar incisors may be used as an objective marker of a successful jaw thrust. Mandibular advancement generates less motion at an unstable C1–C2 level when compared with the CL/HE.[42]

The triple airway maneuver is a two-handed technique that involves applying a simultaneous CL/HE maneuver with a jaw

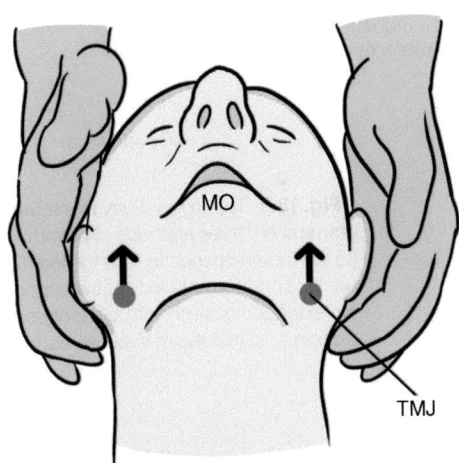

• **Fig. 18.4** The validated jaw thrust is a two-handed technique applied in the transverse plane with the hands at the ascending mandibular ramus advancing the mandible by subluxating bilaterally the temporomandibular joints *(TMJs)*. The objective marker of a maximal mandibular advancement is the distance of 16.2 ± 3.2 mm between the mandibular and the maxillary incisors with an increase in chin–sternum and chin–cervical spine distance. *MO,* Mouth open with the mandibular incisors in front of the maxillary one.

thrust and an open mouth. It is the most efficient technique to relieve airway obstruction in general and relieves UAO at the level of the soft palate (Fig. 18.5).[43]

Elevation of the chin by head extension and mandibular advancement increases the mentum–cervical spine distance, thus enlarging the bony enclosure and increasing the mentum–sternum distance, stretching the anterior neck structures. Airway maneuvers should be maintained throughout the respiratory cycle.

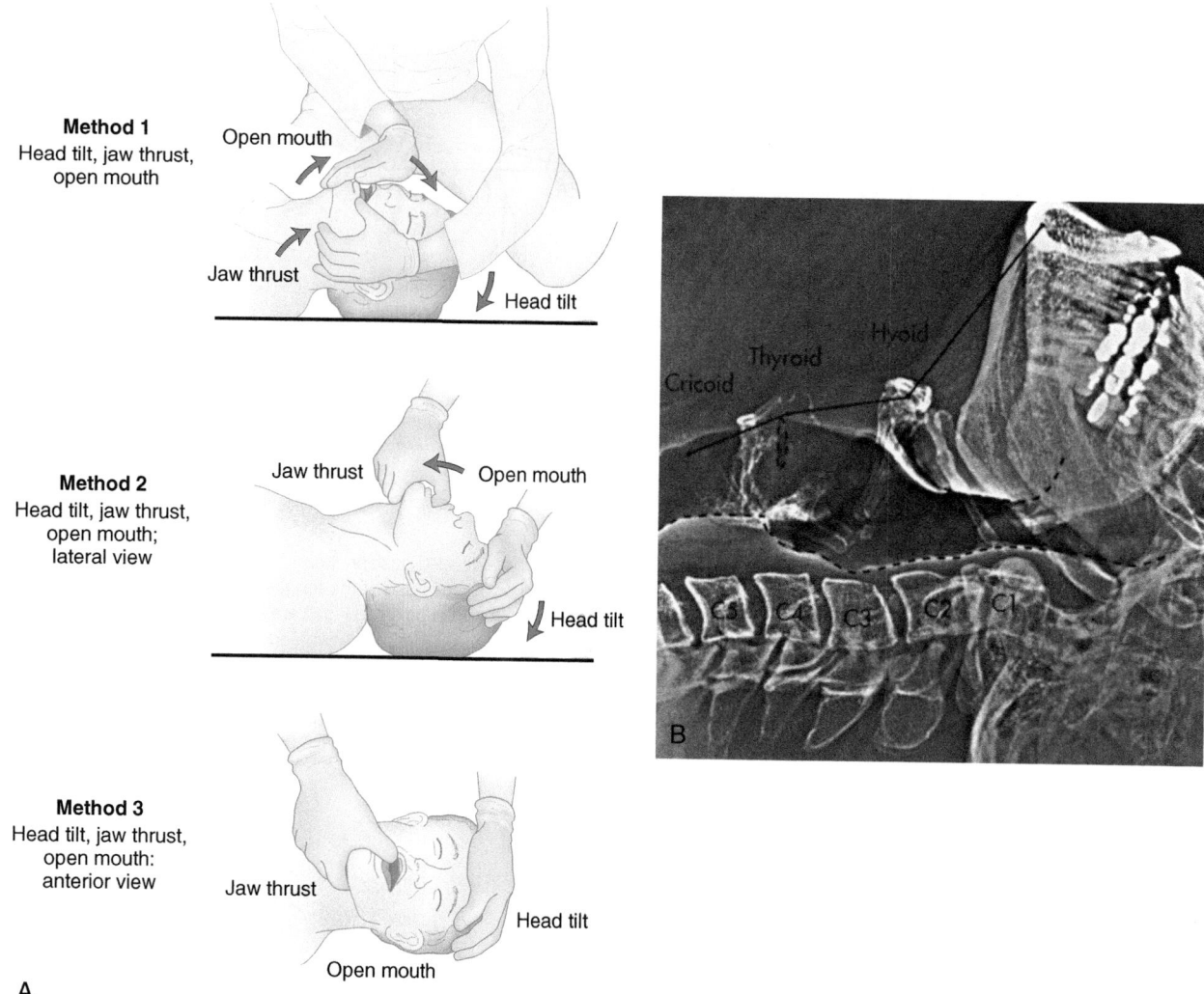

Method 1
Head tilt, jaw thrust,
open mouth

Open mouth

Jaw thrust

Head tilt

Method 2
Head tilt, jaw thrust,
open mouth;
lateral view

Jaw thrust   Open mouth

Head tilt

Method 3
Head tilt, jaw thrust,
open mouth:
anterior view

Jaw thrust

Head tilt

Open mouth

A

B — Cricoid, Thyroid, Hyoid, C5, C4, C3, C2, C1

• **Fig. 18.5** The triple airway maneuver includes the head tilt/chin lift, jaw thrust, and open mouth. (A) Diagrams show three methods of performing the maneuver: (1) the head extended on the atlanto-occipital joint, (2) the mouth opened to take the teeth out of occlusion, and (3) the mandible lifted upward, forcing the mandibular condyles anteriorly at the temporomandibular joint. (B) Lateral xerogram of the head and neck shows the extended position with jaw protrusion. Notice that the mandibular incisors protrude beyond the maxillary incisors and that the mandibular condyles are subluxated anteriorly from the temporomandibular joint.

Resuscitation/Anesthesia Face Mask Design and Techniques for Use

The resuscitation/anesthesia face mask (RAFM) is typically the starting point for linking a positive pressure generating device to a patient's airway. Although FMs have different materials, shapes, types of seals, and degrees of transparency, all are composed of three main parts: a body, a seal (or cushion), and a 22-mm connector (Fig. 18.6). The body is the main structure of the mask and the primary determinant of the mask's shape. As the body of the mask rises above the face (so as not to be completely flush to the face), all FMs increase ventilatory dead space. However, this is rarely clinically significant for spontaneous or controlled ventilation. The seal (or cushion) is the rim of the mask that contacts the patient's face from the bridge of the nose superiorly along the face inferiorly to the tip of the chin. The most common type of seal is an air-filled cushion rim. The connector is positioned at the top of the body and provides a 22-mm female adapter for adult and large pediatric masks or a 15-mm male adapter for small pediatric and neonatal masks to connect to a BVM or a standard ventilator breathing circuit.

A collar with hooks allows a retaining strap to be attached to hold the mask to the patient's face. The precise application of the straps (crossed or uncrossed) is a matter of preference and is usually the result of a trial-and-error process to find the best seal for each individual patient. Mask retaining straps can be placed below the occiput and connected to the mask collar. This technique may compromise the airway patency by flexing the head on the neck and limiting the ability to generate a jaw thrust. The head strap may improve the seal at the expense of the airway patency. A two-handed technique should be used to optimize the seal and the airway maneuver before using a head strap. Also, the presence of the collar defines the dome surface available for any grip dictating and limiting the provider's technique. The collar has been kept on the dome since the 1880s in spite of the fact that it is rarely used. It should be applied only when needed.

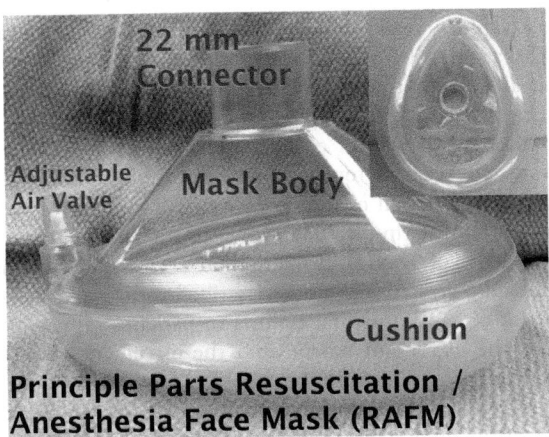

• **Fig. 18.6** Resuscitation/anesthesia face mask (RAFM): anatomy of the principal parts (from superior to inferior). (1) 22-mm female connector; (2) mask body (transparent)—connects 22-mm female connector to mask skirt; (3) Mask skirt (or cushion)—interfaces mask with the face of the patient. Mask skirt can possess an adjustable air valve to tailor the fit to the patient.

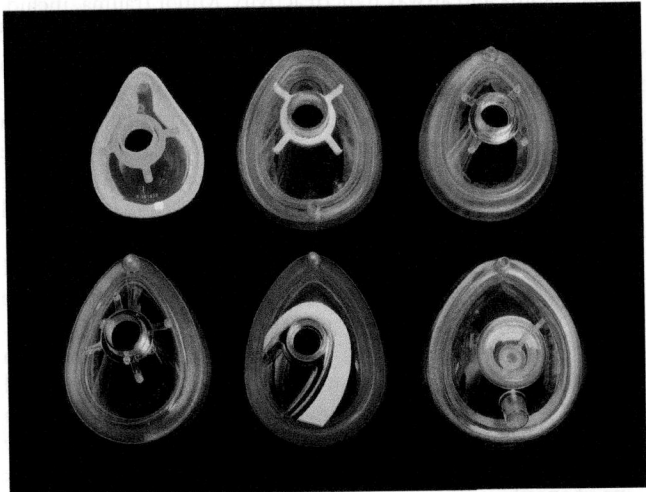

• **Fig. 18.7** Medium-size transparent disposable face masks. *Top row, left to right:* Face mask (FM) without inflatable cushion (Intersurgical Ltd., Wokingham, UK), FM with anterior inflation valve, and FM with posterior inflation valve. *Lower row, left to right:* generic symmetrical mask (King Systems/Ambu, Noblesville, IN, United States), asymmetrical ergonomic face mask (Tuoren Medical Group, Henan, China), and specialty endoscopy mask (VBM Medizintechnik, Sulz a. N., Germany).

The disposable, single-use, transparent plastic RAFM is the most prominently used mask in modern-day hospital and prehospital use (Fig. 18.7). RAFMs are constructed with a high-volume, low-pressure cushion that can be adjusted to seal to a variety of face shapes with the addition or withdrawal of air from the valve present on the mask. Some cushions are factory sealed and lack a valve. RAFMs are not constructed with accommodations for the curve of the chin (as are the "aviator"-style masks that are used for bilevel positive airway pressure therapy) and, as such, can complicate attempts at establishing a proper mask seal during controlled ventilation. The sides of the mask are somewhat malleable to adjust to wide or narrow faces. This can be achieved only with a grip that controls both sides of the face mask and allows the control of the whole mask and lateral pressure on the dome. The asymmetrical ergonomic FM with the connector off-center is

designed to accommodate and to reinforce the one-hand "chin-lift" grip.[44]

The proper use of an FM assumes an optimal first attempt for an effective seal with the patient's face and an airway maneuver for the patency of the UA. The seal should permit maintenance of an airway pressure of 20 to 25 cm H_2O with minimal or no leak. The mask should comfortably fit the hand of the user and the face of the patient. If the mask is too long, the face can be elongated 1 to 2 cm by placing an oropharyngeal airway (OPA). If the mask is too short, it can be moved 1 to 2 cm cephalad along the bridge of the nose to make a good seal at the patient's chin. Careful attention is required to avoid ocular trauma. Several methods are described for holding the mask, but regardless of the precise method chosen, objective monitoring of the technique (seal, airway maneuver) and outcome is necessary.

Artificial Airway Devices to Support Noninvasive Ventilation

Airway devices to support noninvasive ventilation are used in the unexpected difficult mask ventilation (DMV) to supplement an ineffective technique or preemptively with a first attempt in the expected DMV. The next sections address some of the more commonly available devices and discuss techniques for insertion, indications, contraindications, and complications.

Oropharyngeal Airways

The OPA is the most commonly used device to provide a patent UA. The OPA is formed of symmetrical flanges to keep the device stabilized at the lips, a bite block, and a semicircular portion that follows the oropharyngeal anatomy. An air channel is often provided to facilitate oropharyngeal suctioning. It extends from the lips to the laryngopharynx and supports ventilation by opening the mouth and displacing the tongue and soft palate. The OPA bypasses the nasal cavities, nasopharynx, and soft palate obstruction in inspiration and expiration, lifts the tongue and possibly the epiglottis, and supports mandibular advancement. It also lengthens the face by 1 to 2 cm and improves FM fit in edentulous patients. OPAs are manufactured in a wide variety of sizes, from neonatal to large adult, and they are typically made of plastic or rubber (Fig. 18.8). They should be wide enough to contact two or three teeth on the mandible and maxilla, and they should be slightly compressible so that the pressure exerted by a clenched jaw is distributed over all the teeth, whereas the lumen remains patent. The two most popular disposable OPAs are the Guedel (1933) and the Berman (1949) airways. The Guedel airway has a central air channel and is bulkier, whereas the Berman airway has a central support with open sides. Adult sizes are #8 (8 cm), #9 (9 cm), #10 (10 cm), and #11 (11 cm), designated according to the height measured horizontally from the flanges to the distal end of the airway. There may be variations in both shape and length between different OPA manufacturers. Traditionally, the appropriate size is estimated by external measurements, such as the distance from the tragus of the ear to the angle of the mouth or the distance from the incisors to the angle of the mandible. These measurements do not account for internal individual anatomic discrepancies (tongue size, palate height). In average-height adults a size #9 in men and size #8 in women will provide the best fit.[45] An OPA may be too small with the tip at the base of the tongue, pushing the tongue posteriorly, or too long with the tip in the vallecula, pushing the epiglottis into the glottic opening. The OPA is used in approximately 25%

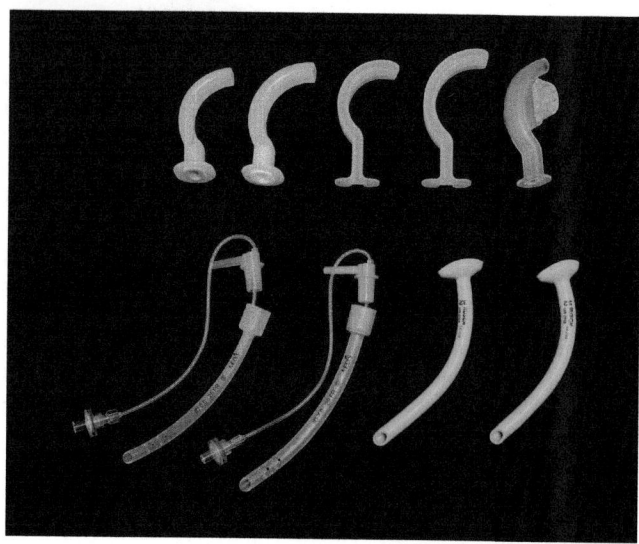

• **Fig. 18.8** *Top row, left to right:* oropharyngeal airway: size #9 Guedel, #10 Guedel, #9 Berman, #10 Berman, specialty oropharyngeal airway with a second bite block for electroconvulsive therapy (Bite-Rite Dupaco Inc., Oceanside, CA). *Lower row, left to right:* nasopharyngeal airway: size #25 and #29 nasopharyngeal airway with $EtCO_2$ connector and oxygen port (Mercury Medical, Clearwater, FL), generic nasopharyngeal airways (Teleflex Inc., Wayne, PA).

of the FMV attempts. In 1991 Marsh and colleagues studied the etiology of OPA obstruction radiographically in patients with a neutral head position. The OPA was impacting the tongue (41%), vallecula (18%), and epiglottic downfolding (13%).[46] There was no way of predicting the site of obstruction from clinical observation. The OPA obstruction could be rectified by airway maneuvers (both CL/HE and jaw thrust), reinsertion, or electing a different size.

The Ovassapian airway has a large anterior flange to control the tongue and a large central opening at the level of the teeth (open posteriorly) to allow a flexible intubation bronchoscope and ETT to be passed through the airway while allowing the ETT to disengage from the airway following tracheal intubation.

The use of an OPA seems deceptively simple, but the device must be used correctly. The patient's pharyngeal and laryngeal reflexes should be depressed before insertion. The mouth is opened, and a tongue blade is placed at the base of the tongue and drawn upward, lifting the tongue off the posterior pharyngeal wall (Fig. 18.9A). The straight tongue depressor may fail to catch the base of the tongue in a supine unconscious patient with a small mouth opening. Alternatively, a curved Yankauer suction may be used to "hook" the tongue and allow the OPA insertion while suctioning the pharynx. The airway is then placed so that the OPA is just off the posterior wall of the oropharynx with it protruding 1 to 2 cm above the incisors (Fig. 18.9B). If the flange is at the teeth when the tip is just at the base of the tongue, the airway is too small, and a larger size should be inserted. The OPA is a passive device: it is the operator's responsibility to implement a mandibular advancement on the bite block. The symmetrical flanges at the lips limit the ability to generate the required maximal mandibular advancement (with the mandibular teeth in front of the maxillary ones) and define a suboptimal design of the bite block realized before the validation of the airway maneuvers in the 1950s (Fig. 18.9C). The routine practice of locking the mandible without advancement

in the "dropped" position on the OPA bite block maintains the mandibular teeth below the maxillary ones, reinforcing an iatrogenic airway obstruction and defining a suboptimal use of the OPA (Fig. 18.10).

An alternative method of placement is to insert the airway backward (convex side toward the tongue) until the tip is close to the pharyngeal wall of the oropharynx. It is then rotated 180 degrees so that the tip rotates and sweeps under the tongue from the side (see Fig. 18.9D). This method is not as reliable as the tongue blade–assisted technique described earlier, and it has the added risk of causing dental trauma in patients with poor dentition. If the UA is not patent after the placement of an OPA, the following situations must be considered. With an OPA that is too small, the pronounced curve may impinge on the base of the tongue, or the tongue may obstruct the native airway distal to the OPA. If a larger OPA still results in obstruction, the curve might have brought the distal end into the vallecula or the OPA might have pushed the epiglottis into the glottic opening or posterior wall of the laryngopharynx. The best treatment for this problem is to withdraw the OPA 1 to 2 cm.

Two major complications can occur with the use of OPAs: iatrogenic trauma and airway hyperreactivity. Minor trauma, including pinching of the lips and tongue, is common. Ulceration and necrosis of oropharyngeal structures from pressure and long-term contact (days) have been reported.[47] These problems necessitate intermittent surveillance during extended use. Dental injury can result from twisting of the airway, involuntary clenching of the jaw, or direct axial pressure. Dental damage is most common in patients with periodontal disease, dental caries, pronounced degrees of dental proclination, and isolated teeth.

Airway hyperactivity is a potentially serious complication of OPA use, because oropharyngeal and laryngeal reflexes can be stimulated by the placement of an artificial airway. Coughing, retching, emesis, laryngospasm, and bronchospasm are common reflex responses. Any OPA that touches the epiglottis or vocal cords can cause these responses, but the problem is more common with larger OPAs. Initial management is to partially withdraw the OPA. If an anesthetic is being administered, deepening the plane of anesthesia (most easily accomplished with an intravenous agent) is often effective in blunting airway hyperreactivity. In cases of laryngospasm it may be necessary to apply mild positive airway pressure and, in trained hands, to cautiously administer small doses of a neuromuscular blocking agent to achieve resolution. A topical anesthetic spray or a water-soluble local anesthetic lubricant reduces the chance of laryngeal activity, but it should be used judiciously or avoided in patients thought to be at increased risk for aspiration. OPA is an underused device. It should be used with the first FMV attempt in obese, OSA, edentulous, and fixed cervical spine patients. FMV with airway adjuncts (OPA and NPA) improves neurologic outcomes of in-hospital cardiac arrest.[48]

Nasopharyngeal Airways

The NPA is a disposable soft tubular device sized in French numbers representing its outer diameter: 24, 28, 30, 32, and 34. The larger the NPA size, the longer the airway. A proximal flange stabilizes the device at the nares while the distal end is beveled (see Fig. 18.8). The NPA supports the nasal route of breathing, treating the obstruction at the nasal cavities, nasopharynx, soft palate, and, if long enough, the base of the tongue. It should be approximately 10 mm above the epiglottis.[49] The NPA size is estimated traditionally by measuring the distance from the tip of the nose to the meatus of the ear, as the length of the device is more

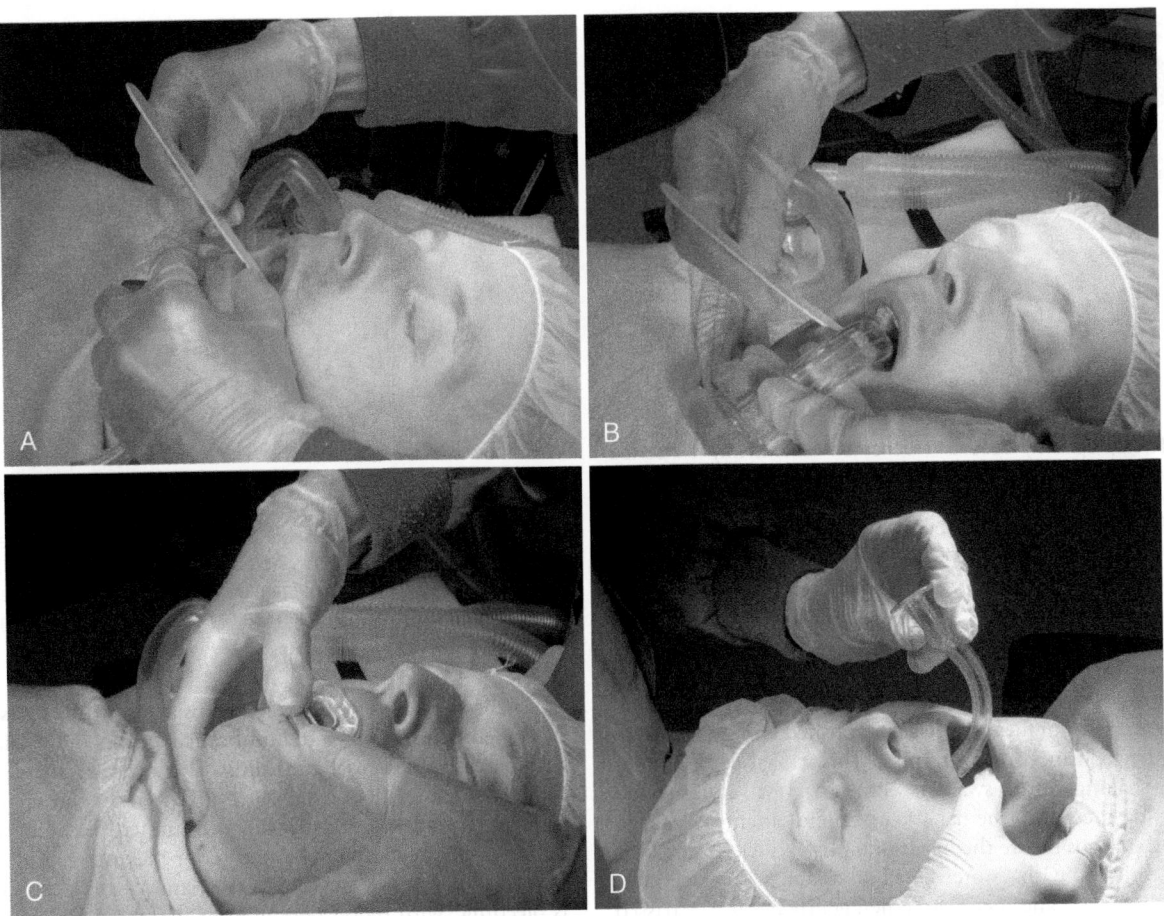

• **Fig. 18.9** Techniques for the insertion of an oropharyngeal airway: standard technique (A–C) and alternative technique (D) without a tongue blade. (A) The tongue blade is placed deep into the mouth and depresses the tongue at its posterior half. The tongue is then pulled forward in an attempt to pull it off the back wall of the pharynx. (B) The airway is then inserted with the concave side toward the tongue until the tube is just off the posterior wall of the oropharynx with it protruding 1 to 2 cm above the incisors. The tongue blade is then removed. (C) A jaw thrust is performed while the thumb taps the airway into place. After the jaw is allowed to relax, the lips are inspected to ensure they are not caught between the teeth and the airway. (D) In an alternative technique the airway is placed in a reverse manner (convex side toward the tongue) and then spun 180 degrees into place so that the lower section of the airway rotates between the tongue and posterior pharyngeal wall.

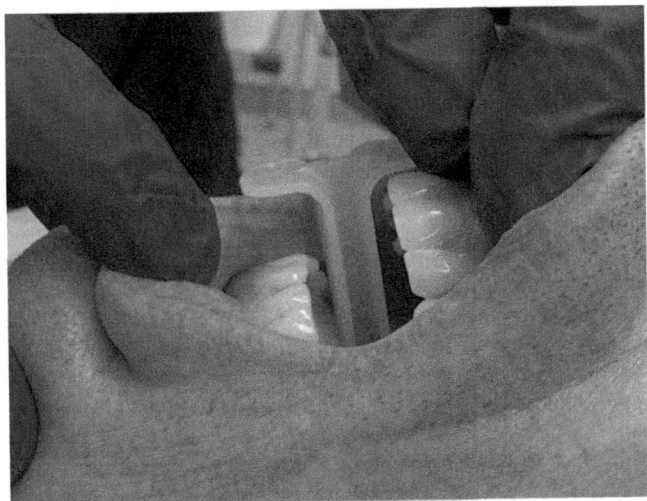

• **Fig. 18.10** Use of the oropharyngeal airway. It is the user's responsibility to implement a mandibular advancement on the bite block. Locking the mandible in the "dropped" position (mandibular incisors posterior to the maxillary ones) defines a suboptimal technique.

important in determining the size than the width. Comparing different sizes of NPAs with the patient's little finger or nose is unreliable.[50] An average-size female requires a size 6 (24 Fr) and a male a size 7 (28 Fr). When in place, an NPA is less stimulating than an OPA and therefore better tolerated in the awake, semicomatose, or lightly anesthetized patient. In cases of oropharyngeal trauma a nasal airway is often preferable to an oral airway. The concavity of the NPA is meant to follow the superior side of the hard palate and posterior wall of the nasopharynx (Fig. 18.11). The tip of the airway is beveled to aid in following the airway and minimizing mucosal trauma as it is advanced through the nasal cavities and the nasopharynx. A narrow NPA is often desirable to minimize nasal trauma but may be too short to reach behind the tongue. The septum is situated medially and the turbinates laterally. The bevel on the nasal trumpet should be oriented facing the turbinates (laterally) so that the leading edge moves along the septum, avoiding the turbinates. A trumpet inserted on the left side can follow its natural curvature into the nose (curvature facing downward), whereas insertion on the right should begin with the trumpet curvature upside down (curvature initially facing upward).

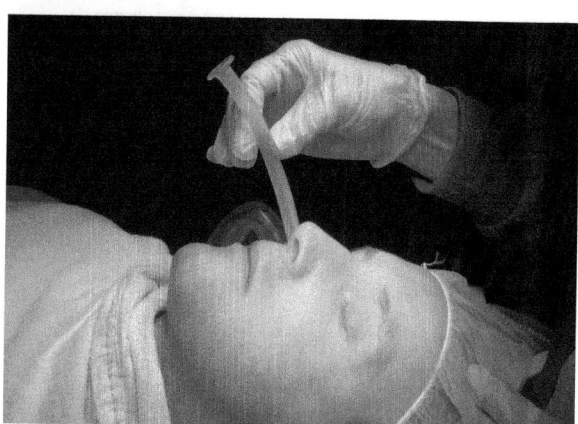

• **Fig. 18.11** Appropriately sized and lubricated nasal airway is inserted with the cut bevel facing the nasal turbinates (laterally) and the overall anatomic curve in alignment with the direction of airflow through the nasopharynx. Should insertion in the opposite nare prove necessary, again, the nasopharyngeal airway is inserted with the cut bevel facing the nasal turbinates to ease the insertion.

Before the insertion of an NPA, the nares should be inspected to determine their size and patency and to evaluate for the presence of nasal polyps or marked septal deviation. Vasoconstriction of the mucous membranes can be accomplished with oxymetazoline or phenylephrine drops or spray. This can also be accomplished by soaking cotton swabs in either of these solutions and then inserting them into the naris (with careful attention paid to removing the swabs before the insertion of the NPA). The NPA is typically lubricated with a water-based lubricant (with or without a water-soluble local anesthetic) and then gently but firmly passed with the concave side parallel to the hard palate through the nasal passage until resistance is felt in the posterior nasopharynx.

When there is resistance to passage, it is sometimes helpful to rotate the NPA bevel toward the septum, bringing the open part of the bevel against the posterior nasopharyngeal mucosa. As the tube makes the bend (indicated by a relative loss of resistance to advancement), it should be rotated back to its original orientation. If the NPA does not advance with moderate pressure, there are two management options: attempt placement of a narrower tube or attempt placement in the other naris. If the tube does not pass into the oropharynx, the clinician may withdraw the tube 2 cm and then pass a suction catheter through the nasal airway as a guide for the advancement of the NPA. If the patient coughs or reacts as the NPA is inserted to its full extent, it should be withdrawn 1 to 2 cm to prevent the tip from touching the epiglottis or vocal cords. When the patient's UA is still obstructed after insertion, the NPA should be checked for obstruction or kinking by passing a small suction catheter through its lumen. If patency of the NPA is confirmed, it is possible that the NPA is too short and the base of the tongue is occluding its tip. Indications for an NPA include the relief of UAO in awake, semicomatose, or lightly anesthetized patients; in patients who are not adequately treated with OPAs; in patients undergoing dental procedures or with oropharyngeal trauma; and in patients requiring oropharyngeal or laryngopharyngeal suctioning. NPAs may work well for patients who are clenching their jaw, which makes inserting an oral airway difficult. The contraindications (absolute or relative) include known nasal airway occlusion, nasal fractures, marked septal deviation, coagulopathy (risk of epistaxis), prior transsphenoidal hypophysectomy or Caldwell-Luc procedures, cerebrospinal fluid rhinorrhea, known or suspected basilar skull fractures, and adenoid hypertrophy.

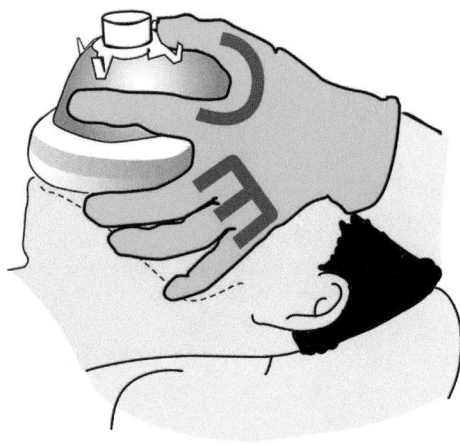

• **Fig. 18.12** The generic E-C one-handed face-mask ventilation technique involves having the thumb and index finger placed on the dome around the collar ("C"), with fingers 3, 4, and 5 spread along the mandible such that the fifth finger anchors the mandibular angle ("E"). The wrist is flexed. The technique is implemented in two steps: first the seal (placing the mask on the face) and then the "airway maneuver" (pulling the mandible into the mask).

The complications of NPAs consist of failure of successful placement, epistaxis as a result of mucosal tears or avulsion of the turbinates, submucosal tunneling, and pressure sores. Epistaxis often becomes evident when the NPA is removed, thereby removing the tamponade. It is usually self-limited. Bleeding from the nares usually is attributable to anterior plexus bleeding, and it is treated by applying pressure to the nares. If the posterior plexus is bleeding (with blood pooling into the pharynx), the physician should leave the NPA in place, suction the pharynx, and consider intubating the trachea if the bleeding does not stop promptly. The patient may be positioned on their side to minimize the aspiration of blood. An otolaryngology consultation may be necessary to further treat posterior plexus bleeding. The management of submucosal tunneling into the retropharyngeal space is to withdraw the airway and obtain otolaryngology consultation.

Face Mask Ventilation Techniques

One-Handed Mask Ventilation Techniques

"E-C" Grip

The "E-C" grip is the generic one-handed FMV technique. This technique has never been validated, and it represents a mix of tradition, personal, and institutional experience. With this technique, the thumb and index finger are placed on the mask dome around the collar (forming the "C"), while fingers 3, 4, and 5 are spread along the mandible (forming the "E") such that the fifth finger anchors on the mandibular angle. The wrist is flexed (Fig. 18.12). This grip often creates an uneven distribution of pressure on the mask dome toward the side of the grip. This, combined with an inability to generate pressure with the "C" portion over the cheeks opposite the grip to improve the mask seal, often lets air leak on the nongrip side of the mask. The strap hooks on the connector limit the surface available for the grip, reinforcing the asymmetry of the "E-C" technique and discouraging a grip on the whole dome. A head strap using the hooks may improve the seal, but will also displace the mandible posteriorly, flex the head on the cervical spine, and limit the ability to generate a mandibular advancement. The traditional practice of observing the patient through a generously

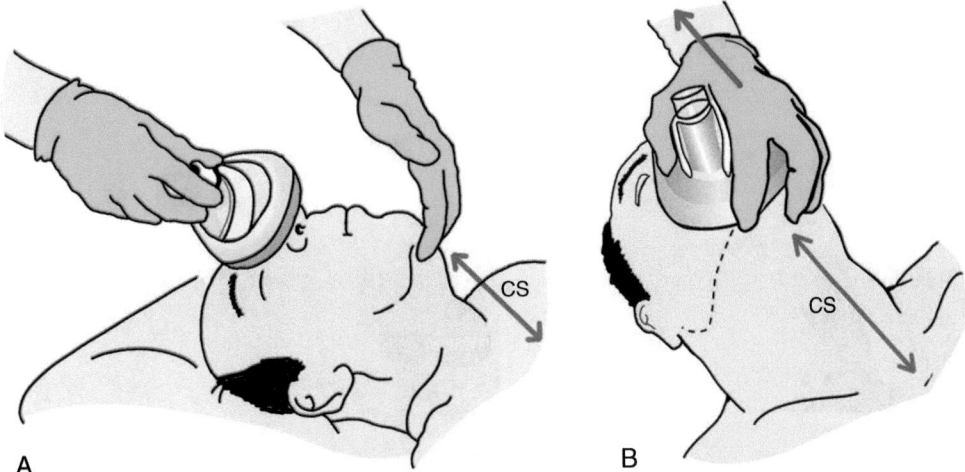

A   B

• **Fig. 18.13** The "chin-lift" grip is a one-handed face-mask ventilation technique implemented in two steps: first the airway maneuver (two-handed CL/HE, Fig. 18.3) and then, while maintaining head extension with the left hand (A), the seal is applied with a grip that controls the whole dome with the web between the thumb and the index finger against the connector (B). The hand is in pronation, and the wrist is straight. *CS,* Chin–sternum.

exposed transparent dome reinforces a limited, suboptimal grip that may promote the very complications the clinician wishes to monitor, such as emesis and cyanosis. The "E" component of the E-C grip is an undefined airway maneuver. The unilateral support of the adult mandible does not generate enough torque for an optimal CL/HE and cannot generate or maintain mandibular advancement in the transverse plane. The concept of the fifth finger generating a jaw thrust at the mandibular angle has been demystified and proven ineffective.[51]

Traditionally, the user's left hand grips the FM with the thumb and index finger around the collar. The left side of the FM fits into the palm, with the hypothenar eminence extending below the left side of the mask. The problem with an FM that is too large for the user is that the hypothenar eminence cannot pull the patient's cheek against the left side of the mask to maintain a seal if pronation is necessary to seal the right side. The nasal portion of the mask is sealed by the downward pressure of the user's thumb. To seal the chin section, the mandible is gripped with the user's fourth and fifth fingers, and the wrist is rotated so as to pull the mandible up into the FM with the fingers while pushing the bridge of the mask down with the thumb.

Traditionally the E-C grip technique is implemented in two steps: first, the "seal" on the face, and then the "lift" of the mandible into the FM.[52] Routinely, practitioners focus on the seal and overlook/neglect the accuracy of the airway maneuver.

"Chin-Lift" Grip

The chin-lift grip is described in the literature but is less seldom used in clinical practice, despite growing evidence of superiority over the one-handed E-C grip.[53–55] After the removal of the hook ring, the web space between the thumb and the index finger is positioned against the mask connector. The remaining three fingers reach for the mentum to implement the CL/HE (Fig. 18.13). The fingers on the mentum maintain the torque in the sagittal plane. The hand is in pronation and the wrist is straight. This is a power grip that generates an even distribution of pressure on the dome, allowing control of the whole mask and side-to-side pressure. There is a space between the first two fingers for patient inspection. The "chin-lift" grip is implemented in reverse order of

the E-C technique: first "lift" the mentum with a validated two-handed CL/HE (see Fig. 18.3), and then, while maintaining head extension with the left hand (Fig. 18.14A), "seal" the FM with a chin-lift grip that controls the whole dome (Fig. 18.14B). This technique gives immediate feedback on the ability to implement a CL/HE: if an airway maneuver cannot be implemented, the insertion of an OPA may be warranted before sealing the FM. The asymmetrical ergonomic FM is designed to implement and reinforce the left-hand "chin-lift" grip technique, allowing improved mask seal and less operator fatigue.[56]

Two-Handed Mask Ventilation Techniques

The two-handed technique includes the features of an optimal FMV attempt: symmetrical pressure of the FM cushion generating an optimal seal and a bilateral jaw thrust generating a validated airway maneuver. The patient's mouth is held open (whether an OPA is used or not). A second assistant is required when BVM or the anesthesia circle system ventilation bag is used for ventilation. Alternatively, a conservatively adjusted ventilator set to pressure control (with appropriate limits and respiratory rate) or an ARMS system may be used by a single operator to permit two-handed FMV.[57] The two-handed FMV technique achieves greater TV during pressure-controlled ventilation than the one-handed E-C technique.[51] Isono recommends routine OR the use of the two-handed triple airway maneuver with pressure-controlled ventilation.[58] The two-handed technique can be implemented with a bilateral "E-C" or "E-V" grip. The latter uses the thenar eminence and thumb to apply downward force on the mask with fingers 2 to 5 reaching for the mandibular angle for a jaw thrust (Fig. 18.14). The "E-V" (thenar) technique may be applied facing the patient. In a mannikin study the bilateral "E-V" was found to be superior to the "E-C" technique and was recommended to the novice.[59]

Measuring Face Mask Ventilation Efficiency

Subjective Markers

Traditional subjective markers indicative of adequate ventilation are the cyclical condensation on the FM dome (not correlated

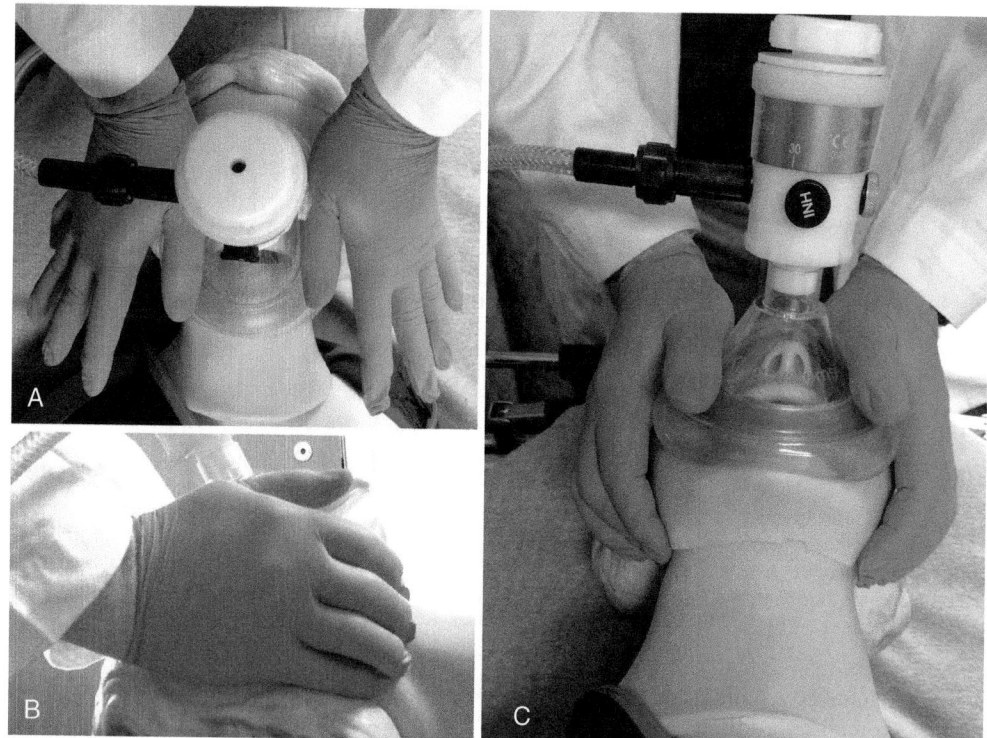

• **Fig. 18.14** Demonstration of hand position to use the "E-V" two-handed mask ventilation technique. (A) The thenar eminence of both hands rests symmetrically over the dome of the body of the mask to provide symmetrical sustained pressure during face-mask ventilation (FMV). Fingers of each hand are free to wrap around the mandible to achieve and sustain airway maneuvers (while fingers 2 to 5 apply a jaw thrust or a triple airway maneuver). (B) Side view of the completed E-V maneuver. (C) Top view of the completed E-V maneuver. Note the natural and relaxed hand and wrist position that is evident during FMV. (Courtesy CPR Medical Devices.)

with TV), chest expansion (difficult to observe in obese patients), bilateral respiratory sounds (unreliable in critical situations, obese patients, and dressed victims), and low resistance to manual inspiration with rapid lung deflation during expiration ("bag compliance" unreliable with BVM resuscitation systems). The commonly held belief that the "educated hand" allows clinicians to detect changes in respiratory compliance and generate appropriate TV was refuted both in pediatric and adult patients.[60,61] Elevation of the chin using both techniques (extension or advancement) stretches the anterior neck structures, and thus the neck skin creases generated by a neutral head position disappear. Possible gastric insufflation of ventilation gases is indicated by epigastric sounds and abdominal distention.

Objective Markers

The ASA difficult airway algorithm states the need for objective markers to define FMV outcome and DMV.[62] Objective markers should be applied to the FMV technique and outcome. The CL/HE technique can be quantified by the increase of the mentum–sternum distance and by the cervical spine extension angle (see Fig. 18.3). Jaw thrust is measured by the increase in mentum–sternum distance and the advancement of the mandibular incisors anterior to the maxillary incisors (see Figs. 18.3 and 18.4). Desired outcomes are normal oxygen saturation and capnography with acceptable airway pressure and satisfactory TV.[63]

FMV failure includes both "impossible" FMV as well as the DMV scenarios that generate "inadequate" ventilation with insufficient oxygenation for the specific clinical setting. Oxygen

desaturation is a late sign of ventilation failure masked by routine preoxygenation. Low TVs in an adult patient (e.g., 3–5 cc/kg) or dead space ventilation (<150 cc) with high airway pressure (e.g., >30–35 cm H_2O) represents a poor outcome and an "inadequate" attempt despite condensation on the mask and a marginal $EtCO_2$ tracing. Impossible FMV is the extreme expression of an inadequate attempt.

The use of objective ventilation parameters in the context of an optimal first attempt allows early acceptance of failure before oxygen desaturation. Implementation of objective markers in the daily routine requires a behavioral adjustment from teachers, researchers, and providers to build a new FMV mental model. The use of objective markers would change the definition and recognized incidence of DMV. The appropriate management of impossible FMV includes the immediate transition to SGA, allowing the patient to emerge from anesthesia if possible and clinically warranted (such as in elective anesthetic cases), administration of neuromuscular relaxant medication if clinically warranted, tracheal intubation, and, if laryngoscopy fails, preparation to perform surgical airway access.

Strategies to Minimize Gastric Insufflation

The goal of an optimal FMV attempt is to keep the airway patent with peak inspiratory flow rates and inflation pressures at a minimum. Gastric insufflation with attendant gastric regurgitation during mask ventilation is the product of high peak inspiratory flow rates and high peak airway pressures, which occur when

BVM or anesthesia circle system bags are squeezed quickly and forcefully. High peak flow rates and inspiratory pressures occur when ineffective airway maneuvers are used during FMV, as the rescuer attempts to compensate for inadequate ventilation and technique with increased driving gas velocity and pressure. Gastric insufflation has been clinically observed with increased inspiratory flow rates, but to date, there is a scarcity of literature to describe its contribution to this problem, because sophisticated flow meter technology currently exists in the spirometric systems of anesthesia machines and is not available for use with BVM systems. Traditionally, gastric insufflation during FMV has been described by measuring the peak airway pressure during mask ventilation, because pressure manometers are widely available (even for BVM systems). The AHA recommendations for mask ventilation during Basic Life Support (BLS) and Advanced Cardiac Life Support (ACLS) have suggested that inspiratory flow rates less than 40 L/min be used to prevent central venous collapse during BLS or ACLS rescue since the 1990s. This recommendation was made by the AHA based on the observed adverse effects of a specific class of ventilation devices that were common in the 1970s through the 1980s, namely, manually triggered Demand Valve resuscitators, the flow rates of which could exceed 120 L/min. As a point of reference, when a BVM is squeezed quickly and forcefully, its inspiratory flow rates will commonly exceed 120 L/min (author's observation with BVM connected to spirometer). ARMS devices control the inspiratory flow to 30 L/min and control inspiratory pressures to ranges that minimize gastric insufflation (although paradoxically, these devices are able to ventilate with peak pressures above 20 cm H_2O without appreciable gastric insufflation; author's observation with the Oxylator ARMS devices).

When gastric insufflation has been studied using inspiratory pressure alone, it has been detected by auscultation starting at an inspiratory pressure of 20 cm H_2O and by ultrasonography at 15 cm H_2O.[64,65] The clinical significance of these numbers is unclear, as there is an overlap between the range of inflation pressures required for adequate ventilation and those producing gastric insufflation. The likely reason for the observation of gastric insufflation in these studies is related to the inspiratory flow rates used during the measurement. There is an increased risk for pulmonary aspiration in patients with a full stomach, hiatal hernia, pharyngeal diverticula, and esophageal motility disorders. Prolonged suboptimal FMV with high peak airway inspiratory flows and pressures may lead to stomach insufflation that will increase intragastric pressure, elevate the diaphragm, restrict lung movements, reduce respiratory system compliance, and further increase the peak airway pressures required for FMV.[66]

Peak airway pressure can be reduced by using a pediatric self-inflatable bag or an adult self-inflating bag with built-in safety features (airway pressure manometers, limited peak airway pressure and peak inspiratory flow).[67] In the operating theater using the ventilator on the anesthesia machine in a pressure-controlled mode (while using two-handed airway maneuvers) controls and reduces the inspiratory peak flow rates, airway pressures, and the gastric inflation risk.[57,68]

Applying "gentle" FMV in rapid sequence induction (RSI) with cricoid pressure may balance the risk of aspiration with the benefit of continuous oxygenation. A "gentle" FMV during anesthesia induction assumes the lowest peak airway pressure that allows for adequate ventilation.[69–71] Cricoid pressure may protect the stomach from inflation but also may be the cause for high airway pressures and laryngeal obstruction.[72] If cricoid pressure is applied and inadequate/impossible ventilation ensues, progressive

release of pressure should be considered until ventilation improves. Recently, gastric distention has been assessed with an ultrasound evaluation.[73] This tool may serve future research questions that aim to evaluate the risk of gastric distention during various airway management procedures.

Difficult Mask Ventilation

FMV difficulty manifests as an inability to generate an adequate seal between the mask and the face and/or the inability to provide a patent airway.[74] DMV definitions were reviewed by El-Orbany and Woehlck[75]; however, Han's subjective DMV progressive scale is used in most FMV studies.[76] The Han FMV grading system defines grade 1 as an easy mask, grade 2 as a difficult mask requiring an OPA or NPA, grade 3 as very difficult mask ventilation requiring two practitioners, and grade 4 as unable to ventilate. DMV incidence reported in the literature for the adult surgical population varies widely from 0.9% to 7.8%, reflecting the lack of a standardized DMV definition, objective markers, and standardized FMV technique.[77–80] The incidence of impossible mask ventilation was reported at 0.07%[79] and 0.16%,[81] and the incidence of DMV and difficult laryngoscopy combination at 0.4%.[82] Joffe and colleagues identified inadequate (3–5 cc/kg) and dead space (<150 cc) ventilation with the "E-C" one-handed technique in 19% of the anesthetized nonparalyzed adults.[51] In the context of the perioperative, emergent, and prehospital use of FMV the incidences of DMV in these settings are quite likely significantly greater than the statistics reported in the published anesthesiology literature. DMV is a "situational interplay" between patient-, operator-, and device-related factors.[83]

Predictors

Patient Factors

Langeron and colleagues, in their seminal article, observed that the presence of two patient-related criteria (age >55 years, BMI >26 kg/m², lack of teeth, presence of a beard, history of snoring) was the most accurate predictor for DMV.[79] Also, in the case of DMV the risk for difficult intubation was increased fourfold.[79] Kheterpal and coworkers identified the following independent predictors of DMV on a case series of 22,660 patients: BMI greater than 30 kg/m², presence of a beard, Mallampati III or IV, age older than 57 years, severely limited mandibular protrusion, and a history of snoring. In this study five independent predictors defined impossible mask ventilation: neck radiation changes, male sex, OSA, Mallampati III or IV, and the presence of a beard. Patients with two, three, or more concurrent risk factors are at markedly increased risk for impossible mask ventilation.[84] The addition of the upper lip bite test as a measure of mandibular movement adds a further useful predictor to the list of DMV predictors. The combination of the upper lip bite test, a history of snoring, and increased neck circumference had a negative predictive value of 95% in Khan's prospective study of DMV.[85] Similar results have been found in more contemporaneous studies.[86,87]

The increased incidence of DMV in obese patients is correlated with male gender, increased neck circumference, limited jaw protrusion, and a Mallampati > III.[88] The association of these independent predictors and the severity of obesity increase the incidence of DMV. Increased fat deposits in the pharynx (soft/solid imbalance), neck (reduced bone mobility), and chest wall (reduced pulmonary compliance) are the hallmarks of obesity. Neck circumference represents regional obesity near the pharyngeal airway

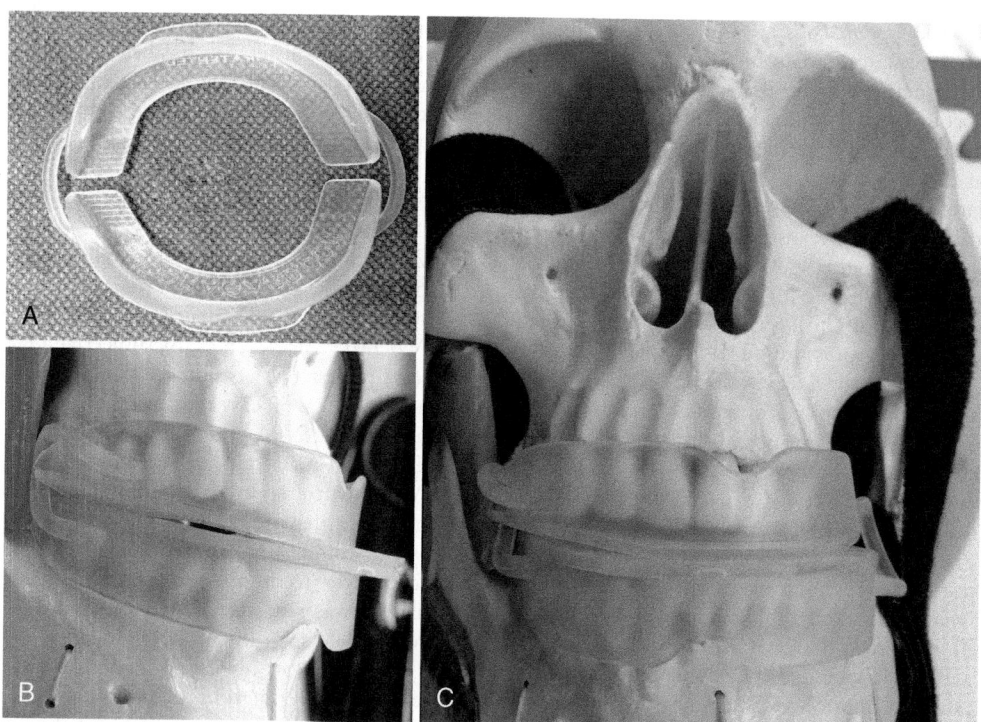

• **Fig. 18.15** The Endoragard Protector as a device to assist face-mask ventilation in edentulous patients. (A) The Endoragard in its open position. (B) The Endoragard from the side position mounted in a skull model. This photo shows the Endoragard's position relative to intact dentition; in the absence of dentition the Endoragard's form will reestablish the upper and lower maxilla form that is normally provided by dentures (or intact dentition). (C) Endoragard from the front, demonstrating its position relative to intact dentition in a skull model. (Courtesy Dux Dental.)

and has a stronger correlation to OSA than the BMI.[89] In a study of the anatomy of the pharynx in patients with OSA as compared with normal subjects Isono and colleagues found that mandibular advancement did not improve the retropalatal airway in obese persons while consistently improving the retroglossal area. Therefore in obese patients it is preferable to bypass the soft palate obstruction with an OPA with the first FMV attempt.[90]

The edentulous patient presents with a lower facial architectural structure collapse because of loss of teeth, bone (alveolar ridge), and muscular tone (buccinators). The air leak during FMV is the result of a suboptimal contact between the RAFM and the cheeks. A large mask can be used in edentulous patients so that the chin fits entirely within the mask with the seal on the caudal surface of the chin. In this configuration the cheeks fit within the sides of the mask, and the sides seal along the lateral maxilla and mandible. These maneuvers to make a difficult mask fit possible are often best sidestepped by endotracheal intubation or the use of an SGA based on clinical judgment. Leaving dentures in place will stabilize the facial anatomy during induction (though with the associated risk of dislodgement with consequent airway obstruction by this foreign body).[91] A potential pitfall of leaving the patient's dentures in place during induction is that the operator will lack useful knowledge about FMV "difficulty" without dentures needed in the postextubation phase. A potential solution to this problem is to substitute a plastic teeth-protection device in place of the patient's dentures to restore structure to the face. The Endoragard Protector (Dux Dental) is a plastic hinged upper and lower teeth protector intended to reduce dental injury from laryngoscopy and intraoral procedures. The device self-centers over the superior and inferior alveolar ridges and provides an

enhanced structure to the upper and lower mandible during FMV (Fig. 18.15). Alternatively, an OPA is needed in a high percentage of edentulous patients without dentures because it stabilizes the oral architecture and the associated tongue enlargement that may overlie the soft palate.[92] Thus the use of an OPA with the first FMV attempt in edentulous patients to reconstruct oral anatomy and support the tongue may be beneficial. Other oral stabilization techniques place the caudal end of the mask between the lower lip and the alveolar ridge while drawing the lip over the mask or place the caudal end above the lower lip while maintaining head extension. Deliberate mouth opening and the use of OPA are part of these techniques.[93] Both techniques can be applied with one or two hands.

Improvements for the DMV in the bearded patient are user/institutional specific: shaving portions of the beard, viscous gel, or transparent dressing (kitchen plastic wrap) applied on the beard or nasal ventilation.[94] In both the edentulous and the bearded patient the focus is on the seal, and an inexperienced operator may compensate for the leak with more pressure on the RAFM, generating neck flexion with attendant iatrogenic airway obstruction.

Airway maneuvers used during DMV may have counterproductive or even deleterious effects if not applied judiciously. The CL/HE maneuver should be used cautiously in the emergent airway prone to atlanto-occipital or atlanto-axial laxity or trauma. Overzealous cricoid pressure application during FMV may result in airway obstruction and inadequate oxygenation.[95]

Provider Factors

DMV may be generated by the operator's lack of skill, knowledge, judgment, or improper use of sedative or induction medications.[75]

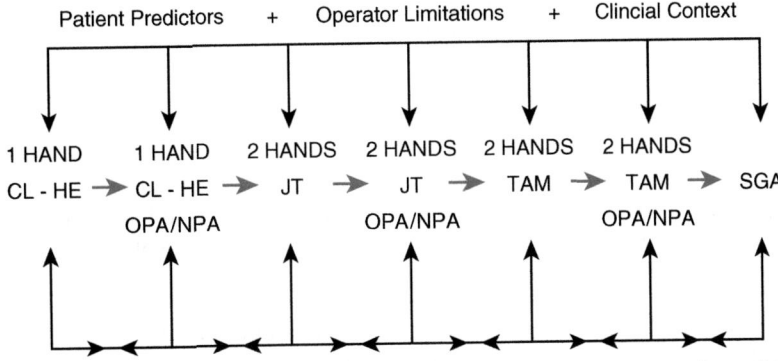

FIRST OPTIMAL VENTILATION ATTEMPT
TAILORED RESPONSE TO:

Patient Predictors   +   Operator Limitations   +   Clinical Context

1 HAND → 1 HAND → 2 HANDS → 2 HANDS → 2 HANDS → 2 HANDS → SGA
CL - HE   CL - HE   JT   JT   TAM   TAM
         OPA/NPA   OPA/NPA   OPA/NPA

• **Fig. 18.16** First optimal ventilation attempt. The traditional progressive face-mask ventilation (FMV) approach (*red arrows*), from simple to complex techniques, deters the operator from tailoring an optimal first response to the predictors of an expected difficult mask ventilation (DMV) producing extended periods of apnea. In a patient with an anticipated DMV, any of the advanced FMV techniques can be used as the first optimal attempt (*black arrows*). In specific clinical circumstances, the first attempt for ventilation with a supraglottic airway is a valid approach. *CL*, Chin lift; *HE*, head extension; *JT*, jaw thrust; *NPA*, nasopharyngeal airway; *OPA*, oropharyngeal airway; *SGA*, supraglottic airway; *TAM*, triple airway maneuver.

Human factors (language barriers, fatigue, stress) and time pressure may have an impact on the FMV outcome as well. The single-hand FMV technique relies on the use of a complex grip as the hand interacts with both the device and the patient. An ergonomic grip with the operator's hand during one-handed FMV assumes a good coupling between the hand and the device, even distribution of pressure across the FM body to the sealing cushion, and a straight wrist to engage the forearm muscles and minimize carpal tunnel pressure. Deviation from the neutral wrist position decreases the grip force and torque.[96] Operator hand size (grip span); preexisting hand, wrist, or upper extremity disability (left carpal tunnel syndrome, arthritis); and poor technique may all contribute to a suboptimal attempt at FMV. Female anesthesia providers are at increased risk for left-side carpal tunnel syndrome.[97] Operators with smaller hands and a weaker grip should acknowledge their limitations with the one-handed technique and develop strategies for alternative management options. The two-handed mask ventilation technique should be practiced in elective operating room cases to maintain proficiency of the operator and familiarity of ancillary staff.

An ergonomic standing posture during FMV assumes an erect spine with minimally flexed knees and minimally extended trunk and head. Strength and stability of the hand/arm can be gained by adducting the arm to the torso. The patient's head positioned at the top of the operating table with the patient's face at or just below elbow height offers comfortable access for the operator.[98] Compensation for table height through postural adjustment is counterproductive. A nonergonomic approach may be unnoticed by the operator but may affect performance in longer and critical attempts at FMV.[99]

Device Factors

An ideal emergency airway management device (e.g., RAFM) should support a first optimal ventilation attempt and compensate for lack of experience. The RAFM and accessory devices are not regulated to conform to set standards regarding ergonomics and construction and present with variations in sizes and design between different brands. There are large disparities in both performance and satisfaction between practitioners with different RAFM designs.[100,101] Current designs, sizes, and shapes of OPAs and NPAs may be suboptimal for maximal clinical effect in the modern day, as the design and dimensions of these devices are decades old, when they served a shorter and leaner population. Most medical institutions offer a minimal assortment of RAFM types and sizes. Poorly fitting sizes of the RAFM, OPA, and NPA or poor technique in utilization may influence the outcome. In this context it is the responsibility of the practitioners to understand and adapt to the limitations of their equipment, their environment, and the particular factors of their patient that will influence the effectiveness of FMV.

A Practical Approach to Difficult Mask Ventilation

Anticipating the degree to which FMV may prove difficult based upon the patient factors (discussed earlier) is important; however, it is not known which patient predictors or combination of predictors define the highest risk of DMV. Unlike current models for predicting difficult tracheal intubation by direct laryngoscopy, the current predictive models for DMV do not guide the operator to specific steps based on preoperative findings. Consequently, it is left to the individual operator to process the information with disappointing results.[102] DMV predictors are collected during a routine airway examination, but practitioners ignore or do not process them for a coherent response. Most clinicians use the traditional progressive FMV approach escalating from the basic one-handed (CL/HE) to advanced techniques: one-handed (CL/HE) with OPA/NPA, two-handed (jaw thrust), two-handed (jaw thrust) with OPA/NPA, and two-handed with triple airway maneuver (Fig. 18.16). This model may lead to an extended apnea time as the operator proceeds diligently from simple to complex maneuvers, extending the overall time of apnea during airway management, leading to hypoxemia.

A proactive DMV approach should ask two questions. The first ("Are the patient's soft tissues prone to collapse?") identifies male patients, increased weight/neck circumference, snoring, OSA, increased age, lack of teeth, and a Mallampati score of III/IV (the "Santa Claus" model). The second ("Is the ability to optimally apply an FM seal and airway maneuver restricted?") explores the following: mandibular protrusion and cervical extension limitations, beard presence, short thyromental distance, lack of teeth, thick neck, history of radiation therapy, operator-specific (small hands, lack of technique), and device-limiting (inappropriate devices) steps. The combination of increased soft tissue collapsibility with limited solid tissue maneuverability and specific non–patient-related variables points to the likelihood and severity of an expected DMV. In an expected DMV, any of the advanced FMV techniques can be used as an optimal first attempt (see Fig. 18.16). The unexpected DMV, just like the unexpected difficult intubation, assumes the use of objective markers for a timely diagnosis and acceptance of failure with an appropriate response. FMV is a dynamic concept, and an unexpected/impossible DMV can develop progressively in the context of an inadequate airway management attempt.

Strategies for an Optimal Attempt at Face Mask Ventilation

An optimal FMV attempt provides adequate oxygenation without stomach inflation and is tailored to the patient's DMV predictors. An optimal first attempt should leave minimal room for subsequent adjustments; that is, it should prove effective on the first attempt and not require multiple adjustments.

Patient Head and Body Position

The patient's head and neck position reflects on the longitudinal tension in the pharyngeal muscles and anterior neck structures. The UA collapsibility can be decreased and the longitudinal pharyngeal tension increased by placing the head and neck in the "sniffing" position with lower cervical flexion, upper cervical extension, and extension of the head on the neck ("passive" UA stretching). The lower cervical spine flexion generated by the sniffing position is needed for maximal extension of the occipito-atlanto-axial complex.[103] Greenberg recommends the placement of a roll under the shoulders of the adult patient, thus further extending the head with a greater opening of the hypopharyngeal structures.[104] Two

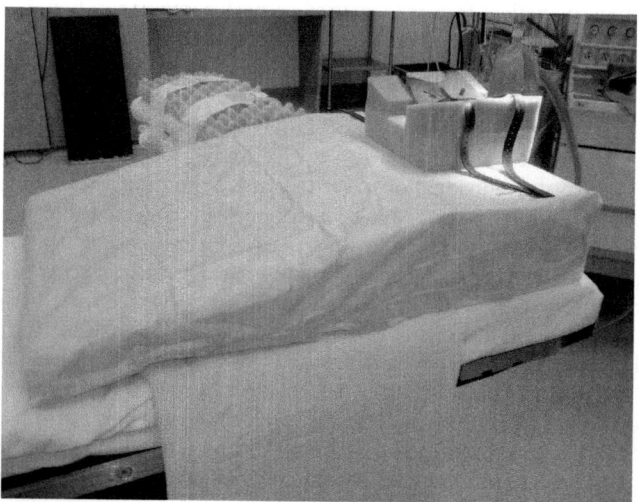

• **Fig. 18.17** Supine and ramped position for a "passive" stretching of the upper airway to optimize a face-mask ventilation (FMV) attempt. The Troop Elevation Pillow (wedge-shaped foam pillow) assists in patient positioning to achieve an advantageous position for FMV as well as invasive airway management. (Courtesy Dr. Craig Troop.)

positions shown to improve the maintenance of the passive pharyngeal airway are the sniffing position in patients with OSA and the Fowler sitting position in morbidly obese patients.[105] In obese and morbidly obese patients the "ramp" position (Fig. 18.17) is implemented with the head elevated beyond the sniffing position by raising the back and the shoulders with regular or manufactured elevation pillows, or in the operating room, using the operating room table control to adjust the table to the "beach chair" position with the head section extended, such that the external auditory meatus is in line with the sternal notch.[106] This position decreases lung and chest wall compliance.

Expected Difficult Mask Ventilation

The traditional gradual FMV approach deters the operator from tailoring the response to specific predictors of DMV and thus can produce extended periods of apnea while the proper response to the DMV case is implemented. Any of the advanced FMV approaches are pertinent first-attempt techniques in a patient with anticipated DMV (see Fig. 18.16). The use of the OPA/NPA is encouraged in patients with predicted soft palate obstruction and large tongue.[107] When both the sniffing position and neck extension are impossible, the application of a two-handed triple airway maneuver with an OPA and pressure-controlled ventilation mode is recommended.[108] Practitioners with small hands should consider a two-handed technique with the first FMV attempt. Current research in mask ventilation has not addressed the category of patients who are at high risk for DMV (e.g., obstetrics, morbidly obese, full stomach, critical airway, prehospital); thus evidence-based strategies for unprotected airway management in these populations is lacking. DMV may be associated with difficult intubation, making the development and implementation of optimal ventilation strategies paramount. Further research in the use of ventilation devices that control inspiratory flow rates, peak ventilatory pressures, and minute ventilation, as well as allow the use of two-handed mask ventilation techniques in these patient populations, is warranted.

Unexpected Difficult Mask Ventilation

When unexpected DMV arises in the context of an optimal attempt, the operator cannot be certain of the contributing factors. Switching from a nasal to an oral ventilation route may be favorable. The insertion of an OPA will bypass two obstruction sites with inconsistent response to airway maneuvers (nasal cavities, soft palate) and support the tongue and mandibular advancement. Many practitioners reach for the OPA late when oxygen desaturation occurs or impossible mask ventilation is confirmed.

Face Mask Ventilation With Neuromuscular Relaxants

Clinicians and researchers are divided based on whether it is necessary to confirm adequate FMV before the administration of muscle relaxants.[109–112] The Difficult Airway Society 2015 guidelines for the management of unanticipated difficult intubation in adults consider that the neuromuscular block facilitates FMV.[113] The traditional practice regarding the use of neuromuscular relaxant medications with the induction of anesthesia to confirm the adequacy of FMV before administration of a muscle relaxant is challenged. Thus this traditional practice is intended to help the practitioner potentially avoid a cannot intubate/cannot oxygenate scenario with the option of "backing out" of the anesthetic and allowing spontaneous ventilation to return. The process of allowing an unventilated unparalyzed patient to wake up after induction may be unpractical and dangerous (such as in the emergency medicine, prehospital, and critical care arenas) as the patient can be exposed to hypoxia, laryngospasm, pulmonary aspiration, negative pressure pulmonary edema, and the need for lifesaving airway techniques in a suboptimal setting.[114] The administration of neuromuscular blockers ensures glottic patency and avoids laryngospasm, facilitates positive pressure ventilation by decreasing pulmonary compliance, and may help intubation and the insertion of SGAs.

The use of sugammadex will consistently reverse rocuronium-generated neuromuscular blockade, but not the effects of induction agents, opioids, and anesthetic gases. As muscle tone recovers following the rapid reversal of neuromuscular relaxants with the patient still anesthetized, effective basic airway management is needed to support the resuming spontaneous ventilation.[115] Poor outcome can manifest as the inability to intubate a paralyzed patient, as well as the inability to oxygenate an unparalyzed "waking" patient. Both events are time sensitive. The decision to administer a neuromuscular blocker at induction should consider the preoperative predictors for DMV and intubation, the general anesthetic technique chosen, and the airway management approaches available and mastered.

Controlled Ventilation by Face Mask

A two-handed mask ventilation technique requires a second assistant to operate a BVM or an anesthesia circle system, unless a mechanical ventilation device is used. This section will discuss specifically the use of a modern anesthesia machine ventilator to control ventilation during mask ventilation. Additionally, we will discuss the use of the standard BVM resuscitator system as well as the use of ARMS, which is a US Food and Drug Administration–approved device that can assume the role of a BVM in elective or emergency scenarios. Controlled ventilation by mask is relatively contraindicated in patients at increased risk for the aspiration of gastric contents; however, this contraindication applies principally to elective anesthetic cases, as mask ventilation is often mandatory in critically ill patients who require advanced airway management because of respiratory failure.

Anesthesia Circle System (Anesthesia Machine)

When used as part of an anesthesia circle system, a face mask can facilitate a patient's spontaneous ventilation as well as various levels and modes of supported or controlled ventilation. When the ventilator of the anesthesia machine is used to support ventilation during FMV, this permits the use of two-handed mask ventilation as well as the proper and efficient use of airway maneuvers to maintain a patent airway. Modern anesthesia machines possess ventilators with multiple ventilatory modes, such as pressure control, volume control, and pressure support, with the ability to administer positive end-expiratory pressure (PEEP). Ventilator settings that are useful in clinical practice are those that limit inspiratory flow rates to less than 40 L/min, limit peak inspiratory pressures to 20 cm H_2O, and achieve a regular and brisk ventilatory rate such that the minute ventilation (which is the product of respiratory rate and TV) equals or exceeds 9 L/min. Fig. 18.18 displays the control panel with the appropriate settings for controlled mask ventilation, specifically pressure control 20 cm H_2O, rate 20

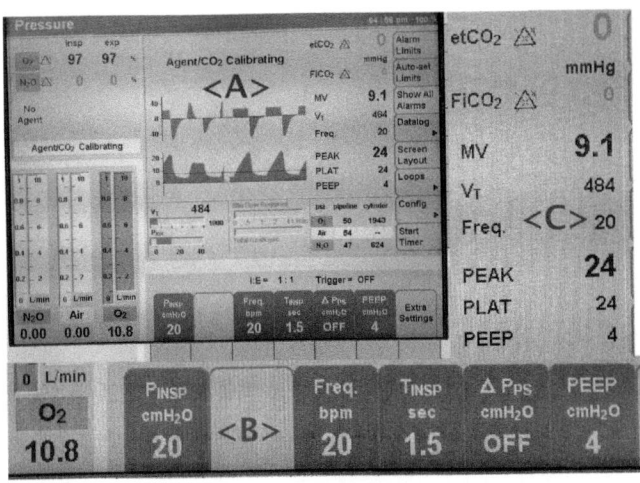

• **Fig. 18.18** Control panel display of a Dräger Apollo Anesthesia Machine adjusted to perform automated face-mask ventilation. The ventilator is specifically adjusted to a pressure control mode (i.e., pressure limited) with an overall minute ventilation of 9 to 10 L/min. Rate is set to 20 breaths per minute; inspiratory to expiratory ratio is set to 1:1 (equal inhalation with exhalation time to decrease the inspiratory flow rates in order to avoid gastric insufflation). Positive end-expiratory pressure is set to 4 cm H_2O to positively affect alveolar recruitment and provide static airway pressure to further maintain airway patency. (Courtesy Dräger.)

breaths per minute, inspiratory to expiratory ratio ratio 1:1, and PEEP 4 cm H_2O (based on the author's clinical experience). The use of PEEP during controlled mask ventilation enhances alveolar recruitment and further serves to complement the airway maneuvers required to maintain a patent airway.

Resuscitator Units

The Air-Mask-Bag Unit

The air-mask-bag-unit, often referenced as an AMBU or BVM, was described in 1955 by Henning Ruben.[116] The BVM provides a simple and effective alternative means of controlled ventilation to the standard anesthesia circle system, should system failure occur during ventilation with these systems, should patient positioning relative to these systems prove difficult or impossible to achieve, or for airway management outside of the operating room. The BVM can be used with an FM, SGA, or ETT. Its main advantages are that it is self-inflating and readily portable, but it lacks the "feel" (airway compliance and resistance) that the clinician has with a circle system, and it requires a compressed oxygen source to deliver oxygen concentrations above that of room air. Although there are various types of BVM systems in use, all incorporate one-way valves to allow PPV and to prevent rebreathing. BVMs are an excellent choice for portable, easy-to-use systems for the delivery of positive-pressure ventilation (PPV) and supplemental oxygen outside of the operating room environment. Understand, though, that the one-way valves in these systems require valve opening to allow oxygen to pass to the patient if used for "preoxygenation."

Automatic Resuscitation Management System

ARMS units, such as the Oxylator FR-300, were developed primarily to facilitate prehospital ventilatory support during resuscitation and transport. The device has largely been compared with

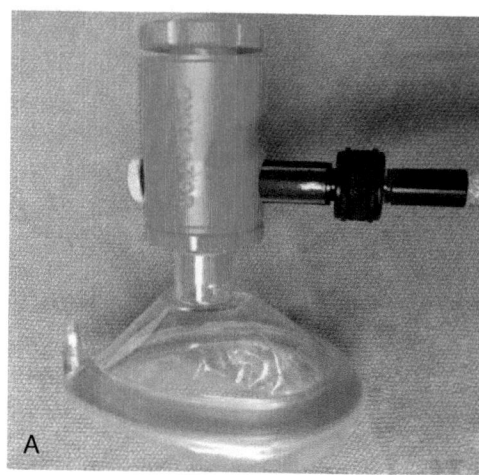
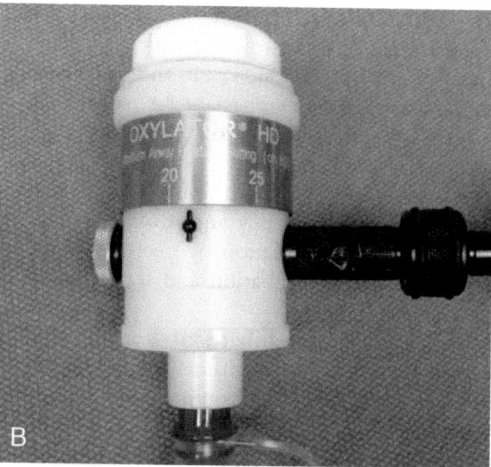

• **Fig. 18.19** (A) Oxylator automatic resuscitation management system (ARMS)—ARMS system with a preset pressure release (i.e., pressure limit) of 20 cm H_2O. May be used in an "Automatic Mode," which will automatically cycle active inspiration phases with passive exhalation phases, or the device can be used in a "Manual Mode," which allows the rescuer to manually initiate (and terminate) the inspiratory phase with the manual press and release of the O_2 release button (colored *gold* in the photo). (B) Oxylator HD—ARMS system with an adjustable pressure release (i.e., pressure limit) between 15 cm and 30 cm H_2O. May be used in an "Automatic Mode," which will automatically cycle active inspiration phases with passive exhalation phases, or the device can be used in a "Manual Mode," which allows the rescuer to manually initiate (and terminate) the inspiratory phase with the manual press and release of the O_2 release button (colored *gold* in the photo). Also capable of providing passive oxygen with an "Inhalator Mode," which passively supplies 15 L/min on activation (separate control knob not visible in photo). (Courtesy CPR Medical Devices.)

BVM, where it provides similar oxygenation with a lowered risk of gastric distention and hyperventilation.[7] The Oxylator ARMS device is a gas-powered, nonelectronic ventilation tool that appears similar in form to its technologic ancestor, the Demand Valve, yet it contains sophisticated technological updates to ensure its flexibility in ventilation patient care. Two-handed mask ventilation is facilitated with the ARMS device, and the technology assists the operator in ensuring that a patent mask seal is maintained during the ventilation cycle with its flow- and pressure-sensitive release valve. The Oxylator device is available in three models: the FR-300, which possess a simple on/off knob interface and limits the inspiratory pressure to 20 cm H_2O (fixed pressure release point), the HD model, which possesses an adjustable pressure release point of 15 to 30 cm H_2O (adjustable with a marked turning bezel), and the EMX model, which possesses an adjustable pressure release point of 20 to 45 cm H_2O (Fig. 18.19). The Oxylator ARMS system possesses a fixed minute ventilation of 10 to 12 L/min; however, a flow-restricting hose can be used to reduce the minute ventilation of these devices to as low as 4.5 L/min. The ARMS systems are primarily prehospital devices; however, they show promise as ventilation devices for in-hospital resuscitation, patient transport, and bi-level positive airway pressure (BiPAP) respiratory support during deep sedation cases (author's own experience). Overall, ARMS systems represent the technological evolution of resuscitators, and their flexibility and durability have been investigated for in-water and underwater use, as well as rescue from mining accidents.[117,118]

Optimal and Safe Face Mask Ventilation Amid a Respiratory Pandemic

The COVID-19 pandemic of late 2019 underscores the importance of safe and effective respiratory care for the safety of both patients and caregivers. Along with the use of proper personal protective equipment and garments for the caregiver, the use of an optimal two-handed FMV technique along with a HEPA filter in-line with the resuscitation bag or device is essential to provide optimal ventilation to the patient, reduce entrainment of air into the patient's stomach, and reduce the leak between the face mask and the patient's airway, which causes the dispersion of infectious droplets and aerosols into the clinical working area. A simulation study utilizing a manikin configured to exhale smoke particles (simulating infectious particles) and quantified by the laser scanning of the clinical work area revealed significant leakage of smoke particles into the area around the manikin's upper torso.[119] The participants utilized the one-handed BVM resuscitator technique (type of mask grip was not specified) and attempted to ventilate the manikin. Smoke particle leakage was noted among all of the participants, with less leakage from more experienced clinicians (e.g., anesthesiologists and intensive care physicians). Smoke particle leakage was substantially reduced when a HEPA filter was added onto the bag-mask system; however, detectable leakage occurred in a downward direction due to subtle mask leaks. It is important to emphasize that one-handed BVM resuscitator use is a suboptimal technique when treating patients with infectious respiratory pathogens. Implementing two-handed FMV on a wide scale would require teamwork among the clinical team, or alternatively, the use of automated resuscitation devices or ventilators to provide consistent ventilation pressures and TVs.

Conclusion

Noninvasive management of the airway by face mask continues to be a vital skill in the care of anesthetized and critically ill patients. Although its use as the primary airway management technique has largely been supplanted by the SGA, it remains an essential part of other approaches to airway management as a transitional technique during induction and emergence or as a backup plan when other techniques fail. With the increasing use of moderate to deep procedural sedation in the operating room, the anesthesiologist is frequently required to employ noninvasive airway maneuvers and artificial airway devices to provide supplemental oxygen and to monitor and support ventilation. Similarly, the practice of noninvasive airway management will benefit emergency medicine and critical care practitioners in assuring adequate oxygenation during invasive airway procedures. Understanding the advantages, disadvantages, and limitations of various airway management techniques continues to be a cornerstone of a safe and effective practice of airway management in anesthesiology, emergency medicine, and critical care medicine, as well as prehospital airway management.

Selected References

12. Nandi PR, Charlesworth CH, Taylor SJ, et al. Effect of general anaesthesia on the pharynx. Br J Anaesth. 1991;66:157–162.
28. Buffington CW, Wells CMQ, Soose RJ. Expiratory upper airway obstruction caused by the soft palate during bag-mask ventilation. Open J Anesthesiol. 2012;2:38–43.
32. Isono S. Obstructive sleep apnea of obese adults. Anesthesiology. 2009;110(4):908–921.
39. Paal P, von Goedecke A, Brugger H, et al. Head position for opening the upper airway. Anaesthesia. 2007;62:227–230.
41. Kuna TS, Woodson LC, Solanki DR, et al. Effect of progressive mandibular advancement on pharyngeal airway size in anesthetized adults. Anesthesiology. 2008;109:605–612.
51. Joffe AM, Hetzel S, Liew EC. A two-handed jaw thrust is superior to the one handed "EC clamp" technique for mask ventilation in apneic unconscious person. Anesthesiology. 2010;113:873–879.
66. Wenzel V, Idris AH, Dorges V, et al. The respiratory system during resuscitation: a review of the history, risk of infection during assisted ventilation, respiratory mechanics, and ventilation strategies for patient with unprotected airway. Resuscitation. 2001;49:123–134.
75. El-Orbany M, Woehlck HJ. Difficult mask ventilation. Anesth Analg. 2009;109:1870–1880.
79. Langeron O, Masso E, Huraux C, et al. Prediction of difficult mask ventilation. Anesthesiology. 2000;92:1229–1236.
81. Kheterpal S, Martin L, Shanks AM, et al. Prediction and outcomes of impossible mask ventilation. Anesthesiology. 2009;110:891–897.

All references can be found online at eBooks.Health.Elsevier.com.

19

Supraglottic Airway Techniques

SONIA VAIDA, HELEN A. LINDSAY, TIM M. COOK, LUIS GAITINI, AND
CARIN A. HAGBERG

CHAPTER OUTLINE

KEY POINTS

- There is a wide range of supraglottic airways (SGAs), and expertise with several devices is necessary to provide optimal airway management to patients in a wide range of settings.
- Although there is an expanding range of indications for use of SGAs, the safety profile for many of them remains undefined. Each practitioner must master the basic skills for optimal use before attempting more advanced techniques. Exercising careful judgment in assessing the suitability of an SGA for a specific patient and clinical environment is also critical.
- Practitioners must understand the advantages and disadvantages of using SGAs. Although the current limitations of SGA research are known, the importance of using an evidence-based approach to select one device over another remains essential.

- Second-generation SGAs have some proven advantages and other potential advantages over first-generation devices.
- SGAs are not intended to replace all functions of the endotracheal tube (ETT) and are primarily suited for use in fasted patients undergoing surgical procedures when there is no specific indication for tracheal intubation.
- Although anesthesiologists are the predominant users of SGAs, use by clinicians with limited anesthetic experience is also indicated for rescue indications, such as cardiopulmonary resuscitation.
- SGAs can be safely used for controlled ventilation in appropriately selected patients and surgical situations, when the correct device is used correctly.
- The risk of aspiration with SGAs is low in expert hands, which is achieved primarily by careful and appropriate case selection,

- expert insertion, and meticulous management of the airway after insertion.
- SGA function is dependent both on its design and correct use. Care and vigilance are required by the user from the point of insertion to removal, with appropriate maintenance of cuff pressures and depth of anesthesia in between. All airway

devices can fail or cause complications, thus being vigilant and prepared for these uncommon events will minimize the risk of patient harm.

- Clinical research is unlikely to ever prove which SGA is safest. Nonclinical information and research must be understood to form a balanced opinion. There remains some art in this science.

Introduction

The classic laryngeal mask airway (cLMA) was developed by Archie Brain and introduced into clinical practice in 1988. In the first article on the cLMA, Brain described the device as "an alternative to either the endotracheal tube (ETT) or the face mask with either spontaneous or positive-pressure ventilation (PPV)."[1] More than three decades later, the cLMA is recognized as one of the most important developments in airway management, becoming the most commonly used airway device for general anesthesia in many countries.[2] Not only has the cLMA revolutionized anesthesia practice, it also continues to fuel ongoing advances in the technology and utility of supraglottic airway (SGA) device design and clinical use.[3]

The cLMA and its variants (together known as LMAs) are the most frequently used and most extensively studied SGAs; however, SGAs with different designs and performance characteristics may provide adequate oxygenation and ventilation in circumstances where an LMA fails. The LMAs and other SGAs have constantly been developed or modified, generally resulting in many improved and safer tools for airway management. Conversely, some SGAs have been released and used in clinical practice and subsequently withdrawn from the market due to poor performance or low utilization.

Selection of an appropriate airway device across and within device subtypes is complex and informed by multiple factors specific to the patient, surgery, and practitioner. With no single ideal airway device, advanced and rescue airway management depends on a repertoire incorporating many airway devices, as recognized in the various international difficult airway algorithms.[4–6] Although some may consider the cuffed ETT the gold standard in providing a secure airway, this should never be assumed to be true when used by someone with inadequate training and judgment to correctly place and remove an ETT. ETTs are typically used without incident; however, complications with their use can occur, ranging from trivial to life-threatening.[7] The use of SGAs should not be considered any differently.

Second-generation SGAs developed in the last two decades have greatly enhanced the safety profile of these devices.[8] For example, since 2015 all Difficult Airway Society (DAS) algorithms on management of the difficult airway have included the recommendation that second-generation SGA devices should be used in the setting of a failed tracheal intubation.[6] Several other organizations are now also adopting this approach.

In this chapter, we outline the design, efficacy, and safety features of SGAs, highlighting fundamental skills required for optimal use and their limitations. A full review of the extensive body of literature and devices (particularly the various disposable laryngeal mask variants) is beyond the scope of this chapter. Rather, we explore current clinical controversies and provide a structure from which to rationalize the use of particular devices for an expanding range of advanced indications. LMA-type and non-LMA-type SGAs are discussed separately.

Terminology and Classification

Terminology

The concept of being supraglottic describes the fact that the ventilation orifice is just above the glottis, in contrast to pharyngeal airway devices, or infraglottic devices that deliver anesthetic gases or oxygen below the vocal cords (e.g., tracheal intubation, transtracheal jet ventilation, cricothyrotomy). Devices stemming from the development of the original cLMA have been variably described as supraglottic airways or devices (abbreviated to SADs or SGAs), extraglottic airways or devices (EADs or EGAs), or periglottic airways or devices.

In 2004, Brimacombe recommended using the term *extraglottic* to highlight that distal extension into the hypopharynx and upper esophagus, below the level of the glottis, is a fundamental safety feature of supraglottic devices.[9] Although each of these variations is based on a sound rationale, for the purposes of simplification we have chosen to use the term because it is still the most commonly used in the literature. It is also noted that the acronym *LMA* (but not the term *laryngeal mask airway*) is trademarked by the manufacturers of the cLMA (Teleflex North America and associated international companies) and should only be used to refer to laryngeal mask airways produced by this company. The acronym *LM* refers to a laryngeal mask manufactured by anyone other than the original manufacturers. Although LMs could superficially be considered LMA imitations, there are design and manufacturing differences among the many products that have been released and withdrawn from the market. Often there is little or no evidence to evaluate the effect of these differences on clinical performance, let alone to compare them with the original cLMA, for which there is a substantive body of performance data.[10,11] As such, discussion of specific LMs is beyond the scope of this chapter.

The classification of SGAs, both the LMA type and the non-LMA type, falls into two broad categories: those based on anatomic or mechanistic features and a pragmatic division into generations.

Pragmatic Classification

The most widely adopted classification was described by Cook in 2009, defining first-generation SGAs as "simple airway tubes" and second-generation SGAs as "those with design features that are intended to reduce the risk of pulmonary aspiration of gastric contents."[12–14]

The utility of this classification is its simplicity and focus on clinical safety, which is perhaps the reason that it has become widely adopted. Its limitations lie with the diversity that remains within each generation. It should also be highlighted that an intentional design does not indicate any substantiation of improved outcomes. As will be described later, the majority of published evidence on SGAs relates to efficacy, whereas clinical decision

TABLE 19.1 Classifications of Currently Available Supraglottic Airway Devices

	First-Generation SGAs	Second-Generation SGAs
Based on the Classic LMA	LMA classic, LMA Unique, LMA Unique with cuff pilot technology, LMA Unique EVO with cuff pilot technology, AES Ultra, AES Ultra clear, Ambu Aura40, Ambu Aura40 Straight, Ambu AuraOnce, Shiley, Soft-Seal, Solus Curve, Solus MRI safe, Solus Standard, Solus Satin,	LMA Proseal, LMA Supreme, LMA Gastro, LMA protector, i-gel, Baska Mask
Based on the ETC - Shiley Esophageal Endotracheal Double Lumen	LT-D	LTS-D, Gastro LT
Based on the Flexible LMA	LMA Flexible, AES UltraFlex, Ambu AuraFlex, Solus Flexible	Ambu AuraGain, Ambu Aura-I
Based on the Intubating LMA	Fastrach ILMA, LMA Classic Excel, air-Q, air-Q disposable, air-Q SP, air-Q SP disposable	air-Q Blocker, Block Buster Intubating Laryngeal Mask Airway, Laryngeal Seal Pro
Other		SLIPA

Adapted from Hagberg CA. Current concepts in the management of the difficult airway. *Anesthesiology News* [Internet]. 2020;17(1). Available at https://www.anesthesiologynews.com/Review-Articles/Article/05-20/Current-Concepts-In-the-Management-of-the-Difficult-Airway-Volume-17-Number-1/58268.

making most commonly focuses on safety. In reality, there is no robust evidence confirming that any SGA is safer than another, and in the absence of this robust evidence, use of "design intent" and "design features" focused on improving safety is a logical and pragmatic compromise (Table 19.1).

Controversially, the term *third-generation SGA* has been used in the literature. At present, the term is used without definition but often implies an improvement or superiority in a new device.[15] The term *third generation* has been proposed to encompass so-called self-pressuring or self-energizing sealers or the additional features of a bite block and novel drain design in the Baska Mask.[16] However, it should be noted that several established second-generation devices have such features, with no evidence that any device termed third-generation has benefits over existing SGAs; the Baska Mask was described as a third-generation device before the publication of any performance data.[15]

Anatomic-Mechanistic Classifications

Anatomic-mechanistic classifications have been recognized as useful for designers of SGAs and are helpful in educating users in the functional benefits and disadvantages of particular designs. However, it is uncertain if they have value to clinicians in their daily practice.

In 2004, Brimacombe proposed a classification based on the presence or absence of a cuff, the route of insertion (oral or nasal), and the anatomic location of the distal portion of the device.[9] Four other potential criteria proposed for consideration included the anatomic location of the distal airway aperture, the ability to use the device for intubation, whether the device is disposable or reusable, and the anatomic location of the cuff if one is present. Although Brimacombe argued the importance of a cuff as a measure of suitability for controlled ventilation, the subsequent efficacy of cuffless designs (e.g., i-gel) has disproven this. The relevance of noting the distal tip location in relation to separation of the respiratory and gastrointestinal tracts is less relevant because most modern SGAs (with the notable exceptions of the Cobra PLA and Tulip) extend into the hypopharynx and upper esophagus. Additionally, tip location is only one element of protection from aspiration, as esophageal seal varies dramatically between SGAs in a cadaver model.[17] In addition, the presence and size of any distal cuff and drain tube are important differentiating features.[18]

Also, in 2004, Miller described an approach based on sealing mechanisms, including cuffed perilaryngeal sealers, cuffed pharyngeal sealers, and cuffless anatomically preshaped sealers, proposing further subdivision based on whether the device is single use or reusable and presence or absence of an esophageal cuff.[19]

In 2014, Miller updated his classification with Michalek, dichotomizing devices into pharyngeal sealers or base of tongue sealers, further classifying "three generations" within each of these groups on the basis of the sealing mechanism used (inflatable, wedge, and self-energizing).[20] Aside from the confusion caused from using the term *generation,* as discussed previously, the current value of a classification system that places the vast majority of devices in the inflatable seal category is yet to be determined.

A further classification used by Hernandez and colleagues in 2012 was also based on cuff design, including those with an inflatable periglottic cuff, no inflatable cuff, a single pharyngeal cuff, or two inflatable cuffs.[21]

Currently, the classifications of SGAs used are potentially confusing and none is perfect. An international consensus classification of SGAs focused on functionality and safety would potentially be of benefit. However, this is currently limited by the paucity of evidence specifying the safety differences among devices and the difficulty in establishing such evidence.

Standards in Evaluation of Supraglottic Airways

Several national and international regulations govern the marketing of medical products.[22] Regulations governing the introduction of new medical devices are much less onerous than those faced when developing and introducing a new drug, which include three phases of clinical trials and mandatory postmarketing surveillance. Rather, when a company obtains a license to market an SGA, it indicates that the manufacturer has assessed the product to be "fit for the purpose" for which it was intended. Although some companies perform extensive laboratory, model, and clinical evaluations before marketing, others invite a select group of hospitals or individuals to perform a trial of the device, and after each use they collect their informal assessment of performance. These practices are far from universal or regulated, and industry reports are not subject to the same rigor as clinical trials, with no requirement to assess clinical efficacy. These issues have long been recognized in the literature.[10,22] Regulatory changes have been proposed in the United Kingdom (UK); however, the DAS recognizes that the logistical and political complexities of engaging in this process make it unfeasible. Rather the DAS proposes that assessment of clinical efficacy should be put in the hands of clinicians by determining purchasing standards.[22]

The development of SGA scoring systems is synergistic with the DAS strategy. Miller was the first to introduce the concept in 2004, using eight desirable objectives to guide device selection for routine use. Although Miller himself recognized the limited data available at this time to accurately inform this process, his work was relevant in highlighting the need for consistency in SGA evaluation.[19] Cook and Kelly similarly used a scoring system to assess seven performance features of SGAs in four clinical situations (routine use, use by a novice at a cardiac arrest, airway rescue by an expert after failed intubation during a rapid sequence induction, and intubation through an SGA after failed intubation), as informed by their knowledge of the literature, judgment, and clinical experience. This summative assessment provided a structure to compare and rationalize the use of six SGAs.[8] However, even 10 years after Miller's efforts, limitations in the current literature base are still open to contrasting interpretations.[23] While recognizing this, the importance of an evidence-based approach to SGA use remains.[22]

This raises important philosophical questions highly relevant to modern medical practice, regarding the minimum level of evidence needed to make a pragmatic decision about the purchase or selection of an airway device.[24] Although a well-designed large double-blind multicenter study provides the most robust assessment of relative efficacy, the associated time, resource, and financial costs may mean it is not always appropriate or possible. Such trials may also establish relative efficacy without determining relative safety, particularly for uncommon events. The difference between *optimal* and *satisfactory* evidence, while balancing the demands of what is *meaningful* as opposed to *achievable*, needs to be considered. The Airway Device Evaluation Project Team (ADEPT) guidelines, produced by the DAS in 2011, argue that a single case-control or historical-control trial is an acceptable minimum standard, while recognizing that it is under the purview of the individual clinician or group to judge if that is "sufficient" for the unique situation being assessed.[22]

While recognizing the limitations and controversies, adoption of the ADEPT guidelines will help to create an infrastructure and motivation to obtain the required evidence, serving to evolve the science and practice of airway device evaluation.[22] This has already been recognized on a national level through guideline development done by the Association of Anaesthetists of Great Britain and Ireland (AAGBI) and the Australian and New Zealand College of Anaesthetists (ANZCA).[25,26]

Laryngeal Mask Airways

As characterized by the prototype LMA, SGAs are minimally invasive and designed to manage the airway of an unconscious patient. An inflatable mask is fitted with a tube that exits the mouth to enable ventilation of the lungs. The mask fits against the periglottic tissues, occupying the hypopharyngeal space and upper esophagus, forming a seal above the glottis rather than within the trachea (Fig. 19.1). Placement is intended to be a less traumatic alternative to tracheal intubation, although more reliable and hands off than face mask ventilation. In the development

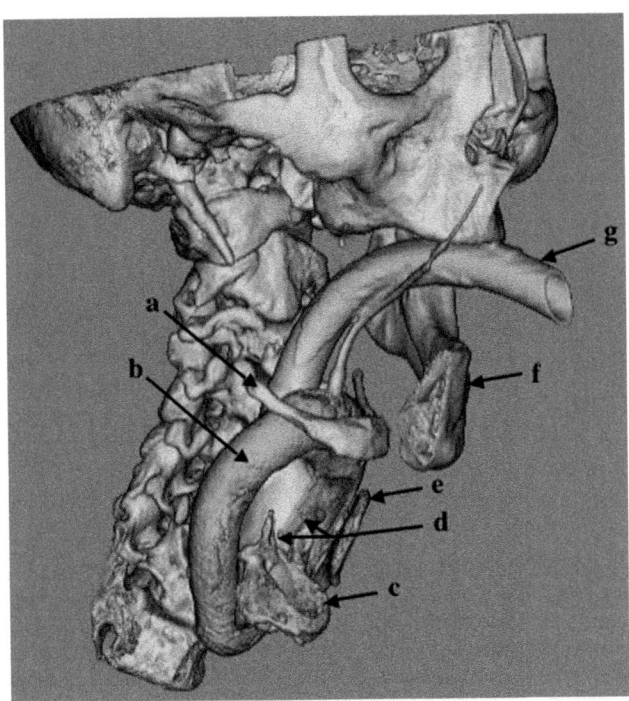

• **Fig. 19.1** Three-dimensional radiologic reconstruction of the human airway with the laryngeal mask airway (LMA) in situ: hyoid bone (a); LMA cuff (b); cricoid ring (c); arytenoid cartilages (d); thyroid cartilage (e), and mandible (f), which are digitally partially removed to demonstrate the position of the LMA; and the LMA's shaft (g). The LMA cuff forms a seal with the periglottic tissues and provides a continuous connection between the natural airway and the device.

of the cLMA, Brain soon realized that despite a range of sizes, one model could not fulfill all clinical needs. Following the cLMA, Brain and the companies he worked with introduced several additional models: LMA Flexible (fLMA), for head and neck anesthesia (Fig. 19.2); LMA Unique (uLMA), a single-use version of the cLMA; Intubating Laryngeal Mask Airway (ILMA, Fastrach), to facilitate blind and flexible scope intubation (Fig. 19.3); LMA Classic-Excel, a cLMA-like device with features to facilitate use of a flexible intubation scope (FIS), released in North America only; ProSeal LMA (PLMA), the first second-generation LMA, with enhanced features to improve efficacy during controlled ventilation and reduce the risk of aspiration (Fig. 19.4); LMA Supreme (SLMA), a single-use second-generation device with features of the uLMA, PLMA, and ILMA (Fig. 19.5); and LMA Protector, a silicone second-generation device dual gastric drainage channels, released in 2016. (Fig. 19.6). The LMA Gastro, released in 2017, is a second-generation SGA specifically designed for upper gastrointestinal procedures (Fig. 19.7). The step changes in design are the fLMA, ILMA, and PLMA, and these are the focus of this chapter with the cLMA.

Important Features

The history of SGAs is one of significant and constant development, from Brain's basic design of the cLMA in the early 1980s to his release of multiple subsequent variants. Each variant on the cLMA was specifically designed to better serve the range of potential roles that Brain envisioned for the LMA devices, as outlined in this chapter's introduction. Concurrent with the development of LMA-type SGAs is an ever-increasing evidence base for their safe

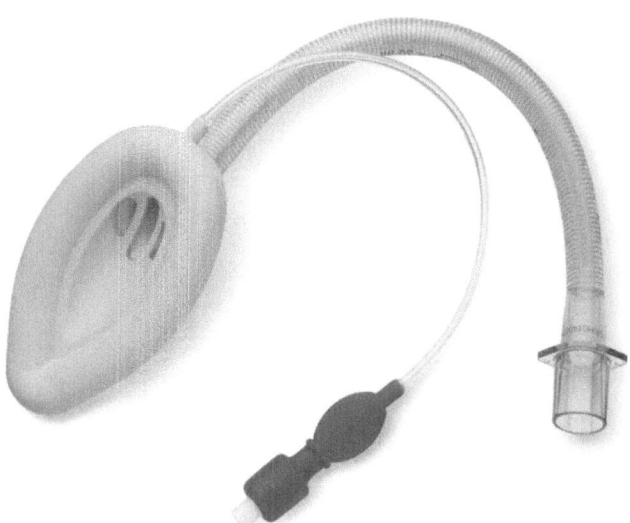

• **Fig. 19.2** The flexible laryngeal mask airway (FLMA), which was introduced into clinical practice in 1994, has a spiral coil built into the shaft to increase the flexibility of the tube and to prevent kinking. This enables the surgeon to manipulate the shaft of the FLMA during surgery and to have good access to the operating field. The FLMA has been used successfully in patients undergoing a variety of head, neck, eye, and oral operations. (Teleflex Medical Europe Ltd., Athlone, Ireland.)

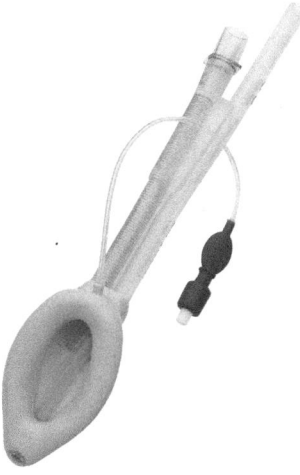

• **Fig. 19.4** The ProSeal laryngeal mask airway was designed to separate the respiratory and gastrointestinal tracts and provide a better seal around the glottis, allowing positive-pressure ventilation in a more reliable manner than the LMA Classic. (Teleflex Medical Europe Ltd., Athlone, Ireland.)

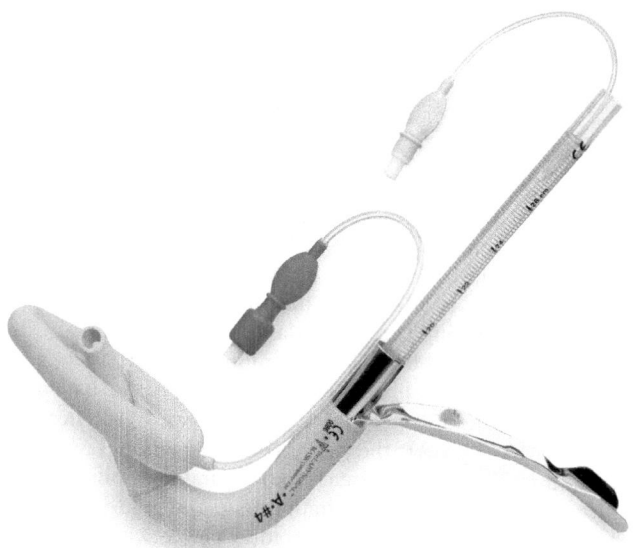

• **Fig. 19.3** The intubating laryngeal mask airway (ILMA) was introduced in 1997. It consists of the mask, which has the same shape as the LMA Classic, and the 13-mm internal diameter stainless steel shaft, which can accommodate an endotracheal tube with an internal diameter up to 8.5 mm. There are three sizes: 3 to 5. A single-use device is available. (Teleflex Medical Europe Ltd., Athlone, Ireland.)

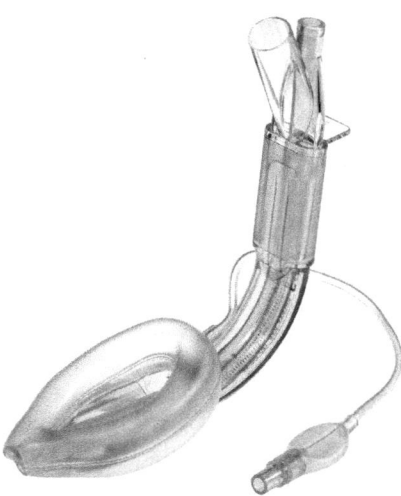

• **Fig. 19.5** The LMA Supreme is made of PVC. It has an integral bite block and fixation tab at the proximal end of the device. Two tubes project from the manifold. The 15-mm-diameter airway tube is designed to connect to the airway circuit. The narrower tube is the proximal end of the drain tube. Two narrow airway tubes run on either side of the drain tube, which passes through the modified cuff. The cuff has no posterior component in contrast to the ProSeal LMA. A pilot balloon is attached to the cuff inflation line. (Teleflex Medical Europe Ltd., Athlone, Ireland.)

use, paralleled by an increasing range of uses, some now widely accepted and some still controversial.

However, despite improvements and the increasing versatility of SGAs, not all design features for a specific purpose are synergistic with one another, meaning no single device can incorporate all roles. For instance, the use of more rigid materials in the tube component of the ILMA and SLMA is intended to improve the ease of insertion, but this also reduces the flexibility required for a device to be useful in head, neck, and shared airway procedures. Similarly, aperture epiglottic bars in the distal orifice of the mask

component of the cLMA reduce the risk of epiglottic obstruction but impair instrumental access to the trachea.

For the various indications for use, there are important design and performance characteristics that must be fulfilled and understood to support optimal device selection and use.

Design Features

In the development of the cLMA, Brain recognized the importance of studying, understanding, and accounting for the anatomic and physiologic principles of the oropharyngolaryngeal complex. The overall size and shape of the tube and mask components vary significantly among SGAs, especially when considering the non-LMA–type SGAs. Not only does this determine the most basic function of how the device passes through the mouth and into its

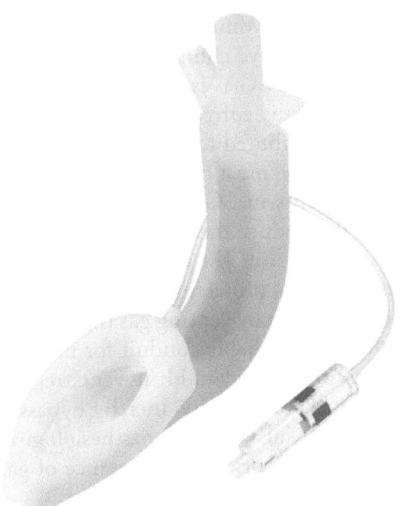

• **Fig. 19.6** The LMA Protector, a silicone, single-use device incorporating features of many earlier LMAs. It has a relatively large central airway tube and two lateral drain tubes. The cuff incorporates a "traffic light" system that enables continuous monitoring of cuff pressure during use. (Teleflex Medical Europe Ltd., Athlone, Ireland.)

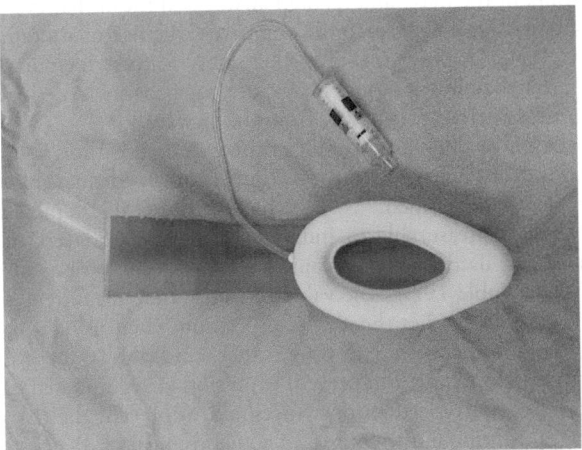

• **Fig. 19.7** Gastro LMA (Courtesy of Dr. Luis Gaitini.)

final position, but it ultimately affects almost all functions of the device, as highlighted in the description of individual devices later in this chapter. With the evolution of second-generation devices, such as the PLMA and SLMA, additional features such as a drain tube, bite block, and fixation tab were developed.[27,28] Within these basic design frameworks, the manufacturing process and materials used can vary.

Differentiation of reusable and single-use devices is also an important design feature. The original SGAs were mostly made of silicone and could be reused in the range of 40 to 60 times after manual cleaning and sterilization.[29,30] Current manufacturer's instructions recommend up to 40 uses.

Although there has been no evidence to prove SGAs are a source of infection, theoretical concerns in the late 1990s about the risk of infectious transmission through the tonsillar bed, particularly small viruslike particles and prion diseases, provided manufacturers with an opportunity to focus on the development of single-use designs. These were mostly made with polyvinylchloride (PVC), and many have been adopted into practice without evidence of clinical efficacy, safety, or equivalent performance compared with

reusable devices. Brimacombe and colleagues described the rush toward single-use LMs as "driven by fears of the unknown and scientific misinformation,"[31] the risks of infection, and financial costs needing to be balanced against the potential risks of using alternative untested equipment.[10]

Efficacy Features

The fundamental purpose of an SGA is to provide a patent airway in the unconscious patient, thus interlinking with multiple safety and efficacy considerations. A minimally effective device will incorporate the following features:
• Easy insertion with a high rate of first-time success;
• A low rate of complications of insertion;
• Maintenance of a patent airway;
• The ability to ventilate the lungs reliably during controlled and spontaneous ventilation;
• Access to the airway;
• Reliable and simple fixation with a low rate of displacement during use;
• Good tolerance during emergence to light planes of anesthesia;
• Simple removal without causing upper airway trauma; and
• Steep learning curve. (Table 19.2)

Insertion Success

A high rate of first-attempt insertion success is an important attribute of any airway device in terms of limiting the risk of upper airway trauma and even more so for rescue indications (see "Rescue Indications") when the time taken to secure the airway is of critical importance. Depending on the clinical environment, qualifying the level of expertise required to achieve this success rate may also be important. The quality of insertion and removal, as determined by the degree of stimulation caused and the depth of anesthesia required, may be relevant to maintaining hemodynamic stability and limiting the risk of coughing and straining. In general, SGA devices have a significant benefit over ETTs at induction and during emergence, as they require lighter levels of anesthesia and are associated with less movement, coughing, breath-holding, laryngospasm, and hypoxia, both during insertion and during removal.[32]

Desirable features and essential safety features for advanced use go beyond these requirements and vary according to the clinical setting. These are discussed in "Advanced Indications."

TABLE 19.2	Desired Features of a Supraglottic Airway
Latex free	
Easy insertion	
High rate of first-time insertion attempt	
Steep learning curve and high retention of skills	
Low rate of complications of insertion	
High airway sealing pressure to enable mechanical ventilation	
Airway access	
Good esophageal seal and drain tube to reduce risk of aspiration	
Conduit for tracheal intubation	
Simple removal	
Good tolerance during emergence from anesthesia	
Minimal upper airway trauma	

Maintaining a Patent Airway and Enabling Ventilation

The primary factors that determine whether an SGA can be used effectively for controlled ventilation are a patent airway and an adequate oropharyngeal seal. For LMAs, this seal is formed when the cuff surrounds the larynx, contacting with the mucosa of the inferior and lateral hypopharynx and the base of the tongue as it projects from the hyoid bone. The important determinants and requirements for this seal are further discussed in "Advanced Indications." However, consider that appropriate use of an SGA for controlled ventilation also depends on the seal formed in the hypopharynx and esophagus, reducing the risk of gastric inflation, and/or the presence of a correctly positioned, patent drain tube for decompression, as discussed further under "Safety Features."

Access to the Airway

There are two key considerations for airway access. First, the ability to access the glottis and trachea determines the utility of the device for assessment and intubation purposes. The diameter, length, and shape of the airway tube and distal orifice components determine whether an FIS and ETT can be passed. For most LMAs, the glottis is visible via the airway tube in approximately 90% to 95% of cases. Although cuff design and alignment of the orifice with the glottis may impact the success of blind and guided intubation techniques, of more importance is the angle at which the airway tube joins the mask portion of the LMA. For all LMAs except the ILMA, the angle is acute and an ETT passed blindly through the LMA will generally pass posterior to the glottis into the esophagus. In contrast, the angle is less acute in the ILMA, and the distal portion of the ILMA airway tube incorporates a ramp that both centralizes the ETT as it leaves the airway tube and increases forward angulation. For many LMAs, blind intubation has success rates around 15% making it both impractical and not recommended as a routine or rescue technique. The ILMA is the exception, with a first-pass success rate of around 75%. In North America, LMA-type and non-LMA-type SGAs are more frequently used as a conduit to tracheal intubation than in most other countries. It is perhaps for this reason that the LMA Classic Excel, which is based on the cLMA design with a removable proximal circuit connector and an epiglottic elevating bar that allows for FIS-assisted intubation, was specifically developed for the North American market.

Second, the clinical usefulness of an SGA for head, neck, and shared airway cases depends on the profile, position, flexibility, and stability of the device once positioned and secured. The provision of a reinforced (flexible) tube in the fLMA provides the greatest versatility for this purpose, with a reduced risk of kinking or dislodgement, with movement of the tube proximally not being transmitted distally. The PLMA also has a flexible tube, but the bulk of its two-tube design and the bite block make it impractical for most intraoral surgery.

Safety Features

In terms of safety considerations, the most pertinent risks with any SGA, including LMA-type SGAs, are aspiration of gastric contents; trauma to the airway; failure of ventilation through airway obstruction or leak; and inability to access the airway, especially if the airway displaces during surgery. The latter two of these have been discussed earlier.

Aspiration Protection

Early in the introduction of the cLMA to clinical practice, concerns were raised about the risk of aspiration as a result of the device stimulating the vomiting reflex and reducing upper esophageal tone.[33] Extensive clinical experience has now clarified that aspiration risk with SGAs is low when patients are correctly selected and the device is correctly placed.[34] Although this high safety margin has contributed to the expanding use of SGAs, the requirements for safe use must be carefully heeded.

Recent developments in SGA design have focused on incorporating features that reduce the risk of aspiration and extend the safe boundaries of their use. The drain tube in second-generation SGAs provides additional protection through several mechanisms: It reduces gastric inflation by venting gas that leaks into the upper esophagus; it provides a reliable conduit for insertion of a gastric tube and drainage of air and fluid; it vents regurgitant matter, directing it beyond the oral cavity, thereby bypassing the larynx; and it provides an early alert to the anesthesiologist of the occurrence of regurgitation because of the presence of gastric contents visible in the drain tube.

In the case of the PLMA, there are several other potentially protective aspects to the design: The higher airway seal reduces the likelihood of leak from the airway, even if airway pressures are high or positive end-expiratory pressure (PEEP) is used; the bulky mask tip creates a high seal with the upper esophagus, meaning that leakage of fluid around the mask tip is less likely; and the larger bulk of the mask and its high airway seal mean that even if regurgitant matter does reach the oral cavity, the risk of aspiration is low. The LMA protector has added safety features including a pharyngeal chamber and dual gastric drainage channels, designed to channel gastric content away from the airway.

Importantly, the efficacy of all of these design features is only realized if the device is correctly positioned and an adequate hypopharyngeal seal is formed.[17,35,36] The hypopharyngeal leak pressure (HLP) is not measurable in individual patients. Cadaver studies have been used to provide indicative values for various SGA designs (see Table 19.3). The value of using these measurements as surrogates to predict the risk of aspiration when using a particular SGA is uncertain. Not only is there uncertainty about the lower threshold required to prevent expulsion of regurgitated gastric contents, but also the upper threshold to prevent the risk of esophageal rupture in the context of active vomiting.[17] Bench-top and cadaver studies have confirmed the high sealing pressure of the PLMA and its ability to protect the larynx from aspiration, even in the face of high rates of "modeled" regurgitation.[37,38]

TABLE 19.3	Currently Reported Data on Esophageal Leak Pressures in Supraglottic Airways
Supraglottic Airway	Esophageal Leak Pressure (cm H$_2$O)
LMA Classic™	≈ 40
Intubating LMA™	≈ 110
LMA ProSeal™	≈ 60–70
LMA Supreme™	≈ 60–70
i-gel™	≈ 15–20
LTS II	≈ 40

From Bercker S, Schmidbauer W, Volk T, et al. A comparison of seal in seven supraglottic airway devices using a cadaver model of elevated esophageal pressure. *Anesth Analg.* 2008;106:445-448. Schmidbauer W, Bercker S, Volk T, Bogusch G, Mager G, Kerner T. Oesophageal seal of the novel supralaryngeal airway device i-gel in comparison with the laryngeal mask airways Classic and ProSeal using a cadaver model. *Br J Anaesth.* 2009;102:135–139.

In terms of clinical outcome literature, the incidence of aspiration with cLMA use is low, between 1:4000 and 1:12,000 for elective surgery, and up to 1:1000 for emergency surgery.[34,39,40] This compares with reported rates of aspiration for the ETT of 1:4000 in elective and 1:900 for emergencies.[40] In an observational study of more than 65,000 patients, cLMA use with mechanical ventilation was not associated with an increased risk of aspiration compared with ETT use,[40] although confounding is likely. When comparing different SGA devices with each other, there is no robust clinical evidence to suggest one is superior to another in terms of aspiration protection, but also insufficient evidence to state that differences do not exist. Large case series have served to highlight common themes associated with aspiration and SGA use, including obesity, use of first-generation devices, use during the maintenance phase with light anesthesia, or controlled ventilation with a poorly positioned device.[7,41]

Although aspiration is uncommon, it is still a highly significant issue, according to the Fourth National Audit Project (NAP4) of the Royal College of Anaesthetists and the DAS, highlighting these three points:

- Aspiration is the most important safety consideration when using an SGA, with 50% of SGA complications related to aspiration.
- Serious morbidity including mortality can result when it does occur, aspiration being the most common cause of death in patients who suffered serious airway complications during anesthesia.
- Of the 17 significant cases of life-threatening aspiration with SGA use (out of the approximately 2 million cases analyzed), most were considered avoidable. The root cause of most cases was poor judgment of both the risk of aspiration and the choice of device to manage the identified risk.[7]

Atraumatic Insertion

Any foreign body or airway device that comes into contact with airway structures has the potential to cause injury and complications. Minor and temporary pharyngeal morbidity related to SGA use most commonly relates to sore throat, dysphonia, and dysphagia, all of which occur less frequently than with ETT use.[42,43] Although a primary mucosal injury may or may not be significant in itself, the potential for secondary complications including bleeding, laryngospasm, and edema is also important.

More serious complications involving vascular and nervous structures are reported, but rare and largely related to compressive injuries as a result of incorrect and prolonged SGA use. When the SGA is not inserted deeply enough or the tube rests on the lateral side of the tongue, blood vessels of the tongue can be compressed and result in tongue engorgement and cyanosis.[44] Compression of the lingual, recurrent laryngeal, or hypoglossal nerve can result in transient or prolonged nerve palsy, with cases of vocal cord paralysis also reported in the literature.[45,46] Other serious but extremely rare injuries reported in the literature include arytenoid dislocation and pharyngeal rupture with subsequent pneumomediastinum or mediastinitis.[47]

The etiology of these complications during SGA use is still poorly understood. Correct insertion techniques and positioning of the device have theoretical value, particularly in preventing compression injury. Animal studies indicate the potential for trauma with prolonged use,[48] as discussed further in "Advanced Indications." Intracuff pressure has been shown to affect the incidence of sore throat and pharyngolaryngeal morbidity[49–51] and may also contribute to compression injury (see "Important Considerations for Safe Use During Maintenance and Emergence"). Ensuring that the SGA is correctly positioned and maintaining

the cuff pressure at no higher than 60 cm H_2O are prudent steps to minimize the risk of such complications.

Indications for Use of Supraglottic Airways

Initially, Brain proposed that "the LMA may have a valuable role to play in all types of inhalational anesthesia" and in some cases of difficult intubation, such that it "may contribute to the safety of general anesthesia."[52–54] Colin Alexander, chairman of one of the first anesthesiology departments to adopt use of the LMA in the UK, concluded that the device "should be considered whenever the indication for tracheal intubation does not include protection of the airway from gastric contents."[55] Such was the impact of the cLMA in the UK that the cLMA had been ordered in all UK hospitals within a year of the first publication describing its use. For release 3 years later in the United States, the US Food and Drug Administration (FDA) added the stricture that "the LMA is not a replacement for the ETT." Subsequent adoption in North America was considerably slower and more circumspect than in the UK. Contrast this with modern anesthetic practice where over 50% of all general anesthetics are managed with an SGA in some counties, and the various advanced indications that have been adopted and continue to be proposed in the literature.[2] This history of initial adoption highlights an important issue in current practice. For the individual clinician, unfamiliarity with a device or technique is a major consideration in determining whether a practice is unsafe in his or her hands. However, this assessment is not necessarily relevant to the practice of individuals who are familiar with a device or technique, or in determining what novel practices should be researched further.

Basic Indications

Routine Use

Early indications for the cLMA when it was a novel device were appropriately cautious. The standard use of the cLMA, as originally designed, was for an anesthetized, American Society of Anesthesiologists (ASA) physical status classification I or II patient, considered low risk for aspiration, with a normal body mass index (BMI), having elective, short, low-risk peripheral surgery. Such caution is also appropriate for the novice user, but these factors relate as much to the skill, experience, and safety of the user as to the inherent utility of the device. SGAs have particular use in the OR for peripheral and ambulatory procedures associated with a low risk of aspiration, as is common in orthopedic, plastics, breast, and urologic surgery. It is also appropriate to use an SGA (particularly a fLMA) in many otolaryngology and maxillofacial procedures.

Suitability of SGA use is not necessarily limited to the OR, especially in pediatrics when the need for cooperation and immobility requires an anesthetic. An SGA can be particularly advantageous when use of a face mask is difficult, inadequate, or not possible or repeated invasive airway management exposes the patient to an increased risk of tracheal ulcerations. Suitable minor pediatric procedures include, but are not limited to, radiologic imaging, cardiology interventions, lumbar puncture or intrathecal therapy, bone marrow aspirations, vascular access procedures, and minor biopsies. Use during transesophageal echocardiography (TEE)[56] (Fig. 19.8) is also described in adults.

Controlled Ventilation

The ability to use SGAs for spontaneous ventilation or PPV was described in Brain's first paper on the cLMA.[1] However, in the first independent trial of the cLMA, concerns about the reliability of applying PPV were raised, in the context of having only a size 3 prototype

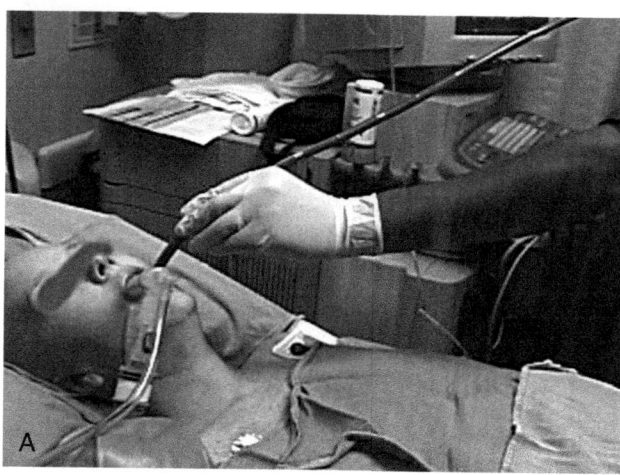
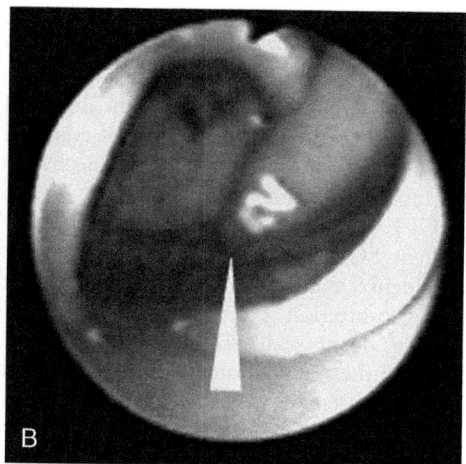

• **Fig. 19.8** Use of the laryngeal mask airway (LMA) during transesophageal echocardiography (TEE) at the University of Texas M.D. Anderson Cancer Center in Houston. The LMA is inserted after TEE placement. (A) The LMA does not interfere with TEE examination. (B) Flexible scope view through the LMA shows the TEE probe *(arrowhead)* inside the LMA bowl.

for a sample of predominantly medium- to large-build British men.[57] Multiple studies involving thousands of adult and pediatric patients have long shown that a cLMA can be used for PPV with efficacy. Such is the clinical experience of controlled ventilation with all types of LMA that it should now be considered mainstream practice.[58–61]

The efficacy of an SGA during PPV is largely dependent on close approximation of the device orifice with the larynx and the presence of an adequate oropharyngeal seal. Given the fact that the seal is created by forces acting between the cuff and surrounding mucosa, it is dependent on multiple factors. Correctly positioning the right-size device and inflation to an appropriate cuff pressure are critical to achieving the best possible seal for a particular device in a particular patient. However, safety depends on correct positioning, avoidance of hypoventilation from leakage, avoidance of gastric inflation, and prevention of regurgitation and aspiration.

As with all LMA practice, careful patient and device selection is the key to safe practice. Controlled ventilation with an SGA can be more difficult or even dangerous in patients with increased BMI, noncompliant lungs, abnormal airways, a full stomach, or gastroesophageal reflux disease. The degree of oropharyngeal seal required for effective and safe use will depend on numerous factors, including device positioning, the patient's lung compliance, and ventilatory requirements, as discussed further in Performance Testing. Among LMAs, the cLMA has the lowest oropharyngeal seal (median 18–20 cm H_2O, see Table 19.3), and in a significant proportion of cases this is inadequate to prevent a clinically significant airway leak. As peak airway pressure rises, an increasing proportion of the leaking gas enters the stomach.[58] In all but the lowest-risk cases, there is an argument for using an LMA with the best oropharyngeal seal, and in most cases a second-generation device likely adds safety. The shape and area of the SLMA cuff provides a better anatomic fit in the pharynx than does the cLMA, whereas the superior silicone-based PLMA cuff with its dorsal component permits for an even higher airway seal.[61,62] With the highest oropharyngeal seal, the PLMA and LMA Protector have the best performance characteristics for controlled ventilation.[62–64]

A patient's physiognomy in terms of the volume and elasticity of their oropharyngeal anatomy also impacts how the SGA interfaces with the airway. Early work published by Brain on the PLMA highlights this fact, noting an increasing oropharyngeal seal with increasing BMI in a small study of 20 female patients

with a BMI of 20 to 35 kg/m².[27] Unpublished work by the authors of this chapter found similar findings in obese patients, as well as a reduced oropharyngeal seal in elderly patients. Similarly, by virtue of affecting airway tone, the administration of neuromuscular blocking agents potentially alters the airway seal and may increase the degree of leak in a small proportion of patients (by 10% in approximately 10% of patients with a PLMA).[65]

Use of a pressure-controlled or pressure-support mode of ventilation is preferable because it reduces peak airway pressure compared with volume-controlled ventilation. PEEP may be applied but is unlikely to be tolerated if there is an inadequate oropharyngeal seal, and may create or worsen airway leak. In contrast, with the optimal oropharyngeal seal of the PLMA, the ability to use PEEP may improve ventilatory performance, particularly in the obese.[66]

Overall, SGAs can be safely used for controlled ventilation in appropriately selected patients and surgical situations, when the correct device is used correctly.

Rescue Indications

Although the ETT is still considered the gold standard for providing a secure airway for PPV and aspiration protection, international resuscitation bodies provide evidence of the ongoing evolution of opinion on using an SGA for airway management during cardiopulmonary resuscitation (CPR) for both in-hospital or out-of-hospital cardiac arrest.[67] The term *rapid sequence airway* (RSA) was introduced in 2007 for using an SGA to secure the airway, as an analogy to rapid sequence induction with an ETT.[68] In this setting, high first-time insertion success (including by inexperienced users), rapid deployment, reliable ventilation (including during chest compressions), and protection from aspiration are all desirable features.

A systematic review of the literature on advanced airway management during adult cardiac arrest serving to inform the International Liaison Committee of Resuscitation (ILCOR) found no high-quality evidence to indicate that ETT improved immediate survival.[69] Although the literature is conflicting and further research is required, ETTs and SGAs are recommended as advanced airway modalities for the purposes of resuscitation, each with its own pros and cons depending on the clinical situation, practitioner experience, and patient condition. Just like tracheal intubation, SGA placement may cause interruption of chest compressions.[70] To date most studies comparing SGAs to ETTs during cardiopulmonary resuscitation have studied non-LMA SGAs. The impact of airway selection on patient survival is an area of active research in both North America and Europe. At present there is no compelling evidence that one type of airway device is superior to another in the setting.

Management of the Unexpected Difficult Airway

During cLMA development, Brain used various prototypes of it to manage expected and unexpected difficult tracheal intubations.[52,54,71] In part, this experience led him to develop the ILMA, which was specifically designed for such management. After the introduction of these devices into practice, there were numerous reports of successful management of difficult airways with cLMAs and ILMAs. Since Benumof's review of the literature in the early 1990s,[72] the cLMA has been well established in the international "unexpected difficult airway" algorithms.[4-6] SGAs have two main roles, first as a rescue device for ventilation and oxygenation after failure of bag-mask ventilation or ETT placement and, second, as a conduit for intubation. SGAs may also be used to secure the airway without first attempting face mask ventilation or tracheal intubation when access is compromised and management with a face mask or ETT would be very difficult, such as when the head and neck are fixed with pins and framework or in the prone position. In modern practice, the cLMA has been replaced by second-generation SGAs as the first choice for airway rescue, and the ILMA has somewhat fallen out of favor due to the complexity of its use compared to alternatives and the potential for complications if used by the untrained.

Advanced Indications

The advanced indications for SGAs are ever expanding, and those discussed here are far from exhaustive.

Management of the Expected Difficult Airway

In addition to the rescue indications already discussed, a well-established body of literature supports the elective use of SGAs in both adult and pediatric patients for oxygenation/ventilation or as a conduit for intubation in the anticipated difficult airway, including in cervical spine instability,[73,74] micrognathia,[75,76] Klippel-Feil syndrome,[77] Treacher Collins syndrome,[78] Pierre Robin syndrome,[79] Goldenhar syndrome,[80] Hurler syndrome,[81] and Down syndrome.[82] However, as highlighted in the NAP4 report, an SGA should not be used solely as a tool to avoid having to manage an expected difficult tracheal intubation, and there should be a clear plan of action for the management of SGA failure.[7]

The cLMA specifically has a substantial body of literature to support its use in the management of a difficult airway. This is likely because it has been available for the longest time and more widely available than other LMAs. Indeed, it is highly unlikely that the cLMA is the SGA of choice for managing most predicted difficulties. Intubation via the cLMA is considered inferior to via the PLMA, ILMA, i-gel, and several other SGAs as a result of the presence of aperture bars, its relatively long length, and the difficulty of removing the cLMA once the ETT is inserted.[8] In terms of blind ETT insertion technique, in one study the cLMA was reported to have first-attempt success of 52% and an overall success rate of 59%,[83] but in practice the success is often markedly lower. Reported success with the uLMA is also notably lower at around 20%.[83,84]

With the ILMA in a study of 254 patients with difficult airways, the overall success rates for blind and FIS-guided intubation (with a maximum of three attempts) were 97% and 100%,

respectively.[85] A 98% success rate was recently reported for FIS-guided tracheal intubation with the LMA protector.[86]

Solutions to overcoming the limitations of the cLMA as a conduit for intubation include using a long ETT or an Aintree Intubation Catheter (AIC; Cook Critical Care, Bloomington, IN). An AIC is a 56-cm-long, uncuffed, semirigid rube with internal diameter 4.7 mm and external diameter 6.3 mm. Use involves a two-stage procedure whereby the AIC is placed over the FIS then railroaded into place before being used as a guide to railroading another ETT of diameter ≥7.0 mm over it and into position. Its use is theoretically more favorable with the PLMA because of its larger airway bowl without aperture bars.[63,87] Case series of AIC use with the cLMA and PLMA have been reported.[88-90] It can also be passed via an SLMA, but the narrow airway lumen, rigid angled airway tube, and presence of an epiglottic fin can trap the AIC in the sagittal plane and this limits the practicality of use with this device.[91] The Classic Excel (as described previously) and particularly the ILMA (described later) are alternative solutions.

Head, Neck, and Shared Airway Surgery

The fLMA is particularly suited for head and neck surgery. For example, the main advantages of using an fLMA for tonsillectomy or adenoidectomy are that it protects the airway from soiling better than an uncuffed ETT,[92] as it is better tolerated with fewer adverse airway events during emergence; it obviates the need for muscle relaxants and it improves OR (OR) turnaround time. However, the fLMA is not universally successful; it must be placed as distally as possible to avoid the proximal part of the cuff interfering with the surgical field, and airway obstruction may occur when adopting the tonsillectomy position in around 5% of cases, particularly when opening the Boyle-Davis gag. Use of an fLMA for these cases, especially in small children, requires skill, good communication, and cooperation between the anesthesiologist and surgeon.

Similarly, the benefits of using an SGA for eye surgery include less change in the intraocular pressure during induction and emergence from general anesthesia, with less hemodynamic stimulation and a reduced risk of coughing and bucking.[60]

Use of an SGA in adult or pediatric dental and oral surgery has also been associated with improved outcomes and reduced airway events, including airway obstruction and oxygen desaturation.[93-95]

Assessment of the Larynx and Respiratory Tree

Head and neck surgery is associated with the risk of traumatizing nerves that control laryngeal motor function. At the end of neck dissection as well as thyroid or parathyroid surgery, if an SGA has not been used throughout the surgery, it can be inserted behind the ETT and inflated before removing the ETT (the Bailey maneuver).[96] While the patient is still anesthetized, spontaneous ventilation is reestablished. An FIS is inserted through the lumen of the SGA to observe the function of the vocal cords.[97] Not only does this provide information to optimize airway management postoperatively, it also enables a smoother emergence from surgery, as SGA use is associated with less risk of coughing and straining.[98] A similar technique can also be used to assess the function of the lower cranial nerves following brainstem surgery (Fig 19.9).

The advantages of using an SGA as a conduit for flexible scope laryngoscopy and bronchoscopy are well described in the literature, especially in pediatric patients.[99-101] In adults requiring stent placement in the tracheobronchial tree, the shaft of the cLMA, i-gel, or others permits use of a 6-mm FIS, with a larger cross-sectional area than a 9-mm ETT typically used. This can enable

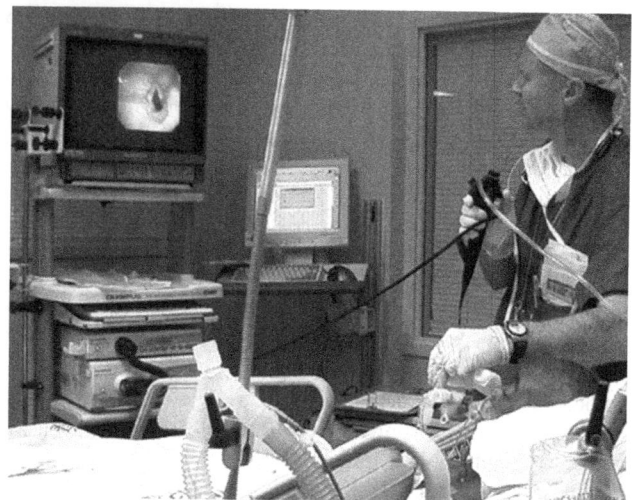

• **Fig. 19.9** A child was admitted to the intensive care unit after brainstem surgery at the University of Texas M.D. Anderson Cancer Center in Houston. Using anesthesia with propofol, the LMA was inserted behind the endotracheal tube (ETT). After successful LMA insertion, the ETT was removed to allow visualization of the vocal cords and evaluation of their function during spontaneous ventilation. This helped the intensivist and the surgeon determine whether the patient would be able to maintain an airway postoperatively.

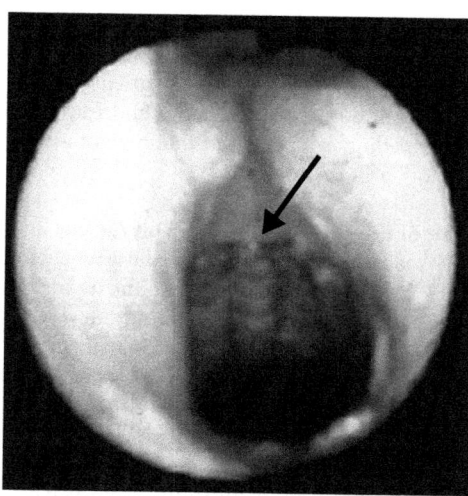

• **Fig. 19.10** Flexible scope view of a tracheal stent *(arrow)* placed high in the trachea (1.5 cm below the vocal cords) through an LMA. The shaft of the LMA permits use of a 6-mm flexible bronchoscope and provides a bigger cross-sectional area than a 9-mm endotracheal tube (ETT), enabling better ventilation during stent placement than an ETT in patients who already have compromised respiratory function.

better ventilation during stent placement and proximal tracheal stent placement without the risk of displacement during extubation (Fig. 19.10).[102]

Surgery in Prone Position

Reports of using an LMA in the prone position were first published in the early 1990s. There are now over 1600 cases in the literature,[103–106] predominantly using the PLMA, with various techniques described (see "Essential Techniques for Optimal Insertion"). Although achievable, and potentially advantageous in terms of reducing positioning injuries and resource (time and manpower) requirements associated with positioning the unconscious patient,[107–108] the current volume of reported cases is inadequate to establish this as a safe or sensible technique, particularly outside centers of expertise.[109]

In a review by Lopez and Valero, first-attempt insertion success was high (97%), with no serious complications. Transient events (including obstruction attributed to kinking, dislodgement, laryngospasm, hypoventilation, and minor leaks) occurred in 0% to 15% of cases, most of which resolved with simple corrective maneuvers.[103] In another randomized controlled trial of 134 patients having spinal surgery of <2 hours' duration, 2 obese patients (BMI 30–33 kg/m^2) had to be turned supine to manage the airway because of an insufficient SGA seal despite successful insertion.[108] This study emphasizes the importance of the need to have a backup plan in the event of difficulty. Additionally, appropriate patient selection is critical to safe use, but data are currently insufficient to fully inform this decision in an evidence-based manner.

Managing the airway in the prone position as a rescue technique, such as in the event of accidental extubation, is also reported in the literature.[110–114] Assuming the necessary skills and familiarity, this approach may be favorable to the more conventional initial response of turning the patient supine, depending on the implications of interrupting surgery and manipulating an open surgical field. Use of a guided insertion technique with the PLMA, SLMA, or a more rigid SGA such as an ILMA, LMA-Protector, or i-gel may be suitable in this setting.

Prolonged Surgery

Cases of various SGAs used without adverse effects up to 9 hours, even 24 hours in the intensive care unit (ICU) setting, are reported in the literature.[115–119] However, a small number of cases offer little perspective on the safety of this practice. The potential complications of prolonged use of SGAs remain largely theoretical; an arbitrary limit of 2 hours was proposed in the literature for first-generation devices in the early 1990s but is likely routinely exceeded.

Concerns about inflation of the stomach are becoming less relevant in the context of modern practice with second-generation devices. However, a porcine study has generated concerns relating to the potential for pressure injuries, with safe use of a PLMA up to 9 hours, but not beyond 12 to 24 hours because of mucosal trauma.[56] It is likely that appropriate monitoring and management of cuff pressure will reduce the risk of such sequelae, and this is certainly prudent where prolonged use occurs.

Minor Laparoscopic Surgery

Safe use of SGAs for gynecological and minor abdominal surgery (e.g., laparoscopic cholecystectomy) is documented in the literature, with several studies showing second-generation LMAs performing equivalently to an ETT.[50,61,98,120–126] However, there are recognized risks with this technique that must be actively managed to ensure safe use. Capnoperitoneum not only increases ventilation pressures but also ventilatory requirements to achieve normocapnia. The need for Trendelenburg positioning or the presence of parenchymal lung disease may further increase ventilation pressures. PEEP may be desirable to optimize lung function. Suggestions for safe use in laparoscopic surgery currently outlined in the literature include appropriate patient selection, use of a second-generation SGA, appropriate positioning, and performance testing, including confirmation before starting the procedure that the oropharyngeal leak pressure is ≥25 cm H$_2$O or ≥8 cm H$_2$O above the peak airway pressure required for normoventilation when supine, and confirmation that the maximal minute ventilation (MMV) is likely to be adequate for the duration of the case (around two times the resting minute ventilation).[127]

With increasing use of laparoscopy for major general surgery, it is quite possible that use of SGAs will become mainstream practice in this area. However, there is currently no evidence base to support or refute this practice. There is a theoretical risk of biliary reflux when the upper abdomen is operated on, especially during biliary surgery including laparoscopic cholecystectomy, but currently there is no evidence that use of a suitable LMA is unsafe in this setting. Confirmation of the absence of gastric inflation before surgery starts is prudent, and passage of an orogastric tube via the drain tube of a second-generation device to empty the stomach is recommended. After emptying the stomach, the orogastric tube should be removed to enable the SGA drain tube to function normally.

Moderately Obese Patients

In NAP4, obese patients (BMI > 35 kg/m^2) were noted to be over-represented in cases of airway complication, particularly those involving use of a first-generation SGA.[7] The relevance of this to second-generation devices is uncertain. Additionally, there is a growing body of literature indicating the potential advantages of using second-generation SGAs in moderately obese patients having peripheral surgery. Zoremba and colleagues studied patients with a BMI between 30 and 35 kg/m^2 having minor peripheral surgery lasting <2 hours and found those managed with a PLMA had significantly superior respiratory variables, including peripheral oxygen saturation and standard lung function tests up to 24 hours postoperatively.[128] There was a lower rate of laryngospasm/bronchospasm in the PLMA group, but this did not reach statistical significance. These findings have been further validated in a subsequent Cochrane systematic review that reported PLMA use was better than an ETT in obese patients in terms of improved oxygenation and reduced coughing. However, in 3% to 5% of cases insufficient ventilation required conversion to an ETT early in the induction phase.[129]

Effective and safe use in the moderately obese does not mean SGAs are safe in severe obesity. Although an evidence base for a safety "cutoff BMI" is lacking (and this is likely to vary with patient, procedure, position, device, and operator experience), as obesity increases lung and chest wall compliance falls, safe apnea time falls and the risk of failure of all airway rescue techniques increases. Risk-benefit analysis should be considered in all obese patients before deciding to use an SGA and in selecting which SGA to use.

Pregnant Patients

Successful and safe use of SGAs (predominantly the PLMA, SLMA, and i-gel) has been reported in both elective and emergent cesarean delivery cases, mostly in fasted nonobese parturients.[130–134] A high first-attempt insertion success rate (98%–99%) was noted, with no reports of aspiration (a single case of regurgitation only), significant hypoxia, or laryngospasm/bronchospasm. A recent systematic review and meta-analysis of 14 studies, including 2236 low-risk patients undergoing cesarean delivery and comparing SGAs and ETT, found similar first-attempt success rates and no difference in adverse events. However, the authors concluded that their analysis was underpowered to detect adverse events and therefore inconclusive.[135] Although to date routine use of second-generation SGAs in obstetric patients is not established practice, this evidence is very important in informing acceptable management of the unexpectedly difficult intubation during cesarean

section.[136] (See Chapter 37 for more on airway management of the obstetric patient.)

Upper Gastrointestinal Procedures

The LMA Gastro is designed to enable simultaneous ventilation of the lungs and upper gastrointestinal access through a 16-mm-internal-diameter endoscopy channel.[137] It was effectively used to perform upper gastrointestinal endoscopy and endoscopic retrograde cholangiopancreatography, peroral endoscopic myomectomy, and percutaneous endoscopic gastrostomies.[137–139] Saxena and colleagues reported the successful insertion of a TEE probe though the endoscopy channel of the LMA Gastro in 9 patients.[140] The Gastro Laryngeal tube, which was released before the LMA Gastro, is a similar device based on the laryngeal tube.

In summary, there are numerous advanced uses of SGAs, many of which would not have been contemplated a decade ago. Some of these remain controversial. In most instances, the second-generation devices are best suited to these advanced uses. The safe limits of use of SGAs have not yet been established. One problem with this is that only by passing beyond our limits is it possible to determine where those limits lie, and this puts patients at risk. A cautious, slowly evolving, evidence-based advance is therefore appropriate, but ultimately the indications for using an SGA will likely increase rather than decrease in the foreseeable future.

Fundamentals of Correct Supraglottic Airway Use

In the NAP4 report, the most common contributory and causal factors in adverse airway events were poor training and judgment. These are arguably the two most important requirements a clinician must fulfill for safe use of SGAs: competency training in specific techniques and adequate knowledge and judgment to select whether to use an SGA and, if so, the correct device for the specific requirements of each case. One would never assume an ETT to be functional in the hands of an untrained individual who cannot avoid dental damage, detect incorrect placement in the esophagus, or judge the appropriate timing for extubation. The approach to safe and effective use of SGAs, particularly for advanced indications, is no different.

In terms of training, size selection, use of the correct insertion technique, and placement tests are critical to ensuring correct positioning and optimal function of an SGA. Performance tests and appropriate vigilance are also important for the full duration of SGA use, including appropriate fixation and positioning throughout the case; careful monitoring of cuff pressure; maintenance of an adequate depth of anesthesia; ensuring optimal conditions and timing for removal; and instituting safe clinical practices universal to all types of airway management. These safe practices include adequate vigilance for prompt identification of an obstructed or displaced airway and making provisions for a backup plan in the event of a complication or failure.

Although the learning curve for proficiency at LMA insertion is estimated at around 70 to 80 cases,[141] the knowledge and abilities required for safe use of an SGA for advanced indications are less clear. Pragmatically, Brain recommended mastering LMA use for basic indications and gradually progressing to more complex uses. Brimacombe reported a short and long learning curve for LMA use, the latter extending to 750 cases.[142] Training in basic SGA insertion techniques and routine use should be an early and fundamental part of every novice anesthesiologist's training. Manikins can be useful as practice trainers before clinical training is undertaken. Learning techniques with the ILMA may be more challenging, but it is a low morbidity procedure and it is a suitable device to use in normal airways, with informed patient consent, to develop the skills and familiarity necessary for success in an emergency situation.

Essential Techniques for Optimal Insertion

Basic LMA Insertion Techniques

The LMA occupies a potential space that is shared by the respiratory and alimentary tracts, which are subject to the control and coordination of several complex reflexes. Although anesthesiologists do not need a detailed knowledge of these specific reflexes to use an LMA, they do need to understand the basic concept behind the recommended insertion technique, which ensures the greatest success and results with the fewest complications. Physiologically, the alimentary tract is capable of accepting (i.e., swallowing) or rejecting (i.e., vomiting) liquids or solids in the form of food. In contrast, the respiratory tract mobilizes defensive responses (e.g., coughing, laryngospasm, bronchospasm) when invaded by liquids or solids (e.g., an ETT). When inserted correctly, the LMA does not stimulate the respiratory tract defenses because the device forms an end-to-end seal against the periglottic tissues.

The recommended standard insertion technique was developed by Brain, over more than a decade of experience. After experimenting with numerous alternative insertion techniques and adjuncts, he realized that his technique was becoming more and more similar to the physiologic act of swallowing food. By studying this mechanism more closely and allowing for the fact that in the anesthetized patient this reflex is generally abolished, the following key points emerged:

1. *Device preparation.* After checking the patency of the device and integrity of the cuff by completely deflating and reinflating the cuff with the maximum recommended volume of air, the device should be fully deflated before insertion. Performing this while pressing the anterior portion of the mask onto a sterile flat surface ensures an appropriately shaped cuff for insertion. The purpose of this process allows the LMA to be presented as a soft foodlike bolus, where any contact pressure generated is distributed widely over the palatal surface, avoiding any localized high-pressure points that could stimulate a rejection reflex depending on the depth of anesthesia. Additionally, when fully deflated, the dorsal surface becomes hollow and can be inverted when pressed into the dome of the hard palate to create a gentle springlike effect, spreading pressure evenly over the hard palate. Partial mask inflation could not achieve this aim because the soft distal end of the mask rolls back. Inserting a fully inflated mask introduces excessive bulk that could stimulate a rejection reflex, much like an excessively large food bolus, with the additional risk of tearing the cuff against teeth. The posterior portion of the device should also be prepared by applying a sterile water-based lubricant just before insertion. Just as lubrication is a key part of deglutition, this is important to aid smooth insertion.

2. *Patient preparation.* Anesthetic technique is important for improving insertion conditions. An adequate depth of anesthesia is required for the patient to tolerate a jaw thrust.[143] For the cLMA, propofol,[144] opioids,[145] local anesthetic spray to the throat,[146] nitrous oxide,[147] and intravenous lidocaine[148] are all associated with improved insertion conditions. Neuromuscular blockade is not routinely required. Correct positioning of the patient's head and neck is also important, with a sniffing position for the cLMA and PLMA, neutral for the SLMA, and either for ILMA. This position can be maintained with use of a pillow and the clinician holding the occiput in the nondominant hand, pressing caudally. By pushing the head of the supine patient in a caudal direction by the clinician's supinated hand, head extension, neck flexion, and mouth opening are simultaneously achieved. This maneuver widens the oropharyngeal angle >90 degrees in the normal subject and draws the larynx away from the posterior pharyngeal wall. Both effects facilitate LMA insertion. Provision of a jaw thrust by an airway assistant can aid smooth passage of the LMA by increasing the pharyngeal space.

3. *Flatten the mask against the hard palate.* This is the first step of LMA insertion. The best way to apply the necessary force is by placing the index finger on the anterior side of the airway tube at its junction with the mask under the deflated proximal rim of the cuff.

4. *Widening the oropharyngeal angle.* This is the first role of the nondominant hand while advancing the LMA with the dominant hand. The nondominant hand should maintain firm caudal pressure on the occiput from the start of insertion until the mask has passed behind the tongue.

5. *Cranioposterior movement of the index finger.* In swallowing, the bolus of food is advanced into the pharynx, esophagus, and stomach through precise coordination of several muscle groups, beginning with the tongue. During LMA insertion, the clinician should use the index finger to advance the mask in the cranioposterior direction, imitating the action of the tongue. This allows a completely deflated LMA tip to slide smoothly along the hard palate, soft palate, and posterior pharyngeal wall while minimizing the contact of the mask with anterior and inferior structures such as the base of the tongue, epiglottis, and laryngeal inlet. The finger must continue to push in a cranioposterior direction even though the anatomy forces the mask and the finger to move caudally. The finger follows the mask as it is advanced along the curve of the airway and inserted to its fullest extent or until resistance is felt as the mask tip enters the upper esophageal sphincter (UES). It is anatomically impossible to perform this action correctly without extending the proximal metacarpophalangeal joint of the index finger and the wrist.

6. *Aiding removal of the index finger.* This is the second role of the nondominant hand. For many operators, the index finger is not long enough to advance the LMA mask into the UES. When the mask is inserted as far as possible, the nondominant hand can then hold the LMA stem and advance the LMA further into place until resistance is felt, as the UES is reached. The index finger should remain in place throughout this to prevent axial rotation. To prevent the mask sliding out of position after it is fully inserted, the nondominant hand should hold the proximal end of the LMA before the index finger is removed. As the index finger is removed, the mask is held steady.

7. *The mask is inflated.* As the mask is inflated, inflation of the tip causes it to slide cranially and out of the mouth. It can be shown anatomically that this results in loss of contact between the mask tip and the UES. However, the LMA should not be held in place during inflation because this can result in the distal end of the mask stretching the UES. All LMAs should be

inflated to a pressure of no more than 60 cm H_2O (see "Important Considerations for Safe Use During Maintenance and Emergence").

8. *Device fixation restores stability of the seal against the UES.* The distal end of the tube is again pressed into the curve of the hard palate to reestablish firm contact between the proximal end of the device and the UES. As this pressure is maintained, the LMA is secured in position either with adhesive tape or a tie. Fixation should exert a modest inward force to maintain the LMA position (e.g., tape can be applied to the maxilla on one side of the patient's face and passed over and under the tube in a single loop before fixing it to the opposite maxilla).

If an LMA is inserted when cricoid force is applied, it is necessary to remove the cricoid force before insertion. Cricoid force obliterates the hypopharyngeal space and the LMA cannot be advanced into position with its tip in the UES. Reapplication of cricoid pressure after insertion significantly impedes ventilation via the cLMA but not the PLMA.[149,150]

Excellent technique is critical to good placement and optimal function of any LMA, but especially the fLMA and PLMA. The standard insertion technique generally results in a reliable airway, a minimal stress response, and an extremely low risk of complications, probably because the LMA's position in relation to the respiratory and alimentary tracts is optimal. Although some report a 10% failure rate as acceptable, good technique and attention to detail are likely to reduce this failure rate considerably. Multiple alternative insertion methods are advocated in the literature, which can create confusion. Many of these approaches were tried and rejected by Brain for being traumatic or unreliable before he described the standard technique. Insertion failure causes harm to individual patients, and poor technique also prevents the acquiring of skills necessary for more advanced clinical applications of LMAs.

Alternatively, an LMA can be inserted with the help of either direct or video-assisted laryngoscopy. This technique may aid insertion and detect malpositioning or incorrect size selection. However, it is not necessary for routine use.

Insertion Techniques for the Proseal and Supreme LMA

The PLMA is more difficult to insert than the cLMA because of its large-size soft cuff and bulky tip, both of which increase the likelihood of posterior folding during insertion. The lack of a rigid backplate in the PLMA also increases the risk of folding compared with the cLMA.

Whichever insertion technique is used, adequate depth of anesthesia, complete mask deflation, posterior mask lubrication, active jaw thrust, and good technique are all important to success.

There are three insertion techniques:

1. *Digital technique.* This is as described for the cLMA earlier, but the index finger may be placed in a small pocket at the base of the airway tube anteriorly.

2. *Insertion tool technique.* The specially designed introducer tool is placed into the pocket at the base of the tube shaft (Fig. 19.11) and proximally clipped onto the PLMA airway tube at the proximal end of the bite block. The introducer tool therefore curves and stabilizes the tube portion of the PLMA and creates an introducing handle. The PLMA is then advanced along the superior posterior aspect of the airway, in a similar manner to insertion of the ILMA (described later). Once the PLMA is correctly positioned, the introducer tool can be easily removed, taking care to avoid the teeth.

When using either the digital or insertion tool techniques, it is useful to insert a finger into the mouth, once the mask is inserted

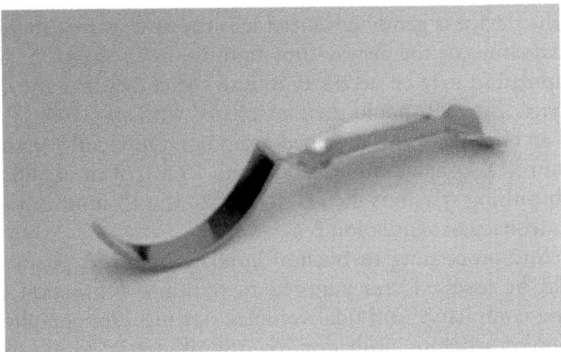

• **Fig. 19.11** Proseal LMA introducer tool. (Teleflex Medical Europe Ltd, Athlone, Ireland.)

toward the posterior aspect of the hard palate, to confirm that the distal tip of the device has not folded over. Avoiding the tip folding over as the mask negotiates the angle between mouth and pharynx prevents the entire mask folding over and malposition (see "Identifying Malposition").

3. *Bougie-guided technique.* A bougie is placed, straight end first, into the esophagus under direct vision with gentle laryngoscopy.[151] This may be done before or after placing the lubricated proximal end of the bougie through the drain tube of the PLMA. The PLMA is then passed into position over the bougie; jaw thrust during insertion improves success. This technique was originally described with a gum elastic bougie (Eschmann tracheal tube introducer) but can also be performed with other bougies. Alternative bougies may be quite rigid, and care must be taken during esophageal placement to avoid trauma.

Although no difference in insertion success has been demonstrated when comparing use of an introducer tool with the digital technique, Brimacombe achieved a 100% first-pass insertion rate when using the bougie-guided technique, in both routine and simulated difficult laryngoscopy, with no increase in airway trauma or sequelae.[87,152] The PLMA has also been successfully passed over nasogastric tubes and flexible intubation stylets, but there is less evidence to support these techniques.[153]

The SLMA, as compared with the PLMA, has some built-in rigidity, so there is no need for an introducer tool. Although the SLMA can be easily inserted over an orogastric tube, it is not easily inserted over a bougie because the curve of the shaft of this device is too acute. The SLMA has a fixation tab proximally, and this is useful for guiding insertion depth, being designed to be approximately 2 cm from the lips.

Insertion Technique for the Intubating LMA

The use of the ILMA is not entirely intuitive. Several high-profile airway misadventures have featured misuse or misunderstanding of best practice with the ILMA, and it is therefore important to understand the correct insertion technique in detail. However, even when used infrequently by emergency physicians, the ILMA provides successful ventilation and oxygenation in 98% of cases and successful insertion of an ETT in 83% of patients.[154]

The ILMA is designed for insertion with the patient's head and neck in the neutral position, though it also works in the sniffing position. As with other LMAs, the use of a jaw lift is recommended during insertion to lift the epiglottis off the posterior pharyngeal wall and increase pharyngeal space. It is useful to place the tip of the handle against the patient's chest and the tip of the mask at the mouth before starting. The ILMA handle is then held, and the device is gently advanced into the airway, rotating along the curvature of the airway tube until it sits in the UES. Some manipulation may be necessary to turn the corner into the upper pharynx. The cuff should then be inflated with air (10 to 20 mL) until an effective seal is obtained or up to an intracuff pressure of 60 cm H_2O. Usually, cuff inflation with 10 mL of air is sufficient. The breathing system is then connected to the 15-mm connector, and adequacy of ventilation is assessed.

Before proceeding to tracheal intubation, ILMA positioning should be assessed and adjusted to optimize ventilation (e.g., highest compliance and tidal volumes, optimal capnography and spirometry). Before intubation, the risk of glottic closure should generally be minimized by administration of a neuromuscular blocking drug, although topical local anesthesia may also be used if paralysis is contraindicated. The patient should be fully preoxygenated. An appropriately sized (generally small) ETT should be selected and prepared by fully deflating the cuff and lubricating the outer surface. The type of ETT is important to success. Using the specially designed ILMA tracheal tube (ILMA-TT, an uncurved, reinforced, flexible silicone ETT with a soft, bullet-shaped tip and longitudinal and transverse markings that guide intubation) will maximize the chances of successful intubation while minimizing the risk of airway trauma. Of note, the ILMA-TT cuff is either low-volume, high-pressure (reusable version) or intermediate-volume, intermediate-pressure (single-use version), and this should be taken into account during its use and after placement.

The ETT connector should be removed (but not discarded) and the ETT inserted through the ILMA to a depth of approximately 12 to 15 cm (or until the horizontal mark on the ILMA-TT enters the ILMA stem). This places the distal tip of the ETT at or just proximal to the opening of the ILMA airway tube within the mask cavity. There is a silicone bar at the end of the airway tube, the epiglottic elevator, which is attached to the ILMA only at one end. Passage of the ETT beyond this point raises the elevator, which displaces the epiglottis from its position protecting the glottic inlet. As the ETT passes through the airway tube a ramp ensures it exits the tube in the midline and deflects it anteriorly toward the glottis. Several acceptable methods can then be used to advance the ETT into the trachea, although the literature supports a flexible scope-guided technique.

Flexible Scope Technique. An FIS is passed through the ETT and into the trachea. There are two techniques, based on whether the scope or tube is inserted first. In the "scope first technique," the FIS is advanced without advancing the ETT and the operator must negotiate the FIS around the epiglottic elevator before entering the glottis. In the "tube first technique," the ETT and FIS are advanced together, raising the epiglottic elevator. The FIS is then advanced through the ETT toward the glottis. The tube first technique requires less skill and is quicker if the glottis is directly behind the epiglottic elevator, but if it is not, it is then difficult to locate the glottis and advance the FIS toward it. If the anatomy is suspected to be difficult or the glottis cannot be seen with a tube first technique, the scope first technique is more likely to be successful in the hands of a skilled operator (Fig. 19.12). When the carina is seen, the FIS can be left in place and the ETT advanced over it using the FIS as a guide. It is here that a smaller ETT has benefits in that it advances more easily. The ETT cuff can then be inflated, the scope removed, and the ETT connector replaced. The FIS-ILMA combination allows a controlled visual technique with success rates up to 100%.[85]

Blind Technique. The recommend technique for blind intubation through the ILMA is the Chandy maneuver.[56] It consists of two steps that are performed sequentially. The first step is important for establishing optimal ventilation and useful for any ILMA technique. It involves rotating the ILMA slightly in the sagittal plane using the metal handle until ventilation is optimal (best compliance and least resistance or leak). The second step is performed just before blind intubation and consists of using the metal handle to lift the ILMA anteriorly away from the posterior pharyngeal wall (but avoiding tilting the mask). This facilitates the smooth passage of the ETT into the trachea (Fig. 19.13). The anesthetic circuit can then be attached to the ETT connector, and capnography may be used as a guide to successful tracheal placement. If resistance to further advancement is encountered, the ILMA should be repositioned. After successful tracheal intubation has been achieved with any of these techniques, the ETT cuff should be inflated, and adequate ventilation should be assessed by observation of bilateral chest movement, auscultation, capnography, or spirometry, as appropriate.

Removal of the ILMA while leaving the ETT in place is the step that most often causes problems. Because the ILMA does cause pressure on the airway if left in place, it should be removed whenever it is possible and safe to do so. When the appropriate position of the ETT is confirmed, the 15-mm connector of the ETT should be removed and the ILMA stabilizing rod used to enable removal of the ILMA. The stabilizing rod is placed, tapered end first, into the proximal end of the ETT until it engages the ETT. The cuff of the ILMA is deflated to enable easier removal. The stabilizing rod is used to maintain the position of the ETT as the ILMA is slowly withdrawn. This should continue until most of the stabilizer is inside the airway tube of the ILMA, but no farther. At this point the stabilizer rod must be removed and the ETT grasped within or as it exits the mouth. ILMA removal can then be completed while the ETT is held gently in place. If the stabilizing rod is left in place while the ILMA is fully removed over the ETT, it is inevitable that the pilot tube of the ETT is avulsed. When this happens, the ILMA-TT cuff deflates and ventilation is no longer possible. Adequate training and correct technique prevent this problem, but if it does occur an 18 G or 20 G cannula or needle attached to a syringe can be inserted into the remaining pilot tube and the cuff reinflated. The 15-mm ETT connector can then be replaced and the correct position of the ETT in the trachea reconfirmed.

Insertion Techniques in the Prone Position

The technique for SGA insertion in the self-positioned prone patient is based on the same technique used in the supine position (as described earlier). The only variation between published techniques relates to the positioning of the patient's head and neck, either extended and elevated in the sagittal plane with the aid of an assistant[155,156] or facing lateral with an optional lateral table tilt.[62,108,157] If the first insertion attempt fails, some authors recommend using a laryngoscope to insert the straight end of a gum elastic bougie into the proximal esophagus to then pass a PLMA into place. This can be left in place during use to enable repositioning if the PLMA partially displaces. Others routinely insert a suction catheter into the esophagus via the gastric drain.[62] The reported success rate for first insertion attempt in the prone position did not differ for the cLMA, the PLMA, and the SLMA.[103] However, performance characteristics would predict that failure rates during use and airway leak may differ between these and other devices.

Predictors of Difficult or Failed Supraglottic Airway Use

Failure to insert and provide ventilation through an SGA (after multiple attempts) is rare, with a quoted incidence between 0.2%

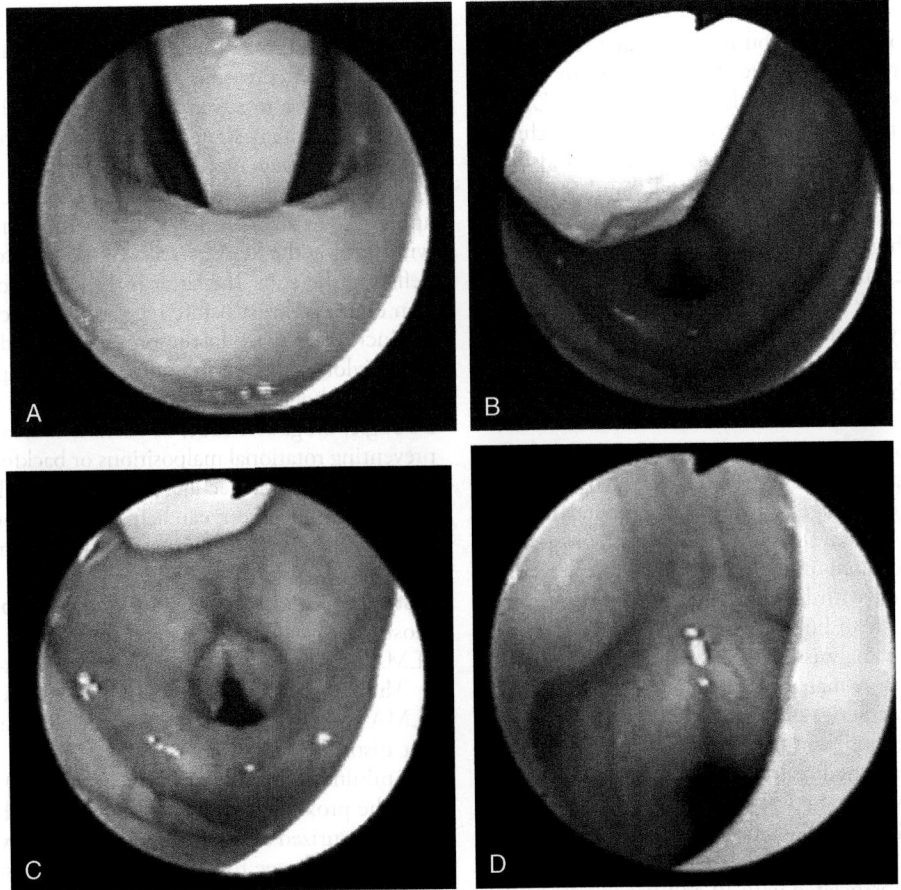

• **Fig. 19.12** (A–D) Flexible scope view of intubation through the intubating laryngeal mask airway (ILMA). (A) Epiglottic elevating bar (EEB) as seen from inside the shaft. (B) The tip of the endotracheal tube (ETT), as it advances through the ILMA, pushes the EEB upward. (C) This movement of the EEB lifts the epiglottis out of the way. (D) It also provides a clear passage for the ETT through the vocal cords.

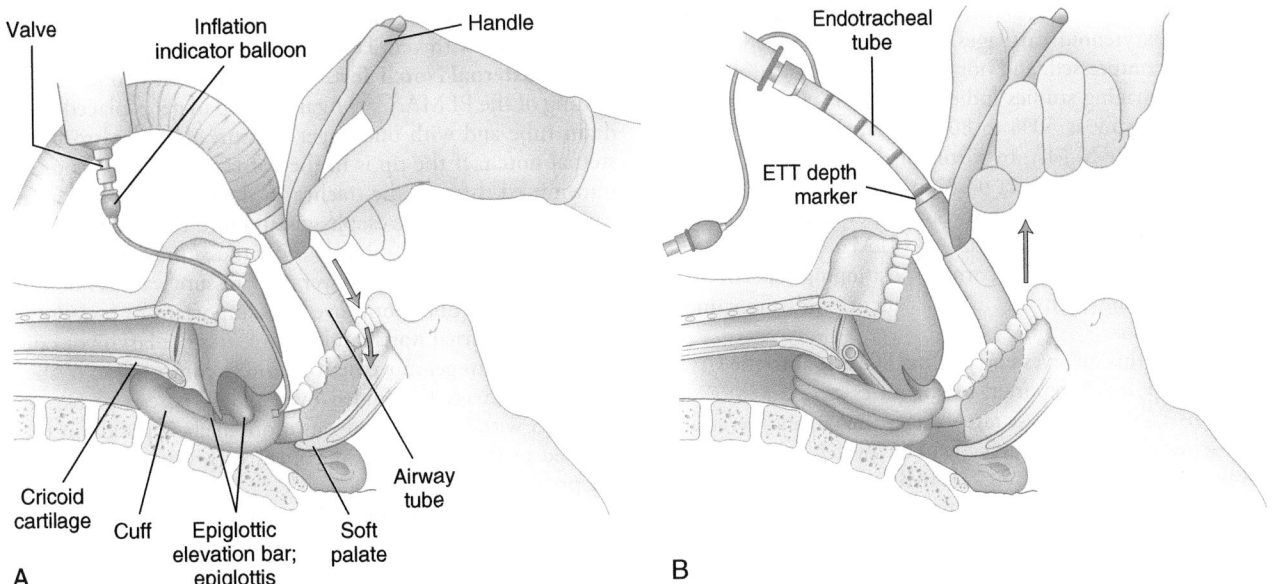

• **Fig. 19.13** The Chandy maneuver consists of two steps that are performed sequentially. (A) The first step is important for establishing optimal ventilation. The intubating laryngeal mask airway (ILMA) is rotated slightly in the sagittal and/or coronal planes using the metal handle until the least resistance to bag ventilation is achieved. (B) The second step is performed just before blind intubation. The metal handle is used to lift away slightly (but not tilt) the ILMA from the posterior pharyngeal wall. This facilitates the smooth passage of the endotracheal tube (ETT) into the trachea.

and 4.7%.[39,158–163] There is a wide variety of definitions of SGA *failure* and a paucity of literature outlining predictors of difficulty, mainly limited to retrospective data analyses. In a large case-control trial of over 15,000 adult patients in the United States, four independent risk factors of uLMA failure included surgical table rotation, male gender, poor dentition, and BMI >30 kg/m^2.[159] Of relevance, those patients in whom uLMA failed also had a threefold increased incidence of difficult mask ventilation. The same research group also completed a similar study of nearly 12,000 pediatric patients using the uLMA and cLMA and identified independent risk factors for failure: patient transport, otolaryngologic surgery, nonoutpatient admission status, prolonged surgery, and a congenital/acquired airway abnormality.[160] Interestingly, none of the risk factors overlapped between the two patient populations.

Another research group from Singapore identified four risk factors for SGA (including cLMA, PLMA, SLMA, ILMA, or i-gel) failure including male gender, age >45 years, thyromental distance <6 cm, and limited neck movement.[161] Subsequent prospective validation of a risk score based on these factors was found to have utility as a screening tool, with high specificity (95%) and negative predictive value (99.6%) but poor sensitivity (23%).[162] In a recent large retrospective analysis including 19,693 adult patients involving an SGA for airway management, use of desflurane and a smaller SGA size were predictive of failure.[163]

In addition to the inherent limitations of observational research, there are fundamental restrictions in the generalizability of this information, not only between SGA devices but patient populations as well. This is highlighted in the findings of a meta-analysis of PLMA failure, noting that there may be increased failure and trauma rates associated with PLMA use in patients of Asian ethnicity, particularly when the size of PLMA is based on gender rather than weight.[164]

Identification of SGA Malposition

For optimal functioning, the tip of the SGA must sit in the hypopharynx and upper esophagus, in the postcricoid region, behind and below the arytenoid cartilages. The larynx should be freely accessible, not compressed, and not obstructed by downfolding of the epiglottis. Imaging studies indicate that SGA malpositioning can occur in as many as 50% to 80% of patients.[165] The PLMA and to an extent the SLMA, by virtue of the presence of a drain tube, can be assessed for correct position of the device or facilitate diagnosis of malposition before use. Such assessments are not feasible with the cLMA, uLMA, fLMA, and ILMA.

Fig. 19.14 illustrates the correct positioning of an SGA (Fig. 19.14A), along with the most frequent, and often undetected, malpositions.

- *Glottic entry.* This involves entry of the SGA tip into the laryngeal entrance. It was reported in one series to occur in 6% of PLMA insertions[166] but was rarely if ever seen in another much larger series.[167] Ventilation is likely to be severely impaired, and airway morbidity is a risk (Fig. 19.14B).
- *Inadequate depth of insertion.* When the SGA is not advanced sufficiently, the tip lies too far proximally, insufficiently sealing the upper esophagus and increasing the risk of a compressive base-of-tongue injury (Fig. 19.14C). Ventilation is impaired by significant leak, and the airway seal is low.
- *Overfolding.* This almost invariably occurs backward with the fold at the midsection of the mask (Fig. 19.14D).

These malpositions are all likely to impact effective ventilation, and multiple safety functions of the device are potentially

impaired, particularly those related to prevention of aspiration and airway trauma. Therefore, it is important that they are identified early and corrected. Correct positioning is especially important before use in advanced settings or in higher-risk patients.

There are many strategies to correct malpositioning once identified. The *up-down and Klein maneuvers* were described for clearing a downfolded epiglottis when using an ILMA, but it is broadly applicable to all SGA devices.[168,169] The former maneuver involves withdrawing the SGA partially (~6 cm) before reinsertion without deflating the cuff. The latter is the same technique with the addition of a jaw thrust before reinsertion, which is particularly useful for increasing space in the oropharynx and the distance between the epiglottis and the posterior oropharyngeal wall.[165] Placement of a second-generation SGA with a drain tube by advancing over a bougie, orogastric tube, or suction catheter is well described for preventing rotational malpositions or backfolding of the tip (as discussed in "Essential Techniques for Optimal Insertion"). Finally, use of a videolaryngoscope can help provide information as to the cause of malposition and therefore the corrective measure required.[165]

Testing to Identify Correct or Incorrect Positioning

Most tests have been designed to use with LMAs, especially the PLMA, but may be suitable for certain non-LMA SGAs.

The Soap or Bubble Test. This test was first described for the PLMA and can be used in SGAs with a drain tube to confirm correct distal tip positioning.[27,170–172] The test involves inserting gel (the minimal amount to seal the drain tube) or soap to form a film over the proximal end of the drain tube. The anesthetic circuit is then pressurized and the drain tube is observed. In essence the test assesses the degree to which the gastrointestinal (drain tube) and respiratory (airway tube) components of the device are separated. If the SGA is correctly positioned, the column of gel will remain undisturbed and the test is negative (Fig. 19.15A). If the SGA is not inserted fully, the drain tube communicates with the respiratory system, causing the gel to be forced out (or the soap film to balloon) (Fig. 19.15B). If the patient is breathing spontaneously and the device is inadequately inserted, the gel (or soap film) will move in time with ventilation.

Suprasternal Notch Test. This test is described to detect overfolding of the PLMA.[172,173] Again a drop of gel is placed inside the drain tube and with one finger pressure is applied to the suprasternal notch. If the tip is in the correct position, this pressure is transmitted through the trachea to the esophagus and a pressure wave rises through the esophagus and into the drain tube. The gel column moves synchronously with the suprasternal notch pressure. If the PLMA is folded over, the pressure wave is not transmitted and the gel does not move. It is important to press low down in the suprasternal notch and not to press the larynx or cricoid as this will lead to gel movement by direct compression of the SGA, even if the mask has folded over. A low false-negative rate was observed with this test and was more likely if the drain tube was blocked or the esophagus was open, with weaker transmission of the pressure changes.[172]

Gastric Tube Insertion. Not only can insertion of a gastric tube through the drain tube and into the esophagus assist with the ease of insertion, but insertion without resistance excludes the possibility that the tip of the airway is twisted or folded.[27] However, this test provides no indication of whether the depth of positioning is adequate.

External Landmarks. Design features such as the positioning of the bite block or fixation tab were intended to help confirm correct insertion depth. When more than half of the bite block on a PLMA

Position	Position and Performance Test Outcomes
Correct placement, with the tip in the hypopharynx 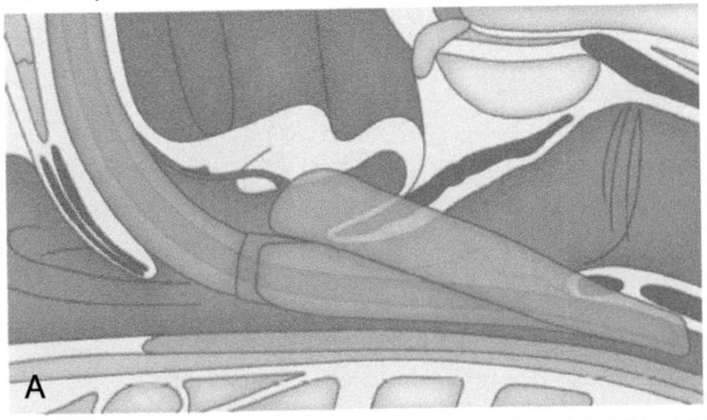 A	Minimal resistance to insertion Bite block >50% beyond the lips A gastric tube passes easily Soap/gel does not move with ventilation or APL closure Soap/gel does not move during chest compression Soap/gel "bobs" with suprasternal pressure Adequate airway seal
Insertion of the tip into the glottis 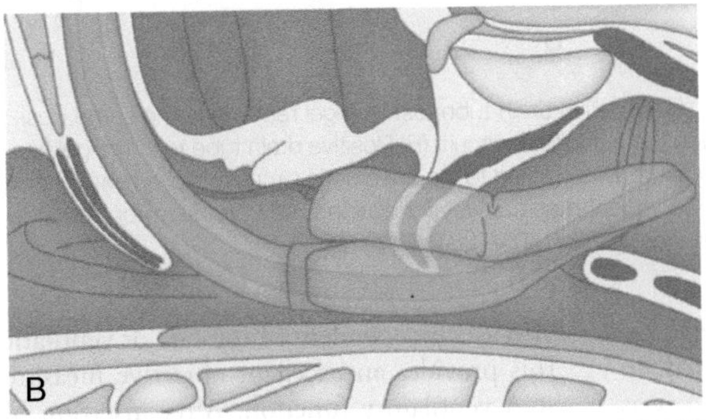 B	Bite block often >50% visible Cannot ventilate the lungs Soap/gel moves during chest compression
The SGA is not inserted deeply enough 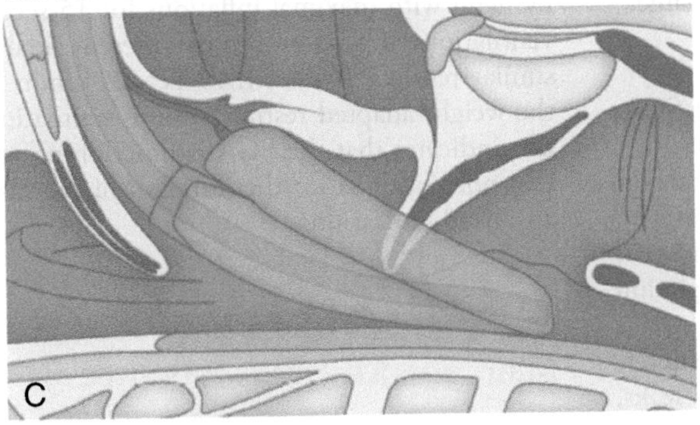 C	Bite block >50% visible Soap/gel moves during ventilation or APL valve closure Low airway seal
Back-folding of the mask 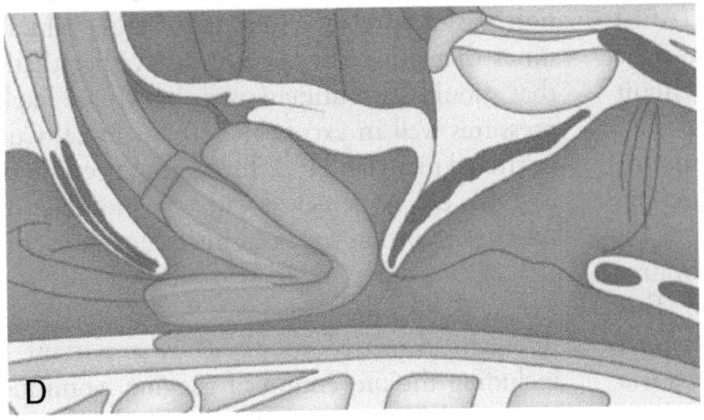 D	Resistance felt during insertion Bite block >50% visible A gastric tube cannot be passed Soap/gel does not move with suprasternal pressure Airway seal may be high or low

• **Fig. 19.14** Assessing for correct placement (A) and malposition of a second-generation supraglottic airway device (B–D). *APL,* Adjustable pressure leak; *SGA,* supraglottic airway device. (Adapted from Bercker S, Schmidbauer W, Volk T, et al. A comparison of seal in seven supraglottic airway devices using a cadaver model of elevated esophageal pressure. *Anesth Analg.* 2008;106(2):445–448.)

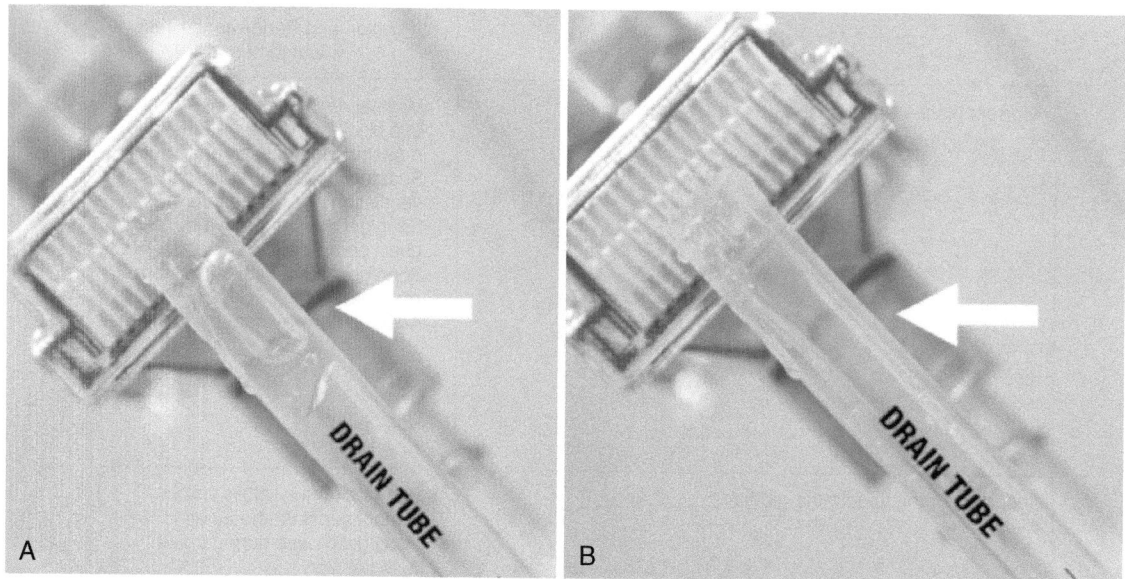

• **Fig. 19.15** The drain tube "bubble" test. (A) Negative drain tube test: the gel remains in the same position *(white arrow)* when pressure is applied to the anesthetic circuit. (B) Positive drain tube test: the gel has been pushed out of the drain tube when pressure was applied to the anesthetic circuit *(white arrow)*. (From Timmermann A, Bergner UA, Russo SG. Laryngeal mask airway indications: new frontiers for second-generation supraglottic airways. *Curr Opin Anaesthesiol.* 2015;28(6):717–726.)

protrudes over the anterior teeth, it must be assumed that the insertion depth is inadequate[174] or the wrong size has been selected. In early pilot studies, when the fixation tab of an SLMA (size 4) was <1.5 to 2 cm from the upper lip, it indicated the size chosen was too small, and more than 3 cm indicated the size chosen was too large.[28]

Performance Testing

Multiple patient and surgical factors can make the use of SGAs for ventilation more demanding, especially in advanced settings. Additionally, insertion of the SGA can cause the glottis to narrow or the epiglottis to fold, partially obstructing the airway.[57,166] Therefore, to confirm adequate opening of the glottis and that appropriate ventilation can be predictably achieved, completion of two performance tests are recommended.

Oropharyngeal Leak Pressure Test. This test is used to determine the maximum airway pressure achievable before air leaks, impairing the ability to ventilate and increasing the risk of gastric inflation. To determine the oropharyngeal leak pressure (OLP), the ventilator is switched off and the adjustable pressure leak (APL) valve is closed to 30 cm H_2O with the fresh gas flow set to 3 L/min (some use 40 cm H_2O and 5 L/min[175]). The airway and circuit pressure will progressively increase until it plateaus or there is an audible leak, which is the point where airway pressure corresponds to the OLP. For use in advanced indications, especially laparoscopic surgery, it is recommended that the OLP should be ≥25 cm H_2O, or ≥8 cm H_2O above the peak airway pressure under pressure-control ventilation at normoventilation in the supine position. This is based on data from nine studies using a PLMA, SLMA, or i-gel in minor laparoscopic surgery, noting that peak airway pressures during normoventilation increased by 2 to 7 cm H_2O after application of pneumoperitoneum.[127]

Maximum Minute Ventilation Test. This test was developed in the early 2000s by Stix and colleagues and is used to determine the achievable maximum minute ventilation (MMV).[176] When an SGA is poorly positioned, the ability to ventilate maximally is affected by both airway leak and slow expiratory flow, such that

MMV is independent of the rate of ventilation and tidal volume. This provides an excellent objective measure of the adequacy of SGA ventilatory function. After insertion of the SGA, the APL valve is closed to 30 cm H_2O, and the patient's lungs are ventilated by hand with maximal inflations for 15 seconds (although more ventilations at a faster rate or different tidal volume will achieve similar results). If the MMV is >12 L/min for adults or double the weight-adapted resting minute ventilation for children, then this indicates that the SGA is functioning well enough to maintain normocapnia for the duration of the case, even under many advanced indications.

Important Considerations for Safe Use During Maintenance and Emergence

Cuff Pressure

Using the manufacturer's "maximum volumes" to guide cuff inflation misinterprets the purpose of these values. These represent volumes that must not be exceeded rather than the "usual volumes" that should be routinely used, which are likely to lead to intracuff pressures well in excess of 120 cm H_2O. Cuff pressure should be restricted to 60 cm H_2O throughout use, especially if it is prolonged, and this can be achieved with a manometer or a built-in cuff pressure monitor that has been introduced to some recent SGAs.[49,177]

Maintenance of Adequate Depth of Anesthesia

Adequate depth of anesthesia is important for multiple reasons, including the prevention of gagging, vomiting, and laryngospasm, particularly during periods of surgical stimulation or before moving the patient.[178]

Management of Regurgitation and Aspiration

Even when appropriate protective measures are taken, regurgitation of gastric contents can occur. Passing a lubricated gastric tube through the drain tube may reduce the risk of aspiration. Once the stomach is emptied, the gastric drain should be removed to enable the drain tube to function as designed. In the event of regurgitation and/or aspiration, the following plan of action should be implemented to reduce potential morbidity: (1) if there is airway obstruction, severe hypoxia or airway displacement, intubation should be considered as an emergency; (2) in the absence of an immediate need to intubate the patient, do not remove the SGA, as there may be a significant amount of regurgitant fluid trapped behind the cuff. The cuff shields and protects the larynx from the trapped fluid, and removing the SGA may worsen the situation; (3) ventilate the patient manually using 100% oxygen and small tidal volumes to minimize the risk of forcing fluid from the trachea into the small bronchi; (4) use suction, ideally under direct vision, to remove any visible gastric contents from the drain tube and oral cavity; (5) temporarily disconnect the circuit to allow assessment and suctioning of the airway tube, while tilting the patient's head down and to the side; (6) use an FIS with suction capability to evaluate the tracheobronchial tree, and remove any remaining fluid; (7) when feasible reinsert a gastric tube and drain any further gastric contents; and (8) if aspiration below the vocal cords is confirmed, consider intubating the patient and institute appropriate treatment protocols.

Optimal Conditions and Timing for Removal

Currently no clear evidence demonstrates whether early (in a deep plane of anesthesia) or late (fully conscious) removal of an SGA is superior. A recent Cochrane review examined this issue, analyzing 15 randomized controlled trials involving more than 2000 adult and pediatric ASA classification I and II patients having elective surgery with a cLMA. Although there was evidence indicating early removal was associated with a reduced incidence of coughing (very low-quality evidence), it was also associated with an increased risk of airway obstruction (low quality), with no difference in the rate of laryngospasm (low quality) or risk of desaturation (very low quality). The quality of data was largely limited because of poor-quality studies and the risk of bias, with inadequacies in blinding and concealment of the random allocation processes.[179] Practical experience indicates that airways should not be removed when the patient is between the states of being anesthetized or awake because complications are more likely to occur.

Summary

The LMA has unequivocally established the precedent that the supraglottic approach to airway management is feasible and preferred in many clinical situations. When the LMA was first introduced, it was an alternative to the face mask. However, by virtue of being a less invasive alterative to the ETT, its clinical applications have far exceeded the original indications. Serious complications associated with LMA use are rare and caused mostly by failed ventilation or pulmonary aspiration.[180] Not only is an SGA the airway management device of choice for the majority of general anesthetics, but its use in managing difficult airways and critically ill patients is also increasingly recognized in international guidelines and in practice.

Non-LMA SGAs

Cuffed Pharyngeal Sealers With Esophageal Cuff

Shiley Esophageal Endotracheal Airway, Double Lumen

The Shiley Esophageal Endotracheal Airway (Medtronic, Minneapolis, MN, USA) is a double-lumen, double-cuff airway

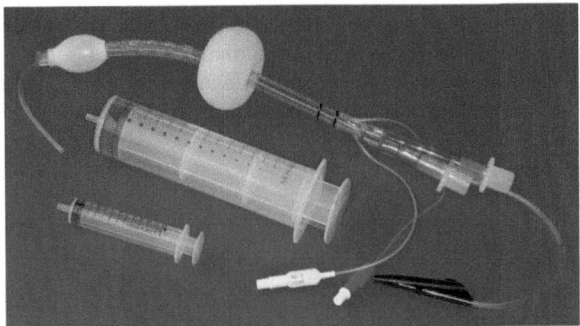

• **Fig. 19.16** The esophageal-tracheal double lumen airway tube has a large syringe for inflation of the oropharyngeal balloon and a small syringe for inflation of the distal cuff.

device for emergency intubation best known as the Esophageal Tracheal Combitube (ETC) or just Combitube (Fig. 19.16). It was designed by Dr. Michael Frass in cooperation with Reinhard Frenzer and Dr. Jonas Zahler in Mödling and Vienna, Austria, in 1983.[181,182] Although of value before the LMA was invented, it is now of mainly historical interest. There are three reasons for this:

- It is associated with a high rate of oropharyngeal trauma.
- It can "fail dangerous" if used incorrectly.
- It has been superseded by more effective and cheaper devices.

The device is designed to permit ventilation of the lungs, regardless of whether its distal tip is positioned in the esophagus or the trachea. It comprises two tubes lying alongside each other, one shorter than the other. A large oropharyngeal balloon is made of latex and located at the midportion of the device, and a smaller tracheoesophageal balloon is located at the device's distal end.[183] The two tube lumens are separated by a partition wall. Proximally, both lumens are opened and linked by short tubes with universal 15-mm connectors. The pharyngeal lumen (1) is blind ended and has eight perforations between the cuffs, whereas the tracheoesophageal lumen (2) extends further and is open (Fig. 19.17). There are two sizes: a 37-Fr small adult (SA) version for use in patients 4- to 6.5-feet tall and a 41-Fr version for use in patients taller than 6.5 feet. In practice the 37-Fr version is sufficient for all but the tallest adults.

The ETC was designed to be inserted blindly, with the patient's head in the neutral position. With the operator behind the patient's head, the lower jaw and tongue are lifted by the thumb and index finger. The tongue is pressed forward by the thumb, and the ETC is inserted along the tongue, in a curved downward movement until the printed ring marks lie between the teeth or the alveolar ridges in edentulous patients (Figs. 19.18A and B). Next, the oropharyngeal balloon is inflated with up to 85 ML of air for the 37-French SA ETC (or up to 100 mL for the 41-French ETC) via the blue pilot balloon, using the 140-mL syringe with the blue color code (Fig. 19.18C). The distal esophageal balloon is then inflated with 10 mL of air, via the white pilot balloon, using the 20-mL syringe. Blind insertion results in esophageal intubation >95% of the time.[182,184] Therefore, test ventilation is recommended first through the longer blue connector (1) (Fig. 19.18D). Air passes out of the perforations between the cuffs, into the pharynx, and then through the glottis into the trachea, because the mouth, nose, and esophagus are blocked by the balloons. Capnography should be used to confirm ventilation of the lungs, and auscultation may be used to confirm breath sounds and the absence of gastric insufflation. In this position, a gastric tube may be passed via the tracheoesophageal tube to enable suctioning and decompression of the stomach.

If ventilation via the pharyngeal lumen fails, it is assumed that the tracheoesophageal tube has entered the trachea (Fig. 19.18E).

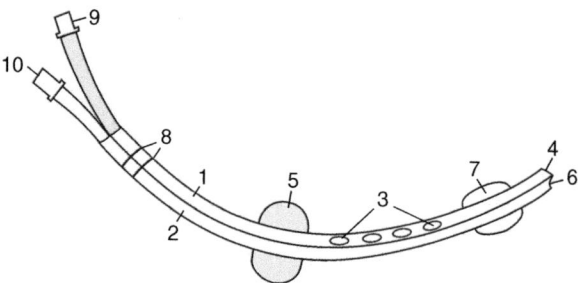

• **Fig. 19.17** Cross-sectional view of the esophageal-tracheal double lumen airway tube: *(1)* pharyngeal lumen (i.e., longer tube with a blocked distal end); *(2)* tracheoesophageal lumen (i.e., shorter tube with open distal end); *(3)* perforations of esophageal lumen 1 in the pharyngeal section; *(4)* blocked distal end of esophageal lumen 1; *(5)* oropharyngeal balloon (yellow); *(6)* open distal end of tracheal lumen 2; *(7)* distal cuff for obturating the esophagus or trachea; *(8)* printed ring marks for indicating the depth of insertion between the teeth or alveolar ridges; *(9)* connector (blue) for the tube leading to esophageal lumen 1; *(10)* connector (transparent) for the tube leading to tracheal lumen 2.

Without changing the position of the ETC, ventilation is changed to the shorter, transparent connector (2), and ventilation of the lungs is again confirmed by capnography. Ventilation is then carried out through this lumen.

If capnography does not confirm ventilation while ventilating through the blue connector, the second most common cause is that the ETC has been inserted too deeply, and the oropharyngeal balloon lies just opposite the laryngeal aperture, occluding the airway.[185]

The operator inserting the ETC may be positioned behind the patient, especially when a laryngoscope is used (Fig. 19.19A), or face to face when the operator stands beside the patient's thorax and faces the patient (Fig. 19.19B), or to the side of the patient's head (Fig. 19.19C). Regardless of the operator's position, the ETC should be inserted with a curved downward-caudal movement.

Indications for Use

The ETC is indicated for emergency airway control, mainly in North America. It can be inserted blindly in patients with limited mouth opening (with an interincisor distance as small as 15 mm) without head or neck movement. It is especially useful in patients with massive airway bleeding or limited access to the airway (eg, a patient who is trapped in a car).[184]

The ETC is contraindicated in patients with intact gag reflexes (irrespective of the level of consciousness), height <6 ft (41-Fr) or

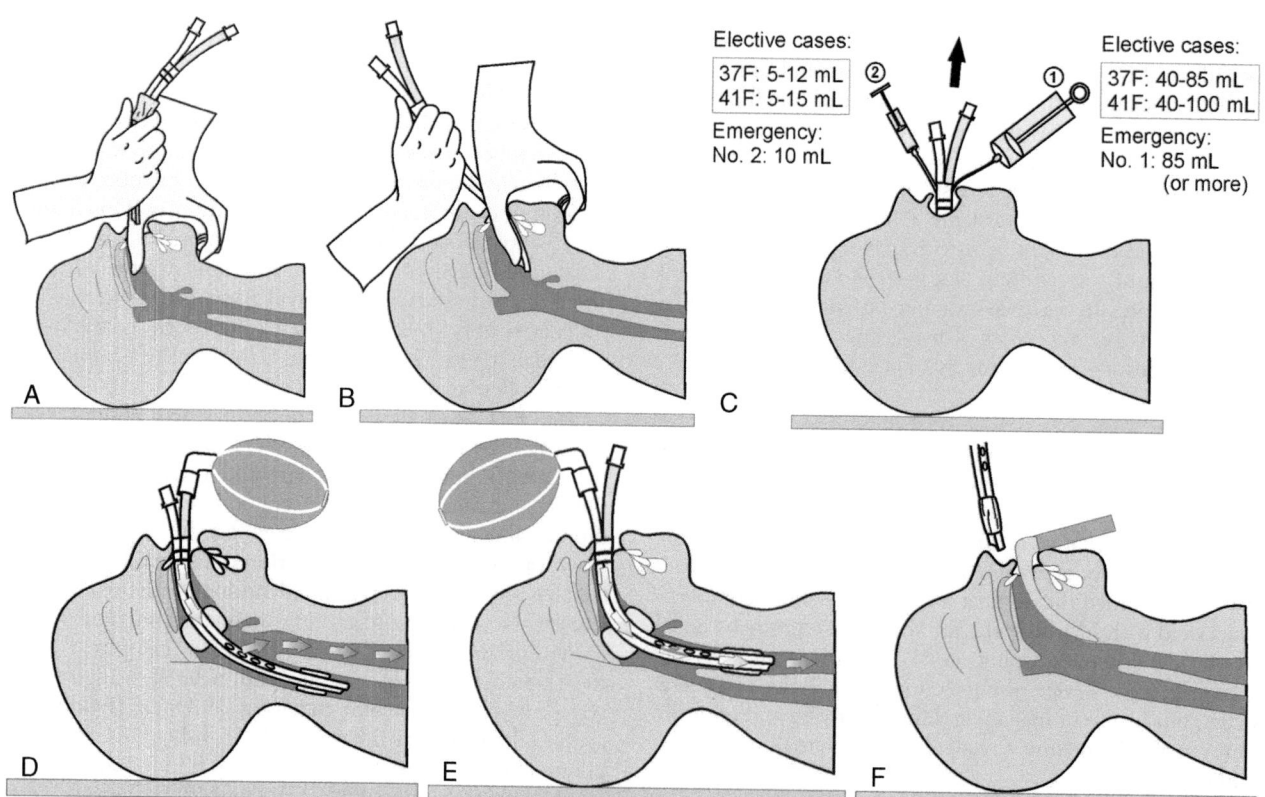

• **Fig. 19.18** Guidelines for insertion of the esophageal-tracheal double-lumen airway tube. .(A) Insertion begins by lifting the chin and lower jaw. (B) The esophageal-tracheal double lumen airway tube is inserted in a downward, curved movement along the tongue. (C) The oropharyngeal balloon is inflated with 85 mL of air, and the distal cuff is inflated with 5 to 10 mL of air. (D) With the esophageal-tracheal double lumen airway tube in the esophageal position, ventilation is performed through the longer no. 1 tube (blue). Air flows through the holes into the pharynx and from there into the trachea (blue arrows). (E) With the esophageal-tracheal double lumen airway tube in the tracheal position, ventilation is performed through the shorter no. 2 tube (transparent). (F). Laryngoscopy facilitated insertion of esophageal-tracheal double lumen airway tube.

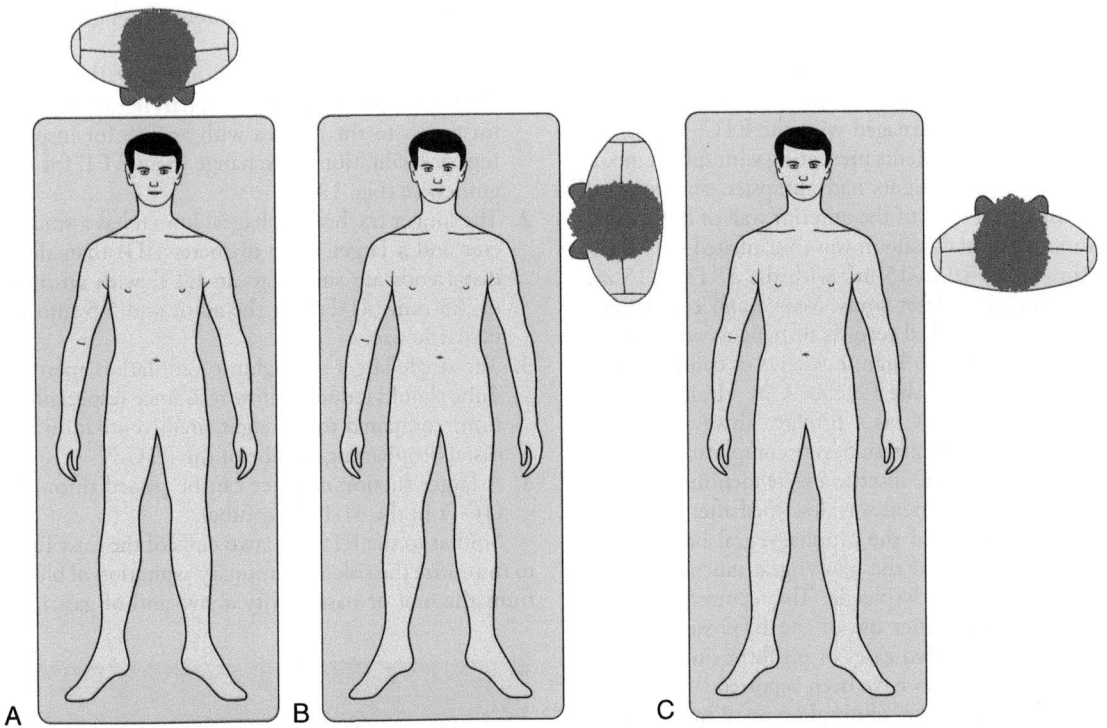

• **Fig. 19.19** Position of the operator during insertion of the esophageal-tracheal double-lumen airway tube. (A) The operator stands behind the patient, especially when using a laryngoscope. (B) The operator stands to the side of the patient's head. (C) The operator stands beside patient's thorax to be positioned face to face.

<4 ft (37-Fr), ingestion of caustic substances, and known upper esophageal pathology.

The ETC is successful in providing airway control when inserted by anesthesiologists after minimal formal training[186] and by relatively inexperienced personnel.[187–190] The reported successful ventilation rate when used as a primary airway device and placed by paramedics or emergency medical technicians (EMTs) during cardiopulmonary resuscitation in prehospital settings varies between 71% and 91%.[186–191] In a small series, the ETC achieved "satisfactory" airway control in 7 of 10 trauma patients, most including facial trauma, after failed rapid-sequence intubation during transport.[192] Timmermann and colleagues[193] prospectively evaluated the airway interventions performed by anesthesia-trained emergency physicians: The ETC or cLMA were used in 2% of cases after failed intubation, with similar success rates.

Insertion of an ETC in s trauma patient whose neck is immobilized in a rigid cervical collar is very difficult, requiring temporary removal of the anterior part of the collar, while the head is maintained in neutral position.[187]

ETC may be used in cases of failed tracheal intubation.[194–197] Mort[198] reported 18 cases of successful use of the ETC to rescue the airway following failed tracheal intubation outside the OR and LMA and failure. In all cases, the ETC tip entered the esophagus.

The ETC has been used as a primary airway device during elective surgery of moderate duration.[199–201] Hartmann and colleagues[200] reported effective and safe airway control with peak inspiratory pressures of 30 cmH$_2$O during laparoscopic gynecological surgery. The authors opted for esophageal insertion of the ETC, under laryngoscopically facilitated vision. Gaitini and colleagues[201] used the ETC as the primary airway for 200 cases of routine surgery lasting 15 to 155 minutes and with both mechanical and spontaneous ventilation. In 97% of patients, excellent oxygenation, ventilation, and respiratory mechanics, as well as hemodynamic stability, were achieved. The authors suggested that after securing the airway with an ETC it may not be necessary to abort the anesthetic or to continue with further airway exchange efforts. In practice modern alternatives and high rates of trauma make the ETC an unlikely tool for routine surgery.

Replacement of the ETC with an ETT

Continued airway management with an ETC that has been placed as a rescue device is a reasonable option in many cases; however, exchange to an ETT may be desirable. Several techniques of ETC-ETT exchange have been described.[202–204] Both direct and video-assisted laryngoscopy have been successfully used to intubate the trachea with an ETC in situ.[184,202] FIS-guided airway exchange can be performed by inserting the FIS alongside the ETC after partially deflating the oropharyngeal balloon. Gaitini and colleagues[203] reported that spontaneous ventilation improved the effectiveness of this exchange technique by making identification and exposure of the epiglottis and larynx easier, as a result of the retention of pharyngeal muscle tone and spontaneous movement of the epiglottis and vocal cords. Although time consuming, this exchange technique enables oxygenation throughout most of the procedure.

If percutaneous tracheostomy is required, the ETC can be left in situ during the procedure.[204] An advantage of this technique is that the trachea is not occupied by an ETT and that ventilation can be continued while the surgical airway is established. A disadvantage is that the trachea is not protected against aspiration of blood generated during the surgical procedure.

Complications

Overinflation of the esophageal balloon can lead to traumatic injuries, such as esophageal lacerations or perforation and airway obstruction.[205–209] In a series of 1139 cases of prehospital cardiac arrests with the airway managed with the ETC, Vezina and colleagues[207] reported eight patients presenting with subcutaneous emphysema. Five of these patients had autopsies, and two had longitudinal transparietal tears of the anterior wall of the esophagus. In these cases, the distal balloon was overinflated with 20 to 40 mL of air (instead of 10 to 15 mL with the 37-Fr or 15 mL with the ETC 41-Fr). In a later study, Vezina and colleagues[208] retrospectively reviewed medical records of patients with cardiac or respiratory arrest reporting a high incidence of complications. The study was performed in the Quebec City Health Region, where paramedics use the ETC as a primary airway device for patients with cardiorespiratory arrest. Severe complications attributed by the authors to the ETC insertion were identified in 12 of 280 patients. Tongue engorgement was described after 4 hours of ETC use.[209] Excessive filling of the oropharyngeal balloon may predispose patients to injury of the pharyngeal mucosa, causing postoperative sore throat and dysphagia. The reported incidence of postoperative sore throat after use of the ETC varies largely between 25% to 48%.[201,210] Two cases of piriform sinus perforation during ETC insertion also have been reported.[211,212] Mercer and Gabbott reported a 45% rate of oropharyngeal trauma when the ETC was used in 40 low-risk elective surgical patients, despite using laryngoscopic insertion to minimize trauma in half of the patients.[213]

Summary

The ETC is a double-lumen/double-balloon SGA designed to work whether the tip is placed in the esophagus or trachea. Inserted blindly, the tip enters the esophagus in most cases. The major indication of the ETC is as a backup device for airway management, and it has been used successfully for rescue ventilation both in and out of hospital settings. It may be particularly useful in patients with a severely soiled airway. Adherence to the manufacturer's guidelines regarding the inflation of the cuffs is very important, and the two lumens are a potential source of confusion during use. There are concerns about trauma during use. In view of the numerous alternatives now available, the use of ETC has significantly reduced in recent years.

EasyTube

The EasyTube (Well Lead, Guangzhou, China) is an SGA similar to the ETC. It was introduced in the European Union in 2003 and approved by the US Food and Drug Administration in 2005. It was developed in an attempt to improve the performance of the ETC.[214] Most characteristics are very similar to the ETC; thus, we only emphasize points of difference between the EasyTube and ETC.

The EasyTube is a latex-free, sterile, single-use, double-lumen tube of similar design to the ETC and is designed to enable lung ventilation when its tip is placed in the esophagus or the trachea (Fig. 19.20). There are two sizes: 28-Fr for pediatric patients 90 to 130 cm tall, and 41-Fr for patients taller than 130 cm. Principles of insertion and use are the same as for the ETC (Fig. 19.21). The pharyngeal and the distal cuffs are inflated with 80 and 10 mL of air, respectively. The EasyTube may be intentionally placed in the trachea using laryngoscopy: a black mark at the distal end of the device indicates correct depth of insertion just below the vocal cords.

The EasyTube has several potential design advantages over the ETC:

1. Its pharyngeal lumen has an orifice (rather than smaller "perforations") just below the oropharyngeal balloon, which allows for access to the trachea with an FIS for inspection, suctioning, or facilitation of exchange to an ETT, for instance using a guidewire (Fig. 19.22).
2. The longer tracheoesophageal lumen has a smaller outer diameter and a larger inner diameter (ID) than the ETC, and its distal ends are similar to an ETT, with an internal diameter of 7.5 mm (41-Fr) for the adult and 5.5 mm (28-Fr) for the pediatric size.
3. The single larger supraglottic ventilation aperture of the EasyTube should reduce airflow resistance (especially during expiration) compared to the eight small ventilation apertures in the distal oropharyngeal tube of the ETC.[215]
4. A larger suction catheter can be passed through both lumens (16-Fr in the 41-Fr EasyTube).

Similar to the ETC, the two cuffs of the EasyTube are designed to minimize the risk of pulmonary aspiration of blood or secretions from the oral or nasal cavity above and of gastric contents from

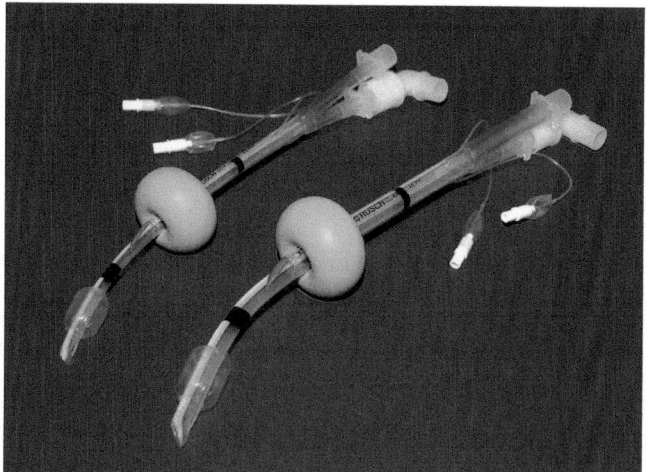

• **Fig. 19.20** Two sizes of the EasyTube: 41 French (large) and 28 French (small). (Courtesy Well Lead Medical Company, Guangzhou, China.)

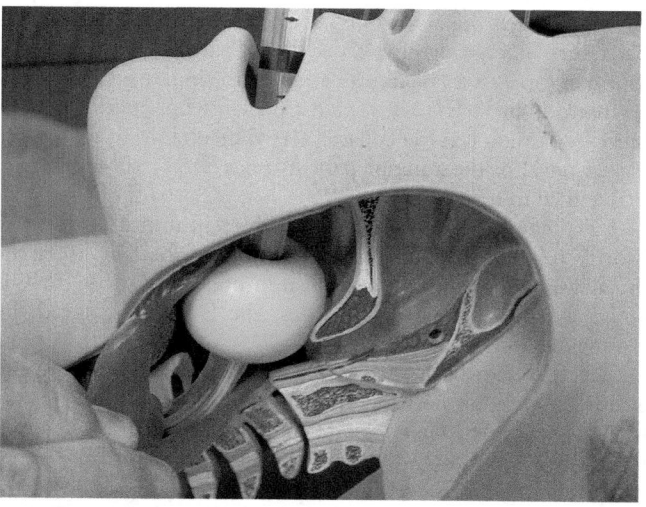

• **Fig. 19.21** The anatomic position of the EasyTube. (Courtesy Well Lead Medical Company, Guangzhou, China.)

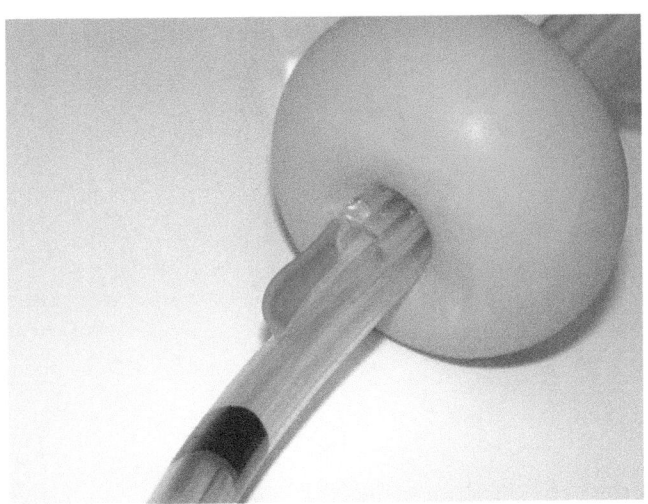

• **Fig. 19.22** Easytube has a pharyngeal lumen that provides a supraglottic ventilation outlet ending just below the oropharyngeal balloon.

below. Bercker and colleagues[17] demonstrated in a cadaver model that both the ETC and the EasyTube are capable of withholding the water pressure up to more than 120 cm H_2O.

Gaitini and colleagues[216] studied 80 patients randomized for use the EasyTube or the ETC by anesthesiologists. Blind insertion led to esophageal placement in all patients. An effective airway was achieved more quickly using the EasyTube (19.4 seconds) than the ETC (30.6 seconds). EasyTube insertion was rated significantly easier than ETC insertion.

Complications associated with the EasyTube are likely to be of a similar nature to the ETC; however, because of the smaller distal tube, the risk of traumatic injury is anticipated to be lower. Similar to other SGAs, high intracuff pressure could result in surrounding oropharyngeal tissue trauma. Frequent intracuff pressure check monitoring using a manometer is recommended to avoid excessive pressure. To date, no major complications associated with the use of the EasyTube have been reported, but there have been few studies reported.

In summary, the major indication for use of the EasyTube is as a backup device for airway management. The EasyTube perpetuates the concept of the ETC but has several advantages, including easier insertion and a shorter time to achieve an effective airway when inserted blindly.

Laryngeal Tube

The Laryngeal Tube (LT) (VBM, Medizintechik, Sulz, Germany) was designed by Volker Bertram as an SGA with high-volume–low-pressure cuffs, offers a good seal, and is easy to insert. The LT was first introduced to the European Union in 2002. In 2004, a disposable version, the LT-D, was launched in the United States by King Systems (Ambu, Noblesville, IN, USA) under the name of King LT. LT and King LT are the same product, but King Systems named the device King LT for marketing reasons.

Terminology associated with the LT is rather confusing. The LT design has undergone multiple changes, and several variants of the device have been developed. The LT Suction (LTS), first launched in 2002 as a reusable device, had a second channel (drain tube) running posterior to the airway lumen, which enabled gastric tube placement. This was followed by a second version (LTS II) and a disposable version (LTS-D). The current versions of the LT are the LTS-D and the LTS, though the current LTS is much more akin to the LTS-II than the original LTS.

Technical Description

The LT was a reusable, single-lumen SGA made from latex-free medical-grade silicon. It comprised a single lumen tube closed at the distal end, with two inflatable interconnected low-pressure cuffs (inflated by a single pilot tube) and a ventilation orifice located between the cuffs (Fig. 19.23). The distal cuff was designed to seal the esophagus and protect against regurgitation, and the proximal cuff, which sits in the oropharynx, was designed to seal the pharynx and stabilize the tube.[217]

The LT-D is made from medical-grade polyvinyl chloride. In addition to the main ventilation outlets, two eyelets were added on each side of the device close to the ventilation orifice (Fig. 19.24). The laryngeal tube suction (LTS) is a further development of the LT. It is made from medical-grade silicon and has an additional, posteriorly placed, gastric channel tube allowing the separation of the respiratory and gastrointestinal tracts. In 2004, the LTS was modified and replaced by the LTS II. The LTS II has a longer shaft, smaller tip, and oval-shaped distal (esophageal) cuff for better adjustment to the esophageal inlet (Fig. 19.25). A gastric tube up to 16 gauge can be passed to drain the gastric contents.

The LTS-D is made from medical grade polyvinyl chloride. It was introduced in Europe in 2005 and in the United States in 2006 (Fig. 19.26). The LTS-D is available in seven sizes (0, 1, 2,

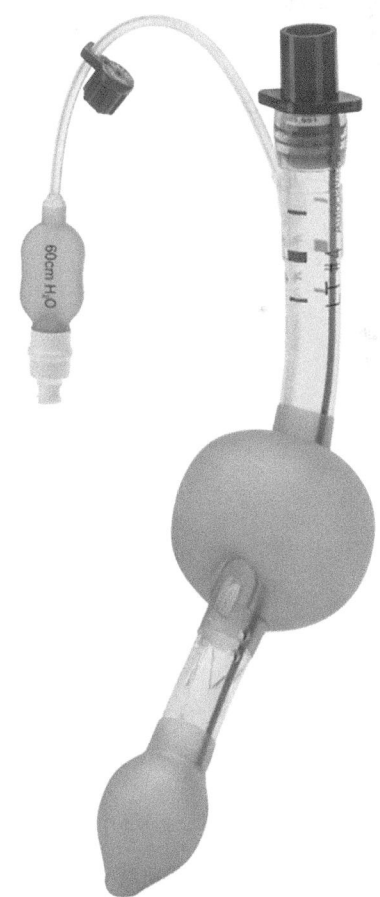

• **Fig. 19.23** A reusable Laryngeal Tube has an airway tube with an approximate angle of 130 degrees and average diameter of 1.5 cm and two low-pressure cuffs (proximal and distal) with an oval aperture placed between them, which allows ventilation. (Courtesy VBM Medizintechnik GmbH, Sulz am Neckar, Germany.)

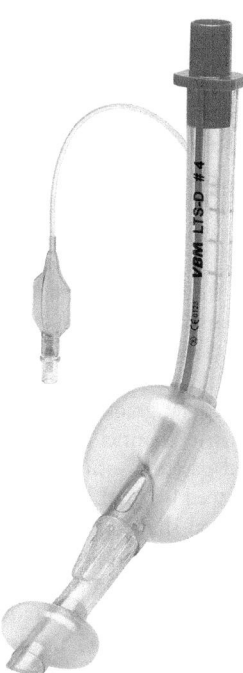

• **Fig. 19.24** Disposable laryngeal tube made from medical-grade polyvinyl chloride. In addition to the main ventilation outlets, it has two eyelets on each side of the device. (Courtesy VBM Medizintechnik GmbH, Sulz am Neckar, Germany.)

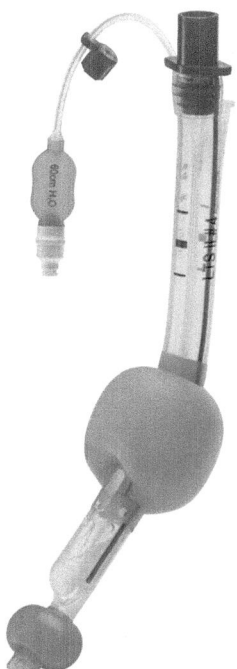

• **Fig 19.25** Laryngeal Tube Suction II multiuse. It is made from silicon and has an additional, posteriorly placed, drain tube. The initial version of the LTS was modified and replaced by LTS II. The LTS II has a longer shaft, smaller tip, and oval-shaped distal (esophageal) cuff for better adjustment to the esophageal inlet. (Courtesy VBM Medizintechnik GmbH, Sulz am Neckar, Germany.)

2.5, 3, 4, and 5). Each size of device has color-coded connectors and correspondent syringes for cuff inflation. In 2014 the LTS-D was further modified, without changing its name, changing its

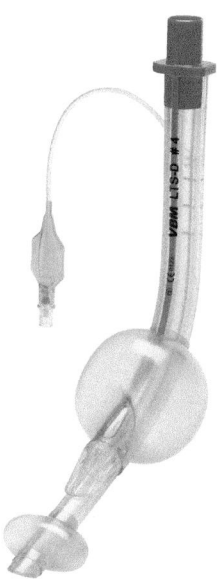

• **Fig. 19.26** Laryngeal Tube Suction Disposable is the disposable equivalent of LTS II. (Courtesy VBM Medizintechnik GmbH, Sulz am Neckar, Germany.)

45-degree curvature to a 60-degree one to better match pharyngeal anatomy. The 2014 version has thinner cuffs and a conical ramp, designed to make the tube slimmer in order to facilitate insertion. The cuffs have been redesigned with the intent of improving airway seal and reducing mucosal pressure. In terms of airway orifices, the new version has two lateral eyelets, four long ventilation slots, and one large ventilation aperture. All sizes have a drain tube, and the proximal aperture of this is funneled to facilitate gastric tube insertion. A gastric tube up to 18-Fr can be passed though the gastric channel (Table 19.4).

As with other cuffed pharyngeal sealers with esophageal cuff SGAs, the LT is contraindicated in patients with intact gag reflexes, upper esophageal abnormalities, known ingestion of caustic substances, and upper airway obstruction.

Insertion of LT

The patient's head can be positioned in the sniffing or neutral position. The LT is inserted blindly into the esophagus by smoothly sliding the distal tip against the hard palate and the hypopharynx, until the teeth are aligned with the black mark on the tube's shaft or until resistance is felt (Figs. 19.27A and B). Application of jaw thrust makes the insertion easier.[218] The cuffs inflation is via a single pilot

TABLE 19.4	Laryngeal Tube Suction Disposable (LTS-D)—Size Selection		
LTS-D Size	**Patient**	**Patient Weight or Height**	**Gastric Tube**
0	Neonate	<5 kg	10 French
1	Baby	5–12 kg	10 French
2	Child	12–25 kg	16 French
2.5	Child	125–150 cm	16 French
3	Adult	<155 cm	18 French
4	Adult	155–180 cm	18 French
5	Adult	>180 cm	18 French

tube and occurs sequentially. Cuffs should be inflated to a pressure of 60 cm H_2O (Figs. 19.28A and B). The maximum inflation volumes (for both cuffs combined) in each size are size 0, 10 mL; size 1, 20 mL; size 2, 35 mL; size 2.5, 40 mL; size 3, 60 mL; size 4, 80 mL; and size 5, 90 mL. A color-coded syringe is provided with the LT for inflation of the cuffs, and the recommended maximum volumes are shown according to the color of the tube connector (e.g., 80 mL with a red mark for the size 4 LT with the red connector). Cuff pressure should be measured with a manometer before use.

Insufficient ventilation may result because of incorrect depth of insertion or placement of the tip into the glottis. Insertion of the tip into the glottic/periglottic structures will cause it to bounce back when released from the intended position and should be repositioned.[219] Axial rotation of the LT may also lead to poor ventilation, and insertion technique should be rigorous to avoid this.

A modified jaw lift technique to insert the LTS has been described by Mahajan and colleagues.[220] The thumb is inserted between the tongue and the floor of the mouth to lift both the jaw and the tongue from the posterior pharyngeal wall, simultaneously pushing the tongue to one side of the oral cavity. In addition, a classic stylet or light wand stylet can be used to facilitate insertion.[221,222] Cricoid force prevents correct insertion of the LT.[223]

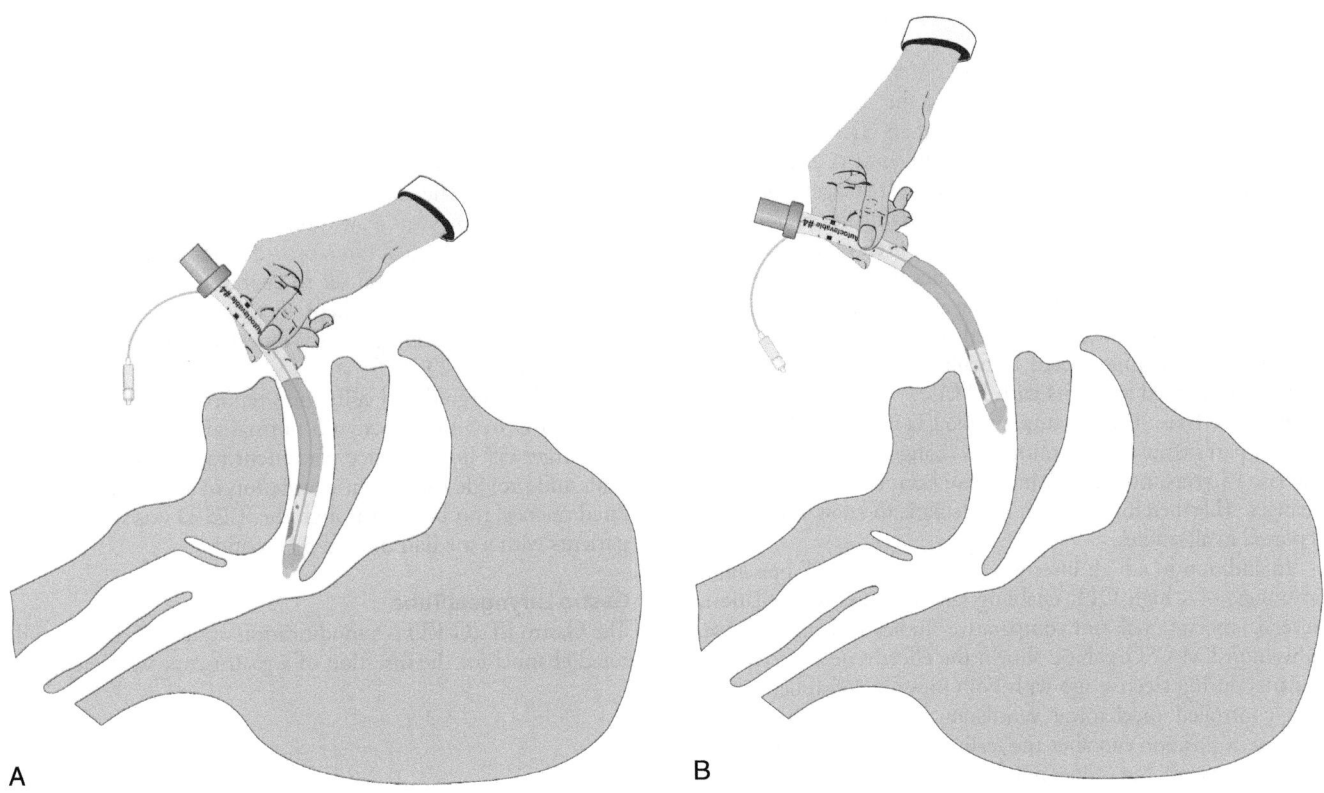

A   B

• **Fig. 19.27** (A, B) Insertion of the Laryngeal Tube. (Courtesy VBM Medizintechnik GmbH, Sulz am Neckar, Germany.)

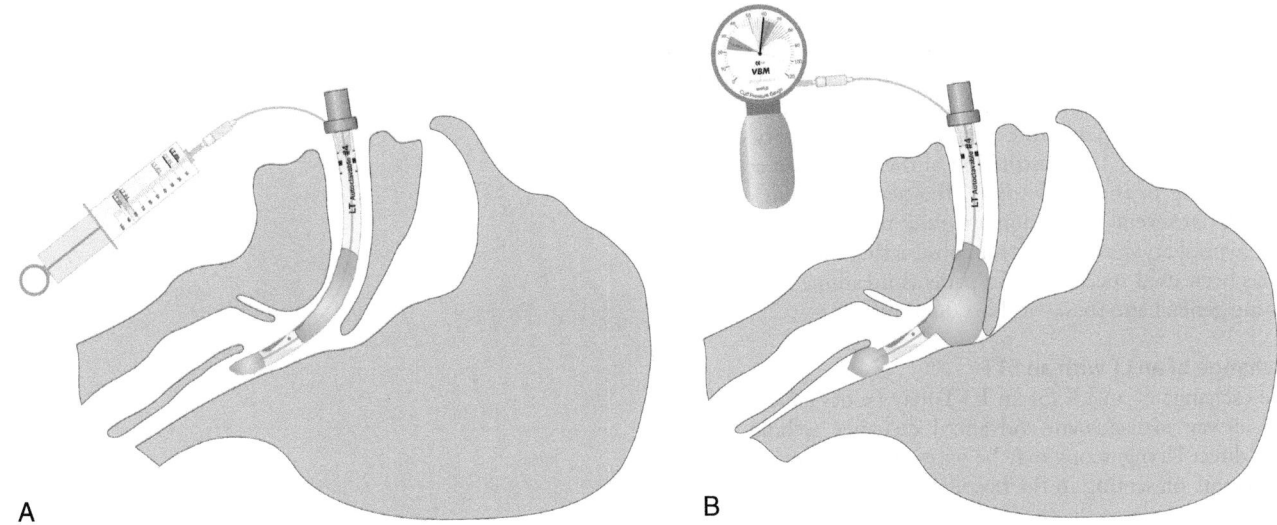

A   B

• **Fig. 19.28** (A, B) Cuff inflation with a syringe or a manometer. (Courtesy VBM Medizintechnik GmbH, Sulz am Neckar, Germany.)

Indications for Use

Emergency Use. The features of the LTs that make it potentially suitable for emergency use are as follows. LTs have a slim design requiring minimal mouth opening (23 mm) for insertion.[224] They are generally easily inserted, including by inexperienced personnel, and achieve an oropharyngeal leak pressure of approximately 25 to 30 cm H_2O with a low risk of aspiration.[225,226] After correct insertion, manual controlled or spontaneous ventilation can be used.

The LT has a well-established role as a primary airway device during cardiopulmonary resuscitation (CPR) requiring minimal disruption of chest compressions during insertion.[227] International guidelines recommend the LT as an alternative device during CPR to secure the airway.[67,228]

In the United States, the Pragmatic Airway Resuscitation Trial (PART) showed a 2.9% improvement in the 72-hour survival rate when laryngeal tubes were used rather than ETTs by paramedics and emergency medical technicians.[229] In some countries, the LT is increasingly used for emergency airway management both as a primary and as a rescue airway, by paramedics and EMTs in prehospital settings. In a meta-analysis of prehospital airway control techniques by Hubble and colleagues, the LT had the highest insertion success rate (96.5%) among alternative airway devices.[230]

LTs have been successfully used as rescue airway devices in patients with an unexpected difficult airway,[231-233] including in situations of failed attempts with LMAs.[234]

Elective Use. The literature on the LTs is complicated to interpret, in part because of the numerous changes to device design over the last 15 years, not all of which have been combined with name changes. This therefore makes it problematic to know what device is reported in all studies.

In addition to a high insertion success rate, the LT presents the advantage of a high OLP, enabling safe mechanical ventilation.[225] Several observational and comparative studies with the LMA and other non-LMA SGAs have shown the effectiveness of certain LT variants during elective use with both pressure-controlled and volume-controlled mechanical ventilation.[225,226,235-237] Changing the head/neck position can alter the sealing capabilities of the LT (and SGAs in general), but it does not appear to affect management using pressure control mechanical ventilation in neutral position.[226,238]

There are conflicting reports regarding the efficacy of LTs during general anesthesia in patients breathing spontaneously. Obstruction of the ventilation aperture by the epiglottis or by axial rotation may occur and is more readily overcome by positive-pressure ventilation than during spontaneous ventilation. Poor performance was noted with the first LT variant, which had only one ventilation aperture and no lateral ventilatory openings. That was attributed to obstruction of the ventilation aperture by downfolding of the epiglottis.[239] The newest version of LT, the LTS-D, has several ventilation apertures that are designed to prevent hypopharyngeal tissues from obstructing the airway inlet and it has been used successfully in patients breathing spontaneously during general anesthesia of short duration.[240]

Exchange of an LT with an ETT

The exchange of an LT for an ETT may be desirable for continued airway management. Advanced exchange techniques other than direct laryngoscopy may be necessary in approximately 80% of patients presenting to the hospital with an inserted LT, due to upper airway edema.[241]

An FIS-facilitated exchange was described by Genzwuerker and colleagues[242] using an Aintree intubation catheter (AIC)

placed in the lumen of the airway tube. The relatively small airway tube and ventilation orifice and the angulation of the LTS-D all present challenges to the use of an AIC. Tube exchange can also be performed with the FIS passed alongside the LT after partial cuff deflation.[243] If it is difficult to access the glottis, the cuffs can be reinflated and ventilation resumed through the LT.

Additional techniques exchange reported in the literature are direct and video-asssited laryngosopy intubation, combined video-assisted laryngoscopy with bougie insertion, combined video-assisted laryngosopy and FIS, and surgical tracheostomy.[244,245]

Intubating Laryngeal Tube Suction Disposable

The Intubating Laryngeal Tube Suction Disposable (iLTS-D) is a modified LTS-D designed to facilitate tracheal intubation (Fig. 19.29). It has a ventilator channel with a 13.5-mm internal diameter, which enables the passage of an ETT, either blindly or with FIS guidance (Fig. 19.30). There are two sizes. The size 2.5/3 is for patients 125 to 155 cm tall and accepts an ETT up to 6.5-mm ID. The size 4/5 is designed for patients taller than 155 cm and allows tracheal intubation with an ETT up to size 8-mm ID. The manufacturer provides an armored ETT with a soft tip and a plastic stabilizer to enable removal of the iLTS-D, while the tracheal tube is kept in place (Fig. 19.31). Manikin studies show encouraging results, especially with blind intubation through the iLTS-D.[246,247]

In 2015, Bergold and colleagues reported the successful use of the iLTS-D in 30 patients with normal airways undergoing elective surgery.[248] Initial device placement took a median of 17 seconds and provided sufficient ventilation in all patients. FIS-facilitated tracheal intubation through the iLTS-D was successful in 29 patients with a median time of 32 seconds.

Gastro Laryngeal Tube

The Gastro LT (G-LT) is a modification of the LTS II, with a dedicated channel for the insertion of a gastroscope while acting as an

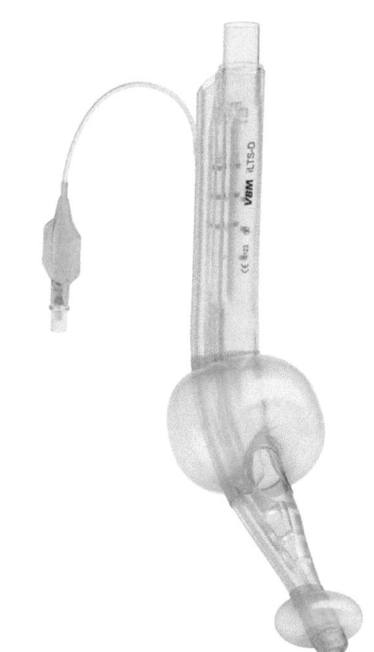

• **Fig. 19.29** Intubating Laryngeal Tube Suction Disposable. (Courtesy VBM Medizintechnik GmbH, Sulz am Neckar, Germany.)

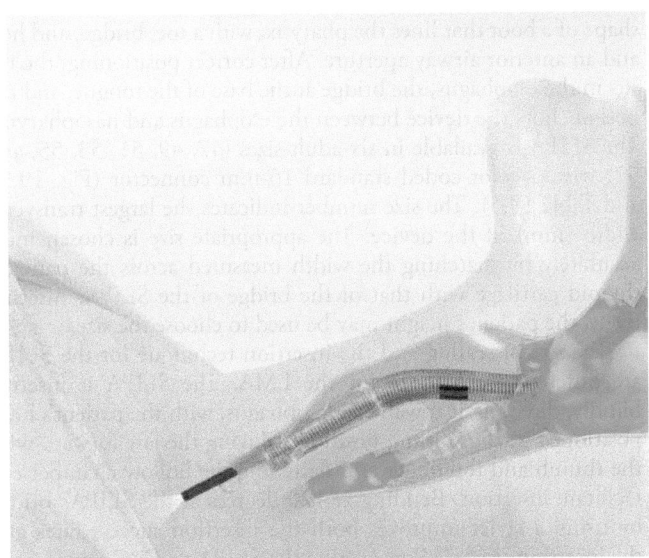

• **Fig. 19.30** Flexible scope intubation through the Intubating Laryngeal Tube Suction Disposable. (Courtesy VBM Medizintechnik GmbH, Sulz am Neckar, Germany.)

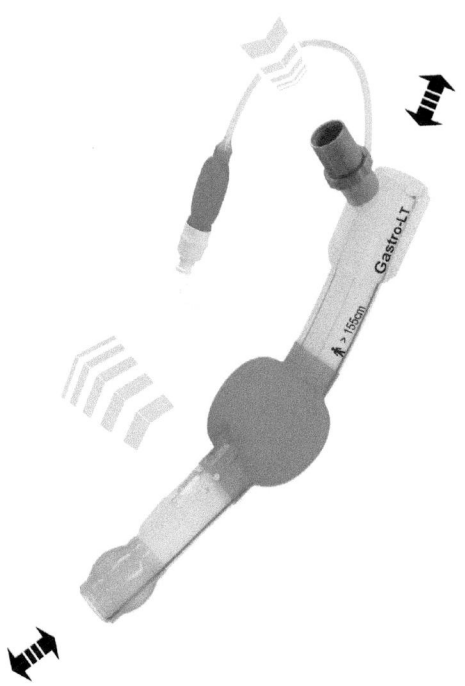

• **Fig. 19.32** The Gastro Laryngeal tube is a modified LTS II, with a dedicated channel for the insertion of a gastroscope. It is made from of silicone and has a built-in bite block to protect the endoscope.

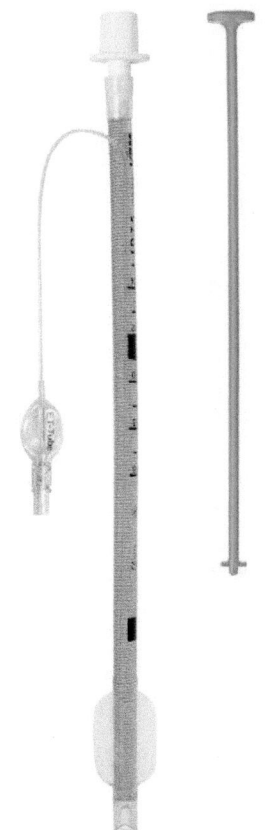

• **Fig. 19.31** Armored tracheal tube and a plastic stabilizer to allow for the removal of the iLTS-D while the tracheal tube is kept in place. (Courtesy VBM Medizintechnik GmbH, Sulz am Neckar, Germany.)

SGA for ventilation (Fig. 19.32). It is made of latex-free medical-grade silicone and has a built-in bite block to protect the endoscope. The endoscopic channel has an internal diameter of 16 mm and enables the insertion and use of a gastrointestinal endoscope with a

maximum external diameter of 13.8 mm (Fig. 19.33). It is coated with a special polymer to minimize friction caused by the insertion and movement of the endoscope. The G-LT is manufactured only in one size and can be used in patients 155 cm tall or taller.

Gaitini and colleagues[249] evaluated the G-LT for effectiveness of airway management and feasibility of performing endoscopic retrograde cholangiopancreatography (ERCP) in 30 patients in the prone position. Oxygenation and ventilation were successful in all patients throughout the procedure, which lasted a mean of 43 minutes. Airway interventions to optimize ventilation were necessary in 12 patients. ERCP was successfully completed in all patients. Fabri and colleagues[250] studied the G-LT to facilitate ERCP and endoscopic ultrasonography in 22 supine patients. The gastroenterologists performing the endoscopies graded the maneuverability of the endoscope as "good" in all patients.

Complications

The LT has an S-shape design, and, therefore, the likelihood of tracheal insertion is very low.

Overinflation of the cuffs may lead to esophageal or oropharyngeal mucosal damage, or it may compromise the circulation of the tongue and produce transient ischemic changes.[251] The intracuff pressure may be increased when using nitrous oxide, which diffuses more rapidly into the cuff than nitrogen diffuses out of the cuff.[252] It is strongly recommended to adhere to the manufacturer's recommendations to inflate the cuffs using a manometer and monitor and adjust the intracuff pressure frequently.

Because of its soft tip and low-pressure cuffs, minor traumatic postoperative complications such as sore throat, hoarseness, dysphagia, dysphonia, and airway bleeding have an acceptably low incidence in the elective setting but may be important in prehospital use. Prehospital use of the LTS-D can cause high incidence of tongue engorgement and glottic edema.[241] Schalk and colleagues[253] prospectively evaluated complications caused by LTs placed in

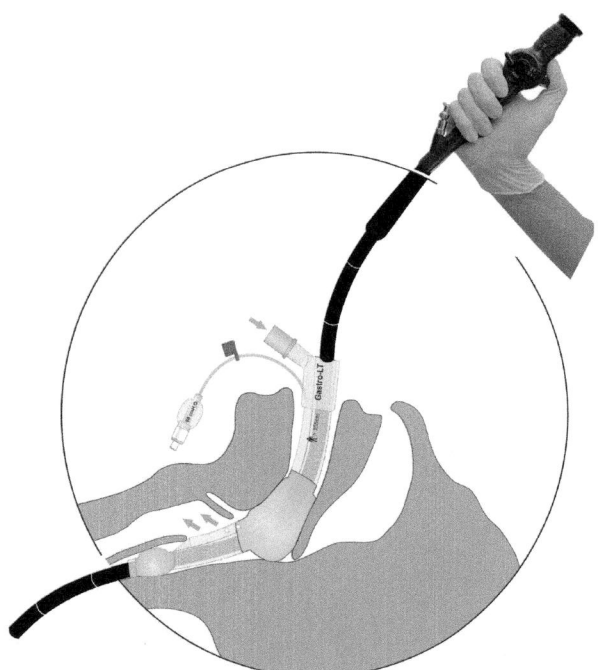

• **Fig. 19.33** An endoscope inserted through the endoscopic channel of the Gastro Laryngeal Tube. (Courtesy VBM Medizintechnik GmbH, Sulz am Neckar, Germany.)

prehospital settings by emergency physicians and paramedics. The authors identified high intracuff pressure (median 100 cm H_2O) at hospital admission, causing tongue swelling in almost 40% of patients. Massive stomach distension was detected in 11% of patients. In these patients first-generation LTs were used.

Hypopharyegeal perforation and damage to the uvula have also been reported.[254,255] The risk of aspiration is minimized by the distal cuff blocking the top end of the esophagus; however, the risk of gastric insufflation and regurgitation exists.[256]

Summary

The LT and variants are easily inserted SGAs. The initial LT has undergone numerous modifications designed to improve performance. Because of easy and fast insertion by inexperienced personnel, the popularity of the LT for emergency airway management in the prehospital environment is increasing in somecountries, both as a primary or rescue airway device after failed endotracheal intubation. Controlled mechanical ventilation is more reliable than spontaneous ventilation. There is a very low incidence of complications, and tracheal misplacement is extremely rare.

Anatomically Preshaped Noninflatable Supraglottic Airways

Streamlined Liner of the Pharynx Airway

The Streamlined Liner of the Pharynx Airway (SLIPA) (Hangzhou Fushan Medical Appliances Co., Ltd., China) was developed by Dr. Donald Miller and launched at the Second All Africa Congress in 2002 and after that in Europe in 2004. It is a disposable, cuffless SGA with a preformed shape of a pressurized pharynx constructed from soft plastic (ethylene-vinyl acetate copolymer) (Fig. 19.34). It is hollow, with a collection chamber (up to 50 mL capacity) designed to act as a reservoir for trapping pharyngeal secretions and potential regurgitated gastric contents. It has a

shape of a boot that lines the pharynx, with a toe, bridge, and heel and an anterior airway aperture. After correct positioning, the toe sits in the esophagus, the bridge at the base of the tongue, and the heel anchors the device between the esophagus and nasopharynx. The SLIPA is available in six adult sizes (47, 49, 51, 53, 55, and 57) with a color-coded standard 15-mm connector (Fig. 19.35 and Table 19.5). The size number indicates the largest transverse width (mm) of the device. The appropriate size is chosen most accurately by matching the width measured across the patient's thyroid cartilage with that of the bridge of the SLIPA. Alternatively, the patient's height may be used to choose the size.

The site of sealing and the insertion technique for the SLIPA are different from those for the LMA. The SLIPA is inserted blindly, directing it toward the esophagus, with the patient's head positioned in the sniffing position. Moving the jaw forward with the thumb and forefinger and flattening the hollow chamber can facilitate insertion. Bending at 120 degrees at the SLIPA's bridge by using a stylet improves both the insertion success rates and the insertion time.[257] Prewarming the SLIPA to 37°C can ease the insertion and reduce the incidence of postoperative sore throat.[258]

SLIPA is indicated for use during anesthesia with spontaneous or mechanical ventilation.

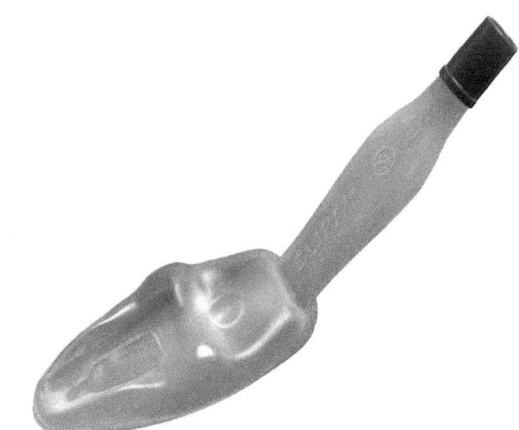

• **Fig. 19.34** Streamlined Liner of the Pharynx Airway (SLIPA) is a disposable, cuffless supraglottic airway.

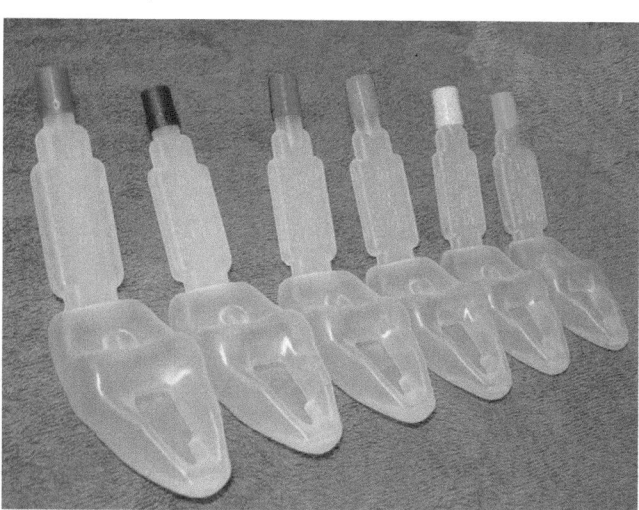

• **Fig. 19.35** Streamlined Liner of the Pharynx Airway (SLIPA): six adult sizes (47–57) with a color-coded standard connector.

TABLE 19.5	SLIPA Size Selection	
SLIPA Size	Patient	Height Range (cm)
47	Very small female	145–160
49	Small female	152–168
51	Medium female	160–175
53	Large female/small male	163–182
55	Medium male	173–193
57	Large male	180–200

SLIPA, Streamlined Liner of the Pharynx Airway.

Evaluations

The manufacturers report that the uniqueness of the SLIPA lies in part with its reservoir chamber, which can act as a sump and potentially reduce the risk of pulmonary aspiration if regurgitation occurs. However, there is no robust evidence to support this claim. Because it can be flattened, it is particularly useful in the case of limited jaw opening. In a laboratory benchtop study, the SLIPA retained up to 50 mL of water within its reservoir at both fast and slow rates of simulated, induced "regurgitation."[259] The first clinical pilot study published in 2002 was performed by Miller and Lavelle[260] in 22 fasted patients undergoing minor elective surgery. The authors reported a 90% success rate of using the SLIPA to establish a patent airway and to maintain oxygenation and ventilation during spontaneous ventilation. Subsequent studies reported high insertion success rates and effectiveness of the SLIPA in providing adequate oxygenation and ventilation (ranging from 92% to 100%).[261–262] Satisfactory oxygenation and ventilation conditions have been reported when using the SLIPA during laparoscopic surgeries.[263,264]

Lim and colleagues[265] described the successful use of the SLIPA as a rescue airway device after LMA failure.

Complications

A significant concern with the SLIPA is an increased incidence of airway trauma as indicated by blood staining of the device after removal and sore throat.[266] Ma and Fang[267] reported two patients presenting prolonged hoarseness following the use of the SLIPA due to arytenoid cartilage dislocation and vocal fold paralysis, respectively.

Summary

Several studies have indicated the effectiveness and safety of the elective use of the SLIPA during spontaneous or mechanically controlled ventilation, including gynecologic laparoscopic surgery. Because it is cuffless, there is potentially enhanced simplicity of use, but this is balanced by complexity of sizing and insertion technique. The SLIPA's reservoir chamber is designed to prevent pulmonary aspiration of regurgitant matter, but its efficacy in this regard is uncertain.

i-gel

The i-gel (Intersurgical, Wokingham, UK) is an anatomically preshaped, single-use SGA device invented by Dr. Muhammed Nasir and marketed in 2007. It is made of medical-grade thermoplastic elastomer gel (styrene-ethylene-butadiene styrene), and it is called i-gel because of the soft gel-like material from which it is made. Pediatric sizes were introduced in 2009.

Technical Description

The i-gel is an anatomically designed SGA, with a stem, a soft mask portion, and a gastric channel (Fig. 19.36). The i-gel's stem is semirigid and wide with an elliptical shape, and it is curved in cross-section and contains a rigid integrated bite block. The airway tube ends in a large ventilation orifice with no bars or grills. The soft mask portion of the device is designed to anatomically fit the pharyngeal, laryngeal, and perilaryngeal structures. An integrated drain tube runs within the wall of the device, from laterally proximal to the posterior distal tip, and accommodates passage of a gastric tube (up to a 14-Fr for size 5 i-gel). A ridge situated at the proximal end of the mask (epiglottic rest) is designed to help prevent ventilation aperture obstruction by a downfolded epiglottis. The first report of the i-gel, by Levitan and Kinkle,[268] evaluated its anatomic position in a series of 73 uses in 63 cadavers. Endoscopy with an optical stylet revealed a full view of the glottis in 44 out of 73 insertions. In all neck dissections performed in 16 cadavers and in 8 radiographs, the bowl of the i-gel covered the laryngeal inlet.

The i-gel is provided in a protective cradle, in seven sizes, for use from neonates to large adults (Fig. 19.37). Appropriate size selection is based on the patient's weight (Table 19.6).

Insertion

Before insertion of the i-gel, lubrication with a water-soluble lubricant is recommended for the back, sides, and front of the mask. The i-gel is inserted with the patient's head and neck in the

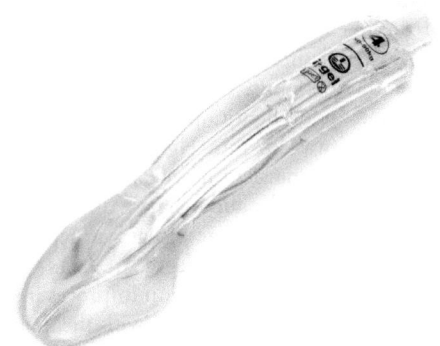

• **Fig. 19.36** The i-gel is anatomically shaped. It has a stem, a soft mask portion, and a drain tube. (Courtesy Intersurgical Company, UK.)

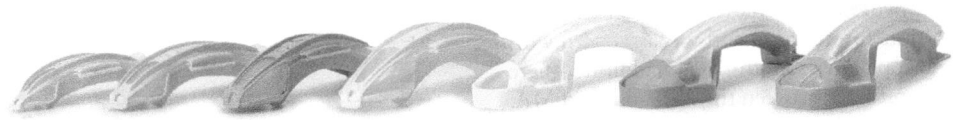

• **Fig. 19.37** i-gel is provided in protective cradles in seven sizes. (Courtesy Intersurgical Company, UK.)

TABLE 19.6   i-gel Size Selection

i-gel Size	Patient	Weight (kg)
1	Newborn	2–5
1.5	Infant	5–12
2	Small child	10–25
2.5	Large child	25–35
3	Small adult	30–60
4	Medium adult	50–90
5	Large adult	90+

sniffing position and the chin gently pressed down. Applying jaw thrust facilitates insertion. The device is advanced along the hard palate until resistance is felt. A black mark near the proximal end of the stem acts as a guide for correct depth of insertion.

Alternatively, a reverse inversion technique can be used, with the i-gel inserted with the concavity facing toward the hard palate and rotated 180% when it reaches the oropharynx.[269] A triple airway maneuver combining head tilt–chin lift, jaw thrust, and open mouth maneuvers was found to be quicker than the standard insertion technique.[270]

Laryngoscopy can also be used to facilitate i-gel insertion.[271] After insertion, the i-gel should be secured with tape from maxilla to maxilla. Cricoid force significantly decreases the success rate of adequate insertion of i-gel but, as its tip is shorter than most SGAs, this may be a lesser effect than for other devices.[272]

Indications for Use

Elective Use. The i-gel is designed for airway management during elective anesthesia with spontaneous and controlled ventilation. Absence of an inflatable cuff makes insertion potentially quicker and easier than cuffed devices. In a large, prospective observational multicenter study, Theiler and colleagues[273] reported 2049 uses of the i-gel. The primary ventilation success rate was 93.4%, and the overall success rate was 96%. Factors associated with primary ventilation failure were male gender, impaired mandibular subluxation, poor dentition, and older age. The mean average leak pressure was 26 mm Hg. Complications included laryngeal spasm (1.2%), transient nerve damage (0.1%), one case of transient vasovagal asystole, and one case of glottic hematoma. A remarkably low incidence of sore throat was reported (2.3%). Head rotation to 30 degrees and 60 degrees reduces OLP, whereas a mild to moderate degree of neck flexion improves it.[274,275]

The good airway leak pressure together with the drain tube may be features that suggest a degree of protection against pulmonary aspiration. Conversely, the i-gel tip is short and creates a low seal with the esophagus (13 cm H_2O compared to the cLMA, 37 cm H_2O, and the PLMA, 58 cm H_2O), which might have a countereffect.[35]

A systematic review and meta-analysis of 31 randomized clinical trials in adult patients comparing the i-gel with multiple types of LMA was performed by de Montblanc and colleagues.[276] The i-gel needed a reduced time for insertion and was associated with a lower incidence of postoperative sore throat. In addition, there was no difference in leak pressure between the i-gel and the LMA. Due to its lack of a cuff, if there is a poor seal after successful insertion (approximately 3% to 5% of cases, perhaps more frequently than for LMAs), the only solutions are to reinsert or change device

size. Multiple articles compare the performance of i-gel with other SGAs, mainly LMAs. A full review of this extensive literature is beyond the scope of this chapter.

Emergency Use. The ease of insertion allied with a steep learning curve has led to recognition of the role of the i-gel in emergency airway management. First responders in rural Germany were able to insert and use an i-gel for airway management during CPR in 88% of patients.[277] As reported by Benger and colleagues, short-term (30 days) and long-term (3 months and 6 months) outcomes and quality of life were similar in patients requiring CPR in prehospital settings with i-gel or ETT used as primary airway devices.[278,279]

The i-gel O_2 Resus Pack is equipped with a supplementary oxygen port, a hook ring for securing of the airway support strap, a sachet of lubricant, and a suction tube.[280] There are multiple reports of i-gel used successfully as a rescue device, including in cases of severe facial trauma,[280] subglottic stenosis,[281] and when a backup airway device is needed after LMA failure.[282]

Conduit for Intubation. Because of its large-diameter lumen, relatively short airway tube, and absence of bars or grills across the distal airway tube or airway orifice, the i-gel can serve as a conduit for tracheal intubation. Table 19.7 shows the ETT sizes that can be passed through each size of i-gel. FIS-guided tracheal intubation via the i-gel has a first-attempt success rate of 96% to 100%,[86,283,284] including in obese patients.[285] Awake i-gel placement followed by asleep FIS intubation was successfully reported in patients with a predicted difficult airway.[286] In contrast, blind intubation through the i-gel has a low success rate.[287]

Complications

Complications of i-gel are relatively infrequent but include tongue trauma,[288] mucosal erosion of the cricoid cartilage,[289] nerve injuries,[290–291] arytenoid dislocation,[292] regurgitation, and aspiration.[293,294]

Summary

The i-gel presents several advantages, including ease of insertion, good performance during spontaneous or controlled ventilation, and a remarkably low incidence of postoperative pharyngolaryngeal complications. Access to the glottis for tracheal intubation is reliable but requires FIS guidance. Its popularity as a conduit for tracheal intubation is increasing. Limitations are its occasional poor seal and its moderate bulky design.

Baska Mask

The Baska Mask (Proact Medical Ltd, Frenchs Forest, Australia) is a single-use SGA device made of medical-grade silicone.[16,295,296] It

TABLE 19.7   Sizing Guidelines for Inserting an Endotracheal Tube Through the i-gel

i-gel Size	Tracheal Tube Size (mm)
1	3.0
1.5	4.0
2	5.0
2.5	5.0
3	6.0
4	7.0
5	8.0

was designed by Drs. Kanag and Meenakshi Baska and marketed in Europe in 2011. Several changes to its design have been made since its launch, making interpretation of the available literature difficult.

The Baska Mask has an oval ventilation tube, with a standard 15-mm connector and an integrated bite block, which runs throughout the entire device (Fig. 19.38). The airway opening is at the distal end of the ventilation tube. A noninflatable expanding membranous cuff inflates and deflates with each positive pressure respiratory cycle, producing the airway seal (Fig. 19.39). There are two drain tubes for gastric fluid drainage, one on each side of the ventilation tube, and both opening on the posterior of the device distally. An inbuilt hand tab is attached to the cuff and can be used to manually increase the angulation of the device to aid insertion. It has a bite block throughout the entire length of the airway tube.[16] The Baska Mask is provided in single-use and reusable versions, and the latter may be used up to 70 times,[16] and it comes in four sizes from small to large adult with color-coded connectors.

Before insertion, the Baska Mask should be checked for integrity by sealing and compressing both ends of the device. The device should be lubricated generously on both sides with water-soluble jelly. A neutral position for the head and neck is preferable. The proximal part of the mask is compressed between the thumb, forefinger, and middle finger and advanced toward the hard and soft palate until resistance is encountered. If necessary, the tab can be pulled to flex the device's tip. The patient's front teeth should be approximately at the part of the tube into which

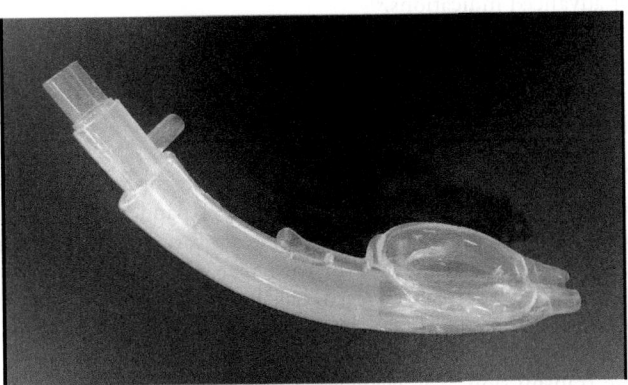

• **Fig. 19.38** Baska Mask. (Courtesy Baska Ltd., Strathfield, Australia.)

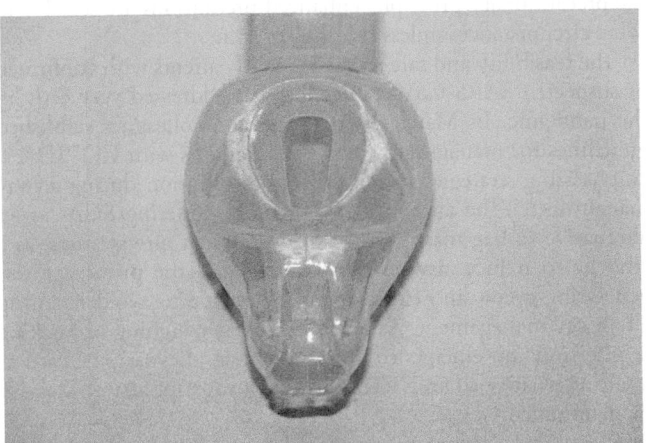

• **Fig. 19.39** Baska Mask—noninflatable expanding membranous cuff. (Courtesy Baska Ltd., Strathfield, Australia.)

the connectors are inserted. If difficulties ventilating the patient are encountered, the insertion depth needs to be adjusted or the Baska Mask replaced with a different size. One of the drain tubes can be connected to a suction device for continuous or intermittent pharyngeal suction during insertion or removal of the device.

The first clinical observational trial with the Baska Mask was performed by Alexiev and colleagues[295] and included 30 women scheduled for elective minor surgery. All insertions were performed by the principal investigator, who had very limited prior experience with the Baska Mask. In 76.7% of patients, the Baska Mask was successfully inserted on the first attempt, with an overall success rate of 96.7%. Mean insertion time was 24 seconds. The learning curve to insert the Baska Mask was short, with notable improvement in performance after the first 10 patients. In another study, also by Alexiev and colleagues,[296] the Baska Mask was compared with what the authors described as "a single-use classic LMA" in 150 females with normal airways. The first-time insertion success rate for the Baska Mask was significantly lower (73%) than that for the LMA (98%). However, the overall success rate was similar: 99% for the LMA and 96% for the Baska Mask. The airway seal pressure was significantly higher with the Baska Mask (40 cm H_2O) compared with the LMA (22 cm H_2O). The authors concluded that in clinical situations where the seal with the glottic aperture takes priority over ease of insertion, the Baska Mask may provide a useful alternative to the LMA. Of note, the Baska Mask has undergone modifications since these early studies, and it is unknown how these impact performance.

The Baska Mask is a new device, and therefore it is premature to discuss potential complications associated with it. Alexiev and colleagues[295] reported that repeated adjustment of the depth of insertion was necessary to obtain a good airway seal. The criteria to choose the correct device size are still not clearly defined.

The uniqueness of the device lies in its noninflatable expanding membranous cuff balloon. There is no pilot tube and no need to inflate the cuff, making insertion easier. Because of its unique design, it may be particularly useful in clinical situations where the airway seal is more important than ease of insertion.

Summary

The introduction and development of a wide variety of non-LMA SGAs have significantly contributed to the range of options available in airway management. Non-LMA SGAs have a well-established role in both elective and emergency airway management, and for some their role outside the OR is expanding, while for others it is decreasing. Limiting the intracuff pressure to 60 cm H_2O significantly increases the safety profile in cuffed SGAs and reduces iatrogenic upper airway trauma. Ideally, the cuff should be inflated using a manometer. This is not applicable in emergency situations, but the intracuff pressure can be adjusted and monitored after insertion, especially for procedures lasting more than 60 minutes. Non-LMA SGAs may offer a viable alternative in the case of LMA failure.

As with LMAs, the development of second-generation non-LMA SGAs is likely to result in reduced risks of regurgitation and pulmonary aspiration. Several non-LMA SGAs are suitable options as a conduit for tracheal intubation, with the i-gel being the most useful. Preference should be given to an FIS-guided intubation technique. Despite the fact that several non-LMA SGAs are easy to insert and learn, adequate skills, clinical judgment, and expertise are needed to ensure proper use. The choice of a specific non-LMA SGA should be determined by a thorough understanding of device performance, limitations, user experience, and proficiency.

TABLE 19.8	Factors to Consider in Selecting the Right Subglottic Airway for a Particular Clinical Case		
Patient Factors		**Surgical Factors**	**Clinician Factors**
• Risk of aspiration • Abnormalities of upper airway anatomy (e.g., a smaller profile SGA for limitations in mouth opening; potential contraindications for use with obstruction of the airway at or above the glottis, or in the presence of potential sources of bleeding) • Lung/chest wall compliance • Ventilatory requirements (e.g., increased with high metabolic requirements) • Body mass index • Special populations including pediatrics, obstetrics		• Location of surgery (e.g., an fLMA for head and neck surgery the aspiration risk of intraperitoneal vs bowel surgery) • Positioning requirements, including the ability to access the airway during the procedure • Duration of procedure	• Training • Experience • Skill • The provision of assistance in the event of airway difficulties

fLMA, Flexible laryngeal mask airway; *SGA*, supraglottic airway.

Choosing to Use an SGA and Choosing Among Them

In the safe use of SGAs, appropriate judgment in the selection of a device is critical and depends on various patient, surgical, and clinician factors, as outlined in Table 19.8. Key details that inform this decision-making process have been addressed elsewhere in this chapter. There remains a strong argument for routine use of second-generation devices.

Since the early development of the cLMA, a substantive body of literature has established the multiple potential advantages that it can provide over the ETT and face mask.[297] In a meta-analysis of 29 randomized prospective controlled trials, appropriate cLMA use was associated with a lower incidence of postoperative hoarse voice, sore throat, nausea, and vomiting, as well as laryngospasm and coughing during recovery, compared with an ETT.[32]

In terms of the evidence base to justify use of the optimal SGA for a particular clinical case, the data are limited. Not only is an evidence base largely nonexistent for some devices, modifications can be made to an original design without product rebranding. These changes mean that the published data based on an older device are not necessarily relevant to the product currently available, and it may be difficult to understand these changes.[297] There is also a significant deficiency in the quality of literature. Despite thousands of studies, there is not only a lack of efficacy research, but there also are less reliable data to determine the complication and safety profile of individual devices.

There are several deficiencies in the literature regarding SGAs. First, it is difficult to power trials when the relevant outcomes and complications are uncommon or rare. Many trials only collect data involving early efficacy (e.g., insertion success and OLP) or minor complications (e.g., sore throat) in low-risk patients who are not generalizable to the expanding repertoire of advanced uses, limiting the use of further meta-analysis.[298] Second, most trials are very small (powered on surrogate measures such as OLP) and fail to collect data relevant to safety issues. Third, the ability to discern the exact cause of SGA failure or complication in a study is often not clear, the response required to correct a device versus human-factor deficiency being starkly different.[297]

Many design features in the second-generation and newer SGAs have identifiable performance advantages, such as higher airway and esophageal leak pressures, which improve certain aspects of efficacy.[77,276] However, whether or not improvements in these performance characteristics translate to improvements in clinical outcomes is uncertain and likely cannot be proven. For the same reasons, the benefits of other features, such as the drain tube designed to reduce the risk of aspiration and help ensure correct positioning, have also yet to show a superior effect in terms of clinical outcomes. Equally, an absence of evidence does not necessarily indicate an absence of impact. It is the opinion of the authors of this chapter that the current knowledge of potential benefit is sufficient to justify routine use of second-generation SGAs, particularly the PLMA and i-gel and especially for advanced indications.[8]

The Role of Supraglottic Airways in a Respiratory Pandemic

On March 11, 2020, the World Health Organization (WHO) declared the coronavirus outbreak to be a pandemic. This has brought unprecedented challenges to healthcare providers in general and to anesthesiologists in particular. COVID-19 is highly contagious. Particular concern has been raised about certain procedures designated as aerosol-generating procedures (AGPs), which have been regarded as high risk in terms of causing disease transmission. The evidence base for many of the interventions listed as AGPs, both in terms of actual generation of aerosols and in being associated, is limited or absent. However, based on the precautionary principle, enhanced precautions are sensible in some circumstances unless risk is disproven.

The feasibility and safe use of SGAs in patients with confirmed or suspected SARS-CoV-2 infection was addressed very early in the pandemic. In March 2020, Cook and colleagues published guidelines for managing the airway in patients with COVID-19, emphasizing strategies to minimize aerosolization during airway maneuvers.[299] The authors recommend considering SGAs as an alternative to bag-mask ventilation in difficult airway cases, as a strategy to reduce airway leak. Coughing is the prime aerosol-generating event, and efforts should be made to avoid it during all airway management. As SGAs cause less coughing or bucking at insertion and emergence from anesthesia, they may be used as a safe alternative to an ETT, providing a superior airway seal can be maintained.

Controlled ventilation with pressures exceeding the OLP increase the risk of airway leak, but it is not known whether this is associated with aerosolization. Airway leak is likely further minimized during

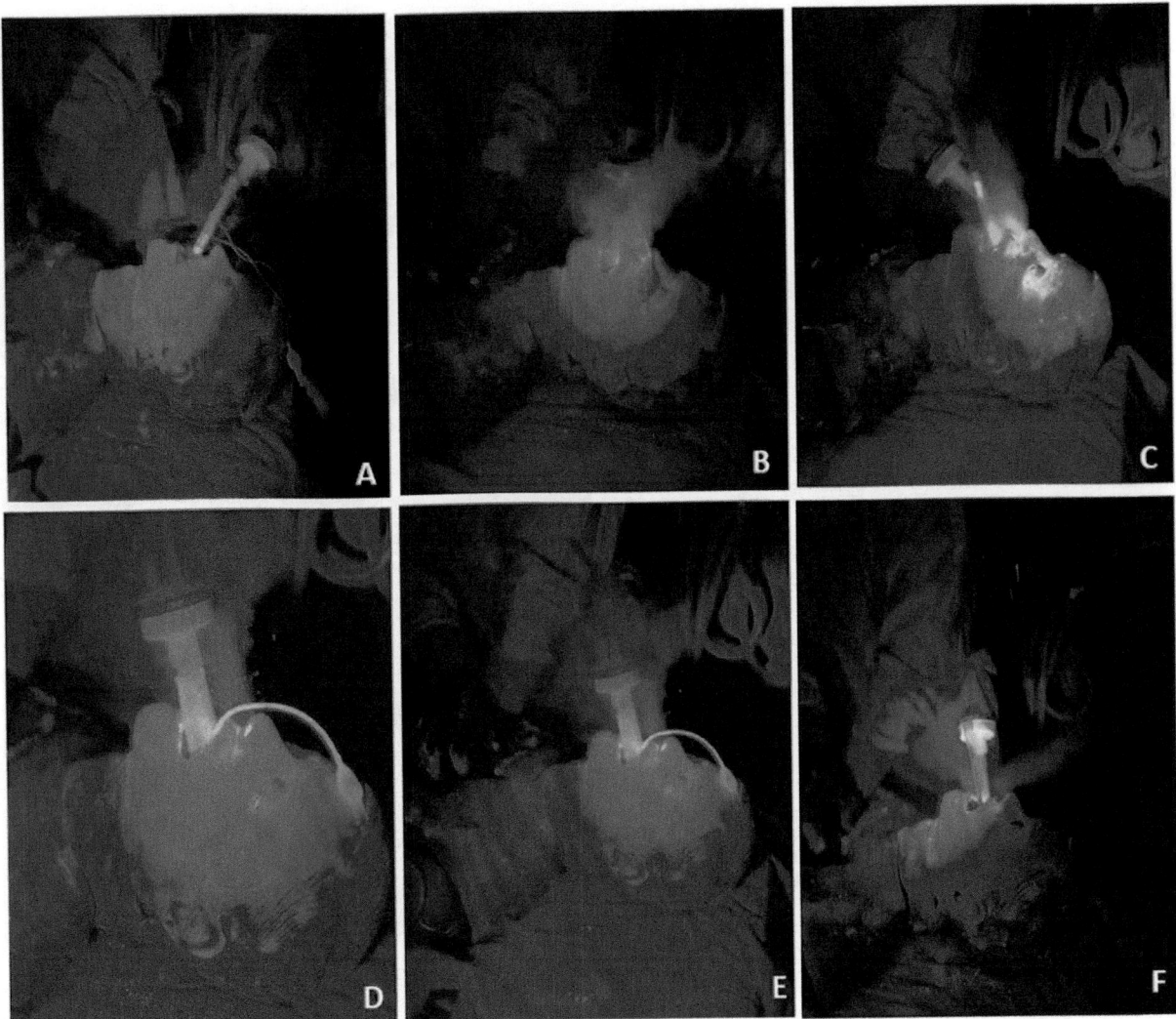

• **Fig. 19.40** Leakage of powder around supraglottic airways in a manikin during simulated cardiac compressions. (A) ETC, (B) LTS-D, (C) LMA Supreme, (D) AuraGain, (E) i-gel, (F) LMA Proseal.

spontaneous ventilation with adequate depth of anesthesia to avoid coughing and bucking.[300] The balance between risk of use of and ETT or SGA during a respiratory pandemic likely has many factors, including many for which there is uncertainty, but because use of an SGA is likely to reduce coughing events overall, it has much in its favor compared to tracheal intubation and extubation.

Clinical evidence around aerosol-generation during SGA use is very limited. Simulation studies are of some value but have important limitations. Somri and colleagues[301] studied the aerosols generated by different second-generation SGAs connected to a high-efficiency particulate air (HEPA) filter during simulated CPR in manikins with an odorless powder that glows when exposed to ultraviolet light. Significant leak was visualized through the mouth and nose of the manikin for all six SGAs studied including the AuraGain (Fig. 19.40A), i-gel (Fig. 19.40B), PLMA (Fig. 19.40C), SLMA (Fig. 19.40D), ETC (Fig. 19.4E), and LTS-D (Fig. 19.40F).[301] The same group investigated the effectiveness of an endoscopic mask (VBM Sulz, Germany) assembled over an SGA (LTS-D) and supported by a harness in reducing airway leak during CPR: This achieved an adequate seal preventing airway leak in a manikin (Fig. 19.41).[302] It is difficult to interpret these studies—manikins cannot simulate the physiology of

aerosol generation, and the simulations described simply demonstrate that the airway was leaking—they do not indicate that in humans aerosols would be generated. In addition, the manikin is no substitute for a human in terms of device performance and airway leak, with SGA performance in many manikins being poor and lacking human verisimilitude.[303]

Changing an ETT to an SGA before extubation while the patient is still under deep anesthesia can minimize coughing and bucking at extubation. However, using an SGA as a bridge for extubation presents the disadvantage of performing an additional airway maneuver.

Overall, we lack clear evidence regarding the risk of aerosol generation or disease transmission during SGA insertion, use, and removal. There is an urgent need to fill this evidence gap with high-quality research.

Conclusion

The family of LMA-type SGAs has dramatically changed practice for both elective and emergency airway management. Since the introduction of the cLMA into clinical practice, numerous SGAs have been developed, some with several features that

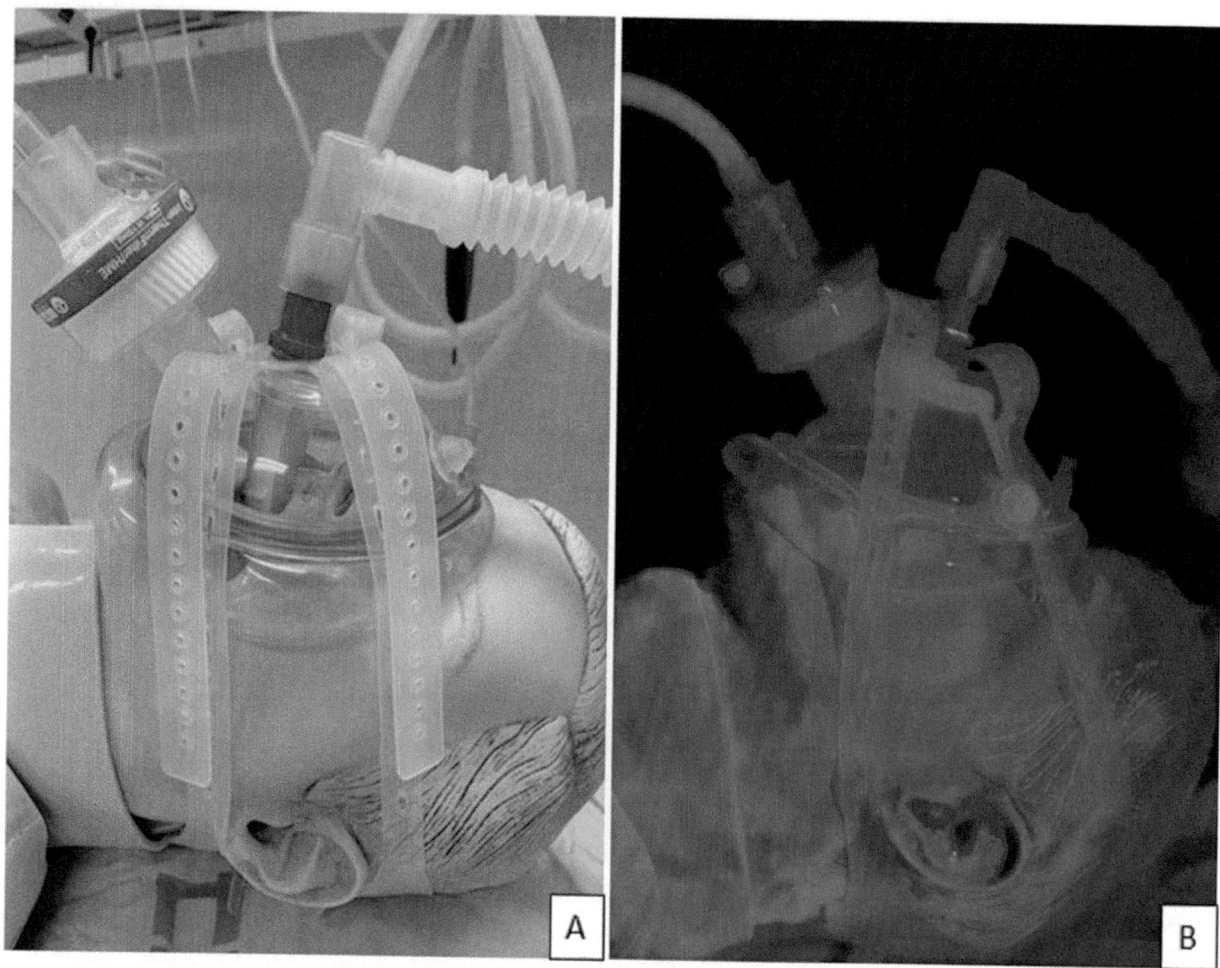

• **Fig. 19.41** (A) Endoscopic mask inserted over LTS-D. (B) The endoscopic mask assembled to the LTS-D prevents powder leak.

enhance safety and utility. Existing literature supports their safe use, emphasizing the importance of appropriate patient selection and atraumatic insertion.

No single airway device meets all the criteria for the ideal SGA, and it is likely that several different airways will always be needed for use in different clinical situations. To be considered competent in airway management, airway providers should be skilled with several devices and techniques.

Although recognizing the current limitations in efficacy and safety data for many SGAs, wherever possible this judgment should be informed by an evidence-based approach. Clinical judgment and expertise are also critical in determining which device is indicated in any situation. Continued research in this field will drive airway management to higher safety standards.

Selected References

7. Cook TM, Woodall N, Frerk C, eds. Fourth National Audit Project of the Royal College of Anaesthetists and the Difficult Airway Society. Major Complications of Airway Management in the UK. Report and Findings. Royal College of Anaesthetists; 2011.

21. Hernandez MR, Klock PA. Ovassapian A. Evolution of the extraglottic airway: a review of its history, applications, and practical tips for success. *Anesth Analg.* 2012;114:349–368

22. Pandit JJ, Popat MT, Cook TM, et al. The Difficult Airway Society 'ADEPT' guidance on selecting airway devices: the basis of a strategy for equipment evaluation. *Anaesthesia.* 2011;66:726–737.

28. Verghese C, Ramaswamy B. LMA-Supreme™—a new single-use LMA™ with gastric access: a report on its clinical efficacy. *Br J Anaesth.* 2008;101:405–410.

32. Yu SH, Beirne OR. Laryngeal mask airways have a lower risk of airway complications compared with endotracheal intubation: a systematic review. *J Oral Maxillofac Surg.* 2010;68:2359–2376.

63. Cook TM, Lee G, Nolan JP. The ProSeal laryngeal mask airway: a review of the literature. *Can J Anaesth.* 2005;52:739–760.

125. Yoon SW, Kang H, Choi GJ, et al. Comparison of supraglottic airway devices in laparoscopic surgeries: a network meta-analysis. *J Clin Anesth.* 2019;55:52–66.

129. Nicholson A, Cook TM, Smith AF, Lewis SR, Reed SS. Supraglottic airway devices versus tracheal intubation for airway management during general anaesthesia in obese patients. *Cochrane Database Syst Rev.* 2013;CD010105.

165. Van Zundert AA, Kumar CM, Van Zundert TC. Malpositioning of supraglottic airway devices: preventive and corrective strategies. *Br J Anaesth.* 2016;116:579–582.

225. Gaitini L, Vaida S, Somri M, et al. An evaluation of the laryngeal tube during general anesthesia using mechanical ventilation. *Anesth Analg.* 2003;96:1750–1755.

All references can be found online at eBooks.Health.Elsevier.com.

20

Laryngoscopic Tracheal Intubation

PAUL A. BAKER AND GEORGE KOVACS

CHAPTER OUTLINE

KEY POINTS

- "Resuscitation Sequenced Intubation" for managing critically ill patients and the physiologically difficult airway has become an accepted term describing the process of intubation and transition to positive-pressure ventilation that poses significant risk to the patient in an at-risk cohort.
- Just as less invasive airway management may be better suited for shockable rhythm cardiac arrests where early return of spontaneous circulation is more likely, there is evidence that for nonshockable rhythms a more advanced airway management such as an endotracheal tube (ETT) is associated with improved outcomes.
- Elective tracheal intubation is indicated for patients requiring anesthesia for major surgery when controlled ventilation, resuscitation, airway access, patient positioning, and duration of surgery are factors in the overall airway plan.
- Avoiding hypoxemia, hypocapnia, and hypotension, and early access to imaging and neurosurgical care are the priorities for managing patients with traumatic brain injury. While early airway, oxygenation and hemodynamic support for trauma may be needed, this does not necessarily mean prioritizing early intubation.

- Tracheal intubation protects against aspiration of gastric contents in anesthetized patients; however, the use of a supraglottic airway (SGA) is not associated with an increased risk of pulmonary aspiration compared with an ETT.
- In 1952, Macintosh wrote "Whatever laryngoscope is used, the principles of laryngoscopy remain the same. If these—namely correct head position and adequate anaesthesia—are ignored, no laryngoscope will give success. The secret of successful intubation lies with the anaesthetist, not with any particular laryngoscope. That good result can be obtained with many different patterns is obvious from the fact that these different types all have their own supporters".
- Tracheal intubation facilitates various types of respiratory therapy, including mechanical ventilation, 100% O_2 for CO poisoning, NO, surfactant, Heliox, and suctioning.
- The risks of tracheal intubation are heightened when airway management is required away from the OR and when multiple tracheal intubation attempts are made.
- The limiting factors for the safe application of tracheal intubation are the skill of the practitioner, the use of patient monitoring, and an understanding of the indications for tracheal intubation.

Introduction

Tracheal intubation (TI) is the placement of an endotracheal tube (ETT) into the trachea as a conduit for ventilation or other lung therapy. The benefits of TI are listed in Box 20.1. Historically, tracheal ventilation arose as a means of resuscitation via a tracheostomy and progressed with the development of the ETT, which protected of the lungs from aspiration. The eventual discovery of inhalation anesthesia facilitated surgical applications requiring a secure airway, controlled ventilation, and lung therapy. This chapter will review these primary indications for TI in the context of resuscitation, prehospital airway management, emergency medicine, intensive care, and anesthesiology. Nontechnical and technical aspects of TI will then be considered.

Tracheal Intubation for Resuscitation

Records of TI date back more than a thousand years to when early experiments were conducted by a Persian physician, Avicenna, who intubated pigs. In 1543, Andreas Vesalius, a Belgian anatomist, performed TI by inserting a cane tube through a tracheostomy into the trachea of a pig. These landmark developments allowed controlled ventilation and laid the foundation for subsequent advances in resuscitation. TI for human resuscitation was first performed in 1754 by an English surgeon, Benjamin Pugh, who orally intubated an asphyxiated neonate with his "air pipe." This was followed in 1788 by Charles Kite, another English surgeon, who reported the use of his curved metal cannula that he introduced blindly into the trachea of several near-drowning victims from the river Thames.[1]

TI is still considered to be the "gold standard" to maintain an airway and provide ventilation in most critically ill patients, but more recent evidence has called into question its prioritization during cardiopulmonary resuscitation (CPR), particularly in the out-of hospital (OH) setting.[2] Previous observational literature involving large patient populations was limited by confounding factors where the airway procedure decision could not be controlled for.[3] Two large prospective randomized trials comparing TI to supraglottic airway (SGA) placement in OH cardiac arrest and one comparing bag-mask ventilation (BMV) to TI favored a less invasive airway approach.[4–6] Physiologically these findings have been explained by the importance of circulating oxygenated blood with uninterrupted high-quality chest compressions to increase coronary perfusion pressure and prioritizing defibrillation for shockable rhythms.[7] This circulation first ("CAB" instead of "ABC") approach emphasizes airway support interventions that are less likely to require any interruption to CPR. This approach is supported in part by literature demonstrating that patients with shockable rhythms managed without an advanced airway (MV) have had better outcomes than those managed with TI.[8] Vigorous, often inadvertent positive-pressure ventilation (PPV) with high

• BOX 20.1   The Benefits of Endotracheal Intubation

1. A patent airway via oral, nasal, or tracheal routes
2. Controlled ventilation with up to 100% oxygen
3. Ventilation with high airway pressure
4. Airway protection from aspiration
5. Removal of secretions
6. Lung isolation
7. Administration of medication including anesthetic gases

rates, pressures, and volumes associated with TI may have negative impact on cardiac arrest patients.[9] Finally, it may be that the technical imperative of performing TI may be distracting from the other priorities in resuscitating a cardiac arrest victim.[2]

Some have questioned the findings from these prospective studies on the basis of the low success rates for TI performed by nonphysician clinicians (paramedics). A recent large German registry dataset compared TI to SGA placement with physician providers using a matched analysis to address known confounders. The study demonstrated improved outcomes with TI during OH cardiac arrest.[10] Additionally, just as less invasive airway management may be better suited for shockable rhythm cardiac arrests where early return of spontaneous circulation is more likely, there is evidence that for nonshockable rhythms a more advanced airway management such as TI is associated with improved outcomes.[8] In a 2019 American Heart Association Focused Update on Advanced Cardiac Life Support, provider experience and training were addressed in the recommendations.[11]

Early intubation for trauma patients in the prehospital setting has yielded mixed results, but for patients with severe injuries managed by skilled emergency medical service (EMS) providers, there appears to be a mortality benefit.[12,13] Much of the literature surrounding airway management for trauma has focused on care of patients with traumatic brain injury (TBI), whether in isolation or as part of a multisystem injury presentation. The most common reason to intubate patients with isolated TBI is for airway protection and/or predicted course (anticipated clinical deterioration). Given the fact that any hypocapnia, hypoxemia, or hypotension is associated with worse outcomes in this patient population, the risks of performing TI early, particularly in a less controlled environment, must be balanced against the benefits of securing the airway.[13–17] The motto of "GCS [Glasgow Coma Scale] less than 8, intubate" is essentially invalidated and much too superficial to be used as decision guidance for a patient with TBI.[18] Skilled provision of prehospital intubation for patients with TBI decreases mortality. This requires care, preparation, and performance of TI to avoid any physiologic derangements.[14–16,19–21] Avoiding hypoxemia, hypocapnia, and hypotension, and early access to imaging and neurosurgical care are the priorities for managing these patients. While early airway, oxygenation, and hemodynamic support for trauma may be needed, this does not necessarily mean prioritizing early intubation.[22]

Resuscitation Sequenced Intubation for managing critically ill patients and the *physiologically difficult airway* has become an accepted term describing at-risk cohorts where the process of intubation and transition to PPV poses significant risk to the patient.[23] The Society for Airway Management recently published consensus recommendations on the Evaluation and Management of the Physiologically Difficult Airway.[20]

The best airway technique for resuscitation depends on the patient's needs and clinical circumstances, the availability of appropriate equipment, and the skill of the rescuer.[6,7] Solutions to these problems involve training in airway management, appropriate selection of airway devices, and patient monitoring.[24] Waveform capnography can supplement clinical assessment of tracheal tube placement during CPR and is the most specific and sensitive method of confirming and monitoring tracheal tube placement during CPR. However, it cannot reliably differentiate tracheal and endobronchial tube placement.[25]

TI for resuscitation of the newborn is indicated if BMV has been prolonged or is ineffective, if chest compressions are to administer tracheal surfactant, or to manage a neonate with a congenital airway anomaly such as congenital diaphragmatic hernia or severe micrognathia. TI may also be indicated for tracheal obstruction as a result of neonatal meconium aspiration; however, routine intubation and suctioning of vigorous infants born through meconium liquor are not recommended.[26,27] Care and experience are required to avoid trauma and esophageal intubation.

Tracheal Intubation for Prehospital Care

Emergency TI in the prehospital environment often occurs in unfavorable conditions on patients who can be critically ill with shock, cardiopulmonary arrest, multisystem trauma, TBI, airway trauma, or uncorrected respiratory failure. The benefit of prehospital intubation (PHI) remains controversial. Conflicting results and opinions in part are related to differences in prehospital provider team makeup.[14,21,28] Outside North America, many prehospital systems use physician-only teams or a team of physician and nonphysician, usually a paramedic or nurse. Most physician prehospital programs are staffed by anesthesiologists and, to a lesser extent, emergency physicians. However, even within nonphysician-staffed prehospital programs, there is considerable variability in team makeup, using some combination of paramedics, nurses, and, in some jurisdictions, respiratory therapists. Most air transport services, in particular helicopter emergency medical services (HEMS), are staffed by specially trained critical care transport personnel consisting of either paramedics, nurses, physicians, or some combination thereof.

The natural history of most survivable illness or injury will be altered based on access to a high level of competent care. Most prehospital systems still consider TI the most definitive form of airway management; however, decision-making in the prehospital environment requires a risk-benefit analysis that must consider clinician skills, equipment access, availability of clinical practice guideline (CPG) support, and other resources, as well as the impact of transport delay. In most ground-based EMS systems in North America, direct laryngoscopy (DL) and intubation are within the scope of practice for a segment of advanced care paramedics; however, performance differences among agencies are quite variable.[31] The decision to perform TI by EMS systems must be supported by training and ongoing experience.[5,11]

While paramedics may be provided with excellent educational and simulation programming, access to operating room and emergency department educational opportunities on patients is increasingly difficult.[3,29] Rates of prehospital intubation are low at 5 to 8 per 1000. EMS calls resulting in many providers performing one or no intubations per year in part explain the low overall success rates in many programs. Additional procedural, equipment, and situational factors, such as having access only to non-RSI drugs, no access to video-assisted laryngoscopy (VAL), limited use of capnography, and the need to perform intubation in a difficult, often austere environment, play a significant role in determining airway management outcomes in the prehospital setting.[30] Many European and Nordic countries use physicians as prehospital providers and have published results demonstrating significantly higher median first-pass intubation success rates for physicians compared to nonphysicians.[31]

The 2016 Scandinavian Society of Anesthesiology and Intensive Care Medicine prehospital airway management guidelines and the more recent publication by the European HEMS & Air Ambulance Committee (EHAC) Medical Working Group on prehospital airway anesthesia are currently the only guidelines that include training recommendations for EMS providers.[31,32] The expectations of these primarily physician-based systems are that prehospital airway-management performance outcomes should be similar to those achieved in a hospital-based critical care environment (emergency department [ED], intensive care unit [ICU]). The authors of these publications work in regions where prehospital airway management is largely provided by physicians, and therefore expectations are high that care standards in the prehospital setting should be equivalent to that provided in a hospital with highly trained emergency/anesthesiology staff. While this may seem a reasonable expectation, existing staffing, logistical, and other system differences around the world make this goal difficult to achieve.

Prehospital care outcomes for critically ill patients are usually time dependent. Delivering prehospital care and airway management to critically ill patients, and then retrieving the patient for hospital care are both time-dependent phases of therapy. This time dependency may be related to both the outgoing and the incoming legs of the transport. The goal of resuscitation is to ensure adequate gas exchange and maintain end-organ perfusion. The technical imperative to get the tube in may not be a patient-centered approach, as an ETT simply provides a conduit for the primary airway management goal of improving and maintaining oxygenation and ventilation. Decisions around *what can be done* and *what should be done* in the prehospital setting will depend on the patient, the illness or injury, system factors (provider skill, scope of practice, equipment access), and geography that influences time to help and time to definitive care.

Tracheal Intubation for Emergency Medicine

Management of the airway in the ED is often a fine balance between urgency and risk. Like the prehospital setting, there are notable differences in who provides/supports airway management in EDs in various regions around the world. Emergency medicine is a relatively new but established specialty for which clinicians must balance disease *prevalence*, life-threatening *acuity*, and *complexity* in systems-based care. Airway management is a necessary, core skill for the specialty, and while the hands-on daily opportunities cannot be compared to those of anesthesiologists, existing registry data support this practice. In a systematic review of over 40,000 intubations from 10 countries over a 15-year period, the reported first-pass success (FPS) rate for ED intubations was 84%.[35] The FPS concept has been challenged from a patient-outcome perspective. It has been demonstrated that as the number of ED intubation attempts increase, so does the incidence of adverse events.[36] More recent data from the National Emergency Airway Registry (NEAR) have demonstrated improving FPS rates in the ED of over 90%.[37] In a recent prospective randomized ED trial by Driver et al. comparing routine use of a bougie with a stylet/ETT combination, FPS in the routine bougie group was 98%.[38] While routine use of the bougie clearly demonstrated benefit in this trial, these patients were managed by an experienced group of EPs performing RSIs using video-assisted DL and who were quite experienced with this approach. It has been suggested that improving results, such as those demonstrated in the Driver et al. study, may be less about the equipment and more about the bundle of optimized airway management care that delivered these high success rates.[16] While some have questioned the benefit of routine use of bundled care and checklists for airway management, there is a growing body of literature supporting their use in the ED.[37,38]

In the Fourth National Audit Project (NAP4) of the Royal College of Anaesthetists (UK) and the Difficult Airway Society (DAS), major airway management complications occurred significantly more often in the ED and ICU compared to the OR.[39] For numerous reasons, airway management of critically ill patients, regardless of location, will be associated with more adverse events compared to the more controlled elective environment of the operating room. The term *difficult airway* (DA) has traditionally referred to anatomic and pathologic challenges surrounding face mask and supraglottic ventilation, laryngoscopy and intubation, and front of neck airway (cricothyrotomy). The incidence of difficulty defined as such in the ED is notably higher than what is reported in the OR. Other factors, however, play a major role in determining ED airway outcome, most important of which is to manage the physiologically difficult airway.[22,23,40] The physiologically difficult airway encompasses a range of homeostatic disorders including but not limited to hypoxemia, shock, and metabolic acidosis, all of which often occur together in critically ill ED patients.[20] Despite the fact that RSI is by far the most commonly performed procedure in EDs around the world and has no doubt been contributory to high FPS rates, the downstream potential morbidity and mortality costs have raised questions about the benefit of RSI for patients in whom physiologic compromise cannot be optimized.[23,40,41] Emergent intubation may be indicated to ensure safe/good outcomes; however, meticulous attention must be paid to identifying and resuscitating these patients in the periintubation period. Performing an RSI might provide optimal laryngoscopy conditions for the provider, but loss of spontaneous ventilation may pose a significant risk in many critically ill patients. The challenge is that the traditional alternative to an RSI—the awake intubation (AI)—frequently will be limited by the patient's limited ability to cooperate and by provider experience. *Delayed Sequence Intubation* (DSI) is a term that refers to pharmacologically facilitated periintubation resuscitation efforts prior to intubation. While it may suggest that an RSI will follow, this intervention may be a helpful bridge to help facilitate an awake approach with topical anesthesia using the technique of preference for the user (DL, VL, or Flexible scope intubation).[42] And so the term *difficult airway* in the ED takes on an expanded definition beyond that described by the patient's native anatomy or acquired pathology in the ED to include the patient's physiology and ability to cooperate with an awake technique. Contrary to popular belief, the need to immediately manage an airway in the ED is relatively uncommon. Rapid, safe ED airway management requires skillful execution of laryngoscopy and intubation using a narrow range of devices in a resuscitated patient—a scope of practice that is well within the discipline of emergency medicine.

Tracheal Intubation for Intensive Care

The most common indications for TI in the ICU are acute respiratory failure, shock, and neurologic disorders.[43] TI is indicated for controlled ventilation in the presence of refractory hypoxemia, often in the presence of multiple organ failure. Predictors of hypoxemic respiratory failure are listed in Box 20.2.

The decision to intubate is usually made on clinical grounds based on the prognosis for the patient's condition. Clinical signs (see Box 20.3) or evolving deterioration in objective criteria may support this decision.

Urgent intubation in the ICU may be required immediately for apnea, airway obstruction, reintubation, or cardiopulmonary arrest. If the patient is unconscious, without airway reflexes, or paralyzed, TI can proceed without pharmacologic support.

RSI, the gold standard technique commonly used in the ED, may not be as applicable for the unstable ICU patient. Preoxygenation of the patient with limited respiratory reserve is compromised by decreased functional residual capacity (FRC) and increased dead space.[46] Commonly used induction agents can adversely affect the unstable patient. In these situations, a non-RSI technique with sedation and local anesthetic might be used.

Noninvasive ventilation techniques have become increasingly popular over the past 20 years with clear indications and a range of masks and interfaces.[45] Indications include patients with cardiogenic pulmonary edema and exacerbations of chronic obstructive pulmonary disease (COPD). Noninvasive ventilation is contraindicated for respiratory arrest or patients who are unable to be mask ventilated.[46] Relative contraindications for noninvasive ventilation that favor TI are listed in Box 20.4.

In the NAP4 of the Royal College of Anaesthetists and the Difficult Airway Society (DAS), 184 patients suffered major complications from airway management (death, brain damage, emergency surgical airway, unanticipated ICU admission, and prolonged ICU stay).[41] Of that number, 36 occurred in the ICU.

• BOX 20.2 Predictors of Hypoxemic Respiratory Failure

1. No or minimal rise in the ratio of Pa_{O_2} to $F_{I_{O_2}}$ after 1 to 2 hours
2. Patients older than 40 years
3. High-acuity illness at admission (simplified acute physiology score >35)[170]
4. Presence of ARDS (acute respiratory distress syndrome)
5. Community-acquired pneumonia with or without sepsis
6. Multiorgan failure

Adapted from Nava S, Hill N. Non-invasive ventilation in acute respiratory failure. *Lancet.* 2009;374:250–259.

• BOX 20.3 Signs of Respiratory Distress and Impending Fatigue

1. Look of anxiety ⟶ Frowning
2. Signs of sympathetic overactivity ⟶ Dilated pupils, forehead sweat
3. Dyspnea ⟶ Decreased talking
4. Use of accessory muscles ⟶ Holds head off pillow
5. Mouth opens during inspiration ⟶ Licking of dry lips
6. Self-PEEP ⟶ Pursed lips, expiratory grunting, groaning
7. Cyanosed lips
8. Restlessness and fidgeting
9. ⟶ Apathy and coma

PEEP, Positive end-expiratory pressure.
Data from references 166–169.

Although less than 20% of the total number of reported cases occurred in the ICU, more than 60% of the ICU cases resulted in death or brain damage compared with 14% in anesthesia. Assessors found a lower standard of airway management in the ICU than in both anesthesia and emergency medicine. The authors recommended the use of an intubation checklist to help prepare the patient, equipment, drugs, and the team before TI. An example of such a checklist appears in Fig. 20.1. The use of capnography for intubation in all critically ill patients was also recommended. The incidence of airway mishaps in the ICU involving TI is relatively low. In a study of 5046 ICU intubated patients, the airway accident rate was 0.7%. Accidents were less common with ETTs than with tracheostomies.[47] Self-extubation is the most common ETT accident, with rates of up to 16%. With strict clinical monitoring and in-service education this rate can reduce to 0.3%. Following unplanned extubation, reintubation rates ranged from 14% to 65%.[47] In a prospective multicenter cohort observational study, the incidence of difficult intubation for obese patients in the ICU was found to be twice as high as a cohort of obese patients intubated in the OR (16.3% vs 8.2%, $p < 0.01$), and severe life-threatening complications related to intubation occurred 20 times more often in the ICU.[48] A standard program of ETT management, including effective fixation techniques, can reduce unplanned extubation rates.[49]

In addition to mechanical ventilation, TI facilitates other types of respiratory therapies. Patients with moderate to severe carbon monoxide poisoning can benefit from 100% oxygen. This concentration of oxygen in normobaric conditions is most reliably achieved through an ETT. Other therapy through an ETT includes synthetic surfactant for premature newborns with established respiratory distress syndrome (RDS). Nitric oxide (NO) is administered to adults, infants, and neonates receiving mechanical ventilation to treat acute lung injury, acute respiratory distress syndrome (ARDS), and RDS. Heliox is a blend of oxygen and helium gas used to improve gas flow to patients with airway narrowing such as in asthma. On the other hand, use of the ETT as a route for emergency drug administration during CPR is no longer recommended because of unpredictable plasma concentrations and the reliability of the intraosseous route.[25]

Clearing secretions by suctioning through the ETT is important to maintain ventilation by avoiding atelectasis and consolidation. Suctioning is associated with several complications such as hypoxemia, cardiovascular instability, elevated intracranial pressure, atelectasis, infection, and trauma to the airway.

• BOX 20.4 Relative Contraindications for Noninvasive Ventilation and Indications for Endotracheal Intubation

1. Medically unstable
2. Agitated and uncooperative
3. Unable to protect the airway
4. Impaired swallow
5. Excessive secretions that are not being adequately managed
6. Multiple organ failure (i.e., two or more)
7. Recent upper airway or upper gastrointestinal surgery
8. Failed noninvasive ventilation

Adapted from Nava S, Hill N. Non-invasive ventilation in acute respiratory failure. *Lancet.* 2009;374:250–259.

Evidence-based recommendations for tracheal suctioning of adult intubated intensive-care patients are listed in Box 20.5.[47]

Tracheal Intubation for Anesthesia

It is reasonable to expect that with advances in device technology and updated practice guidelines, combined with progress in medical education techniques, outcomes from management of the difficult or failed intubation should improve over time. Unfortunately, the results from the latest 2000 to 2012 Anesthesia Closed Claims Project database do not demonstrate that the severity of claims against anesthesiologists were reduced. It was found that patients were more sick than in the previous survey in 1993 to 1999, more difficult TI occurred in nonperioperative locations, there were a higher proportion of deaths than in the previous survey, and a delay occurred in over one-third of patients requiring an emergency surgical airway.[50] There is still an obvious need to improve procedural skill and the response to TI in anesthesia. Conversely, there is some evidence that difficulty with TI may have decreased over time.[51]

Historical Development and Indications

Significant improvements to the design of the ETT have been historically precipitated by evolving surgical techniques. Upper airway surgery performed in the early 19th century led to an increase in postoperative pneumonia caused by aspiration of surgical debris. In 1878, William Macewen first used an ETT in anesthesia for a patient with a tumor of the base of the tongue.[52] Macewen was also concerned with preventing aspiration and in 1880 developed a metal ETT with a sponge collar that he introduced blindly through the mouth for TI. In 1888, O'Dwyer designed a curved metal cannula with a conical end to provide a laryngeal seal. This device helped raise intratracheal pressure to avoid pulmonary collapse during thoracic surgery. In 1895, Alfred Kirstein performed awake DL with the "autoscope."[53] This primitive instrument was the precursor of other laryngoscopes developed by Jackson and others, aiding the utilization of the ETT. World War I precipitated a demand for plastic surgery of the head and neck, which led to oral and nasal ETT designs with pharyngeal or tracheal cuffs by Rowbotham and Magill. Anesthetic management for thoracic surgery led to the next advance in ETT design with the introduction of the first endobronchial tubes in 1932 by Gale and Waters.[1] By this time, the technique of TI was established, prompting the statement by Macintosh that "the ability to pass an ETT under direct vision was the hallmark of the successful anaesthetist."[54]

TI is now used extensively in modern anesthesia for elective and emergency indications both as a primary and rescue airway. Patient characteristics and surgical indications will often dictate the appropriateness of an ETT. Elective TI is indicated for patients requiring anesthesia for major surgery when controlled ventilation, resuscitation, airway access, patient positioning and duration of surgery are factors in the overall airway plan. Specialized ventilation tubes are used for specific indications. Examples include thoracic surgery requiring lung isolation, laryngeal surgery requiring microlaryngoscopy or laser treatment, and nasal intubation for limited mouth opening, oral surgery, and maxillofacial surgery. TI may occur when the primary surgical

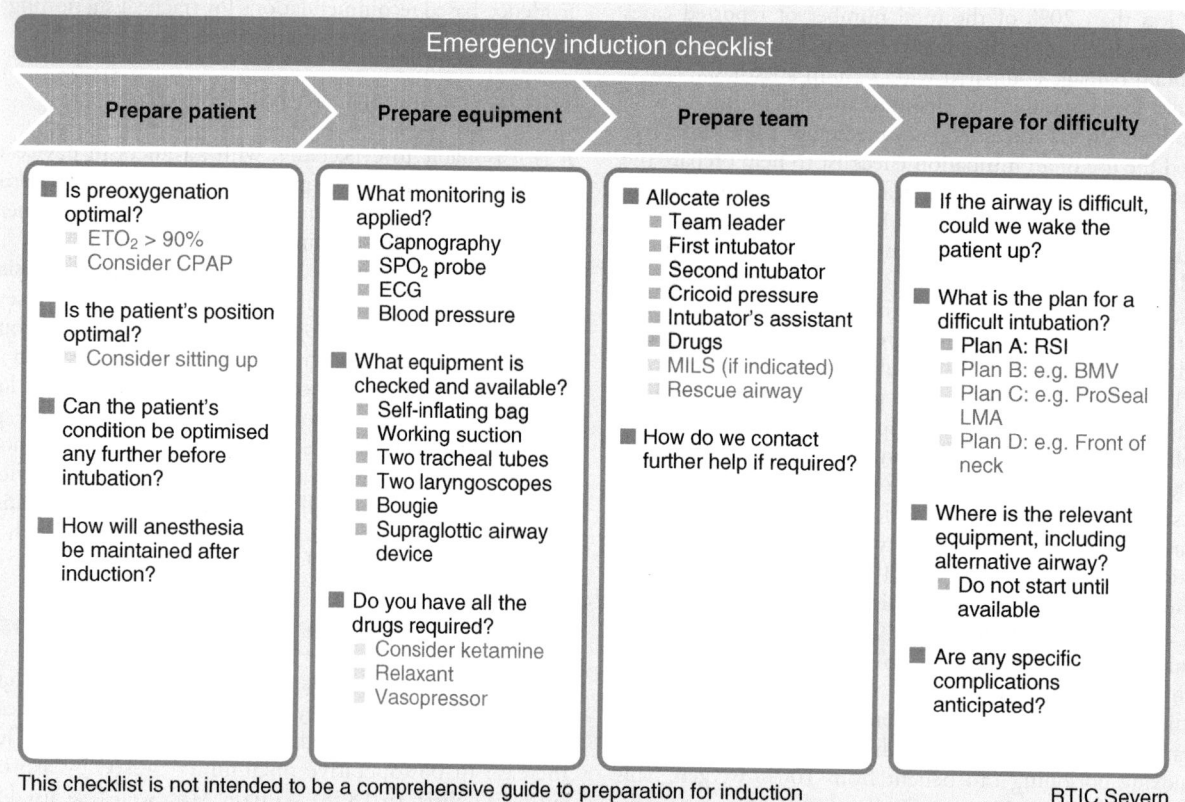

• **Fig. 20.1** A checklist for use before emergency department intubation. *BMV*, Bag-mask ventilation; *CPAP*, continuous positive airway pressure; *ECG*, electrocardiogram; *RSI*, rapid sequence induction. (From the Fourth National Audit Project of the Royal College of Anaesthetists and Difficult Airway Society. Major Complications of Airway Management in the United Kingdom. Report and Findings 2011, Editors Cook TM, Woodall N, Frerk C. With permission from the Royal College of Anaesthetists, London.)

• **BOX 20.5**   **Recommendations for Endotracheal Suctioning of Adult Intubated Intensive Care Patients**

1. Suction no longer than 15 seconds.
2. Perform continuous rather than intermittent suctioning.
3. Avoid saline lavage.
4. Provide hyperoxygenation before and after suctioning.
5. Provide hyperinflation combined with hyperoxygenation routinely.
6. Always use an aseptic technique.
7. Use either closed or open suction systems.

Adapted from Pedersen CM, Rosendahl-Nielsen M, Hjermind J, et al. Review. Endotracheal suctioning of the adult intubated patient—what is the evidence? *Intensive Crit Care Nurs.* 2009;25:21–30.

---

plan changes. An example is conversion of a diagnostic procedure, such as a bronchoscopy to a lung resection. Occasionally, complications arise during a simple anesthetic, necessitating TI during resuscitation, such as major hemorrhage, anaphylaxis, or malignant hyperthermia. Safe airway management should always include a plan B for failed mask or SGA ventilation. Conversion of the airway to TI may occur as plan B following inadequate mask or SGA ventilation. Impossible mask ventilation in anesthesia has an incidence of 0.15% and is associated with neck

radiation changes, male gender, sleep apnea, Mallampati class III or IV, and the presence of a beard.[55] In a study by Kheterpal of 53,041 operations that included an attempt at mask ventilation, 77 patients proved impossible to ventilate (0.15%). Of those 77 patients, 19 (25%) were also difficult to intubate, but 15 of those patients were intubated. Ultimately 74 of the 77 impossible mask ventilation cases were intubated,[55] reinforcing the value of TI for failed ventilation.

The American Society of Anesthesiologists (ASA) "Practice Guidelines for Management of the Difficult Airway" recommends AI for the patient with a known DA.[56] This usually involves TI with a flexible intubation scope (FIS), but other techniques have been described, including retrograde AI,[57] submental AI,[58] AI through an intubating laryngeal mask,[61] awake lightwand,[60] and awake videolaryngoscopy (VL).[61] The outcome of each technique is a secure airway with an ETT.

TI is regarded as the gold standard for protection against aspiration of gastric contents in anesthetized patients[62]; however, evaluation of the cuff seal is important because of the risk of microaspiration of oropharyngeal contents past the cuff. This particularly applies to high-pressure low-volume cuffs.[63] Evidence evaluating the relative risk of an ETT or SGA for pulmonary aspiration is limited. An analysis of the relative risk in 65,712 procedures found that the use of a laryngeal mask airway was not associated with an increased risk of pulmonary aspiration compared with an ETT.[64]

Decisions Before Tracheal Intubation

Before undertaking the technical aspects of TI, consider why, where, how, when, and by whom airway management should be performed.[65] Airway management practice guidelines offer useful advice to inform these decisions.[56,66–70] (See Chapter 11 concerning practice guidelines.) Serious morbidity and mortality can occur when important decisions are overlooked. Poor judgment was the second most common causal and contributory factor (59%) to that after patient factors (77%) in NAP4.[73]

The NAP4 study found that difficult or delayed intubation, failed intubation, and cannot intubate, cannot ventilate (CICV) situations accounted for 39% of events during anesthesia, and CICV accounts for 25% of all anesthesia-related deaths. Obsession with intubation and ignoring other options, such as waking the patient up, has been a fixation error in many cases with adverse outcomes. Having a clear understanding of the indications for TI, devising an airway plan, establishing when and where to proceed, using the technique with the best chance of success, and assembling the necessary skill, equipment, and support are all important requirements for safe TI.

Preparation for Laryngoscopy and Tracheal Intubation

It is wise to spend time preparing for TI. The first attempt at TI has the highest success rate, and diminishing return occurs with each subsequent attempt. Limitations on the number of intubation attempts are recommended by all recent airway management guidelines.[56,66–69] Therefore, it makes sense to make your first attempt be your best attempt. This requires preemptive planning to intubate under optimal conditions.

Equipment

Practice guidelines recommend the presence of a storage unit containing specialized equipment to manage a DA.[56,70] Details of the storage unit and equipment to manage a DA have been reviewed.[72] It is recommended that equipment to manage an emergency airway should be immediately available at all sites where airways are managed.[73] Safety principles for intubation equipment are based on standardization, redundancy, and a culture of safety.[72] Avoid excessive clutter and unnecessary duplication in the airway cart (standardization). This principle promotes familiarization with equipment across an organization and aids teaching and learning. Redundancy ensures the safety of backup in the event of failure (e.g., spare laryngoscopes, a range of sizes, alternative designs such as Macintosh, Miller, McCoy, videolaryngoscope). A culture of safety includes education, checklists, updating of equipment, sterilization, and backup plans. Equipment must comply with performance standards and should be checked regularly to ensure that it is fit for purpose.[73] A list of appropriate equipment for performing TI appears in Box 20.6.

Laryngoscopy

The objective of DL is to expose laryngeal anatomy and provide illumination of the larynx for subsequent TI. In the hands of an experienced practitioner, 82% of laryngoscopies reveal an easy view of the larynx, a restricted view in 16%, and a difficult view in 2%.[75] In difficult laryngoscopies, the larynx can easily be missed if the epiglottis is distorted or masked by adjacent mucosa. In these conditions, optimum illumination from the laryngoscope is important to provide good optical conditions. A study of visual acuity during DL at different illuminance levels demonstrated that visual acuity improved up to 700 lux illuminance, and subjectively anesthesiologists favor illuminance of 2000 lux. The International Organization for Standardization specifies illumination from hook-on laryngoscopes shall exceed 500 lux for at least 10 minutes of testing (ISO 7376:2009).[76]

Assessment

Airway management guidelines recommend taking a history, examining the patient, reviewing the clinical record, and performing other tests to assess the airway before airway management.[56,66,65] Several bedside screening tests have been described to identify patients with features of difficult DL and difficult TI. Unfortunately, bedside tests, such as the modified Mallampati test, thyromental distance measurement, sternomental distance measurement, and mouth opening, lack accuracy as stand-alone tests to predict difficult TI.[77,78] Combining bedside tests and examining multiple physical features improve the chances of predicting a DA, but not enough to perform as reliable predictive tests. Several studies have examined risk factors associated with airway management techniques and patient factors.[79] This information can be useful when planning to manage a patient's airway, but it is wise to plan for the unexpected DA because only 50% of DAs are anticipated preoperatively.[71,80] A New Zealand study found evidence of airway assessment in 68% of anesthetic records, but only half of the patients with a DA were anticipated preoperatively.[80] Also, evidence derived from airway assessment is often disregarded. Of 15,499 patients from the Danish Anaesthesia Database with a past history of either a difficult or a failed intubation, 24% with a previous difficult intubation were given a general anesthetic for subsequent anesthesia. Thirty percent of those with a previous failed intubation were also given a general anesthetic for a subsequent procedure.[81] Although repeating a general anasthetic in the face of a previous DA is not necessarily doomed to failure, the likelihood of difficulty is high, particularly if the same conditions apply. This reinforces the importance of detailed documentation following the management of a DA, including information about the patient positioning and specific details about the equipment used.

Assistance

It is important for the airway practitioner to have a trained assistant. It has been shown that an assistant improves safe management of simulated crises.[82] Given the unpredictable nature of a difficult intubation, the assistant should be briefed about an airway plan, and ideally that briefing should take place at the sign-in (preinduction) stage of the WHO Surgical Safety Checklist.[66,83] Assistants must understand their role and be familiar with their environment, particularly the availability of equipment and the contents of the airway cart.[84]

Positioning

"Some of the chief difficulties which arise during intubation for anaesthetic purposes may be traced to a faulty position of the patient's head."

Sir Ivan Magill, 1930[87]

Preoxygenation and Ventilation

1. Oxygen (O_2) source
2. Ventilation bag or anesthesia circuit (for positive-pressure ventilation)
3. Appropriately sized face mask
4. Appropriately sized oropharyngeal and nasopharyngeal airways
5. Tongue blade

Endotracheal Tubes

1. Bougie with coude tip
2. Appropriately sized ETTs (at least two)
3. Malleable stylet
4. Syringe for tube cuff, 10 mL
5. Jelly and/or ointment, 4% lidocaine (Xylocaine)

Drugs

1. Intravenous anesthetics and muscle relaxants (ready to administer)
2. Reliable, free-flowing intravenous infusion (some pediatric exceptions)
3. Topical anesthetics and vasoconstrictors (for nasotracheal intubation)

Laryngoscopy

1. Working suction apparatus with tonsil tip
2. Assortment of Miller blades with functioning battery handle
3. Assortment of Macintosh blades with functioning battery handle
4. Bolsters (folded sheets, towels) for positioning of head and shoulders

Fixation of the Endotracheal Tube

1. Tincture of benzoin
2. Appropriate tape or tie
3. Stethoscope
4. End-tidal carbon monoxide (EtCO$_2$) monitor
5. Pulse oximeterETT, Endotracheal tube.

ETT, Endotracheal tube.

For more than a hundred years, opinions have varied about the best position for DL. Early pioneers of indirect laryngoscopy included Johan Czermak in 1865 and Alfred Kirstein (the inventor of the first laryngoscope, or autoscope) in 1895. To indirectly examine the anterior commissure of the vocal cords, Czermak and Kirstein positioned the patients on a chair in a sitting position with the neck of the patients flexed and head extended. Images of these patients undergoing awake laryngoscopy show their head in a "sniffing position," and in the case of Czermak, external laryngeal manipulation (ELM) was applied. In 1915, Chevalier Jackson, a prominent surgeon and bronchoscopy specialist from Boston, stressed the importance of raising the head 10 cm away from the bed in a neck flexion position to align with the axis of the trachea, neck, and thorax.[86] Sir Ivan Magill, in 1930, described the position for TI in the recumbent position. He recommended a pillow behind the occiput to slightly extend the head on the atlas, bringing the mandible into a position approximately at right angles to the table. "These …are the positions …adopted by a man standing in the normal erect position when he scents the air."[85,87] In 1944, Freda Bannister and Ronald Macbeth proposed the three-axis theory, whereby the mouth and the pharyngeal and laryngeal axes are brought into near alignment by neck flexion and extension around the atlanto-occipital joint.[88]

A new concept of two curves consisting of a primary oropharyngeal curve and a secondary pharynx-glotto-tracheal curve was proposed by Greenland et al. in 2010.[89] Using MRI studies and changing different head and neck positions, the primary curve and the proximal section of the secondary curve maximally approximated the line of sight in the sniffing position. Other positions that included extension, head lift, and a neutral position were less effective. This provided objective evidence to support the sniffing position during DL, with neck flexion of 35 degrees and face plane extension of 15 degrees.

The importance of head elevation has been confirmed by Hochman et al. who found that full laryngeal exposure during straight blade laryngoscopy was achieved by increasing head elevation into a flexion–flexion position.[90] Levitan et al. termed this position "head elevation laryngeal position," or HELP, because the atlanto-occipital joint is not truly flexed.[91] The HELP position has proven to be particularly beneficial in obese and pregnant patients undergoing DL, using the ramped position with the external auditory meatus and sternal notch aligned horizontally.[92,93]

Other patient positions help to optimize laryngoscopy and TI. Bed height elevation to achieve patient's forehead at the xiphoid process of the anesthesiologist will provide better views of the larynx[94] (Fig. 20.2). Moving the patient to the head of the bed provides a more comfortable position for the laryngoscopist. Semi-seated (Fowler's) position or reverse Trendelenburg position helps postpone hypoxia with prolonged apnea in obese and nonobese patients. Using a 20-degree head-up position in nonobese anesthetized apneic patients can prolong nonhypoxic time, exceeding that of patients in a supine position or those with positive end-expiratory pressure (PEEP).[95] Children undergoing laryngoscopy and TI have different requirements for head positioning because of changes in relative head size with maturity. A newborn may benefit from a small pillow behind the shoulders during laryngoscopy, to help align the oral, pharyngeal, and tracheal axes. An infant may not require anything behind the occiput or shoulders, and a small pillow behind the head is not required until the child grows, often until 8 years old.

Preoxygenation

Preoxygenation and the administration of oxygen throughout TI are recommended by current airway management guidelines.[56,66,68] These techniques increase oxygen reserve in the lungs and therefore increase the duration of apnea without desaturation (DAWD) reaching ≤90% prolonging the time for laryngoscopy and TI before the onset of hypoxia.[96] Without oxygen, following the induction of anesthesia and the onset of apnea, oxygen desaturation occurs rapidly once the oxygen saturation falls to 94%, particularly if the airway is obstructed during apnea.[97] The DAWD to ≤90% depends on the preoxygenation technique, oxygen reserve at the start of apnea, oxygen consumption (increased in obese and pregnant patients), and the amount of oxygen required to maintain Spo$_2$ at 90%. In a theoretical healthy adult that time is 6.9 minutes with 100% oxygen therapy, and 1 minute if the patient is breathing air. Preoxygenation is indicated for all patients before the induction of anesthesia because a DA is unanticipated in 50% of patients.[80] Specific individual indications for preoxygenation include patients with anticipated difficult mask ventilation and/or difficult intubation, double lumen tube insertion, obese patients, pregnant patients, and patients with coexisting lung disease.

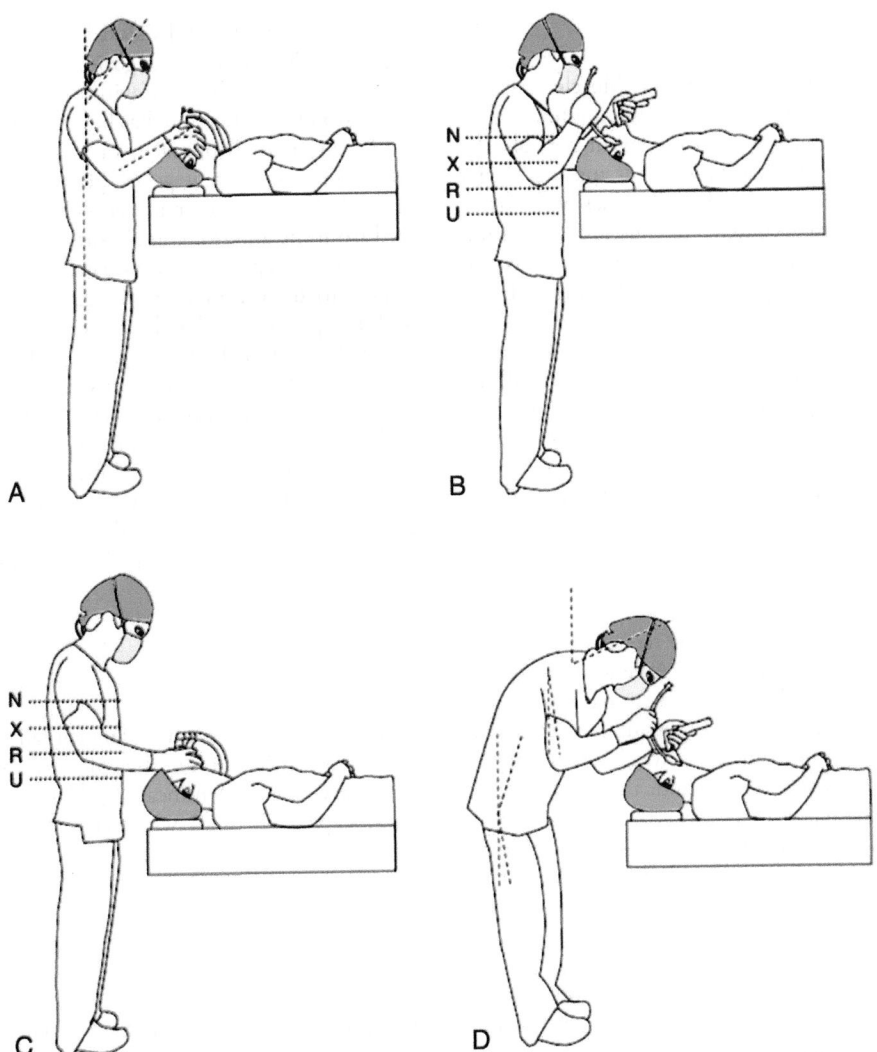

• **Fig. 20.2** Illustration of the nipple level (A and B) and the umbilicus level (C and D) operating table height during mask ventilation (A and C) and tracheal intubation (B and D). The measured angles of arm elevation, neck, low back, knee flexion, and wrist deviation are indicated with dashed lines. The levels of landmarks are marked as dotted lines. *N*, Nipple; *R*, lowest rib margin; *U*, umbilicus; *X*, xiphoid process. (Adapted from Lee H-C, Yun M-J, Hwang J-W, Na H-S, Kim D-H, Park J-Y. Higher operating tables provide better laryngeal views for tracheal intubation. *Br J Anaesth.* 2014;112:749–755, with permission from Oxford University Press.)

Preoxygenation technique involves tidal volume breathing (TVB), with 100% oxygen through a sealed face mask for 3 minutes. A fast technique of equivalent efficacy to TVB involves 8 deep breaths of 100% oxygen for 60 seconds. The endpoint for these techniques is an end-tidal oxygen concentration of 90% ($FE_{O_2} = 0.9$). Another fast technique using four deep breaths of 100% oxygen over 30 seconds is inferior to the TVB for 3 minutes and 8 deep breaths and is not recommended.[96,98] Failure to reach $FE_{O_2} = 0.9$ can be attributed to a decreased fresh gas flow, low FI_{O_2}, inadequate preoxygenation time, and leaks around the mask. The DAWD depends on the quality of the preoxygenation technique, the lung FRC, and oxygen consumption. Preoxygenation can be optimized by sitting the patient up to increase FRC. Application of PEEP has been studied in this context, and several studies show improved denitrogenation conditions and prolonged DAWD with PEEP.[99]

The use of nasal cannula to extend oxygenation into the postinduction phase of anesthesia is recommended during laryngoscopy and TI. Dry nasal oxygen at 15 L/min can achieve near 100% FI_{O_2} but has limitations for preoxygenation because of patient intolerance due to nasal desiccation; it can be tolerated in adults up to 10 L/min.[165] Despite this limitation, this technique is effective at prolonging apnea time after the administration of sedatives and muscle relaxants.[99] This technique has been given the acronym NO DESATS for "nasal oxygen during efforts securing a tube."[100] Preoxygenation can comfortably start with 2 L/min nasal oxygen, and the flow can increase to 15 L/min after induction. In contrast, the use of high-flow nasal oxygen (HFNO) up to 70 L/min for conscious adult patients is well tolerated, as demonstrated in a series of patients receiving HFNO during AI.[101] HFNO has also been used effectively in the ICU during difficult TI and as a primary oxygenation mechanism for prolonged periods of apnea during surgery.[102,103]

Medications

Anesthesia can influence laryngoscopy and TI. Muscle relaxants make TI easier and less traumatic.[104] This principle applies to children[105] and adults.[106] The choice of muscle relaxant may also be important. The time to oxygen desaturation after apnea is longer after rocuronium than after succinylcholine. This has been attributed to increased metabolism secondary to muscle fasciculation with succinylcholine.[107] The time to oxygen desaturation was also prolonged if succinylcholine was preceded by lidocaine and fentanyl.[107]

In the event of a failed intubation, a safe option may be to rapidly wake up the patient, provided the clinical scenario allows for safe return of spontaneous ventilation. The sedative used as an induction agent may stilll have residual significant effect depending on the timing of the reversal agent being administered. This can be achieved with 16 mg/kg sugammadex if the muscle relaxant was rocuronium.

Morbidity, Mortality, and Tracheal Intubation

The incidence of laryngeal morbidity can be reduced by improving the conditions of TI. According to the American Society of Anesthesiologists closed claims database, the larynx is the most common site of injuries to the airway, occurring in 33% of all airway claims.[110] Laryngeal injury includes vocal cord paralysis, hematoma, and hoarseness. Risk factors include tracheal tube size, tube design, and cuff pressure.

Repeated intubation attempts are associated with significant morbidity, including hypoxia, regurgitation and aspiration of gastric contents, bradycardia, and cardiac arrest.[110] Numerous publications have identified this relationship, which has resulted in recommendations to limit the number of intubation attempts.[56,66,67] Failed intubation, unrecognized esophageal intubation, aspiration of gastric contents, and airway trauma caused by intubation adjuncts, such as airway exchange catheters, also have potential to cause serious morbidity or mortality.[39]

Dental damage is among the most common causes of complaints against anesthesiologists and has an incidence ranging from 1:150 to 1:1000 TIs; however, some believe these numbers are underreported. Preoperative dental examination and use of a dental guard can protect the teeth from damage and reduce the incidence of damage by up to 90%. Despite this, the use of a dental guard is very low based on the belief that it will increase the difficulty of an intubation. This belief may be ill founded. A study of 80 patients found that intubation time increased by only 7 seconds when a dental guard was in place.[110]

Laryngoscopy Assessment

Various methods have been described to score the quality of the laryngeal view and TI. These scores can be used for research purposes and dissemination of airway information. The scores do not necessarily correlate with a difficult intubation, and the laryngeal score may vary, depending on the device and technique used for laryngoscopy and the subjective opinion of the observer. This raises issues of validity and reliability.

The best known scoring system for DL was described by Cormack and Lehane (CL), who originally proposed it to assist training and help decision-making during laryngoscopy.[111] This is a 4-point scale that has since been applied to different forms of DL and VL.[112] Since the first description, this score has undergone

modification with subdivisions plus an attempt to simplify the 4-point scale into three categories of easy, restricted, and difficult[75] (Fig. 20.3). Problems exist with the CL score because it is poorly understood and therefore has low reliability as a scoring system.[113]

An alternative approach was described by Levitan et al., who suggested the percentage of glottic opening (POGO) score[114] (Fig. 20.4). This score represents the portion of the glottis visualized from the anterior commissure to the interarytenoid notch. A score of 0% represents no visualization of the glottis, and 100% applies to an entire view of the glottis. This score has good intra- and interphysician reliability.

An Intubation Difficulty Scale (IDS) was described by Adnet et al.[115] The IDS is a comprehensive scale that incorporates the CL score, an intubating difficulty scale, and a scoring system. The IDS includes practical details of TI, such as cord mobility, lifting force, laryngeal mobility, number of attempts, number of operators, use of ELM, and use of alternative devices. A score of 0 (zero) indicates an easy intubation, less than 5 is slight difficulty, and greater than 5 reflects moderate to major intubation difficulty.

Techniques for Laryngoscopy and Tracheal Intubation

Laryngoscopy and TI can be conceptualized into five steps: mouth opening, identification of the epiglottis, tongue control, exposure of the larynx with identification of laryngeal landmarks, and TI.[116] These steps apply to DL with a curved blade, with a straight blade, and VL.

Macintosh Laryngoscopy and Tracheal Intubation

Macintosh designed his curved laryngoscope blade based on two observations[117]—first, that laryngoscopy could be achieved by passing the laryngoscope only until the epiglottis came into view,[118] and second, a curve in the blade improved the view of the larynx.[119]

The gentle continuous curve of the Macintosh blade is designed to push the base of the tongue upwards. This has the effect of flattening the primary oropharyngeal curve, described by Greenland, which helps achieve a straight line of sight from the eye to the larynx. The tip of the blade is designed to be placed in the vallecula, tensioning the hyoepiglottic ligament and thereby indirectly lifting the epiglottis. Various modifications of the Macintosh blade have been designed changing proximal blade height (Fig. 20.5) (American, "English" Macintosh or E Mac, and German), tip movement (McCoy), handle angle (Polio), and size from 1 to 4.

The Macintosh blade is the most popular laryngoscope in the world and has a number of advantages.[119] Success with this blade is high, with only a 1% to 3% failure rate.[121,122] The Macintosh blade is less stimulating than a straight blade because it does not touch the under glottic surface of the epiglottis. It was originally believed that the lingual surface of the epiglottis was innervated by the glossopharyngeal nerve and the glottic surface was innervated by the vagus. It is now known that both sides of the epiglottis are densely innervated by both vagus and glossopharyngeal nerves; however, the glottic surface is more sensitive, with more nerve endings than the lingual surface.[123] Macintosh laryngoscopy is relatively easy to learn, which made it an instant success. When Macintosh invented his blade in 1943, intubation occurred without muscle relaxants,

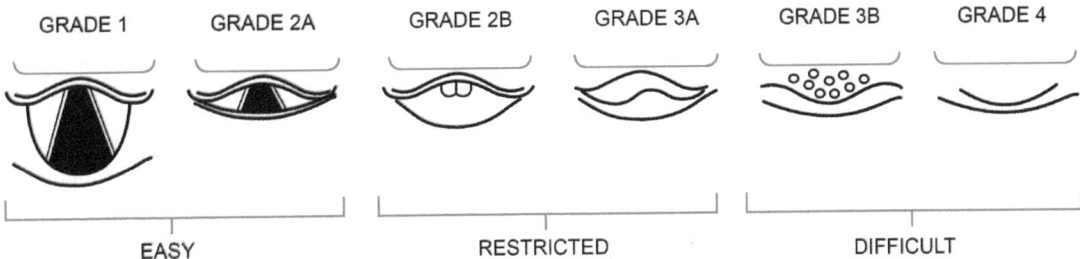

• **Fig. 20.3** Cormack and Lehane classification and new classification of view at laryngoscopy. Views are divided into easy, restricted, and difficult categories. (Courtesy Cook TM. A new practical classification of laryngeal view. *Anaesthesia.* 2000;55:274–279, with permission from John Wiley and Sons.)

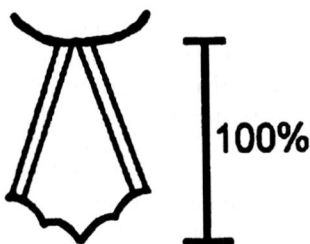

• **Fig. 20.4** The percentage of glottic opening (POGO) score. (From Levitan RM, ed. *The AirwayCam Guide to Intubation and Practical Emergency Airway Management.* Airway Cam Technologies Inc; 2004;94. With permission from Dr RM Levitan.)

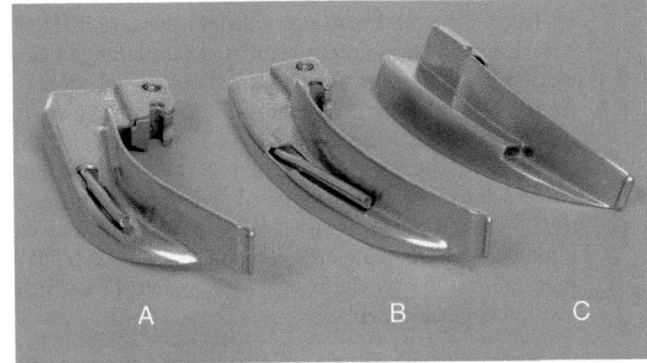

• **Fig. 20.5** American (A), "English" or E Mac (B) and German (C) Macintosh laryngoscope blades. (A and B from Welch Allyn, Skaneateles Falls, NY. C from Heine USA Ltd, Dover, NH.)

and straight blade laryngoscopy had become difficult due to a poor midline approach adopted by some individuals.[120]

There are some disadvantages of the Macintosh blade: The curvature of the Macintosh laryngoscope can intrude into the line of site when laryngoscopy is difficult[124] and the base of the tongue can be compressed distally producing posterior displacement of the epiglottis.[125]

Technique

1. Examine the patient and determine the suitability for curved blade laryngoscopy (can be beneficial with reduced upper airway space, such as a small narrow mouth, palate, and oropharynx).
2. Select the appropriate-length blade. The thyromental distance (TMD) can be used to indicate blade length selection. If the TMD = 5 cm, use a 2 Macintosh blade[127]; if the TMD = 6 cm, use a 3 Macintosh; and if the TMD is greater than 7 cm, use a 4 Macintosh blade. Historically, the first adult Macintosh blade was a size 3, which was tested by Macintosh during his gynecology lists in 1943. It therefore should be considered a blade suitable for women and is inappropriate for larger patients. Complaints about inferior laryngoscopy using the size 3 blade on men led to the development of the size 4 blade in 1951.[120]
3. Position the patient into a "sniffing" position, aiming to align the external auditory meatus with the sternal notch (HELP position). This is achieved by extending the patient's head 80 degrees at the atlanto-occipital joint and flexing the neck forward approximately 35 degrees (Fig. 20.6).
4. Open the mouth. One method is the "scissor" technique, which uses the first and third fingers of the right hand to part the lips and separate the maxilla and mandible (Fig. 20.7).

An intraoral crossed scissor-type maneuver can be achieved by fully separating the incisor teeth with the fingers, which rotates the temporomandibular joint (TMJ). The mandible is then moved anteriorly using digital pressure behind the mandibular incisors. Alternatively, push the occiput with the right hand to maximize extension of the patient's head. This widens mouth opening and increases the space between the palate and the tongue[127] (Fig. 20.8).

5. Consider using a dental guard.
6. While holding the handle of the laryngoscope in the left hand close to the blade, introduce the blade slowly down the midline, sequentially exposing and identifying the tongue, the uvula, and then the epiglottis. Careful identification of the epiglottis is a critical step for successful laryngoscopy.
7. Insert the blade to the right of the tongue, pushing the tongue to the left.[117] This maneuver controls the tongue with the flange of the blade.
8. Position the tip of the blade in the vallecula and then change the angle of lift to 45 degrees (Fig. 20.9).
9. The vocal cords are exposed by distracting the tongue and jaw upward and indirectly elevating the epiglottis. The laryngoscopist achieves this with an upper arm action involving shoulder and elbow movement (avoid excessive wrist movement, which can cause dental damage). Correct positioning of the blade is more important than brute force. Proper insertion and lifting of the laryngoscope is crucial for good laryngoscopy[128] (Fig. 20.9).
10. Delivery of an appropriately designed tracheal tube occurs under direct vision down the right side of the laryngoscope.

The success of TI can be enhanced by various techniques.

a. Tube selection. A tube with a small external diameter is easier to intubate, giving a clearer unobstructed view of the glottis than a larger tube. Smaller tubes tend to be less traumatic and smaller beveled tubes are less likely to cause hold-up on the arytenoids. Some specialized tubes with modified tip designs avoid problems with hold-up, including the Parker Flex-Tip tubes (Parker Medical, Highlands Ranch, CO) and Intubating LMA tubes (Teleflex Medical, Morrisville, NC).

b. ELM of the thyroid cartilage with the laryngoscopist's right hand, or an assistant's hand, can improve the view of the larynx during laryngoscopy (Fig. 20.10). This technique is enhanced by VAL where the assistant can view the result of ELM. The backward-upward-right-pressure (BURP) maneuver and cricoid pressure can make the laryngeal view worse.[131] If this occurs, the pressure should be released.

c. In 1949, Sir Robert R Macintosh described the use of a urinary gum elastic bougie as an ETT introducer.[130] This application lead to Venn's design in 1970 of the current Eschmann ETT introducer.[131] Taking advantage of the 35-degree coudé tip, the bougie can be manipulated blindly under the epiglottis to achieve TI. The ETT is then railroaded over the bougie to complete TI with the laryngoscope held in place.

d. A malleable metal stylet can also enhance the chances of successful placement of an ETT. Care is required to avoid trauma caused by the stylet to the pharynx, larynx, trachea, or esophagus. Ensure that the stylet is positioned at least 2 cm from the tip of the ETT.[116] Intubation is enhanced by a "straight to cuff" configuration with a distal bend of 35 degrees[132] (Fig. 20.11).

e. An ETT must be correctly placed in the trachea. Immediate confirmation of tube placement is essential to avoid endobronchial, esophageal, or incorrect TI. In an adult, the tip of the tube ideally is placed between 2 and 4.5 cm from the carina. This avoids the tube entering the bronchus during neck movement, or proximal displacement of the tube that can result in unwanted extubation or tube cuff located at the vocal cords giving rise to gas leaks. Correct tube placement can be guided by tube markers, which are more reliable than formula-based nasotracheal methods for pediatric nasotracheal intubation.[133] The cuffed ETT should be checked deflated at 20 cm H_2O pressure for a leak around the cuff (fit) and then inflated and maintained with a manometer and pressure set at 20 cm H_2O pressure (seal)[134] (Fig. 20.12). Care is required to select the ETT with the appropriate diameter, particularly for pediatrics. For this age group, a wide variety of external-cuff diameters are available for different tube designs and

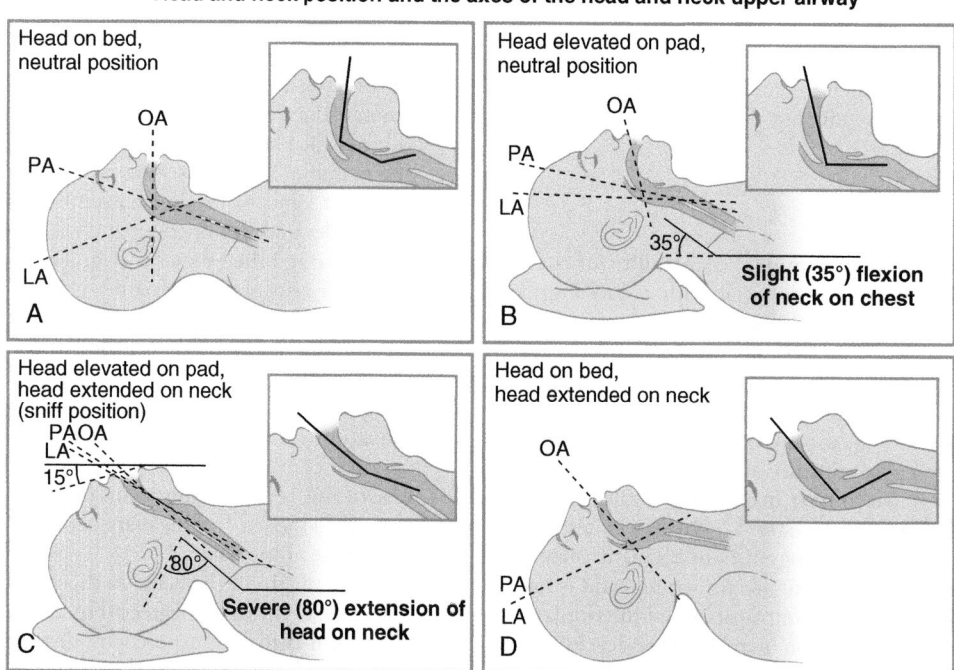

Head and neck position and the axes of the head and neck upper airway

• **Fig. 20.6** Schematic diagrams show the alignment of the oral axis *(OA)*, pharyngeal axis *(PA)*, and laryngeal axis *(LA)* in four different head positions. Each head position is accompanied by an inset that magnifies the upper airway (oral cavity, pharynx, and larynx) and superimposes *(bent bold line)* the continuity of these three axes within the upper airway. (A) The head is in the neutral position with a marked degree of nonalignment of the LA, PA, and OA. (B) The head is resting on a large pad that flexes the neck on the chest and aligns the LA with the PA. (C) The head is resting on a pad (which flexes the neck on the chest). Concomitant extension of the head on the neck brings all three axes into alignment (sniffing position). (D) Extension of the head on the neck without concomitant elevation of the head on a pad, which results in nonalignment of the PA and LA with the OA. (From Benumof JL, ed., *Airway Management, Principles and Practice.* Mosby; 1996, p. 263.)

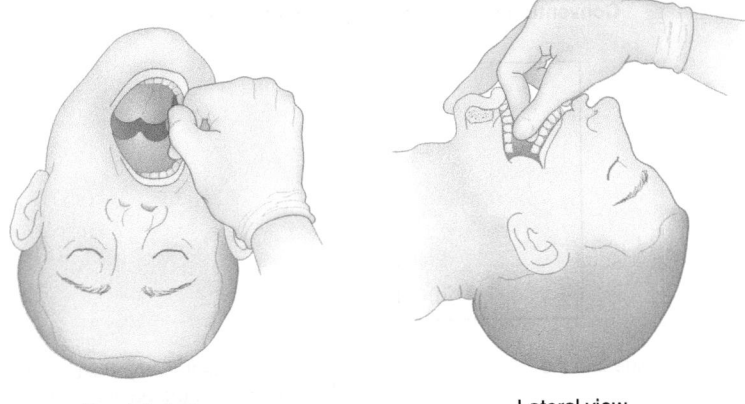

Frontal view   Lateral view

• **Fig. 20.7** The mouth can be opened wide by pressing the thumb of the right hand on the right, lower, posterior molar teeth in a caudal direction while the index finger of the right hand simultaneously presses on the right, upper, posterior molar teeth in a cephalic direction (intraoral technique). Gloves should be worn during laryngoscopy because the hands may come into contact with the patient's secretions.

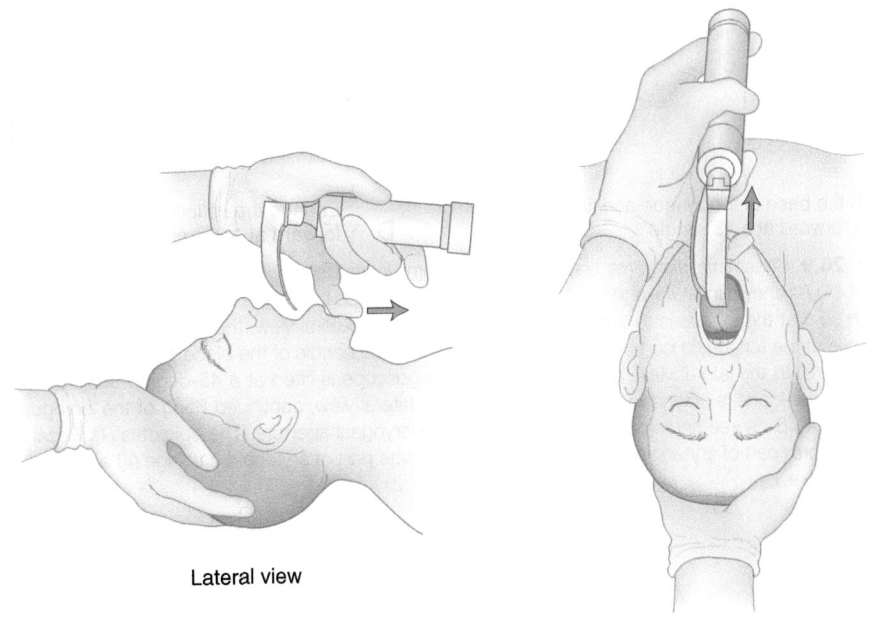

Lateral view   Frontal view

• **Fig. 20.8** The mouth can be opened wide by extending the head on the neck with the right hand while the small finger and medial border of the left hand simultaneously push the anterior aspect of the mandible in a caudal direction (extraoral technique). As the blade approaches the mouth, it should be directed toward the right side of the mouth. Gloves should be worn during laryngoscopy because the hands may come in contact with the patient's secretions.

manufacturers. Ideally, a high-volume, low-pressure, short cuff length should be chosen, with tracheal tube markers to ensure that the tube cuff is not inflated in the subglottic region.[134] Oversize ETTs and excessive cuff pressure can lead to significant morbidity, including tracheal tears.[135] In pediatrics, microcuff ETTs provide a high-volume, low-pressure, short, distally placed cuff.[138] A tube marker at the vocal cords level clearly identifies correct intubation depth and position.[136]

Note; Esophageal intubation is a life-threatening complication of TI that can occur with any intubation, even when performed by experienced practitioners. Confirmation of TI must be confirmed by capnography or indirect observation of the trachea down the ETT with a flexible bronchoscope. (Other methods of intubation confirmation are discussed in Chapter 30.)

   f. Securing the tracheal tube is essential to avoid tube migration or unplanned extubation and reintubation. In the ICU, tracheostomy and tracheal tube displacement are leading causes of morbidity and mortality.[39] Obese or mobile patients are particularly at risk. Capnography in the ICU is recommended for all intubations in critically ill patients, irrespective of location. (in ICU, ED, or on a ward room) Similarly continuous capnography is recommended for all ICU patients with tracheostomies or tracheal tubes during ventilation.[39]

Conventional Laryngoscopy with a Curved Blade

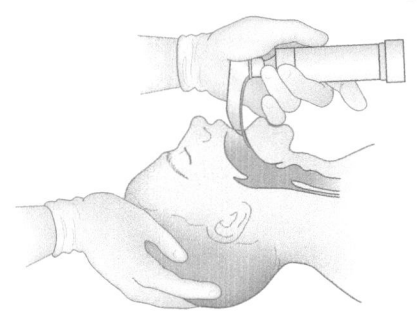
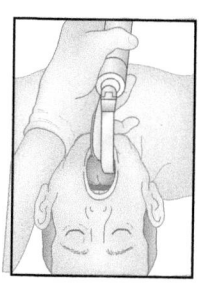

A Insert the laryngoscope blade into the right side of the mouth

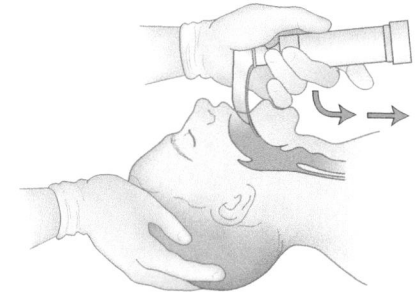

B Advance the laryngoscope blade toward the midline of the base of the tongue by rotating wrist

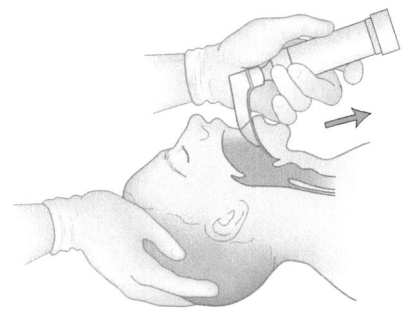

C Approach the base of the tongue and lift the blade forward at a 45° angle

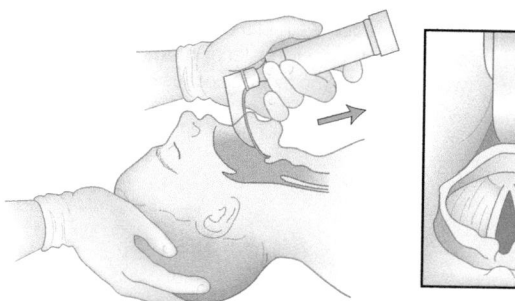

D Engage the vallecula and continue to lift the blade forward at a 45° angle

• **Fig. 20.9** Schematic diagrams show how to perform laryngoscopy with a Macintosh blade (curved blade). (A) As shown in lateral and frontal views, the laryngoscope blade is inserted into the right side of the mouth so that the tongue is to the left of the flange. (B) In the lateral view, the blade is advanced around the base of the tongue, in part by rotating the wrist so that the handle of the blade becomes more vertical *(arrows)*. (C) In the lateral view, the handle of the laryngoscope is lifted at a 45-degree angle *(arrow)* as the tip of the blade is placed in the vallecula. (D) In the lateral view, continued lifting of the laryngoscope handle at a 45-degree angle results in exposure of the laryngeal aperture. The epiglottis *(1)*, vocal cords *(2)*, cuneiform part of arytenoid cartilage *(3)*, and corniculate part of arytenoid cartilage *(4)* are identified in the frontal view.

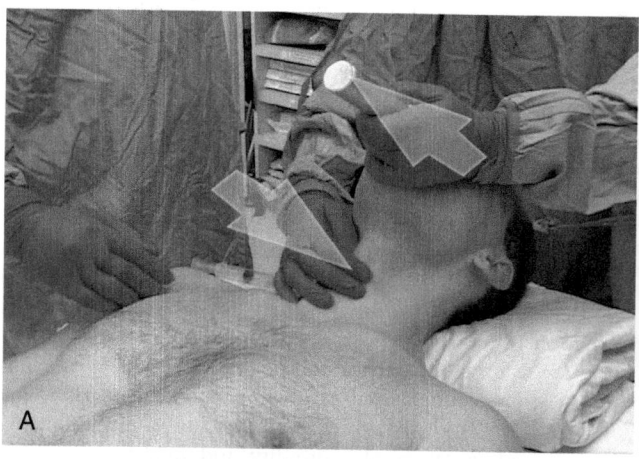
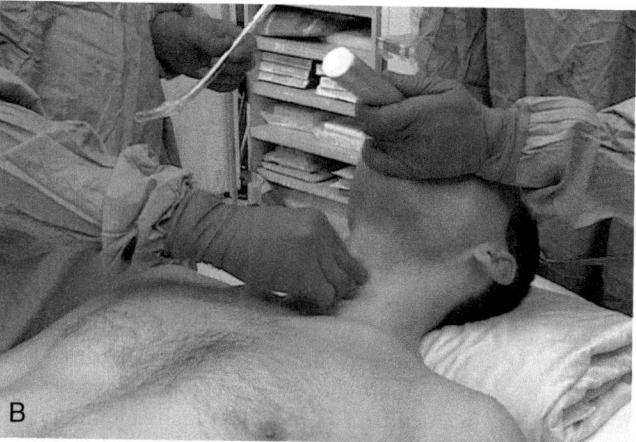

• **Fig. 20.10** (A) External laryngeal manipulation (ELM) by the laryngoscopist—bimanual laryngoscopy. Operator's right hand presses on anterior neck, most commonly at thyroid cartilage, while directly observing the effect on the laryngeal view. (B) Once the view has been optimized by the laryngoscopist, an assistant takes over maintaining external laryngeal manipulation at the optimal spot, freeing the operator's right hand to place the tracheal tube. (From Levitan RM, ed. *The Airway Cam Guide to Intubation and Practical Emergency Airway Management.* Airway Cam Technologies Inc; 2004: 106. With permission from Dr RM Levitan.)

Reliable tube fixation techniques are essential to avoid unwanted ETT migration or extubation.[137] Acceptable techniques can be utilized and written into departmental protocols (Figs. 20.13 and 20.14). Adhesive tape applied to the tube and the face is the most common form of tube fixation. Tincture of benzoin applied to the skin prior to taping can improve the bond between the tape and the skin. Tape must be changed after 2 days of intubation.

A cotton tie may be used to secure the tube in patients with beards. Intubated patients in a prone position can inadvertently extubate due to the weight of the circuit loosening of the tape due to oral secretions and oral secretions and loosening the tape. In this situation taping may require reinforcement with a cotton tie. Patients with a shared airway, including gastroscopy, ear, nose, and throat surgery, plastic surgery, dental surgery, or maxillofacial surgery, are at risk of inadvertent extubation. In some cases, special approaches, such as submental intubation, may be required. Other unusual tube-securing techniques may be indicated, such as wiring the tube to the teeth or suturing the tube to adjacent tissue. Patients being transported may benefit from a commercially available tube holder.

Straight Blade Laryngoscopy

When Miller developed his blade in 1941, it was designed to overcome a number of faults present in other existing straight blades.[138]

- Miller reduced the proximal portion of the blade, compressing the C-shaped cross-section into a modified D shape. This allowed intubation of patients with a small mouth opening and helped prevent dental trauma.
- A distal curve starting 2 inches from the tip replaced the more distal curve, providing a positive and improved lift action of the epiglottis.
- The tip was narrowed to improve blade maneuverability.
- The base of the Miller blade was rounded to prevent the tongue being pushed into the floor of the mouth.
- The length of the blade was said to be adequate and adaptable for all patients except infants.

The intubation technique in 1941 was paraglossal, as described by Jackson and Magill.[85,139] Miller suggested using

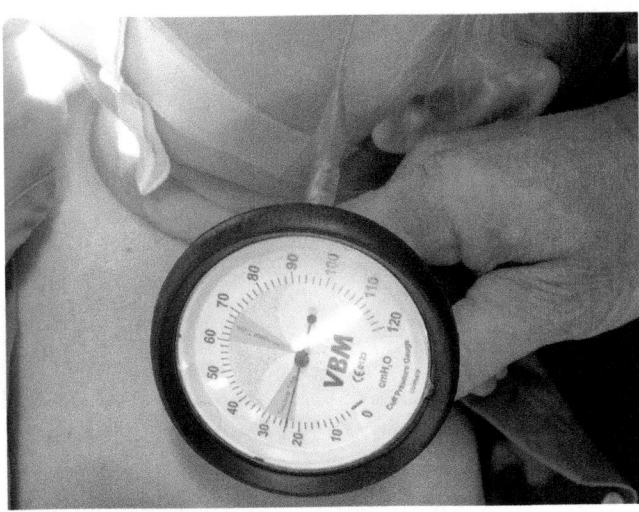

• **Fig. 20.12** A cuff manometer designed to accurately inflate and maintain cuff pressure. (Image Courtesy VBM, Einsteinstrasse 1, DE-72172 Sulz a.N., Germany. www.vbm-medical.de.)

a stylet to overcome reduced mouth space. The Miller blade is now the most commonly used straight laryngoscope blade and is produced by many manufacturers with a range of modifications and designs. Not all Miller blades are identical. Poorly designed Miller blades are available with the light at the leading edge of the left flange, which promotes embedding of the blade into the tongue, resulting in poor illumination of the larynx. Other Miller blades are available with the bulb on the right side, which interferes with the line of sight.[140] Modern blades are equipped with glass rods and a light-emitting diode (LED) light source in the handle, which can include rechargeable batteries. These laryngoscopes are capable of emitting a bright light in excess of 2000 lux (Fig. 20.15).

Technique

The paraglossal straight laryngoscope technique (PGSLT) was preferred by Jackson and Magill and more recently was described by Henderson.[141]

- The blade is passed from the right corner of the mouth.
- Insertion is along a groove between the tongue and the tonsil.
- Leftward and anterior pressure of the blade sweeps and holds the tongue to the left (Fig. 20.16).
- The blade is advanced, the epiglottis is identified, and the blade is positioned posterior to the epiglottis, holding it out of view (Fig. 20.17).
- The blade is lifted anteriorly, elevating the epiglottis and exposing the glottis.

Bonfils made a number of suggestions to achieve a straight intubation axis despite distorted anatomy. He suggests pressure on the cricoid, pushing the larynx to the side, hyperextending the neck, adjusting the degree of flexion, pushing or rotating the head to the left side, or appropriate bending of the ETT with a stylet.[142] An assistant can also retract the right corner of the mouth to enlarge the view and intubation space.[141] Advancing the straight blade into the esophagus and withdrawing until the glottis comes into view is potentially traumatic to the arytenoids and aryepiglottic folds, and hence this technique is discredited.[143]

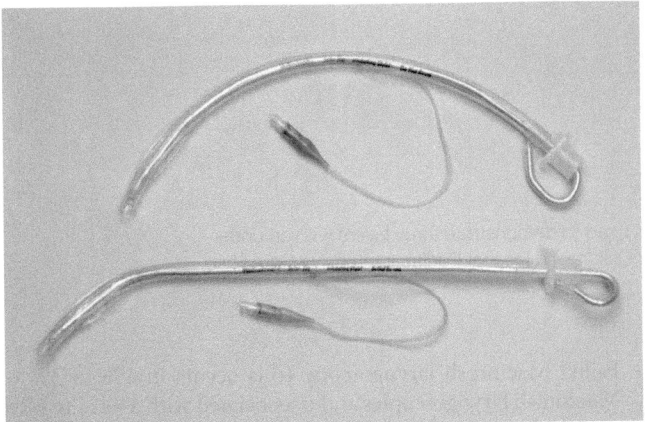

• **Fig. 20.11** Stylet shaping. A straight-to-cuff configuration with stylet and tube improves the line of site for the laryngoscopist, who can observe down the length of the straight tube to the tip. The alternative arcuate curve interferes with the line of sight. (Courtesy Covidien, a Medtronic company, Mansfield, MA. www.medtronic.com.)

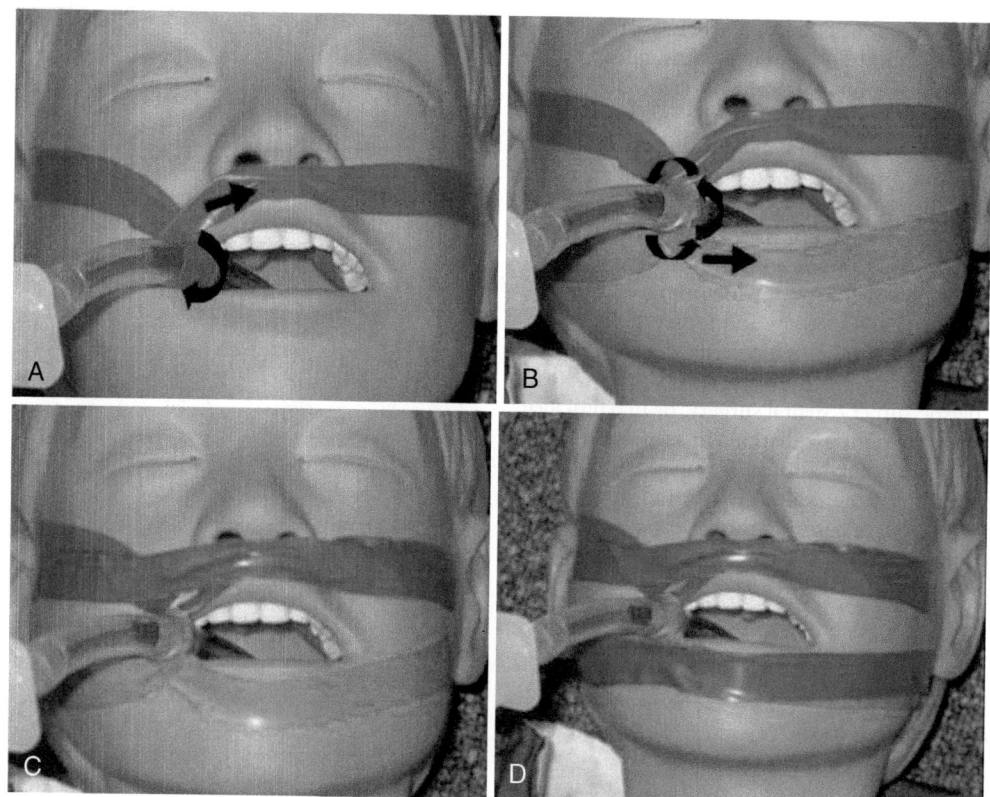

• **Fig. 20.13** Oral pediatric tube fixation (colored tape is used to demonstrate three layers with an underlying silk tie). (Reproduced with permission from Starship Children's Hospital Pediatric Intensive Care Unit. Auckland, New Zealand.)

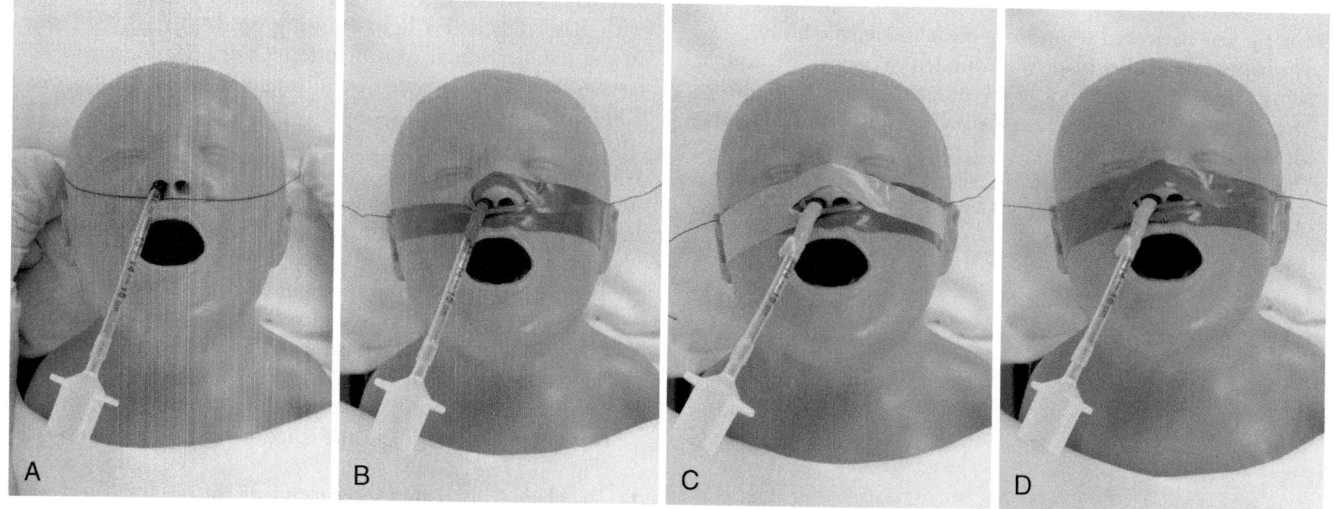

• **Fig. 20.14** Nasal pediatric tube fixation (colored tape is used to demonstrate three layers with an underlying silk tie). (Reproduced with permission from Starship Children's Hospital Pediatric Intensive Care Unit. Auckland, New Zealand.)

Indications

PGSLT is particularly useful for cases where the line of sight from the prominent part of the maxilla to the larynx is obstructed:
- Buck teeth
- Overriding teeth
- Large tongue
- Large floppy epiglottis

- Failed Macintosh laryngoscopy (this occurs in 1% to 3% of Macintosh laryngoscopies and is associated with a 44% to 68% straight blade success rate[141])

Difficulties

Difficulties with PGSLT can be attributed to poor technique and laryngoscope design:

- Poor alignment of the tip to the glottis
- Inadequate control of the epiglottis
- Soft tissue obscuring the light source
- Inadequate oral space provided for ETT intubation
- Poor control of the tongue

Opinions about the use of curved blades and straight blades during pediatric anesthesia vary. Two studies involving children ≤2 years old compared the Macintosh and Miller blades.[144,146] In both studies, children with known DAs were excluded. In these studies, the views by DL were equivalent for each type of blade; however, the methodology varied, and different placements of the laryngoscopes occurred. A PGSLT approach was not specified. In a case series of six infants with Pierre Robin syndrome, all children were successfully intubated with a PGSLT approach after conventional laryngoscopy failed.[146] There are many pediatric laryngoscope blades, including the pediatric straight McCoy size 1 (based on the Seward straight blade), Anderson-Magill, Robertshaw, Seward, Wis-Hipple, Henderson, Dörges, and Flagg. Availability, personal preference, and skill will determine the selection of blade.

In 1952, Macintosh wrote, "Whatever laryngoscope is used, the principles of laryngoscopy remain the same. If these—namely correct head position and adequate anaesthesia—are ignored, no laryngoscope will give success. The secret of successful intubation lies with the anaesthetist, not with any particular laryngoscope. That good result can be obtained with many different patterns is obvious from the fact that these different types all have their own supporters."[147]

Nasal Intubation

There are a number of indications for nasal intubation, including limited mouth opening, distorted oral anatomy, oral surgery, and

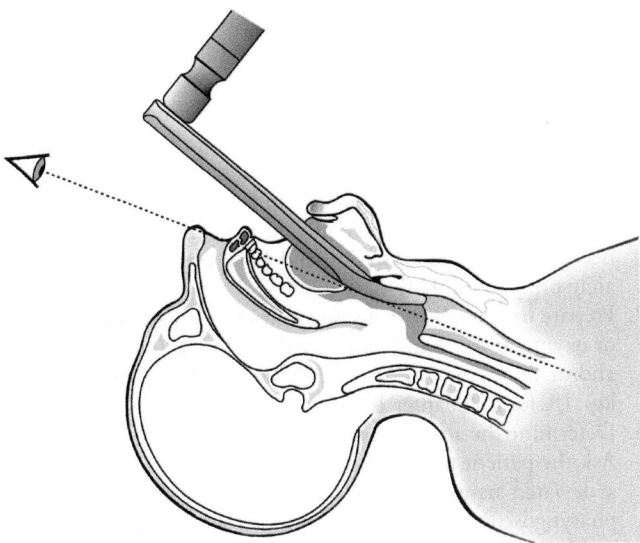

• **Fig. 20.16** Use of Miller blade in the paraglossal technique of laryngoscopy. Note that the blade is at the right side of the tongue, which bulges on the left side of the blade. The position of the laryngoscope close to the midline would be satisfactory when intubation is easy. The line of sight shown (over the molars) is that sought when intubation is more difficult and is achieved by rotating the head to the left and moving the heel of the laryngoscope to the right. (From Henderson JJ. The use of paraglossal straight blade laryngoscopy in difficult tracheal intubation. *Anaesthesia.* 1997;52:552–560, with permission from John Wiley and Sons.)

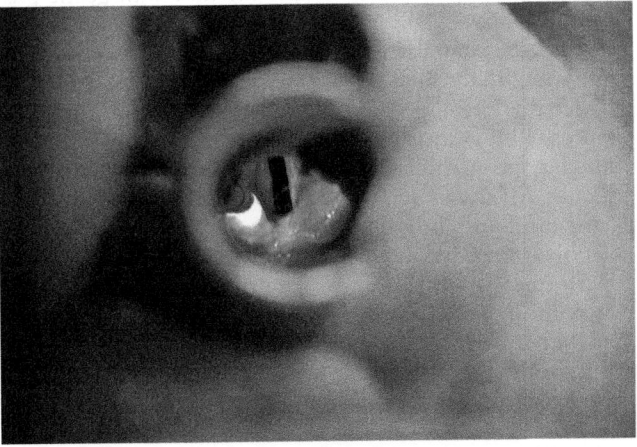

• **Fig. 20.17** Paraglossal straight blade laryngoscopy with a Wisconsin blade. (From Levitan RM, ed. *The Airway Cam Guide to Intubation and Practical Emergency Airway Management.* Airway Cam Technologies Inc., 2004:166. With permission from Dr RM Levitan.)

emergency awake blind nasal intubation. Nasal intubation is relatively contraindicated for patients with a coagulopathy because of the risk of epistaxis. Also, base of skull fractures associated with facial trauma are a relative contraindication to nasal intubation due to the small risk of intracranial intubation.

There are advantages of nasotracheal versus oral intubation: a favorable anatomic route to the larynx, relative ease to anesthetize the nose, less potential for a gag reflex, and after intubation a nasal tube is well tolerated. Disadvantages include a risk of epistaxis, bacteremia, rigors, pyrexia, lower respiratory tract infections, discomfort during awake nasal intubation, and the nasal ETT can get held up on the epiglottis.[148,149]

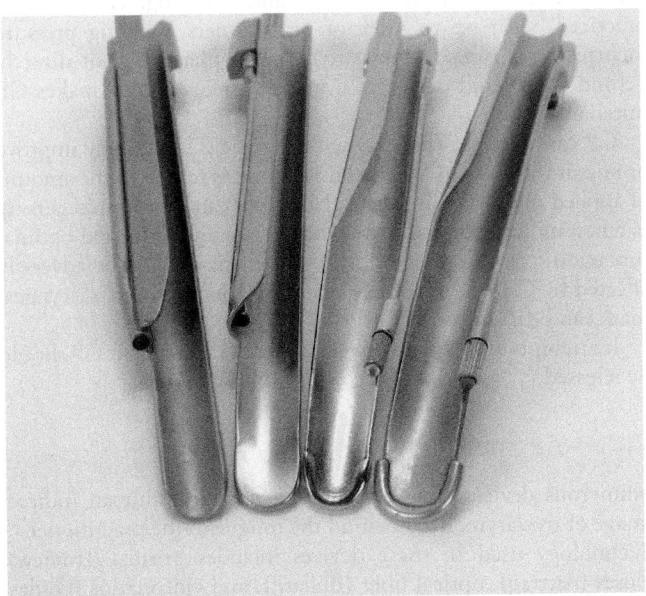

• **Fig. 20.15** Miller blade designs showing variation in tip designs and light location. (From Levitan RM, ed. *The Airway Cam Guide to Intubation and Practical Emergency Airway Management.* Airway Cam Technologies Inc; 2004:190. With permission from Dr RM Levitan.)

Preparation

1. Select an appropriate nasotracheal tube. To minimize the risk of epistaxis, use a tube with a relatively small diameter (for adults, 6.5 to 7.0 mm internal diameter). A Parker Flex-Tip tracheal tube is less painful and traumatic following nasotracheal intubation compared with a standard polyvinyl chloride (PVC) Magill tube.[150] The tube can be softened in warm water and lubricated with water-soluble jelly (not lignocaine jelly because of the risk of drying and ETT obstruction) immediately prior to intubation.
2. Prepare the nostril with a vasoconstrictor (phenylephrine 0.5% or oxymetazoline) and local anesthetic for AI (lignocaine spray and/or ointment 5% or jelly 2% within dose limits of 5 mg/kg). (Refer to Chapter 13.)
3. Determine the appropriate nostril with the maximum patency. Ask the patient to sniff through respective nostrils. Inspect for a deviated nasal septum. Examine the nostrils with a nasopharyngoscope looking for a deviated septum, hypertrophied turbinates, or distal bone spurs. If the nostrils appear to have equal patency, choose the left nostril because the ETT tip of a standard PVC Magill tube runs down the septum, avoiding the lateral turbinates.

Intubation

1. Oxygen can be delivered through the advancing ETT or via buccal cannula during nasal intubation.
2. To minimize the risk of posterior pharyngeal trauma and perforation, insert a soft, lubricated nasopharyngeal suction catheter through the nose prior to the ETT insertion. This can act as a guide for the ETT. Advance the tube with gentle pressure. After passing the nasopharynx, direct the base of the ETT toward the contralateral nipple, which moves the tip of the ETT toward the midline.
3. Once the ETT passes the nasopharynx, the tip of the tube needs to lift away from the posterior pharyngeal wall toward the larynx. A specialized Endotrol tube (Mallinckrodt, St. Louis, MO) can achieve this lift. Alternatively, the ETT cuff can be slightly inflated. If the ETT is held up at the larynx, it can be obstructed by the epiglottis. In that case perform a jaw thrust and rotate the tube bevel so that it is pointing anteriorly.[149] For hold-up on the anterior commissure or cricoid cartilage, flex the head, rotate the tube, and readvance. If the ETT is held up in the piriform fossa, rotate the ETT in the contralateral direction and readvance.[151,152]
4. For a blind nasal intubation, if the patient is breathing spontaneously, a BAMM (Beck Airflow Airway Monitor [Great Plains Ballistics, Lubbock, TX]) attached to the 15-mm ETT connector will sound an audible whistle during the patient's expiration as the tube tip approaches the glottis.
5. For intubation under DL, the larynx can be exposed by the laryngoscope and the ETT can be advanced down the trachea under direct vision. If the ETT is held up, gently guide the ETT through the larynx under direct vision using Magill forceps. Care is required to avoid cuff rupture with the Magill forceps.
6. Nasal intubation can be achieved with an indirect technique using a nasotracheal Airtraq (Pradol Meditec, Vizcaya, Spain). A randomized controlled trial showed superior intubating success for predicted DAs when the nasotracheal Airtraq was compared to the Macintosh laryngoscope.[153]
7. Confirm TI by capnography, ensure that the ETT is intubated to the correct length at the nares (26 cm mark for women and 28 cm for men), and secure the ETT to the nostril and maxilla with adhesive tape.

Rapid Sequence Induction

For the patient with a full stomach at risk of regurgitation and aspiration, for whom AI is not an option, the common airway technique is a rapid sequence induction (RSI). As the name suggests, the emphasis of this technique is rapid intubation to minimize the time between loss of consciousness and secure placement of an ETT. The "classical" recommended techniques include preoxygenation, rapid injection of predetermined doses of rapidly acting anesthetic and muscle-relaxant drugs, application of cricoid pressure (CP), cessation of PPV, and intubation with an appropriate-size cuffed ETT. This induction technique is widely practiced in emergency medicine, ICU, and anesthesia. The technique is used for a number of conditions that are associated with a risk of aspiration, including trauma, emergency surgery, obstetrics, obesity, diabetes, and bowel obstruction.

RSI with CP was proposed by Sellick in 1961.[154] The technique as described by Sellick involves "occlusion of the upper esophagus by backward pressure on the cricoid ring against bodies of the cervical vertebrae to prevent gastric contents from reaching the pharynx."[154] Since then the technique has changed. Sellick originally recommended ventilation after induction, but fears about inflating the stomach during this phase led to cessation of ventilation prior to intubation. This has now reversed, and it is considered acceptable to carefully use PPV after induction.[166] The current recommendation for CP is to apply 10 N (Newtons) of pressure on the cricoid cartilage when the patient is awake and increase that pressure to 30 N upon loss of consciousness.

Cricoid pressure has received criticism for many reasons. Some believe that there is a lack of scientific evidence to support CP, with the only effectiveness being demonstrated on cadavers. The lower esophageal pressure is decreased during CP, and the technique can initiate nausea and vomiting. CP is poorly practiced, with up to 48% of practitioners applying pressure incorrectly. It is also known that the esophagus is not directly behind the cricoid cartilage in many patients, which makes CP unreliable.[155]

CP can interfere with laryngoscopy and TI.[156] It may improve or impair the view on DL, and this impact is related to the amount of applied pressure. CP greater than 40 N can compromise airway patency and occlude the airway. Bag-mask ventilation and optimal supraglottic airway device (SAD) placement can also be adversely affected by CP.[157,158] Flexible scope intubation through a laryngeal mask can be impaired by CP.[159]

If attempts at laryngoscopy are difficult during RSI, CP should be released.[66,160]

Video-Assisted Laryngoscopy

Numerous devices have been designed to transmit an indirect image of the larynx from behind the tongue to the practitioner.[167] Technology used in these devices includes prisms (Truview), lenses (Airtraq), optical fiber (Bullard), and video chips (Glidescope, McGrath, C Mac and Pentax AWS) that are integrated into a rigid indirect laryngoscope (RIL). Subtle differences in design can have an impact on the best technique to achieve a laryngeal view.[127]

VAL (also see Chapter 23) usually results in a satisfactory indirect view of the larynx, but intubation times can be longer and intubation may be more difficult than for DL. A systematic review and meta-analysis of VAL for patients with cervical spine immobilization found that the Airtraq device reduced the risk of intubation failure, but other devices showed no benefit compared to a Macintosh laryngoscope and DL.[161]

Levitan describes three distinct steps involved in VAL:[162]

1. Placement of the videolaryngoscope up to the larynx. This step occasionally requires manipulation of the patient's head and neck, and application of a jaw thrust to create space for the advancing laryngoscope.[127]
2. Delivery of the tracheal tube to the larynx. This maneuver could depend on the optimum placement of the laryngoscope blade and the method used to elevate the epiglottis. Some blades are based on a Macintosh design and therefore the tip of the blade is placed in the vallecula. Other blades trap the epiglottis as in straight blade laryngoscopy. Some blades incorporate a channel to direct the ETT to the glottis (Airtraq, Pentax AWS, King vision). Utilizing indirect technology, an indirect view of the vocal cords is usually achieved, but delivery of the ETT may not follow. With unchanneled blades, tube delivery may require an angulated stylet and vertical retraction of the blade to create manipulation space for the ETT and correct alignment of the approaching ETT to the glottis.
3. TI is the final step. This can be the most difficult step and may be facilitated by head and neck positioning. Use of a hyperangulated stylet and ETT can result in impingement of the tube tip against the cricoid ring, requiring withdrawal of the ETT and stylet, then rotation of the ETT off the stylet.

VAL often results in a superior view of the larynx, but subsequent maneuvers may be required to achieve TI. New VAL skills that differ from those used for DL are required.

Conclusion

The benefits of TI apply to patients in many clinical situations. Although recent developments of SGAs have provided a useful alternative, particularly for day surgery procedures or for inexperienced practitioners in emergency situations, TI is still the first choice in many situations. The limiting factors for the safe application of this important technique are the skill of the practitioner, the use of patient monitoring, and an understanding of the indications for TI. The ability to safely perform TI remains one of the most important skills for airway specialists.

Selected References

20. Kornas RL, Owyang CG, Sakles JC, Foley LJ, Mosier JM, Society for Airway Management's Special Projects C. Evaluation and Management of the Physiologically Difficult Airway: Consensus Recommendations from Society for Airway Management. *Anesth Analg.* 2020;14:14.
23. Mosier JM, Joshi R, Hypes C, Pacheco G, Valenzuela T, Sakles JC. The physiologically difficult airway. *West J Emerg Med.* 2015;16(7):1109–1117.
31. Crewdson K, Lockey DJ, Roislien J, Lossius HM, Rehn M. The success of pre-hospital tracheal intubation by different pre-hospital providers: a systematic literature review and meta-analysis. *Crit Care.* 2017;21(1):31.
35. Driver BE, Prekker ME, Reardon RF, Fantegrossi A, Walls RM, Brown CA 3rd. Comparing emergency department first-attempt intubation success with standard-geometry and hyperangulated video laryngoscopes. *Ann Emerg Med.* 2020;76(3):332–338.
39. Cook TM, Woodall N, Harper J, Benger J, Fourth National Audit P. Major complications of airway management in the UK: results of the Fourth National Audit Project of the Royal College of Anaesthetists and the Difficult Airway Society. Part 2: intensive care and emergency departments. *Br J Anaesth.* 2011;106(5):632–642.
40. Sakles JC, Pacheco GS, Kovacs G, Mosier JM. The difficult airway refocused. *Br J Anaesth.* 2020;125(1):e18–e21.
65. Baker P. Preparedness and education in airway management. *Anesthesiol Clin.* 2015;33(2):381–395.
72. Bjurstrom MF, Bodelsson M, Sturesson LW. The difficult airway trolley: A narrative review and practical guide. *Anesthesiol Res Pract.* 2019;6780254. doi:10.1155/2019/6780254.
109. Mort TC. Emergency tracheal intubation: complications associated with repeated laryngoscopic attempts. *Anesthesia and Analgesia.* 2004;99(2):607–613, table of contents.
119. Scott J, Baker PA. How did the Macintosh laryngoscope become so popular? *Paediatric Anaesthesia.* 2009;19(suppl 1):24–29.
141. Henderson JJ. The use of paraglossal straight blade laryngoscopy in difficult tracheal intubation. *Anaesthesia.* 1997;52(6):552–560.

All references can be found online at eBooks.Health.Elsevier.com.

21

Nonvisual Techniques of Tracheal Intubation

OLIVER J. POOLE, KATHRYN SPARROW, AND ORLANDO HUNG

CHAPTER OUTLINE

KEY POINTS

- Blind intubation techniques have proven to be effective, safe, and simple techniques, especially in a timely manner during emergency situations where fogging, presence of blood, secretions, and vomitus can create impossible conditions for the direct or indirect laryngoscopic visualization of the glottis or when alternative options are either unavailable or not functional. Successful nonvisual intubation depends largely on the clinician's preparation, experience, and skill.
- Blind digital intubation may be considered in situations where positioning for conventional intubation is not possible.
- Pulling of the tongue forward by an assistant during the digital technique facilitates traction on the epiglottis, thereby improving the overall chances of successful digital intubation.

- Blind digital intubation may be facilitated by the use of a tracheal introducer, which produces confirmatory tracheal clicks prior to the railroading of the endotracheal tube (ETT) and can facilitate intubation using various devices and techniques.
- The use of a stethoscope, BAAM, Endotrol ETT, lighted stylet, and cuff inflation are all helpful adjuncts and maneuvers to improve the success rate of blind nasal intubation.
- If not contraindicated, neck flexion (if ETT is caught anteriorly on epiglottis) or extension (if ETT keeps entering the esophagus) can help the clinician successfully intubate a patient during blind nasal intubation.
- Retrograde intubation may be considered in a "CANNOT intubate, CAN oxygenate" (CICO) scenario.

Introduction

The technique of the placement of an endotracheal tube (ETT) in the trachea for ventilation and oxygenation is more than a thousand years old. It was first performed on pigs by the Arab Avicenna between 980 and 1037.[1,2] However, modern methods of laryngoscopic tracheal intubation did not emerge until early in the 20th century following the introduction of a flexible metal tube by Kuhn[3] and the laryngoscope by Jackson.[4] Over the years, direct laryngoscopic intubation has been shown to be an effective, safe, and relatively easy technique. Using a laryngoscope to obtain line of sight to the laryngeal inlet has become the conventional method of tracheal intubation in the operating room, intensive care unit, and emergency department. Unfortunately, even in the hands of experienced laryngoscopists, this approach to intubation has limitations, especially in the presence of specific anatomic variations, such as a receding mandible, prominent upper incisors, restricted mouth opening, or limited movement of the cervical spine. The incidence of difficult and failed intubation employing this technique can be as high as 21%, particularly in emergency situations.[5] In the obstetrical population the incidence of failed direct laryngoscopic intubation has been reported to be between 0.05% and 0.35%.[6] Many predictors of difficult direct laryngoscopic intubation have been suggested in the literature over the past few decades.[7,8] Unfortunately, almost all univariate predictors have low positive predictive value[9] and the use of multivariate predictors appears to improve the positive predictive value of these airway assessment tools for direct laryngoscopy.[10–12] Moreover, studies have shown that considerable experience is required before a trainee becomes proficient in direct laryngoscopic intubation. Konrad et al. and Mulcaster et al. have constructed learning curves demonstrating that a 90% probability of success requires between 47 and 57 direct laryngoscopic intubations in patients.[13,14]

These difficulties and failures associated with direct laryngoscopic intubation have driven the development of many alternative intubation devices and techniques, such as rigid and flexible endoscopes, video laryngoscopes, and optical intubating stylets. All these devices have gained a measure of popularity. Unfortunately, these devices are substantially more expensive than the laryngoscope. Furthermore, the cleaning and sterilization processes of some of these devices, such as the flexible intubation scope (FIS), require an average of 50 to 60 minutes to complete, hindering their availability and practicality in emergency airway management and in prehospital care.

Given that direct and indirect laryngoscopic visualization of the glottis may not be possible, especially in a timely manner during emergency situations where fogging, presence of blood, secretions, and vomitus are frequent, several devices and techniques have been developed to enable the clinician to pass the ETT "blindly" or "nonvisually" into the trachea. It is precisely these kinds of difficulties that have motivated the search for nonvisual techniques, such as digital intubation, blind nasal intubation, and retrograde intubation, all of which have proven to be simple, effective, and safe techniques.

These nonvisual techniques are particularly useful in low- and middle-income countries with limited resources. Our experience in Rwanda as part of the Global Outreach Program funded by the Canadian Anesthesiologists' Society[15] confirmed the clinical utility of these nonvisual techniques. The availability of contemporary airway management devices in Rwanda proved difficult because either they were cost prohibitive or there was no service for the devices should they become nonfunctional. Therefore in the setting of countries with limited resources inexpensive nonvisual techniques may play an important role when faced with a failed tracheal intubation under direct laryngoscopy. While some may find nonvisual techniques obsolete,[16] we believe that the basic principle of airway management is to provide adequate oxygenation and ventilation to patients and this should depend on the context as well as the tools available to clinicians in their particular environment.[17]

Digital Intubation

History

Although likely first described by Herholt and Rafn[18] in 1796 for drowning victims, digital intubation did not receive much attention in the medical literature until its revival in emergency medicine and prehospital care by Stewart in the mid-1980s.[19,20] Notable publications on the topic over the years have portrayed the technique as an acceptable alternative to conventional direct laryngoscopic intubation, particularly when the conventional technique is contraindicated, has failed, or is not possible because of a lack of equipment. In 1880 Macewen[21] described the technique of utilizing a curved metal tube in awake patients, and Sykes[22] recommended the routine use of the digital technique in anesthetic practice in the 1930s. Siddall[23] and Lanham[24] considered the technique to be a last-ditch effort following failure of conventional intubation methods.[19] The technique has been described in neonatal resuscitation[25–27] and as an adjunct in blind nasotracheal intubation.[28] Currently, there is widespread variation in awareness, expertise, and application of the technique in anesthesia, emergency medicine,[29,30] and prehospital care. Unfortunately, digital intubation is now often forgotten when the time comes to think about alternate techniques in the case of an emergency,[31] despite a recent cadaver study establishing that the overall success after three attempts may be as high as 90%,[32] when performed by emergency medicine residents and staff. Although advances in airway management equipment and expertise have made the routine use of digital intubation obsolete, it remains a valuable skill for some patients, especially in the emergency setting[19] or under circumstances with limited resources and in which the clinician cannot be positioned at the head of the patient, rendering direct laryngoscopic intubation impossible.

Indications

The use of the digital technique is neither aesthetically pleasing and easily accomplished nor entirely safe. Placing the fingers far enough down a patient's throat to elevate the epiglottis and guide an ETT into the trachea has implications related to the selection of patients and the manual dexterity and anatomic features of the clinician. The technique has received some popularity in the prehospital care environment, where difficult positioning of the patient, poor lighting conditions, disrupted anatomy, potential cervical spine instability, and unknown infectious status are the norm.

Successful digital intubation demands that the patient be unconscious to tolerate the intense oropharyngeal stimulus without triggering a gag reflex and to prevent bite injuries to the clinician. The risk of infectious disease transmission must always be borne in mind. Neuromuscular blockade facilitates the technique, although its use should be considered carefully in patients with anatomically difficult or disrupted airways. The skill level of the clinician, coupled with previous experience in using the technique of digital intubation, is an important prerequisite for success. The importance of practicing this technique in nonemergency situations cannot be overemphasized.

Digital intubation may be indicated as follows:

1. When equipment for tracheal intubation is unavailable or not functional.
2. When the positioning of the patient or the clinician prevents traditional laryngoscopic intubation.
3. When other methods have failed or are likely to fail and the skill and experience of the clinician make the digital technique a reasonable alternative.
4. When there is a potential or actual cervical spine instability and the clinician selects the digital technique based on the risk–benefit analysis. Although there is no evidence to suggest that the technique of digital intubation will alter the neurologic outcome of a patient, there may be less cervical spine motion during intubation with the digital technique as compared with the conventional direct laryngoscopic intubation without in-line immobilization.
5. When adequate visualization of the airway to allow conventional intubation is not possible because of the presence of copious secretions, blood, or vomitus in the oropharynx or because of traumatic injury of the upper airway anatomy.

Technique of Digital Intubation

Preparation

As with any intubation technique, preparation involves assembling the necessary personnel and equipment, including emergency drugs, rescue airway devices, an oxygen source, and adequate suction, to optimize success and preserve ventilation and oxygenation. An appropriately sized ETT is selected. The use of a stiff but malleable stylet improves maneuverability and facilitates glottis passage of the ETT during the intubation. What follows is a classic description of the technique.[33] The lubrication of the stylet with a water-soluble lubricant ensures easy retraction following the placement of the tip of the ETT in the glottis opening. The stylet is inserted into the ETT so that the distal end of the stylet is at the level of the Murphy eye. With the stylet in place, the distal half of the styletted ETT unit is bent to a "U" shape (Fig. 21.1). The proximal half of the styletted ETT is then bent 90 degrees to the dominant side of the clinician to allow the manipulation of the styletted ETT by the dominant hand during intubation (Figs. 21.2 and 21.3). The degree of bend at the tip of the styletted ETT should be individualized and is dependent on the clinician's experience.

The tip of the ETT should also be well lubricated with a water-soluble lubricant. In the uncommon event that the intubation is performed in an awake patient, especially an uncooperative patient, a wedged bite block should be placed between the patient's molars on the opposite side to where the clinician stands to minimize the risk of injury to the clinician's fingers.

Positioning

Depending on the environment, in general, the patient should be placed supine with the head in a slight sniffing position (except in

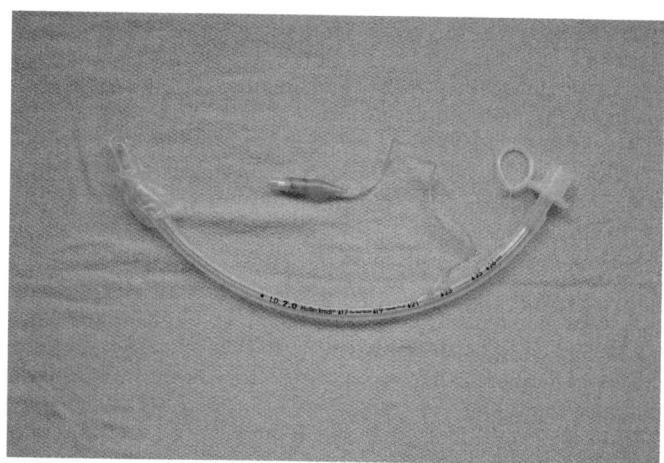

• **Fig. 21.1** With the stylet in place, the distal half of the ETT is bent to a U shape.

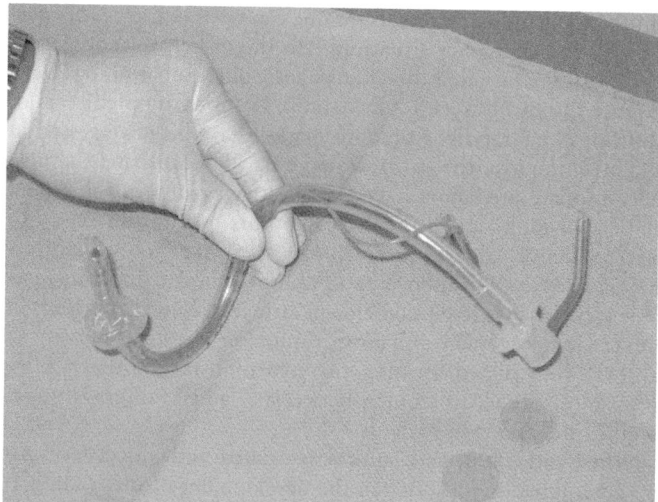

• **Fig. 21.2** The proximal half of the ETT is bent 90 degrees toward the dominant side of the clinician.

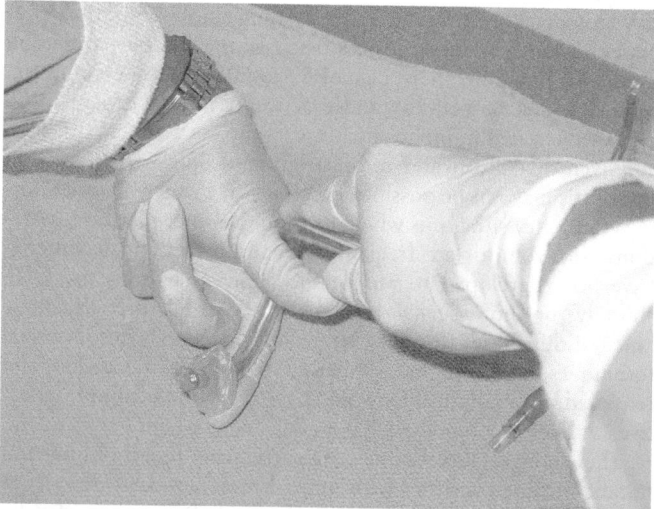

• **Fig. 21.3** Final configuration of the styletted ETT allows improved control of the ETT with both hands. During the intubation, the index finger of the dominant hand can help advance the ETT while the index and middle fingers of the nondominant hand guide the tip of the ETT into the glottis.

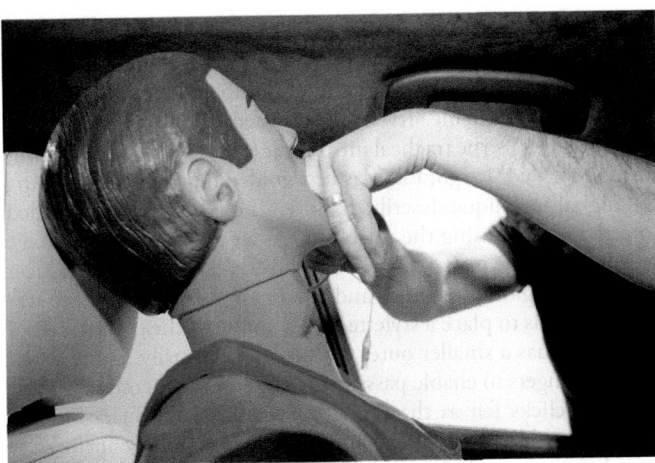

• **Fig. 21.4** Digital intubation of a trapped driver on the left side of the vehicle. The left hand of the clinician palpates the epiglottis while the right hand delivers the ETT.

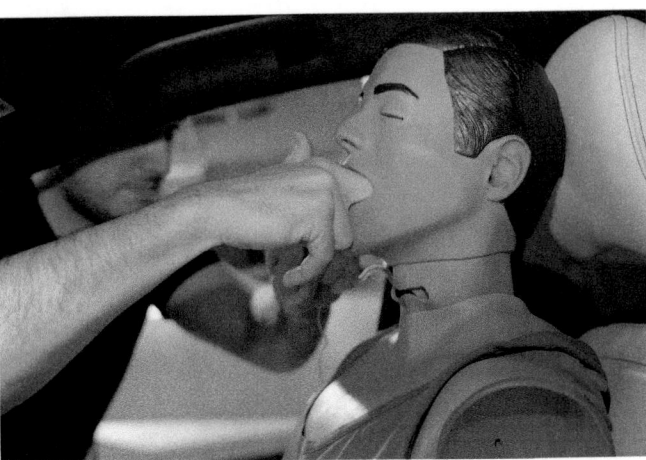

• **Fig. 21.5** Digital intubation of a trapped driver on the right side of the vehicle. The right hand of the clinician palpates the epiglottis while the left hand delivers the ETT.

patients with cervical spine instability). The clinician stands (or kneels if the patient is on the ground) beside the patient and faces the head so that the nondominant side of the clinician is closest to the patient. An assistant can help to facilitate the intubating procedure. In-line immobilization should be performed in the setting of cervical spine instability. Cricoid pressure should be applied where clinically indicated.

Digital intubation is a technique that may be considered in the prehospital setting for an unresponsive patient who is trapped in the seat of a crashed motor vehicle. This is an environment where the patient is likely to be in a sitting position, making traditional laryngoscopy challenging. The airway is likely to be bloody, which can impair glottic visualization with video laryngoscopy, and more advanced airway equipment may not be available. Digital intubation is a simple technique that allows the clinician to manage the airway while facing the patient or standing at the opening of the driver's door. The location of the driver's seat may influence which hand the clinician uses to palpate the epiglottis versus that used to deliver the ETT. The driver sits on the left side of the car in North America, making it easier for the clinician to place the fingers of the left hand into the oropharynx and deliver the ETT with the right hand. This approach would be ergonomically awkward in countries where drivers are seated on the right side of the car, and reversing the roles of the hands should be considered (Figs. 21.4 and 21.5)

Technique

Pulling the tongue forward by an assistant facilitates the palpation of the epiglottis, thus improving the success rate for digital intubation. This can be achieved by applying suction tubing to the tip of a 20-mL syringe with the plunger removed (Fig. 21.6). The tongue will be sucked into the open end of the barrow of the syringe, allowing it to be grasped gently by an assistant with a piece of gauze. Traction on the tongue moves the epiglottis slightly cephalad, enhancing its palpability and facilitating the placement of the tip of the ETT into the glottic opening. The clinician then inserts the index and middle fingers of the nondominant hand into the oral cavity and slides the palm down along the surface of the tongue (Figs. 21.7 and 21.8). The tip of the middle finger touches the tip of the epiglottis, which is then directed anteriorly (Fig. 21.8). The ease of palpating and lifting the epiglottis depends

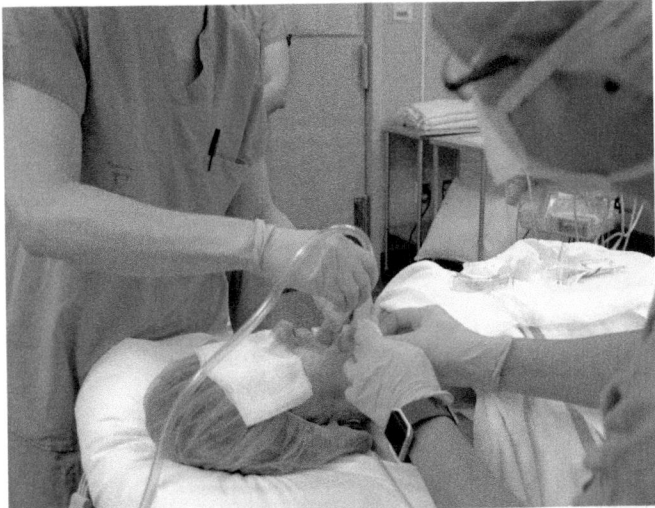

• **Fig. 21.6** Anterior displacement of the tongue can be facilitated by applying suction tubing to the tip of a 20-mL syringe with the plunger removed. The tongue is sucked into the open end of the syringe, allowing it to be grasped gently by an assistant with a piece of gauze.

on the length of the clinician's fingers, the height of the patient, the anatomy of the oropharynx, and the presence or absence of teeth.

Once the epiglottis is identified and directed anteriorly, the styletted ETT is inserted through the corner of the mouth. The styletted ETT glides along the groove between the middle and index fingers on the palmar surface of the nondominant hand (Fig. 21.8). While firm anterior pressure is maintained against the epiglottis with the middle finger, the styletted ETT is advanced slowly into the glottic opening by the dominant hand. The index finger may be used to guide the tip of the styletted ETT into the glottic opening (Fig. 21.8). In general, the middle finger of the nondominant hand lifting the epiglottis has to be moved laterally to allow passage of the styletted ETT.

The ETT should be stabilized while withdrawing the stylet, and the ETT is then slowly advanced into the trachea. During the intubation, the styletted ETT should never be advanced forcefully against resistance. Correct tube placement is confirmed by

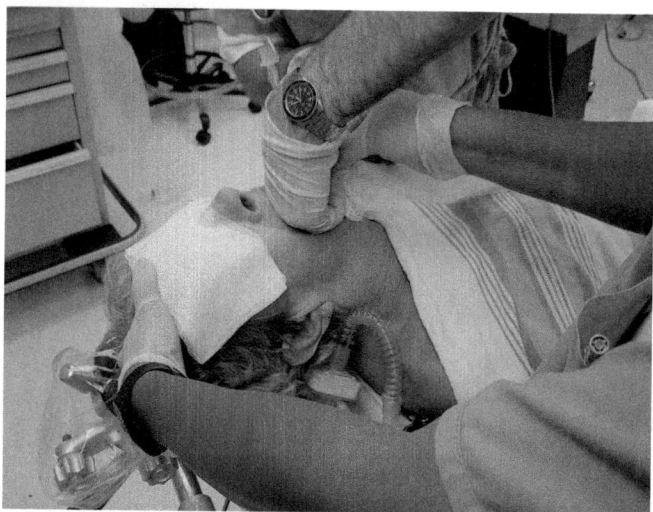

• **Fig. 21.7** Insertion of the index and middle fingers of the nondominant hand into the oral cavity with the palm facing down.

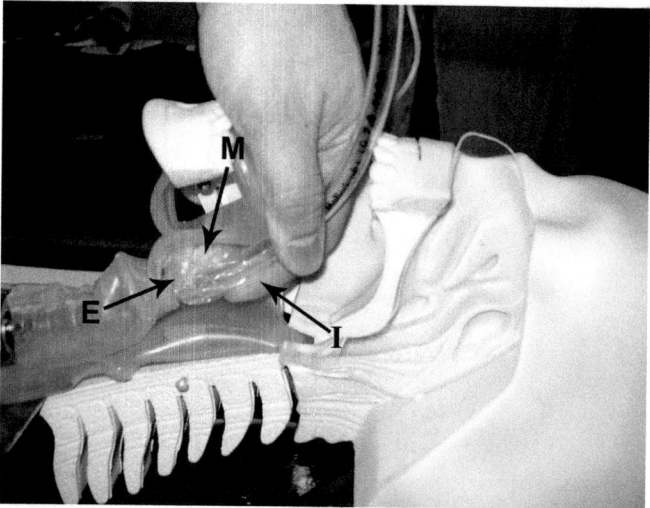

• **Fig. 21.8** View of the larynx (of a manikin) demonstrating the guidance of the ETT into the glottic opening by the tip of the index (*I*) and middle (*M*) fingers of the nondominant hand. The fingers are advanced to the point where the middle finger (*M*) can palpate the tip of the epiglottis (*E*) and push it anteriorly.

conventional techniques, such as end-tidal CO_2 detection. Occasionally, the tip of the epiglottis cannot be palpated. An upward (cephalad) and backward (posterior) pressure applied anteriorly to the larynx by an assistant may be helpful. Alternatively, the index and middle fingers of the nondominant hand may be used to keep the styletted ETT in the midline while observing tissue movement in the anterior neck during gentle rocking of the styletted ETT back and forth to locate the glottic opening.

An alternative technique described by Cook begins with the placement of the tips of the index and middle fingers of the nondominant hand in the hypopharynx, posterior to the larynx.[34] The ETT held in the dominant hand is then passed into the pharynx. The volar surfaces of the fingers serve as a "basketball backstop" to guide the ETT held in the dominant hand through the glottic opening. If required, the index finger of the nondominant hand may be flexed to help guide the ETT through the glottis.

Tracheal Introducer–Assisted Digital Intubation

Rich reported the use of a tracheal introducer (commonly known as a "bougie") in facilitating a digital intubation technique in an unanticipated difficult airway after several failed direct laryngoscopy attempts.[35] The tracheal introducer (e.g., SunMed ETT Introducer, SunMed, Largo, FL) was first guided into the trachea using the digital technique described above. The ETT was then guided into the trachea using the introducer as a conduit. The advantage of this technique is that it is easier to advance a tracheal introducer through the glottic opening and then pass the ETT into the trachea than it is to place a styletted ETT in the trachea. The tracheal introducer has a smaller outer diameter and is easily manipulated with the fingers to enable passage through the vocal cords. In addition, the clicks felt as the tip of the tracheal introducer brushes over the tracheal rings after flattening the angle of the introducer once it goes through the glottis, together with the "hold-up," assist in the confirmation of tracheal placement. The ETT with the malleable stylet is more rigid and perhaps more likely to cause blunt trauma to the upper airway, especially if repeated manipulation is necessary for successful entry into the trachea.

Neonatal Digital Intubation

Blind digital intubation in neonates has not gained widespread acceptance as a primary technique of intubation. Moura and da Silva[36] performed a randomized control trial comparing neonatal direct laryngoscopic intubation to the digital method of intubation. They determined that neonatal digital intubation had a higher success rate and a shorter intubation time. A single experienced clinician was responsible for performing all the steps of the procedure, which was identified as a study limitation. It has been used in several low- and middle-income countries where experience with and access to conventional laryngoscopes are limited.[26] Hancock and Peterson have employed the blind digital intubation technique in neonatal resuscitation and accidental extubation situations.[25] The clinician uses the gloved index finger of the nondominant hand to identify the epiglottis and glottic opening. The index finger is then used to guide the ETT through the glottic opening. The thumb of the nondominant hand can be used to apply external cricoid pressure. A styletted ETT is recommended. The fifth finger of the nondominant hand can be used in very small neonates. Advantages of the digital technique in neonates include reduced lip and gum trauma, controlled palpation of anatomic landmarks, and easy access to the airway in various transport scenarios, without the need to adjust lines and monitor equipment in unstable patients. The technique can also be used to confirm accidental extubation of the trachea. Caution should be exercised when airway pathology is suspected. The digital intubation of neonates and infants can be considered in situations in which other visual techniques have failed, when available equipment has failed, or when inadequate access may preclude the conventional laryngoscopic technique.

Combined Techniques

The technique of digital intubation has been combined with the Beck Airway Airflow Monitor (BAAM, Great Plains Ballistics, Lubbock, TX) (Fig. 21.9) and the Endotrol Endotracheal Tube (Mallinckrodt Medical, Argyle, NY) (Figs. 21.10 and 21.11) to facilitate tracheal intubation in several situations where direct laryngoscopy has failed.[37,38] The BAAM was initially developed to facilitate blind nasotracheal intubation techniques under spontaneous ventilation. The BAAM produces a characteristic whistling

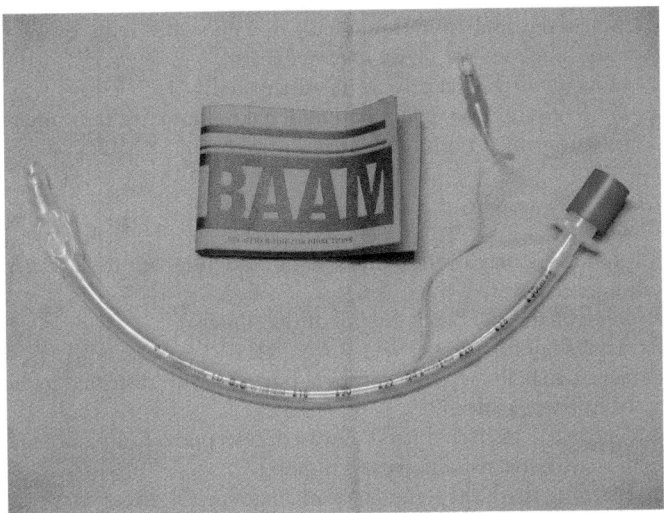

• **Fig. 21.9** The BAAM placed at the connector of the ETT.

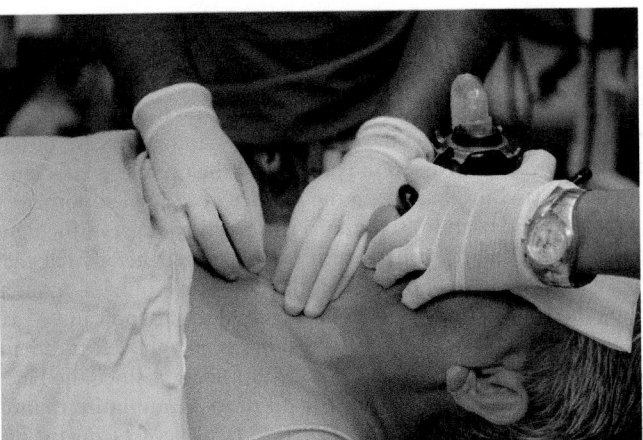

• **Fig. 21.10** The Endotrol Endotracheal Tube.

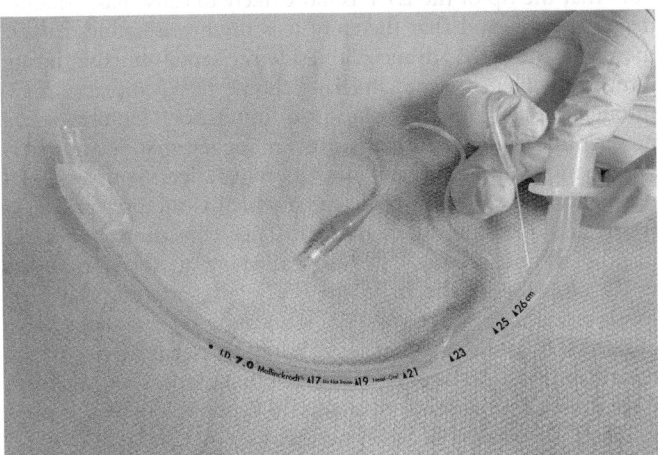

• **Fig. 21.11** Pulling the ring of the Endotrol Endotracheal Tube exaggerates the natural curvature.

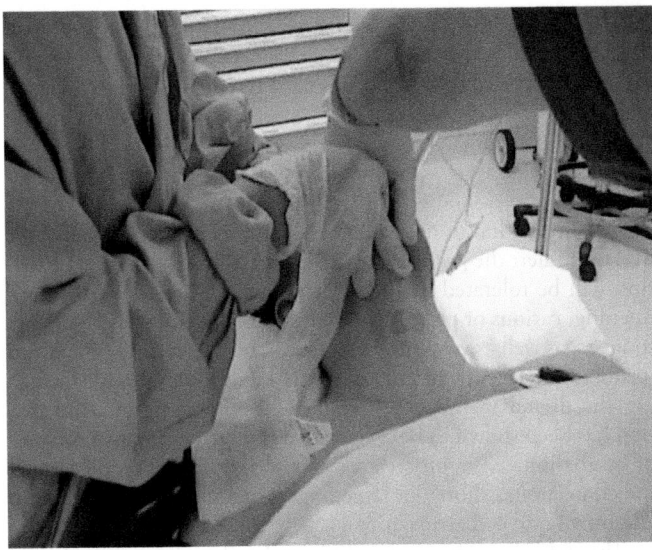

• **Fig. 21.12** Digital intubation using a lighted stylet. The light glow from the anterior neck can be used to confirm the correct placement of the ETT tip into the glottis.

sound during inspiration and expiration if the tip of the ETT is positioned within the air column leaving or entering the trachea. The device has also been shown to be effective in guiding nasotracheal tube placement in situations in which external cardiac massage is being applied.[38]

The Endotrol ETT's (Figs. 21.10 and 21.11) unique design allows the clinician to bend the distal tip anteriorly by pulling on a plastic ring attached to a wire that runs along the concave curvature of the ETT. This motion allows better alignment of the distal tip of the ETT with the glottic opening.

In tracheal intubation using an FIS it can be difficult to advance the ETT into the trachea. Asai and colleagues reported the use of the digital technique to help guide a 39-French double-lumen tube off the FIS into the trachea of a patient undergoing an anterior thoracic laminectomy procedure.[39] Additionally, Parker Flex-Tip ETTs, which have a flexible, curved, centered, and tapered distal geometry, allow for the easier passage of the ETT off the FIS and into the glottis and can be utilized to minimize trauma to either the vocal cords or nasal turbinates.

Light-guided tracheal intubation using the Trachlight (Laerdal Medical, Wappingers Falls, NY) can be difficult in patients with a long and floppy epiglottis.[40] This difficulty can be overcome by using the combined light-guided digital intubating technique. During the intubation, the middle finger of the nondominant hand can be used to lift the epiglottis off the posterior wall of the pharynx to allow the ETT with the Trachlight to go underneath the epiglottis into the glottic opening. The light glow from the anterior neck can be used to confirm the correct placement of the ETT tip into the glottis (Fig. 21.12). Over the past two decades, one of the authors (OH) has performed >20 intubations using this combined light-guided digital intubating technique. The lighted stylet–guided digital intubation technique has been described in newborns and infants with difficult airways.[41]

Nasotracheal intubation in the pediatric population can be combined with a digital technique to facilitate atraumatic passage of the tube behind the soft palate and entrance into the trachea.[42] However, this has not been systematically studied in a randomized control trial.

Clinical Utility

Blind digital intubation is a relatively simple technique that requires minimal equipment and can be learned easily. The 2013 iteration of the American Society of Anesthesiologists (ASA)

Practice Guidelines for Management of the Difficult Airway[43] still lists blind oral intubation as an alternative approach to difficult intubation when bag-mask ventilation remains adequate but tracheal intubation is unsuccessful.

Limitations

Digital intubation in uncooperative patients is generally difficult. The more alert the patient is, the less likely it is that digital intubation will be tolerated or successful. Patients with limited mouth opening, carious or prominent dentition, small mouths, and large tongues, as well as very tall patients, can be predictably difficult to intubate the trachea regardless of the method employed, including the digital method. With practice, however, digital intubation has been shown to be an effective and safe alternative method of intubation.[38] The procedure can also be difficult to perform if the clinician has short[44] or large fingers in relation to the patient's anatomy (e.g., pediatric patients).

The risk of injury to the clinician by the patient's teeth and body fluids is real.[29] This risk can be minimized by selecting unconscious or paralyzed patients or by placing a bite block between the patient's molars. In our experience double-gloving provides a wider margin of safety in protection against barrier interruption, injury from teeth, and the potential for disease transmission.

As with other techniques of intubation, complications, such as trauma to the upper airway, can occur during digital intubation. However, trauma can be minimized by advancing the ETT gently during intubation. Other potential complications of digital intubation, including esophageal or endobronchial intubation, can be minimized by a good technique, gentle manipulation, employing tracheal placement confirmation techniques, such as end-tidal CO_2 detection if available, and auscultation. The induction of emesis is also a possible complication.[44]

Digital intubation is a "blind" technique and therefore is relatively contraindicated in patients with upper airway abnormalities resulting from infectious diseases (e.g., retropharyngeal abscess), neoplasms, foreign bodies, caustic and thermal burns, and anaphylaxis.

Blind Nasal Intubation

History

First reported in 1902 by Kuhn,[45] the blind passage of an ETT into the trachea while attempting intubation via the nasal route was then observed by Stanley Rowbotham[46] in 1920. Sir Ivan Magill[47] then popularized the technique of blind nasal intubation in the 1930s. This method of tracheal intubation has been proven to be lifesaving in many difficult airway situations and it was used in 2014 as a Plan A in managing a difficult airway case electively[48] because the FIS was not functioning properly. Blind nasal intubation has also been taught in low- and middle-income countries[15] as a difficult airway management technique where FISs and video laryngoscopes may be too expensive to obtain and maintain.

Indications

The maintenance of spontaneous ventilation is necessary for blind nasal intubation. The experience and skill of the clinician are key determinants for success with this technique.

The following is a list of indications for blind nasal intubation:
a. Elective oral, pharyngeal, and dental surgery

b. When the oral route is difficult or impossible (e.g., limited mouth opening or severe masseter spasm)
c. Difficult airway (elective or unanticipated)
d. When equipment required to undertake alternative techniques is unavailable or not functional.

Contraindications

The following may contraindicate blind nasal intubation, although most are relative:
a. Inadequate experience or skill of the clinician
b. Basal skull fractures
c. Severe maxillofacial and/or nasal fractures with distorted nasal or midface anatomy
d. Known or suspected nasal obstruction secondary to pathology (e.g., massive nasal polyps or tumors)
e. Bleeding diathesis secondary to hematological disease or anticoagulant medication
f. Acute epiglottitis

Nostril Selection

Since the majority of clinicians are right handed, most would favor the use of the right hand to advance the ETT through the right nostril while using the left hand to perform a jaw lift or feel the anterior neck to assess the position of the tip of the ETT during blind nasal intubation. In the absence of a septal abnormality (e.g., a septal deviation) traditional teaching also suggests the right nostril over the left for nasal intubation.[49] It is generally felt that the left-facing bevel of the ETT is the main cause of nasal trauma. The mucosa over the turbinates is highly vascular and can be easily traumatized. It is likely that the mucosa over the left turbinate is particularly at risk during left-sided intubation since the bevel tends to impact directly against it. In order to minimize trauma most clinicians would insert the ETT with the bevel facing the flat nasal septum rather than facing the irregularly shaped turbinates along the lateral wall of the nasal cavity. However, others consider that the tip of the ETT is more likely to cause nasal trauma than the bevel and that therefore it is more reasonable to have the tip of the ETT advance alongside the septal mucosa during intubation. Hence some clinicians choose to advance the ETT through the left nostril during nasal intubation. Unfortunately, no scientific evidence currently exists to suggest that one nostril is safer than the other for nasal intubation in patients with a normal nasal anatomy.[50] Instead of debating which is the preferred nostril to minimize the risk of injury, it is perhaps more important to properly prepare the ETT (e.g., selecting an appropriate-size ETT, removing all the air in the ETT cuff, softening the ETT in warm saline or water as well as lubricating the external surface of the ETT) and the patient (e.g., apply a vasoconstrictor to the nostrils prior to performing the nasal intubation), resist excessive force during intubation, and change to a different nostril or use a smaller ETT when it becomes necessary.

Technique

Preparation

In elective situations the nares are best prepared with a vasoconstrictor (although there is little evidence that this maneuver reduces bleeding or enhances success rates) and a local anesthetic such as lidocaine, if needed for an awake patient. In emergency situations with life-threatening hypoxemia this may not be possible. The potential for severe epistaxis with airway hemorrhage must always be borne in mind. Rescue airway equipment, including extraglottic devices and surgical airway kits, should be readily available. Vital sign monitors should be placed on the patient, and, if possible, denitrogenation should be achieved prior to any airway intervention. Cervical spine precautions should be instituted as indicated. The maintenance of spontaneous ventilation is necessary for successful blind nasotracheal intubation. Some clinicians fully insert their little finger to gently dilate the nostril, minimize bleeding on tube insertion, and identify midnaris or posterior naris anatomic abnormalities that would preclude the use of that nostril.

Positioning

The patient's head should initially be placed in a neutral position.

Technique

First, an appropriate-size ETT is inserted into the naris and gently advanced. Avoid excessive force if resistance is met. This may mean that the tip of the ETT has entered the depression in the nasopharynx where the eustachian tube enters. If resistance occurs, the clinician should consider switching to the alternative nostril. A prominent anterior arch or tubercle of C1 is a common point of obstruction to nasal ETT passage. This obstruction can be relieved by inserting the index finger into the oral cavity reaching under the soft palate to sweep the ETT free of the bony obstruction.[51]

During nasal intubation under direct laryngoscopy, the ETT is often seen slightly off the midline when approaching the glottis through the nasal route. This can be corrected by slightly rotating the ETT medially when the ETT is approaching the glottis.

Listen for breath sounds as the ETT is advancing toward the glottis opening. One of the authors (OH) has successfully used a stethoscope attached to the ETT adaptor to auscultate for breath sounds during the procedure. The BAAM (Fig. 21.9) providing an auditory cue in the form of a to-and-fro whistle to facilitate nasotracheal intubation coupled with an Endotrol ETT (Figs. 21.10 and 21.11) has been reported.[38] Careful inspection of the anterior neck can also provide useful visual clues to the location of the tip of the ETT. The tip of the ETT can be felt if it is in a pyriform fossa.[45] A supralaryngeal bulge can be seen if the ETT is caught between the epiglottis and the base of the tongue (vallecula).[45] Occasionally, if the tip of the ETT repeatedly impinges the epiglottis anteriorly, it may be necessary to flex the neck slightly to aid in the passage of the ETT through the glottic opening and into the trachea.

When the ETT enters the larynx, a cough reflex can be elicited and advancement toward the carina can be suspected when a slight motion of the trachea externally is observed.[45]

The ETT can also rest on the vocal cords without entering the larynx. Slow counterclockwise rotation of the ETT can help advance the tip beyond the vocal cords.[45]

In the event that the ETT enters the esophagus repeatedly the ETT can be withdrawn to the hypopharynx and inflation of the cuff of the ETT will elevate the tip of the ETT tip toward the glottic opening.[52] If not contraindicated, neck extension is employed if the ETT repeatedly passes posterior to the glottis into the esophagus. The Endotrol ETT described above may also be used in this situation.[38] Clearly, this maneuver should not be performed in patients with known or suspected cervical pathology.

If a BAAM is not available, a small square of tissue paper can be taped to the 22-mm connector of the ETT. The tissue paper can be visualized fluttering with spontaneous respiration when the ETT

is directed at the glottic opening. Correct ETT placement should be confirmed by the detection of end-tidal CO_2 and auscultation.

Blind nasal intubation can be highly successful and easy to perform. In 1998 Van Elstraete and colleagues[53] compared the success rate of blind intubation using a cuff inflation technique with nasotracheal intubation using an FIS in 20 ASA I and II adult patients breathing spontaneously under general anesthesia without cervical spine injury but immobilized with a rigid cervical collar. Overall success was the same (95%), but the mean times to intubate were different (21 vs 60 seconds; $p < 0.001$) in favor of blind nasal intubation. More attempts were necessary with the blind technique compared to the flexible bronchoscope technique. Therefore in experienced hands blind nasotracheal intubation can be as successful as using a flexible bronchoscope, even when the cervical spine is immobilized.

Light-Guided Blind Nasal Intubation

Light-guided blind nasal intubation has also been performed successfully using a lighted stylet.[54,55]

Complications

In 1980 Danzl and Thomas[45] studied 300 consecutive nasotracheal intubations in an emergency department for a variety of indications (drug overdose, trauma, respiratory failure, cardiac failure, and neurological conditions). The overall success rate of the blind nasal intubation technique was 92%, with a 3% complication rate. Direct laryngoscopy with the Magill forceps was used for 24 patients, where the blind technique alone was unsuccessful. Complications included five significant epistaxes (one requiring nasal packing), two cuff punctures (probably in the 26 patients necessitating the use of Magill forceps), one partial avulsion of turbinate mucosa, and one superficial cellulitis over the cricothyroid membrane (translaryngeal anesthesia was used in 86% of patients). At least one other report of accidental turbinectomy[56] has been published in the literature.

Softening the ETT in warm saline or water reduced the incidence[57,58] and severity[58] of epistaxis following nasotracheal intubation in patients scheduled for elective surgery. A clot can form from the epistaxis and occlude the ETT if it is not suctioned thoroughly after final positioning.[59]

Clinical Utility

The 2013 revision of the ASA Practice Guidelines for Management of the Difficult Airway,[43] as well as the Canadian Airway Focus Group recommendations,[60] still list blind nasal intubation as an alternative approach to difficult intubation when face-mask ventilation is adequate but tracheal intubation is unsuccessful.

Limitations

Blind nasal intubation is performed by listening to the breath sounds. Therefore it can only be performed in patients with spontaneous ventilation. It cannot be used to intubate the trachea of an apneic patient or rescue a failed airway of a patient under general anesthesia with muscle relaxation.

Blind nasal intubation is commonly performed out of necessity in an emergency situation and is rarely performed electively. Because of the lack of opportunities, it can be difficult to teach blind nasal intubation to trainees. The need for spontaneous ventilation during the blind nasal technique creates a challenge when

TABLE 21.1	Equipment Necessary to Facilitate Light-Guided Retrograde Intubation	
Equipment	**Function**	
Chlorhexidine or other antiseptic solutions	To minimize risk of infection	
An appropriately sized endotracheal tube (ETT)	Intubation	
An 18-gauge needle or intravenous Angiocath	Cricothyroid membrane puncture	
A 5-mL syringe with 3 mL of saline or lidocaine 1% if for awake intubation	Aspiration of free air and topicalization of the tracheal mucosa	
A 21-gauge epidural catheter (Portex) or a 110-cm-long guide wire (0.038 in. diameter)	To guide the ETT into the trachea	
A 70-cm tapered anterograde guide catheter is required for the guide wire technique	To facilitate ETT insertion into the trachea	
Magill forceps and a laryngoscope	To retrieve the epidural catheter from the oropharynx	
Two hemostats	To hold the epidural catheter or guide wire	
4 × 4 gauze	To hold the tongue forward during intubation	
Water-soluble lubricant	To lubricate the tip of the ETT	

using a manikin for teaching purposes. The authors have experience teaching this technique to trainees in Rwanda, where there is a paucity of advanced airway technology, such as video laryngoscopes and FISs. Developing competence in "low-tech" techniques in such settings can be lifesaving. Zhang et al.[15] taught the blind nasal technique described in this chapter using manikins by having an instructor perform bimanual compression of the artificial lungs to simulate spontaneous respiration. All 37 participants at the workshop were able to successfully perform blind nasal intubation on a manikin using a BAAM whistle with simulated spontaneous ventilation.

Retrograde Intubation

History

In 1960 two surgeons, Butler and Cirillo,[61] reported the first retrograde intubation in surgical patients through an existing tracheotomy opening to allow a better surgical exposure in lower neck surgeries. The technique was subsequently modified in 1963 by Dr. Waters, a British anesthetist working in Africa, who performed a cricothyroid membrane puncture using a Tuohy needle[62] in patients with trismus. Waters inserted an epidural catheter through the Tuohy needle and advanced it cephalad so that the catheter was brought out through the nose by a hook. An ETT was then advanced over the epidural catheter into the trachea while pulling both ends of the catheter taut. After the ETT entered the trachea, the catheter was cut and pulled out through the oral cavity. He also advocated the use of this technique for patients without trismus in whom a difficult intubation is encountered. The catheter would then be picked up in the pharynx with forceps. He even described an awake version of the technique.

"Classic" Technique

Preparation

Although a preassembled kit is commercially available, the list of equipment necessary for the retrograde intubation is summarized in Table 21.1.

Positioning

In contrast to the sniffing position advocated for laryngoscopic intubation, the patient's head and neck should be in a neutral or,

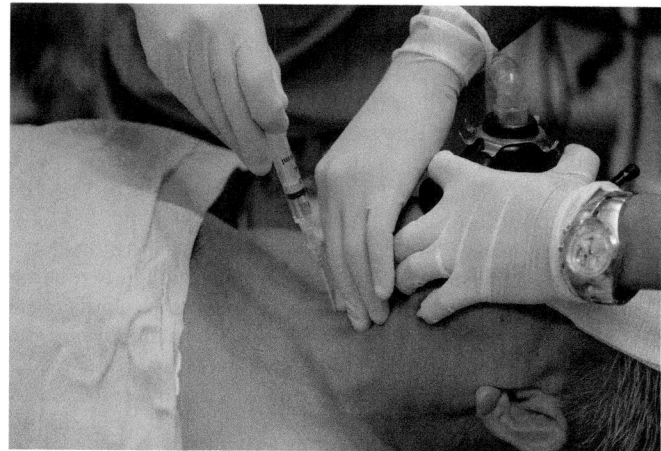

• **Fig. 21.13** Puncture of the cricothyroid membrane at a 90-degree angle to the skin in the midline position.

if there are no contraindications, in a relatively extended position to facilitate locating and puncturing the cricothyroid membrane. In obese patients or patients with an extremely short neck placing a pillow under the shoulders and neck may be useful.

Technique

This technique can be used in patients who are awake under topical anesthesia with sedation or under general anesthesia.[63,64] Although a cricothyroid membrane puncture can be performed using a blunt-tip Tuohy needle, the Angiocath is less traumatic and substantially easier to use. The cricothyroid membrane is punctured at a 90-degree angle to the skin using the 18-gauge Angiocath (or needle) in the midline position (Fig. 21.13). Considering that the identification of the cricothyroid membrane by palpation is successful only 25%–72% of the time, depending on the gender and size of the patients,[65–70] the use of ultrasound may be helpful to identify the cricothyroid membrane in some patient populations (e.g., obese patients or patients with a thick neck) provided time is available.[71] Correct tracheal placement can be confirmed by aspirating a free stream of air bubbles in a fluid-filled syringe. Upon entering the tracheal lumen, the Angiocath needle is removed, leaving the catheter behind. The fluid-filled syringe is reattached to the Angiocath and aspiration of air bubbles will reconfirm intratracheal placement. For awake

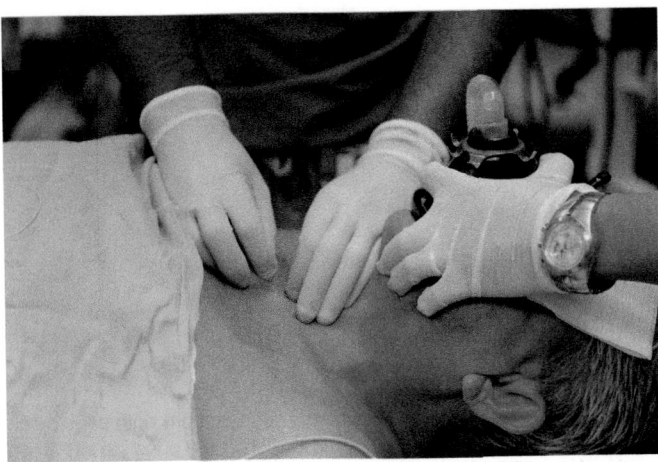

• **Fig. 21.14** The Angiocath catheter is angled at 45 degrees in a cephalad direction through which a 21-gauge epidural catheter can be inserted and advanced cephalad into the oropharynx.

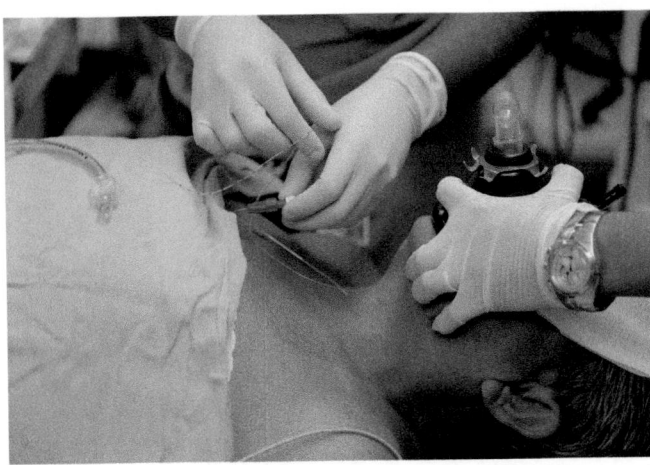

• **Fig. 21.16** After the Angiocath is removed from the anterior neck puncture site, the epidural catheter connector is attached to the distal end of the epidural catheter to avoid accidentally pulling the epidural catheter through.

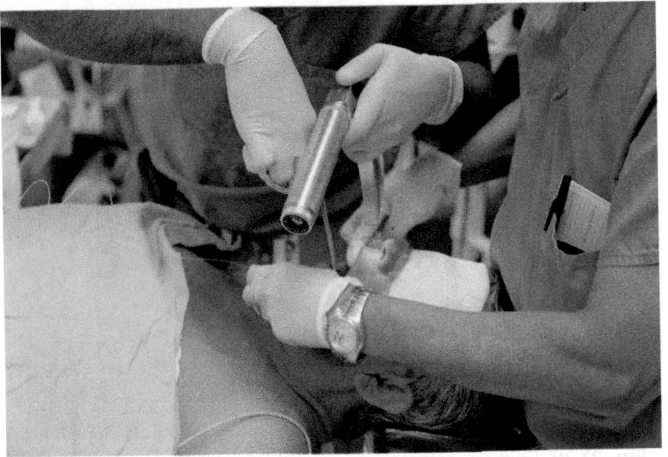

• **Fig. 21.15** The epidural catheter is retrieved from the oral cavity using the Magill forceps.

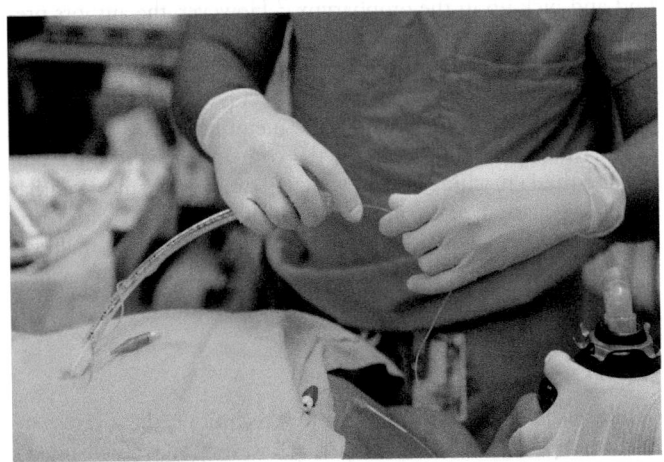

• **Fig. 21.17** Insertion of the epidural catheter into the ETT.

intubation, 3 mL of 1% lidocaine can be instilled intratracheally through the Angiocath. The Angiocath catheter is then angled at 45 degrees in a cephalad direction through which a 21-gauge epidural catheter (or a guide wire) can be inserted and advanced cephalad into the oropharynx (Fig. 21.14). The epidural catheter can be readily retrieved from the mouth using the fingers or the Magill forceps (Fig. 21.15). After the removal of the Angiocath catheter from the anterior neck, and to avoid accidentally pulling the epidural catheter (or the guide wire) through, the epidural catheter connector (or a hemostat) is attached to the distal end of the epidural catheter or guide wire close to the skin entry point (Fig. 21.16). The epidural catheter or guide wire is then inserted into the ETT (Fig. 21.17). The lubrication of the tip of the ETT will facilitate its entry into the glottic opening. To elevate the tongue and epiglottis away from the posterior pharyngeal wall, the tongue of the patient can be gently pulled forward by an assistant if the procedure is performed under general anesthesia or in patients who are unconscious. While pulling the epidural catheter or the guide wire taut from both ends by an assistant (Figs. 21.18 and 21.19), the ETT is inserted into the

oropharynx in the midline position to ensure that the ETT will be aligned with the glottis. When the tip of the ETT enters the glottic opening, a resistance can be felt. If the clinician is using a lighted stylet, a glow will be seen at the anterior neck, just below the thyroid prominence (Fig. 21.19). Now, the tension of the epidural catheter at the distal end should be relaxed so that the ETT can be advanced further into the trachea. The distal end of the epidural catheter will become shorter as the ETT pushes the catheter further down the trachea. For the guide wire technique, the guide wire should be removed before advancing the ETT into the trachea. If the wire is not removed, the ETT cannot advance past the puncture site because of the stiffness of the guide wire. While leaving the epidural catheter inside the ETT, the anesthesia circuit can be connected to the ETT to allow end-tidal CO_2 detection and confirm correct placement. While the epidural catheter can be easily removed through the cricothyroid membrane (Fig. 21.20), removal through the mouth end of the ETT may minimize puncture wound contamination by oral flora.[64]

The use of a guide wire rather than an epidural catheter has been suggested to improve success because it is believed that its

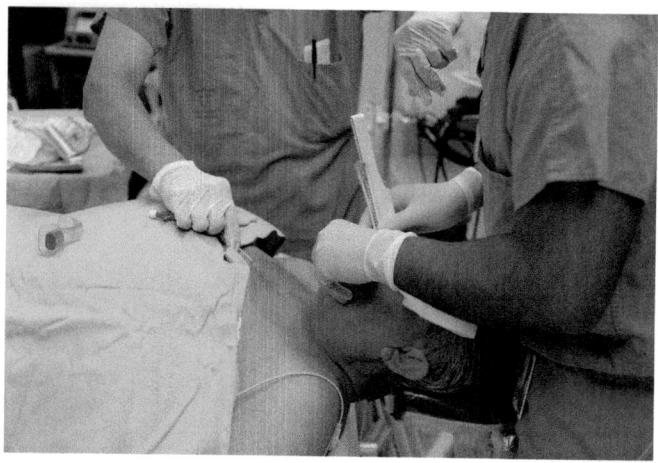

• **Fig. 21.18** With the epidural catheter pulled taut from both ends by an assistant, the ETT is inserted into the oropharynx in the midline position (here shown using a Trachlight for a combined technique).

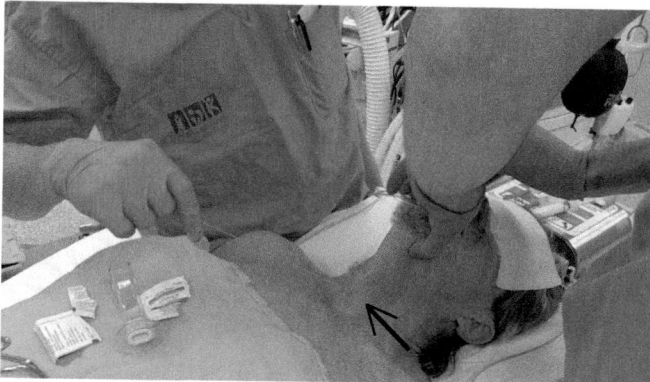

• **Fig. 21.19** With the epidural catheter pulled taut from both ends by an assistant, a circumscribed glow (*arrow*) is seen at the puncture site when the tip of the ETT is just beneath the cricothyroid membrane using the lighted stylet (Trachlight).

passage through the vocal cords is easier and that it is easier to find and pick up in the oropharynx.[72] However, the authors prefer an epidural catheter because it is substantially cheaper and perhaps less traumatic. In addition, the flexibility of an epidural catheter permits the ETT to advance deeply into the trachea past the puncture site at the cricothyroid membrane because it bends easily. Moreover, it fits between the connector of the ETT and the anesthesia machine circuit, which permits mechanical ventilation, oxygenation, and confirmation of ETT position within the trachea prior to the removal of this guide. In the case of malposition one can pull out the ETT and repeat the attempt of tracheal intubation while avoiding catheter reinsertion.

Other Techniques

While retrograde intubation is a simple technique, the success rate of tracheal intubation is unacceptably low. In a study involving 35 cadavers Lenfant et al.[73] reported a success rate of 69% using the conventional guide wire technique. The investigators suggested that failures were likely due to incorrect positioning of the ETT. In addition, because of the short distance between the cricothyroid membrane and the vocal cords, the depth of insertion of the ETT through the glottis opening is shallow (<10 mm in adults[64]), and accidental extubation can easily occur during the removal of the guide wire with this technique.

A number of technique modifications have been suggested to improve the success rate of retrograde intubation. These include the insertion of a tapered hollow catheter through the guide wire so that it can go further down the trachea beyond the cricothyroid membrane while removing the guide wire[73]; the insertion of the epidural catheter (or guide wire) through the Murphy eye of the ETT[74] from outside to inside to increase the depth of ETT insertion inside the trachea; the use of a subcricoid puncture[75] for the same reason; a pulling rather than a guided technique[76]; and employing a multilumen catheter guide.[77] To increase the stiffness and allow easier negotiation of the ETT through the oropharynx into the trachea, a tapered tip anterograde guide catheter (e.g., pediatric tube changer) placed over the guide wire has been suggested to improve the effectiveness of retrograde intubation.[64,78] Although these modifications are useful, they do not overcome the difficulty of determining the location of the tip of the ETT during

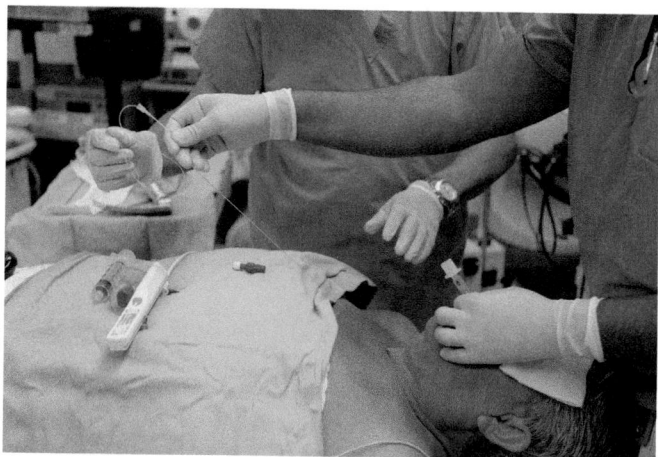

• **Fig. 21.20** Epidural catheter removed through the cricothyroid membrane while maintaining the ETT in place.

intubation. Simultaneous visualization of the ETT passage can be achieved if a flexible endoscope is placed through the nose into the nasopharynx beforehand.

Retrograde intubation using a guide wire passed retrograde through the working channel of an FIS has also been shown to be effective as the tip of the ETT can be guided into the glottis under indirect vision.[79–81] However, the FIS is expensive and the retrograde passage of the guide wire through the working channel of the bronchoscope can potentially damage the internal lining of the channel.[82] In addition, visualization of the laryngeal structures through a bronchoscope can also be difficult in the presence of blood and secretions.

The tip of the ETT can also be guided into the trachea using transillumination. The placement of the bulb of a lighted stylet at the tip of the ETT during retrograde intubation may assist in ETT advancement. A bright circumscribed glow can be readily seen in the anterior neck when the tip of the ETT enters the glottis opening and advances to the cricothyroid membrane puncture site (Fig. 21.19), potentially improving the success rate of the technique. The light-guided retrograde intubating technique using the flexible Trachlight (without the stiff internal stylet) has been shown to be effective and safe in patients with cervical spine instability.[63] Sharma[83] has also described a modification to this technique to add the possibility of EtCO$_2$ monitoring.

Ultrasound-guided retrograde intubation[84] and retrograde intubation while an extraglottic device is in place[85] have been recently described.

Clinical Utility

While retrograde intubation is not mentioned in the 2015 revised Difficult Airway Society guidelines for management of unanticipated difficult intubation in adults,[86] the ASA Difficult Airway Algorithm[43] lists retrograde intubation as a suitable option. However, it is our opinion that retrograde intubation can play an important role in the management of both anticipated and unanticipated difficult airway provided oxygenation of the patient can be readily achieved, i.e., in a CICO scenario, because retrograde intubation takes time. Our view is in agreement with the 2013 Canadian Airway Focus Group revised guidelines,[87] which state that retrograde intubation is not recommended in CICO scenarios, as it takes longer than cricothyrotomy.

Retrograde intubation can be performed either under general anesthesia or awake with skin infiltration and topical anesthesia.[63,64] Successful retrograde intubation has been described in numerous recent publications[84,85,88-93] and in many older ones cited by a review from Dhara.[64] This technique has also been used in patients with cervical spine instability.[63] Marchello et al.[93] recently described the elective use of retrograde tracheal intubation to manage the airway of a 72-year-old male with a pleomorphic adenoma of the lower jaw, extending into the oropharynx and rhinopharynx. The intubation was successfully performed under procedural sedation with the maintenance of spontaneous breathing using the technique described previously. The guide wire made it naturally into the nasal cavity, so nasal intubation was performed. Once the trachea was intubated, the ETT was retrieved in the oral cavity and a submental intubation was performed to allow surgical exposure.

Contraindications to performing retrograde intubation include difficult subglottic access, coagulopathy, infection or tumor around the puncture site,[64] and poorly palpable landmarks.[94]

Complications

While retrograde intubation is an effective intubating technique, it has some complications. These include sore throat, hoarseness, bleeding (puncture site and peritracheal hematomas), subcutaneous emphysema, upper airway obstruction (secondary to subcutaneous emphysema), pneumothorax, pneumomediastinum, pretracheal abscess, and trigeminal nerve trauma.[64] Fortunately, most of these complications are minor and self-limiting. It should be emphasized that, compared to the Tuohy needle, the use of an 18-gauge Angiocath or needle has been found to make the cricothyroid membrane puncture substantially easier to perform and less traumatic. In addition, to avoid wound contamination by the oral bacterial flora, the epidural catheter or guide wire should be removed from the cephalad end wherever possible following intubation.[64]

Conclusion

Although tracheal intubation under direct vision using a laryngoscope remains the conventional method of tracheal intubation, it is challenging in a small percentage of patients. Many alternative techniques, including video-assisted laryngoscopy, have been developed over the last several decades to improve the intubation success rate. However, these techniques often require expensive equipment and specialized skills and are sometimes not particularly useful for patients in an emergency with limited resources and in the presence of blood and secretions.

Nonvisual intubating techniques play an important role in airway management. Over the last several decades, these nonvisual techniques have been demonstrated to be effective and safe in securing an airway. However, as with all technical skills, one must recognize that there is a learning curve and that it requires regular practice.

Selected References

11. Karkouti K, Rose DK, Wigglesworth D, Cohen MM. Predicting difficult intubation: a multivariable analysis. *Can J Anaesth*. 2000;47:730–739.

14. Mulcaster JT, Mills J, Hung OR, et al. Laryngoscopic intubation: learning and performance. *Anesthesiology*. 2003;98:23–27.

40. Hung OR, Pytka S, Morris I, et al. Clinical trial of a new lightwand device (Trachlight) to intubate the trachea. *Anesthesiology*. 1995;83:509–514.

43. Apfelbaum JL, Hagberg CA, Caplan RA, et al. Practice guidelines for management of the difficult airway: an updated report by the American Society of Anesthesiologists Task Force on Management of the Difficult Airway. *Anesthesiology*. 2013;118:251–270.

55. Hung OR, Pytka S, Morris I, Murphy M, Stewart RD. Lightwand intubation: II—Clinical trial of a new lightwand for tracheal intubation in patients with difficult airways. *Can J Anaesth*. 1995;42:826–830.

60. Law JA, Broemling N, Cooper RM, et al. The difficult airway with recommendations for management: part 2. The anticipated difficult airway. *Can J Anesth*. 2013;60(11):1119–1138.

64. Dhara SS. Retrograde tracheal intubation. *Anaesthesia*. 2009;64:1094–1104.

69. Lamb A, Zhang J, Hung O, et al. Accuracy of identifying the cricothyroid membrane by anesthesia trainees and staff in a Canadian institution. *Can J Anaesth*. 2015;62:495–503.

71. Kristensen MS, Teoh WH, Rudolph SS. Ultrasonographic identification of the cricothyroid membrane: best evidence, techniques, and clinical impact. *Br J Anaesth*. 2016;117 Suppl 1:i39–i48.

82. Ovassapian A, Mesnick PS. The art of fiberoptic intubation. *Anesthesiol Clin North Am*. 1995;13:391–409.

86. Frerk C, Mitchell VS, McNarry AF, et al. Difficult Airway Society 2015 guidelines for management of unanticipated difficult intubation in adults. *Br J Anaesth*. 2015;115:827–848.

87. Law JA, Broemling N, Cooper RM, et al. The difficult airway with recommendations for management—Part 1—difficult tracheal intubation encountered in an unconscious/induced patient. *Can J Anaesth*. 2013;60:1089–1118.

All references can be found online at eBooks.Health.Elsevier.com.

22

Intubating Introducers and Lighted and Optical Stylets

KATHRYN SPARROW, OLIVER J. POOLE, AND ORLANDO HUNG

CHAPTER OUTLINE

KEY POINTS

- The Eschmann Introducer (EI) is best used when the epiglottis can be seen under direct laryngoscopy (DL) (Cormack and Lehane [CL] grade 3 view). The coudé tip can be hooked under the epiglottis, and then the EI is advanced blindly through the glottis. The success of this maneuver can be improved if the EI has been preshaped into a curve.
- The "hold-up" is a more reliable sign than the tracheal "clicks" for confirming the correct placement of the EI into the trachea.
- To facilitate the advancement of the endotracheal tube (ETT) over the EI after tracheal placement, the tongue and epiglottis should be elevated by a jaw lift or, preferably, by a laryngoscope.
- To have a clear passage to the glottic opening during lighted-stylet intubation, it is necessary for the clinician to perform a jaw lift, which will elevate the tongue and epiglottis away from the posterior pharyngeal wall to facilitate placement of the tip of the ETT posterior to the epiglottis and into the glottic opening.
- Because the lighted stylet uses the principle of transillumination of the soft tissues of the anterior neck without visualization of laryngeal structures, it should not be used in patients with known abnormalities of the upper airway, such as tumors, polyps, infection, or trauma of the upper airway.
- Although a jaw lift can be used to elevate the tongue and epiglottis away from the posterior pharyngeal wall during tracheal intubation using an optical stylet, it may be best to use the device in combination with other airway devices, such as a Macintosh laryngoscope or a videolaryngoscope (VL).

Introduction

Tracheal intubation performed by either direct or indirect (video-assisted) laryngoscopy has been shown to be effective, safe, and relatively easy. Unfortunately, even in the hands of experienced direct laryngoscopists, accurate and timely placement of an endotracheal tube (ETT) remains a significant challenge in some patients. This is particularly true in "unprepared" patients or patients requiring emergency intubation. When using any standard laryngoscope, obtaining line-of-sight to the patient's larynx can prove difficult in the presence of specific anatomic variations, such as a receding mandible, prominent upper incisors, restricted mouth opening, or limited movement of the cervical spine. It has been estimated that between 1% and 3% of surgical patients have difficult airways (DAs), making direct laryngoscopic intubation difficult and sometimes impossible.[1] In the obstetric population, the incidence of failed direct laryngoscopic intubation has been reported to be between 0.05% and 0.35%.[2] Many predictors of difficult direct laryngoscopic intubation have been suggested in the literature over the past few decades.[3,4] However, the sensitivity and specificity of these tests remain relatively low.[5–7] Therefore all clinicians must be prepared to deal with the prospect of both anticipated and unanticipated difficult direct laryngoscopies.

Given that visualization of the glottis may not be possible using both direct and indirect laryngoscopy, especially in a timely manner during emergency situations, many devices have been developed to aid the practitioner to pass the ETT into the trachea. During the past few decades, intubating guides, such as stylets, tracheal introducers, lighted stylets, and optical stylets have proven to be simple, effective, and safe. This chapter will briefly review the principles and techniques of tracheal intubation using these airway adjuncts.

Although many types of intubating guides, lighted stylets, and optical stylets have been commercially available for many years, this chapter will focus on devices proven in the medical literature to be effective and safe. It should be emphasized that this is not an exhaustive review of all commercially available intubating stylets and that the concepts and techniques discussed may be applicable to other similar devices.

Intubating Introducers and Stylets

Eschmann Introducer

In 1949, Macintosh first described the use of a "gum elastic introducer" as an aid to passing ETTs. Using an introducer in this fashion, however, did not become widespread until the development of the Eschmann Introducer (EI) by Venn in 1973 (currently sold as Portex Venn Introducer, Smiths Medical, UK). Venn's design has several key features. First, it is relatively long at 60 cm (Fig. 22.1A), allowing the introducer to be placed between the vocal cords before advancing the ETT over its distal end. It has been suggested that a naked introducer allows better dexterity and tactile sensation to the user compared with an introducer on which an ETT has been preloaded.[8] Second, the EI has a coudé tip (a 40-degree bend) for "hooking" under the epiglottis. The material from which the EI is made—a combination of a polyester core and resin covering—contributed to its success.[8] The EI is malleable, firm enough to direct, yet flexible enough to yield on contact. Furthermore, it is a multiuse device that can be sterilized between uses. The EI is commonly referred to as a *gum elastic bougie*, despite not being made of gum elastic (rubber) and not being a bougie at all (a bougie being a dilating device).[9,10]

Although an EI can be used to direct the ETT toward an anterior or narrow larynx, its real strength lies as a tool to facilitate intubation when the laryngeal aperture cannot be seen at laryngoscopy (e.g., a grade 3 laryngoscopic view as described by Cormack and Lehane [CL]).[11] A randomized clinical trial by Driver and colleagues concluded that use of the EI led to a significantly higher first-attempt intubation success rate with a Macintosh laryngoscope blade than a styleted ETT (96% vs 82%) in patients with a DA.[12]

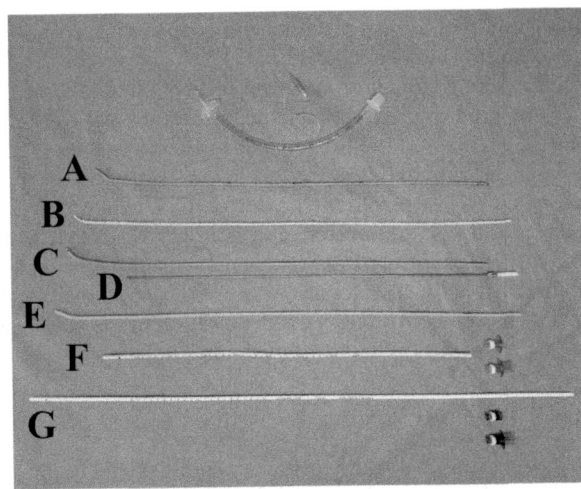

Fig. 22.1 Tracheal introducers. (A) Eschmann Introducer with a coudé tip (currently sold as the Portex Venn Introducer, Smiths Medical, UK); (B) Muallem Tracheal Stylet (VBM Medizintechnik, Sulz am Neckar, Germany); (C) hollow Frova Intubation Introducer (Cook Inc., Bloomington, IN); (D) rigid Frova Intubation Introducer internal cannula (Cook Inc., Bloomington, IN); (E) SunMed Endotracheal Tube Introducer (SunMed, Largo, FL); (F) Cook Aintree Catheter (Cook Inc., Bloomington, IN); (G) Cook Airway Exchange Catheter (Cook Inc., Bloomington, IN).

If the epiglottis cannot be seen at all (i.e., a grade 4 CL laryngoscopic view), it is the view of the authors that the EI should not be used, as the likelihood of successful intubation with the EI is unacceptably low. In cases where the epiglottis can be seen, the coudé tip can be hooked under the epiglottis, and the EI is then advanced blindly through the glottis. As the introducer is advanced farther, tracheal "clicks" are felt approximately 90% of the time if the EI is correctly placed,[13] whereas no "clicks" will be observed if the EI has been advanced into the esophagus. The authors believe that "clicks" are more likely to be perceived if, once the tip of the EI is through the vocal cords, the introducer is advanced at a shallow angle relative to the patient. This ensures that the tip of the introducer will contact the cartilaginous rings on the anterior tracheal wall as it advances, producing the "clicking" sensation. One can imagine that "clicks" are less likely to be felt if the only contact between the trachea and the EI is along the posterior tracheal wall or along the trachealis muscle. Additional clues to confirm tracheal placement include the perception that the EI slightly deviates to the right as it is advanced into the right main bronchus and a "hold-up" that is felt at the 30- to 35-cm mark as the EI becomes lodged in a distal airway. In contrast, if it is placed in the esophagus, the entire EI could be advanced without encountering any resistance (reportedly a 100% reliable sign),[13] although theoretically it would be possible for a pharyngeal pouch to "hold up" the introducer if one were present.[14] Some authors have cautioned against the use of the "hold-up" sign, believing that it increases the risk of airway trauma. If "clicks" are felt, then the "hold-up" test is usually not required.[13]

After tracheal placement, an ETT is advanced over the EI into the trachea. A jaw lift by the nondominant hand of the clinician or, preferably, insertion of a laryngoscope will facilitate the advancement of the ETT over the EI by elevating the tongue and epiglottis. If difficulty persists while advancing the ETT, rotating the ETT 90 degrees counterclockwise will turn the ETT bevel posteriorly and minimize the risk of it impinging on the structures of the glottic opening.[15] Following intubation, the position of the

ETT is confirmed using conventional methods, such as end-tidal CO_2 monitoring and auscultation.

The EI is long enough to be useful for nasal intubations[16] and can also be used to place supraglottic airways (SGAs) or double-lumen tubes (DLTs). The long length of the EI enables it to be used as an airway exchange device: It can be placed down the lumen of a correctly placed ETT, which can be removed over the introducer and discarded before a new airway is advanced in its place. During the entire maneuver, the EI remains within the trachea, thereby guiding correct placement of the new airway device. After the EI is removed, as always, the position of the new airway should be confirmed by standard methods.

Other Types of Intubation Guides

Over the past several decades, many intubating guides of different sizes, shapes, lengths, and materials have been developed. All the designs serve a function similar to the EI, but many have additional features. Some are single-use devices to address concerns regarding the possibility of prion transfer between patients with multiuse airway equipment.

The risk to patients of using suboptimal airway equipment with limited clinical evaluation is very real. Clinicians should be wary of new equipment and always insist on only using instruments that have proven to be effective and safe.[17] Careful review of product monographs is suggested for using the correct-size ETT with intubating guides.

- The Muallem Stylet (VBM Medizintechnik, Sulz am Neckar, Germany) (Fig. 22.1B) is a malleable, single-use, 65-cm-long tracheal introducer with a soft tip. Unfortunately, there is no published data comparing this device with other intubating guides.
- The Frova single-use intubating introducer (Frova Intubating Introducer; Cook Inc., Bloomington, IN) is firmer than the EI, has a 35-degree coudé tip, two side ports, and a hollow lumen (Fig. 22.1C). It comes with a Rapi-Fit connector that connects directly to standard ventilatory equipment, such as an Ambu bag or anesthetic circuit, enabling the Frova introducer to also serve as a conduit for oxygen delivery and/or ventilation. The Frova may be connected to an esophageal detection device; thus, correct placement can be confirmed before advancing an ETT.[18] The rigid removable internal cannula (Fig. 22.1D), designed to increase the stiffness of the Frova, has limited clinical indications and may increase the risk of trauma. The Frova introducer has two sizes: a 14-French, 70-cm-long adult version for use with ETTs 6.0 mm or greater internal diameter (ID); and an 8-French, 35-cm-long pediatric version for ETTs 3.0- to 5.5-mm ID. First-pass success rates with the Frova introducer are similar to those of the EI and are substantially better than the Portex introducer, which is a similarly shaped single-use device.[19] Presumably, this success is attributed to the increased malleability of the EI and Frova, enabling preshaping of the device, compared with the Portex introducer.[19]
- The Endotracheal Tube Introducer (SunMed, Largo, FL) is another example of a single-use version of the EI (Fig. 22.1E). It is similar to the EI in size and shape but 10 cm longer (i.e., 70 cm long). Like the Frova, it is stiffer than the EI. There are 10 cm markings on the proximal end of the SunMed Introducer to indicate the depth of insertion. Although it is marketed as a single-use disposable device, resterilization is possible.

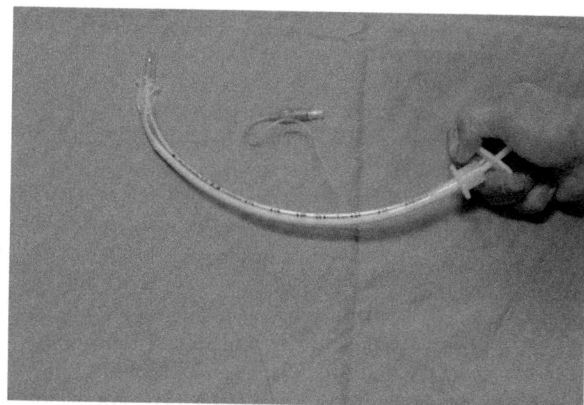

• **Fig. 22.2** The Schroeder Directional Stylet (currently sold as the Parker Flex-It Articulating Stylet, Parker Medical, Highlands Ranch, CO) can be used to elevate the tip of the endotracheal tube by wrapping all four fingers around the proximal tracheal tube and using the thumb to depress the proximal end of the stylet.

- The Schroeder Oral/Nasal Directional Stylet (Parker Flex-It Directional Stylet; Parker Medical, Englewood, CO) is a disposable articulating stylet that requires no bending before intubation. Inserting the stylet into an ETT allows the clinician to elevate the tip of the ETT by wrapping all four fingers around the proximal tracheal tube and using the thumb to depress the proximal end of the stylet (Fig. 22.2). Although the stylet is suitable for both oral and nasal intubation, it has been reported to be somewhat awkward to use, and the curvature created is not at the tip but rather over the distal half of the tube.[20] However, it has been reported to be effective for difficult, as well as for blind, intubations.[21]
- The Introes Pocket Bougie (BOMImed, Winnipeg, Manitoba, Canada) is made of Teflon and therefore requires no lubrication. The Pocket Bougie is curved and malleable with a soft, rounded tip. There has been no published data comparing this unique device with other intubating guides.
- The Flexible Tip Bougie (Sharn Anesthesia Inc., Tampa, FL) is a steerable introducer that uses an innovative sliding mechanism capable of producing both anterior flexion and retroflexion. It has an atraumatic silicone tip that reduces the risk of tracheal trauma (Fig. 22.3).

The effectiveness of intubating guides in patients with a DA has been well established.[22,23] Most of these studies, however, used the EI. With only a few exceptions, there is currently little data to support the use of the newer devices for tracheal intubation, particularly in patients with a history of DA. It should be emphasized that most of these new intubating guides and stylets are disposable and designed for single use. In contrast, the EI is more cost-effective because it is reusable.

Endotracheal Tube Exchangers

ETT exchangers, or airway exchange catheters (AECs), are ETT guides designed to facilitate exchanging an ETT, DLT, or SGA. Although the EI can be used as an ETT exchanger, several devices have been developed specifically for this purpose.

- The Cook Airway Exchange Catheter (Cook Inc., Bloomington, IN) is a hollow, flexible, straight tube designed as an ETT exchanger. It is 83-cm-long and available in 11-French, 14-French, and 19-French sizes to accommodate ETTs 4.0 mm or more, 5.0 mm, and 7.0 mm IDs, respectively. A 45-cm-long,

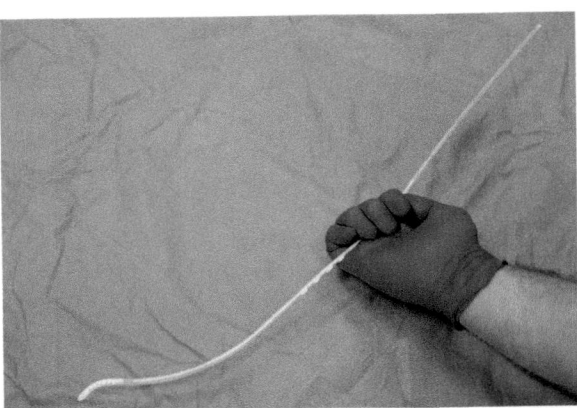

• **Fig. 22.3** The Flexible Tip Bougie. Through the motion of the thumb, the tip of the bougie can be either flexed or extended.

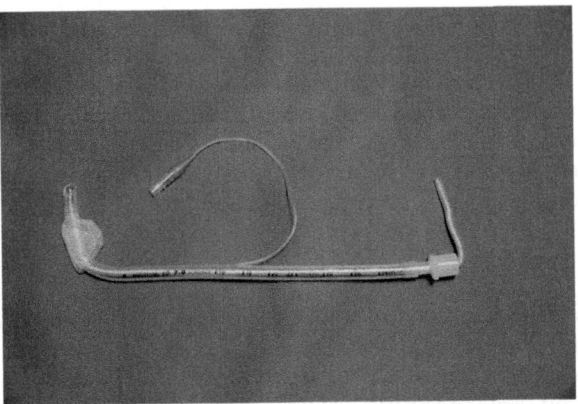

• **Fig. 22.4** A styletted endotracheal tube (ETT). The stylet remains "straight-to-cuff" at which point the ETT can then be bent to the desired angle like a "hockey stick."

8-French version is available for ETTs 3.0 mm or more. The extra firm (EF) model, available in 11-French and 14-French sizes, has a soft, atraumatic tip and a stiff proximal portion that is useful for exchanging DLTs.

• The Aintree Intubation Catheter (Cook Medical Inc., Bloomington, IN) is a shorter (56 cm), hollow, flexible, straight catheter designed to accommodate passage of a flexible intubation scope (FIS) with a maximum outer diameter of 4.2 mm (Fig. 22.1F). It can be used for uncomplicated ETT exchange or to exchange an SGA for an ETT 7.0 mm or more ID. Additionally, the Aintree Catheter can be advanced over a pediatric (11-French) AEC to provide additional stiffness to facilitate advancement of an ETT.

• The Sheridan Tube Exchanger (Sheridan Catheter Corp., Oregon, NY) serves a similar function as the Cook AEC.

Many AECs are hollow and include adaptors that allow connection to an oxygenation source, such as the anesthesia circuit or jet ventilation. In a review by Duggan and colleagues, it is recommended that, should a patient decompensate with an AEC in-situ, reintubation should be the primary management strategy due to the risk of failure or barotrauma.[24] Supplemental oxygen can be provided using standard techniques prior to tracheal intubation or between attempts, but should not be attempted through the AEC.

Stylets

ETT stylets are plastic-coated metal rods that can be placed inside the lumen of an ETT before intubation to stiffen and/or preshape the ETT. Unlike the EI and other introducers, the stylet should not protrude past the tip of the ETT to avoid trauma to the airway. Water-based lubricant should be used, and easy passage of the stylet in and out of the ETT should be demonstrated before use. The best shape for a stylet-shaped ETT depends upon the clinician's preference and the patient's position and anatomy, as well as the type of laryngoscope used. However, Levitan has shown that the line of sight to the larynx can be improved if the stylet remains "straight-to-cuff,"[25] at which point the ETT can be bent to the desired angle like a "hockey stick"[25] (Fig. 22.4). An angle of 35 degrees or less reduces the risk of traumatic injury. Once the ETT has passed through the vocal cords, the stylet should be withdrawn as the ETT is advanced into the trachea.

In a randomized trial, Gataure and colleagues compared the efficacy of the EI versus the malleable stylet in 100 anesthetized patients with simulated difficult (CL grade 3 view) direct laryngoscopy (DL). The EI had a success rate of 96% after two attempts, compared with 66% in the stylet group.[26]

Use With Video-Assisted Laryngoscopy

Video-assisted laryngoscopy (VAL) has changed the way in which patients with anticipated difficult DL are managed. Videolaryngoscopes (VLs) can be divided into those that feature classically shaped laryngoscope blades and those that feature highly curved or hyperangulated blades. Classically shaped blades feature a Macintosh-type design that allows the operator to visualize the glottis either directly or indirectly via an image displayed on the video screen. Hyperangulated VLs, such as the GlideScope (Verathon, Bothell, WA) and the C-MAC D-Blade (Karl Storz, Tuttlingen, Germany) depend on visualization of the glottis on the video screen, converting the passage of the ETT into an indirect approach.[27] One common issue with VAL, especially when using a hyperangulated blade, is difficulty placing the ETT through the glottis despite excellent glottic visualization.

The routine use of a styletted ETT has been advocated when indirect laryngoscopy is performed with a VL.[28–30] The use of a malleable stylet or bougie is usually required for the hyperangulated VLs. A nonstyletted ETT can be used for VLs with Macintosh-type blades; this is generally based on the preference of the operator.[31] Benefits of a bougie-based technique versus a styletted ETT remain unclear.[32]

In addition to malleable stylets, device-specific rigid stylets are available. The GlideScope manufacturer has produced a GlideScope-specific rigid stylet, the GlideRite stylet (Verathon Seattle, WA; Fig. 22.4). This rigid stylet is reusable, with processing required between each use. Several studies have shown conflicting results regarding time to intubation and overall success rates when comparing the GlideRite stylet with malleable stylets.[33–35]

As with DL, multiple studies have been performed to determine the best angle for a styletted ETT to be used with VAL.[33,35,36] Various configurations have been advocated, including a corkscrew configuration,[37] a "hockey stick" of 90 degrees, other different angles,[38] and a stylet angle that mimics the curvature of the VL blade.[29]

Despite the good visualization of the glottis achievable with VAL, there is often difficulty encountered with ETT delivery. When using a hyperangulated VL, advancement of the ETT past the vocal cords may be difficult as the anteriorly directed ETT often abuts and is held up by the anterior tracheal wall. This has led to some practitioners advocating a "reverse loading" approach for preparation of the styletted ETT[38,39] or the use of a straight ETT.[40–43] Because of small, mostly simulation-based studies, the ideal ETT stylet angle is not known. In agreement with previously published reports,[35,38] the authors of this chapter generally use a saline- or sterile-water-warmed, reverse-loaded, 90-degree-angled ("hockey stick") ETT when performing VAL.[44]

Complications

Despite widespread use, complications associated with the use of an ETT introducer, tube exchanger, or stylet are rare. Since the advent of VAL, multiple case reports have been published regarding soft tissue and pharyngeal injuries in which contribution from a styletted ETT could not be ruled out.[45–49] These cases highlight the importance of vigilance and awareness of ETT location with initial placement and advancement when using an introducer or styletted ETT for VAL. Reports of trauma during airway management frequently come from cases in which multiple attempts at securing the airway have occurred and multiple devices were used, making it difficult to attribute damage to a single device. Because of the firmer material, single-use ETT introducers exert more pressure at the tip when compared with the multiuse EI[19]; whether this corresponds to greater risk of airway trauma remains unknown.[18] However, as with all airway devices, excessive force should always be avoided. Holding an ETT introducer close to the coudé tip (e.g., with Magill forceps) increases the pressure exerted at the tip and is therefore not recommended.

Following tracheal intubation, all introducers and stylets should be inspected to ensure that no part of the device has been left behind. One case report describes the tip of an EI becoming detached and lodged in a patient's airway,[50] whereas a similar case describes how the plastic coating peeled off a stylet, blocking the ETT lumen.[51] An unusual case report described an ETT involuting at its tip as the EI was withdrawn, thereby lodging the EI firmly within the ETT and necessitating removal of both devices.[52] Routine generous lubrication of intubating guides should reduce the likelihood of such complications.[53]

Clinical Utility

Intubating introducers, stylets, and tube exchangers have been used successfully to facilitate tracheal intubation for many decades. The tracheal introducer is an inexpensive, reliable, and familiar tool used by anesthesiologists and, more recently, by emergency physicians and in the prehospital setting.[54–56] Although the popularity of these nonvisual intubating techniques may decrease as VAL is more frequently used, these devices may still play an important role in video-assisted intubation as a number of studies have reported the efficacy and usefulness of stylets and introducers to assist intubation using VLs.[57,58]

Lighted Stylets

Tracheal intubation using the transillumination technique was first described by Yamamura and colleagues in 1959 when they reported the use of a lighted stylet for nasotracheal intubation.[59] Modern lighted stylets use the principle of transillumination of the soft tissues of the anterior neck to guide the tip of the ETT into the trachea. This method takes advantage of the anterior (superficial) location of the trachea relative to the esophagus. When the tip of an ETT with a lighted stylet enters the glottic

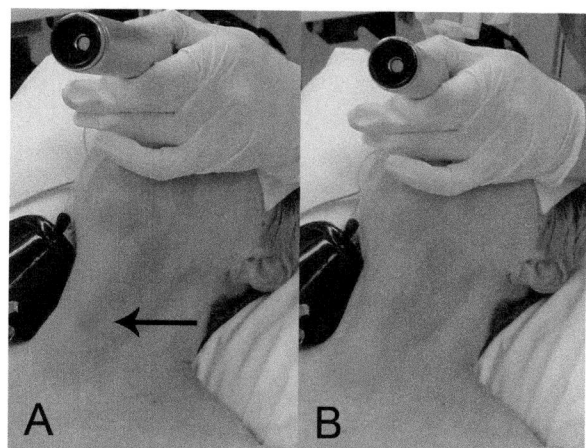

• **Fig. 22.5** (A) When the tip of the endotracheal tube (ETT) with the lighted stylet is placed at the glottic opening under direct laryngoscopy, a well-defined circumscribed glow *(arrow)* in the anterior neck just below the thyroid prominence can be readily seen. (B) If the tip of the ETT is in the esophagus, the transmitted glow is diffuse and cannot be detected easily under ambient lighting conditions.

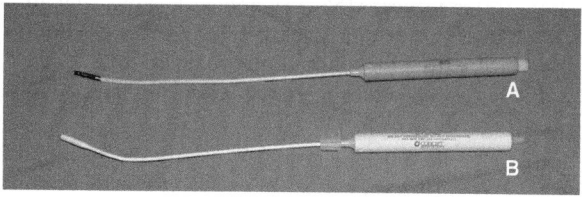

• **Fig. 22.6** Different lighted stylets: (A) Flexi-lum; (B) Tubestat. (Alero Inc., Chino, CA.)

opening, a well-defined circumscribed glow can be readily seen slightly below the thyroid prominence (Fig. 22.5A). However, if the tip of the ETT is in the esophagus, the transmitted glow is diffuse and cannot be detected easily under ambient lighting conditions (Fig. 22.5B). If the tip of the ETT is placed in the vallecula, the light glow is diffuse and appears slightly above the thyroid prominence. Using these landmarks and principles, the practitioner can guide the tip of the ETT easily and safely into the trachea without the use of a laryngoscope.

During the past three decades, several versions of the lighted stylet have been introduced, including the Surch-Lite (Bovie Medical Corporation, Clearwater, FL), Flexi-lum (Concept Corporation, Clearwater, FL; Fig. 22.6), Tube-Stat (Concept Corporation, Clearwater, FL; Fig. 22.6), and the Trachlight (Laerdal Medical Corp., Wappingers Falls, NY; Fig. 22.7). Over the years, these devices have proven to be effective and safe in placing an ETT both orally and nasally.[60–65]

Compared with the other devices, the Trachlight has a longer and flexible wand with a retractable metal wire stylet and an improved light source. These features add flexibility, broaden the utility of the device for both oral and nasal intubation, make intubation easier, and permit the evaluation of the position of the tip of the ETT after intubation. To date, the Trachlight has been the most popular and well-studied of the lighted stylets. Although the Trachlight is no longer manufactured, a new version of the lighted stylet similar to the Trachlight is currently in development.[66,67] One of the authors of this chapter (Orlando Hung) was involved in the design and development of the Trachlight; for these reasons, much of what follows reflects this experience and bias toward the

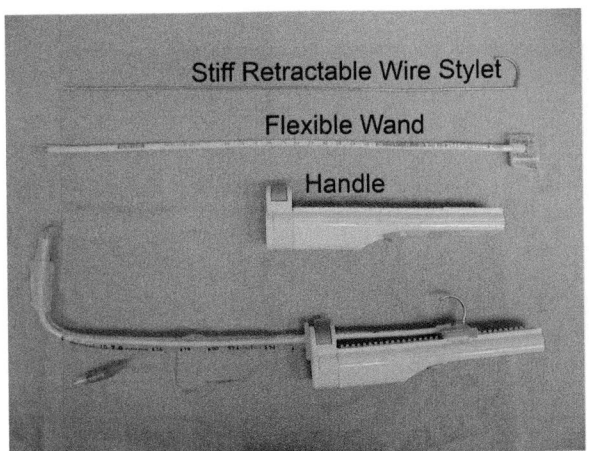

• **Fig. 22.7** The Trachlight consists of three parts: a handle, a flexible wand, and a stiff retractable wire stylet. With the lighted stylet placed inside the endotracheal tube (ETT), the endotracheal tube-lighted stylet unit is bent at a 90-degree angle just proximal to the cuff of the ETT in the shape of a "hockey stick" (Laerdal Medical Corp., Wappingers Falls, NY).

Trachlight. Nevertheless, the concept and principles of intubation using transillumination are applicable to all other lighted stylets.

For oral intubation, the lighted stylet is best used to shape the ETT into the form of a "hockey stick" (see Fig. 22.7). This configuration directs the bright light of the bulb against the anterior wall of the larynx and trachea. In addition, the "hockey stick" configuration enhances maneuverability during intubation and facilitates placement of the ETT through the glottic opening. However, a "hockey stick" is an awkward-shaped object to advance into the trachea. Thus, if the Trachlight is used for intubation, once the tip of the ETT-lighted stylet (ETT-LS) unit has passed through the glottic opening, the internal wire stylet should be retracted about 10 cm. This makes the distal end of the ETT-LS unit malleable and enables advancement into the trachea safely and without difficulty.

The glow emitted from the Trachlight can now be seen to migrate down the patient's neck and may be used to confirm correct placement of the ETT. When the glow reaches the sternal notch, the tip of the ETT is located about halfway between the vocal cords and the carina.[68] The lighted stylet is then removed, leaving the ETT in place.

Lighted-Stylet Intubation: Detailed Technique

Preparation

The importance of this frequently overlooked or rushed step cannot be overstated. Proper preparation will make the use of lighted stylets much easier and will increase the likelihood of successful intubation.

The wand of the lighted stylet should be well lubricated with a water-soluble lubricant to facilitate removal following tracheal placement of the ETT. If the Trachlight is used, the internal wire stylet is best lubricated using a silicone-based lubricant. This ensures its easy retraction during intubation. Once the wand is inserted into the ETT, the lightbulb should be placed close to, but not protruding beyond, the tip of the ETT.

With the lighted stylet in place, the ETT-LS unit is bent at a 90-degree angle just proximal to the cuff of the tube in the shape of a "hockey stick." Even though the degree of bend should be individualized to the patient, a 90-degree bend generally makes

the intubation considerably easier and is the authors' preference for most oral intubations. When the tip of the ETT is in the glottic opening, the 90-degree bend projects the maximum light intensity toward the surface of the skin, producing a well-defined circumscribed glow through the soft tissues of the neck. In contrast, if the lighted stylet is bent to 45 degrees, the maximum light intensity will be directed down the trachea, and the glow will not be so readily seen. For obese patients or patients with short necks, a more acute bend (greater than 90 degrees) provides better transillumination. The exact point at which to make the bend in the lighted stylet has been debated, although it is our experience that between 6.5 and 8.5 cm from the distal tip is generally suitable for most patients. A study by Chen and colleagues suggested that the bent length of the lighted stylet should be adjusted according to the patient's thyromental distance (TMD) after demonstrating that a shorter bent length (6.5 cm) was more suitable for patients with a shorter TMD (<5.5 cm).[65] It stands to reason that the shape of the lighted stylet should be individualized to the patient's anatomy.

Finally, the tip of the ETT should be coated with a water-soluble lubricant to facilitate its passage into the trachea.

Positioning

In the hospital setting, the clinician usually stands at the head of the table or bed. It is also possible to use the lighted stylet from the front or side of the patient, making it a useful tool in the prehospital environment. Depending on the clinician's height, it may be advisable to lower the height of the table or use a footstool to allow maximal visualization of the anterior neck of the patient during intubation. In contrast to the technique for laryngoscopic intubation, the patient's head and neck should be in a neutral or relatively extended position rather than in the "sniffing" position; the epiglottis is in close contact with the posterior pharyngeal wall when the head is in the sniffing position, making it more difficult for the lighted stylet to pass posterior to the epiglottis. In contrast, the epiglottis is lifted off the posterior pharyngeal wall when the head is extended, thereby facilitating entrance of the ETT into the glottic opening.

Control of Ambient Light

Compared with its predecessors, the light emitted by the Trachlight is extremely bright with a directed beam that enhances soft tissue transillumination of the neck. In most cases, tracheal intubation can be performed easily under ambient lighting conditions. In fact, in a large clinical study, tracheal intubation using the Trachlight was successfully performed under ambient light in 85% of the cases.[68] In very thin patients or in children, it is possible to mistakenly interpret an esophageal intubation as an intratracheal placement, although the glow generated from inside the esophagus is more diffuse in character. Dimming the room lights should be done only when absolutely necessary, such as in the case of obese patients or patients with thick necks. In the emergency department or prehospital setting when controlling the ambient lighting is not possible, it may be helpful to shade the neck with a towel or hand.

Intubation Technique

Oral Intubation

As with other intubation techniques, proper denitrogenation should precede airway management. Full muscle relaxation is recommended if clinically appropriate. In a study of 176 patients, Masso and colleagues showed that muscle relaxation is associated with a lower failure rate, decreased intubation time, and fewer

(A)   **(B)**

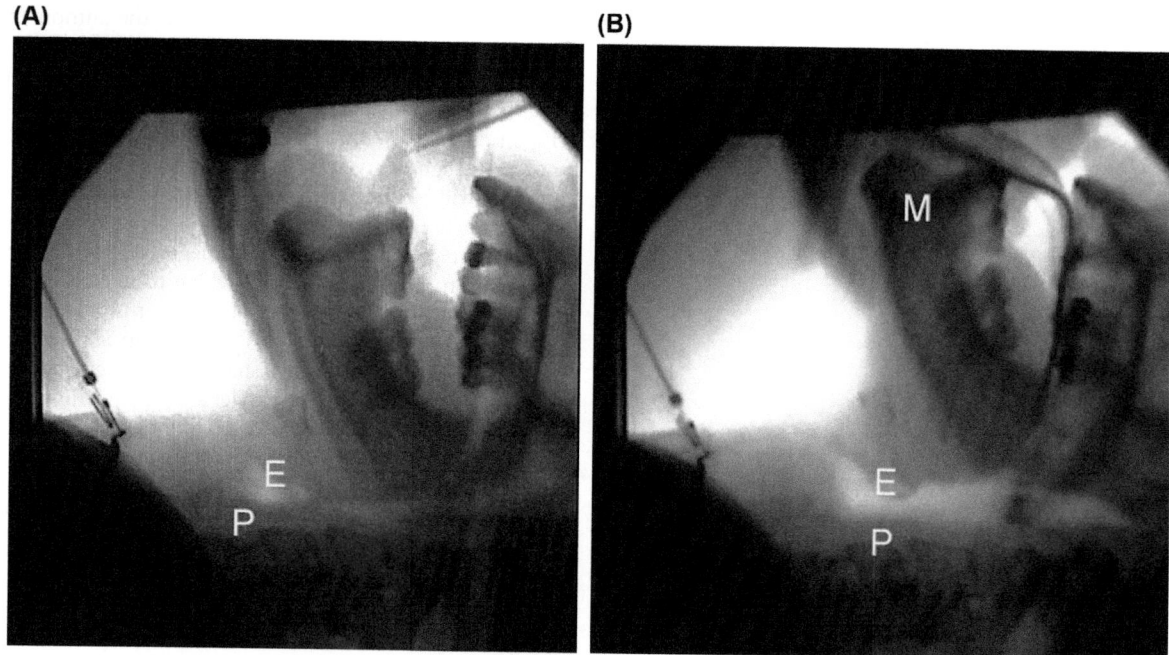

• **Fig. 22.8** Lateral radiographic view of the upper airway of an anesthetized patient. (A) The tongue falls posteriorly, pushing the epiglottis *(E)* against the posterior pharyngeal wall *(P)*. (B) A jaw (or mandible *[M]*) lift can elevate the tongue and the epiglottis *(E)* off the posterior pharyngeal wall *(P)* with an open passage for the endotracheal tube-lighted stylet unit to enter the glottic opening.

attempts when performing lighted-stylet orotracheal intubation.[69] When a patient is under anesthesia and lying supine, the tongue falls posteriorly, pushing the epiglottis against the posterior pharyngeal wall (Fig. 22.8A). To have a clear passage to the glottic opening during intubation, it is necessary for the clinician to grasp the jaw or mandible and lift upward using the thumb and index finger of the nondominant hand (Fig. 22.8B). This lifts the tongue and epiglottis away from the posterior pharyngeal wall to facilitate placement of the tip of the ETT posterior to the epiglottis and into the glottic opening. The nondominant hand must be kept close to the corner of the mouth to ensure an unobstructed path in the midline for the lighted stylet.

With the light switched on, the ETT-LS unit is held by the dominant hand and inserted into the midline of the oropharynx. The midline position of the ETT-LS is maintained while the device is advanced gently along an imaginary arc in the sagittal plane, thereby moving the light source closer to the larynx. The practice of blindly placing the ETT-LS in the oropharynx while looking for a glow in the anterior neck is ill advised and may increase the risk of pharyngeal trauma. Instead, under visual guidance, the ETT-LS should be able to be placed and angled so that the tip is very close to the larynx before beginning to look for transillumination of the anterior neck tissues. The ETT-LS should always be manipulated gently.

Once the clinician is satisfied that the tip of the ETT-LS is close to the larynx, the clinician looks to see a glow in the anterior neck. Now the dominant hand can be used to slowly rotate the lighted stylet slightly to the right or left; these movements are exaggerated at the tip of the ETT-LS. By watching the transillumination in the patient's neck moving from side to side, the degree of rotation required to ensure that the tip of the lighted stylet is exactly midline can be established. Once in the midline, a faint glow seen above the laryngeal prominence indicates that the tip of the ETT-LS is located in the vallecula. A jaw lift, or retraction of the tongue,[70] helps to

elevate the epiglottis and enhance the passage of the ETT-LS under the epiglottis, while rocking the handle backward advances the tip of the lighted stylet toward the vocal cords. When the tip of the ETT-LS enters the glottic opening, a well-defined, circumscribed glow can be seen in the anterior neck slightly below the laryngeal prominence (Fig. 22.5A). However, the ETT-LS cannot be readily advanced into the trachea because of the preshaped "hockey stick" configuration of the lighted stylet (Fig. 22.9A).

If the Trachlight is being used for intubation, retracting the stiff internal wire stylet approximately 10 cm makes the distal portion of the ETT-LS unit more pliable, allowing advancement into the trachea with reduced risk of trauma (Fig. 22.9B). Advancement of the pliable ETT-LS unit into the trachea before removing the lighted stylet will improve the success rate of intubation. This is analogous to the successful placement of an intravenous catheter by advancing the angiocath together with the needle a few millimeters into the vein once the needle tip enters the vein; this ensures that the catheter is inside the vein before removing the needle from the angiocath. As the ETT-LS is advanced into the trachea, the transillumination glow can be seen migrating down the neck. When the glow begins to disappear at the sternal notch (Fig. 22.10), the tip of the ETT is approximately 5 cm above the carina in the average adult.[71]

The lighted stylet can then be removed from the ETT. The ETT cuff is inflated, and correct tracheal tube placement is confirmed by standard means, such as chest auscultation and capnography. Although structural damage to the lighted stylet during intubation would be an unlikely event, it is good practice to always examine the device for structural integrity post intubation, lest a foreign body be inadvertently left in the airway.

Occasionally, the circumscribed glow cannot be readily seen in the anterior neck because of anatomic features, such as morbid obesity or a short neck. Neck extension as described above may be helpful. Placing a support under the shoulders may further assist

(A) **(B)**

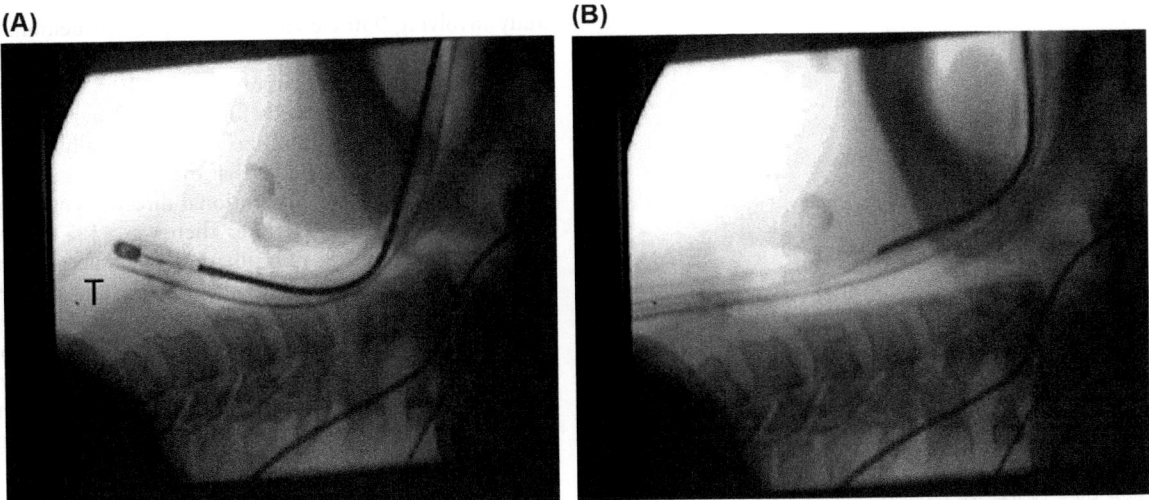

• **Fig. 22.9** (A) This lateral radiographic view of the upper airway of an anesthetized patient shows that when the tip of the endotracheal tube-lighted stylet unit is placed at the glottic opening, the endotracheal tube cannot be advanced readily into the trachea *(T)* because of the preshaped "hockey stick" configuration of the Trachlight (Laerdal Medical Corp., Wappingers Falls, NY). (B) With the stiff internal wire-stylet retracted approximately 10 cm, the distal endotracheal tube-lighted stylet unit becomes more pliable, allowing easy advancement of the endotracheal tube into the trachea.

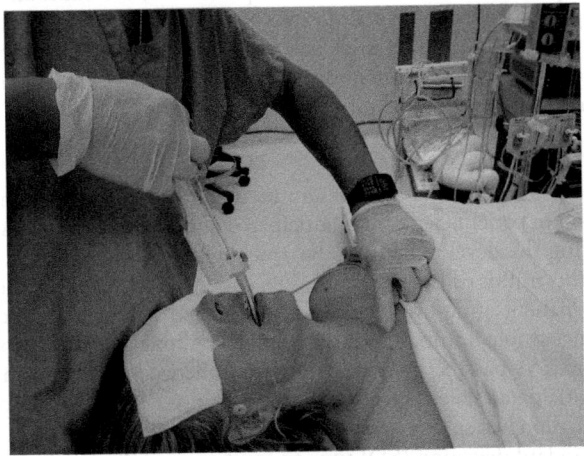

• **Fig. 22.10** Following retraction of the stiff internal wire stylet, the endotracheal tube-lighted stylet unit becomes pliable, permitting the endotracheal tube (ETT) to be advanced farther into the trachea. The ETT is advanced until a well-circumscribed glow is seen at the sternal notch.

neck extension.[72] Retraction of the breast or chest wall tissues caudally together with indentation of the tissues around the trachea by an assistant enhances transillumination of the soft tissues in the anterior neck. Dimming the ambient light is required only on some occasions.

If tracheal intubation is performed using a different lighted stylet, once the tip of the ETT-LS enters the glottis opening, the lighted stylet must be retracted slightly to allow the ETT to advance. However, advancing the ETT into the trachea can sometimes be difficult. This may be because the tip of the ETT may be caught at the vestibular folds or may be abutting the anterior wall of the larynx or trachea. This hold-up can usually be overcome by rotating the ETT 90 degrees or more clockwise or counterclockwise. The tip of the ETT will then be pointing sideways or downward, disengaging the hold-up and allowing entrance of the ETT into the trachea. Alternatively, grasping the anterior larynx

with the nondominant hand with an upward lift will help the tip of the ETT to come off the vestibular folds or tracheal ring.

Nasal Intubation

Most of the lighted stylets other than the Trachlight are too rigid for nasal intubation. Light-guided nasotracheal intubation using the Trachlight is particularly useful when nasal intubation is indicated, such as in emergency situations in patients with a limited mouth opening or cervical spine instability. Although similar to oral intubation, the technique for Trachlight nasal intubation differs in a few important ways.

Complete removal of the internal stiff wire stylet from Trachlight makes the ETT-LS unit pliable enough for atraumatic nasotracheal intubation. If a preshaped nasal ETT is used, the internal stiff wire stylet of the Trachlight can be retracted halfway (about 15 cm). This "unbends" the proximal curvature of the tube (Fig. 22.11), making lighted stylet nasal intubation with a preshaped nasal ETT easier.

Application of a vasoconstrictor nasal spray to the nasal mucosa before intubation may minimize bleeding. If time permits, the ETT-LS should be immersed in warm sterile water or saline to soften the ETT and further reduce the risk of mucosal damage during nasal intubation. Water-soluble lubricant is applied to the nostril to facilitate entry of the ETT-LS through the nose.

As with oral intubation, the head is placed in a neutral or extended (not sniffing) position. The Trachlight is switched on once the tip of the ETT-LS has been advanced into the oropharynx and positioned in the midline; it is then advanced gently, using the light glow as a guide. A jaw lift is necessary to lift the epiglottis from the posterior pharyngeal wall (Fig. 22.12). However, without the stiff internal wire stylet in situ, difficulty may be encountered controlling the tip of the ETT during light-guided nasal intubation. In particular, because of the natural curvature of the ETT, the tip commonly courses posteriorly into the esophagus. Various maneuvers may help bring the tip of the ETT anteriorly during intubation. One such maneuver is to flex the neck of the patient while advancing the ETT-LS slowly. In the event that flexing the neck of

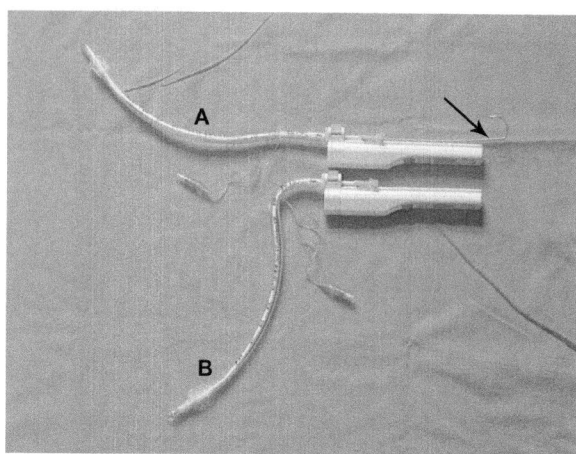

• **Fig. 22.11** If a preshaped nasal endotracheal tube (ETT) is used, the stiff internal wire stylet of the Trachlight *(arrow)* can be retracted halfway (about 15 cm) to allow unbending of the proximal curvature of the ETT (A) or removed altogether (B) (Laerdal Medical Corp., Wappingers Falls, NY).

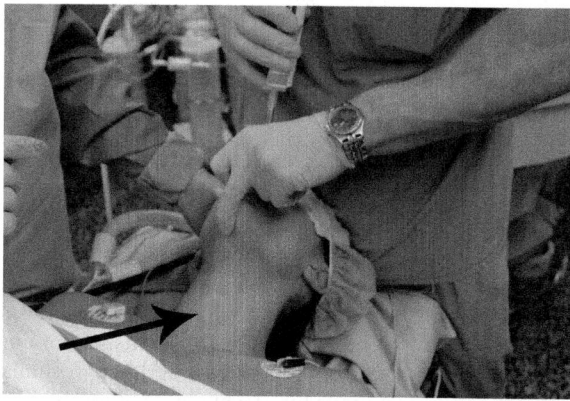

• **Fig. 22.12** During nasotracheal intubation using the Trachlight, the jaw is grasped and lifted upward with the nondominant hand, elevating the tongue and epiglottis away from the posterior wall of the pharynx to facilitate the placement of the tip of the endotracheal tube into the glottic opening. When the endotracheal tube-lighted stylet unit enters the glottic opening, a well-defined circumscribed glow *(arrow)* is seen in the anterior neck just below the thyroid prominence (Laerdal Medical Corp., Wappingers Falls, NY).

the patient is contraindicated, inflating the ETT cuff slowly with up to 20 mL of air will help to elevate the tip of the ETT and align it with the glottis during intubation.[73] Alternatively, an ETT with a controllable tip (e.g., the Endotrol tube; Mallinckrodt Medical, Argyle, NY) can be used for nasotracheal intubations and directed toward the glottis.[74] In some difficult circumstances, nasotracheal intubation can be performed effectively and safely with the internal stiff wire stylet in place.[75,76] Although there may be an increased risk of nasal trauma with the wire stylet in place, this technique may be associated with fewer head and neck manipulations and better control of the tip of the ETT.

Clinical Utility of Lighted Stylets

Use in Routine Practice

Tracheal intubation using a lighted stylet is easy to learn. The Trachlight has a learning curve of approximately 10 to 30 intubations.[77,78] Once mastered, the Trachlight is quick to use. A large

study involving 950 elective surgical patients demonstrated that Trachlight intubation was statistically significantly faster than direct laryngoscopic intubation (15.7 ± 10.8 seconds for Trachlight vs 19.6 ± 22.7 seconds for laryngoscopy),[68] although such a small time difference is unlikely to be clinically significant. The same study also demonstrated that the Trachlight appears to compare favorably with the conventional direct laryngoscopy regarding effectiveness and failure rate. There was a 1% failure rate with the Trachlight, and 92% of intubations were successful on the first attempt, compared with a 3% failure rate and an 89% success rate on the first attempt using a standard Macintosh laryngoscope. There were significantly fewer traumatic events and sore throats in the Trachlight group compared with laryngoscopy patients. Tsutsui and Setoyama reported similar findings in a study with 511 patients.[79] Trachlight intubation appeared to be highly effective (99%) with the majority of intubations successful after one attempt (93%). Unsuccessful intubation after three attempts occurred in 3 patients (1%).

Other lighted stylets have been less well studied. However, in 1991 a letter to the editor reported 1200 TubeStat intubations in one institution over a 2-year period. In this series, the TubeStat was used without laryngoscopic assistance. Whereas most intubations were undertaken with the patient under general anesthesia, some intubations were performed under topical anesthesia in anticipation of a DA. The authors reported that the TubeStat had a high success rate after failed direct laryngoscopic intubation and a low failure rate when used as a first-choice device. The authors concluded that "in the majority of elective cases, TubeStat intubation is our method of choice."[80]

Difficult Airway

The Trachlight has also proven to be useful for nasal or oral intubation in patients with both anticipated and unanticipated DAs.[81] During the development of the Trachlight, a study reported the clinical utility of the device in 265 patients with DAs; of these, 206 patients (Group 1) had a documented history of difficult laryngoscopic intubation or anticipated difficult laryngoscopy, whereas 59 patients (Group 2) were anesthetized patients with an unanticipated failed direct laryngoscopic intubation. In Group 1, intubation was successful in all but two of the patients with a mean ± standard deviation (SD) time to intubation of 25.7 ± 20.1 seconds. The two patients who were not successfully intubated with the Trachlight (a morbidly obese patient weighing 220 kg and a patient with severe flexion deformity of the cervical spine) were intubated successfully using an FIS. Orotracheal intubation was successful in all patients in Group 2 using the Trachlight with a mean ± SD time to intubation of 19.7 ± 13.5 seconds. Apart from minor bleeding (mostly from nasal intubation), no serious complications were observed in any of the study patients.

Other investigators have also reported successful use of the Trachlight for tracheal placement in patients with a DA. These include patients with a history of limited mouth opening,[76] thoracolumbar kyphosis,[82] severe burn contractures,[83] pediatric tongue-flap surgery,[84] Pierre-Robin syndrome,[85] other pediatric craniofacial abnormalities,[86] and cardiac patients with a DA.[87]

The Trachlight also can be used for patients with cervical spine abnormalities. In a randomized crossover trial of 36 healthy patients, Turkstra and colleagues compared cervical spine motion produced by Macintosh laryngoscopy, the GlideScope VL, and the Trachlight while manual in-line stabilization was applied.[88] Using video fluoroscopy, these investigators showed that the GlideScope and Trachlight methods of intubation produced roughly half as much cervical spine motion as Macintosh laryngoscopy. This study, and another by Huang and colleagues,[89] found Trachlight intubation to be considerably faster than GlideScope intubation in healthy anesthetized patients with simulated in-line cervical spine stabilization. In Huang's randomized study of 60 patients, time to intubate was 15 ± 5 seconds in the Trachlight group versus 33 ± 9 seconds in the GlideScope group ($p < 0.05$).[89] In a prospective, randomized crossover trial of 20 patients, the Trachlight produced as little cervical spine motion as intubation using a flexible bronchoscope in anesthetized, paralyzed adults with normal cervical spines.[90] A prospective randomized trial of 148 patients with cervical spine abnormalities compared airway management with the Trachlight versus the Fastrach intubating laryngeal mask airway (LMA). This study found the Trachlight to be considerably quicker (23 ± 9 seconds vs 71 ± 24 seconds) and more reliable (97.3% vs 73.0% were successfully intubated after a maximum of two attempts) than the Fastrach LMA in this patient population.[91]

The utility of lighted stylets for the management of patients with predicted DAs is not limited to the Trachlight. In 2009, Rhee and colleagues randomized 60 patients with high Mallampati scores (III or IV) to receive tracheal intubation using either a standard laryngoscope or the Surch-Lite lighted stylet. Successful tracheal intubation in the Surch-Lite group was significantly higher after one attempt (97% vs 80%) and significantly quicker.[92]

Hemodynamic Effects

Although many studies have reported the comparative hemodynamic changes associated with Trachlight intubation and direct laryngoscopic intubation, results have been inconsistent. Several studies involving only a small number of patients ($n = 26–60$) have shown no statistical differences in the hemodynamic changes following tracheal intubation using either the lighted stylet or the laryngoscope.[93–97] However, most of these studies did not perform a power analysis to determine the appropriate sample size for the study, thus running the risk of falsely accepting the null hypothesis. Although Siddiqui's study comparing conventional DL with the Trachlight and GlideScope was powered to detect clinically significant changes in blood pressure (BP) and heart rate (HR), there was no significant difference in BP and HR between the groups.[96] One study did not include a standardized general anesthetic technique.[93]

These findings were not consistent with the results of other studies demonstrating lower hemodynamic responses following tracheal intubation using a lighted stylet compared with a laryngoscope.[79,98–100] In a large study ($n = 511$), Tsutsui and colleagues reported that Trachlight intubation was associated with less elevation of BP during intubation compared with laryngoscopic intubation.[79] During the development of the Trachlight, a study involving 450 elective surgical patients showed that the increase in mean arterial blood pressure (MAP) and HR following intubation was significantly less using the Trachlight than with DL.[98] Unfortunately, in this study the anesthetic technique employed was not standardized. In Rhee's study involving 60 patients with high Mallampati scores (III and IV), patients who were intubated by DL had significantly higher increases in MAP and HR following intubation than those in the Surch-Lite lighted stylet group.[92]

In a small study ($n = 40$), Nishikawa et al. showed that the lighted stylet technique significantly attenuates hemodynamic changes after intubation in comparison with the laryngoscopic technique in normotensive patients.[99] However, they did not find any significant difference in hemodynamic changes between the two techniques in patients with hypertension. These results were in contrast to the findings of another comparative study of the hemodynamic changes between three intubating techniques using either a Macintosh laryngoscope, a Trachlight, or a Fastrach intubating LMA.[100] The investigators reported that both the Fastrach and the Trachlight attenuate the hemodynamic stress response to tracheal intubation compared with the Macintosh laryngoscope in hypertensive, but not normotensive, patients.

In a randomized controlled trial of 80 patients with coronary artery disease, Montes et al. compared hemodynamic responses to intubation with the Trachlight versus DL.[101] Although the results were not significantly different, the Trachlight group trended toward lower BP and HR during the intubation period.[101] Clearly, future studies involving a large number of patients are necessary to clarify these conflicting data regarding the hemodynamic stimulation associated with tracheal intubation using a lighted stylet.

Pediatric Patients

The pediatric Trachlight has been used both orally and nasally,[102] including in pediatric patients with DAs.[84,103] In 2008, Xue et al. published a case series of four children with craniofacial abnormalities who were unable to be intubated via DL (all children had CL grade 4 views of the larynx) or with a FIS.[86] These four children were successfully intubated within 30 seconds with the Trachlight. The small body of published pediatric Trachlight experience suggests that some adjustments to technique may be necessary. Suggestions include (1) bending the Trachlight to 60 to 80 degrees instead of the usual 90 degrees to better suit the pediatric anatomy, (2) the distance before the bend in the Trachlight should reflect the shorter length of the pediatric airway, (3) small distances mean that transillumination should be expected soon after insertion of the Trachlight, and (4) transillumination is so readily seen through the relatively small amount of tissue that transillumination from the esophagus can be more readily mistaken for that from the trachea, although experience will enable the clinician to tell the difference.[86]

Synergy With Direct Laryngoscopy

No airway management technique is 100% successful, and attempts at intubation with a lighted stylet can certainly fail. In a study with 950 patients, all Trachlight failures were resolved with DL.[68] Similarly, all failures of DL were resolved with the Trachlight. These results suggest that a success rate approaching 100% can be achieved in tracheal intubation with the use of a technique combining the two methods.

Using the two techniques simultaneously may be particularly useful for an unanticipated difficult laryngoscopic intubation (e.g., patients with a CL grade 3 laryngoscopic view).[11] While maintaining the grade 3 view with the direct laryngoscope in situ, the practitioner can use an ETT-LS with a 90-degree bend. Under direct visualization, the tip of the ETT-LS can be hooked under the epiglottis. If the tip of the ETT is placed at the glottic opening, a well-defined circumscribed glow can be seen in the anterior neck slightly below the laryngeal prominence. However, if a glow is not seen, the ETT-LS should be repositioned until a glow can be seen in the anterior neck.[104] Since the development of the Trachlight, the authors have had more than a dozen failed intubations using either the Trachlight or Macintosh laryngoscope. But in each of these failures, tracheal intubation was successful using the Macintosh laryngoscope together with the Trachlight. Other investigators have also reported the successful use of this combined technique. Agro and colleagues reported successful tracheal intubation in 350 surgical patients with a simulated DA using the Macintosh laryngoscope together with the Trachlight.[105]

Use With Other Airway Devices

In addition to its use together with DL, the Trachlight has been combined successfully with other intubating techniques. These include intubation through the LMA Classic,[106,107] intubation through the Fastrach intubating LMA,[108] with the Bullard laryngoscope,[109,110] and with a retrograde intubation technique.[111]

Percutaneous Tracheotomy

The Trachlight can be used to identify the intratracheal position of the tip of the ETT during percutaneous tracheotomy.[112] This simple technique can help to avoid puncturing the ETT and/or cuff, thus ensuring adequate ventilation and oxygenation during the procedure. This technique is also inexpensive and minimizes the risk of damaging equipment such as a flexible bronchoscope. If it is used properly, it is possible that this simple light-guided technique can also be used to accurately determine when the tip of the ETT is above the tracheotomy site as the ETT is pulled back during a surgical tracheotomy.

Limitations

Although lighted stylets have been demonstrated to be safe and effective for oral and nasal intubation, the technique requires transillumination of the soft tissues of the anterior neck without visualization of the laryngeal structures. Therefore, they should not be used in patients with known abnormalities of the upper airway, such as tumors, polyps, infection (e.g., epiglottitis or retropharyngeal abscess), and trauma of the upper airway, or if there is a foreign body in the upper airway. In these cases, other alternatives, including direct or indirect laryngoscopy, should be considered. Lighted stylets should also be used with caution in patients in whom transillumination of the anterior neck may be inadequate, such as patients who are grossly obese or patients with limited neck extension. Additionally, this technique should not be attempted with an awake uncooperative patient unless a bite block is used to prevent damage to the device or injury to the practitioner. A bench-top study showed that repeated cleaning of the Trachlight was shown to decrease the light intensity from the device.[113]

Complications

Since its introduction in 1995, the Trachlight has been used extensively in many countries. Although there are potential risks of airway injury during tracheal intubation using a blind intubating technique, there are very few case reports of complications.

In 2001, Aoyama and colleagues reported that the epiglottis of a patient was partially pushed into the laryngeal inlet, along with the ETT, following Trachlight intubation.[114] To investigate the potential risk of laryngeal injury during Trachlight intubation, the investigators used a nasally placed flexible bronchoscope. They reported that during placement of the ETT using the Trachlight, structures around the glottic opening, including the epiglottis and the arytenoids, could be transiently displaced. In some instances, the epiglottis was pushed into the glottic opening. Fortunately, the epiglottis usually spontaneously returned to the correct anatomic position. The investigators suggested that there are potential risks of laryngeal injury in addition to the down-folding of the epiglottis during the ETT placement using the Trachlight. Such occurrences, however, have not been observed to cause permanent damage, and the reduction in the incidence of sore throat in patients intubated using the Trachlight compared with DL would suggest such reports are of little clinical significance.[68]

Although rare, subluxation of the cricoarytenoid cartilage has also been reported by a study using an older version of a lighted stylet, the Tubestat.[115] However, because of the retractable wire stylet, the risk of damaging the arytenoid cartilages during Trachlight intubation is low.

In 2008, Zhang and colleagues reported a case in which the part of the silicon sheath that protects the Trachlight wand and bulb broke off from the device during intubation and was left behind within the lumen of the ETT.[116] This is the only such published case involving the Trachlight, although there are four similar case reports of instrument disarticulation with other lighted-stylet devices.[117–119] In Zhang's case, "the wand was withdrawn from the ETT with some difficulty." Softening the ETT before intubation by placing it in warm saline will make the ETT more malleable, whereas lubricating the Trachlight wand with a water-based lubricant makes disengaging the Trachlight from the ETT unit much easier. These steps, together with the mindset that undue force should always be avoided, will likely reduce the risk of structural damage to the Trachlight. Nevertheless, it is good practice to always examine the Trachlight post intubation for structural integrity.

Noguchi and colleagues reported that the application of 8% lidocaine in a pump spray as a lubricant for the Trachlight resulted in the disappearance of the print markings of the device.[120] However, lidocaine jelly and glycerin showed no effect on the print marks. The investigators suggested that lidocaine pump spray should not be used as a lubricant on the Trachlight.

Although lighted stylets have been shown to be effective and safe intubating devices, their potential risks and complications, as well as their indications, must be kept in mind.

Optical Stylets

Optical stylets are metallic stylets that, when inserted into an ETT, allow the clinician to view the advancement of the tip of the ETT via an eyepiece or video monitor. Optical stylets historically used fiberoptic bundles; modern optical stylets, including the Clarus Video System (CVS; Clarus Medical LLC, Minneapolis, MN), use video-chip technology. Many optical stylets with varying external diameter, angulation, image resolution, source of illumination, display capabilities, and flexibility have been introduced.[121] It is helpful to classify these devices as nonmalleable (rigid) or malleable (semi-rigid) optical stylets. Of the commercially available optical stylets, the rigid Bonfils Retromolar Intubation Fiberscope (Karl Storz Endoscopy, Culver City, CA) is the only nonmalleable optical stylet. Malleable optical stylets that will be reviewed in this chapter include the Shikani Optical Stylet (Clarus Medical LLC, Minneapolis, MN), the Levitan FPS (first-pass success) Scope (Clarus Medical LLC, Minneapolis, MN), and the CVS. Other optical stylets, including the Visual Intubating Stylet and the Reusable Video Stylet (Bedsdata, Shenzhen, China), Discopo Visual Stylet (Kangmin Medical Technology Co. Ltd, Changsha, China), and the AincA Video Stylet (Richards Medical Equipment Inc., Wheeling, IL) will not be discussed in this chapter because of limited available clinical data.

Potential advantages of optical stylets include portability, a potentially lower cost than FISs, and the ability to be used on their own or in conjunction with other airway devices. All devices require disinfection as per the manufacturer's guidelines and are generally less prone to damage than flexible endoscopes. In the hands of experienced clinicians, optical stylets allow for easy

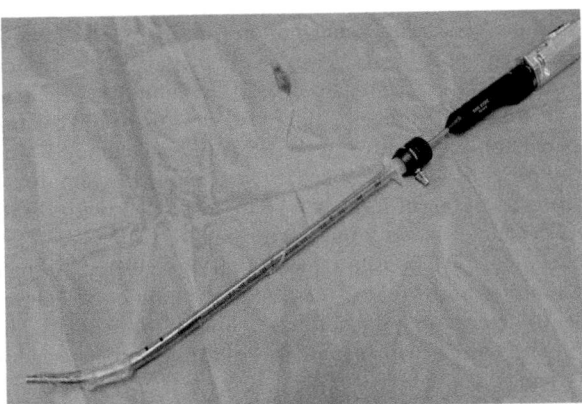

• **Fig. 22.13** The Bonfils Retromolar Intubation Fiberscope (Karl Storz, Tutlingen, Germany) is the only available nonmalleable optical stylet. There are options for a battery pack for portability or light cables for connecting to a monitor display.

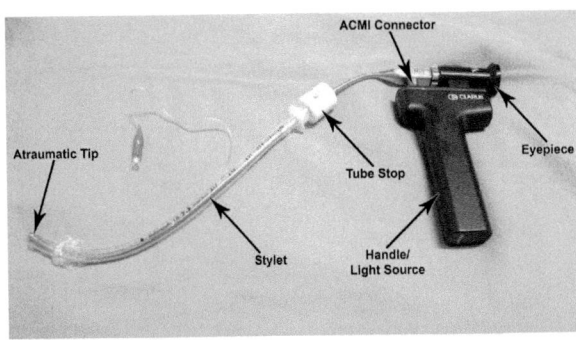

• **Fig. 22.14** The semi-malleable Shikani Optical Stylet (Clarus Medical, Minneapolis, MN) has a bending tool that allows for viewing angle adjustment. There is an eyepiece for viewing, or a camera may be attached with an adaptor for viewing on a larger screen.

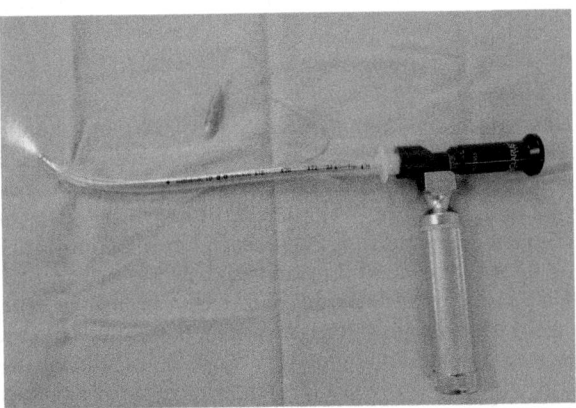

• **Fig. 22.15** The semi-malleable Levitan optical stylet (Clarus Medical, Minneapolis, MN) can be shaped to 90 degrees. However, a 25- to 35-degree angle is recommended.

maneuverability to the glottis and high rates of successful tracheal intubation. Like lighted stylets, optical stylets have also been associated with an attenuated hemodynamic response when compared with DL.[122,123] Challenges when using optical stylets include difficulty visualizing airway structures because of the presence of blood or secretions in the airway. Some optical stylets are short, requiring the ETT to be cut to a specific length before use, and proper preparation is required so that the rigid tip of the stylet remains within the ETT to minimize trauma to the airway. Case reports have documented successful use of these devices in patients with altered or distorted upper airway anatomy in the hands of skilled clinicians. However, one must be aware of the rigidity of the distal tip when using optical stylets in these patient populations.[124,125]

Types of Optical Stylets

• The Bonfils Retromolar Intubation Fiberscope is the only available nonmalleable optical stylet (Fig. 22.13). This rigid scope is available in two different diameters: 3.5 mm (pediatric) and 5.0 mm (adult). The scope's shaft is 35 or 40 cm in length and is angled at 40 degrees at the distal segment with a viewing angle of 90 degrees. Different scope models allow viewing through an eyepiece or have an available attachment for a camera head. ETTs up to 39 cm in length with 5.5 mm or greater ID can be used with the adult version of the Bonfils scope. The ETT is secured to the optical stylet with a standard 15-mm adapter. There are options for a battery pack for portability or light cables for connecting to a Storz-based monitor display. The manufacturer states that oxygen should only be administered through the available insufflation channel at gas flow rates not exceeding 3 to 6 L/min because of a published complication of subcutaneous emphysema when higher flow rates were administered.[126] Local anesthetic may also be administered through the insufflation channel.
• The semi-malleable Shikani Optical Stylet has a stylet length of 37.9 cm and a diameter of 5.0 mm (Fig. 22.14). It can accept an ETT with an ID 5.5 mm or greater. A bending tool allows the stylet to form up to a 120-degree angle, and the viewing angle is 70 degrees. There is an oxygen port for insufflation via the ETT that can be attached to an adjustable tube stop, and there is no working channel. There are multiple options for light sources: a fiberoptic connector, LED, a GreenLine laryngoscope handle, or a light cable. There is an eyepiece for

viewing, or a camera may be attached with an adapter for viewing on a larger screen.
• The Levitan FPS was designed by Dr. Richard Levitan (Fig. 22.15). His original article described the scope as having the ability for fiberoptic augmentation of emergency laryngoscopy.[127] The semimalleable stylet can be shaped to 90 degrees; however, a 25- to 35-degree angle is recommended. Because of a stylet length of 30 cm and a fixed 15-mm tube connector, the ETT must be cut to 27.5 cm. The 5.0-mm stylet can accommodate an ETT 5.5 mm or greater ID. There is an available oxygen insufflation port, and the light source can be provided by an LED light or a GreenLine laryngoscope handle.
• The CVS is a video-based optical stylet (Fig. 22.16). There is a 4-inch LCD screen that can be variably angled for operator comfort during use. It has a stylet length of 31.7 cm. The manufacturer specifies that the stylet diameter of 5.0 mm can accommodate both cut and uncut ETT size ranges of 5.5 to 9.0 mm as there is a fixed tube stop adapter. The CVS has two light sources: a white LED for visualizing the airway and an additional red LED for transillumination through the patient's skin.

Clinical Utility of Optical Stylets

Clinical scenarios that lend themselves to optical stylet use are similar to the scenarios already discussed with the lighted stylet:

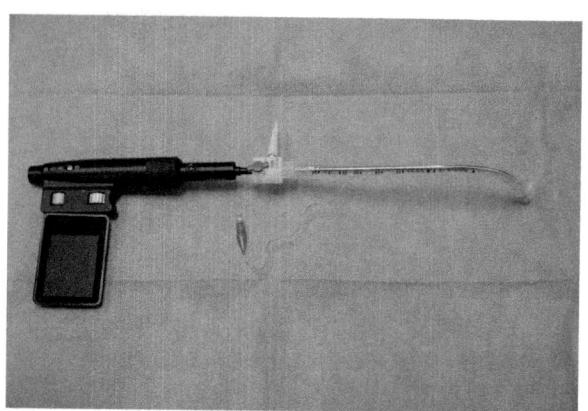

• **Fig. 22.16** The Clarus Video System (Clarus Medical, Minneapolis, MN) is a video-based optical stylet with a 4-inch LCD screen on the handle. An additional red LED can be used for transillumination through the patient's skin.

patients with limited mouth opening, cervical spine abnormalities, or DAs. Optical stylets have the added benefit of being able to confirm placement within the trachea.

VAL or DL may be very difficult or impossible in patients with limited mouth opening requiring endotracheal intubation. A light-guided nasotracheal intubation has already been described, though there is concern that this blind technique may cause tissue damage or be challenging in certain patient populations.[128] Lee and colleagues completed a randomized controlled trial involving 80 patients with limited mouth opening who required nasotracheal intubation for oromaxillofacial surgery.[129] Under general anesthesia, patients were randomly assigned to tracheal intubation using either an FIS or the Trachway (Biotronic Instrument Enterprise Ltd., Tai-Chung, Taiwan), an optical stylet similar to the CVS. The authors concluded that the Trachway nasotracheal intubation was quicker and easier than the FIS group. The mean total intubation time was 35.4 seconds in the Trachway group compared with 71.8 seconds in the FIS group. In addition to being statistically significant, the authors found this to be clinically significant. A two-person intubation technique was required for the majority of the flexible scope intubations, and the authors suggest that this may have factored into the increased time required for intubation. However, the Trachway group experienced more bleeding from the nostril (38% vs 28%) and blood accumulation in the oropharyngeal space (35% vs 25%) when compared with the FIS group. Unfortunately, the authors did not comment on the quality of visualization of the airway in the presence of blood during the intubation attempts in either group.

Optical stylets have been studied for use in patients with cervical spine instability. Two studies have documented less cervical spine movement with optical stylets compared with the DL.[130,131] Twenty-four healthy patients were enrolled in a crossover randomized controlled trial by Turkstra and colleagues with manual inline stabilization maintained during tracheal intubation.[131] This study showed that on average, cervical spine motion was 52% less ($p < 0.02$) at the occiput-C1, C2–C5, and C5-thoracic motion segments with the Shikani Optical Stylet compared with Macintosh DL. However, laryngoscopy with the Shikani took longer when compared with the Macintosh group (28 ± 17 seconds vs 17 ± 7 seconds, $p < 0.01$). Rudolph and colleagues similarly showed a prolonged intubation time with the Bonfils when compared with the Macintosh laryngoscope.[130] Another study was

able to show less cervical spine motion with the Bonfils in healthy volunteers compared with Macintosh DL laryngoscope, although time to intubation was not recorded.[132] Echoing the results of a previous study examining the Bonfils scope,[133] Kim and colleagues compared the CVS with the Pentax-AWS (a channeled VL) in healthy patients.[134] Cervical collars were applied to simulate DA conditions. The mean intubation time was longer with the Pentax-AWS (30.4 ±16.5 seconds) compared with the CVS (18.9 ± 15.2 seconds; $p = 0.003$). Interestingly, hemodynamic parameters were similar in both groups. The clinical significance of these small studies in determining the optimal technique for management of patients presenting with potential or documented cervical spine injury remains unresolved.

Optical stylets have also been used in patients with DAs.[132] In a randomized crossover study of 34 patients with a simulated CL grade 3A view, Greenland and colleagues showed similar success rates when the Levitan FPS was compared with a single-use tracheal introducer ("bougie") for tracheal intubation.[135] Although the mean insertion time for the Levitan FPS (13.3 to 21.1 seconds) was statistically longer than that for the tracheal introducer group (8.6 to 8.9 seconds), the investigators felt that this difference was not clinically relevant. Of note were three cases of prolonged intubation in the Levitan FPS group (50–52 seconds) because of the presence of significant amounts of secretions. These results were consistent with simulated difficult CL grades in manikin studies.[136,137] Kok and colleagues completed a randomized controlled study of 94 patients with simulated DAs by application of manual in-line stabilization.[138] This group reported that indirect laryngoscopy with the Levitan FPS in conjunction with the Macintosh laryngoscope in simulated DAs did not improve the safety or efficacy of tracheal intubation as measured by CL grade. Although there were higher POGO (percentage of glottic opening) scores with the Levitan FPS, this did not translate into easier or faster intubations for participants. In another study, the Bonfils had a high success rate after failed DL: Tracheal intubation was successful in all but one patient. Intubation time was clinically acceptable despite a grade 4 CL laryngoscopic view in 76% of the patients.[134]

Optical stylets have also been used for double-lumen tube (DLT) insertion. In a prospective randomized controlled trial, Yang and colleagues were able to demonstrate that DLT intubation with the OptiScope (Pacific Medical, Seoul, Korea), another optical stylet similar to the CVS, was faster and more successful after one attempt and caused less trauma when compared with the Macintosh laryngoscope.[139] Recently, there have been a multitude of published case reports highlighting the use of the CVS or Trachway in DA settings.[124,125,140–142]

Because fogging, secretions, or blood can cause difficulty with visualization when using optical stylets, this can make the application of simulation-based manikin studies challenging in real-life DA scenarios. The manufacturers of all the optical stylets offer instructions for intended use. Although there is a paucity of supporting evidence, the instructions suggest that these optical stylets can be used in a variety of situations, such as confirmation of cricothyrotomy placement, use in combination with VAL to confirm tracheal placement, and intubation via SGAs.[143] Be aware of the maneuvers that can increase the chance for success when using these devices. This concept is highlighted by Jagannathan and colleagues when describing the use of the Shikani for intubation of seven children with DAs via an SGA.[144] All seven patients required jaw thrust and anterior laryngeal pressure to facilitate intubation using the Shikani. Performance of a jaw lift has also been supported as improving time to successful intubation.[145]

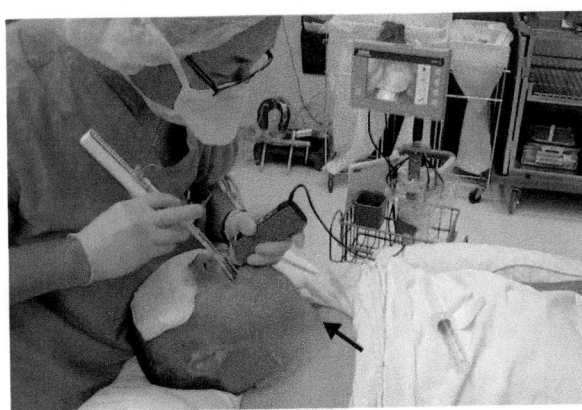

• **Fig. 22.17** Combination techniques with video-assisted laryngoscopy (VAL), seen here with the Karl Storz C-MAC (Karl Storz, Tutlingen, Germany) and the Trachlight (Laerdal Medical Corp., Wappingers Falls, NY) (or other optical and video stylets), are useful when a Cormack-Lehane grade 3 laryngoscopic view is encountered. The clinician can use an endotracheal tube-lighted stylet unit (ETT-LS) with a 90-degree bend. Under VAL, the tip of the ETT-LS can be "hooked" under the epiglottis. If the tip of the ETT-LS is placed at the glottic opening, a well-defined circumscribed glow can be seen in the anterior neck slightly below the laryngeal prominence (arrow).

Combination Techniques

Our ability to visualize and manage the airway has changed dramatically in the era of VAL. However, these devices have limitations: fogging, bleeding, and secretions can make visualization of the airway challenging. In addition, as our ability to see the airway improves with more angulated VLs, our ability to advance the ETT through the glottis opening may become more challenging. Lighted stylets and optical stylets can be easily used in combination with DL or VAL (Fig. 22.17).[146] Transillumination in the setting of a bleeding airway, real-time tracheal confirmation of ETT placement in a patient with a challenging laryngoscopic view, or intentional restriction of the glottic view to minimize cervical spine movement are all applications for these combination techniques. Interestingly, a combination technique was encouraged in the original description of some of these airway devices, such as the Levitan FPS,[127] and more studies are required in this area.

Conclusion

Difficult laryngoscopic intubation has led to the development of many alternative techniques for placing an ETT. An intubating guide, such as the reusable and malleable EI or "gum elastic bougie," has been shown to be a safe, effective, and quick method of guiding an ETT into the trachea when the laryngeal aperture cannot be well seen under direct vision using a laryngoscope. Use of the EI is well supported by many reports and 60 years of clinical use. Some newer single-use tracheal introducers, such as the Frova Intubation Introducer, have also performed well in studies, although they tend to be stiffer and less malleable than the EI. The longer and larger-diameter ETT exchangers are introducers specifically designed to be securely placed in the trachea so that ETTs can be advanced over them into the trachea. ETT exchangers are

useful when a secure airway must be exchanged or temporarily removed but DL is likely to be difficult. Stylets that enable stiffening and reshaping of an ETT before intubation have been used for many years but are not well studied. Limited evidence suggests that these stylets are not as effective as introducers when used for the management of DAs. More recently, introducers and stylets have been used to facilitate VAL.

Transillumination of the soft tissues of the neck using a lighted stylet has been shown to be an effective intubation technique for decades. Although many versions of lighted stylets are available, the Trachlight has incorporated many design modifications to facilitate both oral and nasal intubation in both awake and anesthetized patients. It has been demonstrated as an effective and safe intubating device in a large variety of surgical patients, including those with documented DAs. However, lighted stylets should not be used in patients with anatomic abnormalities of the upper airway. Optical stylets are being used with more frequency in patients with DAs and will likely become more frequently used in combination with other airway devices. As with any intubation technique, regular use of and practice with these intubating devices will improve performance and may also reduce the likelihood of complications.

Selected References

24. Duggan LV, Law JA, Murphy MF. Brief review: supplementing oxygen through an airway exchange catheter: efficacy, complications, and recommendations. *Can J Anaesth.* 2011;58(6):560-568.
25. Levitan RM, Pisaturo JT, Kinkle WC, Butler K, Everett WW. Stylet bend angles and tracheal tube passage using a straight-to-cuff shape. *Acad Emerg Med.* 2006;13:1255-1258.
32. Batuwitage B, McDonald A, Nishikawa K, Lythgoe D, Mercer S, Charters P. Comparison between bougies and stylets for simulated tracheal intubation with the C-MAC D-blade videolaryngoscope. *Eur J Anaesthesiol.* 2015;32:400-405.
33. Turkstra TP, Harle CC, Armstrong KP, et al. The GlideScope-specific rigid stylet and standard malleable stylet are equally effective for GlideScope use. *Can J Anaesth.* 2007;54:891-896.
36. McElwain J, Malik MA, Harte BH, Flynn NH, Laffey JG. Determination of the optimal stylet strategy for the C-MAC videolaryngoscope. *Anaesthesia.* 2010;65:369-378.
44. Hung OR, Tibbet JS, Cheng R, Law JA. Proper preparation of the Trachlight and endotracheal tube to facilitate intubation. *Can J Anaesth.* 2006;53:107-108.
81. Hung OR, Pytka S, Morris I, Murphy M, Stewart RD. Lightwand intubation: II. Clinical trial of a new lightwand to intubate patients with difficult airways. *Can J Anaesth.* 1995;42:826-830.
88. Turkstra TP, Craen RA, Pelz DM, Gelb AW. Cervical spine motion: a fluoroscopic comparison during intubation with lighted stylet, GlideScope, and Macintosh laryngoscope. *Anesth Analg.* 2005;101:910-915.
96. Siddiqui N, Katznelson R, Friedman Z. Heart rate/blood pressure response and airway morbidity following tracheal intubation with direct laryngoscopy, GlideScope and Trachlight: a randomized control trial. *Eur J Anaesthesiol.* 2009;26:740-745.
144. Jagannathan N, Kho MF, Kozlowski RJ, Sohn LE, Siddiqui A, Wong DT. Retrospective audit of the air-Q intubating laryngeal airway as a conduit for tracheal intubation in pediatric patients with a difficult airway. *Paediatr Anaesth.* 2011;21:422-427.

All references can be found online at eBooks.Health.Elsevier.com.

23

Video-Assisted Laryngoscopy

MICHAEL F. AZIZ AND ANSGAR M. BRAMBRINK

CHAPTER OUTLINE

KEY POINTS

- The opportunity to take still pictures or video-record airway management stands to alter the approach to the medical record.
- For the novice practitioner or for patients predicted to be difficult to intubate by direct laryngoscopy (DL), video-assisted laryngoscopy (VAL) improves intubation success rates.
- When DL fails, VAL provides a high likelihood of success as a rescue technique.
- VAL may be as useful as a flexible technique for awake airway management.
- The use of VAL outside of the operating room (OR) has grown substantially, and its use is supported by many observational studies; however, prospective randomized trials to support this practice are still limited.

- Despite high success rates, VAL can fail. Several important predictors of failure have been identified.
- The use of VAL may require less suspension pressure to achieve an adequate laryngeal view during intubation compared with DL; however, the ability to reduce cervical motion while applying manual in-line stabilization has not yet been determined conclusively.
- VAL is associated with an increased risk of pharyngeal injury.
- The literature is mixed in terms of supporting one specific device or design feature; however, clinical experience with any given device is a key variable that predicts performance.

Introduction

Video-assisted laryngoscopy (VAL) refers to the use of a video component, such as a fiberoptic bundle or video chip, to facilitate laryngoscopy and tracheal intubation. The video component can be used alongside a typical rigid laryngoscope blade to augment a direct laryngeal view, that is, video-assisted direct laryngoscopy using a standard blade. Alternatively, video-assisted indirect laryngoscopy using a nonstandard blade (e.g.,

an acute-angle or hyperangulated blade) can be used for a technique that is entirely video-image based. VAL is useful for the potentially difficult airway (DA) because the video view may magnify the laryngeal exposure and overcome difficulties with the alignment of the visual and tracheal axes. This chapter will focus on the scientific evidence regarding the use of VAL in various practice environments, its limitations and problems, unique complications associated with VAL, and some device-specific considerations.

Brief History

The concept of VAL was introduced many years ago with devices such as the Bullard laryngoscope and the WuScope; it was initially considered a niche technology in the hands of a few airway management experts. At that time, most practitioners used flexible fiberoptic bronchoscopes as the standard approach to the DA. VAL suddenly became more popular in the early 2000s with the advent of new video technologies. Specifically, the application of light-emitting diode (LED) light, liquid-crystal display (LCD) screens, and complementary metal–oxide–semiconductor (CMOS) video chip technology has made VAL more portable, easier to use, and more economically feasible. Since then, VAL has been intensely studied, and today solid evidence directs current practice toward the best use of the available devices. However, more questions are continuously generated that guide current investigation. Overall, VAL consistently provides an improved view of the larynx compared with direct laryngoscopy (DL) and exceptionally high intubation success rates.

Image Recording

Video or still picture recording is now an option on most videolaryngoscopes (VLs), providing opportunities for education, clinical assessment, and documentation of airway management that is unavailable with conventional laryngoscopy. First, reviewing video clips or still images taken during VAL will benefit those who are less experienced with identifying laryngeal structures. Similarly, such materials can be displayed before any clinical experience as part of didactic instruction or for students to review their own performance together with a mentor. Second, upon review of such material, clinicians may discover complications that were not noticed while performing the procedure itself. For example, injury to airway structures or an aspiration event may be discovered upon review of video footage and thus may prompt further patient assessment and appropriate interventions. Furthermore, preexisting pathologies such as a laryngeal tumor or lesion may be discovered and lead to further diagnostic evaluation. Third, video recordings during VAL allow unbiased documentation of the airway management procedure. The traditional intubation note, which contains a narrative of the technique used, typically the Cormack-Lehane (CL) score achieved but without further detail about the endotracheal tube (ETT) passage, relies entirely on the practitioner's self-report. In contrast, video recordings of the intubation procedure will document both laryngeal exposure and ETT passage. Although this may seem rather futuristic today, video documentation of tracheal intubation is feasible and may soon become the standard way of documenting airway management and part of the electronic medical record of each patient.

Clinical Scenarios

Undifferentiated Airway

It is unclear whether the use of VAL improves intubation success in routine (not difficult) airway management in the hands of experienced airway practitioners. Compared with DL, the laryngeal view is improved when using VAL.[1-3] The improved view may be attributed to a magnified video view, the anterior curvature of the laryngoscope blade, visual axis extension, or a reduced need to align a direct visual axis. Although DL is associated with failure when a laryngeal view cannot be achieved, VAL frequently

overcomes the obstacle of an inadequate laryngeal view. However, the improved laryngeal view does not necessarily translate to increased intubation success. As the success rate for DL in normal airways is very high, it remains to be determined whether or not the use of VAL would further improve intubation success compared with DL in routine airway management.

When managing normal airways, VAL tends to be a slower intubation technique. There may be several reasons why practitioners require more time until successful intubation when using a VAL, including visual attention in two different places, difficult ETT passage, or lack of experience with a newer technique. However, whether longer intubation times associated with VAL cause an increased incidence of oxygen desaturation or intubation failure has never been confirmed.

The management of the routine airway by anesthesiologists has raised interesting questions, and many argue that VAL may not be helpful for the routine airway based on the evidence reviewed above. However, most of these studies investigated the role of acute-angle VLs for routine airway management. In contrast, VAL with standard laryngoscope blade designs offers the benefits of two worlds: the familiarity of the use and simplicity of ETT passage combined with the availability of a video image if needed in an unanticipated DA. Interestingly, a recent systematic review highlights that VAL reduces intubation failure across study cohorts.[4]

In summary, VAL improves the laryngeal view for routine airway management and likely reduces intubation failure, but large studies confirming improved success rates for routine airway management in experienced practitioners' hands are lacking.

Novice Practitioner

VAL offers benefits for practitioners who have less experience with airway management. Compared with DL, intubation success rates are higher with VAL in novice practitioners' hands.[5,6] This benefit is achieved with both video-assisted standard and nonstandard laryngoscope blades. Additionally, instructor-guided laryngoscopy using a video device also appears to accelerate DL skills.

A long-standing concern regarding VAL is that its routine use for any potentially DA scenario might impair DL skills. Indeed, using VAL as the first choice for airway rescue as well as for patients with predicted difficult intubation will lessen the exposure to difficult DL over time. Nevertheless, the use of VAL can also be part of the solution: regular training using video-assisted devices that feature standard blades allows a trainee laryngoscopist to perform the laryngoscopy under direct vision while an instructor looking at the screen can use that information to teach DL skills. As such, it has become common practice for many instructors to use standard blade VAL when working with novice laryngoscopists.

A number of experts believe that VAL is easier to learn than other intubation techniques. To date, however, competence with various techniques has not been studied rigorously. Many trials with VAL are difficult to interpret because it is unclear if practitioners in the studies had adequate competence with each particular device. On the other hand, it is useful to understand if the early adoption of a technique can maintain or improve existing success rates with conventional DL. In a longitudinal observational trial Cortellazzi and colleagues determined the number of intubation attempts required to achieve more than 90% reliability of first-attempt intubation success with a CL grade 1 view with the GlideScope.[7] They observed that 76 intubations were necessary for this level of proficiency. These findings are novel because they suggest that competency with VAL may require as much training as needed to become proficient with DL; others found that 57 DL attempts are necessary to achieve intubation success rates greater than 90%.[8]

In summary, novices have higher intubation success with VAL compared with DL, but the learning curve for either technique appears not to be different as both techniques require about the same number of procedures before proficiency is achieved. Furthermore, experience with one VAL technique may not translate to similar performance with another VAL technique.

Predicted Difficult Intubation

Patients with predictors of difficult laryngoscopy likely realize more benefit when VAL is utilized. Although the majority of related trials were not powered to effectively compare success rates, a few demonstrated a reduction in intubation difficulty scale (IDS) scores with better views when VAL was used.[9,10] Only a handful of clinical studies so far have defined "intubation success" as the primary end point in comparing VAL with DL; in a randomized crossover study intubation success rates were higher with the Pentax-AWS than with DL in patients under simulated difficult intubation conditions created by manual in-line stabilization.[11] Others observed an increased success rate of tracheal intubation in patients with higher Mallampati scores when VAL was studied in a large randomized controlled trial.[12] Another randomized controlled trial explored VAL success in a large group of practitioners while applying broader inclusion criteria for DA. These authors demonstrated higher intubation success on the first attempt with a video-assisted direct laryngoscope compared with DL.[13] Together, the available data suggest that VAL indeed improves intubation success in patients with predicted DA, and the most recent American Society of Anesthesiologists (ASA) Guidelines for Management of the Difficult Airway reflect this evidence.[14] Nevertheless, additional well-designed trials are needed to understand whether the same is true for different intubation environments and other VAL devices.

Unanticipated Difficult Intubation

Case reports have confirmed that VAL can be used to rescue an intubation that has failed with DL.[15–18] In a large, two-center database evaluation of 71,570 perioperative intubations VAL rescued failed DL in 94% (224/239) of cases.[19] In a study of another VAL technique 99% (268/270) of intubations were successfully rescued after practitioners failed to achieve an adequate laryngeal view with DL.[20] These studies provide strong evidence because these rescue successes reflect the use of different VLs by a large number of practitioners in diverse patient populations. Compared to other techniques used to rescue failed DL, VAL is associated with a higher rescue success rate than other commonly employed techniques.[21] It underscores the particular benefit of having VAL available for the unanticipated DA at every site that may encounter such patients. Furthermore, as repeated DL attempts are associated with morbidity and mortality,[22,23] the use of VAL as the next step after failed DL may help to further improve intubation safety for affected patients, as reflected in the most recent guidelines.[14] Nevertheless, other airway management techniques (e.g., flexible scope intubation [FSI]) retain an important role for airway rescue when primary techniques have failed. Therefore experts agree that practitioners always should use the airway devices with which they feel most comfortable and have the highest proficiency.

Video-Assisted Laryngoscopy for Awake Airway Management

Awake VAL has been evaluated in direct comparison to awake FSI in the scenario of potential DA.[24] Findings demonstrated similar performance with both techniques; however, the validity of the findings is somewhat limited because patients were sedated rather than "awake," patients were excluded when presenting with neck pathologies, and the study design allowed post-randomization exclusion.[25] In another study of awake nasal intubation with flexible bronchoscopy versus VAL both techniques also performed similarly.[26] In this study patients in both interventional groups were sedated with the goal of avoiding recall of the procedure. As such, findings from both studies may not apply to the true "awake" intubation. Nevertheless, one study demonstrated lower sedation requirements for awake VAL than FSI.[27] Despite these limitations, awake VAL may be a technique that can be acquired and maintained more easily than flexible bronchoscopy and may change the practice of awake intubation in the future. Accordingly, the Difficult Airway Society's recent guidelines on awake tracheal intubation include VAL as an acceptable approach.[28]

This technique, however, likely requires some careful practice and prior experience with VAL. Because the vallecula may be quite sensitive, adequate topicalization and/or patient sedation may be necessary before inserting a laryngoscope in this location. Furthermore, the practitioner should be careful not to apply too much suspension pressure on this location because it is poorly tolerated. Lastly, ETT passage may require careful attention. A rigid stylet may be used within the ETT for unchanneled devices, while channeled devices should be carefully manipulated such that the ETT passes gently into the trachea without traumatizing laryngeal or tracheal structures.

Video-Assisted Laryngoscopy Outside of the Operating Room

Early investigations in various clinical environments outside of the operating room (OR) suggest a potential benefit when VAL is used. These environments are challenged with both DA scenarios and practitioners who perform tracheal intubation less frequently than their colleagues in the ORs. In critical care and emergency medicine environments VAL is associated with a higher intubation success rate in patients with a broad selection of indicators.[29–33] Confirming these observations, one randomized controlled trial recently found higher intubation success with VAL compared with DL in critically ill patients.[34] In contrast, in the emergency medicine environment one randomized trial found no difference between VAL and DL.[35] In fact, intubation time was longer and survival worse in a subgroup of head-injured patients when VAL was applied; however, only limited conclusions can be drawn from the above studies because they involved select patient populations and a small number of practitioners. Two large randomized trials also failed to confirm the benefit of VAL over DL in the ICU.[36,37] In the larger study patients in the VAL arm suffered more hypoxemia and more frequent severe life-threatening complications.[36] These comparative trials all have study limitations as patient inclusion, practitioner experience, and intubation technique are difficult to optimize in these study settings. Nonetheless, the assimilation of current data continues to suggest that VAL does not yet demonstrate improved patient outcomes outside of the OR.[38]

In obstetric patients VAL has been used for emergency airway management, potential difficult intubations, and rescuing failure of DL.[39] This distinctive airway management setting is typically challenged by its remote location from other ORs, a patient population prone to having a DA, and, often, a need for tracheal intubation under the most pressing circumstances (i.e., for emergent crash cesarean section). Therefore it has been recommended that VAL be available for all obstetric general anesthetics.[40] This unique environment is discussed in further detail in Chapter 37.

Finally, in prehospital emergency medicine VAL is associated with a reduction in the number of intubation attempts and a shorter laryngoscopy time than DL.[41,42] However, most studies so far have had a retrospective design; therefore the interpretation of the results requires some caution. Likewise, four prospective randomized trials have failed to demonstrate any benefit of VAL compared with DL, and intubation success was worse.[43–46] Nevertheless, as above, the interpretation of these results is limited: in one of the studies practitioners received little training in the instrument studied, the Airtraq, which so far is not well established in this practice environment. The failure of the GlideScope and AWS to perform well in this environment, however, was surprising and was attributed to difficulties with ETT passage despite an adequate laryngeal view or contamination of the lens from oral substances. Nevertheless, prospective randomized studies are difficult to perform in this clinical environment. Finally, the practice environments of these trials (Europe and Asia) may not reflect clinical practice in other regions of the world with vastly different emergency medical systems.

In summary, VAL is becoming more accepted in clinical practice environments outside of the OR, but studies have not yet ubiquitously confirmed the benefits of this technique. Observational data suggest benefits when using VAL, but so far, the results of prospective randomized trials have been mixed. More prospective randomized controlled trials are needed to determine the potential superiority of VAL over DL in any of these practice environments.

Difficulty or Failure With Video-Assisted Laryngoscopy

Despite the many benefits established for VAL and the DA, it too can fail. One potential scenario is the inability to achieve a laryngeal view. However, a frequent and more perplexing scenario is that of an adequate laryngeal view but an inability to pass the ETT into the trachea. This difficulty may occur with any of the VAL devices, whether they feature conventionally designed blades, acutely curved blades, or a channel to guide the ETT. For the GlideScope, an acute-angle VL, we recently identified neck pathologies from tumor, radiation, or surgical scar as specific predictors of failure.[19] Other predictors included a short thyromental distance, obese neck, and limited cervical motion. In a separate study we identified otolaryngologic patients, those with limited mouth opening, and patients placed in the supine position as predictors of difficult acute-angle VAL.[47] These findings suggest that, particularly for the otolaryngologic patient population, FSI remains an important technique that should be mastered when providing anesthesia to these patients, as neck pathologies also are predictors for difficult bag-mask ventilation and difficult DL. In another study a pathologic upper lip bite test was identified as the strongest predictor for difficult VAL with the GlideScope.[48] Others have used the el-Ganzouri risk stratification index[49] and have shown that it also predicts difficulty with VAL.[50] Together, these studies indicate that certain objective predictors can be used to determine which patients

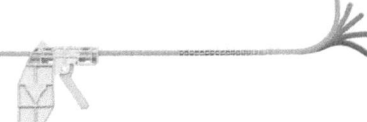

• **Fig. 23.1** The Total Control Introducer. (Courtesy Through the Cords LLC, Salt Lake City, UT.)

should be reserved for alternate techniques such as awake FSI. Interestingly, many of the classic predictors of difficult DL have not been identified as predictors of difficult VAL. Specifically, obesity and high Mallampati score have never been identified as independent predictors of difficult VAL. Thus VAL remains a highly viable alternative in patients with predictors for difficult DL who have no predictors of difficult VAL. Additionally, patients with multiple predictors of difficult DL who also have, for example, pathology of the neck are likely to also be at risk for difficult or failed VAL.

When using acute-angle VAL, maneuvering the ETT into the glottic opening may be impaired when the blade is inserted too deep with the epiglottis lifted. In this situation an excellent laryngeal view may be achieved, but ETT passage is difficult because the larynx is suspended too anteriorly. Evidence suggests that a deliberately restricted view when utilizing acute-angle VAL is associated with easier tracheal intubation.[51] By pulling the laryngoscope back such that the epiglottis falls, the laryngeal view may be less optimal, but the trajectory for ETT passage may improve, allowing successful intubation (Video 23.1).

Beyond strategies to manipulate the VAL, several experts have discussed strategies to manipulate the ETT. When the glottis is well visualized, the fundamental challenge becomes guiding the tube through different angles. Specifically, the ETT needs an anterior trajectory as it enters the oropharynx toward the glottis but needs to take a posterior turn as it enters the trachea. These multiple turns can be achieved by using a stylet that is subsequently withdrawn upon glottic entry. Alternatively, several bougie and stylet designs are coming to market that aim to achieve these goals (Fig. 23.1); however, evidence to support their use is limited.

Although it is a highly successful technique, VAL can still fail. VAL failure may simply be attributed to an inadequate laryngeal view or may occur despite an adequate view of the glottis opening. Patients with neck pathologies, such as a tumor, previous cervical scar, or radiation, deserve careful attention as VAL is associated with an increased risk of failure.

Suspension Pressure During Video-Assisted Laryngoscopy

The risk for the traumatic effects of laryngoscopy can be assessed by using pressure transducers applied to areas of interest within the airway. Using such measurement techniques demonstrates less pressure exerted on the maxillary incisors during routine intubation using video-assisted direct laryngoscopes versus conventional direct laryngoscopes.[52] When measuring the pressure exerted on the tongue, less force is required with the GlideScope compared with DL.[53] Similar results have been demonstrated with the Airtraq device.[54] Interestingly, suspension pressure and cervical motion are not directly associated when using VAL.[54]

It remains to be determined whether the reduced suspension forces exerted with VAL are the cause for the reduced hemodynamic response that is sometimes observed with VAL compared

TABLE 23.1	Studies of Video-Assisted Laryngoscopy on Intubation Performance for the Patient Maintained in Manual In-Line Stabilization				

Author	Device	Control	Sample Size	Outcome Assessed	Major Findings
Malik et al.[9]	GlideScope Pentax-AWS	DL	120	Laryngeal view IDS Intubation time Success rate	Improved laryngeal view and IDS Slower intubation time No difference in success
Maharaj et al.[93]	Airtraq	DL	40	IDS Intubation attempts Laryngeal view	Reduced number of intubation attempts. Improved IDS Improved laryngeal view
Smith et al.[63]	WuScope	DL	87	IDS Laryngeal view Intubation attempts	Improved IDS and laryngeal view. No difference in success or number of attempts
Malik et al.[61]	Pentax-AWS	DL	90	IDS Laryngeal view	Improved IDS and laryngeal view
Enomoto et al.[11]	Pentax-AWS	DL	203	Laryngeal view Intubation time Success rate	Improved laryngeal view, increased success rate, faster intubation time
Liu et al.[67]	Pentax-AWS	GlideScope	70	IDS Intubation time Success rate within a defined time interval	Faster intubation time, lower IDS, improved laryngeal view, and higher intubation success with Pentax-AWS
McElwain[66]	Airtraq C-MAC	DL	90	IDS Success rate Laryngeal view Hemodynamic stability	Reduced IDS, improved laryngeal view with Airtraq

DL, Direct laryngoscopy; *IDS,* intubation difficulty scale score.

with conventional DL. Several reports, however, demonstrate similar hemodynamic responses with both VAL and conventional DL.[55–57] Likewise, both FSI and VAL produce comparable hemodynamic responses.[58] Other studies have demonstrated a reduction in hemodynamic stimulation and reduced bispectral index scores during VAL versus conventional DL.[59,60]

In summary, VAL is associated with less suspension pressure than DL, but it is not clear whether or not this is associated with less hemodynamic stress or cervical spine dislocation. The reduced suspension pressures may make VAL a feasible strategy for awake airway management, as mentioned earlier.

Video-Assisted Laryngoscopy for the Immobilized Cervical Spine

Although VAL improves tracheal intubation success in many challenging airway scenarios, the benefits of VAL in patients at risk for cervical spine injury require specific consideration. Several studies have tested the role of VAL for airway management in the context of acute neck injury or suspected unstable cervical spine by simulated manual in-line stabilization to determine if VAL can improve intubation success under these conditions (Table 23.1). Consistently, the data shows that the laryngeal view is improved with VAL compared with DL when the cervical spine is immobilized.[9,11,61–64] Accordingly, overall intubation conditions (using the IDS score)[65] were rated as better with VAL compared with DL.[66] One study demonstrated improved intubation success rates with VAL compared with DL in this setting.[11] Similarly, performance was improved with a channeled device compared with an unchanneled device under these conditions.[67]

However, VAL may not completely resolve all intubation challenges during cervical immobilization. We recently found that limited cervical spine mobility either as a preexisting condition or from the application of manual in-line stabilization is an independent predictor of VAL failure (relative risk 1.76; 95% CI: 1.01, 3.06).[19] In conclusion, although VAL provides benefit in terms of ease of intubation and may improve intubation success compared with DL, its use cannot guarantee success in patients with existing cervical spine pathology or procedural precautions. Accordingly, and as further emphasized in Chapters 34 and 39, when airway management is required in patients with presumed cervical spine injury, it is recommended that the cervical spine be kept immobilized and the procedure be performed with manual in-line stabilization using the device that the practitioner is most familiar with.

Cervical Spine Motion During Video-Assisted Laryngoscopy

Based on the improved visualization of the glottic opening, VAL may also reduce cervical motion during tracheal intubation. Several studies have addressed this relevant issue by using fluoroscopy during the intubation procedure (Table 23.2). Without the application of manual in-line stabilization, less cervical extension may be necessary with VAL compared with DL.[64,68–71] However, when manual in-line stabilization was applied, results were inconsistent, with some studies showing less extension in certain cervical segments with VAL,[54,72–75] whereas others observed no differences in cervical motion between VAL and DL.[76]

It remains unclear whether the choice of the airway management device in patients at risk for cervical spinal cord injury

TABLE 23.2	**Studies of Cervical Motion While Using Video Laryngoscopes**				
Study	Device	Control	Cervical Precautions	Fluoroscopy	Major Findings
Hastings et al.[70]	Bullard	DL	None	In selected patients at C0–C4. Angle finder used in the entire sample	Reduced extension across C0–C4
Robitallie et al.[76]	GlideScope	DL	MILS	Continuous C0–C5 during several time points	No decrease in cervical movement
Maruyama et al.[68]	Pentax-AWS	DL and McCoy	None	C1/C2, C3/C4	Reduced extension at adjacent vertebra
Hirabayashi et al.[69]	Pentax-AWS	DL	None	C0–C4	Reduced extension at all segments
Turkstra et al.[75]	GlideScope Lightwand	DL	MILS	C0–C5	Reduced C2–C5 motion with GlideScope. Reduced motion across all segments with Lightwand
Watts et al.[72]	Bullard	DL	One arm with MILS, one arm without	C0–C5	Reduced cervical extension in the Bullard + MILS arm
Maruyama et al.[68]	Pentax-AWS	DL	MILS	C0–C4	Reduced cumulative cervical motion
Turkstra et al.[74]	Airtraq	DL	MILS	C0–thoracic	No difference at C1–C2 segment; less extension at C2–C5 and C5–thoracic
Hindman et al.[54]	Airtraq	DL	No MILS	C0–C5	Less extension at C2–C5
El-Tahan et al.[64]	King Vision	DL	No MILS	C0–C5	Less extension at C0–C1, C3–4, C4–5, and cumulatively

DL, Direct laryngoscopy; *MILS*, manual in-line stabilization.

affects long-term neurologic outcomes. Thus as of today, the best approach appears to be using the technique with the highest likelihood of success while maintaining manual in-line stabilization during the entire procedure. Although awake FSI may cause the least stress to the cervical spine, this procedure requires specific skills and a cooperative patient. When performed in an anesthetized patient, FSI often requires jaw thrust, which in turn may cause critical traction in the cervical spine. In contrast, VAL may be easier to learn than FSI and clearly improves intubation conditions compared with DL. As such, it is now more frequently used for tracheal intubation in patients with cervical spine precautions.

In summary, it remains unclear whether VAL reduces cervical motion during airway management across cervical segments when manual in-line stabilization is performed. However, less manipulation of the neck is typically required to achieve good intubation conditions with VAL than with DL.

Combination Techniques With Video-Assisted Laryngoscopy

Several adjuncts can be used to further improve ETT passage while performing VAL. In a large series of video-guided intubations a bougie was applied in 2% of cases to achieve successful intubation.[19] In another large study in emergency medicine the use of a bougie technique resulted in an impressively high first attempt success rate of 96%, mostly with VAL.[77] Others have used additional video-guided devices to facilitate ETT placement. In one study a flexible intubation scope (FIS) was used along with VAL to determine if intubation could be further improved.[78] In cases where the procedure failed using VAL with a rigid stylet tracheal intubation was rescued by adjunctive FIS guidance; however, adding an FIS-guided approach to VAL extended the

time needed for successful intubation.[78] Such a combination of techniques requires multiple practitioners to operate the different instruments but offers several interesting procedural options. The intubation may be primarily guided by the FIS, while VAL is used to keep the oropharynx patent. Alternatively, tracheal intubation may be primarily guided by the VL, while the FIS is merely used as a malleable ETT introducer. Finally, a combination of the two approaches may allow for a more complete visualization of the intubation procedure to reduce the risk of trauma to sensitive airway structures. There are several new ETT stylets or bougies specifically designed to facilitate VAL by articulating to meet an anterior airway that are also capable of deflecting down to enter the trachea (see Fig. 23.1). Evidence to support the use of these new tools to ease intubation difficulty is currently lacking.

Injury Associated With Video-Assisted Laryngoscopy

The risk for injury associated with VAL is different from that of DL. Possible injury of the pharynx or soft palate may be of the greatest concern. Several publications have documented pharyngeal perforation by ETTs during VAL, even when performed by experienced practitioners.[19,79–81] Nevertheless, this injury may be prevented by applying a few precautions: the risk is the highest when the ETT is first advanced into the airway. The practitioner should give direct visual attention to the ETT as it enters the oropharynx until the tip of the ETT begins to curve around the laryngoscope and can be seen on the video screen. In addition, some VLs have a wider profile than standard direct laryngoscopes and should be advanced into the airway with caution as maneuverability may be limited (see Chapter 48).

Comparison of Video-Assisted Laryngoscopy Devices

Device Considerations

The ideal VAL device depends on the goal of the clinical environment in which it is used. Generally, devices can be divided into those with standard (Macintosh or Miller) blade designs versus those with nonstandard blade designs that have an acute angle or curvature. Devices may further be categorized by the presence of a preformed channel within the device to guide the passage of the ETT. This section will briefly describe only a few of the devices in each category, which may serve as examples for others.

A few notable considerations may be used to help choose one device over another. The need for sterile processing is a burden in certain clinical environments, especially outside of the OR. Therefore it makes more sense in some of these environments to pursue disposable equipment. This equipment may come as a completely disposable unit versus a portion of the blade and handle that is disposed of separately from a reusable video component.

Another important consideration is the position of the screen. A screen that is incorporated directly into the handle allows for easy portability and a video view that is aligned with the intubation itself. A screen separated by a cord allows for a larger video screen that can be carried in a bag or on a pole. The larger screen allows for better optics and larger magnification. Although the screen is then removed from the intubation line of sight, it does allow for others to better participate in and help guide the intubation procedure.

Further considerations include the size and weight of the device. Lighter devices are more suitable for air medical units where ounces are an important consideration to flight. Smaller units also are more practical for traveling bags used for resuscitation, such as a "code bag." However, smaller devices are more prone to theft and misplacement and are found to need more frequent replacement compared with larger devices, especially those attached to a pole.

Lastly, cost remains a major barrier to the broad implementation of VAL across airway management procedures around the world. Considerations to take into account include expected frequency of use, per-use cost, repair or replacement costs, and scope of coverage for the device(s), such as how many units for how many intubating locations. Not surprisingly, the most popular devices and those associated with the most outcome data are some of the more costly devices. Newer devices have emerged in the market with a clear goal of offering more competitive pricing. As noted earlier, it is not clear that outcomes are identical by class effect. So the reduced cost of some devices may come at the expense of worse initial performance because of unfamiliarity. The good news is that video-chip technology and LCD screens are becoming less costly. These changes may bring down the cost of VAL units in the future.

Unfortunately, there is very limited data effectively comparing these devices against each other. In one trial of routine elective airway management the channeled devices were associated with shorter intubation times than the unchanneled devices.[82] However, in another trial comparing two VALs in routine airway management the McGRATH MAC performed better in terms of first-attempt success rate and intubation time compared with the channeled King Vision device.[83] In a trial comparing two similar acute-angle VALs the authors failed to demonstrate the noninferiority of the C-MAC D-Blade to the GlideScope in terms of first-attempt intubation success in a DA population.[81] Nevertheless, success rates for both groups were very high, and the absolute difference in success rate was less than 3%, which was attributable to relative inexperience with a newer device. In another trial of patients with predicted difficult laryngoscopy several parameters of intubation difficulty were better during VAL with the C-MAC compared with the McGRATH Series 5.[84] The interpretation of these varying study results suggests that experience with a given technique may be more important than the device design features. Nonetheless, in a large systematic review of VAL versus DL with a broad patient inclusion a subgroup analysis revealed that only a standard-blade VL (C-MAC) demonstrated a reduced failure rate compared to DL, while the three nonstandard-blade VLs (GlideScope, Pentax-AWS, and McGRATH Series 5) demonstrated no difference.[4]

Unchanneled Blade Designs

Storz C-MAC

Karl Storz (Tuttlingen, Germany) were the first to bring video-assisted DL to the market. The current-generation VL, marketed as the C-MAC system, carries direct laryngoscope blade designs from sizes for infants to large adults (Fig. 23.2). These systems have disposable or reusable options. The system can be carried on a moving pole, airway cart, or portable bag. The system is even more versatile with the Pocket Monitor device that carries the video screen attached directly to the laryngoscope handle.

The intubation technique for the standard blade Storz C-MAC system is identical to that of DL. The blade is inserted, and the tongue is swept to the left. The tip of the blade is positioned into the vallecula, and suspension is applied until a laryngeal view is achieved, either directly or on the video screen. This technique offers a familiarity that is difficult to achieve with techniques that rely on indirect laryngeal views alone.

Evidence suggests that the video view achieved with the Storz system is superior to the view achieved with DL alone.[13,85] Therefore the benefit of video-assisted DL likely extends beyond teaching environments to facilitating intubation and improving intubation success in the airway predicted to be difficult to intubate by DL alone.

C-MAC D-Blade

The D-Blade was introduced in 2010 to complement its C-MAC system (see Fig. 23.2). The D-Blade is acutely curved in a fashion similar to the GlideScope and requires indirect laryngoscopy. The technique for insertion is similar to that used in the GlideScope (midline insertion). This blade is attached to modules for a portable setup in a bag or with the monitor attached directly to the handle. The blade is also available in a disposable form.

The D-Blade itself has been tested in several trials. One clinical series showed it to improve the laryngeal view to a CL grade of 1 or 2A in 20 out of 20 patients who had a CL grade of 3 or 4 with DL.[86] Another randomized trial aimed to determine if the D-Blade was "noninferior" to the GlideScope in terms of first-attempt intubation success; however, the trial did not produce that result despite a high success rate for both devices.[81]

GlideScope

The GlideScope (Verathon Medical, Bothell, WA) was the first of the newer-generation VALs to market. The novel feature, which has persisted over time, is the acute-angle indirect approach to laryngoscopy. Initially, the GlideScope used reusable plastic blades with options for larger monitors or more portable smaller monitors (Fig. 23.3). The blades have transitioned to reusable titanium or disposable plastic blades (Fig. 23.4).

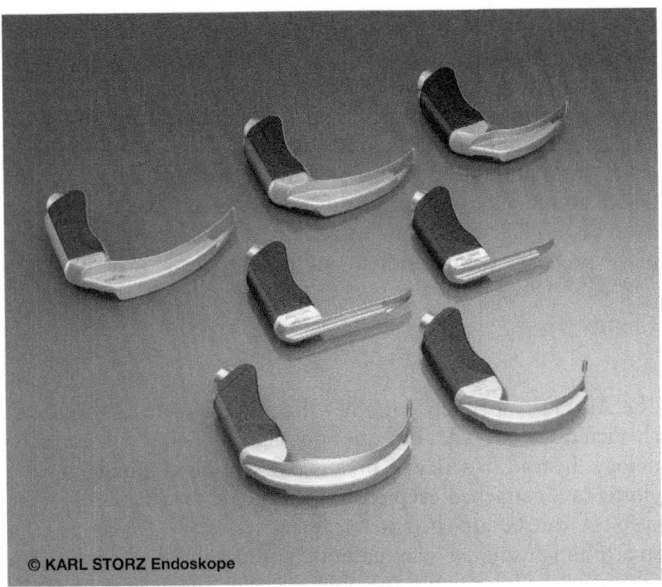

• **Fig. 23.2** The Storz C-MAC video laryngoscope. (Courtesy Karl Storz Endoscopy-America, Inc., El Segundo, CA.)

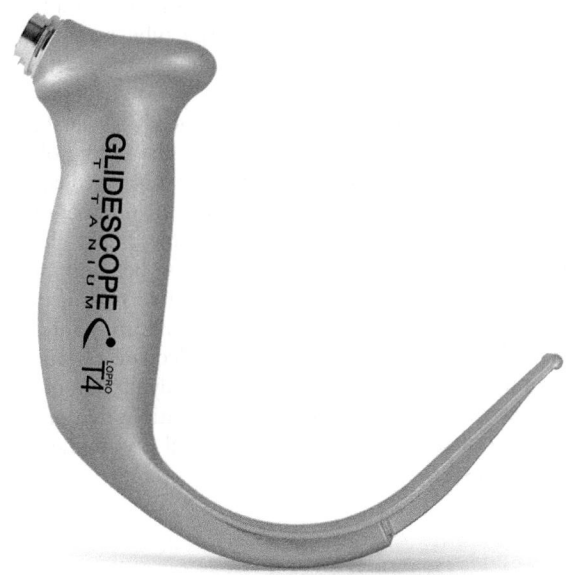

• **Fig. 23.3** The GlideScope system with titanium blades. (Courtesy Verathon Medical, Bothell, WA.)

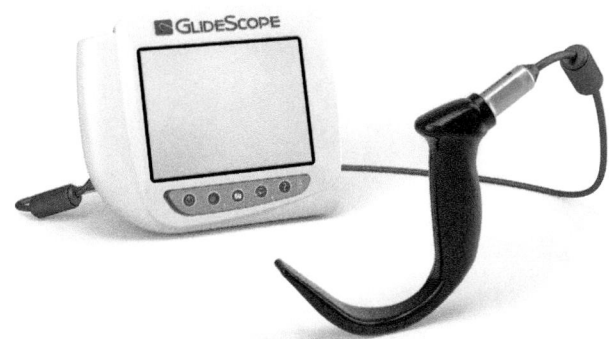

• **Fig. 23.4** The GlideScope AVL system with disposable blades. (Courtesy Verathon Medical, Bothell, WA.)

Unlike DL, the GlideScope is inserted using a midline approach. The blade may need to be turned for insertion if there is inadequate oral space for insertion or if a large chest impedes the position of the handle. The blade is advanced under direct vision until it begins to turn around the tongue. At this point, the practitioner will need to look at the video view as the laryngoscopy is all indirect. The tip of the blade is positioned in the vallecula. The tube is then passed initially under direct vision into the mouth until it is seen turning around the tongue. Then the video screen is used to guide the final intubation into the trachea. Because this turn comes at an acute angle, a specific rigid stylet (the GlideRite stylet) has been designed for use with the GlideScope that matches this angle to facilitate tube passage. However, a 90-degree bend on a malleable stylet has been shown to be similarly effective in facilitating tube passage with the GlideScope.[87]

The GlideScope has been studied in all airway management scenarios, as described in previous sections, and is likely the most studied VL. Positive, meaningful outcomes have been described with its use in prehospital, intensive care, emergency medicine, obstetrics, and DA management in the OR.

GlideScope Direct

The GlideScope Direct is a Macintosh design blade. The laryngoscope is attached to a monitor via a cord that can be mounted on a pole or in a bag (Fig. 23.5). The device may be used like others in this section for video-assisted DL and in a teaching setting.[88] The laryngoscopy technique is also identical to DL.

McGRATH MAC

The McGRATH MAC is a portable video-assisted DL device. It is a small, very portable device with a video screen attached to the laryngoscope, and it has several disposable blade options (Fig. 23.6). The unit is battery powered and automatically shuts down when left on. The laryngoscopy technique for the standard blades is identical to that used in DL as described above. Compared with other VLs, the cost of the units is relatively low.

Evidence suggests that laryngoscopy is improved with this video augmentation compared with standard DL for double-lumen tube placement.[89] However, using the DL feature of this device without the video augmentation may not be adequate because IDS scores are worse with the McGRATH MAC direct

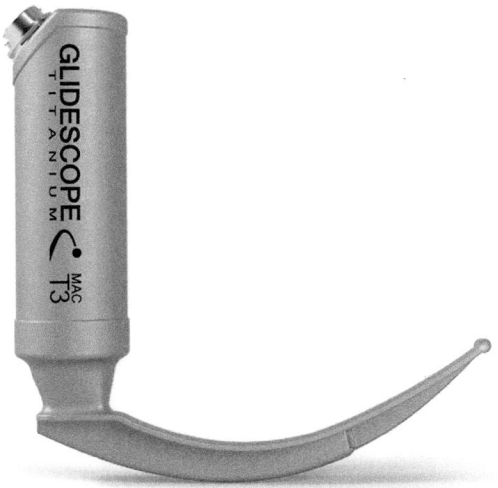

• **Fig. 23.5** The GlideScope Direct system with Macintosh blade design. (Courtesy Verathon Medical, Bothell, WA.)

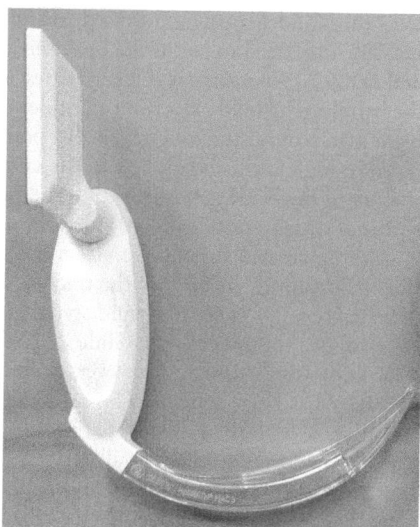

• **Fig. 23.6** The McRATH MAC. (Courtesy Medtronic, Minneapolis, MN.)

view than with standard DL or the use of the video component of the McGRATH MAC.[83]

McGRATH X-Blade

The McGRATH X-Blade is a disposable blade equipped with the same device as the McGRATH MAC. As it also is acutely curved, the intubation technique resembles that of the GlideScope. To date, evidence on performance is limited to small series.[90]

King Vision

The King Vision is a VL system that is portable, has an attached monitor, and uses disposable blades that are either channeled or unchanneled (Fig. 23.7). The technique for insertion is also midline under direct visualization until the laryngoscope turns around the tongue. At this point, the video is used to further direct the laryngoscope tip into the vallecula. The ETT is then placed under video visualization using a styletted tube or through the channel.

The King Vision has been evaluated in the prehospital environment. In this challenging situation observational data suggest a higher first-attempt intubation success rate with the King Vision compared with DL.[42] For routine airway management in the OR,

video-assisted DL may be easier for experienced practitioners than the King Vision.[83] When comparing the channeled system to the unchanneled system, the unchanneled system leads to shorter intubation times.[91] This device has seen clinical expansion in North American prehospital airway management; the relatively lower cost, portability, and disposable blade options make this device an attractive option in this environment. Further research is needed to determine how this device compares with other VLs in the prehospital environment and other settings.

Channeled Devices

Airtraq

The Airtraq is a small, portable, channeled system that often is characterized as a VAL but does not actually employ video technology. Instead, a series of prisms reflect a lighted image of the glottis to an attached eyepiece within the device (Fig. 23.8). The eyepiece can be attached to a camera for video display or to a smartphone using an adapter along with an installed application to project the image onto the phone screen. The devices are available as single-use devices or multiple-use devices with single-use external covers. There are no completely reusable Airtraq systems.

The technique for insertion is midline. The glottic opening is centered in the prism or camera view, and the tube is advanced through the channel into the glottis. The tube must then be detached from the channel system by pulling both the tube and Airtraq in opposite directions horizontally.

The literature has established the Airtraq as a valuable DA management tool in the OR. Particularly in the setting of cervical spine immobilization, the Airtraq offers an improved laryngeal view, eases intubation difficulty, and reduces the number of intubation attempts compared with DL (see Table 23.1). However, the literature is yet to demonstrate that these benefits translate well outside of the OR. In the only randomized trial of prehospital airway management the Airtraq was significantly inferior to DL.[43] The difference is attributable to inadequate training and clinical competence with the device before studying it in the field. However, there may be device design considerations that make the Airtraq more difficult to use in the prehospital environment than other techniques.

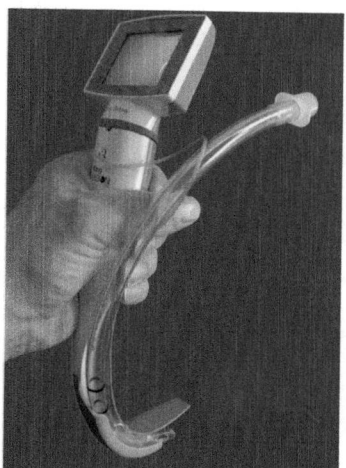

• **Fig. 23.7** The King Vision video laryngoscope with channeled blade feature. (Courtesy Ambu USA, Columbia, MD.)

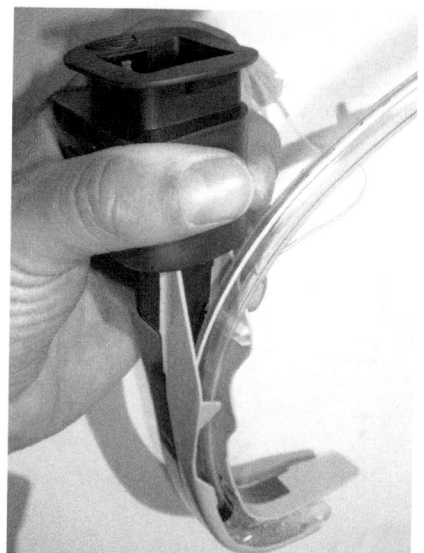

• **Fig. 23.8** The Airtraq system. (Courtesy Teleflex, Wayne, PA.)

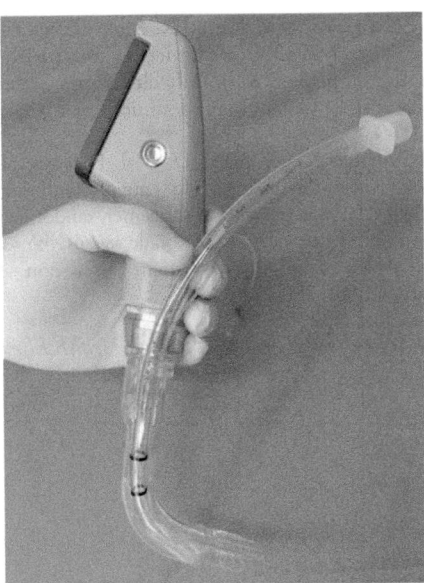

• **Fig. 23.9** The Pentax-AWS. (Courtesy Hoya, Tokyo, Japan.)

Pentax-AWS

The Pentax-AWS is another small, portable, channeled system with disposable blade components (Fig. 23.9). However, unlike the Airtraq, it is truly video powered, and the video component is reusable. The video screen is attached to the handle and can swivel so that changes in the angle of insertion of the blade can be properly followed on the video screen. The technique for insertion is midline, and the video component places a target mark to be aligned with the laryngeal structures. The ETT is then advanced into the trachea and slipped out of the channel to allow the removal of the device.

The literature supports the use of the Pentax-AWS for anticipated DA management and to rescue failed DL.[10,20] In particular, the Pentax-AWS has been shown to be very useful for the patient immobilized with cervical spine precautions (Table 23.1). Beyond manikin studies, the device has not been tested robustly outside of the OR in settings such as prehospital or emergency airway management.

Practitioners in the United States have grown increasingly concerned about the fact that the disposable portion of the blade does not also cover the handle. More and more, oversight groups look for individualized processing of all components of airway management, but the video component of the Pentax-AWS is left exposed without the means to undergo proper cleansing by some standards. As a result, some centers are looking instead for systems where the entire device is either disposable or can be processed using accepted sterile processing standards.

Future Directions With Video-Assisted Laryngoscopy

Future research is poised to address some new questions. In particular, very few studies have compared VAL types and designs to determine ideal device characteristics. Some limited data suggest that devices with channeled components (i.e., with a preloaded ETT) result in faster and easier intubation than unchanneled devices[82] However, other studies have found

opposite results.[83,91] Furthermore, questions surrounding blade design continue to arise. For example, video-assisted direct laryngoscopes (i.e., the Macintosh blade design) have the potential benefit of familiarity, simple ETT passage, and a narrow blade profile. On the other hand, acutely curved blade designs may further augment the laryngeal view for the anterior airway beyond what may be achieved with a video-assisted direct laryngoscope. Thus far, studies have not shown a clear difference in success rate among various blade design types.[81,92] A commonly asked question is whether or not VAL will replace DL. Today, two major barriers preclude this advancement. First, the cost of care is still prohibitive. However, as video technology becomes more widespread, costs may decline and may better balance the increased costs of routine DL because of processing requirements. Second, for routine airway management in the hands of experienced laryngoscopists, DL appears to be easier than acute-angle VAL. Because most VAL systems employ an acute blade, it appears that this design will remain preferential for the potential DA, for novice practitioners, and outside of the OR but not for routine airway management in the OR by experienced practitioners. However, VAL appears to be a useful tool for any patient and at any time and may further reduce the risk of an unanticipated difficult intubation[4]. Future research stands to address the device concerns and variability mentioned above and better tackle the question of potential benefits, especially outside of the OR.

Conclusion

VAL has altered the approach to airway management. Across various patient and practitioner populations, an improved and magnified laryngeal view is associated with improved intubation conditions and/or ultimately improved intubation success rates. Nevertheless, intubation with VAL can be difficult. Experience may overcome many of the technical barriers to difficulty with VAL; however, specific patient, practitioner, and environmental circumstances can make VAL challenging.

The use of VAL has grown outside of the OR and is now used for awake airway management or together with other airway management techniques, such as FSI. Future studies may seek to address the optimal device design features for individual populations of patients and practitioners.

Selected References

13. Aziz MF, Dillman D, Fu R, Brambrink AM. Comparative effectiveness of the C-MAC video laryngoscope versus direct laryngoscopy in the setting of the predicted difficult airway. *Anesthesiology* 2012;116:629–636.
14. Apfelbaum JL, Hagberg CA, Caplan RA, et al. Practice guidelines for management of the difficult airway: an updated report by the American Society of Anesthesiologists Task Force on Management of the Difficult Airway. *Anesthesiology* 2013;118:251–270.
19. Aziz MF, Healy D, Kheterpal S, Fu RF, Dillman D, Brambrink AM. Routine clinical practice effectiveness of the Glidescope in difficult airway management: an analysis of 2,004 Glidescope intubations, complications, and failures from two institutions. *Anesthesiology* 2011;114:34–41.
21. Aziz MF, Brambrink AM, Healy DW, et al. Success of intubation rescue techniques after failed direct laryngoscopy in adults: a retrospective comparative analysis from the multicenter perioperative outcomes group. *Anesthesiology* 2016;125:656–666.

24. Rosenstock CV, Thøgersen B, Afshari A, Christensen A-L, Eriksen C, Gätke MR. Awake fiberoptic or awake video laryngoscopic tracheal intubation in patients with anticipated difficult airway management: a randomized clinical trial. *Anesthesiology* 2012;116:1210–1216.

34. Silverberg MJ, Li N, Acquah SO, Kory PD. Comparison of video laryngoscopy versus direct laryngoscopy during urgent endotracheal intubation: a randomized controlled trial. *Crit Care Med.* 2015;43:636–641.

47. Aziz M, Bayman E, Van Tienderen M, et al. Predictors of difficult videolaryngoscopy with GlideScope® or C-MAC® with D-blade: secondary analysis from a large comparative videolaryngoscopy trial. *Br J Anaest.* 2016;117:118–123.

77. Driver BE, Prekker ME, Klein LR, et al. Effect of use of a bougie vs endotracheal tube and stylet on first-attempt intubation success among patients with difficult airways undergoing emergency intubation: a randomized clinical trial. *JAMA* 2018;319: 2179–2189.

81. Aziz MF, Abrons RO, Cattano D, et al. First-attempt intubation success of video laryngoscopy in patients with anticipated difficult direct laryngoscopy: a multicenter randomized controlled trial comparing the C-MAC D-Blade versus the GlideScope in a mixed provider and diverse patient population. *Anesth Analg.* 2016;122(3):740–750.

All references can be found online at eBooks.Health.Elsevier.com.

24

Flexible Scope Intubation Techniques

KARIEM EL-BOGHDADLY AND IMRAN AHMAD

CHAPTER OUTLINE

KEY POINTS

- A proactive low threshold for FIS (Flexible Intubation Scopes) use is important when considering a DA. Rigid VAL, Optical Laryngoscopes, or stylet use when FISs are indicated can worsen already grim situations and impede FIS rescue.
- FIS instruments are frequently very delicate and expensive. However, balance FIS expenses against costs of multidevice airway rescue attempts; cardiac, airway, brain, psychological, and other system injuries; and litigation and reputation damages.
- For planned intraoral local anesthesia (LA), consider giving an antisialagogue at least 15 to 20 minutes beforehand. Supplemental oxygen, sedative, opioid, and/or LA use depends on the patient's situational urgency and respiratory status. Adequate LA helps prevent discomfort, psychological distress, hemodynamic changes, and lack of cooperation. If you are unfamiliar with an ATI technique, then we recommend the use of the Difficult Airway Society awake tracheal intubation (DAS ATI) guidelines as a source of recommendation for the best techniques for the procedure[18]
- During FIS techniques, single or combined supplemental oxygenation modes may be advantageous: high-flow nasal cannula, an oral catheter, nasopharyngeal airway, mask, mask plus continuous positive airway pressure (CPAP) (oral or nasal), or transtracheal oxygen therapy (TTO). Rarely, give oxygen via working channels as needed, if flows are appropriate and the

view is definitely above the esophagus/stomach or a very narrowed glottis/trachea.
- After laryngeal entry, follow three directions successively with an FIS to reach the trachea through nasal or oral routes. In the supine patient these are downward to the posterior oropharyngeal or nasopharyngeal wall, upward to the anterior vocal cord commissure, and downward to the wider posterior glottic entrance.
- The number one cause of flexible bronchoscopic intubation (FSI) failure is inexperience as a result of insufficient training and practice. Performing FIS examination/intubation on healthy asleep patients is ethical. A routine equivalent to one use per week provides competence after 50 uses and expertise after 100 to prepare for successful FIS management when really needed.
- Inferior preparation of patients, equipment, and personnel leads to difficulty in FSI use, if not failure. Optimize and individualize psychological preparation, antisialagogues, sedatives, opioids, equipment, and local anesthetics for each patient. Advise and show untrained personnel tongue pull, jaw thrust, midline maintenance of intubating oral airways, and FIS working channel local anesthetic injection maneuvers.
- Keep options for combined FIS and the use of other airway devices, well prioritized for difficult intubation (DI), uncertain

device placement, and rescue. Multimodal approaches are likely to impact patients with fluid-soiled upper airways and edema or many airway pathologies.

- Uncommonly, the FIS can be at a disadvantage, having little innate ability to gently move larger soft tissue structures which may be present in the airway or in soiled airways secondary to

its small viewing tip diameter. With other devices, FIS combinations may overcome these difficulties.

- Patients with preexisting upper airway obstructive narrowing may have difficulty with nonhollow objects placed in the area. Avoid obstruction by speeding up maneuvers after respiratory tract entrance if change to a smaller FIS is unlikely to help.

Introduction

Whereas experts continue to consider flexible bronchoscopic intubation (FSI) as the "gold standard" for difficult airways (DAs), this chapter aims to address both the fundamentals and the advancements in this technique and associated technologies. The fundamentals we describe aim to equip the airway practitioner with the knowledge to be able to understand and implement safe and effective use of FSI techniques, either awake or asleep, regardless of the clinical setting.

The first observations on the movement of the vocal cords were published by Manual P Garcia (a singing teacher) in 1854, who used a head-strap mirror to reflect sunlight onto an intraoral dental mirror. The Royal Society in London named him the "first laryngoscopist."[1] Using a blind digital technique, William Macewen completed the first tracheal intubation under general anesthesia (GA) and the first awake intubation for surgery and anesthesia in 1878.[2] An accidental intratracheal esophagoscope insertion in 1895 prompted Alfred Kirstein to use one to perform the first "direct" laryngoscopy and invent a laryngoscope-like "autoscope."[3]

Bronchoscopy began to develop in 1887, when Gustav Killian extracted a foreign body from a farmer's respiratory tract with a rigid bronchoscope. Chevalier Jackson modified it with a distal tungsten lightbulb and a working channel in 1904, resulting in a greater success rate of endotracheal intubation attempts.[4]

In 1966 Shigeto Ikeda proposed ideas for the construction of a flexible fiberoptic bronchoscope (FOB) to two companies, Machida Endoscope and Olympus.[5] Meanwhile, in 1967 Peter Murphy ingeniously used a choledochoscope for tracheal intubation.[6] In 1968 Machida produced an extremely "bendable" guided FOB, featuring an eyepiece for seeing images transmitted along 15,000 glass fibers (14 μm in diameter, each), which Ikeda then passed through a rigid bronchoscope. Later that year, Olympus produced a more maneuverable FOB with a working channel. At the International Congress on Disease of the Chest, Ikeda's new FOB distal airway pictures were instantaneously news-making revelations. He demonstrated stand-alone FOB insertion for tracheal intubation in many countries and published his experiences in 1971.[7]

Over time, clinicians used FOB for diagnostic purposes, routine clinical practice intubations, and, eventually, DA management.[8–12] The inherent superiority of the FOB forged its place as the first choice for difficult intubation (DI) and cervical spine risk cases and as a diagnostic/therapeutic tool for DA instrumentation, hypoxemia, high airway pressure, obstructive sleep apnea (OSA), infection, foreign bodies, airway stenosis, tracheomalacia, pulmonary tumors, and other abnormalities. Raj and colleagues promoted

FOB assistance for double-lumen tube (DLT) placement. Ovassapian and colleagues further delineated advantages during one-lung isolation in 1987,[10,13] whereas Benumof and colleagues compared right and left DLT bronchial insertions to explain why the relationship of bronchial anatomy to DLT construction inevitably resulted in less successful right-sided DLT positioning.[14]

In the 1980s the Asahi Pentax Company's integration of FOBs with preexisting charge-coupled devices (CCDs) permitted video monitor airway viewing and heightened the educational and clinical utility of FOBs.[15] Further developments rapidly ensued, with multiple sizes of FOBs, the addition of working channels allowing diagnostic or therapeutic use (beyond simply visualization), the addition of light-emitting diodes (LEDs), and full-color imaging. The most recent technological advancements in this space, and perhaps the most significant, include the introduction of micro video complementary metal–oxide–semiconductor (CMOS) chips for transmission. This has entered the market of "single-use devices," resulting in entirely disposable nonfiberoptic intubation scopes[16] or reusable flexible bronchoscopes with disposable, sheath-like protective barriers, with the former gaining increasing traction.

Ovassapian and colleagues were pioneers in FOB educational promotion through workshop training and simulation, popularizing effective techniques.[17] Currently, the FSI is the "gold standard" for DI and part of a growing trend for combination with other airway devices in a multimodal approach to DA management.[18]

Terminology

Throughout this chapter, several terms are used that are increasingly being implemented in routine clinical practice. Flexible bronchoscopes are named so as they have at least one flexible portion, usually the tip, and are long enough to visualize the division of the trachea into the two main bronchi. As the use of fiberoptic technology is decreasing and the utilization of CMOS technology for flexible bronchoscopes grows, the term FOB should only be reserved for the former. Flexible scope intubation (FSI) as a term should be used when describing the tracheal intubation of a patient with an FIS. This can also be achieved in an awake, spontaneously breathing patient, in which case this is called awake tracheal intubation (ATI). When performed with a flexible intubation scope (FIS), this is referred to as ATI:FIS, and when performed with a videolaryngoscope (VAL), this is termed ATI:VAL.

Note that various terms for those who are considered airway providers will also be used synonymously in this chapter, including airway expert, specialist, endoscopist, operator, manager, or caregiver.

How They Work, How to Choose, and What to Do With Them

FISs, whether fiberoptic or not, are available from various manufacturers: Olympus (Olympus America, Center Valley, PA, USA), Karl Storz (Karl Storz GmbH & Co. KG, Tuttlingen, Germany), Pentax (Pentax Medical, Montvale, NJ, USA), Ambu (Ambu A/S, Ballerup, Denmark), Verathon (Verathon Medical, Bothell, WA), and Cogentix Medical (Minnetonka, MN, USA) (Fig. 24.1).

Note that for simplicity, whether fiberoptic or not, any such flexible scope will be referred to as an FIS unless otherwise indicated. Likewise, flexible bronchoscope intubation will have an FSI acronym.

Most reusable FISs cost thousands of dollars. They are quite delicate, except for nonfiberoptic ones, which are somewhat less harmed by bending. Disposable FISs are much cheaper per unit cost; however, there is some conflicting evidence on their cost-effectiveness as compared to reusable FISs. According to Tvede and colleagues,[19] single-use FISs are not cost-effective if used more than 22.5 times per month. At that time, with expensive video monitors, reusables cost $219 per use, whereas disposables cost $252. This reusable cost was very much improved (<$160 per use) with an FIS care training program similar to that instituted by Lunn and colleagues, reducing normal repair costs of $51 per use by 84% to $8.[20] Mouritsen and colleagues performed a detailed microcosting analysis of reusable versus single-use FISs in a London teaching hospital.[21] The total per-unit cost of a single-use FIS was £220. When taking the potential costs of cross-contamination and infection of patients into account, this cost was estimated to be £511 per patient, compared to the unit cost of £200 for the single-use devices, which have no risk of cross-contamination if they are only used once.

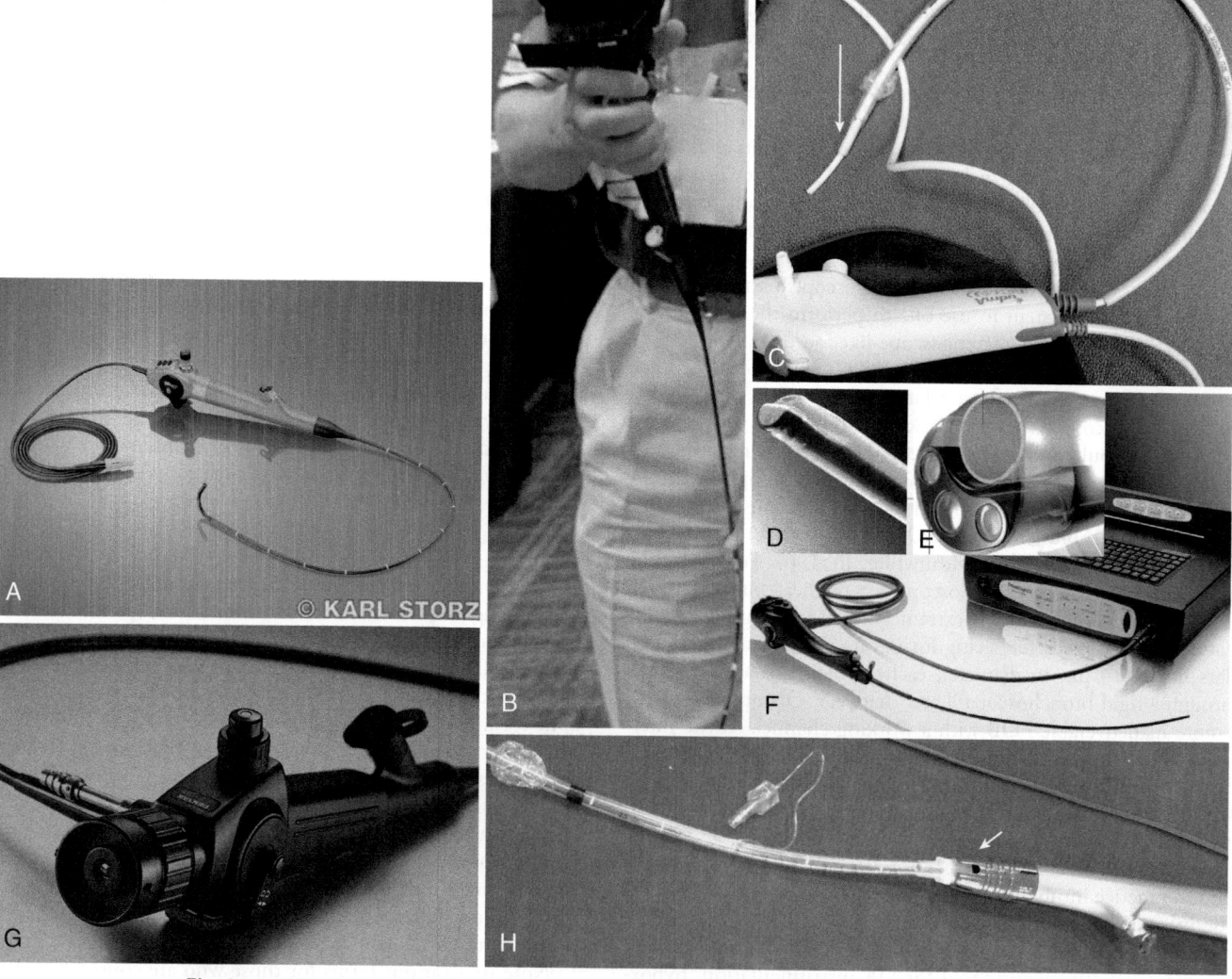

• **Fig. 24.1** (A) Heat-treated flexible intubation scope (FIS) for smoother endotracheal tube passage (Karl Storz GmbH & Co. KG, Tuttlingen, Germany); (B) Olympus MAF—completely portable, autoclavable FIS (Olympus America, Center Valley, PA); (C) Ambu disposable FIS (Ambu A/S, Ballerup, Denmark) with an Aintree catheter (Cook Medical Inc., Bloomington, IN), to reduce diameter difference between an endotracheal tube and the FIS; (D) Cogentix disposable sheath cover; (E) FIS tip of its insertion tube; (F) nondisposable FIS equipment (Cogentix Medical, Minnetonka, MN); (G) Pentax FIS (Pentax Medical, Montvale, NJ); (H) FIS with an endotracheal tube holder.

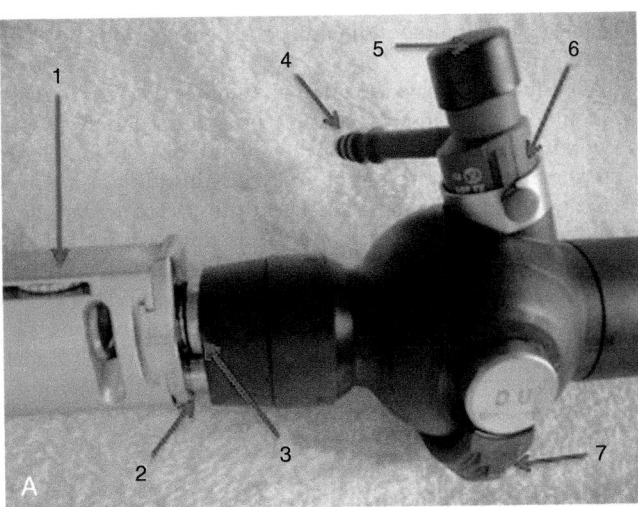 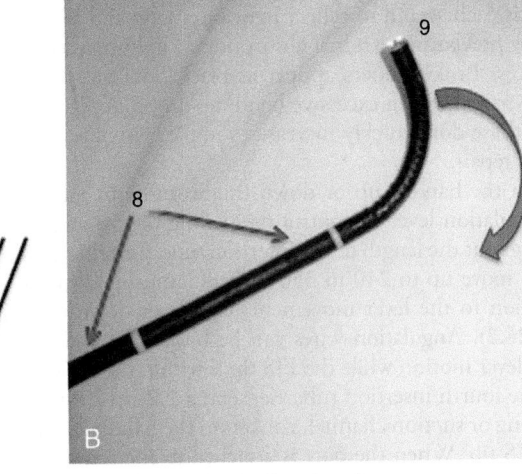

• **Fig. 24.2** (A) Flexible bronchoscope (FIS) handle (control section) design. *1,* Focus-adjusting ring; *2,* light source connection; *3,* video output connection; *4,* suction port; *5,* valve; *6,* working channel; *7,* angulation control lever. (B) FIS insertion tube leading to flexible tip: *8,* insertion tube; *9,* flexible tip.

Flexible Bronchoscope Design

All FISs have certain commonalities. There are three main parts: handle, insertion tube, and flexible tip (Fig. 24.2). The handle has a battery-operated light source (allowing more portability) or an optical cable connection to an external light source. The handle's "visual section" is the location of an eyepiece and lens, a video output adapter, or an actual video screen with an integrated camera (depending on the model). FISs with a CCD or CMOS camera chip at the tip have a wide-angle image and higher picture resolution compared with models having a narrower field of view and less optical detail (Fig. 24.3). Video FISs are more useful clinically, particularly in teaching, as the instructor can view the endoscopist's moves onscreen.

Many FISs have a visible black notch in the eyepiece at the 12 o'clock position to aid altered patient orientation (e.g., facing a sitting patient). Some models can rotate notches to give any desired orientation. Near the handle, an adjustable focusing ring or diopter can be fine-tuned to sharpen the image. This should be done prior to use to ensure the image is optimized. Some models have a venting ethylene oxide sterilization cap nearby.

The handle is attached to the insertion tube (second component) for entry into the patient. Its outer diameter (OD) determines minimum endotracheal tube (ETT) internal diameters (IDs) through which FISs can easily pass, usually a 0.3- to 0.5-mm difference. Insertion tubes average 50 to 65 cm in length with a flexible inner stainless steel mesh and a flexible water-impermeable outer plastic wrap.

Four specific elements traverse the length of fiberoptic insertion tubes in many reusable FISs (Fig. 24.4). The first element allows light transmission toward the tip via one or two "noncoherent" fiberglass light guide bundles. A high degree of light intensity is focused within proximal light guide bundles, whereas heat filters or reflecting mirrors prevent damage to other insertion tube components.

The handle's lens and the tip's objective lens are perpendicular to the insertion tube's longitudinal axis, enabling transmission of identical, completely spatially oriented patient images between the lenses via "coherent" fiberoptic bundles. These involve 10,000 to 50,000 glass fibers, as small as 8 to 9 μm in diameter. As a

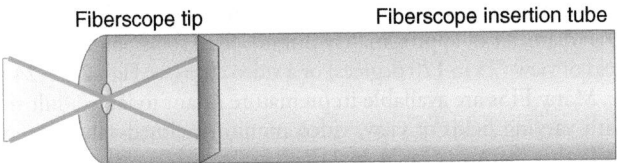

Legend:

▷ Field of view

◯ Lens

▧ CCD chip

✕ Light rays of image entering fiberscope

• **Fig. 24.3** Flexible scope tip mechanics: field of view. Insertion tip transmission of light through a lens to the charge-coupled device (CCD) chip.

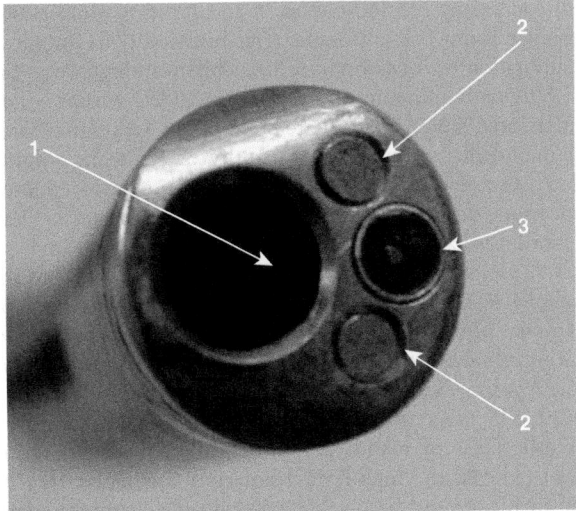

• **Fig. 24.4** Flexible scope tip components. *1,* Working channel; *2,* two angulation wires; *3,* cladded fiberoptic-lighted bundle.

reference, human hairs are 17 to 180 μm. A secondary layer surrounds each strand to reflect light internally and maintain intensity by preventing external absorption or light reflection off lateral surfaces. Broken fibers appear as black dots on the eyepiece or video screen. From excessive bending, dropping, or external pressure, these dots quickly increase to impair visual acuity and incur costly repair.

On the handle, up or down thumb motions move a bending or angulation lever to control the pulling of two angulation wires throughout the length of the insertion tube. Levering causes the FIS tip to move up to 240 to 350 degrees (amusingly, in the opposite direction to the lever movement [e.g., lever down = tip up]) (see Fig. 24.2). Angulation wires can be broken by excessive pressure (e.g., lever motion while the FIS tip is within the ETT lumen).

The fourth insertion tube element, a 1.2- to 2.8-mm-diameter working or suction channel, runs from the handle's suction port to the FIS tip. When the port is attached to suction or oxygen tubing, the nearby spring valve is opened by index finger pressure for suctioning or oxygen administration. Alternatively, a syringe with medication can be attached to this port or a biopsy/injection port below (present in some models). When injecting, the endoscopist must ensure the suction is off to prevent loss of medication.

The distal FIS segment is a hinged, bendable tip with an objective lens (diameter of approximately 2 mm), fixed focal point, and short field of view (75 to 120 degrees) or a video chip (see Figs. 24.2–24.4).

Many FISs are available in premature infant to large adult sizes with varying fields of view, video monitors, closed-valve systems, and other features (Table 24.1).

Flexible Bronchoscope Cleaning

Almost half a million bronchoscopies are performed per year in the United States.[22] Whenever equipment is reused among different patients, there is a concern about avoiding communicable disease transmission. From 2000 to 2007, the American Association for Respiratory Care (AARC), American College of Chest Physicians (AACP), American Association for Bronchology and Interventional Pulmonology (AABIP), and Association for Professionals in Infection Control (APIC) issued guidelines and consensus statements to assist in the prevention of FIS-associated infection or contamination.[23–25]

Although there are no reports of infection or cross-contamination caused by FIS intubation in an operating room (OR) or emergency room (ER), sporadic references testify to instances of contamination or infection after bronchial washing/lavage. Since the 1970s, contamination sources have included sentinel patients, contaminated water, inadequate sterilization techniques (attributed to insufficient quality or quantity of sterilizing solution), repeated use of cleaning fluid or brushes, automated endoscope reprocessors, and FISs with design errors or damage.[26–28] Valves and working channels are the most suspected areas for ineffective FIS sterilization. Multiple organisms have been found, including *Pseudomonas aeruginosa*, nontuberculous mycobacteria, *Serratia marcescens*, *Mycobacterium tuberculosis*, *Stenotrophomonas maltophilia*, *Legionella pneumophila*, *Rhodotorula rubra*, *Klebsiella* species, *Proteus* species, and fungi.[23–30]

With FIS usage, the involved clinical sites automatically fall under the aegis of mandatory universal precautions. Constant vigilance in care and high-level disinfection are imperative. Once used, an FIS should be directly handed off to trained assistants or placed in marked vertical holding tubes for rapid pickup (e.g., ProShield, Seitz Technical Products, Avondale, PA). To prevent

damage, holding tubes should be long enough to handle FISs up to 65 cm.

Disinfection may take up to 45 minutes (Fig. 24.5). Assistants should carefully insert a cleaning brush into portals to span the working channel's length for the removal of secretions according to the manufacturer's and/or health care institution's instructions. Next, the entire FIS must be diligently inspected for damage, tears, indentations, or abnormalities. A leak test to detect holes in the insertion tube sheath is essential, and detected failures necessitate sending them for repairs without sterilization. Suction and biopsy ports must be disassembled. Nondisposable parts must be gently placed in glutaraldehyde, peracetic acid, orthophthaldehyde, hydrogen peroxide gas plasma, or another manufacturer-indicated solution. The working channel must be syringe-flushed with disinfectant according to instructions.[31–33] The Olympus model BF Q180 is autoclavable.

After the completion of sterilization, all parts must be removed to prevent caustic damage. The FIS should be gently washed and thoroughly rinsed with sterile water, including through the working channel to prevent residual chemical toxicity. It is mandatory to dry the channel by suctioning or purging with solutions (e.g., 70% alcohol) and compressed air, per instructions.

Most bacteria, fungi, and viruses, including human immunodeficiency virus (HIV) and hepatitis, are susceptible to sterilization processes. In patients with contagious diseases (e.g., tuberculosis) FISs may require lengthy ethylene oxide sterilization and aeration procedures for up to 24 hours, with the venting cap secured to a venting connector. In cases of suspected prion infection (e.g., Creutzfeldt-Jakob disease) or highly dangerous diseases (e.g., Ebola) avoiding FIS usage or using a disposable system is recommended.[23–25]

Presently, routine surveillance cultures are not recommended by the AARC, AACP, AABIP, or APIC because of a lack of criteria to determine the testing frequency, relevance when positive results occur, courses of action, and costs of testing procedures.[32,33] However, bioburden testing is recommended whenever unusual rates of infection are found.[34]

During handling and sterilization, keeping the FIS straight is extremely important. Once cleaned, it is preferably stored suspended by its handle in a moderately lighted, climate- and humidity-controlled, safe location. Close proximity to radiation should be avoided because of deleterious effects on FIS material.[35]

Deciding on Disposables or Partially Disposables

Because efforts toward the production of a truly autoclavable FIS (e.g., Bronchosteril Endoscope, Andromis, Geneva, Switzerland) did not lead to a widely accepted device, other solutions aimed at the prevention of cross-contamination were developed.

Partial Disposable—EndoSheath on a Nondisposable Flexible Fiberoptic Scope

The Slide-On EndoSheath is a clear, durable, presterilized flexible thermoplastic elastomer with a working channel (variable size) that snugly fits only its own adult nonchanneled PrimeSight FIS or FIS system. It potentially prevents the transmission of 27-nm-sized organisms and permits FIS availability in one-third of the time needed for sterilizing other FISs.[36,37] The length of time to check for breaches is unknown but can be done by instilling a methylene blue dye in the used sheath and sinking it in a water bowl. There are no studies on breach probability. Without breaches, this FIS is US Food and Drug Administration (FDA) approved for a

TABLE 24.1   Comparison of the Specifications of Multiple Flexible Intubating Scopes

Models	Unique Qualities	Light Source	External Diameter (mm)	Working Channel (mm)	Working Length (cm)	Tip Field-of-View Range (Degrees)	Range of Motion Up/Down (Degrees)
Olympus							
LF-V	Fib; CCD	Electric	4.1	1.2	60	120	120/120
LF-DP, LF-GP, LF-TP	Fib	Battery/electric	3.1–5.2	1.2–2.6	60	90	120–180/120–130
LF-P	Fib; neonate	Electric	2.2	—	60	75	120/120
MAF-GM, MAF-TM	Fib/hybrid video; built-in screen; camera	Battery	4.1–5.2	1.5–2.6	60	90	120–180/130–180
BF-XP60, BF-3C40, BF-MP60, BF-P60, BF-IT60, BF-XT40	Fib; designed for therapeutic application	Electric	2.8–5.9	1.2–3	Up to 55–60	90–120	180/130
BF-H190, BF-1TH190, BF-Q190, BF-P190, BF-XP190	HD and SD CCD video scopes for diagnostic therapeutic apps	Electric	2.8–6.0	1.2–2.8	60	110–120	180–210/130–130
BF-Q180-AC	Completely autoclavable; some have CCD; often for therapeutic applications (including intubation)	Electric	5.3–5.5	2.0		120	180/130
Ambu							
Ambu aScope	CMOS; disposable no suction	Battery	5.3	0.8	63	80	120/120
Ambu aScope Slim	CMOS; disposable suction +	Built-in LED	3.8	1.2	60	80	150/130
Ambu aScope 3	CMOS; disposable suction +	Built-in LED	5	2.2	60	80	150/130
Karl Storz							
K.S. 1130 AB	Fib; CCD	Battery/electric	5.5	2.3	65	115	140/140
K.S. 11301 BN	Fib; CCD	Battery/electric	4	1.5	65	115	140/140

Anticipating two more sizes (2.8 mm and 6.4 mm).
Expecting validation for the hands-free, brush-free EVOTECH system for reprocessing.
Video screen (4:3) format provides an overview of the working area (pixel-free and moiré-free).

Models	Unique Qualities	Light Source	External Diameter (mm)	Working Channel (mm)	Working Length (cm)	Tip Field-of-View Range (Degrees)	Range of Motion Up/Down (Degrees)
Pentax							
FI-7BS, FI-7RBS	Fib; neonate; eyepiece; CVS	Battery	2.4	—	60	95	130/130
FI-9BS, FI-9RBS	Fib; eyepiece; CVS	Battery/electric	3.1	1.2	60	90	130/130
FI-10BS/FI-10RBS	Fib; eyepiece; CVS	Battery/electric	3.5	1.4	60	90	130/130
FI-13BS, FI-16BS	Fib; eyepiece; CVS	Battery/electric	4.2	1.8	60	95	160/130
FI-16BS/FI-16RBS	Fib; eyepiece; CVS	Battery/electric	5.2	2.6	60	95	160/130
EB-1570K	CCD; CVS	Electric	5.1	2.0	60	120	210/130
EB-1970K	CCD; CVS	Electric	6.2	2.8	60	120	180/130
Cogentix Medical							
BRS-4000	Fib; disposable EndoSheath with suction	Battery	Insertion tube, 4.1	1.5–2.8	57	95	215/140
BRS-5100	CVS		Insertion tube, 4.1	1.5–2.8	60	110	215/140

Bronchoscopes have three different channel sizes, namely, 1.5 mm, 2.1 mm, and 2.8 mm, with progressively more suction. Enables one bronchoscope to fit through small to larger endotracheal tubes.
CCD, Digital cameras using charge-coupled devices; *CVS,* closed valve system (allows fluid injection without siphoning into suction); *CMOS,* digital cameras using complementary metal–oxide–semiconductors; *Fib,* fiberoptic scope (per company description); *HD,* high-definition resolution; *SD,* Standard-definition resolution.

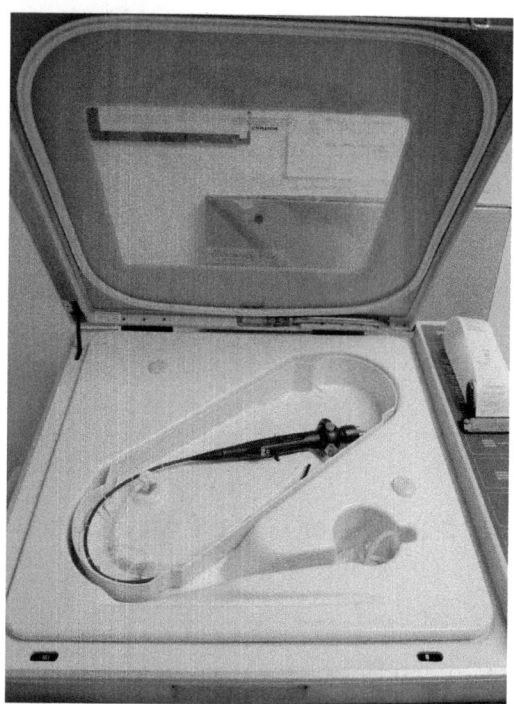

• **Fig. 24.5** Steris (Steris Corporation, Mentor, OH) machine for the sterilization of a flexible bronchoscope. The working channel is flushed out before being carefully placed within the sterilizer.

wipe-down cleaning with the company's product, making FOB damage unlikely. Advertised claims for all its various endosheathed devices (including uroscopes) boast "over 5-million sold, zero reported cross-contaminations." It may reduce costs by requiring fewer FISs and limiting sterilization equipment or personnel needs. This is uncertain because its FIS has a 9-year lifetime, compared with FISs with up to a 15-year lifetime.[36,37] Presently, use is aimed more at intensive care units (ICUs), but other areas are possibilities; however, the use of these sheaths is becoming more and more obsolete due to the introduction of single-use FISs.

Fully Disposable—Flexible Bronchoscopes

The Ambu aScope is a fully disposable, sterile, battery-operated non-FOB with a working channel. It has a CMOS chip, a steering button lever to flex the tip, and a distal LED (Fig. 24.1). Images are transmitted along the insertion tube's cable to a small portable monitor by way of a video connection cable at the handle. Its total disposability may be advantageous for patients with highly contagious diseases (e.g., Creutzfeldt-Jakob, Ebola), immunosuppressed patients, or in insufficiently funded sites.

Initial Ambu aScope 2 studies revealed little difference in intubation success rates for normal or DA patients, whereas optic quality and intubation times were better with reusable FISs,[38] although since that study, they do now have a high-quality 12.8-in fully high-definition monitor. Kristensen and colleagues found the button system easy but had worse secretion problems compared with reusable FISs.[39] The Ambu lens needed cleaning twice as often, with two completely blurred episodes after lidocaine instillation requiring FIS replacements.

Studies by Tvede (with his magic number of <22.5 cases/year for disposables to be less expensive), Aïssou, and Reynolds perceived almost no cost saving with it.[40,41] McCahon and colleagues paper might seem at odds to these studies, as their UK FIS costs per patient were almost double the Danish or French costs and more than triple Liu's US and Reynolds' Canadian costs.[41–43] Mouritsen and colleagues' systematic review and cost-effectiveness analysis found that single-use FISs are cost-effective and associated with a lower risk of infection. No comparative studies have better results for the Ambu aScope 3, with the exception of perhaps cost benefit.[21]

Two other single-use FISs are now available, the GlideScope BFlex and the Storz single-use video endoscope (Fig. 24.6).

The BFlex is fully disposable and comes in three sizes (3.8 mm, 5.0 mm, and 5.8 mm), all three of which have working channels with 50-mm interval markings on the insertion tube. The internal CMOS camera offers excellent image clarity and the FIS connects via magnetic GlideScope QuickConnect technology to the GlideScope Core monitor, enabling the added advantage of a dual view with the GlideScope videolaryngoscope for viewing multimodal airway procedures. At the time of writing this chapter, there is no published data on this device comparing its performance to other single-use or reusable FISs.

The Storz single-use video endoscopes are also sterile packed and consist of a CMOS sensor and LED illumination to provide high-resolution images with good lighting conditions when attached to the C-MAC monitor or the Tele Pack. There are four sizes available (2.9 mm, 3.5 mm, 5.2 mm, and 6.5 mm), all of which have a working channel and working length of up to 65 cm.

Many professionals are concerned with the hazards of nonrecyclable product use; however, the materials in the aScope 4 Broncho generate less CO_2 emissions and utilize fewer scarce resources. All three companies involved in producing single-use FIS are working toward reducing CO_2 emissions, reducing PVC packaging, and increasing to 100% recyclable and compostable packaging.

Rationale for Flexible Bronchoscope Intubation

Airway management failure is the bane of closed claims analyses. From 1975 to 1985, 34% of claims were attributed to DA; 70% involved death or brain damage.[44] Between 1985 and 1992, 62% concerned death/brain damage after induction, whereas from 1993 to 1999, 35% suffered this outcome.[45] In another analysis, between 2000 and 2012, difficult tracheal intubation claims were more likely to end in death than between 1993 and 1999 (73% vs 42%). However, permanent brain damage was similar between both time periods of the analyses.[46]

Direct laryngoscope (DL) use had a DI incidence of 1% to 13%.[47–51] Shiga and colleagues' meta-analysis of studies on 50,760 patients estimated average DI occurrence at 5.8%,[52] a range of 4.5% to 7.5%,[53,54] and an even greater incidence in obstetric or obese patients.[53,55,56] Benumof's estimate of "cannot intubate, cannot mask ventilate" frequency was verified by Heidegger and associates at 0.007%.[57,58] The overall published incidence of difficult face mask ventilation ranges between 0.66% and 2.5%,[59–61] difficulty in placement or ventilation with supraglottic airways (SGAs) is between 0.5% and 4.7%[62–66] and difficulty with tracheal intubation has been reported between 1.9% and 10%.[67–69]

Despite the plethora of intubation devices such as intubating SGAs, lighted stylets, video-assisted laryngoscopes (VALs), optical laryngoscopes (OLs), and optical stylets and greater intubating success rates, FISs still have a place in the management of DAs in the form of ATI. Rosenblatt and colleagues' survey of US anesthesiologists revealed a strong preference for FIS when managing patients with known DAs.[70] Avarguès and colleagues' survey of French

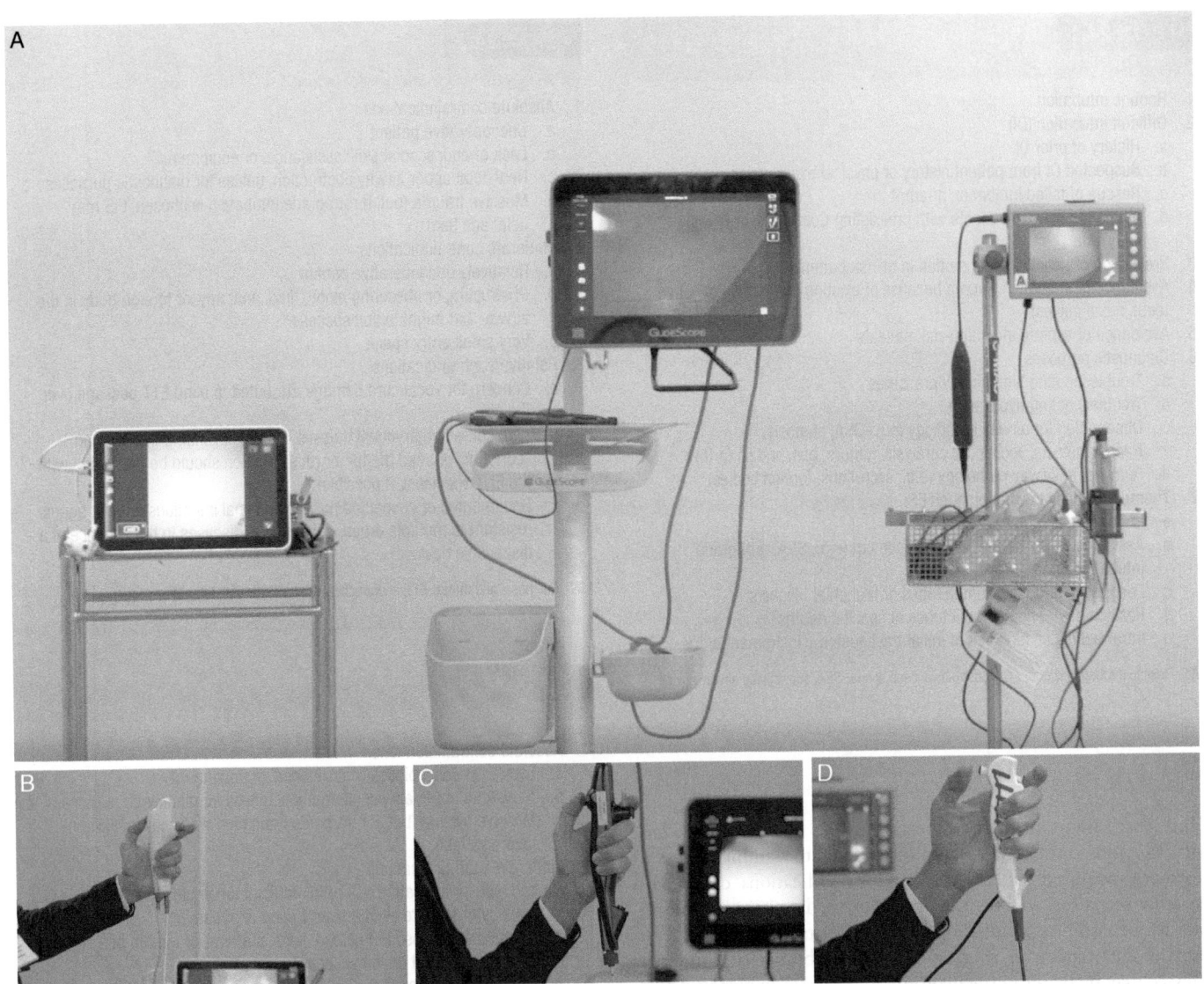

• **Fig. 24.6** Disposable flexible scopes. (A) Screens (*left* to *right*) for Ambu Scope (Ambu A/S, Ballerup, Denmark), GlideScope (Verathon, Seattle, WA), and Storz (Karl Storz GmbH & Co. KG, Tuttlingen, Germany). (B) Ambu Scope handle. (C) B Flex disposable flexible scope handle. (D) Storz disposable flexible scope handle.

anesthetists in 1999 revealed that 64% of responders voiced the need for more ATI training.[71] In the revised 2013 Difficult Airway Algorithm (DAA) 69.7% of expert panelists formulating the American Society of Anesthesiologists (ASA) practice guidelines for DA management strongly agreed that FISs should be used for emergency noninvasive intubations. They also agreed that FISs should be readily available in most DA situations.[72] In a 2009 review of existing DA management algorithms Frova and Sorbello affirmed that the FIS was universally recognized as the gold standard in awake, sedated, or anesthetized DI patients.[73] No clearly validated predictive assessment tool developed specifically for ATI exists; therefore ATI must be considered in the presence of any predictors of DA management done during the airway assessment.[18]

FISs have greater capability to rescue most airway device failures, including recently developed inventions, and facilitate successful airway management (either alone or in a multimodal approach), as illustrated by 13 DAA references, citing 87% to 100% success rates in DA patients.[72–75]

Unique FIS characteristics compared with any other airway device include flexibility and ability to navigate along the most tortuous airways; least need for cervical motion, which is ideal for cervical spine risk cases; functional capability in any body position, oral or nasal route, and age; association with the most hemodynamic stability with the ideal local anesthesia (LA); and topicalization and capability in multimodal, troubleshooting, diagnostic, or therapeutic scenarios.

Criteria for Use

An ATI approach is usually chosen to avoid failure from an asleep intubation technique. An ATI technique should always be considered in the presence of predictors of DA management.[18] For asleep FIS tracheal intubations, most anesthesiologists follow certain criteria, although many routinely employ this device. Asleep indicators include awake criteria (only if no adversity is likely) and more, as listed in Box 24.1.

1. Routine intubation
2. Difficult intubation (DI)
   a. History of prior DI
   b. Suspected DI from patient history or physical examination
   c. Rescue of failed intubation attempt
   d. Intubation need in patients with preexisting Combitube or Rüsch EasyTube
3. Prevention of cervical spine motion in at-risk patients
4. Avoidance of intubation trauma because of existing anatomy (e.g., loose teeth, nasal polyps)
5. Avoidance of aspiration in high-risk patients
6. Diagnostic purposes
   a. Troubleshooting high airway pressures
   b. Troubleshooting hypoxemia
   c. Observation for airway pathology (e.g., OSA, stenosis, tracheomalacia, vocal cord paralysis, tumors, pus, and so forth)
   d. Removal of airway pathology (e.g., secretions, foreign bodies)
7. Therapeutic uses beyond planned FSI
   a. Endotracheal tube exchange
   b. Assistance with airway device placement (e.g., SGA, retrograde intubation, etc.)
   c. Positioning of double-lumen tubes or bronchial blockers
   d. Positioning of endotracheal tubes at specific depths
   e. Intratracheal observation of initial tracheostomy instrument entry

FIS, Flexible intubation scope; *OSA*, obstructive sleep apnea; *SGA*, supraglottic airway device.

Contraindications

The most important contraindication to FIS use is usually a lack of FIS endoscopist skill because of inadequate training or loss of formerly acquired skills. Relative contraindications depend on specific scenarios, such as the lack of trained assistance, unavailability of equipment, uncooperative patients, degree of known airway tract narrowing (Fig. 24.7), or advisability that a different device may be better (a tracheotomy for excessively bleeding massive facial trauma). Contraindications for awake and asleep FIS intubation are listed in Boxes 24.2 and 24.3, respectively.

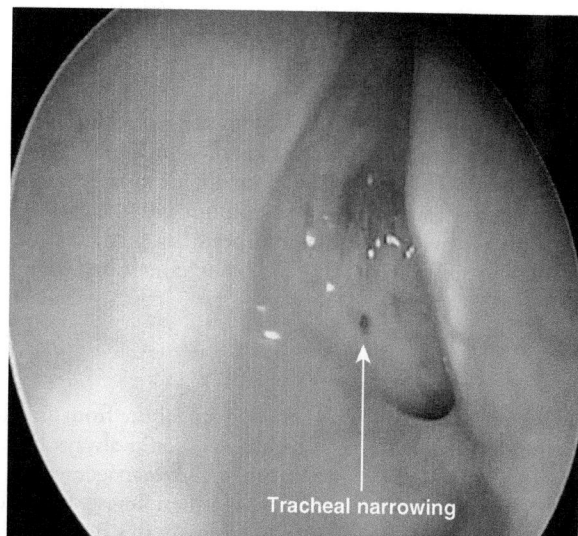

• **Fig. 24.7** Severe subglottic stenosis appears as a pinpoint tracheal opening (*arrow*).

1. Absolute contraindications
   a. Uncooperative patient
   b. Lack of endoscopist skill, assistance, or equipment
   c. Near-total upper airway obstruction, unless for diagnostic purposes
   d. Massive trauma (but, if retrograde intubation is chosen, FIS may help; see text)
2. Moderate contraindications
   a. Relatively uncooperative patient
   b. Obstructing or obscuring blood, fluid, anatomy, or foreign body in the airway that might inhibit success
   c. Very small entry space
3. Relative contraindications
   a. Concern for vocal cord damage attributed to blind ETT passage over the FIS
   b. With some perilaryngeal masses, blindly advancing the ETT can "cork out" or seed the tumor (this situation should be discussed with the ENT specialist, if possible)
   c. Documented or suspected nonconventional infectious agents, agents resistant to multiple drugs, or infectious diseases in the absence of a disposable device

ENT, Ear, nose, and throat; *ETT*, endotracheal tube; *FIS*, flexible intubation scope.

1. Absolute contraindications
   a. Lack of endoscopist skill, assistance, or equipment
   b. Near-total upper airway obstruction, unless for diagnostic purposes
   c. Massive trauma (but, if retrograde intubation was chosen, FIS may help; see text)
2. Moderate contraindications
   a. Too high an aspiration risk or too difficult an airway
   b. Inability to tolerate even a short period of apnea
   c. Obstructing or obscuring blood, fluid, anatomy, or foreign body in the airway that might inhibit success
   d. Very small entry space
3. Relative contraindications
   a. Concern for vocal cord damage that might be caused by blind ETT passage over the FIS
   b. With some perilaryngeal masses, blindly advancing the ETT can "cork out" or seed the tumor (this situation should be discussed with the ENT specialist, if possible)
   c. Documented or suspected nonconventional infectious agents, agents resistant to multiple drugs, or infectious diseases in the absence of a single-use device

ENT, Ear, nose, and throat; *ETT*, endotracheal tube; *FIS*, flexible intubation scope.

Equipment

Fiberoptic and Nonfiberoptic Flexible Bronchoscope Inner Workings

FIS specifications and characteristics are presented in Table 24.1. Some have eyepieces or video attachments and varying degrees of portability. Olympus developed a very portable MAF-GM FIS system featuring a lithium rechargeable battery with a fixed, rotatable video screen by the handle, all totally immersible for sterilization. Its CCD camera has a memory card and an xD chip for still photography and video recording. One model is autoclavable.

Flexible Bronchoscope Intubation Cart

Preparation is the springboard for FSI success. Mobile FSI carts must be readily and rapidly transportable for routine or emergency use. Carts can be used for institutional education programs or teaching workshops. Logical, instantly recognizable content arrangement must be uniform across facilities. Preferably, carts have two widely separated tubular structures for hanging clean or used FISs (Fig. 24.8). Typically, they include a light source, video monitor (ideally), endoscopy masks, intubating oral airways (IOAs), bite blocks, atomizers, tongue blades, cotton-tipped swabs, gauze, soft nasal airways, alcohol wipes, bronchoscopy swivel adapters, and local anesthetics. Organizational updates lie within the anesthesiology purview

Optionally, FSI cart setups can exist within a DA cart, having items needed to follow the DAA (VAL and screen, SGAs, intubating SGAs, ETT introducers/exchangers, and invasive airway rescue sets).[76,77] With the increased availability, accessibility, and reduced cost of single-use FIS compared to reusable FIS, many institutions have these on their carts as there is no need to sterilize the bronchoscopes and they can be rapidly assembled if required in an emergency.

Ancillary Equipment

Bronchoscopy Swivel Adapters and Endoscopy Masks

Bronchoscopy swivel adapters are used for diagnostic examinations, therapeutic maneuvers, or intubation. They can rotate when placed between the ventilating system and a mask, SGA, or ETT. They resemble elbow adapters equipped with a flip-cap port on top, covering a centrally open diaphragm (Fig. 24.9). This facilitates FIS passage with virtually no leak during uninterrupted ventilation. Swivel adapters only permit very small ETT passage (sizes ≤5.5 mm;

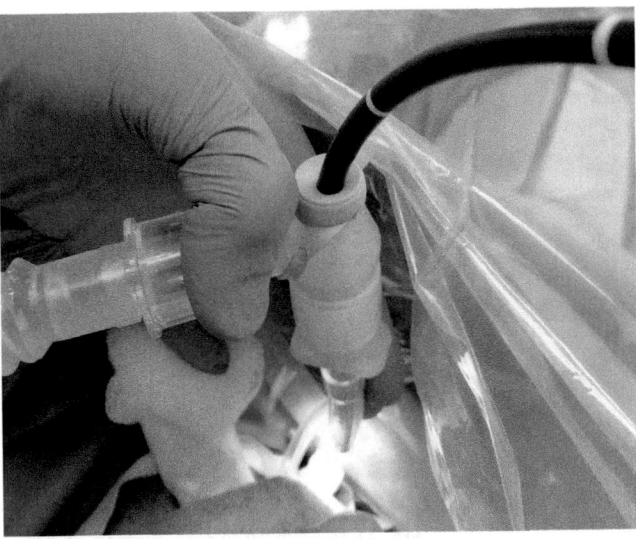

• **Fig. 24.9** Bronchoscopy swivel adapter with a snug flexible bronchoscope diaphragm, permitting ventilation with no leakage.

uncuffed 6.0 mm is very snug). Apart from a ventilation connection, endoscopy masks have more than one larger opening whose design function may be similar to a swivel adapter port (Fig. 24.10). This allows FIS or FIS and ETT (≤8.0 mm) passage during continuous mask ventilation. Some have recessed valvelike openings.

Intubating Oral Airways

For conscious or unconscious patients, IOAs are conduits to keep an FIS midline during oral intubation (Fig. 24.11). They must not be placed too deeply into small mouths.

The ideal IOA (1) protects the FIS from damage; (2) keeps it midline; (3) keeps tissues away; (4) permits FIS maneuverability within; (5) has an ideal length to approach the glottis; (6) allows the passage of larger ETTs; (7) possesses a breakaway quality for easy removal; (8) avoids tissue discomfort (minimizing gagging) or trauma to tissues or ETT cuffs; and (9) has the ability to assist with mask ventilation. If no IOA is used in awake patients (because of unavailability, endoscopist preference, or inadequate mouth opening), a bite block between the molars or incisors may prevent FIS damage.

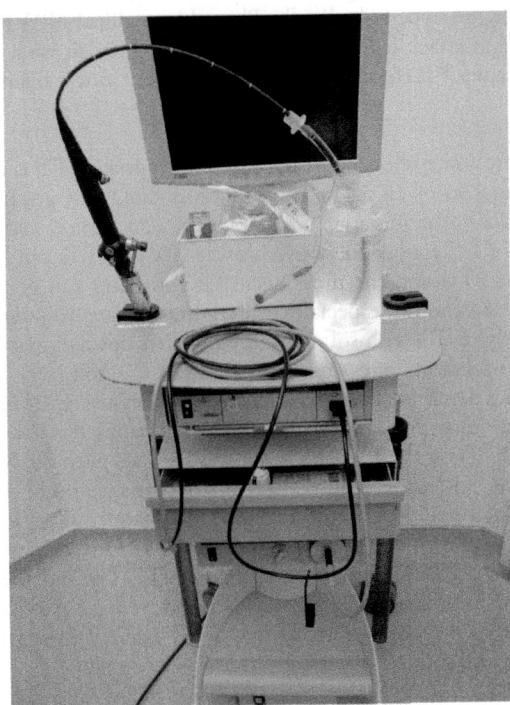

• **Fig. 24.8** Mobile airway cart with a video screen and supplies underneath. The flexible intubation scope (FIS) is braced in the clean container on the left, and a holding tube for the used FIS is located on the right. The FIS insertion section lies within an endotracheal tube in a warm saline solution.

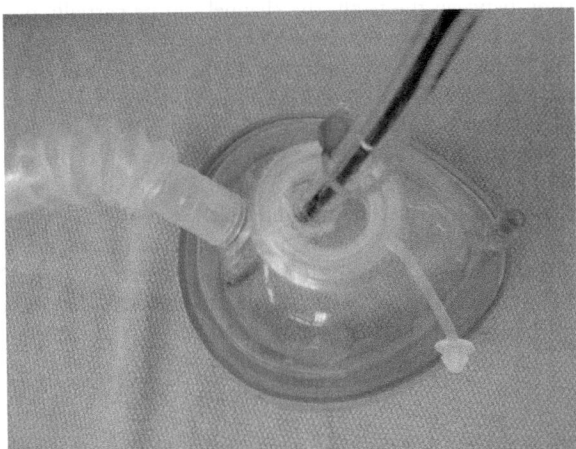

• **Fig. 24.10** Endoscopy mask with connector tubing for ventilation (on the *left*) and a snug diaphragm (on *top*) for the passage of a fiberoptic bronchoscope within an endotracheal tube.

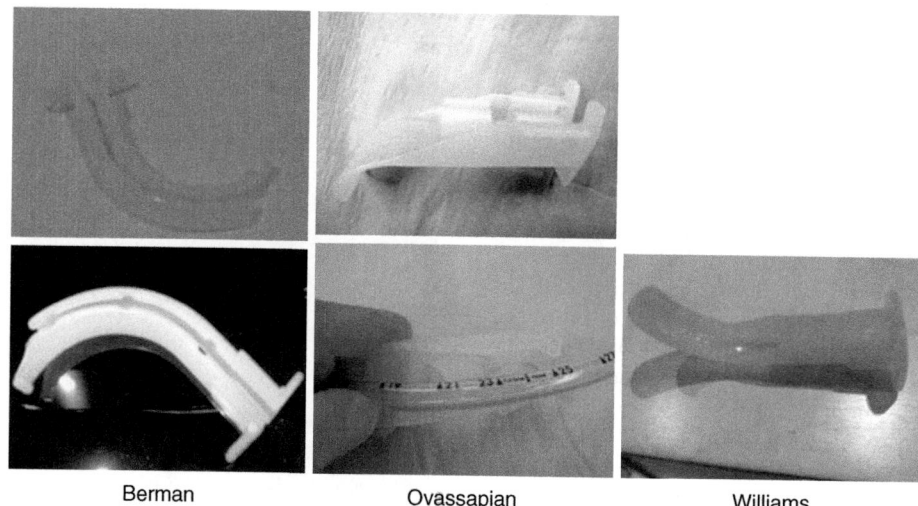

| Berman | Ovassapian | Williams |

• **Fig. 24.11** From left to right, Berman intubating pharyngeal airway (Teleflex Medical Research, Triangle Park, NC); Ovassapian intubating airway (Teleflex Medical Research, Triangle Park, NC); and Williams airway intubator (SunMed Medical Systems LLC, Grand Rapids, MI).

Most studies comparing IOAs involve non-DA patients.[78] All are disposable, except the aluminum Patil-Syracuse oral airway (Anesthesia Associates, Inc. [AincA], San Marcos, CA).

The Berman Intubating Pharyngeal Airway (Teleflex Medical Research, Triangle Park, NC) in neonatal, child, and adult sizes admits ETTs up to 8.5 mm. Its full-length tubular shape does not help FIS maneuvering, but its wide lateral perforated slits break away from postintubation ETTs (although possibly difficult, particularly with periglottic ETT impingement). Kept midline, it provides a better lead to the glottis if the length is appropriate.[79] If too long, distally, it may lie in the vallecula; 1- to 2-cm withdrawal may rectify the situation. This device has largely been superseded by newer IOAs.

The proximal channel of the Ovassapian Fiberoptic Intubating Airway (Teleflex Medical Research, Triangle Park, NC) permits the passage of ETTs up to 9 mm. It has flexible lateral walls and a posterior opening for easy ETT removal. Its distal half has a wide, flat, open, curved area designed to keep the tongue and soft tissues away, make it easier to stay midline, and permit free FIS movement. A marker line drawn lengthwise down the middle of its concave surface aids FIS orientation upon entry.[80] During ETT insertion between the teeth, the channel can be partially opened to avoid tearing the cuff on its corners.

The Williams Airway Intubator (SunMed Medical Systems, Grand Rapids, MI) has two adult sizes, allowing the passage of an ETT up to 8.5 mm. It has a closed channel proximally and a curved section distally with a scalloped opening on the lingual surface to permit FIS movement. If kept midline and its length is appropriate, it may be the best guide to the larynx.[81] If the length is too long, visualization can be problematic. With smaller sizes, cuff damage is more frequent for ETTs larger than 7.0 mm. During removal, which may be difficult, the enclosed channel part should have been liberally prelubricated.[82] Afterward, reconnect the ETT to its 15-mm ETT connector.

Unexpected Adaptations of Short, Soft Nasopharyngeal Airways

Two nasopharyngeal airway (NPA) techniques may be employed during ATI. One simplifies nasal ATI by making a breakaway NPA with a single full-length slit to permit breakaway capability, as reported by Lu and colleagues.[83] Lubricate the breakaway NPA inside and outside, gently insert it into the largest naris to an appropriate depth, and guide the FIS through it toward the glottis. After maximal entry into the trachea, an assistant strips the NPA away. Advance the FIS until two to three rings above the carina and railroad the ETT into the trachea.

The second technique is where the NPA is used as a conduit for oxygen delivery and possibly for inhalation of volatile anesthetic gases during FSI (most commonly in pediatric patients).[84,85] This is particularly advantageous in spontaneously breathing patients after cutting a Murphy eye-type hole distally. Place this modified NPA into one nostril, and attach it to a supported breathing circuit via a 15-mm ETT adapter.[86] Perform ATI through a different airway opening.

Endotracheal Tubes: What Is Best?

The appropriate selection of the most appropriate ETT is integral to the success of an ATI. Consideration should be given to the appropriate tube material, size, tip shape and design, and length of the ETT. Regular polyvinylchloride (PVC) ETTs can be used for FSIs. However, the most distal ETT tip area can get caught on the arytenoids, especially the right, causing impingement. Previously, ETTs with soft centrally directed tips had greater successful intubation rates than PVC ETTs.[87–89] However, Joo and colleagues demonstrated no difference in success rates or manipulation instances required during ATI when comparing these two types of ETTs if the PVC ETT tip was inserted with the Murphy eye facing anteriorly with respect to the patient's body to avoid arytenoid contact.[90] It represented a 90-degree counterclockwise rotation of the ETT from its normal position during direct laryngoscopy (Fig. 24.12). Reinforced Parker Flex-Tip and the ETTs used with intubating laryngeal mask airways have good clinical evidence to be superior to regular PVC ETTs and are recommended over them.[91–97]

Awake Tracheal Intubation in Adults

The principles of ATI can be broken down into four key elements: oxygenation, topicalization, sedation, and procedural setup and performance (Fig. 24.13).

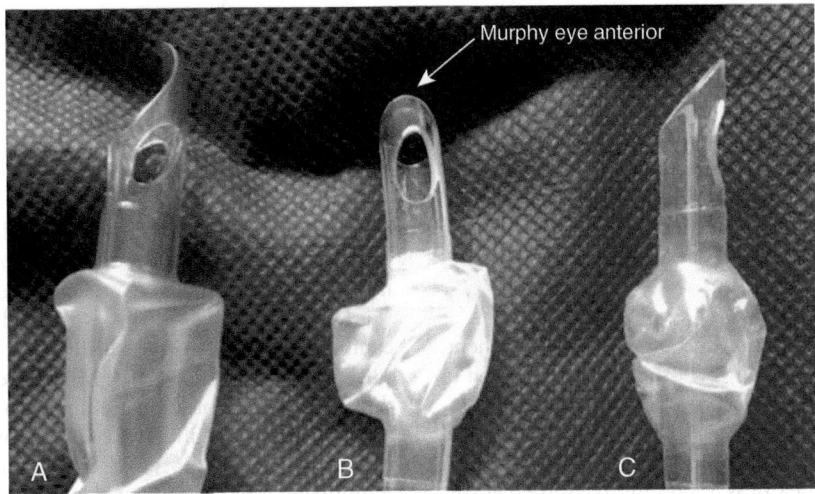

Murphy eye anterior

• **Fig. 24.12** (A) Centrally directed endotracheal tube with a Parker Flex-Tip. (B) Rotation 90 degrees counterclockwise. (C) Common rigid laryngoscope intubating direction.

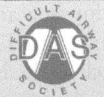
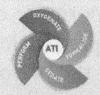

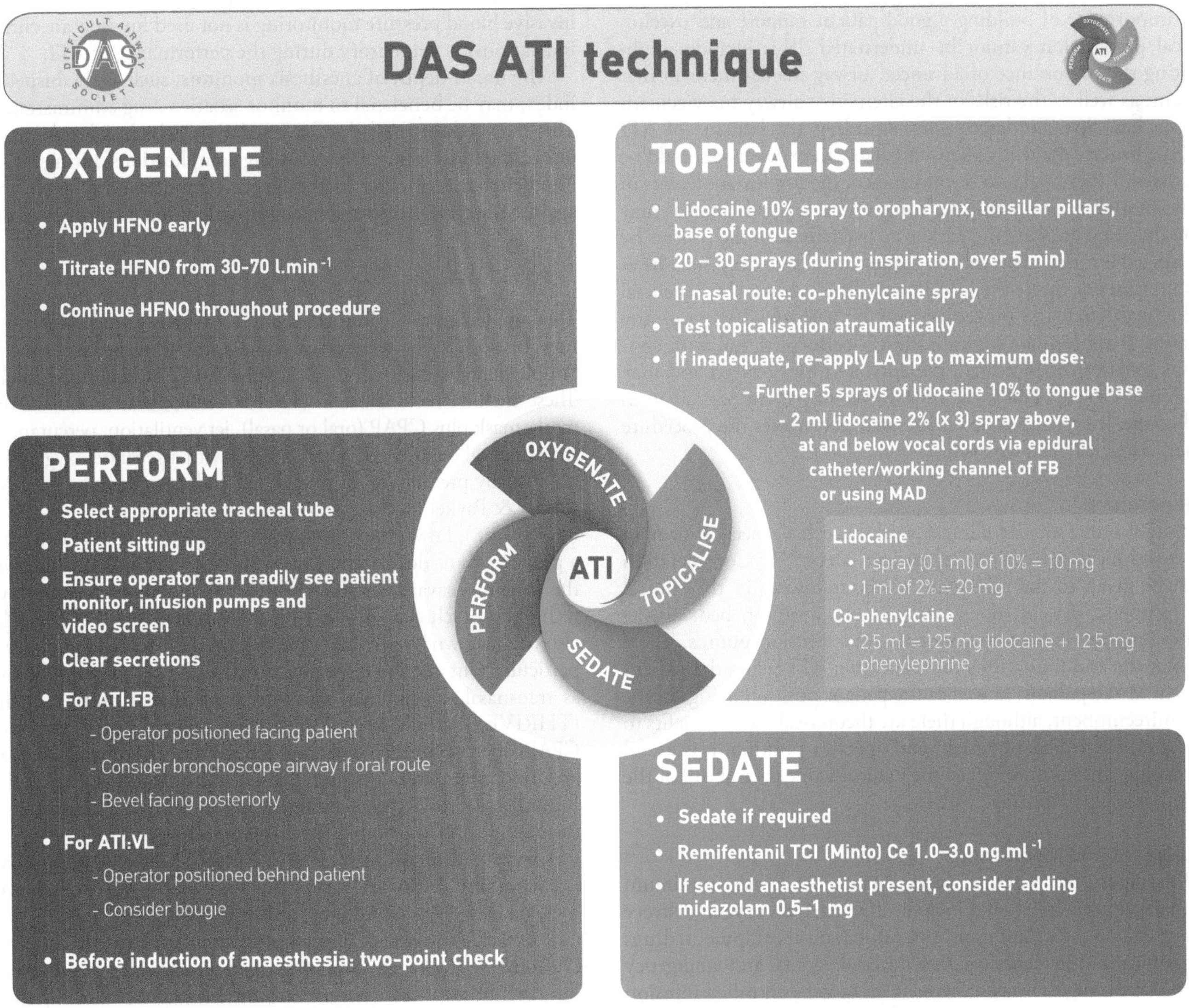

DAS ATI technique

OXYGENATE

- Apply HFNO early
- Titrate HFNO from 30-70 l.min^{-1}
- Continue HFNO throughout procedure

TOPICALISE

- Lidocaine 10% spray to oropharynx, tonsillar pillars, base of tongue
- 20 – 30 sprays (during inspiration, over 5 min)
- If nasal route: co-phenylcaine spray
- Test topicalisation atraumatically
- If inadequate, re-apply LA up to maximum dose:
    - Further 5 sprays of lidocaine 10% to tongue base
    - 2 ml lidocaine 2% (x 3) spray above, at and below vocal cords via epidural catheter/working channel of FB or using MAD

    Lidocaine
    - 1 spray (0.1 ml) of 10% = 10 mg
    - 1 ml of 2% = 20 mg

    Co-phenylcaine
    - 2.5 ml = 125 mg lidocaine + 12.5 mg phenylephrine

PERFORM

- Select appropriate tracheal tube
- Patient sitting up
- Ensure operator can readily see patient monitor, infusion pumps and video screen
- Clear secretions
- For ATI:FB
    - Operator positioned facing patient
    - Consider bronchoscope airway if oral route
    - Bevel facing posteriorly
- For ATI:VL
    - Operator positioned behind patient
    - Consider bougie
- Before induction of anaesthesia: two-point check

OXYGENATE

PERFORM — ATI — TOPICALISE

SEDATE

SEDATE

- Sedate if required
- Remifentanil TCI (Minto) Ce 1.0–3.0 ng.ml^{-1}
- If second anaesthetist present, consider adding midazolam 0.5–1 mg

• **Fig. 24.13** The Difficult Airway Society awake tracheal intubation (ATI) technique. *Ce,* Effect-site concentration; *FIS,* flexible intubation scope; *HFNO,* high-flow nasal oxygen; *LA,* local anesthetic; *MAD,* mucosal atomizing device; *TCI,* target-controlled infusion; *VAL,* video-assisted laryngoscopy. (© Difficult Airway Society 2019.)

Procedural Setup

ATI is associated with greater physical and psychological stress on operators than any other airway management intervention.[98] These stressors may adversely impact performance and increase the risk of complications.[99] Thus effective communication, teamwork, and patient and operator preparation are critical. Moreover, having competent assistance, available expertise and support, and an environment that is geared toward safety is essential.[100]

Location

Planning for the appropriate location and prerequired equipment, drugs, and staffing is essential. Ideally, ATI should be performed in the OR environment as this affords access to DA carts, skilled assistance and nursing, proximity to other anesthesiologists, and surgical skills, as well as providing adequate space for ATI to be performed. Early communication with the OR is important to ensure that sufficient time is planned for DA management. External pressure from nonairway managers must be limited gently but firmly.

Patient Preparation

The importance of building a good patient rapport and psychological preparation cannot be understated. This includes highlighting the importance of advanced airway management in that patient, as well as the risks of the alternative airway management approaches. Specific descriptions regarding the benefits of ATI and the process that the patients are likely to experience should be discussed. Patients should be informed of the unpleasant flavors of local anesthetic; comparing to "tonic water" or "old banana" may be useful. Encouraging the patient to participate in the process by advising them that they will be requested to take deep breaths at certain times or gargle then swallow at others. It may be beneficial to highlight that the procedure may be performed without any sedation if appropriate topicalization is performed, but with conscious sedation, if indicated, patients are often relaxed and may not remember it. Finally, the importance of patient participation and cooperation cannot be understated as it makes the procedure easier, faster, and less worrisome.[101]

Ergonomics

The ergonomics of the clinical workspace have been shown to affect technical procedures and patient safety.[102,103] Consideration must be given to the placement of the following in the clinical environment: patient, operator, assistant, monitor, bed, airway trolley, anesthetic machine, suction, and infusion pumps. There are benefits and limitations to performing ATI facing the patient or behind the patient, as well as the patient position being supine or semirecumbent, although there are theoretical safety benefits to the latter. Regardless of patient and operator position, it is useful to consider the ergonomics of the clinical workspace ahead of the arrival of the patient (Fig. 24.14).

Equipment and Monitoring

Unless emergency circumstances dictate otherwise, minimum standard equipment should include a DA cart; an oxygen delivery system; suctions; patient monitors; resuscitation equipment; drugs (for topicalization, sedation, GA, reversal agents, and emergency drugs); and drug delivery systems (e.g., target-controlled infusion devices). Equipment for primary and alternative airway management strategies should also be discussed, available, and checked.

Monitoring physiological parameters reduces risks and alerts operators regarding impending complications.[104–106] Frequently occurring complications that may be avoidable during ATI that may be detected by monitoring are airway obstruction and hypoventilation, which may arise due to oversedation.[107–109] Thus continuous pulse oximetry should be utilized as a standard. End-tidal carbon dioxide pressure (P_{ETCO_2}) monitoring may be beneficial with alarm parameters set for P_{ETCO_2} and respiratory rate. There have been modifications to existing devices that can be used to attach one end of the CO_2 analyzer line from the nasal cannula to the circle breathing circuit, minimizing the burden of disconnecting sampling lines at crucial times during the ATI process (Fig. 24.13). However, this is dependent on the use of a nasal cannula for oxygenation, which might not be ideal. Attachments to high-flow nasal oxygen (HFNO) devices have now been produced, are affordable, and are simple to use, and they may provide an opportunity to undertake continuous waveform capnography in this setting (Fig. 24.15). Regardless of the strategies employed, monitoring for respiratory depression is important during the process of ATI.

Cardiac dysrhythmias or hypotension may occur after the administration of sedation or topicalization agents,[110–112] and therefore noninvasive blood pressure monitoring cycling frequently (if invasive blood pressure monitoring is not used for separate clinical indications) is mandatory during the performance of ATI.

The use of depth of anesthesia monitors, such as the bispectral index, may be beneficial to monitor sedative drug administration. This may reduce the risk of oversedation, which is known to be one of the most frequently occurring complications during ATI.[107] The benefits of the use of the bispectral index must be weighed against the risks of increasing cognitive load on airway operators.

Oxygenation

The supplementary administration of oxygen during ATI should now be seen as mandatory, regardless of the technique selected. Supplemental oxygenation can involve single or combined modes. These include nasal cannula (12–15 L/min), oral cannula, NPA, mask, mask plus CPAP (oral or nasal), jet ventilation, percutaneous transtracheal oxygen therapy (TTO)—with a separate oxygen supply (usually preexisting for oxygen-dependent patients), or HFNO (Fisher & Paykel Healthcare, Auckland, New Zealand) (Fig. 24.16) (Video 24.8). Low-flow (≤30 L/min) techniques are associated with a greater risk of desaturation than high-flow techniques, and with the increasing availability of HFNO, this is rapidly becoming the technique of choice. Along with delivering oxygen, HFNO has also been shown to provide some carbon dioxide clearance as well, particularly in the apneic patient, where the technique is known as transnasal, humidified, rapid-insufflation ventilatory exchange (THRIVE). In addition, HFNO may provide flow-dependent CPAP, open soft-tissue passages, reduce dry gas mucosal damage and discomfort, and assist in the dispersion of local anesthetic.[113–115] Regardless of the oxygen strategy implemented, it should be commenced as soon as possible once patients attend the OR.

Oxygen insufflation at 3 to 5 L/min via the working channel in adults during ATI was previously proposed to stave off hypoxia, help clear secretions, and prevent fogging.[57,116,117] Benumof described this technique and recommended it be used very cautiously.[57] If oxygen flow into a patient exceeds gaseous escape into the atmosphere, serious barotrauma might occur, especially with airway narrowing or laryngospasm. Pneumothorax has been reported in pediatric patients with oxygen at excessive adult flow rates.[118,119] Acute cervical, facial, and thoracic emphysema were reported in a patient.[120] Documented gastric rupture with

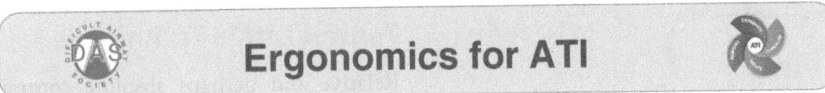

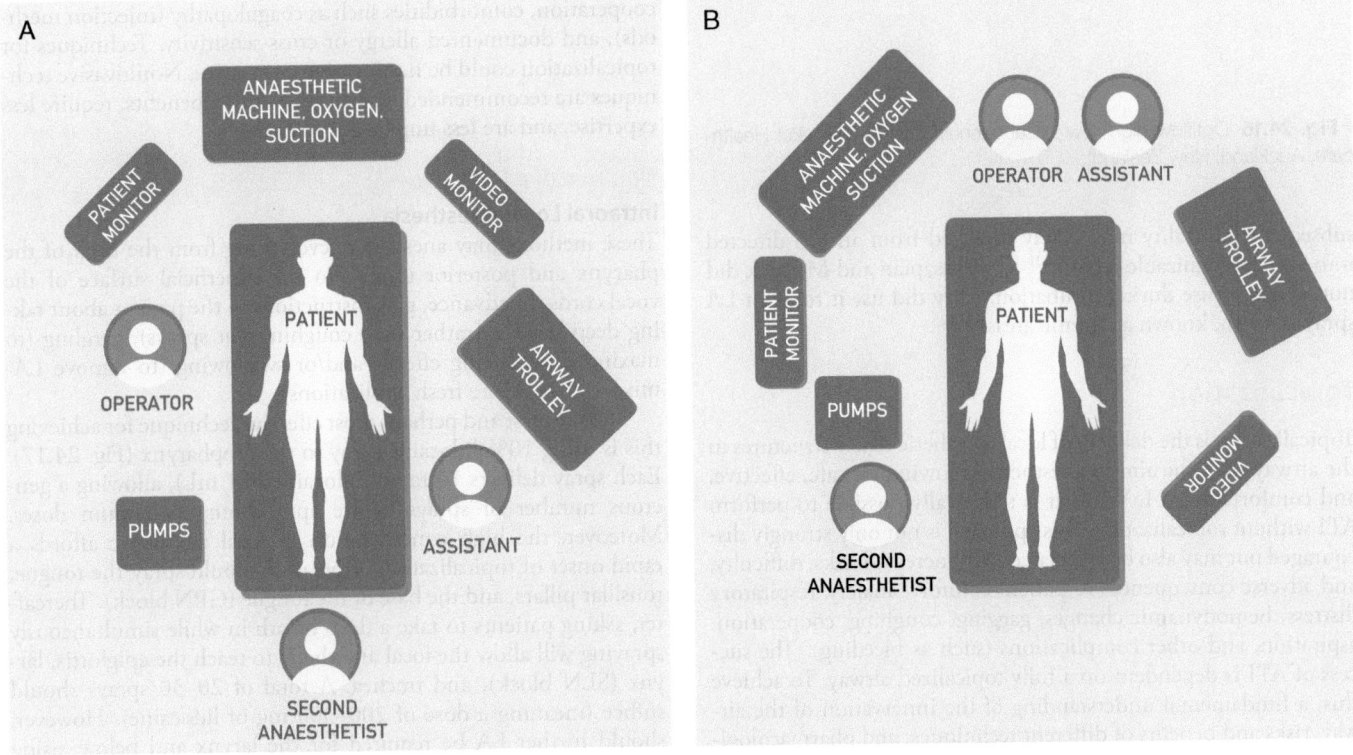

• **Fig. 24.14** Examples of ergonomics for awake tracheal intubation (ATI). The primary operator should have a direct line of sight of the patient, video monitor, and patient monitor, as well as immediate access to infusion pumps, anesthetic machine, suction, and oxygen delivery device. If a second anesthesiologist is present, they should be positioned with a direct line of sight of the patient and have immediate access to infusion pumps, as well as be able to access all other equipment. The assistant's primary position should be with immediate access to the airway trolley and in proximity to the operator. (A) Awake tracheal intubation performed with the operator positioned facing the patient who is in a sitting up position. (B) Awake tracheal intubation performed with the operator positioned behind the supine/semirecumbent patient. This figure forms part of the Difficult Airway Society guidelines for ATI in adults and should be used in conjunction with the text. (© Difficult Airway Society 2019.)

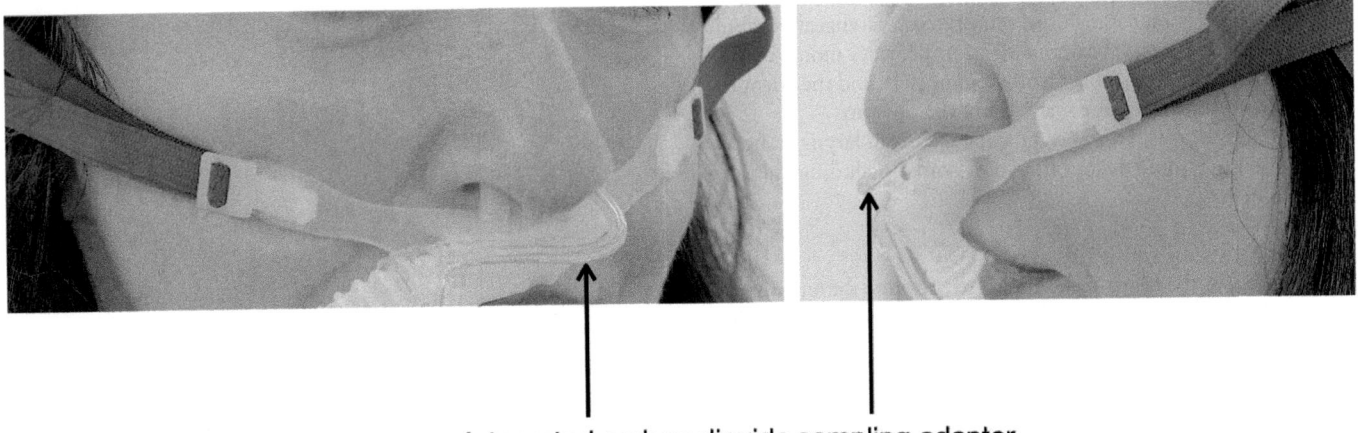

Integrated carbon dioxide sampling adaptor

• **Fig. 24.15** Example of integrated carbon dioxide sampling adapter on high-flow nasal cannulas.

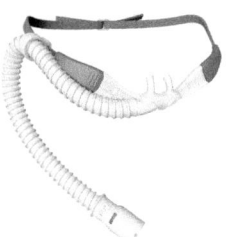

• **Fig. 24.16** Optiflow high-flow nasal cannula (Fisher & Paykel Healthcare, Auckland, New Zealand).

subsequent mortality most likely occurred from an FIS directed into an unrecognizable region.[121–123] Ovassapian and Mesnick did not advise its use during intubation. They did use it to assist LA spray in open, known anatomic areas.[124,125]

Topicalization

Topicalization is the delivery of local anesthetic to key structures in the airway with the aim to anesthetize allowing for safe, effective, and comfortable ATI. While it is technically possible to perform ATI without topicalization, this approach is not only strongly discouraged but may also be associated with increased risks, difficulty, and adverse consequences to patient comfort, anxiety, respiratory distress, hemodynamic changes, gagging, coughing, cooperation, aspiration, and other complications (such as bleeding). The success of ATI is dependent on a fully topicalized airway. To achieve this, a fundamental understanding of the innervation of the airway, risks and benefits of different techniques, and pharmacological principles of local anesthetics is required.

Innervation of the Orotracheal Airway

Cranial nerve IX, the glossopharyngeal nerve (GPN), supplies sensory innervation to the soft palate, the posterior third of the tongue, the tonsils, and most of the pharyngeal mucosa.[126,127] Some fibers also supply the lingual surface of the epiglottis.[128] It controls the afferent component of the gag reflex. Cranial nerve V, the trigeminal, gives sensory supply to the anterior two-thirds of the tongue, but this area rarely needs anesthesia.

Cranial nerve X, the vagus, forms part of the pharyngeal plexus, giving motor function to the soft palate and pharyngeal muscles. Its superior and inferior laryngeal branches carry sensory supply to the laryngopharynx. The superior laryngeal nerve (SLN) has an internal division for sensory supply to the tongue base, vallecula, epiglottis, piriform recesses, supraglottic mucosa, and laryngeal vestibule above the vocal cords. Its external division provides motor control to the adductors/tensors, the cricothyroid muscle, and the cricopharyngeal part of the inferior constrictor of the pharynx.

The inferior branch of the vagus, the recurrent laryngeal nerve, receives sensory input below the vocal cords, including the subglottic mucosa.

Innervation of the Nasotracheal Airway

Cranial nerve V, the trigeminal, supplies sensation to the anterior half of the NP via its first branch. The second branch of the trigeminal nerve forms part of the sphenopalatine ganglion, innervating some of the anterior, superior, and central regions.[126,127] Cranial nerve IX, the GPN, supplies parasympathetic innervation, while the carotid plexus supplies sympathetics.[129] Cranial nerve VIII, the facial nerve, has parasympathetic function and forms part of the sphenopalatine ganglion to assist in the control of nasopharyngeal reflexes.

Topicalization Techniques

Relative and perhaps absolute contraindications to techniques include local infection, anatomic abnormalities, lack of patient cooperation, comorbidities such as coagulopathy (injection methods), and documented allergy or cross-sensitivity. Techniques for topicalization could be noninvasive or invasive. Noninvasive techniques are recommended as they carry safety benefits, require less expertise, and are less unpleasant to patients.

Noninvasive Techniques

Intraoral Local Anesthesia

These methods may anesthetize everything from the back of the pharynx and posterior tongue to the superficial surface of the vocal cords. In advance, give instructions to the patient about taking deep breaths (rather than coughing out sprays), gargling (to maximize local drug effect), and/or swallowing (to remove LA-mixed saliva before fresh applications).

The simplest and perhaps most effective technique for achieving this is using 10% lidocaine spray to the oropharynx (Fig. 24.17). Each spray delivers 10 mg of lidocaine (0.1 mL), allowing a generous number of sprays before approaching maximum doses. Moreover, the high concentration of local anesthetic affords a rapid onset of topicalization. Operators should spray the tongue, tonsillar pillars, and the base of the tongue (GPN block). Thereafter, asking patients to take a deep breath in while simultaneously spraying will allow the local anesthetic to reach the epiglottis, larynx (SLN block), and trachea. A total of 20–30 sprays should suffice (meaning a dose of 200–300 mg of lidocaine). However, should further LA be required for the larynx and below, using the effective and inexpensive MADgic atomizer (Teleflex Medical, Morrisville, NC, USA) curved to allow careful placement above the glottis with 1–4 mL of lidocaine sprayed and gargled may further contribute to SLN block. This combined technique can often be used as the sole topicalization strategy if delivered appropriately and has been advocated by the Difficult Airway Society (UK).

Other approaches include a lollipop method with 3 cm of 2% to 5% lidocaine paste on one end of a tongue depressor, or a direct toothpaste method (gel down the middle of the tongue)

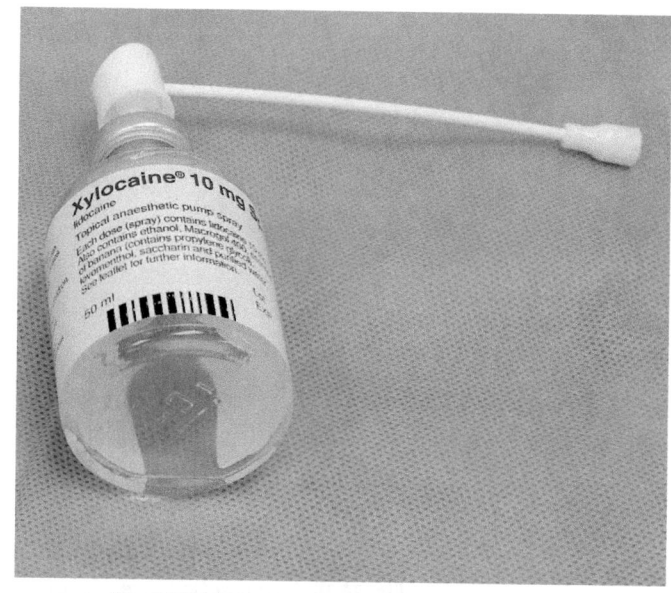

• **Fig. 24.17** Lidocaine 10% bottle with attached spray.

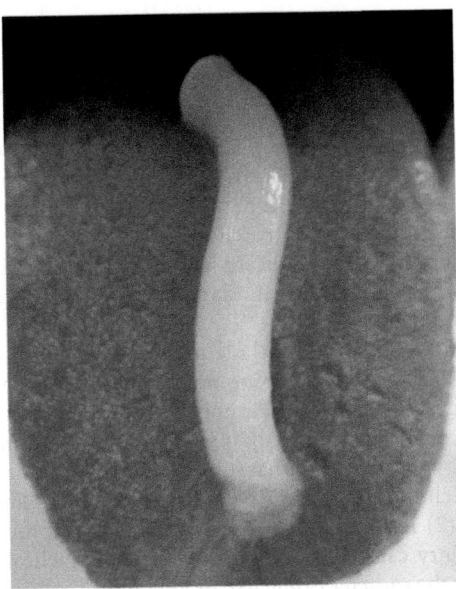

• **Fig. 24.18** Intraoral anesthesia: the 5% lidocaine toothpaste method.

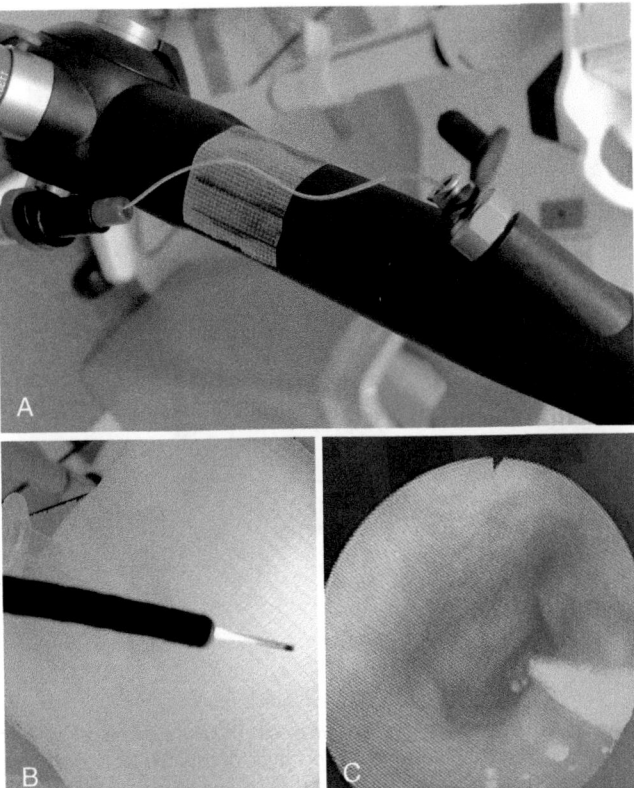

• **Fig. 24.19** (A) Proximal epidural catheter taped to the handle by working channel. (B) Distal catheter 1 cm out from the tip. (C) Drop of lidocaine from initial "spray as you go."

(Fig. 24.18), leaving drugs to dissolve over 5 to 10 minutes. Alternatively, let a Tessalon Perles (benzonatate) dissolve in the middle of the tongue (may need to bite it slightly, once).

Aerosol/Nebulized Method

This is an alternative to the simple spraying of local anesthetic described above. The advantage of the aerosol method is that 5 mL of 4% nebulized lidocaine can potentially anesthetize the entire airway without needling or much cooperation if given by mask. If it works, nebulized lidocaine is the best method to avoid coughing during LA administration; however this technique is time consuming, has variable effectiveness, and is associated with variable local anesthetic absorption; thus higher doses are required.[110,130]

"Spray as You Go" Technique

This method is for patients with incomplete or no GPN, SLN, and/or transtracheal block(s). Quick pulses of 1 mL of 2% to 4% lidocaine from a syringe attached to the FIS working channel are injected onto areas requiring further LA. It is best to avoid using suction concomitantly as this will lead to reduced local anesthetic dispersion. To avoid obscured movement views from reactions to sprays, attach the syringe to a three-way stopcock on a taped epidural catheter (0.5- to 1-mm diameter; single distal hole) threaded through the suction port until extending 1 to 2 cm beyond the FIS tip (Fig. 24.19). Epidural catheters mimic the effect of small pediatric FIS channel diameters, causing jet-like flows that require smaller 0.2-mL pulses.

Invasive Techniques

External Approach to Superior Laryngeal Nerve Block

We do not recommend the routine use of invasive approaches to airway topicalization beyond expert hands. This is because they have been associated with higher plasma concentrations of local anesthetic, local anesthetic systemic toxicity, and lower patient comfort,[131–133] as well as carrying risks of causing hematomas, potentially worsening airway compromise, and increasing the complexity of the entire procedure. Moreover, the effectiveness of minimally invasive techniques means that the necessity for invasive approaches is less apparent. Finally, the use of landmark

approaches, while useful, is probably now superseded by ultrasound-guided techniques, allowing the visualization of structures of interest that one hopes to either access or avoid. However, it is useful for readers to have a full understanding of the benefits and landmark-guided techniques of invasive approaches.

The SLN approach is particularly advantageous if intraoral chances of success are less, including in patient situations with no oral cavity entry and that only permit a few quick peritonsillar sprays (e.g., limited cooperation); to rescue failed gel, spray, aerosol, or nebulized internal SLN block; if coughing or hemodynamic changes from FIS "spray as you go" are inadvisable; or to prevent severe laryngospasm episodes that might have been experienced previously with intraoral LA.

The easiest technique is with 6 mL of 1% lidocaine in a 10-mL syringe attached to a 21- or 22-gauge needle as an injection system while aiming for a hyoid cornu (Fig. 24.20). After the needle tip hits the bone, shift the nondominant hand to brace the system at the hub against the neck. Aspirate gently. If no blood returns, inject 3 mL slowly. Repeat on the other side. Constant aspiration and bracing are vital and easily avoid intravascular injection (especially intracarotid), similar to regional blocks (e.g., interscalene). This approach has a lower incidence of complications, such as laryngospasm or gagging, compared with topical LA techniques.

An uncommon intraoral SLN block method involves putting pressure in the piriform fossa with a lidocaine-soaked gauze on a forceps, requiring up to 20 minutes to take effect.

Transtracheal Block

Of all the invasive topicalization techniques, this is probably the most. Of course, transtracheal blocks (TTBs) provide excellent

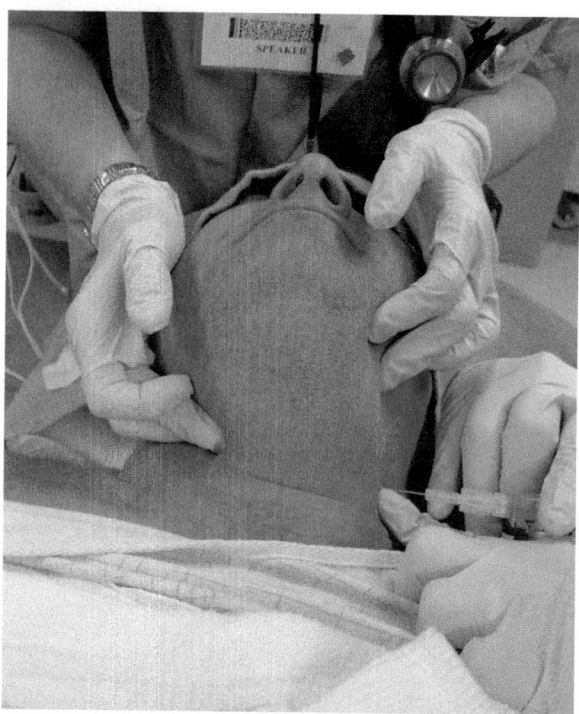

• **Fig. 24.20** Superior laryngeal nerve block. The assistant holds pressure on the right hyoid cornu while the operator directs the local anesthetic 22-gauge needle at the left hyoid cornu.

intratracheal anesthesia. However, other benefits include developing expertise in locating the cricothyroid membrane (CTM) by manual assessment (an immediate test for accuracy is the aspiration of many bubbles) or ultrasound (which is more accurate than manual palpation alone (Fig. 24.21).[134,135]

This skill extends to emergency cricothyrotomy situations, with potential life-saving benefits. Poor ability to detect the CTM was evident in the 4th National Audit Project (NAP4), which reported a 43% to 64% cricothyrotomy failure rate in emergencies.[136] Before this, Elliott and colleagues demonstrated that

accurate CTM assessment by the equivalent of experienced residents and attending faculty was only 30%, with poorer estimates mostly dependent on female gender or obesity.[137] Aslani and colleagues later pointed out that 46 of 56 female patients had an incorrect evaluation of the CTM up to 1.6 cm laterally, 2.5 cm superiorly, and 4 cm inferiorly.[138] One in 16 obese patients had correct identification. These results indicate that, as frequently as possible, clinicians should be encouraged to perform TTBs. The use of ultrasound is a significant advancement in this setting, and success rates have increased substantially with the assistance of this imaging modality.[134,135]

Tips for TTB success include the following: with two hands, aspirate gently with a posterior aim to enter the CTM, to avoid vocal cords; keep aspirating air until after maximal patient exhalation, brace, and continuously inject. It causes a minimal cough, followed by a huge breath that spreads the LA and more coughing. Needle technique advantages: (1) is faster than an angiocatheter method; (2) has fewer steps; (3) is less likely to provoke coughing or injury caused by hitting the posterior tracheal wall while threading the catheter (some like to fully thread it like an IV); and (4) is more successful (needles are shorter, less flexible, and, even if pulled out of the trachea, can be advanced easily). Using a needle rather than an angiocatheter is advocated by various authors.[139]

Is coughing during TTB a problem in cervical spine–risk patients? According to Todd[140] and Crosby,[141] the answer is no. They advise that concern about TTB is unfounded; because of those who coughed, none has ever been shown to develop secondary neurologic damage.

Which technique(s) is/are best? With regard to the occurrence of coughing during FIS insertion, in comparison studies between TTB and "spray as you go," patients in the TTB group reacted far less, according to Webb and colleagues.[142] Gupta and colleagues demonstrated a better result with TTB as well, when comparing it with nebulized LA.[143] This study was associated with much less gagging and laryngospasm in the TTB group, even though a lidocaine gargle had been used for everyone. Others have also found that a combination translaryngeal, SLN, and GPN block was better than nebulization, with fewer reactions, less grimacing, or fewer hemodynamic changes.[144,145] El-Boghdadly et al.

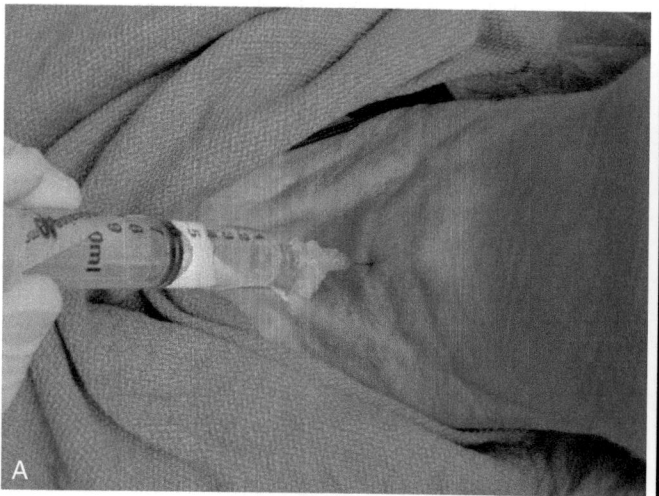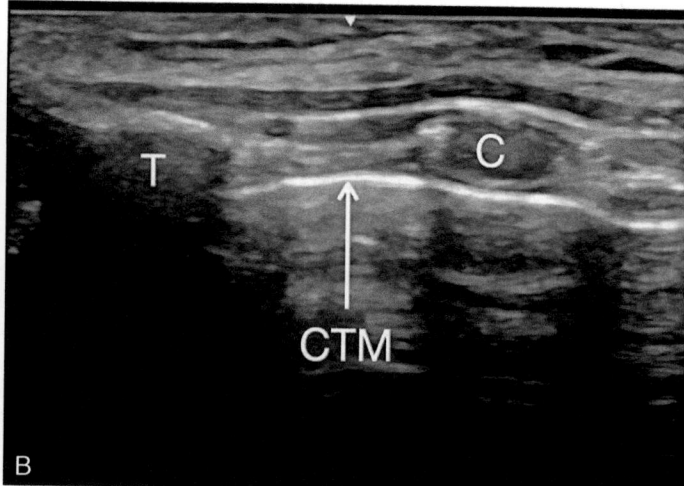

• **Fig. 24.21** (A) Transtracheal block. The operator braces his or her hand on the patient's chest while aspirating for air through the cricothyroid membrane. (B) Sagittal plane ultrasound image of the cricothyroid membrane, where left is cranial and right is caudal. *C,* Cricoid cartilage; *CTM,* cricothyroid membrane; *T,* thyroid cartilage;.

demonstrated that the use of a spray-only technique in conjunction with MADgic glottic spraying is associated with a high success rate and low complication rate.[107] It is therefore our opinion, as well as that of the Difficult Airway Society,[146] that this noninvasive approach should be the most widely practiced, with more advanced techniques reserved for specialist hands (Video 24.1).

Nasopharyngeal Topicalization Techniques

The route for tracheal intubation should factor in patient anatomy, surgical access, and extubation plan. For example, in patients with limited mouth opening the nasal approach may be the only option, while in patients having nasal surgery, the oral approach may be the preferred route. There is also no evidence favoring the superiority of the oral route when compared with a nasal route, or vice versa.[147,148] Therefore the nasal approach remains an invaluable route for tracheal intubation that readers should be familiar with.

Topicalization involves the administration of both a local anesthetic agent to render the nasopharynx (NP), posterior pharyngeal wall, and periglottic area insensate and a vasoconstrictor to reduce the risk of bleeding and maximize the caliber of the NP. Oropharyngeal topicalization is still required to ensure the larynx and trachea are also anesthetized. This is most easily achieved with the use of co-phenylcaine spray, which is composed of 2.5-mL lidocaine 5% with phenylephrine 0.5%. This can be delivered using a nasal mucosal atomizing device (Fig. 24.22). First, one should select the nasal passage with the greatest luminal size by asking the patient to sniff through each nare; the one with the least subjective restriction to inspiration should be used in the first instance unless otherwise indicated. Regardless of luminal caliber, when topicalizing, apply them to both nasal passages to avoid delays in having to anesthetize the other side if the first is too small. Then co-phenylcaine is sprayed synchronously to a deep "sniff" by the patient to ensure appropriate dispersion. It is usual for patients to experience a "trickle" of the local anesthetic spray in the back of

their throat. This approach is simple, rapid, and well tolerated by patients.

There are alternative approaches to nasopharyngeal topicalization. For example, one may use two Q-tips per nostril dipped in either phenylephrine, in oxymetazoline mixed with lidocaine, or in plain cocaine. Apply every single swab in succession to the outermost part within the nostril, using a fingertip on the stick end to gently push inward perpendicularly to the facial plane until feeling slight resistance (Video 24.4). By the fourth Q-tip, vasoconstriction onset will allow sequential pushing farther in with each in a similar fashion until a point of no resistance posteriorly. This facilitates gauging the NP caliber for ETT passage. Midway through the process, pulse in 0.2 mL of solution with a 20-gauge angiocatheter (needle removed) in each of three different directions per nostril to minimize trauma. This uses a total of 2 mL of solution (e.g., 80 mg of 4% cocaine). It is notable that the use of cocaine for this purpose is reducing given that it is associated with cardiovascular complications and does not lead to a superior effect when compared with phenylephrine or oxymetazoline.[149–152]

Alternative techniques involve using NPAs coated in lidocaine gel and phenylephrine. Some suggest that inserting progressively larger NPAs can mechanically dilate the NP passage. However, Adamson and colleagues reported that this method only caused increased trauma, hemorrhage, and delay of intubation,[153] and therefore this practice should be avoided.

Local Anesthetic Drug Choices

LA dosing for various airway blocks is listed in Table 24.2. It is not recommended to use LA brands containing benzocaine because of methemoglobinemia risk (Hurricaine, Exactacain).[154–156] Although methemoglobinemia instances were much more frequently reported in patients undergoing transesophageal echocardiography, some occurred among FSI-managed patients after

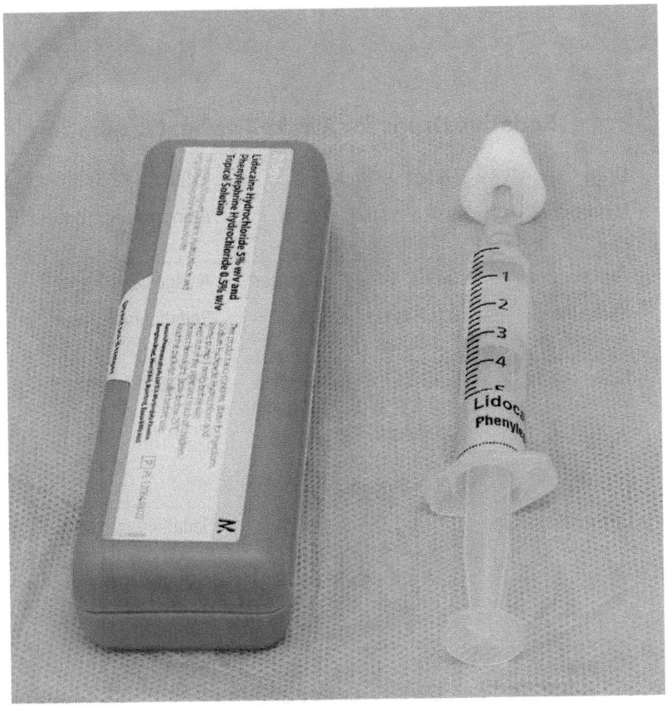

• **Fig. 24.22** Co-phenylcaine box drawn up into a 5-mL syringe with an attached nasal mucosal atomizer.

TABLE 24.2	Oropharyngeal Local Anesthesia	
Drug	**Form**	**Appropriate Blocks**
Lidocaine	Pacey's paste (slurry): 7 mL 2% solution + 7 mL 2% viscous in two syringes with 3 mL air each + sweetener (mix back and forth via three-way stopcock); should be swished intraorally in 2 aliquots	
	2%–4% solution	All blocks except as listed below
	1% solution	Preferred for SLN neck blocks
	4% solution	Preferred for transtracheal blocks
	2% viscous lidocaine	Intraoral or nasopharyngeal
	2%–5% gel/ointment/paste	Intraoral
Tessalon Perle (benzonatate)	200-mg capsule	Intraoral

SLN, Superior laryngeal nerve.

unlimited, continuous spraying.[156] Lidocaine is the most commonly used LA for topicalization in this setting and is associated with a safer and more predictable cardiovascular and systemic toxicity risk profile.[157] The dose of topical lidocaine should not exceed 9 mg/kg lean body weight, as higher doses are associated with a significantly increased risk of toxicity.[158] The total dose of all local anesthetics delivered, regardless of the route (e.g., regional anesthesia or surgical infiltration), must also be considered. In terms of selecting the appropriate concentrations of local anesthetic to use there has been some evidence that lower concentrations of lidocaine are as effective as higher concentrations, but higher concentrations may be associated with more rapid onset of airway anesthesia.[159-161] A high index of suspicion of the rare possibility of local anesthetic systemic toxicity should be in place[162] (Box 24.4).

Sedation

ATI may be safely and effectively performed without sedation.[110,111] However, its use may reduce patient anxiety and discomfort and increase procedural tolerance. Sedatives have both desirable (e.g., amnesia) and detrimental effects (e.g., oversedation), and the risks of the latter may lead to respiratory depression, airway loss, hypoxia, aspiration, and cardiovascular instability. It could therefore be beneficial to have an independent anesthesiologist delivering, monitoring, and titrating sedation. Targeting a Ramsay sedation scale level 3 or 4 is ideal (Box 24.5). A single-sedative strategy is likely to be the safest approach, but if multiple agents are used, this is further reason to have an independent practitioner taking responsibility for safe sedation.

The choice of appropriate sedative drugs is critical. Remifentanil and dexmedetomidine are associated with high levels of patient satisfaction and low risk of oversedation and airway obstruction when used for ATI.[163] Dexmedetomidine provides sedation, analgesia, hemodynamic stability, antisialagogue effects, and amnesia.

It is administered as a 0.7- to 1.0-μg/kg bolus over 10 minutes, followed by a 0.5- to 1.0-μg/kg/h infusion. Remifentanil provides analgesia and antitussive effects and is administered as a 0.05- to 0.1-μg/kg bolus followed by a 0.03- to 0.1-μg/kg/min infusion. Alternatively, a target-controlled infusion of 1–3 ng/mL using a Minto model may be used.

Propofol is associated with a significant risk of respiratory depression and unresponsiveness, with there being a fine line between nonsedative effects and respiratory depression. More precisely titrated sedation may be administered with target-controlled infusions. Propofol and remifentanil have been studied most extensively.[164] Mean target plasma concentrations for propofol and remifentanil were 1.3 μg/mL (standard deviation, 0.2 μg/mL) and 3.2 ng/mL (SD, 0.2 ng/mL), respectively. Rai and colleagues found no difference in patient satisfaction between the two while noting better ATI conditions and a higher recall incidence with remifentanil than with propofol.[165] Similar results were reported by Cafiero and colleagues.[166] Surprisingly, with remifentanil alone, up to 100% of patients had a recall of events, usually not perceived as unpleasant. In cervical trauma patients a remifentanil effect site concentration as low as 0.8 ng/mL was effective for ATI.[167] Very short induction and recovery times with remifentanil may represent a major advantage. Possibilities of increased thoracic wall rigidity and laryngospasm should be kept in mind.[168]

Other sedatives may be used but are associated with inferior safety and efficacy when compared with dexmedetomidine and remifentanil (Table 24.3).

Antisialagogues

Antisialagogues have traditionally been used to reduce secretions to improve FIS views, dilute LA, and reduce the risk of laryngospasm. However, their use is not mandatory in ATI as they may be associated with undesirable clinical consequences and must be administered well in advance of the ATI (Table 24.4).

BOX 24.4 Nasopharyngeal Drug Therapy Before Intubation Using a Flexible Intubation Scope

Vasoconstriction
  Phenylephrine 0.5% spray
  Oxymetazoline 0.05% spray
Local anesthesia
  Lidocaine 2%–4% spray, gel, viscous, paste
Both vasoconstriction and local anesthesia
  Cocaine 4% with a maximum dose of 1.5 mg/kg104
  Mixture of 2%–4% lidocaine (3 mL) + 0.5% phenylephrine (1 mL) or 0.05% oxymetazoline (1 mL)

BOX 24.5 Ramsay Sedation Scale

1. Patient is anxious and agitated, restless, or both.
2. Patient is cooperative, oriented, and tranquil.
3. Patient responds to commands only.
4. Patient exhibits brisk response to light glabellar tap or loud auditory stimulus.
5. Patient exhibits a sluggish response to light glabellar tap or loud auditory stimulus.
6. Patient exhibits no response.

TABLE 24.3 Sedative Drugs for Awake Tracheal Intubation

Drug	Dose	Effects
Midazolam	0.015- to 0.03-mg/kg boluses	Amnesia/sedation
Fentanyl	0.7- to 1.5-μg/kg boluses	Analgesia/antitussive
Ketamine	0.07- to 0.15-mg/kg boluses	Sedation/analgesia
Remifentanil	0.05- to 0.1-μg/kg bolus; 0.03- to 0.1-μg/kg/min infusion Or TCI 1–3 ng/mL	Analgesia/antitussive
Dexmedetomidine	0.7- to 1.0-μg/kg bolus over 10 min, followed by 0.5- to 1.0-μg/kg/h infusion	Sedation/analgesia/ hemodynamic stability/ antisialagogue/ amnesia
Propofol	25- to 75-μg/kg bolus; 25- to 75-μg/kg/min infusion	Sedation

TABLE 24.4	Antisialagogues for awake tracheal intubation				
Drug	Onset	Duration of Action	Terminal Elimination Half-life	Dosing	Notes
Glycopyrrolate	20 min (IM)	30–60 min	40–80 min	0.2–0.4 mg	Administer 30–60 min preprocedure
	3–5 min (IV)	30–60 min	40–80 min	0.1–0.2 mg	May produce significant tachycardia
Atropine	20 min (IM)	30–60 min	2 h	0.3–0.6 mg	Administer 30–60 min preprocedure—less commonly used than glycopyrronium bromide due to tachycardia
	2–3 min (IV)	30–60 min	2 h	0.2–0.3 mg	May produce significant tachycardia
Hyoscine	30 min (IM) 5–10 min (IV)	4 h	5 h	0.2–0.6 mg	Administer 30–60 min preprocedure Longer-lasting systemic effects than glycopyrrolate and atropine May produce tachycardia, dizziness, and sedation

Procedural Performance

Preparation for ATI should follow sequentially, while adjustments are made according to individual concerns (see Box 24.6). The use of a checklist is beneficial (Fig. 24.23), and constant communication with patients is mandatory. After timely antisialagogue administration (if used), early application of oxygen, and administration of LA with or without sedatives, move the bed/table to its lowest setting, if supine. If ATI is performed facing the patient, sit the patient upright while elevating the legs slightly to reduce the risk of the patient drifting down the bed. Ramping patients with blankets is possible but not ideal (Fig. 24.24).[169] A step stool may be useful to keep the FIS straight and reduce strain on the operator's arms.

Throughout the process, operators must constantly think about optimizing the key elements of ATI: oxygenation, topicalization, sedation, and procedural performance. Oxygen should be up-titrated throughout the procedure, and if using HFNO, this should increase to 60 L/min. Careful, accurate, and dose-calculated LA should be administered without rush while appropriate and titrated sedation delivered simultaneously, if used. Once the planned topicalization strategy is complete, the sensation of the oropharynx should be tested with a Yankauer sucker, which would also simultaneously clear secretions. A wide-bore soft suction catheter may be advanced in the midline through the oropharynx and then further advanced into the trachea by asking the patient to inspire while advancing the catheter. This will allow both the assessment of the extent of topicalization and suctioning secretions. If the patient gags, GPN anesthesia is lacking, whereas if coughing occurs, SLN anesthesia is inadequate, presenting a good opportunity to apply further LA.

Oral Approach

For an oral route, the patient can be asked to open their mouth and protrude their tongue, after which a bronchoscope airway (VBM Medical Inc., Noblesville, IN) or a Berman IOA can be inserted in the midline. If the patient is unable to protrude their tongue, an assistant can grasp the anterior and posterior surfaces of the tongue with gauze to gently pull it outward but not tear the frenulum linguae.[170] This often lifts the tongue off the palate and elevates the epiglottis (Fig. 24.25).

Many experts recommend holding the FIS handle with a non-dominant hand, because thumb pressures on the lever and forefinger depression of the suction valve are not as intricate movements as directing the bronchoscope tip with the dominant hand.[171] To prevent the ETT from sliding down, gently snug it fully up the bronchoscope, tape it in place with the connecter, or use an ETT-holding element if the bronchoscope has one (Fig. 24.26). Before you begin, gently warm the tip of the bronchoscope on the patient's tongue to reduce the risk of misting, then ensure the tip is wiped clean. Control the bronchoscope as it advances through the mouth, keeping it midline with the dominant hand's thumb and first two fingers, similar to a pen. Brace the fourth and fifth fingers on the IOA, lip, or cheek to avoid tremulous motion and eye injuries.

To reduce endoscopist fatigue, employ a gentle curve in the bronchoscopy by bending the handle control arm's elbow very near to one's anterolateral rib cage so that the handle hand is relaxed by the shoulder unless the arm-straight-out style is preferred.

Insert the bronchoscope into the patient's mouth, down the IOA, while keeping the demarcation between IOA and mucosa colors in the center of view. Use the lever to look up or down while turning the bronchoscope (using both hands in unison) to

• BOX 24.6 General Plan of Patient Preparation for Awake Flexible Scope Intubation

1. Check FIS equipment.
   - Choose FIS diameter closest in size to ETT diameter (keep lubricant available).
   - Attach to electricity and light source, adjusting according to FIS instructions.
   - Test FIS lever, tip motion, clarity, and focus by looking at nearby printed object.
   - Choose ETT size at least one-half size smaller if a difficult airway is present.
   - Use defogger as needed and insert FIS and ETT into warm irrigation bottle.
2. Interview and examine patient; discuss the plan (psychological preparation).
3. Administer antisialagogue at least 15 minutes before giving topical oral LA.
4. Administer sedative intravenously if not contraindicated, and possibly LA.
5. Administer sodium citrate if small aspiration risk is present.
6. If patient is going to the operating room, on arrival, place monitors.
7. Administer oxygen by cannula, unless patient is healthy and listening to Spo₂ preferred.
8. Start or finish LA administration, and titrate sedatives/opioids as indicated.
9. Position the patient: if supine, lower the bed maximally. If sitting, locate equipment where optimal, keeping in mind that some FISs have adjustable arrow indicators.

ETT, Endotracheal tube; *FIS*, flexible intubation scope; *LA*, local anesthetic.

1. Location ....

2. Appropriate staff present

   Anaesthetic assistant ☐   Second anaesthetist ☐
                                              monitoring, sedation, anaesthesia

   Other ....

3. Team briefed

   Procedure outline ☐   Role allocation ☐

   Plan for failure ☐

4. ATI device selected, prepared and checked

   Tube *(type/size)* ....

Flexible bronchoscope ☐	Videolaryngoscope ☐
Route	**Device/blade**
Optional adjuncts	**Optional adjuncts**
Oral airway ☐ Suction ☐	Stylet ☐
SAD ☐ Mucosal atomiser ☐	Suction ☐
	Bougie ☐
Aintree catheter ☐ Epidural catheter ☐	Mucosal atomiser ☐
Device check	**Device check**
Focus ☐ Tube correctly loaded ☐	Lubricated ☐
White balance ☐ Image orientation ☐	Anti-fog/wiped ☐
Lubricated ☐	Tube correctly loaded ☐
Anti-fog/wiped ☐ Battery/power ☐	Battery/power ☐

5. Oxygenation ....

6. Sedation *(if required)* ....

7. Topicalisation

Nose .... Oropharynx .... Larynx .... Trachea ....

Vasoconstrictor *(if required)* .... Antisialagogue *(if used)* ....

> **Maximum** lidocaine dose
> ____ kg × 9 mg.kg^{-1} = ____ mg
>
> **Planned** lidocaine dose
> ____ sprays of 10%   ____ mg
> ____ ml of 2%   ____ mg
> ____ ml of 4%   ____ mg

8. Setup position

Operator ☐	Patient ☐	Monitor ☐	Suction ☐
Pumps ☐	Step ☐	Airway Trolley ☐	Bed ☐

• **Fig. 24.23** Example of a checklist for awake tracheal intubation produced by the Difficult Airway Society. (© Difficult Airway Society 2019.)

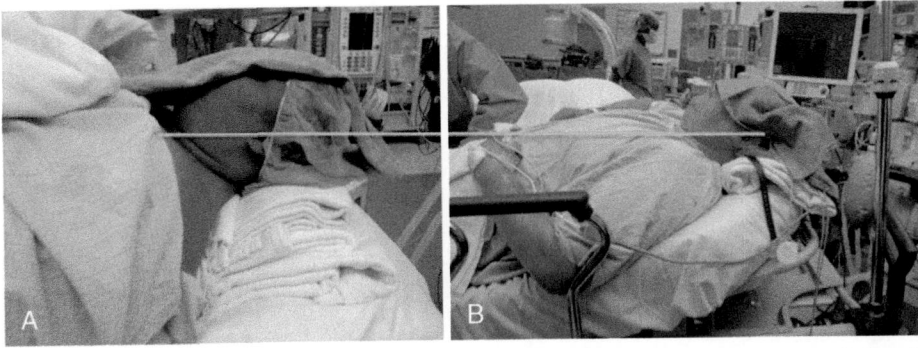

• **Fig. 24.24** Comparison of positions for intubation in patients with increased body mass index. (A) Ramping with multiple blankets, which need to be situated and then removed after intubation. (B) More simplistic back-up bed position. Reverse Trendelenburg or back-up positions are used to align the external auditory meatus with the sternal notch (*blue line*). Following intubation, the bed is easily returned to normal.

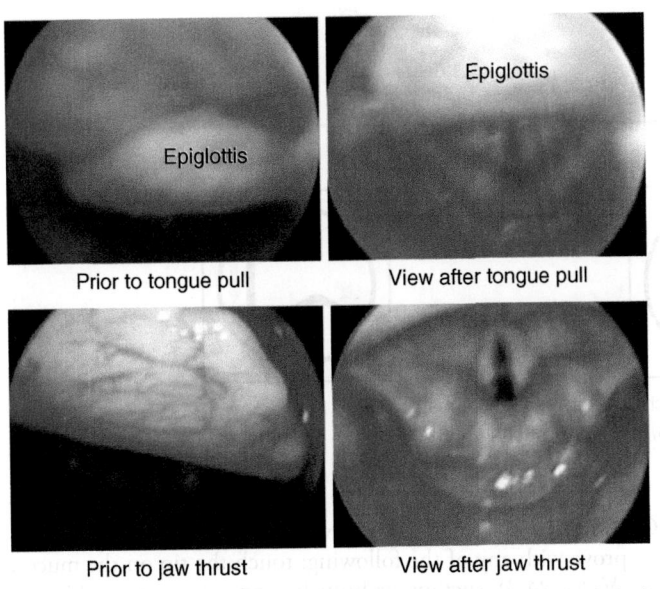

Epiglottis

Epiglottis

Prior to tongue pull   View after tongue pull

Prior to jaw thrust   View after jaw thrust

• **Fig. 24.25** Effects of tongue pull and jaw thrust on epiglottic and glottic views.

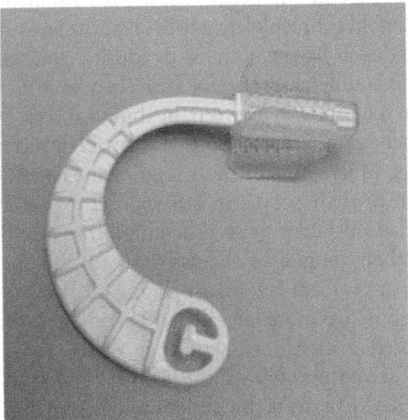

• **Fig. 24.26** BiteGard for dental and fiberoptic bronchoscope protection is inserted between the premolars.

look left or right; always keeping known anatomy in the center. Go around obstacles, such as secretions, or suction them. Slowly insert the bronchoscope perpendicularly toward the pharynx 6 to 8 cm, past the palate and the uvula, and move the lever to look for the epiglottis and glottis. Jaw thrust or asking the patient to phonate and protrude their tongue often helps lift the epiglottis.[172,173] For severely limited mouth opening, retromolar entry is often possible. Then consider the three successive directions.

Three Successive Directions for Flexible Bronchoscope Guidance

Airway specialists are familiar with the upper airway configuration, as routinely observed with a laryngoscope. On the other hand, the different axes successively followed plus the structures involved during bronchoscopic intubation and their reciprocal spatial organization are less emphasized in classic teaching programs. Moreover, many medical textbook sketches or drawings are inaccurate, depicting the upper airways as a regularly curved line joining the oropharynx or NP to the carina. This is misleading, because three successive directions must be followed to reach the trachea from the nasal or the oral route.[169] These successive directions in the supine patient are (1) downward to the oropharyngeal or nasopharyngeal posterior wall; (2) upward to the vocal cords' anterior commissure; and (3) downward again into the laryngeal and tracheal lumen to the carina (Fig. 24.27). That is: down, up, and down again (Video 24.2).[171] These same movements are applicable regardless of patient position.

When performing an orotracheal flexible bronchoscopy, it can be difficult to stay in the median sagittal plane, particularly when pharyngeal obstructive flaccidity is present. The difficulty may be overcome with an IOA, assistant aid, or FIS insertion through an SGA while aiming downward to get to the point of upward tip flexion to view the glottis.

During the second phase, while slowly advancing toward the anterior commissure, the posterior part of the glottic aperture will come into view. Continue toward the anterior commissure by keeping the tip of the device in a sharp upward/anterior path. In the absence of anatomic distortions resist the temptation to push the bronchoscope unswervingly in this direction. When the anterior commissure is very close, angle the tip in the third direction, downward toward the widest opening of the larynx. This maneuver aligns the bronchoscope with the anatomic axis of the larynx successively in its supraglottic and infraglottic segments, avoiding contact damage to the mucosa and arytenoid cartilages.

Follow the third direction into the trachea until the tip lies two to three rings above the carina. Do not provoke coughing by being too close to it (often is not anesthetized), but ensure you are able to visualize the carina.

At this point, stop looking at the screen/eyepiece. Instead, look at the patient to judge when the ETT tip is near the larynx. Hold

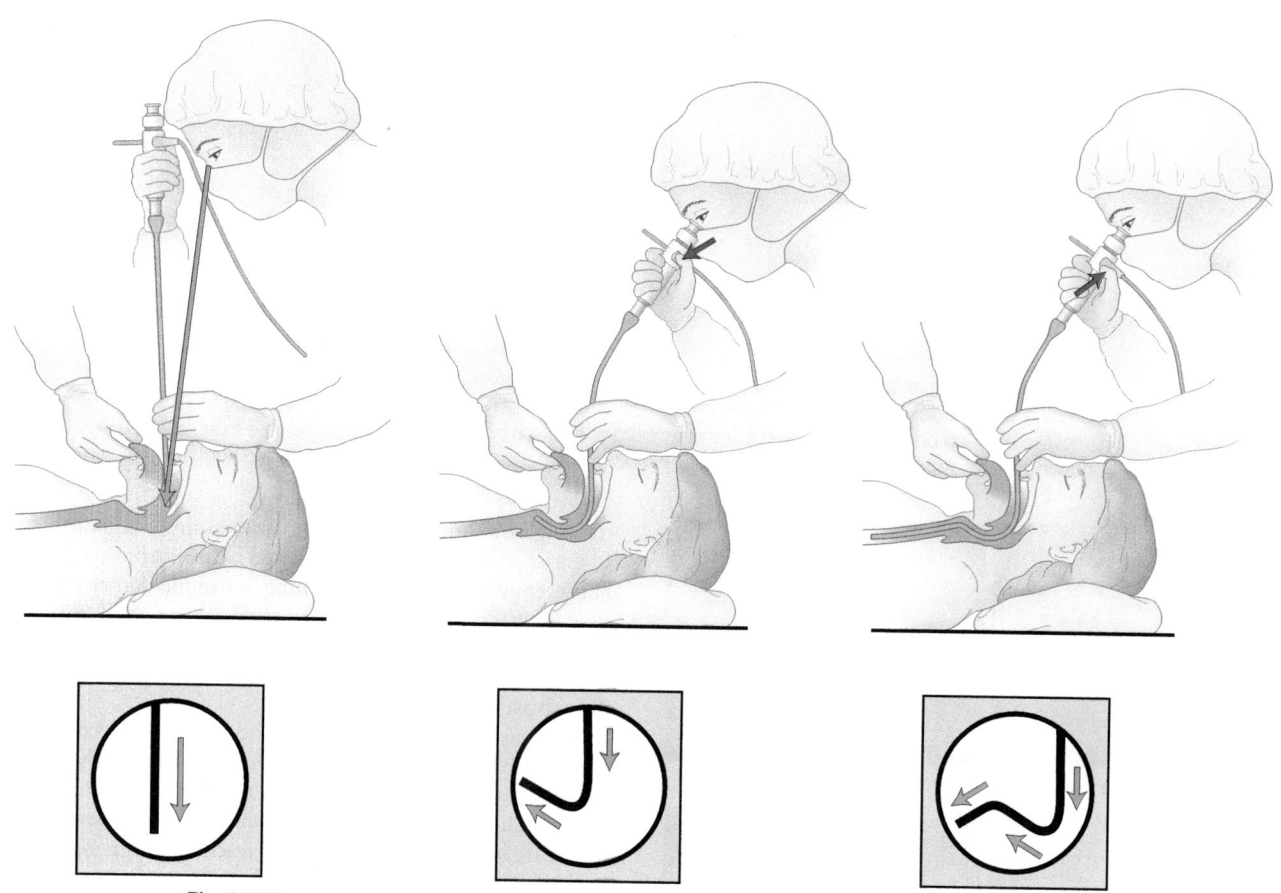

• **Fig. 24.27** Three directions in the anatomic approach to flexible scope intubation (*left to right*): downward into the pharynx, upward through the vocal cords, and downward into the trachea.

the bronchoscope immobile in your left hand and, with your right hand, slide the ETT forward with the Murphy eye oriented anteriorly if using a PVC ETT (a 90-degree rotation) to prevent it from getting hung up on the arytenoids (statistically, most frequent on the right).[170,174] Ask the patient to take a deep breath to open the vocal cords widely, and advance the ETT as you are rotating it. After judging that it is beyond the vocal cords, observe the screen to slide the ETT two to three rings above the carina. Gently inflate the ETT, stabilize it, and remove the bronchoscope by putting it straight into the used vertical holder or hand it to an assistant. Attach the ventilating system, check for P_{ETCO_2}, and secure the ETT. A two-point check is advocated before induction of anesthesia: (1) visualizing the ETT in the trachea and (2) confirming P_{ETCO_2}. Without either of these checks, proceeding with GA might not be safe.

At any point from the mouth to the trachea, if nothing is recognizable, back up slightly to look around with slow lever motions until anatomic structures are familiar, then proceed again. For very difficult ETT insertions, it is worthwhile to recheck the secured ETT with the bronchoscope, especially after patient positioning, which may cause ETT movement.

Here are some scenarios and suggestions on how to deal with issues.

Question. What do I do when the patient is too sleepy before the FIS insertion and I can't grab the tongue? Reduce the level of sedation and ask the patient to stick out their tongue. You may also consider applying large suction tubing to it. Slowly draw it out, until grasped with gauze.

Question. The bronchoscope view isn't clear. Is it fog? It may improve with any of the following: touch the tip on the mucosa (Video 24.3); suction via bronchoscope or separate tubing, or both; check the focus dial or eyepiece. If unsolved, remove the bronchoscope and clean the tip by carefully holding the tip tightly near its end and gently wiping it with alcohol.

Question. What if I can't look laterally because the lever only moves the tip up and down? Rotate both hands equally, clockwise for right (if supine) and counterclockwise for left. Then lever it. As an alternative, loosen the handgrip between the thumb and two fingers on the distal bronchoscope insertion section to avoid bronchoscope torque and damage while simultaneously rotating the handle.

Question. The bronchoscope tip is stuck on the posterior pharynx. What do I do if I can't get by the epiglottis? Ask the patient to stick out their tongue or the assistant to pull the tongue out more and/or perform jaw thrust (Fig. 24.25). As an alternative, try moving the tip more laterally and caudally to angle in under the epiglottis or assist with another airway device to lift the epiglottis (see combo with DL [25], ETT [24], stylet).

Question. What do I do if the patient keeps gagging or coughing as the bronchoscope advances? Consider correcting inadequate LA blocks, or use the "spray as you go" technique.

Question. What do I do if the patient has too many secretions and/or blood and I can't see? Use one or two suctions continuously. Direct a straightened FIA midline and posterior, equal to two-thirds of the mouth-to-ear distance. Turn the room lights down or off, angle the tip caudally, and use FIS light transillumination, similar to a lighted stylet (Fig. 24.28). Once

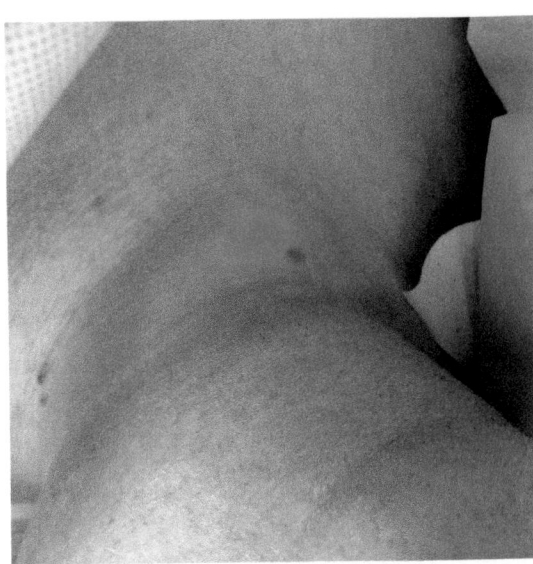

• **Fig. 24.28** Flexible intubation scope as a lighted stylet, used when no video is available for teaching or in soiled situations, shows brightness near the glottis.

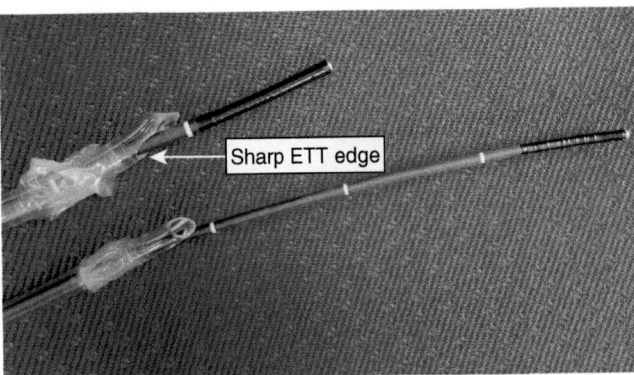

Sharp ETT edge

• **Fig. 24.29** Pediatric and adult flexible intubation scope (FIS) exiting endotracheal tube (ETT) through the Murphy eye. FIS withdrawal can result in a cut FIS sleeve by the ETT edge.

in the trachea, suction via the bronchoscope until tracheal or carina reaction is observed or those structures are visualized. If unsure, insert an epidural catheter down the working channel for Petco$_2$ analysis. There are a number of alternatives. (1) Use a VAL for ATI instead, allowing a wider field of view, easier ability to suction, and a lower probability of the image becoming obstructed. (2) Insert a second-generation SGA to seal the periglottic area. Suction the ventilating lumen of the SGAs, ventilate, and check the Petco$_2$ waveform. Advance a bronchoscope until near the carina. (3) Insert a long (≥80 cm) guidewire into the bronchoscope to extend it 3 cm past its tip. Tape it proximally. Tape the ETT to the FIS so that the FIS tip ends just before the ETT tip. With simultaneous oral suctioning, the FIS may stay clear of the soiling, and the wire may be directed to the glottis. Once it goes 8 cm past the glottis, quickly advance the FIS and then the ETT. Rapidly inflate and suction the ETT. (4) Use retrograde-flexible scope–assisted intubation (see Combinations). (5) At any point, if oxygenation, ventilation, or aspiration threatens, consider a surgical airway.

Question. What do I do if the bronchoscope passes the glottis and I can see rings? The airway is getting very narrow and the patient is getting agitated and desaturating a bit. It may be a compromised airway. Tracheal stenosis or obstructive pathology causes inadequate room around the bronchoscope for ventilation. Do not insufflate oxygen through the bronchoscope in case ventilation volumes cannot exit (pneumothorax risk). Speed up the process to intubation and remove the FIS as soon as possible. Alternatively, if an adult FIS was used, remove it and use a pediatric one.

Question. What do I do if the bronchoscope is clearly right above the carina but I can't slide the ETT into the trachea? Withdraw the ETT 1 to 2 cm, keep the convex side right, and advance with a rotational movement while asking the patient to take a deep breath. If unsuccessful, apply tongue pull/jaw thrust, repeat, and/or rotate the ETT 180 degrees clockwise the other way. Han's study found that these maneuvers could double success rates for first-attempt ETT passage with an FIS; oddly, sometimes, even releasing jaw thrust helps.[175] Alternatives include try-

ing slight cricoid pressure or neck flexion[126]; removing the FIS and trying a smaller ETT or a centrally curved, soft-tip ETT; inserting a pediatric FIS on an Aintree Intubation Catheter (Cook Medical Inc., Bloomington, IN) and sliding the ETT over both (lessens diameter disparity); or using a nasotracheal approach.

Question. I pushed the ETT forward after successfully placing an FIS. Despite every maneuver, the ETT wouldn't enter. What should I do? Back the bronchoscope out. If more than minimal resistance is felt, withdraw the bronchoscope/ETT carefully as a unit. The bronchoscope may have exited through the Murphy eye. Strong attempts at removing the FIS can damage the outer skin as a result of catching sharp Murphy eye edges (Fig. 24.29). However, the ETT may be too big. In this case remove the scope and start again using a different approach.

Nasotracheal Bronchoscopic Intubation Technique

Use a lubricated ETT at least a half-size smaller than that used for the oral route. A north-facing, ivory PVC Portex® nasal tube (Smiths Medical, Minneapolis, MN) and a microlaryngeal tube are safe, easy to insert, and effective ETT options for nasotracheal intubation. Preblock preparation is similar to that done orally, although antisialagogues are not as important if intraoral LA is not used. Insert a well-lubricated FIS one of three ways: (1) initially for a distance of 12 to 15 cm while steering through the darkest regions within the nasopharynx (NP) until the glottis is seen; (2) through an inserted, lubricated breakaway NPA until as close as possible to the carina (then direct an assistant to remove the NPA and advance the FIS more); or (3) after placing an ETT into the posterior NP. The last method is least preferred because of Mishra and colleagues' report of a fourfold risk for epistaxis and FIS exiting through the Murphy eye.[176]

After locating the carina, the procedure is similar to oral FSI except for ETT rotation. Direct the ETT leading edge along the septum to help prevent evisceration of the turbinates. On the right, keep the convex side facing anteriorly until arriving at the posterior NP. Then rotate it 180 degrees. On the left, keep the convex side posterior. Either way, when close to the glottic entry, rotate ETTs 90 degrees over the bronchoscope to avoid impingement.

Alternatively, insert a PVC ETT with a lubricated, slightly protruding nasogastric or suction tube to fill its lumen to prevent the leading ETT edge from causing injury (Fig. 24.30).

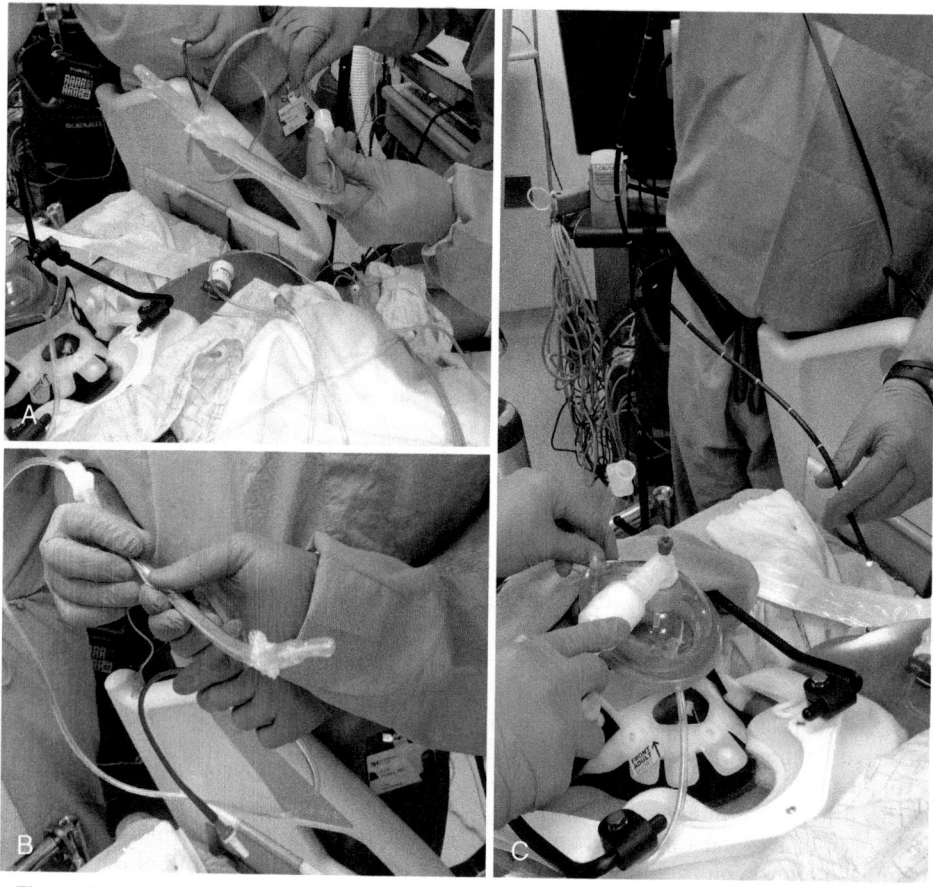

• **Fig. 24.30** (A) Cervical spine risk patient with halo; nasogastric tube within a preformed nasal endo-tracheal tube (ETT). (B) Lubricant applied. (C) Postinsertion ETT left in place for flexible bronchoscope insertion.

Oral or Nasal Flexible Bronchoscopic Intubation in Asleep Patients

During Routine General Anesthesia

There are two types of asleep FSIs: elective and indicated. A purely elective FSI can always be used in patients with normal airways. It is considered acceptable and ethical because it can be used routinely by many professionals, and patients need not be informed beforehand.[177]

Indicated asleep FSI may be chosen only if face-mask ventilation (FMV) is expected to be relatively easy in patients with an amalgam of mild to moderate tracheal intubation risk with or without comorbidity risk that could be adversely impacted by difficult alternative airway device management and an ATI is deemed inappropriate.

Preparation steps have been described previously. Because tissue laxity can obscure the airway, choose a half-size-smaller ETT and a partially head-up position. Preoxygenate with 5 to 10 cm HO CPAP. After the induction of anesthesia, muscle relaxant administration, and FMV is established, request the assistant to perform tongue pull, hold the IOA (if oral approach), and/or perform jaw thrust, and keep track of time. Proceed with FSI as described (Videos 24.3 and 24.5). Between attempts, return to FMV and check anesthetic/relaxant levels. Alternatively, use an FSI combination method (see combo with many devices: e.g., SGA [25], DL [25], VAL [26]). The use of high-flow nasal oxygenation during asleep FSI is increasingly being used as this prolongs the safe apnea time and may also increase airway patency at high flows, making FSI easier.

Flexible Scope Intubation in Unconscious, Unanesthetized Patients

For emergency intubation in unconscious, unanesthetized patients, ideally, all equipment is available. VAL is the ideal approach in this setting, but in the scenario of failed VAL or limited access to the oropharynx FSI may be indicated. Only the most experienced bronchoscopists should make attempts. Give descriptive directions to assistants who are often inexperienced in urgent cases. Assume a full stomach, use supplementary oxygen, consider cricoid pressure if this is local standard practice, and maximize helpful airway maneuvers.

Combination Techniques: Devices Combined With Flexible Intubation Scopes

Awake or under GA, an FIS can be combined with almost every airway device to accomplish multiple goals: intubation, diagnosis, therapy, and rescue.

Intubation: An SGA helps seal off laryngeal areas from extrinsic blood and accomplish ventilation in patients with intraoral bleeding and the potential for difficult FMV and/or intubation. Its blind ETT insertion success rate is moderately high (90% to 96.2% for up to three attempts or adjusting maneuvers).[178–180] An FIS-SGA combination, however, changes this to a controlled visual technique with success rates up to 100% in Ferson and colleagues' study.[181]

Diagnosis and therapy: During prone spinal surgeries, FIS examination through a swivel adapter can be used to determine the causes of rising airway pressures and sometimes help in treating them: e.g., suctioning secretions, repositioning endobronchial ETTs, or changing kinked ETTs (Fig. 24.9). For flexible bronchoscopy procedures such as endobronchial ultrasound (EBUS), bronchial and tracheal biopsies, and dilatations, an SGA can be placed, either awake or asleep, and then used as a conduit for the FIS via a swivel connector. This also allows for assisted ventilation during the procedure if required.

Rescue: In morbidly obese patients under GA common failed DL intubation scenarios occur, with Cormack-Lehane grade 3 and 4 views, despite the use of intubation guide catheters or bougies. Multiple attempts and tissue trauma result in deteriorating conditions, especially if FMV worsens. Sometimes, trying solo FIS or VAL rescues might be impeded. In combination, a DL or VAL can be used to elevate tissues away from the FIS path. The multimodal approach to the airway is increasingly accepted as flaws and inadequacies of individual airway devices or techniques become more apparent, and their failures, when used alone, are more frequently reported.[182–187]

Superficial Devices

Endoscopy Masks

During ATI, endoscopy masks provide oxygen administration and CPAP in respiratory-compromised patients, when a nasal cannula, nasal CPAP, or high-flow nasal oxygen (HFNO) is insufficient or impossible (Fig. 24.10). LA can be given during intermittent mask lifts while continuing supplementary oxygenation devices (especially high flow).

Prepare an ETT-loaded FIS with the 15-mm connector removed and kept safe. For oral intubation, insert the ETT-FIS unit through the mask port and IOA toward the larynx. After tracheal intubation, remove the FIS and mask and join the ETT and connector to the respiratory system. Alternatively, if urgent ventilation is needed, remove the mask later.

During asleep FSI, this mask affords more time, particularly during elective use. After induction, FMV, and IOA insertion, request an assistant to hold the mandible and strapped mask with 100% oxygen. With muscle relaxants, the assistant must be competent to maintain PPV. With no muscle relaxants, ensure relatively deep anesthesia (to prevent laryngospasm), or use a "spray as you go" LA method and follow the technique.

For nasotracheal intubation, initially insert the FIS well ahead of the ETT through the port. An ETT inserted beforehand or simultaneously may limit FIS maneuverability if the FIS route exiting the ETT is at odds with the direction of nasal passage entry and is therefore not recommended.

Bronchoscopy Swivel Adapters

For intubation purposes, under oxygen-enrichment conditions similar to those for an FIS–endoscopy mask, a successful combination is possible by using an FIS and a swivel adapter attached to a mask or SGA. Begin by inserting a pediatric FIS within an Aintree intubation catheter (ID 4.7 mm, OD 6.3 mm) through the swivel adapter port while the patient is breathing spontaneously or being ventilated (Fig. 24.31). Once the FIS enters the trachea and nears the carina, slide the Aintree over it two to three rings above the carina. Hold the Aintree securely while noting the depth of insertion, and remove the FIS. Slide a lubricated ETT (≥6.5 mm)–loaded FIS through the Aintree into the trachea, near

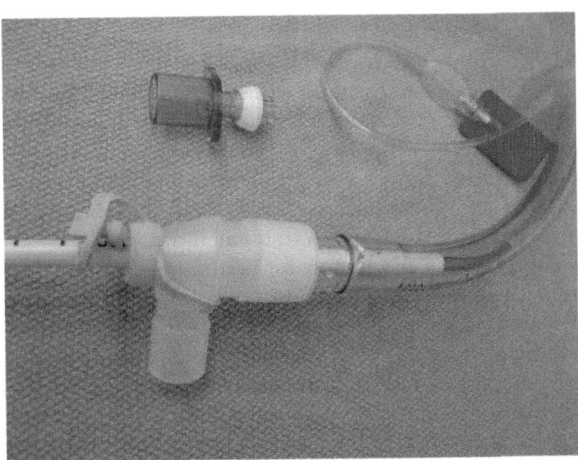

• **Fig. 24.31** Combination of a flexible intubation scope with an Aintree catheter (Cook Medical Inc., Bloomington, IN) through an MC-3125 bronchoscopy suction swivel adapter (Medicomp, Princeton, MN).

the carina. Pass the ETT over the Aintree until it lies nearby. Firmly hold the ETT to remove the FIS and Aintree. ETTs greater than 5.5 mm cannot easily fit through the adapters. It is possible, but the FIS must be small enough to lie within the small lubricated ETT. In adults this means using something like a microlaryngeal tube (MLT) (Rüsch Incorporated, Duluth, GA) ETT (≤5.5 mm).

Short, Soft Nasopharyngeal Airways

The role of the breakaway NPA in combination with FSI was detailed earlier (see nasotracheal bronchoscopic intubation technique).

The modified NPA technique has been described to serve as a conduit for GA gases and oxygenation. Especially in children, it is not unusual to see this technique used on one nostril while FSI is pursued through a different orifice, perhaps even through a breakaway NPA on the opposite side.

Supraglottic Airways

FSI-SGA combinations assist tracheal intubation and diagnostic/therapeutic SGA maneuvers. When used in the context of difficult mask ventilation, SGAs can restore ventilation and are embedded in all DAAs. The FSI-SGA combination for intubation can be used in awake patients or under GA, as described above.[181] The FIS-SGA combination has been successfully employed with multiple SGA brands (Fig. 24.32).

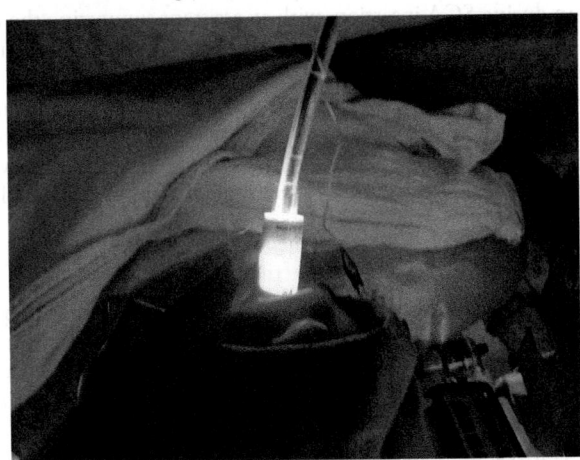

• **Fig. 24.32** Intubating with the combination of a flexible intubation scope within an Ambu Aura-i intraoperatively (Ambu A/S, Ballerup, Denmark).

Supraglottic Airways and Multiple Endotracheal Tube Techniques

Not all lubricants have equal efficacy. Some viscous lidocaine and any bacitracin, neomycin, and polymyxin B ointments are more adept at achieving a far greater degree of slickness than common surgical lubricants. If an FIS-SGA combination technique is intended for intubation, ascertain first that the lubricated ETT size traverses easily back and forth through the SGA.

Many SGAs have indicators for maximum ETT size, and the larger ones permit the entry of an adult-sized FIS. Compare the ETT length with that of the SGA, because the distance from the periglottic opening of the SGA's bowl to the patient's vocal cords may be 3.5 cm or more. Inattention to lengths may result in a scenario of an ETT that is too short. In adults MLTs can avoid this because of their greater lengths and larger cuff sizes with respect to MLT diameter.

With the LMA SGA, the alignment of the ETT bevel in a transverse plane or preemptive cutting of the aperture bars will avert situations in which FIS and ETT tips abut or straddle the bars.

Administer LA for SGA placement and intubation in awake patients. For asleep patients, induce with muscle relaxant and insert the SGA. FIS-SGA intubation is similar in both conditions. Obtain an optimal P_{ETCO_2} waveform with good chest excursion. Disconnect the SGA, and slide an ETT-loaded FIS through it until the glottis is visualized. Place the FIS tip near the carina and deeply advance the ETT. Remove the FIS and observe P_{ETCO_2}. Remove the 15-mm connector and use a small pusher ETT to enter two-thirds down the SGA tube length against the original ETT while withdrawing the SGA just until part of the first ETT is grasped in the oropharynx. Remove the pusher ETT and SGA. Reconnect the 15-mm connector and ventilate.

SGA removal is not mandatory if concerns dictate otherwise, as long as the ETT is well below the vocal cords. However, the SGA cuff should be deflated, if it exists.

An easier strategy for planned FSI through an SGA involves using a prepared ETT-SGA unit. Insert a lubricated ETT so that its tip lies 1 to 2 cm above an SGA bowl. Inflate the ETT cuff. Advance the ETT-SGA unit into the patient, similar to a solo SGA. Ventilate through the ETT part. After good P_{ETCO_2} waveforms are obtained, insert an FIS after removing the 15-mm connector. Once the carina is found, deflate the ETT cuff to intubate.

An FIS-SGA combination can assist the successful placement of the SGA itself. Place an FIS tip barely inside the bowl for observation during SGA insertion, with an assistant supporting the FIS handle and pulling the tongue. The SGA insertion converts into a visual one. Corrections are made more easily.

FISs have been used to diagnose SGA problems (e.g., causes of high airway pressure or leakage from malplacement, often as a result of infolding of periglottic structures into the SGA bowl).

As discussed previously, a swivel adapter and Aintree or MLT can aid FIS through an SGA.

Supraglottic Airways and Aintree Catheters

As described in the sections on SGAs and multiple ETT techniques and swivel adapters, extrapolation can be made for FIS with an ETT and Aintree-loaded FIS via a correctly seated SGA with or without a swivel adapter. This combination can avert diameter discordance between pediatric FISs and adult ETTs. After the FIS, Aintree, and ETT are near the carina, remove the FIS and Aintree. Confirm ETT ventilation and complete the technique as described (Fig. 24.33).

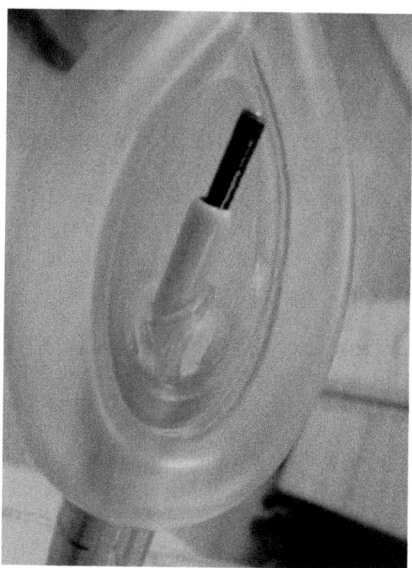

• **Fig. 24.33** Combination of a flexible intubation scope (FIS), Aintree catheter (Cook Medical Inc., Bloomington, IN), and endotracheal tube in a laryngeal mask airway (Teleflex Medical, Morrisville, NC).

Likewise, FISs may have a role at the end of surgery if extubation success is questionable. In this case inserting an FIS with an Aintree catheter through the existing ETT allows leaving a secured Aintree as an airway bridge after FIS and ETT removal. If reintubation is needed, an ETT-loaded FIS can be reinserted around the Aintree. Patients can be remarkably tolerant of bridges, especially with intermittent lidocaine instillation.

Supraglottic Airways and Guidewires

For more obscured glottic openings, sometimes a thin guidewire can assist entry. Place a long guidewire (110–145 cm, diameter 0.38–0.97 mm) down the FIS working channel. Insert this through the SGA with or without a swivel adapter. In adults leave 8 cm of wire in the trachea. Hold the wire firmly, and extract both FIS and SGA. Subsequently, thread the wire's cephalad end into the tip of an ETT-loaded FIS or ETT–Aintree–loaded pediatric FIS until it exits the working channel by the handle port. This could constitute FIS–ETT–Aintree–wire–SGA, a quintuple combination. With the FIS, visually follow the wire into the trachea, and make appropriate insertions for intubation. Wires are especially useful for FSI for SGAs with small openings, such as King LTD (Fig. 24.34).

Intubating Supraglottic Airways

Reports of FSI through the LMA prompted the silicon-covered, steel-body Fastrach creation. Its moveable single epiglottis deflector bar eliminates aperture bar hang-ups. Its own centrally curved, soft-tip ETT more readily traverses the glottic aperture compared with non–90-degree-rotated PVC ETTs. A number of SGA models have larger tube diameters for FSI. The Ambu Aura-i (Ambu A/S, Ballerup, Denmark) is a soft, rounded PVC SGA designed with a less J-curve than the Fastrach and a bite block area indicating the maximum ETT size (Fig. 24.35).

Studies have shown that SGA models have varying capabilities for ventilation, blind intubation success, and FSI-SGA success.[182–187] In a study by Erlacher and associates 180 patients

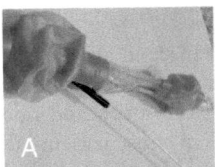

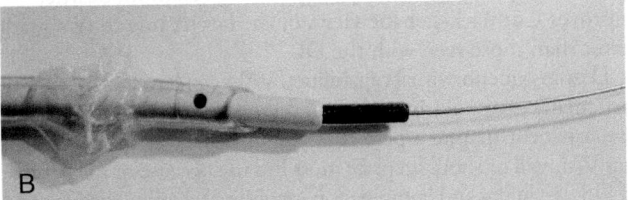

• **Fig. 24.34** (A) A pediatric flexible intubation scope (FIS) and wire down the working channel can be inserted into the King LTD (Ambu A/S, Ballerup, Denmark); (B) after FIS and supraglottic airway removal and wire bracing, an endotracheal tube which is loaded FIS is threaded along the wire for intubation (Cook Medical Inc., Bloomington, IN).

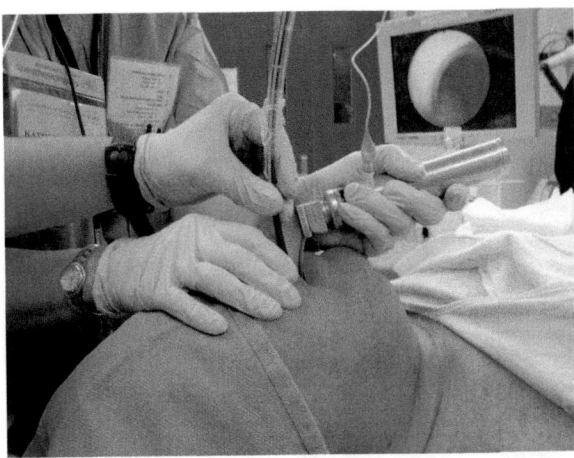

• **Fig. 24.36** Fiberoptic intubation assisted by a rigid laryngoscope with a video view of the trachea.

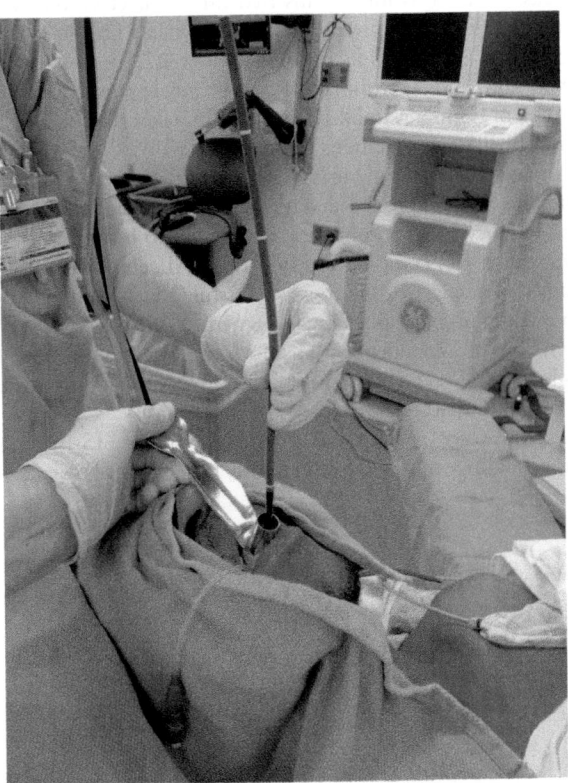

• **Fig. 24.35** Intubating with a combination of a flexible intubation scope through a Fastrach.

were intubated blindly through Cobra PLUS (Pulmodyne, Indianapolis, IN), air-Q (Mercury Medical, Clearwater, FL), or Fastrach devices with success rates of 47%, 57%, and 95%, respectively.[188] Of the approximately 60 patients for whom blind intubation failed, the overall success rate for the FIS-SGA combination was more than 98%.

Direct Laryngoscopes

Just as DL can fail occasionally, when an FIS is used as a solo airway device, impediments may prevent glottic entry, for example, a nonmobile or floppy posteriorly directed epiglottis, periglottic mass, or upper airway edema. DL can lift the mandible and move

obstructing tissues away (Fig. 24.36). The FIS-DL technique requires two endoscopists or one endoscopist and a very knowledgeable assistant. Clinical situations, knowledge, and technical abilities of personnel involved dictate who handles different roles in combination techniques.[189] FIS-DL may have an advantage of reduced nociceptive intubation stress, because of less DL blade pressure exertion than might have been needed during solo DL use in DA cases.

Successful FIS-DL combinations for controlled extubation/reintubation have been reported in DA ICU patients.[190]

Unsoiled Airway Conditions

The FIS-DL technique can proceed in two ways: first, use the DL to obtain the best view while moving blocking structures away. Turn over DL control to keep it braced, and suction as needed. While looking directly intraorally with the DL, insert the FIS in the created space until its tip is under the epiglottis (similar to inserting an ETT). Once beyond the epiglottis, advance by using FIS optics, and continue with FSI, basically using the FIS as a modified bougie or stylet.

Alternatively, hold the DL immobile and insert the FIS as far as possible under DL light. Then monitor via the FIS while maneuvering the insertion portion and directing the assistant to move FIS controls for FSI. Also, consider giving instructions for Yankauer suction use or other tools to move structures out of the way (e.g., the epiglottis).

Soiled Airway Conditions

For FSI, two suctions are frequently needed. If an errant ETT is in the esophagus, consider leaving it there as an outlet if the gastroesophageal tract is the source of soiling. Bloody soiling near the glottis can be cleared by using a suction catheter or nasogastric tube directed from outside to inside through an ETT Murphy eye. After exiting the ETT tip, they can also act as guide tubes toward the glottis (Fig. 24.37). Or, if more is needed, place a bigger suction by connecting an ETT (without its 15-mm adapter) to large suction tubing that has or has not been cut off (depending on the ETT size); the suction must be halted immediately if glottic entry occurs to avoid pulmonary injury (Fig. 24.37).

As described previously, a 110- to 145-cm guidewire with 2 to 3 cm extending from an FIS whose tip is nestled just within the ETT tip (for protection against soiling) can be used in case a

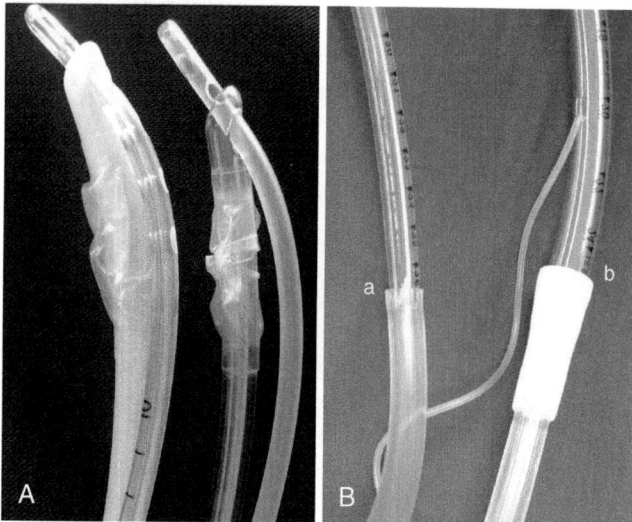

• **Fig. 24.37** (A) Small and large endotracheal tube (ETT) with a nasogastric tube (*left*) and suction catheter (*right*) directed through the Murphy eye. (B) Small and large ETT with direct fitting into cut-off (*left, a*) and uncut (*right, b*) suction tubing.

glimpse of the glottis is sufficient for wire passage, after which the ETT-loaded FIS could be threaded over it (Fig. 24.38). If vision clears, any of the ETTs are viable options for intubation.

Alternatively, begin the process of getting the best DL view possible next to an ETT-loaded FIS while directing suctioning deeply, and look for bubbles as a guide to the glottis.

Alternatively, use the transillumination method with the loaded FIS, or if impossible to visualize how to direct the FIS, insert a second-generation SGA or an intubating SGA. Suction through it (and the gastric port, if present), ventilate, and proceed to intubate through it with the FIS. At any point, undertake surgical management as the best option.

Video-Assisted Laryngoscopes

VALs are devices that have established their place in airway management and DAAs. Many VALs give clear images as a result of wide-angle camera capability, exceptionally clear optics, and video monitoring. Learning curves are very fast. In most patients the up to 60-degree–angled GlideScope VAL (Verathon, Seattle, WA) improves Cormack-Lehane views of the larynx one to two grades better than those seen with the DL.[191–194]

Despite superior visual capabilities, VALs can have failures.[186,192,195] Particularly disappointing are instances when it is impossible to intubate a patient despite a perfect laryngeal view.[186,192,195] It is unlikely that VAL will or should replace most FIS use because of the nature of an FIS: flexibility and combination capabilities. Unlike the FIS, VALs are unable to act as physical guides for railroading ETTs into the trachea or assist diagnostically or therapeutically in subglottic areas.

In addition, pharyngeal perforation from the ETT tip, although rare, has been reported with two excellent, extensively employed VAL brands thus far. Undoubtedly, with increasing use, all VAL will be associated with this complication. The cause is simple to understand. Whereas the ETT is initially inserted under direct vision, at some point, its tip is pushed ahead blindly until finally seen again on the video screen.[196–199] Hugging the tongue with the ETT while curving it centrally and caudally within the airway greatly lessens this possibility. This type of trauma is unlikely with an FIS when the ETT railroads over it. The FIS has limitations compared with VAL devices because of its narrow-angled field of view, shorter focal distance, greater chance of obscured optics in soiled airways, inability to open the airway, and lesser tendency to remain midline in the path to intubation.[200] Ideal circumstances can combine an FIS with a VAL, employing strengths of both to make intubation more successful (Video 24.6) and a situation of extraordinary airway management. With FIS-VAL, the oropharynx can be kept open, with tissues lifted away from the epiglottis and glottis. VAL view of the FIS position plus simultaneous the FIS view of anatomy foster success.

The VAL can monitor ETT passage over the FIS in the glottic area, aiding in the resolution of ETT impingements. This

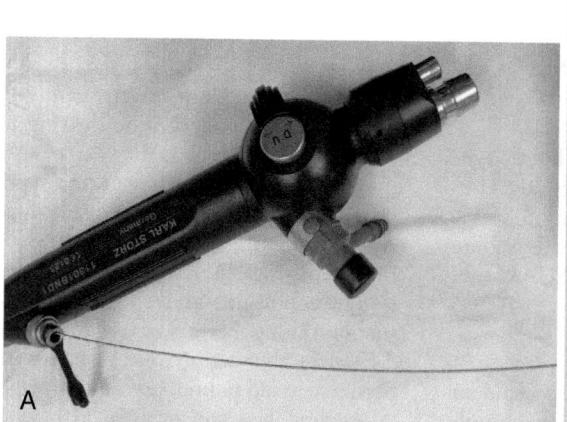

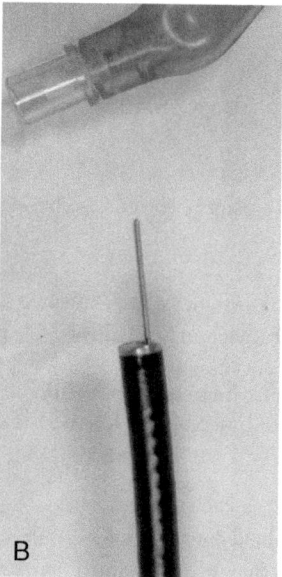

• **Fig. 24.38** (A) A 110-cm wire extending from bronchoscope tip. (B) Proximal end of the wire exiting from the lower working channel port.

combination requires both an endoscopist and a very knowledgeable assistant for rescue techniques in DA patients, such as a failed intubation after VAL-precipitated papillomatous bleeding.[74,201] Subsequently, FIS-VAL usage resulted in success with no further injury.

FIS VAL also permits better observation of FIS manipulation by operators to enhance FSI teaching and maximize learning.[202]

Nonchanneled Video-Assisted Laryngoscopes

Assistance for intubation by combining an FIS and a nonchanneled VAL is similar to that of the combined FIS-DL method. Situate FIS and VAL screens near one another (if separate). Seek an intubatable VAL view. Proceed similarly to either of the FIS-DL methods described previously (Fig. 24.39). Likewise, use techniques similar to those for FIS-DL soiled airways.

Here are some scenarios and suggestions on how to deal with issues.

Question. What do I do when VAL brightness is causing my view to be whited out while looking down the FIS? Dim the brightness of the VAL model (if it possesses this feature) to prevent excessive glare (Fig. 24.40). Otherwise, insert the VAL to best view and insert the FIS until it just whites out. Power the VAL off and use the FIS to view the anatomy. Power it back on intermittently, as needed.

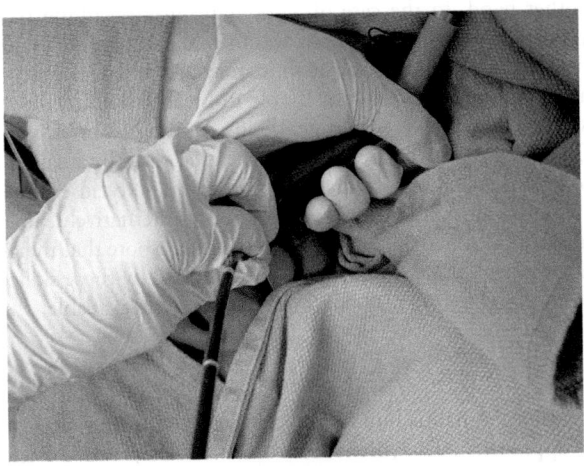

• **Fig. 24.39** Intubating with a combination of a flexible intubation scope (Karl Storz GmbH & Co. KG, Tuttlingen, Germany) and a GlideScope video laryngoscope (Verathon, Seattle, WA).

Question. It is impossible to get the FIS tip to go under the epiglottis. What do I do? It may be too flimsy to execute this maneuver in comparison to epiglottic bulk or immobility (especially if using a pediatric FIS in an adult). Request tongue pull, jaw thrust, or both. Observe via the VAL until the tip gets near the epiglottis. A somewhat lateral FIS approach may be beneficial. Advance the ETT just past the FIS tip to slide the firmer ETT tip under the epiglottis. Advance the FIS out the ETT to the glottis. Note that inflating the ETT may lift its tip off the pharyngeal wall if it is too posterior.

Question. I have a dyspneic patient, stabbed very low in the midneck, with moderate subcutaneous emphysema. Intermittently, he's coughing up lots of blood. The surgeons aren't quite sure of the anatomy or if tracheostomy is possible. Should I choose DL or VAL? Neither, unless it's a dire emergency. Beyond locating the glottis, the ETT route is blind with these techniques. ETTs exiting tracheal tears can result in massive emphysema. An FIS or combination technique might be better, allowing the FIS to bypass the hole, even if it ends up endobronchial.

Channeled Video-Assisted Laryngoscopes

Visualization of the larynx may be perfect with a channeled VAL and yet still result in failure. In that case, perfect view or not, insert the FIS into the channeled ETT. If needed, slightly withdraw the VAL/OL for FIS maneuverability and direct the FIB to the glottis for intubation (Fig. 24.41), essentially using it as a maneuverable bougie.

Special Flexible Bronchoscope Uses

Attempts at airway control are periodically pursued with suboptimal equipment or techniques. Before embarking on these procedures, make sure that capable personnel, oxygen delivery methods, monitoring equipment, and emergency airway equipment are readily available, especially for DA patients and those unable to tolerate short periods of apnea. Keep alternative management plans in mind, and in risky situations consider preemptively marking the location of the CTM, applying antiseptic solution, and draping a sterile towel on the neck in readiness for surgical access.

Facilitating Endotracheal Tube Exchange

Patients may require the exchange of existing ETTs attributed to incorrect ETT size, cuff leakage, ETT obstruction, a need for a different type of ETT, or a need for an alternative route of entry for the ETT. Asking for experienced assistance is recommended.

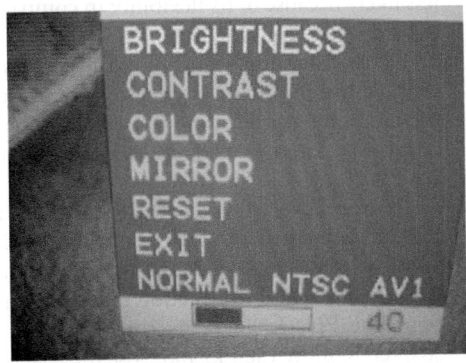

Controlled VL brightness permits good
FOB viewing

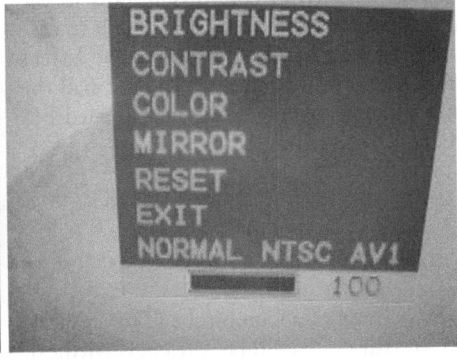

Excessive VL brightness may impair
FOB viewing

• **Fig. 24.40** Controlled brightness with the GlideScope video laryngoscope prevents glare during combined flexible intubation scope (FIS) viewing (Verathon, Seattle, WA).

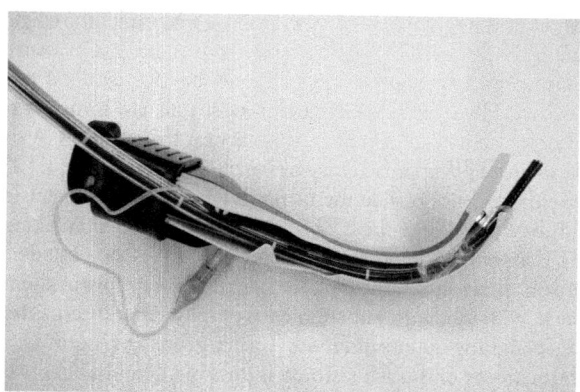

• **Fig. 24.41** Combination of a flexible intubation scope with an endotracheal tube within an Airtraq optical laryngoscope (Teleflex Medical, Morrisville, NC).

Frequently, Cook airway exchange catheters have been used to blindly carry out this process by passing the exchange catheter deeply into the existing ETT (which is then removed) and railroading a new ETT over it. However, these two methods are less successful in DA situations, which become fraught with airway losses, morbidity, and mortality. A retrospective review by McLean and colleagues showed a failure rate of 13.8%, injury rate of 7.8%, and pneumothorax incidence of 1.5%.[203] Often, for anticipated DI or cases intolerant of apnea, the exchange needs almost simultaneous extubation of the old and intubation with the new. Not uncommonly, DL or VAL are used to observe the removal of the old ETT from within the glottis while the replacement is introduced sequentially.

The use of an FIS to facilitate ETT exchange results in a more controlled, successful completion of that goal. An Aintree catheter has the benefit of allowing FIS passage within to turn a blind technique into a visual one. The ETTs must be at least 6.5-mm ID to allow for the passage of the Aintree.

When using the FIS–Aintree technique, ensure that the Aintree is sufficiently long to allow the removal of the old ETT while keeping the Aintree in the trachea. Insert an FIS–Aintree down the old ETT, remove only the FIS and ETT, and reintubate with a new ETT-loaded FIS. When using the FIS–wire technique, insert a wire-loaded FIS near the carina via the old ETT. Remove the FIS and old ETT, leaving the wire in the trachea. Insert an ETT-loaded FIS down the wire and intubate. Alternatively, use side-by-side FIS-ETT or FIS–wire techniques: insert either an ETT-loaded FIS or an ETT–wire–loaded FIS under visual control into the trachea along the anterior commissure next to the old ETT. When the FIS tip reaches the old cuff, deflate it to ease FIS or wire entry until either the former's FIS tip or the latter's wire rests near the carina. Remove the old ETT and railroad the new ETT in the former instance, or thread the ETT-loaded FIS over the wire.[204]

Intubation in the Presence of Preexisting Combitube or Rüsch EasyTube

There are reasons for the removal of a Combitube (Tyco Healthcare, Mansfield, MA) or Rüsch EasyTube (Teleflex Medical, Research Triangle Park, NC) in exchange for an ETT. These devices are very large, with limited timelines for remaining in patients because of direct pressure effects on esophageal or airway structures. Also, in situ tracheal suctioning can be difficult because

of inherent bulk or the 5% chance of tracheal intubation during blind insertion.

If possible, undertake endotracheal intubation before their removal if insertions occurred in emergency circumstances (full stomach risk) to prevent regurgitation and aspiration. Some caregivers approach intubation by shifting them leftward, deflating the intraoral cuff, and using a DL or VAL to intubate. This is not easy. Ovassapian and colleagues found that their bulk even hindered FIS manipulation. Surprisingly, FIS usage enjoys a high intubation success rate because the device often causes upward lifting of the epiglottis, making laryngeal targeting easier.[205]

To use the FIS-ETT and/or Aintree and/or wire combination, load one or two or all three on the FIS (as described previously). Use preoxygenation and whatever is needed to prevent combativeness. Partially deflate the oral cuff to "just sealing" with continued ventilation to allow the combination to pass. Proceed with FSI. After intubation, remove the FIS, suction the device's esophageal side, and remove it.

If the device is in the trachea, use a technique similar to one in the ETT exchange section.

Troubleshooting Blind Nasotracheal Intubation

The 80% success rate of blind nasal intubation (with a warmed ETT) can be improved upon by using a visual FIS technique. On the other hand, in the case of a spontaneously breathing patient with obstructive nasopharyngeal and/or oral pathology, FIS movements next to anatomic abnormalities may precipitate visual confusion during the glottic search. If able to breathe well through one passage, switch to a very slow, gentle insertion of a lubricated nasal ETT while listening to breath sounds, similar to a blind nasal intubation. As they intensify, indicating glottic proximity, insert the FIS for visual confirmation and complete FSI. Alternatively, an FSI-breakaway NPA may be of aid. However, please note that the blind intubation technique should only be performed by those skilled in the technique or if there are no intubation devices available.

Use Similar to a Lighted Stylet

In experienced hands blind lighted stylet intubation success rates may approach 90% (Bovie Aaron Surch-Lite; Bovie Medical Corporation, Clearwater, FL). Used in an identical manner in a darkened room, an FIS improves intubation success rate toward 100%, especially when it is possible to visualize through it.[206] Importantly, trauma from an FIS extended beyond the ETT is less likely because of its flexibility in comparison with an extended lighted stylet (Fig. 24.28).

FIS transillumination can aid in locating the trachea for surgeons during difficult tracheostomies.[207] Airway specialists prefer the use of airway ultrasound more because of additional anterior neck information, avoidance of surgery damage to the FIS, and less hypercarbia.[208,209]

If unavailable, to protect the FIS, employ a dual-device method: FIS and lighted stylet. Under GA, insert the FIS through an ETT swivel adapter. If anyone notes transillumination, or if the endoscopist sees tracheal indentation from a clamp pressed on the neck, brace the FIS. To mark its entrance, put a tape into the swivel adapter. Remove the FIS and close the adapter. Measure the lighted stylet tip next to the length from the FIS tip to the tape and mark the stylet here. Gently insert the lighted stylet to the same depth through the adapter and turn it on intermittently to assist surgeons. Awake patients will need airway anesthesia to tolerate the procedure.

One-Lung Isolation Assistance (See Also Chapter 26)

For one-lung ventilation (OLV), the FIS-DLT combination is uniquely suited to diagnosing correct DLT positioning and aiding the removal of tracheobronchial secretions, pus, or blood. For some bronchial blocker (BB) systems, FIS is actually an integral part of their insertion technique.

Troubleshooting Double-Lumen Tubes

The blind technique for OLV involves DLT intubation with DL or VAL, followed by a 90-degree rotation, advancement until resistance is felt, and OLV confirmation by auscultation.[210] Patients required ample repositioning in 78% and 83% of left-sided and right-sided DLTs, respectively, according to Alliaume and colleagues.[211]

Using a narrow FIS down the tracheal side helps ensure that just a little dome of the endobronchial tube cuff remains near the carina (Video 24.7). Klein and colleagues noted that only 33% of these patients needed subsequent repositioning 0.5 cm or greater.[212]

Right upper lobe (RUL) collapse has been reported in 10% to 90% of cases with right DLTs. Campos and colleagues described a modified technique in 20 patients: insert the DLT just beyond the vocal cords, advance slightly and rotate 90 degrees right, and use exquisitely careful endobronchial FIS observation of DLT target points.[213] The result was 0% RUL collapse.

For DI cases, intubate with an FIS-DLT unit by extending it from the endobronchial side.

Troubleshooting Bronchial Blockers

BBs have different features such as nylon wire loops that couple to the FIS, wheel devices, torque rotation capability, preshaped bent tips, or nothing.

For those BBs designed to incorporate FIS during placement, use the FIS to position a large ETT two to three rings above the carina. Techniques for BB passage vary according to manufacturers' instructions. BBs requiring tethering to an FIS are inserted through three-port adapters (included with some BBs) or swivel adapters for simultaneous ventilation. Once passed, remove the FIS as directed. Whether situated with FIS aid or not, use the FIS to monitor for correctly inflated balloon depth: 2 cm below the carina on the left, 1 cm on the right.

For some BBs, FIS use is diagnostic, just as it is for 6-French or 8-French styletted Fogarty venous embolectomy catheters used as blockers.

Facilitating Retrograde Intubation

The blind technique of normal retrograde intubation (RI) can be used electively or to rescue intubation failures from other devices. It is especially useful for soiled or severely abnormal airways. Unless the caregiver is very experienced, it is rarely used for urgent, dire circumstances because of time factors. For RI, insert a guidewire through a needle or angiocatheter directed cephalad from the CTS or the cricotracheal space until it exits the mouth or nose or is grasped with a clamp. Also, clamp it at skin level 2 cm outside the neck. To decrease diameter disparity, railroad a narrow Teflon guide catheter and ETT into the trachea while maintaining cephalad wire tension. Then release the neck wire clamp to permit intubation. The ETT may get hung up by the larynx because of diameter discordance or the wire's acute tracheal entrance angle.

The FIS-RI combination facilitates a visual component to RI to improve success and speed up completion in some difficult RI cases. Perform steps identically until able to thread the cephalad wire end through an ETT-loaded (Aintree-loaded) FIS, to exit out the handle port. While clamped, maintain wire tension (Fig. 24.38) and advance the FIS into the glottis. After tracheal entry, release the neck clamp and advance the FIS while observing the wire flip inward (slowly withdraw it cephalad, as needed). Proceed to the carina and railroad the ETT.

Flexible Scope Oxygen Insufflation (Rarely Recommended)—Supplements Preferred

Oxygen insufflation at 3 to 5 L/min via the working channel in adults during FSI was proposed to stave off hypoxia, help clear secretions, and prevent fogging.[57,116,117] Benumof described this technique and recommended it be used very cautiously.[57] If oxygen flow into a patient exceeds gaseous escape into the atmosphere, serious barotrauma might occur, especially with airway narrowing or laryngospasm. Pneumothorax has been reported in pediatric patients with oxygen at excessive adult flow rates.[118,119] Acute cervical, facial, and thoracic emphysema were reported in a patient.[120] Documented gastric rupture with subsequent mortality most likely occurred from an FIS directed into an unrecognizable region.[121–123] Ovassapian and Mesnick did not advise its use during intubation. They did use it to assist LA spray in open, known anatomic areas.[124,125]

Supplemental oxygenation can involve single or combined modes. These include nasal cannula (12–15 L/min), oral cannula, NPA, mask, mask plus CPAP (oral or nasal), jet ventilation, percutaneous TTO therapy—with a separate oxygen supply (usually preexisting for oxygen-dependent patients), or high-flow nasal cannula methods, such as Optiflow HFNO (Fisher & Paykel Healthcare, Auckland, New Zealand) (Fig. 24.16) (Video 24.8). Pressure effects from airway CPAP and HFNO can dilate soft tissue passages ahead of the FSI.

THRIVE is a recent concept that uses HFNO systems to accomplish flow-dependent dead space flushing during apneic oxygenation to maintain adequate saturations for extended durations. It may potentially slow P_{ETCO_2} rises. THRIVE's humidified systems (60–70 L/min) prevent dry gas mucosal damage and discomfort and the high flow rates can improve airway patency.[113,114,214]

Despite opposition to oxygen insufflation through the FIS, it may be invaluable.[215] Hung and colleagues described a patient undergoing prone craniotomy, with a pin system keeping the neck flexed.[216] Intraoperatively, the ETT was totally dislodged. SGA insertion was futile while prone because of a very enlarged tongue plus neck flexion. Nasotracheal FSI was chosen with reverse Trendelenburg and a left-sided tilt. The endoscopist (sitting on the floor) gave periodic FIS oxygen insufflation and passive mask oxygen flow. The oxygen saturation was greater than 90% during the ordeal, for almost 6 minutes.

Flexible Scope Intubation in Infants and Children (See Also Chapter 36)

Pediatric settings are replete with examples of beneficial multimodal approaches to the DA. To think that intubation criteria and FSI techniques in infants and children are the same as in adults, except the subjects are smaller, ignores the major differences in these two patient groups, anatomically, physiologically, and psychologically.

FSI criteria are almost identical to those for adults; however, they are expanded to embrace numerous congenital syndromes plus hereditary and acquired diseases with localized and/or wide-ranging anatomic and systemic effects (Box 24.7).[217,218] Normally, younger pediatric patients may be more sensitive to drugs (periodically, the opposite). Those with listed problems can be highly sensitive, with a greater likelihood of DA, reactive airways, bronchospasm, aspiration, cough, increased secretions, sleep apnea, declining respiratory function, and postextubation failure. In Altman and colleagues' study 37% of patients with congenital syndromes had multiple airway abnormalities, with three times more laryngeal abnormalities than tracheal ones.[217] Reflux occurred in 28%. Stridor was the most common (74%) symptom, followed by episodes of cyanosis, apnea, and failure to thrive. Tracheotomy was required in 19%.

Patients with listed problems often have difficult FMV, while OPA insertion may worsen the situation if the tongue buckles posteriorly or if a long epiglottis is folded downward.[218] Those with lingual enlargement, limited oropharyngeal access, small mandibles, or cervical spine limitations can be extremely poorly suited to DL and possibly VAL use. Even trauma morbidity can pose greater impediments. FIS flexibility, low profiles, and success often justify the choice of FSI for challenging pediatric cases.

Preparing for Oral Flexible Bronchoscopic Intubation in Awake Pediatric Patients

The approach for oral FSI in more mature or older awake pediatric patients is similar to that in adults. In less mature or younger cases differences are striking in terms of equipment, monitoring, psychological preparation, drugs, and technique.

Equipment and Monitoring

These may be unique because of the inclination toward hypoxia, bradycardia, and DA. DA carts may be needed more often. Although FISs service patients down to premature infants with ETTs 2.5-mm ID (see Table 24.1), the smallest FIS sizes may lack working channels if the OD is less than 2.8 mm. Transnasal and foot (infant) oximetry probes are more common in children.

Psychological Preparation

For receptive children, psychological preparation is useful, and guardian presence may contribute to patient cooperation and understanding. Plans for awake airway control are often abandoned in others, if success is doubtful.

Pharmacologic Therapy: Rationale

Antisialagogues, sedatives, opioids, LA, and/or vasoconstrictors can be administered according to dosing considerations and observations of clinical effects. Before instrumentation, antisialagogues should be given either IV or IM (if IV is not established). In younger patients atropine is preferred to prevent bradycardia because of airway stimuli. Short-acting sedatives or opioids are preferred to avoid desaturation from respiratory depression or obstruction. Fear often increases drug resistance until a point when significant respiratory deterioration transpires. Drug doses used for pediatric patients are listed in Table 24.5. Maintenance of spontaneous ventilation, sedation, analgesia, and/or amnesia is the objective (unless contraindicated).

IM ketamine is especially suited for infants, small children, and patients who are mentally handicapped because respiratory function tends to stay adequate with fewer adverse outcomes, as detailed by Hostetler and colleagues.[219] Transient apneas, with less than 40 to 60 seconds duration, can sometimes occur.[219,220] No difficulties as a result of increased airway reactivity with ketamine have been documented during FSI.[220] Antisialagogues usually offset ketamine's propensity for salivation and possible laryngospasm. Nevertheless, always suction the airway before FSI.

Dexmedetomidine's analgesic and lesser respiratory depressive effects make it more attractive than propofol. Both are titratable sedatives with rapid onset and awakening.

Highlighting Differences in Pediatric Airway Anatomy

The airways of the adult, child, and infant are compared in Chapter 36. Anatomic differences include the following: pediatric patients have relatively larger tongues, a more rostral larynx, and

---

• BOX 24.7 Summary of Abnormal Anatomic Conditions Affecting the Pediatric Airway

Nasopharyngeal abnormalities: choanal atresia, nasopharyngeal masses, deviated septum

Abnormalities with resultant smaller oropharyngeal access: underdevelopment of the mandible; limitation of mouth opening or temporomandibular joint impairment; macroglossia, glossoptosis, tonsillar enlargement, intraoral masses, cleft abnormalities

Prominent or abnormal mandible or midface hypoplasia

Enlarged mandible or facial feature distortion

Epiglottic abnormalities: epiglottitis, bifid epiglottis, anomalous epiglottis

Glottis abnormalities: laryngomalacia, cysts, arthrogryposis multiplex congenital, interarytenoid web, cri du chat, anterior laryngeal masses, Plott syndrome

Tracheal abnormalities: subglottic stenosis, webs, atresia, cysts, hemangiomas, tracheoesophageal fistulas, vascular rings, external compression

Bronchopulmonary abnormalities: asthma, bronchiolitis, cysts, infection

Cervical spine impairment: spine inflexibility or laxity, encephalocele, neck or posterior cerebral masses

---

TABLE 24.5 Pediatric Drug Doses Assisting Flexible Scope Intubation

Drug	Dose
Atropine	0.02 mg/kg IV or IM
Glycopyrrolate	0.004 mg/kg IV or IM
Fentanyl	0.5 µg/kg IV increments
Ketamine	0.5 mg/kg IV increments (4–5 mg/kg IM if lesser airway difficulty)
Ketamine	2 mg for each 1 mL propofol infused as a propofol drip at 50–200 µg/kg/min
Midazolam	10–20 µg/kg IV increments (0.4–0.5 mg/kg intranasal-use 0.5% solution)
Propofol	0.5–2.0 mg/kg IV bolus; infused as a drip at 50–200 µg/kg/min
Remifentanil	Infused as an IV drip at 0.05–0.1 µg/kg/min
Dexmedetomidine	0.5–0.7 µg/kg IV bolus × 10 min; infused as a drip at 0.5–1.0 µg/kg/min

IM, Intramuscular; *IV*, intravenous.

more inclined vocal cords.[218,221–225] In contrast to adults, the larynx in newborns is relatively smaller in comparison to their bodies, softer, and more sensitive. The newborn larynx lies at C4 and moves to C6 to C7 by puberty (Table 24.6). The infant cricoid cartilage is elliptical anteroposteriorly. Although not as narrow as the larynx, it is not distensible. Thus the cricoid cartilage is often the narrowest "limiting" part of infant airway anatomy, although variations occur. The infant omega-shaped epiglottis is floppier, longer, more tubular, and often directed posteriorly in comparison to adults. The innervation of the airway is similar, except that the left recurrent laryngeal nerve has a relatively longer course around the aortic arch and may be more prone to pathology.

Local Orotracheal Anesthesia Techniques

LA techniques can make ATI a very quiet, efficient procedure. Even under GA, LA application reduces hemodynamic responses and reflexes, particularly prominent in pediatric cases. LA techniques are similar to those in adults, with exceptions mostly involving younger patients.

Oral techniques may work well for patients able to cooperate, especially aerosolized LA for patients familiar with inhalers. The external approach for an SLN block is less preferred because of the dangers of closer anatomic proximity. For TTB, the cricothyroid area is smaller and harder to palpate in infants younger than 6 months. The needling of small tracheas, even in older children, is not recommended. Intratracheal drops of blood may compromise airways more significantly.

Local Anesthetic Drug Choices

Pharmacologic doses and volumes should be tapered according to patient size. Review all suggested LA doses before administration (Table 24.7) and avoid benzocaine.

TABLE 24.6	Changing Levels of the Larynx From Fetus to Puberty	
Age	Spinal Level (Cervical Vertebrae)
Fetus	C2 and C3
Newborn	C4
Age 6 years	C5
Puberty	C6–C7

TABLE 24.7	Aerosolized Lidocaine: Suggested Dosing According to Weight	
Weight (kg)	Volume of 4% Lidocaine (mL)	Volume of Saline (mL)
10–14	0.5	2
15–19	1.0	2
20–24	1.5	3
25–29	2.0	4
30–34	2.5	0
35–39	3.0	0
40–44	3.5	0
≥45	4.0	0

Positioning Infants and Small Children

Usually, the head and neck can remain neutral. Place a towel under the upper thorax for slight neck extension if large heads tend to produce neck flexion while supine. Adjust table or bed heights to keep the FIS relatively straight. Swathe infants in a towel or sheet with sufficient length for one end and then the other to be wrapped over the baby's arms and stuffed under the back. No ventilatory restriction results from this technique, in contrast to entire body wraparounds.

Endotracheal Tubes: Cuffed Versus Uncuffed

The choice of an uncuffed ETT for patients younger than 8 years of age had been traditional for decades, owing to various concerns. One was that smaller-ID, high-volume, low-pressure cuffed ETTs might be needed because of the added bulk of a deflated cuff. ETT downsizing prompted worry about increased resistance to ventilation. In actuality, the trachea is relatively large for a pediatric body habitus, and this concern is not a factor if ETT sizes are chosen appropriately for age and dimensions.[226]

Two other concerns were that cuff pressure might result in a higher incidence of subglottic ischemia with stenosis, and although the ETT tip was in the trachea, its cuff might cause damage if left between vocal cords, particularly in the smallest children.[227] More recent literature, including extensive comparisons of morbidity and outcomes in surgical and ICU patients, has refuted some of these ideas.[227–231] The elliptical cricoid shape might necessitate larger uncuffed ETTs (than cuffed) to minimize leak and result in worse pressure in the subglottic area.[225] Weiss and associates studied two groups of patients undergoing surgery with cuffed ETTs (Microcuff PET with distance markings [Microcuff GmbH, Weinheim, Germany]) versus uncuffed ETTs (multiple brands).[229] Among 2246 children (mean age <2 years, ASA physical status class I or II), the incidence of repeat laryngoscopy in the cuffed ETT group was 15 times lower with less trauma because there were fewer too small or too large ETTs. The incidence of stridor between groups was almost identical (4.4% and 4.7%, respectively). Always monitor ETT intracuff pressures to a maximum of 20 to 25 cm H_2O.[232]

Orotracheal Flexible Bronchoscopic Intubation Technique

FSI techniques for infants and children are aided by procedures and airway maneuvers similar to adults (e.g., tongue pull). Supplemental oxygen is advised. Endoscopy masks (e.g., VBM) are available in infant and child sizes (Fig. 24.42), with a central endoscopy port that is more likely to provide access to either oral or nasal FSI approaches in patients with closer anatomy. Likewise, for some techniques, regular masks with a bronchoscopic swivel adapter can be used.

After antisialagogue dosing, insert an IOA such as the VBM Bronchoscope Airway (VBM Medical Inc., Noblesville, IN), available in newborn and child sizes. This IOA is superficially three-quarters enclosed with an open side. Its distal half gives way to a completely curved open spatula-like area, similar to the Ovassapian. A bite block is another choice. Gently brace the insertion hand on the patient's face to keep the FIS midline, a critical step in dealing with smaller anatomy. As always, strive to maintain recognizable structures central. Hold the FIS and carry out the procedure as described for adults.

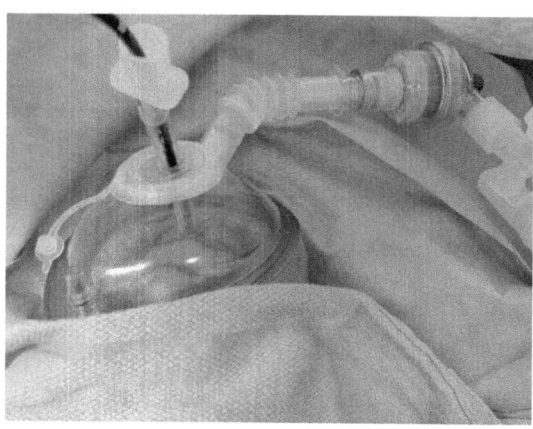

• **Fig. 24.42** Combination of a flexible intubation scope with an endotracheal tube through an endoscopy mask.

Two-Stage Flexible Scope Intubation Technique

Some patients have airways too small to permit an FIS through the needed ETT. In these cases FSI can be carried out in two stages. First, thread a guidewire from a Cook PAEC (Cook Pediatric Airway Exchange Catheter) set down the FIS working channel. The PAEC is available in sizes 8 French or greater (2.7 mm) with a length of 83 cm. Allow only up to 1 cm of wire to exit beyond the FIS tip. Insert them into the oropharynx. After glottic visualization, advance the wire into the trachea for a distance approximating the length to the carina. Remove the FIS. For the second stage, railroad the PAEC and/or ETT over the wire.

Nasotracheal Flexible Scope Intubation Technique

For oral or nasal FSI in younger patients, it is almost always advised to introduce it before the ETT, because ETT size may limit full FIS maneuverability. Similar to adults, rout out nasal anomalies. Give appropriate antisialagogues (mainly to avoid bradycardia), sedatives and/or opioids, LA, and vasoconstrictors. Phenylephrine or oxymetazoline and ETT warming may reduce the incidence and severity of epistaxis by over 40%.[233,234]

This technique is similar to that for adults. In children blind ETT introduction before the FIS is associated more with epistaxis because of the possible hypertrophied adenoids, especially between ages 2 and 6 years. Endoscopy masks, swivel adapters, modified NPAs, and breakaway NPAs may be used.

Here is a scenario and suggestions on how to deal with issues.

Question. The ETT is optimally sized for the nasal passage, but what do I do if I can't get the FIS through it? If its size fits, insert the ETT through one nostril, and the FIS through the other or into the oropharynx. Observe the ETT in the posterior pharynx to advise an assistant on how to move it, the head, or the neck to complete the FSI. As an alternative, if its size fits, use a wire-loaded FIS in the NP for the two-stage approach.

Oral or Nasal Flexible Scope Intubation in Asleep Pediatric Patients

Patients Under Routine General Anesthesia

Give anticholinergic agents and vasoconstrictors as indicated. Optimize equipment, including FIS combinations. Make the first choice the best technique possible to avoid desaturation, particularly in smaller or high-risk patients, whether or not difficult FMV or DI is expected. Have two suctions available for regurgitation threats. Experienced assistants in FMV are needed. Induce GA and give 100% oxygen by FMV. If FSI through an endoscopy mask is not planned, lift the face mask for short intermittent periods to minimize reflexes by applying preemptive airway LA or using "spray as you go." Carry out short FSI attempts with prompt returns to intermittent FMV to avert desaturation. Combinations, such as FIS-SGA or FIS-intubating SGA, are more likely to result in success.

General Anesthesia Using Short, Soft Nasopharyngeal Airways

A breakaway NPA may be used in older children to assist FSI, as detailed earlier. For small, spontaneously breathing patients, join a 15-mm ETT connector to a lubricated modified NPA (with a precut Murphy eye–type hole distally).[83-85,235] Place it in the smaller nostril, and attach it to a supported anesthetic circuit for continued inhalation anesthesia and oxygen supply.[86] Proceed with FSI orally or nasally.

Alternatively, gently use a smaller lubricated ETT orally or nasally attached to a circuit for gas supply while executing FSI at another orifice. Close orifices to minimize atmospheric pollution.

Here is a scenario and suggestions on how to deal with the issues.

Question. This small child has an easy FMV but probably a DI. The mouth opening is too small for an appropriately sized ETT. There's no endoscopy mask. One nasal passage is blocked. How am I going to keep her asleep while I do any intubation through any route? Find out if the retromolar space permits an ETT-loaded FIS for oral FSI. Supply anesthetic gases and oxygen through a modified NPA. Alternatively, see if the mouth (perhaps retromolar) is big enough for a smaller ETT used as a gas supply conduit while closing all orifices, except the patent nasal one that can be used for FSI.

Advantages of Flexible Bronchoscopes

A universally documented fact is that the long FIS history of helping accomplish numerous types of airway management and rescuing failed devices supports its place as the gold standard for DA management. Its innate ability to enter through very limited airway openings, glide by aberrant structures, and follow airway contour in any body position, body habitus, or age is unique to this device. Its multimodal ability to be combined with almost all airway tools, including surgical ones, is incomparable. It can be life-saving and even life altering by accomplishing safe airway management or diagnostic and therapeutic maneuvers that permit GA for operations on patients for whom airway control would otherwise be impossible, even surgically, such as those with chin-on-chest ankylosing spondylitis (Fig. 24.43).

Confirmation Accuracy of the Location of Respiratory Tract Intubation

Its ability to supply visual verification of detailed respiratory tract anatomy among airway devices provides the greatest degree of certainty of respiratory tract intubation and OLV.

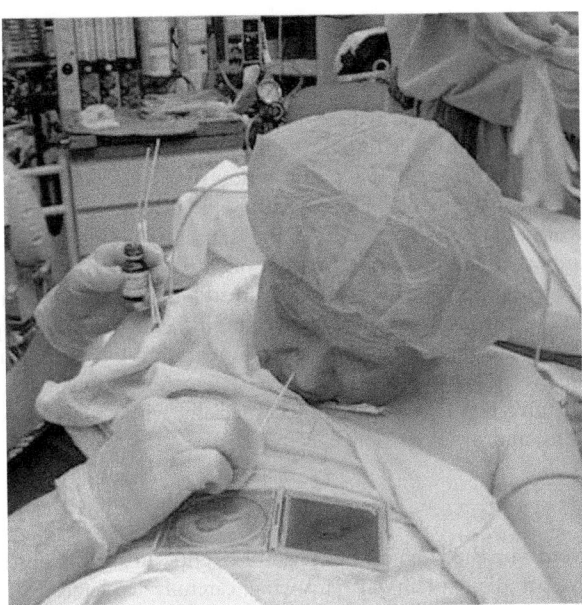

• **Fig. 24.43** Nasal application of local anesthetic in anticipation of awake flexible scope intubation in a patient with severe "chin on chest" ankylosing spondylitis, ideally managed with the use of a flexible intubation scope.

Faster Learning Curve—Faster Time to Intubate Very Difficult Airways

When novices learn to use devices for intubation, shorter learning curves and faster speed to gain expertise are always more desirable, and FSI is one of the fastest. In contrast, recall how many difficult attempts at DL intubation were encountered during training, even after dozens of patient intubations often followed by an attending physician's effortless success. Studies support faster learning curves for FSI.

Heidegger and colleagues found that novice residents reached a half-life in ability after 10 FSI attempts (94% success rate after 25 cases).[58] Johnson and colleagues demonstrated 90% FSI success after 10 patients among novices, 100% after 15 cases.[236] In contrast, Erb and colleagues estimated that up to 100 DL cases were needed for a good competence level.[237] VAL has an initial short learning curve. However, its more successful rate for the intubation learning curve is long (i.e., great view, but cannot intubate). Cortellazzi and colleagues noted that trainees with DL experience needed VAL assistance after numerous intubations, "only reaching a 90% probability of optimal VAL on their 76th attempt."[238]

Less Patient Trauma or Side Effects

Ovassapian and colleagues pointed out that when combined with excellent LA, patients had almost no cardiovascular changes during ATI.[17] Various GA studies have indicated no hemodynamic differences between DL and VAL intubation in comparison with FSI.[239–241]

The FIS is unlikely to cause more damage to the NP, lips, teeth, oropharynx, and trachea than other airway devices. Heidegger and colleagues demonstrated that postintubation laryngeal injury incidence was 8.5% after ATI using FIS (centrally directed soft-tip ETT) versus 9.3% after asleep DL (PVC ETT), with 4% postoperative hoarseness in both groups.[242]

Note that silicone or armored ETTs cause less pressure and injury, whereas centrally directed softer tips reduce perilaryngeal impingement,[243] similar to a 90-degree counterclockwise rotation for PVC ETTs (Fig. 24.44).

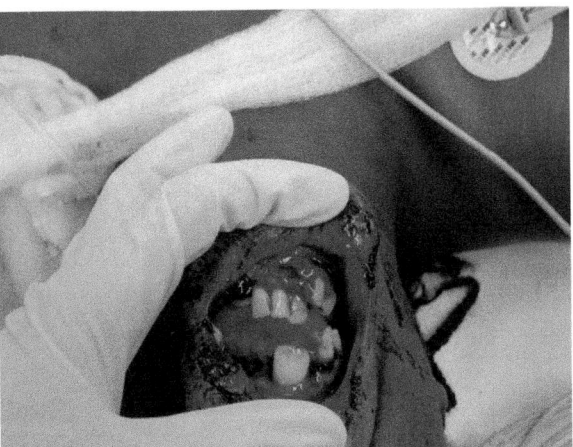

• **Fig. 24.44** Flexible scope nasotracheal intubation is planned for a patient with multiple loose and displaced teeth secondary to an automobile injury.

Minimal Cervical Spine Motion

FSI and blind nasal intubation are associated with the least amount of cervical spine motion (Box 24.8) compared with other devices, including VAL (e.g., 95% less motion than DL laryngoscopy).[244] Note that no intubation device has been proven to cause or prevent secondary neurologic deficits in high-risk cervical spine cases (Fig. 24.45).[140,141]

• **BOX 24.8** Cervical Spine Risk and Airway Management: Literature Support[a]

Todd M. Cervical spine mechanics, instability and airway management. Ovassapian Memorial Lecture. Presented at the Society for Airway Management Annual Meeting, Chicago, September 2010.

Wong DM, Prabhu A, Chakraborty S, et al. Cervical spine motion during flexible bronchoscopy compared with the Lo-Pro GlideScope. Br J Anaesth. 2009;102:424–430.

Crosby E. Considerations for airway management for cervical spine surgery in adults. Anesthesiol Clin. 2007;25:511–533.

Crosby E. Airway management in adults after cervical spine trauma. Anesthesiology. 2006;104:1293–1318.

Brimacombe J, Keller C, Künzel K, et al. Cervical spine motion during airway management: a cinefluoroscopic study of the posteriorly destabilized third cervical vertebrae in human cadavers. Anesth Analg. 2000;91:1274–1278.

Crosby T. Tracheal intubation in the cervical spine injured patient. Can J Anaesth 1992;39:105–109.

Meschino A, Devitt H, Koch J, et al. The safety of awake tracheal intubation in cervical spine injury. Anesthesiology. 1992;39:114–117.

Suderman V, Crosby T, Lui A. Elective oral tracheal intubation in cervical spine-injured adults. J Anaesth. 1991;38:785–789.

Crosby E, Lui A. The adult cervical spine: implications for airway management. Can J Anaesth. 1990;37:77–93.

Graham J. Complications of cervical spine surgery: a five-year report on a survey of the membership of the Cervical Spine Research Society by the Morbidity and Mortality Committee. Spine. 1989;14:1046–1050.

Grande CM, Barton CR, Stene JK. Appropriate techniques for airway management of emergency patients with suspected spinal cord injury. Anesth Analg. 1988;67:714–715.

[a]Suggested reading for a more in-depth determination of at-risk cervical spine considerations regarding airway management

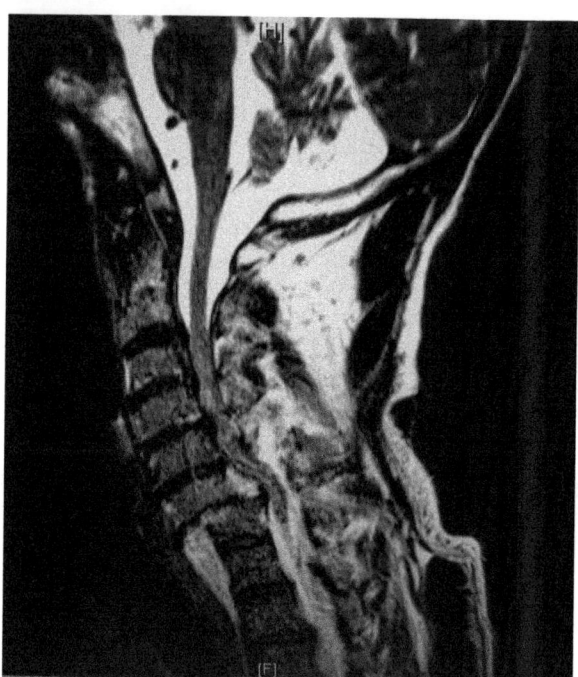

• **Fig. 24.45** Patients with cervical spine risk are least in danger of cervical motion if a flexible intubation scope is used for intubation.

More Diagnostic Capabilities

The FIS is very capable of investigating airway status, vocal cord motion for recurrent laryngeal nerve injury, tracheal motion for tracheomalacia, high airway pressure, endobronchial intubation, DLT positioning for one-lung isolation, quality of a bronchial or tracheal suture, foreign bodies, a malpositioned SGA, airway injury, and so forth.[245]

More Therapeutic Capabilities

The FIS can be therapeutic by aiding the removal of blood, secretions, or foreign bodies, etc., placement or adjustment of numerous devices, exact positioning of an ETT to bypass obstructive pathology, and exchanging ETTs or tracheostomy tubes.[246]

Disadvantages of Flexible Bronchoscopes: Are They Significant?

This section only details problems related to direct FIS effects, not to those common to non-FIS devices or methods (e.g., ETT tracheal wall cuff pressure).

Unsuccessful Intubation

Causes and solutions to eliminate unsuccessful FSI:

To avoid failed FIS entry into the trachea, use more head-up positions, optimize assisting maneuvers, and think of using combinations such as DL or VAL to move away obstructing anatomy.
To decrease the possibility that an ETT railroaded blindly over an FIS can get hung up, use centrally directed, softer-tip or 90-degree rotated PVC ETTs.[89,242,243] Reduce diameter disparity by using closer FIS and ETT sizes or adding circumferential fillers such as an Aintree. Additionally, use a DL, VAL, OL,

optical stylet, or another FIS to observe the ETT tip to indicate changes needed in ETT direction or patient position.
To avoid flipping of the FIS, ensure that the FIS tip is positioned near the carina, and reduce diameter disparity (Video 24.9).
To prevent FIS from exiting through the Murphy eye (Fig. 24.29), insert the FIS first. If ETT insertion-first is needed, however, search for the two ETT tip openings and exit the distal one.
To avoid FSI adversity in soiled airways, use suctioning, FIS-SGA, and other combinations (see the soiled FSI section).
To prevent mistaking the esophagus for the trachea, always search for the carina or bronchi. Rarely, after FIS entry into the esophagus in smaller pediatric patients, indentation-like rings attributed to close proximity of the trachea or distal esophageal rings can give this false impression, especially with fogging, secretions, and/or inexperience.

Worsening Respiratory Tract Obstruction

To avoid worsened clinical signs from FIS entry in areas of obstructive pathology or airway narrowing, carefully accelerate FSI. Alternatively, withdraw and use a narrower FIS, if not used initially.

Fragility and Expense

To dramatically reduce repair costs, avoid FIS bending, tapping FIS tips on a pad to clean them, moving angulation levers with the FIS tip inside the ETT, bite injury from the absence of bite blocking aids, pinching in slammed drawers, dropping, or excessive advancement or withdrawal resistance. Ensure that it easily traverses the ETT to prevent intussusception of its outer cover. Care must also be taken when using an FIS with DLTs to confirm correct placement; these lumens are narrower and there is a risk of shearing damage to the flexible tips when withdrawing the FIS from the DLT.
To cut FIS costs, form an FIS team promoting departmental education, training, and discussions. This can reduce FIS costs to only $89 per use.
To decide if disposables are cheaper, the magic number is less than 22.5 FIS uses per month.[19]

Space Logistics for Storage and Use

To shrink FIS equipment, innovations in development are helping. Bulky FIS video monitoring towers have downsized considerably or have been eliminated as a result of cable adapters that can be attached to surgical OR monitors, battery-operated systems, attached video screens, smaller stand-alone screens, and lighter FISs. Adequate storage space is still needed to hang clean and used instruments or to supply disposables (Fig. 24.8).
To ease usage impeded by their space occupation at patient sites, logistic help must be sought.

Time to Intubation

To make FSI faster, not slower, in normal airways compared with other devices,[239] practice. Surprisingly, FSI may require only slightly more time. Some can perform FSI in 10 to 30 seconds.

In DA circumstances FSI is often the fastest method. Tawfeek and colleagues observed intubation times in 100 DA patients. They found that FISs were almost twice as fast (79.9 ± 27.2 sec) as DLs (128 ± 93.7 sec).[247] Heidegger and colleagues examined a mixed patient population with mixed operators. They reported 92.3%

success rates for 955 nasotracheal intubations within 3 minutes and 90% for 657 orotracheal intubations within 2 minutes.[147] Rosenstock and colleagues compared FIS versus McGRATH VAL on 93 anticipated DI patients, noting time ranges of 33 to 424 seconds and 20 to 678 seconds, respectively: no interquartile range (IQR) difference.[248]

Complications

Under GA, hemodynamic changes from intubation or tongue pull/jaw thrust during FSI were less than or similar to those from DL or VAL use. All changes during FSI, RV, and VAL intubations decreased after preemptive LA use.[17,239–241]

To minimize nasopharyngeal injuries, laryngospasm, bronchospasm, and injuries related to ETT passage near the larynx or arytenoids, administer LA and improve techniques regarding disparate diameters, ETT tip recommendations, ETT rotation, and so forth. Postoperative sore throat, dysphonia, and dysphagia in non-DA patients after FSI have a similar incidence to those after DL use, although dental and soft tissue oral injury is more common with DLs.[47,58,176,247]

Preventing and Overcoming Flexible Intubation Scope Failure

Conquering Inexperience

The number one cause of FSI failure is inexperience from insufficient training and practice. Some experienced clinicians think FSI is harder to learn and give up attempting, whereas others discourage FIS use because of institutional concerns about costs. This results in less advancement and a loss of experience. Incredibly, some have advocated saving FIS costs by only using FIS on DA patients while forgetting that any FIS cost is infinitely cheaper than costs resulting from airway loss, such as patient morbidity and mortality, litigation, psychological trauma, time, equipment, personnel used in rescue, and damage to reputation. Success is achieved by knowing FIS indications and contraindications, looking for practice opportunities in normal airways, and having a proactive low threshold for FSI in DA or DA-related patients. FSI attempts following indiscriminate DL or VAL use are hindered by bloodied or edematous anatomy, engendering bleak hopes of success.

To develop FSI competence, perform FIS uses (examinations or intubations) as often as possible and consider joining our ENT colleagues in their clinics or our respiratory physicians in their bronchoscopy lists.

Preventing Insufficient Preparation

To deter defeat, avoid suboptimal preparations for patients, plans, or equipment.

Maximizing Assistance

Being ready to seek help is good; especially, consult experienced endoscopists for harder cases. Show less-experienced assistants exactly how to execute maneuvers (auditory and visual explanations are best) and explain why they are done.

Rescuing Insufficient Local Anesthesia

Test LA efficacy, even after nebulization, by suctioning toward the larynx for GPN (gagging) and SLN (coughing) blocks. If inadequate, repeat the LA topicalization or use the "spray as you go" method, up to a maximum of 9 mg/kg total dose. No cough during a TTB injection marks it as a suspect. Inject 1 mL of an equal amount of LA drug transtracheally as a test. If a cough occurs, inject the rest.

Combination Subsets of Plans A, B, and C

Consider expanding each plan A, B, and C, to employ combination techniques. Even for the preparation of patients, equipment, and assistants, there should be alternative ideas. For example, fogging may occur with an eyepiece FIS, but the poor view may also be a result of the endoscopist's exhaled breath on it.[204]

Dodging Discordance Diameters

Avoid impingement and flippage problems due to diameter discordance, as discussed (Fig. 24.46).

Practicing Tips for Novices, Intermediates, or Experts

It has been 50 years since Shigeto Ikeda decided not to be stagnant in his practice. He catapulted a facet of airway control away from a steel 1940s-style DL towards an excellent alternative device, the FIS, constantly evolving in its design to rescue DL and more modern airway device failures. Thanks to the FIS, many surgeries were not postponed or canceled, teeth were not dislodged, surgical airways were avoided, complications were minimized, brain deaths did not occur, lives were saved, and caregivers suffered less psychological stress.

If Ikeda could imagine a better way to help patients, then perhaps in this era, all airway caregivers in anesthesiology, emergency medicine, or critical care medicine can resolve to master an FIS that promises 95% intubation success for novices by the 10th patient on the first attempt while speeding up to only an average

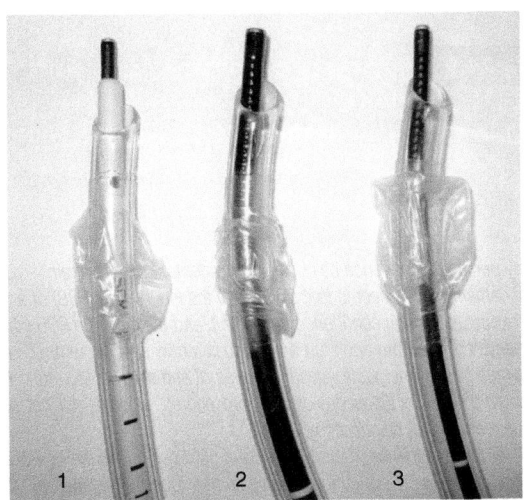

• **Fig. 24.46** Diameter differences should be minimized: *1*, pediatric flexible intubation scope (FIS) within Aintree within endotracheal tube (ETT); *2*, adult FIS within ETT; *3*, pediatric FIS within ETT (Cook Medical Inc., Bloomington, IN).

of 91 seconds.[236] In a survey conducted in 23 medical schools in 2007, 94% of responders characterized FSI as a basic residency skill.[177] FIS strategy acquisition leads to appropriate decisions in stressful situations and the ability to act as a team leader in any medical setting while fending off ill-advised cost-cutters.

A Spectrum of Games, the Web, and Workshops for Learning

Whether inexperienced or not, anyone can take charge; set priorities to become a competent, complete airway management specialist; and enjoy the challenge of overcoming DAs rather than dreading them. The FIS may seem formidable, but it is not. Similar to excelling in a field of study, artistic endeavors, sports, or computer games, FIS proficiency only requires practice.

Box 24.9 presents a personal quotation authored by Dr. Ovassapian for use at the Annual Meeting of the ASA's two-day Basic and Advanced Adult Flexible Fiberoptic Intubation Workshop. It has been cited at each subsequent workshop since 2007. This workshop provides hands-on dexterity experience, with devices from every distinct airway model type listed in the following section. Workshops are wonderful resources; instructors give succinct explanations and their best tips to everyone.

Make time to work with an FIS for half an hour. Watch videos on YouTube. Look up fiberoptic intubation or airway anesthesia. Then request an FIS in-service from a colleague or instructor. Additionally, there are all other resources available, such as online educational resources (see later), journal articles, books, and FIS workshops.

A Gamut of Free to Intricately Designed Dexterity Practice

Manikin Heads and Full Bodies

Practicing on intubation manikin heads or simple or complex full-body simulation models (medium to moderately expensive) is interesting, but after a short time, it may seem unchallenging or simplistic even if turned laterally or upside down. FSI workshops improve manual dexterity and develop confidence, that is, feelings of competence. This is what concerns people the most.

For the artistically inclined, Di Domenico and colleagues have made wire papier-mâché respiratory tract models that have been used successfully by participants to gain dexterity.[249]

Dexterity Models and Sophisticated Simulators (see also Chapter 50)

Many dexterity models are available. Research shows that higher benefits are derived from practice with them than after didactic lectures. Some are free (Video 24.10), whereas others cost thousands of dollars.

This learning type is part or partial task training, involving the deconstruction of a complex psychomotor task, FIS, into several elementary tasks. An example of one part learned through simulation is to follow the three directions of entering the oropharynx, traversing the larynx, and advancing into the trachea (downward, upward, and downward again). The acquisition of multiple partial tasks results in the integration of all the different acquired steps.[250]

High-Fidelity Inanimate Airway Models

High-fidelity dexterity models are anatomically realistic looking, made to mimic the airway down to the bronchial tree (Fig. 24.47). The Laerdal Airway Management Trainer (moderate) and SimMan (expensive) (Laerdal Medical, Wappingers Falls, NY) have many programmable pathologic states on their computers to coincide with physical patient simulators changes, such as tongue obstruction or laryngospasm. Solo FIS use, combinations, and BB insertion are possible. The CLA Broncho Boy series (moderate) (CLA, Coburg, Germany) simulates pathology, including a fluorescing tracheobronchial tree for autofluorescence bronchoscopy.

Computer-Based Bronchoscopy Simulators

The virtual fiberoptic intubation (VFI) program (free) developed by Diemunsch is a computer-generated model to improve the understanding of airway anatomy (including distant bronchioles), FSI technique, and dexterity (Fig. 24.48).[251] It is graphically represented with and without multiple types of pathology in clinical scenarios for practice on any computer. Three separate images simultaneously give a better understanding of the overall anatomy: (1) a transparent reconstructed image derived from computed tomography or magnetic resonance imaging scans; (2) the scans themselves; and (3) simulated airway imagery through which an FIS can be directed. Insertion through graphic oropharyngeal or nasopharyngeal routes can be chosen. With each scenario, movable computer controls can initiate predesigned motions to

---

| • **BOX 24.9** | **A Quotation Repeated Yearly Since 2007 During Presentations to the Annual Meeting of the American Society of Anesthesiologists' Basic and Advanced Adult Flexible Fiberoptic Intubation Workshop** |

"In my personal experience by observing residents, following their advancement, etc., it seems that 50 uses of the Fiberscope (FOB) of any kind give residents enough confidence in use of it, and they use the FOB when they leave the program and start a new job in a new environment. The number 50 comes from some gastrointestinal literature and surgical literature that indicated after 50 colonoscopy or other procedures residents did well on independent use of colonoscopy.

After this experience, if the FOB is used 50 times for awake or asleep intubation, for airway evaluation, Double Lumen Tube placement, etc., this will give them enough experience for independent use of the FOB with an acceptable success rate."

—**ANDRANIK OVASSAPIAN, MD**

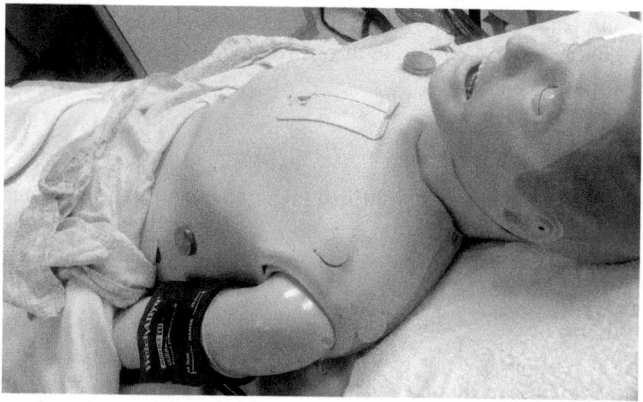

• **Fig. 24.47** High-fidelity dexterity model: Laerdal SimMan simulator (Laerdal Medical, Wappingers Falls, NY).

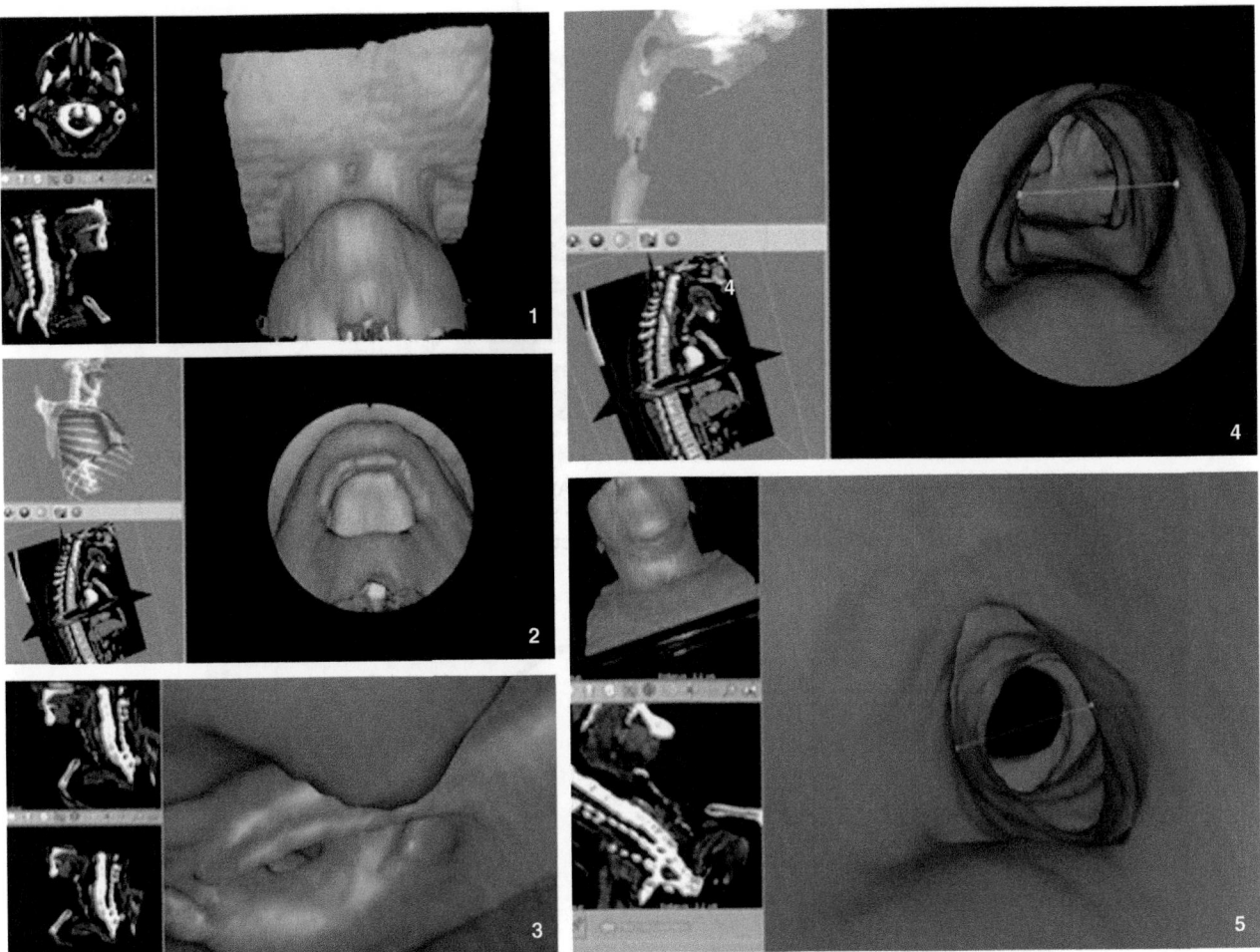

• **Fig. 24.48** Virtual fiberoptic intubation (VFI) images: *1,* comparison with radiologic scans; *2,* transparent anatomic and radiologic comparison with pharyngeal entry; *3,* posterior nasopharyngeal view of uvula above and posterior larynx below; *4,* carina comparison with imaging planes; *5,* intratracheal view.

advance the FIS. The computer-generated picture of anatomy as seen from the FIS point of view can be compared synchronously with the other images to elucidate spatial relationships. The VFI program does not need expensive or elaborate simulation setups, takes up no space, and is available in DVD form at no cost from the Karl Storz Company.

The ORSIM Bronchoscopy Simulator (Airway Simulation Ltd., Auckland, New Zealand) involves a briefcase-size portable device with three parts: a replica video bronchoscope (its insertion tube is shortened), a desktop sensor (with a hole in it for the FIS tip entry), and a computer with a software program (Fig. 24.49). Depicted are multiple relatively realistic-looking, airway scenarios that can be undertaken while the participant experiences the feel of actually moving FIS handle controls for desired navigational maneuvers.

The Endoscopy AccuTouch System (moderate) (Immersion Medical, Gaithersburg, MD) has a similar short FIS, computer system with a software program, and face-like physical control area (with a hole for FIS insertion). Operators get a realistic feel of bronchoscopy control, performing bronchial lavage, and taking biopsies.[252,253]

Surprisingly, Chandra and colleagues demonstrated that Accu-Touch simulator training did not bring additional benefits compared with the low-cost, low-fidelity choose-the-hole model.[254]

Low-Fidelity Training Models

Commercially available low-fidelity models, such as choose-the-hole models (relatively cheap), Dexter (moderate) (Dexter Endoscopy, Wellington, New Zealand), and the Oxford Fibreoptic Teaching Box (relatively cheap) (Pharmabotics Ltd., Winchester, UK), require no computers (Fig. 24.50). They are semianatomic or nonanatomic, modular systems featuring multiple paths, bifurcations, conduits, and/or maps by which an FIS can be directed toward targets. Naik and colleagues found that in human subjects, trainees using the choose-the-hole model (three wooden panels with holes for FIS insertion in different directional sequences) had better success than those only receiving didactic lectures. Time spent in visualization down to the carina in the model group tended to be faster, although not significantly different (both groups also practiced on models in addition to their teaching sessions[255]).

Self-Made Models

The low-fidelity Gil 5-Minute Fiberoptic Dexterity Model can be practiced with any FIS and requires only 5 minutes to make (https://youtu.be/e3TUsr6mLFI; Fig. 24.51). This model can be assembled from scrap pieces of readily available OR/ICU/ER materials (i.e., tape, pieces of ventilation hose, ETTs, suction tubing, etc.). Tape elements down securely in any dexterity

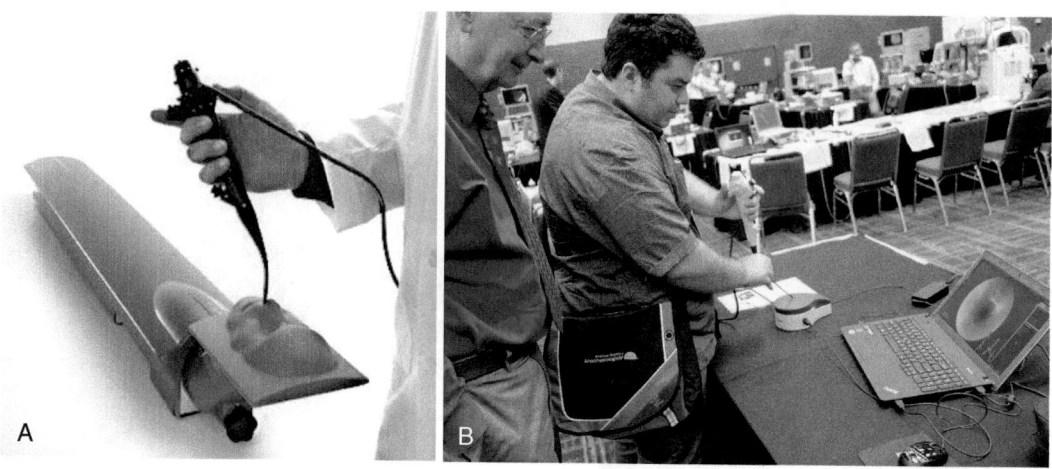

• **Fig. 24.49** Computer-based bronchoscopy simulators: (A) Endoscopy AccuTouch System (Immersion Corporation, Gaithersburg, MD); (B) ORSIM Bronchoscopy Simulator. (From ION Design, LLC; website: http://www.idsa.org/awards/idea/medical-scientific-products/immersion-medical-accutouch%C2%AE-endoscopy-simulator.)

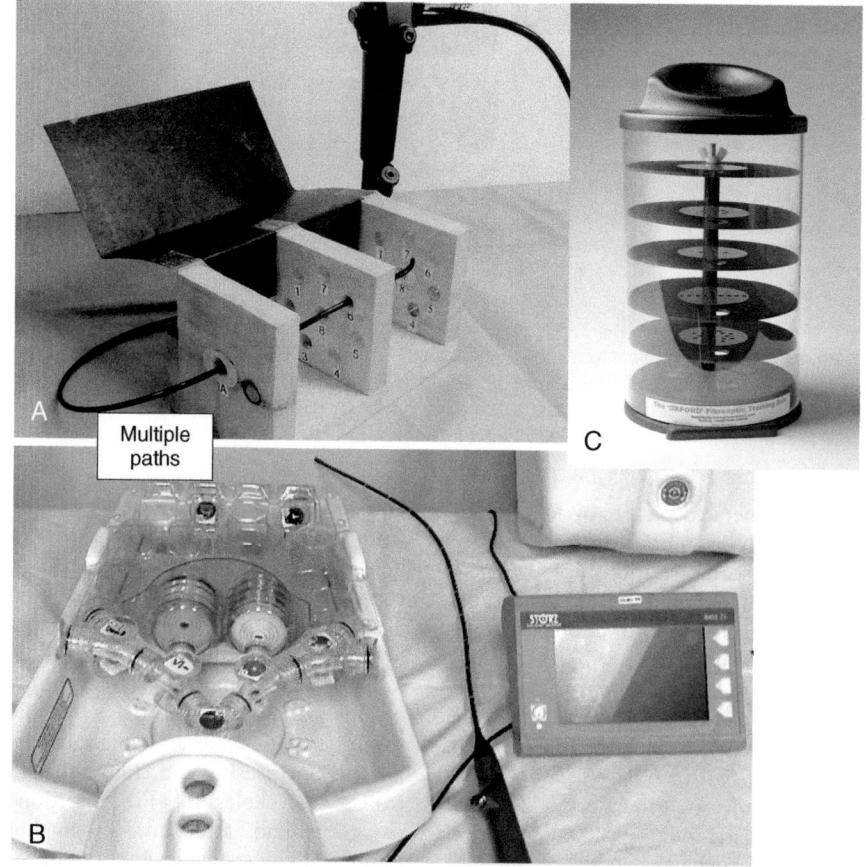

Multiple paths

• **Fig. 24.50** Low-fidelity dexterity models: (A) Choose-the-hole model (designed by Dr. Arthur Frederick David Cole, University of Toronto, Ontario, Canada); (B) Dexter (Dexter Endoscopy, Wellington, New Zealand); (C) Oxford Fibreoptic Teaching Box (Pharmabotics Ltd., Winchester, UK).

course layout with multiple targets, look at it, and then cover it with a towel. Practice underneath for 10 minutes or more with an FIS while using actual clinical hand positions and bracing under the towel. The dexterity challenge involves choosing more distal routes: going through each modeled bronchus and aiming for particular tubular targets (Video 24.10). If desired, add difficulty by slightly changing the directions of elements or placing something underneath them to produce small vertical misalignments between bronchi and targets.

The Living Human Experience: The Best Care

How much model/simulator practice is needed? The end point is when FIS maneuvers are easily carried out as intended without excessive repeats.

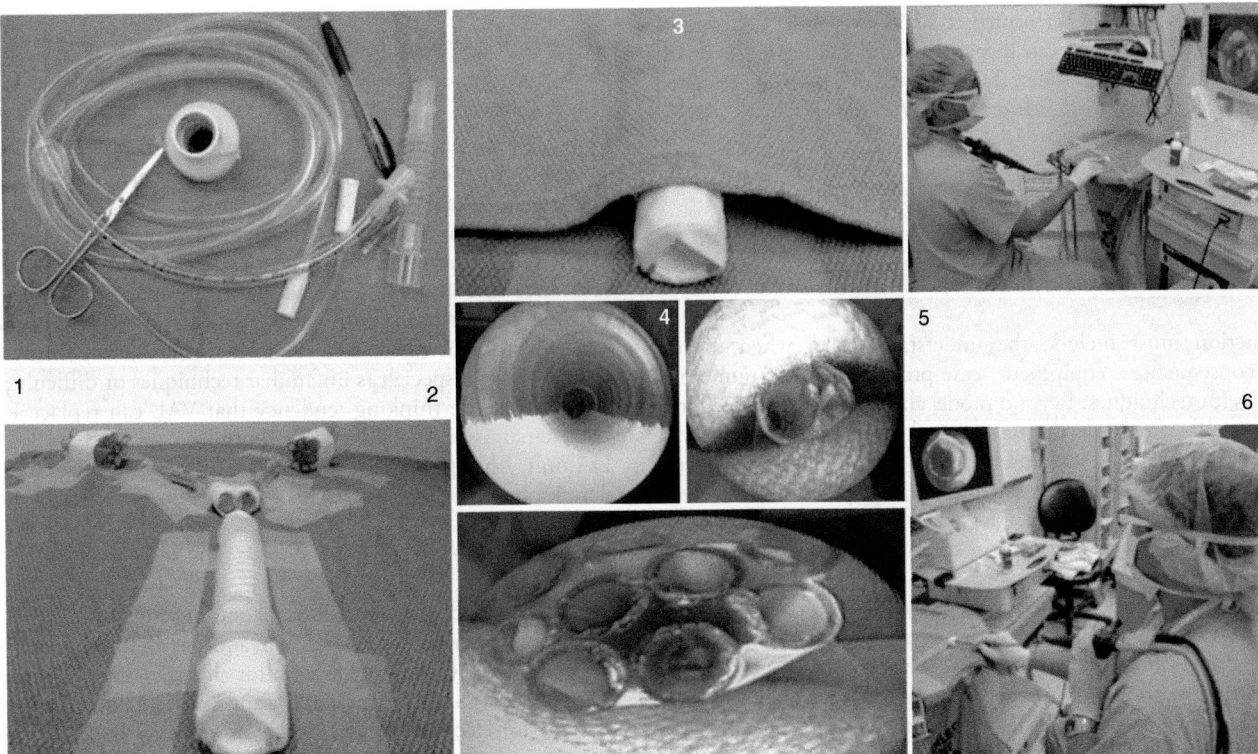

• **Fig. 24.51** Gil 5-Minute Dexterity Model: *1,* simple discarded or inexpensive materials for model construction; *2,* model shown to the trainee with the "trachea" leading to "carina" leading to two sets of targets; *3,* covered model; *4,* fiberoptic views seen—flexible corrugated tubing "trachea" with "membranous" posterior tape, "carina," and one set of suction tubing "targets"; *5,* trainee visualizing one set of targets, with correct hand position and care of the flexible intubation scope evident; *6,* trainee successfully entering the chosen target.

No models compare with the reality of using an FIS to see vibrant, living, anatomically accurate tissue in a living patient. It is easiest to practice in patients under GA by selecting younger, healthy patients having elective surgery. This aids visual reality and dexterity required for DA patients.

McNarry and colleagues' survey of trainees revealed that 82.7% believed there was no ethical concern in performing FIS examination or intubation in patients under GA without the patient's prior knowledge or consent.[177] Many anesthesiologists routinely choose FIS for ordinary planned OR intubations in non-DA cases. Even more use FIS for all nasotracheal intubations.

Project a positive and professional attitude toward colleagues, ancillary personnel, and institutional controllers when discussing plans to become proficient in FIS usage. This will alleviate their concerns, enlist their support, and save the costs of failed intubation.

Examination Experience With Already Intubated Healthy Patients
Under sufficiently deep GA with or without muscle relaxation in healthy patients, use extreme gentleness with the smallest lubricated FIS to inspect the oropharynx and NP. Do not use a vasoconstrictor or exert the slightest force on the NP against resistance to avoid epistaxis during a pure examination technique. Take 2 to 3 minutes to insert the FIS down the ETT (with or without a swivel adapter) to the carina.

Asleep Patients Using Endoscopy Mask or Swivel Adapters
Deeply anesthetized relaxed patients can be examined and perhaps even intubated with an FIS through an endoscopy mask, face

mask, or SGA (with or without a swivel adapter) if an assistant monitors ventilation, vital signs, and time. Pressure-assist ventilators can facilitate solo techniques.

Practice Troubleshooting High Airway Pressures, Low Saturations, Uncertain Endotracheal or Supraglottic Airway Positions, or One-Lung Isolation
Use an FIS–adapter combination to check for ETT obstruction, secretions, or ETT, SGA, and DLT positioning. This adds to dexterity and expertise.

Choose Handling Routine General Anesthesia and Intubation
Practice on a dexterity model for 15 minutes beforehand. Less experienced operators should keep choosing younger, healthier patients. Inform staff that only 2 minutes and one or two attempts will be taken for FIS laryngoscopy with or without FSI after induction, muscle relaxants, and 100% oxygen FMV. Video screens improve staff understanding and cooperation. Enlist an assistant for tongue pull/jaw thrust maneuvers, keeping the IOA midline, and monitoring oxygenation, vital signs, and the clock. After 2 minutes, if the trachea is entered, railroad the ETT. If it has not been entered, return to FMV and give anesthetic agent as needed. If stable, try again (may need suction), or use a common fallback intubation technique (e.g., DL). Initially, be content with FIS laryngoscopy.

Advance to Awake Tracheal Intubation Experiences
Awake techniques require consent and are not recommended for developing experience or dexterity, except under experienced

direction. After having performed 10 to 20 FSIs under GA, undertake awake approaches even in patients with moderate DA, with a degree of confidence. Enlist the assistance of a more experienced caregiver, especially for LA and sedation/opioids.

Generous Instructor Teaching and Learning Experience

Instruction

Instruction must include the understanding of when to use FIS, consequences, equipment, case preparation, and numerous choices for techniques. Beyond model and dexterity practice, proficiency only progresses through clinical teaching. Instructors can select easy airway patients under GA for novice FIS operators and assist with optimized management plans, equipment, and maneuvers, as well as for those with advanced levels of experience. For advanced operators, combination techniques and other tips can also be employed regularly.

With novices, many instructors choose the oropharyngeal route with an IOA or especially the nasotracheal route with a breakaway NPA, often leading the FIS directly to the larynx in 10 seconds.

Instructors and operators needing experience should be heartened, knowing that the FIS learning curve is short. Delaney and colleagues' study of ER trainees performing nasotracheal intubation correlated with Johnston's, with marked improvement after 10 patients.[256]

The presence of FIS teams increases understanding and promotes research.

Assessing Knowledge, Planning, and Technical Proficiency

Trainee proficiency evaluation involves determining the knowledge of and performance with indications and contraindications for FIS use, patient assessment and preparation, informed consent, administration of drugs, equipment preparation and use, monitoring, positioning, and direction of assistants. This can be gauged by clinical observation and written testing.

Often, a clinical observation method assesses only a simplistic recording of FSI totals. Nevertheless, noted in Dr. Ovassapian's quotation (see Box 24.9) of 50 FIS examinations/intubations to provide competence and the ability to perform independent FSI was the idea that 15 to 20 should be asleep FSI and 15 to 20 should be awake FSI. Competency of FIS use in DA cases is more difficult to determine, but Dr. Ovassapian also documented that for the myriad purposes and techniques described in this chapter, one could achieve an expert level after 100 or more FIS cases.

Aside from pure numbers to determine proficiency, it has been evaluated in several studies. Chandra and colleagues detailed proposed items to be recorded for this determination, including success or failure, time needed, a validated global rating scale, and a performance checklist.[254]

A didactic learning and testing site was mentioned earlier (see section on games), called the Essential Bronchoscopist. It is free of charge in an assessment question-and-answer form in five languages: English, French, Japanese, Portuguese, and Spanish (http://bronchoscopy.org/).

Tips on Using Flexible Bronchoscopes in Any Clinical Setting

Concerns about lack of FIS training or inadequate proficiency can be overcome easily whether one works in private practice or a teaching hospital. Inexperienced operators should convey the need for several minutes of FIS practice instead of the 20- to 60-minute DA rescue scenarios that may have dangerous consequences. Any resistance to FIS usage needs to have some push-back. Negative attitudes toward trying to develop more FIS experience are at odds with what nonairway personnel consider when taking time to deal with their own specialty's unfamiliar techniques or difficult problems. Avoid the thinking tendency that VAL can replace FIS in most circumstances or that FIS should be reserved for extreme DA only. That perspective stunts development and promotes the deterioration of endoscopy skills.

Skill Retention Tips

To prevent psychomotor skill deterioration, follow three tips: (1) engage in dexterity model, manikin, and/or FIS internet activities; (2) enroll in a systematic program for all facets of FIS instruction (such as the ASA DA workshop); and (3) designate a single day as a day for elective FIS use, weekly or monthly (≥12 per year) to accustom staff to a routine, and improve or maintain skills (even in institutions with few indicated FIS cases) (Box 24.10).

Conclusion

Airway loss is a two-word phrase that chills the hearts of all professional airway caregivers. Closed claims analysis and numerous reviews reveal the importance of mastering critical techniques of airway management.[45,136,257] The FIS justifies the training needed to develop and maintain expertise. FIS cost is small compared with the time and money spent during DA rescue attempts by using cheaper airway devices. Catastrophic airway failure expenses can easily eclipse the cost of a full complement of FIS systems. There has been some debate on whether the FIS has been superseded by other newer technologies for the management of DAs, such as VAL[258]; however, retrospective and prospective case series have demonstrated its high success rate and favorable patient outcome.[107,108]

> **• BOX 24.10   Steps to Introduce Flexible Scope Intubation Techniques Into a Practice**
>
> Step 1: Go to the websites and read the literature; DVDs and videos are also available.
> Step 2: Attend workshops on use of flexible intubation scopes (FISs) or use the FIS representatives to provide in-service training, or both.
> Step 3: Practice on simulated anatomical and dexterity models.
> Step 4: Have all equipment prepared ahead of time.
> Step 5: Look for proper prospects—healthy, young patients undergoing general anesthesia whose surgical sites are far removed from the airway.
> Step 6: Use the FIS to examine and to observe normal anatomy in anesthetized patients, not plastic models.
> Step 7: Enlist surgeons, nurses, and technical colleague to help, by emphasizing a better equation: Experience = Success + Safety.

Every comprehensive airway management text in anesthesiology, critical care, or emergency medicine places an extremely high value on this technique, making it not optional but recommended as the gold standard for anyone viewed as an airway management professional.

The Difficult Airway Society (DAS) November 2015 guidelines for management of unanticipated DI in adults stresses the immediate use of a second-generation SGA device to maintain oxygenation should difficulty occur. These guidelines specifically state: "It is recommended that the number of airway interventions are limited" and "blind techniques using a bougie or through SGAs have been superseded by video- or fiber-optically guided intubation."[259] In other words, direct visual control is advised. This guideline concept challenges traditional ideas that the FIS is not indicated as a second-line device after a failure of laryngoscopy or in emergency airway management.

Whether DI is unanticipated or anticipated, it is obvious that a blind technique through an SGA is not recommended in a setting where oxygenation may be precarious and that a combination with an FIS in a multimodal approach is often the technique of choice.

Acknowledgments

The framework and building blocks of this chapter were initially written by Dr. Katherine S.L. Gil and Dr. Pierre A. Diemunsch, to whom we are deeply grateful. Their clarity and depth of knowledge permeate throughout this chapter.

Selected References

18. Ahmad I, El-Boghdadly K, Bhagrath R, et al. Difficult Airway Society guidelines for awake tracheal intubation (ATI) in adults. *Anaesthesia.* 2020;75(4):509–528.

21. Mouritsen JM, Ehlers L, Kovaleva J, Ahmad I, El-Boghdadly K. A systematic review and cost effectiveness analysis of reusable vs. single-use flexible bronchoscopes. *Anaesthesia.* 2020;75(4):529–540.

46. Joffe AM, Aziz MF, Posner KL, Duggan LV, Mincer SL, Domino KB. Management of difficult tracheal intubation: a closed claims analysis. *Anesthesiology.* 2020;818–829.

58. Heidegger T, Gerig H, Ulrich B, Kreienbühl G. Validation of a simple algorithm for tracheal intubation: daily practice is the key to success in emergencies—An analysis of 13,248 intubations. *Anesth Analg.* 2001;92:517–522.

107. El-Boghdadly K, Onwochei DN, Cuddihy J, et al. A prospective cohort study of awake fibreoptic intubation practice at a tertiary centre. *Anaesthesia.* 2017;72(6):694–703.

114. Patel A, Nouraei SAR. Transnasal Humidified Rapid-Insufflation Ventilatory Exchange (THRIVE): a physiological method of increasing apnoea time in patients with difficult airways. *Anaesthesia.* 2015;70(3):323–329.

189. Kaplan MB, Hagberg CA, Ward DS, et al. Comparison of direct and video-assisted views of larynx during routine intubation. *J Clin Anesth.* 2006;18:357–362.

208. Gadkaree S, Schwartz D, Gerold K, et al. Use of bronchoscopy in percutaneous dilational tracheostomy. *JAMA Otolaryngol Head Neck Surg.* 2015;30:1–7.

163. Johnston KD, Rai MR. Conscious sedation for awake fibreoptic intubation: a review of the literature. *Can J Anesth.* 2013;60(6):584–599.

259. Frerk C, Mitchell VS, McNarry AF, et al. Difficult Airway Society 2015 guidelines for management of unanticipated difficult intubation in adults. *Br J Anaesth.* 2015;115(6):827–848.

All references can be found online at eBooks.Health.Elsevier.com.

25

Combination Techniques

PIERRE DIEMUNSCH AND CARIN A. HAGBERG

CHAPTER OUTLINE

KEY POINTS

- Combining airway techniques takes advantage of the respective strengths of each device while minimizing their specific shortcomings when used alone.
- The multimodal approach is appropriate in the use of various airway devices, including oxygenation tools.
- The multimodal approach is useful for teaching, clinical practice, and maintenance of knowledge in airway management.

- The most common examples of advantageous combinations in the field of airway management are the facilitation of flexible scope intubation (FSI) with video-assisted laryngoscopy and the use of a supraglottic device as a guide for FSI.
- Using THRIVE (transnasal humidified rapid insufflation ventilatory exchange), oxygenation is of paramount interest in association with FSI.

Introduction

The technical approach to airway management is one of the core medical techniques, and tracheal or bronchial intubation is a major concern in anesthesia (both operating room and procedural areas), the intensive care setting, and during resuscitation. The importance of the subject is reflected by the number of societies dedicated specifically to airway management, such as the Society for Airway Management (SAM), the Difficult Airway Society (DAS), and the European Airway Management Society (EAMS), in addition to intensive care and pulmonology societies, anesthesiology and perioperative medicine societies, and societies specializing in otorhinolaryngologic and thoracic surgery, which also incorporate airway management.

The field has evolved considerably in recent decades, as evidenced by the programs of the many specialized airway meetings. The first change was to emphasize that airway management is not an end in and of itself but rather a means of delivering oxygen to a patient. Likewise, decisive progress has been made in the prevention of hypoxemia, which may occur to varying degrees during the performance of tracheal intubation. Major advances have been made regarding ventilation, from the introduction of supraglottic airways (SGAs) and the general acceptance of high-flow apneic oxygenation to the concept of protective ventilation. The second substantive change in the field of airway management was to not only focus on the predictive signs of difficult intubation but to better address all forms of difficulty with airway management.

Current thinking focuses primarily on what to do in the event of difficulty rather than simply knowing that something will have to be done.

These major developments have been underpinned by the advent of mechanical, optical, and ultrasound-based techniques, which, as unimaginable as it might seem today, did not come into use until recently,[1] as well as the widespread introduction of new methods in initial and continuing education, and the production of recommendations and of intelligent and intelligible algorithms resulting from reflection rather than the mere sequential alignment of existing means.

Therefore the "stop and think" approach, which is a necessary part of the overall strategy to resolve difficult situations,[2] was applied to the specific matter of selecting the appropriate tools. It became apparent that, despite the progress brought about by the new systems, none of them were infallible, and it would be more beneficial to use them together rather than separately. This conclusion underpins the multimodal approach to upper airway management.[3]

The 2013 ASA Practice Guidelines for Management of the Difficult Airway have recently been revised and published in Anesthesiology 136.[4] The new guidelines include the use of combination techniques in both the adult and pediatric algorithms, either when the patient is awake or after induction of anesthesia, as part of the airway management strategy. The airway practitioner's assessment and choice of techniques should be based on their prior experience, available resources (including equipment), availability and competency of help, and the context in which airway management will occur. As with all techniques, experience and practice in nonemergent settings stand to optimize success in all environments.

The consultants and members of participating organizations in the most recent guideline development strongly agree with the recommendation to identify a preferred sequence of noninvasive devices to use for airway management if a noninvasive approach is selected. The consultants strongly agree, and members of participating organizations agree or strongly agree, that if difficulty is encountered with individual techniques, combination techniques may be performed.

Combining systems is a general approach that can involve most of the medical tools available to us, particularly regarding flexible or rigid, steerable or nonsteerable airway management devices, either with or without optical properties. Thus the multimodal airway management strategy consists of using the specific advantages of one medical device to mitigate the limitations of another. Additionally, the placement of pressure on the thyroid cartilage (backward, upward, rightward pressure [BURP] maneuver) or the utilization of special endotracheal tubes (ETTs) (e.g., Endotrol, Parker Flex-Tip, etc.) may facilitate tracheal intubation when utilizing any combination technique.

The most prominent example in the literature is the use of a videolaryngoscope (VL) to facilitate intubation with a flexible intubation scope (FIS), which may result in improved intubation success. In a recent randomized controlled trial comparing video-assisted laryngoscopy (VAL) itself or combined with flexible bronchoscopy, Mazzinari and colleagues reported a greater first-attempt success rate with the combination technique than with VAL alone.[5] It is this technique that this chapter will present in detail.

Other multimodal approaches are based on a combination of flexible scope intubation (FSI) with direct laryngoscopy (DL), second-generation SGAs, specially designed face masks (e.g., the VBM Endoscopy Mask), retrograde intubation, jet ventilation, or percutaneous tracheostomy. The use of conduits such as SGAs or endoscopy masks differs from those aimed solely at facilitating tracheal intubation in that they optimize the safety of the procedure by maintaining the delivery of oxygen to the patient. The combination of THRIVE (transnasal humidified rapid insufflation ventilatory exchange) and bronchoscopy can be included in the same group. A detailed and comprehensive review of multimodal procedures incorporating FSI can be found in Chapter 24.

The multimodal approach, which is particularly useful in the clinical setting, is also suitable for FSI training where textbook knowledge is combined with computer-based virtual reality training and simulation training, encompassing the development of nontechnical and team working skills, before a trainee ultimately engages in clinical practice under the guidance of a tutor.

Additionally, there are other combination techniques that do not involve FSI, including DL or VAL in combination with an optical stylet, an intubation/extubation catheter, or retrograde intubation; SGA placement in combination with an optical stylet, an intubation/extubation catheter, or retrograde intubation; and DL or VAL in combination with SGA placement.

Difficulty With the Use of Flexible Endoscopy in Clinical Practice

Despite the increase in the number of available airway devices and techniques, awake FSI remains the standard method for airway management in the event of foreseeable difficulties in mask ventilation and tracheal intubation. The possibility of abandoning awake FSI in favor of VAL has been discussed but is no longer regarded as a serious option in the most recent literature.[5–8] On the contrary, the extension of FSI indications to unexpected emergency situations was highlighted in the UK's National Institute for Health and Care Excellence (NICE) Medical Technologies Guidance (MTG14) on the single-use aScope (Ambu, Ballerup, Denmark), which is described as "specially recommended for unexpected difficult airways."[9]

Despite anesthesiologists being required to master FSI,[10,11] opportunities for practice are limited: the absolute number of patients with predicted difficult airway management is low, and teaching FSI in patients with normal airways may be considered ethically arguable.

FSI teaching has been further limited by the availability and fragility of equipment, hygiene issues, and the risk of transmitting infectious diseases through nonconventional agents (i.e., prions), in particular.

Previous reports have suggested that many anesthesiologists have completed their initial training without acquiring FSI skills properly.[12] In addition to the problems surrounding initial training, as many airway practitioners have few opportunities to practice flexible endoscopy, they are in real danger of losing their skills. There are various solutions to these training issues; the advent of single-use endoscopes has largely resolved the problems relating to equipment availability and hygiene. Extending the indications for FSI beyond the scope of difficult airway management, and the classic indication of cervical spine instability, seems advisable for many patients with normal airways who could benefit from the avoidance of stress related to DL (neonates or adult patients with hypertension, diabetes, and coronary artery disease, in particular). Finally, initial training and the practical implementation of FSI in a clinical setting are largely facilitated by the multimodal approach.

Learning the Multimodal Airway Management Concept With Virtual Reality

The acquisition of both tracheal and bronchial endoscopy skills is based primarily on an understanding of the three clearly defined steps of the procedure (the "down–up–down" steps, as described elsewhere[5,13]) and on initial learning using a virtual reality simulator or navigator according to a *partial-task training program*.[14,15] Different types of simulators are available at various prices,[16–19] and it is well established that simulation actually optimizes the subsequent practice of FSI.[20] The benefit of so-called "high-fidelity" simulators lies in the realism of the simulated procedure; their main limitations are their purchase cost and the cumbersome logistics essential to their implementation. "Low-fidelity" simulators, such as homemade wooden panels with a selection of holes to choose from, or the Gil 5-Minute Dexterity Model, are inexpensive and their educational effectiveness is comparable to that of high-fidelity devices.[21] However, they still require a logistic infrastructure, including (1) premises, (2) a real FIS with connectors and a display screen, and (3) a team of motivated instructors. They do not allow trainees to familiarize themselves with the endoscopic anatomy of the human upper airways.

Virtual FSI software overcomes these limitations by enabling users to browse inside a three-dimensional reconstruction of human computed tomography (CT) or magnetic resonance images. It has proven its relevance in facilitating flexible endoscopy learning and was developed using the multimodal bronchoscopy model.[22] For instance, the VFI (Virtual Fiberoptic Intubation) program (Karl

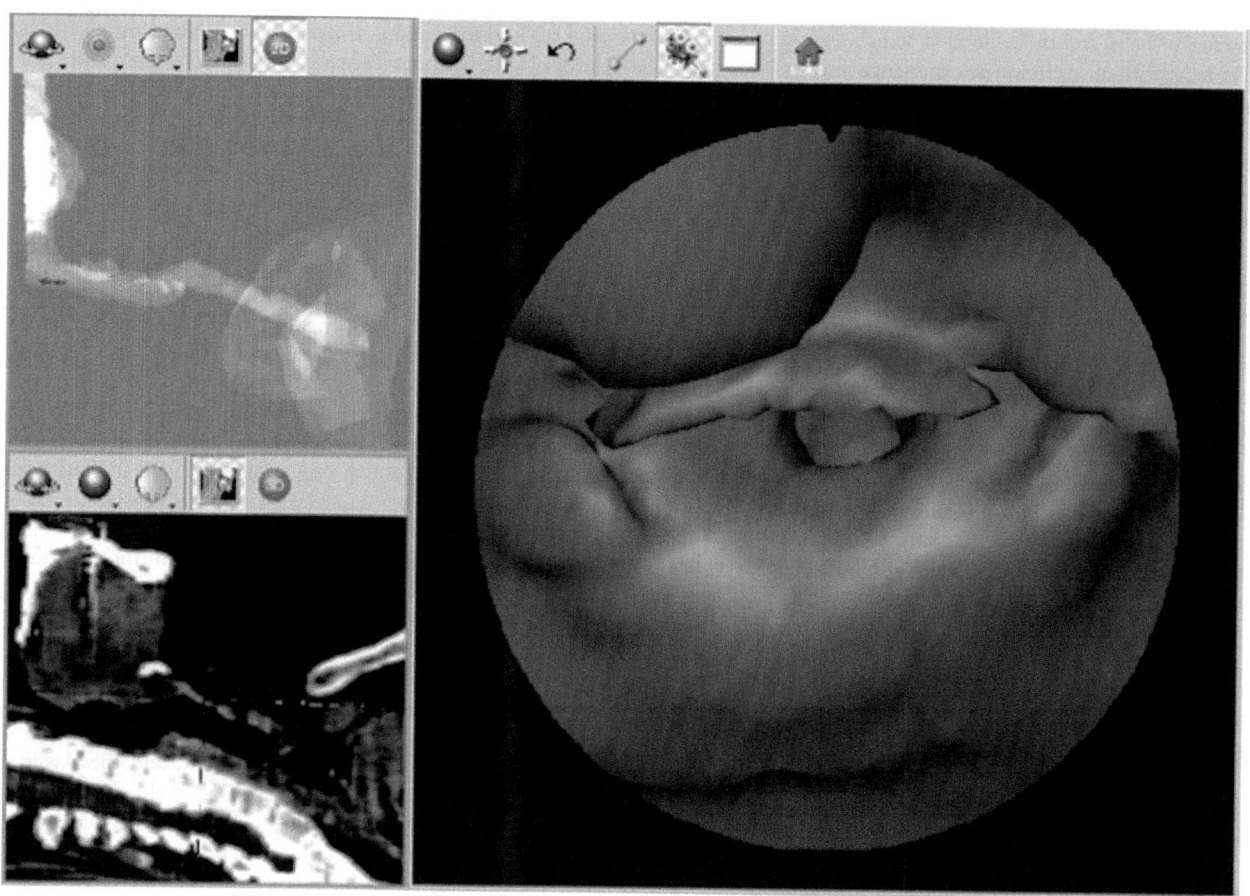

• **Fig. 25.1** The VFI simulation program (Karl Storz, Tuttlingen, Germany). The two lateral screens show a three-dimensional reconstructed image of the entire airway and the corresponding CT image, while the main panel provides the image collected by the virtual FIS. The *red arrow* identifies where the tip of the virtual endoscope sits in the upper airway (in this example in the nasopharynx just above the uvula). (Courtesy P. Diemunsch, MD, PhD.)

Storz, Tuttlingen, Germany) provides a three-dimensional reconstructed image of the entire airway and the corresponding CT image on two panels alongside the main panel, which provides the image collected by the virtual FIS (Fig. 25.1). The location of the tip of the virtual FIS is indicated on the two imaging panels with a red arrow. Using a computer mouse, the trainee can perform a virtual progression through the airways from either the mouth or the nose to the trachea. The trainee benefits from a partial task schedule since they can first familiarize themselves with the airway anatomy, as visualized endoscopically, which can be quite different from the distorted direct laryngoscopic view. They can then acquire endoscopic psychomotor skills easily, since they can constantly follow both the position of and the view from the FIS tip. Indeed, this is the ideal preparation for the clinical multimodal VL-FIS approach to intubation, where the anesthesiologist can follow the position of the FIS on a VL screen as the FIS provides the main endoscopic view on its own screen and is progressively introduced toward the carina (see below).

Limits of Video-Assisted Laryngoscopy When Used Alone

The introduction of VAL was a decisive step forward in terms of both direct intubation and facilitating the endoscopic approach.

However, this combination of techniques is still underutilized. The excellent performance of VAL used alone could, paradoxically, explain this state of affairs. VAL used in isolation has become an integral part of the recent recommendations of learned societies concerning difficult intubation in anesthetic practice and resuscitation.[23,24] It is important to emphasize that VAL is nevertheless associated with a significant risk of failure when used alone. VAL cannot reliably and completely replace flexible endoscopic techniques (see above).

The GlideScope (Verathon, Seattle, WA) is one of the most widely used VLs and owes its dominant position to its long existence. The latest version (Spectrum) comes with single-use blades. The McGRATH (Medtronic, Boulder, CO, USA) has a small screen attached to the handle, a single-use blade, and a shock-absorbent casing. Its main advantage is that it is ready to use almost immediately, since it does not need to be connected to a light source, remote screen, or power outlet. It therefore seems to be particularly suited to emergency situations or unexpected difficult intubations, where no special equipment has been prepared in advance. A highly angulated blade designed specifically for difficult intubation (X-Blade) is available. The C-MAC (Karl Storz, Tuttlingen, Germany) offers an optional compact video system suitable for both prehospital and outpatient facility care.

The GlideScope, McGRATH, and C-MAC are examples of VLs that do not have a guide channel for the intubation tube.

They are therefore associated with a risk of misplacement, as the tube is partially inserted blindly. The risk is greater when the tube is mounted on a rigid stylet, as is often recommended. Using a long, angle-tipped catheter, such as the Frova Intubating Introducer (Cook Medical, Bloomington, IN), could be an alternative option for orotracheal intubation with this type of VL.

Other VLs have a guide channel that allows the intubation tube to be inserted toward the glottis without the risk of traumatic misplacement. The King Vision, with its aBlade, can be included in this category (Ambu, Copenhagen, Denmark). Likewise, the Airtraq (Prodol Meditec, Bilbao, Spain) has a guide channel for the tube and a screen attached to its handle. Like the Mc GRATH, these devices are ready to use immediately. The Airway Scope (Pentax, Tokyo, Japan) is another portable VL. Its single-use blade has a guide channel. Although any of the VLs offers its own unique advantages, VLs in general provide several advantages to the clinician managing the airway, namely, an improved view of the glottis, decreased cervical spine motion, and the ability to improve instruction to a trainee.

Supraglottic Devices and Multimodal Airway Management

Many SGAs have attempted to reproduce or even improve the performance of Brain's original LMA (Teleflex, Wayne, PA). Their advantages are variable and often debatable; some were quickly withdrawn from the market. The LMA CTrach, which was an intubating LMA with a removable screen and an optical system for viewing the glottis (Teleflex, Wayne, PA), was particularly suitable for intubation but is no longer available. The i-gel (Intersurgical, Wokingham, UK) was a significant breakthrough. It is a single-use SGA device made of a gel-like thermoplastic elastomer, which is characterized by its ability to adapt to the laryngeal anatomy without cuff inflation and an airway shaft that facilitates insertion, to ensure stability in the mouth, and to facilitate intubation with a standard-sized ETT. Second-generation SGAs have a drain channel for an orogastric suction tube, a tube shaped channel to guide the ETT to the glottis, a cuff to ensure a high seal pressure, and a built-in bite block.

In difficult intubation algorithms SGAs are placed immediately in the second line (Plan B) after intubation failure under DL or videolaryngoscopy. Once an SGA is in place, other methods and/or devices may be used in combination with these devices to either effectively ventilate the patient or secure a more definitive airway. It is no longer recommended to subsequently attempt blind tracheal intubation through an SGA. On the contrary, intubation should be carried out under visual control, aided by an FIS to guide the ETT.[25] This recommendation by both the ASA and the DAS is the first formal framework for the implementation of a multimodal FSI strategy. It has also been reported in pediatric practice.[26–28] An advantage with any of these devices is that the larynx is effectively "sealed" off from blood or secretions, and they achieve ventilation in patients who may be difficult to mask-ventilate, difficult to intubate, or have significant intraoral bleeding.

In regard to multimodal FSI, we can illustrate the value of SGAs by considering them as a conduit equivalent to a nasopharyngeal airway placed in the mouth or oropharynx. Like a nasal airway, the SGA naturally directs the FIS to the glottis and it can be used to help ventilate the patient. This conduit spares the natural nasal fossae, does not contain fragile turbinates or mucosa, does not bleed, and easily accommodates an ETT loaded onto

a flexible scope to guide it.[29] Alternatively, an airway exchange catheter (such as the Aintree Intubation Catheter, Cook Medical, Bloomington, IN) may be loaded onto the FIS. Placed in the trachea, it can serve as a guide for the ETT and resolve the issue of the relative lengths of the ETT and the SGA.[30–32]

Video-Assisted Laryngoscopy and Flexible Scope Intubation

Rigid VLs have been proposed for the management of difficult intubations because they provide better glottic exposure and improve the Cormack-Lehane laryngoscopic grade compared to DL.[33,34] However, it is sometimes difficult to advance the ETT toward the glottis and complete the intubation procedure. Such failures illustrate the difference between the two components of a successful intubation: (1) obtaining a clear view of the glottis and (2) passing the ETT between the vocal cords. During DL with a Macintosh-type blade, the success of the visual component (laryngoscopy) usually predicts that of the mechanical component (insertion of the ETT), because the former already requires mechanical alignment of the pharyngeal and laryngeal axes. On the other hand, VAL primarily improves the visual component by means of an optical device, particularly when a highly curved blade (e.g., the McGRATH X-Blade or the C-MAC D-BLADE) or an acutely angled blade is used. It has no effect on the mechanical difficulties that may be encountered during ETT insertion due to the patient's specific anatomic characteristics; the VL may provide a very clear image of the posterior passage of the tip of the ETT, behind the corniculate cartilages and the arytenoids. Clinical cases illustrating this difficulty have been reported for several types of VL, with or without a guide channel. These particularly frustrating failure situations are not unusual.[35] Of interest is the description of the predictive factors of difficult VAL by Aziz.[36] There is a very real risk that VAL has been used in the belief that it could resolve all difficult intubation situations alone, when a flexible device, such as an FIS with a steerable tip, was indicated.

Another risk associated with the use of VAL is specific to devices that do not have a guide channel for the ETT. Indeed, even if the glottis is clearly visible on the VL screen, there is a blind portion midway through the supraglottic path taken by the ETT, when the tip of the ETT escapes direct external visual control but cannot yet be seen on the VL screen. Some manufacturers recommend using a preformed rigid stylet to reduce failures. Besides the fact that they are not always effective, these stylets can cause pharyngeal injuries, including to the soft palate,[37–41] the tonsillar pillars,[42] and other structures in this region.[43] Such injuries are caused by forcing the stylet through the operator's "blind spot"; there is a major risk of blind spot injury, particularly where a pharyngeal tumor is present.

For safety and efficacy reasons, it is preferable to replace the rigid stylet with a flexible, atraumatic stylet or, better still, with a combination of VAL and an FIS to benefit from the advantages of both techniques.[44,45] After the induction of general anesthesia and face mask oxygenation, or after appropriate topical anesthesia, the clinician performing the intubation starts by placing the VL in the patient's mouth until the best possible view of the glottis is obtained. The primary operator then takes the FIS from his assistant, holding the distal end as if it were an ETT (Fig. 25.2). The primary operator begins to insert the FIS under direct external vision and then, under indirect videolaryngoscopic guidance, brings it as close as possible to the glottic orifice. The assistant, who

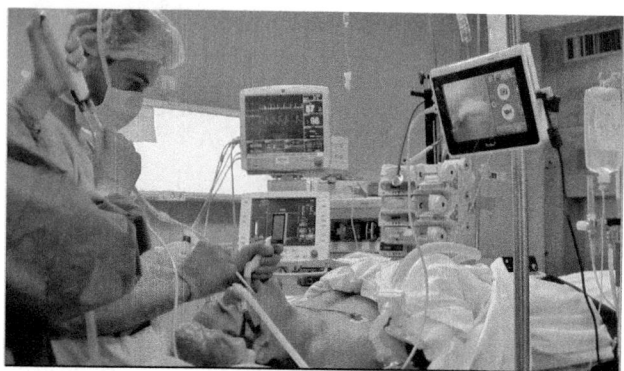

• **Fig. 25.2** Multimodal bronchoscopic intubation using video-assisted laryngoscopy and a flexible intubation scope: primary technique (see text). (Courtesy P. Diemunsch, MD, PhD.)

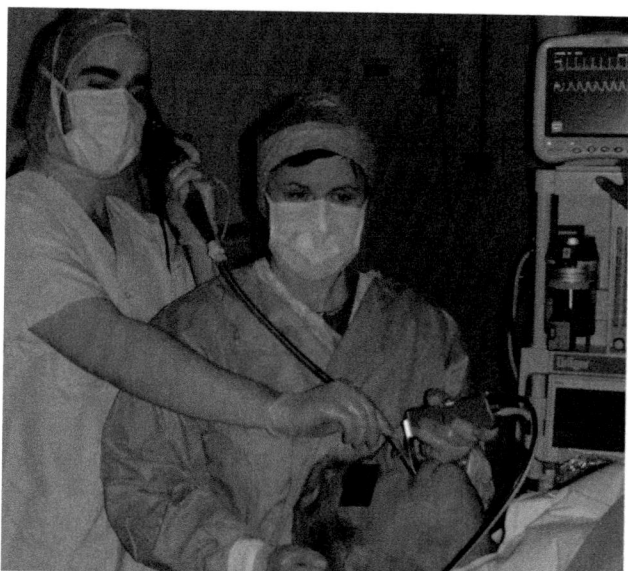

• **Fig. 25.3** Multimodal bronchoscopic intubation using video-assisted laryngoscopy and a flexible intubation scope: alternate technique (see text). The primary operator performs the endoscopy while the assistant facilitates the procedure with a videolaryngoscope. The operator may stand lateral to or, as here, behind the assistant. (Courtesy P. Diemunsch, MD, PhD.)

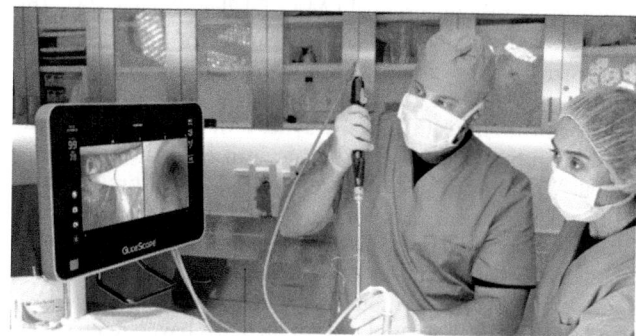

• **Fig. 25.4** The GlideScope Core dual-screen system allowing for simultaneous videolaryngoscopy and bronchoscopy. (Courtesy Verathon Inc., Bothell, WA, USA)

may be a less experienced provider, holds the handle of the FIS and actuates the control lever. On the operator's instructions, the assistant presses the control lever on the handle of the FIS in order to bend its tip upward. This maneuver displays the glottis on the FIS screen, even if it is not visible on the VL screen. Then the primary clinician, under double visual (videolaryngoscopic and FIS) control, inserts the FIS through the glottis and into the trachea until it is just above the carina, directing the assistant to angle the tip of the FIS as appropriate throughout the procedure (upward until the anterior commissure of the vocal cords is reached, then downward toward the carina while remaining as centered as possible in the tracheal lumen). The primary operator then performs tracheal intubation by advancing the ETT previously mounted over the FIS until its tip is correctly positioned above the carina.[46] The VL also provides a view of the tube's passage into the laryngeal inlet. This may help to resolve any difficulties at this point. When appropriate, the nasal route is also possible.[47]

This technique is the one we prefer, but the primary clinician may choose to perform the traditional FSI procedure with the ETT loaded onto the FIS while the assistant operates the VL (Fig. 25.3). In this case the operator can track the position of the FIS tip as it advances on the VL screen. It is the primary operator who will successively direct the FIS down to the posterior wall of the oropharynx, then upward to the anterior commissure of the vocal cords, and finally downward toward the carina while remaining as perfectly centered in the tracheal lumen as possible. The rest of the procedure is identical to the one previously described. This alternative technique is ideal for experienced endoscopists, although it is slightly less ergonomic than the first, as both the operator and the assistant are standing next to the patient's head. The combined use of DL and FSI has also been reported in intensive care patients and as a means to support the learning of FIS-aided intubation skills.[48]

In our experience VAL considerably facilitates FSI by keeping the oropharynx open and preventing lateral deviations of the FIS.[49] The operator uses both the external view of the FIS tip on the VL screen and the internal view of the airway on the FIS screen. Every step of the FSI procedure is carried out under visual control, and using a combination of both techniques can also reduce the pressure exerted by the VL blade on the base of the tongue, thereby reducing the associated stress.[50] This combined technique has been demonstrated to be effective, particularly with the C-MAC and the McGRATH,[46] and device manufacturers have begun to provide systems reflecting the increased interest in combined techniques such as the GlideScope Core (Verathon Inc., Bothell, WA), which has a large dual-view screen to facilitate multimodal airway management

(Fig. 25.4). The combined technique can be used regardless of the VL and FIS chosen[51]; when the FIS is used in combination with a channeled VL, the FIS can either be inserted within the lumen of the ETT or next to the device. It is suitable as a "best first attempt" in the event of predicted difficulty and has regularly been used with success following failed intubation attempts with VL or FIS alone.[52] VAL can also diagnose problems with ETT entry into the glottis during FSI, as the combination technique provides the advantage of the visualization of the passage of the ETT over the FIS into the glottis and identifies, as well as helps resolve, any passage difficulties. Additionally, if the procedure is captured by camera or videography, these images/videos can be uploaded into the electronic medical record for viewing by future care providers (Fig. 25.5).

Conclusion

A constructive approach to the problem of difficult intubation consists of combining available techniques to take advantage of their respective strengths rather than using them individually in a manner that does not minimize their specific shortcomings. This multimodal approach is used in many settings, such as balanced

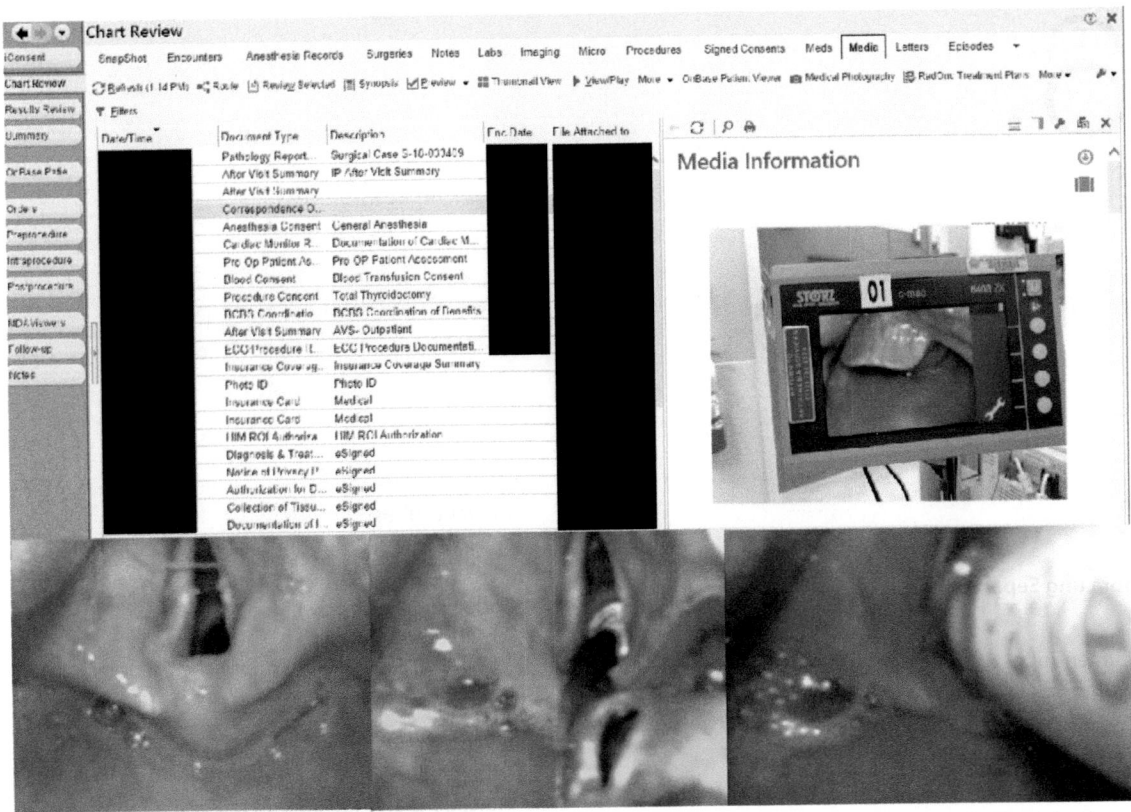

• **Fig. 25.5** Images in an electronic health record providing details of a combination videolaryngoscope and flexible scope intubation.

anesthesia, multimodal analgesia, and the management of hypertension or infections. The multimodal management of difficult intubation is an increasingly popular solution among clinicians. It can be applied to a large number of devices intended for airway visualization and intubation and patient oxygenation.[53]

The multimodal approach is particularly useful for the vast majority of practitioners who only occasionally perform bronchial endoscopy. It is part of the holistic care of our patients and applies to medical training, the facilitation of clinical technical procedures, the prevention of complications, and the avoidance of failures.

Each airway device has unique properties that may be advantageous in certain situations yet limiting in others. Specific airway management techniques are greatly influenced by individual disease and anatomy, and successful management may require combinations of devices and techniques. Thus clinicians should gain the knowledge of combination strategies, such as those outlined in this chapter, to increase their success in the use of these airway devices and techniques. As with any intubation technique, practice and routine use will improve performance and may reduce the likelihood of complications.

Additional material (Videos 25.1 and 25.2) is available as an example of multimodal airway management.

Selected References

1. Hagberg C. Current concepts in the management of the difficult airway. *Anesthesiology News.* 2018;15:1–32.

9. National Institute for Health and Care Excellence: NICE—guidance MTG 14. *Medical Technologies Advisory Committee Meeting:* 21 February 2013. Updated June 2019. nice.org.uk.

14. Jirapinyo P, Abidi WM, Aihara H, Zaki T, Tsay C, Imaeda AB, Thompson CC. Preclinical endoscopic training using a part-task simulator: learning curve assessment and determination of threshold score for advancement to clinical endoscopy. *Surg Endosc.* 2017;31:4010–4015.

20. Boet S, Bould MD, Schaeffer R, Fischhof S, Stojeba N, Naik VN, Diemunsch P. Learning fibreoptic intubation with a virtual computer program transfers to "hands on" improvement. *Eur J Anaesthesiol.* 2010;27:31–35.

23. Quintard H, l'Her E, Pottecher J, et al. Intubation and extubation of the ICU patient. Guidelines. *Anaesth Crit Care Pain Med.* 2017; 36:327–341.

36. Aziz M. Routine clinical practice effectiveness of the Glidescope in difficult airway management. *Anesthesiology.* 2011;114:34–41.

44. Greib N, Stojeba N, Dow WA, Henderson J, Diemunsch PA. A combined rigid videolaryngoscopy-flexible fibrescopy intubation technique under general anesthesia. *Can J Anaesth.* 2007;54:492–493.

49. Boet S, Bould D, Diemunsch P. Combined rigid videolaryngoscopy-flexible bronchoscopy for intubation. *Korean J Anesthesiol.* 2011;60:381–382.

52. Liew GHC, Wong TGL, Lu A, Kothandan H. Combined use of the Glidescope and flexible fibrescope as a rescue technique in a difficult airway. *Proc Singapore Healthc.* 2015;24:117–120.

All references can be found online at eBooks.Health.Elsevier.com.

26

Lung Isolation Techniques

EDMOND COHEN

CHAPTER OUTLINE

KEY POINTS

- Lung isolation should only be performed by well-trained and experienced practitioners who understand the significant risks and benefits of such techniques.
- Indications for lung isolation include protection of the healthy lung from contamination in the case of infection or hemorrhage; control of ventilation distribution; and bronchopulmonary lavage.
- Relative indications for lung separation are mainly for surgical exposure.
- Double-lumen tubes (DLTs) come in sizes 28, 32, 35, 37, 39, and 41 French, and the appropriate length is based on height, build, and airway examination. Positioning should be confirmed by flexible scope visualization, selective ventilation auscultation, or radiographic studies.
- DLTs are advantageous because they provide the capability of independent bilateral lung ventilation, bronchial suctioning, lung deflation, and stability, but they have the disadvantages of difficult tube placement, large size, rigidity, and difficulty in management for prolonged ventilation.
- For patients with difficult airways, anatomic anomalies, tracheal obstructions, tracheal-vascular distortions, or the need for

segmental lung isolation, the use of one-lung ventilation (OLV) isolation devices should be strongly considered.
- Disadvantages of OLV isolation techniques include difficulty with lung deflation, difficulty suctioning the isolated lung, difficulty with stability and positioning, and inability to independently ventilate the isolated lung portion.
- Univent tubes are single-lumen tubes (SLTs) with an external bronchial blocker attachment; they can be used as an effective device for lung isolation, including large segmental-lobar isolation.
- Bronchial blockers come as stand-alone devices and can be used with SLTs or DLTs that have a low-volume, high-pressure cuff system; they may be used paraxially or axially for whole or segmental lung isolation.
- Pediatric lung isolation techniques are similar, if not identical, to those used for adults, although SLT techniques are often used. However, pediatric anatomy and physiology differ from those of adults in terms of positioning and ventilation.
- Successful lung isolation and protection are vastly improved with the use of a flexible scope.

Introduction

The physiology, indications, and techniques of lung isolation and one-lung ventilation (OLV) are discussed in this chapter. Lung isolation is most commonly used during thoracic, esophageal, and some cardiac procedures; however, it can often be useful and potentially lifesaving in other situations like massive hemoptysis. Modern disposable double-lumen tubes (DLTs), single-lumen tubes (SLTs) with built-in endobronchial blockers (Univent), new endobronchial blockers, and enhanced video technology are making lung isolation and OLV safer to perform. Knowledge of these topics is requisite for an anesthesia provider.

Physiology

The most common physiologic problem with OLV is the presence of a large intrapulmonary shunt through the collapsed nonventilated lung. This shunt may result in hypoxia with severe irreversible end-organ damage. Most anesthesia providers aim to maintain arterial oxygen saturation above 90% (Pao_2 >60 mm Hg because hemoglobin saturation and O_2 content drop sharply below this value as a result of the characteristics of the O_2 dissociation curve).

In most surgical cases patients are placed in lateral decubitus position with the ventilated lung dependent. The physiologic goal is to promote blood flow to the nonsurgical, dependent lung. By reducing the pulmonary vascular resistance (PVR) of the dependent lung to minimal levels, improved ventilation-perfusion (V/Q) matching may occur. Excess positive end-expiratory pressure (PEEP), high airway pressures, hypoxia, hypercapnia, and hypovolemia may contribute to an increase in PVR of the dependent lung, thereby increasing the shunt fraction. Improvement of the shunt fraction can be accomplished by decreasing the blood flow and/or supplying O_2 to the nondependent lung.

Hypoxic pulmonary vasoconstriction is a powerful protective reflex that increases the PVR of the hypoxic alveoli and lung, thus diverting blood to the well-oxygenated areas of the lung. It is therefore useful to limit agents that inhibit hypoxic pulmonary vasoconstriction, such as nitrates and high concentrations of volatile agents.

The supplementation of O_2 to the nondependent lung may also alleviate hypoxia. This can be accomplished via apneic oxygenation by the application of an external continuous positive airway pressure (CPAP) circuit to the nondependent lung or simply by trapping partial inflations of the nondependent lung. The goal is to allow enough O_2 into the nondependent lung to reverse hypoxia while not obscuring the surgical field.

Indications for Lung Separation

The current indication for lung separation distinguished between lung isolation or lung separation. Lung isolation includes protecting and isolating the nondiseased lung from the pathology of the diseased lung to maintain adequate gas exchange. Lung isolation may be lifesaving by simply preventing drowning or severe contamination of the ventilated lung by the nondependent lung. Lung protection will prevent further deterioration of overall pulmonary function. As depicted in Box 26.1, these cases include hemoptysis, empyema, or any contaminant in the noninvolved lung that can lead to severe atelectasis, pneumonia, sepsis, and inadequate ventilation. A large bronchopleural or bronchocutaneous fistula can lead to little or no ventilation. In this situation the decreased resistance to flow in the affected lung results in most of the positive-pressure

---

> ● **BOX 26.1** Indications for One-Lung Ventilation
>
> **Lung Isolation**
>
> Isolation of one lung from the other to avoid spillage or contamination
> 1. Infection
> 2. Massive hemorrhage
>
> Control of the distribution of ventilation
> 1. Bronchopleural fistula
> 2. Bronchopleural cutaneous fistula
> 3. Surgical opening of a major conducting airway
> 4. Giant unilateral lung cyst or bulla
> 5. Life-threatening hypoxemia related to unilateral lung disease
>
> Unilateral bronchopulmonary lavage
> 1. Pulmonary alveolar proteinosis
>
> **Lung Separation**
>
> Surgical exposure—high priority
> 1. Thoracic aortic aneurysm
> 2. Pneumonectomy
> 3. Thoracoscopy
> 4. Upper lobectomy
> 5. Mediastinal exposure
>
> Surgical exposure—medium (lower) priority
> 1. Middle and lower lobectomies and subsegmental resections
> 2. Esophageal resection
> 3. Procedures on the thoracic spine
>
> Pulmonary edema after cardiopulmonary bypass
> Hemorrhage after the removal of totally occluding, unilateral, chronic pulmonary emboli
> Severe hypoxemia related to unilateral lung disease

ventilation (PPV) being directed toward the diseased lung. This results in minimally ventilating the normal lung and producing inadequate gas exchange. Conversely, a relatively noncompliant transplanted lung cannot compete with the better compliance of the native lung, and, as a result, the healthy transplanted lung can be severely underventilated. Another scenario involves a lung with bullous or cystic disease or a lung with tracheobronchial disruption.[1] Tension pneumothorax or tension mediastinum could result during these scenarios from elevated airway pressures that are often observed with OLV in the lateral decubitus position.

Patients with alveolar proteinosis may require unilateral bronchopulmonary lavage, which involves multiple instillations of large fluid volumes into the target lung with subsequent drainage of the effluent fluid.[2-4] Lung isolation and protection are mandatory to avoid lung cross-contamination and drowning caused by the large volume of fluid required to perform the lavage.

Lung separation involves facilitating surgical exposure by providing a still operating field, avoiding lung trauma, and improving gas exchange. Operations such as the repair of thoracic aneurysms, pneumonectomy, pulmonary lobectomies (especially of the upper lobe), video-assisted thoracoscopic surgery (VATS), esophageal surgery, and anterior spinal surgery all benefit from the optimized surgical exposure afforded by OLV (see Box 26.1). Lung protection further improves recovery by minimizing lung instrumentation and trauma to the nonventilated, nondependent lung. In cases of unilateral lung trauma, oxygenation and recovery may be optimized with OLV by improving V/Q matching.

Most procedures in which OLV is used are for lung separation, while only a few require isolation for lung protection. This distinction of lung isolation versus lung separation is important when selecting the method to provide OLV. In cases where lung protection is necessary, DLTs are preferable to endobronchial blockers (BB) because the low-pressure, high-volume cuff of the BB would not provide a protective seal to prevent contamination of the dependent lung. In addition, once the balloon of the blocker is deflated, the nondiseased lung is subjected to contamination from the pathology of the diseased lung. The use of blockers limits the ability for robust suctioning and removal of debris or thick pus before balloon deflation.

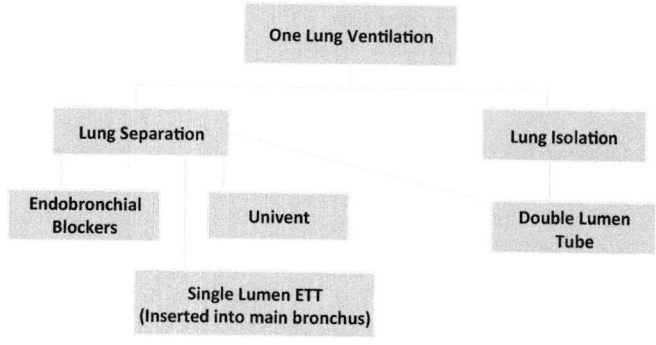

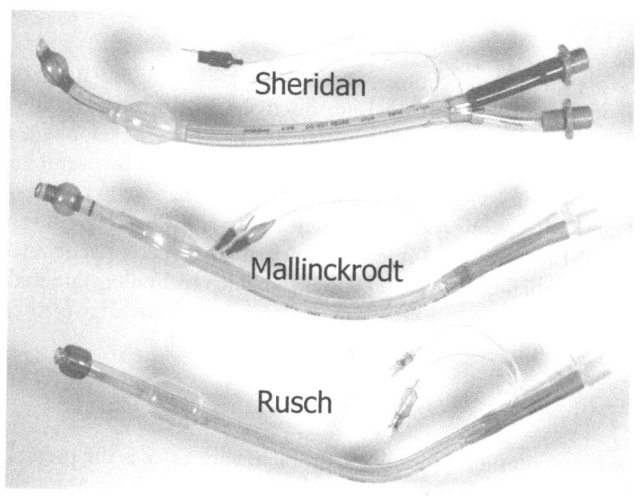

Techniques

Double-Lumen Tubes

Anatomy

DLTs are essentially two tubes bonded together with a design that allows each tube to ventilate a specified lung. DLTs are right-sided or left-sided devices. Left-sided DLTs have a bronchial port that extends into the left main stem bronchus and a tracheal port that is designed to sit above the carina. In right-sided DLTs the bronchial port extends into the right main stem bronchus, and the tracheal port sits above the carina. The cuff of the right-sided DLT may be at an oblique angle to facilitate ventilation of the right upper lobe bronchus at the Murphy eye (Fig. 26.1).

The original DLTs were reusable, Robertshaw-design red rubber tubes with high-pressure cuffs that became stiff and brittle over time, making placement more difficult and traumatic. Modern DLTs are made of nontoxic polyvinyl chloride (the Z-79 marking) and are disposable (Fig. 26.2). As the plastic warms up from the surrounding body temperature, the DLT conforms to the anatomy of the patient. This increased malleability, however, makes it more difficult to reposition the same tube. Current DLTs employ high-volume,

low-pressure, color-coded cuffs. The bronchial cuff and its pilot balloon/connector are blue. The tracheal cuff and its pilot balloon/connector are clear or white. Cuff inflation pressure requires a balance between preserving an adequate seal and maintaining mucosal perfusion. Measured cuff pressures between 15 and 30 mm Hg achieve these goals.[5–8] In cases involving the use of nitrous oxide the cuff pressures should be checked periodically as the nitrous oxide will diffuse into the cuff and increase the pressure in the balloon.

DLTs come in various French sizes, namely, 28, 32, 35, 37, 39, and 41. French equals approximately 0.33-mm measurement of the outer diameter (OD). In most adult men a 39- to 41-French DLT fits well, having an adequate length and appropriate diameter while providing the capability of suctioning or intubation with a fiberoptic bronchoscope (FB). A 35- to 37-French DLT fits most adult women. A 32-French will fit a small adult, while a 28-French will be adequate for an adolescent. A left-sided DLT size can also be estimated by using tracheal width measurements obtained from imaging. A radiopaque line may be seen at the end of each lumen to allow for radiographic positioning. A Y-adapter for the proximal end allows ventilation of both lumens through a single circuit. The cross-section of the DLT is designed as one D-shaped lumen and one crescent-shaped tracheal lumen. Left- and right-sided DLTs are curved at the distal end to enable advancement into the respective main stem bronchus. DLTs from different manufacturers have their own characteristic feel and slight modifications to the basic design described. The depth required for insertion of the DLT correlates with the height of the

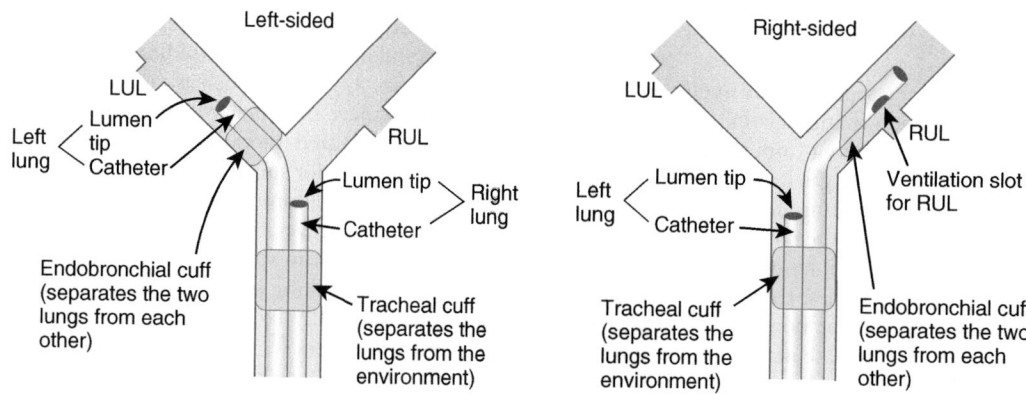

• **Fig. 26.1** Essential features and parts of left-sided and right-sided double-lumen tubes. *LUL,* Left upper lobe; *RUL,* right upper lobe. (From Benumof JL. *Anesthesia for Thoracic Surgery.* Philadelphia: Saunders; 1987.)

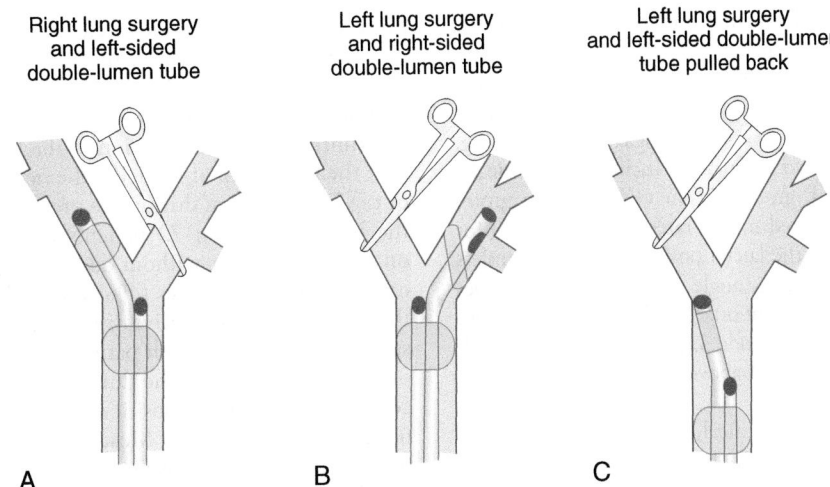

Right lung surgery
and left-sided
double-lumen tube

Left lung surgery
and right-sided
double-lumen tube

Left lung surgery
and left-sided double-lumen
tube pulled back

A   B   C

• **Fig. 26.2** Use of left-sided and right-sided double-lumen tubes (DLTs) for left and right lung surgery is indicated by the clamp. (A) When surgery is performed on the right lung, a left-sided DLT should be used. (B) When surgery is performed on the left lung, a right-sided DLT may be used. (C) However, because of uncertainty about the alignment of a right upper lobe ventilation slot to the right upper lobe orifice, a left-sided DLT can be used for left lung surgery. If left lung surgery requires a clamp to be placed high on the left main stem bronchus, the left endobronchial cuff should be deflated, the left-sided DLT pulled back into the trachea, and the right lung ventilated through both lumens (using the DLT as a single-lumen tube). (From Benumof JL. *Anesthesia for Thoracic Surgery*. Philadelphia: Saunders; 1987.)

patient. For any adult 170 to 180 cm tall, the average depth for a left-sided DLT is 29 cm. For every 10-cm increase or decrease in height, the DLT is advanced or withdrawn 1.0 cm.[9]

Advantages

When properly positioned, the DLT allows independent ventilation of each lung in unison or separately. This is a great advantage in cases in which each lung needs to be ventilated using different modalities. Treatment and prevention of desaturation are also easier with DLTs, because CPAP or partial lung inflation is easy to perform on the surgical lung while the opposite lung is ventilated normally. Suctioning and flexible bronchoscopy are facilitated by the relatively large luminal accesses into each main stem bronchus. Access beyond each main stem bronchus also allows for the egress of gases and lung deflation for surgical exposure. Other advantages include the solid structure and improved cuff seals of the DLTs, which prevent easy dislodgment after proper positioning and is the tube of choice for cases of lung isolation to prevent contamination from the diseased lung.

Disadvantages

The most significant disadvantages of the DLT are related to its bulky size and stiffness. Intubation with a DLT is often more difficult than with an SLT depending upon the mouth opening and the size of the tongue.[6] Intubation is even more complex in patients with difficult airway anatomy.[10] In cases of a distorted or compressed tracheobronchial tree the placement of a DLT may be impossible because of its size and rigidity. DLT size can contribute to airway damage during placement or when the device is left in place for a long period. Because of some difficulty managing DLTs in the intensive care unit (ICU) with regard to weaning and pulmonary toilet, they are often exchanged for SLTs. The process of exchanging a DLT for an SLT can be dangerous, especially after procedures in which airway edema and secretion accumulation has occurred. Although DLT lumens are relatively large, flexible bronchoscopy may be cumbersome because of the extended length of each tube and the narrowed crescent shape of the tracheal lumen.

Multiple ports and connections further require a good working knowledge of the DLT anatomy to prevent errors in ventilation and management.

Novel Double-Lumen Tubes

The Silbroncho Tube (Fuji Systems Corporation, Tokyo, Japan)

The Silbroncho DLT is made of silicone material reinforced with a wire-reinforced endobronchial tip that allows the tube to be inserted at a >50-degree angle without risk of kinking. The short endobronchial cuff tip can provide a greater margin of safety to avoid obstruction of the left upper lobe bronchus. It is useful in left upper lobectomy for those presenting for a repeated thoracic procedure. The expansion of the left lower lobe will cause an upward rotation of the left upper lobe bronchus to >50-degree takeoff.[11,12] Because the short endobronchial tip is positioned 20 mm below the tracheal carina into the left mainstem bronchus,

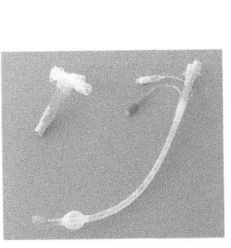

Silbroncho®
(Fuji, Tokyo)

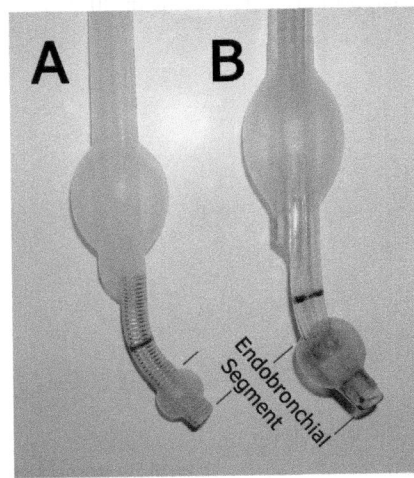

the outer balloon of the endobronchial lumen is seen below the tracheal carina, preventing dislodgement of the tube.

A recent study by Kwon et al.[13] involving 108 patients requiring OLV, comparing a displacement of the polyvinyl chloride (n = 54) to silicone Silbroncho left-sided DLT (n = 54) during lateral positioning, showed that both DLTs produced comparable incidence of clinically significant displacement (DLT group 35.4% vs Silbroncho group 34.6%). Both devices also required similar rates of repositioning for successful lung separation after the lateral position. Therefore unless the main bronchus is at a >50-degree angle, there are no advantages to using the Silbroncho over a conventional DLT for lung separation. The sizes of the Silbroncho DLT include 33, 35, 37, and 39 French (Unnumbered figure above). Figure A above (Unnumbered) shows a left-sided Silbroncho DLT.

The Papworth BiVent tube (P3 Medical, Bristol, UK) is a divided SLT with a distal end that forms a forked tip designed that rests on the carina and contains a premeasured blocker intended to be inserted into the operative side. Unlike the DLT, this tube eliminates the need for endobronchial intubation. Ghosh et al.[14] demonstrated that the Papworth BiVent tube provides satisfactory operating conditions and can enable the inexperienced provider to achieve lung isolation without the need for endoscope-guided blocker placement.

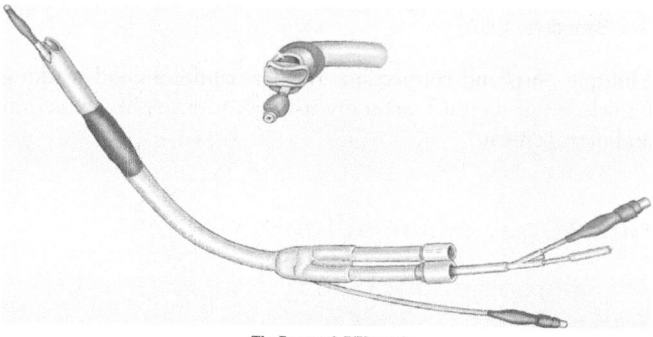

The Papworth BiVent tube

VivaSight Double-Lumen Tube

ET View DLT (Ambu Inc., Columbia, MO) has an integrated high-resolution camera.[15] The main advantage of the VivaSight DLT is the continuous real-time view of the DLT position, which allows an earlier identification and correction of intraoperative endobronchial displacement.[16,17] The below unnumbered figure shows the VivaSight DLT with the embeded camera.

In a prospective single-center study by Massot et al. of 76 patients, 99% had correct position of the VivaSight DLT after intubation. Malpositions were present in 40 patients (53%) intraoperatively;

however, these malpositions were easily corrected via the guidance of the embedded camera of the VivaSight DLT view without the need for a flexible bronchoscope.[18]

Adequate visualization may decrease the need for the use of FB to confirm the proper position of the DLT. Several studies evaluated the possibility of reducing the need for the FB confirmation of the DLT position during the procedure. Rapchuk et al. placed the VivaSight-DL in 72 patients and achieved lung separation on the first attempt without additional manipulation in 85% of cases. In only three cases (4%) was an FB required to reposition the tube after intraoperative dislodgement.[19] Levy-Faber et al. prospectively studied 71 adult patients using either the VivaSight DL or conventional DLT. The duration of intubation and the visual confirmation of tube position was significantly reduced while using the VivaSight-DL. Most importantly, none of the patients who underwent study using the VivaSight-DL required FB during the course of the procedure.[20] Schuepbach et al. enrolled 40 adult patients scheduled for thoracic surgery randomized to conventional DLT or the VivaSight DLT. They evaluated the time to intubation, insertion success without flexible bronchoscopy, frequency of tube displacement, ease of insertion, quality of lung collapse, and airway injuries. The VivaSight DLTs were correctly inserted during all intubation attempts and were significantly faster compared with the conventional DLT (63 vs 97 seconds). When malpositioning of the VivaSight DLT occurred, it was easily remedied without the need for FB, even in the lateral position. Both devices were comparable with respect to postoperative coughing, hoarseness, and sore throat.[21]

Whether the use of the VivaSight DLT is associated with reduced cost-effectiveness as measured by the number of times that flexible scope confirmation of the tube placement during intubation or surgery was avoided was evaluated. In a randomized controlled trial of 52 patients flexible scope confirmation of tube placement was only necessary for two (6.66%) procedures when using VivaSight-DL. The cost of using VivaSight-DL was $299 per procedure versus $347 for a conventional DLT with a reusable FB.[22] The VivaSight SLT was also used to guide bronchial blocker placement to achieve lung separation in a patient with a middle tracheal tumor during tracheal resection.[23] The VivaSight SLT provided a real-time and continuous monitoring of the position of the bronchial blocker without the need for flexible bronchoscopy. It can be particularly useful during a right-side blockage with an endobronchial blocker, where the cuff position can be continually monitored for potential dislocation.

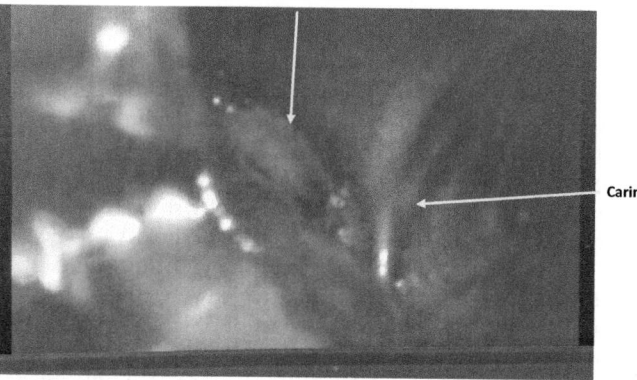

A VIEW THROUGH THE TRACHEAL LUMEN

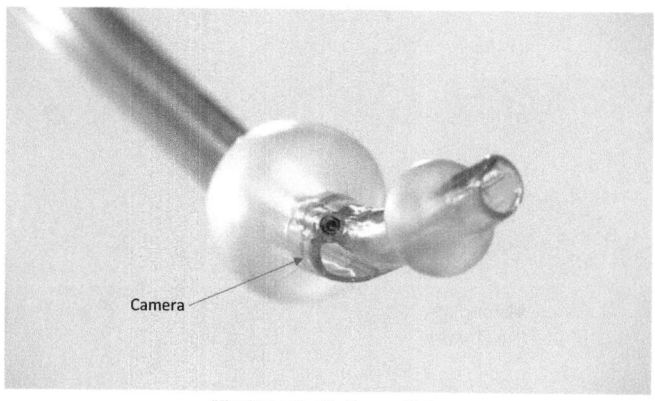

VivaSight Double-Lumen Tube

One of the limitations of the VivaSight is the presence of secretions on the tip of the camera; using a suction channel and flushing it with normal saline can alleviate the problems. Unfortunately, all previous studies have shown more hoarseness and discomfort with the use of the VivaSight DLT. The practitioner should be aware that connecting the camera for prolonged periods of time in vitro may lead to the melting of the portion of the tube near the light source. The VivaSight-DL DLT is only available for a left-sided DLT version and is placed similarly to a conventional DLT.

However, despite the reduced need for flexible bronchoscopy, one must be available in every case. Furthermore, significant variances in the cost of maintaining an FB at different institutions may affect unit cost.

The ECOM DLT is capable of continuously measuring the patient's cardiac output (CONMED Corporation, Utica, NY). The ECOM DLT has seven silver-doped plastic electrodes on the bronchial cuff in close contact with the ascending aorta, which allows direct monitoring of impedance changes from the ascending aorta in real time.[24] The technology has already been described 20 years ago by Wallace et al[25]; however, the translation of the technology into

clinical practice is recent. The system is based on the principle that the fluctuations in the volume of the flow through the aorta allow for the estimation of cardiac output by measuring the change in resistance from the impedance system and calculating the stroke volume of each cardiac contraction. At the present time, there is a study that clinically validates these measurements by using the ECOM DLT. However, based on the original ECOM endotracheal tube (ETT), it appears to be promising to derive hemodynamic parameters while in use in thoracic surgical patients. The SLT ECOM was evaluated in off-pump coronary artery bypass grafting that was compared with a standard of care in that specific surgical setting and found to be associated with a significant reduction in the rate of admission to the ICU and an improvement in immediate outcome.[26]

Tubes Selection

Right-Sided Versus Left-Sided Double-Lumen Tubes

To minimize tube displacement, some practitioners elect to intubate the nonoperated bronchus (i.e., using a left-sided DLT for a patient undergoing right lung surgery) (Fig. 26.2).[27] However, controversy exists regarding left lung procedures because of the anatomic variability of the right upper lobe take-off. The bronchial port of a right-sided tube may be difficult to position for adequate lung isolation and ventilation of the right upper lobe bronchus. This can result in difficulties during surgery, including severe hypoxia during isolated right lung ventilation.[28]

Most anesthesia providers prefer to use left-sided DLTs for all lung surgeries; however, there are insufficient data to support actual increased safety, as opposed to the perception of safety when intraoperative hypoxia, hypercapnia, and high airway pressures are used as criteria.[29,30] If manipulation of the left main stem bronchus is required, such as in left pneumonectomy, the left-sided DLT can be withdrawn and repositioned with the bronchial port above the carina. For operations of tumor in the left main stem, including sleeve resection, a right-sided DLT must be used (Fig. 26.3).

Contraindications for the use of a DLT include anatomic barriers that make positioning improbable or dangerous, such as

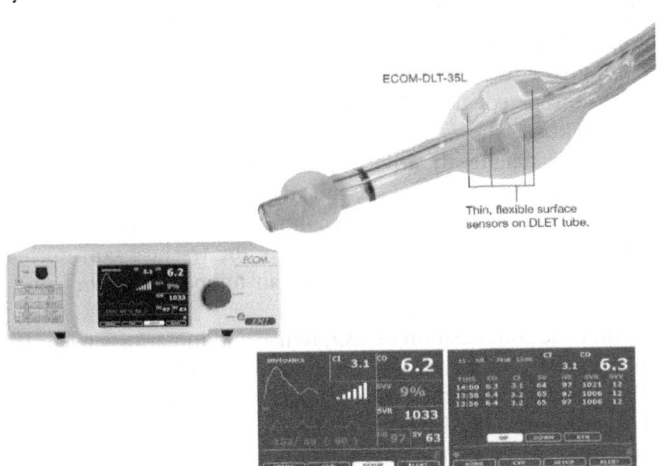

The ECOM DLT

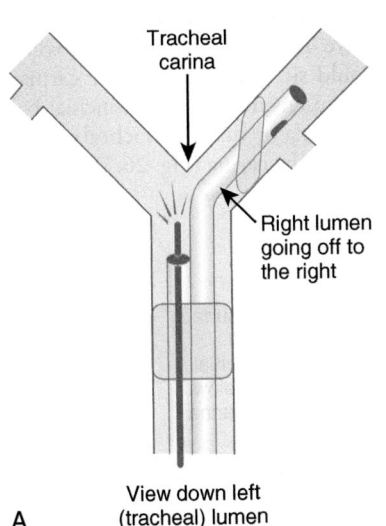

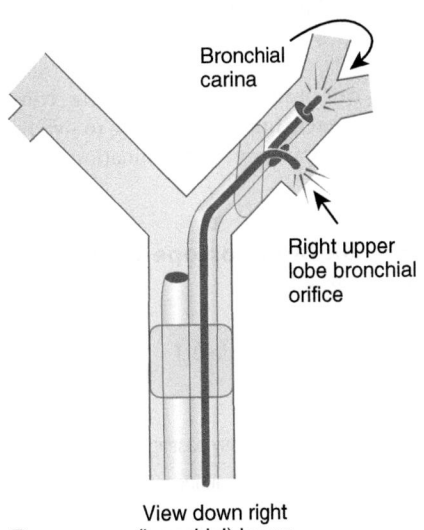

• **Fig. 26.3** Schematic diagram portrays the use of a flexible bronchoscope (FB) to determine the precise position of a right-sided double-lumen tube. (A) When the FB is passed down the left (tracheal) lumen, the endoscopist should see a clear, straight-ahead view of the tracheal carina and right lumen going off into the right main stem bronchus. (B) When the FB is passed down the right (bronchial) lumen, the endoscopist should see the bronchial carina in the distance; when the FB is flexed laterally and cephalad and passed through the ventilation slot of the right upper lobe, the bronchial orifice of the right upper lobe should be visible. (From Benumof JL. *Anesthesia for Thoracic Surgery*. Philadelphia: Saunders; 1987.)

carinal or bronchial lesions, strictures, and aberrant bronchus.[6,31,32] Right-sided DLTs may be indicated in cases with tortuosity and compression of the trachea or left main stem bronchus vascular compression by aortic aneurysm, which can make the placement of a left-sided DLT impossible or potentially rupture the aortic aneurysm. Newly designed DLTs may be applicable for patients with special conditions, including those with unusual anatomic variability.[33]

Double-Lumen Tube Size

A properly sized DLT is one in which the main body of the tube passes without resistance through the glottis and advances easily within the trachea and in which the bronchial component passes into the selected bronchus without difficulty or resistance. A DLT that is too small in size requires a larger endobronchial cuff volume for effective blockade, with potential for mucosal damage. An undersized tube, in addition, would increase the incidence of malposition or can result in a DLT that is too short to be properly positioned in the target bronchus, resulting in failure to achieve lung separation. In addition, an undersized DLT might present a higher resistance to gas flow and increase intrinsic auto-PEEP as compared with the wider lumen of larger DLTs. An oversized DLT can potentially produce trauma to the airway; therefore it is important to select the appropriate size for the patient to prevent complications.

The ideal size of a DLT is one that results in a near-complete seal of the bronchial lumen without inflation of the cuff. The high inflation pressures of a small tube can cause as much mucosal damage as forcing too large a tube into a small bronchus.[34] Even when height- and weight-based size estimates are used, it is impossible to choose the correct size of the tube every time.[35] Commonly, a 39-French or 41-French DLT is selected for men and a 37-French or 39-French DLT for women of average height and build. The intentional use of smaller DLTs has not had significant clinical benefits.[36] A flexible bronchoscope may be passed through the bronchial lumen to assess the appropriate diameter and length of the DLT during placement (Table 26.1).

Positioning

Malposition of the DLT can lead to life-threatening consequences. Ventilation can be severely impaired, leading to hypoxia, gas trapping, tension pneumothorax, cross-contamination of lung contents, and interference with surgical procedures. Multiple studies have shown that DLTs, if blindly positioned, are often malpositioned.[31,35] On the basis of these studies, direct visualization with an FB should be used routinely for the confirmation of positioning. Various techniques using an FB are discussed in the following sections.

Placement of the Double-Lumen Tube

DLTs are placed similarly to SLTs but with some additional maneuvers and considerations. DLTs are larger in diameter and stiffer and longer than SLTs, making them more difficult to place. They should never be forced into position. For laryngoscopy, the shoulder of a Macintosh blade provides better tongue displacement and more space through which to insert the tube than a Miller blade. The use of a video laryngoscope has also been described as effective and potentially time saving.[36,37] The bronchial tip of the DLT is placed through the cords, and the stylet is then removed to prevent trauma. After the bronchial portion has passed the cords, the DLT must be rotated 90 degrees toward the selected side of the bronchial lumen to sit properly. If resistance is encountered on rotating or advancing the tube, the use of a smaller tube needs to be considered. The average depth of insertion is 29 cm for an individual who is 170 cm tall. For every 10-cm increase or decrease in height, the tube depth is increased or decreased by 1 cm, respectively.[31] When the tube depth is reached, the tracheal cuff is inflated, and the patient is connected to the ventilator. Care must be taken not to tear or puncture the tracheal cuff during intubation. Covering the teeth with an unopened alcohol swab can minimize cuff damage.

After the confirmation of CO_2 return and initiation of ventilation, an FB is placed through the tracheal lumen (Fig. 26.4). The FB is advanced, and the carina is identified. The bronchial lumen of the tube must be visualized entering the appropriate main stem bronchus (i.e., the bronchial lumen should be in the left main stem bronchus for a left-sided DLT). The semilunar view of the blue bronchial balloon should be inflated under direct vision and should lie just distal to the carina. Direct visualization of the balloon inflation helps to confirm tube position and size. Some DLTs have an indicator line just proximal to the bronchial cuff that should sit at the level of the carina. Direct visualization is necessary to ensure that the bronchial balloon does not herniate over the carina or that the tracheal portion of the DLT does not encroach on the carina (Fig. 26.5).

TABLE 26.1	Relation of Flexible Bronchoscope Size to Double-Lumen Tube Size		
FB OD Size (mm)	DLT Size (F)	Fit of FB Inside DLT	
5.6	All sizes	Does not fit	
	41	Easy passage	
	39	Moderately easy passage	
4.9	37	Tight fit, needs lubricant,[a] hand push	
	35	Does not fit	
3.6–4.2	All sizes	Easy passage	
Approximately 2.0	All sizes	Most operating rooms need special arrangements to obtain this size FB	

[a]The lubricant recommended is a silicon-based fluid made by the American Cystoscope Makers Inc.

DLT, Double-lumen tube; F, French measurement (1 F = OD in mm × 3); FB, flexible bronchoscope; OD, outer diameter.

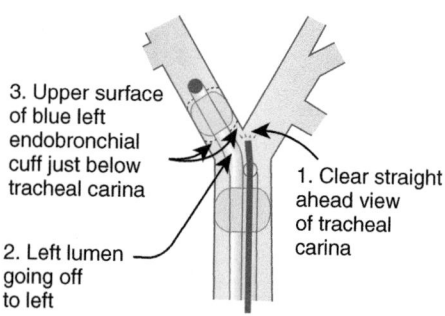

3. Upper surface of blue left endobronchial cuff just below tracheal carina

1. Clear straight ahead view of tracheal carina

2. Left lumen going off to left

• **Fig. 26.4** Use of a flexible bronchoscope down the right lumen to determine the precise position of a left-sided double-lumen tube. The endoscopist should see a clear, straight-ahead view of the tracheal carina (1); the left lumen going off into the left main stem bronchus (2); and the upper surface of the blue left endobronchial cuff just below the tracheal carina (3). (From Benumof JL. *Anesthesia for Thoracic Surgery*. Philadelphia: Saunders; 1987.)

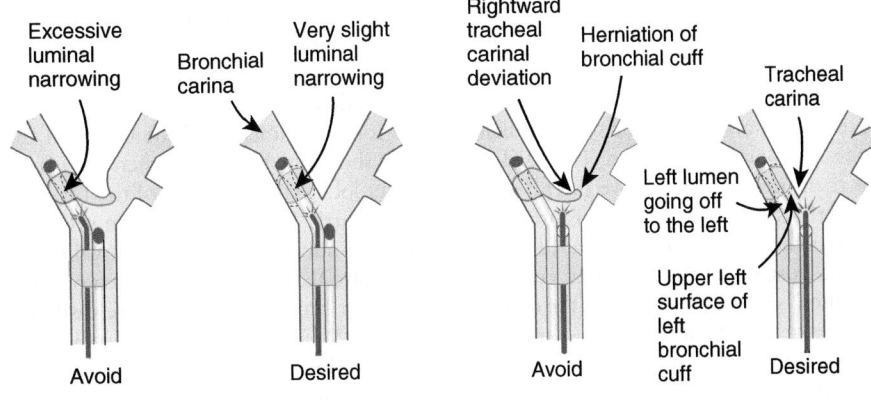

Excessive luminal narrowing

Bronchial carina

Very slight luminal narrowing

Rightward tracheal carinal deviation

Herniation of bronchial cuff

Tracheal carina

Left lumen going off to the left

Upper left surface of left bronchial cuff

Avoid   Desired

Avoid   Desired

View down left (bronchial) lumen

View down right (tracheal) lumen

• **Fig. 26.5** Desired views and views to be avoided when using a flexible bronchoscope (FB) to determine the position of a left-sided double-lumen tube (DLT). *Left,* When an FB is passed down the left lumen of a left-sided DLT, the endoscopist should see a slight left luminal narrowing and a clear, straight-ahead view of the bronchial carina in the distance. Excessive left luminal narrowing should be avoided. *Right,* When the flexible FB is passed down the right lumen of the left-sided DLT, the endoscopist should see a clear, straight-ahead view of the tracheal carina; the left lumen going off into the main stem bronchus; and the upper surface of the blue, left endotracheal cuff just below the tracheal carina. Excessive pressure in the endobronchial cuff, as manifested by tracheal carinal deviation to the right and herniation of the endobronchial cuff over the carina, should be avoided. (From Benumof JL. *Anesthesia for Thoracic Surgery.* Philadelphia: Saunders; 1987.)

Determination of right versus left main stem bronchus is done via the visualization of the anterior and posterior aspects of the trachea. The anterior of the trachea is identified by the tracheal rings, which extend throughout the anterior two-thirds of the trachea. Posteriorly, the trachea consists of the membranous component with longitudinal striations. After the anterior and posterior aspects of the trachea are identified, right and left orientations are obvious. The most appropriate determination of the right versus

left bronchus is identifying the right upper lobe orifice. It may be necessary to suction the DLT before the insertion of the FB. Lubrication and antifogging agents applied to the FB can facilitate manipulation and visualization. The appropriate use of antisialagogues can also be useful to limit secretions before DLT placement.

An alternative method of DLT placement is to use the FB as an intubating stylet to guide the bronchial tip of the DLT directly into the correct main stem bronchus (Fig. 26.6). This is

Use of Fiberoptic Bronchoscope to Insert Left-Sided Double-Lumen Tube

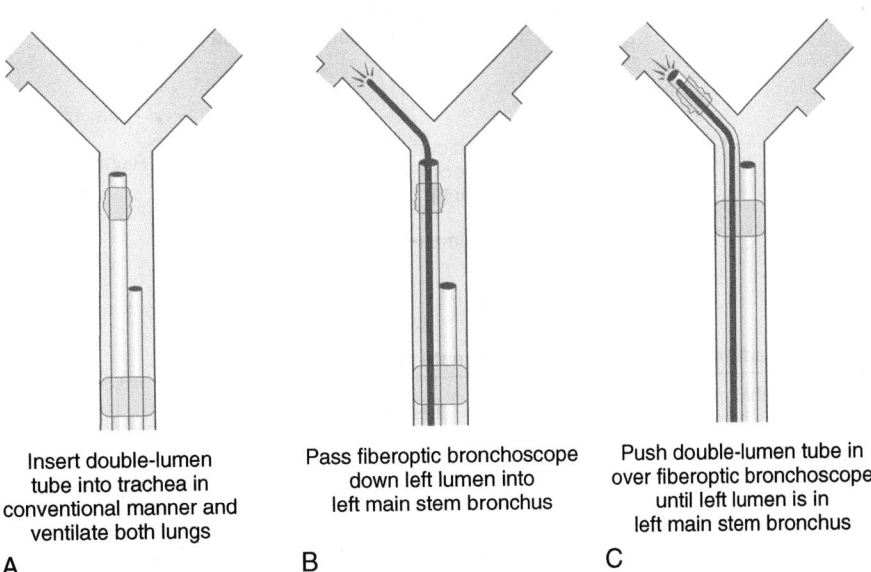

Insert double-lumen tube into trachea in conventional manner and ventilate both lungs

A

Pass fiberoptic bronchoscope down left lumen into left main stem bronchus

B

Push double-lumen tube in over fiberoptic bronchoscope until left lumen is in left main stem bronchus

C

• **Fig. 26.6** (A) A double-lumen tube (DLT) can be put into the trachea in a conventional manner, and both lungs can be ventilated by both lumens. A flexible bronchoscope (FB) may be inserted into the left lumen of the DLT through a self-sealing diaphragm in the elbow connector to the left lumen; this allows continued positive-pressure ventilation of both lungs through the right lumen without creating a leak. (B) After the FB has been passed into the left main stem bronchus, (C) it is used as a stylet for the left lumen; the FB is then withdrawn. The final precise positioning of the DLT is performed with the FB in the right lumen (see Figs. 26.19 and 26.20). (From Benumof JL. *Anesthesia for Thoracic Surgery.* Philadelphia: Saunders; 1987.)

accomplished by inserting the FB through the bronchial port of the DLT after the bronchial tip has passed the vocal cords. The FB is then advanced down the trachea while identifying the anterior-posterior and right-left orientation. The FB is advanced further to identify the carina and the right and left main stem bronchi and then advanced into the appropriate bronchus. The DLT is advanced over the FB. It is then necessary to remove the FB after confirming that the bronchial tip is not obstructed and is proximal to the secondary bronchial branches. The FB is then placed in the tracheal lumen to confirm the position of the bronchial cuff and to ensure that the tracheal lumen is not encroaching on the carina. This technique allows for assessment of the carina and tracheal rings and allows placement in tortuous airways. However, it takes more time to perform, and, in some patients with poor pulmonary reserve this extra time can lead to desaturation.

Confirmation of Proper Placement

Many maneuvers have been described to assess the proper position of a DLT,[38,39] including the visualization of chest excursion while alternately clamping and unclamping the tracheal and bronchial ports, auscultation of lung fields while alternately clamping and unclamping the tracheal and bronchial ports (Fig. 26.7), and radiographic confirmation.[40,41]

The simplest maneuver to check the tube would be to clamp first the tracheal lumen and observe the chest rising to determine if the bronchial lumen is on the selected side. If both hemithoraces are rising, the tube is too shallow in the trachea. Following auscultation and physical examination, subsequent viewing with an FB demonstrated that 48% of the tubes were malpositioned by the clinician assessment alone. When using a left-sided DLT, the FB is usually first introduced through the tracheal lumen to visualize the carina and to ensure that the bronchial cuff has not herniated. The upper surface of the blue endobronchial cuff should be just below the tracheal carina; the blue bronchial cuff of the DLT is easily visualized. The FB is then passed through the bronchial lumen to identify the left upper lobe bronchial orifice. When a right-sided DLT is used, the carina should be visualized through the tracheal lumen, and the orifice of the right upper lobe bronchus should be identified when the FB is passed through the right upper lobe ventilating slot of the DLT.

Pediatric FBs are available in several standard sizes: 5.6-, 4.9-, and 3.6-mm OD. The 4.9-mm OD bronchoscope can be passed through DLTs that are 37 French or larger. A 3.6-mm or smaller-diameter bronchoscope is more easily passed through all sizes of DLTs.[42-44] DLT placement must be rechecked when the patient is repositioned, because the movement of the tube is common. Training in the use of FB may be achieved during the evaluation of any SLT-intubated patient and through the use of airway simulation and mannequins.[45]

Malposition and Complications

The use of a DLT is associated with a number of problems, the most important of which is malpositioning (see Fig. 26.7)[46,47] by various means:

a. The DLT may be accidentally directed to the side opposite the desired main stem bronchus. In this case the lung opposite the side of the connector clamp will collapse. Inadequate separation, increased airway pressures, and instability of the DLT usually occur. Because of the morphology of the DLT curvatures, tracheal or bronchial lacerations may result. If a left-sided DLT is inserted into the right main stem bronchus, it obstructs ventilation to the right upper lobe. It is essential to recognize and correct such a malposition as soon as possible.

b. The DLT may be passed too far down into the right or the left main stem bronchus. In this case breath sounds are greatly diminished or not audible over the contralateral side. The tube

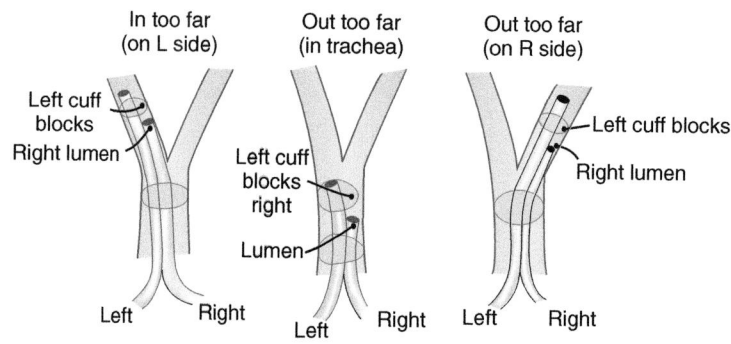

Left Sided Double-Lumen Tube Malpositions

Procedure	Breath sounds heard		
Clamp right lumen; both cuffs inflated	Left	Left and right	Right
Clamp left lumen; both cuffs inflated	None or faint right	None or very	None or faint left
Clamp left lumen; deflate left cuff	Left only or left and faint right	Left and right	Right only or right and faint left

• **Fig. 26.7** Three major malpositions involving a whole lung are possible for a left-sided double-lumen tube. The tube can be in too far on the left (i.e., both lumens are in the left main stem bronchus), out too far (i.e., both lumens are in the trachea), or down the right main stem bronchus (i.e., at least the left lumen is in the right main stem bronchus). In each of these malpositions the left cuff, when fully inflated, can completely block the right lumen. Inflation and deflation of the left cuff while the left lumen is clamped create a breath sound differential diagnosis of tube malposition. *L*, Left; *R*, right. (From Benumof JL. *Anesthesia for Thoracic Surgery*. Philadelphia: Saunders; 1987.)

should be withdrawn until the opening of the tracheal lumen is above the carina.

c. The DLT may not be inserted far enough, leaving the bronchial lumen opening above the carina. In this position good breath sounds are heard bilaterally when ventilating through the bronchial lumen, but no breath sounds are audible when ventilating through the tracheal lumen because the inflated bronchial cuff obstructs gas flow from the tracheal lumen. The cuff should be deflated and the DLT rotated and advanced into the desired main stem bronchus.

d. A right-sided DLT may occlude the right upper lobe orifice. The mean distance from the carina to the right upper lobe orifice is 2.3 ± 0.7 cm in men and 2.1 ± 0.7 cm in women. With right-sided DLTs, the ventilatory slot on the side of the bronchial catheter must overlie the right upper lobe orifice to permit ventilation of this lobe. However, the margin of safety is extremely small and varies from 1 to 8 mm.[35] It is difficult to ensure proper ventilation to the right upper lobe and avoid dislocation of the DLT during surgical manipulation.

e. The left upper lobe orifice may be obstructed by a left-sided DLT. Traditionally, the take-off of the left upper lobe bronchus was thought to be at a safe distance from the carina and that it would not be obstructed by a left-sided DLT. However, the mean distance between the left upper lobe orifice and the carina is 5.4 ± 0.7 cm in men and 5.0 ± 0.7 cm in women.[48] The average distance between the openings of the right and left lumens on the left-sided disposable tubes is 6.9 cm. An obstruction of the left upper lobe bronchus is possible while the tracheal lumen is still above the carina. There is also a 20% variation in the location of the blue endobronchial cuff on the

disposable tubes because this cuff is attached to the tube at the end of the manufacturing process (Fig. 26.8).

f. Bronchial cuff herniation may occur and obstruct the contralateral bronchial lumen if excessive volumes are used to inflate the cuff. The bronchial cuff has also been known to herniate over the tracheal carina and, in the case of a left-sided DLT, to obstruct ventilation to the right main stem bronchus.

g. A rare complication with DLTs is tracheal laceration or rupture from the stiff tip of the bronchial lumen (Fig. 26.9). Overinflation of the bronchial cuff, inappropriate positioning, an oversized DLT, and trauma because of intraoperative dislocation resulting in bronchial rupture have been associated with the use of the Robertshaw tube and the disposable DLT.[49] The pressure in the bronchial cuff should be assessed and decreased if the cuff is overinflated. If lung isolation is no longer necessary, the bronchial cuff should be deflated to avoid excessive pressure on the bronchial walls. The bronchial cuff should also be deflated during any repositioning of the patient unless lung separation is absolutely required during this time.

The use of a bronchial blocker versus DLT was evaluated in a prospective trial of 60 patients. OLV was achieved with an endobronchial blocker or a DLT. Postoperative hoarseness and sore throat were assessed at 24, 48, and 72 hours after surgery. Bronchial injuries and vocal cord lesions were examined using visualization with an FB immediately after surgery. Postoperative hoarseness occurred significantly more frequently in the double-lumen group than in the blocker group (44% vs 17%). Similar findings were observed for vocal cord lesions (44% vs 17%). The incidence of bronchial injuries is comparable between groups.[50]

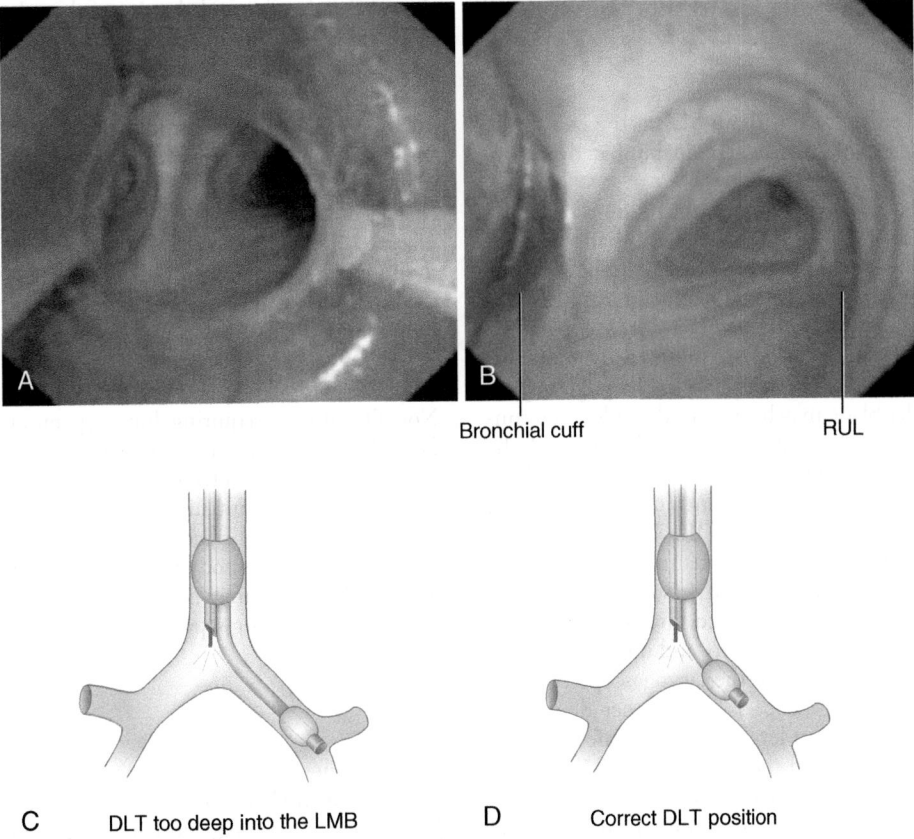

• **Fig. 26.8** Fiberoptic bronchoscopy for a left-sided double-lumen tube (DLT). (A and C) The DLT is too deep into the left main bronchus (LMB). (B and D) Correct DLT position. *RUL*, Right upper lobe.

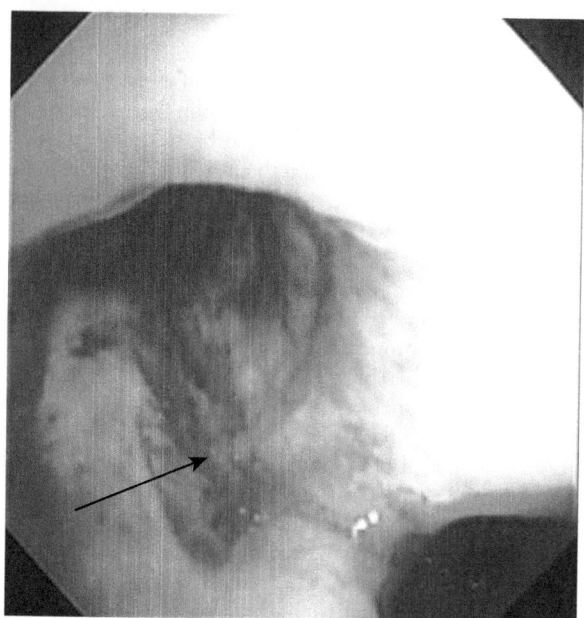

• **Fig. 26.9** Injury (*arrow*) to the main left bronchus.

The most common minor complication is sore throat and temporary hoarseness. Other complications include laryngeal and bronchial injury, tracheobronchial tree disruption,[51] inadvertent suturing of the DLT to thoracic structures, and direct vocal cord injury.[52] Although most of the complications, except malpositioning, have been reported in the older-style DLTs (e.g., Carlens, Robertshaw), the newer designs can also pose risks.[53–55]

Exchanging the Double-Lumen Tube for a Single-Lumen Tube

Procedure

It is desirable to replace the DLT with an SLT at the end of the surgical procedure if the patient is to remain intubated postoperatively.

The replacement of a DLT with an SLT can be life-threatening and must be performed with great caution. Before changing out a DLT, the anesthesia provider must prepare for reintubation. The patient should be well preoxygenated and paralyzed. An SLT with stylet, face mask, and suction must be readily available. Individual bronchial suctioning may be considered, followed by bronchial cuff deflation and suctioning of the oropharynx. Laryngoscopy is then performed; a Miller blade may be preferred to allow the control of the epiglottis. If the DLT and larynx are well visualized, the blade can be passed into the larynx just past the vocal cords. After the laryngoscope is positioned, an assistant (upon instruction) deflates the tracheal cuff of the DLT. The DLT is retracted under constant direct vision. When the DLT is removed, the assistant hands the SLT over to the right hand of the person who maintains a view of the larynx. The SLT is then placed directly into the larynx. It is vital not to lose sight of the larynx and not to reposition the laryngoscope blade. The choice of the laryngoscope blade or even the use of a video laryngoscope is practitioner dependent and should be directed by comfort level and airway safety considerations. When the SLT is beyond the cords, the cuff is inflated, the patient is ventilated, and CO_2 confirmation is obtained. If, on the initial laryngoscopic inspection of the airway, the vocal cords are too edematous, bloody, or difficult to visualize, the tube exchange should be aborted.

Airway Exchange Catheters

Alternative techniques of tube exchange involve the use of airway exchange catheters (AECs). Of those available, the Cook AECs (CAECs; Cook Critical Care, Bloomington, IN USA) are easy to use and allow ventilation, if the need arises. The technique involves placing an AEC through the existing DLT and then removing the DLT. Either the tracheal or bronchial port may be used. Although the bronchial port may provide more stability, it requires full extraction of the DLT to get hold of the AEC distally. Care must be taken to keep the AEC in place as the DLT is removed. After the DLT is removed, the SLT is guided over the AEC into the trachea. Then the AEC is removed while the SLT is kept in place. The cuff is inflated, and ventilation with confirmation of CO_2 is then obtained.

AECs are easy to dislodge at any point during the attempted exchange. The fit between the exchanger and the SLT is often such that the SLT becomes caught at the level of the vocal cords. Rotating the SLT can overcome this obstruction, but it can also cause dislodgment of the ETT and the AEC.

A combination technique using a tube exchanger under direct vision may be a safer approach. With this technique, the larynx and the DLT are visualized while an AEC is inserted through the DLT. The AEC is seen passing into the distal airway; then, under direct vision, the DLT is withdrawn and the AEC position is confirmed. The SLT is then advanced over the AEC while the larynx is visualized. The tube is guided under direct vision into the larynx, and the AEC is removed. Proper placement is determined by using CO_2 detection and bilateral lung auscultation.

Several tube exchangers are commercially available from Cook Critical Care (Bloomington, IN) and Sheridan Catheter Corporation (Argyle, NY). The depth is marked in centimeters on these tube exchangers. They are available in a wide range of ODs and are easily adapted for oxygen insufflation or jet ventilation. The size of the tube exchanger and the size of the tube to be inserted should be tested before use in a patient. The 11-French tube changer can pass through a 35- to 41-French DLT, whereas the 14-French tube exchanger does not pass through a 35-French DLT.

To prevent lung laceration, the tube exchanger should never be inserted against resistance. Because the first-generation tube exchanger tips were very stiff, there was a risk for tracheal or bronchial laceration. A tube exchanger with a soft flexible tip, also manufactured by Cook Critical Care (Bloomington, IN), may be safer to use for the exchange of DLTs. A laryngoscope should always be used to facilitate the passage of a tube over the airway guide and past the supraglottic tissues.

Contraindications

Not all patients requiring lung separation are candidates for a DLT. Contraindications to the placement of a DLT include (1) known or anticipated technical difficulty in DLT placement, such as dangerous/difficult airway anatomy, small airways or small patient, and view obstructed by bleeding, opaque secretions, and masses and (2) a hemodynamically unstable patient; complex airway manipulation may not be desirable. For these patients, alternative means of lung separation are discussed.

Univent Tubes

Anatomy

The Univent tube (Fuji Systems, Tokyo, Japan) is a Silastic SLT with a built-in chamber that allows the advancement of the integrated blocker (see Fig. 26.10).[56–58] The integrated blocker has a small lumen along its entire length that facilitates lung deflation and allows very limited suctioning. At the distal tip of the blocker is a

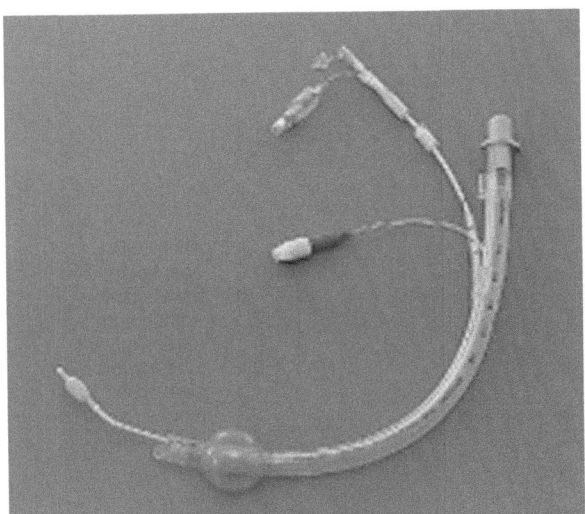

• **Fig. 26.10** Univent single-lumen tube and bronchial blocker system. (Courtesy LMA North America, Inc., San Diego, CA.)

small balloon, and the proximal end of the blocker section contains a lumen cap. This cap needs to be engaged when the blocker balloon is deflated during full-lung ventilation. Failure to engage the cap when the blocker balloon is deflated results in a circuit leak. Univent tubes are available in many sizes (Table 26.2), all designated by internal lumen size. Because of the thickness of the tube wall and the integrated blocker chamber, the outer size of these devices is much larger than that of a similarly designated SLT. For example, a 7.5-mm Univent tube has an 11.2-mm OD, compared with the 10.2-mm OD of a 7.5-mm SLT. Despite the larger size, these tubes are very useful.

Positioning

Before the Univent tube is placed, it must be prepared. Preparation involves the removal of the distal and proximal tension wires that help keep the Univent's shape during storage. The cuffs of the bronchial blocker and the main tube should be checked and deflated. After the tip of the bronchial blocker is bent to the shape of a hockey stick, it is retracted into the blocker chamber so that its distal tip is flush with the main tube. The tube is then inserted into the trachea with the tracheal balloon just distal to the cords. The main tube cuff is then inflated and secured at a distance of at least 2 to 3 cm between the distal tip of the main tube and the carina (Fig. 26.11) so that the curved shape of the blocker can be maintained and manipulated as it is advanced beyond the tip of the main tube. Failure to provide this adequate distance between the tip of the main tube and the carina makes directional control of the bronchial blocker very difficult.

Because the material of the Univent tube makes the passage of a nonlubricated FB difficult, the scope should be well lubricated before it is inserted into the main segment of the tube. It is often helpful to attach some type of self-sealing diaphragm device between the Univent tube and the elbow connection of the circuit. This allows continuous ventilation while the blocker is being positioned with the FB. The FB is advanced beyond the distal tip of the tube, and the anterior tracheal rings are identified, allowing proper orientation of the right and left main stem bronchi. The blocker portion of the tube is then visually advanced while the main tube position is maintained (see Fig. 26.11).

The placement of the blocker into the desired main stem bronchus is achieved by advancing the blocker with a clockwise or a counterclockwise rotation. If this maneuver is not sufficient to align the blocker into the desired bronchus, the entire Univent tube may be rotated in the desired direction to assist blocker orientation. The blocker is advanced into the correct location, and the locking cuff at the proximal end of the blocker is secured. Note the distance marker on the blocker. If lung isolation is desired, the blocker cuff is inflated (best performed under direct FB visualization), and the proximal cap of the blocker may be disengaged to enhance lung deflation (see Fig. 26.11). Blind placement of the blocker is often unsuccessful. Blind placement may result in trauma to the tracheobronchial tree, resulting in complications including bleeding or even tension pneumothorax. Limitations of the Univent tube are summarized in Table 26.3. The solutions related to Univent blocker issues may be applicable to other types of bronchial blockers.

Endobronchial Blockers

In modern thoracic anesthesia lung separation can be achieved with an endobronchial blocker.[59–62] Inflation of the cuff at the

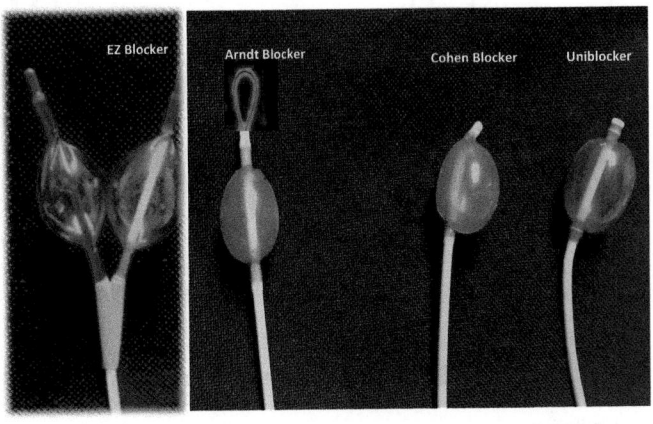

TABLE 26.2	**Comparative Tube Sizes**				
Univent ID (mm)	Univent Gauge (F) of Single Main Lumen[a]	Univent OD (mm) Lateral/AP[b]	Equivalent SLT OD (mm)	Equivalent DLT (F)
7.5	31	11.0/12.0	9.6	35
8.0	33	11.5/13.0	10.9	37
8.5	35	12.0/13.5	11.6	39
9.0	37	12.5/14.0	12.2	41

[a]Marked on the tube.

[b]The AP diameter is greater than the lateral diameter because of the bronchial blocker lumen.

AP, Anteroposterior; *DLT*, double-lumen tube (Broncho-Cath); *F*, French measurement (1 F = OD in mm × 3); *ID*, internal diameter; *OD*, outer diameter; *SLT*, single-lumen tube (Shiley).

Data from MacGillvray RG. Evaluation of a new tracheal tube with a moveable bronchus blocker. Anaesthesia. 1988;43:687; Slinger P. Con: the Univent tube is not the best method of providing one-lung ventilation. J Cardiothorac Vasc Anesth. 1993;7:108–112.

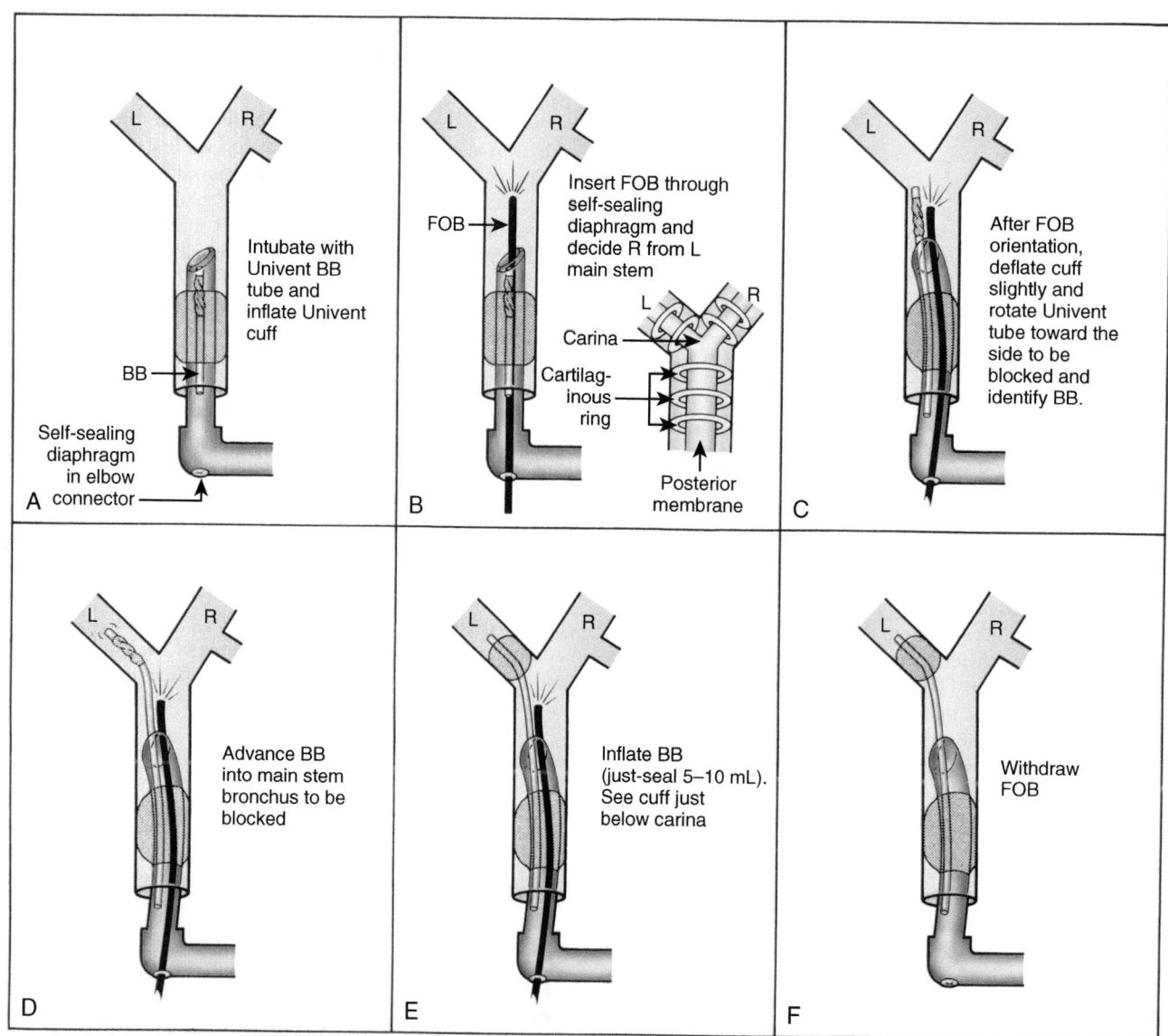

• **Fig. 26.11** (A–F) Sequential steps of a flexible scope aided method of inserting and positioning the Univent bronchial blocker (BB) in the left main stem bronchus. Ventilation of one or two lungs is achieved by inflating or deflating, respectively, the bronchial blocker balloon. *FOB*, Flexible bronchoscope; *L*, left; *R*, right. (From Benumof JL. *Anesthesia for Thoracic Surgery*. Philadelphia: Saunders; 1987.)

TABLE 26.3

Univent Bronchial Blocker Tube: Limitations and Solutions

Limitation	Solution
Slow inflation time	Deflate the bronchial blocker cuff, and administer a positive-pressure breath through the main single lumen. Then carefully administer one short, high-pressure (20–30 psi) jet ventilation.
Slow deflation time	Deflate the bronchial blocker cuff, and compress and evacuate the lung through the main single lumen. Then apply suction to the bronchial blocker lumen.
Blockage of bronchial blocker lumen by blood or pus	Suction, use a wire stylet, and then suction.
High-pressure cuff	Use a just-seal volume of air.
Intraoperative leak in bronchial blocker cuff	Ensure the bronchial blocker cuff is positioned below the carina. Increase the inflation volume, and rearrange the surgical field.

distal end of the blocker blocks ventilation to that lung. All modern blockers have a lumen that permits suctioning of the airway distal to the catheter tip, and, depending on the clinical circumstance, oxygen can be insufflated through the catheter lumen.

The main advantage of these blockers is that they can be placed through a conventional SLT. When a blocker is placed in the right main bronchus, it is usually positioned proximal to the carina to block the right upper lobe. Because the blocker balloon requires a high distending pressure, it has the potential of slipping out of the bronchus into the trachea as a result of changes in position or surgical manipulation. That movement can result in obstructing ventilation and losing the seal between the two lungs. The loss of lung separation can be a life-threatening situation if it is performed to prevent the spillage of pus, blood, or fluid from bronchopulmonary lavage. For that reason, bronchial blockers are not recommended in cases in which lung protection is required.

Indications

Indications for the use of a bronchial blocker are shown in Box 26.2. Because the blocker is placed through an SLT, it avoids the use of a DLT in a patient with a difficult airway. The use of a bronchial blocker also eliminates the need to change a DLT to an SLT at the conclusion of the procedure should the patient require ventilatory support in the ICU or if the surgeon elects to perform pulmonary toilet through a 6.0 FB. This is important because the airway after the procedure may be different from that in the initial period as a result of secretions and edema. In the past Fogarty vascular embolectomy catheters were used for lung separation, but there is no place for their use in the current practice of thoracic anesthesia. The balloon of the Fogarty is high pressure and low volume, and there is no lumen to allow the egress of gas from the lung to facilitate deflation. The characteristics of bronchial blockers are summarized in Table 26.4.

> ### BOX 26.2 Indications for the Use of Endobronchial Blockers
>
> Lung isolation versus lung separation
> Video-assisted thoracoscopy, increased number of patients who require one-lung ventilation
> To avoid the need for tube exchange
> Patients with difficult airways
> 1. Patients after laryngeal or pharyngeal surgery
> 2. Patients with a tracheotomy
> 3. Patients with distorted bronchial anatomy (e.g., aneurysm compression, intraluminal tumor)
> 4. Patients who require nasotracheal intubation
> 5. Patients with an immobility or kyphoscoliosis
> Surgical procedures not involving the lung
> 1. Esophageal surgery
> 2. Spinal surgery that requires a transthoracic approach
> 3. Minimally invasive cardiac surgery
> Special management circumstances
> 1. Video-assisted thoracoscopy in which a quick look or wedge resection of the chest is planned
> 2. Possible segmental blockade in a patient unable to tolerate one-lung ventilation
> 3. Morbidly obese patients
> 4. Small adult or pediatric patients
> 5. Patients who require intraoperative lung isolation
> 6. Patients who arrive in the operating room intubated from the intensive care unit

INDICATIONS FOR ENDOBRONCHIAL BLOCKERS

DLT is Mandated
- Lung Isolation (Empyema, Hemoptysis, Large bullae, Lung Lavage)
- Lesion in the mainstem bronchus
- Sleeve resection
- Tracheal bronchus

DLT is Preferred
- Thoracic Aneurysm
- Bilateral lung intervention :
  - Lung transplant
  - Bullectomy
  - Sympathectomy
- Right upper lobectomy
- Cost

Coaxial Stand-Alone Endotracheal Blockers

Arndt Endobronchial Blocker

A snare-guided bronchial blocker, the Arndt Endobronchial Blocker (Cook Critical Care, Bloomington IN), has a wire-guided catheter with a loop snare (Fig. 26.12). An FB is passed through the loop of the bronchial blocker and then guided into the desired bronchus. The blocker is then slid distally over the flexible bronchoscope and into the selected bronchus. Flexible scope visualization confirms blocker placement and bronchial occlusion (Fig. 26.13).

This balloon-tipped catheter has a hollow lumen of 1.6 mm (in the largest version), which allows suction to facilitate the collapse of the lung and insufflation of oxygen to the nondependent lung. The balloon is available in a spherical or elliptic shape. The set contains a multiport adapter (Fig. 26.14) that allows uninterrupted ventilation during the positioning of the blocker. The wire may then be removed,

TABLE 26.4 Characteristics of Endobronchial Blockers

Characteristics	Arndt Blocker	Cohen Blocker	Uniblocker	EZ-Blocker
Size	9 F, 7 F, 5 F (pediatric)	9.0 F	9.0 F, 5.0 F (pediatric)	7.0 F
Guidance feature	Wire loop to snare the FB	Deflecting tip	Prefixed bend	Double-lumen bifurcated tip
Recommended ETT size (mm)	9-F 8.0 ETT 7-F 7.0 ETT 5-F 4.5 ETT	8.0 ETT	8.0 ETT	8.0 ETT
Central lumen	1.8 mm	1.8 mm	2.0 mm	1.4 mm (divided in half)
Murphy eye	Only in the 9-F device	Yes	No	No
Disadvantages	BB not visualized during insertion	Expensive	No steering mechanism; prefixed bend	Each lumen is too small; impossible to suction

BB, Bronchial blocker; *ETT,* endotracheal tube; *F,* French measurement (1 F = OD in mm × 3); *FB,* flexible bronchoscope.

and the 1.6-mm lumen may be used as a suction port or for oxygen insufflation. In the first generation of this device it was not possible to reinsert the string after it had been pulled out, losing the ability to redirect the bronchial blocker if necessary. External reinforcement of the wire allows its reintroduction through the lumen. The smallest

recommended SLT size for use with an Arndt blocker is 5.5 for the 7 French and 7.5 for the 9 French. A disadvantage of the Arndt blocker is that it is advanced blindly over the FB into the desired main bronchus. In some cases the tip of the blocker may get caught at the main carina or at the Murphy eye of the SLT. This blocker is also available in a 5.0-French size for the pediatric population.

Cohen Flexitip Endobronchial Blocker

The Cohen Flexitip Endobronchial Blocker (Cook Critical Care, Bloomington, IN) is designed for use through an SLT with the aid of a small-diameter (4.0-mm) FB (Fig. 26.15).[63] The blocker has a rotating wheel that deflects the soft tip by more than 90 degrees and easily directs it into the desired bronchus. The blocker cuff is a high-volume, low-pressure balloon inflated through a 0.4-mm lumen inside the wall of the blocker. Its pear shape provides an adequate seal of the bronchus. It takes 6 to 7 mL of air to seal the bronchus with the cuff. The distinctive blue cuff is easily recognizable via FB visualization. It is best to inflate the cuff under direct vision by the FB, which is particularly important during right-sided blockade. In this case the cuff is inflated near the carina, and proper position and cuff inflation are critical. The 9-French blocker has a central main lumen (1.6 mm) that allows limited suctioning of secretions and insufflation of oxygen to the collapsed lung.

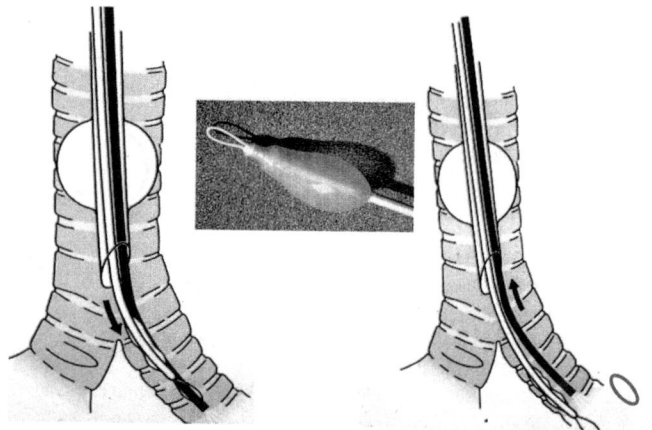

• **Fig. 26.12** Arndt endobronchial blocker. (left and right figures courtesy of Cook Medical.)

Left-side blockade

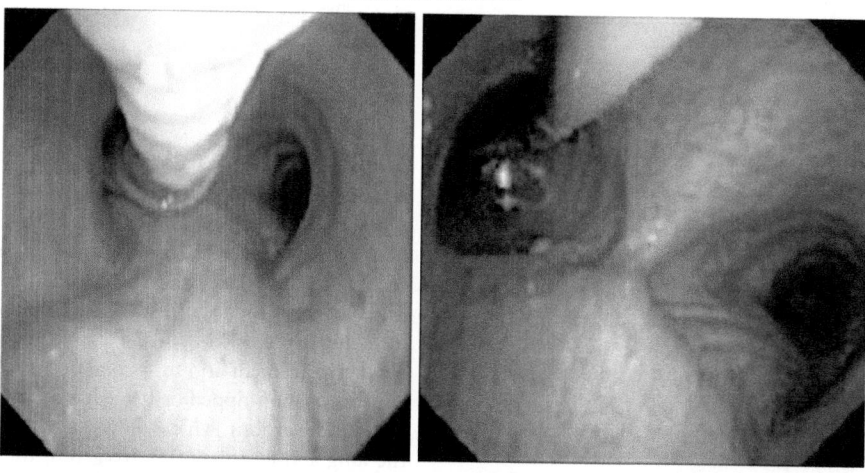

Right-side blockade

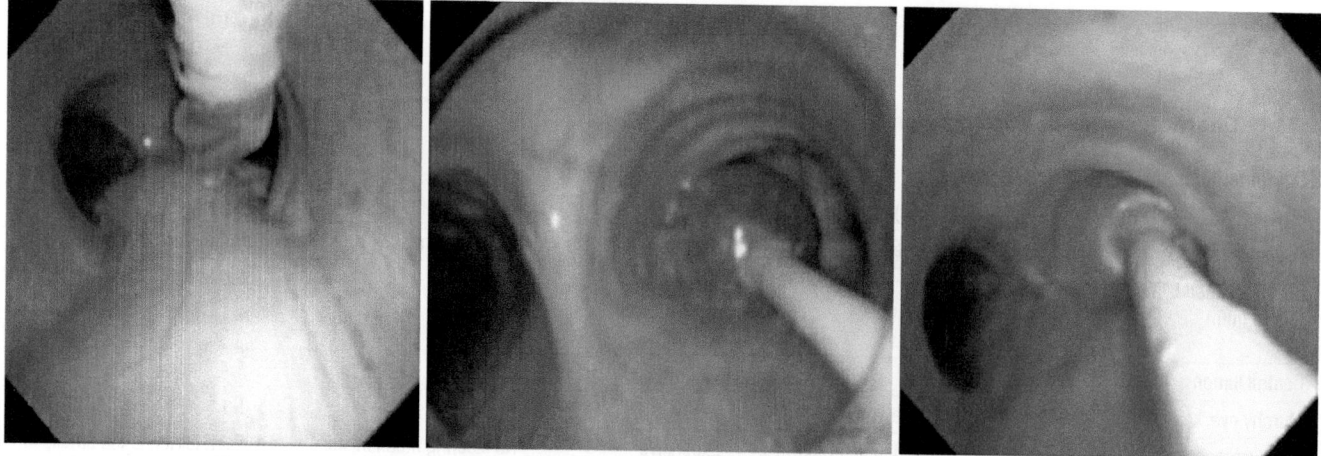

• **Fig. 26.13** *Top,* Left main stem bronchus bronchial blocker in position before (*left*) and after (*right*) "just-seal" inflation. *Bottom left,* Right main stem bronchus bronchial blocker in the entering position. *Bottom center,* Bronchial blocker is too deep, occluding only the bronchus intermedius. *Bottom right,* Bronchial blocker in the right main stem bronchus with a just-seal inflation.

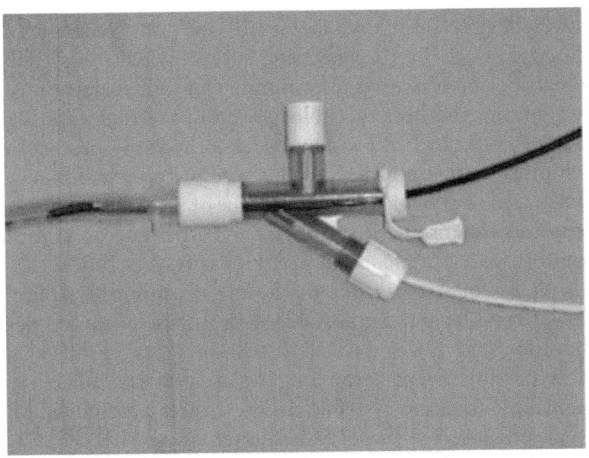

• **Fig. 26.14** Multiport adapter for the Arndt Endobronchial Blocker.

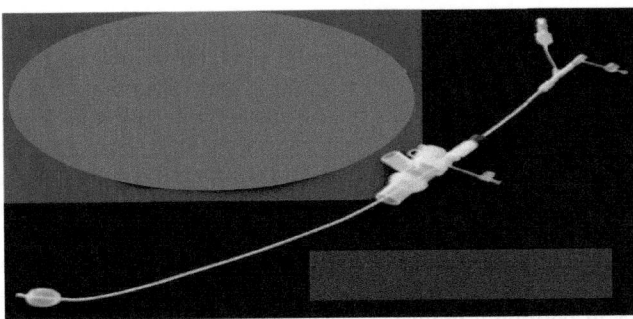

• **Fig. 26.16** Uniblocker is a 9-French, balloon-tipped, angled blocker. (Courtesy Fuji Systems Corporation, Tokyo, Japan.)

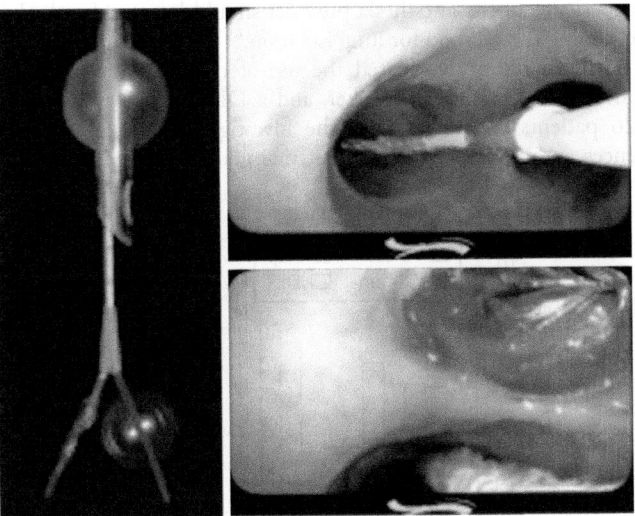

• **Fig. 26.17** EZ-Blocker: device, insertion, and deployment.

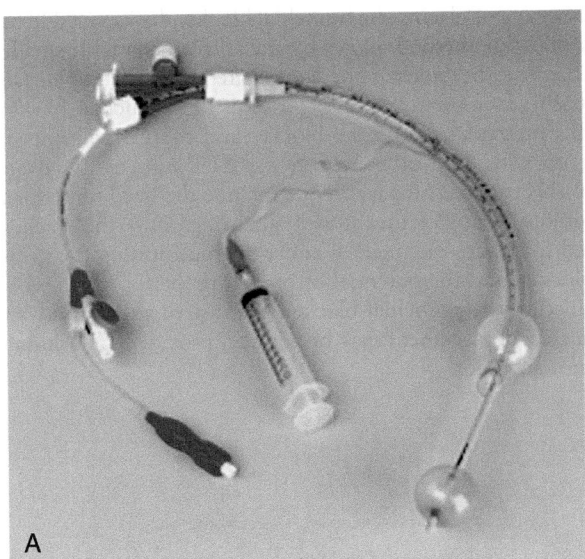

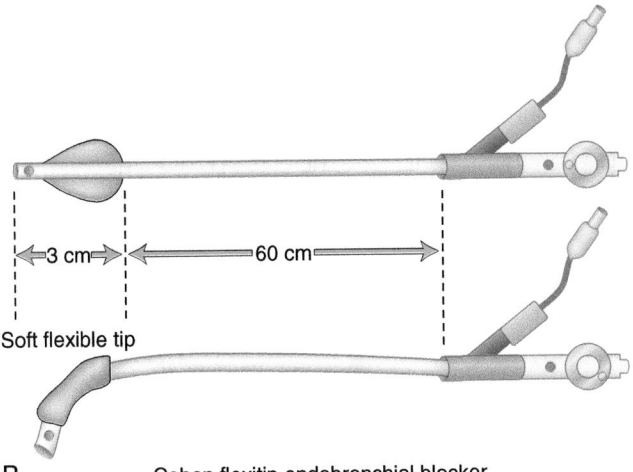

B   Cohen flexitip endobronchial blocker

• **Fig. 26.15** Cohen Flexitip Endobronchial Blocker. (A) Equipment. (B) Diagram.

Uniblocker

Fuji Systems introduced a 9-French, balloon-tipped, angled blocker with a multiple-port adapter that is essentially the same design as the Univent tube blocker, but it can be used as an independent blocker passed by means of a special connector through a standard ETT (Fig. 26.16). It has a prefixed bend, like a hockey stick, to facilitate insertion into the desired bronchus. This blocker is also available in a 5.0-French size for the pediatric population.

EZ-Blocker

The latest addition to the endobronchial blocker design is the EZ-Blocker (IQ Medical Ventures, Rotterdam, Netherlands). It is a 7-French, four-lumen, 75-cm, disposable endobronchial blocker used to facilitate selective lung ventilation (Fig. 26.17). It has a symmetrical, Y-shaped bifurcation, and both branches have an inflatable cuff on each arm and a central lumen. The bifurcation resembles the bifurcation of the trachea. During insertion through a standard ETT, each of the two distal ends is placed into a main stem bronchus. The selected lung is isolated by inflating the blocker's balloon to the least volume necessary to occlude the main stem under FB visualization. This device should offer an advantage during bilateral procedures, because each lung can be deflated without the need for repositioning the blocker. The clinical experience with this device is increasing.

The effectiveness of lung isolation with three devices, namely, the left-sided Broncho-Cath DLT, the Univent torque-control blocker,[64] and the wire-guided Arndt, has been compared in a prospective, randomized trial. There was no significant difference in tube malpositions for the three devices, but it took longer to position the Arndt blocker (86 vs 56 seconds) than the left-sided DLT and the Univent. Excluding the time for tube placement, it also took longer for the lung to collapse in the Arndt group (26 minutes) compared with the DLT group (18 minutes) or the Univent group (19.5 minutes). Unlike the other two groups, most of the Arndt patients required suction to achieve lung collapse. After lung isolation was achieved, overall surgical exposure was rated excellent for the three groups (Fig. 26.18). One minute longer to position a bronchial blocker or 6 minutes longer to collapse the lung with the bronchial blocker is clinically insignificant considering the length of the thoracic procedure. The risk–benefit ratio and the patient safety profile for each patient and the clinical experience of the anesthesia provider should be considered when choosing the method for lung isolation.[65]

Another study evaluated the use of the Cohen blocker, the Arndt blocker, the Uniblocker, and a DLT in four groups with 26 patients in each group. The investigators found no differences among the groups in the time taken to insert these lung

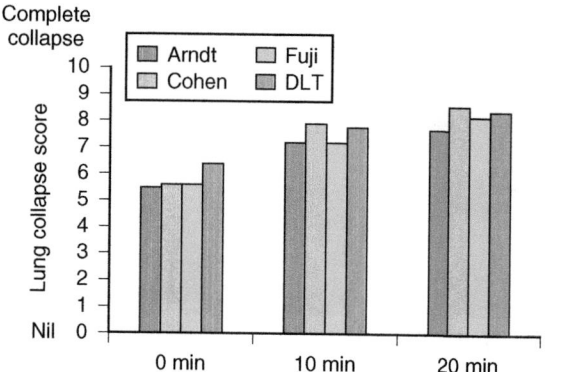

• **Fig. 26.18** Comparison of lung collapse times for three bronchial blockers and a double-lumen tube.

isolation devices or in the quality of the lung collapse.[66] The grading was done by the operating surgeons, who were blinded to which device was used. The number of cuff dislocations was higher among the bronchial blocker groups, which was highest with the Arndt blocker, possibly because the study protocol used the elliptical cuff. Regardless of the type of bronchial blocker or DLT selected to provide OLV, the choice of technique depends on the clinical circumstances, the physician's experience, and the level of comfort with a particular device. However, the clinician should not limit his or her practice to the use of only one device but rather be versatile and comfortable with the use of several devices in the "tool box."

It is possible to perform lung isolation if specialized endobronchial blockers are available. In these cases a bronchial blocking device is inserted through the lumen of an SLT (Fig. 26.19) or outside the SLT between the tracheal cuff and the trachea (Fig. 26.20). Placement is confirmed by FB. Any device that has a balloon-tipped catheter can be used as a bronchial blocker (see Fig. 26.19).[67] The most common devices used are Fogarty embolectomy catheters and the 5.0-French Cook bronchial blockers most frequently used for pediatric patients.[68]

Paraxial Endotracheal Blockers

The advantage of placing the bronchial blocker device outside the SLT is that this method allows blocker placement with smaller ETTs because the blocker does not share the ETT lumen (see Fig. 26.20). It is often easier to position the bronchial blocker with this method, because the blocker and the FB will not get caught up with each other within the ETT lumen. Disadvantages of this paraxial tube technique include the need to perform laryngoscopy to place the bronchial blocker into the trachea, the need to deflate the tracheal cuff while positioning the bronchial blocker, and the potential of rupturing the ETT cuff while manipulating the bronchial blocker. Because of these disadvantages, a coaxial placement may be advised, provided ETT lumen size is not an issue.

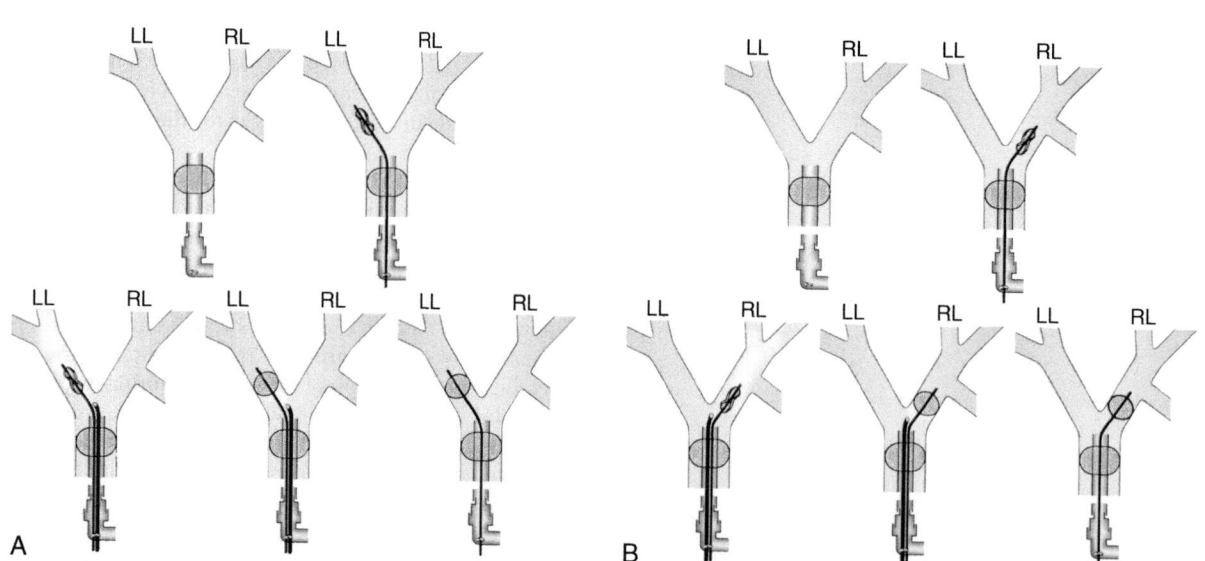

• **Fig. 26.19** Sequence for lung separation with a single-lumen tube (SLT) and a bronchial blocker within the SLT. (A) Left lung (LL) bronchial blocker. (B) Right lung (RL) bronchial blocker. The bronchial blocker (Fogarty embolectomy catheter) is placed in the correct main stem bronchus under fiberoptic vision. (From Benumof JL. *Anesthesia for Thoracic Surgery*. Philadelphia: Saunders; 1987.)

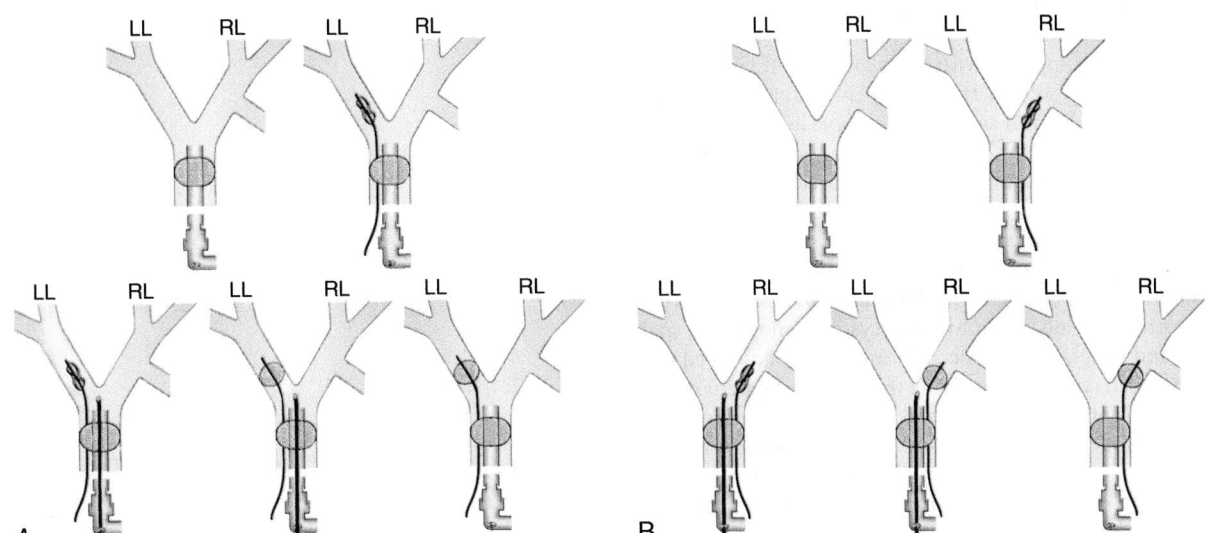

• **Fig. 26.20** Separation of two lungs with a single-lumen tube (SLT), flexible bronchoscope (FB), and a left lung (A) and a right lung (B) bronchial blocker that is outside the SLT. The SLT is inserted, and the patient is ventilated (*upper left diagrams*). The bronchial blocker is passed alongside the indwelling endotracheal tube (*upper right diagrams*). The FB is passed through a self-sealing diaphragm in the elbow connector to the endotracheal tube and is used to place the bronchial blocker into the appropriate main stem bronchus under direct vision (*lower left diagrams*). The balloon on the bronchial blocker is inflated under direct vision and is positioned just below the tracheal carina (*lower middle diagrams*). During the insertion and use of the FB (*lower panels*), the self-sealing diaphragm allows the patient to continue to receive positive-pressure ventilation around the FB but within the lumens of the ETT. *LL,* Left lung; *RL,* right lung. (From Benumof JL. *Anesthesia for Thoracic Surgery*. Philadelphia: Saunders; 1987.)

Pediatric Lung Isolation

Ventilation/Perfusion During Thoracic Surgery

As discussed previously, ventilation is normally distributed preferentially to dependent regions of the lung so that there is a gradient of increasing ventilation from the most nondependent to the most dependent lung segments. Because of gravitational effects, perfusion normally follows a similar distribution, with increased blood flow to dependent lung segments. Ventilation and perfusion are normally well matched. During thoracic surgery, several factors act to increase V/Q mismatch. General anesthesia, neuromuscular blockade, and mechanical ventilation cause a decrease in the functional residual capacity (FRC) of both lungs. The compression of the dependent lung in the lateral decubitus position can cause atelectasis. Surgical retraction or OLV, or both, can result in the collapse of the operative lung. Hypoxic pulmonary vasoconstriction, which acts to divert blood flow away from the nonventilated lung, thereby minimizing V/Q mismatch, may be diminished by the use of inhalational anesthetic agents and intravenous vasodilating drugs. These factors apply to infants, children, and adults. The overall effect of the lateral decubitus position on V/Q mismatching is different in infants than in older children and adults.

In adults with unilateral lung disease oxygenation is optimal when the patient is placed in the lateral decubitus position with the healthy lung dependent and the diseased lung nondependent.[69] Presumably, this is related to an increase in blood flow to the dependent, healthy lung and a decrease in blood flow to the nondependent, diseased lung resulting from the hydrostatic pressure (or gravitational) gradient between the two lungs. This phenomenon promotes V/Q matching in the adult patient who is undergoing thoracic surgery in the lateral decubitus position.

In infants with unilateral lung disease, on the other hand, oxygenation is improved when the healthy lung is nondependent.[70] Several factors account for this discrepancy between adults and infants. Infants have a soft, easily compressible rib cage that cannot fully protect the underlying lung. The FRC is closer to the residual volume, making airway closure likely to occur in the dependent lung even during tidal breathing.[71] When the adult is placed in the lateral decubitus position, the dependent diaphragm has a mechanical advantage because it is "loaded" by the abdominal hydrostatic pressure gradient. This pressure gradient is reduced in infants, reducing the functional advantage of the dependent diaphragm. The infant's small size also results in a reduced hydrostatic pressure gradient between the nondependent and dependent lungs. Consequently, the favorable increase in perfusion to the dependent, ventilated lung is reduced in infants.

Infants' increased O_2 requirement, coupled with a small FRC, predisposes them to hypoxemia. The O_2 consumption in infants is normally 6 to 8 mL/kg/min, compared with a normal O_2 consumption in adults of 2 to 3 mL/kg/min.[72] For these reasons, infants are at increased risk for significant O_2 desaturation during surgery in the lateral decubitus position.

Indications and Techniques for Single-Lung Ventilation in Infants and Children

Before 1995, almost all thoracic surgery in children was performed via thoracotomy. In most cases anesthesia providers ventilated both lungs with a conventional ETT, and surgeons retracted the operative lung to gain exposure to the surgical field. Over the past decade, the use of VATS has dramatically increased in both adults and children. Reported advantages of VATS include smaller chest incisions, reduced postoperative pain, and more rapid postoperative recovery compared with thoracotomy.[73–75] Advances in surgical technique as well as technology, including high-resolution microchip cameras and smaller endoscopic instruments, have facilitated the application of VATS in smaller patients.

VATS is being used extensively for pleural debridement in patients with emphysema, lung biopsy, or wedge resections for interstitial lung disease, mediastinal masses, or metastatic lesions. More extensive pulmonary resections, including segmentectomy and lobectomy, have been performed for lung abscess, bullous disease, sequestrations, lobar emphysema, cystic adenomatoid malformation, and neoplasms. In selected centers more advanced procedures have been reported, including the closure of patent ductus arteriosus, repair of hiatal hernias, and anterior spinal fusion.

VATS can be performed while both lungs are being ventilated with the use of CO_2 insufflation and placement of a retractor to displace lung tissue in the operative field. However, OLV is extremely desirable during VATS because lung deflation improves the visualization of thoracic contents and may reduce lung injury caused by the use of retractors. Although a recent report did not show improved outcomes with OLV compared with double-lung ventilation during thoracoscopic surgery in children, OLV is routinely used in many pediatric centers in the United States and around the world.[76,77] There are several different techniques that can be used to provide OLV in children.

Single-Lumen Tube

The simplest means of providing OLV is to intubate the ipsilateral main stem bronchus with a conventional SLT.[67] When the left bronchus is to be intubated, the bevel of the ETT is rotated 180 degrees, and the head is turned to the right.[78] The ETT is advanced into the bronchus until breath sounds on the operative side disappear. An FB may be passed through, or alongside, the ETT to confirm or guide placement. When a cuffed ETT is used, the distance from the proximal cuff to the tip of the tube must be shorter than the length of the bronchus so that the proximal cuff is not in the trachea.[79] Ideally, the distance from the distal cuff to the tip of the ETT is shorter than the main stem bronchus so that the orifice of the upper lobe bronchus is not occluded (Fig. 26.21). This technique is simple and requires no special equipment other than the optional use of an FB. This may be the preferred technique of OLV in emergency situations such as airway hemorrhage or contralateral tension pneumothorax.

If a smaller, uncuffed ETT is used, it may be difficult to provide an adequate seal of the intended bronchus. This may prevent the operative lung from adequately collapsing or fail to protect the healthy, ventilated lung from contamination by purulent material from the contralateral lung. The use of a cuffed tube may cause tracheal obstruction, especially in infants and young children. The practitioner is unable to suction the operative lung using this technique. Hypoxemia may occur because of obstruction of the upper lobe bronchus, especially when the short right main stem bronchus is intubated.

Variations of this technique have been described, including the intubation of both bronchi independently with small ETTs.[80–83] One main stem bronchus is initially intubated with an ETT, after which another ETT is advanced over an FB into the opposite bronchus. This technique is limited because of concern regarding vocal cord and airway mucosal injury and the need to use very small ETTs.

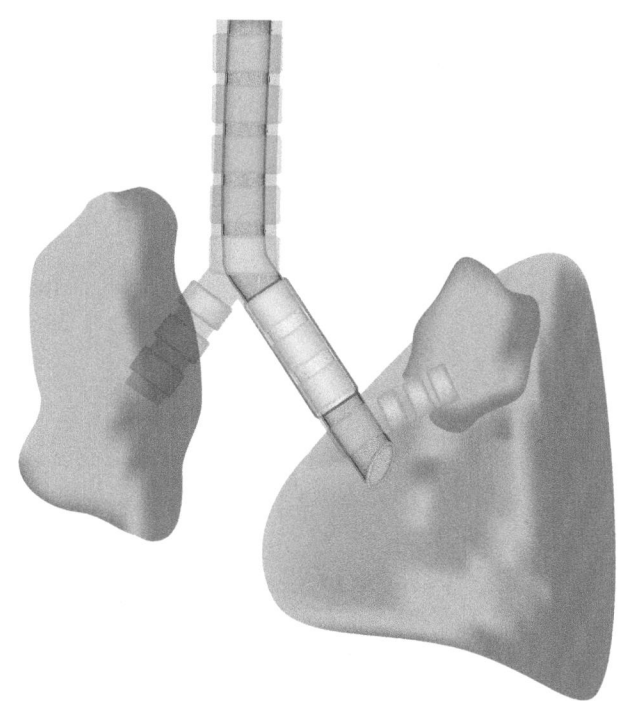

• **Fig. 26.21** Occlusion of upper lobe bronchus when the conventional, cuffed endotracheal tube is used for SLV. When a cuffed ETT is used for SLV, the distance from the proximal cuff to the tip of the ETT should not exceed the length of the main stem bronchus. Otherwise, either the cuff will reside in the trachea, risking tracheal obstruction, or the tip of the ETT will occlude the upper lobe bronchus, causing atelectasis of the upper lobe of the lung on the ventilated side.

Balloon-Tipped Bronchial Blockers

A Fogarty embolectomy catheter or an end-hole, balloon wedge catheter may be used for bronchial blockade to provide OLV.[84–86] The placement of a Fogarty catheter is facilitated by bending the tip of its stylet toward the bronchus on the operative side. An FB may be used to reposition the catheter and confirm appropriate placement. Various methods have been described to facilitate the positioning of these catheters outside of an ETT. In one method the bronchus on the operative side is initially intubated with an ETT.[87] A guidewire is then advanced into that bronchus through the ETT. The ETT is removed, and the bronchial blocker is advanced over the guidewire into the bronchus. An ETT is then reinserted into the trachea alongside the blocker catheter. The catheter balloon is positioned in the proximal main stem bronchus under flexible scope visual guidance. With an inflated bronchial blocker balloon, the airway is completely sealed, providing more predictable lung collapse and better operating conditions than with an ETT in the bronchus.

A potential problem with this technique is the dislodgment of the bronchial blocker balloon into the trachea. The inflated balloon blocks ventilation to both lungs and prevents the collapse of the operated lung. The balloons of most catheters currently used for bronchial blockade have low-volume, high-pressure properties, and overdistention can damage or even rupture the airway.[88] One study, however, reported that bronchial blocker cuffs produced lower ratios of cuff-to-tracheal pressure than DLTs.[89] When closed-tip bronchial blockers are used, the operative lung cannot be suctioned, and CPAP cannot be provided to the operative lung if needed.

Adapters that facilitate ventilation during the placement of a bronchial blocker through an indwelling ETT have been used.[90,91] A 5-French endobronchial blocker that is suitable for use in children with a multiport adapter and FB has been described (Cook Critical Care, Bloomington, IN.)[92] The risk of hypoxemia during blocker placement is diminished, and repositioning of the blocker may be performed with FB guidance during surgery. Even with an FB with a 2.2-mm OD, the indwelling ETT must have an ID of 5.0 mm or larger to allow the passage of the catheter and FB. This technique typically is limited to children older than 18 months and up to 2 years of age.

Univent Tube

As described earlier in this chapter, the Univent tube is a conventional ETT with a second lumen containing a small tube that can be advanced into a bronchus.[57,92,93] A balloon located at the distal end of this small tube serves as a blocker (see earlier). Univent tubes require an FB for successful placement. Univent tubes are available in sizes as small as 3.5- and 4.5-mm ID for use in children older than 6 years of age.[94] Because the blocker tube is firmly attached to the main ETT, the displacement of the Univent blocker balloon is less likely than when other bronchial blocker techniques are used. The blocker tube has a small lumen, which allows the egress of gas and can be used to insufflate O_2 or suction the operated lung.

A disadvantage of the Univent tube is the large amount of cross-sectional area occupied by the blocker channel, especially in the smaller tubes. Smaller Univent tubes have a disproportionately high resistance to gas flow.[95] The Univent tube's blocker balloon has low-volume, high-pressure characteristics, and mucosal injury can occur during normal inflation.[96,97]

Double-Lumen Tubes

All DLTs are essentially two tubes of unequal length molded together. The shorter tube ends in the trachea and the longer tube in the bronchus. Marraro described a DLT for infants that consists of two separate uncuffed ETTs of different lengths attached longitudinally.[98] This tube is not available in the United States. DLTs for older children and adults have cuffs located on the tracheal and bronchial lumens. The tracheal cuff, when inflated, allows PPV. The inflated bronchial cuff allows ventilation to be diverted to either lung or both lungs and protects each lung from contamination from the contralateral side.

The smallest cuffed DLT is 26 French (Rusch, Duluth, GA) and may be used in children as young as 8 years of age. For children 10 years of age or older, DLTs are also available in sizes of 28 and 32 French (Mallinckrodt Medical, St. Louis, MO).

DLTs are inserted in children using the same technique as is used in adults.[99] The tip of the tube is inserted just beyond the vocal cords, and the stylet is withdrawn. The DLT is rotated 90 degrees to the appropriate side and then advanced into the bronchus. In the adult population the depth of insertion is directly related to the height of the patient.[100] No equivalent measurements are yet available in children. If an FB is used to confirm tube placement, one with a small diameter and sufficient length must be available.[101]

A DLT offers the advantage of the ease of insertion as well as the ability to suction and oxygenate the operative lung with CPAP. Left-sided DLTs are preferred to right-sided instruments because of the shorter length of the right main bronchus. Right-sided DLTs are more difficult to position accurately because of the greater risk of right upper lobe obstruction.

DLTs are safe and easy to use. There have been very few reports of airway damage from DLTs in adults and none in children. Their high-volume, low-pressure cuffs should not damage the airway if they are not overinflated with air or distended with nitrous oxide while in place.

There is significant variability in overall size and airway dimensions in children, particularly in teenagers. For average-sized children 8 to 10 years of age, a 26-French DLT may be appropriate. However, in patients 11 to 14 years of age the appropriate DLT size may range from 26 to 32 French. The estimation of the appropriate-sized cuffed ETT may be used to correlate OD measurements for proper DLT selection in these age groups. Difficulty in the selection of DLT size contributes to the use of other single-lung ventilation OLV techniques. Ultimately, proper evaluation of the patient with knowledge of anesthetic and surgical procedure requirements will determine proper modality selection and patient safety.

Conclusion

The anesthesia provider caring for patients who require OLV and lung isolation faces many challenges. An understanding of the primary underlying lesion, as well as associated anomalies that may affect perioperative management, is paramount. A working knowledge of respiratory physiology and anatomy is required for the planning and execution of appropriate intraoperative care. Familiarity with a variety of techniques for OLV suited to the patient's needs allows maximal surgical exposure while minimizing trauma to the lungs and airways.

Selected References

13. Kwon NK, Jung SM, Park SJ, et al. Comparison of displacement of polyvinyl chloride and silicone left-sided double-lumen tubes during lateral positioning. *Korean J Anesthesiol*. 2019;72:32–38.

15. Campos JH, Hanada S. DLT with incorporated fiberoptic bronchoscopy. In: Rosenblatt WH, Popescu WM, eds. *Master Techniques in Upper and Lower Airway Management*. Liam Rzosenblatt 1st ed, Wolters Kluwer, 2015, pp. 250–251.

19. Rapchuk IL, Kunju SAM, Smith IJ, Faulke DJ. A six-month evaluation of the VivaSight™ video double lumen endotracheal tube after introduction into thoracic anaesthetic practice at a single institution. *Anaesth Intensive Care*. 2017;45(2):189–196.

22. Larsen S, Højberg J, Tove H, Sauer N, Andersen C. A cost-effectiveness analysis comparing the VivaSight double-lumen tube and a conventional double-lumen tube in adult patients undergoing thoracic surgery involving one-lung ventilation. *Pharmacoecon Open*. 2020;4:159–169.

31. Brodsky JB, Benumof JL, Ehrenwerth J, et al. Depth of placement of left double-lumen endobronchial tubes. *Anesth Analg*. 1991;73:570–572.

35. Benumof JL, Partridge BL, Salvatierra C, et al. Margin of safety in positioning modern double-lumen endotracheal tubes. *Anesthesiology*. 1987;67:729–738.

36. Amar D, Desiderio DP, Heerdt PM, et al. Practice patterns in choice of left double-lumen tube size for thoracic surgery. *Anesth Analg*. 2008;106:379–383.

40. Benumof JL. The position of a double-lumen tube should be routinely determined by fiberoptic bronchoscopy. *J Cardiothorac Vasc Anesth*. 1993;7:513–514.

41. Cohen E, Neustein SM, Goldofsky S, et al. Incidence of malposition of polyvinylchloride and red rubber left-sided double-lumen tubes and clinical sequelae. *J Cardiothorac Vasc Anesth*. 1995;9:122–127.

44. Campos JH, Hallam EA, Ueda K. Training in placement of the left-sided double-lumen tube among non-thoracic anaesthesiologists. Intubation model simulator versus computer-based digital video disc, a randomised controlled trial. *Eur J Anaesthesiol.* 2011;28:169–174.

62. Campos JH. Update on selective lobar blockade during pulmonary resections. *Curr Opin Anaesthesiol.* 2009;22:18–22.

66. Narayanaswamy M, McRae K, Slinger P, et al. Choosing a lung isolation device for thoracic surgery: a randomized trial of three bronchial blockers versus double-lumen tubes. *Anesth Analg.* 2009;108:1097–1101.

76. Dingemann C, Zoeller C, Bataineh Z, Osthaus A, Suempelmann R, Ure B. Single- and double-lung ventilation in infants and children undergoing thoracoscopic lung resection. *Eur J Pediatr Surg.* 2013;23(1):48–52.

All references can be found online at eBooks.Health.Elsevier.com.

27

Rigid Bronchoscopy

SOHAM ROY, IRVING BASAÑEZ, AND RONDA E. ALEXANDER

KEY POINTS

- Open communication between the surgeon and the anesthesiologist is of the highest importance during rigid bronchoscopy.
- Inspect the equipment before the procedure; ensure that the bronchoscopes, light sources, light carriers, and connectors are all in working order.
- Check that instruments (suction, graspers, telescopes) are the appropriate length for the selected bronchoscopes.

- Have a backup set that is a size smaller than what you plan to use with appropriate instruments at the ready.
- For pediatric patients, calculate the safe maximum dose of each topical medication (e.g., lidocaine), and restrict their presence in the operative field.
- Place dental/gingival protection, and never leave the bronchoscope on the teeth.
- Advance the scope only when there is an identifiable lumen.

Introduction

Rigid bronchoscopy is a surgical technique that is used to visualize the oropharynx, larynx, vocal cords, trachea, and proximal pulmonary branches. The origin of rigid bronchoscopy can be traced back to Hippocrates (460–370 BCE), who advised introducing a pipe into the larynx in a suffocating patient to assess the airways.[1] Because of limitations in light delivery, the field was largely dormant until the 1800s, when incandescent lightbulbs were invented. The development of local anesthesia in 1880 also made bronchoscopy more tolerable. In 1897 Gustave Killian passed an endoscope through the larynx and removed a piece of pork bone from the right mainstem bronchus using cocaine as topical anesthesia.[1] Chevalier Jackson further advanced the field of rigid endoscopy by improving lighting, developing auxiliary instrumentation for the removal of foreign objects, and implementing rigid bronchoscopy training programs.[2] As a result of these and other efforts, he is recognized as the father of contemporary rigid endoscopy.[3] Since Jackson's time, instrumentation has continued to advance, such that current rigid instrumentation and ventilation systems allow for more precise assessment of and intervention within the respiratory tract.[3] HH Hopkins of England invented the first conventional lens system by using glass rods instead of small lenses, which produced a significantly brighter image, occupied less space, and allowed for greater visualization of an object in a single field.[1] This provided the basis for modern fiberoptic bronchoscopy.

Indications and Contraindications

The tracheobronchial tree can be directly observed using either rigid or flexible bronchoscopy. Although the advent of flexible bronchoscopy has given physicians improved access to more distal portions of the tracheobronchial tree with a more rapid learning curve and less patient discomfort compared with rigid bronchoscopy,[2] there are still clinical situations in which rigid bronchoscopy is more appropriate. The larger working port and defined structure of the instrument make rigid bronchoscopy useful for surgical interventions within the airway, such as the removal of foreign bodies and masses.[4] At the same time, the bronchoscope can be used to establish and maintain the airway in patients presenting with ventilation difficulty, including obstructing masses, external compression, and hemorrhage.[4] In contrast to the flexible apparatus, the rigid bronchoscope has a ventilation port that can be connected directly to the anesthesia circuit, allowing for ventilation while airway procedures are performed. In fact, earlier

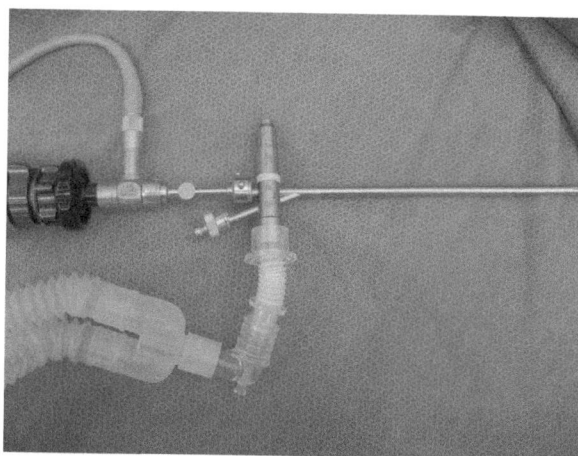

• **Fig. 27.1** Bronchoscope with attachments to the anesthesia circuit.

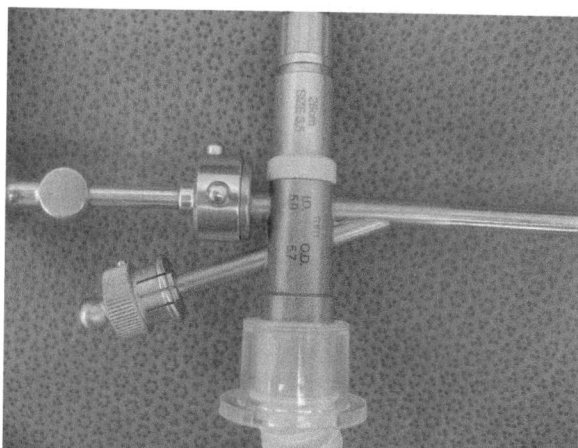

• **Fig. 27.2** Close-up view of a ventilating bronchoscope. The anesthesia circuit attaches inferiorly, the prismatic light source superiorly, and the suction port at an angle.

iterations of the American Society of Anesthesiologists (ASA) Practice Guidelines for Management of the Difficult Airway included the use of rigid bronchoscopy under techniques for difficult ventilation; however, it was removed from the 2013 revision.[5] Other instances in which rigid bronchoscopy may be preferred include deep and/or large diagnostic biopsies when a fiberoptic specimen would be inadequate, dilatation of stenosis, bronchial stenting, reduction of fractures, application of laser therapy or cryotherapy, tumor removal, and diagnosis of vascular rings. A summary of the indications for rigid bronchoscopy is presented in Box 27.1.

There are few contraindications to rigid bronchoscopy. In practice, most of the factors limiting rigid bronchoscopy are related to the need for general anesthesia, such as an unstable cardiovascular or respiratory status.[6] One absolute contraindication to rigid bronchoscopy is an unstable cervical spine, because of the hyperextension of the head required during the performance of the procedure. In this instance, flexible bronchoscopy is indicated to avoid further spinal injury. Other contraindications include laryngeal stenosis that prevents the passage of the bronchoscope, limited range of motion of the mandible, severe kyphoscoliosis, uncontrolled coagulopathy, and extreme ventilatory/oxygenation demands.[7,8]

Instrumentation

The Storz endoscope with the Hopkins rod-lens optical system, introduced in 1966, is the most widely used rigid bronchoscopy system and has largely replaced the Jackson and Holinger endoscopes.[9] This rod-lens system provides better illumination, greater visualization, and angled views. The bronchoscope is a hollow, rigid metal tube that is tapered and beveled on the distal end and has a series of ports on the proximal end that serve different purposes. There are side holes at the distal portion of the bronchoscope to allow for ventilation just proximal to the tip.[10] The beveled edge of the distal tip is used to facilitate the introduction of the bronchoscope into the airway and for the dissection of planes during the resection of tumors. At the proximal end, the inferior port may be connected to the anesthesia circuit, allowing ventilation and oxygenation, while the superior port connects to the prismatic light deflector and light source (Figs. 27.1 and 27.2). The central, in-line port is the working channel used for the insertion of instruments such as telescopes, biopsy forceps, laser

fibers, balloon devices, cryotherapy probes, and stents. The port can be left open to allow room air into the system, or it can be closed to prevent the leakage of air or anesthetic gases, depending on the ventilation strategy and anesthetic technique being used. Bronchoscopes vary in size, in length, and in internal and external diameter. The size of the instrument must be tailored to the individual patient; Table 27.1 depicts the different sizes of the Storz bronchoscopes that are typically appropriate based on the patient's age. The ideal size is one that will maximize the surgeon's view while causing the least trauma to the airway.[9] Telescopes with different angles (0, 30, and 70 degrees), lengths, and diameters may be inserted through the main working port to visualize areas that are difficult to see with the rigid bronchoscope alone, namely, the right and left upper bronchial orifices and the right middle bronchial orifice.[9] Illumination can be provided either through a light carrier rod that goes down a channel in older endoscopes, through the telescope, or by means of a port that attaches to a prismatic light deflector that subsequently attaches to a light source in newer endoscopes (Figs. 27.3 and 27.4). This last configuration has the advantage of providing both proximal and distal illumination.

Rigid bronchoscopy should be performed either in an operating room (OR) or an endoscopy suite. As with all procedures that require general anesthesia, the room should be equipped with equipment for oxygen saturation monitoring, carbon

Size	Length (cm)	ID (mm)	OD (mm)	Age
2.5	20	3.5	4.2	Premature
3.0	20, 26	4.3	5.0	Premature, newborn
3.5	20, 26, 30	5.0	5.7	Newborn–6 months
3.7	26, 30	5.7	6.4	6 months–1 year
4.0	26, 30	6.0	6.7	1–2 years
5.0	30	7.1	7.8	3–4 years
6.0	30, 40	7.5	8.2	5–7 years
6.5	43	8.5	9.2	Adult

TABLE 27.1 Suggested Bronchoscope Sizes (Brand: Karl Storz) According to Patient Age

ID, Internal diameter; *OD,* outer diameter.
Modified from Tom LWC, Potsic WP, Handler SD. Methods of examination. In: Bluestone CD, Stool DE, Alper CM, et al., eds. *Pediatric Otolaryngology.* 4th ed. Philadelphia: Elsevier; 2003.

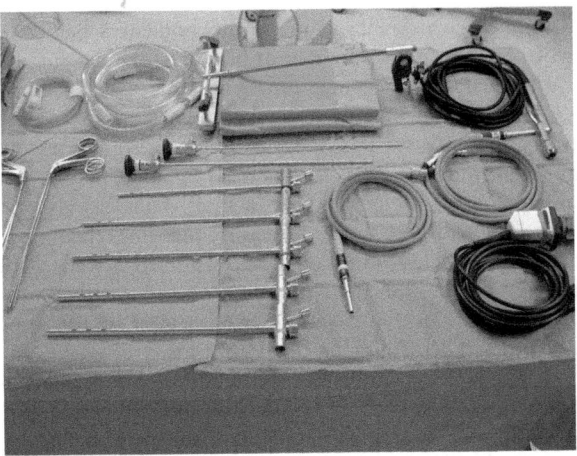

• **Fig. 27.5** Additional setup including graspers and suction.

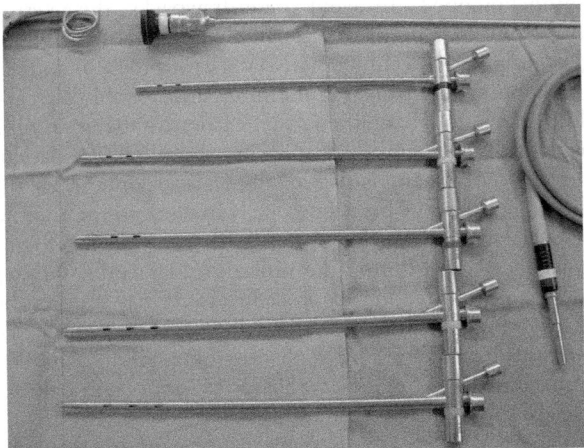

• **Fig. 27.3** Bronchoscopes of varying sizes in an example setup.

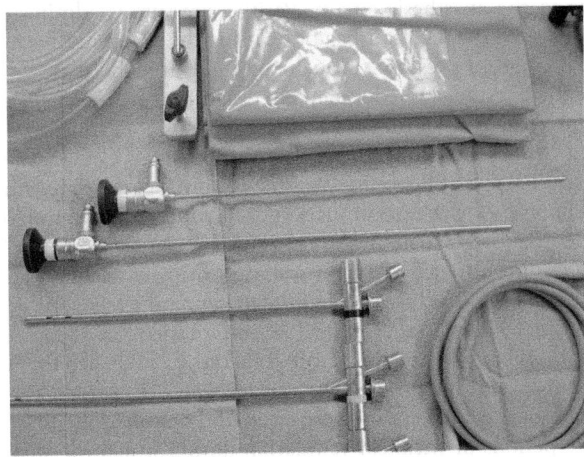

• **Fig. 27.4** Optical telescopes for visualization through bronchoscopes.

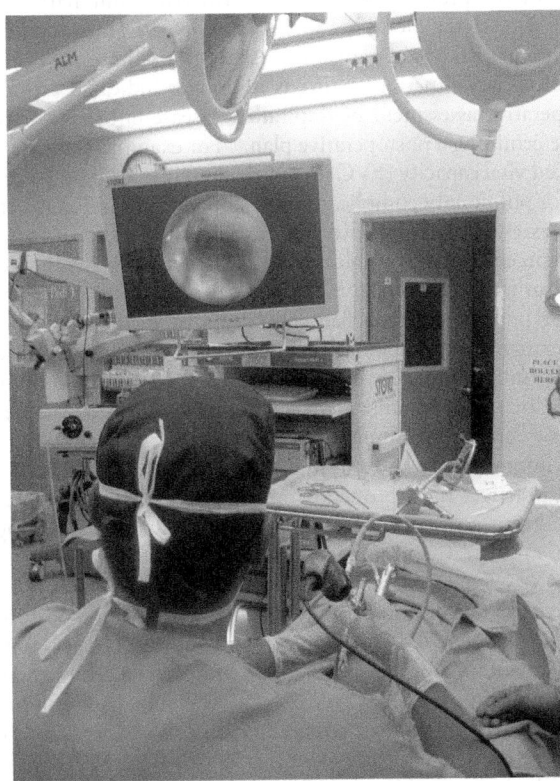

• **Fig. 27.6** Bronchoscopist's view during a procedure. The monitor is shared so that it may be viewed simultaneously by the bronchoscopist and the anesthesiologist.

Optional items include a flexible bronchoscope that can be passed through the rigid bronchoscope for further examination of the lower tracheobronchial tree. Video capability is also desirable but not required (Fig. 27.6).

Preoperative Considerations

Because rigid bronchoscopy is typically performed under general anesthesia, preprocedural evaluation should include the standard considerations for this technique. A thorough history should be taken to assess previous cardiac disease (e.g., recent myocardial infarction or documented dysrhythmias) or pulmonary disease

dioxide (CO_2) monitoring, blood pressure monitoring, and electrocardiography. A full set of ventilating bronchoscopes and a backup light source should be available. The standard adult-size rigid bronchoscope is 8 mm in diameter and 40 cm long. Other instruments such as graspers, biopsy forceps, optical forceps, and suction devices should also be available to the surgeon (Fig. 27.5).

(e.g., asthma), which may require bronchodilators before bronchoscopy.[4] To minimize the risk of bleeding, the patient should have a normal platelet count; unless an abnormal bleeding history is known, a preoperative coagulation workup is typically not necessary. In patients with suspected bleeding disorders functional coagulation studies, such as thromboelastography, may be useful. Because patients with uremia have qualitative platelet abnormalities that can predispose them to excessive bleeding, creatinine and blood urea nitrogen values should be considered as well.[4] Patients should also be questioned about aspirin or anticoagulant use and the timing of the last dose. Additional laboratory studies and tests may be ordered depending on the patient history.

A 12-lead electrocardiogram is required for patients with cardiac risk factors, such as smoking, diabetes mellitus, arterial hypertension, or hypercholesterolemia, and for those with a significant cardiac history. A chest radiograph may provide information regarding congestive heart failure, pulmonary consolidations, or the presence of chronic obstructive pulmonary disease (COPD). Arterial blood gas analysis can be performed to evaluate the patient's acid-base status in the setting of pulmonary disease.

Pulmonary function testing is no longer indicated as routine preoperative assessment of respiratory disease but may be useful for determining a postoperative plan.[11] For example, patients with a forced vital capacity (FVC) of less than 20 mL/kg are at increased risk for pulmonary complications postoperatively and may benefit from extended postoperative monitoring.[10] In addition, patients with forced expiratory volumes of less than 50% are at risk for hypercarbia and hypoxia.[12] The clinical predictors of perioperative or postoperative cardiac complications include unstable or severe angina, decompensated congestive heart failure, significant dysrhythmias, and severe valvular disease.[13] Cardiac conditions should be evaluated and medical therapies optimized before the surgery. Perhaps the simplest way to assess the patient's overall cardiopulmonary status is to inquire about exercise tolerance.

In practice, rigid bronchoscopy is often performed urgently or emergently with limited preoperative evaluation or testing to secure an airway, so patient characteristics predictive of cardiopulmonary complications, difficult intubation (DI), and difficult mask ventilation (DMV) also impact perioperative and postoperative management. DI is associated with morbid obesity; limited range of motion of the head, neck, and jaw; receding mandible; overjetting ("buck") teeth; high Mallampati classification; decreased thyromental or sternomental distances; and a history of DI.[5,14,15] The five independent risk factors for DMV have been established as age older than 55 years, body mass index greater than 26, presence of a beard, edentulism, and a history of snoring.[14] A careful evaluation of the patient's jaw and neck mobility should be made because severe cervical spine disease is an important contraindication to rigid bronchoscopy.

Anesthesia for Bronchoscopy

Because of the nature of the procedure and sharing of the airway, the anesthesiologist and surgeon must be in constant communication during a rigid bronchoscopy procedure. The goals for anesthesia during bronchoscopy include the provision of amnesia and analgesia, muscle relaxation as needed to accomplish the exposure, blunting of respiratory tract reactivity and reflexes, maintenance of adequate oxygenation, and achieving prompt emergence at the conclusion of the procedure. General anesthesia is typically used to prevent unnecessary patient movement and possible unintentional damage to the airway. This can be accomplished with deep

inhalational anesthesia, total intravenous anesthesia (TIVA), or a combination of inhalational and intravenous anesthesia with or without neuromuscular blocking drugs (NMBDs) depending on the specifics of the patient and procedure along with the preferences of the surgeon and anesthesiologist.

As previously described, rigid bronchoscopes have ventilating ports that can be attached to the anesthesia circuit directly, allowing anesthetic gases and oxygen to flow continuously during the procedure. This is the most common and straightforward manner in which to keep a patient adequately ventilated during rigid bronchoscopy, although spontaneous ventilation, positive-pressure ventilation (PPV), apneic oxygenation, jet ventilation, or negative-pressure ventilation (NPV) may also be employed.

Traditionally, particularly in the pediatric population, inhalational anesthesia with spontaneous respiration has been used during rigid bronchoscopy. Disadvantages of inhalational anesthesia with spontaneous respiration include difficulty in maintaining an adequate plane of anesthetic depth and anesthetic pollution of the surgical environment from a gas leak around the bronchoscope.[16] To avoid these drawbacks, the anesthetic is often converted to TIVA after induction. Malherbe and colleagues proposed a technique of TIVA with propofol and remifentanil and spontaneous respiration as a reasonable alternative to deep inhalational anesthesia that carries no major complications.[16] In the spontaneous respiration technique the patient is not given NMBDs and is allowed to breathe spontaneously. The ventilating port of the bronchoscope is attached to the anesthesia circuit with 100% O_2 flow (see Fig. 27.1), allowing for continuous ventilation during the procedure. However, the depth of anesthesia required for the procedure itself may suppress both cardiac output and the respiratory drive, making spontaneous respirations inadequate.[17] Also, the instrumentation required for the procedure itself can increase airway resistance and reduce the efficacy of spontaneous respirations.[18]

When PPV is used, it is typically achieved by terminating spontaneous respiration with NMBDs or high-dose opioids and, subsequently, connecting the ventilating port of the bronchoscope to the anesthesia circuit. Positive pressure is administered by squeezing the reservoir bag or by using the mechanical ventilator, forcing gas pressure through the rigid bronchoscope.[19] This technique results in reduced atelectasis, improves oxygenation, and compensates for the increased airway resistance caused by the instrumentation within the rigid bronchoscope.[18] One disadvantage of PPV is that it requires that the proximal eyepiece remain in place, preventing the use of suction or other instrumentation during ventilation.[20] There is also usually some gas leak during PPV owing to the absence of a tight seal, decreasing efficiency. Finally, the size of the bronchoscope and the presence of a telescope in the lumen increase resistance to airflow and increase dead space ventilation, making ventilation more difficult. PPV is therefore best suited to diagnostic procedures.

In apneic oxygenation the surgeon and anesthesiologist coordinate periods of withheld ventilation during which the surgeon works. The patient is first hyperventilated to produce significant hypocarbia. Under direct visualization, a catheter is then passed to the carina, and the flow rate of oxygen is set. The period of time in which the surgeon can work is determined by the rise in CO_2, after which the patient is allowed an equivalent amount of time during the next ventilation cycle to return to baseline. The partial pressure of CO_2 (Pco_2) is expected to rise continuously at a rate of 3 mm Hg per minute. This technique is to be avoided in patients who have a history of CO_2 retention (e.g., COPD), and intraprocedural awareness has also been reported more frequently with this technique.

Jet ventilation is usually used during laser procedures, and it is provided by the use of a jet ventilator with a jet injection cannula (JIC), also known as a Saunders injector.[21] This technique is used to overcome the hypoventilation caused by air leaks during PPV.[22] The cannula has three lumens, two of which open proximally and deliver the jet ventilation, while the distal lumen measures airway pressure.[21] The JIC is 3 mm in diameter, can have various lengths, and is made of stainless steel and therefore has a lower risk of endotracheal ignition.[21,22] The JIC is usually introduced distal to the lesion being accessed to provide optimal ventilation. High-pressure oxygen (50 psi) is delivered to the airway at high velocities, creating a Venturi effect[16] and entraining a column of air from outside the injector to flow into the airways and expand the lungs. Exhalation is passive and relies on the collapse of the airway once the pressure is removed. Sufficient time and an open pathway for air egress must be ensured during this technique to prevent stacked breaths and progressive hyperinflation. This method is contraindicated in foreign body removal, because the high-flow air may dislodge the foreign body and cause a complete obstruction.[18] Of note, jet ventilation does not prevent acidemia or hypercarbia and may increase the risk of air embolism, pneumothorax, and particle dissemination into the lungs and distal airways.[20] Also, in patients with poor lung compliance ventilation may be inadequate with this technique.[10]

NPV, compared with spontaneous assisted ventilation, reduces the administration of opioids, shortens recovery time from anesthesia, and prevents hypercarbia.[20] It can be accomplished by a poncho-wrap connected to a negative-pressure ventilator, with a 2-L/min oxygen flow, a negative pressure of –25 hPa, a respiratory rate of 15 breaths per minute, and an inspiration/expiration ratio of 1:1. NPV may be safer in patients with poor tolerance to hypercarbia, such as those with myocardial ischemia.[20]

Intravenous and topical medications can be used provided the patient's history reveals no prior adverse reactions and if the potential benefit outweighs the expected risks. Opioids are often used for analgesia, sedation, and reduction of the cough reflex. However, because they depress the respiratory drive, they should be used with caution in patients who have signs of airway obstruction or a foreign body. The addition of an opioid to a propofol-based anesthetic has been demonstrated to depress average oxygen saturation as measured by pulse oximetry (Spo_2; 96.4 ± 1.1 vs 97.8 ± 1.6, $p < 0.01$).[23] The degree of cough (measured using a 100-mm visual analog scale), however, was not different between the groups (73.4 ± 22.7 vs 72.2 ± 18.5, respectively). The intrinsic antitussive properties of propofol may obviate the need for opioids in many patients.

Anticholinergics are often used to reduce airway secretions and have been shown to enhance the absorption and prolong the analgesic action of topical analgesics such as lidocaine, which are administered to the airways to reduce reactivity, prevent bronchospasm, and dampen the systemic reaction to airway manipulation.[24] Intravenous anticholinergics are also commonly used to prevent the parasympathetic-mediated bradycardia and hypotension that can occur during rigid bronchoscopy.[11] Their routine use remains debatable.[25] A steroid such as dexamethasone can be used to decrease intraoperative and postoperative edema that can result from airway instrumentation.

For emergence from anesthesia, all anesthetic gases are turned off, NMBDs are reversed, and the patient is ventilated until spontaneous respirations resume. Topical lidocaine may again be administered to prevent laryngospasm and diminish coughing.[12]

Surgical Technique

The surgeon should verify that the necessary instrumentation is available before induction of anesthesia is initiated. In all patients bronchoscopes one and two sizes smaller than the preselected one should be available in case the airway encountered is smaller than anticipated.[9] The surgeon should also select the appropriate length of instruments that will be used during the procedure and ensure that they are functioning properly.

After informed consent for the procedure is obtained, the patient is taken to the OR/endoscopy suite. The patient should be positioned with the neck flexed on the body and the head extended at the neck.[9] This position is referred to as the "sniffing position" and is used to position the trachea anteriorly.[4] A shoulder roll to elevate the shoulders and a foam donut to stabilize the head are usually placed in adults and older children; in younger children a small donut for the head is often sufficient. The goal is to align the oral, pharyngeal, and tracheal axes to facilitate the insertion of the bronchoscope. The patient's teeth should be protected with rubber or thermoplastic guards, and the eyes should be protected with lubricant and tape.[4,12]

The anesthesiologist may induce anesthesia with either mask ventilation or intravenous agents, after which the surgeon begins the endoscopy by examining the oral cavity, oropharynx, and supraglottic larynx.[12] The vocal folds are identified and may, at this point, be sprayed with a topical agent such as lidocaine to diminish airway reactivity and laryngospasm. In both children and adults a slotted laryngoscope can be used in combination with a telescope to examine the larynx and the airway before the rigid bronchoscope is inserted. This facilitates the evaluation of the larynx without the risk of blind, unintentional dislodgement of a high airway foreign body.[12] Oxygen can also be insufflated via a flexible large-bore catheter into the laryngeal inlet during the preliminary examination to allow the surgeon additional working time (Fig. 27.7).[12]

Whereas in older children and adults the bronchoscope may be advanced directly into the trachea without laryngoscopic assistance, in younger children it is easiest and safest to use a laryngoscope to guide the rigid bronchoscope.[9] The laryngoscope is introduced in the usual fashion into the vallecula until the glottis is in the field of vision. The rigid bronchoscope is then introduced within or adjacent to the lumen of the laryngoscope down to the level of the true vocal folds.[9] If the glottis is not open, then the patient is not sufficiently relaxed, and additional intravenous

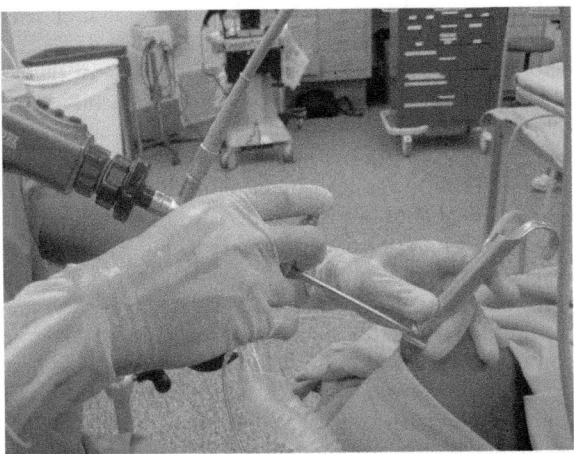

• **Fig. 27.7** Bronchoscope in position for ventilation during a procedure.

anesthetic or NMBD should be administered.[3] The rigid bronchoscope is then rotated 90 degrees to align the leading edge with the axis of the vocal folds as the bronchoscope passes through the glottic opening into the subglottis. This provides the path of least resistance and minimizes the risk of glottic injury.[7] A slight twisting motion may be required to advance the bronchoscope into the subglottis[9]; it can then be rotated back to its original orientation (see Video 27.1). Although the beveled tip of the rigid bronchoscope is conventionally directed anteriorly, some surgeons advocate placing the tip along the posterior wall of the trachea to prevent injury to the membranous trachea.[8]

In older children and adults laryngoscopy is not always required. The patient's maxilla is grasped with the left hand while support is provided for the rigid bronchoscope, and the dentition is protected by the thumb of the surgeon's nondominant hand as a reinforcement of the dental guard placed at the outset.[4,9] The bronchoscope is passed into the oral cavity in a plane perpendicular to that of the patient, and the posterior pharynx can be visualized. The bronchoscope is then rotated to a plane parallel with the airway axis. After visualization of the epiglottis, the tip of the bronchoscope is used to displace the epiglottis and tongue anteriorly. This maneuver requires gentle rocking of the bronchoscope on the thumb (not on the teeth) and brings the vocal folds into the field of vision.[4] Once the laryngeal inlet is exposed, the glottis can be approached, and the subglottis may be entered, as previously described.[9]

For the intubated patient, the rigid bronchoscope may be advanced alongside the endotracheal tube and then passed through the glottic opening as the tube is removed under direct visualization. If the larynx has been surgically removed or closed, the rigid bronchoscope should only be placed through the laryngostoma.[8]

Once the bronchoscope has been successfully introduced into the trachea, the sniffing position can be converted to cervical hyperextension by removing the supporting pillow and/or donut from under the head and lowering the headboard to extend the neck.[4,26] This maneuver is typically used in adults. The nondominant hand then holds the bronchoscope while the dominant hand is used for instrumentation of the airway for the duration of the procedure.[4] If any resistance is felt during the procedure, the surgeon should always reevaluate the patient's head and positioning, jaw opening, and bronchoscope size, as well as ensure that the patient's lips are not caught. At this point, the anesthesia circuit may be attached to the bronchoscope through the side port, and the oxygenation catheter can be removed (Fig. 27.8). Unless TIVA is being used, the lens cap to the main working port should be maintained in place to prevent the leakage of anesthetic gas through the proximal end of the bronchoscope.

Before any intervention, an initial examination of the airway should be performed, with photo or video documentation, when available. The subglottis and trachea are examined, and any masses or mucosal discolorations should be thoroughly investigated (see Video 27.2).[9] Even after premedication with an anticholinergic agent, secretions are frequently encountered during bronchoscopy and can be suctioned by introducing a rigid or flexible suction cannula into the main working port. Flexible suction catheters can also be inserted through a smaller side port to prevent loss of the closed anesthesia circuit.[12] Care must be taken not to suction the airways excessively, because this may lead to mucosal edema and inflammation and worsen the respiratory status of the patient. This effect can be mitigated by premedicating the patient with a steroid, such as dexamethasone.

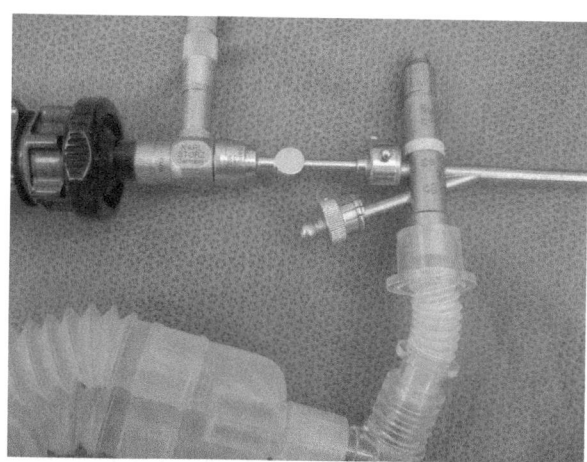

• **Fig. 27.8** Rigid ventilating bronchoscope with a telescope attached to a camera posteriorly.

The bronchoscope is then advanced to the level of the carina. The appearance and movement of the carina are noted during respirations. Decreased movement of the carina can be an indicator of hilar lymphadenopathy.[9] To advance the rigid bronchoscope to the main stem bronchus, the head should be slightly turned to the side opposite the intended bronchus. The distal airways may be evaluated by inserting different-angled telescopes to view the tracheobronchial tree. The 30- and 90-degree telescopes are especially useful to examine the segmental orifices of the upper lobes, in particular the right upper lobe, which is often in a difficult location to access.[3,7] The distal tracheobronchial tree can also be examined by inserting a flexible bronchoscope through the rigid bronchoscope.[7]

After the preliminary evaluation of the airway is completed, any necessary intervention may be initiated. For diagnostic bronchoscopy, bronchial brushings, washings, and biopsies are performed, in that order.[3] If any bleeding is encountered, it can be controlled with electrocautery or topical application of vasoconstrictive agents such as epinephrine, oxymetazoline, or phenylephrine.[3] Of note, phenylephrine may result in pulmonary edema or cardiac depression and should be used very cautiously. The surgeon should communicate with the anesthesiologist regarding any topical medications used during the procedure. Depending on the anesthetic technique selected, it may be necessary to periodically pause and seal the working port to minimize leakage of anesthetic gases into the OR environment and to allow for adequate ventilation. After the procedure is completed, secretions should be thoroughly suctioned to prevent atelectasis.[12] Once the patient has been prepared for postbronchoscopy ventilation, the bronchoscope can be removed under direct vision, if the oxygen saturation is greater than 90%.[3,12] Bronchospasm and temporary hypoxia are not uncommon after the withdrawal of the bronchoscope, and the anesthesiologist must be ready to support ventilation via mask ventilation or endotracheal intubation until spontaneous ventilation resumes.[3,12]

Complications

The complications that may occur during or after rigid bronchoscopy can often be avoided via a thorough preoperative evaluation and proper technique.[3] These include damage to dentition, arytenoid dislocation, respiratory depression, laryngospasm, bronchospasm, subglottic edema, hypoxia, dysrhythmias, mucosal or parenchymal bleeding, perforation, pneumothorax, pneumomediastinum, and death.[3,9,27] In pediatric rigid bronchoscopy reported complication rates range from 1.9% to 4%[27]; in adults rates from 5% to 13.4% have been reported.[28,29] Patients with an increased preoperative risk, neoplastic disease, the presence of a foreign body, or carinal involvement should be monitored closely because these conditions are particularly associated with an increased complication rate in adults.[29] The three risk factors identified by Hoeve and colleagues for an increased complication rate in children are a history of tetralogy of Fallot, need for biopsy or drainage of a lesion during bronchoscopy, and a history of foreign body aspiration.[27]

It is imperative that patients be evaluated preoperatively for poor dentition because loose teeth are at risk for damage or dislodgement during the procedure. If cervical spine disease with a contracted neck is present, rigid bronchoscopy may not be safely performed; a limited range of cervical motion precludes the safe advancement of the scope into the airway, resulting in complications ranging from dental injury to perforation of the posterior pharynx, membranous trachea, or distal airway.[26] Such perforation of the airway may result in pneumomediastinum or pneumothorax but can be avoided by choosing an alternative method for examining the airway (e.g., flexible bronchoscopy) in appropriate patients.[16]

Hemorrhage can occur during bronchoscopy, especially during deep tissue biopsies. It may be controlled by the use of the bronchoscope to apply pressure to the bleeding site, thorough suctioning, local application of epinephrine, or intravenous vasopressin. The patient's greatest danger when this occurs is aspiration rather than hemorrhagic shock.[27]

Bronchospasm and laryngospasm occasionally occur intraoperatively. Their incidence can be reduced by maintaining an adequate depth of anesthesia and via the topical application of a local anesthetic, such as lidocaine. Other agents, including opioids and beta-blockers, can be used to blunt the hemodynamic response to airway stimulation.[16]

Late complications of rigid bronchoscopy include airway edema, pneumothorax, and atelectasis.[12] Laryngeal edema is usually more serious in children, because their airway lumen is smaller and resistance increases exponentially with any airway swelling.[12] This condition can be improved with the administration of humidified oxygen, aerosolized racemic epinephrine, and systemic steroids. If the patient does not respond to medical management, tracheal intubation may be necessary. If severe, potentially obstructive laryngeal edema is identified intraoperatively, consideration should be given to leaving the patient intubated until the edema resolves. Laryngeal edema may be reduced by using premedication with intravenous steroids.[16] Pneumothorax may result from barotrauma in cases of jet ventilation or high ventilation pressures.[10,12]

Rigid bronchoscopy requires excellent communication between the anesthesiologist and the surgeon. Failure to communicate may lead to inadequate control of the airway and can result in hypercarbia, hypoxemia, or death, especially in patients with impending complete airway obstruction.[26] This can be prevented by having all parties involved in the surgery familiarize themselves with the procedure before starting. A contingency plan must be in place in the event the airway is lost. This may entail preparation for tracheostomy or extracorporeal membrane oxygenation in an absolute emergency.

Foreign Body Removal

The removal of aspirated foreign bodies remains one of the primary indications for rigid bronchoscopy, especially in children, in whom the use of flexible bronchoscopy is comparatively risky.

In 2013 the total number of deaths caused by the aspiration or ingestion of foreign objects, including food, totaled 4864.[30] Most deaths resulting from foreign body aspiration occur before hospital arrival.[31] The incidence of foreign body aspiration peaks in older infants and toddlers, with 74% of cases occurring in children 3 years of age or younger.[32] The male-to-female ratio is about 2:1 in children.[32] In adults the peak incidence occurs in the sixth decade of life.[33]

The clinical progression of foreign body aspiration occurs in three stages. The initial stage is usually characterized by a choking episode followed by coughing, gagging, and even obstruction of the airway.[32] In a series of 100 cases published by Barrios and colleagues a history of a choking crisis was the clinical parameter with the highest sensitivity (97%) for foreign body aspiration; it also had a fair specificity (63%).[34] Chest radiographs may appear normal, and symptoms can be minimal even in the presence of an aspirated foreign body.[31,34] In cases of suspected foreign body aspiration rigid bronchoscopy remains the gold standard for both diagnosis and treatment. Whereas atelectasis is more common in adults, air trapping is more common in children.[33] The most common location for the foreign object to be present also differs among adults (right bronchial tree) and pediatric patients (central airway). The second stage is usually asymptomatic, because the initial symptoms frequently resolve because of a fatigued cough reflex.[32] As many as 50% of initial presentations of foreign body aspiration go undiagnosed for longer than 7 days,[29] and this is more likely to occur in adults.[33] The third stage indicates a complication from foreign body aspiration, which can be associated with pneumonia, hemoptysis, bronchiectasis, chronic cough, lung abscess, fever, or malaise.[32]

Radiographic evaluation includes anteroposterior and lateral views of the extended neck and chest. It is imperative that both inspiratory and expiratory views be obtained whenever possible to evaluate for unilateral air trapping.[32] The four main types of obstruction at a bronchial orifice are bypass-valve obstruction, check-valve obstruction, stop-valve obstruction, and ball-valve obstruction.[32] In bypass-valve obstruction the obstruction is incomplete and will result in a normal radiographic evaluation. In check-valve obstruction commonly seen acutely, the foreign body permits airflow into the lung segment but blocks the airflow out of the lung segment. This results in a mediastinal shift away from the obstruction on an expiratory film. Stop-valve obstruction is seen when a foreign body has been present for an extended period; it is characterized by no airflow into, and the subsequent collapse of, the affected lung segment. The rarest type of obstruction, the ball-valve type, permits airflow out of the lung segment but not into it. This phenomenon results in atelectasis and a mediastinal shift toward the obstructed segment on an expiratory film. Other studies (e.g., fluoroscopy or videofluoroscopy) have been used when the diagnosis is uncertain.[31,32]

The management of an aspirated foreign body depends on the clinical picture. If an acute complete obstruction is suspected, rigid bronchoscopy must be performed promptly. More frequently, however, the patient presents in the second or third stage, when there is adequate time to plan a successful and safe bronchoscopy. If possible, the procedure should be scheduled when experienced personnel are available, the instruments have been appropriately selected, and the patient is fasted appropriately to prevent the aspiration of gastric contents.[19,32] Advanced planning for the procedure includes determining the nature of the foreign object to guide the selection of instruments for its retrieval.

Controversy remains regarding the anesthetic approach during bronchoscopy for foreign body aspiration. Those who advocate spontaneous ventilation argue that PPV may precipitate an acute obstruction with clinical deterioration,[18,32] whereas others advocate for controlled ventilation with neuromuscular blockade to prevent the patient from moving and decrease the probability of airway trauma. A retrospective series of 94 cases showed no difference in adverse events with either ventilatory management approach,[18] whereas a prospective study by Chen and colleagues consisting of 384 children found that patients managed with TIVA and spontaneous ventilation had increased intraoperative body movement, longer duration of emergence from anesthesia, a lower percentage of successful foreign body removal, and more postoperative laryngospasm.[35] Chen's study also identified five risk factors for intraoperative hypoxemia ($Spo_2 \leq 90\%$): younger age, plant seed as the type of foreign body, longer operative time, presence of pneumonia before the procedure, and spontaneous ventilation. Manual jet ventilation was found to decrease the risk of intraoperative hypoxemia. The factors associated with postoperative hypoxemia were plant seed as the foreign object and prolonged emergence from anesthesia. Patients with these characteristics should be closely monitored after the procedure.

If the foreign body is small enough, it can be removed through the lumen of the main working port. However, the objects are often larger and must be removed with the bronchoscope as a unit. Once the object is within the forceps, it is dislodged from the airway and the bronchoscope is advanced to cover the foreign object, preventing it from being stripped off the forceps during withdrawal.[32] The removal of the bronchoscope may compromise the airway; thus as mentioned previously, communication during withdrawal is critical. Vegetable foreign bodies should be grasped lightly or retrieved with strong suction to avoid fragmentation of the foreign body into the distal airways.[32] After the removal of the object, bronchoscopy should be repeated to ensure that no residual or additional foreign body remains and to assess the patency of the airway distal to the previous obstruction. Bleeding is usually controlled with thorough suctioning and vasoactive agents. If residual granulation tissue is present and is the source of bleeding or residual obstruction, it may be resected at the repeat bronchoscopy.[32]

Conclusion

Despite the advances that have expanded the applications for flexible bronchoscopy, rigid bronchoscopy remains an essential tool in the surgeon's armamentarium. Rigid bronchoscopy is preferred when the airway is in peril and for procedures in which direct manipulation of the airway is needed. The most common indications are foreign body aspiration and massive hemoptysis, but it is also employed to secure or assess an otherwise unstable airway. The wide lumen of the bronchoscope allows for the instrumentation of the airway, which is required for endoscopic airway procedures, such as biopsies and laser therapy. Typically performed with the patient under general anesthesia, there are many different ventilation techniques that can be safely adopted.

The risk of complications increases significantly with inexperienced personnel, and the American College of Chest Physicians recommends that trainees perform at least 20 procedures under supervision to obtain basic competency and at least 10 procedures per year to maintain competency.[7] The importance of communication between the bronchoscopist and the anesthesiologist cannot be overstated. When applied appropriately, rigid bronchoscopy can be a life-saving intervention in airway management.

Selected References

2. Hass AR, Vachani A, Sterman DH. Advances in diagnostic bronchoscopy. *Am J Respir Crit Care Med.* 2010;182:589–597.
7. Ernst A, Silvestri GA, Johnstone D. Interventional pulmonary procedures: Guidelines from the American College of Chest Physicians. *Chest.* 2003;123:1693–1717.
8. Shepherd RW, Beamis JF. Understanding the basics of rigid bronchoscopy. *J Respir Dis.* 2006;27:100–113.
17. Litman RS, Ponnuri J, Trogan I. Anesthesia for tracheal or bronchial foreign body removal in children: an analysis of ninety-four cases. *Anesth Analg.* 2000;91:1389–1391.
18. Farrell PT. Rigid bronchoscopy for foreign body removal: anaesthesia and ventilation. *Paediatr Anaesth.* 2004;14:84–89.
23. Yoon HI, Kim JH, Lee JH, et al. Comparison of propofol and the combination of propofol and alfentanil during bronchoscopy: a randomized study. *Acta Anaesthesiol Scand.* 2011;55:104–109.
27. Hoeve LJ, Rombout J, Meursing AE. Complications of rigid laryngobronchoscopy in children. *Int J Pediatr Otorhinolaryngol.* 1993;26:47–56.
28. Lukomsky GI, Ovchinnikov AA, Bilal A. Complications of bronchoscopy: comparison of rigid bronchoscopy under general anesthesia and flexible fiberoptic bronchoscopy under topical anesthesia. *Chest.* 1981;79:316–321.

All references can be found online at eBooks.Health.Elsevier.com.

28

Percutaneous Emergency Airway Access

LAURA F. CAVALLONE, DAVIDE CATTANO, AND ALBERTO G.G. PIACENTINI

CHAPTER OUTLINE

KEY POINTS

- Clinicians should quickly recognize severe airway obstruction and hypoxia to allow fast intervention, which should include a rapid progression to emergency invasive airway access as opposed to multiple attempts to intubate the trachea.
- Proper identification of airway anatomy is the first step in successful performance of percutaneous invasive airway techniques and the avoidance of complications.
- The airway practitioner should always consider the danger of piercing the posterior wall of the trachea and midline neck blood vessels during percutaneous invasive airway techniques.
- Cricothyrotomy, whether by surgical or percutaneous technique, is the technique of choice to secure the airway in cannot intubate/cannot oxygenate (CICO) emergencies and in impending airway obstruction.
- Training should be maintained by performing at least one procedure twice each year on live or cadaveric models or specialized manikins.

- Providers may become and remain skilled in accessing the cricothyroid membrane (CTM) by routinely using the transtracheal block to anesthetize the airways in the context of awake and spontaneous breathing flexible intubation scope (FIS)-assisted intubations.
- Translaryngeal insufflation of oxygen requires a high-pressure oxygen source unless catheters greater than 3 mm in inner diameter (ID) are used.
- Ventrain and other similar devices (as they become available) that assist exhalation with active aspiration may be safer to use in situations of complete upper airway obstruction when transtracheal jet ventilation (TTJV) appears to be the only option available. However, more data are needed on the safe use of these devices, which are still not widely available.
- Only commercial-grade devices should be used for these life-saving techniques.

Introduction

Attempts at using a surgical technique to bypass an obstructed upper airway and restore breathing have been described in several ancient cultures since the Egyptian First Dynasty (c. 3200 BCE).[1] In modern times (1546), the Italian physician Antonio Musa Brasavola performed the first recorded tracheostomy on a patient who was dying of suffocation due to a submandibular abscess.[2,3] Over the next two centuries, tracheostomies continued to be performed in similar emergent situations; however, these procedures never gained popularity as they were poorly understood and associated with a low rate of success and a high rate of severe complications. In America, tracheostomies were not introduced until the 19th century.[3] Famously, the first president of the United Sates, George Washington, died on December 14, 1799, of complications of an upper respiratory tract infection; three physicians at his bedside debated whether an emergent tracheotomy could save his life but eventually decided not to perform one as it was deemed too dangerous.[3,4] Throughout the 19th century, these procedures, although seen as "life-saving," continued to be rarely performed with no standardized surgical technique or a clear understanding of the etiology of the most severe complications. In 1909, Dr. Chevalier Jackson, a laryngologist at the Jefferson Medical School in Philadelphia, first described the surgical techniques and critical considerations related to performing "high tracheostomies," or cricothyrotomies, opening the way to a better understanding of the causes of failure and complications of these delicate procedures.

Today, emergency airway access through the cricothyroid membrane (CTM), otherwise referred to as emergent cricothyrotomy, is considered an essential rescue technique in the "cannot intubate/cannot oxygenate" (CICO) situation. Although advancements in modern airway management have made resorting to invasive procedures a rare event, the CICO scenario still occurs.[5] Unfortunately, although cricothyrotomy is considered the rescue technique of choice in perioperative CICO situations, this procedure still carries a high failure rate when performed by anesthesiologists rather than head and neck surgeons. Lack of training or availability of appropriate equipment may be to blame, but more research is needed to better understand and address issues in this area. By equipping the clinician with minimally invasive, effective alternatives to routine upper airway management, the potential for rescuing a failed airway and preventing devastating adverse outcomes is substantially increased.

Adverse outcomes related to respiratory events account for one of the two largest classes of injury in the American Society of Anesthesiologists (ASA) Closed Claims Project. As reported in the 2006 Closed Claims analysis,[6] the two major categories of anesthesia-related events or mechanisms causing death or brain damage between 1975 and 2000 were respiratory and cardiovascular. Between 1986 and 2000, more than 1411 damaging events associated with death and permanent brain damage were reported, of which 503 events (36%) were respiratory in nature. Three mechanisms of injury were responsible for most of the adverse respiratory events: difficult endotracheal tube (ETT) placement (23%), inadequate ventilation (22%), and esophageal intubation (13%).[6] Airway management-related and respiratory events remained the most represented category of complications overall in an analysis of 4549 anesthesia claims from 1990 to 2007 in the same database.[7] In an analysis of claims against the National Health System in England between 1995 and 2007,[8] airway and respiratory claims accounted for 12% of anesthesia-related claims, 53% of deaths, 27% of costs, and 10 of the 50 most expensive claims in the dataset. These claims most frequently described events at induction of anesthesia, involved airway management with an ETT, and typically led to hypoxia with subsequent death or brain injury. Similarly, an analysis of closed civil legal cases between 2007 and 2016 from the Canadian Medical Protective Association involving specialist anesthesiologists found 46 of the 406 (11%) cases to be airway related. In this case series, faulty judgment, inappropriate evaluation of the airway, and lack of proper planning for difficulty were common errors encountered that led to failed airway management and subsequent patient harm, brain injury, or death.[9] Clinicians involved in airway management, and in particular anesthesiologists, must be acutely aware of the dire consequences of failing to plan appropriately and not acquiring or maintaining the necessary skills and equipment to deal with airway emergencies.

In the operating room (OR), intensive care unit (ICU), other hospital areas, and the prehospital setting, three difficult situations can be observed during attempts to control the airway: (1) the airway can be easily controlled by mask ventilation, but tracheal intubation is not possible; (2) the airway cannot be mask ventilated but can be intubated; and (3) rarely, the airway cannot be mask ventilated or intubated (i.e., the CICO scenario). Between 5 and 35 of every 10,000 patients (0.05% to 0.35%) reportedly cannot be tracheally intubated, and approximately 0.01 to 2.0 of every 10,000 patients are difficult to both mask ventilate and intubate.[10,11]

The ASA, Difficult Airway Society, and Advanced Trauma Life Support guidelines, as well as other expert organizations, concur that, although invasive airway access is rarely practiced, any clinician who practices advanced airway management must possess this skill.[5,12,13] The ASA Guidelines for Management of the Difficult Airway provide a difficult airway (DA) algorithm and propose strategies for evaluating, preparing for, and managing a patient with a DA. This algorithm describes emergency and nonemergency pathways for managing the airway if intubation fails and suggests that equipment suitable for "emergency surgical airway access" (i.e., surgical or percutaneous tracheostomy or cricothyrotomy) be among the contents of a readily available portable storage unit for DA management.[12]

Surgical cricothyrotomy has long been a standard of emergency invasive airway rescue; however, its use has declined, in part because of advances in noninvasive airway devices such as supraglottic airways (SGAs) and video laryngoscopes (VLs), the adoption of rapid sequence intubation (RSI) in the emergency department, and increased requirements for trainee supervision.[14] Percutaneous techniques for invasive airway access, the focus of this chapter, increasingly replaced surgical cricothyrotomy for many years; this is likely because many anesthesiologists prefer percutaneous to surgical techniques given the familiarity with similar techniques for other procedures (e.g., central venous catheterization). However, a return to greater use of open surgical techniques has recently been widely advocated, based on a higher success rate,[13,15] particularly after the Fourth National Audit Project of the Royal College of Anaesthetists and the Difficult Airway Society (NAP4) called attention to the high failure rate of percutaneous cricothyrotomies performed by anesthesiologists.[16] Whether the failures described in NAP4 were caused by anesthesiologists' lack of training, the use of inappropriate equipment, equipment design problems, or technical failures needs further study.[16]

Definitions and Classifications

Cricothyrotomy and Percutaneous Dilatational Cricothyrotomy

Cricothyrotomy is a technique for providing an opening in the space between the anterior inferior border of the thyroid cartilage and the anterior superior border of the cricoid cartilage for the purpose of gaining access to the airway. This area is the most accessible part of the respiratory tree below the glottis.[17,18] Based on the urgency of the clinical situation, the procedure can be performed emergently or electively. Emergent cricothyrotomy may be done in the prehospital setting, emergency room, ICU, or OR. Elective cricothyrotomy is usually performed before a surgical procedure in the OR. Depending on the technique used, the procedure may also be classified as surgical or nonsurgical. The nonsurgical approach can be achieved by needle puncture or percutaneously over a guidewire, with or without a CTM incision.[19]

A practical classification of cricothyrotomy techniques includes three categories. The first category includes narrow-bore (≤9-French or 3-mm inner diameter [ID]) cannula-type devices placed directly through the CTM using an over-the-needle

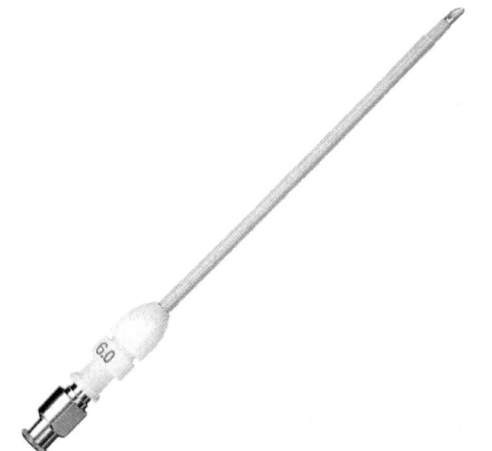

• **Fig. 28.1** Cook Transtracheal Airway Catheter. (Courtesy Cook Medical, Bloomington, IN.)

technique; the cannula is then used for transtracheal catheter ventilation or, more accurately, transcricoid ventilation.[20] The Cook Transtracheal Airway Catheter (Fig. 28.1) and the Ravussin cannula (Fig. 28.2) are examples of these devices. Devices such as the Arndt cricothyrotomy catheter are narrow bore (Fig. 28.3) but are inserted as described for the second category.

The second category includes techniques that require the introduction of a guidewire inserted through a needle or catheter and followed by dilation of the cricothyroid space (i.e., a Seldinger technique). The needle or catheter placement may be preceded by an incision of the skin and of the CTM. An airway catheter is introduced over the dilator threaded over the guidewire. These techniques allow insertion of an airway considerably larger than the initial needle or catheter, often of sufficient ID to allow ventilation with conventional ventilation devices, suctioning, and spontaneous ventilation. These techniques are known as percutaneous dilatational cricothyrotomy (PDC).

The third category is surgical cricothyrotomy, which involves the use of a scalpel and other surgical instruments to create an opening between the skin and the cricothyroid space. It is discussed in Chapter 29.

Transtracheal Jet Ventilation

The term *transtracheal jet ventilation* (TTJV) is used to describe a ventilation technique in which rapid access to the airway at the level of the CTM is followed by jet ventilation through a narrow-bore cannula or catheter. TTJV is primarily used as an emergency technique, but it has also been used electively as a bridge to more secure airway control and in the context of upper airway surgery. A number of different terms and acronyms are used in the literature to describe this same technique. Terms such as *percutaneous* (or simply *trans-*), *laryngeal* (versus *tracheal*), and *insufflation* or *oxygenation* (versus *ventilation*) may all be appropriate.

The Cannot Intubate/Cannot Oxygenate Scenario

A CICO emergency has been defined as the inability to restore alveolar oxygenation by means of any nonsurgical technique (i.e., face mask, ETT, or SGA device).[21] It is a primary responsibility of physicians skilled in advanced airway management to be able

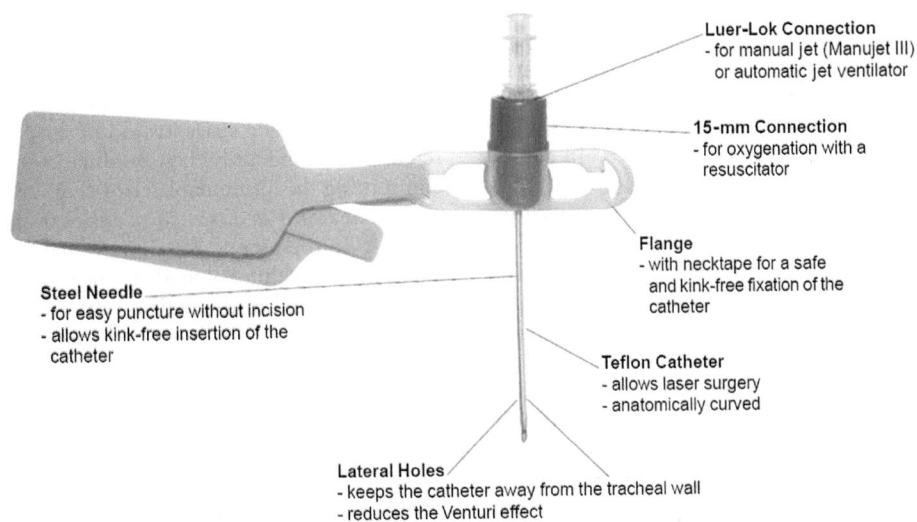

Luer-Lok Connection
- for manual jet (Manujet III) or automatic jet ventilator

15-mm Connection
- for oxygenation with a resuscitator

Flange
- with necktape for a safe and kink-free fixation of the catheter

Steel Needle
- for easy puncture without incision
- allows kink-free insertion of the catheter

Teflon Catheter
- allows laser surgery
- anatomically curved

Lateral Holes
- keeps the catheter away from the tracheal wall
- reduces the Venturi effect

• **Fig. 28.2** Ravussin cannula. (Courtesy VBM Medical, Noblesville, IN.)

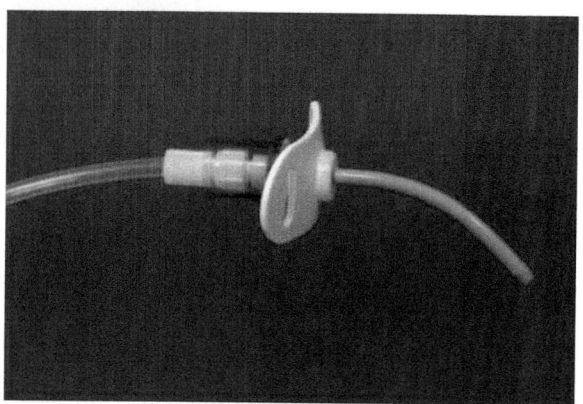

• **Fig. 28.3** Arndt Emergency Cricothyrotomy Catheter. (Courtesy Cook Medical, Bloomington, IN.)

to promptly recognize and manage a CICO scenario by means of an invasive airway access technique. A typical pattern of events and pitfalls has been recognized in the development of CICO, where several attempts to intubate the trachea by multiple providers initially occur in a cannot intubate/*can* oxygenate scenario.[22] This situation deceptively encourages providers to persist with attempts to secure the airway by intubation or SGA positioning until inflammation and edema of the airway lead to obstruction and impossibility to oxygenate.

Following a high-profile case of perioperative death in a CICO scenario that developed in this manner,[23] several national and international airway societies have revised airway management guidelines to emphasize a final common "emergency" pathway that culminates in emergency invasive airway access.[12,13,21] The importance of avoiding delays in addressing the CICO scenario with an emergency invasive airway is also stressed in the Vortex approach. The Vortex approach is a cognitive aid, or high-acuity implementation tool, designed to support teamwork and decision-making during airway emergencies. It is based on the analogy of a funnel, which represents the diminishing time and options available as one spirals deeper into the emergency, after exhausting all viable options (see Chapter 11).[24] Once emergency invasive airway access has been obtained, oxygenation and ventilation through a narrow-bore catheter presents challenges and risks of complications that will be discussed in detail later in this chapter.

Anatomy and Physiology

The safe and rapid performance of cricothyrotomy requires a thorough knowledge of cricothyroid anatomy (Fig. 28.4A) and its relation to other structures in the anterior neck.[18,25–29] In adults, the CTM is approximately 10 mm long and 22 mm wide and is composed mostly of yellow elastic tissue. It covers the cricothyroid space and is located in the anterior neck between the thyroid cartilage superiorly and the cricoid cartilage inferiorly. The cricothyroid space can be readily identified by palpating a slight dip or indentation in the skin immediately below the laryngeal prominence.

The CTM consists of a central anterior triangular portion (the conus elasticus) and two lateral parts. The thicker and stronger conus elasticus narrows above and broadens below, connecting the thyroid to the cricoid cartilage. It lies subcutaneously in the midline and is often crossed horizontally in its upper third by the superior cricothyroid vessels. Characteristically, the CTM does not calcify with age and lies immediately underneath the skin.

Variations in the anatomy and dimensions of the CTM are common. The anterior cricothyroid space is trapezoidal and has a cross-sectional area of approximately 2.9 cm². The mean distance between the anterior borders of the inferior thyroid cartilage and the superior cricoid cartilage is 9 mm (range, 5 to 12 mm), whereas the width of the anterior cricothyroid space ranges from 27 to 32 mm. The cricothyroid space is not much larger than 7 mm in its vertical dimension, and that space may be narrowed further by contraction of the cricothyroid muscle. The vertical distance between the undersurface of the true vocal cords and the lower anterior edge of the thyroid cartilage is between 5 and 11 mm. The vertical height of the CTM from the superior border of the cricoid cartilage to the inferior border of the thyroid cartilage in the midline varies from 8 to 19 mm (mean, 13.69 mm), a somewhat greater distance that can probably be explained by the fresh rather than fixed state of specimens.

The arterial and venous vessel patterns in the neck area surrounding the CTM also vary considerably. Although the arteries always lie deep to the pretracheal fascia and are easily avoided during a skin incision, veins may be found in the pretracheal fascia and between the pretracheal and superficial cervical fascia. Vascular structures may cross vertically and anterior to the CTM, predisposing them to damage during cricothyrotomy. A small cricothyroid artery, which is a branch of the superior thyroid artery, commonly crosses the upper portion of the CTM, anastomosing with the artery on the other side.

To minimize the possibility of bleeding, the CTM should be incised at its inferior third portion. The two lateral parts are thinner, lie close to the laryngeal mucosa, and extend from the superior border of the cricoid cartilage to the inferior margin of the true vocal cords. On either side, the CTM is bordered by the cricothyroid muscle. Lateral to the membrane are venous branches from the inferior thyroid and anterior jugular veins. Because the vocal cords usually lie 1 cm above the cricothyroid space, they are not commonly injured, even during emergency cricothyrotomy.[30] The anterior jugular veins run vertically in the lateral aspect of the neck and are rarely injured, but branches may occasionally course over the cricothyroid space and be damaged during the procedure.

External visible and palpable anatomic landmarks are used to locate the CTM. The laryngeal prominence (i.e., thyroid cartilage or Adam's apple) and the hyoid bone above it are readily palpable. The CTM usually lies 1 to 1.5 fingerbreadths below the laryngeal prominence. The cricoid cartilage is usually felt below the CTM.

The importance of these landmarks is emphasized because of the disastrous consequences of placing a cricothyrotomy tube into the thyrohyoid space instead of the cricothyroid space. Conscious effort to identify these landmarks reduces the possibility of committing this preventable error (Fig. 28.4B and C). When the normal anatomy is distorted, identification of these landmarks is difficult. In these cases, the suprasternal notch may be used as an alternative or additional marker. The small finger of the right hand should be placed in the patient's suprasternal notch, followed by placement of the ring, long, and index fingers adjacent to each other in a stepwise fashion up the neck, with each finger touching the one below it. When the head is in the neutral position, the index finger is usually on or near the CTM.

The use of ultrasonography has been proposed to improve identification of landmarks, as well anatomic variations and vascular structures (see Chapter 3).[31,32] However, in emergencies, its utilization and practical usefulness are debatable, depending on immediate availability and providers' skill.

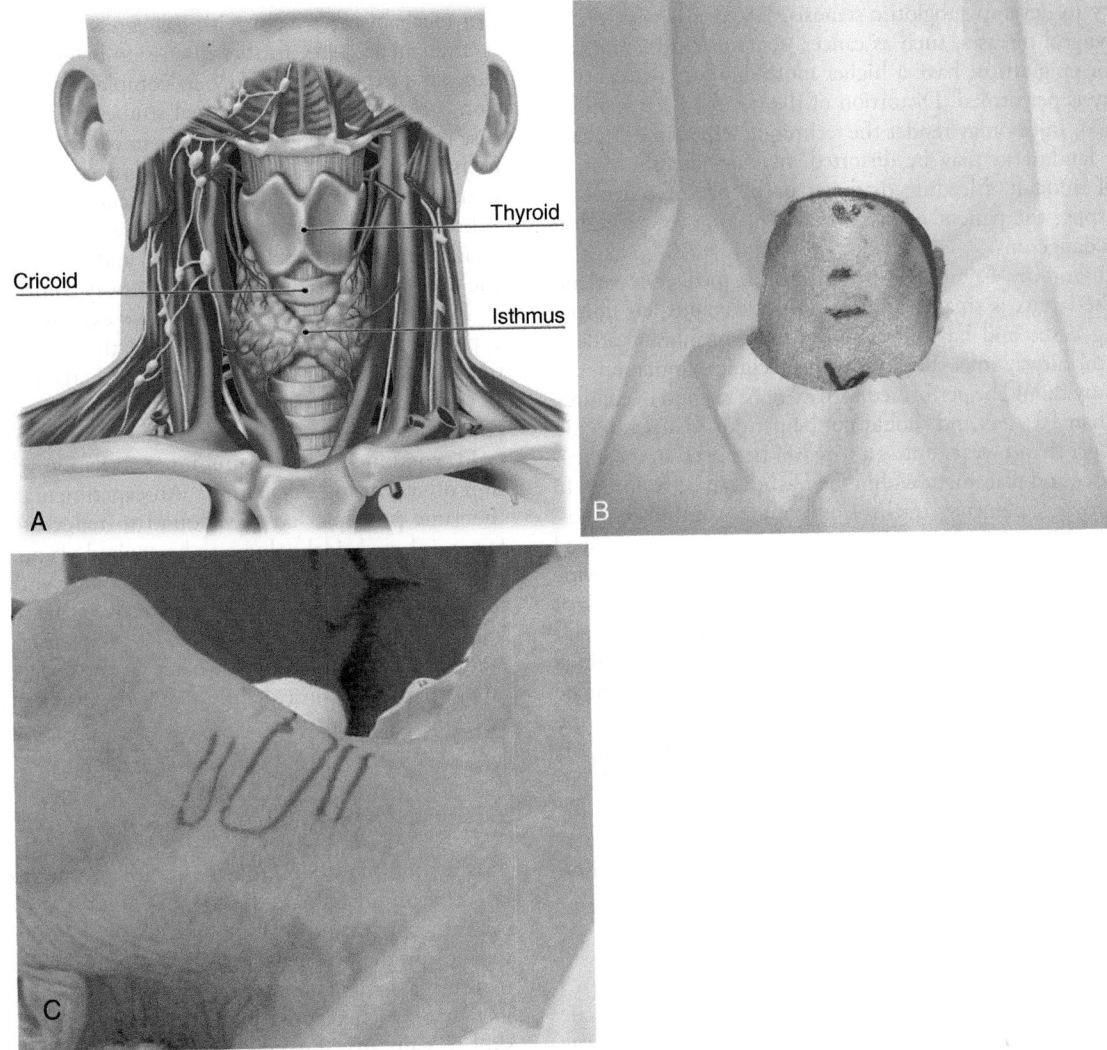

• **Fig. 28.4** (A) Dissection anatomy of the anterior neck. (B) External landmarks. From cephalad to caudad, the thyroid notch, inferior border of the thyroid cartilage, superior border of the cricoid cartilage, and sternal notch are marked. (C) External landmarks. From cephalad to caudad, the hyoid bone, thyroid cartilage, and cricoid cartilage are marked. ([A] From De Leyn P, Bedert L, Delcroix M. Tracheotomy: clinical review and guidelines. *Eur J Cardiothorac Surg.* 2007;32:412–421.)

Indications and Contraindications

Cricothyrotomy

Cricothyrotomy is considered by many to be the standard approach to airway management when orotracheal or nasotracheal intubation approaches have failed and oxygenation and ventilation are not achievable by other means.[10,12] In the emergency room or prehospital setting,[33,34] cricothyrotomy is indicated for immediate airway control in patients with maxillofacial, cervical spine, head, and/or neck trauma and in patients in whom tracheal intubation is impossible to perform or contraindicated. It is also used for the immediate relief of upper airway obstruction. In the OR and in the ICU, the technique is indicated when conventional methods of intubation fail, such as in patients with traumatic facial injuries in whom other techniques of airway access are difficult or impossible to perform. Cricothyrotomy can also be used as an alternative to tracheostomy in patients with recent sternotomy who require invasive airway access because the incision does not communicate with the mediastinal tissue planes. A cricothyrotomy catheter may be fitted with a Luer-Lok connection (for jet ventilation) or with an anesthesia circuit-size (15 mm) connector for thoracic and other procedures involving the airways, especially the trachea, larynx, epiglottis, and base of the tongue.

Emergency cricothyrotomy has largely replaced emergency tracheostomy in the emergency department because of its simplicity, rapidity, and minimal morbidity, whereas debate continues on the value of percutaneous techniques as opposed to surgical approaches.[35,36] The performance of emergency tracheostomy is limited and indicated only when laryngeal trauma may be accompanied by local edema, hemorrhage, subcutaneous emphysema, and damage to the thyroid or cricothyroid cartilage, precluding the performance of a cricothyrotomy.

Absolute and relative contraindications to cricothyrotomy are rare, considering that it is a life-saving, emergency procedure in a CICO scenario. Patients who have been intubated translaryngeally for more than 3 days (or 7 days or longer, according to different investigators) should not undergo cricothyrotomy because of the propensity to develop subglottic stenosis.[104-106] Those with preexisting laryngeal diseases, such as cancer, acute or chronic inflammation, or epiglottitis, have a higher morbidity rate when cricothyrotomy is performed. Distortion of the normal neck anatomy by disease or injury may render the technique impossible. Normal anatomic landmarks may be distorted, making identification of the CTM difficult. Bleeding diatheses or history of coagulopathy predispose the patient to hemorrhage, making the procedure extremely dangerous.

Cricothyrotomy is difficult to perform in pediatric patients because the larynx is smaller and the airway contains less fibrous supporting tissue and has only loose mucous membrane attachments in the airway inlet. Because of this technical limitation, cricothyrotomy should be performed with extreme caution in children younger than 10 years and should not be performed at all in children younger than 6 years unless a wire can be placed in the cricothyroid space and placement within the trachea can be verified.[37] In this age group, emergency tracheostomy under controlled conditions is the preferred choice.[38] Johansen and colleagues described an exceedingly high failure rate (83%) in an experimental swine model of the juvenile population, likely attributable to the lack of circumferential support offered by the immature cricoid cartilage.[39]

Physicians who are unfamiliar or inexperienced with the technique are discouraged from performing the procedure without adequate supervision from a more senior or knowledgeable member of the medical team. Inexperience has been implicated as the most important factor contributing to cricothyrotomy complications.[40] Accuracy in identifying anatomic landmarks significantly depends on the physician's experience but is poor overall, justifying the percutaneous technique in emergency conditions but supporting the use of ultrasound or video-enhanced visualization during elective procedures.

Transtracheal Jet Ventilation

The most common indications for performing TTJV are rescue oxygenation in a CICO situation (emergent indication), airway rescue in complete upper airway obstruction (emergent indication), supplemental oxygenation during difficult tracheal intubation (elective indication), and ventilation during upper airway surgery (elective indication). Here, we will briefly discuss the emergent indications of TTJV use.

Rescue Oxygenation in a CICO Scenario

The primary indication for TTJV through a narrow-bore cannula is rescue oxygenation in an emergent CICO scenario. However, in a CICO scenario complicated by upper airway obstruction, TTJV may have relative or absolute contraindications, depending on the location and degree of obstruction. Barotrauma as a result of air trapping is the major risk associated with the use of TTJV and manifests when the gas that is insufflated at high pressure does not have a path for egress due to an obstructed upper airway. A recent systematic review of the use of TTJV in CICO emergencies concluded that TTJV in this scenario is associated with a high risk of device failure and barotrauma, suggesting that support for the use of this technique in the CICO emergency should be reconsidered.[15]

Airway Rescue in Complete Upper Airway Obstruction

TTJV in the setting of complete airway obstruction can lead to a dramatic increase in intrathoracic pressure, resulting in barotrauma and hemodynamic collapse. Because of these potentially fatal complications, TTJV is considered contraindicated in this setting, although it may be appropriate as a temporary last resort measure

if a mechanism to assist with gas egress in the exhalation phase is implemented (see further discussion below). Data are sparse in support of the use of TTJV in complete upper airway obstruction, primarily based on animal studies,[41-43] lung models,[44-45] or case reports of emergent situations in which the technique proved useful despite significant safety concerns for the high risk of barotrauma.[46] Low-flow translaryngeal rescue insufflation of oxygen of as little as 2 L per minute has been shown to maintain oxygenation in a large animal model (34-kg pigs) and may be a short-term rescue option when definitive surgical airway control is anticipated.[41]

Recently, the concept of an active expiratory phase has been applied to TTJV by introduction of the Ventrain system (Ventinova Medical B.V., Eindhoven, Netherlands), a rescue oxygenation device with expiratory assistance based on the Venturi effect.[47] Expiratory ventilation assistance devices, such as the Ventrain, combine high-pressure lung ventilation with active aspiration of gas during exhalation.[48] An experimental device based on the same principle has been found to reduce the time required for an injected tidal volume to be expired via a narrow-bore cannula and also increase the effective minute ventilation.[44] Expiratory ventilation assistance is less effective when the upper airway is unobstructed, possibly because of preferential entrainment of ambient air into the TTJV catheter via the lower-resistance upper airway path and, consequently, reduced removal of alveolar gases.[49]

Percutaneous Dilatational Cricothyrotomy

Principles and Planning

This section focuses on techniques for percutaneous dilatational cricothyrotomy (PDC), which is fast and usually easy to perform, even on patients with short necks or with spinal injury. Cricothyrotomy may be performed for elective airway management in trauma patients with technically challenging neck anatomy in lieu of tracheostomy because it does not require a surgeon's skill to gain airway access and has fewer operative and postoperative complications.[50-52] Several commercially available devices use this technology. These devices have in common the insertion of an airway catheter over a dilator, which is usually introduced over a guidewire. The guidewire is inserted through a needle or over-the-needle catheter (i.e., Seldinger technique) after making an initial skin incision. This technique, often used for the insertion of catheter-introducer sheaths and central lines, is familiar to anesthesiologists. An airway over a dilator and guidewire is preferable because of the inherent safety of this technique and the ability to insert an airway of far greater diameter than the initial catheter.

Some devices allow insertion of the dilator directly over a needle or directly into a skin incision (e.g., the QuickTrach [VBM Medical, Noblesville, IN] or the PCK Portex Cricothyrotomy Kit [Smiths Medical, Minneapolis, MN]). Although they lack the step of introducing a guidewire, they are included in this discussion because they require a skin incision and a dilator for insertion of the airway. These devices are technically faster to use in theory but overall are less safe, carrying a higher complication rate (e.g., multiple attempts, inability to advance the cannula, false passage) than the Seldinger technique.

The guidewire technique seems to offer several advantages over direct dilatational or over-the-needle techniques that, although they may be faster to perform, have a greater reported rate of difficulties and complications. Complications have included failure to gain airway access, multiple attempts at cannulation, mediastinal injury, esophageal injury, pneumothorax, and severe bleeding. The wire-guided technique, on the other hand, has the disadvantage of potential wire kinking. Several animal and cadaver-based studies have compared the safety and efficacy of the percutaneous over-the-needle and wire-guided techniques.[53–58] yet randomized, controlled clinical studies are lacking. An over-the-needle, wire-guided dilation technique may be adaptable to various practitioners (with different training time and specialties) and could still be relatively quick to perform. Over-the-needle techniques that do not use a guidewire, may be justified in emergency situations and remote locations where the availability of the system or the need to treat a severely damaged airway outweighs the potential complications. On the other hand, use of these systems in less emergent situations may be questionable, especially by first-time users.

In the past few years, many changes in airway management have occurred as a result of better airway equipment availability and implementation of airway protocols. Cricothyrotomy is rare, even in emergency airway conditions, if an airway protocol is used (assuming no major neck trauma).[59,60] However, a careful reading of the literature shows a significant number of complications that may indicate an underuse of invasive techniques and argue for their earlier use, depending on the level of training, the setting, and clinical conditions. Appropriate training is fundamental to maintain proficiency in the technical skills required to perform these invasive procedures safely, rapidly, and effectively.

Insertion Techniques

Skin Incision Before Needle Insertion

When performing a wire-guided PDC technique, for two reasons it is not usually recommended to make an incision before introducing the catheter. First, the catheter is more likely to kink when the needle is removed, making it difficult to pass the guidewire. Second, there have been reports of an inability to advance the dilator because the skin incision was not next to the guidewire; extending the incision to the guidewire will solve the problem. Anesthesiologists and critical care physicians usually make a skin incision after wire introduction. In that case, a firm incision into the CTM next to the wire, which is carefully done to avoid cutting the wire, is recommended. Predilating the incision before inserting the airway cannula can help with placement, reducing the likelihood of the cannula impinging on tissue (i.e., the gap between the airway cannula and dilator).

Vertical Versus Horizontal Incision

It is unclear whether a horizontal or vertical skin incision is superior. The literature is evenly divided on this matter but usually refers to surgical cricothyrotomy. It can be argued that a vertical incision is better during emergency cricothyrotomy because it can be extended superiorly or inferiorly if the relationship between the skin and CTM changes (as frequently happens). A horizontal stab through the CTM in the inferior third is recommended to ease placement of the dilator and avoid the cricothyroid arteries, which often anastomose in the midline superiorly.

Over-the-Needle Catheter Versus Introducer Needle

Inserting the guidewire through a needle versus an over-the-needle catheter tends to be superior when a skin incision is not used, but the two techniques have a similar success rate if an incision is used initially. It appears that catheters tend to kink when attempts are made to pass the entire length of the catheter into the airway.

Specific Cricothyrotomy Sets

Melker Emergency Cricothyrotomy Catheter Set

The Melker emergency cricothyrotomy catheter set (Cook Critical Care, Bloomington, IN) uses a skin incision followed by insertion of a guidewire and insertion of a dilator and airway catheter (i.e., cricothyrotomy tube). The Melker set is available in 3.5-, 4.0-, and 6.0-mm-ID uncuffed airway catheter sizes with lengths of 3.8, 4.2, and 7.5 cm, respectively, and in a 5-mm-ID cuffed airway catheter that is 9 cm in length. The kit contains a scalpel blade, a syringe with an 18-G over-the-needle catheter and/or a thin-walled introducer needle, a guidewire, a dilator of appropriate length and diameter, and a polyvinyl airway catheter with or without a cuff (Fig. 28.5). A universal kit combines open cricothyrotomy and percutaneous tools in a single tray. Detailed insertion instructions for this type of device are available from the manufacturer's website and brochure. A description of the Melker insertion technique (Fig. 28.6) follows (always refer to manufacturer instructions for proper use):

1. Position the patient supine and, if there is no contraindication, slightly extend the neck by using a roll under the neck or shoulders. If cervical spine injury is suspected, properly immobilize the head and neck and maintain a neutral neck position.
2. Open the prepackaged cricothyrotomy set, and assemble the components. Whenever possible, use aseptic technique and local anesthetic.
3. Identify the CTM between the cricoid and thyroid cartilages by palpation, as described above, or by ultrasonography (USG) if the equipment and an experienced provider are available.
4. Carefully palpate the CTM and, while stabilizing the cartilage, make a vertical or horizontal skin incision using the scalpel blade. Make a stab incision (vertical or horizontal) through the lower third of the CTM. An adequate incision eases introduction of the dilator and airway. The incision can follow the placement of the guidewire (see later discussion).
5. Attach the supplied syringe to the 18-G introducer needle-plastic catheter (over-the-needle technique) system, or, alternatively, attach the syringe to the introducer needle only (having removed the plastic catheter). Insert the syringe needle-catheter or syringe-needle assembly, and advance it through the incision into the airway at a 45-degree angle to the frontal plane in the midline in a caudal direction. When advancing the needle forward, entrance into the airway can be confirmed by aspiration with the syringe, resulting in free air return or air bubbles in a saline-filled syringe.
6. Remove the syringe and needle, leaving the plastic catheter or introducer needle in place. Do not attempt to advance the plastic catheter completely into the airway, which may result in kinking of the catheter and an inability to pass the guidewire. Advance the soft, flexible end of the guidewire through the catheter or needle several centimeters into the airway.
7. Remove the plastic catheter or needle, leaving the guidewire in place. Make a skin incision if not done previously.
8. Advance the handled dilator inside the airway catheter, tapered end first, into the connector end of the airway catheter until the handle stops against the connector. Use of lubrication on the surface of the dilator may enhance the fit and placement of the emergency airway catheter.
9. Advance the emergency airway access assembly over the guidewire until the proximal stiff end of the guidewire is completely through and visible at the handle end of the dilator. Always visualize the proximal end of the guidewire during the airway

insertion procedure to prevent its inadvertent loss into the trachea. Maintaining the guidewire position, advance the emergency airway access assembly over the guidewire with an in-and-out motion.

10. As the airway catheter is fully advanced into the trachea, remove the guidewire and dilator simultaneously.

11. If a cuffed tube is inserted, inflate it with 10 mL of air with the syringe provided.

12. Fix the emergency airway catheter in place with the cloth tracheostomy tape strip in a standard fashion.

13. Using its standard 15- to 22-mm adapter, connect the emergency airway catheter to an appropriate ventilatory device.

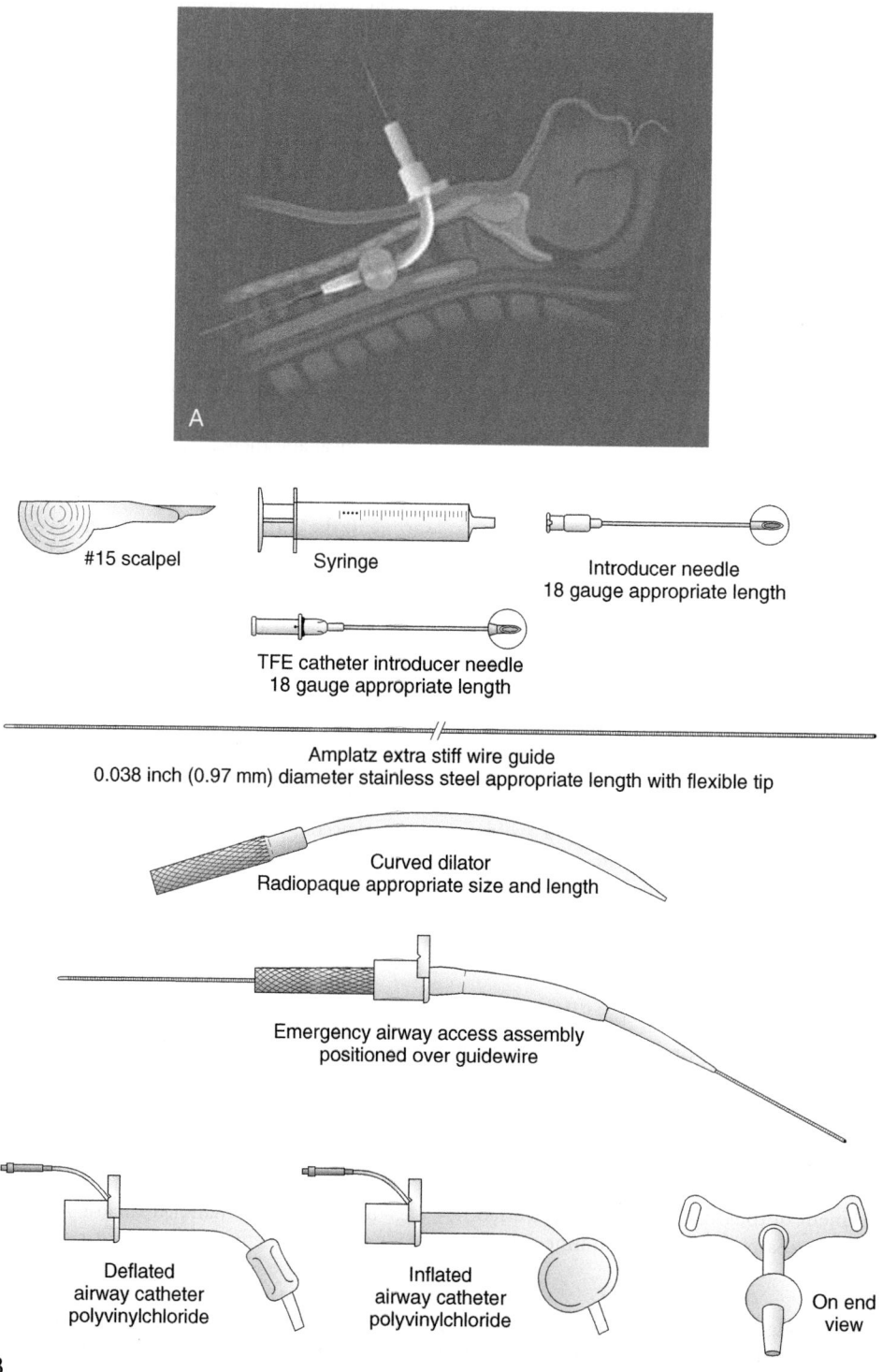

• **Fig. 28.5** (A) Melker cuffed cannula inserted in a model. (B) Melker cricothyrotomy kit contents. (Courtesy Cook Medical, Bloomington, IN.)

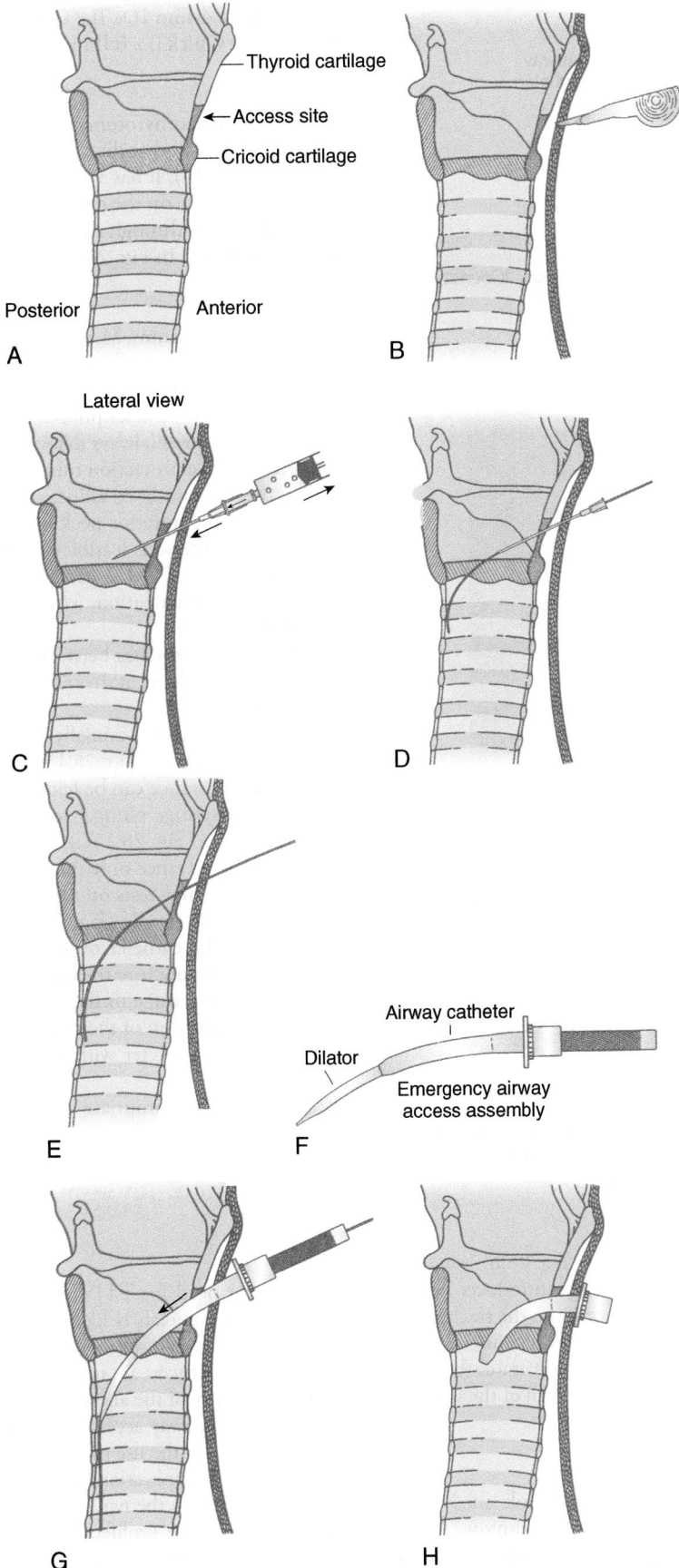

Lateral view

Thyroid cartilage

Access site

Cricoid cartilage

Posterior   Anterior

A

B

C

D

Airway catheter

Dilator

Emergency airway
access assembly

E

F

G

H

• **Fig. 28.6** (A–H) Melker insertion technique. See text for details. (From Melker emergency cricothyrotomy sets: suggested instructions for placement, instruction pamphlet. Cook Critical Care, Bloomington, IN.)

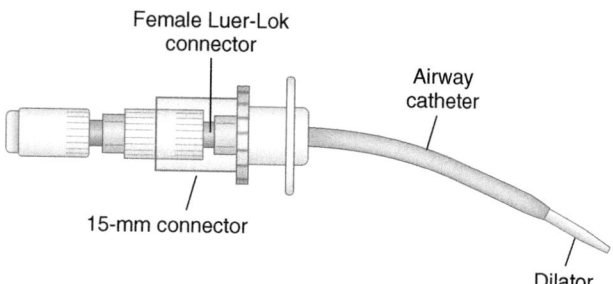

• **Fig. 28.7** Arndt cricothyrotomy cannula schematic. (Courtesy Cook Medical, Bloomington, IN.)

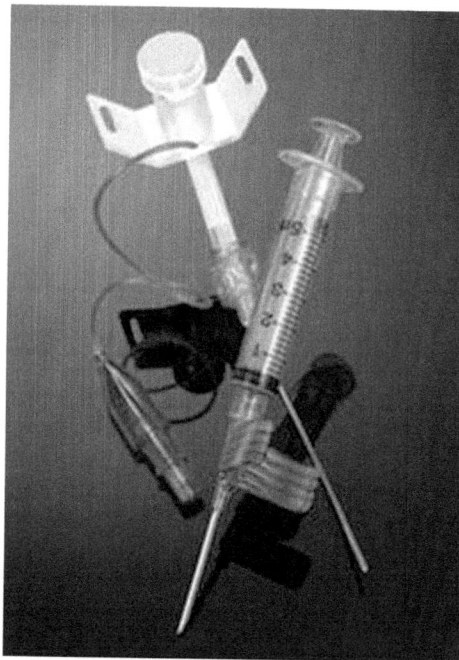

• **Fig. 28.8** Pertrach cannula with splitting introducer needle. (Courtesy Pulmodyne, Indianapolis, IN.)

Arndt Emergency Cricothyrotomy Catheter Set

The Arndt cricothyrotomy catheter (Cook Medical, Bloomington, IN) is technically a percutaneous dilatational wire-guided cannula designed for TTJV (Fig. 28.7; see also Fig. 28.3).

Pertrach Emergency Cricothyrotomy kit

The Pertrach (Pulmodyne, Indianapolis, IN; Fig. 28.8) is a direct dilatational device that uses a special splitting introducer needle. After the distal end of the dilator is advanced into the trachea, the introducer needle is split and removed (Fig. 28.9). A useful training video available from the manufacturer demonstrates the insertion technique and clearly explains the mechanism of the splitting introducer needle.[61]

Rüsch QuickTrach

The Rüsch QuickTrach (VBM Medizintechnik, Sulz am Necker, Germany) offers a single-step, over-the-needle technique that is preceded by a skin incision. A removable stopper is used to prevent too deep an insertion and to avoid the possibility of perforating the posterior tracheal wall. A conical needle tip allows for the smallest necessary stoma and reduces the risk for bleeding. The adult version has a 4-mm ID. The QuickTrach I is cuffless (Fig. 28.10), whereas the QuickTrach II has a cuff over the cannula (Fig. 28.11).

Portex Cricothyroidotomy Kit

The Portex Cricothyrotomy Kit (PCK; Smiths Medical, Minneapolis, MN) is another directly dilating, over-the-needle device for PDC (Fig. 28.12). It has a Veress needle system, which is designed to detect pressure on the posterior wall of the trachea. The PCK is inserted directly through the CTM after a skin incision; insertion details are shown in Fig. 28.13.

Cricath

The Cricath (Ventinova Medical B.V., Eindhoven, Netherlands) is a minimally invasive, small-bore, cannula-over-needle system for percutaneous cricothyrotomy (Fig. 28.14). It has an ID of 2 mm and a length of 7 cm. A description of the Cricath insertion technique (Fig. 28.15) follows (always follow manufacturer instructions):

1. Remove the protection tube from the catheter, fill the syringe with sterile water or saline, and attach it to the catheter.
2. Prepare the anterior neck of the patient (aseptic technique, local anesthetic as feasible and necessary).
3. Identify the CTM, located between the cricoid and thyroid cartilage by palpation, as described above (Fig. 28.15A, see also Fig. 28.4.)
4. Stabilize the trachea between thumb and index finger.
5. Hold the catheter at the transparent needle hub or water-filled syringe.
6. Insert the catheter caudally by puncturing the CTM with the tip of the needle (Fig. 28.15B). When entering the trachea, a loss of resistance can be felt.
7. Pull the syringe plunger to confirm the catheter position in the trachea (Fig. 28.15C). Air should be aspirated.
8. Carefully advance only the catheter into the trachea caudally until the flange rests on the neck (Fig. 28.15D).
9. Remove the needle (Fig. 28.15E). Do not reinsert the needle into the catheter once the needle is withdrawn. It may damage or puncture the catheter wall.
10. Attach the syringe to the catheter and aspirate again to confirm the position of the catheter.
11. Secure the catheter with the supplied strap or other means (Fig. 28.15F).
12. Connect an appropriate ventilation device (e.g., Ventrain) to the catheter (Fig. 28.15G).

Transtracheal Jet Ventilation

Principles and Planning

An emergent need for TTJV may be anticipated, but it is rarely expected. No clinician is likely to induce anesthesia when complete loss of airway control is the outcome. However, although most patients' airways are managed without critical incident, it is the responsibility of the anesthesiologist to plan for the scenario in which invasive airway access becomes necessary.

Preparation for the use of TTJV may be the single most important aspect of its application; willingness to use it is the next. Most anesthesiologists, by the nature of their training, prefer noninvasive methods. Given the proliferation of SGAs and advanced tracheal intubation techniques during the past 30 years, it is not surprising that surgical and percutaneous airway rescue procedures, even when performed properly, are often applied too late in the lost airway scenario to effect a change in outcome and prevent death or brain

Procedural sequence

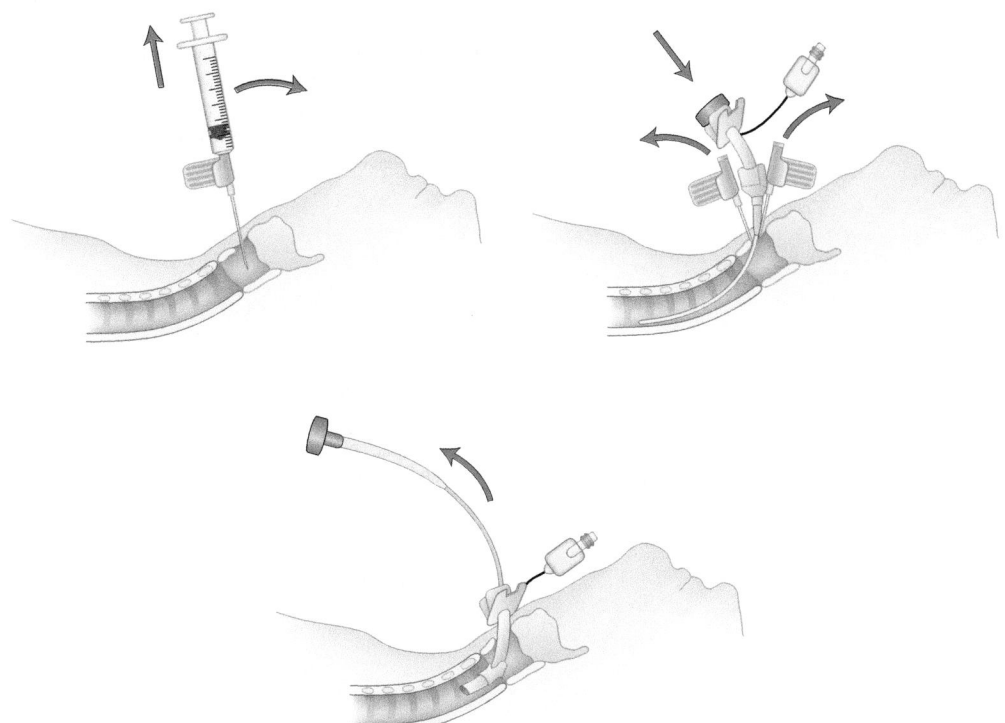

• **Fig. 28.9** Pertrach cannula insertion technique.

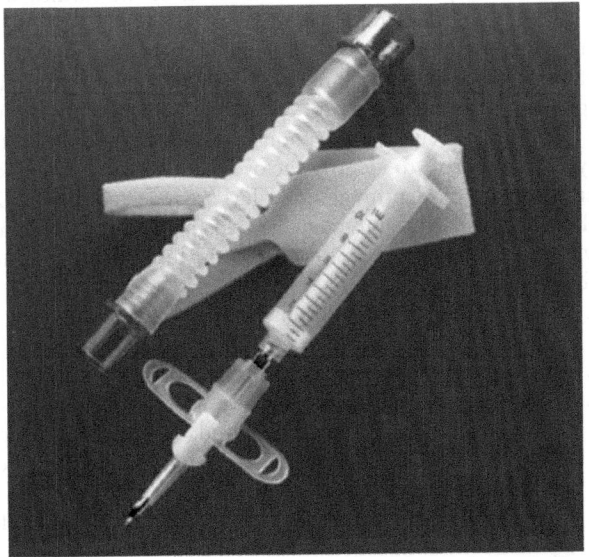

• **Fig. 28.10** QuickTrach I cricothyrotomy set. (Courtesy Teleflex Medical, Research Triangle Park, NC.)

death.[21,22,62] Obstinate persistence with laryngoscopy and unsuccessful SGA ventilation must be avoided; evidence attests that this is not only futile but also contributes to worsened outcomes.[21,22,62]

Equipment

Historically, a variety of catheter-over-needle devices have been employed for TTJV.[63–65] The literature on TTJV techniques covers a number of commercial and OR-rigged devices.[66–70] Although

OR-rigged setups may resemble working systems, performance in a true clinical emergency is unknown.[71] The great advantage of using a preassembled, commercially made TTJV system is the quality assurance associated with a commercial product.

The size of the TTJV cannula is important for the success of oxygenation. Cannulas smaller than 3-mm ID (8 G) are unreliable for oxygenation and ventilation unless high-pressure regulator systems are used and there is egress for exhaled gas; catheters smaller than 14 G are unreliable even with the use of high-flow regulators. The ideal characteristics of a TTJV system are listed in Box 28.1.

Several cannulas are commercially available for TTJV. The Cook emergency transtracheal airway catheter (Cook Critical Care,

---

• **BOX 28.1** **Characteristics of an Ideal Transtracheal Jet Ventilation Device**

- Validated in clinical or laboratory studies
- Minimum cannula size: 14 G
- Low-compliance tubing, fixed component joints
- Ability to connect to a high-pressure (50 psi) oxygen source
- Ability to connect to anesthesia circuit or self-inflating bag (if ≥3 mm ID)
- Kink resistant
- Intratracheal pressure measurable
- EtCO$_2$ measurable
- Flow controllable
- Pressure regulation provided
- Available preassembled
- Available sterile

EtCO$_2$, End-tidal carbon dioxide concentration; *ID*, internal diameter.

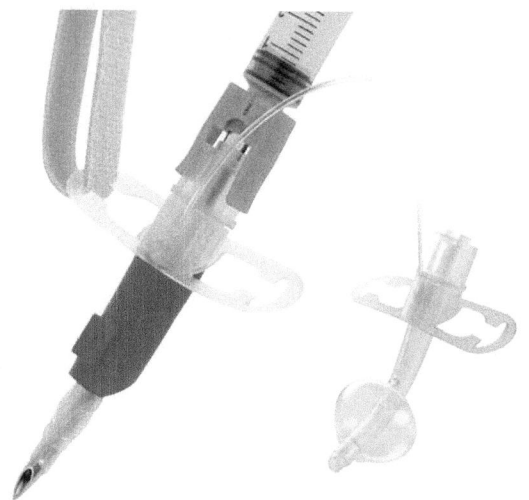

• **Fig. 28.11** QuickTrach II cricothyrotomy set. (Courtesy VBM Medical, Noblesville, IN.)

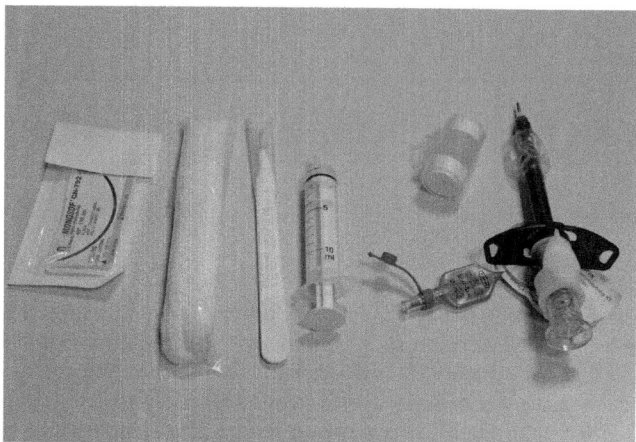

• **Fig. 28.12** Portex cricothyroidotomy kit. (Courtesy Smiths Medical, Minneapolis, MN.)

Bloomington, IN) is a 6-French, 5- or 7.5-cm, wire-reinforced, kink-resistant cannula. The proximal end has a female Luer-Lok–type adapter (see Fig. 28.1). The Ravussin jet cannula (VBM Medizintechnik, Sulz am Necker, Germany), available in 13-G or 14-G sizes, has rings for securing the cannula to the patient, both Luer-Lok and 15-mm proximal adapters, and a preformed curve (see Fig. 28.2). The Arndt emergency cricothyrotomy catheter (Cook Critical Care, Bloomington, IN) is a precurved, 9-French, 6-cm-long cannula made of a kink-resistant material; unlike the other catheters, it is inserted with the use of an over-the-wire Seldinger technique (see Fig. 28.3).

Insertion Techniques

The CTM is the established access point for insertion of a cannula-over-needle for TTJV because of several advantages. The cricoid is the only completely circumferential cartilage in the airway. The mature cricoid cartilage lends rigidity to the larynx, making it resilient to the anteroposterior pressure of an inserted cannula-over-needle, resulting in a reduced risk of trauma.[57] The posterior wall of the cricoid cartilage extends inferiorly from below the level of the CTM; this provides a solid backstop for the placement of a TTJV cannula, reducing the chance of injury to the posterior trachea and esophagus.

- 1 operator's fingerbreadth below thyroid notch (adult)
- 1 patient's fingerbreadth below thyroid notch
- Second skin crease lies over cricoid cartilage
- 4 operator's fingerbreadths above sternal notch (adult)
- 2 cm below thyroid notch (adult)

- Personal protective equipment
- Skin marking pen
- Antiseptic solution, sterile drapes
- Needle cricothyrotomy catheter
- Luer-Lok syringe (5–10 mL)
- Scalpel for small vertical skin incision
- Saline
- Local anesthetic with epinephrine 1:200,000
- Fine-gauge needle (22 G to 25 G)

Several reports have described intentional and unintentional placement of a TTJV cannula at the level of the trachea when the CTM was difficult to identify. Salah and colleagues, in a swine cadaveric airway study, noted increased trauma to the tracheal anatomy with some, but not all, percutaneous techniques, emphasizing the preference for CTM access.[72] Identification of the CTM among clinicians is poor, with one study showing that only 30% were able to identify the overlying surface landmarks.[27] Many methods of identifying the CTM are reported (Box 28.2).

Box 28.3 lists the equipment needed for insertion of a translaryngeal cannula for TTJV. The standard insertion technique is as follows:

1. Position: A right-hand-dominant operator stands on the patient's left side.
2. Antiseptic solution should be applied if time permits.
3. The translaryngeal cannula-over-needle is readied with a 5- to 10-mL syringe, with or without fluid. Note that, if not pre-shaped by the manufacturer, a small-angle bend (15 degrees) can be made 2.5 cm from the distal end.[73]
4. The CTM is palpated with the neck of the patient extended, unless a contraindication to cervical extension exists.
5. Local anesthetic with epinephrine can be injected into the skin to reduce bleeding if time permits.
6. The skin is punctured in the midline over the lower third of the surface landmarks of the CTM.
7. Initially, the axis of the cannula-over-needle is oriented at a 90-degree angle to the imagined location of the cervical spine.
8. As downward pressure is exerted, constant negative pressure is applied to the syringe plunger. Large-bore needles can be difficult to pass through the skin; a small vertical incision through the skin can be made with a scalpel blade to facilitate passage.
9. Entrance into the larynx is signaled by air aspiration. A 13-G or 14-G needle entering the airway will allow for the effortless aspiration of air.

10. The syringe is oriented 30 degrees cephalad, and the cannula is advanced off the needle and into the airway.
11. When the hub of the cannula reaches the skin and the needle has been fully removed and safely discarded, air should once again be aspirated from the in situ cannula to confirm the intratracheal location.
12. The transtracheal cannula should be manually held in place until a definitive airway is established.

Transtracheal Jet Ventilation Techniques and the Ventrain System

Transtracheal ventilation through a narrow-bore catheter (as small as 2 mm ID) can be provided with different techniques, all of which must be utilized with some caveats and are at high risk of significant complications. Conventional TTJV has been administered with manual injectors (manual jet ventilation technique) or via

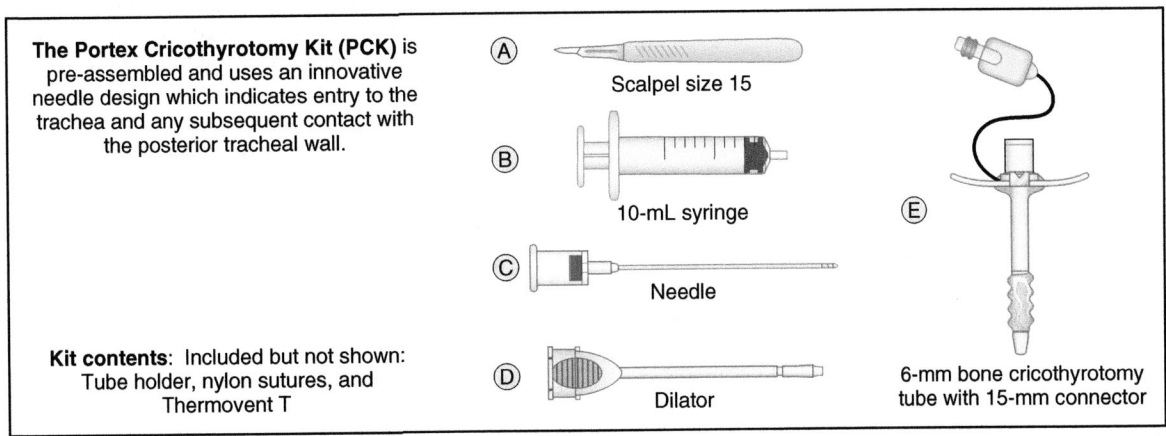

The Portex Cricothyrotomy Kit (PCK) is pre-assembled and uses an innovative needle design which indicates entry to the trachea and any subsequent contact with the posterior tracheal wall.

Ⓐ Scalpel size 15

Ⓑ 10-mL syringe

Ⓒ Needle

Ⓓ Dilator

Ⓔ 6-mm bone cricothyrotomy tube with 15-mm connector

Kit contents: Included but not shown: Tube holder, nylon sutures, and Thermovent T

Portex® PCK

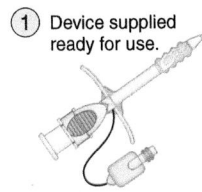

① Device supplied ready for use.

② Stabilize the trachea between thumb and forefinger and locate the cricothyroid membrane between the thyroid and cricoid cartilage.

- Thyroid cartilage
- Cricothyroid membrane
- Cricoid cartilage
- Cricotracheal ligament
- Tracheal cartilage
- Sternal notch

③ Make a 2-cm-long horizontal skin incision with scalpel through the skin only. An adequate length of incision eases introduction of device. Confirm correct location of cricothyroid membrane before progressing further.

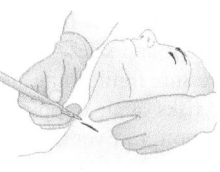

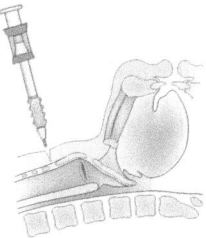

④ Position the needle tip above cricothyroid membrane, perpendicular to the skin.

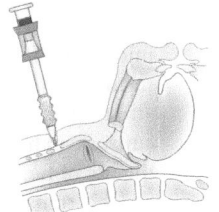

⑤ Insert the device while constantly observing the red indicator flag in the needle hub. This indicates contact of the needle tip with tissue.

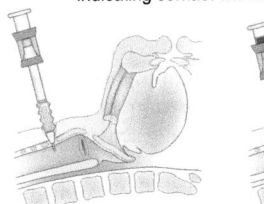

⑥⑦ Advance the device until the red indicator flag in the needle hub disappears, confirming entry into the trachea. Carefully continue insertion until the red indicator is seen again, indicating contact with the posterior cartilage.

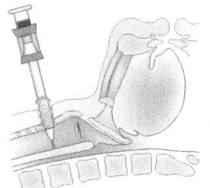

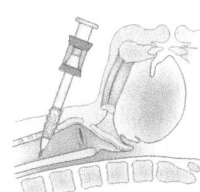

⑧ Angle the device caudally and advance it 1-2 cm into the trachea. Remove needle.

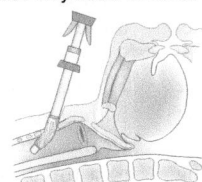

⑨ While holding the dilator stationary, slide cricothyrotomy tube off dilator fully into the trachea. Slight twisting of the dilator within the tube may assist removal.

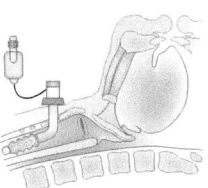

⑩ Once tube has been fully inserted, remove the dilator completely to establish an airway.

• **Fig. 28.13** Portex cricothyroidotomy kit insertion technique. (Modified from Smiths Medical, Minneapolis, MN.)

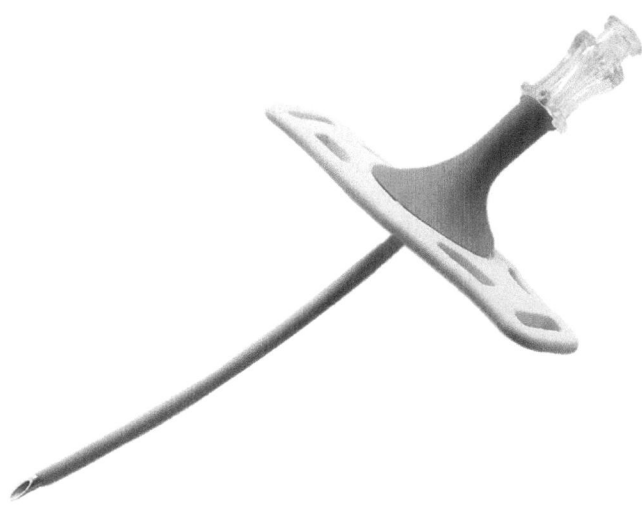

• **Fig. 28.14** Cricath adult percutaneous cricothyrotomy cannula. (Courtesy Ventinova Medical, Eindhoven, Netherlands.)

automatic jet ventilators (automatic jet ventilation), using a driving pressure between 20 and 50 psi. Both manual and automatic jet ventilation may be administered at high and low frequency, typically with small tidal volumes (1 to 3 mL/kg) in the high-frequency jet ventilation (HFJV) mode, and with varying ratios of inspiratory and expiratory times, to allow for appropriate passive gas exhalation from the lungs. However, in the presence of a narrow-bore catheter and complete airway obstruction, the risk of barotrauma with these techniques remains high. Automatic jet ventilators are equipped with alarms and safety mechanisms that prevent insufflation above a set pressure limit in the airway; these safety features, while reducing the risks of air trapping and barotrauma, can impede effective oxygenation and ventilation. More recently, the Ventrain system, which provides flow-controlled ventilation (FCV) has become available (Fig. 28.16). This system creates a continuous flow of gas in and out of the lungs and applies the Venturi effect to support active exhalation, thus reducing the risk of barotrauma while providing high-pressure ventilation. The Venturi effect is an application of the Bernoulli principle, which states that an increase in the speed of a fluid (a gas in this case) leads to a decrease in pressure. In the Venturi application, the gas passing through a narrowing in a tube increases its speed, creating a decrease in pressure. In the Ventrain system, this negative (subatmospheric) pressure created in a narrow passage in the system is used to suction air out of the airway during the expiratory phase, creating actively assisted exhalation, as opposed to passive exhalation (Fig. 28.17).[74]

In a pig model, Ventrain has been shown to be safer and more effective than manual jet ventilation in providing transtracheal ventilation and oxygenation through a small-bore (2 mm ID) catheter in open, partially obstructed, as well as completely obstructed, upper airways.[47] These encouraging findings, however, should not falsely reassure clinicians that the use of narrow-bore catheters to provide transtracheal oxygenation and ventilation, while an important last resort remedy in selected emergency scenarios, is a foolproof technique in any circumstance.[75] Also of note, the Ventrain system does not have a pressure-release valve and is currently not equipped with any alarm; therefore, as for jet ventilation techniques, the primary safety mechanism during ventilation with this device is observation of rising of the chest during inspiration and falling during exhalation, which may be difficult to appreciate in an emergency.[76]

Ultimately, the safe delivery of oxygenation and ventilation in an emergency CICO scenario relies on appropriately trained clinicians who are skilled in the use and familiar with the application of proven techniques and reliable devices.

Postoperative Considerations

Cricothyrotomy

Although it can be performed electively with limited indications,[20,77] cricothyrotomy is usually performed emergently to secure a DA. When cricothyrotomy is performed under less than ideal circumstances, it should be considered a temporary measure, and when the patient is stabilized, tracheal intubation with or without a flexible intubation scope (FIS) or a tracheostomy should be performed. Needle cricothyrotomy should not be performed unless it is the only option, as a last resort, and it should be converted to a safer, more effective airway as rapidly as possible. Seldinger and surgical techniques should be performed preferentially in CICO scenarios. Flexible tracheoscopy by FIS should be used to inspect the site of the cricothyrotomy and to confirm the catheter/cannula stable position in the airway before transporting the patient.

The cricothyrotomy site should be examined frequently for signs of infection, and all patients should have a careful neurologic and airway evaluation before discharge from the hospital to ensure that there has been no damage to the vocal cords or other nearby structures. There is no consensus on what workup is necessary after emergency cricothyrotomy, but any complaints by the patient of difficulty swallowing or phonating should be carefully evaluated. While complication rates from properly performed emergent cricothyrotomy seem to be acceptably low, large clinical studies to confirm this claim are needed.[83,84]

Cuff Pressure

Cricothyrotomy tube cuffs are used to create a seal against the tracheal mucosa, thereby minimizing aspiration and facilitating positive-pressure ventilation by preventing leakage of air. Tracheal stenosis from low-volume, high-pressure, low-compliance cuffs was a major complication of tracheostomy during the 1960s. These cuffs may exert pressures as high as 180 to 250 mm Hg on the tracheal mucosa, far in excess of the normal capillary perfusion pressures of 20 to 30 mm Hg. The result is a time-related, progressive ischemic injury ranging from inflammatory changes to chondronecrosis and tracheal stenosis or tracheomalacia. With the accumulated evidence attesting to the deleterious effects of low-volume, high-pressure cuffs, there has been a gradual shift in the past few decades toward the use of high-volume, low-pressure cuffs because they are safer.

The transition to high-volume, low-pressure cuffs decreased the incidence of cuff-related tracheal stenosis by 10 fold because of the ability of the cuff to seal the airway at pressures below the mucosal capillary perfusion pressure. These cuffs inflate symmetrically, adapt to the tracheal contour, and allow pressure distribution over a wide area. The risk of overinflation with resultant high cuff pressures may be minimized by the following: having a pressure-controlled cuff with a pressure pop-off valve that prevents inflation beyond 20 mm Hg (although less than 20 mm Hg has been associated with increased risk of leakage of bacterial pathogens around the cuff into the lower respiratory tract),[78] regular measurement of intracuff pressure with a manometer attached to a three- or four-way stopcock (the latter gives more accurate results), and cuff deflation for as long as safely possible in patients who do not require mechanical ventilation.

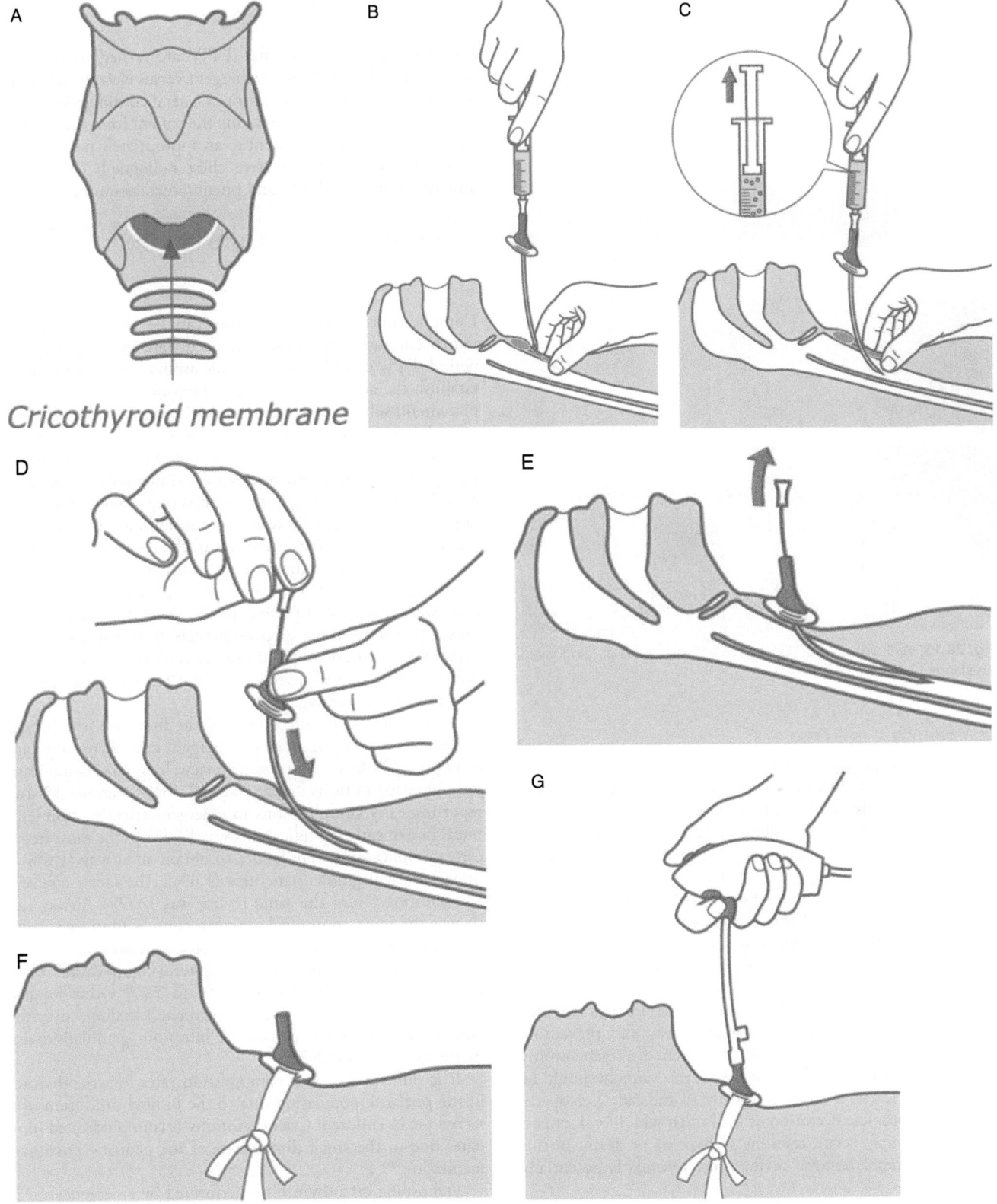

• **Fig. 28.15** (A–G) Cricath insertion technique. See text for details. (Courtesy Ventinova Medical, Eindhoven, Netherlands.)

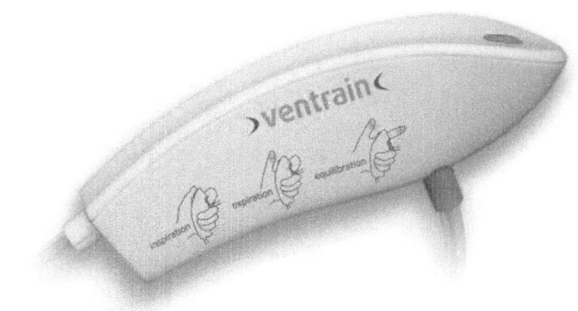

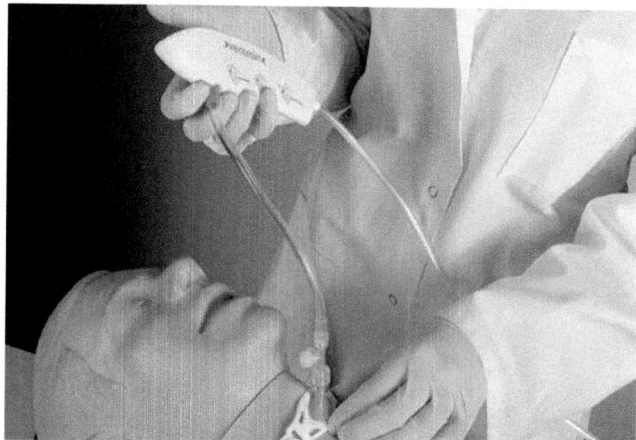

• **Fig. 28.16** Ventrain system. (Courtesy Ventinova Medical, Eindhoven, Netherlands.)

Suctioning and Tube Care

Hypoxia, cardiac dysrhythmia, injury to the tracheobronchial tree, atelectasis, and infection have been associated with suctioning. These events can be minimized by close attention to technical details. Factors that may contribute to hypoxia include suctioning of oxygen-rich air for too long and the use of inappropriately large catheters. This can be prevented by applying suction for less than 2 seconds with a catheter less than half the size of the tracheostomy tube and ventilating the patient with 100% oxygen for at least 5 breaths before and after suctioning. A strictly aseptic technique using disposable catheters is mandatory to reduce the risk of cross-contamination.

Meticulous care of the tracheostomy tube and peristomal area is important for maintaining a patent airway and preventing infection and breakdown of the skin. Placement of a tracheostomy tube with an inner cannula is mandatory. This cannula should be removed and cleared several times daily in the early postoperative period. Complete occlusion of the lumen with blood, crusts, and secretions may occur, resulting in hypoxia or death; in this circumstance, rapid removal of the inner cannula is potentially life-saving.

Bacterial colonization of the peristomal area may also occurs. The wound should be cleaned of accumulated secretions and crusts with hydrogen peroxide to prevent breakdown of the skin and progression from wound colonization to infection. The skin under the tracheostomy neck plate should be kept dry with a thin, nonadherent dressing. Petroleum-based products should be avoided on open wounds because they may stimulate granulation tissue formation.

Transtracheal Jet Ventilation

Postprocedural concerns after TTJV are related to the type of scenario in which it is used (emergent versus elective) and depend strictly on the patient's condition. General considerations include securing the airway before moving the patient from the emergency room or admitting the patient to an appropriately monitored unit and obtaining a postoperative chest radiograph to ensure the absence of pneumothorax and pneumomediastinum.

Complications and Outcome Data

Cricothyrotomy

Complications of cricothyrotomy can be categorized as those that occur early and those that occur late in the postoperative period. Early complications include asphyxia related to failure to establish the airway, hemorrhage, improper or unsuccessful tube placement, subcutaneous and mediastinal emphysema, prolonged procedure time, pneumothorax, and airway obstruction. Esophageal or mediastinal perforation, vocal cord injury, aspiration, and laryngeal disruption may also occur.[79] Long-term complications include tracheal and subglottic stenosis (especially in the presence of preexisting laryngeal trauma or infection), aspiration, swallowing dysfunction, tube obstruction, tracheoesophageal fistula, and voice changes.[80] Voice change is the most common complication, occurring in up to 50% of cases.[81] Voice problems include hoarseness, weak voice, or decreased pitch. Voice dysfunction may be caused by injury to the external branch of the superior laryngeal nerve, decreased cricothyroid muscle contractility, or mechanical obstruction related to narrowing of the anterior parts of the thyroid and cricoid cartilages.[82]

In a recent systematic review of the literature, the incidence of short-term complications of emergent cricothyrotomy ranged from 0% to 31.6%.[83] In the same review, long-term complications were reported to be as low as 0% to 7.86%.[83] Among 13 studies reporting early complications in emergent cricothyrotomies, the mean rate of early complications was 13.4%.[84] The most frequent early complications were failure to obtain an airway (1.6%) and injury to cartilaginous structures (1.6%). The mean rate of late complications from the same review was 13.6%. Airway stenosis was the most common long-term complication, occurring at a low rate (1.1%).[84] However, subglottic stenosis following emergent cricothyrotomy as the main long-term complication has been reported at rates ranging from 2.9% to 5%.[83] Other long-term complications observed were peristomal bleeding, dysphonia, aspiration pneumonia, peristomal infection, granulation tissue, dysphagia, and air leak.[83,84]

It is difficult to assess complication rates for cricothyrotomy in the pediatric population due to the limited utilization of this technique in children. Cricothyrotomy is contraindicated in neonates due to the small dimensions of the neonatal cricothyroid membrane.[103]

Prehospital cricothyrotomy performed by emergency medical services (EMS) personnel carries a higher risk of morbidity than the in-hospital procedure. In an early study, Spaite and Joseph reported an overall acute complication rate of 31% in 16 emergency patients.[34] Failure to secure the airway accounted for the major complication rate (12%). Minor complications included right mainstem intubation, infrahyoid placement, and thyroid cartilage fracture. Sixty surgical cricothyrotomies performed by trained aeromedical system personnel had a complication rate of

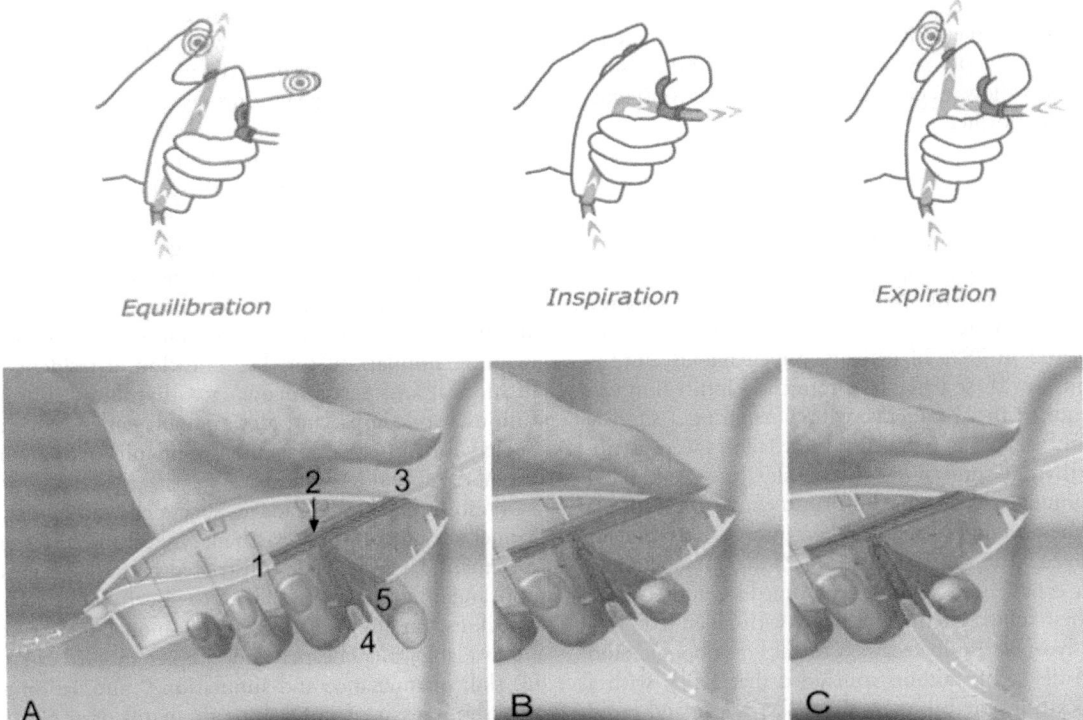

Equilibration   *Inspiration*   *Expiration*

• **Fig. 28.17** Ventrain internal mechanism and functionality. (1) inlet hose connection to hospital oxygen gas flow, (2) narrow diameter to increase gas velocity, (3) outlet gas flow, (4) connection to patient, (5) equilibration opening. (A) Equilibration is achieved by removing the index finger from the equilibration opening and the thumb from the outlet gas flow. During equilibration, there is no significant positive or negative pressure at the catheter tip, resulting in a safety mode. (B) Inspiration is achieved by placing the index finger on the equilibration opening and the thumb on the outlet gas flow. (C) Exhalation is achieved by maintaining the index finger on the equilibration opening and removing the thumb from the outlet gas flow. (Courtesy Ventinova Medical, Eindhoven, Netherlands.)

8.7%.[85] These complications included significant hemorrhage or soft tissue hematoma and incorrect placement.

All of the aforementioned complications are from surgical or mixed surgical and percutaneous cricothyrotomy studies. Complications associated specifically with percutaneous cricothyrotomy include difficulties with insertion, esophageal or mediastinal misplacement, and bleeding.[86]

In a cadaveric porcine airway model that compared the performance of a kit for percutaneous technique with the bougie-assisted cricothyrotomy technique (BACT), securing the airway with the percutaneous kit was significantly faster than with BACT, but tracheal laceration occurred in six (30%) of the percutaneous procedures and in none of the BACT procedures.[87] In a live porcine model of a simulated cardiac arrest comparing BACT and percutaneous cricothyrotomy, BACT was significantly faster than percutaneous cricothyrotomy. However, while there was no difference in overall success rate, more attempts were needed in the percutaneous technique group, and trauma to the posterior tracheal wall was 5 times more frequent in the percutaneous cricothyrotomy group compared to the BACT group.[88] These findings seem to point to an overall higher complication rate associated with percutaneous techniques.

The risk of infection requires special and separate consideration. Colonization of the surgical wound after cricothyrotomy occurs within 24 to 48 hours with primarily gram-negative organisms, including *Klebsiella*, *Pseudomonas aeruginosa*, *Escherichia coli*, and occasionally *Staphylococcus aureus*.[89,90] Wound edges may demonstrate mild erythema, and yellow or green secretions from the area may be copious, particularly in the first 7 to 10 days. These findings are more marked after standard open tracheostomy than after percutaneous cricothyrotomy and tracheostomy, probably because of the very small incision and tight tract in the latter techniques. Frequent and meticulous wound care with mechanical debridement, if necessary, is the best way to deal with this situation. Progressive cellulitis, despite aggressive local care, indicates infection, usually polymicrobial, and warrants systemic antibiotics. Management involves replacing the tracheostomy tube with an ETT (as feasible) and aggressive wound debridement and cleaning with antiseptic dressings. Rarely, local flaps may be necessary to provide soft tissue coverage for vital structures.

Colonization of the wound, along with mechanical irritation from the tube, cuff, and tube tip, means that there is always some degree of localized, reversible tracheitis, which often manifests by increased secretions. Progression of this situation may lead to loss of tracheal support, resulting in tracheal stenosis or tracheomalacia. Full-thickness loss may result in life-threatening complications such as tracheal-esophageal or tracheal-innominate fistula. Selecting appropriate tube sizes, materials, and cuffs can minimize mechanical irritation. The cuff should be inflated only when necessary. The known bacterial colonization of polyvinyl chloride devices makes a strong argument in favor of more frequent tube changes, perhaps weekly, in ventilator-dependent, critically ill patients.

It is important to remember that cricothyrotomy, especially when performed in emergent situations, should be considered a temporary measure at higher risk of complications, and, as soon as patient conditions allow, tracheal intubation or elective tracheostomy should be performed.

Transtracheal Jet Ventilation

In a retrospective chart review, Patel described a 53-month experience with patients in acute respiratory failure in the ICU.[91] In 352 patients requiring tracheal intubation, 29 emergent percutaneous TTJV attempts were made. Successful cannulation of the airway was achieved in 79% of patients. Subcutaneous emphysema occurred in 2 of these patients. Orotracheal intubation was subsequently required in 22 patients, with 1 requiring a surgical tracheostomy. TTJV failed in 6 patients; these failures were attributed to recent thyroid surgery (n = 1), obesity (n = 2), kinking of the TTJV cannula (n = 2), and misplacement of the cannula (n = 1). Subcutaneous emphysema was seen in only 1 patient for whom TTJV failed. The other patient who suffered subcutaneous emphysema experienced severe pneumomediastinum treated with bilateral chest tubes. Of the 6 patients with failed TTJV, 2 were subsequently orally intubated with the aid of a bougie, and the remaining 4 died. The authors concluded that TTJV with a large-bore angiocath inserted through the CTM is safe and rapid in providing immediate oxygenation and should be considered as a temporary life-saving procedure in emergent situations when conventional methods to provide adequate gas exchange are unsuccessful.[91]

More recently, Duggan and colleagues conducted a rigorous systematic review to determine the complication rates of TTJV in CICO emergencies compared with non-CICO emergency settings or the elective surgical setting.[15] In this analysis of the literature, complications were categorized as device failure, barotrauma (including subcutaneous emphysema), and miscellaneous. Device failure was defined by the inability to place and/or use the TTJV device.

Among the more than 44 studies (428 procedures) included in the review, device failure occurred in 42% of CICO emergency situations vs in 0% of non-CICO emergencies and 0.3% of elective procedures. Barotrauma occurred in 32% of CICO emergencies vs in 7% of non-CICO emergencies and 8% of elective procedures. The total number of procedures with any complication was 51% of CICO emergencies vs 7% of non-CICO emergencies and 8% of elective procedures. In several instances, TTJV-related subcutaneous emphysema impeded subsequent attempts at securing the airway. In consideration of the high rate of complications with use of TTJV in CICO emergencies, the authors of this review conclude that guidelines and recommendations supporting the use of TTJV in CICO should be reconsidered.[15]

Training Models

Because PDC is rarely performed, there exists a need for quality teaching and training aids.[92,93] Although the technique closely mimics over-the-wire vascular insertion methods, it is sufficiently different that anesthesiologists should ideally practice it on a regular basis.[94] Simple and inexpensive models can be made for training residents and inexperienced personnel, as well as maintaining the skills and proficiency of trainees and experts.

Of the available animal models, dogs appear to be most similar to humans. The canine CTM, neck muscles, and cricothyroid

area are similar to those in humans. The tracheal dimensions of a 25-kg dog are comparable with those of the adult human.[95] Cricothyrotomy has been performed on other animals, including pigs, sheep, and goats. In pigs, attempts to pass a needle or over-the-needle catheter into the cricothyroid space may result in hitting cartilage. The space can be entered by directing the needle cephalad, not caudad. Dissection of the larynx reveals a projection on the inferior surface of the thyroid cartilage that articulates with the cricoid cartilage. This cornu has been previously described and must be removed to perform cricothyrotomy studies.[82] The pig trachea model (professionally isolated and prepared) is used for airway training and is combined with manikin simulations for the education of residents and faculty in surgical and percutaneous cricothyrotomy in teaching institutions, workshops, and airway management courses (e.g., the Society for Airway Management Difficult Airway Workshop and the ASA Annual Meeting).

Fresh or embalmed cadaver specimens can be used.[54,96–98] The former are superior because the laryngeal structures of embalmed specimens are somewhat constricted because of muscle contraction, and it may be more difficult to discern the cricothyroid space. Manikins can also be an acceptable model, and several products are available, but cheaper and simpler models can also be used for skill maintenance and simulation.[99] Simulation and practice workshops are used in teaching programs or as part of dedicated airway management courses or meetings.[40,100–102]

Lastly, providers may become and remain skilled in accessing the CTM by performing the recurrent laryngeal nerve block (transtracheal block) to anesthetize the airways in the context of awake and spontaneous breathing, FIS-assisted intubations, or other indications.

Conclusion

In the 1970s, after a 50-year hiatus, cricothyrotomy became recognized as an important procedure for emergency airway management. Despite considerable evidence that cricothyrotomy can be life-saving and has an acceptable low complication rate, controlled clinical trials comparing various techniques have not been, and are unlikely to be, performed. This is largely the result of the infrequency with which physicians and other health care providers encounter patients requiring emergency cricothyrotomy. The lack of opportunity to perform cricothyrotomy or other emergency airway procedures is a problem for anesthesiologists, who are recognized airway experts. Although the opportunity to perform a cricothyrotomy is rare, it must be performed expeditiously and correctly when required. The authors believe that PDC should be easy for anesthesiologists to learn because it is similar to the Seldinger technique for insertion of catheters and sheaths, a technique used on a daily basis. Anesthesiologists should be well trained in emergency airway techniques and have appropriate equipment available at all times. Although anesthesiologists practice primarily in the OR, they are likely to be called on to perform emergency airway procedures in other settings.

Continuous advancements in the field have expanded the availability of safer techniques and devices to assist clinicians in the management of airway emergencies; however, the only way to improve patient outcomes in these emergency situations is to ensure that clinicians who routinely perform airway management are appropriately trained and familiar with the equipment available to them.

Selected References

4. Abou-Foul AK. A lesson on human factors in airway management learnt from the death of George Washington. *Otolaryngol Head Neck Surg.* 2020;163(5):1000-1002.

12. Apfelbaum J L, Hagberg CA, Caplan RA, et al. Practice guidelines for management of the difficult airway: an updated report by the American Society of Anesthesiologists Task Force on Management of the Difficult Airway. *Anesthesiology.* 2013;118(2);251-270.

13. Frerk C, Mitchell VS, McNarry AF, et al. . Difficult Airway Society 2015 guidelines for management of unanticipated difficult intubation in adults. *Br J Anaesth.* 2015;115(6):827-848.

15. Duggan LV, Ballantyne Scott B, Law JA, Morris IR, Murphy MF, Griesdale DE. Transtracheal jet ventilation in the 'can't intubate can't oxygenate' emergency: a systematic review. *Br J Anaesth.* 2016. 117(suppl 1):i28-i38.

22. Cook TM. Strategies for the prevention of airway complications: a narrative review. *Anaesthesia.* 2018;73(1):93-111.

23. McClelland G, Smith M. Just a routine operation: A Critical discussion. *J Perioper Prac.* 2016;26(5):114-117.

24. Chrimes N. The Vortex: a universal 'high-acuity implementation tool' for emergency airway management. *Br J Anaesth.* 2016;117(suppl 1):i20-i27.

47. Paxian M, Preussler NP, Reinz T,Schlueter A, Gottschall R. Transtracheal ventilation with a novel ejector-based device (Ventrain) in open, partly obstructed, or totally closed upper airways in pigs. *Br J Anaesth.* 2016;115(2):308-316.

57. Salah N, El Saigh I, Hayes N, McCaul C. Airway injury during emergency transcutaneous airway access: a comparison at cricothyroid and tracheal sites. *Anesth Analg.* 2009;109(6):1901-1907.

74. Doyle DJ. Ventilation via narrow-bore catheters: clinical and technical perspectives on the Ventrain ventilation system. *Open J Anesthesiol.* 2018;12:49-60.

83. Macedo MB, Guimaraes RB, Ribeiro SM, Sousa KM. Emergency cricothyrotomy: temporary measure or definitive airway? A systematic review. *Rev Col Bras Cir.* 2016;43(6):493-499.

All references can be found online at eBooks.Health.Elsevier.com.

29

Surgical Airway in Emergent and Nonemergent Contexts

LAURA V. DUGGAN, LIANE B. JOHNSON, MARK KASTNER, AND MICHAEL ALFRED GIBBS

CHAPTER OUTLINE

KEY POINTS

- For anatomic reasons, emergency surgical airway in the hands of advanced airway managers will usually be a cricothyrotomy.
- The critical step in cricothyrotomy is recognizing when it is required. Decision-making should not be left solely to the airway manager—those not directly involved in airway management may better recognize an emerging cannot ventilate/cannot oxygenate (CVCO) situation.
- We have chosen CVCO in this chapter to reflect two quantitative measurements that can be verbalized by team members, usually in the order they occur (e.g., "I notice the waveform capnography is flat, and the oxygen saturation is now going down to the mid 80s. I'll get out the supraglottic device and cricothyrotomy set"). This deemphasizes the need for the airway manager to have the insight into their cognitive errors including perseveration of tracheal intubation attempts.
- Due to the infrequent need to perform cricothyrotomy, skills maintenance requires regular practice, coaching, and keeping the technique as simple as possible. Similar to Advanced Cardiac Life Support (ACLS) and Advanced Trauma Life Support (ATLS), infrequent high-acuity emergencies require a standardized predictable approach.
- Due to its unpredictable nature, cricothyrotomy supplies should be stocked in every location in which advanced airway management

occurs (e.g., in every trauma room, not just on one central cart). Equipment is simple; #10 scalpel, bougie, and 6.0 tracheal tube. These should be stocked together and clearly labeled.
- The cricothyroid membrane is difficult to palpate in females, as well as in patients with a thick or short neck. There is a high failure rate of cricothyrotomy techniques that rely on accurate identification of the cricothyroid membrane (e.g., wire-guided cricothyrotomy).
- Evidence of repeated success supports simplicity of choice and technique. The use of a scalpel, bougie, and tracheal tube emphasizes simplicity. Landmarking is key to success, and when faced with challenging dissection or excessive bleeding, the index finger can be used to internally palpate and confirm airway anatomy prior to horizontally incising the cricothyroid membrane. The index finger can then serve as a guide for insertion of the bougie followed by the tracheal tube.
- Suctioning the tracheal tube immediately for blood after insertion is recommended. Waveform capnography is the gold standard of the tracheal tube being in the airway, even in the setting of cardiac arrest. Confirm intratracheal placement with waveform capnography. Bronchoscopic assessment is a helpful as a visual adjunct to tracheal tube placement and positioning. Obtain a chest x-ray to assess tracheal tube placement and possible barotrauma, including pneumothorax.

Introduction

Nonemergent and emergent surgical airway approaches differ in context, anatomic approach, equipment, and training. Nonemergent surgical airway generally takes the form of open tracheotomy or percutaneous tracheostomy in the hands of a surgeon or intensivist with expertise in these techniques. The decision to perform a nonemergent surgical airway is, by definition, scheduled with a robust multidisciplinary airway plan. Elective tracheotomy is not without its dangers; poor physiologic reserve, difficult surgical access, and the inability to easily reintubate the patient may all result in an elective tracheostomy becoming emergent. In contrast, an emergent surgical airway generally takes the form of cricothyrotomy, often in the hands of advanced airway managers whose experience of cricothyrotomy often consists of simulation only. The decision to perform an emergency cricothyrotomy must be made expeditiously in the setting of possible hypoxic brain damage or death, if not performed imminently. The power of a team approach harnessed during these emergent situations may be lifesaving.

The term *surgical airway* should not be misinterpreted as needing to be performed by a surgeon. Any advanced airway manager (those performing airway management beyond mask ventilation) should have the skills to perform an emergency surgical airway (cricothyrotomy) when required. The indications, methods, and complications of achieving a successful surgical airway in emergency and non-emergency contexts is the focus of this chapter.

Most nonemergent surgical airways will be in the form of either tracheotomy (open surgical technique) or tracheostomy (percutaneous technique). Most critical care patients requiring tracheostomy will undergo bedside percutaneous tracheostomy with bronchoscopic guidance by a critical care physician. Patients with difficult anatomy are usually transferred to the operating room for open tracheostomy performed by surgeons skilled in this technique. This selects for the most difficult cases being transferred to the operating room. Anesthesiologists involved in these procedures should be well versed with the steps involved, engage in open communication with the surgery team, and be prepared with alternative oxygenation techniques should any of the emergencies reviewed in this chapter occur.

Patients requiring nonemergent surgical airway procedures often have an orally or nasally placed tracheal tube in situ. Although many airway managers will not perform a surgical airway in a nonemergent context, many will be called upon to assist or support oxygenation and ventilation during the tracheostomy. It is important to understand the anatomy, steps involved, and potential pitfalls. Communication and understanding of the sequential steps involved on both sides of the drape will prevent a nonemergency situation from devolving into an emergency. Oral/nasal tracheal tube withdrawal should only occur following confirmation of proper placement of the new surgical airway. The surgical airway should be confirmed by waveform capnography. If there is no waveform despite suctioning through the surgical airway, the creation of a false passage should be assumed. False passage occurs when surgical dissection diverges from the airway into anterior neck tissues. False passage creation is associated with hypoxia, cardiorespiratory instability, and loss of the airway if not managed correctly. Other rare immediate complications include airway fire in the presence of a combustible gas (such as a high Fio_2 escaping from the tracheal incision, a spark from electrocautery, and ignition of drapes, towels or gauze) or uncontrolled bleeding from an overlying thyroid gland or important vessels that cross the midline, such as the innominate artery. Finally, barotrauma or pneumothorax can result due to

tube migration, high pressure/high flow ventilation, or accidental trauma to the pleura from challenging surgical dissection in the mediastinum or lung apices in the lateral neck.

Establishing an emergency surgical airway is often a second- or third-line choice to secure an airway after tracheal intubation (TI) attempts have failed. It is important to consider, particularly in the setting of obstructing airway pathology, if performance of a surgical airway whilst the patient is awake should be the first choice of securing the patient's airway. A styleted tracheal tube or flexible bronchoscope through the patient's native narrowed airway may completely obstruct the airway. This may lead to patient panic, loss of cooperation, and the change from a semiurgent situation into a less-controlled emergency.

Advanced airway managers, regardless of specialty, will be usually involved in performing an emergency cricothyrotomy at least once in their career, usually during a cannot ventilate/cannot oxygenate (CVCO) situation.

Waveform capnography and pulse oximetry provide objective physiologic assessments of patency from the patient's mouth to alveoli and of oxygenation of circulating blood, respectively. Both are essential parts of advanced airway management. We have used the term *CVCO* in this chapter to reflect the temporal sequence of these two objective findings; nonreassuring waveform capnography (due to upper airway obstruction) usually precedes the patient becoming hypoxemic. The term CVCO, unlike cannot intubate/cannot oxygenate (CICO), deemphasizes failure of TI as a criterion for diagnosing the CVCO airway emergency. In retrospective and prospective observational studies, CVCO has been associated with perseveration of TI attempts. If this life-threatening emergency situation can be recognized by any member of the healthcare team based on objective criteria, the decision to adjust the action becomes independent of the primary airway manager's insight to a failure of airway management. Team members should be empowered to state when waveform capnography is no longer a square wave or is completely absent, as well as pulse oximetry falling. This level of engagement and situational awareness allows the entire team to mobilize and prepare for immediate surgical airway.

A *failed airway* is not defined as the need for a surgical airway. A failed airway is:

1. not recognizing the need for surgical airway, or
2. not performing a surgical airway in a timely manner, or
3. not being adequately practiced in the technique.

In a coordinated manner, the team should ensure the following: adequate patient paralysis, optimal two-handed, two-person with oral airway bag-valve-mask (BVM) technique, and insertion of a supraglottic device while positioning and preparing for a surgical airway, usually in the form of a cricothyrotomy.

The ideal cricothyrotomy technique should be as simple as possible with equipment that can be stocked and maintained in every airway management location. It should be practiced and refined on a regular basis. It should have a high first-pass success rate that is not dependent on fine motor skills, which often deteriorate due to the airway manager's own physiologic stress response. For these reasons, the authors recommend a scalpel-bougie-ETT cricothyrotomy for the performance of a surgical airway in a CVCO emergency for all non-surgeon airway managers.

Surgical Airway

Surgical airway is the term used to encompass placing a breathing tube through the cricothyroid membrane (CTM) (cricothyrotomy) or between or through tracheal rings (tracheotomy). The term should not imply that it is performed only by surgeons. The term denotes the use of a scalpel to create an artificial conduit for oxygen provision (oxygenation) and carbon dioxide elimination (ventilation). No matter what approach is taken, the operator should expect blood to obscure the surgical field; palpation is the primary sense that will be used to successfully establish a surgical airway in an emergency.

There are a multitude of subtle variations of both tracheostomy and cricothyrotomy techniques that share the same goal following incision of the skin and soft tissue followed by the use of a tracheal tube through the CTM or tracheal rings to oxygenate and ventilate the patient.

History of Surgical Airways

Emergency surgical airway as a lifesaving procedure has been performed for thousands of years. The first depictions of surgical tracheostomy were found on Egyptian tablets dating from 3600 BCE. In the second century AD, Galen suggested tracheostomy, using a vertical incision, as an emergency treatment for airway obstruction. Vesalius published the first detailed descriptions of tracheostomy in the 16th century, using a reed to ventilate the lungs. Ironically, his alleged resuscitation through tracheostomy and ventilation of a Spanish nobleman led to condemnation by the Spanish Inquisition and his ultimate death. Such condemnation may be reenacted to a degree in contemporary practice, whereby the performance of a surgical airway may be met with a retrospective and harsh critique!

Dr. Chevalier Jackson published a landmark article on tracheostomy in 1921,[1] enumerating the surgical principles still relevant today. Cricothyrotomy, which Jackson called high tracheostomy, was condemned as the cause of subglottic stenosis. It is now clear that subglottic stenosis developed due to underlying inflammation of the respiratory mucosa, usually from an infectious cause (often diphtheria), rather than the site of incision. However, knowledge translation of this evidence has taken decades and is only now leading to a paradigm shift supporting the safety of cricothyrotomy.

The dangers of cricothyrotomy were not widely reconsidered until 1976, when Brantigan and Grow published a retrospective study of cricothyrotomy for long-term airway management in 655 patients.[2] Only 5 patients (0.76%) developed subglottic stenosis. More recently, a 2019 systematic review analyzed the short- and long-term complications of cricothyrotomy (n = 1219) and tracheotomy (n = 342) procedures performed during emergency situations, the most common reason being trauma.[3] All studies included were retrospective. Early complications occurred in 4.8% of cricothyrotomies, the most common being failure of the technique (1.6%) and damage to cartilaginous structures (1.6%). By comparison, early complications occurred in 9.1% of emergency tracheotomies, the most common being hemorrhage (5.6%) and pneumothorax/subcutaneous emphysema (2.9%). Subglottic stenosis occurred in 1.1% of patients who underwent cricothyrotomy *regardless of whether early conversion to tracheotomy was performed* versus 7.0% of patients undergoing tracheostomy.

In conclusion, not every cricothyrotomy performed requires immediate conversion to tracheotomy to prevent subglottic stenosis. The exception to this remains what Chevalier Jackson observed 100 years ago: in the face of inflammatory or infectious airway pathology, conversion as soon as possible to performing tracheostomy is advised, ideally within 24 hours.

Incidence of Surgical Airway

The incidence of surgical airway varies depending on the clinical context.[4] For example, in critical care where prolonged ventilatory support is anticipated,[5] the incidence of tracheostomy can range from 7% to 24% depending on available resources and patient population. In emergencies, such as on the battlefield and in the prehospital setting, frequencies range between 0.5% and 18.5%.[6] In the emergency department, a rate of 0.9% to 2.8% has been observed.[7] In the operating suite, the incidence is much lower at 0.002% to 0.39%.[8]

Types of Surgical Airway

Surgical airway encompasses both cricothyrotomy and tracheotomy.[9] Principles of the ideal surgical airway procedure can be found in Table 29.1. An anatomic comparison of cricothyrotomy versus tracheotomy can be found in Table 29.2. Surgical cricothyrotomy and surgical tracheotomy refer to the use of a scalpel and other surgical instruments to create an opening through the anterior neck and into the airway, through the CTM or through/between tracheal rings, respectively. In adults, these techniques allow the insertion of a cuffed tube. The 2019 American Society of Anesthesiologists (ASA) airway-related closed claims review reported protracted delays in performing a surgical airway due to, among other reasons, the belief that a surgeon was required.[10] Therefore, the authors support the use of the term *surgical airway* to encompass both cricothyrotomy and tracheotomy, with one or both being in the skill set of any advanced airway manager. Surgical airway may be further subclassified according to the technique used: (1) surgical, (2) percutaneous, (3) dilatational, and (4) cannula based.

Tracheostomy

For a tracheostomy, an incision is made below the cricoid cartilage (the most distal cartilage of the larynx), usually between two tracheal rings, but minor variations and preferences exist based on surgical training and clinical experience (Bjork flap, cruciate incision, ring excision) and placement of a tracheostomy tracheal tube.[11] In the adult population, tracheostomy involves an initial horizontal skin incision, followed by sharp vertical dissection to divide the midline fascia between the strap muscles and to identify the thyroid isthmus, which is then retracted or divided to expose the trachea. Prior to incising the trachea, a tracheal hook is applied to the larynx at the cricoid ring and tractioned rostrally to provide inline stabilization of the larynx during insertion of an appropriately sized tracheostomy tube. The experienced operator will create the smallest possible horizontal incision in the trachea to accommodate the optimally sized tracheotomy tube to minimize the risk of tracheal transection leading to rapid intrathoracic retraction of the distal limb of the trachea due to negative intrathoracic pressures.

Percutaneous tracheostomy involves initial horizontal skin and soft tissue incision to facilitate a puncture and dilatation procedure into the trachea. Once again, an appropriately sized tracheostomy tube should be selected based on patient need and anatomic characteristics. Several commercial devices are available.[12]

Cricothyrotomy

Cricothyrotomy is an incision made between the laryngeal structures of the thyroid and cricoid cartilages, through the CTM, with subsequent placement of a tracheal tube.

Open cricothyrotomy is generally preformed in emergency situations and involves an initial vertical midline skin and soft tissue

TABLE 29.1	Principles of the Ideal Emergency Front-of-Neck Airway Technique
Principle	**Explanation**
There is an acceptable first-pass success rate.	Analogous to the literature for tracheal intubation (TI), it is not an unreasonable expectation that surgical airway has a first-pass success rate of 85% or greater.[59]
Landmarks are preserved.	The chosen technique should not impair the ability to perform a second technique should the first technique fail. Published evidence in adults from the American Society of Anesthesiologists (ASA) closed claims,[10,60] as well as a systematic review of transtracheal jet ventilation techniques used in cannot ventilate/cannot oxygenate (CVCO) emergencies,[61] document a high rate of cannula misplacement. Subcutaneous emphysema leading to obliteration of landmarks and failure of subsequent open scalpel-based surgical airway rescue attempts was documented frequently.
There is minimized risk of creating a false passage.	False passage occurs when surgical dissection diverges from the airway into anterior neck tissues (Fig. 29.1A). Palpation and stabilization techniques can minimize this risk while providing tactile feedback. Advancement of the bougie without resistance also suggests proper placement in the airway. Tracheal "clicks" felt through the bougie as it slides over the tracheal rings although specific are not sensitive.[62] Preloading the ETT alters tactile feedback from the bougie and impedes the proper mechanics of ETT insertion. Therefore this technique is not recommended.
Equipment should be minimal, familiar, and immediately available.	Multiple technique choices and a multitude of devices may lead to delay in initiating a surgical airway due to device choice confusion and construction failure (Fig. 29.4). Equipment should be as simple as possible, at a cost that permits availability in every airway management location versus only centralized in difficult airway carts (Fig. 29.3). Packaging should be clear and unambiguous. There may be merit in labeling equipment with icons rather than written descriptors to enable healthcare workers to understand the contents despite their own physiologic and cognitive stress responses (Fig. 29.3).
Equipment cost should allow for simulated cricothyrotomy practice by advanced airway practitioners on a regular basis.	The equipment used in a CVCO emergency should be the same equipment used during practice sessions. Intermittent observation/coaching of technique improves performance compared to repetition alone.[63]
The need for fine motor skills is minimized.	The stress response of the airway manager cannot be overstated and is a key factor in performance outcome in cricothyrotomy during a CVCO emergency. Fine motor skills decay when the heart rate >115 beats per minute[46]; therefore, techniques depending on fine motor skills (e.g., connecting various pieces of equipment) are discouraged.
Many CVCO emergencies are due to airway obstruction at or above the laryngeal inlet.	Surgical airway should allow for both inspiration and expiration of the full tidal volumes to avoid breath stacking and potential barotrauma.
The cricothyroid membrane (CTM) is not a palpable structure; the cartilaginous structures that surround it are. Surgical airway choice should not rely on accurate palpation of CTM (i.e., the absence of cartilaginous structures) prior to initiation of cricothyrotomy. Palpation of the surrounding laryngeal structures surrounding the CTM (thyroid and cricoid cartilages) is useful.	Techniques that require precise, rapid identification of the CTM (e.g., cannula or wire-guided techniques) have a lower first-pass success rate versus scalpel-based techniques.[29] Gender, body mass index (BMI), and patients with a short and/or thick neck have been associated with poor CTM identification based on palpation.[64]

incision (Figure 29.2A), followed by a horizontal incision through the full width of the CTM. Unike tracheosotmy, complete transection of the CTM and muscles anteriorly will not lead to transection of the airway for several reasons. The larynx consists of a cartilaginous skeleton, with supportive ligaments and muscles. The cartilaginous skeleton includes the thyroid, cricoid, epiglottis, and arytenoid cartilages. The larynx is anchored in the neck. By contrast, the trachea is much more mobile, is more "slinky" in its anatomy, and moves considerably with intrathoracic pressure changes, or space occupying lesions such as hematoma and infection of the lateral neck. The cricoid and thyroid cartilages are also coupled by two posterolateral cricothyroid joints. Functionally, these joints allow for anterior widening or narrowing of the cricothyroid space, which in the day to day contribute to changes in pitch on vocalization. When establishing a surgical airway via cricothyrotomy, after incising the CTM and muscles will engage the joints and open this space to facilitate placement of a tracheal tube to secure the airway. A tracheal hook is not required. Avoiding the need for a tracheal hook simplifies cricothyrotomy equipment.

Percutaneous cannula cricothyrotomy relies on accurate identification of the CTM and involves initial puncture simultaneously through the skin and CTM or skin incision followed by cannula placement through the CTM. Oxygenation occurs through the cannula by pressure- or flow-determined oxygen provision through oxygen tubing. Ventilation (exhalation) does not occur through the cannula. Percutaneous wire-guided cricothyrotomy relies on accurate identification of the CTM and uses a Seldinger technique, in which the cannula technique (described in the preceding paragraph) is followed by wire insertion, dilatation, and insertion of the device. The device is large enough to provide both oxygenation and ventilation.

TABLE 29.2 Cricothyrotomy versus Tracheotomy		
	Cricothyrotomy	**Tracheotomy**
Location of tracheal tube insertion	Larynx lies between the thyroid and cricoid cartilages.	Between tracheal rings inferior to larynx
Overlying tissues	Larynx is the most anterior superficial structure of the airway.	Increasing depth as the trachea dives posteriorly from its proximal origin at the first tracheal ring to its entry into the thoracic inlet
Bleeding	Anterior thyroid artery; possible pyramidal lobe of the thyroid in 5% to 30% of people.	Anterior jugular veins Thyroid gland High-riding innominate artery
Stability of structures	The larynx, because of complexity and interattachment of its components, is more anchored in the neck, thus far less mobile than the trachea.	More mobile in the neck compared to the larynx, requiring more instruments, expertise to identify, and traction of the trachea
Extra equipment	Engaging the cricothyroid joints laterally by insertion of a finger widens the cricothyroid space.	Need for tracheal hook
Risk of airway transection	Transverse incision CTM does not result in airway separation due to the presence of the bilateral cricothyroid joints. Posterior wall of the airway cannot be severed without hefty deliberate effort as it is protected by the long, thick, posterior plate of the cricoid cartilage.	Transverse incision between tracheal rings may leave just the posterior membranous tracheal attachment, which can easily tear with placement of the tracheal tube, leading to impressive intrathoracic retraction of the distal limb of the trachea.

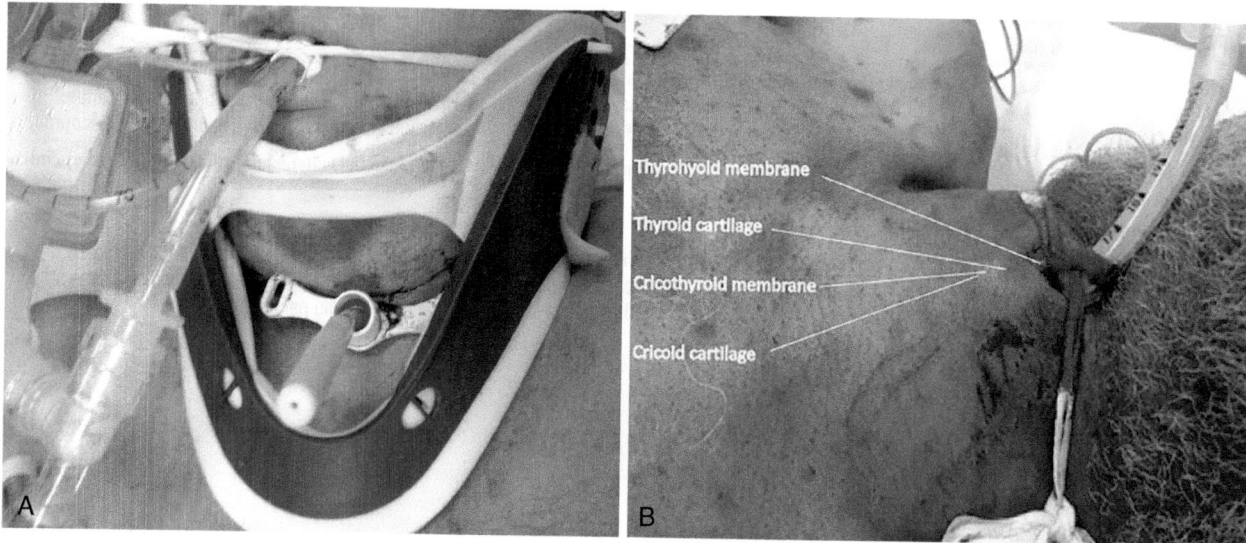

Fig. 29.1 (A) Wire-guided (Seldinger) technique leading to a false passage into the left neck soft tissues. The tip of the dilator of the cricothyrotomy device abutted but did not damage the left subclavian artery, allowing nonsurgical removal. (B) Endotracheal tube placed through the thyrohyoid membrane, superior to the thyroid cartilage, therefore above the vocal cords, making this a supraglottic airway device. (Courtesy of A, Dr. Laura Duggan and B, Dr. Sid Khosla.)

Since 2010,[13] ultrasound localization studies have shown that accurate identification of the CTM by palpation is generally poor among anaesthesia providers[14] and has the lowest reliability in obese females.[15] In an emerging airway obstruction, the fine motor dexterity required to accurately perform this refined procedure is more likely to end in failure than success. Another drawback is understanding that in a situation of upper airway obstruction, with no airflow in or out, use of a small cannula in the airway below the obstruction may indeed provide a path for oxygenation, but if sufficient exhalation time or space for outflow is not created, then barotrauma remains a real and dramatic risk to further exacerbate the dire situation, provoking cardiovascular collapse and failure of salvage open techniques due to tissue destruction.

Indications for Nonemergency Surgical Airway

There are a multitude of indications to perform a nonemergency surgical airway, usually in the form of a tracheostomy or tracheotomy. Most indications are due to the anticipated course of disease (e.g., respiratory failure due to primary lung disease, inadequate respiratory mechanics due to head injury, head and neck cancers requiring staged surgical procedures). Placement of a tracheostomy has several benefits, including decreased sedation with improved swallowing and laryngeal function.[12]

In patients with COVID-19 disease and respiratory failure, or any other respiratory-borne infection, healthcare professionals' safety also must be prioritized. There is currently no evidence suggesting a benefit of open tracheotomy over percutaneous techniques.[16] Current evidence suggests tracheostomy placement at 10 to 14 days of ventilation shows earlier discharge from critical care but no change in mortality.[17] If full personal protective equipment (PPE) is worn, there is no difference in healthcare provider infection for those performing or assisting in the tracheotomy procedure, but data are heterogeneous.[17] Although initial guidelines suggested a delay for tracheotomy of 14 to 21 days to reduce viral shedding to enhance healthcare workers safety,[18] this has now been revised to 10 to 14 days.[19] Additional safety measures for this high-risk, aerosol-generating procedure will include a negative pressure room; full PPE, including powered air-purifying respirators (PAPRs) (if available); full neuromuscular paralysis of the patient; and placement of a cuffed tracheostomy tube.[18,19] A predetermined checklist and sequence of events are followed to minimize the need for urgent communication (e.g., correcting equipment deficits) due to the impediment of communication when full PPE is in use. Planning and multidisciplinary rehearsal are essential prior to the procedure.[20]

Care of the patient with a tracheostomy is beyond the scope of this chapter, but standard care and emergency management require essential knowledge of it. Excellent articles are included in the references.[21,22]

Indications for Emergency Surgical Airway

Performance of a surgical airway technique during a CVCO emergency is a core skill for all advanced airway managers.

By definition, CVCO is the inability to ventilate and oxygenate the patient despite optimal attempts at all three of the following:

1. BVM using a two-handed two-person technique with an appropriately sized oral airway
2. Insertion of an appropriately sized supraglottic airway (SGA)
3. TI attempts, 2–3 in number, usually with both direct and video-assisted laryngoscopy

The number of attempts at 2 and 3 above are limited to two or three, depending on the algorithm and guidelines used.[9,23,24] Under certain circumstances, the airway team may deem attempts at BVM, SGA placement, and TI to be futile and

immediate; surgical airway may be the first choice of technique. An example of this situation is acute obstructing airway pathology from various conditions, such as head and neck cancer, Ludwig's angina, severe angioedema, or facial trauma. Context, such as an entrapped prehospital patient, may also influence the decision to directly move to a surgical airway. These may be referred to as the "inevitable" surgical airway.[25]

Essential Anatomy for Emergency and Nonemergency Surgical Airway

Many emergent surgical techniques, including surgical airway, involve surgical fields that may obscured rapidly by blood. For this reason, surgical airway should be considered a primarily tactile, not visual, procedure. Therefore, an understanding of the anatomy involved and regular practice primarily using haptic (identification by palpation) input may be lifesaving (Figure 29.2B).

Hyoid Bone

The horseshoe-shaped hyoid bone is the most cephalad rigid structure in the anterior neck and anchors the larynx to the floor of the mouth. The height of the hyoid bone in the anterior neck is variable and may be palpated above, below, or at the same level as the mentum. The hyoid bone suspends the larynx by the thyrohyoid membrane and muscle. Most importantly, misidentifying the hyoid bone as the thyroid cartilage can result in insertion of a tracheal tube through the thyrohyoid membrane above the vocal cords (Fig. 29.1B),[3] with the tracheal tube essentially becoming a supraglottic device. This error also risks trauma to the true vocal folds, further obstructing the airway, and gastric insufflation, restricting inspiratory tidal volumes and increasing aspiration risk. Waveform capnography may be present, but may have a varied pattern.

Thyroid Cartilage

The thyroid cartilage, located between the hyoid bone superiorly and the cricoid cartilage inferiorly, is the largest structure of the larynx. The thyroid cartilage consists of two laminae fused in the

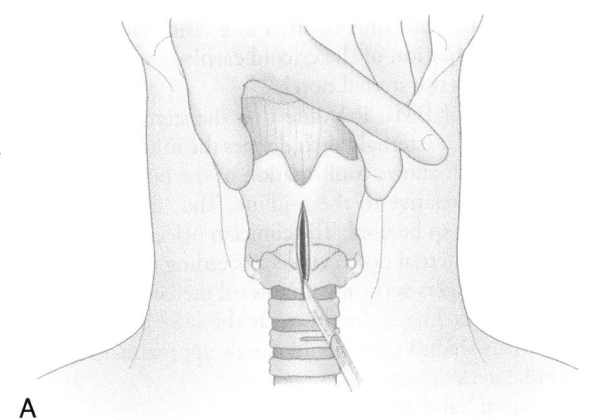

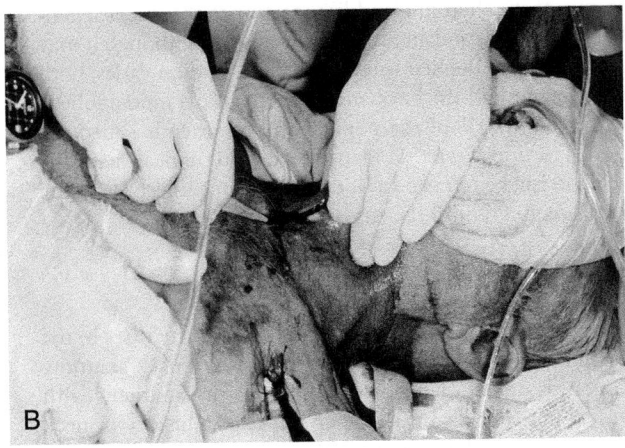

A   B

• **Fig. 29.2** A vertical skin incision is made down to, but not through, the airway. Blood may obscure visualization of structures; the airway manager should be comfortable with palpating structures. ([A] Modified from and [B] from Walls RM, Luten RC, Murphy MF, Schneider RE. Manual of Emergency Airway Management. 2nd ed. Lippincott Williams & Wilkins; 2004.)

midline anteriorly to form the laryngeal prominence, also called the thyroid notch or Adam's apple. The angle of this fusion is more acute in males, creating a readily palpable prominence. Hormonal influence determines the growth and structural development of the laryngeal cartilages, and as such the thyroid notch is not as easily identifiable in women, irrespective of body habitus.[26] The true vocal cords are located just below the midpoint between the thyroid notch and the inferior margin of the thyroid cartilage. The true vocal cords are well protected by the thyroid cartilage, minimizing risk of injury during a cricothyrotomy. Bilateral cricothyroid muscles fuse to the underlying CTM. Anterior jugular veins can be present in the superficial fascial layer over the thyroid cartilage and may lead to significant bleeding within the surgical field, hence the need to identify structures by palpation in the surgical field when visualization is not possible (Fig. 29.2B).

Cricoid Cartilage

The cricoid cartilage is the only complete cartilaginous ring in the upper airway and defines the inferior aspect of the larynx (Fig. 29.2A). It is shaped like a signet ring; with a taller lamina fused posteriorly, and much shorter lamina fused anteriorly. The arytenoid cartilages sit on top of the posterior cricoid lamina via synovial articulations. The cricoid ring is attached to the inferior aspect of the thyroid cartilage by the CTM anteriorly and by the cricothyroid joints bilaterally. These articulations of the thyroid and cricoid cartilages together form an enclosed "cartilaginous box" with a potential entry point anteriorly through the CTM (Fig. 29.2A). This cartilaginous box is bordered by the cricothyroid joints bilaterally, the tall cricoid lamina posteriorly, the inferior border of the thyroid cartilage superiorly, and the superior border of the cricoid cartilage inferiorly.

The CTM is a fibroelastic membrane attached inferiorly to the thyroid cartilage and superiorly to the cricoid ring. It has a height between 0.5 and 1.0 cm vertically and a width of 2.0 to 3.0 cm horizontally. Once the CTM is incised, the posterior cartilaginous wall of the cricoid cartilage can be palpated through the CTM as a "hard stop" posteriorly within the surgical field. Finger palpation is a helpful confirmatory step prior to bougie insertion.

Thyroid Gland

The isthmus of the thyroid gland lies anterior to the trachea, generally between the second and third tracheal rings, although it may extend superiorly to the first ring. Its size and location varies; both its average height and thickness are 1.25 cm. A pyramidal lobe is present in 5% to 30% of the population and extends superiorly over the CTM and larynx. If identified in the surgical field, the thyroid gland can be retracted as it can bleed impressively. Pressure is all that is required until the airway is secured.

Surface Anatomy Landmarking

Landmarking refers to identifying the underlying structures in the neck. Although many resources regarding anterior neck anatomy include photos of well-defined neck anatomy, it is patients with obesity; features such as a thick, short neck; or a history of neck radiation or surgery that are more often associated with CVCO emergencies. Palpation of the CTM was first questioned by the important 2010 milestone article by Elliott et al.,[13] who found a 30% accuracy at identifying the CTM when 18 anaesthesia consultants or trainees assessed six participants with varied body mass

index (BMI). This sobering finding sparked a spate of literature. Regardless of specialty[15] and operator confidence, CTM palpation of females, regardless of BMI, is less than 50%.[27,28] Given the unreliability of identifying the CTM, it is not surprising that techniques relying on its cutaneous identification (e.g., wire-guided cricothyrotomy) have a lower success rate than those scalpel-based procedures that confirm anatomy after skin and subcutaneous tissue incision (Fig. 29.4).[29]

Perhaps palpating a membrane is the wrong approach. The negative space structures, such as the thyrohyoid membrane and the CTM, can be much more challenging to identify compared to palpating the surrounding cartilaginous structures. For this reason, we recommend palpation and identification of the cartilaginous structures prior to vertical neck incision. Cutaneous attempts at identifying the CTM prior to neck incision waste valuable time. Identification of the CTM should not be sought until after vertical neck incision.

During cricothyrotomy, an airway manager should remain at the head of the bed to continue oxygenation attempts via BVM or SGA insertion. A second airway manager should move to the side of the bed to initiate a surgical airway. An SGA may provide more benefit than simply an oxygenation device, early data show an inserted SGA may assist in laryngeal landmarking and anchoring of the laryngeal structures.[30]

Positioning the patient with their head in neutral position and the mentum above the level of the sternal notch will provide the optimal skin tension to palpate the underlying structures. However, the optimal position to perform a surgical airway is with the patient's neck extended. Ultrasound studies show that, with neck extension, the CTM may move superiorly, inferiorly, and remain in the same location depending on a multitude of factors including gender and neck dimensions.[31]

The following techniques should not further delay action but, rather, should enhance the efficiency and confidence of the provider tasked to perform the surgical airway. We recommend that advanced airway managers incorporate these physical exam maneuvers into their everyday practice. When required to perform the rare surgical airway, palpation will not delay but, rather, will enhance the confidence of the clinician as to location of their initial vertical neck incision.

1. Visual identification of neck creases[32]

   Most adults have three main horizontal neck creases. The midline of the second neck crease generally overlies the cricoid cartilage and can thus be used as a visual landmark for rapid, directed palpation of the cricoid cartilage.

2. Palpation at the sternal notch[33]

   Regardless of BMI, it is rare that the sternal notch cannot be identified. The sternal notch defines the midline. Identifying the sternal notch allows confirmation of the position of the trachea and larynx relative to the midline. The "finger stacking" technique can then be used: The clinician places the tip of their fifth digit in the sternal notch while proceeding to stack their remaining three fingers vertically up toward the larynx. The upper edge of the index finger should be at the level of the cricoid cartilage. This second step should closely approximate the visualized middle neck crease.

3. Laryngeal handshake[34]

   First described by Levitan, the "laryngeal handshake" is a technique that can be done concurrently with finger stacking. Using the nondominant hand, the arc-shaped hyoid bone is identified by bilateral palpation of the greater horns, which are then balloted back and forth as a confirmatory maneuver with the thumb and middle finger. The index finger can then palpate down the laryngeal structures, identifying the firm and raised positive spaces of the thyroid notch and cricoid cartilage. The laryngeal handshake can then be used to confirm that the visual identification of the cricoid via the neck creases and the finger stacking technique all coincide with the same point of confluence at the cricoid cartilage.

The laryngeal handshake is an essential component of the surgical steps for the cricothyrotomy as it immobilizes the larynx and allows for tactile feedback and reconfirmation of laryngeal landmarks once the incision is made.

Special Challenges in the Obese Patient

It is important to highlight the unique challenges of airway emergencies in the obese patient. As of 2022, obesity (BMI >30 kg/m²) affected 19% of the world's population, with 36% of the US population being obese.[35,36] Obesity is associated with many airway management–related complications and the increased need to rapidly deploy advanced airway rescue techniques, including a surgical airway. CVCO emergencies occur more often in male patients with thick, short necks; central obesity; and a history of obstructive sleep apnea; therefore, difficult surgical airway is the rule rather than the exception.[37]

Several specific obesity-related anatomic and physiologic challenges also complicate management. It is difficult to maintain oxygenation of the obese patient due to restrictive pulmonary function and ventilation/perfusion mismatch. Rapid desaturation will result in increased airway management urgency and potential need to provide cardiovascular support (e.g., atropine, epinephrine) to prevent asystole. Although the use of ultrasound in a CVCO emergency remains of questionable benefit, it is a very reasonable adjunct in the planning stages of airway management[38] of the obese patient, providing preinduction identification of airway structures to determine depth from skin to larynx and to identify the key landmarks should an emergency occur.[39–41]

Which side of the bed to stand on to perform a surgical airway with the best ergonomics depends on the airway manager. Akin to which hand drives a flexible scope, the choice of side and mechanics of the procedure must be practiced, and the ergonomics that work best for the operator should be decided upon long before the need to perform a surgical airway. This procedure and positioning as an airway manager should be practiced routinely to establish familiarity with the required dexterity and economy of motion to create a fluid transition to establishing a cricothyrotomy. From an ergonomic and anatomic perspective, most right-handed clinicians will be more comfortable on the patient's right side, and vice versa for left-handed clinicians. Following this positioning recommendation, the larynx would most readily be stabilized from above, creating many ergonomic advantages. First, stabilizing the larynx with the thumb and middle finger of the nondominant hand (laryngeal handshake) at the level of the thyroid cartilage is more secure than trying to stabilize the larynx from below. Second, the nondominant hand can maintain extension of the mandible with the hypothenar eminence resting on the chin. Third, the surgical airway incision can be made vertically downward toward the sternal notch, away from the airway manager's hand, rather than incising vertically upward and contending with the mandible and impeding smooth uniform hand motion if performed from the opposite side of the bed. There is always the potential for hands to cross no matter which side one

prefers, but frequent practice is essential to maximize efficiency and economy of motion. The benefits described would equally apply to the left-handed provider stepping to the left side of the patient.

In conclusion, being intimately familiar with laryngeal anatomy is essential when performing a surgical airway. As a rule, blood will be in the field. In the setting of upper airway obstruction, patients may breath stack and build up positive intrathoracic pressure. As the CTM is opened, it is not uncommon to have blood spray at the airway manager. This sensory-rich experience relies on interpreting with your mind's eye what you feel with your fingers.

Cricothyrotomy

An advanced airway manager may perform a cricothyrotomy once in their careers. Therefore, much of the published literature outside surgical fields is based on surveys and opinions or animal and nonanimal models. Given its infrequency, randomized trials of various techniques are not practical. Most patient-based research consists of retrospective or prospective case series.[29,42] Given the paucity of CVCO events requiring surgical airway, there is questionable utility of surveys that assess comfort or preference of a procedure that many airway practitioners have never performed. This leads to some controversy and confusion over which technique offers the highest first-pass success, shortest time to reoxygenation and reventilation, along with acceptable complication rates.

Until the previous decade, there was a paucity of patient-based evidence. Evidence regarding procedural human factors also plays a procedural role in decision-making. As this is a rare life-threatening event, stocking of equipment should prioritize those methods with these traits:

1. High first-pass success
2. Do not depend on visual input but can succeed via structural recognition by palpation to overcome the loss of visual cues in a blood-covered field
3. Do not depend upon accurate identification of the CTM prior to skin incision
4. Equipment stocked, at reasonable cost, in all airway management locations
5. A low risk of creating subcutaneous emphysema, which would obliterate neck landmarks leading to grave difficulty in securing the airway with an open technique

Recently, larger case series have been published evaluating success rates and complications using various cricothyrotomy techniques in actual CVCO emergencies.[29,43–45] It has been argued that anesthesiologists may be hesitant to use a scalpel; however, there can be little argument that all airway managers are motivated to perform the cricothyrotomy technique that has the highest success and lowest complication rates.[46] With the proper training, this hesitation can be overcome by dedicated simulation training on a regular basis. As with any procedure, without regular practice the confidence and the ability to landmark and to perform cricothyrotomy will not be adequate for patient care.[47]

Scalpel-Finger-Bougie Technique

A variant of the traditional surgical cricothyroid technique involves use of a bougie to guide introduction of an ETT into the trachea.[48] This technique is the preferred technique for surgical airway in the 2015 Difficult Airway Society guidelines.[9]

Assurance of neuromuscular blockade and oxygenation attempts though positive-pressure ventilation should continue. Following the landmarking techniques previously described, the patient's neck should be extended, if possible, to optimize access and tissue tension. A roll under the shoulders may be helpful to further optimize access to the anterior neck. Although many advocate for the use of prep solution and local anaesthesia prior to emergency surgical airway access, both require at least a 5-minute wait to achieve efficacy. According to manufacturer's instructions, the prep solution must be left to dry before an incision is made. Without drying, prep solutions render the surgical field slippery, making it that much more difficult to palpate and stabilize laryngeal structures. In a similar vein, injection of local anaesthesia distorts the subcutaneous tissues and may obscure palpation of landmarks more than it will provide localized vasoconstriction. It is inevitable that an emergent surgical airway will bleed, often spraying blood at the operator when the CTM is opened (due to positive intrathoracic pressure). The airway is not a sterile environment, and as such the procedure should never be delayed for either sterilization of the skin or injection of local anaesthetic.

Once landmarked and properly positioned, a midline vertical incision through the patient's skin and underlying soft tissue should be made over the larynx. Although it is difficult to state a specific incision size, it is not unreasonable to begin with at least a 4 to 6 cm incision,[49] centering the incision over the cricoid cartilage. This is a very rough estimate. Thicker necks will require a longer, more generous skin and subcutaneous fat incision as the incision tends to "cone down" as one cuts deeper through the tissues. Subcutaneous fat will not simply 'fall away' with incision but contains septa requiring repeated incisions through the fat itself in larger-necked patients. A larger belly blade, such as a number 10 or 15, would be an optimal blade choice, enhancing efficiency of every incision stroke. Although other blades will cut skin and other structures, an 11 blade is not made to cut thick layers of skin and tissue but, rather, is a precision blade for tiny, often delicate detail work and is

therefore ergonomically difficult. A 20 blade is large, generally used for pathology specimens, and would be cumbersome to use in an emergency. For these reasons, and its ubiquitous availability, a standard number 10 scalpel blade may be the best choice.

Once the skin and soft tissue have been incised, the CTM should be more palpable and recognized as the structural depression between the thyroid and cricoid cartilages. Care should be taken to ensure the membrane is *not* so superior (under the chin) that it may be the thyrohyoid membrane (Fig. 29.1B). Once the CTM is identified, a horizontal stab incision is made through the entire thickness and width of the membrane. This horizontal stab may result in an immediate spray of blood due to patient breath stacking from upper airway obstruction. Spraying of blood is a positive sign that the airway has been entered below the glottis. Universal precautions, including goggles or a visor along with a face mask, are recommended.

The next step may have some variation, dependent on the advanced airway practitioner's comfort and experience in performing a surgical procedure. The scalpel may be anchored laterally at the margins of the cut CTM to engage the cricothyroid joints and, thus, further open the cricothyroid space. If the practitioner is less confident or needing to identify a landmark internally, the scalpel can then be replaced by the airway manager's index finger in the cricothyroid space. Alternatively, the scalpel can be replaced by the airway manager's index finger to allow tactile confirmation of the cricothyroid space. Finger insertion will allow confirmation of airway access by palpation of the posterior wall of the cricoid cartilage and tracheal rings inferiorly. Given most practitioners' once-in-a-career experience of performing a cricothyrotomy. Given most practitioners' once-in-a-career experience of performing a cricothyrotomy, it is prudent for safety reasons to remove the scalpel from the field as soon as possible. Finger insertion will allow confirmation of airway access by palpation of the posterior wall of the cricoid cartilage and tracheal rings inferiorly. Insertion of a finger can also dilate the cricothyroid

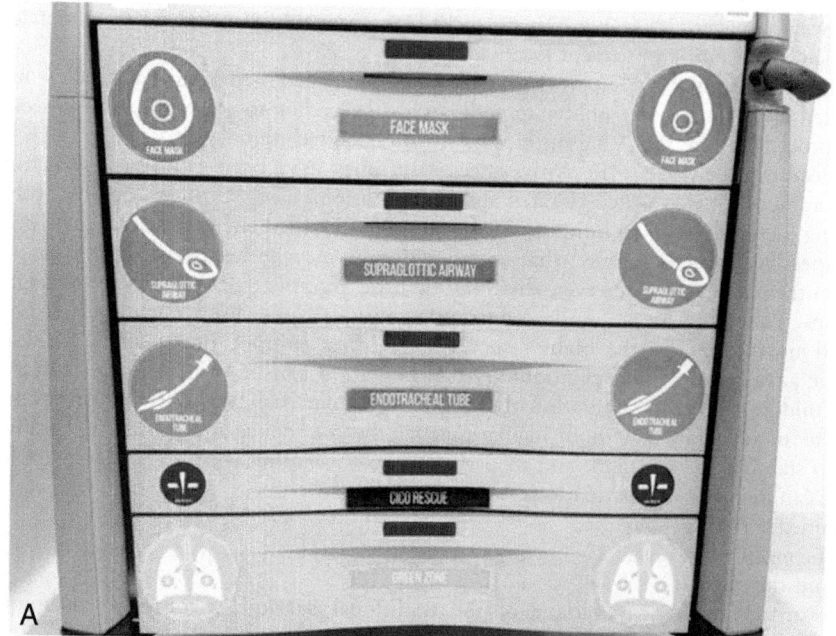
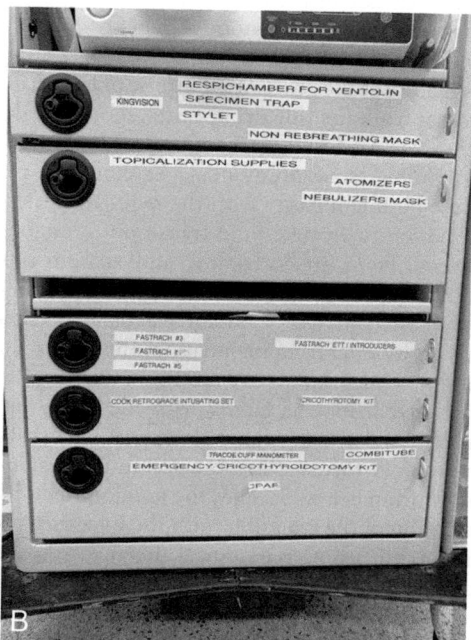

• **Fig. 29.3** (A) Icons and minimizing writing may assist team members locate appropriate equipment rapidly during an airway emergency. (Photo courtesy Dr. N. Chrimes.) (B) Versus writing alone.

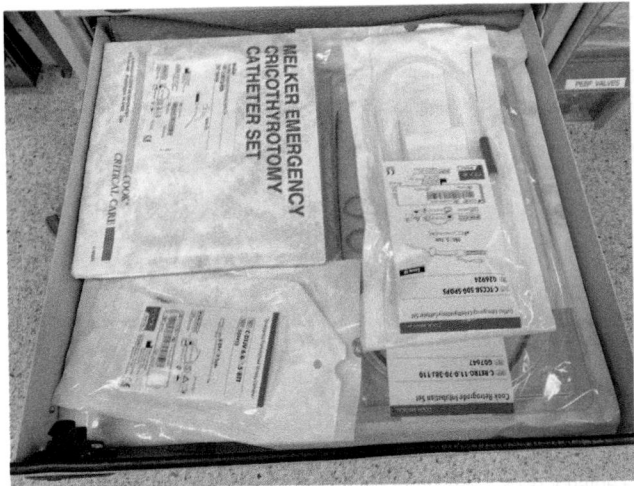

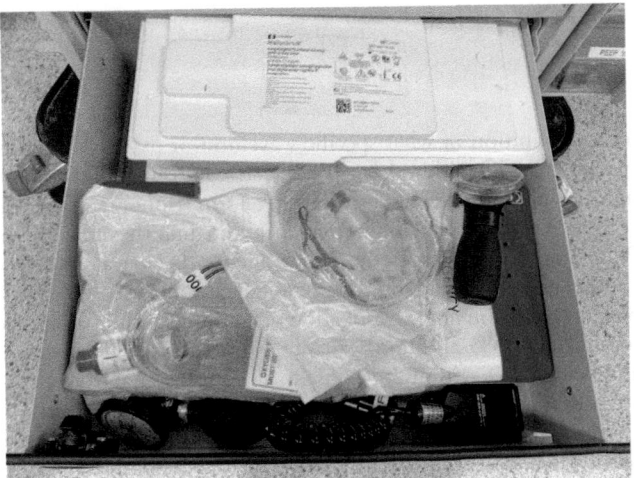

• **Fig. 29.4** Multiple choices of cricothyrotomy equipment may lead to device confusion and/or delay in initiation of the procedure. (Photo Courtesy of Dr. Laura Duggan.)

space by engaging the cricothyroid joints. The finger then serves as a guide for the bougie, which should now be inserted far enough that approximately 10 to 15 cm are in the patient's trachea. The bougie should pass freely; if resistance is met, depending on the angle of insertion this may indicate that either the bougie is in a false passage or is catching on the posterior tracheal wall. Palpation and insertion of the index finger into the cricothyroid space may greatly reduce the risk of these complications, especially when faced with an inability to visually identify the opening into the airway due to excessive soft tissue or bleeding.

A 6.0 cuffed ETT is then introduced over the bougie into the trachea. After tracheal tube insertion, the bougie is then removed, the ETT cuff is inflated, and confirmation of correct tracheal tube placement is made using waveform capnography. Even in cardiac arrest, an attenuated but reassuring square waveform should be visible.[50] Lack of waveform capnography would suggest some kind of lower airway obstruction. Suctioning of the ETT should be done immediately to ensure that blood has not clotting in or below the ETT from the potential for blood to pool in the distal airway. Bronchoscopy should also be considered, not only to confirm ETT placement but also to rule out an endobronchial tube insertion and to visually ensure that no blood clots remain in the airway. A chest

x-ray should be performed to rule out pneumothorax and, in the absence of bronchoscopic evaluation, can also be used to confirm ETT position in the trachea. The healthcare team should be aware that negative pressure pulmonary edema may occur after airway obstruction.[51] Securing of the ETT is akin to securing a chest tube and is best performed with a large figure-eight silk stitch once tracheal tube patency and placement have been confirmed.

Post-Cricothyrotomy Care

The long-term care of a surgical airway is beyond the scope of this chapter. However, appropriate attention to the surgical airway site should be continued once the patient is stabilized. Consulting the usual surgical airway practitioners as soon as possible, if they were not yet involved in the case, can lead to an assessment of the precise placement of the airway and determine whether the airway should be relocated to minimize the risk of developing long-term complications.

Contraindications to Cricothyrotomy

Although cricothyrotomy has been discussed at length, it should not be considered a panacea. Certain anatomic or physiologic conditions may contraindicate the performance of a cricothyrotomy. As noted in "History of the Surgical Airway," infection in the airway leading to airway obstruction can be temporized with a cricothyrotomy that should be converted to a tracheostomy within 24 hours. Cricothyrotomy depends on both the larynx and trachea being intact and contiguous. Fractures of the thyroid or cricoid cartilages are an absolute contraindication to cricothyrotomy (Fig. 29.5A, B, C). Attempts at cricothyrotomy when fractures of the larynx exist can result in transection of the airway and complete airway loss. Penetrating neck injuries showing signs of breaching the airway (e.g., subcutaneous emphysema) should be approached with caution as trauma may have occurred below the level of the larynx.

Human Factors in Surgical Airway Performance

"Human factors mean making it easy to do the right thing."
Martin Bromiley

"Making it easy to do the right thing" includes having easily understandable images instead of labels with words on difficult airway carts (Fig. 29.3) decreasing the need to assemble rarely used equipment during an emergency (Fig. 29.4), and decreasing the choices of equipment that may lead to confusing devices (Fig. 29.4). It is important to add new equipment to a difficult airway trolley when evidence deems it useful; however, it is even more important to remove equipment when it is deemed not to be useful. Moreover, by simplifying equipment, it becomes feasible to stock and maintain CVCO airway equipment (SGAs and surgical airway equipment; a #10 scalpel, bougie, and a 6.0 ETT) in every airway management location.

Management of CVCO emergencies have been included in airway guidelines since 1993 (ASA guidelines)[52]; focus has mainly centered on honing the airway manager's decision-making and technical skills. These 1993 airway guidelines were a huge step forward in patient care, as they provided a generalizable algorithm of decision-making during a high-stress situation where there previously were none. We now know relying solely on the skill set of the individual clinician to perform advanced airway management while maintaining situational awareness, engaging in clear closed-loop

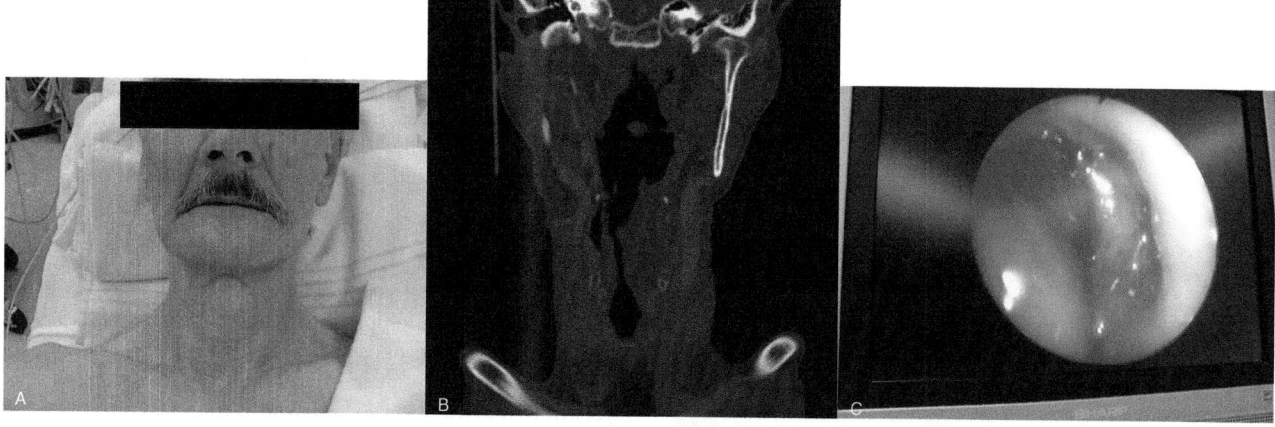

• **Fig. 29.5** (A) Blunt force trauma to the larynx resulting in shortness of breath lying down. No supplemental oxygen required. Tenderness on palpation of the anterior neck but no subcutaneous emphysema. (B) Coronal reconstruction CT scan reveals fractures of both thyroid and cricoid cartilages with a 4-mm-diameter airway. Should the patient deteriorate, a cricothyrotomy would be potentially lethal.

communication, and avoiding cognitive pitfalls and biases in decision-making during a CVCO emergency are fraught with error. No airway manager can manage a CVCO emergency alone.

Over 20 years later, the Difficult Airway Society was the first organization to include human factors in its 2015 guidelines for difficult management.[9] In 2021, the Canadian Airway Focus group emphasized the need to utilize the observations of all healthcare team members during airway emergencies.[23]

"The best people sometimes make the worst mistakes."

James Reason

The essential role human factors play in CVCO emergencies was highlighted by the heartbreaking death of Elaine Bromiley. She presented for an elective sinus operation in 2005 and died of hypoxemic brain injury. Involved in her care were multiple anaesthetists and an otolaryngologist, all with extensive experience and skills in airway management. None recognized the evolving CVCO emergency; none performed a surgical airway despite failure of BVM and SGA, and all perseverated with numerous attempts at TI despite both nonreassuring waveform capnography and ongoing hypoxemia.[53]

Perseveration has been elegantly defined as "the consistent application of any airway management technique or tool in three or more attempts without deviation of change, or return to a technique or tool that was previously unsuccessful."[10] Other healthcare professionals in the room recognized the CVCO emergency, but communication of their concerns was not heard, not understood, and/or not acted upon by the airway practitioners. The group of individual airway mangers simply lost situational awareness and, with it, effective communication and the ability to create a shared mental model with others in the room who saw more clearly what was occurring.[54]

In the enquiry that followed, multiple individuals involved discussed what they should have done and could not understand why they didn't act in a way they believed they should have.[55]

Recognizing an Evolving CVCO Emergency

A CVCO emergency is based on the objective data from waveform capnography and pulse oximetry, respectively. However, there is no set definition of what specific waveform or oxygen saturation specifies CVCO within these two objective measurements. It is not unreasonable to think that a flat waveform capnography signals complete obstruction somewhere between mouth and alveolus. Pulse oximetry values should also influence the airway manager's choice and speed of action: Decreasing below 90% to 92% should prompt attention and investigation of equipment and patient factors, below 85% additional airway assistance should be sought, and below 70% without response to all conventional oxygenation attempts a surgical airway should be initiated.

Elective, otherwise well patients comprise a surprisingly high proportion of anesthesia airway-related closed legal claims in Canada and the United States. Slow change blindness,[49] or the failure to obtain or understand information that is developing over time, versus a situation that occurs suddenly, may be a contributing factor. Readers are referred to the video *Change Blindness* to assess their own slow change blindness.[56] Context may also play a role; one may not expect airway difficulty in an elective patient with a reassuring preoperative airway exam.[57]

Calling for help upon early signs of trouble and engaging the helper in active, out-loud problem solving may be a useful mitigating strategy. However, this requires the primary airway manager to realize that they require help. Creating and adhering to standard operating procedures, or SOPs, and bypassing the need for a single person to make the decision to seek assistance may thereby be lifesaving (e.g., "The oxygen saturation is now 80%; insert an SGA and prepare the neck for cricothyrotomy."). SOPs decrease decision-making and cognitive load and do not rely solely on the primary airway manager to recognize or respond appropriately to the developing airway emergency. This approach, used in the London Air Ambulance Service, has resulted in very high cricothyrotomy success.[43]

Although some clinicians are concerned that adopting SOPs may reduce their autonomy, evidence that SOPs save lives is already recognized by most, if not all, healthcare institutions worldwide. The World Health Organization's surgical safety checklist SOP, including a discussion involving all healthcare team members and the patient prior to initiation of a procedure, halved inpatient mortality (1.5% to 0.8%) regardless of country.[58] As airway societies worldwide revise their guidelines to include various aspects of human factors, there is increased awareness that simplicity and the creation of SOPs will assist in predictable teamwork and may very well save lives.

Future Directions

Institutional readiness for a surgical airway event is comprised of multiple spheres: equipment availability, predictability, and generalizability in all airway management locations; individual and team practice of decision-making and motor skills; individual and team prediction and recognition of an emerging CVCO situation; and individual and team communication drills with standardized documentation to further enhance healthcare provider communication. Institutional support for the timely use of a surgical airway in CVCO emergencies is essential. Analogous to advanced cardiac life support or advanced trauma life support, team training in a simulation environment with clear roles, communication, and decision nodes may make the difference between life and death. Given the infrequency of surgical airway events, simulation of these events as a team, preferably as regular in situ simulation to discover possible weaknesses in the hospital system, is encouraged. Debriefing for quality improvement is invaluable, and exploring the experiences of patients and members of the healthcare team alike for research and teaching purposes is extremely helpful.

Conclusion

Emergency surgical airway management is a skill required of all advanced airway practitioners. Because it is rarely encountered, it is critical that the practitioners are trained in appropriate procedural skills to perform the technique in a critical situation. Emergency surgical airway management should usually be via cricothyroidotomy. These authors advocate training in the scalpel-bougie-finger technique as it is simple, easily trained, and associated with a high success rate. The most important aspect of surgical airway management is identifying when it should occur. The CVCO event may not be immediately recognized by the airway manager; the whole team should be empowered to declare such a surgical airway emergency. It is imperative that airway practitioners are sufficiently trained in identifying the CVCO event, understand the value and limitations of surface airway anatomy, learn the cricothyroidotomy technique, and rehearse team performance in simulated environments.

Selected References

3. DeVore EK, Redmann A, Howell R, Khosla S. Best practices for emergency surgical airway: a systematic review. *Laryngoscope Investig Otolaryngol.* 2019;4(6):602-608. doi:10.1002/lio2.314.

9. Frerk C, Mitchell VS, McNarry AF, et al. Difficult Airway Society 2015 guidelines for management of unanticipated difficult intubation in adults. *Br J Anaesth.* 2015;115(6):827–848, editorials: aev298, aev404. doi:10.1093/bja/aev371.

10. Joffe AM, Aziz MF, Posner KL, Duggan LV, Mincer SL, Domino KB. Management of difficult tracheal intubation. *Anesthesiology.* 2019;131(4):818-829. doi:10.1097/ALN.0000000000002815.

13. Elliott DSJ, Baker PA, Scott MR, Birch CW, Thompson JMD. ORIGINAL Accuracy of surface landmark identification for cannula cricothyroidotomy. *Anaesthesia.* 2010;65(9):889-894. doi:10.1111/j.1365-2044.2010.06425.x.

23. Law JA, Duggan LV, Asselin M, et al. Canadian Airway Focus Group updated consensus-based recommendations for management of the difficult airway: part 1. Difficult airway management encountered in an unconscious patient. *Can J Anesth.* 2021;68(9):1373-1404. doi:10.1007/s12630-021-02007-0.

29. Duggan LV, Lockhart SL, Cook TM. The Airway App: exploring the role of smartphone technology to capture emergency front-of-neck airway experiences internationally. 2018. Available at https://associationofanaesthetists-publications.onlinelibrary.wiley.com/doi/10.1111/anae.14247. https://doi.org/10.1111/anae.14247.

31. Dixit A, Ramaswamy KK, Perera S, Sukumar V, Frerk C. Impact of change in head and neck position on ultrasound localisation of the cricothyroid membrane: an observational study. *Anaesthesia.* 2019;74(1):29-32. doi:10.1111/anae.14445.

39. Kristensen MS, Teoh WH, Rudolph SS. Ultrasonographic identification of the cricothyroid membrane: best evidence, techniques, and clinical impact. *Br J Anaesth.* 2016;117:i39-i48. doi:10.1093/bja/aew176.

40. Siddiqui N, Yu E, Boulis S, You-Ten KE. Ultrasound is superior to palpation in identifying the cricothyroid membrane in subjects with poorly defined neck landmarks. *Anesthesiology.* 2018;129(6):1132-1139. doi:10.1097/ALN.0000000000002454.

43. Aziz S, Foster E, Lockey DJ, Christian MD. Emergency scalpel cricothyroidotomy use in a prehospital trauma service: a 20-year review. *Emerg Med J.* 2021;38(5):349-354. doi:10.1136/emermed-2020-210305.

50. Scarth E, Cook T. Capnography during cardiopulmonary resuscitation. *Resuscitation.* 2012;83(7):789-790. doi:10.1016/j.resuscitation.2012.04.002.

53. Bromiley M. *Just a Routine Operation.* YouTube. 2015. https://www.youtube.com/watch?v=JzlvgtPIof4.

All references can be found online at eBooks.Health.Elsevier.com.

30

Confirmation of Tracheal Intubation

TRACEY STRAKER, MAGED SOLIMAN, AND FELIPE URDANETA

CHAPTER OUTLINE

KEY POINTS

- Clinical signs to determine proper endotracheal tube (ETT) placement and positioning have limitations.
- Secondary confirmatory methods must be used in routine and emergent settings to minimize the chances of ETT misplacement or improper ETT depth.
- Exhaled CO_2 detection, especially by waveform capnography, is the most sensitive method to detect proper ETT placement in the respiratory tract.
- Exhaled CO_2 determines tracheal placement of the ETT but does not eliminate the possibility of endobronchial intubation.
- Exhaled CO_2 detection sensitivity decreases in cases with low or no pulmonary blood flow, such as during cardiac arrest.
- After nonelective intubations outside the operating room, when the ETT will remain in place for an undetermined length of time,
the use of chest x-ray (CXR) is recommended to confirm proper ETT depth.
- The use of ultrasonography as a confirmatory method of proper tracheal tube placement and depth is gaining popularity and has many advantages over traditional radiologic methods.
- Bilateral breath sounds do not always mean equal breath sounds and do not eliminate the possibility of an endobronchial intubation.
- A normal end-tidal CO_2 (EtCO$_2$) and capnogram waveform cannot exclude the possibility of endobronchial intubation. An increased EtCO$_2$, reduced EtCO$_2$, or abnormal capnogram should encourage consideration of endobronchial intubation in the differential diagnosis of hypoxia or increased peak inspiratory pressures.

Introduction

A fundamental tenet of elective and emergent airway management with tracheal intubation is the timely placement of the endotracheal tube (ETT) through the glottic opening, followed by confirmation of proper tube position. Inadvertent ETT misplacement, malposition, or dislodgment can have profound adverse clinical consequences. ETT misplacement occurs most commonly when inexperienced providers carry out intubation. However, it can even occur to seasoned veterans, especially in emergencies when airway management is performed in less-than-optimal conditions—for example, in the critically ill (including patients in cardiac arrest), in out-of-hospital intubations, and when difficulty visualizing the larynx is encountered.[1]

Unrecognized esophageal intubation (EI) is the most severe complication of attempted tracheal intubation. All practitioners who perform advanced airway maneuvers experience EIs during their careers. Most EIs are immediately and easily recognized. When accidental EI is not promptly recognized, it can result in grave consequences: rapid, irreversible clinical deterioration, esophageal perforation (especially with traumatic intubation attempts), cerebral anoxia, and death.[2,3] If the ETT is inserted too deeply into a mainstem bronchus, complications range in severity from mild hypoventilation and atelectasis of the nonventilated lung, to hyperinflation and pneumothorax of the ventilated lung with subsequent development of hypoxemia and hemodynamic instability. The ETT may also not be placed deeply enough (i.e., pharyngeal placement), which predisposes to emesis, aspiration, and laryngospasm. In every instance where advanced airway maneuvers and tracheal intubation are performed, there should be a plan for assessment of tube placement and determination of tube depth, as well as proper documentation of both activities.

An ideal, "silver bullet" method or device to detect successful tracheal intubation does not exist. There is no method sufficiently reliable to confirm proper ETT placement and position in all patients and all circumstances. Properly placed ETTs may become displaced at any time; therefore, constant vigilance and reconfirmation of tube position may be needed. Of the available techniques to detect ETT placement, some are primarily intended to detect and confirm the ETT presence in the respiratory tract and rule out EI, whereas others are meant to establish correct ETT depth within the trachea. Some techniques have a dual role.

This chapter will review past and current knowledge of malpositioning of ETTs and the currently recommended techniques for primary and secondary determination of their adequate placement and positioning. Emphasis has been placed on more recent evidence because monitoring and detection methods have advanced considerably since the introduction in 1986 of the American Society of Anesthesiologists (ASA) Standards for Basic Monitoring, including oxygenation, ventilation, circulatory, and temperature monitors. Exhaled carbon dioxide (CO_2) as a monitor for proper ETT placement and ventilation has been widely adopted. It is espoused by both the American Heart Association (AHA) and the European Council on Resuscitation.[4,5,6] Placement and positioning of double-lumen tubes are discussed elsewhere.

Overview

Tracheal intubation is considered the gold standard for advanced airway management. It can be performed in controlled settings, such as the operating room, or emergently, in and out of the hospital, in different circumstances, including trauma. Tracheal intubation is performed in all patient age groups by a diverse group of medical and paramedical providers with different skills, abilities, and procedural experience. Given the variety of circumstances, it is no surprise that the incidence of ETT malposition at the time of intubation or as a result of dislodgment after placement has been reported to be in the 4% to 26% range, with an incidence of accidental EI of 2.7% to 25%.[7,8] With significant advancements in airway management in the past three decades, and the introduction of mandatory ETT confirmation methods, the incidence of misplacement and malposition of ETT, including accidental EI, has decreased in all but the emergency setting and pediatrics. Airway management in the emergency setting is often performed in uncontrolled circumstances, in combative or intoxicated patients, or in tight spaces with decreased visibility. Transportation to or

within a medical facility also predisposes to malposition or displacement of ETTs.[1,9–12] Pediatric and neonatal patients have proportionately shorter tracheas and therefore are particularly vulnerable to ETT misplacement and dislodgment, even with mild head flexion and extension.[13–16]

Reports of Incidence of Endotracheal Tube Malposition

In recent decades, there has been considerable interest in understanding and attempting to limit the impact of adverse events related to airway management. Several large-scale efforts have been conducted since advanced airway maneuvers became popular in the second half of the 20th century. These efforts have been extensively studied and reported, mainly by the ASA Closed Claims Project in the United States, the Australian Incidence Monitoring Study in Australia (AIMS), the Canadian Medical Protective Association (CMPA), the Denmark National Board of Patients' Complaints (NBPC), and more recently the Fourth National Audit Project (NAP4) of the Royal College of Anaesthetists and the Difficult Airway Society.[17–22] Major complications in airway management are rare but carry a high degree of mortality. They cover a broad spectrum of injuries ranging from mild, transitory, nonlife-threatening reversible issues to irreversible ones, such as brain damage and death. They are frequently associated with medicolegal issues and costly malpractice claims.

There are two primary sources of information for studies of airway-related complications: litigation-based retrospective reviews and critical incident analyses. These resources share the same goal of identifying problem areas related to different aspects of anesthetic care and analyzing patterns of injury so that strategies for prevention can be devised.

The nature of anesthesia malpractice claims has changed considerably since the 1970s. Modern respiratory monitoring (i.e., capnography for ventilation and pulse oximetry for oxygenation) was introduced in 1986 and adopted as part of the standard of care. In 1993, the ASA Task Force on Management of the Difficult Airway introduced Practice Guidelines for Management of the Difficult Airway. Since the introduction of the guidelines, significant complications, such as death and brain damage, have declined. Respiratory and airway-related events continue to be an important source of adverse events, according to the latest ASA closed claims analysis published in 2011, representing events from 1970 through 2007. Respiratory management issues, including airway management, accounted for 17% of claims in 2011, compared with 34% in Caplan's original report in 1990.[23] The most common respiratory events leading to anesthesia claims since 1990 were difficult intubation, inadequate oxygenation or ventilation, and pulmonary aspiration.[24] In the original report, accidental EI (the most severe and lethal of all adverse events related to ETT misplacement) was reported in 18% of cases, and was considered the third most common event related to airway management. Since that time, EI has decreased to 5%, which is a significant improvement and a practice management success.[25]

Almost any practitioner who has attempted tracheal intubation has experienced incidents of EI. This is for the most part harmless; what is of concern and a significant cause of litigation is placing an ETT in the esophagus and not recognizing it promptly before undue harm occurs. Unrecognized EI continues to be a problem because of its associated lethality and liability, especially in cases outside the operating room, in the emergency department, and in critical care and trauma settings. EI also has been reported consistently in all databases: The 2005 CMPA report showed that in 9 of the 16 cases where airway management was a central issue of litigation, EI occurred; the AIMS study revealed that there were 35 incidents of EI, which constituted 1.75% of all adverse events reported; NAP4 included 11 EIs resulting in 6 deaths.[26,27] Failure to detect adequate ETT placement and exclusion of EI constitute avoidable diagnostic errors that are usually caused by failure to adequately interpret clinical signs and confirm ETT placement with secondary methods.

Primary Endotracheal Detection Techniques

No technique for confirmation of tracheal intubation is 100% reliable in all circumstances and age groups; therefore, the use of multiple available confirmatory methods is recommended when attempting to confirm the placement of ETTs. Even though the clinical determination of proper ETT placement should be performed in all instances, none of the primary clinical modalities (visualization of the ETT passing through the vocal cords, auscultation of bilateral breath sounds, humidification of the ETT, chest wall movement, and lack of abdominal distention) alone or in combination are sufficiently accurate to determine proper ETT placement and position, and, given their subjectivity, they must be accompanied and supplemented by rapid secondary point-of-care methods and techniques.

Endotracheal Tube Visualization

Visualization of the ETT passing through the vocal cords during any type of laryngoscopy is a primary technique to determine proper placement of the ETT but is fallible, does not determine proper positioning, and does not exclude dislodgement either before or after the ETT has been secured. Visualization of the ETT as it passes through the vocal cords is an operator-dependent method, and the success and effectiveness vary depending on the skill and experience of the provider performing the laryngoscopy. It is less accurate in cases of difficult laryngoscopy when there is a limited view of the glottic opening as a result of anatomic distortion or the presence of secretions, vomitus, or blood.[28] It may be more accurate with the use of indirect laryngoscopy (e.g., video-assisted laryngoscopy [VAL]) given the improved glottic view compared with line-of-sight techniques such as direct laryngoscopy (DL). The benefits of VAL are more prominent when dealing with difficult intubations and in cases with limited glottic visualization (i.e., Cormack-Lehane grades III or IV). The improved view afforded by VAL can turn blind intubation into successful intubation under visual control (Fig. 30.1). In a recent meta-analysis, De Jong and colleagues compared DL with VAL in the critical care setting. They reported a reduction of difficult intubation by 29%, a decrease in the incidence of Cormack-Lehane grade III or IV views by 26%, and a decrease the incidence of EI by 14%.[29] Mosier and colleagues compared VAL use with DL and found that the first-attempt success rate for VAL was 78.6% versus 60.7% and that the use of VAL reduced the EI rate from 12.5% with DL to 1.3%.[30] Kory and colleagues reported a 14% incidence of EI with the use of DL compared with 0% for VAL in a cohort of critical care patients.[31]

Auscultation

Routine auscultation at one or two points on each side of the chest and over the epigastrium is recommended to establish

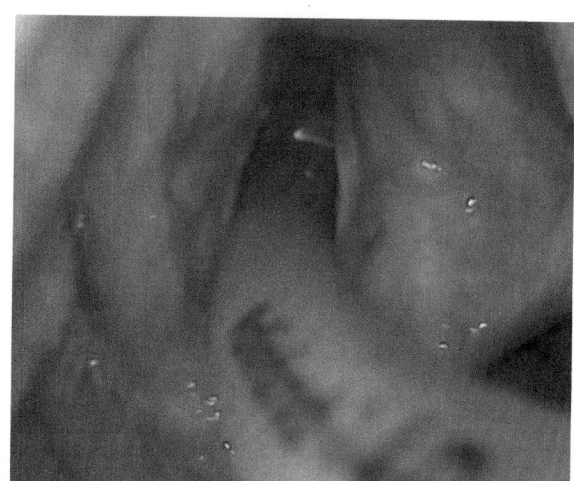

• **Fig. 30.1** Indirect (videolaryngoscopic) view of the glottic opening with the endotracheal tube and cuff visible beyond the vocal cords.

proper ETT placement and position. Auscultation is widely used and is a cost-effective and straightforward method to confirm ETT placement; however, it also has its limitations. Anecdotal reports show that errors during auscultation constitute a significant source of litigation and a cause of undetected accidental EI. In the 1990 ASA closed claims analysis, Caplan noted that auscultation was reported as normal in 48% of cases involving EI.[17] Normal breath sounds can be transmitted to the epigastric area, and gastric sounds can be transmitted to the chest wall, resulting in false-negative and false-positive readings, respectively.[32] Esophageal sounds (sounds generated when the ETT enters the esophagus) can be transmitted to the chest wall of smaller patients because of the anatomic proximity of the esophagus and trachea in children[28] and may be misinterpreted as pulmonary in origin. Normal breath sounds can also be easily transmitted to the epigastrium (mainly when uncuffed ETTs are used), potentially leading to an erroneous diagnosis of EI.[15] In cases of hiatal hernia, gastric pull-through, diaphragmatic hernia, or gastric distention, the presence of gastric viscera in the thoracic cavity can predispose practitioners to a false determination of respiratory tract placement after EI.

Auscultation is also limited in detecting mainstem intubation; breath sounds from one lung can be transmitted to the opposite side of the chest in the case of mainstem intubation.[33] Other limitations of auscultation include its operator dependency, and its greater accuracy when performed by experienced providers. In a study set in the intensive care unit (ICU), Knapp and colleagues demonstrated that experienced examiners were correct in all attempts at auscultation to determine the presence of the ETT in the trachea or in the esophagus, but inexperienced examiners were incorrect in 32% of cases.[34] Auscultation is limited in noisy environments or when dealing with morbidly obese, cachectic, or pediatric patients. Air rescue missions, because of the high ambient noise and the requirement to wear helmets during flight, demand specialized equipment. In two reports by Grmec, auscultation was less sensitive and specific to detect proper ETT placement than end-tidal CO_2 (EtCO$_2$) during emergency intubations in the field.[89] Although it is encouraged that all providers attempt to detect proper ETT placement with the help of auscultation, it is recommended that other secondary methods be performed routinely given the inherent limitations of this method.

Condensation in the Endotracheal Tube

Although the presence of water vapor condensation is a sign many intubation practitioners routinely rely upon, and it may indicate the presence of the ETT in the respiratory tract, it is not a reliable indicator to rule out EI or to confirm adequate ETT depth within the trachea. Cases of ETT humidification despite EI have been reported,[32] and the presence of ETT fogging cannot establish correct midtracheal positioning of an ETT. In an animal study, Kelly and colleagues detected ETT humidification in 83% of tubes placed in the esophagus and concluded that the presence of condensation should not be used as the sole clinical indicator to determine correct ETT placement.[35]

Abdominal Distention and Chest Wall Movement

Abdominal distention versus symmetric chest movements with positive pressure ventilation can distinguish between esophageal and tracheal intubation in normal circumstances; however, in obese patients, obstetric patients, patients with large breasts, patients with chest wall pathology, or when there is an alteration of lung compliance, neither abdominal distention nor chest wall movement is a reliable clinical sign of adequate ETT placement and position. Likewise, as can occur with auscultation (see Auscultation), the presence of gastric viscera in the thoracic cavity can lead to thoracic movement despite EI, which can therefore be misinterpreted as proper ETT placement.[36] Gastric distention could occur during mask ventilation and be subsequently mistaken for EI after intubation. Prior placement of a gastric drainage tube (i.e., an oral or nasogastric tube) can lead to decompression and, therefore, decrease the reliability of gastric distention as a clinical sign of accidental EI.

Secondary Endotracheal Detection Techniques

Several other methods and secondary adjuncts have been developed because of limitations with clinical primary detection methods for proper ETT placement. Some of these techniques are used more to determine proper ETT placement, others to determine ETT position, and some serve both purposes. Secondary techniques for the determination of endotracheal placement include detection of the presence of CO_2 in exhaled gases, the use of esophageal detection devices, transtracheal illumination, pulse oximetry, imaging techniques (e.g., chest x-ray [CXR] and tracheal ultrasonography [USG]), and flexible bronchoscopy.

Carbon Dioxide in Exhaled Gases

Confirmation of proper ETT placement should be completed in all patients at the time of initial intubation. Physical examination methods, such as auscultation of the chest and epigastrium, visualization of thoracic movement, and fogging in the tube, are not sufficiently reliable to confirm ETT placement. Similarly, pulse oximetry and chest radiography are not reliable as sole techniques to determine ETT location. Exhaled CO_2 detection is the most accurate method to evaluate ETT position in patients with adequate tissue perfusion. Capnography is a noninvasive, versatile monitoring modality that allows fast and reliable insight into ventilation, circulation, and metabolism. Detection and measurement of exhaled CO_2 are used to detect EI (or the

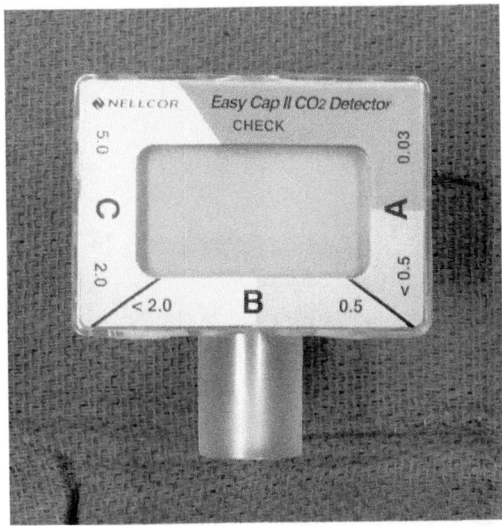

• **Fig. 30.2** Colorimetric CO_2 detector with purple coloring indicating an end-tidal CO_2 concentration less than 0.5%, or 3 mm Hg.

proper placement of alternative advanced airway devices such as supraglottic airways) and for continuous assessment of the ventilatory status of both intubated and nonintubated patients. If used continuously, capnography can detect ETT dislodgement or migration after head movement or rotation or when the patient is repositioned or moved.[37] It also provides information regarding how effectively CO_2 is being transported in the blood and how effectively normal metabolic processes produce it. When CO_2 is absent as measured by end-tidal capnography, it may mean the ETT is in the wrong position (EI) or pulmonary blood flow is absent or low, as can occur during shock, cardiac arrest, or cardiopulmonary resuscitation (CPR) with inadequate chest compressions.

Exhaled CO_2 concentration reaches a maximal level at the end of exhalation; this maximum concentration is referred to as the $EtCO_2$. Exhaled CO_2 can be measured by colorimetry, capnometry, and capnography. CO_2 monitors are either quantitative or qualitative. Qualitative devices report a range in which the $EtCO_2$ falls (e.g., 0 to 15 mm Hg or 15 to 303 mm Hg) instead of a precise value, as with quantitative devices.

The most used qualitative capnometry device is the colorimetric $EtCO_2$ detector. This device is used for initial confirmation of ETT placement when waveform capnography is not available, such as in prehospital or emergency settings (Fig. 30.2). Colorimetric devices have a transparent plastic dome over a filter paper specially treated with a pH-sensitive indicator that changes color when exposed to CO_2. Upon exposure to exhaled air, it will turn purple for $EtCO_2$ less than 0.5% or 3 mm Hg; tan for $EtCO_2$ in the 0.5% to 2% or 3- to 15-mm Hg range; and yellow for $EtCO_2$ greater than 2% or 15 mm Hg (Fig. 30.3). Colorimetric devices are considered less accurate compared with waveform capnography, and their use is a Class IIa recommendation by the AHA and European Resuscitation Council.[4–6,38–40]

Quantitative devices measure expired CO_2 either as a number (capnometry) or as a number and a waveform (capnography). A normal capnogram has a roughly rectangular-shaped pattern with four distinct phases (Fig. 30.4). There is normally a 0- to 5-mm Hg gradient between exhaled CO_2 and the arterial concentration of CO_2 ($Paco_2$), which corresponds to the alveolar dead space. Waveform capnography is considered the most reliable method to confirm

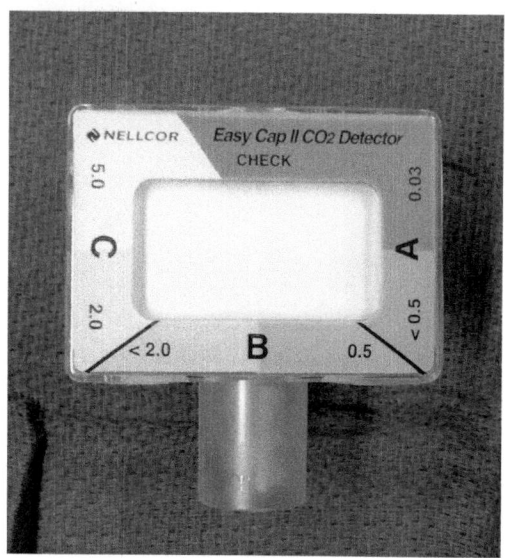

• **Fig. 30.3** Colorimetric CO_2 detector with yellow coloring indicating an end-tidal CO_2 concentration greater than 2%, or 15 mm Hg.

and monitor ETT placement, and since 2010 is considered a Class 1 recommendation by the AHA during CPR [4,5,38,39]

Following intubation, a normal four-phase capnogram typically indicates that the ETT is through the glottic opening. A normal capnogram does not indicate whether the ETT has been placed at an adequate depth in the midtrachea above the carina, because an ETT placed in a mainstem bronchus can still produce a normal waveform. In cases where the ETT has been placed in the hypopharynx, a normal-appearing waveform may be present for a few breaths, but the waveform changes over time and is likely to become erratic, a result of displacement of the ETT. The absence of $EtCO_2$ or a flat-line waveform generally indicates esophageal placement. Other conditions, such as cardiac arrest, also produce a flat waveform capnogram that must be ruled out by other means. Inadequate pulmonary blood flow, as can occur

with poor chest compressions during CPR, severe bronchospasm, ETT obstruction by a foreign body, blood clot, or large mucous plug, and malfunction of the monitor or tubing can all produce a flat waveform capnogram. Asai and Shingu reported an unusual case of a normal capnogram despite EI after attempted nasotracheal intubation in a patient with a cuffed oropharyngeal airway (COPA) placed before the induction of anesthesia. Initially a normal capnogram waveform suggested successful tracheal intubation; however, the waveform disappeared once the oropharyngeal airway cuff was inflated. In this case, the mechanism was thought to be expired CO_2 pooling in the pharynx as a result of obstruction by the COPA, which was then aspirated into the esophagus during spontaneous ventilation.[41]

In patients not in cardiac arrest, the use of qualitative colorimetric and quantitative exhaled CO_2 detection has been reported to be 100% sensitive and 100% specific for confirming ETT placement in the respiratory tract and ruling out placement of the tube outside the trachea. The sensitivity for determination of correct ETT placement in cardiac arrest patients ranges from 62% to 100%.[42-44] The sensitivity of waveform capnography decreases after a prolonged cardiac arrest. In this scenario, pulmonary blood flow is considerably reduced, even with high-quality CPR, and this accounts for failure to detect exhaled CO_2 despite a correctly placed ETT. However, providers should never assume that a flat capnogram is due to very low pulmonary flow and should instead rule out EI by other primary and secondary methods; if the ETT is in the esophagus, the provider should reattempt intubation of the trachea.

Quantitative capnography has a higher sensitivity than qualitative readings during low perfusion states and CPR because the exhaled CO_2 concentration can fall below the colorimetric threshold. Also, colorimetric and nonwaveform CO_2 detection techniques are not sufficiently accurate to be used as continuous ETT monitors.[44] Although $EtCO_2$ detection has a high positive predictive value during normal perfusion states, the positive predictive value is lower during cases of low or no perfusion, and CO_2 can be detected even in the setting of EI (e.g., in cases of ingestion of large amounts of carbonated liquids or antacids shortly before cardiac

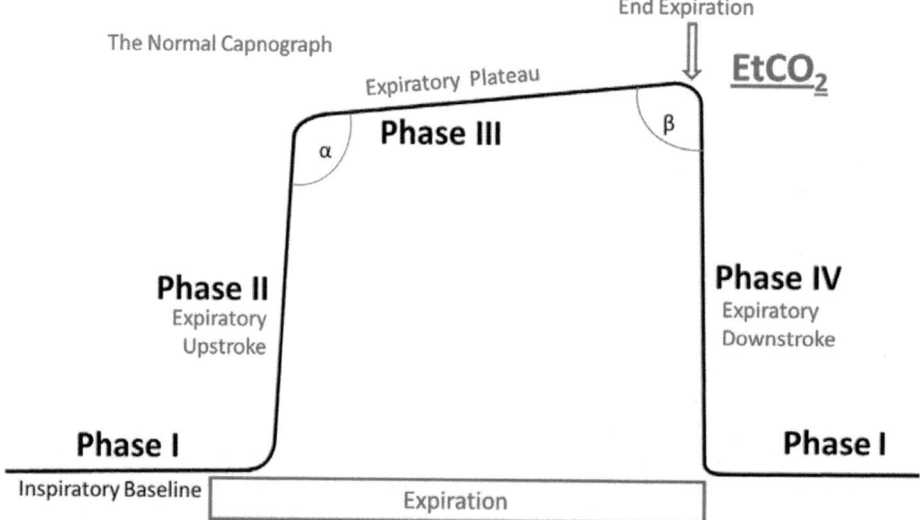

• **Fig. 30.4** A normal capnogram waveform with four distinct phases. (From Manifold CA, Davids N, Villers LC, Wampler DA. Capnography for the nonintubated patient in the emergency setting. *J Emerg Med.* 2013;45(4):626–632.)

arrest or during instances of prolonged mask ventilation with gastric insufflation and distention).[45] In all patients, but specifically in cardiac arrest patients, alternative objective methods for ETT placement and position should be used because there are known limitations to detection of exhaled CO_2.

The International Liaison Committee on Resuscitation (ILCOR) Advanced Life Support Task Force recommends using waveform capnography to confirm and continuously monitor ETT position during CPR in addition to clinical assessment (strong recommendation, low-quality evidence). Waveform capnography is prioritized, given it also has other potential uses during CPR, such as monitoring ventilation rate, assessing the quality of CPR, and predicting the return of spontaneous circulation. If waveform capnography is not available, a nonwaveform CO_2 detector, esophageal detector device (EDD), or USG, in addition to clinical assessment, is an alternative to capnography.[6,40] Even though these recommendations have been in effect since 2010, Turle and colleagues, in a recent study in the United Kingdom, reported that capnography was not available in 67% of hospital wards and one of the ICUs surveyed.[46]

Esophageal Detector Device

The EDD is a complementary device that has been mainly used in the prehospital setting for detecting CO_2 in exhaled gases in order to rule out EI. It is an inexpensive, easy to use, requires no power source, and can be used in all levels of light and during emergencies both in and out of the hospital. It is essentially a self-inflating bulb designed to detect the presence of the ETT in the trachea and not in the esophagus. The EDD is not as reliable as $EtCO_2$ determinations for verifying tracheal intubation in patients with adequate tissue perfusion and therefore is more useful during CPR when exhaled CO_2 might be affected by a lack of pulmonary perfusion. The EDD is unaffected by ingested carbonated beverages and antacids, by the presence of a nasogastric tube, or by ETT cuff deflation.

Originally, the EDD consisted of a 60-mL syringe with an adapter for the 15-mm ETT connector. After tracheal intubation, and before initiating positive-pressure ventilation, aspiration of gas with minimal resistance when withdrawing the syringe plunger would indicate that the ETT was placed correctly in the lungs. In EI, withdrawal of the plunger would cause apposition of the walls of the esophagus, occluding the lumen around the ETT and creating negative pressure and resistance as the plunger is pulled back.

The EDD was modified by replacing the syringe with a self-inflating bulb; the bulb has a capacity of 75 to 90 mL. After intubation, the device, fitted with a standard ETT adapter, is connected to the ETT, and the bulb is compressed. If the ETT is in the trachea, inflation of the bulb will occur; if the ETT is in the esophagus, the bulb will remain collapsed.[47] Reinflation of the bulb within 5 seconds is considered a positive result for tracheal intubation; inflation between 5 and 30 seconds is considered delayed although still consistent with endotracheal placement; and a lack of inflation, or inflation taking longer than 30 seconds, is indicative of EI.[48] This technique has been further modified by compressing the bulb before, rather than after, connecting it to the ETT. If the bulb is compressed after connection to the ETT, a volume of gas is introduced into the airway before the self-inflating bulb generates negative pressure, which could lead to a false-positive result.[49] In one of the original studies, Wee reported excellent performance of the EDD with 99 out of 100 first-attempt

correct identifications of ETT placement (51 esophageal and 48 tracheal), and a mean time to correct diagnosis of 6.9 seconds (range: 5–16 seconds).[50] In a study of 500 patients, Zaleski and colleagues determined that the sensitivity and specificity of the EDD was 100%.[48]

Problems with the use of the EDD have been reported as mainly attributable to false-negative results (i.e., the ETT is placed within the respiratory tract, but the device fails to detect it). False-negative results have been seen in infants in whom the tracheal wall is not held open by cartilaginous rings,[15,51] in patients with marked reduction of functional residual capacity (e.g., the morbidly obese), in obstetrics during cesarean section, and in the presence of pulmonary edema, adult respiratory distress syndrome, and severe bronchospasm.[52] Slow or absent reinflation of the bulb has been described if the ETT bevel is placed at the carina or if the ETT is in a mainstem bronchus. False-positive results (i.e., the ETT is placed in the esophagus but the bulb inflates) have been seen in cases when bag-mask ventilation before intubation has resulted in gastric distention and insufflation[53] or when the EDD is incompletely attached to the ETT, allowing air to enter the bulb.[54]

Currently, the EDD should be used only as an adjunct to other methods for ETT confirmation. According to the AHA and ILCOR Resuscitation Guidelines, it can be used as the initial method for confirming ETT placement, in addition to clinical assessment, in victims of cardiac arrest when waveform capnography is not available (Class IIa recommendation).[4,38]

Transtracheal Illumination

Although lighted stylets have traditionally been used as guides for intubation, transillumination can also be used to detect tracheal intubation and exclude EI. With transillumination, if a lighted stylet is placed in the trachea during or after tracheal intubation, the stylet should emit an intense, midline glow in the anterior neck above the suprasternal notch; if the lighted stylet is placed in the esophagus, the light will either be diminished or absent, or the beam will be diffuse or dull. Typically, light transmission is dependent on the intensity of the light, ambient light conditions, the proximity of the tissue to the light source, and the thickness and color of the tissue itself. In the presence of a large neck, a large goiter, neck swelling, limited neck extension, dark skin, or bright ambient light, the intensity of the transilluminated light may be affected, and therefore the accuracy and sensitivity of the technique are limited. Evidence of the effectiveness of transillumination as a technique to distinguish between tracheal and esophageal ETT placement is limited. Mehta studied tracheal transillumination in 420 patients; he graded the technique as excellent in 81% of patients and good in 19%. Transesophageal illumination could not be demonstrated in any patient. He concluded that the method was simple, effective, and reliable for the recognition of tracheal intubation.[55]

Knapp and colleagues studied four different ETT detection methods: auscultation, $EtCO_2$, EDD, and transillumination. Of all the techniques, transillumination had the highest incidence of false results as interpreted by both novice and experienced providers.[34] False-positive results have also been reported in thin patients. With the introduction of newer intubation devices such as videolaryngoscopes, lighted stylets are used less commonly, especially in the hospital setting. Several commercially available stylets have been discontinued, and evidence for the effectiveness of newer, currently available devices is limited.

Pulse Oximetry

Oxygen saturation by pulse oximetry (SpO_2) monitoring is not a confirmatory method for ETT placement and position, but it is discussed here because it is part of standard respiratory monitoring that can provide valuable information. With the adoption in 1986 of modern standards for respiratory monitoring by the ASA to improve patient safety, the use of pulse oximetry and the identification of CO_2 in expired gases became standard respiratory monitors in surgical patients. Initially, these monitors were used primarily in the hospital setting and in the operating room, but since then their use has extended beyond the operating room and hospital; they have been advocated by members of ILCOR when airway management is performed in both hospital and out-of-hospital settings. Desaturation, as indicated by pulse oximetry, is a relatively late manifestation of incorrect ETT placement; therefore, it should be used as a complementary respiratory monitor to $EtCO_2$ and to determine the level of oxygenation. Without pulse oximetry, hypoxemia may not be clinically apparent until it is profound and tissue hypoxia has begun; this would lead to an unacceptable delay in the diagnosis of accidental EI. Normal pulse oximetry readings immediately after intubation should not be taken as evidence of successful tracheal intubation. The use of SpO_2 monitoring has not decreased the incidence of difficult intubation or the incidence of medical liability associated with cases of EI. SpO_2 monitoring during advanced airway maneuvers must be complemented by other primary and secondary methods of confirmation of tracheal intubation, particularly the detection of expired CO_2.[15]

Chest Radiography

Radiography of the chest, or CXR, is used to detect proper ETT depth and perhaps dictate the need for ETT repositioning; however, unless fluoroscopic equipment is immediately available with no delay in obtaining the images, CXR is not a technique for immediate confirmation of tracheal intubation. CXR is time-consuming, not foolproof, and should not be relied upon to diagnose EI, even in the critical care setting.

Ultrasonography

The use of quantitative capnography has been recommended as the gold standard for confirming proper ETT placement; however, it has multiple limitations: false-positive readings when the tip of the ETT is in the hypopharynx and false negatives in cardiac arrest, low cardiac output, or low or absent pulmonary blood flow, which may lead to the unnecessary removal of a well-placed ETT. Capnography also requires administering positive-pressure ventilation to confirm that the ETT is in place, which may lead to abdominal distention, emesis, aspiration, or esophageal rupture in case of EI. Unlike capnography, confirmation of ETT placement via USG is independent of adequate pulmonary blood flow and CO_2 in exhaled gas and can be used directly without ventilation.

USG has several advantages for imaging of the airway, particularly in emergency settings: It is portable, safe, and quick and allows dynamic real-time visualization as the tube enters the trachea or esophagus; it also has no limitations of use in noisy environments. Tracheobronchial USG has excellent specificity for EI detection. USG offers two methods of assessing proper ETT tube placement: direct and indirect. The direct method involves assessing the trachea with USG to confirm the presence of the ETT within the

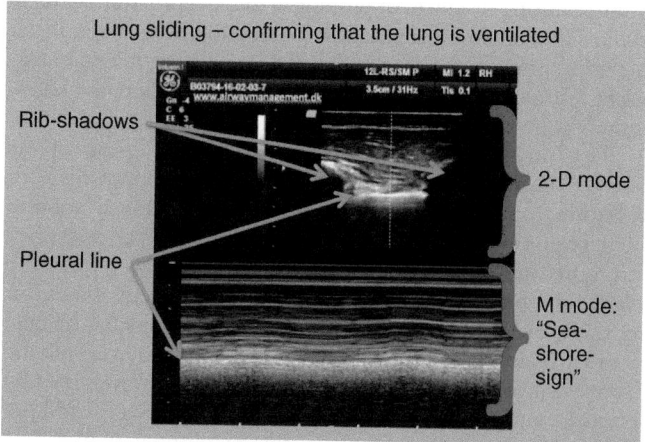

• **Fig. 30.5** Ultrasound showing bilateral "lung-sliding," a sign of normal endotracheal tube placement and positioning. (Image courtesy Dr. Michael Seltz-Kristensen.)

airway. The indirect method to assess proper ETT placement is to determine pleural and diaphragmatic movements indicating lung expansion. Bilateral lung sliding and equal diaphragmatic movement synchronized with ventilation can be seen if the ETT is in the trachea (see Chapter 3). Unlike the direct tracheal USG method, the indirect method can confirm ETT position by distinguishing between tracheal and endobronchial intubation (Fig. 30.5).

A recent meta-analysis of direct and indirect ultrasonographic methods for assessing ETT placement found a high diagnostic sensitivity (93%) and specificity (97%); therefore, these techniques are very useful for identifying EI, particularly in situations where capnography may be unreliable. Attending physicians demonstrated superior sensitivity (98%) compared with resident physicians (92%); a lower sensitivity was found in the emergency department than in other settings.[56] In one of the included studies, the Tracheal Rapid Ultrasound Examination (TRUE), which uses a transducer placed transversely over the suprasternal notch, had an overall accuracy of 98.2% with a median time to perform the exam of 9 seconds.[57] In a recent study with 115 patients, the overall accuracy of ultrasound to confirm tracheal intubation by indirect methods (pleural sliding) was 88.7% with a positive predictive value of 94.7%.[58]

The use of USG or any other technique as a sole test for detection of EI is not recommended. USG is not foolproof and has several limitations: It is an operator-dependent technique because the accuracy and speed of obtaining and interpreting images vary among providers; the equipment is expensive and fragile and must be immediately available and turned on because of the need for the machine to warm up; it requires training and experience; and no clear guidelines for training requirements or certification have been established or adequately studied, given its recent adoption. USG also requires a second provider to perform the examination during the intubation attempt because the sensitivity of real-time imaging is higher than determining placement after intubation.[59] Current evidence on the use of USG is promising and exciting, but there is insufficient evidence to endorse its widespread use and implementation to detect proper ETT placement.

Flexible Bronchoscopy

Flexible bronchoscopy is perhaps the gold standard for confirming proper ETT placement and position; it is the only direct method for accomplishing this and is independent of physiologic parameters. This technique is mainly used in the operating room to confirm proper positioning of double-lumen tubes used for lung isolation, but it is also used for single-lumen tubes in the operating room, critical care unit, emergency department, and out-of-hospital settings. One advantage of bronchoscopic direct examination of the airway is that it is not only used to confirm ETT placement and position but can also be used to examine a patient's airway for evidence of trauma, aspiration, or the presence of foreign bodies. Visualization of tracheal rings and positioning the ETT tip at least 2 cm, but no more than 6 cm above the carina (with the head in a neutral position), is one of the more accurate methods for adequate ETT placement in adult patients. For emergent intubations, this method is only convenient if the bronchoscopy equipment is readily available. The presence of blood or secretions can decrease the technique's effectiveness, but the identification of tracheal rings can usually still be accomplished.

Several alternative video-enabled airway devices have been used to confirm ETT placement. Weiss in 1998 described the technique of video-intuboscopy using a malleable metallic element with a thin fiberoptic component bound by a plastic case and forming an optical stylet. It had the advantage of not only helping to guide the laryngoscopic intubation procedure but also to provide instant confirmation of ETT placement.[60] Sum Ping and colleagues used the Rapiscope device (Cook Critical Care, Bloomington, IN) to verify ETT placement, and determined that the technique was 100% sensitive and 96% specific with a mean time to recognize structures of 22 seconds.[61] Angelotti and colleagues evaluated the use of the FAST Clarus Plus Scope, a portable fiberoptic bronchoscope, by critical care transport nurses unfamiliar with flexible bronchoscopy. Use of the device was compared with humidification of the ETT and by $EtCO_2$ detection. Sensitivity of the FAST Clarus Plus Scope was found to be 87%, and sensitivity reached 100% when all three modalities were used.[62] The lack of 100% sensitivity with the flexible bronchoscope indicates that the technique requires training and experience; however, the largest obstacle to its routine use is the cost of the delicate equipment and the need for sterilization after use. More recently, disposable single-use flexible intubation scopes have been introduced that are portable, lightweight, and cost-effective. The advantages of these devices include eliminating repair and reprocessing costs and the lack of a need for cleaning, thereby reducing the risk of cross-contamination.[63,64] Additionally, a new ETT with an integrated high-resolution imaging camera allows for monitoring and surveillance of patency and position of the ETT during and after intubation.[65,66] The most significant limitation of this device is that the distal tip's camera cannot be manipulated as with an endoscopic device, which may result in difficulty maneuvering through obstructions or getting rid of secretions, which can impact its optics.

Techniques to Determine Endotracheal Tube Insertion Depth

Successful tracheal intubation does not end once the tube has been placed into the trachea. Accurate depth of ETT placement within the trachea is vital to avoid accidental extubation or endobronchial intubation. In pediatric patients, because of the relatively short length of the trachea, proper positioning is not only difficult

but critical. In the initial ASA closed claims analysis by Caplan and colleagues, endobronchial intubation was responsible for 1% of respiratory adverse events.[17]

Proper ETT placement has been defined as the presence of the ETT tip between 2 and 6 cm above the carina with the patient's head in a neutral position.[67] Inappropriate positioning of the ETT in the mainstem bronchus may result in several physiologic manifestations, including atelectasis, shunting, hypoxemia, tachycardia, hypertension, bronchospasm, and tension pneumothorax.[68] Several techniques have been used to verify ETT insertion depth. These techniques may be used before, during, or after intubation to ensure proper ETT positioning.

Tracheal Tube Markings

Using the depth markings present on all modern ETTs is the most common method of ensuring proper ETT positioning in the trachea. Before intubation, the ETT can be placed alongside the patient's face and neck so that the tip of the ETT is in the suprasternal notch; the centimeter marking where the tube intersects the teeth for oral intubation or the naris for nasal intubation is noted and secured at that depth after intubation. Alternatively, in patients of standard height (158 to 174 cm for females, 168 to 184 cm for males), securing the ETT at the incisors at a depth of 21 cm in females and 23 cm in males has been shown to reduce the likelihood of endobronchial intubation.[69] A study of 160 patients found that 55% of inexperienced anesthesia practitioners misdiagnosed endobronchial intubation when using only auscultation of breath sounds for verification of tube insertion depth. The greatest sensitivity for diagnosing endobronchial intubation in both experienced and inexperienced providers was achieved by combining the average tube insertion depth based on gender (20 to 21 cm for females, 22 to 23 cm for males) and auscultation.[70]

Formulas

Several formulas have been used to determine the correct placement and insertion depth of an ETT. Cherng and colleagues surmised that there was a significant correlation between body height and proper ETT position. Using linear regression, a formula for optimal orotracheal tube insertion depth was developed.[71]

$$\text{Distance from 5 cm above the carina to the right mouth angle (cm)} = \frac{\text{body height (cm)}}{5} - 13$$

The most common formula used for approximation of proper ETT depth for nasotracheal intubation is the Chula formula:

$$\text{Depth of ETT at right naris (cm)} = \frac{\text{body height (cm)}}{10} + 9$$

The mean depth of the nasotracheal tube at the right external naris calculated by the Chula formula was 25.4 cm in males and 24.4 cm in females.[72] The investigators of this study subsequently looked at whether the Chula formula could be modified to assess orotracheal ETT depth of insertion, and the following formula was developed:[73]

$$\text{Depth of ETT at right upper incisor (cm)} = \frac{\text{body height (cm)}}{10} + 4$$

The manubriosternal joint (MSJ) is in the same transverse (horizontal) plane as the tracheal carina. Lee and colleagues compared the straight length from the upper incisor to the MSJ in an extended neck position and the length from the upper incisor to the carina in the neutral position. Verification of ETT depth was performed with flexible bronchoscopy. A formula for the regression line was derived. It was concluded that a valid prediction of airway length from the upper incisor to the carina in the neutral position can be established by the straight length from the upper incisor to the MSJ in the extended position in adults.[74,75]

$$\text{Depth of ETT at right upper incisor (cm)} =$$
$$0.868 \times (\text{Incisor to MSJ length [cm]}) + 4.26.$$

Cuff Palpation

Cuff palpation is used to establish proper ETT depth, rather than endotracheal placement and the exclusion of EI. Because the proper depth of an ETT cannot be accurately established in all patients by using the distance markings on the side of the ETT, palpation and ballottement of the ETT cuff between the cricoid cartilage and the suprasternal notch has been proposed as a method to confirm proper ETT position. The technique involves placing two or three fingers above the suprasternal notch, followed by several rapid inflations of the ETT cuff with up to 10 mL of air. If the ETT is positioned correctly, an outward bulge is felt by the palpating fingers in the neck. Ledrick and colleagues reported that the technique was simple to use, reproducible, and sensitive but nonspecific.[76] The advantage of this technique is that it is easily performed and does not require any special equipment or dexterity. The disadvantage is that the use of a high-volume, low-pressure cuff may make palpation more difficult despite correct placement; false-negative determination is common in patients with thick necks or in the presence of a neck mass or swelling. Pollard used a modification of the technique using intermittent squeezing of the pilot balloon with the thumb and index finger while sensing the transmitted pulsations in the neck at the suprasternal notch. Using their method, they achieved an average distance from the tip of the ETT to the carina of 3 cm (range: 2–5 cm) in women and 3.4 cm (range: 2–6 cm) in men.[77]

An alternative method of determining adequate ETT depth that involves cuff palpation is to push on the anterior neck and feel for transmitted pressure in the pilot balloon. When the ETT is at the correct depth in the trachea, maximal impulses in the pilot balloon should be felt when pushing between the cricoid cartilage and suprasternal notch. Likewise, this technique does not rule out EI and is only for determining ETT depth once tracheal intubation has been established.

Positioning Under Direct Visualization

Studies have shown that placing the upper margin of the cuff of a 7.0- or 8.0-mm internal diameter ETT 2 cm below the vocal cords places the distal end of the ETT approximately 4 cm above the carina. This technique has been validated except in cases of a short neck.[77] This method is limited to instances when the view of the glottic opening is adequate. It serves as an initial method to determine ETT position but does not identify migration or movement. If there is head flexion, extension, or rotation, the ETT may migrate into the mainstem bronchus or above the vocal cords, depending on the position in the trachea. There is approximately a 4-cm movement of the ETT toward the carina when the head is moved from full extension to full flexion.[78] The average movement of the ETT when the head is moved from the neutral position to full flexion or full extension is 1.9 cm. If the ETT is properly placed in the middle of the trachea, it is unlikely to result in endobronchial intubation or extubation. Lateral head movement moves the ETT 0.7 cm cephalad.[79] Bed positioning may also impact ETT positioning. The Trendelenburg position may cause endobronchial intubation by the upward movement of the abdominal organs and carina; reverse Trendelenburg leads to the opposite scenario.[68] Insufflation of the abdomen during laparoscopic procedures in reverse Trendelenburg has a similar effect on ETT positioning as the Trendelenburg position.[80]

Auscultation and Chest Wall Movement

The same previously described limitations to the use of auscultation and observation of chest wall movement for determination of tracheal intubation apply for proper ETT position and depth within the trachea.[70] In pediatric patients, one method to detect proper ETT depth involves deliberate mainstem intubation and auscultation of the left side of the chest while slow withdrawal of the ETT is performed. The tube is secured 2 cm shallower than when equal breath sounds are first heard. In a study of 60 pediatric patients, Mariano and colleagues compared this method to both external ETT markings and ETT depth based on formulas and found it more accurate (73% vs 53% and 42%, respectively). However, even with the most accurate of the three methods, ETT malposition still occurred in 27% of cases, an unacceptably high incidence.[73] A confounding factor is the Murphy eye of the ETT. The Murphy eye is a 1.0-cm opening approximately 0.8 cm from the tip located on the ETT's right side. The function of the Murphy eye is to allow ventilation of the lungs if the bevel becomes obstructed, as well as ventilation of the right upper lobe in case of a right mainstem intubation.[81] The Murphy eye also allows retrograde ventilation of the left lung because there is airflow between the ETT cuff and the right mainstem bronchus, which may lead to bilateral breath sounds even in the setting of an endobronchial intubation.[33,80]

Alternative methods to traditional auscultation with a stethoscope have been explored. Electronic stethoscopes placed over the chest wall and epigastrium increase the volume of the breath sounds.[12] They are specifically recommended for air rescue missions when traditional auscultation is markedly limited or impossible.

The observation of asymmetric chest wall movement and chest excursion during positive-pressure ventilation as a sign of endobronchial tube placement has been described in pediatrics. However, in adult patients, particularly in the obese or in female patients with large breasts, chest excursion as a clinical sign of deep intubation is markedly limited. It is not discouraged that providers attempt to detect proper ETT placement solely based on clinical grounds; rather, it is recommended that secondary methods also be used routinely given the inherent limitations of clinical methods.

Transtracheal Illumination

The transillumination technique can be used to detect proper depth of ETT placement, but it is not a precise method. It has been suggested that when a lighted stylet is placed inside the ETT, if the point of maximal illumination is distal to the cricoid cartilage, then the ETT is usually placed above the carina. In a study by Mehta using this method, the mean distance between the tip

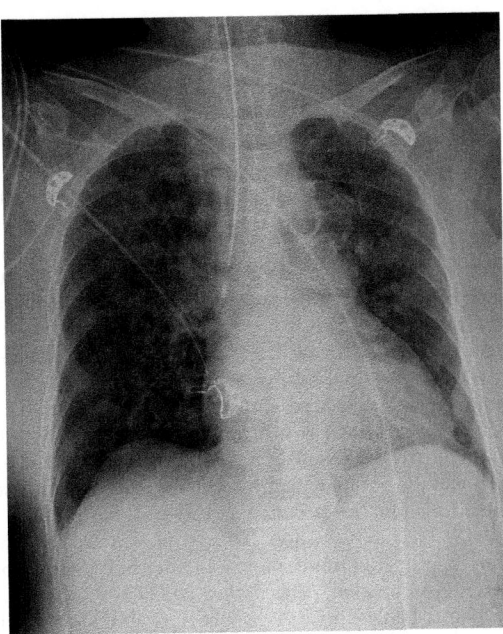

• **Fig. 30.6** Adult chest x-ray showing a right mainstem endobronchial intubation.

of the tracheal tube and the carina varied between 3.7 and 4 cm.[55] As is the case when using this method to rule out EI, light transmission is dependent on the intensity of the light, ambient light conditions, the proximity of the tissue to the light source, and the thickness and color of the tissue itself. In the presence of a thick neck, large goiter, neck swelling, dark skin, bright ambient lighting, or limited neck extension, the intensity of the light may be affected, and therefore the accuracy and sensitivity of the technique are limited. In a study of 80 pediatric patients, Yamashita and colleagues compared transillumination with deliberate mainstem intubation for achieving proper ETT position. Transillumination was the superior technique (80% vs 65%), but the sample size was too small to detect a statistically significant difference.[82]

Flexible Bronchoscopy

As described, bronchoscopic examination is a highly accurate method for determining proper ETT positioning within the trachea, but the technique is constrained by the need for specialized equipment and training. The availability of flexible bronchoscopic equipment outside the operating room and critical care settings can be limited. When using flexible bronchoscopy to determine accurate ETT positioning, the carina must be properly identified. To ensure that intermediate bronchi are not mistaken for mainstem bronchi, the right upper lobe bronchus should be located. As previously described, new ETTs with an integrated high-resolution imaging camera at the tip allow for continuous monitoring and surveillance of patency and position of the ETT.[63,66]

Chest Radiography

The use of CXR or fluoroscopy for confirmation of adequate ETT depth is used mainly in emergency airway management and in ICUs where prolonged intubation is anticipated. ETT misplacement is very common in these settings in both adult and pediatric populations. In a study of 1081 patients, Geisser and colleagues demonstrated the incidence of ETT malposition as determined by

CXR to be 18.2%, with a 5.2% incidence of mainstem intubation (Fig. 30.6)[61]

In pediatric patients, because of a shorter trachea, the incidence of malposition, particularly after emergency intubation, has been reported to be as high as 35% despite standard clinical determination of ETT position in patients younger than 1 year of age. In one study, the overall incidence of malposition was 18%, and the incidence decreased with advancing age, although it remained at 10% until the age of 10.[15] More recently, Kerrey and colleagues found an incidence of endobronchial intubation of 19% in pediatric patients and demonstrated that CXR had excellent correlation with diaphragmatic USG; however, CXR results were obtained a median of 8 minutes later than by USG.[62]

Wang and colleagues compared the actual results of repositioning of ETTs based on CXR findings and external ETT markings at the incisors. ETT position by a second CXR was compared with the proposed intervention (either advancement or withdrawal of the ETT). In 47% of the advancing group and 50% of the withdrawal group, the desired ETT position change was not achieved. In three cases, the ETT moved in the opposite direction than planned. The authors concluded that CXR is justified in the critical care setting after initial placement and after repositioning the ETT and that determination of adequate ETT depth is of paramount importance.[83,84] In a study of 77 pediatric patients requiring critical care transport (34 of them neonates), the incidence of initial ETT malposition was 47% based on CXR. When determining ETT depth by external markings, and based on neonatal and pediatric resuscitation guidelines, the rate of malposition was 35.3% in neonates and 27.8% in pediatric patients. Therefore, it was concluded that postintubation CXRs are informative in the pediatric/neonatal critical care transport population and should be obtained when feasible.[85]

The radiographic image usually obtained in emergency situations is the single anteroposterior (AP) chest view. In this AP view, determining the correct ETT location can be difficult because of superimposition of the trachea over the esophagus. The features of EI are more readily appreciated when a lateral view of the chest is observed; however, this view is often difficult to obtain. Radiographic clues that the ETT is outside the trachea include the presence of gastric distention and esophageal air, marked deviation of the trachea with an overinflated cuff, and the radiolucent ETT seen outside the tracheobronchial tree.

Ultrasonography

As described, USG offers two methods for assessing proper ETT tube placement. The indirect method, which assesses pleural and diaphragmatic movements indicating lung expansion, can assess proper ETT positioning. Bilateral lung sliding and equal diaphragm movement synchronized with ventilation can be seen if the ETT is appropriately placed in the trachea and can distinguish between tracheal and endobronchial intubation. In a study in neonates, Dennington and colleagues compared the accuracy of USG with CXR to establish proper ETT depth. The correlation of the two techniques was 68%, but USG was faster and avoided additional radiation exposure and no patient repositioning, which is a predisposing factor for further displacement of ETTs.[86,87] Kerrey and colleagues compared CXR with USG in 127 adult patients. The agreement between the two modalities was 83%; the sensitivity of USG for tracheal placement was 91%, with a specificity for mainstem intubation of 50%.[88] Further study is needed to establish the clinical utility of USG to determine proper ETT position.

Conclusion

Tracheal intubation is a two-part procedure: correct placement of the tube in the trachea and confirmation of proper ETT depth. Tracheal tube malposition is common, especially when advanced airway maneuvers are performed in emergency circumstances or pediatrics, and can lead to severe adverse consequences. The most severe form of ETT malpositioning is unrecognized EI, which, if not promptly corrected, will lead to anoxic brain injury and death.

A variety of methods and techniques are used to confirm proper ETT placement. No single technique is sufficiently sensitive or specific to detect ETT placement in all patients, age groups, and circumstances. A combination of techniques should be used for confirmation of tracheal tube placement. Secondary confirmatory techniques should complement primary detection methods. Detection of exhaled CO_2 by waveform capnography is considered the most sensitive method to confirm that the ETT is in the respiratory tract. Nonwaveform CO_2 detectors can be used when waveform capnography is not available, but they are less accurate. During conditions of little or no pulmonary blood flow (e.g., during cardiac arrest), the sensitivity of exhaled CO_2 is diminished. In these cases, other modalities, such as the use of the EDD or USG, are valid alternatives for determining proper ETT placement.

Establishing and maintaining proper ETT position in the trachea is also of the utmost importance. Similar approaches and techniques are used to determine proper ETT depth. Superficial placement may predispose to accidental extubation, especially if the head or patient is moved, whereas deep placement will predispose to endobronchial intubation. Endobronchial intubation leads to atelectasis of the contralateral lung and hyperinflation of the ipsilateral lung, leading to pneumothorax in extreme cases, with the associated adverse hemodynamic and respiratory consequences. Once correct ETT placement and position have been established, proper securing methods must be applied to prevent further movement of the ETT. If there is a clinical deterioration or if the patient's position, the patient's head, the ICU bed, or the operating room table has been modified, a high index of suspicion for ETT malposition must be maintained, and confirmatory methods should once again be used to determine proper ETT depth.

Selected References

14. Harris EA, Arheart KL, Penning DH. Endotracheal tube malposition within the pediatric population: a common event despite clinical evidence of correct placement. *Can J Anaesth.* 2008;55(10):685–690.
25. Bailie R, Posner KL. New trends in adverse respiratory events from the closed claims project. *A.S.A. Newsl.* 2011;75(2):28–29.
30. Mosier JM, Whitmore SP, Bloom JW, et al. Video laryngoscopy improves intubation success and reduces esophageal intubations compared to direct laryngoscopy in the medical intensive care unit. *Crit Care.* 2013;17(5):R237.
37. Silvestri S, Ralls GA, Krauss B, et al. The effectiveness of out-of-hospital use of continuous end-tidal carbon dioxide monitoring on the rate of unrecognized misplaced intubation within a regional emergency medical services system. *Ann Emerg Med.* 2005;45(5):497–503.
46. Turle S, Sherren PB, Nicholson S, Callaghan T, Shepherd SJ. Availability and use of capnography for in-hospital cardiac arrests in the United Kingdom. *Resuscitation.* 2015;94:80–84.
58. Sim S-S, Lien W-C, Chou H-C, et al. Ultrasonographic lung sliding sign in confirming proper endotracheal intubation during emergency intubation. *Resuscitation.* 2012;83(3):307–312.
70. Sitzwohl C, Langheinrich A, Schber A, et al. Endobronchial intubation detected by insertion depth of endotracheal tube, bilateral auscultation, or observation of chest movements: randomized trial. *BMJ.* 2010;341:c5943.
83. Geisser W, Maybauer DM, Wolff H, Pfenninger E, Maybauer MO. Radiological validation of tracheal tube insertion depth in out-of-hospital and in-hospital emergency patients. *Anaesthesia.* 2009;64(9):973–977.
85. Sanchez-Pinto N, Giuliano JS, Schwartz HP, et al. The impact of postintubation chest radiograph during pediatric and neonatal critical care transport. *Pediatr Crit Care Med.* 2013;14(5):e213–e217.
88. Kerrey BT, Geis GL, Quinn AM, Hornung RW, Ruddy RM. A prospective comparison of diaphragmatic ultrasound and chest radiography to determine endotracheal tube position in a pediatric emergency department. *Pediatrics.* 2009;123(6):e1039–e1044.

All references can be found online at eBooks.Health.Elsevier.com.

PART 5

Difficult Airway Situations

31

Prehospital Airway Management

DARREN ALAN BRAUDE AND MICHAEL THOMAS STEUERWALD

CHAPTER OUTLINE

KEY POINTS

- Noninvasive ventilation (NIV) is widely used in the prehospital setting and may be considered in patients with altered mental status when closely attended.
- Supine patients undergoing medication-facilitated airway management (MFAM) should be moved off the ground (e.g., to the stretcher) before intubation whenever possible.
- Patients being intubated on the ground should have their positioning optimized, and video-assisted laryngoscopy (VAL) used whenever possible.

- Strong consideration should be given to supraglottic airways (SGAs) for invasive airway management of entrapped patients.
- Sedation-only intubation is not recommended.
- For prehospital patients in cardiac arrest, either an SGA or tracheal intubation performed without stopping chest compressions is a reasonable option.

Overview of the Prehospital Care Environment and Structure

Different Types of Emergency Medical Service Systems and Providers

It is impossible to consider airway management in the out-of-hospital environment without understanding emergency medical service (EMS) systems and providers. EMS systems are generally designed to stabilize emergency conditions and facilitate rapid transport to an appropriate receiving hospital or to transport patients between hospitals. Although there are international and regional differences, prehospital care in the United States is commonly provided by professionals at the emergency medical responder (EMR) through paramedic levels. These caregivers may be cross-trained as firefighters or devoted entirely to medical care.

Interfacility transport of critically ill and injured patients is often performed by specialty teams, whether traveling by ground ambulance, airplane, or helicopter. In the United States, these teams are most commonly composed of paramedics and nurses, although respiratory therapists, advanced practice providers, and physicians may also be team members. In other countries, it is much more the norm for physicians to be integrally involved in critical care transport.

The amount of training required to achieve certification at each level of EMS licensure is highly variable from region to region and country to country. In the United States, it commonly takes 50 to 100 hours for an EMR, 150 to 200 hours for an emergency medical technician (EMT), 150 to 250 hours for an advanced EMT (AEMT), and 1000 to 1500 hours, possibly with an associate's or bachelor's degree, for a paramedic. The specific amount of time spent on airway training and the scope of practice of the certified or licensed practitioner are also highly variable. Typically, an EMR and EMT are limited to basic measures to remove a foreign body, providing supplemental oxygen, and performing bag-mask ventilation (BMV). Advanced EMTs can place supraglottic airway devices (SGAs), whereas paramedics can deliver noninvasive ventilation (NIV) and perform endotracheal intubation (ETI).

Many paramedics are also credentialed to perform percutaneous or surgical cricothyrotomies, and some may be able to perform medication-facilitated airway management (MFAM). EMS physicians are likely able to perform the broadest scope of prehospital airway management. The wide variability in scope of practice is noteworthy because some jurisdictions may allow EMTs to provide continuous positive airway pressure (CPAP) and place SGAs, whereas in others, paramedics neither intubate nor perform cricothyrotomies.

Unique Considerations

The prehospital setting presents unique challenges to all patient care, not the least of which is airway management. The patient's disease process is often undifferentiated, resources and equipment may be more limited than in the hospital setting, and there may be issues of patient access, lighting, adverse weather, confined space, turbulence or road vibration, and safety of the provider. When these factors are taken in aggregate, it is unreasonable to expect that out-of-hospital airway management will look identical to in-hospital airway management. Physicians who are not specifically trained in out-of-hospital care or do not have substantial experience in this setting may be particularly challenged when trying to translate their hospital practice to this unique environment.

EMS is an American Board of Emergency Medicine (ABEM)-approved subspecialty, with board certification available to physicians after a minimum 1 year of fellowship that includes a substantial clinical prehospital care component. The subspecialty is open to physicians from any primary specialty although most EMS fellowships are restricted to graduates of emergency medicine residencies. EMS physicians in the United States primarily serve in administrative roles as medical directors although direct patient care by EMS physicians is seen in a few systems, bringing an advanced level of airway management practice and oversight. Internationally, direct patient care by physicians is much more common.

EMS Airway Education and Training

Initial Intubation Training

The best methods for teaching airway procedures have not been definitely established, but it is clear that a sufficient number of procedures are required to attain proficiency. Studies have shown that it takes about 15 intubations in the operating room (OR) to achieve a 90% chance of success on the next attempt, although it is likely that this is skewed because the supervising anesthesiologists and anesthetists probably selected easier cases for the students.[1] Interestingly, even 30 intubations do not predict 90% success in the challenging prehospital environment.

There is extensive debate regarding whether or not live intubations are essential for initial airway training. For a variety of issues, including learner saturation, fewer intubation procedures in the surgical environment, and concerns about liability, fewer supervised live intubations in the OR are available. As a result, many EMS students are trained largely on manikins and simulators. The US Committee on Accreditation of Educational Programs for the Emergency Medical Services Professions (CoAEMSP) recommends a combination of a minimum of 50 "airway encounters" across all age ranges with 100% success in their last 20 attempts at airway management. CoAEMSP states that airway management "may be accomplished using any combination of live patients, high definition fidelity simulations, low fidelity simulations, or cadaver labs."[2] Although discouraged, it is possible for a paramedic student to complete initial training without a single live intubation. On the other hand, the province of Alberta, Canada, requires 30 intubations of which 20 have to be supervised in the OR. Overall, we believe there is great value in spending time in the OR with an experienced anesthesia practitioner, but not just for intubations. There is equal or greater value, in our opinion, to supervised BMV and SGA placement, as well as the academic discussions that often ensue.

Skill Retention

Initial training is only half the battle. Once working, opportunities for intubation skill maintenance are often limited because of the increased use of NIV and SGAs, as well as the increased number of providers deployed to EMS.[3] Patient survival has been correlated to the number of intubations that the treating paramedic had performed in the previous 5 years.[4] As a result, many agencies set requirements for a minimum number of encounters and success, often relying on low-fidelity simulation. The Committee on Accreditation of Medical Transport Systems (CAMTS) requires three adult, pediatric, and infant intubations per quarter, or a total of 36 intubations per year, all of which may be simulated. Despite this mandate, a number of studies have shown relatively poor first-pass success by nonphysician EMS providers in both the air medical and ground environments utilizing rapid sequence intubatin (RSI), as well as ground-based environments primarily intubating patients in cardiac arrest.[5-8] This suggests that the CAMTS standards may be insufficient to maintain competence in these challenging settings. It is incumbent on each provider, agency, and system to set its own standards to ensure patient safety and optimize success. Anesthesia providers are strongly encouraged to help provide initial and ongoing learning opportunities in the OR for EMS providers in their catchment areas.

Quality Assurance and Improvement

Whatever the levels of training or particular skills employed within an EMS system, medical directors, educators, and administrators should monitor performance and look for opportunities for improvement. Historically, the most common airway metric has been overall intubation success rate, but this may not be the best measure of quality. Take this scenario: System A has a 99% overall success rate but only a 40% first-pass success rate, and

20% of cases become hypoxic or require three or more attempts, whereas system B has an 80% first-pass success rate with an overall success rate of 90% and no hypoxia by moving to an SGA after two failed attempts. By the classic metric of overall intubation success, system A has better performance than system B, yet many would argue that system B is practicing better prehospital medicine.

Because true outcome data are often hard to obtain, EMS systems that perform MFAM should at a minimum be measuring known surrogate markers of outcome in patients with head injury, such as hypoxemia, hypotension, and hyperventilation. One proposed quality assurance metric is Definitive Airway Sans Hypoxia/Hypotension on First Attempt (DASH-1A).[9] This metric requires the collection of objective data from monitors that record data points every few seconds. One landmark study from San Diego demonstrated very high rates of desaturation when such data collection methods were used.[10] An aggressive continuous quality improvement program in a large air medical system has been shown to improve first-pass success and minimize complications.[11]

Of course, focusing on intubation excludes the much larger population of patients managed with basic life support (BLS) maneuvers. One method to "level the playing field" in quality assurance is direct subjective observation of patient care in the field by medical directors, EMS physicians, and supervisors.

Airway Management Issues by Specific Clinical Situation

Cardiac Arrest

In the majority of advanced life support (ALS) EMS systems worldwide, MFAM is not authorized and invasive airway management is primarily performed during out-of-hospital cardiac arrest (OHCA) resuscitation. Some systems exclusively utilize SGAs because of low intubation success rates in this patient population, and to avoid lengthy interruptions in chest compressions. Other systems and experts strongly believe intubation is better for OHCA management and that high first-pass success rates can be still be favorable, especially with the use of video-assisted laryngoscopy (VAL).

Two large studies now shed light on this issue. A multicenter US trial cluster randomized over 3000 patients in OHCA to airway management with either tracheal intubation or a laryngeal tube. First-pass success was 51.6% with intubation and 90.3% for the laryngeal tube. Survival at 72 hours and neurologic status at discharge were both improved in those patients managed with a laryngeal tube.[6] Another multicenter trial in the UK cluster randomized almost 9300 patients with OHCA to airway management with either tracheal intubation or an i gel, an SGA.[12] Airway management was successful within two attempts (first attempt not reported) for 79% of intubations and 87.4% of SGAs. Favorable functional outcomes were not different between the two groups at 30 days. Interestingly, aspiration rates were not different between patients managed with an SGA or intubation in either of these trials, suggesting that many patients had aspirated prior to airway management and/or that SGAs do provide some aspiration protection. Taken together, these two large studies support SGAs as primary airways in OHCA, especially if intubation success rates are comparable. Systems that can obtain higher first-pass success rates despite the challenges of airway management in OHCA, including patients positioned on the floor with ongoing chest compressions, may wish to continue that practice. The AHA

ACLS updates from 2019 indicate that either approach is acceptable with a 2a level of evidence.[13]

These studies also serve to refute suggestions that SGAs impair blood flow to the brain as seen in a swine managed with SGAs (LT, LMA-Flexible) compared to ETI during induced cardiac arrest.[14] This assertion was countered by a case series of 17 perfusing patients undergoing neck imaging while ventilated with various SGAs.[15] Two blinded neuroradiologists were unable to detect any evidence of mechanical carotid compression in any of these patients, suggesting that there are important differences in swine and human anatomy. Offsetting these concerns is the greater interruption of CPR often inherent with ETI compared with SGA placement.[16]

Interestingly, there is evidence for improved outcomes for OHCA patients managed with BMV over any type of invasive airway[17-20]; however, a randomized controlled trial (RCT) was inconclusive.[21] These results are potentially confounded by those patients who had return of spontaneous circulation very early and resumed spontaneous breathing, a group of patients with excellent prognosis. Two studies, however, have also found improved outcomes for patients who underwent BMV after failed intubation or SGA insertion.[17,18] This may reflect something inherently detrimental from invasive airways, or it may be that it is simply easier to overventilate with an invasive airway compared to BMV.[22] There is not yet enough evidence to abandon invasive airway management altogether, but we should definitely focus on strategies to avoid overventilation and subsequent impairment of venous return and cardiac output.[22]

Trauma

Critically injured patients often present with secretions, blood, or vomit in their airway; hypoxemia; and/or cervical spine injury, making airway management exceedingly complex and difficult. Initial focus should, therefore, be on basic measures, such as positioning, suctioning, oxygen administration, and BMV. Concerns for cervical spine injury should not preclude allowing patients to sit upright, if best for the airway. A surgical airway should be considered immediately for patients who have catastrophic injuries that preclude airway management via the mouth or when the patient has trismus and providers do not have access to MFAM.

MFAM practitioners may consider RSI or rapid sequence airway (RSA; see "Rapid Sequence Airway") for severely injured patients who are not moribund, if it does not create substantial delays. Median prehospital scene times of 42 and 68 minutes have been reported, which raises the question of whether such delays are preventable and/or justifiable.[23,24] Results from prehospital studies of MFAM in patients with severe traumatic brain injury are very mixed, ranging from worse outcomes to improved outcomes, as compared with BLS management.[25-31] Only one RCT has been performed,[29] which reported improved outcomes with RSI, but these results have recently been questioned.[32] Outcomes seem to be most closely tied to severity of injury and management of ventilation and hypoxemia on hospital arrival than on a specific mode of positive-pressure ventilation (PPV).[33,34] In patients with severe head injury, the emphasis must be on avoiding hypoxemia, hyperventilation, and hypotension regardless of how the airway is managed.[35] There is no compelling evidence to support more widespread use of MFAM in this patient population.

It is worth noting that trauma patients who will tolerate invasive airway management without medications are usually in cardiac arrest or a moribund peri-arrest state. These patients generally have poor outcomes regardless of airway management and should be transported without delay, if resuscitation and transport are indicated.[26,36–39]

Pediatric Intubation

The weight of evidence, including RCTs, indicates that out-of-hospital intubation of the pediatric patient does not improve survival in cardiac arrest when compared with BMV, although prehospital pediatric intubation has not been adequately compared with SGAs.[40] Some EMS jurisdictions, such as Los Angeles and Orange counties in California and the entire state of New Mexico, have restricted pediatric intubation by paramedics.

Reasons why pediatric intubation may be particularly challenging in this setting include anatomic differences that are unfamiliar to providers, the added stress involved with critical pediatric patients, and limited provider exposure to these procedures during initial training and ongoing clinical practice. In air medical transport, only 5% of intubation cases may be for patients 14 years of age or younger.[5] A ground-based RSI study in a large metropolitan area with a population over 2 million reported only 299 prehospital intubation cases in 6.3 years; their first-pass success was 66% overall, 53% for infants, and 56% for children in cardiac arrest.[41] This region reports that, on average, paramedic students perform six pediatric intubations during training, which we suspect far exceeds the national average. Another ground-based pediatric RSI study from Australia[42] reports much higher success rates, but only 109 procedures were performed over 9 years despite a population of over 6 million and an outcome benefit could not be determined. Evidence suggests that physician-based prehospital teams have higher success rates and fewer complications when performing prehospital pediatric intubations, although such teams are uncommon in the United States.[43]

Given the infrequent need for this procedure, the difficulty maintaining competence, and the excellent pediatric SGAs now available, it is reasonable for systems and medical directors to withhold pediatric intubation pending further research. Systems that continue to perform pediatric intubation, and particularly pediatric MFAM, should carefully track their success rates, complications, and outcomes and create processes to ensure the safety of this vulnerable population.

Medication-Facilitated Airway Management

This is a complex procedure performed in very ill patients. Even under the most controlled circumstances, there are significant risks. When performed under less-than-ideal conditions, the potential for adverse events greatly increases. Those agencies that perform prehospital MFAM must be trained constantly and consistently to stay proficient. Teams should also look for system-level solutions to increase operator efficiency and mitigate risk. For example, the most common patient to undergo MFAM in most prehospital agencies is the adult male with trauma; therefore, the ventilator can be set up at the beginning of the shift for this hypothetical patient to minimize the need for adjustments. Having all other airway equipment checked and ready in a familiar location also improves efficiency during these high-stakes situations. Specific prehospital criteria to predict difficult intubation, such as the HEAVEN assessment, have also been developed and validated.[44]

Because MFAM is a team effort and there may be only one or more advanced crew members on scene, it is very beneficial to train the first responding personnel as assistants. These other providers, regardless of level of training, may be used to assist with external laryngeal manipulation, in-line cervical spine stabilization with jaw thrust, passing tubes over a bougie, monitoring oxygen saturation, and other tasks. It is also helpful to train first responders to provide estimated patient weight, which may allow for medications and ventilators to be prepared prior to arrival at the scene. One ground-based EMS system requires a minimum of three paramedics to perform an MFAM procedure, although this is not generally possible in most jurisdictions.[23]

Rapid Sequence Intubation

The data supporting prehospital RSI are mixed—from worse outcomes to improved outcomes—with the vast majority of studies looking specifically at the moderate to severe traumatic brain injury population.[25–29,30,31,33,45–49] One of the seminal articles on this topic came from Dunford and colleagues looking at prehospital RSI of patients in San Diego County with head injury and a Glasgow Coma Scale (GCS) score less than 8, using continuously recording pulse oximeters.[10] The authors reported a remarkable and concerning degree of hypoxemia despite extensive education and a close degree of medical director involvement. Follow-up demonstrated that the patients did better if they came by air than by ground, even when controlling for transport time.[50] Eventually they were able to discern that the major clinical factor at play was hyperventilation.[51] The patients with normal end tidal carbon dioxide ($EtCO_2$) on arrival to the hospital had the best outcomes, and these were most often the patients who came by air: the flight crews all had capnography, ventilators, and training in how to use them to maintain appropriate $EtCO_2$ as compared with the ground crews who had none of the above at the time.

It is very hard to analyze a skill to determine the outcome benefit when it is confounded by multiple variables and used by diverse providers in unique systems in a heterogeneous patient population. It may be that RSI is most beneficial in a specific subset of patients or only when performed by a specific set of providers, but that is not yet clearly established. In particular, we have no evidence regarding outcomes from prehospital RSI in patients with medical conditions or multisystem trauma. On balance, until more evidence becomes available, it seems reasonable to assume that some patients will benefit from prehospital RSI, as long as it can be done meticulously, regardless of the level of provider training. The protocol described by Jarvis et al. provides an example of such high standards, although their scene times were quite long.[23] It also appears that allowing patients to become hypoxemic, hypocarbic, or hypotensive during or after intubation can offset the potential benefit of airway security.

There is recent interest in prehospital use of delayed sequence intubation (DSI) techniques during which ketamine is given first to facilitate preoxygenation followed by administration of the paralytic. This was originally described only for patients with refractory hypoxemia[52] but has also been reported for patients without hypoxemia.[23,24] Neither of these studies provide any data on outcomes or complications, such as aspiration. DSI cannot yet be recommended as evidence based at this time, but it is a reasonable approach for consideration by medical directors.

Rapid Sequence Airway

RSA, as originally defined, is an alternative MFAM strategy in which the same preparation and pharmacology as RSI are used for the immediate planned placement of an SGA, preferably with gastric suctioning capability.[53] This concept has also been termed RSI with a King LT in two reports.[54,55] Although this approach has also been reported in the hospital setting for preoxygenation, it has been employed primarily in EMS settings.[56,57] The advantages of RSA are that it is faster with higher first-pass success than intubation, especially when employed in tight spaces, such as aircraft or by crews with less intubation experience.[58] The disadvantages are the increased risk of aspiration, although many newer SGAs offer more protection than might be expected and many patients undergoing these procedures in the field have already aspirated.[59] A recent series of 68 cases showed a 94% success rate and aspiration rates comparable to other methods of emergency airway management.[60] This approach should be subjected to more rigorous academic evaluation before it can be uniformly recommended but is worth considering on a case-by-case basis.

Sedation-Facilitated Intubation

Sedation-facilitated intubation (SFI) describes the use of an induction agent, often midazolam or etomidate, without the subsequent use of a paralytic. This technique is likely more commonly used in EMS than in hospitals, although data are lacking. SFI is usually used in EMS by medical directors and providers who wish to avoid the obvious risk of chemical paralysis in uncontrolled settings. Although well intended, this technique may be more dangerous than managing the patient with BLS techniques or RSI. The evidence would suggest that success rates with SFI are substantially lower than with RSI. The National Emergency Airway Registry (NEAR) data demonstrated that RSI had a first-pass success rate of 91% compared with SFI, which was 76%.[14] This is a large and important difference when considering the potential increase in complications with multiple attempts. A prehospital trial comparing etomidate and midazolam for SFI reported an overall success rate of only 76%.[61] Another small air medical trial found 92% success with RSI but only 25% success when only etomidate was used.[62]

An even greater concern than lower success rates with SFI is the increased risk of massive emesis and aspiration. When critically ill or injured patients with a full stomach are given an induction agent, they may retain enough gag reflex to allow for active vomiting when stimulated but not enough reflex to prevent aspiration. One study reported gagging in up to 65% of the patients and vomiting in up to 13%.[61] If the provider or medical director does not have confidence in the ability to intubate, then the better practice is to emphasize good BLS and transport. It is unclear if the use of ketamine carries a lower risk of aspiration than the agents that have been studied for SFI. For now, this approach cannot be widely recommended.

Airway Management Issues by Specific Setting

Ground Versus Air/Critical Care Transport

Airway management by critical care transport teams represents a hybrid between traditional EMS (usually provided by EMTs and paramedics with limited equipment and experience, often without medication assistance, and entirely in the field) and hospital-based care (provided by nurses and physicians, with the latest in technology and pharmacology, in a controlled environment). Critical

care teams (CCTs) may consist of any combination of paramedics, nurses, respiratory therapists, advanced practice practitioners, and physicians. In the United States, a nurse-paramedic model is the most prevalent, whereas internationally physician-based teams are more common. These teams usually have additional airway training and certification, have a broad range of available pharmacology, often have access to VAL, and often may perform airway procedures in the field, in an ambulance, in an aircraft, or at a sending facility. Data suggest that critical care and physician-based teams perform more airway procedures with higher success rates.[41,43,63–69] There is limited evidence that the performance of these advanced procedures or the use of air medical transport improves patient outcomes.[25,45-47,70–75]

Historically, the medical directors of these CCT teams have strongly discouraged the performance of airway procedures en route, which requires a lower threshold for invasive procedures and longer scene times before transport. The conventional thinking has been that airway management en route is more technically challenging and less likely to be successful. While this is still largely the industry standard, some programs and medical directors are now becoming more accepting, or even encouraging, of en route airway management, although the approach may need to be modified as a result of space/access constraints in aircraft and the number of hands available to assist. A physician-based helicopter emergency medical service (HEMS) service found equivalent success and complications whether the airway procedure was performed prior to flight or during flight, although these intubations were classified as nonemergent.[76]

Performing a standard RSI procedure with only two crewmembers, one of whom may have limited access to the patient if remaining seatbelted, is challenging. An RSA technique, in which an SGA is placed with the aid of an induction agent and paralytic agent, may be preferable in this unique situation, depending on aircraft, crew, and patient factors.[53,58] On the other hand, performing an airway procedure before transport in the emergency department (ED) or intensive care unit (ICU) of a smaller sending facility may mimic traditional hospital-based airway procedures in terms of personnel and space.

Urban Setting

Urban EMS systems usually have short transport times to an appropriate receiving hospital. In the time it takes to perform a protracted airway intervention, the patient could be in the resuscitation bay of the ED. In these systems it often makes more sense to focus on life-saving basics—positioning, oxygen delivery, NIV, BMV, SGAs, and foreign-body removal—than it does to focus on intubation, especially medication-facilitated intubation. The evidence of a survival benefit from MFAM in the prehospital setting has not been demonstrated outside of helicopter emergency medical services, and even then the majority of evidence suggests worse outcomes.

Austere Environment

A small percentage of civilian EMS (i.e., search and rescue, National Park Service, etc.), and a larger percentage of military EMS, occurs in what would be considered austere environments with severely limited resources. These environments present entirely new considerations. On the one hand, the delayed transport time may warrant more airway interventions, whereas on the other hand equipment is often limited as a result of space and weight considerations. There is also a tremendous variability in training of providers. Civilian search-and-rescue teams are often trained only to the EMR or EMT levels, although intermediate and ALS providers, including physicians, may be available. In the US Army, the typical combat medic is an EMT with the addition of limited advanced skills, such as intravenous access and needle thoracostomy, whereas many US Special Forces teams travel with paramedics, if not more advanced providers, trained to an expanded scope of practice including RSI.

Infectious Diseases/COVID

The COVID-19 pandemic has highlighted the risk to EMS providers from aerosol-generating airway procedures. In the early days of the pandemic, a myriad of conflicting recommendations could be found. For example, the American Hospital Association (AHA) was recommending intubation over SGAs to minimize the risk of ongoing aerosol generation while many medical directors were encouraging SGAs over intubation to minimize the amount of initial exposure time.[77] With time, most systems have chosen to focus on appropriate PPE rather than changing airway practice. A limited number of prehospital-specific airway management recommendations have now been released with more likely to appear.[78]

If a patient has arrested from COVID, then the risk for aerosol is significant and the benefit of any resuscitation is likely limited, so it makes sense to pause CPR during airway management to avoid aggressive aerosol generation. If any system gets to the point of implementing true crisis standards of care for patients, then it may be appropriate to withhold resuscitation.

Simple use of in-line HEPA filters during mask ventilation has become the norm in most hospital settings but not yet in many EMS systems. This would seem to be a simple infection control measure when available. Another airway issue that has arisen for EMS providers, medical directors, and administrators is the use of nebulizers. Early on, many EMS agencies stopped all use of nebulizers. Many agencies have now resumed the practice whenever it is felt to be in the patient's best interest, as long as the provider has appropriate personal protective equipment (PPE), along with limiting the number of providers in the ambulance and encouraging ventilation.

Likewise, continuous positive airway pressure (CPAP) was initially felt to be high risk for aerosol generation; however, our comfort with this technique in the prehospital arena is growing similar to in the hospital setting. One needs to distinguish CPAP delivered with a mask that vents exhaled gases from CPAP delivered via a ventilator circuit with all exhaled gases directed through a HEPA filter. A patient in respiratory distress breathing rapidly through a nonrebreather mask with an overlying procedure mask is likely still generating aerosol in the immediate environment; therefore, judicious use of NIV seems beneficial to patients and of manageable risk to the EMS providers.

PPE has been shown to limit transmissibility to EMS providers working in a ground-based urban/suburban system to less than 0.5%.[79] Critical care transport of the patient with infectious respiratory illnesses adds additional risk to the provider because of typically longer exposure times than with initial transport from scene to hospital. A recent paper from the Four Corners region of the United States during the first few months of the COVID-19 pandemic had average patient contact times of 140 minutes.[80] Fortunately, despite nearly 3000 hours of exposure to COVID positive and suspected positive patients, most of whom were not intubated, less than 2% of crewmembers developed symptomatic infections attributed to work exposure.

Application of Airway Techniques in the Prehospital Environment

Bag-Mask Ventilation

Although BMV is a fundamental airway skill taught to EMS providers of all levels starting at the EMR level, it can be very difficult to perform in the prehospital setting for a variety of complex reasons. Patients often present with multiple predictors of mask ventilation difficulty, access and positioning may not be optimal, personnel may be limited, and, perhaps most important, the procedure is often relegated to the least experienced provider. Strategies to mitigate these issues include emphasizing optimal technique including proper positioning, use of appropriate airway adjuncts and the two-person technique whenever possible, use of a transport ventilator, and assigning an experienced responder to perform or supervise this critical skill. When difficulty is encountered with achieving an adequate mask seal (e.g., due to blood/secretions, trauma, obesity, facial hair, etc.), early consideration should be given to bypassing these anatomic difficulties with an SGA.

Noninvasive Positive-Pressure Ventilation

One of the most significant advances in the EMS management of medical patients over the past decade has been the introduction of NIV. Outside of some critical care transport teams, prehospital NIV is almost exclusively CPAP rather than bi-level positive airway pressure (BiPAP). CPAP is primarily an ALS skill, although it has been extended to the EMT-Intermediate and EMT-Basic levels in some jurisdictions. Numerous products are now available to provide CPAP in the prehospital setting, from simple single-use devices to complex ventilators (Fig. 31.1). A disposable BiPAP device is now available as well, which may increase the use of this modality (Mercury Medical, Clearwater, FL). CPAP is most commonly used as a bridge to facilitate transport to the hospital for patients with pulmonary edema, pneumonia, or chronic obstructive pulmonary disease (COPD) exacerbations and has been used quite extensively with the COVID-19 pandemic. CPAP is also used in some systems as a preoxygenation strategy, as an alternative to intubation in patients with predicted intubation difficulty, in patients anticipated to require only short-term positive pressure while other therapies have an effect, and for patients with a Do Not Intubate order.

Meta-analyses have come to different conclusions on whether prehospital CPAP improves outcomes and decreases intubation rates.[81–83] The vast majority of patients included in CPAP trials have (or are presumed to have) pulmonary edema or COPD exacerbations; it is unclear whether CPAP is safe in conditions such as pneumonia, with only one small study looking at this specifically.[84] Even when protocols restrict CPAP to patients with suspected pulmonary edema or COPD, it is inevitable that patients with other conditions will end up being treated, as diagnostic discrimination in the prehospital setting by paramedics is poor.[85]

The greatest challenge to applying CPAP in the prehospital setting is coaching a hypoxic, hypercarbic, and anxious patient to wear the requisite tight-fitting mask through the initiation

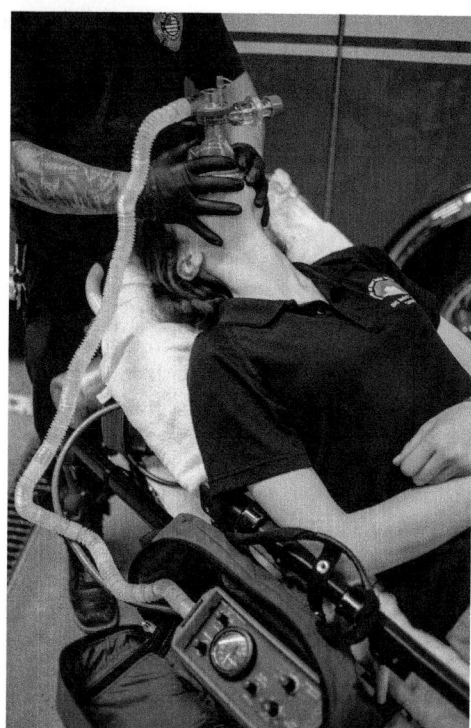

• **Fig. 31.1** A simple transport ventilator can facilitate very effective one-person mask ventilation.

process, especially in a loud and chaotic environment. Despite these barriers, there is now an established track record of success in many systems proving that it can be done. Ideally, one provider will be dedicated to coaching the patient through the first several minutes of use; the person chosen for this "coaching" task does not have to be the most experienced airway practitioner, but they must be able to work effectively with the patient.

One area of controversy lacking sufficient literature guidance is the use of CPAP in patients with altered mental status. Despite long-standing instruction to the contrary, it is our opinion and experience that CPAP can be applied safely in selected patients with altered mental status in the prehospital setting when other options are limited, as long as the providers are constantly attending and monitoring the patient while positioned close enough to immediately remove the mask in the event of vomiting.

Another challenge with the use of NIV that is unique to the EMS settings is the limited availability of oxygen and compressed gases. EMS personnel must have appropriate training and expertise to determine the rate of oxygen consumption with their particular NIV device and patient-specific demands and be able to calculate the amounts of gas and, consequently, time that remain. There is wide variability in oxygen consumption among commercially available devices, requiring extra attention for rescuers who may be inexperienced with this mode of airway and ventilation support.

Given that CPAP is noninvasive, affordable, and likely safe in any condition for short periods, and because alternatives such as MFAM are not widely available and/or associated with more serious risks, we strongly recommend making prehospital CPAP widely available. Systems may attempt to restrict use of CPAP to patients with suspected pulmonary edema or COPD exacerbations based on the available literature, or they may reasonably extend the technology to any cause of respiratory failure. The use

of CPAP in the setting of altered mental status should also be considered in the prehospital setting when better alternatives are not available, and the patient is closely observed one on one at all times during transport.

Blind Nasotracheal Intubation

Blind nasotracheal intubation (BNTI) has all but disappeared from hospital-based practice but persists in some EMS jurisdictions, particularly as an alternative to surgical airways when MFAM is not indicated or not part of the scope of practice. Advantages to BNTI include the ability to keep the patient in a seated position and avoid the inherent risks of sedation and paralysis. Disadvantages to BNTI include the lower success rate, requirement to use a smaller ETT, need to exchange for oral intubation at the hospital in most cases, and the potential to cause elevated intracranial pressure (ICP) and epistaxis.[86–88] BNTI may also induce vomiting. Many cases that were historically managed with BNTI may now be managed with NIV to either delay intubation or avoid the need for invasive airway management altogether.

Tracheal Intubation

Tracheal intubation has been considered a core paramedic and EMS physician skill for decades. Evidence supporting use of this procedure is limited at best, particularly in regard to patient outcome. When ALS-level prehospital care was added to the Province of Ontario, Canada, there was no survival advantage for medical cardiac arrest patients undergoing tracheal intubation and there were worse outcomes for trauma patients.[89,90] Although intubation was only part of the ALS "bundle," it was one of the predominant procedures performed. Other reviews and meta-analyses have not found advantages to intubation over alternative techniques.[47,91,92]

Techniques for intubation are similar to those in more conventional environments. However, when access is limited or patients cannot be optimally positioned, practitioners should have a low threshold for use of SGAs, at least until the patient is moved to a better position and/or location. Regardless, we strongly advocate for thorough preparation of materials at the start of each shift, as well as immediately before any procedure, to include use of a checklist. It is worth noting that the use of checklists in hospital-based intubation has had mixed results, but this has not been well studied in the prehospital environment where practitioners may have much less overall airway experience and are often working with unfamiliar teams.[93–95]

Video-Assisted Laryngoscopy

Use of VAL in emergency medicine has exploded over the past several years.[96] Although the data on VAL use in the prehospital environment are more limited, current evidence suggests that VAL is an important tool for management of the airway in the field. Wayne and colleagues compared the GlideScope Ranger with direct laryngoscopy (DL) in a ground-based EMS system and found that paramedics were able to intubate faster and with fewer attempts with the GlideScope compared with DL.[97] Jarvis and coworkers compared the King Vision with DL in their EMS system.[98] They found an increased first-pass success when the King Vision was used compared with DL (74% vs 44%), as well as an increased overall success rate with the King Vision (92% vs 65%). Boehringer and coworkers found that when the C-MAC Pocket Monitor was incorporated into their aeromedical flight program, first-pass success improved from 75% to 95% and overall success improved from 95% to 99%.[99] However, despite many positive studies for VAL in the prehospital and emergency environment, prospective randomized studies have had mixed results. One concern with more widespread use of prehospital VAL is the perceived high prevalence of secretions, blood, and/or emesis that might obscure the optics; direct sunlight also appears to impair visualization of the video monitor.[100] Interestingly, trauma airways in the ED were more successfully managed with VAL than with DL, suggesting that blood and emesis may not cause obscuration of the camera as frequently as once thought.[101] We suggest that VAL is reasonable to use even if encountering blood or vomitus is likely, as long as suction is available and the provider has had deliberate training on mitigating those factors. Further, standard-geometry VAL may also be favorable when camera obscuration is at all possible, as reversion to DL can be easy and immediate.

It is likely that over time use of VAL in the field will increase, especially as the cost of this technology becomes lower. However, VAL should not be seen as the panacea for poor first-pass intubation rates, although it may be part of a comprehensive program. Many EMS systems, especially those that do not use MFAM, may expect the most improvements by focusing on optimal BMV and SGAs than by introducing VAL. VAL is covered more broadly in Chapter 23.

Intubation of the Supine Patient

Managing patients who are supine on the floor or ground is clearly more challenging than managing those on an adjustable stretcher or hospital bed. For MFAM procedures, it is best to move the patient onto the transport stretcher before the procedure (Fig. 31.2) because this will both facilitate a better intubation position and eliminate one additional movement of the intubated patient, each of which comes with a risk of tube dislodgment. For patients in cardiac arrest, movement to the stretcher requires interruption of chest compressions and also creates the potential for risk when resuscitative measures are terminated on scene and the patient must be removed from the stretcher. Therefore, patients in cardiac arrest are usually managed on the floor or ground, which often favors SGA placement, although standard geometry or hyperangulated VAL may help overcome the challenge of the nonstandard positioning.

Common body positions for the airway manager in these cases are kneeling or prone, although some literature would recommend the left lateral decubitus and straddling positions (Figs. 31.3, 31.4, and 31.5).[102,103] It is unclear if any of these studies apply to VAL; most likely they do not. The straddling position requires the laryngoscope to be held in the right hand, which is very unnatural for most experienced airway practitioners. When laryngoscopy is not possible in a kneeling position, and the left lateral decubitus position is not feasible as a result of space constraints, we prefer a two-person technique (Fig. 31.6), whereby an assistant rather than the primary airway practitioner straddles the patient in a position of mechanical advantage. The primary airway practitioner still places the laryngoscope in the mouth, sweeps the tongue if appropriate, and guides the blade around the base of the tongue, before handing it off to the assistant; the practitioner can then direct fine movements before passing the tube from the conventional orientation. It is still very important to employ simple

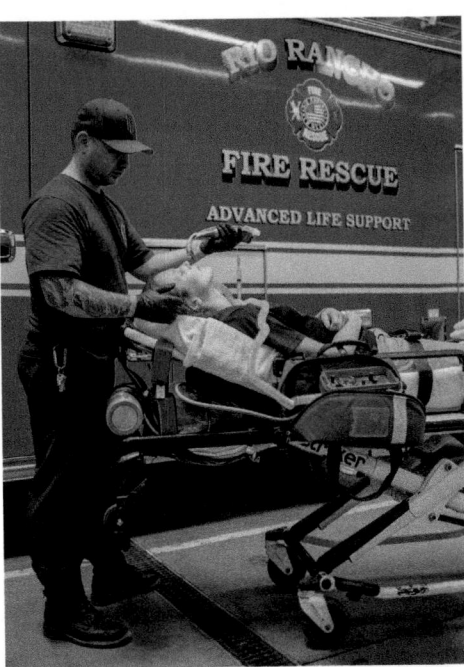

• **Fig. 31.2** Transfer of the patient to the stretcher before intubation allows the patient to be positioned at an optimal height for laryngoscopy and also minimizes movement of the intubated patient, which reduces the risk of accidental tube dislodgment.

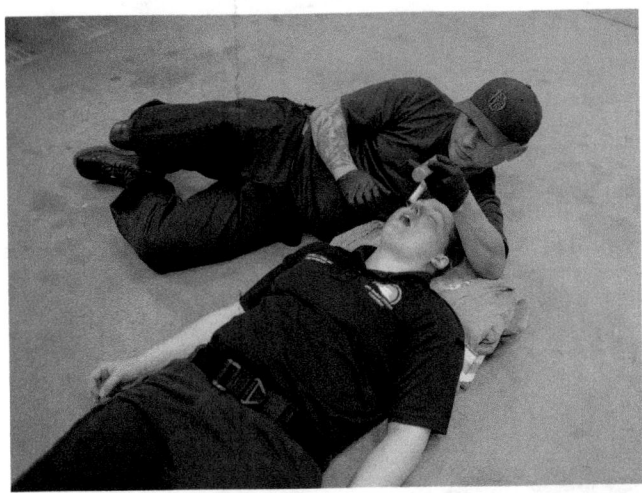

• **Fig. 31.3** Intubation of a patient on the ground with the operator in the left lateral decubitus position.

positioning measures such as lifting the head into a sniffing position with towels or anything available on scene.

Another unique consideration for prehospital intubation is the effect of direct sunlight on laryngoscopy, in particular VAL. Recent data suggest that sunlight can adversely affect the success of VAL in the prehospital environment by impairing visualization of the video monitor.[100] Strategies to mitigate this effect include using other practitioners as a human shade or placing an opaque object such as a blanket over the head of the intubator and patient (Fig. 31.7). Use of standard-geometry VAL devices may also make these situations more favorable: if vision becomes impaired because of glare, a reversion to DL can hypothetically be made.

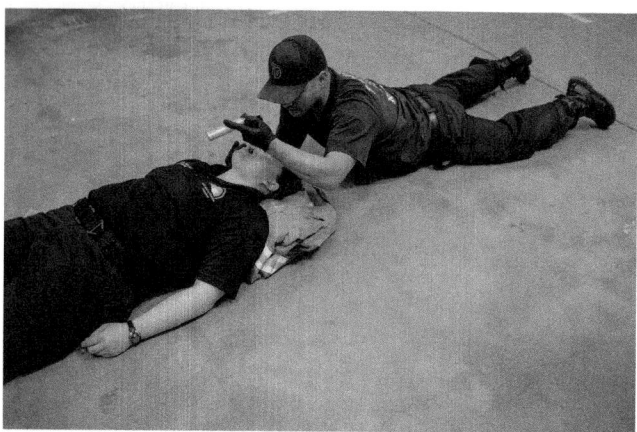

• **Fig. 31.4** Intubation of a patient on the ground with the operator in the prone position.

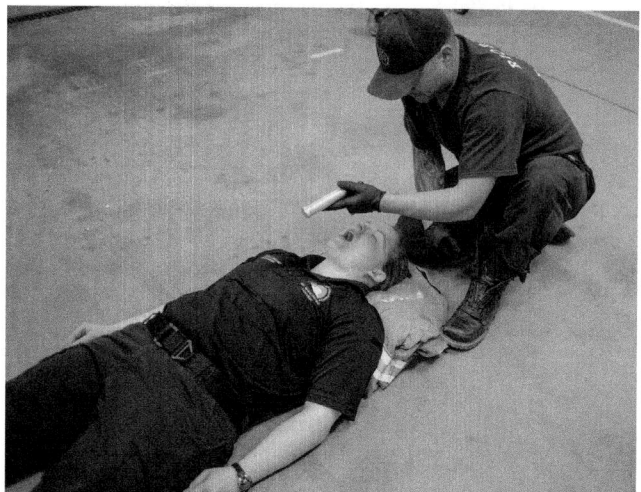

• **Fig. 31.5** Intubation of a patient on the ground with the operator in the kneeling position.

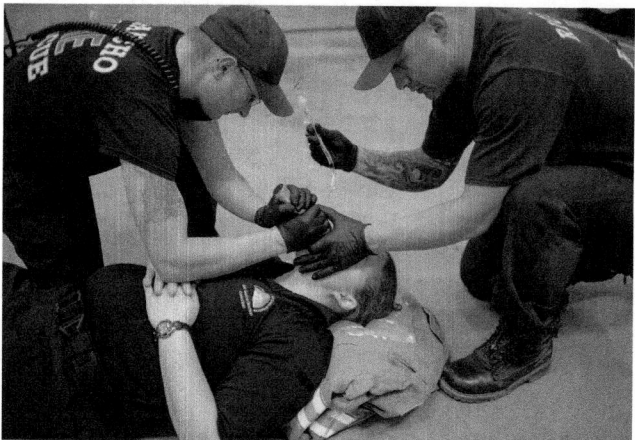

• **Fig. 31.6** Two-person technique: intubation of a patient on the ground.

Entrapped Patients

Patients may become entrapped in a variety of positions and situations, but the most common scenario is a seated patient in a motor vehicle. Patients who are entrapped without a gag reflex have a very poor prognosis from the outset, and airway interventions

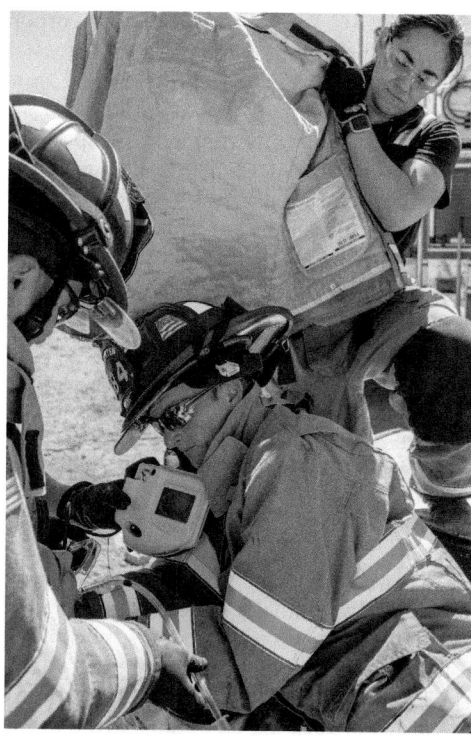

• **Fig. 31.7** This patient is being intubated while entrapped in a vehicle after the roof has been flapped back, which allows the intubator to assume a position behind and above the patient. An assistant is also seen applying shade for the operator to improve visualization of the video laryngoscope screen.

should be as rapid as possible without endangering the rescuer to allow focus on extrication. When evaluated in manikins, intubation is possible in these circumstances,[104,105] but in our experience placement of an SGA with gastric decompression capacity (second-generation SGA) usually makes the most clinical sense. We are more likely to opt for tracheal intubation when there is exceptional access to the patient, such as when the vehicle roof has been cut and peeled back but the lower body remains entrapped. Alternatives to traditional laryngoscopy techniques include the face-to-face technique and positioning the intubator above the patient, both of which can be performed with VAL (Fig. 31.8). Much like the straddling position for intubating the supine patient, face-to-face intubation requires very unfamiliar movements that must be extensively practiced if they are to be attempted clinically.

Managing entrapped patients who are still maintaining their own airways but appear to be deteriorating or who are no longer able to maintain satisfactory oxygenation is even more complicated. Although many of these patients would be obvious candidates for RSI in other circumstances, the risk-to-benefit ratio is clearly different when the patient is entrapped. RSI is particularly risky in this setting because (1) the intubation itself is usually more difficult because of positioning and time constraints, (2) rescue techniques such as BMV and surgical airways may be equally difficult to perform, and (3) the patient may not tolerate the hemodynamic effects of RSI medications and positive-pressure ventilation well. It is usually best to delay the procedure until after extrication if at all possible. If the provider and incident commander determine that airway control cannot or should not be delayed, and there is sufficient safe access to the patient

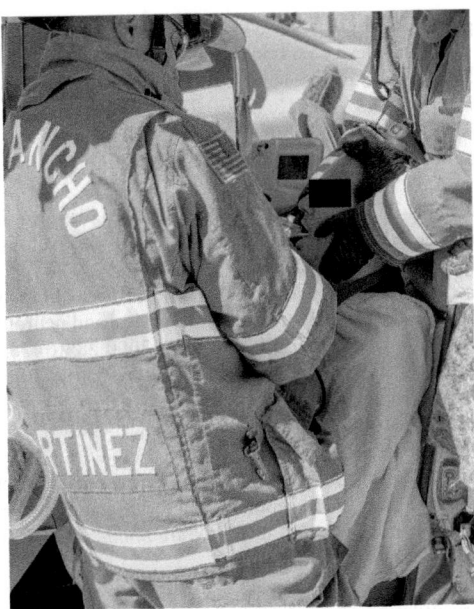

• **Fig. 31.8** Face-to-face video-assisted laryngoscopy with a seated and entrapped patient.

to perform the procedure, it is prudent to take as much time as possible to be confident of preparations. Rushing into an airway procedure on an entrapped patient without all equipment available, along with well-developed first attempt and backup plans, can be disastrous. RSA may also be considered as an alternative to RSI in this setting.[53]

Whether the airway is managed with an ETT or an SGA, continuous capnography is imperative to monitor for device dislodgment during extrication. Rather than managed with manual ventilation, the patient should be placed on a portable ventilator as soon as possible, which will maintain much more consistent ventilation and keep one additional person out of the way of those performing the extrication.

Cricothyrotomy

Prehospital cricothyrotomy (PC) is an infrequent procedure, generally occurring in less than 2% of airway encounters but up to 10% in one air medical study.[106] Techniques available include an "open" or "surgical" approach (with or without bougie assistance), needle cricothyrotomy, and various hybrid "percutaneous" or "minimally invasive" approaches. There is a wide range of EMS practice across jurisdictions, recognizing that surgical airways are generally restricted to patients older than 8 to 12 years. Some regions do not allow any PC, some allow only surgical PC for adults, others allow only needle PC for pediatrics, others allow needle or other less invasive approaches only for both adults and pediatrics, and some allow all age-appropriate techniques. A prehospital meta-analysis found a remarkably higher success rate for surgical cricothyrotomy compared with needle cricothyrotomy.[107] The Fourth National Audit Project (NAP4) looked at major airway complications during anesthesia in Great Britain and found a 60% failure rate for less invasive techniques and concluded "anesthetists should be trained to perform a surgical airway."[108] Other studies have also demonstrated higher complications in the less invasive approaches, which may seem counterintuitive.[109]

Based on our experience and the available evidence, we recommend that all paramedics be trained and allowed to perform

surgical airways (with a strong preference for bougie-aided techniques) in the appropriate age groups and circumstances, as dictated by local medical direction. An analysis of the National EMS Information System (NEMSIS) database revealed only 47 pediatric needle cricothyrotomy procedures across 40 states in 1 year.[110] Success rates and outcomes are not available, but it is unlikely that all were successful or that all patients had survivable conditions from the outset. Local medical directors and administrators must decide on a case-by-case basis if continued training in pediatric needle cricothyrotomy is justifiable.

Future Directions

Approaching the Airway as Continuum of Care

Airway management in EMS has traditionally been treated as a distinct environment, unrelated to hospital care, and supervised in isolation by EMS medical directors and administrators. The reality is that most patients undergoing prehospital airway management become ED patients and subsequently ICU and/or OR patients. It is not uncommon for providers in these settings to be called to manage patients with devices in situ that they are unfamiliar with or that they believe to be suboptimal. Although EMS physicians, particularly those with subspecialty board certification, should always be considered the ultimate experts regarding any decisions affecting the prehospital environment, it is ideal that decisions about prehospital airway management practices and equipment be made in consultation with providers from all disciplines in the hospital who will later ultimately be managing these patients. For example, when selecting an SGA for prehospital use, one of the myriad of factors to be considered are the thoughts of those providers who may be called upon to later exchange the device for an endotracheal tube.

Awake Techniques

Awake intubation is frequently an active consideration for the management of patients with predicted difficult airways in the hospital setting. EMS providers commonly face similar clinical scenarios, yet awake intubation techniques are very rarely included in prehospital scopes of practice and training, outside of teams that staff with experienced physicians. It is not hard to envision circumstances, however, when delaying the intubation to arrival at the hospital may not represent ideal patient care. This is particularly true for critical care transport teams that might be faced with the decision to either attempt high-risk MFAM using an RSI approach in predicted very difficult intubation or placing a tenuous nonintubated patient in an ambulance or aircraft for prolonged transport. In the future, medical directors should consider training critical care transport crews in simplified approaches to awake intubation including VAL with topical anesthesia and flexible scope intubation.

Flexible Scope Techniques

Similar to the preceding discussion regarding awake airway techniques, endoscopic techniques have rarely been included in prehospital education and guidelines, first and foremost because of high cost. Now that disposable, flexible, video-based intubating bronchoscopes have become available, it is reasonable to consider them for teams staffed with experienced physicians who already may be very comfortable with their use.[111] These tools may be ideal for use in conjunction with many SGAs to facilitate intubation through them, as well as for the awake procedures previously referenced.

Conclusion

The prehospital environment presents unique clinical challenges that may be overcome with education, research, specific techniques, and appropriate use of technology. It is helpful for all airway practitioners to at least be familiar with these considerations so that they are better prepared to advise EMS physicians and systems, assist with the education of EMS providers, and assume care of prehospital patients.

Selected References

1. Wang HE, Seitz SR, Hostler D, Yealy DM. Defining the learning curve for paramedic student endotracheal intubation. *Prehosp Emerg Care.* 2005;9(2):156–162.
6. Wang HE, Schmicker RH, Daya MR, et al. Effect of a strategy of initial laryngeal tube insertion vs. endotracheal intubation on 72-hour survival in adults with out-of-hospital cardiac arrest: a randomized clinical trial. *JAMA.* 2018;320(8):769–778.
9. Powell EK, Hinckley WR, Stolz U, et al. Predictors of difficult airway sans hypoxia/hypotension on first attempt (DASH-1A) in traumatically injured patients undergoing prehospital intubation. *Prehosp Emerg Care.* 2020;24(4):470–77.
10. Dunford JV, Davis DP, Ochs M, Doney M, Hoyt DB. Incidence of transient hypoxia and pulse rate reactivity during paramedic rapid sequence intubation. *Ann Emerg Med.* 2003;42(6):721–728.
12. Benger JR, Kirby K, Black S, et al. Effect of a strategy of supraglottic airway device vs. tracheal intubation during out-of-hospital cardiac arrest on functional outcome: the AIRWAYS-2 randomized clinical trial. *JAMA.* 2018;320(8):779–791.
23. Jarvis JL, Gonzales J, Johns D, Sager L. Implementaiton of a clinical bundle to reduce out-of-hospital peri-inutbaiton hypoxia. *Ann Emerg Med.* 2018;72(3):272–279.
30. Gravesteijn BY, Sewalt CA, Nieboer D, et al. Tracheal intubation in traumatic brain injury: a multicenter prospective observational study. *Br J Anaesth.* 2020;125(4):505–517.
40. Gausche M, Lewis RJ, Stratton SJ, et al. Effect of out-of-hospital pediatric endotracheal intubation on survival and neurological outcome: a controlled clinical trial. *JAMA.* 2000;283(6):783–790.
44. Kuzmack E, Inglis T, Olvera D, et al. A novel difficult-airway prediction tool for emergency airway management: validation of the HEAVEN criteria in a large air medical cohort. *J Emerg Med.* 2018;54(4):395–401.
49. Dumont TM, Visioni AJ, Rughani AI, Tranmer BI, Crookes B. Inappropriate prehospital ventilation in severe traumatic brain injury increases in-hospital mortality. *J Neurotrauma.* 2010;27(7):1233–1241.
51. Davis DP, Dunford JV, Poste JC, et al. The impact of hypoxia and hyperventilation on outcome after paramedic rapid sequence intubation of severely head-injured patients. *J Trauma.* 2004;57(1):1–8, discussion: 8–10.
60. Braude D, Dixon D, Torres M, Martinez JP, O'Brien S, Bajema T. Brief research report: prehospital rapid sequence airway. *Prehosp Emerg Care.* 2020;22:1–5.

All references can be found online at eBooks.Health.Elsevier.com.

32

Cardiopulmonary Resuscitation and Airway Management

BASMA MOHAMED AND LAUREN C. BERKOW

CHAPTER OUTLINE

KEY POINTS

- Cardiac arrest is a leading cause of mortality.
- Current AHA Guidelines recommend chest compressions before initial airway management.
- Ventilation and oxygenation during CPR can be performed via bag mask ventilation or an advanced airway device (either an endotracheal tube or a supraglottic airway).
- Interruptions in chest compressions should be minimized during airway management.
- Hyperventilation should be avoided during CPR.
- Ventilation plays a larger role in pediatric and neonatal resuscitation and high levels of supplemental oxygen should be avoided in neonates.

Introduction

Cardiac arrest is one of the leading causes of mortality in the United States. Most cardiac arrests occur outside the hospital, usually in the home, and 50% of arrests are unwitnessed. In-hospital cardiac arrests (IHCA) have a more favorable outcome than out-of-hospital cardiac arrests (OHCA). The average survival to discharge for adult OHCA patients who receive cardiopulmonary resuscitation (CPR) ranges from 3.4% to 22%,[1] with a 10.4% survival rate after initial hospitalization and 8.2% survival rate with good functional outcome. Among adults admitted to hospitals, 1.2% suffer from IHCA, and of those, 25.8% were discharged from the hospital, and 82% of those survivors had good functional status.[2] Early CPR and defibrillation are recognized as the most important treatment steps for cardiac arrest, but adequate oxygenation and ventilation are also important for providing oxygen to vital organ systems. Although earlier American Heart Association (AHA) CPR guidelines focused on the airway and ventilation as first steps in resuscitation, more recent versions have placed a stronger emphasis on rapid return of circulation.

The most common etiology of cardiac arrest in adult patients outside the hospital setting is cardiac in nature, most often ventricular fibrillation.[3] In the hospital, however, cardiac arrest may be because of cardiac or pulmonary causes.[4] Most first responders outside the hospital are not trained in advanced airway management; therefore, the AHA CPR guidelines related to airway management are different for lay rescuers than for in-hospital providers.

Basic Life Support and Cardiopulmonary Resuscitation Guidelines

The initial 2005 AHA guidelines for basic life support (BLS) and CPR recommended the sequence of airway, breathing, and circulation (A-B-C).[5] Thus, the first steps in the 2005 BLS guidelines were opening the airway, checking for breathing, and providing 2 rescue breaths if adequate breathing was not detected. The third step was to initiate chest compressions (Fig. 32.1). To check for breathing, lay rescuers and healthcare providers were advised to "look, listen, and feel." Healthcare providers were then advised to check for a pulse after delivering the initial rescue breaths to a nonresponsive, nonbreathing individual.

The 2005 AHA CPR guidelines recommended 2 rescue breaths, each given over 1 second, with sufficient tidal volume to produce visual chest rise. If an advanced airway was in place, the guidelines recommended 8 to 10 breaths per minute without synchronizing breaths between chest compressions.

Changes to AHA Guidelines 2010–2015

Updated BLS and CPR guidelines were released by the AHA in 2010 and in 2015 with significant changes.[6–9] Table 32.1 summarizes these guidelines. The recommended sequence was changed to circulation, airway, and breathing (C-A-B). In conditions of low blood flow (e.g., cardiac arrest), oxygen delivery to the brain and heart is limited primarily by blood flow rather than arterial oxygen content.[10] Using cardiac-only resuscitation and minimizing delays or interruptions in chest compressions can improve survival.[11] Evidence does not show any difference in survival rates between chest compressions delivered alone and chest compressions combined with positive-pressure ventilation (PPV).[11–13] The 2010 AHA guidelines recommended that chest compressions be initiated before rescue breaths or advanced airway placement, with rescue breaths provided after the first cycle of chest compressions. "Look, listen, and feel" was removed from the 2010 algorithm. The AHA released updated guidelines in 2015, but the C-A-B sequence remained unchanged, with a continued focus on early initiation of quality chest compressions before airway management.[9] The BLS components listed in Table 32.1 from the 2010 AHA guidelines were not changed in the 2015 update.

The recommended compression-to-ventilation ratio and ventilation rate with an advanced airway in place, as outlined in Table 32.1, remained unchanged in the 2015 guidelines. The 2015 AHA guidelines also recommended that in a patient with a witnessed OHCA and a shockable rhythm, PPV may be delayed for up to three cycles of chest compressions. This recommendation was based on recent evidence that neurologic survival and survival to hospital discharge are improved with this delayed ventilation strategy.[14,15]

The 2015 guidelines recommended that lay rescuers check for absence of breathing or gasping only after checking for patient response and activating emergency response, whereas the recommendation to healthcare providers is to check for lack of breathing and absence of pulse simultaneously (Table 32.2). The 2015 guidelines also recommended that emergency dispatchers become trained to recognize that abnormal or agonal breathing patterns are associated with a high likelihood of cardiac arrest. The misinterpretation of agonal gasps or abnormal breathing as normal may delay the onset of chest compressions.[16,17]

Although the optimal oxygen concentration to be delivered during CPR has not been defined, current AHA guidelines recommend initial delivery of 100% oxygen during resuscitation. After return of spontaneous circulation (ROSC), the 2010 guidelines recommended titration of oxygen administration to maintain oxygen saturation level of 94% or greater to avoid hyperoxia when appropriate monitoring is available. The 2015 guidelines added to this recommendation that the highest available oxygen concentration should be administered after ROSC to avoid hypoxia until arterial oxygen saturation or partial pressure of arterial oxygen can be measured.[18] Box 32.1 summarizes the changes pertaining to airway management during CPR that were introduced in the 2010 AHA guidelines, and Box 32.2 summarizes the additional changes introduced in the recent 2015 AHA guidelines.

AHA Updated Guidelines 2015–2020

Since 2015, the AHA has released yearly focused updates based on updated evidence, as well as updated guidelines in 2020 that incorporated updated recommendations from the previous focused updates.[2,19] The 2020 guidelines stress that if a patient demonstrates agonal breathing or gasping respiration, lay rescuers should assume the patient is in cardiac arrest and begin CPR.[2] The steps and recommendations provided in Tables 32.1 and 32.2 remain unchanged in the updated 2020 guidelines.

The 2019 focused update provided updated recommendations for the use of advanced airway devices and stressed the need for training and use of capnography, and these recommendations are incorporated into the 2020 updated guidelines as well[2,19] (Box 32.3). Both the 2019 and 2020 guidelines also support previous versions to avoid interruptions in chest compressions for airway management, suggesting that advanced airway management

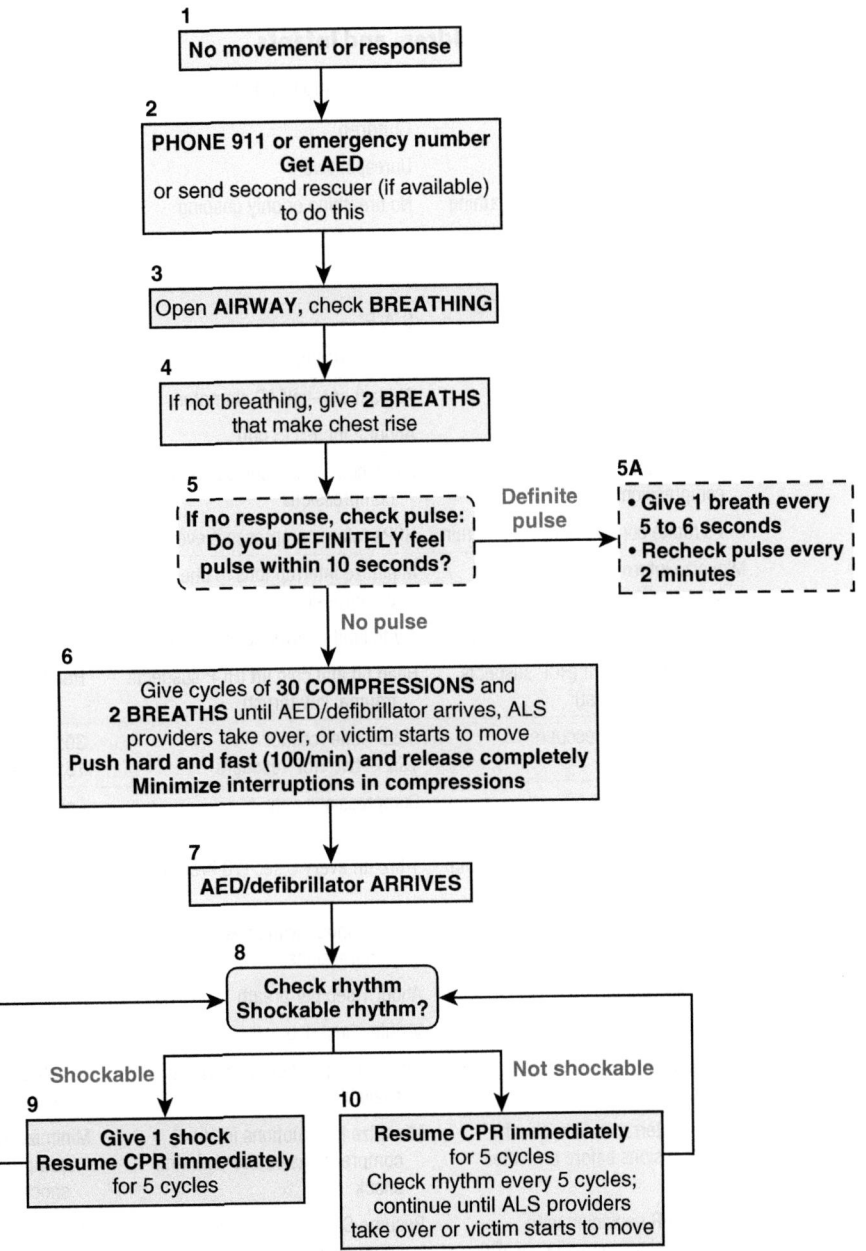

1
No movement or response

2
PHONE 911 or emergency number
Get AED
or send second rescuer (if available)
to do this

3
Open **AIRWAY**, check **BREATHING**

4
If not breathing, give **2 BREATHS**
that make chest rise

5
If no response, check pulse:
Do you DEFINITELY feel
pulse within 10 seconds?

Definite
pulse →

5A
• Give 1 breath every
  5 to 6 seconds
• Recheck pulse every
  2 minutes

No pulse

6
Give cycles of **30 COMPRESSIONS** and
2 BREATHS until AED/defibrillator arrives, ALS
providers take over, or victim starts to move
**Push hard and fast (100/min) and release completely
Minimize interruptions in compressions**

7
AED/defibrillator ARRIVES

8
**Check rhythm
Shockable rhythm?**

Shockable   Not shockable

9
**Give 1 shock
Resume CPR immediately**
for 5 cycles

10
Resume CPR immediately
for 5 cycles
Check rhythm every 5 cycles;
continue until ALS providers
take over or victim starts to move

• **Fig. 32.1** The 2005 Adult Basic Life Support (BLS) Health Care Provider Algorithm. *AED,* automatic external defibrillator; *ALS,* advanced life support; *CPR,* cardiopulmonary resuscitation. (From Emergency Cardiovascular Care (ECC) Committee, Subcommittees, and Task Forces of the American Heart Association. 2005 American Heart Association Guidelines for Cardiopulmonary Resuscitation and Emergency Cardiovascular Care. *Circulation.*, 2005;112(suppl):IV1–IV203)

can be delayed until after two rounds of chest compressions or even until after ROSC if bag-mask ventilation is adequate. The 2020 updated adult BLS algorithm for healthcare providers is shown in Fig. 32.2. The only change in this algorithm from the 2010 and 2015 versions is the simplification to provide rescue breathing every 6 seconds or 10 breaths per minute. The 2020 updated AHA guidelines also recommend that either a supraglottic airway (SGA) or an endotracheal tube (ETT) can be considered as an advanced airway technique and that an SGA may be preferred over an ETT in settings with minimal training opportunities or low intubation success rates (Fig. 32.3).

Initial Airway Management During Cardiopulmonary Resuscitation

Rescue Breathing

Initial rescue breathing during CPR should be provided through a mouth-to-mouth method, mouth-to-barrier device, or bag-mask ventilation (if available). If the mouth is not accessible or the patient has a tracheal stoma, mouth-to-nose or mouth-to-stoma ventilation may be necessary. Each rescue breath should be given over 1 second with a sufficient tidal

TABLE 32.1 Basic Life Support Components for Adults, Children, and Infants

Component	RECOMMENDATION		
	Adults	Children	Infants
Initial response	Unresponsive	Unresponsive	Unresponsive
	No breathing or no normal breathing (i.e., only gasping) No pulse palpated within 10 sec for all ages (HCP only)	No breathing or only gasping	No breathing or only gasping
CPR sequence	C-A-B	C-A-B	C-A-B
Compression rate	At least 100/min	At least 100/min	At least 100/min
Compression depth	At least 2 inches (5 cm)	At least one-half AP diameter About 2 inches (5 cm)	At least one-half AP diameter About 1.5 inches (4 cm)
Chest wall recoil	Allow complete recoil between compressions	Allow complete recoil between compressions	Allow complete recoil between compressions
	HCPs rotate compressors every 2 min	HCPs rotate compressors every 2 min	HCPs rotate compressors every 2 min
Compression interruptions	Minimize interruptions in chest compressions	Minimize interruptions in chest compressions	Minimize interruptions in chest compressions
	Try to limit interruptions to <10 sec	Try to limit interruptions to <10 sec	Try to limit interruptions to <10 sec
Airway	Head tilt and chin lift (HCP suspects trauma: jaw thrust)	Head tilt and chin lift (HCP suspects trauma: jaw thrust)	Head tilt and chin lift (HCP suspects trauma: jaw thrust)
Compression-to-ventilation ratio (until advanced airway placed)	30:2—one or two rescuers	30:2—one rescuer 15:2—two HCP rescuers	30:2—one rescuer 15:2—two HCP rescuers
Ventilations when rescuer untrained or trained and not proficient	Compressions only	Compressions only	Compressions only
Ventilations with advanced airway (HCP)	1 breath every 6 sec (10 breaths/min)	1 breath every 6 sec (10 breaths/min)	1 breath every 6 sec (10 breaths/min)
	Asynchronous with chest compressions	Asynchronous with chest compressions	Asynchronous with chest compressions
	About 1 sec per breath	About 1 sec per breath	About 1 sec per breath
	Visible chest rise	Visible chest rise	Visible chest rise
Defibrillation	Attach and use AED as soon as available	Attach and use AED as soon as available	Attach and use AED as soon as available
	Minimize interruptions in chest compressions before and after shock	Minimize interruptions in chest compressions before and after shock	Minimize interruptions in chest compressions before and after shock
	Resume CPR beginning with compressions immediately after each shock	Resume CPR beginning with compressions immediately after each shock	Resume CPR beginning with compressions immediately after each shock

A, airway; *AED*, automated external defibrillator; *AP*, anterior-posterior; *B*, breathing; *C*, circulation; *CPR*, cardiopulmonary resuscitation; *HCP*, healthcare provider.
(Modified from American Heart Association: Highlights of the 2010 American Heart Association Guidelines for CPR and ECC. Available at https://www.ahajournals.org/doi/10.1161/circulationaha.110.970889?cookieSet=1#d3e854.)[6]

volume to produce a visible chest rise. If a pulse is present, 1 rescue breath should be given every 6 seconds (or 10 breaths per minute) to maintain oxygen levels, and the pulse rechecked every 2 minutes. Once CPR is initiated, 2 ventilations should be provided after completing 30 compressions (30:2 compression-to-ventilation ratio). Trained lay rescuers or healthcare providers should initiate rescue breathing. An untrained lay rescuer should provide chest compressions only and not initiate rescue breathing.

The airway should be opened by a head-tilt–chin-lift maneuver, unless a cervical spine injury is suspected. If a cervical spine injury is suspected, a jaw thrust should be performed with the head maintained in a midline position.

Airway Adjuncts

Oropharyngeal airways can assist bag-mask ventilation by displacing the tongue, which can occlude the airway. Oropharyngeal airways are recommended for unconscious patients and should be placed by rescuers trained in their use.

Nasopharyngeal airways are better tolerated in conscious patients than are oral airway adjuncts, and they can assist ventilation by

TABLE 32.2   Basic Life Support Sequence from the 2020 AHA BLS Guidelines

Step	Untrained Lay Rescuer	Trained Lay Rescuer	Healthcare Provider
1	Confirm scene safety.	Confirm scene safety.	Confirm scene safety.
2	Check for patient response.	Check for patient response.	Check for patient response.
3	Shout for help, phone 911, or ask bystander to phone 911. Keep phone at side of patient, with the phone in speaker mode.	Shout for help, activate emergency response system. Keep phone at side of the patient if possible.	Shout for help, activate resuscitation team (resuscitation team can also be activated immediately after pulse/breathing check).
4	Follow the instructions provided by telecommunicator.	Check for absence of breathing or presence of gasping only. If none, begin chest compressions.	Check for absence of breathing or presence of gasping only while simultaneously checking for pulse. AED and emergency equipment should be retrieved immediately after breathing and pulse check.
5	Follow telecommunicator instructions to look for absence of breathing, identify gasping only.	Answer questions and follow instructions from telecommunicator.	Begin CPR immediately, use AED/defibrillator when available.
6	Follow instructions of telecommunicator.	Send a second person, if available, to retrieve an AED.	When a second rescuer arrives, provide two-person CPR and use AED/defibrillator.

AED, automated external defibrillator; *CPR*, cardiopulmonary resuscitation.
(Modified from Kleinman ME, Brennan EE, Goldberger ZD, et al. Part 5: Adult basic life support and cardiopulmonary resuscitation quality: 2015 American Heart Association guidelines update for cardiopulmonary resuscitation and emergency cardiovascular care. *Circulation*. 2015;132(Suppl 2):S414–S435 and Panchal AR, Bartos JA, Cabañas JG et al. Part 3: Adult Basic and Advanced Life Support: 2020 American Heart Association Guidelines for Cardiopulmonary Resuscitation and Emergency Cardiovascular Care. *Circulation*. 2020 Oct 20;142(16_suppl_2):S366-S468.. Available at https://cpr.heart.org/en/resuscitation-science/cpr-and-ecc-guidelines/adult-basic-and-advanced-life-support#IoR22 [accessed November 2020].)

• BOX 32.1   2010 Adult Advanced Cardiac Life Support Guidelines: Changes in Airway Management

Management
1. The basic life support sequence changed from A-B-C to C-A-B for adults, children, and infants. Initiate chest compressions *before* ventilations.
2. Use of cricoid pressure during ventilations is not recommended.
3. Instruction to "look, listen, and feel for breathing" was removed from the algorithm.
4. Excessive ventilation should be avoided.
5. Continuous quantitative capnography is recommended to confirm endotracheal tube placement.
6. Oxygen concentration is weaned after return of spontaneous circulation to maintain oxygen saturation at 94% or greater.

A, Airway; *B*, breathing; *C*, circulation.

• BOX 32.3   2020 Adult Basic and Advanced Cardiac Life Support Guidelines: Additional Changes in Airway Management Since 2015

1. If a patient demonstrates agonal breathing or gasping respiration, lay rescuers should assume the patient is in cardiac arrest and begin CPR.
2. Rescue breathing was simplified to 10 breaths/minute.
3. Either bag-mask ventilation or an advanced airway may be considered during CPR in any setting.
4. Either a supraglottic airway (SGA) or an endotracheal tube (ETT) can be considered as an advanced airway technique,
5. In settings with minimal training opportunities or low intubation success rates, an SGA may be preferred.
6. Waveform capnography should be used to confirm and monitor ETT placement, including during transport.

CPR, cardiopulmonary resuscitation, *ETT*, endotracheal tube; *SGA*, supraglottic airway.

• BOX 32.2   2015 Adult Advanced Cardiac Life Support Guidelines: Additional Changes in Airway Management

1. Positive-pressure ventilation can be delayed for up to three cycles of CPR in OHCA patients with a shockable rhythm.
2. Passive ventilation techniques are not routinely recommended during conventional CPR but may be considered by EMS systems when performing continuous chest compressions.
3. Manual in-line stabilization, rather than an immobilization device, is recommended when cervical spine injury is suspected.
4. The use of ultrasound was added as method for confirming endotracheal tube placement.

CPR, cardiopulmonary resuscitation; *EMS*, emergency medical service; *OHCA*, out-of-hospital cardiac arrest.

---

relieving nasopharyngeal obstruction. Nasal airway adjuncts should be placed by a rescuer trained in their use, and they should be avoided if a basilar skull fracture or coagulopathy is suspected. Case reports have described intracranial placement of the nasopharyngeal airway in the presence of a basilar skull fracture, so an oral airway is preferred in these patients.[20,21] Incorrect placement of an oropharyngeal or nasopharyngeal airway may worsen airway obstruction.

Advanced Airway Management During Cardiopulmonary Resuscitation

The primary goal of airway management during CPR should be to provide adequate oxygenation and ventilation. If bag-mask ventilation is adequate and an advanced airway strategy will interrupt chest compressions, current AHA guidelines suggest that insertion

Adult Basic Life Support Algorithm for Healthcare Providers

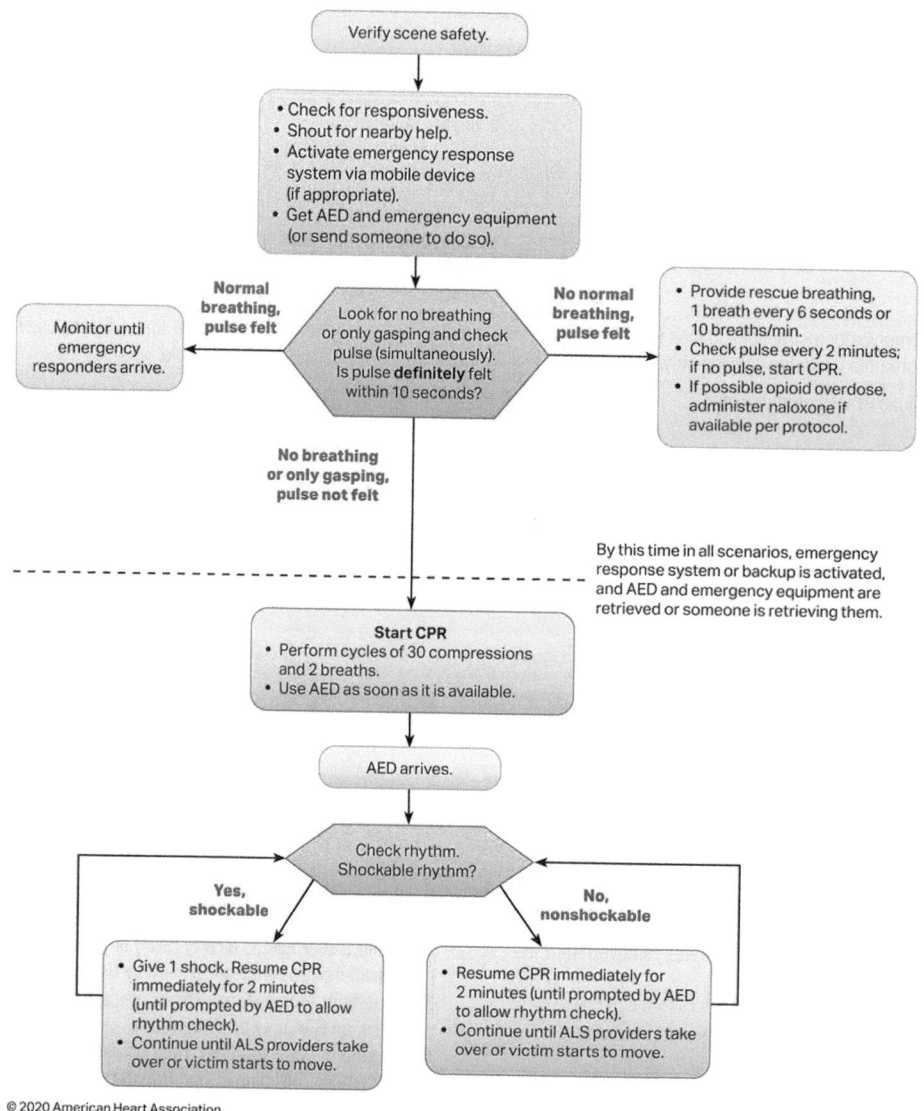

© 2020 American Heart Association

• **Fig. 32.2** The Adult Basic Life Support Algorithm for Healthcare Providers—2020 Update. *AED,* Automatic external defibrillator; *ALS,* advanced life support; *CPR,* cardiopulmonary resuscitation. (Reprinted with permission *Circulation.* 2020;142:S366-S468 ©2020 American Heart Association, Inc.)

of an advanced airway can be deferred until either ROSC occurs or the patient fails to respond to chest compressions and defibrillation. If bag-mask ventilation is not adequate, however, an advanced airway should be placed.[2]

Trained healthcare providers should perform tracheal intubation during CPR while minimizing interruptions in chest compressions. Tracheal intubation performed by direct laryngoscopy may be more difficult if performed during chest compressions. Prolonged attempts at tracheal intubation should be avoided, especially if chest compressions are halted during attempts. Placement of an endotracheal tube (ETT) or another advanced airway device has not been associated with any improvement in ROSC. Tracheal intubation attempts by inexperienced providers may result in complications, such as failed intubation or esophageal intubation.[22]

After ETT placement, ventilations are delivered without interruption of chest compressions at a rate of 1 breath every 6 seconds. Certain resuscitation medications can be delivered through the ETT (Box 32.4). Secretions can be removed from the airway through the ETT, and the ETT cuff may provide a barrier against aspiration. Per the 2020 updated AHA advanced cardiovascular life support (ACLS) guidelines, in order to use advanced airway devices effectively, healthcare providers should maintain their knowledge and skills through frequent practice. In addition to mastering bag-mask ventilation, providers should master an advanced airway strategy and a second (backup) strategy for use.

More recent studies comparing the use of an SGA versus an ETT demonstrate no difference in survival or neurological outcome between the two techniques.[2] Therefore, the most

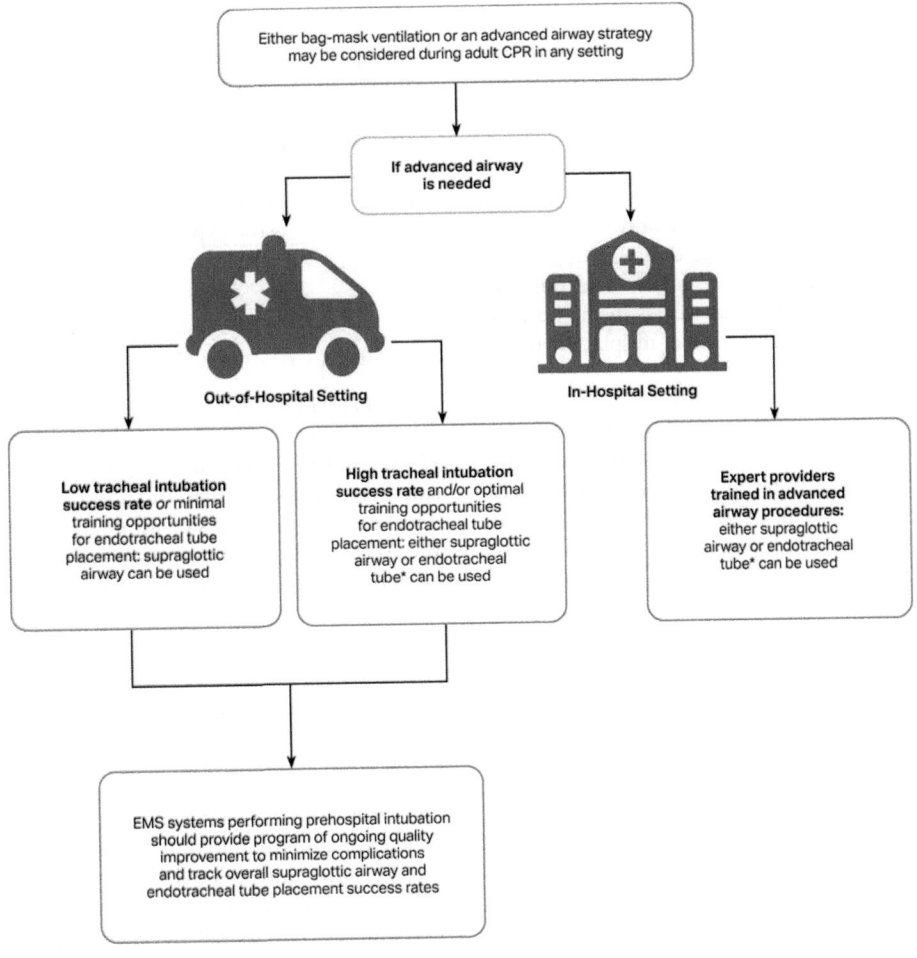

• **Fig. 32.3** Schematic representation of ACLS recommendations for use of advanced airways during CPR. (Reprinted with permission *Circulation*. 2020;142:S366-S468 ©2020 American Heart Association, Inc.)

<table>
<tr><td>• BOX 32.4</td><td>Resuscitation Medications That Can Be Delivered Through an Endotracheal Tube</td></tr>
</table>

Administer two to three times the intravenous dosage, followed by 10 mL of normal saline:

Lidocaine
Epinephrine
Atropine
Vasopressin
Naloxone

---

recent guidelines recommend that providers can use either advanced airway technique during CPR in any setting (OHCA or IHCA). Since the success of advanced airway placement is highly dependent on provider skill set, either bag-mask ventilation or an advanced airway is considered acceptable during CPR. If an advanced airway is used, an SGA can be used in settings with low intubation success rate or minimal training for ETT placement, whereas in settings where ETT placement success is high with optimal training, either an SGA or ETT can be used. See Fig. 32.3 for the current recommendations related to advanced airway management in patients with cardiac arrest.

Confirmation of Endotracheal Tube Placement During Cardiopulmonary Resuscitation

The 2005 CPR guidelines recommended the use of exhaled carbon dioxide (CO_2) detectors or esophageal detectors for confirmation of ETT placement, in addition to clinical assessment by auscultation and direct visualization. Exhaled CO_2 detectors may produce a false-negative result because of decreased blood flow and CO_2 delivery to the lungs, pulmonary embolus, pulmonary edema, or severe airway obstruction.[23] False-positive readings have been detected when the stomach contains large amounts of carbonated liquids.[24]

Since 2010, the updated CPR guidelines recommend the use of continuous waveform capnography for confirmation of ETT placement during CPR, although the use of exhaled CO_2 detectors or esophageal detectors is considered acceptable if waveform capnography is not available. It should be noted, however, that the specificity and sensitivity of continuous waveform capnography may decrease during prolonged resuscitation and decreased perfusion. Since 2015, the updated guidelines also recommend the use of ultrasound, if available, as a method to confirm ETT placement. On ultrasound imaging, correct ETT placement can be confirmed by observing the lung sliding against the pleura.[25] The current guidelines recommend using continuous waveform capnography for monitoring the placement of an advanced airway device not only upon placement of the airway device in the field but also during any patient transfers in the field, as well as in the hospital to minimize the risk of unrecognized tube misplacement or displacement.[2,19]

Capnography can also be useful both to assess the effectiveness of CPR and as a prognosticator of ROSC.[2] A sudden and sustained increase in capnography (typically greater than 40 mm Hg) has been demonstrated to be an indicator of ROSC. Conversely, failure to achieve an end-tidal CO_2 of greater than 10 mm Hg after 20 minutes of CPR is one of several indicators that can be used to guide termination of resuscitation efforts.

Thoracic impedance measurement may aid in detection of esophageal intubation, but evidence is insufficient to recommend its use for confirmation of ETT placement. Thoracic impedance is significantly higher during inspiration than during expiration, and changes in impedance, which can be measured by defibrillation pads, occur only if the ETT is correctly placed.[26]

Supraglottic Airway Devices

All of the AHA CPR guidelines (2005–2020) support the use of an SGA device as an alternative to tracheal intubation. Because intubation through an SGA does not require glottic visualization, placement may be faster than tracheal intubation, and it may result in shorter no-flow times (i.e., period when chest compressions are halted for other interventions).[27,28] The most recent updates state that if an advanced airway is placed, either an ETT or an SGA may be considered, based on the skill of the provider, and that an SGA may be preferred in settings with a low tracheal success rate or minimal training.[19] SGA placement should be considered an option if tracheal intubation fails and in situations where the success rate of ETT placement is low[2,19] (Fig 32.3). Ventilations are delivered through an SGA device in the same ratio as they are through an ETT (i.e., 1 breath every 6 seconds without interruption of chest compressions). The use of capnography to confirm and monitor the placement of an SGA has undergone limited evaluation, and its utility will depend on the airway design.[2] Effective ventilation through an SGA device should result in a capnograph waveform similar to that seen with an ETT during CPR and upon ROSC.

If available, newer SGA devices that provide a conduit for intubation can be considered. Preliminary evidence supports their use in the prehospital environment, especially if intubation is difficult.[29,30]

Role of Advanced Airway Devices

Advanced airway management techniques, such as flexible scope intubation (FSI) and video-assisted laryngoscopy (VAL) have not been widely studied as intubation techniques for airway management during CPR. Preliminary evidence suggests that VAL may be an acceptable alternative to conventional laryngoscopy, especially for difficult intubations, and may achieve intubation in less

time than conventional direct laryngoscopy.[31–33] Recent evidence also suggests that patients can be intubated via VAL without interruptions in chest compressions.[34,35] However, advanced airway devices may not be easily accessible in the prehospital environment. Additionally, inadequate light conditions and the lack of electricity may limit the usefulness of VAL outside the hospital setting. The advanced airway device used should depend on availability, as well as the experience of the provider.

Use of Cricoid Pressure During Cardiopulmonary Resuscitation

The 2005 AHA CPR guidelines recommended the use of cricoid pressure by a third rescuer, if the victim is deeply unconscious. However, some evidence suggests that applying cricoid pressure may impede ventilation and interfere with the placement of advanced airway devices or intubation.[36,37] Therefore, since 2010, the AHA CPR guidelines recommend against the routine use of cricoid pressure as part of airway management during CPR.[2]

Alternative Methods of Oxygen Delivery During Cardiopulmonary Resuscitation

Oxylator

The Oxylator (CPR Medical Devices, Ontario, Canada) is a fixed-flow automatic resuscitation management system with an adjustable pressure limit. Several models exist, including the Oxylator EMX, which is recommended for prehospital use (Fig. 32.4). The Oxylator delivers oxygen flow at 30 L/min until an adjustable maximum pressure (up to 45 cm H_2O) is reached, at which point passive exhalation occurs to an airway pressure of 2 to 4 cm H_2O. The device allows manual (rescuer-initiated) and automatic inhalation modes. The Oxylator works with medical oxygen or hospital air supply, tank, or compressor; it does not require electricity; and it can be connected to a face mask, SGA, or ETT (Video 32.1).

Potential advantages of the Oxylator over bag-mask ventilation include consistent ventilation and oxygenation to a set pressure; possible avoidance of hyperventilation, excessive ventilation, or gastric insufflation; and early detection of airway obstruction.[38] Use of the Oxylator in the automatic mode can free the CPR

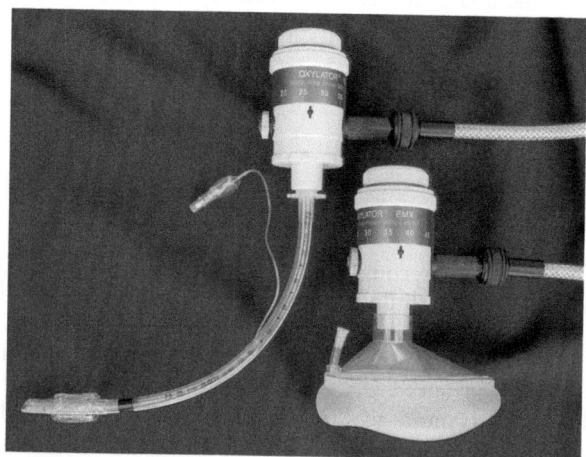

• **Fig. 32.4** The Oxylator EMX is a positive-pressure resuscitation and inhalation system. (Courtesy Lifesaving Systems, Inc., Roswell, GA.)

provider to focus on other resuscitation tasks. The Oxylator may be useful in austere environments in which access to the patient's head and airway may be limited.

ResQPOD

The ResQPOD (Zoll Medical Corporation, Chelmsford, MA, USA), designated as an AHA Class 2A recommendation for patients in cardiac arrest, is an impedance threshold device. By regulating thoracic pressure during ventilation, the device increases blood flow to the heart and brain, increases systolic blood pressure, and increases the success rate of defibrillation. By preventing excess air from entering the thorax during ventilation, the device increases thoracic negative pressure and increases blood flow to the heart. It is placed proximal to a face mask, SGA, or ETT and connects to the source of ventilation (Fig. 32.5). The ResQPOD also contains timing-assist lights to guide proper ventilation rates and prevent hyperventilation. Use of this device during CPR has improved survival rates.[39]

Passive Oxygen Insufflation

Oxygen can be delivered passively through an oropharyngeal airway, face mask, SGA, or modified endotracheal tube (Boussignac endotracheal tube, Vygon Corporation, Montgomeryville, PA, USA). The Boussignac tube contains capillaries through which oxygen is delivered by continuous insufflation, generating a constant positive alveolar pressure. The proximal end of the tube remains open to allow exhalation (Fig. 32.6). The changes in intrathoracic

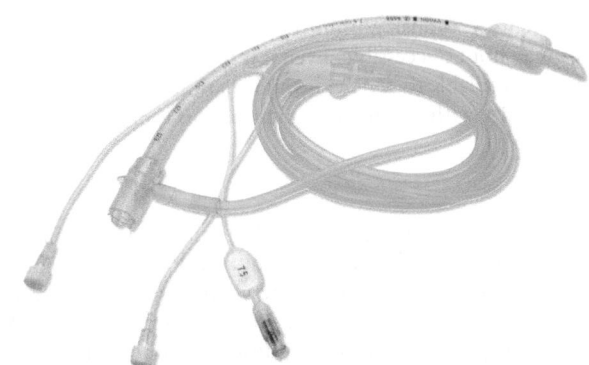

• **Fig. 32.6** The Boussignac endotracheal tube contains capillaries through which oxygen is delivered by continuous insufflation, generating a constant positive alveolar pressure. (Courtesy Vygon, Ecouen, France.)

pressure that occur during chest compressions trigger passive inhalation and active exhalation, allowing adequate gas exchange.

Passive oxygen delivery does not require the use of a rescuer to deliver ventilations, minimizes interruptions in chest compressions, and may reduce the risk of barotrauma caused by excessive ventilation. Evidence shows passive oxygen delivery to be as effective as bag-mask ventilation or mechanical ventilation through an ETT.[14,40] In the 2010 AHA guidelines, passive oxygen delivery is described as an alternative to, but not a replacement for, ventilation during CPR. In the updated 2015 AHA guidelines, as well as more recent updates, passive ventilation techniques are not recommended for routine use during conventional CPR but may be considered as part of a bundle of care when continuous chest compressions are applied.[2,41]

Airway Management Postintubation and after Return of Spontaneous Circulation

Post-ROSC care has focused on identifying the cause of cardiac arrest, management of multiorgan system failure, post-ROSC hypothermia protocols, and prognostication for survival. The AHA guidelines also address elements related to airway management, oxygenation, and ventilation after ROSC. In regard to oxygenation, and in order to avoid hypoxemia in adults with ROSC after cardiac arrest, it is reasonable to use the highest available oxygen concentration until arterial oxyhemoglobin saturation or PaO_2 can be measured.[2,42] Once arterial oxygenation can be measured, supplemental oxygen delivery should be titrated to maintain an SpO_2 range of 92% to 98% and a PaO_2 >100 to avoid oxygen toxicity. Capnography can be useful after ROSC to confirm proper airway device placement, during conversion of an SGA to an ETT if needed, and to optimize ventilation. Ventilation at 10 breaths per minute is recommended to maintain normocarbia ($EtCO_2$ of 30–40 or $PaCO_2$ of 35–45). Mild hypocapnia may be considered as a temporizing measure to manage elevated ICP, whereas permissive hypercapnia may be considered in the setting of lung injury.[42]

Challenges of Airway Management During Cardiopulmonary Resuscitation

When a patient requires CPR in an emergency, immediate airway management is required. In the prehospital setting, no general medical history or intubation history is available to guide airway

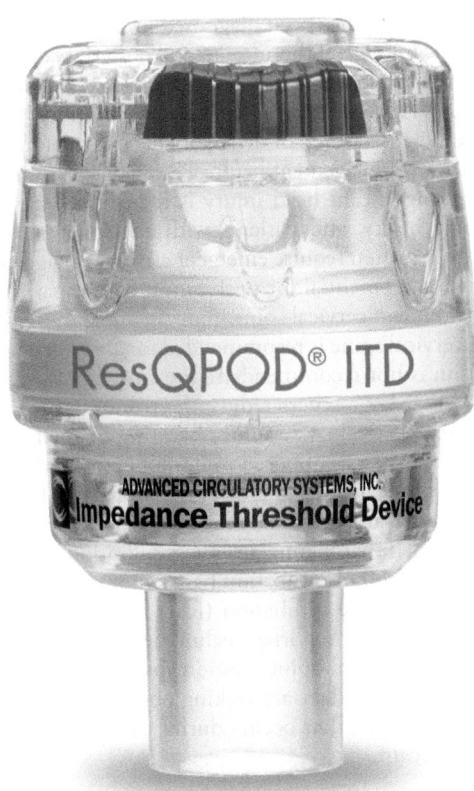

• **Fig. 32.5** The ResQPOD is an impedance threshold device that provides perfusion on demand (POD) by regulating pressures in the thorax during states of hypotension. (Used with permission from ZOLL Medical Corporation.)

management decisions. Within the hospital, patient information may or may not be accessible. Even if it is available, adequate time may not be available to review the information. Knowledge of previous difficulty with ventilation or intubation is often unknown.

Access to the Airway

Access to the airway during CPR may be limited in prehospital and hospital settings. Outside of the hospital, CPR may be required in whatever location or situation the victim presents, and access may be limited by the outside environment or accident scene. Airway access may also be challenging inside an ambulance or helicopter. Other equipment required to resuscitate the patient and treat life-threatening injuries may also limit access to the patient. Within the hospital, access to the patient's airway may be limited by equipment, invasive lines or monitors, or the small size of many hospital rooms and intensive care suites. For patients under airborne and contact isolation (severe acute respiratory syndrome [SARS], coronavirus, active tuberculosis, Ebola), care providers may need to use respirators and PPE during airway management. Hospitals with high-risk contact isolation units may consider using completely disposable airway devices to reduce the risk of cross-contamination and avoid the need for sterilization. During mass casualty disasters and pandemics, the use of PPE or chemical protection gear may make airway management more difficult.[43,44]

Infection Risk During CPR and Airway Management

Recent epidemics and pandemics involving viruses that cause SARS, such as the 2019 novel coronavirus (COVID-19), have highlighted concerns about aerosolization of infectious viral particles during airway management and CPR, both of which are considered aerosol-generating procedures.[45] To help rescuers treat individuals with cardiac arrest while maintaining their own safety, the AHA in collaboration with other societies recently published guidance for basic and advanced life support in adults, children, and neonates with suspected or confirmed COVID-19.[46] It is unclear whether chest compressions and defibrillation cause aerosol generation or transmission of airborne and droplet viral infections, so it is still recommended that lay rescuers (most likely household contacts), as well as healthcare providers, start chest compressions and defibrillation as early as possible to increase chances of survival.[46] It is recommended that healthcare providers don PPE prior to CPR and airway management, although defibrillation prior to donning PPE may be considered if the benefits to the patient outweigh the risk.[46] The use of these guidelines highlights the need for a certain set of precautions whenever there is risk of airborne transmission of a highly infectious disease. In addition to the aerosol risks associated with chest compressions, PPV and advanced airway placement add further aerosolization risk. These resuscitation efforts often require multiple providers in close proximity to the infected patient, and high stress events may create inconsistencies in infection-control measures.

See Box 32.5 for a list of recommendations adapted to reduce exposure risk. These recommendations focus on reducing the provider exposure to infection, as well prioritizing oxygenation and ventilation strategies with lower aerosolization risk. Early donning of PPE and clear communication of the patient's infectious status are important strategies to reduce risk. Viral filters should be used during all methods of ventilation (bag-mask ventilation or an advanced airway

> • **BOX 32.5** **Interim Guidance Recommendations for CPR in the Setting of High Infectious Risk (such as COVID-19, SARS, Ebola)[46]**
>
> - Early chest compressions and defibrillation are still recommended for lay providers and healthcare providers.
> - Avoid close proximity to nose and mouth when checking for breathing.
> - Healthcare providers should don personal protective equipment (PPE) prior to chest compressions and defibrillation. Defibrillation prior to PPE can be considered if patient benefit outweighs provider risk.
> - Minimize personnel in the room during resuscitation efforts.
> - Use a viral (HEPA) filter between the self-inflating bag and airway device to minimize viral spread.
> - Consider SGA over bag-mask ventilation to reduce aerosol spread. Use tight mask seal if mask ventilation is performed.
> - Most experienced providers should perform airway management. Consider the use of videolaryngoscopy to remain further away from the patient's mouth. Use a cuffed ETT (adults and children).
> - Pause chest compressions during airway interventions to reduce aerosol spread.
>
> *COVID*, coronavirus; *CPR*, cardiopulmonary resuscitation; *ETT*, endotracheal tube; *HEPA*, high-efficiency particulate air; *PPE*, personal protective equipment; *SARS*, severe acute respiratory syndrome; *SGA*, supraglottic airway.

device). Advanced airway management should be performed by the most experienced provider to minimize the number of attempts and delays in compressions. The use of video-assisted laryngoscopy is also recommended to decrease proximity to the patient.

Cervical Spine Injury

Cervical spine injury has been diagnosed in 2% to 5% of patients after traumatic injury.[47] If the anterior and posterior columns of the cervical spine are injured, the injury is considered unstable.[48] Most trauma patients are placed in a cervical collar until cervical injury is ruled out; however, some of these patients may require CPR and emergent airway management before a radiologic examination can be obtained. Significant head injury is associated with traumatic cervical spine injury, and patients with a Glasgow Coma Scale score of 8 or less often require emergent airway management.[49]

To reduce the potential for neck movement in patients with a suspected or known cervical spine injury, manual in-line stabilization of the cervical spine is recommended for airway management. Neck traction is not recommended. The current AHA guidelines recommend that lay rescuers reduce the risk of harm in patients with suspected cervical spine injury by using manual in-line stabilization techniques, as opposed to immobilization devices.[2] The presence of a cervical collar increases the difficulty of intubation. Therefore, if necessary, the collar may be removed for airway management, provided that manual in-line stabilization is maintained.

No single method of intubation has been proven to be the safest, but rapid sequence intubation (RSI) by direct laryngoscopy is the most commonly reported technique. Evidence shows that some degree of cervical spine motion occurs with all methods of intubation,[50,51] but data are lacking about whether the small amount of movement that occurs during airway management is clinically significant.

Equipment Challenges

In the prehospital environment, airway management must be provided with the equipment that is available. Depending on the resources, a full complement of airway equipment, including oxygen supplies, may or may not be available. Equipment also may be unavailable within the hospital if airway management is required in a location remote from the operating room or intensive care setting. The type of airway management provided may be dictated by the available supplies and equipment, and adjunct airway devices for difficult airway management may not be quickly accessible. In emergent situations, bag-mask ventilation should be initiated and maintained until additional airway equipment becomes available.

Controversies

Role of Hyperventilation

Evidence suggests that hyperventilation may decrease overall survival and should be avoided.[52] Excessive ventilation should also be avoided because of the risk of gastric insufflation, regurgitation, or aspiration. Hyperventilation increases intrathoracic pressure and results in reduced coronary perfusion pressures.[53]

When to Secure the Airway

Existing information is inadequate to guide the ideal timing of advanced airway device placement. However, evidence supports the practice of initiating chest compressions early, before the start of airway management. Rescuers should use airway management strategies that minimize interruptions in resuscitation. Newer, advanced airway devices that can be placed quickly and that do not require direct visualization of the vocal cords may achieve this goal. Studies to date that have compared the use of bag-mask ventilation with advanced airway devices have found no difference in survival or favorable neurologic outcome, and the most recent updates to the AHA guidelines recommend that the choice of airway device and method of ventilation be based on the skill and experience of the airway provider.[41,54] The current 2020 AHA guidelines recommend either the use of bag-mask ventilation or an advanced airway strategy during CPR for adult cardiac arrest in any setting (Fig. 32.3).[2] These recommendations were informed by randomized controlled trials and systematic reviews that showed no difference in survival or neurological function between groups treated with an advanced airway versus bag-mask ventilation.[2,19,54,55]

Supraglottic Airway Device Versus Endotracheal Intubation as an Advanced Airway Technique

The 2015 AHA CPR guidelines recommended using either an SGA device or an ETT for advanced airway management. Although some observational studies show that the time to insertion may be faster with an SGA,[56,57] most evidence to date shows no difference between SGA use and ETT use in ROSC, neurologic survival, or survival to hospital discharge.[58–63] Whereas faster placement of an SGA may result in shorter low-flow times and fewer interruptions in chest compressions,[27,28] an ETT remains the preferred route for administration of resuscitation medications if intravenous access is not present.[64,65] Ultimately, the choice of advanced airway device should be based on availability, as well as on the expertise of the individual advanced airway provider.

Pediatric Basic and Advanced Life Support and Resuscitation

The AHA pediatric basic and advanced life support guidelines apply to infants (age less than 1 year) and children up to the age of puberty.[66,67] Unlike in adults, the most common cause of cardiac arrest in the pediatric patient is asphyxia; however, the resuscitation sequence used (C-A-B) and the compression rate are the same as those for adult cardiac arrest. The pediatric OHCA average survival rate to hospital discharge is 11.4%, but outcomes differ by age (17.1% in adolescents, 13.2% in children, and 4.9% in infants).[67] Pediatric IHCA incidence is 12.66 events per 1000 hospital admissions, with an overall survival to hospital discharge rate of 41.1%.[68] Favorable neurological outcome has been reported in up to 47% of survivors to discharge.[67] Because respiratory causes (asphyxia) are a common etiology for cardiac arrest in infants and children, ventilation during resuscitation may be more important in children than in adults, and has been associated with improved outcomes.[69]

The pediatric BLS algorithm is almost identical to the adult algorithm except for recommendations that chest compressions should be started in pediatric patients if the pulse is less than 60 beats per minute. In infants and children with a pulse but absent or inadequate respiratory efforts, it is reasonable to provide rescue breaths at a rate of 1 breath every 2 to 3 seconds (20–30 breaths/min).[67] This respiratory rate of 20 to 30 breaths/minute should also be employed during CPR.

The 2020 updated Pediatric Basic and Advanced Life Support Guidelines include updated recommendations for advanced airway management.[67] They recommend that bag-mask ventilation is a reasonable strategy compared to an ETT or SGA, since advanced airway placement may interrupt chest compressions and may be difficult for providers who do not routinely intubate infants and children. If an ETT is used, a cuffed ETT is recommended since it improves capnography accuracy, reduces the need for ETT changes, and improves tidal volume delivery. Routine use of cricoid pressure during intubation is not recommended for children, and monitoring of exhaled CO_2 is recommended with an advanced airway to confirm correct placement, as well as monitoring during transport. As in adults, excessive hyperventilation and interruptions in chest compressions during ventilation and airway management should be avoided. Titration of supplemental oxygen after cardiac arrest and ROSC should target an oxygen saturation of 94% to 99%, similar to the adult ACLS recommendations, but the pediatric ACLS guidelines suggest targeting normocapnia as well.[66,67] See Box 32.6 for a summary of recommendations related to airway management during pediatric resuscitation.

• BOX 32.6 *Airway Management During Pediatric Resuscitation*

1. For infants and children with a pulse but absent or inadequate respiratory efforts, give 1 rescue breath every 2 to 3 seconds.
2. When performing CPR with an advanced airway, target a respiratory rate of 1 breath every 2 to 3 seconds (20–30 breaths/min).
3. Either bag-mask ventilation or an advanced airway can be considered for ventilation during CPR.
4. The use of cuffed ETTs and capnography is recommended. Correct tube size selection is important, and cuff inflation pressure should not exceed 20 to 25 cm H_2O.
5. Routine cricoid pressure is not recommended during intubation.
6. Avoid excessive ventilation, and target normocapnia.

BMV, bag-mask ventilation; *CPR*, cardiopulmonary resuscitation; *ETT*, endotracheal tube.

Neonatal Resuscitation Algorithm

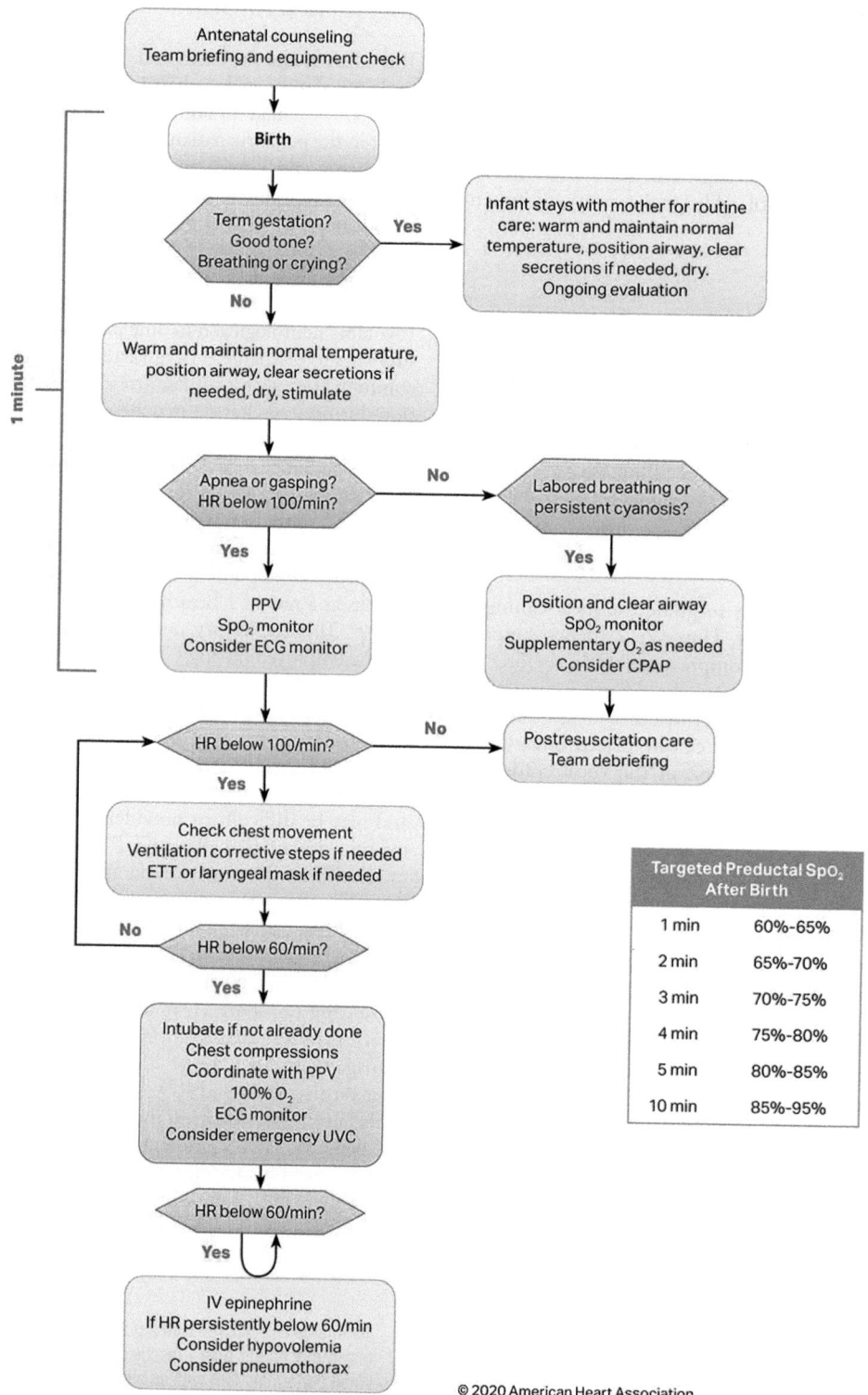

Targeted Preductal SpO₂ After Birth	
1 min	60%-65%
2 min	65%-70%
3 min	70%-75%
4 min	75%-80%
5 min	80%-85%
10 min	85%-95%

© 2020 American Heart Association

• **Fig. 32.7** Neonatal Resuscitation Algorithm—2020 Update. *ECG*, electrocardiography; *ETT*, endotracheal tube; *HR*, heart rate; *IV*, intravenous; *O₂*, oxygen; *PPV*, positive-pressure ventilation; *SpO₂*, oxygen saturation; *UVC*, umbilical venous catheter. (Reprinted with permission *Circulation*. 2020;142:S524-S550 ©2020 American Heart Association, Inc.)

Neonatal Basic and Advanced Life Support and Resuscitation

Although up to 10% of newborn infants require assistance with ventilation at birth, fewer than 1% require extensive CPR.[70] If a term newborn presents with good tone, breathing, and crying, usually no interventions are needed (Fig. 32.7).

The first steps of neonatal resuscitation include warming the infant, placing the infant in a "sniffing" position, clearing secretions as necessary, and stimulating the infant to breathe. The 2020 updated Neonatal Advanced Life Support Guidelines do not recommend routine oral, nasal, or oropharyngeal suctioning, unless PPV is required and the airway appears obstructed.[70] For nonvigorous newborns delivered through meconium-stained amniotic fluid who have evidence of airway obstruction during PPV, intubation and tracheal suction may be beneficial, but routine laryngoscopy and tracheal suctioning in these newborns are not recommended.

If breathing is labored or the infant is cyanotic, low levels of supplemental oxygen (21%–30%) or continuous positive airway pressure (CPAP) should be administered and titrated to pulse oximetry. Administration of higher supplemental oxygen doses (>65%) is not recommended and has been associated with higher mortality.[70] If the infant is apneic or persistently bradycardic (HR less than 100/min), PPV with 20 to 25 cm H_2O peak inflation pressure should be applied via bag-mask ventilation or a T-piece resuscitator at a rate of 40 to 60 breaths per minute.[70] The use of PEEP can also be considered, but excessive peak inflation pressures (higher than 30) may be harmful and should be avoided. When delivering PPV, it is reasonable to use an inspiratory time of 1 second or less. The use of sustained inflation can be harmful and should not be performed. An increase in heart rate is an indicator of effective ventilation.[70]

If bag-mask ventilation is inadequate or the heart rate remains below 100 beats per minute despite adequate ventilation, an advanced airway (uncuffed endotracheal tube or supraglottic airway) should be placed and chest compressions initiated. An advanced airway is the preferred method of ventilation during CPR, and placement should be confirmed by auscultation as well as capnography. Once chest compressions are initiated, 100% oxygen should be delivered, and a compression-to-ventilation ratio of 3:1 should be used.

Early assistance with ventilation and oxygenation is the most important step in neonatal resuscitation. Equipment and trained personnel who can provide advanced airway management should be available in the labor and delivery suite, especially if perinatal risk factors, such as prematurity, are present.[71]

Clinical Pearls

- The current AHA CPR guidelines recommend beginning chest compressions before initial airway management (i.e., circulation, airway, and breathing).
- Ventilation and oxygenation during CPR can be performed via bag-mask ventilation or via an advanced airway device (ETT or SGA).
- Hyperventilation during CPR should be avoided because it may reduce overall survival.
- Newer advanced airway devices, such as video-assisted laryngoscopes, are acceptable alternatives to conventional laryngoscopy for intubation during CPR. The advanced airway device used should depend on availability and on the experience of the provider.

- Interruptions in chest compressions should be minimized during transition from mask ventilation to an advanced airway device.
- Limited access to the patient may make airway management and resuscitation during disasters more challenging.
- In any setting with high infection risk, appropriate PPE should be worn during resuscitation and airway management strategies should be adapted to minimize aerosol risk.
- Ventilation plays a larger role in pediatric and neonatal resuscitation.
- High levels of supplemental oxygen should be avoided when providing assisted ventilation during neonatal resuscitation.

Conclusion

The updated CPR guidelines stress initiation of chest compressions before airway management. Either bag-mask ventilation or an advanced airway device can be considered for ventilation and oxygenation during CPR. The choice of the advanced airway device should depend on provider training and availability. Advanced airway devices, such as SGAs, can be considered if access to the patient is limited or endotracheal intubation fails. Ventilation plays a larger role in resuscitation of children and neonates than in adult CPR. Airway management during CPR is often guided by the resources available to the provider, which may be limited.

Selected References

2. Panchal AR, Bartos JA, Cabañas JG, et al. Part 3: adult basic and advanced life support: 2020 American Heart Association Guidelines for Cardiopulmonary Resuscitation and Emergency Cardiovascular Care. *Circulation*. 2020;142(16 suppl 2):S366-S468. doi:10.1161/CIR.0000000000000916.

11. SOS-KANTO Study Group. Cardiopulmonary resuscitation by bystanders with chest compression only (SOS-KANTO): an observational study. *Lancet*. 2007;369(9565):920-926. doi:10.1016/S0140-6736(07)60451-6.

41. Link MS, Berkow LC, Kudenchuk PJ, et al. Part 7: adult advanced cardiovascular life support: 2015 American Heart Association Guidelines Update for Cardiopulmonary Resuscitation and Emergency Cardiovascular Care. *Circulation*. 2015;132(18 suppl 2): S444-S464. doi:10.1161/CIR.0000000000000261.

48. Crosby ET. Airway management in adults after cervical spine trauma. *Anesthesiology*. 2006;104(6):1293-1318. doi:10.1097/00000542-200606000-00026.

66. Atkins DL, Berger S, Duff JP, et al. Part 11: pediatric basic life support and cardiopulmonary resuscitation quality: 2015 American Heart Association Guidelines Update for Cardiopulmonary Resuscitation and Emergency Cardiovascular Care. *Circulation*. 2015;132(18 suppl 2):S519-S525. doi:10.1161/CIR.0000000000000265.

67. Topjian AA, Raymond TT, Atkins D, et al. Part 4: pediatric basic and advanced life support: 2020 American Heart Association Guidelines for Cardiopulmonary Resuscitation and Emergency Cardiovascular Care. *Circulation*. 2020;142(16 suppl 2):S469-S523. doi:10.1161/CIR.0000000000000901.

69. Aziz K, Lee HC, Escobedo MB, et al. Part 5: neonatal resuscitation: 2020 American Heart Association Guidelines for Cardiopulmonary Resuscitation and Emergency Cardiovascular Care. *Circulation*. 2020;142(16 suppl 2):S524-S550. doi:10.1161/CIR.0000000000000902.

All references can be found online at eBooks.Health.Elsevier.com.

33

Austere Environment and Disaster Preparedness

JOSEPH H. MCISAAC III, NATHAN D. MARK, AND HEATHER K. HAYANGA

KEY POINTS

- Mass casualty events and the practice of anesthesia in austere environments are situations for which anesthesiologists should be prepared.
- Proper triage techniques can help prevent misallocation of resources and also can help alleviate psychic trauma on healthcare professionals.
- Anesthesiologists are willing to respond to disasters but desire further education and training in preparation for them.
- A mass casualty event resulting from communicable disease, whether from SARS, influenza, or another novel viral strain, will remain a threat indefinitely.

- Patients afflicted by chemical, biological, or radiological exposures may also present with concomitant traumatic injuries.
- Airway management in a challenging environment requires creativity from airway practitioners.
- Performing a surgical airway may be the best approach to airway management in an austere environment because of combat, positional constraints, or associated craniofacial trauma.
- Infrastructure resiliency and training and maintenance of skills that may not be practiced routinely are integral to disaster preparedness planning.

Introduction

We live in an unpredictable world and uncertain times. The threat of disaster, natural or man-made, causing a mass casualty scenario is forever looming underneath the surface of our otherwise casual routines. Although there are many definitions of the word *disaster*, the most commonly used medical definition of a disaster is an "event that results in a number of casualties that overwhelms the existing healthcare system."[1] Typically, disasters also degrade the fundamental infrastructure necessary for a viable economy and civil society. This disruption magnifies the impact of the event by widening the gap between needed and available resources.

In most parts of the world, natural disasters, such as floods, major storms, earthquakes, wildfires, tsunamis, and epidemics, occur at higher frequencies than man-made disasters, such as wars or technological events.[2] Catastrophic events can be viewed by

scale (local vs regional), proximity (happens locally vs somewhere else), time scale (discrete vs continuous), degree and type of infrastructure degradation (minimal vs total; physical destruction vs loss of personnel), and casualty spectrum[3] (Box 33.1).

Epidemiology: Natural Versus Man-Made Disasters

Disasters are not uniformly distributed in time or geographic location. According to the Center for Research on the Epidemiology of Disasters (CRED), 396 disasters related to natural hazards were reported in 2019, and one-third of all disasters reported in the database are technological and related to industrialization. These disasters culminated in the deaths of tens of thousands of individuals, hundreds of millions of dollars' worth of damage, and countless lives affected or displaced.[4,5] The greatest impacts are felt in the countries with the lowest levels of technological development.

As clinicians, we are increasingly likely to encounter mass casualty situations and/or deliver care in austere environments. For instance, climate change is likely to accelerate and increase the frequency of all types of disasters, with human consequences ranging from famine, to pandemic spread of disease, to acts of terrorism and war. As a result of increased ease of world travel, recent years have witnessed the rapid spread of infectious disease resulting in potentially fatal consequences on a large scale. Diseases, such as influenza, SARS coronavirus 2 (SARS-CoV-2), and the Ebola

virus, continue to threaten populations and test the containment and treatment strategies of our healthcare infrastructure. We are living in a time when terrorism, mass shooting, natural disaster, and infectious disease are always on the horizon, threatening to overcome our present healthcare resources (Fig. 33.1).

Triage Techniques

By definition, a mass casualty incident is one in which the number of injured individuals exceeds the available healthcare resources. In such a scenario, it is imperative to ensure that the patients in the direst need of attention receive help first. It naturally follows that the patients with clearly unsurvivable injuries are categorized to receive comfort measures but not necessarily life-saving resources. Therein lie the art and science of disaster triage. Simply put, triage is the act of sorting patients to maximize incremental survival and most efficiently use resources.[6–8] Triage is also used as a clinical decision-making tool and to minimize moral and intellectual distress among care personnel.[9] **S**ort-**A**ssess-**L**ifesaving interventions-Treatment/**T**ransport (SALT) and **S**imple-**T**riage-**A**nd-**R**apid-**T**reatment (START) are two systems commonly used in the United States (Figs. 33.2 and 33.3). Most triage techniques

---

Natural Versus Man-Made

Locally contained versus widespread
Happens locally (to you) versus responding to a disaster at a distance
  (somewhere else)
Infrastructure degradation (minimal versus total)
Time scale: discrete vs continuous event
Casualty spectrum (medical vs surgical disease)

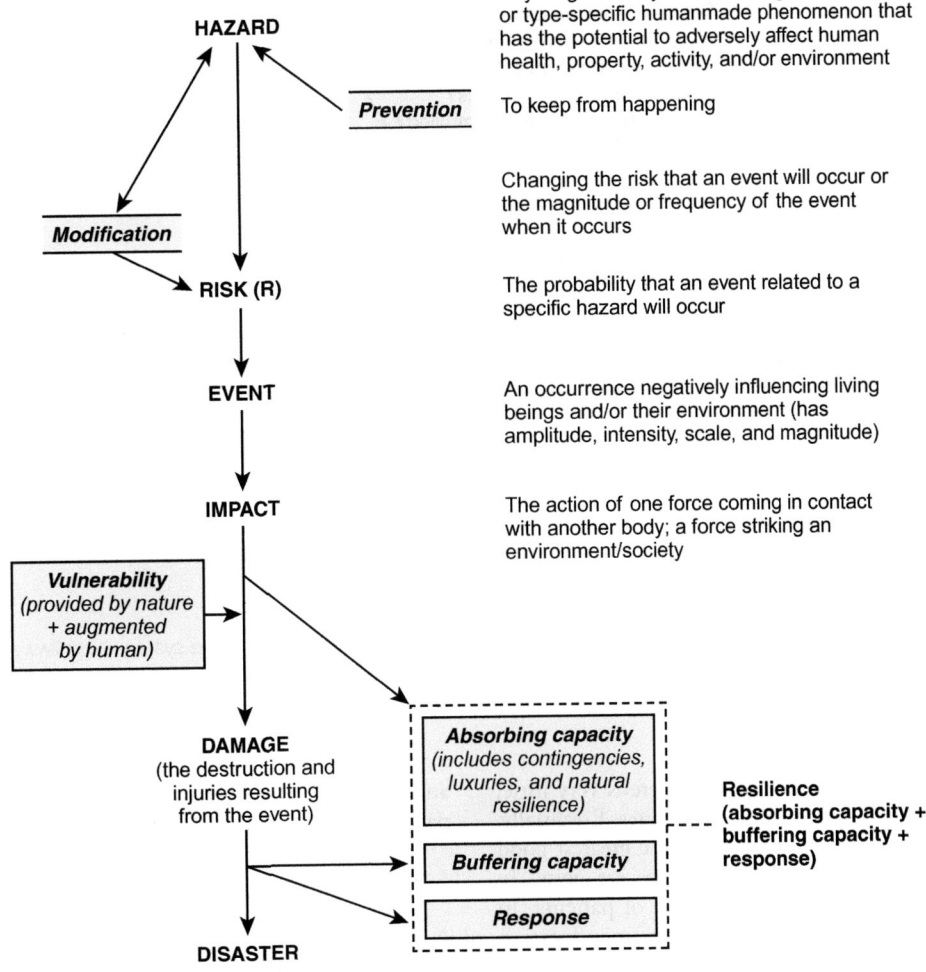

HAZARD — Anything that may cause a danger; a natural or type-specific humanmade phenomenon that has the potential to adversely affect human health, property, activity, and/or environment

Prevention — To keep from happening

Modification — Changing the risk that an event will occur or the magnitude or frequency of the event when it occurs

RISK (R) — The probability that an event related to a specific hazard will occur

EVENT — An occurrence negatively influencing living beings and/or their environment (has amplitude, intensity, scale, and magnitude)

IMPACT — The action of one force coming in contact with another body; a force striking an environment/society

Vulnerability (provided by nature + augmented by human)

DAMAGE (the destruction and injuries resulting from the event)

Absorbing capacity (includes contingencies, luxuries, and natural resilience)

Buffering capacity

Response

Resilience (absorbing capacity + buffering capacity + response)

DISASTER

• **Fig. 33.1** Disaster nomenclature. Standardized definitions of terms used to communicate by the various disciplines involved in disasters. (Modified from Task Force for Quality Control of Disaster Medicine (TFQCDM)/World Association for Disaster and Emergency Medicine (WADEM): Health disaster management: guidelines for evaluation and research in the Utstein style. Chapter 3: Overview and concepts. *Prehosp Disast Med.* 2002;17(suppl 3):31-55. Available at https://wadem.org/wp-content/uploads/2016/03/chapter_3.pdf.)

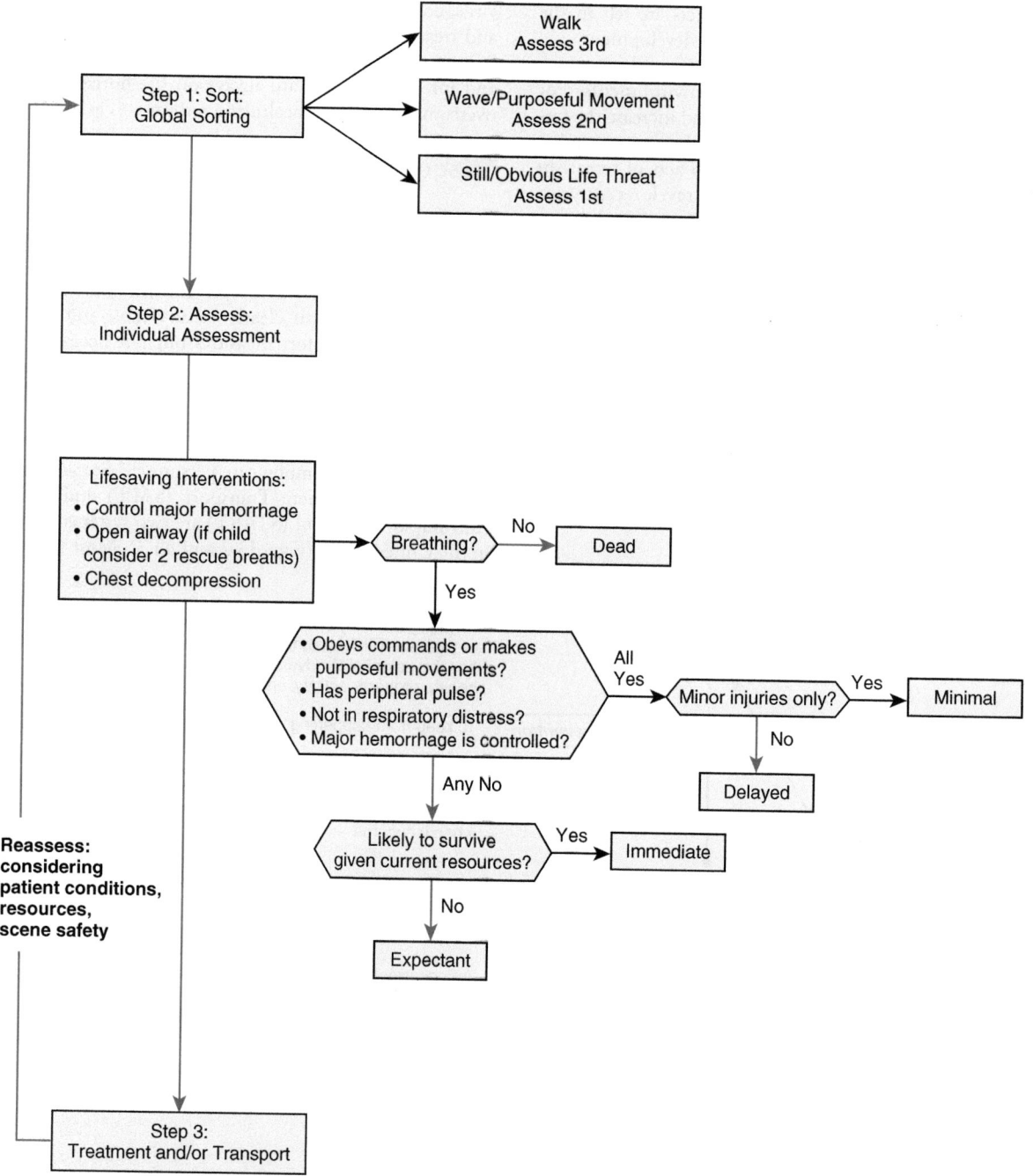

• **Fig. 33.2** Sort, assess, life-saving interventions, treatment/transport (SALT) triage system. http://www. remm.nlm.gov/salttriage.htm (Adapted from Lerner EB, Cone DC, Weinstein ES, et al. Mass casualty triage: an evaluation of the science and refinement of a national guideline. *Disaster Med Public Health Prep.* 2011;5(2):129-137.)

have their origins in military practice though there is very little, if any, scientific validation to any of these techniques. Essentially, triage is conducted with the purpose of doing the greatest good for the largest number of people. All techniques are going to have some error, such as over- or under-triaging of patients. In cases where patients are over-triaged, there may be misallocation of resources, where patients with relatively minor injuries may receive higher than necessary levels of care.[9,10] Under-triaging of patients may lead to potentially avoidable morbidity and mortality. Regardless of the technique used for triage, it should be performed by a person or team that has received appropriate training

and practice. Triage may have to be repeated when circumstances, patients' conditions, and resource availability changes.

Mass Trauma

A variety of types of incidents can overwhelm the medical care infrastructure. A large-scale trauma, as can occur as a result of natural or man-made disasters, is one category of incidents. In these circumstances, first responders on the scene and emergency room physicians are likely to perform the initial triage and medical stabilization of casualties, with many patients requiring prehospital

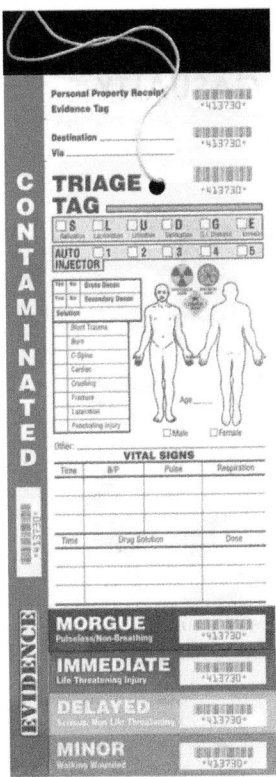

• **Fig. 33.3** Example of a triage tag. (Courtesy Disaster Management Systems, Inc., Pomona, CA.)

airway management, including tracheal intubation. Most anesthesiologist roles will likely be in the realm of operating room (OR) management and critical care, although this is institutionally dependent. Nonetheless, as initial responders start to become overwhelmed, it may be increasingly important for anesthesiologists to participate in the first response.

Recent research has demonstrated that approximately 50% of airway-compromised trauma patients require some sort of advanced airway management technique.[11,12] Furthermore, burn patients, those with extensive craniofacial trauma, and patients with neck injuries often require advanced and early securing of the airway to prevent or minimize hypoxia-induced end-organ and brain injuries. Aspiration of gastric contents and blood in trauma patients are also of concern and may have some bearing on the airway management technique chosen. In some nations, the use of supraglottic airway (SGA) devices for prehospital airway intervention is the norm. An SGA may actually provide some degree of airway protection from contamination from the upper airway, but it will not protect the airway against the regurgitation of gastric contents.[13]

Anesthesia care personnel must be flexible enough to provide surgical-level care for large numbers of patients. This may require alteration of anesthetic plans that allow for patients to breathe with a natural airway if invasive airway management is not available (Ketamine is an excellent choice).[14,15] Regional anesthesia and total intravenous anesthesia may be employed when there is tenuous access to electricity.

Operating Room Checklist for Mass Casualty

The Joint Commission (TJC) (formerly the Joint Commission on Accreditation of Healthcare Organizations [JCAHO]) and

governmental policies require all U.S. hospitals to have disaster plans prepared and tested twice per year. The most accepted standard for hospital disaster response is the hospital incident command system (HICS).[16] HICS consists of a command and control framework headed by the incident commander and prioritized task lists for each designated subordinate. Modeled on military combat systems and perfected by the California Fire Service, HICS is a time-tested system.

Literature about the management of mass casualty scenarios at the anesthesia department level is scarce. Previous literature has suggested that the majority of attending and resident anesthesiologists believe that their hospital or residency program, respectively, should incorporate disaster training, with 1 hour per 3 months of dedicated education about preparedness being most frequently desired.[17]

Anesthesia and OR management in a mass casualty scenario must follow the overall principles of hospital preparedness.[18] Namely, there must be integration of all surgical specialties, anesthesia, nursing, and support staff. There must be the ability to accommodate the "surge"—in other words, the OR should be able to expand beyond normal services to meet increased demand. In order to satisfy medical and surgical needs, identification of the types of injuries of the at-risk population should be accomplished rapidly. Of utmost importance are coordination and communication among all levels and aspects of surgical care, including surgeon, blood bank, anesthesiologist, patient transport, nursing, central supply, and more. Herein lie some of the most difficult challenges and hence the importance of preparedness. The OR disaster plan must also include surveillance, defined objectives, management of the response, and identification of clinical and administrative leaders (Fig. 33.4).[19]

According to the American Society of Anesthesiologists (ASA) Committee on Trauma and Emergency Preparedness, the priorities of the OR chief during a mass casualty situation should include the following:

1. All surgical teams should be notified and instructed to finish elective cases as soon as possible. Elective cases that have not been started should be placed on hold.
2. Assign available staff to set up for emergency/trauma cases.
3. Coordinate with anesthesia technicians to ensure adequate supplies are on hand.
4. If airborne infectious disease is suspected or there is the potential for chemical or radiological contamination, isolation and/or personal protection measures should be implemented.
5. All members of the anesthesia department should be aware of their department's respective disaster plan.
6. You may refer to the *Manual for Anesthesia Department Organization and Management* for a more comprehensive description of responsibilities.[20]

Biological Threats

In a world with multidrug-resistant organisms, increased ease of world travel, population overcrowding, and other factors,[21] the threat of a mass casualty event resulting from communicable disease is real. In 1918, influenza A was responsible for 657,000 deaths in the United States alone and 50 million deaths worldwide. In 1957, the Asian flu killed 70,000 people in the United States. In 2003, severe acute respiratory syndrome (SARS), which involved 29 countries, infected more than 8,000 people, and killed approximately 900. Another novel form of coronavirus, SARS coronavirus 2 (SARS-CoV-2), first reported in December 2019

OPERATING ROOM PROCEDURES FOR MASS CASUALTY

MANAGEMENT STEP BY STEP

Objective

To be able to manage the flow of patient care in the OR's during a mass casualty situation.

Steps (Indicate date and time for each item)

☐ **Refer to facility's Operations Manual**

Open up appropriate annex

☐ **Activate call-in tree**

Assign an individual to activate. Use clerical personnel or automatic paging system, if available

☐ **Assess status of operating rooms**

Determine staffing of OR's 0-2, 2-12, and 12-24 hours. Hold elective cases.

☐ **Alert current ORs**

Finish current surgical procedures as soon as possible and prepare to receive trauma

☐ **Assign staff**

Set up for trauma/emergency cases

☐ **Anesthesia Coordinator should become OR Medical Director**

Work with OR Nursing Manager to facilitate communication and coordination of staff and facilities

☐ **Report OR status to Hospital Command Center (HCC)**

Enter telephone, email address of HCC

☐ **Ensure adequate supplies**

Coordinate with anesthesia techs/supply personnel to ensure adequate supplies of fluids, medications, disposables, other

☐ **Contact PACU**

Accelerate transfer of patients to floors/ICUs in preparation for high volume of cases

☐ **Anesthesiologist should act as liaison in Emergency Department (ED)**

Send an experienced practitioner to the ED to act as a liaison (your eyes & ears) and keep communications open to Anesthesia Coordinator

☐ **Consider assembly of Stat Teams**

Combination of anesthesia, surgical, nursing, respiratory personnel to triage, as needed

☐ **HAZMAT/WMD event**

Review special personal protective procedures, such as DECON & isolation techniques. Consider if part of the OR or hallways should be considered "hot" or should have ventilation altered. Good resources include CHEMM/REMM websites

☐ **Coordinate with blood bank**

Verify blood availability

☐ **Coordinate with other patient care areas**

ICUs, OB, Peds, etc. to ensure continuity of care for new and existing patients

Developed by the Committee on Trauma and Emergency Preparedness

• **Fig. 33.4** Operating room mass casualty management checklist. (From https://www.asahq.org/about-asa/governance-and-committees/asa-committees/committee-on-trauma-and-emergency-prepared-ness-cotep/emergency-preparedness.)

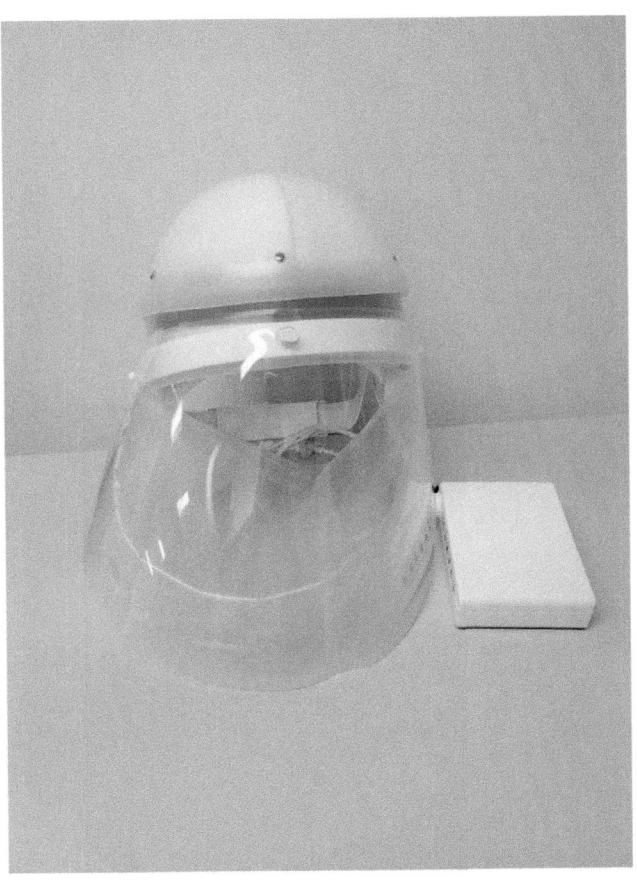

• **Fig. 33.5** Powered air-purifying respirator (PAPR).

and frequently cited as the coronavirus 2019 (COVID-19) pandemic, has been responsible for more than 64 million cases and 1.4 million deaths to date worldwide, at the time of this writing.

Tracheal intubation and extubation are aerosol-generating procedures and may pose significant exposure risk to personnel if proper precautions are not taken.[22] This became evident in the death of at least one anesthesiologist during the SARS epidemic in 2003, and it has become a primary focus of disaster response during COVID-19. Whenever the agent is unknown or highly lethal with exposure to relatively low infectious particle numbers (eg, Ebola), all caregivers should wear powered air-purifying respirators (PAPRs) and several waterproof barriers (impermeable suit, multiple layers of gloves) (Fig. 33.5). Hot, warm, and cold zones should be established with strict adherence to protocols. Aerosol-generating procedures can be conducted under a tent of clear plastic, ideally with air evacuation, to reduce the spread of particulates and droplets. Video laryngoscopy can be used to increase the distance between the patient and the anesthesiologist's face.[23,24] It is wise to stockpile personal protective equipment (PPE) to ensure availability when supply chains are disrupted.

Epidemic Versus Pandemic

According to Morens and colleagues in "What Is a Pandemic?" a pandemic is a disease with wide geographic extension, sometimes to nonadjacent regions, sometimes globally.[25] Pandemic spread of disease is usually traceable, either from widespread person-to-person transmission or from a variety of vectors. Most have high attack rates and are explosive in their spread. Pandemics often result from novel variants of existing organisms in populations

where immunity is low. Contagiousness, infectivity, and severity are also key features of impact.[25] As previously noted, increased ease of transportation, population overcrowding, and geopolitical circumstances leading to infrastructure degradation all contribute to the increased risk of pandemic spread of disease. When such conditions are met, the number of casualties can be staggering and, as such, can put a severe strain on a hospital drug supply and staffing resources.

Those healthcare professionals who have a role in airway management and critical care, such as anesthesiologists, are ideally suited for confronting pandemics that have respiratory sequelae, such as influenza, Ebola, and novel coronavirus-induced SARS (COVID-19).

Chemical Threats

Although accidental or unintentional release of toxic industrial compounds (TICs) is more likely, events in Syria (2015) and the United Kingdom (2018) demonstrate that the threat of terrorists using a weaponized chemical is a significant one. Chemical weapons can be classified as corrosives, asphyxiants, or metabolic poisons. The use of chemical weapons, even in small quantities, can have catastrophic effects on the health of large populations. Chemical weapons can be prepared with minimal infrastructure and from easily obtainable items, and they are easily concealable. They can behave as a force multiplier in an "asymmetric conflict."[26] This is certainly a growing concern for the emergency preparedness of the community and, in particular, anesthesiologists. The very nature of chemical weapons as nerve intoxicants mandates the participation of anesthesiologists in the care of casualties and preparedness planning for such an event.[27]

Nerve agents were developed in the 1930s in Germany from organophosphate-based pesticides. Organophosphates inhibit the action of acetylcholinesterase, thereby dramatically increasing the amount of acetylcholine (ACh) available to interact with postsynaptic nicotinic and muscarinic receptors. It so happens that acetylcholinesterase is a remarkably efficient enzyme, capable of hydrolyzing 10,000 ACh molecules in a single second. It naturally follows that inhibition of this enzyme floods the system with ACh and results in a full-blown cholinergic crisis (Box 33.2).

Nerve agents are typically divided into two types, G-type and V-type, based on their volatility and boiling points. The G-type nerve agents are highly volatile liquids that vaporize sufficiently at room temperature to yield a dense vapor. Their primary absorption route is by inhalation. These substances are easy to transport, spread quickly, and thus are well suited for terrorist attacks.[26] The

---

• **BOX 33.2** **Cholinergic Toxidrome of Nerve Agents[a]**

D Diarrhea
U Urination
M Miosis
M Muscle Weakness
B Bradycardia
B Bronchoconstriction
E Emesis
L Lacrimation
S Salivation
S Sweating

[a]Mental confusion may also occur with some agents.

V-series nerve agents are mostly absorbed transcutaneously and have a slower onset but can be just as lethal. A new class of nerve agent, the Novichoks, require prolonged supportive care and large amounts of anticholinergics.[28]

The casualties of exposure to these agents will present with a variety of cholinergic symptoms and a range of severity that depends on proximity to the source and duration of exposure. All organ systems can be affected, but not all will be present in all patients. In those with minimal exposure, the only symptoms may be miosis and rhinorrhea. Patients with moderate exposure may present with dyspnea, chest pain, and muscle weakness. More severe cases experience respiratory difficulty arising from bronchospasm, increased secretions, and diaphragmatic weakness. The skin will be diaphoretic. Nausea and vomiting will be present. Anticonvulsant therapy may be required. However, random contractions of large muscle groups should be differentiated from true seizure activity. Hemodynamic compromise may be present as tachycardia or bradycardia with concomitant blood pressure changes.

Medical management must first be directed at preventing the spread of contamination to rescuers and healthcare professionals. Triage techniques should be able to differentiate mild exposure and severe exposure as treatment and resource allocation will be at a premium. Decontamination of victims exposed to vapor may merely consist of removing the victim(s) to a well-ventilated place away from the source. Liquid droplet exposure will require more extensive decontamination, consisting of removal of clothing and perhaps rinsing off.[29]

Tracheal intubation is required for apneic patients and those in respiratory distress and also serves to isolate the lungs from further inspiration of toxic vapors. Lung isolation also can be achieved with a good mask seal, a bag valve mask connected to an oxygen source or compressed air, and a suitable high-efficiency particulate air (HEPA) filter (Fig. 33.6).[30,31]

Definitive medical care will require a nerve agent antidote. Atropine can be used to antagonize the muscarinic effects of ACh. Notably, atropine has a short half-life and will have to be redosed every few hours. The dosage of atropine is titrated to the effect of improving respirations and drying secretions. Convulsions resulting from the ensuing cholinergic toxidrome can be treated with benzodiazepines. Oximes, such as pralidoxime, obidoxime, and HI-6, given early in the course of poisoning, displaces the nerve agent from the enzyme complex and thereby helps to regenerate functional acetylcholinesterase.

Radiation Exposure

A mass casualty scenario arising from radiation exposure is also of increased concern given the current geopolitical climate around the world. Hospitals and state and local agencies need to have radiologic emergency medical response plans. These plans should include guidelines for the treatment of contaminated and injured patients. It should also include methods to minimize exposure to healthcare personnel.

According to Bushberg and colleagues, there are many possible causes of radiation-induced injury in the civilian population. These include, but are not limited to, (1) placement of a sealed radioactive source in a public location, (2) use of a radiologic dispersion device (RDD), (3) attack on or sabotage of a nuclear facility, and (4) detonation of a nuclear weapon (atomic bomb).[32] There are also radiation emergencies that are not caused by terrorism, such as accidental exposures from medical facilities

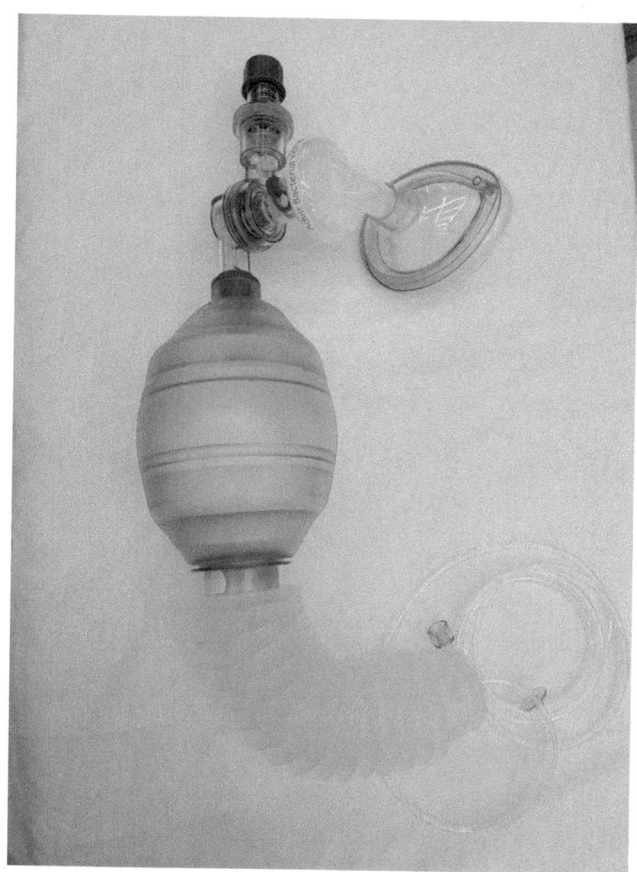

• **Fig. 33.6** Bag valve mask with high-efficiency particulate air filter.

and nuclear reactor accidents. All of these scenarios are rare but potentially catastrophic. Between 1980 and 2013, 634 radiation overexposure accidents were reported worldwide, resulting in 190 radiation-related deaths.[33]

Radiation is part of the natural environment to which people are exposed regularly, and, to a large degree, it is harmless. Ionizing radiation, such as alpha, beta, gamma, and x-rays, can cause harmful changes in DNA, such as cancer, and kill cells.[34] However, being exposed to radiation does not necessarily imply that one has been contaminated. Radioactive contamination signifies that there is radioactivity in a place where it should not be, such as inside the human body or on clothing or skin. Contaminated patients require care to limit the spread of radiation or radioactive substances.

As many radiation-exposed patients may suffer from concomitant traumatic injuries or serious medical comorbidities, it is also important to understand the risk to healthcare workers. In most cases, the amount of radiation present in the victim will not be enough to adversely affect healthcare professionals. According to sources from the Armed Forces Radiobiology Research Institute, 90% of radioactive contamination is removed when the clothes are removed. Universal precautions are generally enough to protect healthcare workers, with the one variant of wearing two sets of gloves. The outer pair can be changed as needed to avoid cross-contamination. This concept underlines the fact that medical and/or surgical care should never be delayed for reasons of decontamination.[34] Resuscitation and stabilization of the patient are the primary objectives. This is starkly different from the care of victims of either chemical or biological warfare in that decontamination may be an integral part of their care or that they may pose a significant risk to healthcare workers. Furthermore, compared to detecting biological or chemical contamination, radioactive contamination is easy to detect with a Geiger counter or similar device.[35]

Airway Management in Austere Environments

Anesthesia may have to be provided in challenging environments or in situations that are considered austere. These situations can challenge the ingenuity and resourcefulness of the most talented anesthesiologists. In such circumstances, anesthesia personnel may be forced to put best "principles before preferences" of medical care, as was described by Frame S, and Salomone JP. *Pre-hospital trauma life support.* Norman E, Ed. McSwain. Mosby-Year Book; 1994.

In his article "Anesthesia and Resuscitation in Difficult Environments," Boulton[14] described four broad types of challenging environments:

1. Planned but isolated situations. This could include the provision of anesthesia on deployment at sea or on an expedition. There is likely to be limited personnel support, requirements of portability of equipment, and issues of resupply.
2. Extreme urgency. This type of scenario may involve, for example, a casualty trapped at the scene of an accident.
3. Disaster or battle conditions. In this type of scenario, the healthcare team may be well equipped initially, but maintaining staffing or supplies may prove difficult as there may be sudden changes in numbers of victims.
4. Remote locations in the hospital setting, such as the MRI suite or bedside in the intensive care unit (ICU). (In this section, austere environments will not refer to this type of situation.)

As noted, austere environments are those in which there are staffing constraints and potential equipment shortages. Availability of electricity and lighting, access to oxygen and monitoring, and adequate patient positioning may also be limiting. In the majority of situations encountered by anethesiologists and considered to be austere, the patients will be victims of traumatic injury, which may or may not involve biological or chemical exposure. As will be described, any mass casualty situation can turn an otherwise well-equipped, well-staffed facility into an austere environment.

Airway management in the austere environment can pose a particular challenge but is also the paramount priority in managing patients and is often the difference between life and death. At times, noninvasive airway management techniques, such as nasopharyngeal airways or manual maneuvers to maintain airway patency, will suffice. A conscious patient should be allowed the opportunity to maintain their own airway by finding a position of comfort, such as leaning forward and letting blood drain from the oropharynx. In such circumstances, supine positioning may compromise an otherwise intact, albeit tenuous, airway.[36] In the unconscious, hypoxic, or hemodynamically unstable patient, one may opt for performing direct laryngoscopy with orotracheal intubation. However, this may prove extremely difficult in the setting of airway or facial trauma, blood in the pharynx, edema, or combat. Other airway adjuncts must be at hand in these situations. SGA devices and video-assisted laryngoscopy (VAL) can all be useful in various circumstances. Each of these devices will have its own advantages and disadvantages. Not every clinical scenario can possibly be covered in this section, so in-depth knowledge and practice with an ASA difficult airway algorithm are requisite.[37]

Regardless of the difficult airway algorithm used, all come to the final point of performing a surgical cricothyrotomy.[37] In an austere environment, the use of an endotracheal tube (ETT) or an SGA may not be appropriate because of tactical, situational, or supply constraints.[38] Indications for a surgical airway become broader in the austere environment. Severe facial, oropharyngeal trauma, as well as edema of the glottis, are the most common indications for cricothyrotomy. The challenges of combat, low light, complicated positioning, or prolonged extrication may necessitate surgical versus conventional airway management.[38] Many techniques are described for performing a surgical airway,[39] but it is very difficult to scientifically verify the superiority of one technique over another, especially in an austere setting. One example described by Markarian and colleagues[40] is a simple three-step approach that may be appropriate, referred to as "scalpel-bougie-tube":

1. Make a midline longitudinal incision with #20 blade over the cricothyroid membrane, and use the nondominant index finger to palpate the membrane.
2. Make a 5-mm transverse incision through the membrane, and insert a gum elastic bougie into the trachea.
3. Place a 6.0 cuffed ETT over the bougie, and slide it into the trachea; remove the bougie; and secure the ETT.

General anesthesia with inhalation anesthetics may prove very cumbersome in austere conditions. Consideration should be given to regional anesthesia and IV anesthetics. Ketamine, in particular, offers the advantages of spontaneous ventilation, preservation of airway reflexes, and potent analgesia. However, ketamine may cause excessive salivation, which could compromise airway management conditions. Ketamine also has the ability to cause less hypotension in the hypovolemic patient because of a rise in circulating catecholamines. However, in the trauma patient, total catecholamines may be depleted, and ketamine may act as a direct myocardial depressant. Thus, ketamine, although a potential useful adjunct, must be administered, if appropriate, with caution.

Surge Management

A hospital can quickly become overwhelmed but must have the ability to absorb the surge of victims of mass casualty events.[41] The "surge capacity" of a hospital is the institution's ability to expand services quickly to meet a greatly increased medical care demand. This can prove to be extremely challenging from a financial and infrastructural point of view. Hospitals will need to rapidly augment the number of ICU beds available by expanding existing ICUs into other areas, such as postoperative care units and emergency departments or other areas with expanded monitoring capabilities. For the COVID-19 pandemic, guidance was created on purposing anesthesia machines as ICU ventilators.[42] Draw-over anesthesia circuits can be used in low-resource environments to provide inhalational anesthesia without the need for oxygen or electrical power (Fig. 33.7).

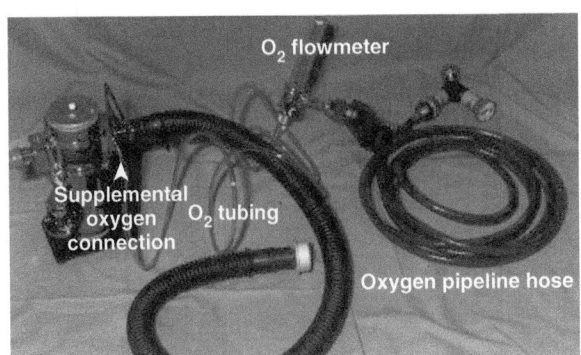

• **Fig. 33.7** Omeda Universal Portable Anesthesia Complete (U-PAC) drawover anesthesia system. (Courtesy GE Healthcare, Fairfield, CT.)

Surge capacity also implies existence of a plan to ensure adequate staffing. In a study of attending and resident anesthesiologists, the majority reported that all attendings share an obligation to be involved in disaster planning, response, and recovery efforts. Greater than 70% were willing to respond to a natural disaster or pandemic influenza regardless of severity, and the majority were willing to do so in any medical capacity or whatever capacity they might be needed. Those who reported knowing one's role in disaster response and feeling psychologically prepared were found to be more willing to respond.[17] Staffing demand can be estimated from medical surge–planning software. Organization among hospital administration, emergency departments, the OR, and infrastructure maintenance is crucial to absorbing the surge of victims in a mass casualty situation. Furthermore, hospitals must develop contingency plans in coordination with local and state governments to meet the needs of mass disaster or pandemic circumstances.

Personal Protective Equipment

Personal protective equipment (PPE) is used by medical personnel to prevent occupational exposure to infectious, radiologic, or chemical agents. Gloves, gowns, and masks are a normal part of responders' daily lives under universal precautions. High-risk infections, such as tuberculosis, require the use of HEPA filtration masks, most commonly the N95 mask, a filter found to remove at least 95% of airborne particles during worst-case testing (Fig 33.8).[22] A PAPR has approximately 100 times the effectiveness of the N95. When used together, a protection factor approaching 10,000 times that of a paper surgical mask can be achieved. Negative-pressure isolation rooms and wards are used to keep airborne infection risks contained (Fig. 33.9). As such, with the COVID-19 pandemic, performing aerosol-generating

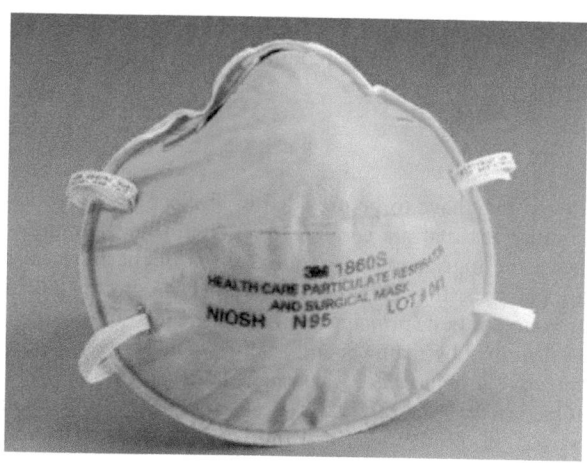

• **Fig. 33.8** N95 mask. Filters 95% of suspended particulate material. (Courtesy 3M Company.)

procedures, such as tracheal intubation and extubation, in an airborne-infection isolation room with negative pressure rather than in a positive-pressure operating room has been recommended.

Distinguishing between decontamination and isolation is important. Infectious patients cannot be decontaminated because the infection is internal. Patients with external chemical and radiologic contamination should be decontaminated to minimize their exposure to the agent and the exposure of the treating staff. The best universal decontamination strategy includes removal of clothing and washing with copious amounts of water (with or without soap). This goal can be accomplished for mass casualties through a formal decontamination system or by any improvised method. Employing a method for assessing the effectiveness of

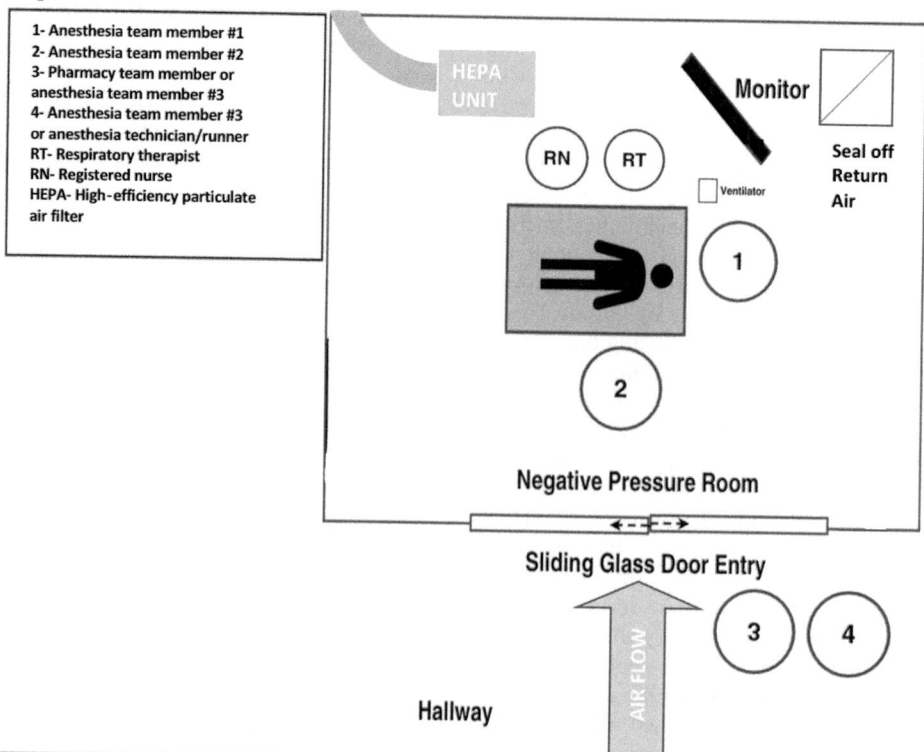

• **Fig. 33.9** Example of tracheal intubation scenario in a patient room temporarily outfitted as negative pressure isolation room.

decontamination (eg, testing patients after decontamination with a Geiger counter, a chemical meter, or a surrogate tracer) can increase confidence in the system, but studies have consistently shown several orders of magnitude of contamination reduction using only clothing removal and shower. The main exception to this rule is a gross level of contamination by persistent chemicals used by the military, such as thickened nerve agents and some vesicants. These scenarios are more likely to occur in large-scale chemical warfare. First responders at the hospital level typically wear level-C PPE, whereas first responders at a site of high agent concentration often wear level-A or level-B PPE.

Use of PPE imposes a burden on the caregiver. In addition to the psychological impact and heat stress, impediments to vision, hearing, communication, and manual dexterity are measurable. Suyama and colleagues found for a non–PPE-wearing operator needle-to-skin time favored intravenous placement over intraosseous, but an intraosseous approach provided faster vascular access when wearing PPE.[43] The effect of PPE on airway management seems less clear. Although Greenland and colleagues[44] found that PPE affected bronchoscopy but not intubation, Castle and colleagues[45] found that chemical-biologic-radiologic-nuclear (CBRN) PPE significantly impaired intubation but not LMA placement while kneeling, sitting, or lying on the floor.

Infrastructure Resiliency

Disaster preparedness must consider infrastructure resilience. This can be accomplished through hardening of existing infrastructure, such as utilities and communications, or through the acquisition of alternatives. Examples of alternatives are power sources, such as solar-powered, mechanical-powered, and steam-powered engines; amateur radios as a substitute for standard communications; and food prepared for long-term storage. As seen during the COVID-19 pandemic, stockpiling of PPE is necessary to ensure safety of hospital personnel when previously intact supply chains may falter.

Simulation and Training

An integral part of preparedness is training and maintenance of skills that may not be practiced frequently. Computer-based and real-life simulation scenarios can greatly aid in the ability of healthcare professionals to meet the needs of mass casualty situations. Simulation can aid in the development and implementation of triage and care protocols for situations that clinicians do not encounter regularly. Simulation also serves to mentally prepare healthcare professionals for stressful and potentially overwhelming situations. Computer-based simulations can help hospitals prepare the response for pandemic mass casualties by illustrating the disparity between available and needed resources. Ideally, training opportunities in donning and doffing of PPE should occur regularly to minimize unintentional exposure.

Conclusion

Disaster preparedness involves coordination among all levels of hospital management and care, as well as governmental agencies. Mass casualty scenarios arising from terrorism, industrial accidents, weather-related phenomena, or pandemic spread of disease can place great strain on existing healthcare supply and staffing infrastructure. Optimizing patient and population outcomes depends heavily on practitioners who are ideally suited for mass casualty planning.

Selected References

8. Kennedy K, Aghababian R, et al. Triage: techniques and applications in decision making. *Ann Emerg Med.* 1996;28(2):136–144.
9. Christian M, Sprung C, King M, et al. Triage: care of the critically ill and injured during pandemics and disasters: chest consensus statement. *Chest.* 2014;146(4).
14. Boulton TB. Anesthesia and resuscitation in difficult environments. *Int Anesthesiology Clin.* 1973;11:143–238.
16. California Emergency Medical Services Authority. Hospital Incident Command System – current guidebook and appendices. Available at https://emsa.ca.gov/disaster-medical-services-division-hospital-incident-command-system.
17. Hayanga H, Barnett D, Shallow NR, et al. Anesthesiologists and disaster medicine: a needs assessment for education and training and reported willingness to respond. *Anesth Analg.* 2017;124(5):1662–1669.
18. Tobin J, Grabinsky A, McCunn M, et al. A checklist for trauma and emergency anesthesia. *Anesth Analg.* 2013;117(5):1178-1184.
20. thesiologists Committee on Trauma and Emergency Preparedness. Emergency preparedness for anesthesiologists. Available at https://www.asahq.org/about-asa/governance-and-committees/asa-committees/committee-on-trauma-and-emergency-preparedness-cotep/emergency-preparedness.
23. American Society of Anesthesiologists. COVID-19 information for professionals. Available at https://www.asahq.org/about-asa/governance-and-committees/asa-committees/committee-on-occupational-health/coronavirus.
26. Macintyre A, Christopher G, Eitzen E, et al. Weapons of mass destruction events with contaminated casualties, effective planning for healthcare facilities. *JAMA.* 2000;283(2):242–249.
34. Bui E, Bellal J, Rhee P, Diven P, Pandit V, Brown, CVR. Contemporary management of radiation exposure and injury. *J Trauma Acute Care Surg.* 2014;77(3):495–500.
37. Apfelbaum J, Hagberg C, Caplan RA, et al. Practice guidelines for management of the difficult airway: an updated report by the ASA task force on management of the difficult airway. *Anesthesiology.* 2013;118:251–270.
38. Dessert MJ, Bennet B. Optimizing emergent surgical cricothyrotomy for use in austere environments. *Wilderness Environ Med.* 2013;24(1):53–66.

All references can be found online at eBooks.Health.Elsevier.com.

34

Airway Management in Trauma

RON E. SAMET, CALEB B. HODGE, AND THOMAS E. GRISSOM

CHAPTER OUTLINE

KEY POINTS

- Although many trauma patients may initially appear to maintain and protect their airway, they remain at risk of progressive airway obstruction or multisystem traumatic comorbidities necessitating frequent reevaluation.
- Intubating a trauma patient should be part of an overall team-based approach to resuscitation. Although intubation may not be necessary to maintain airway patency, the patient's expected clinical course or need for emergent surgical intervention may prompt intubation.
- The gag reflex should not be used to gauge airway protection in a trauma patient. If these patients do vomit, they should be rolled with the board into a lateral decubitus position.
- Current evidence supports a strategy of not immobilizing the cervical spine in patients with isolated penetrating trauma, who do not have signs of neurologic compromise.
- Advent of the videolaryngoscope has changed the management of difficult airways (DAs). Improved glottic visualization, comparable success rates, and growing experience support its use as an early rescue tool and principal intubating device in the trauma patient.

- Use of cricoid pressure (CP) most likely does not prevent aspiration and may make intubation more difficult. Although it may decrease gastric distention during bag-valve-mask (BVM) and can provide tactile feedback during intubation attempts, it should be discontinued during intubation attempts if any difficulty is encountered.
- Predictors of a DA, such as those contained in the modified LEMON criteria, should be applied in a timely fashion to the trauma patient.
  - Use of propofol or high-dose benzodiazepines may produce more hemodynamic instability in the hypovolemic, hypotensive trauma patient and should be used with caution.
- Point-of-care ultrasound (POCUS) airway and lung exams are increasingly playing a role in the airway management of the acutely injured patient.
- A variety of effective rescue airway devices are available for use in trauma patients. Airway specialists should become familiar and practice with several of them to maximize the options available in case of a failed airway.

Introduction

Because of the need for urgent and decisive decision-making in a dynamic environment, airway management in the trauma patient can be particularly challenging. The presence of hemodynamic instability, potential for direct airway trauma, and need for cervical spine immobilization in the face of competing surgical priorities requires a rapid evaluation for the potentially difficult airway (DA), development of an airway management plan (including rescue techniques in the event of failure), and a willingness to act quickly, often with incomplete information. Intubation approaches commonly used in the elective setting can be difficult or impossible to apply in patients with massive oropharyngeal hemorrhage, traumatic airway injury, or combative behavior because of altered mental status. Nevertheless, sound airway management principles common to all intubations remain the key to success.

Although the need to intervene will be apparent in most cases, the "stable" trauma patient can remain at risk of progressing to respiratory failure or airway loss. An expanding subdural hematoma can lead to a reduced level of consciousness and loss of airway protective mechanisms. The patient with a blunt or penetrating neck injury who appears stable during the primary survey may have an expanding neck hematoma that progresses to complete airway obstruction. Similarly, the patient with a high cervical spine injury may have adequate spontaneous ventilation during the initial evaluation but will remain at risk of progressing to respiratory failure because of fatigue and extension of the initial level of injury. These considerations mandate frequent airway and respiratory reevaluation of the trauma patient at risk of deterioration. The anticipated clinical course should then guide the decision to intubate in patients who do not have an immediate problem with airway protection, ventilatory effort, or oxygenation.

Consideration should also be given to anticipatory airway management in patients who are likely to require a near-term operative intervention, where early intubation allows for a more controlled and planned approach to their overall management. For example, a patient involved in a motor vehicle crash with bilateral lower extremity fractures, intractable pain, and agitation can be intubated early in his or her course to facilitate thorough radiologic evaluation and fracture reduction with improved sedation and pain management before going to the operating room (OR). These decisions should be made after discussion with both the trauma and operative teams to ensure perioperative considerations such as consent, timing, and patient optimization are addressed in a timely fashion.

Not all trauma patients, however, will require emergent intubation during their acute resuscitation and evaluation. Trauma patients frequently undergo surgery that is not related to their acute resuscitation but is required during the first few days of their hospital stay. Burn debridement and grafting, fracture fixation, complex wound revision and repair, and other procedures are often required hours or days after the patient has been stabilized and more acute, life-threatening problems have been controlled. Decision-making in this setting is easier with respect to airway management because the decision to intubate is driven by the need for surgery and anesthetic management; however, careful preoperative assessment remains essential. In addition to the usual comorbidities that can make airway management difficult, trauma patients often have other complicating factors, such as direct airway injury, underlying pulmonary injury, hemodynamic instability, or brain injury with elevated intracranial pressure (ICP). This combination of considerations can make airway management in this intermediate-time window anything but routine. A careful approach, including detailed consideration of possible DA management protocols and relevant comorbidities, is essential.

Finally, traumatized patients frequently require multiple operative repairs or revisions before and during the rehabilitation phase. Delayed operations are often performed between 1 and 6 months after injury and may involve many of the considerations outlined previously. However, these patients are usually stable, and most have already undergone procedures that require tracheal intubation, with most airway difficulties being previously identified. Although the management of these patients raises important issues, this chapter focuses on the acute trauma patient and issues related to airway management in this setting.

General Considerations

Challenges in the Emergency Department or Trauma Resuscitation Unit

Victims of trauma present with a spectrum of injuries, ranging from minor, localized injuries to catastrophic, multisystem trauma, and present unique challenges for the individual providing airway support and management. Although many of these patients do not require intubation outside of the OR, those requiring intubation in the emergency department (ED) or trauma resuscitation unit (TRU) can be some of the most challenging airway cases because of limited time for evaluation, immobilization, combativeness, direct airway trauma, presence of blood or vomit, or a combination of these factors. Emergency intubations outside the OR are generally associated with a higher frequency of difficult intubation and an increased complication rate,[1,2] and, in many cases, the usual paradigms of airway management used in elective perioperative care are not applicable. Care of the acute, severely injured trauma patient is best done using a team approach with a clearly designated team leader, who controls the decision-making, sequence, and flow of the entire resuscitation to include airway management considerations.

In the late 1990s, anesthesiologists performed the majority of trauma airway management in the United States both inside and outside the OR, with emergency medicine (EM) physicians handling the majority of nontrauma cases in the ED.[3] More recently, multiple studies examining the impact of transitioning to a primarily EM-based airway management system for trauma have shown no adverse impact on complication or success rates.[4–7] Currently in the United States, trauma patients are intubated primarily by EM physicians, although patients with direct trauma to the airway or with obvious signs of a DA may be managed best using a team approach, with EM physicians, anesthesiologists, and surgeons working in concert to achieve the best possible results. This includes determining algorithm-based backup plans and the appropriate location to proceed with advanced airway techniques in complex cases. Internationally there is considerable variation in the primary airway providers and capabilities available for the trauma patient.[8–10]

An emergency trauma intubation in the ED generally requires more assistance than an intubation performed under controlled conditions. Multiple providers are required to ventilate the patient, hold cricoid pressure (CP) if applied, administer medications, and provide manual in-line stabilization (MILS) of the cervical spine, as necessary. Fig. 34.1 is an illustration of this approach. In addition, more assistance may be required to control a patient who is combative because of intoxication, traumatic brain injury (TBI), or other causes of altered mental status associated with agitation. The immediate presence of a surgeon or other physician who can expeditiously perform a surgical airway is also desirable. Even if a surgical airway is not required, additional experienced hands may prove useful during difficult intubations. The surgeon may wish to be present during laryngoscopy if there has been trauma to the face or neck or to personally visualize the upper airway when video-assisted laryngoscopy (VAL) is employed. Alternatively, the views obtained during intubation can frequently be recorded with most VAL devices and reviewed later by the managing surgical service.

Indications for Airway Management

Airway management decisions in the trauma patient are frequently driven by considerations beyond identification of the need for an operative intervention. The decision regarding when and how to

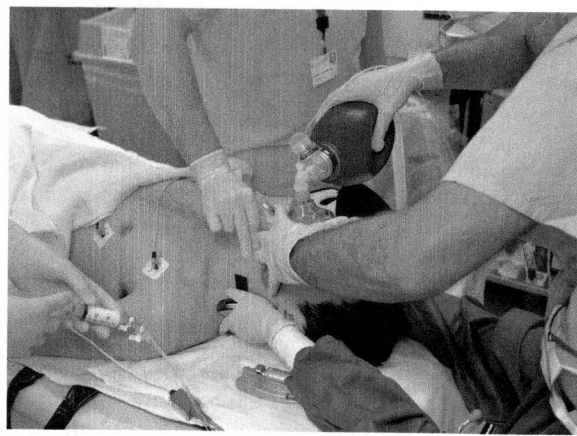

• **Fig. 34.1** Rapid sequence induction and intubation integrating manual in-line stabilization of cervical spine, application of cricoid pressure, preoxygenation, and administration of induction agents.

control a patient's airway is based on a complex series of considerations related to the patient's specific injuries and overall condition, the likelihood of clinical deterioration, and the need for transport to locations in the hospital where airway control is desirable based on these and other factors (e.g., interventional radiology suite). Although the need for emergent or semiurgent intubation is obvious in many patients, it is less intuitive in others. The Eastern Association for the Surgery of Trauma (EAST) has published practice management guidelines addressing emergency tracheal intubation following traumatic injury, including indications for intubation; this information is summarized in Table 34.1. The main indications for emergent intubation can be addressed by asking the following questions during the initial and subsequent evaluations:

• Is there a failure to maintain or protect the airway?
• Is there a failure of oxygenation or ventilation?
• Is there a need for intubation based on the anticipated clinical course?[11]

The requirement to proceed with intubation, based on a failure to maintain an airway, will be clinically apparent in most cases.

In some patients, however, the potential for rapid loss of an initially intact airway may drive the decision to intubate. Examples of this include a penetrating neck injury with an expanding neck hematoma or an inhalational injury with anticipation of progressive airway edema. The need to proceed with intubation for airway protection, however, may be less clear. Loss of the ability to protect the airway can occur because of several mechanisms, including altered mental status secondary to TBI, hemorrhagic shock, or ingestion of drugs or alcohol. When determining need for intubation, consideration should be given to possible effects of prehospital medications such as ketamine, opioids, and naloxone. For example, patients who receive relatively large doses of ketamine in the field will likely exhibit altered mental status and increased secretions despite maintaining airway reflexes, and these signs may factor into a decision to intubate. One of the most common approaches to determining the ability of a patient to maintain his or her airway is to calculate the patient's Glasgow Coma Scale (GCS) score. A GCS score of 8 or lower in the absence of a rapidly reversible cause has been used as an indicator of coma and a general requirement for intubation in the setting of trauma. This cutoff has been promulgated through the Advanced Trauma Life Support (ATLS) program, although patients with a higher GCS score may still require intubation in the setting of an altered neurologic assessment.[12] In a retrospective review of 1000 consecutive patients intubated after injury, Sise and colleagues found that twice as many patients were intubated for the discretionary indication of altered mental status (GCS score >8) than those with a GCS score of 8 or less, suggesting that other factors contributed to the decision to establish a definitive airway.[13]

Basic testing for the presence of adequate airway protection in the initial assessment can be accomplished by asking the patient to phonate. Phonation requires an unobstructed upper airway and the ability to execute complex, coordinated maneuvers. Observation of the patient's ability to swallow and handle secretions is also useful during the primary survey. The ability to sense the pooling of secretions in the posterior pharynx and to perform the coordinated series of neurologic and muscular maneuvers to swallow requires a high degree of function and demonstrates a

TABLE 34.1   **Eastern Association for Trauma Indications for Tracheal Intubation**

Strong Indication	Discretionary Indication
Airway obstruction	Facial or neck injury with potential for airway obstruction
Hypoventilation	Moderate cognitive impairment (GCS score >9–12)
Persistent hypoxemia ($Sao_2 \leq 90\%$) despite supplemental oxygen	Persistent combativeness refractory to pharmacologic agents
Severe cognitive impairment (GCS score ≤8)	Respiratory distress (without hypoxia or hypoventilation)
Severe hemorrhagic shock	Perioperative management (e.g., pain control, painful preoperative procedures)
Cardiac arrest	Spinal cord injury (complete cervical injury at C5 level or above) with any evidence of respiratory depression
Smoke inhalation with any of the following: -airway obstruction -severe cognitive impairment (GCS score ≤8) -major burn (≥40% BSA) -major burns and/or smoke inhalation with prolonged transport time -impending airway obstruction	

BSA, Body surface area; *GCS,* Glasgow Coma Scale; *Sao₂,* arterial oxygen saturation.
Data from Mayglothling J, Duane TM, Gibbs M, et al. Emergency intubation immediately following traumatic injury: an Eastern Association for the Surgery of Trauma practice management guideline. *J Trauma Acute Care Surg* 2012;73:S333-S340

greater likelihood of airway protection.[14] Hospitalized patients with secretions pooling in the back of their mouths and demonstrated swallowing dysfunction are known to be at greater risk for aspiration and pneumonia although this has not been studied in the acute trauma setting.[15]

The loss of the gag reflex may seem like a reasonable test as another indicator of inadequate protective airway reflexes and indication for intubation; however, it should not be assessed in a critically injured, immobilized trauma patient. Insertion of a tongue blade or other device to stimulate the patient's posterior oral pharynx can cause the muscles of the soft palate and pharynx to contract collectively because of the reflex, and vomiting is easily provoked with potential aspiration of gastric contents. This can be made worse by vocal cord paralysis or depression of the gag reflex by sedatives where the glottis does not completely close with stimulation of the reflex.[16–18] Additionally, the gag reflex is much less reliable than phonation and swallowing, and it is absent in up to 25% of the normal adult population.[19] Generally, the presence of a gag reflex does not equate to airway protection, and its absence does not necessarily indicate a need to intubate.

The ability of a patient to maintain appropriate oxygenation and ventilation can be assessed clinically and evaluated by pulse oximetry and capnography. Although arterial blood gas analysis can be useful in evaluating the trauma patient with respect to adequacy of resuscitation efforts in the setting of severe shock, it will have little or no role in the decision to intubate during the acute resuscitation. Evaluation of the patient's respiratory effort and magnitude of injuries in the context of pulse oximetry readings is more important to the intubation decision than arterial blood gas values. Patients with compromised ventilation or oxygenation, particularly those with suspected brain injury,[20] should receive supplemental oxygen (O_2), and all reversible issues should be addressed. Hemothorax, pneumothorax, and opioid overdose are examples of potentially reversible conditions that compromise oxygenation and ventilation. However, most cases of hypoxemia or hypoventilation in multitrauma patients are multifactorial and do not respond to simple interventions. In these cases, early intubation is typically indicated.

Most trauma patients will maintain and protect their airways and exhibit adequate or correctable oxygenation and ventilation during their initial assessment. In these cases, it is the anticipated clinical course that guides the decision to intubate. A patient may appear stable at the time of evaluation, but deterioration can be predicted as a natural course of the injuries. For example, the patient with burns from a closed-space fire with significant inhalation of superheated air (see Chapter 35) may present with a somewhat hoarse voice or a simple cough but an otherwise patent airway. Failing to recognize the possibility of progressive obstruction of the airway attributed to toxic and thermal insults and to intervene in a timely fashion can lead to disaster. Although the patient may not meet the criteria for emergency intubation related to airway maintenance, oxygenation, or ventilation at admission, the likelihood of deterioration may be sufficient to warrant intervention, including intubation and/or direct examination via fiberoptic nasoendoscopy.[21] It is the predictability of the deterioration that determines the decision to intubate. Similarly, the patient presenting with multitrauma, complicated pelvic fracture, open femur fracture, and hypotension is inevitably intubated, even though there is no immediate threat to airway patency or oxygenation. The need for advanced imaging, aggressive pain control, and operative repair of obvious injuries dictates that the patient be intubated early and in a more controlled fashion than trying to

manage a chaotic intubation in the computed tomography (CT) scanner.

Trauma patients may be aggressive, threatening, or combative because of anxiety, pain, fear, intoxication, TBI, or some combination of these. Attempts should be made when reasonable to determine and address the cause of the behavior both pharmacologically and nonpharmacologically, prior to consideration of induction and intubation. Induction and intubation are typically performed if the patient is at risk for self-harm or harming others due to their behavior when more conservative measures have failed. Similarly, if patient behavior prevents further work-up of life-threatening injuries, then intubation may be required. For example, a patient who will not remain still for a necessary CT scan despite conservative measures may need induction and intubation. Apart from patient behavior posing a risk of self-injury, injury to others, or prevention of a needed timely work-up, intubation is rarely required for behavior alone and every attempt should be made to control behavior without intubation where possible. Management of the combative patient is discussed in further detail in the section Management of the Combative Patient later in this chapter.

The decision to intubate is a critical resuscitative decision and can greatly influence subsequent management. Airway management in trauma patients can provoke anxiety because airway difficulty is often exaggerated by the need for cervical spine immobility, presence of direct airway trauma, compromise of hemodynamic status, and propensity for clinical deterioration. Early definitive airway management must be performed in a logical and safe fashion to support evaluation and resuscitative efforts for these patients. Decision-making must be based on a consistent series of principles that accounts for the patient's current condition, likelihood of deterioration, planned diagnostic and therapeutic interventions (including transport and surgery), preinjury comorbidity, as well as the resources and expertise available in the resuscitation area.

Principles of Airway Management in the Trauma Patient

Prevention of Aspiration

All trauma patients are at higher risk for aspiration given intoxication, trauma-induced reduction or absence of gastrointestinal motility, and unknown time of last food intake. Additionally, pharyngeal hemorrhage because of maxillofacial trauma, secretions, and foreign bodies may increase the risk. Reasonable precautions should be taken to prevent aspiration of gastric contents during overall trauma management and airway procedures. The initial intubation method depends on the constellation of patient injuries, hemodynamic status, and available equipment and expertise. Most patients, however, will undergo rapid sequence induction and intubation (RSI) with the intent of mitigating the risk of vomiting and aspiration during the procedure and securing the airway in a rapid, controlled fashion.

The application of CP held throughout laryngoscopy to prevent passive aspiration remains a controversial component of RSI. The use of CP was widely accepted dogma in trauma for many years based on the belief that it could prevent aspiration via passive regurgitation through compression of the upper esophagus against the anterior cervical vertebral bodies. More recently, this belief has been challenged.[22–26] Advanced imaging suggests the cervical esophagus is positioned lateral to the cricoid ring in many patients and may not be compressed during application of CP.[27] This relationship is exaggerated by posterior pressure, although the hypopharynx posterior to the cricoid ring may still be compressed by CP.[28] Misapplication of CP is common and can result in more difficult mask ventilation, direct laryngoscopy (DL), supraglottic airway (SGA) placement, and tracheal tube passage,[29-31] although a recent meta-analysis suggests CP may overall have little impact on intubation outcomes.[32] Cervical spine motion may also occur during application of CP, although cadaveric work suggests that movement is relatively limited and can be reduced further with posterior manual support.[33]

Controversy regarding the risk-benefit assessment for the continued use of CP in patients undergoing RSI is reflected in published guidelines from multiple organizations that have recommended eliminating its use or considering it an optional measure.[34-38] The use of CP in the trauma patient was recently addressed in the EAST practice management guidelines for emergency tracheal intubation immediately following traumatic injury.[34] Based on evidence that CP may worsen the laryngoscopic view, impair bag-valve-mask (BVM) ventilation efficiency, and not reduce the incidence of aspiration, the use of CP was removed as a level 1 recommendation. Similarly, the Scandinavian Society of Anaesthesiology and Intensive Care Medicine in its Clinical Practice Guidelines on General Anaesthesia for Emergency Situations determined that the use of CP is not mandatory and leaves its use up to individual judgment.[35] This trend has continued in other areas of emergent airway management with the 2020 American Heart Association Guidelines for Cardiopulmonary Resuscitation and Emergency Cardiovascular Care recommending against the routine use of CP during laryngoscopy and BVM ventilation.[39] These recommendations are reflected in recent surveys of anesthesiologists, emergency medicine physicians, and surgeons showing significant variability in the use of CP during RSI of patients requiring emergent intubation.[22,25,40,41] In a recent national survey of teaching hospitals in the United States, however, 91% of participants indicated the continued use of CP as part of their modified RSI technique.[42] In support of CP, the most recent guidelines of the American College of Surgeons' ATLS course and the Difficult Airway Society 2015 unanticipated difficult intubation guidelines in adults include CP as a component of RSI.[12,43]

Although there is no universal agreement on the role of CP for aspiration prevention during RSI in the trauma patient, application of CP by trained personnel can still be useful during airway management. Correctly applied CP has been shown to reduce gastric insufflation during BVM ventilation[44,45] and may provide tactile feedback during endotracheal tube (ETT) placement. The most recent Cochrane Collaboration review concludes that the lack of randomized controlled trials addressing this question provides no strong evidence for or against the assumption that CP protects against aspiration; however, nonrandomized controlled trials suggest that CP may not be necessary for safe RSI performance.[23] If the decision is made to use CP, it should be altered or removed to facilitate ventilation, laryngoscopy, or ETT/SGA placement if they are noted to be difficult. Securing the airway and providing ventilation should take precedence over the potential risk of aspiration in the trauma setting given the current level of evidence for CP during RSI.

In addition to the risk of aspiration during trauma RSI, other factors including patient positioning and other airway manipulation may influence the chance of aspiration. Placing patients in a 20- to 40-degree head-up position during RSI is theorized to capitalize on gravitational forces to reduce passive regurgitation above

the upper esophageal sphincter.[46] Caution must be exercised, however, in extreme shock states, as this positioning can decrease preload. If the patient vomits while immobilized on a spine board, the patient and the board should be rolled together into the right lateral decubitus position to permit suctioning and evacuation of the vomitus from the mouth. Recurrent vomiting is a relative indication for early intubation in patients who require immobilization and may be unable to manage the vomitus attributed to alterations in swallowing or level of consciousness. Because most patients may only require immobilization during transport, early evaluation should allow for discontinuation shortly after arrival at the ED. When applying awake intubation techniques, adequate sedation and topical anesthesia should be used to prevent gagging and emesis. If the patient vomits during awake intubation, there may be an increased risk of aspiration because of supraglottic and vocal cord topical anesthesia. Prompt suctioning and repositioning of the patient, if necessary, should help reduce aspirate volume.

Pharmacologic Considerations

In the trauma patient, use of RSI remains the most employed approach to facilitating intubation. As previously described, the primary objective of this technique is to minimize the time interval between loss of protective airway reflexes and tracheal intubation with a cuffed ETT. Following preoxygenation adjusted as needed for urgency and patient condition, rapid-acting induction and neuromuscular blocking (NMB) agents are administered to facilitate the procedure. Some providers, including the authors, routinely perform modified RSI (gentle mask ventilation after rapid sequence induction) in nearly all acute trauma patients as hypoxia and hypercarbia may be more detrimental to the patient condition than the risk of aspiration. This can be particularly important in patients with significant hypoxia prior to induction or in patients with suspected TBI due to difficulties with establishing adequate preoxygenation.[47] The optimal medications for RSI in the setting of trauma would include the following properties: rapid onset and short duration of action, negligible hemodynamic effects, minimal side-effect profile, and rapid reversibility.[48] Unfortunately, the perfect combination of drugs does not exist, leaving the provider with the necessity to make decisions based on specific drug considerations and patient factors. A lack of randomized controlled trials in the trauma population provides no additional insight into the best induction agent for specific subpopulations.

Induction Agents

The most used induction agents in the trauma patient are etomidate, ketamine, and propofol.[49-51] Other less commonly used agents described in the literature include remifentanil, thiopental (no longer available in the United States), and midazolam.[52] If the patient is not completely obtunded and unresponsive, it is recommended to use an induction agent to decrease the likelihood of awareness and recall. Trauma patients are frequently hypovolemic, even if their initial mean arterial blood pressure is normal. Drug selection must go hand in hand with volume resuscitation and other resuscitative measures, such as tube thoracostomy, control of external hemorrhage, and pelvic stabilization. The individual decisions related to the choice of agents are discussed throughout this chapter, but a few general points are emphasized here.

Induction agents should be chosen to provide the best possible intubating conditions with the least likelihood for adverse hemodynamic consequences. The most used induction agent in the United States in the ED/TRU setting is etomidate.[52,53] Etomidate administered in a range of 0.2 to 0.3 mg/kg is associated with hemodynamic stability and has an onset/duration profile similar to that of succinylcholine. Its safety for use in RSI in trauma patients has been challenged, although these studies are largely retrospective with the potential for selection bias and other methodologic deficiencies.[54,55] Etomidate is associated with transient adrenocortical suppression after a single dose; however, this appears not to be clinically significant when a single dose is used for induction for intubation in both trauma and mixed surgical-medical patients undergoing RSI.[56,57] Etomidate can cause myoclonic jerks during its onset, but use of a rapidly acting NMB agent mitigates this effect substantially.

Ketamine is also a frequently used induction agent for hypotensive trauma patients because of its centrally mediated increase in sympathetic tone and catecholamine release.[58] Sympathomimetic-induced normotension may effectively mask hypovolemia and give the trauma team a false sense of security, so it is worth alerting other providers when ketamine is used so this can be accounted for. Its use in patients with concomitant TBI has been questioned based on older reports of associated ICP elevation.[59] More recent analysis, however, suggests that the preservation of cerebral perfusion by maintenance of mean arterial blood pressure in hemodynamically unstable patients is more important than any theoretical risk to the brain caused by ketamine's tendency to increase cerebral activity and ICP.[60] Some investigators have also raised concern that the psychotropic effects associated with ketamine may increase the risk of acute and posttraumatic stress disorders in trauma patients[61,62] although this was not found in a study examining its intraoperative use in burn patients[63] or combat casualties. Of more concern is the potential for barriers to use based on institutional dispensing, tracking, and documentation procedures preventing timely access to ketamine. When these barriers exist, limiting its availability, ketamine in the emergency setting may not be as readily available as other induction agents. Overall, ketamine continues to be a very commonly used drug for RSI in the ED and TRU.

Other induction agents, such as propofol, sodium thiopental, and high-dose benzodiazepines, must be used with caution in the trauma patient because they have a greater tendency to cause hypotension. Whereas propofol is the most common induction agent in the nonemergent patient presenting to the OR, it also reduces systemic vascular resistance and induces myocardial depression, making it less appropriate in the hypotensive and hypovolemic trauma patient. Pharmacokinetic and pharmacodynamic studies in a swine hemorrhagic shock model suggest a significant reduction in propofol dosage of more than 80% to achieve the targeted effect site concentration.[64,65] Unfortunately, there is no corresponding clinical data on the impact of reduced propofol dosing in the setting of hemorrhagic shock on recall and awareness. Patients in shock with an immediate need for intubation should be given a reduced dosage, regardless of the induction agent. This may need to be further reduced because of age and additional comorbidities.

It is worth mentioning that the positive-pressure ventilation necessitated by concomitant sedative and paralytic use may be enough to cause cardiovascular collapse in severely hypovolemic trauma patients in whom the increase in intrathoracic pressure and resultant decrease in preload is not tolerated. As such, it is paramount that resuscitation occurs prior to or at least concurrently with induction.[66]

Neuromuscular Blocking Agents

The selection of an NMB agent as a component of RSI is not altered by the presence or absence of trauma. Succinylcholine and rocuronium are reasonable choices for RSI with several caveats.[67–69]

In a Cochrane systematic review, rocuronium produced slightly inferior intubation conditions compared with succinylcholine for RSI, although this included studies utilizing a dosage as low as 0.6 mg/kg.[67] It also results in significant prolongation of neuromuscular relaxation. In the setting of an altered level of consciousness and suspected TBI where early clinical examination may impact overall management decisions, succinylcholine may be the preferred agent. If TBI is not suspected and the patient requires a CT scan or placement of invasive lines, the prolonged relaxation with rocuronium can facilitate these activities. With the availability of sugammadex, a rapid-onset selective binding agent for rocuronium, RSI with rocuronium followed by reversal with sugammadex allows for more rapid return of spontaneous ventilation than with succinylcholine.[70]

Other Pharmacologic Agents

During RSI, other pharmacologic agents such as lidocaine, atropine, and opioids have been proposed to be useful in attenuating negative physiologic responses that may occur during intubation. For many years, lidocaine was proposed to attenuate elevations in ICP associated with intubation by blunting the sympathetic response. This practice is controversial, with limited evidence to support the preinduction administration of lidocaine in the trauma patient with suspected TBI.[48] Several minutes are required after lidocaine administration for it to be effective, which may not always be possible with a trauma RSI.[71] In infants and in children receiving succinylcholine, atropine at a dose of 0.01 mg/kg is recommended to blunt vagal stimulation and bradycardia. Similar to lidocaine, there is significant controversy regarding the necessity of atropine in this population with insufficient high-quality evidence to support indiscriminate use in the pediatric trauma population.[72] The presence of hypotension and hypovolemia, which can contribute to the negative feedback loop of hypoperfusion and cardiac dysfunction in the setting of bradycardia, may influence the decision to pretreat these patients with atropine, particularly in the presence of succinylcholine use.

Short-acting opioids, such as fentanyl, are frequently used to blunt the hemodynamic response to intubation. In the trauma patient, this must be done with caution given the possibility of hypovolemia and exaggeration of the blood pressure response to RSI. In addition, rapid administration of opioids may induce respiratory depression leading to hypoventilation that can both limit efforts at preoxygenation and cause increased ICP. Finally, some clinicians advocate the use of α-adrenergic agents, such as phenylephrine or epinephrine, as a pretreatment before RSI in the hemodynamically unstable patient. There are no trials examining the clinical impact of this practice, so this will be a clinical decision for the practitioner based on assessment of the patient's vital signs, volume status, and cardiac function at the bedside.[73] This presumes that appropriate resuscitation is ongoing at the time of RSI.

Choice of Technique and the Difficult Airway

For the trauma patient, the choice of intubation technique must consider the injury pattern, underlying physiologic state of the patient, potential difficulties, urgency, and availability of various devices and surgical backup in a timely fashion. While awake flexible scope intubation (FSI) is often proposed as the safest method for patients with possible cervical spine injuries in a cervical collar and a suspected full stomach, RSI or modified RSI with DL or VAL remains the preferred method for most trauma intubations for several reasons, including those discussed earlier. In addition, unrelaxed patients present the potential for significantly more cervical spine motion because of coughing, bucking, gagging, or other movement during an awake intubation attempt. In a published report of 17,583 ED intubations from the National Emergency Airway Registry, including 5451 trauma intubations, 85% were done with RSI.[7]

Whether patients present with an anatomically DA or a DA due to an acute trauma, early recognition is essential.[74,75] A thorough airway assessment is ideal before RSI in the multitrauma patient but may not be possible in the trauma bay. Acquired characteristics, such as airway trauma, cervical spine immobility, hemodynamic compromise, and other potentially life-threatening injuries, can exacerbate inherent DA markers, necessitating rapid decision-making without a complete evaluation. Thus, the use of rapidly identified and easily obtained factors associated with difficult intubation in the ED setting would be optimal in identifying the subset of highest risk patients.

The modified LEMON criteria (Box 34.1) have been shown to have a high sensitivity and a reasonable negative predictive value in several studies.[74,76] The original criteria included the Mallampati score, but this was dropped because of difficulty in obtaining valid assessments in the emergent airway management setting and poor correlation with a difficult intubation grade.[77] Although the tool is overly sensitive at the cost of specificity, focused application of the criteria in the trauma setting should alert the provider to the more high-risk patient. For example, visual inspection (L for Look in LEMON criteria) is even more critical with patients with a mechanism suggestive of or obvious signs of head and neck trauma. Prior to induction, and with maintenance of in-line neck stabilization, the front of the collar should be briefly removed to assess anterior neck trauma and swelling that can make for a DA.

Other chapters discuss various airway techniques, development of an airway management plan, and algorithms for management of the DA. The remainder of this section will address trauma-specific considerations of an airway management plan starting with the DA. The American Society of Anesthesiologists (ASA) originally developed its first practice guidelines for management of the DA in 1993.[78] Since then, these guidelines have been updated twice, in 2003 and 2013,[79,80] following an extensive analysis of the scientific literature, thorough review of new evidence, and collected opinions of both experts and randomly selected ASA members. Similarly, other societies have promulgated recommendations for management of the DA.[81] Although the 2013 ASA DA algorithm and guidelines for management of the DA proposed by the ASA

• BOX 34.1   Modified LEMON Mnemonic

L Look externally:
   facial trauma
   large incisors
   beard or moustache
   large tongue
E Evaluate the 3-3-2 rule:
   mouth opening = 3 fingerbreadths
   hyoid-mental distance = 3 fingerbreadths
   thyroid-to-mouth distance = 2 fingerbreadths
M Mallampati score: no longer counted in total score
O Obstruction: presence of obstructing airway
N Neck mobility: decreased
Total maximum airway assessment score = 9, minimum = 0.

From Hagiwara Y, Watase H, Okamoto H, et al. Prospective validation of the modified LEMON criteria to predict difficult intubation in the ED. *Am J Emerg Med.* 2015;33:1492–1496.

DA task force continue to serve as an excellent starting point for trauma airway management, modifications in the trauma setting remain necessary.

In the setting of a difficult trauma airway, several issues should be considered. First, there may be limited time for evaluation as stated previously, making it necessary to proceed without a full airway assessment. Even in the setting of a likely DA, the presence of hemodynamic instability (e.g., shock) or lack of cooperation (e.g., intoxication, TBI, combativeness) will override or limit some airway management options. Second, waking up the patient or canceling the procedure is rarely an option because the need for emergent airway control will likely remain. Finally, several conditions associated with trauma (discussed later in more detail) may further alter the airway management plan.

Modifications to the ASA DA algorithm for trauma have been proposed by the ASA Committee on Trauma and Emergency Preparedness, although insufficient outcome data have ever been collected to demonstrate the success of one technique over another.[82] The modifications consist of a general algorithm for DA in the trauma patient (Fig. 34.2) with additional recommendations for specific trauma conditions, including closed head injury, airway disruption, cervical spine injury, oral/maxillofacial trauma, and potential airway obstruction.

In addition to RSI with DL, the use of VAL for airway management in the trauma patient provides additional functionality. Although it is susceptible to lens contamination from secretions and blood, glottic visualization nearly always improves. There has been a significant interest in the use of VAL in the ED for both the trauma and nontrauma population.[83,84] As a result, it is now commonly employed in many centers with results comparable with DL.[85] A recent meta-analysis examined the use of DL compared to VAL outside of the OR, concluding that VAL is associated with fewer esophageal intubations with a greater first-pass success in the intensive care unit and among less experienced clinicians.[86] VAL appears to be playing an increased role in trauma airway management; however, the importance of other adjuncts should not be forgotten. It cannot be overemphasized that the bougie intubating stylet is arguably the most important DA adjunct during DL. The combination of DL and bougie may be the optimal approach to successful first-pass success in the trauma airway with anything less than a grade 1 Cormack and Lehane (CL) laryngeal view. The bougie stylet is low profile, allows less cervical movement, as well as a "blind" insertion under the epiglottis during poor view attempts.[87] Most importantly, rapidly progressing down the DA algorithm with the use of supraglottic airway devices, then cricothyrotomy can be lifesaving and should be employed quickly when traditional techniques fail.

In summary, when dealing with the difficult trauma airway, a team approach is the best solution in any scenario. The most experienced airway operator should be present to increase the first-attempt success rate because the first attempt is always the best. In managing the severely traumatized patient, gather the necessary equipment and personnel resources, have a clear definition of airway failure, and proceed quickly with backup plans such as those detailed in Fig. 34.2.

Management of the Combative Patient

Trauma patients, particularly those who are intoxicated, have sustained a head injury, or have an underlying psychiatric condition, are frequently agitated or combative on arrival at the ED. In some cases, this agitation is a result of an overwhelming combination of

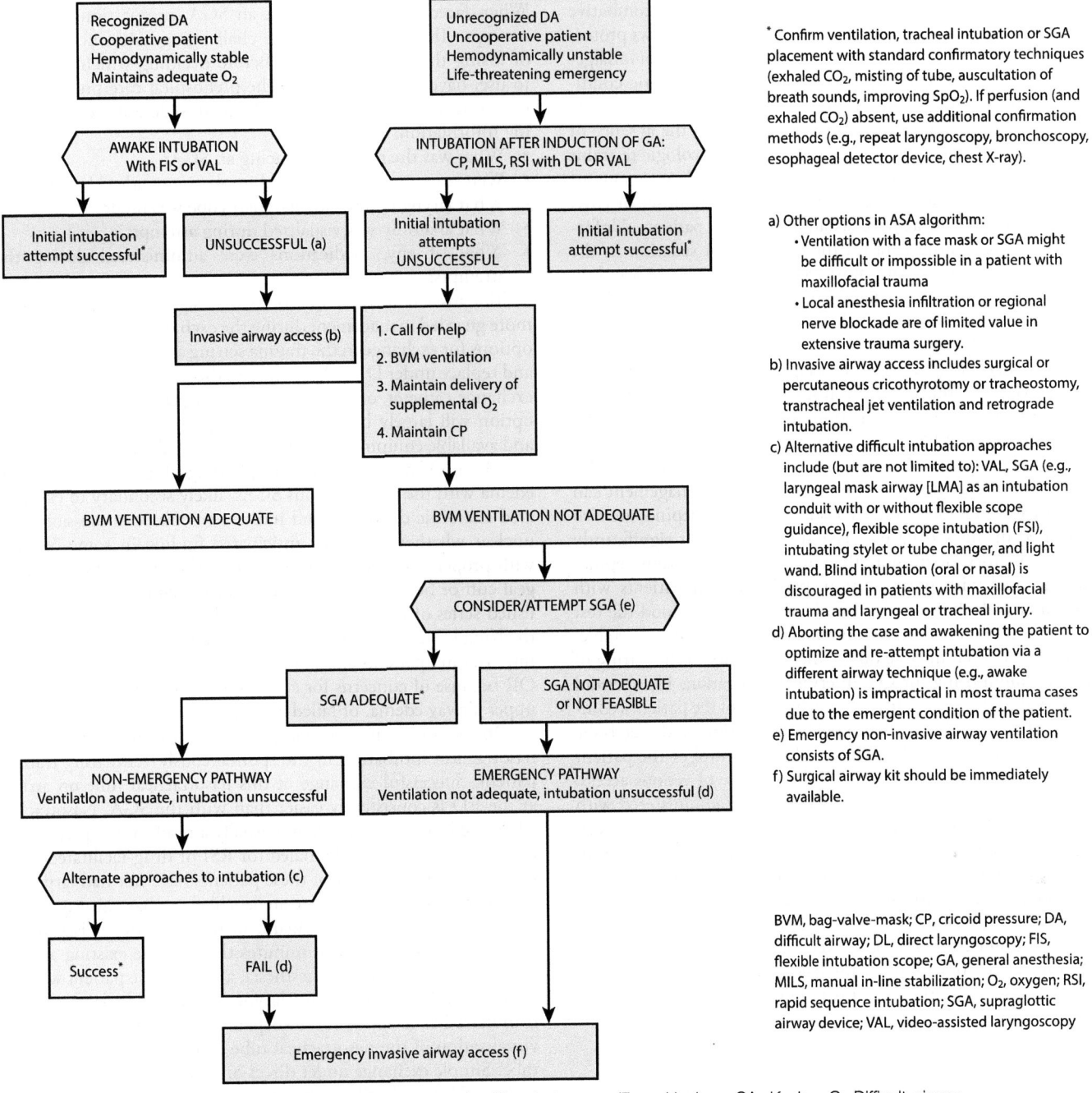

* Confirm ventilation, tracheal intubation or SGA placement with standard confirmatory techniques (exhaled CO_2, misting of tube, auscultation of breath sounds, improving SpO_2). If perfusion (and exhaled CO_2) absent, use additional confirmation methods (e.g., repeat laryngoscopy, bronchoscopy, esophageal detector device, chest X-ray).

a) Other options in ASA algorithm:
  • Ventilation with a face mask or SGA might be difficult or impossible in a patient with maxillofacial trauma
  • Local anesthesia infiltration or regional nerve blockade are of limited value in extensive trauma surgery.
b) Invasive airway access includes surgical or percutaneous cricothyrotomy or tracheostomy, transtracheal jet ventilation and retrograde intubation.
c) Alternative difficult intubation approaches include (but are not limited to): VAL, SGA (e.g., laryngeal mask airway [LMA] as an intubation conduit with or without flexible scope guidance), flexible scope intubation (FSI), intubating stylet or tube changer, and light wand. Blind intubation (oral or nasal) is discouraged in patients with maxillofacial trauma and laryngeal or tracheal injury.
d) Aborting the case and awakening the patient to optimize and re-attempt intubation via a different airway technique (e.g., awake intubation) is impractical in most trauma cases due to the emergent condition of the patient.
e) Emergency non-invasive airway ventilation consists of SGA.
f) Surgical airway kit should be immediately available.

BVM, bag-valve-mask; CP, cricoid pressure; DA, difficult airway; DL, direct laryngoscopy; FIS, flexible intubation scope; GA, general anesthesia; MILS, manual in-line stabilization; O_2, oxygen; RSI, rapid sequence intubation; SGA, supraglottic airway device; VAL, video-assisted laryngoscopy

• **Fig. 34.2** Difficult airway management algorithm in trauma. (From Hagberg CA, Kaslow O. Difficult airway management algorithm in trauma updated by COTEP. *ASA Newsletter.* 2014;78:56-60.)

confusing sensory inputs. Intoxication, head injury, disorientation, and severe pain can contribute to combative or agitated behavior. It is also possible that the patient's altered mental status may be because of a medical condition contributing to the initial injury. Hypoglycemia, stroke, syncope, and seizure should be considered when the patient's mental status is significantly altered or when prehospital reports suggest a minor mechanism or minimal vehicular damage.

Initially, attempts should be made to reassure and help the patient orient to the chaotic environment of the resuscitation room. Patients who remain agitated and physically aggressive present a risk to themselves and the resuscitation team. Delays in examination and care delivery as well as inability to observe cervical spine precautions can disrupt the initial evaluation and treatment plan. Combativeness is often cited as an indication for

intubation of the trauma patient.[13] This practice, however, may contribute to increased lengths of stay, higher incidence of pneumonia, and worsened discharge status.[88] Alternative measures should be attempted to control or limit the impact of agitation and combativeness although many patients will still require intubation and sedation to facilitate the initial work-up and treatment. Physical and chemical restraints are often necessary to facilitate an orderly, efficient, and safe trauma assessment. Combative patients are commonly restrained on a long spine board with a cervical collar, tape, and sandbags, but these constraints are temporary, and the patient's ability to move and to exert significant forces on the potentially injured spine often warrants further action.

The decision regarding whether to sedate or intubate a patient for behavioral control should be made based on the patient's overall injuries. If intubation is inevitable, even without combative behavior, early intubation is the best approach. RSI allows protection of the cervical spine, provision of adequate sedation/analgesia, and treatment of multiple injuries under less chaotic conditions. If the patient's overall injuries are deemed to be relatively modest and intubation would not be indicated in the absence of the combative behavior, intravenous (IV) pharmacologic restraint without intubation is the preferred approach. When venous or intraosseous access cannot be established, the intramuscular (IM) route can be used to achieve sedation in many patients. Unfortunately, there is little data on the effect of IM sedation in the acutely injured patient, and most recommendations are based on literature addressing the management of the patient with medical-related or psychiatric-related behavioral disturbances.

When the IV route is available, repeated doses of a butyrophenone, such as haloperidol, can rapidly achieve control of the agitated patient without compromising respiration or significantly altering the neurologic examination. In the hemodynamically stable patient, 5 mg of haloperidol can be given IV in repeated doses every 5 minutes, with observation for effect.[89] Most patients calm rapidly under the influence of haloperidol, and management can then proceed in a more orderly fashion. Benzodiazepines are also often used in this setting but have the potential for significantly more respiratory depression than haloperidol. Benzodiazepines must be used with great caution, particularly in patients with concomitant alcohol intoxication. Haloperidol has stood the test of time in trauma patients, who remain hemodynamically stable, and it can be given in large doses when necessary in the setting of adequate monitoring for QT interval prolongation. Haloperidol does not alter the need to investigate the cause of the patient's combative behavior with CT, neurologic examination, and metabolic testing, but it does rapidly help to achieve control of the patient and permit ongoing evaluation. In the absence of venous access, droperidol, ketamine, and midazolam can be administered with caution by the intramuscular (IM) route.[90–92] Ketamine has seen a significant resurgence for treatment of agitation and delirium in both the prehospital and ED settings,[93] although use by prehospital personnel may contribute to a higher frequency of intubation on arrival at the hospital.[94] Droperidol has also seen resurgence for this indication despite the controversial black box warning about QT interval prolongation, as for haloperidol, recommended by the U.S. Food and Drug Administration.[95]

Confirming or Replacing the Field-Placed Airway

In many settings, prehospital providers work under protocols that allow for advanced airway management, including intubation and/or placement of an SGA. It is recommended that the individuals responsible for airway management at the ED level be familiar with the protocols and devices available in their region to facilitate early assessment and airway exchange if indicated. All intubations done in the field should be immediately confirmed using capnometry. In the event of cardiac arrest and inability to confirm correct placement by observation of end-tidal carbon dioxide (EtCO$_2$), DL or VAL can be employed to visualize position of the ETT. When a supraglottic device is used in the prehospital setting, the positioning and ability to ventilate should be confirmed by capnometry, presence of breath sounds, and chest movement. If there is adequate ventilation, replacement of the SGA can be delayed during the initial evaluation.

Because the SGA is not considered a secured definitive airway, it should be changed out to a cuffed ETT as soon as practical.

When faced with changing out an SGA, preparation is the key concept. This procedure can be challenging, with increased risk of losing the patient's airway. Before deciding which technique to use, have a discussion with the prehospital care provider who managed the patient's airway in the field to determine the following information:

- What was the reason for placing an SGA?
- Were attempts at oral or nasal intubation made? How many?
- What laryngoscope/videolaryngoscope was used?
- What anatomy was visualized during attempts?
- What, if any, medications were administered during the attempts?

The answers to these questions may suggest a DA prompting more guarded management during the exchange process. The three options for exchange in the trauma setting are (1) remove the SGA and replace under DL or VAL, (2) use the SGA to place an ETT or exchange catheter, or (3) proceed to a surgical airway. The second option will largely be guided by the specific SGA, channel size, and available equipment.[96–99] One proposed algorithm is shown in Fig. 34.3. Of note are reports of pharyngeal, glottic, and lingual edema with the use of various SGAs, likely secondary to exaggerated anatomic distortion and indirect vascular compression. It is unclear whether this is an anticipated finding in some patients with proper placement and inflation of the proximal oropharyngeal cuff or because of overinflation of the cuff. In the only published series of patients presenting with prehospital placement of the King LT (S)-D (King Systems; Noblesville, IN, USA), seven of nine trauma patients ultimately underwent tracheostomy in the OR because of concerns for concomitant facial trauma, observed upper airway edema, or failed attempts at DL.[96]

On occasion, prehospital personnel will perform a blind nasotracheal intubation in the spontaneously ventilating trauma patient. Successful exchange of this nasotracheal tube on arrival at the ED is consistently easier than with the SGA. Nasotracheally placed tubes in the field are usually a result of the prehospital providers not being credentialed for RSI or drug-facilitated intubation. As a result, most of these patients have not had laryngoscopy performed and therefore are less likely to have airway edema from intubation attempts. Again, in this scenario, it is prudent to preoxygenate for several minutes through the existing airway, ensure adequate sedation/anesthesia, and relax the patient with an NMB agent before attempting laryngoscopy. A videolaryngoscope is preferred as it allows for an expanded view of the glottis with visualization of the nasotracheal tube before removal of the nasal tube. Simple exchange under direct or video visualization with an oral ETT is usually all that is required. A bougie should be readily available in these situations for rapid placement into the glottis with various sized ETTs readily available. If the glottis cannot be adequately visualized with laryngoscopy, it is recommended that the nasotracheal tube be left in place for a period to allow for either a controlled tracheostomy or swelling to improve and then an exchange for an oral tube made at a later time.

Point-of-Care Ultrasound and Airway Management

The early evaluation of the traumatically injured patient increasingly relies on imaging to guide early management and operative decisions. These principles apply to airway management under the concept of rapid point-of-care ultrasound (POCUS) airway and lung scanning. With the almost universal availability of ultrasound in most EDs, airway providers should be able to integrate

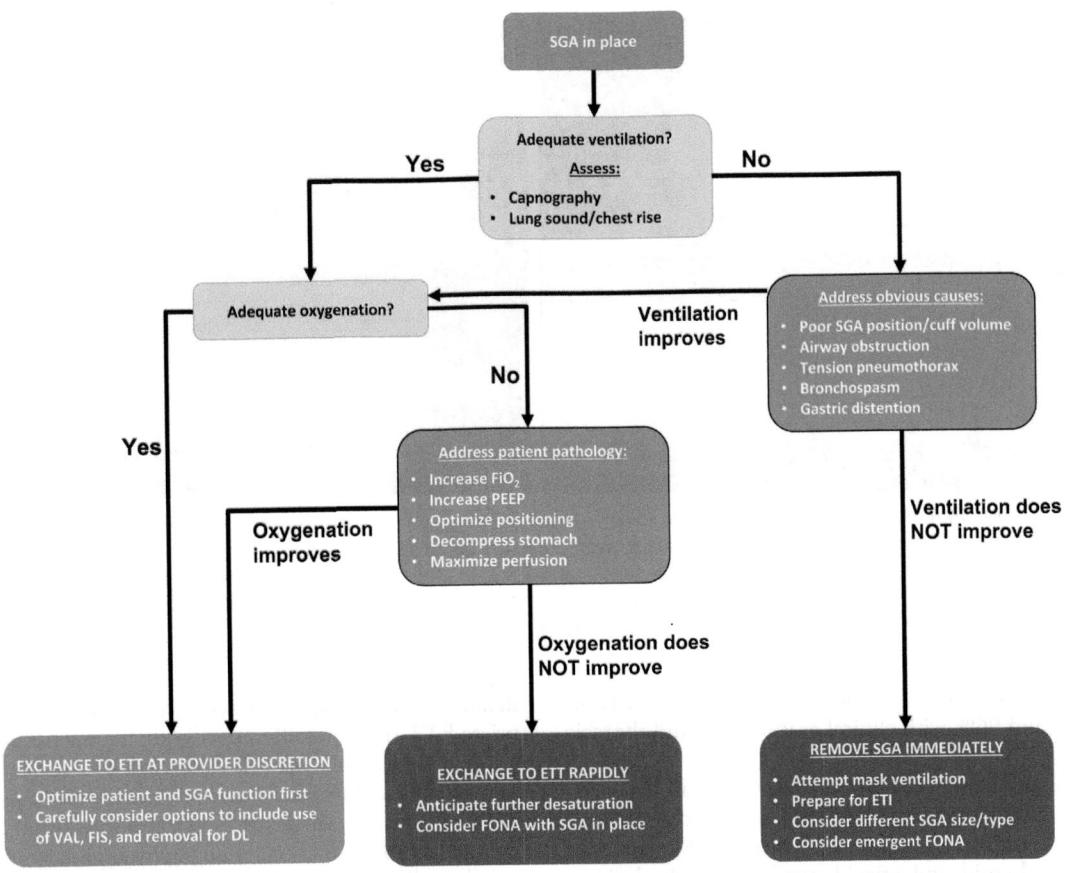

DL, direct laryngoscopy; ETI, endotracheal intubation; FiO$_2$, fraction of inspired oxygen; FIS, flexible intubation scope; FONA, front-of-neck airway; SGA, supraglottic airway device; PEEP, positive end-expiratory pressure; VAL, video-assisted laryngoscopy

• **Fig. 34.3** Algorithm summarizing approach to managing field-placed supraglottic airway. (From Braude D, Steuerwald M, Wray T, Galgon R. Managing the out-of-hospital extraglottic airway device. *Ann Emerg Med.* 2019;74(3):416-422.)

POCUS into their trauma airway management protocols. This starts with the Extended-Focused Assessment with Sonography in Trauma (E-FAST) examination, which expands the traditional Focused Assessment with Sonography in Trauma (FAST) examination to detect an acute pneumo- or hemothorax.[100] In nonpathologic states, visceral and parietal pleurae slide against each other during the respiratory cycle. This manifests as a "lung sliding" sign seen in sonographic Brightness mode (B-mode) . In Motion mode (M-mode), normal sliding appears as "sand-on-the-beach" with the movement artifact at the pleural line having a speckled appearance below the nonmoving muscle and fascial layers of the chest wall (Fig 34.4A). In a pneumothorax, the air trapped between the visceral and parietal pleurae attenuates the ultrasound waves and leads to the absence of lung sliding. These signs are replaced by the presence of a "stratosphere" or "barcode" sign in M-mode which suggests that sonographic detection of lung movement is impaired at the location of insonation. Concerns for a pneumothorax should prompt investigation for a lung point (a single image where the junction between lung sliding and absent lung sliding is present) visceral and parietal surfaces and be pathognomonic for a pneumothorax (Fig. 34.4B). As most acute trauma patients present to the ED in the supine position, exploration for sonographic evidence of a pneumothorax must be assessed at the least dependent part of the thoracic cavity located in the

anterior midclavicular line. Even small pneumothoraces, unable to be appreciated by supine anterior-posterior chest radiography, can be appreciated using ultrasound. The more lateral and posterior a lung point is observed defines a pneumothorax of increasing size, which would prompt a more aggressive approach to decompressive thoracostomy.

In application, the E-FAST examination has been determined to be much more sensitive for detection of pneumothorax than chest radiographs in trauma with near 100% specificity.[101–103] It also provides results sooner than the chest radiograph. It is now considered to be the best modality for rapid diagnosis and treatment of pneumothorax in trauma. High-frequency linear probes, typically used to establish central venous access, provide great resolution and accuracy in identifying lung sliding and are often readily available. As evidence, Hyacinthe and colleagues evaluated 119 patients admitted with chest trauma and compared clinical examination and chest x-ray (CXR) with clinical examination and thoracic ultrasound for the detection of hemothorax, pneumothorax, and lung contusion.[101] When compared with follow-up CT examination, they found clinical examination and ultrasound to be significantly better than clinical examination and CXR for both pneumothorax and lung contusion evaluation, with no significant difference between the two for hemothorax evaluation. For hemothorax detection, the sensitivity and specificity for clinical

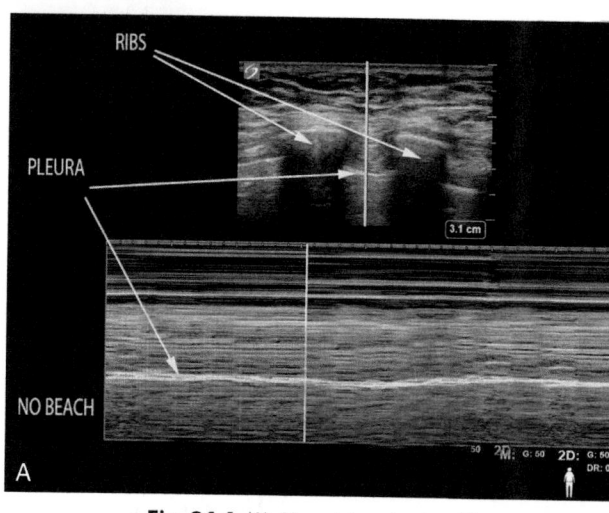
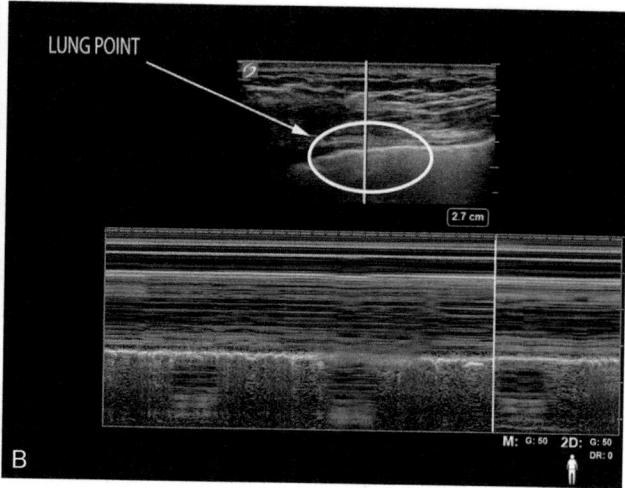

• **Fig. 34.4** (A) Absent beach sign. The granular beach is not seen because the sound waves echo off the highly reflective pleura/air interface, creating a reverberation artifact and continuation of waves consistent with a pneumothorax. (B) Lung point. In the two-dimensional image at the top, the separation of the visceral and parietal pleura is seen. This separation intermittently causes the beach sign to be lost as seen in the M-mode image at the bottom suggesting the presence of a pneumothorax.

examination and CXR were 17% and 94%, respectively, compared with 37% and 96% with clinical examination and thoracic ultrasound.

Ultrasound is also being used for other aspects of airway management.[104] Ultrasound evaluation of the anterior cervical area allows accurate location of important structures. Superficially, the hyoid bone, thyroid and cricoid cartilages, tracheal rings, and cricothyroid membrane can be easily identified. The deeper structures of the epiglottis and vocal cords can often be identified as well. The ability to identify the cricothyroid membrane and tracheal rings quickly and accurately for emergent surgical airway procedures is not a simple task in some patients, and ultrasound can better define the anatomy (Fig. 34.5). In patients where a thick, burned, or irradiated neck would otherwise make this an extremely difficult task, ultrasound examination shows tremendous benefit. Ultrasound can also help determine the inner

diameter of the subglottic trachea, allowing selection of an appropriate ETT size especially in pediatric trauma patients.[105]

Trauma patients may also develop or present in cardiopulmonary arrest. In these situations, ultrasound can be helpful in determining tracheal versus esophageal intubation and is recommended as an adjunct to capnography, especially in patients who may have little or no $EtCO_2$.[106] Later, at the point of extubation, ultrasound examination may be helpful in predicting postextubation stridor[107] and has been proposed as a modality to assess diaphragmatic function and thickening as a predictor of extubation success.[108] As bedside POCUS exams continue to be developed and integrated into medical algorithms, it is anticipated that POCUS airway and lung exams will play an increasing role in acute trauma and emergency care.[109]

Specific Clinical Considerations in Trauma

Direct Airway Trauma

Direct trauma to the airway can be broadly classified as blunt or penetrating injury. Each of these categories can be considered in the context of direct injury to the airway itself versus compromise or threat to the airway caused by the proximity of an injury in the neck. Injury to the airway can occur at one or more levels. Maxillofacial trauma can compromise the upper airway; direct injury to the neck can compromise the airway from the hypopharynx to the trachea; and injuries to the thorax can disrupt the lower trachea, main stem bronchi, or other smaller bronchi. Although the frequency of these injuries in the traumatized patient is relatively low (1%–2%), mortality because of traumatic injury is high because of early airway loss or associated injuries.[110] They also represent a disproportionate percentage of trauma patients who require a planned or emergent FONA. The overall approach to airway management is dictated by the clinical presentation of the patient and the best judgment of the operator.[111]

General principles for evaluation of the traumatized airway include frequent clinical assessment because airway compromise attributed to edema, tissue disruption, and hematoma can worsen over time. Evaluation of traumatic airway injury can incorporate

• **Fig. 34.5** Cricothyroid membrane. The thyroid and cricoid cartilages are typically easy to identify with a high-resolution (high-frequency) probe. The hyperechoic cricothyroid membrane is located between the two structures.

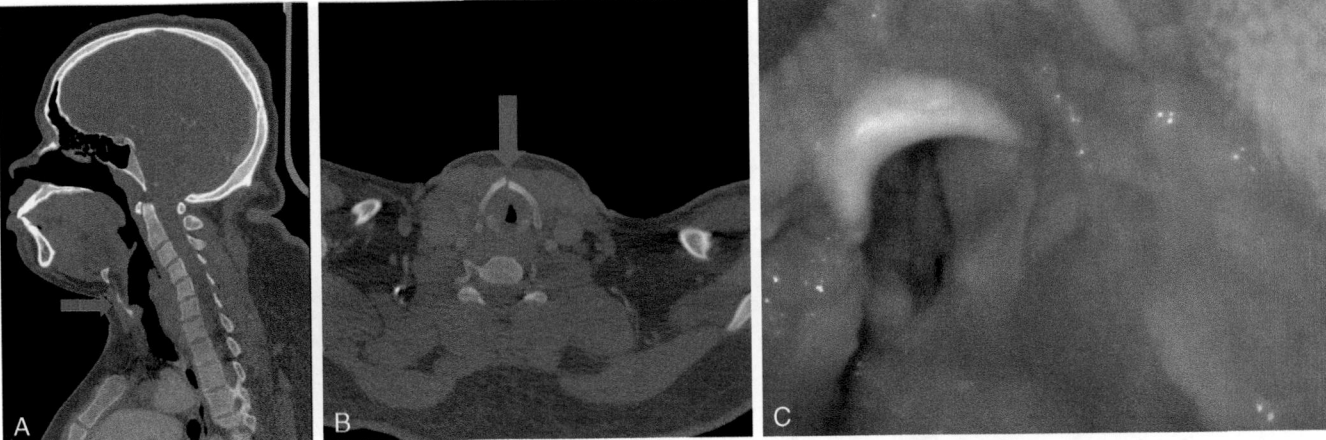

• **Fig 34.6**   Example of blunt force trauma to neck with resulting thyroid and cricoid cartilage fractures and airway compromise. (A) Sagittal view of neck with thyroid cartilage fracture (*red arrow*) and significant edema/hemorrhage narrowing visible airway. (B) Transverse view of the neck at the level of the fracture (*red arrow*) showing compromised airway. (C) View of vocal cords showing significant subglottic edema and airway narrowing.

DL, VAL, flexible bronchoscopy, nasal endoscopy, or ultrasound imaging, with or without sedation and topical anesthesia. In the stable patient not requiring emergent intubation or after the airway is secured, CT and magnetic resonance imaging (MRI) with contrast can be accomplished to provide additional information regarding structural injury and potential for airway compromise[112] (Fig. 34.6). Patients at greatest risk for need of intubation or surgical intervention include those who present with (1) self-inflicted and/or penetrating mechanism, (2) hyoid/thyroid fractures, and/or (3) respiratory distress.[113] An excellent review by Jain and colleagues provides an in-depth discussion on this topic.[114]

Penetrating Neck Trauma

Penetrating neck injuries range in scope from stab or other puncture wounds to major lacerations from both low-velocity and high-velocity projectile injury. The consequences of these injuries can vary significantly. The patient with a stab wound to the neck usually has identifiable anatomy and can undergo airway evaluation and early intubation under controlled circumstances. Patients with high-velocity injuries often have significant vascular and aerodigestive tract injuries with anatomic distortion making airway management a challenge. These injuries mandate urgent airway evaluation, but the presence of other surgical priorities can make this difficult.[115]

Penetrating neck wounds can be described according to anatomic zones that can influence the diagnostic, surgical, and airway management approach (Fig. 34.7). Zone 1 extends from the clavicles to the level of the cricoid cartilage. Zone 2 extends from the cricoid cartilage to a line drawn through the angles of the mandible. Zone 3 is the area above the angles of the mandible. This classification is most useful for low-velocity penetration, such as from a stab or long-distance birdshot, but it has also been applied to high-velocity injuries, such as rifle wounds.[116] Zone 1 is dominated by the major vascular structures at the root of the neck, specifically the carotid arteries, internal jugular veins, subclavian arteries and veins, and innominate arteries and veins. Zone 1 injuries are relatively uncommon (<10% of penetrating neck injuries) but are often associated with major vascular injuries or injuries to the dome of the lung.[117] Patients with zone 1 injuries may require emergency airway management because of direct airway compromise from hemorrhage or an anticipated clinical course

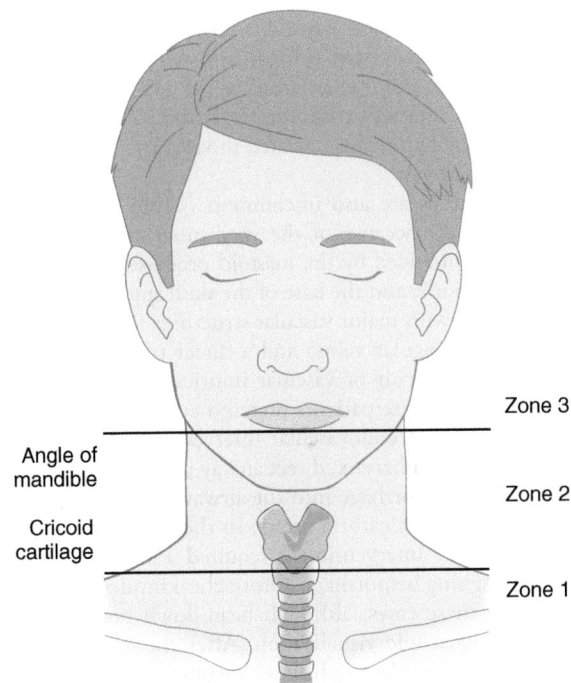

Angle of mandible

Cricoid cartilage

Zone 3

Zone 2

Zone 1

• **Fig. 34.7**   Zones of the neck.

predicted by the profound shock that typically develops. There is little literature to guide the selection of airway management techniques for zone 1 penetrating injuries, and most information is limited to small subsets of larger series that are dominated by zone 2 injuries. The approach to airway management is dictated more by the nature of the threat to the airway than by the location of the inciting wound. The overall approach to airway management in penetrating neck injuries is outlined below.

Zone 2 is the most common location for penetrating neck injuries, accounting for most reported cases.[118] Zone 2 injuries require emergency airway intervention in approximately one-third of the cases, with a large proportion of the remainder undergoing subsequent intubation related to evaluation or surgical repair. The area of concern in zone 2 extends from the anterior margins of the paravertebral muscles bilaterally. In this area, major vascular

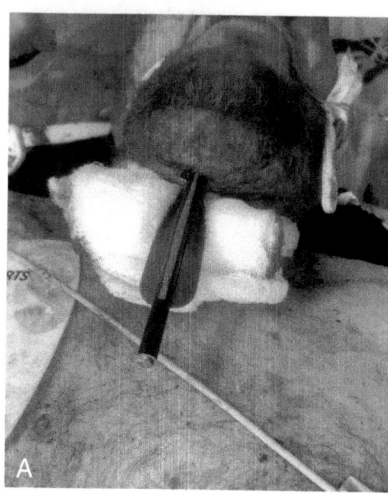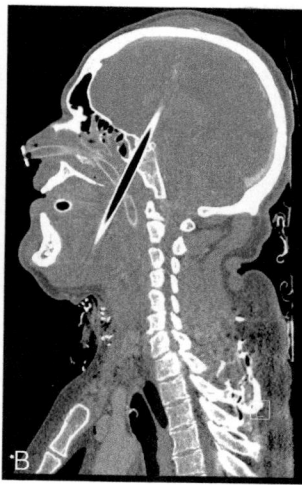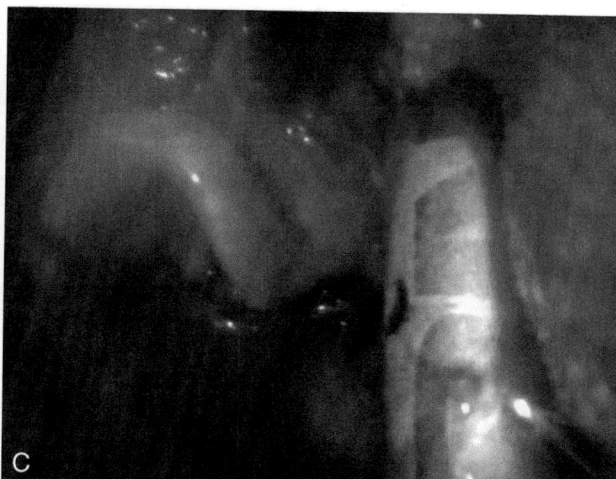

• **Fig. 34.8** (A) Penetrating injury with arrow involving zones 2 and 3 with concomitant traumatic brain injury. (B) Sagittal image showing penetration through oral cavity and posterior nasopharynx. (C) View of vocal cords showing arrow shaft.

structures (e.g., common carotid arteries and internal jugular veins) and their associated sympathetic ganglia, hypopharynx, esophagus, larynx, and trachea are all at risk (Fig. 34.8). The most common cause of airway compromise in zone 2 injuries is external distortion by hemorrhage related to vascular injuries or direct injuries to the airway.[119]

Zone 3 injuries are also uncommon (<10% of all penetrating neck injuries) because of the very small area involved and the protection provided by the mastoid processes posteriorly, the mandible anteriorly, and the base of the skull superiorly. The area, however, is rich with major vascular structures (i.e., carotid arteries and internal jugular veins) and a direct path for pharyngeal injuries. Surgical repair of vascular injuries in this area is difficult, and most of these patients undergo evaluation by angiography and subsequent endovascular intervention. Because zone 3 injuries involve the pharynx, direct airway compromise is uncommon except by hemorrhage into the airway from a through-and-through injury to the carotid artery. In these rare circumstances, immediate airway intervention is required and may be difficult because of ongoing hemorrhage. Orotracheal intubation is usually successful in these cases, although head-down positioning may improve laryngoscopic visualization. After the airway is secure, the mouth can be packed tightly with gauze to control the internal hemorrhage while direct external pressure is simultaneously applied as the patient is transported for surgical or angiographic interventions.

The approach to the airway in the patient with penetrating neck trauma is guided by the same principles as outlined earlier in this chapter. The tougher management decisions involve the patient who has evidence of injury to the neck but does not have an obviously compromised airway at the initial evaluation and does not require immediate intubation. It is in these cases that judgment, consultation with the trauma team, and solid planning are most important. Considerations for airway management in the setting of penetrating neck injuries have been proposed based on the zone of injury, external evidence, and stability of the patient (Box 34.2). Combination approaches such as the use of VAL and FSI may also be appropriate in some cases. In the stable patient without evidence of airway compromise, however, current management recommendations allow for continued observation during their evaluation.[120]

There are two specific considerations to address in those patients not requiring immediate airway management. The first is whether there is evidence of an aerodigestive tract injury, such as subcutaneous crepitus, dysphagia, or hematemesis. In severe cases, particularly patients with injury to both vascular and aerodigestive tract structures, obstruction can occur rapidly, requiring emergency FONA.[121] In initially stable patients, it is sometimes difficult to determine whether the esophagus or airway is involved, and early direct or fiberoptic examination of the airway is indicated. The decision must be made whether an awake examination of the airway is warranted in concert with other surgical priorities.[120] The risk lies in blind insertion of an ETT into a false passage distal to the area being visualized and is more likely to occur with zone 1

• **BOX 34.2**   **Airway Management Considerations in the Setting of Penetrating Neck Injury**

Zone I Injury

- Direct intubation through a large defect
- Tracheostomy
- Thoracotomy in complete tracheal transection

Zone II Injury

- Plan for CT scan to exclude distal airway injury if there is no impending obstruction of the airway
- Oral intubation by RSI for injuries proximal to the larynx
- Flexible scope intubation for injuries distal to the larynx
- FONA for injuries distal to the larynx

Zone III Injury

- Oral intubation by RSI for small defects
- FONA for gross disruption

For Any Large Airway Defect

- Direct intubation through the defect

CT, Computed tomography; *FONA*, front-of-neck airway; *RSI*, rapid sequence induction and intubation.
From Mercer SJ, Lewis SE, Wilson SJ, et al. Creating airway management guidelines for casualties with penetrating airway injuries. *J R Army Med Corps.* 2010;156(suppl 1):S355–360.

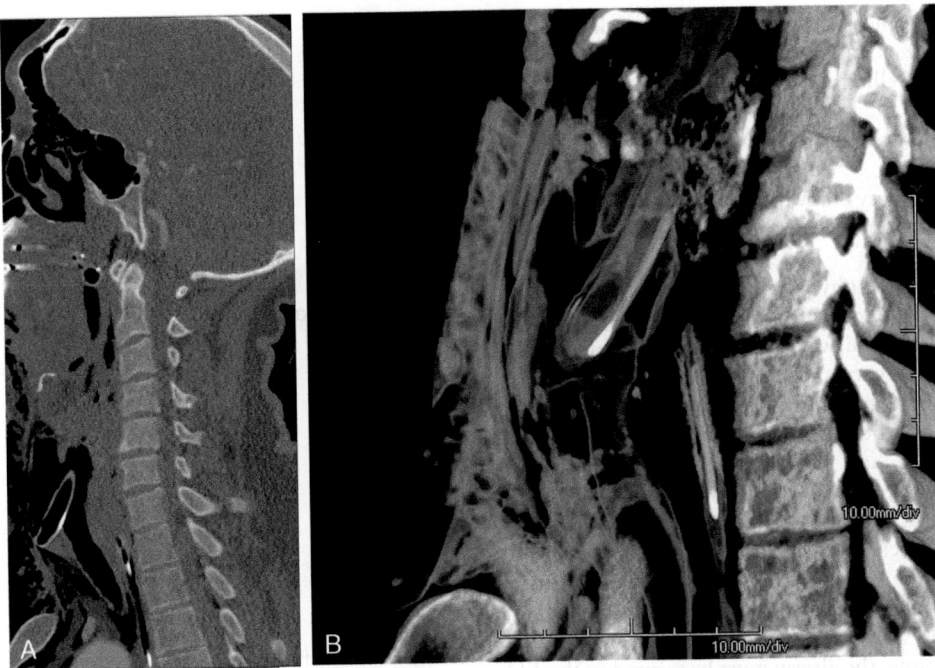

• **Fig. 34.9** Transection of trachea in high-velocity motor vehicle crash. (A) Sagittal view of neck showing endotracheal tube entering anterior defect of trachea at the level of the cricoid cartilage. (B) Magnified view of 3D reconstruction of tracheal defect showing tip of endotracheal tube outside of airway but with Murphy eye within lumen allowing for ventilation.

and 2 injuries (Fig. 34.9). In many cases, airway control is first established through RSI, and then evaluation using flexible endoscopy and/or esophagoscopy can be performed. In some cases, an awake approach is preferred with sedation and topical anesthesia to facilitate the evaluation. Preparation of an ETT (e.g., 6.0-mm to 7.0-mm inside diameter) mounted on the bronchoscope before initiating endoscopy facilitates prompt intubation if the injury is found to be significant. If an injury is found and the scope can be placed successfully distal to it, the patient can be gently intubated over an FIS with placement of the balloon below the level of injury. Although tracheostomy may be necessary in these cases, temporary oral tracheal intubation over an FIS ensures airway control and minimizes the subsequent leakage of air into the tissues. If no airway injury is identified and there is no evidence of increase in the subcutaneous emphysema in the neck during spontaneous or assisted ventilation, the injury is likely esophageal.

The second consideration is whether there is evidence of significant vascular injury to the neck. A hematoma of any size, ongoing external hemorrhage, or displacement of airway structures can serve as evidence of direct vascular injury. If direct vascular injury is suspected, active airway management should be undertaken.[122,123] Most of these patients present early, when anatomy is preserved and orotracheal intubation is more likely to be straightforward. Waiting to determine whether the hematoma is expanding is dangerous because hemorrhage into the neck can continue in deeper tissue planes, distorting and displacing the airway. Early intubation can typically be accomplished using RSI following careful examination for DA attributes. Early intervention allows the operator to intubate in a controlled fashion rather than to rush to secure an emergency airway later in the patient's course when airway obstruction is imminent or has already occurred.

If there is doubt regarding the anatomy using the oral route and time permits, three approaches can be considered. The first option is to perform oral RSI under a double setup with preparations and personnel in place to perform an immediate surgical airway if orotracheal intubation is not successful. This approach should only be undertaken if preintubation assessment indicates that orotracheal intubation, although potentially difficult, is still likely to be successful. Similarly, there must be confidence that BVM ventilation will be successful, if required. If visualization is suboptimal during conventional DL, the use of a bougie or VAL can be considered.

The second option is to perform FSI under sedation and topical anesthesia, as previously described. This allows the operator to use the FIS to identify and enter the airway, even if the anatomy has become distorted. If this is done early in the patient's course, there is typically sufficient time and control to yield a high success rate. However, a distorted and bloodied airway makes FSI technically challenging, and the most experienced operator should perform the procedure.

The third option is to proceed directly with a planned surgical airway. This requires that the airway be identifiable with clear landmarks to permit a surgical approach. Local anesthetic infiltration and direct transcricothyroid puncture for instillation of local anesthesia into the airway are likely to make the procedure easier to perform (see Chapter 29). In patients with penetrating cervical tracheal injuries, the insertion of a tracheostomy tube through the wound is the best way to secure the airway and spares tissue for future repair if this is deemed feasible and necessary.

Blunt Neck Trauma

Most of the management issues related to penetrating neck trauma apply to management of the patient with blunt neck injury. The primary difference is related to the inability to precisely localize the injury. Initial evaluation of the patient with a blunt neck trauma should include identification of bruising or ecchymosis related to the external injury. The oropharynx should be inspected to ensure that there is no injury to the tongue or dentition. The external neck should then be palpated carefully, with temporary removal of the front of a neck collar while in-line neck stabilization is provided, from the mandible to the clavicle focusing on:

- Identification of swelling, hemorrhage, or subcutaneous emphysema
- Evaluation for tenderness (if possible) of the neck, particularly the airway structures
- Evaluation of the anatomy of the upper airway for direct airway injury and for the anatomic landmarks in the event a FONA is required (see Chapter 29)

Because subcutaneous emphysema may be occult, it requires careful palpation. Extensive ecchymosis or swelling should prompt consideration of impending airway compromise, and urgent airway intervention may be necessary.[124] Infrequently, direct blunt neck trauma can cause laryngeal fracture or tracheal injury (Fig. 34.6A).[125] In these cases, there is usually subcutaneous air, often accompanied by swelling, and pain elicited by palpation of the anterior airway. When a cervical airway injury is suspected, the best approach is prompt transfer to the OR for surgical exploration of the anterior neck and establishment of the airway by tracheostomy distal to the level of injury. Often, however, airway management must be undertaken before the surgery, and careful awake FSI with an FIS after inhalational induction may be the best choice. If, for example, the airway must be secured in the ED before transportation to a higher level of care, the same approach is used, substituting IV sedation and topical anesthesia for inhalational anesthesia.

Airway management in the blunt trauma patient is complicated by the potential for cervical spine injury. Up to 50% of patients with blunt airway injury are found to have a concomitant spine injury.[126] This necessitates the inclusion of cervical spine precautions during all airway procedures. In clothesline-type injuries where the neck is struck by a transverse fence wire or similar object, the central neck area may be significantly but deceptively disrupted from the impact.[121] Although these injuries can be dramatic and often require immediate airway management, the airway itself is often intact, signified by identification of intact structures and the absence of air bubbling or gurgling during negative-pressure or positive-pressure ventilation. Early intubation from above, preferably with an FIS, is best in these cases. If the airway has been breached and gurgling or subcutaneous air is evident in the tissues of the neck, positive-pressure BVM ventilation is not likely to be successful and may result in insufflation of large amounts of air into the soft tissues of the neck, further compromising the airway and attempts at securing it. The best approach in these cases is to attempt to secure the airway over an FIS using sedation and topical anesthesia, with a plan to progress directly to a cricothyrotomy or emergency tracheostomy, if FSI is unsuccessful.

Maxillofacial Trauma

Mandibular fractures are usually isolated injuries, but they can occur in the setting of multitrauma, particularly in the setting of a motor vehicle collision or severe assault. Patients with bilateral mandibular body fractures are especially at risk for tongue base prolapse. Placing the patient in a sitting or lateral position or initiating tongue retraction with a heavy suture or towel clamp will allow ventilation until a definitive airway is secured.[127] Although most patients with mandibular fractures present with limitation of mouth opening secondary to pain, individuals with fractures of the angle of the mandible or the mandibular condyles may have mechanical restriction that will not improve with sedation and/or muscle relaxation. These types of injuries should be induced with caution and backup plans in the event mouth opening does not improve.

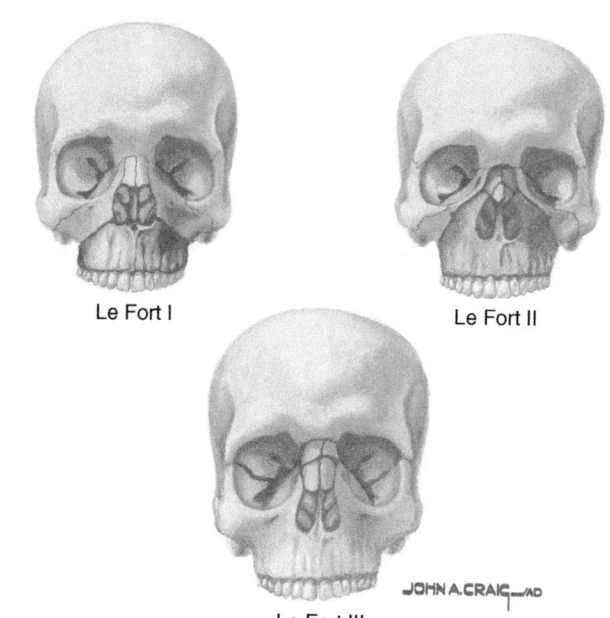

Le Fort I

Le Fort II

Le Fort III

• **Fig. 34.10** Le Fort classification. (From the Netter Collection of Medical Illustrations: Website. Available at http://www.netterimages.com. Copyright Elsevier Inc. All rights reserved.)

Midfacial fractures can cause unilateral or bilateral Le Fort I, II, or III and associated fractures (Fig. 34.10). Le Fort I fractures rarely cause airway compromise. If the fracture fragment has displaced posteriorly, it can be pulled forward easily by gripping the upper incisors or alveolar ridge. Le Fort II fractures similarly do not compromise the airway unless extensive hemorrhage is present. The fracture fragment, although free floating, rarely displaces posteriorly enough to compromise the airway. In the absence of hemorrhage, the mouth and oral pharynx are usually patent and functional. However, Le Fort III fractures can significantly compromise the upper airway because of posterior displacement of the entire central face, compromising the oral and nasal pharynx. Bleeding from facial fractures may also complicate airway management. Swallowing or suctioning of blood clears the airway and is facilitated with the patient in the sitting position. However, gastric distention and irritation from swallowing of blood may increase the likelihood of regurgitation and aspiration. Venous bleeding can be controlled by packing and fracture reduction. In all cases, careful oral inspection and suctioning to determine the patency and adequacy of the oral cavity, followed by early intubation for airway protection, if indicated, is advisable.[128]

Cervical Spine Injury

Unstable injury to the cervical spine presents a particular hazard with respect to airway management because of the potential to cause or exacerbate spinal cord injury (SCI) during intubation. Cervical SCI usually occurs when there is high-energy transfer, such as in a motor vehicle collision, but it can occur with relatively minor trauma in patients with significant degenerative disease of the cervical spine, such as rheumatoid arthritis or osteopenia. Motor vehicle collisions are the greatest cause of spinal injury, accounting for about 50% of these injuries, followed by falls, athletic injury, and interpersonal violence.[129]

In the ED, all patients who have been subjected to significant blunt trauma should be assumed to have a cervical spine injury until it has been excluded. Penetrating trauma can also cause spinal injury, but creation of an unstable spinal injury without concomitant SCI is exceedingly rare. With penetrating injury, SCI is usually apparent with neurologic deficit present below the level of injury. Barring this finding, cervical spine immobilization in a patient with isolated penetrating trauma is typically unnecessary and may even be harmful.[130,131]

One of the significant challenges related to airway management in patients with blunt trauma is the inability to rule out a cervical spine injury before intubation is required. Fortunately, most patients with a cervical spine injury do not require intubation during the acute phase of resuscitation, allowing time for evaluation. However, those who have the most severe trauma are likely to require intubation, and this is the population who is at highest risk for spinal injury.[132] It has been estimated that 2% to 14% of all patients with serious blunt trauma have a significant cervical spine injury.[133,134] If there is no emergent need for advanced airway management, the patient should undergo thorough evaluation per established protocols to clear the cervical spine. Currently, evidence demonstrates that plain cervical radiographs are insufficient to indicate the absence of cervical spine injury. Published guidelines now recommend the use of a validated clinical examination with the addition of high-quality CT in the obtunded patient.[135]

Airway management in the patient with known cervical spine injury, detected by neurologic compromise or radiologic evidence, demands particular attention. Aside from exacerbating the injury and worsening the neurologic function due to cervical spine movement during intubation, one must beware of impending airway obstruction or a DA given the proximity of the anterior cervical spine to airway structures. A trauma mechanism significant enough to cause a cervical spine injury likely induces prevertebral bleeding and edema formation, which in severe cases can compress the pharynx and narrow or displace the airway (Fig. 34.11). As this process is occult and slow to progress at times, vigilance in monitoring and frequent reassessment of the patient are essential. Not uncommonly, these patients are scheduled for lengthy MRI imaging in remote locations in the hospital, and it may be prudent to prophylactically intubate them prior to their departure from the ER or TRU.

Regardless of the technique chosen, airway management in known cervical spine injuries must be undertaken with strict attention to cervical spine immobilization. This is best performed by a second individual whose sole function is to maintain the alignment of the head, neck, and torso using MILS. The choicest immobilization technique is one that allows the person performing the immobilization to have direct contact with the head and the torso. In one method, the assistant approaches the head from the thorax, resting his or her forearms on the upper chest and clavicles and passing the wrists and hands up alongside the neck bilaterally, so that the hands (with fingers spread) can grip and immobilize the occipital-parietal area of the head (Fig. 34.12A). This allows the assistant to prevent and detect any change in the angle of the head on the neck or the neck on the body during laryngoscopy and intubation. The assistant must provide direct feedback to the intubator of any motion.

In another method, the assistant crouches below the operating table, usually to the intubator's left side. The assistant then reaches up over the head of the table and immobilizes the base of the occiput with the heels of both hands. The fingers extend down alongside the neck to the top of the patient's shoulders, permitting the assistant to immobilize the head and neck and allowing detection of movement (Fig. 34.12B).

MILS often worsens the laryngoscopic view and can lead to longer intubation times, failure to secure the airway, or increased applied pressure by the intubating provider resulting in more pressure transmitted to the cervical spine. One must balance the benefits of MILS against the risk for hypoxemic injury if intubation and adequate ventilation cannot be accomplished. Therefore, as was noted for CP, MILS may be altered or discontinued if its use impedes tracheal intubation.[136]

When it comes to selecting the appropriate technique to facilitate intubation, the same caveats apply regarding patient condition and urgency. With the stable, cooperative, and well-topicalized patient, an awake FSI will induce the least amount of cervical spine rotation. This is frequently impossible to accomplish in the setting of acute trauma, and its use will be limited by patient factors and operator experience. In more emergent situations, DL with MILS continues to be an appropriate choice for intubation. Alternatively, multiple VAL devices compare favorably with DL for first pass and overall success in normal patients intubated with MILS or other forms of cervical immobilization.[137] One device, the Airtraq (Prodol Meditec, Vizcaya, Spain), is the only one shown to have a statistically higher first-pass success rate. The amount of observed cervical spine movement with both direct and indirect techniques varies among studies and test conditions.[138–140] To date, no studies have been done in patients with known cervical injuries, making it difficult to extrapolate these results to the clinical setting.

Intubation should usually be performed with the anterior portion of the cervical collar open because it may limit mouth opening and affect laryngoscopy. Leaving the collar intact has not been shown to reduce significant cervical spine movement during intubation and is not a substitute for MILS.[141] Although an emergent FONA can be performed through the openings in most cervical collars, it is often technically challenging, and it is preferable to remove the anterior half of the collar before undertaking FONA management.

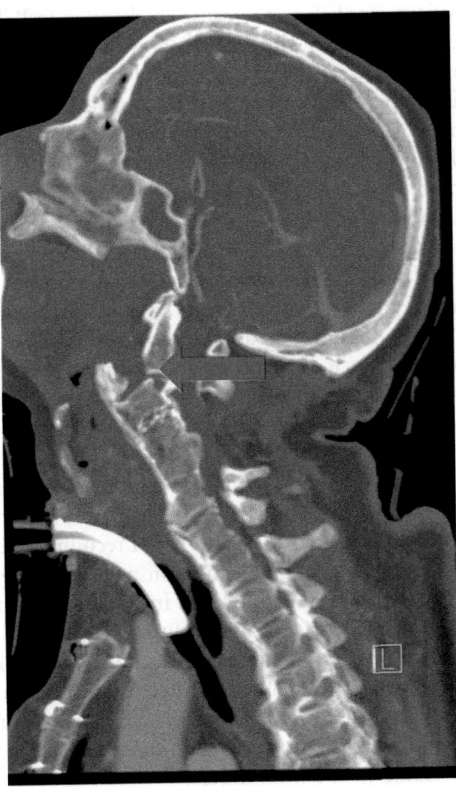

• **Fig. 34.11** Severe cervical fracture (*red arrow*) resulting in occlusion of upper airway resulting in emergent front-of-neck airway.

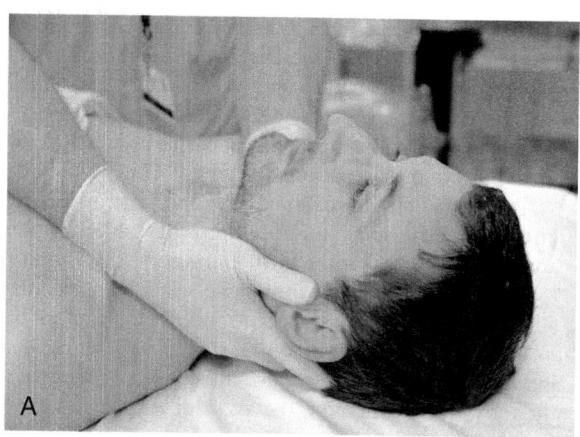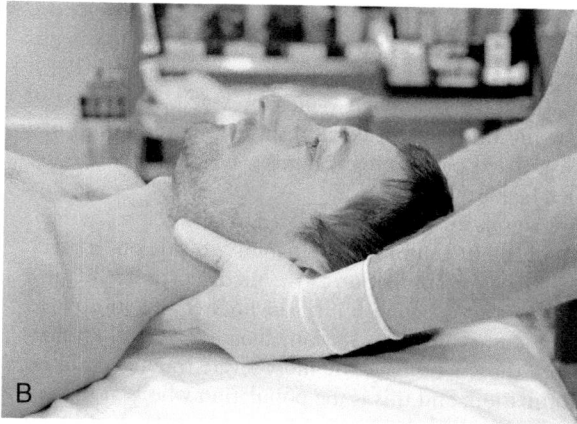

• **Fig. 34.12**   (A) Manual in-line stabilization (MILS) of the cervical spine applied from below. (B) MILS of the cervical spine applied from above.

Traumatic Brain Injury

Intracranial injury commonly occurs with blunt and penetrating forms of trauma. As discussed, alteration in consciousness (i.e., GCS of 8 or lower) continues to be the primary indicator for early intubation in these patients. In the absence of a rapidly reversible cause (e.g., opioid overdose, hypoglycemia), a sustained low GCS risks inadequate airway protection and the potential for deterioration, and thus demands airway securement. The primary consideration regarding airway management in the patient with some form of intracranial injury is the avoidance of hypotension, hypercapnia, and hypoxemia while avoiding practices that are likely to increase ICP. To a large degree, these considerations focus on appropriate drug selection and preoxygenation because there are few airway-specific concerns with isolated TBI other than an increased association with SCI.

Airway management in the patient with intracranial injury is dictated by an often-conflicting series of choices between limiting the adverse responses in the brain related to intubation and limiting the hemodynamic consequences of sedation and analgesia. In patients with an elevated ICP, stimulation of the upper airway structures by a laryngoscope or other device results in an increase in ICP.[142] This increase is primarily because of two mechanisms. First, an increase in sympathetic adrenergic stimulation results in elevation in heart rate and blood pressure, which translates to an elevation in ICP made worse in the setting of altered cerebral autoregulation.[143] Second, a direct reflexive increase in ICP is caused by laryngeal stimulation, although the mechanism is not precisely defined.[144]

To blunt this response, anesthetic induction agents are administered during intubation. This must be done with consideration for the patient's volume status, comorbidities, and overall injury pattern because a single episode of hypoxemia or hypotension (systolic blood pressure <90 mm Hg) is associated with worsened outcomes in patients with TBI.[145] The majority of this data is based on vital signs obtained in the field or arrival at the ED, and it is less clear whether a single episode of transient hypotension related to medications administered for intubation has the same association.[146] Nonetheless, general practice continues to focus on aggressive treatment of hypotension through resuscitation and use of pressors as indicated by overall patient condition.

Selection of the induction agent should take into consideration this need for hemodynamic stability. Propofol produces significant vasodilation, even in the nontrauma patient, and is the most likely induction agent to produce hypotension during induction. Given the association of hypotension and worsened outcomes in the setting of TBI, it should be used with caution in this patient population. Etomidate appears to be the most commonly used agent as a result of a better hemodynamic profile, but a hypertensive response can still be seen during intubation that may have a negative impact on ICP.[147] Historically, it was believed that ketamine raised ICP in head-injured patients based on studies in patients with obstructive cerebrospinal fluid outflow pathology.[148] More recently, review of the available data shows no detrimental effects with the use of ketamine in patients with TBI.[59,149] Hence, there is now support for use of ketamine in head-injured patients because of its favorable hemodynamic and pharmacologic profiles.

Choice of NMB agents in TBI has also been a topic of debate. Succinylcholine, which is the most common choice for RSI of the multitrauma patient, was believed to cause an elevation in ICP, although this has been disputed.[150] This exacerbation of the ICP elevation by succinylcholine, however, is likely to be of no clinical significance. The benefit of rapid airway control, with avoidance of hypoxemia and maintenance of normocarbia, far outweighs the risk of a mild increase in ICP following administration of succinylcholine.

Rocuronium is appropriate when there is a contraindication to succinylcholine or where sugammadex is readily available. It achieves intubation conditions within about 1 minute without an associated rise in ICP.[151] Without reversal agents at hand, however, the duration of paralysis when 1.0 mg/kg of rocuronium is administered is up to 45 minutes and may impact clinical decision-making in the absence of an obtainable neurologic assessment.[152] For this reason, succinylcholine, with its ultra-rapid onset and shorter duration of action, remains the most used drug for emergency intubation of patients with suspected TBI and ICP elevation. Evidence is poor supporting the administration of a defasciculating dose of a nondepolarizing NMB before succinylcholine to attenuate any increase in ICP and is not recommended.

In addition to appropriate induction and NMB agent selection, other pharmacologic adjuncts to intubation may play a role in achieving optimal intubation conditions for the TBI patient. As noted, the preinduction administration of lidocaine in trauma patients with suspected TBI has limited utility in blunting the ICP response to intubation.[48] Several minutes are required after lidocaine administration for it to be effective, which may not always be possible with a trauma RSI.[71]

The sympathetic response to intubation has been extensively studied, and synthetic opioids and beta-blockers have been shown to attenuate the reflex sympathetic response to laryngoscopy. Administration of a beta-blocker to a trauma patient may worsen hemodynamic instability and is rarely desirable, except in certain cases of isolated head trauma. Similarly, administration of full sympathetic-blocking doses of the synthetic opioids,[153] such as fentanyl, can have adverse effects, particularly in patients with hypovolemia, who depend on sympathetic drive. Fentanyl, in a dose of 2 to 3 µg/kg as a pretreatment agent, has been shown to attenuate the reflex sympathetic response to laryngoscopy and should have minimal adverse cardiovascular effects.[153] Care must be used, however, to ensure that the patient has sufficient hemodynamic stability to tolerate even this small dose.

Given the importance placed on avoiding hypoxemia in the setting of TBI, emphasis should be placed on achieving adequate preoxygenation. Many patients with TBI are combative and will not be cooperative with preoxygenation. In this group of patients, it may be beneficial to use a small dose of sedation to allow the patient to tolerate preoxygenation before the intubation attempt. This technique has been described as a "delayed sequence intubation" where a low dose of ketamine or other sedative is administered to allow for better tolerance of attempts at preoxygenation.[154] The use of sedation, however, must be measured against the potential for respiratory depression, relative urgency of airway control, and hemodynamic status.

In summary, when RSI is planned, and there is no contraindication, IV fentanyl in addition to a standard, albeit lower-dose, IV anesthetic induction agent should be considered before the administration of succinylcholine. Laryngoscopy and intubation should be as gentle and atraumatic as possible to minimize laryngeal stimulation and potential worsening of the hemodynamic and ICP response to intubation. Studies comparing intubation over a stylet with DL indicate that the placement of the ETT into the trachea is more stimulating than the laryngoscopy itself.[155]

Intraocular Injury

Most patients with open globe injuries can be intubated in the OR under controlled conditions. Penetrating globe injuries are typically isolated and caused by impalements (e.g., sticks, toys, woodshop splinters) or low-velocity missiles (e.g., BBs, pellets). Decisions related to overall management of the patient's multiple injuries should take precedence over management of the eye injury. The greatest controversy revolves around the use of succinylcholine for RSI in the patient with an open globe injury because of an associated increase in intraocular pressure (IOP) with its use and concern for extrusion of ocular contents.[156,157] Despite this concern, reports have been very limited for attributing vitreous humor extrusion to the use of succinylcholine for RSI.[158] In contrast, the increases in IOP seen with increased venous pressures associated with coughing, straining, or bucking during intubation under suboptimal conditions are significantly higher than those observed after administration of succinylcholine. The priority in airway management should then focus on optimization of intubating conditions and the prevention of increased intrathoracic

and venous pressures during induction and laryngoscopy. In this setting, the increase in IOP with succinylcholine use for RSI can be significantly attenuated by a defasciculating dose of a nondepolarizing NMB agent given 3 minutes before induction combined with an adequate dose of the selected anesthetic induction agent.[159] Alternatively, the use of rocuronium at a dose of 1.2 mg/kg IV for RSI can eliminate the need for succinylcholine and provide excellent intubation conditions, albeit with a longer duration of action.

Conclusion

The trauma airway is a subset of the DA. The need to integrate airway management into a dynamic environment with ongoing evaluation and resuscitation potentially complicated by hemodynamic instability, cervical spine immobilization, and/or direct airway trauma can be very challenging. At the same time, fundamental principles of DA management must be applied to the trauma patient with the realization that rarely will one be able to "wake" up the patient and start over. The foundation for success is an orderly approach, including prioritization of resuscitation steps, evaluation of the specific characteristics of the DA, careful selection of pharmacologic agents, early use of video or optically enhanced airway tools, and coordination with other members of the resuscitation team.

Selected References

13. Sise MJ, Shackford SR, Sise CB, et al. Early intubation in the management of trauma patients: indications and outcomes in 1,000 consecutive patients. *J Trauma.* 2009;66:32–39, discussion 39–40.
23. Algie CM, Mahar RK, Tan HB, et al. Effectiveness and risks of cricoid pressure during rapid sequence induction for endotracheal intubation. *Cochrane Database Syst Rev.* 2015;(11):CD011656.
34. Mayglothling J, Duane TM, Gibbs M, et al. Emergency intubation immediately following traumatic injury: an Eastern Association for the Surgery of Trauma practice management guideline. *J Trauma Acute Care Surg.* 2012;73:S333–S340.
47. Casey JD, Janz DR, Russell DW, et al. Bag-mask ventilation during tracheal intubation of critically ill adults. *N Engl J Med.* 2019;380(9):811–821.
67. Tran DTT, Newton EK, Mount VA, et al. Rocuronium versus succinylcholine for rapid sequence induction intubation. *Cochrane Database Syst Rev.* 2015;(10):CD002788.
69. Guihard B, Chollet-Xemard C, Lakhnati P, et al. Effect of rocuronium vs succinylcholine on endotracheal intubation success rate among patients undergoing out-of-hospital rapid sequence intubation: a randomized clinical trial. *JAMA.* 2019;322(23):2303–2312.
82. Hagberg CA, Kaslow O. Difficult airway management algorithm in trauma updated by COTEP. *ASA Newsl.* 2014;78:56–60.
112. Bagga B, Kumar A, Chahal A, Gamanagatti S, Kumar S. Traumatic airway injuries: role of imaging. *Curr Probl Diagn Radiol.* 2020;49(1):48–53.
114. Jain U, McCunn M, Smith CE, et al. Management of the traumatized airway. *Anesthesiology.* 2016;124:199–206.

All references can be found online at eBooks.Health.Elsevier.com.

35

Airway Management in Burn Patients

SARAH A. LEE, SAM R. SHARAR, AND HERNANDO P. OLIVAR

CHAPTER OUTLINE

KEY POINTS

- The priorities and approaches to airway management in the burn patient are different in the acute, subacute, and chronic phases of burn injury.
- Airway edema results from thermal and inhalation injury, and rapidly increases with fluid resuscitation.
- Induction drugs that cause vasodilation or decreased cardiac output can result in hemodynamic instability in burn patients, even though the dose requirements may be augmented.
- Succinylcholine is contraindicated following the initial 48 to 72 hours after injury due to life-threatening hyperkalemia risk. Succinylcholine can be administered again once the patient's wounds have healed, mobility and muscle tone have returned, and critical illness has resolved.
- Face burns, neck burns, and airway edema can make mask fit and mask ventilation very difficult.

- Postburn contractures can restrict mouth opening and limit neck flexion in patients during the chronic phase of burn injury. A thorough airway exam—particularly observing circumoral and pharyngeal tightness and wound contractures—is important in airway management.
- Cuffed endotracheal tubes (ETTs) are recommended in pediatric burn patients, as airway and ventilatory mechanics can quickly change during the acute phase of burn injury and exchanging the endotracheal tube to maintain adequate ventilation poses significant risk.
- Identification of burn patients at high risk for failed extubation and difficult reintubation is critical so that the appropriate personnel and equipment are present and an interdisciplinary care plan is in place, should extubation fail.

Introduction

Burn injury results in approximately 40,000 hospitalizations and over 3000 fire and smoke inhalation deaths each year in the United States.[1] Airway evaluation of burn patients assesses the extent of both direct burn injury and inhalation airway injury, the latter of which can present insidiously. Airway management of burn patients presents unique complexity, because the burn patient's airway is continuously evolving from the time of injury throughout the period of recovery, and the challenges faced during the acute, subacute, and chronic periods postinjury are uniquely different.

Burn Injury and the Airway

The severity and prognosis of burn injury are typically assessed by estimating the total body surface area (TBSA) burned, the depth of burn, and the presence or absence of inhalation injury. The classification of burns, based on depth, is shown in Table 35.1. Generally, burns are considered severe when partial- and full-thickness burn TBSA is greater than 25%.[2]

The extent of direct thermal injury to the airway depends on the type of inhaled air. Dry air has a low specific heat capacity and loses heat rapidly, limiting damage to the supraglottic airway (SGA). The efficiency of the nares and pharynx in thermoregulating

TABLE 35.1	Classification of Burns			
Degree	Depth	Tissue Involved	Appearance	Spontaneous Recovery Time
1st	Superficial	Epidermis	Dry, red, blanches	3 to 6 days
2nd	Superficial partial thickness	Superficial dermis	Moist, weeping, blisters, blanches	7 to 20 days
2nd	Deep partial thickness	Deep dermis	Moist or waxy dry, blisters unroof, nonblanching	Longer than 21 days
3rd	Full thickness	Entire dermis	Dry, waxy, charred, inelastic	No
4th		Involves muscle, tendon, bone	Dry, waxy, charred, inelastic	No

inhaled gases as well as the the glottis's protection of the lower airway also play a role in limiting thermal injury to the upper airway. In contrast, wet air (steam) has a larger heat capacity, fast thermal transmission, and slow heat elimination, characteristics that predispose to lower airway injury.[3]

Common signs on physical examination suggesting inhalation injury include facial burns, singed facial and nasal hair (Fig. 35.1), oropharyngeal ulceration, mucosal edema, and cough producing carbonaceous sputum. Studies have shown that the incidence of difficult intubation in patients with face and neck burns is more than twice that of the general population.[4]

Phases of Burn Injury

Burn injuries and their care are typically described in three phases: acute, subacute, and chronic. The acute phase of burn injury describes the 48-hour postinjury period when a classic systemic inflammatory response is present and requires critical interventions, including airway management and aggressive fluid resuscitation. Inhalation injury may be present as a result of damage to both the upper and lower airway by steam, smoke, and/or toxic chemicals; its presence predicts increased incidence of respiratory failure and mortality.[5] Cardinal features of upper airway injury during this phase include stridor, dysphonia, dysphagia, and glottic and periglottic edema. Upper airway narrowing is augmented by accumulation of extravascular fluid/edema with the rapid administration of resuscitation fluids.

Subglottic or lower airway inhalational injury during the acute phase results from a constellation of pathophysiologic changes. Tracheobronchial epithelial damage leads to impaired mucociliary function, mucosal edema and sloughing, and increased airway secretions, all of which lead to lower airway obstruction, atelectasis, and consequent ventilation/perfusion (V/Q) mismatch. Toxic inhalation products in smoke trigger increased bronchial blood flow that, in combination with fluid resuscitation and compromised capillary membrane integrity, leads to further bronchial edema. Nitric oxide is also released with inhalation injury and impairs hypoxic pulmonary vasoconstriction, further contributing to physiologic shunt and V/Q mismatch. Lower airway injury during the acute phase of injury generally presents as bronchospasm from the inhalation of aerosolized irritants. Therefore, bronchodilator therapy is often required, and administration of epinephrine may be necessary if bronchospasm is refractory to other treatments.[6]

The presence of circumferential full-thickness thoracic burns can also produce oxygenation and ventilation difficulties in the acute phase of burn injury. Such injuries reduce thoracic compliance and create a restrictive lung defect. This defect is worsened with large volume burn resuscitation, and limits chest wall excursion with either spontaneous or positive-pressure ventilation. Treatment of this restrictive defect involves chest wall escharotomies.

The subacute phase of burn injury begins approximately 3 to 5 days after injury, when burn wound excision and grafting procedures typically begin. The subacute phase is often marked by worsening pulmonary function and respiratory distress due to further accumulation of mucosal debris and secretions, and infectious complications (e.g., wound infection, pneumonia). It is estimated that pneumonia and bronchitis occur in up to half of severely burned patients 1 week postinjury.[7]

The chronic phase of burn injury occurs weeks to years after the initial insult. By this point, lower lung injury is generally resolved; however, new airway management issues can arise because of unpredictable fibrous tissue deposition and scarring that lead to skin contractures. Contractures of the neck and mouth can distort upper airway anatomy, cause severely constricted mouth opening, and limit neck movement, particularly neck extension. During this

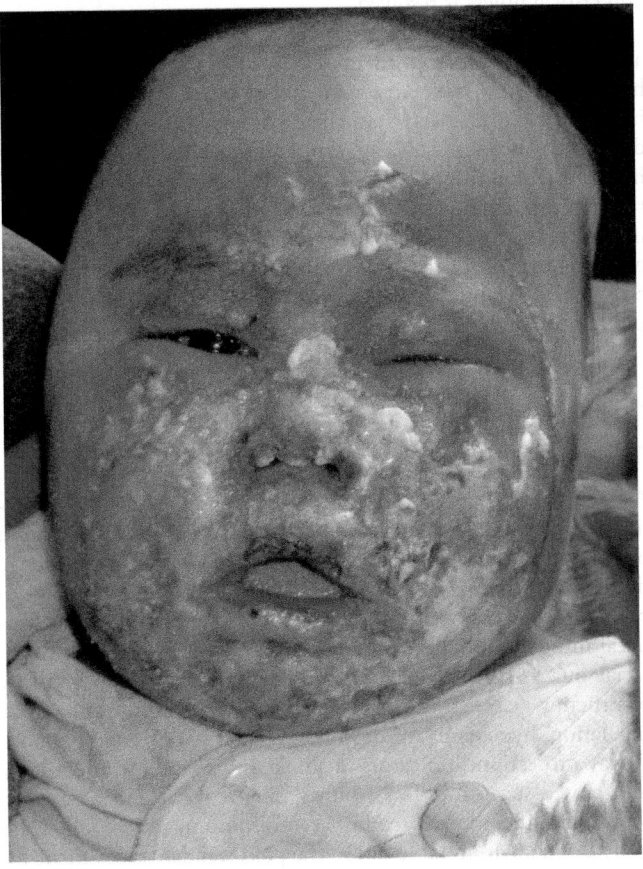

• **Fig. 35.1** Perioral facial burns and soot are potential indicators of inhalation injury associated with smoke inhalation or flame burn.

phase, patients can also develop tracheal stenosis as a consequence of prolonged tracheal intubation and/or tracheostomy placement. Chest wall contractures can result from spontaneously healed or grafted circumferential truncal burns and create a restrictive lung defect due to decreased chest wall compliance.

Carbon Monoxide and Cyanide Toxicity

Major early complications of inhalation injury include tissue hypoxia results from carbon monoxide (CO) and/or cyanide toxicity. Because CO binds to hemoglobin with an affinity that is 200-fold greater than oxygen, the resulting carboxyhemoglobin (COHb) both decreases oxygen-carrying capacity and shifts the hemoglobin dissociation curve to the left, impairing oxygen release to tissue. Together with CO-mediated disruption of intracellular cytochrome physiology, COHb results in metabolic acidosis and cellular hypoxia, particularly in neural tissues. Neurological deficits and cardiac dysrhythmias can occur when COHb levels exceed 15%, and hypoxic brain injury and cardiac arrest can occur with COHb levels above 50%.[8] A high incidence of delayed neurologic complications is reported among patients who have suffered CO toxicity.[9] Standard pulse oximetry monitors overestimate arterial oxygenation and are unreliable in patients with CO toxicity because COHb confounds oxyhemoglobin light absorption in these devices. Co-oximetry is generally required to distinguish between oxyhemoglobin and COHb light absorption, in order to accurately measure arterial oxygen saturation.

Patients with suspected CO toxicity should be given 100% facemask oxygen while plasma COHb levels are obtained, even in patients without obvious signs or symptoms of inhalation injury. If CO toxicity is severe, hyperbaric oxygen treatment is possible, although it is often logistically not feasible, and a recent Cochrane review failed to demonstrate clear efficacy.[10]

Similarly, cyanide toxicity can occur when plastic combustion products are inhaled and, similar to CO, can result in metabolic acidosis and tissue hypoxia. Immediate administration of high oxygen concentrations is imperative, and in extreme circumstances treatment with sodium thiosulfate may be necessary, although there is a paucity of clinical trial evidence. Amyl nitrate and sodium nitrite form methemoglobin and are therefore generally avoided in inhalation injury.[11]

Specific Airway Management Considerations in Burn Patients

Pharmacologic Considerations in Burn Patients

When providing airway management in burn-injured patients, specific attention must be paid to the pharmacokinetic and pharmacodynamics changes that accompany burn injury, and therefore affect drug and dose choices. In the acute phase, burn patients are typically intravascularly volume depleted with impaired cardiac contractility, such that administration of vasodilatory induction agents can potentially result in profound hypotension. Ketamine and etomidate are preferred to more vasodilating drugs such as propofol, in order to maintain hemodynamic stability. Ketamine has the added benefit of maintaining respiratory drive and pharyngeal tone, as well as decreasing airway resistance, if airway management is difficult enough to warrant maintenance of spontaneous ventilation. Dexmedetomidine may also be useful because it provides relative hemodynamic stability while maintaining

respiratory drive, allowing sedation with spontaneous ventilation in patients with potential airway difficulty.[12] During the acute phase, burn patients are also hyperdynamic with increased drug clearance. Moreover, burn-induced increases in capillary endothelial permeability result in decreased intravascular protein content, increased free fraction of unbound drugs, and a subsequent increase in volume of distribution of many drugs. Therefore, an increased dose of plasma-bound drugs (e.g., propofol) may be necessary to achieve desired therapeutic effect.[13]

The use of neuromuscular relaxants in burn patients requires careful consideration. Burns result in the upregulation of both junctional and extrajunctional acetylcholine (ACh) receptors in skeletal muscle. When succinylcholine is administered, the increased number of ACh receptors, coupled with burn-induced decreases in plasma pseudocholinesterase concentrations, results in an acute increase in circulating potassium levels. If severe, such hyperkalemia can lead to cardiac arrest. The degree of hyperkalemia is related to a number of factors including extent of injury, dose of succinylcholine, duration of patient immobility, critical illness, and other comorbidities.[14] Accordingly, the onset and duration of hyperkalemia risk in burn patients after receiving succinylcholine cannot be definitively predicted. Generally, it is considered safe to use succinylcholine during the acute phase of injury, but wise to avoid its use beyond 48 to 72 hours after injury. The upregulation of ACh receptors persists until wound healing has occurred and the patient is mobile. Case reports describe persistently upregulated ACh receptor levels for up to 1 year after injury, although the clinical significance of these levels is unclear.[15] Current clinical practice suggests that succinylcholine only be used when wound healing is complete, muscle function and mobility have returned, and critical illness is resolved.

Because of these significant changes in ACh physiology, and when combined with increased drug clearance during the hyperdynamic phase, burn patients are resistant to nondepolarizing muscle relaxants.[16,17] In these patients, generous intubating doses of rocuronium (1.2 mg/kg) still typically result in delayed intubation conditions.[18] Therefore, the recommended dose of rocuronium required to perform a rapid sequence induction (RSI) in burn patients is increased to 1.2 to 1.5 mg/kg. The duration of action of nondepolarizing muscle relaxants is also decreased in burn patients, who generally require more frequent redosing when prolonged paralysis is desired.

Airway Management During the Acute Phase of Burn Injury

As stated in the Advanced Trauma Life Support (ATLS) guidelines, airway management is the first priority in the acute period of burn injury, and may take place in the prehospital, emergency department, intensive care, or operating room settings. Factors to consider when assessing patients who may require immediate tracheal intubation include presence of severe burns (>25% TBSA), facial burns, perioral edema, signs of impending upper airway obstruction (e.g., stridor, hoarseness), signs of significant smoke inhalation, hypoxemia, or declining mental status rendering poor airway protection. Indicators of smoke inhalation include history of a closed-space fire, facial burns, singed facial and nasal hair, soot in mouth and nares, carbonaceous sputum, and COHb levels >10%, as shown in Table 35.2. The gold standard assessment for lower airway inhalation damage is bronchoscopy (carbonaceous deposits, mucosal ulceration, and erythema), although the

TABLE 35.2	Indicators of Smoke Inhalation Injury

- History of closed-space fire
- Facial burns
- Singed facial and nasal hair
- Soot in mouth and nose
- Carbonaceous sputum
- Carboxyhemoglobin >10%

diagnosis is frequently made by clinical features alone (as described previously).

Developing guidelines for prehospital airway management in burn-injured patients has proven to be complex and requires balancing avoidance of catastrophic outcomes during transport (e.g., complete airway obstruction) with procedural risks of tracheal intubation performed by less experienced operators.[19] Thus, factors including distance and/or travel time to hospital and skill level of first responders responsible for intubation, all of which are highly variable, must be considered. Although evidence suggests that the inability to secure the airway is the foremost complication during prehospital transport, a recent study suggests that more than one-third of tracheal intubations performed in burn patients prior to hospital arrival are unnecessary, with over 50% of patients extubated within the first 24 hours after admission.[20,21] Guidelines for prehospital airway management in burn patients are suggested in Table 35.3.

As mentioned, burns to the neck and face confer a significantly increased risk of difficult tracheal intubation. A detailed airway examination is crucial, with particular attention to cervical neck mobility, tightness and mobility of neck and submandibular tissue, and evidence of tongue and oropharyngeal swelling. Facial burns or the presence of burn dressings should also be noted, as these may interfere with mask ventilation. Extensive thoracic burns, particularly circumferential eschars, can also severely limit chest wall compliance, create a restrictive lung defect, and hinder mask ventilation. In the acute phase, most burn patients are at significant risk for aspiration, both because they are rarely fasted and because underlying trauma and stress slow gastric emptying. Therefore, the airway exam (as described previously) will inform the decision for managing the airway awake or sedated/unconscious. If mask ventilation and tracheal intubation are predicted to be favorable, an RSI can be performed. Neck burns may preclude the proper use of cricoid pressure. Moreover, cervical in-line stabilization may be necessary if the patient has suffered from concomitant trauma that places the cervical spine and spinal cord at risk.

For tracheal intubations occurring within 48 hours of the initial injury, use of succinylcholine offers the benefit of faster return of muscle function and spontaneous ventilation in the event that tracheal intubation is not possible. All appropriate backup equipment should be immediately available, including oral and nasal airways, SGA, videolaryngoscope, bougie, and FIS, with transtracheal and/or surgical airway tools readily available. Regardless of technique, one must always anticipate a "failure to intubate" situation and follow the American Society of Anesthesiologists difficult airway algorithm. During the acute phase, tracheostomy is considered only in cases where multiple attempts at tracheal intubation have failed.

Airway Management During the Subacute Phase of Burn Injury

Airway management in the subacute phase is typically performed for operative procedures or ventilation in the ICU, ensuring that unintentional extubation is avoided and ongoing pulmonary disease is appropriately managed. During the subacute phase, residual airway edema following massive initial fluid resuscitation can contribute to difficulties with both mask ventilation and tracheal intubation. In addition to the thorough airway examination described previously, mouth opening and circumoral soft tissue compliance must be evaluated, as airway edema, healing burns, and recent facial grafts can limit both of these features. Such findings may limit standard facemask placement and require alternate methods of oxygen or anesthetic gas delivery (Fig. 35.2).

TABLE 35.3	Guidelines for Tracheal Intubation in the Prehospital Setting

- Patient safety should not be compromised, and patient status is the ultimate determinant of tracheal intubation need.
- Standard indications for tracheal intubation should be followed, including (but not limited to) shortness of breath, wheezing, stridor, hoarseness, combativeness, or decreased level of consciousness.
- Contact should be made with the regional burn center as soon as possible to discuss the events surrounding the burn and need for tracheal intubation.
- For patients who are clinically stable with no signs or symptoms of compromised airway, tracheal intubation prior to transport generally is indicated by the following conditions:
  - Burns sustained from causes other than flame injury
  - Burns that do not occur in enclosed spaces
  - Burns that are less than 20% total body surface area (TBSA)
  - Burns that do not include full-thickness burns to the face
  - Patients within reasonable time/distance to a burn center

Modified from Romanski KS, Palmieri TL, Sen S, et al. More than one third of intubations in patients transferred to burn centers are unnecessary: proposed guidelines for appropriate intubations of the burn patient. *J Burn Care Res.* 2016;37:e409–414

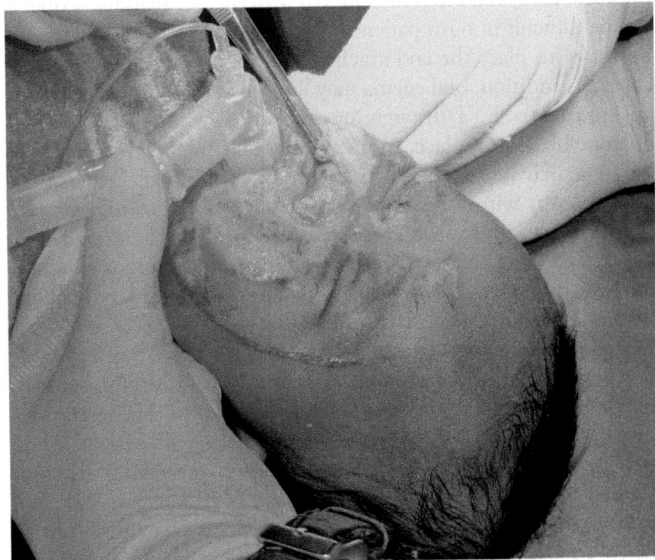

• **Fig. 35.2** Freshly debrided wounds around the mouth present challenges for mask ventilation during operative procedures.

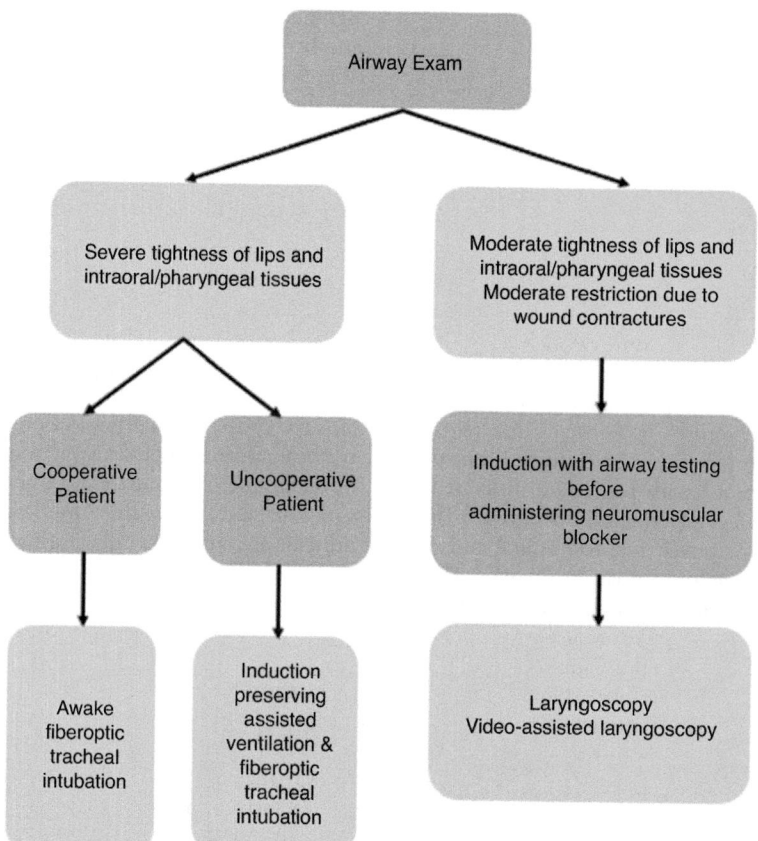

• **Fig. 35.3** Recommended algorithm for airway management of burn patients. (From Kaiser HE, Kim CM, Sharar SR, et al. Advances in perioperative and critical care of the burn patient: anesthesia management of major thermal burn injuries in adults. *Adv Anesth.* 2013;31:137–161.)

Among the standard airway management techniques described previously, several deserve special mention. First, in burn-injured patients with peri- and intraoral edema, the videolaryngoscope allows for visualization of the vocal cords past these swollen tissues, and also allows for glottic visualization at a more acute angle when neck range of motion is limited by burn injuries. While a view of the vocal cords can often be achieved with the videolaryngoscope, it can be difficult in burn patients to achieve the anatomic alignment necessary to place the endotracheal tube (ETT) through the vocal cords. In addition, oral edema may limit the amount of space available to pass the ETT through the oropharynx while the videolaryngoscope blade is in place. In these situations, tracheal placement of a bougie may be beneficial. Alternatively, combining video-assisted laryngoscopy with FSI can be very useful, as the former negotiates the proximal airway, while the flexible tip of the latter can then be used to enter the glottis. This combination technique generally requires two operators to facilitate holding the videolaryngoscope blade while simultaneously manipulating the FIS.[22]

If on initial assessment the airway anatomy appears unfavorable (e.g., severe limitation of mouth opening and/or intraoral space), it is crucial to maintain spontaneous ventilation during tracheal intubation. The degree of sedation required will depend upon patient cooperation; if possible, performing an awake FSI is considered the safest method. Alternatively, FSI can be performed on sedated, but spontaneously breathing, patients who are too combative or agitated to tolerate the procedure awake. Topical airway anesthesia is typically employed, as associated head and neck burns may obscure anatomic landmarks necessary for superior laryngeal

nerve blocks or transtracheal local anesthetic injection. In patients with supraglottic or glottic swelling, use of a Parker Flex Tip endotracheal tube (differentiated from a standard ETT by the acute curvature of the tip) can facilitate advancement of the ETT over the FIS. In deeply sedated or unconscious patients, an intubating SGA permits spontaneous ventilation and facilitates placement of the ETT either blindly or using a flexible scope through the SGA.[23] Fig. 35.3 offers a suggested airway management algorithm for burn-injured patients that focuses on assessment for abnormal circumoral and pharyngeal anatomy (Fig. 35.4) and is a complement to the ASA difficult airway algorithm.

Securing the ETT can prove challenging in patients with facial burns, particularly if the tube is in close proximity to the surgical site. Where tape is inadequate, the tube can be tied circumferentially around the patient's head, though this may still interfere with the surgical site. Other methods to secure the ETT include looping a nasogastric tube through the nostrils and around the hard palate, wiring the tube to the teeth, or suturing it to the mandible, septum, or nares. One such example involves securing the ETT onto a standard dental arch bar that has been fixed onto two maxillary premolar/molar teeth on each side. Another example involves placing an 8-mm intermaxillary fixation screw onto the maxilla and palatine bone above tooth buds and then using a 26-gauge wire to stabilize the ETT onto the screw (Fig. 35.5).

As mentioned, respiratory deterioration can occur during the subacute phase due to pneumonia or adult respiratory distress syndrome and is demonstrated by decreased pulmonary compliance, worsening hypoxia, and worsening Pao_2/Fio_2 ratio. Chest x-ray

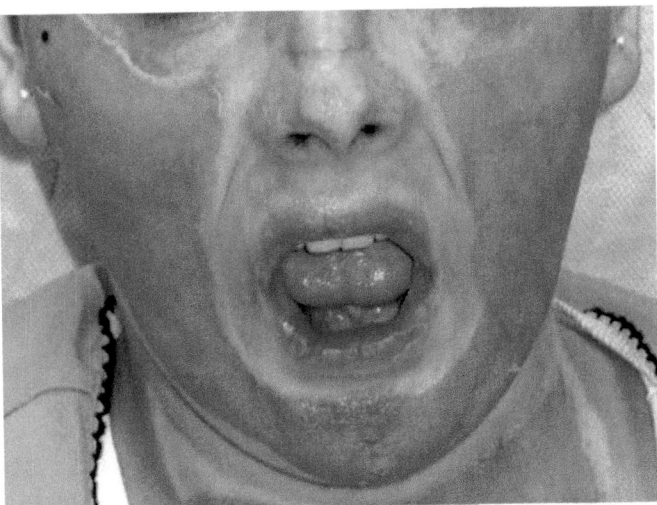

• **Fig. 35.4** The burn airway evaluation includes the assessment of tightness of lips and intraoral and pharyngeal tissues, as contractures and fibrous scarring can severely restrict mouth opening.

(CXR) may reveal focal or bilateral pulmonary infiltrates, pleural effusions, and diffuse pulmonary edema. The current recommendation is to employ lung-protective ventilation techniques by limiting tidal volumes to 6 mL/kg, maintaining moderate levels of positive end-expiratory pressure (PEEP) and titrating Pao_2 and Fio_2 obtained on serial arterial blood gases.

Aggressive pulmonary toilet is often necessary, as secretions and endobronchial debris can be copious. Frequent suctioning plays an important role in maintaining airway patency in intubated patients in the ICU and also in the OR. Excessive secretions can potentially obstruct the ETT, particularly in small children with narrow diameter tubes, and can create a potentially life-threatening scenario of emergent reintubation in a patient with a difficult airway. Therapeutic bronchoscopy may also be helpful. A significant number of patients will development pneumonia, and early detection and treatment with antibiotics based on sputum culture are critical.[9] Elective tracheostomy during this phase may be considered for patients for whom long-term tracheal intubation is expected, once neck edema has subsided and provided it is not in the direct area of burn injury. The timing of this decision is controversial and should be made on a case-by-case basis and weighed against its risks, such as subglottic stenosis.[24,25]

Airway Management During the Chronic Phase of Burn Injury

During the chronic phase of burn injury, patients may return for a variety of single or sequential reconstructive surgical procedures and may present some of the greatest challenges in airway management. Postburn and postgraft scarring and fibrosis result in contractures that can severely limit mouth opening (especially circumoral scarring), neck extension, and mandibular mobility (Fig. 35.6). In patients whose airway assessment suggests potential difficulty with mask ventilation or tracheal intubation, it is often safest to maintain spontaneous ventilation throughout tracheal intubation. Use of sedatives that maintain respiratory drive and airway patency, as described previously, can provide conditions that allow for awake or sedated spontaneously ventilating intubation. It is important to anticipate and prepare for difficult mask ventilation if the patient stops spontaneously breathing. Strategies

include having two people available to perform two-handed mask ventilation, ensuring that oral/nasal airways and SGAs are immediately available and, in extreme cases, having the surgeons present for emergent tracheostomy if necessary.

Tracheal intubation with spontaneous respiration can be performed using an FIS with topicalization of the airway using aerosolized lidocaine and/or a transtracheal nerve block (assuming neck anatomy is not distorted by burn scar). It is important to note that a large tongue, especially in combination with a limited mouth opening, can limit airway access. For these situations, a tongue depressor, Ovassapian airway or manual retraction of the tongue together with forceful lower-jaw lift may prove very helpful. If there is significant oral swelling, the combined use of a videolaryngoscope and FIS is often very effective, as described previously.

For patients presenting with severe postburn neck contractures which prevent neck extension, surgical release of neck contractures performed under mask general anesthesia or intravenous sedation prior to tracheal intubation has been described. One study reviewed 15 patients who underwent sternomental contracture release while spontaneous ventilation was maintained, using ketamine and/or inhalation anesthesia. In every case, contracture release resulted in successful tracheal intubation by direct laryngoscopy without airway complications.[26]

Burn patients with a history of prolonged tracheal intubation or tracheostomy are at increased risk for developing subglottic stenosis. A history of dyspnea on exertion or stridor on physical exam can indicate the presence of subglottic stenosis. For these patients, one should anticipate a smaller airway caliber and have an array of smaller ETTs ready in the event that it is difficult to advance the standard-size tube beyond the subglottis during laryngoscopy.

Tracheal Extubation in Burn Patients

In addition to standard extubation criteria, the extubation of burn patients requires special attention, because of the potential increased difficulty of airway management. Thus, it is important to take extra caution and preparation during the extubation period, as reintubation may be necessary, and inability to reintubate can be catastrophic. This is particularly true for patients with previously difficult airway management, those whose anatomy has changed since their last airway management (e.g., fresh face or neck skin grafts, new contractures), or those with increased body mass index. To facilitate safe extubation in this high-risk group, at the University of Washington Harborview Level I trauma/burn center we have developed guidelines to identify at-risk patients and increase both awareness and preparedness when an at-risk patient is being extubated. When a high-risk patient is extubated, an anesthesiologist is called to bedside, a difficult airway cart is present, and a plan for airway management is clearly communicated among the multidisciplinary team prior to extubation. Fig. 35.7 is an example of an algorithm that is used for risk stratification of potentially difficult airways during extubation, including burn-injured patients.

Assessment for readiness to extubate is also important and requires special consideration in burn-injured patients. In addition to demonstrating adequate spontaneous ventilator mechanics (e.g., passing a spontaneous breathing trial) and satisfactory gas exchange, it is important to ensure that upper airway edema resulting from inhalation injury and/or massive fluid resuscitation has resolved, such that there is adequate airway patency. A number of techniques to assess airway edema have been described, including testing for presence of an air leak around the ETT during

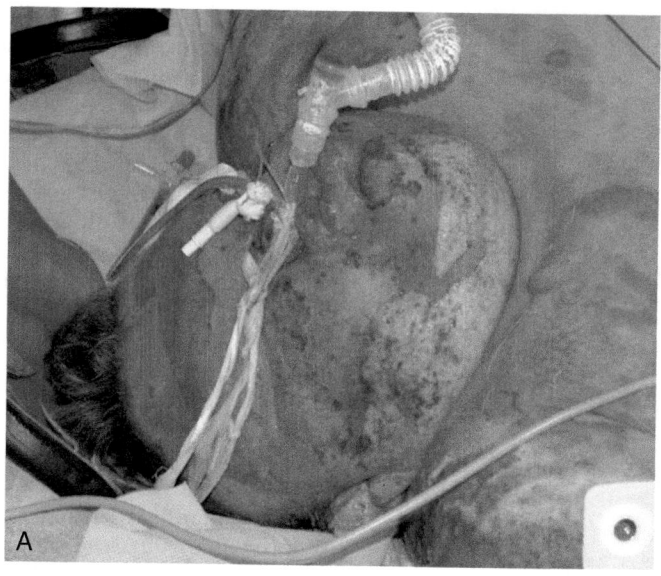

A

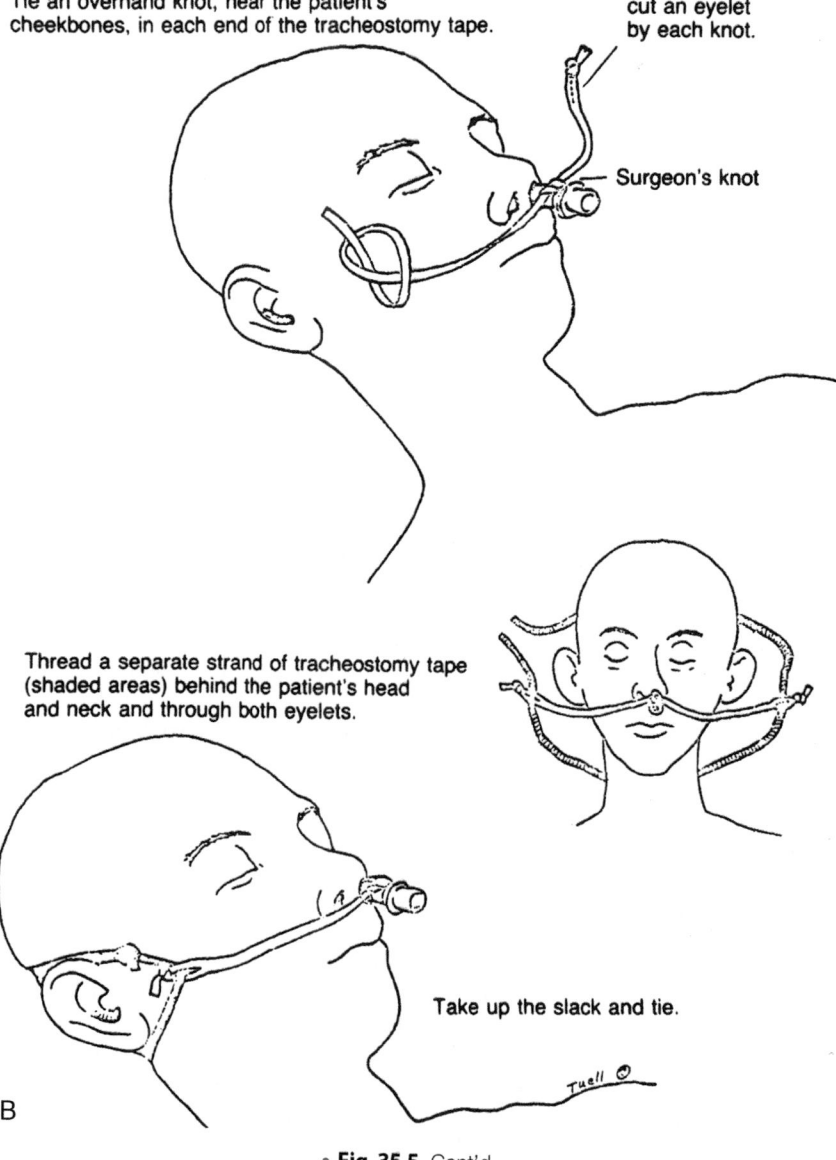

Tie an overhand knot, near the patient's
cheekbones, in each end of the tracheostomy tape.

With scissors,
cut an eyelet
by each knot.

Surgeon's knot

Thread a separate strand of tracheostomy tape
(shaded areas) behind the patient's head
and neck and through both eyelets.

Take up the slack and tie.

B

• **Fig. 35.5** Cont'd

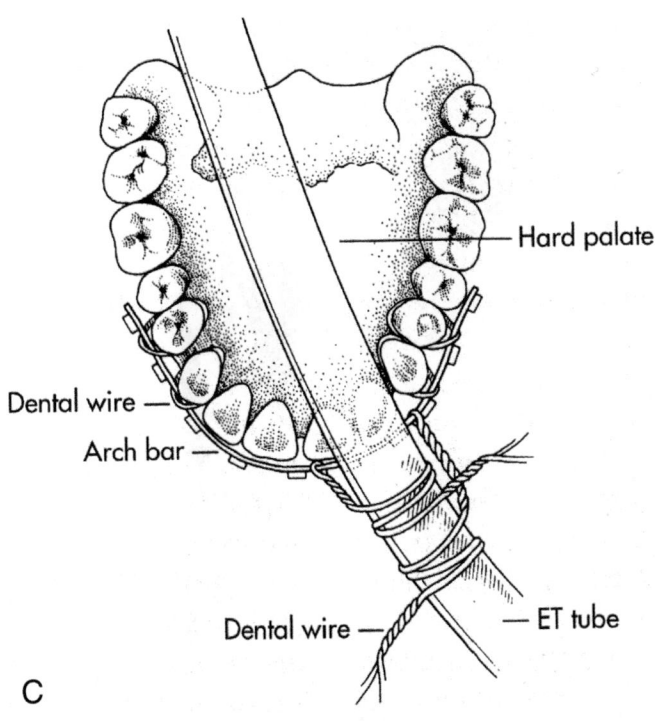

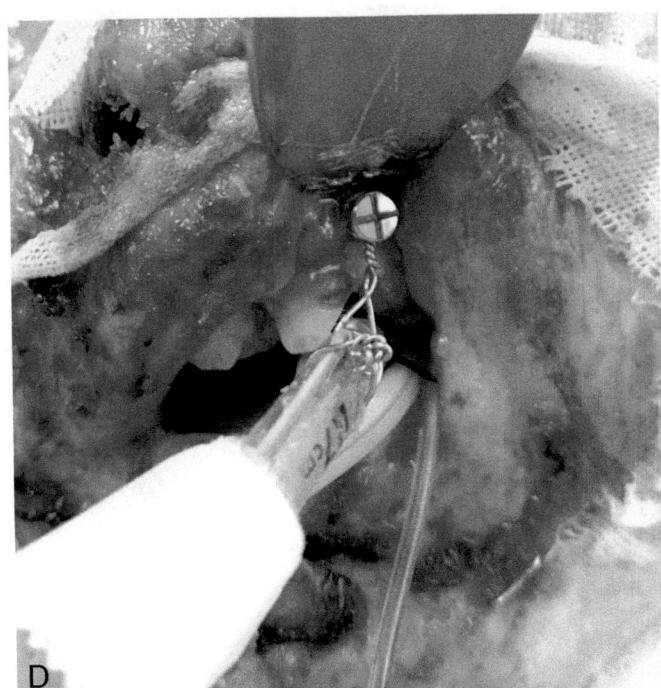

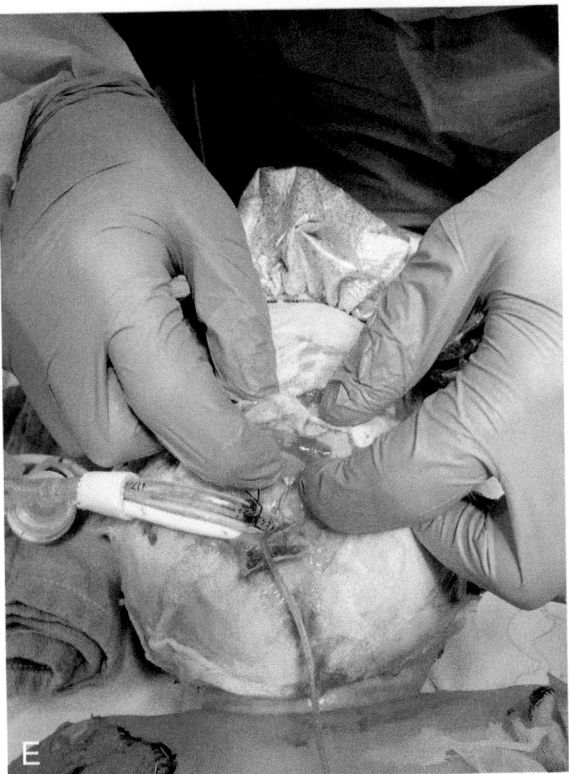

• **Fig. 35.5** Methods for securing the endotracheal tube in patients with facial burns include tying the tube circumferentially around the patient's head (A, B), wiring the tube to the patient's teeth (C), attaching the tube onto a dental arch bar (C), or wiring the tube to a screw placed into the maxilla (D, E). (photos courtesy of Jasjit Dillon, MD, University of Washington.)

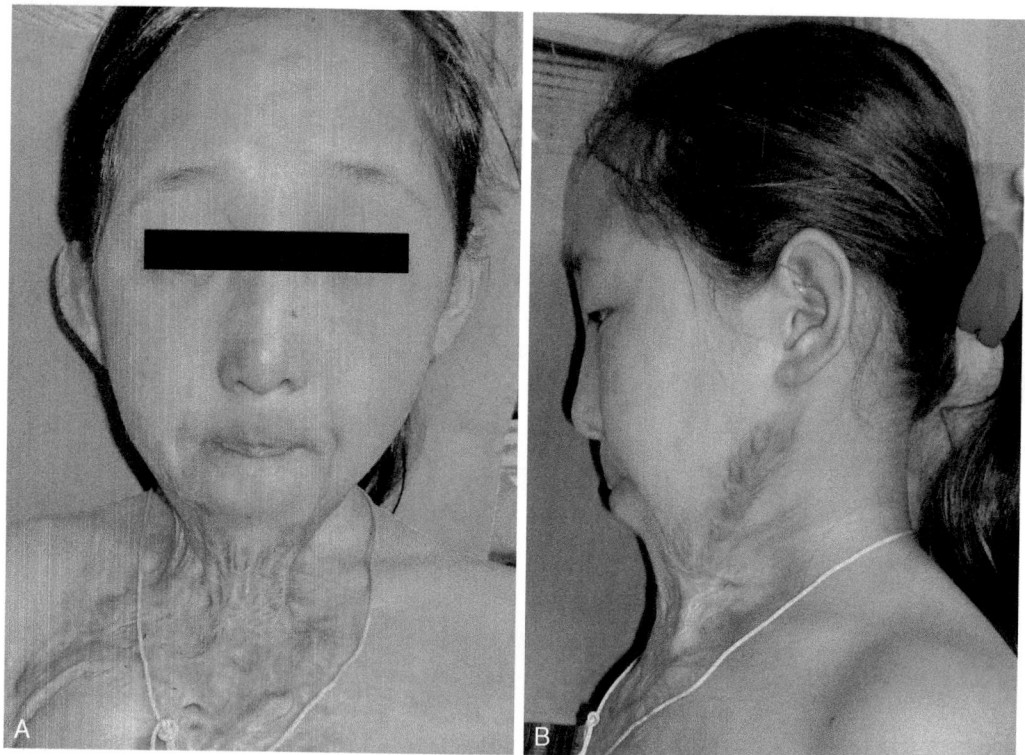

• **Fig. 35.6** Severe scarring and fibrous tissue deposition weeks to years after burn injury can produce skin contractures that limit neck extension and mandibular mobility.

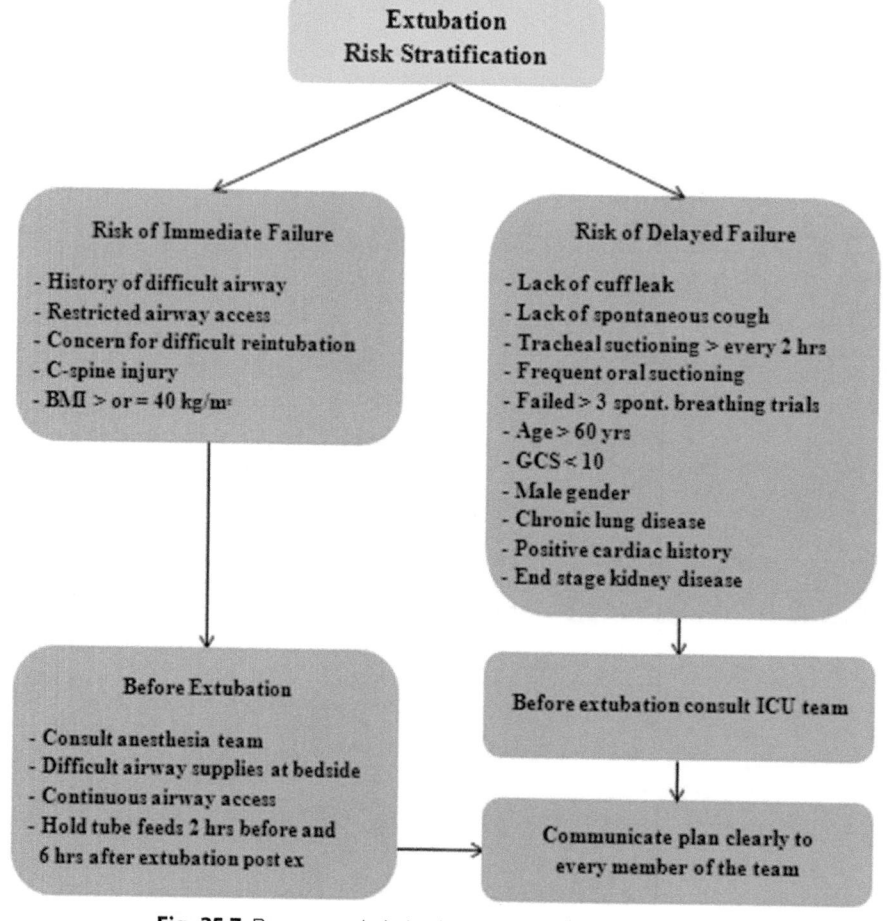

• **Fig. 35.7** Recommended algorithm for extubation risk stratification. *BMI*, Body mass index; *GCS*, Glasgow Coma Scale.

sustained inspiratory pressures between 20 and 30 cm H_2O, and direct visualization of pharyngeal and vocal cord edema surrounding the ETT using a videolaryngoscope. In addition, patients must be able to clear and manage airway secretions, which can be problematic if secretions are copious and/or the patient is unable to mount an adequate cough. Moreover, one must ensure that the patient's chest wall (particularly with burn injury of the thorax) and pulmonary compliance are not so significantly impaired as to cause excessive work of spontaneous breathing.

Airway Management of Pediatric Burn Patients

The pediatric burn patient poses specific challenges to airway management, due to differences in anatomy and physiology from those of adults. Smaller children and infants tend to have larger tongues, shorter jaws, a longer palate and epiglottis, narrower cricoid cartilage, and an increased risk for laryngospasm.[27] Edematous injury to pediatric patients' already relatively larger tongue and longer epiglottis can cause precipitous upper airway obstruction, undermine mask ventilation, and make tracheal intubation difficult. Because the pediatric airway is significantly narrow, even small decreases in tracheal diameter from edema and mucous production result in large increases in airway resistance, as demonstrated by Poiseuille's Law.[28]

Infants are prone to desaturate more rapidly because of their increased oxygen demand and their decreased functional residual capacity (FRC), posing obvious risk in burn patients given their potential difficulties with mask ventilation and intubation, as described previously. In addition, ventilation in pediatric burn patients is often more difficult as baseline pulmonary compliance is already lower than in adults and is further undermined by pulmonary injury and edema. Burn-injured children are, therefore, more susceptible to rapid deterioration, and because initial airway evaluation is often a poor predictor of eventual airway obstruction, earlier tracheal intubation during the acute phase is commonly recommended.

Evaluation and management of the airway in burned pediatric patients involves intentional evaluation and planning. Although uncuffed ETTs were at one point favored, cuffed tubes are now recommended because they create both a variable and more reliable seal to allow for adequate positive-pressure ventilation in the settings of evolving airway edema/diameter and changes in pulmonary compliance. Clinical outcome studies have demonstrated that use of uncuffed tubes in pediatric burn patients leads to increased incidence of tidal volume loss and inadequate ventilation, and increased rates of reintubation, which can be very difficult in children with face/neck burns.[29,30]

To avoid development of tracheal stenosis in these intubated children, an air leak should be audible at 20 to 25 cm H_2O and regularly monitored. FSI can be performed in children using small-caliber or "spaghetti" bronchoscopes, but their smaller size and decreased rigidity make it more difficult to navigate through swollen pharyngeal tissue and to facilitate tube placement. Additionally, smaller scopes do not have suction capability to remove copious burn-induced airway secretions and mucous that can hinder visibility.

The challenge of managing airways in burn-injured children is demonstrated in the numerous case reports describing different combinations of methods used to secure the airways.[26] One such method—the "flex-flex" method—offers potential benefit in management of anterior pediatric airways, particularly when neck extension is limited and/or mouth opening is small.[31] The technique involves positioning the patient's head in neck flexion, and then further flexing the head of the bed. This extreme flexion position can allow for a direct view of the vocal cords with a long straight blade and does not require a large mouth opening.

Among more rarely used techniques, tracheostomy is considered in extreme cases when tracheal intubation is considered impossible or very unsafe, and anatomy is amenable; however, studies of early elective tracheostomy have failed to demonstrate outcome benefits in burn children.[24] Of note, one case report describes the successful use of extra-corporeal membrane oxygenation (ECMO) in a severely burn-injured infant who had airway distortion and neck contractures too severe to secure the airway by traditional methods.[32]

Conclusion

Airway management in burn patients poses unique challenges attributed to the often profoundly distorted airway anatomy, as well as the impaired respiratory mechanics and physiology. A thorough understanding of the different phases of burn injury and recovery allows one to anticipate the specific challenges presented during each phase and to tailor management appropriately.

Selected References

2. Kaiser HE, Kim CM, Sharar SR, et al. Advances in perioperative and critical care of the burn patient: anesthesia management of major thermal burn injuries in adults. *Advances in Anesthesia.* 2015;31:137–161.

4. Esnault P, Prunet B, Cotte J, et al. Tracheal intubation difficulties in the setting of face and neck burns: myth or reality? *Am J Emerg Med.* 2014;32:1174–1178.

8. Bitter EA, Shank E, Woodson L, et al. Acute and perioperative care of the burn-injured patient. *Anesthesiology.* 2015;122:448-464.

9. Sheridan RL. Airway management and respiratory care of the burn patient. *Int Anesthesiol Clin.* 2000;38:129-145.

14. Martyn JA, Richtsfeld M. Succinylcholine-induced hyperkalemia in acquired pathologic states: etiologic factors and molecular mechanisms. *Anesthesiology.* 2006;104:158-169.

21. Romanski KS, Palmieri TL, Sen S, et al. More than one third of intubations in patients transferred to burn centers are unnecessary: proposed guidelines for appropriate intubations of the burn patient. *J Burn Care Res.* 2015. [Epub ahead of print]

26. Caruso TJ, Janik LS, Fuzaylov G. Airway management of recovered pediatric patients with severe head and neck burns: a review. *Paediatr Anaesth.* 2012;22: 462-468.

27. Cote CJ, Todres ID. The pediatric airway. In: Cote CJ, ed. *A Practise of Anesthesia for Infants and Children.* 5th ed. Elsevier Saunders; 2013: 238-243.

30. Sheridan RL. Uncuffed endotracheal tubes should not be used in seriously burned children. *Pediatr Crit Care Med.* 2006;7(3):258-259.

31. Hochman II, Zeitels SM, Heaton JT. Analysis of the forces and position required for direct laryngoscopic exposure of the anterior vocal folds. *Ann Otol Rhinol Laryngol.* 1999;108(8):715-724.

All references can be found online at eBooks.Health.Elsevier.com.

36

Airway Management in Pediatric Patients

RANU R. JAIN AND STACI D. CAMERON

CHAPTER OUTLINE

KEY POINTS

- The first attempt at the pediatric airway should be the best attempt and includes proper preparation of equipment and positioning.
- The pediatric airway anatomy is different in children, whose larynx is located higher in the neck with a relatively larger tongue. Children have a differently shaped epiglottis, and their vocal cords are angled.
- The newborn rib cage is oriented parallel, and the intercostal muscles are not as effective at increasing intrathoracic volume with inspiration as are those of adults.
- The work of breathing for each kilogram of body weight is similar in infants and adults.
- The oxygen consumption of a full-term newborn (6 mL/kg/min) is twice that of an adult (3 mL/kg/min), which results in an increased respiratory rate.
- An infant's tidal volume is relatively fixed.
- Minute alveolar ventilation in infants is more dependent on increased respiratory rate than on tidal volume.
- Functional residual capacity (FRC) of an infant is similar to FRC of an adult when normalized to body weight because the ratio of alveolar minute ventilation to FRC is doubled (with hypoxia or apnea or under anesthesia), the infant's FRC is diminished, and desaturation occurs more precipitously.
- Continuous apneic oxygenation should be utilized during intubation of the neonate and small infants.
- In infants, most airflow resistance occurs in the bronchial and small airways.
- Resistance to airflow is inversely proportional to the radius of the lumen to the fourth power for laminar flow and to the radius of the fifth power (r^5) for turbulent flow.
- There is lateral displacement of the airway in 45% of the population under 8 years of age.
- Radiographic evaluation may be extremely helpful to diagnose a difficult airway (DA) in a child.
- Radiographs of a child's upper airway (AP and lateral films, fluoroscopy) may show site and cause of airway obstruction.
- When necessary, magnetic resonance imaging (MRI) and computed tomography (CT) of pediatric patients provide more detailed information if time permits.

Introduction

One of the most challenging aspects facing anesthesiologists is maintaining the technical skills necessary for the management of the difficult airway (DA). The American Society of Anesthesiologists (ASA) guidelines define a DA as the clinical situation in which a conventionally trained anesthesiologist experiences difficulty with any of the following: face-mask ventilation of the upper airway, layrngoscopy, ventilation using a supraglottic airway (SGA), tracheal intubation, extubation, or invasive airway.[1] Recent reports demonstrate how important skilled airway management is to the practice of pediatric anesthesia. Data from the ASA pediatric closed claims database demonstrate a greater frequency of adverse respiratory events in the pediatric population.[2] In the pediatric closed claims analysis, respiratory events accounted for 43% of all adverse events, most frequently related to inadequate ventilation (20%). Esophageal intubation, airway obstruction, and difficult intubation (DI) combined accounted for 14% of the remaining adverse respiratory events. In the pediatric perioperative cardiac arrest (POCA) registry, 20% of all cardiac arrests were attributed to the respiratory system.[3] Airway obstruction and DI were responsible for 27% and 13% of these events, respectively. Incidence of difficult mask ventilation in nonobese children is 2.1%. Most of the patients who experience arrests from airway obstruction or DI have an underlying disease or syndrome. Unless otherwise indicated, throughout this chapter "patient" refers to the pediatric patient.

In addition, infants and small children display anatomic differences compared with adults. Knowledge of these differences, as well as congenital syndromes and different disease states, is required for management of the DA. Airway management in the pediatric patient may require general anesthesia (GA) before intubation attempts, which might not be a primary approach in a cooperative adult patient. Practice guidelines should be followed when managing the difficult pediatric airway in order to minimize adverse events.

Anatomy of the Pediatric Airway

The pediatric airway, particularly in infants, is different from the adult airway. Understanding these differences is important when managing the pediatric airway. The following is a brief review of the anatomy of the normal pediatric airway.[4–7]

Larynx

The larynx is situated more cephalad at the third and fourth cervical vertebrae (C3–C4) level in the infant and migrates to the adult C5 level by 6 years of age.[6] Because the infant's larynx is more rostral (higher), the tongue is located closer to the palate and more easily opposes the palate. As a result, airway obstruction may occur during induction or emergence from anesthesia. A common misnomer is that the infant's larynx is more anterior, when it is really more rostral or superior in the neck, compared with the adult larynx. In syndromes associated with mandibular hypoplasia, such as Pierre Robin, the larynx is actually positioned more posteriorly than normal. This results in a greater acute angulation between the laryngeal inlet and the base of the tongue. In this circumstance, direct visualization of the glottis may be difficult or impossible. Because of the cephalad position of the larynx and the large occiput, the sniffing position does not assist in visualization of the pediatric larynx.[4,7] Elevating the head only moves the larynx into a more anterior position. Infants should be positioned with the head and shoulders on a flat surface with the head in a neutral position and the neck neither flexed nor extended[5] (Fig. 36.1). A small roll can be placed under the infant's shoulders to achieve a more neutral position (Fig. 36.2).

Epiglottis

The infant epiglottis is long, stiff, and often described as Ω or U shaped.[6] It projects posteriorly above the glottis at a 45-degree angle. Because the epiglottis is more obliquely angled, visualization of the vocal cords may be difficult during direct laryngoscopy. It may be necessary to lift the tip of the epiglottis with a laryngoscope blade to visualize the vocal cords. Straight laryngoscope blades are often preferred for this reason. If the patient is not paralyzed, use of a Macintosh blade is less stimulating because it is not necessary to lift the epiglottis.

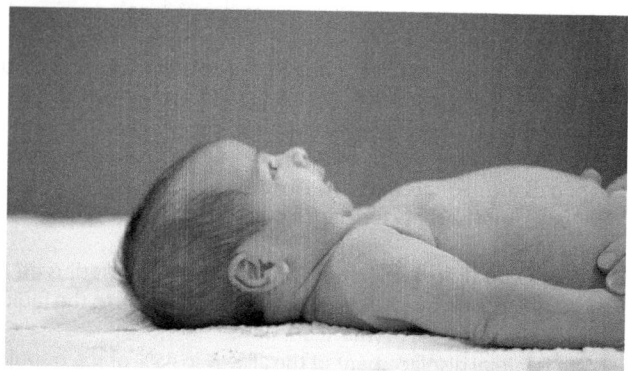

• **Fig. 36.1** Infants should be positioned with the head and shoulders on a flat surface with the head in a neutral position and the neck neither flexed nor extended.

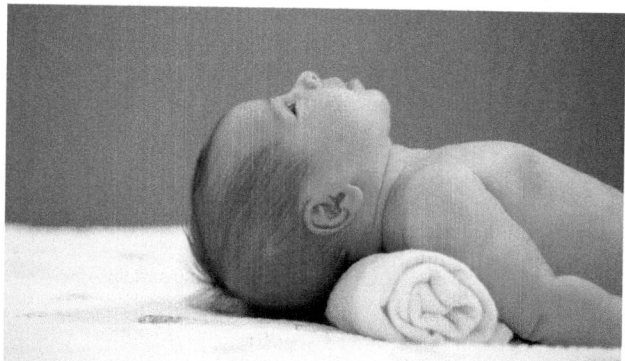

• **Fig. 36.2** A small roll can be placed under the infant's shoulders to achieve a more neutral position.

Subglottis

Historically, it was thought that the cricoid cartilage was the narrowest portion of the infant's airway, causing the larynx to be funnel shaped; however, recent studies demonstrate that the glottic opening and the subvocal cord level are the narrowest portions of the infant's airway, and the airway is more cylindrical in shape.[7-9] Tight-fitting endotracheal tubes (ETTs) that compress the mucosa at this level may cause edema and increase resistance to flow. Resistance to flow is inversely proportional to the radius of the lumen to the fourth power (r^4). One millimeter (1 mm) of edema can reduce the cross-sectional area of the infant trachea by 75%, versus 44% in the adult trachea.

Evaluation of the Pediatric Airway

No completed studies have evaluated the predictors of DI in children. Physical examination to predict the potential DA should be guided by the knowledge of normal anatomy and the syndromes associated with the DA.

The evaluation of the pediatric airway should begin with a history and physical examination of the head and neck. The examinations mostly involve subjective experience, and consistent evaluation criteria should improve the ability to predict the DA. Clues to a potential DA include snoring, noisy breathing, difficulty breathing with feeding or an upper respiratory tract infection, decreased neck mobility and extension, small mouth opening, and recurrent croup. Review of previous anesthesia records should be performed, if available. If a DA is encountered,

documentation of events and the ability to mask ventilate are helpful for future caregivers. A prior uneventful anesthesia does not guarantee success the next time.[4,7]

Knowledge of syndromes that may adversely affect the airway is crucial to the management of the difficult pediatric airway. The presence of one anomaly mandates a search for others. A common feature in patients with many of these syndromes is micrognathia. Micrognathia creates more difficulty with displacement of the tongue during direct laryngoscopy, thus increasing the chance that the glottis will be difficult to visualize.[4,7] The ability to intubate often changes as the child grows. Intubation often becomes easier with syndromes associated with micrognathia (e.g., Pierre Robin) as the patient ages. In mucopolysaccharide disorders or abnormalities involving the cervical spine (e.g., Klippel-Feil syndrome), intubation may become more difficult as the child ages.[5]

Abnormalities of the ear or the presence of ear tags has been suggested as an indicator of DI.[5] In one study, bilateral microtia was associated with an increased incidence of DI (42% vs 2% in unilateral microtia). Mandibular hypoplasia was associated with bilateral microtia 10 times more than with unilateral microtia (50% vs 5%), thus allowing bilateral microtia to be used as an indirect predictor of DI.[8]

Physical examination must focus on the head, neck, and cervical spine. Many evaluations used to predict DA in adults have not been extrapolated to the pediatric population. Cooperation of the patient is necessary for precise evaluation. In the young or uncooperative child, appropriate evaluation is limited. Preliminary data indicate that the Mallampati classification may be an insensitive predictor of DI in the pediatric population.[9] Pediatric anesthesiologists are at a disadvantage because they are anesthetizing patients with less objective airway information available. This underscores the need for a skilled approach to the difficult pediatric airway.

Evaluations should focus on the size and shape of the mandible, size of the mouth and tongue, absence or prominence of teeth, presence of loose teeth, and the neck length and range of motion. Berry suggests that the appropriate thyromental distance in infants is one finger breadth (1.5 cm).[10] Lateral examinations of the head and neck may provide clues to the presence of micrognathia. Mandibular enlargement has also been identified as a risk factor for DI.

Cherubism is a childhood disease consisting of painless mandibular enlargement with or without maxillary involvement that progresses rapidly in early childhood and then regresses during puberty. In cherubism, the potential displacement space is encroached on by mandibular enlargement.[11] Palpation of the soft tissue of the potential displacement area may reveal the problem.

Diagnostic Evaluation

Magnetic resonance imaging (MRI) and computed tomography (CT) may be extremely helpful in the evaluation of airway pathology. Flexible endoscopy may be of benefit before intubation when visualization of vocal cords is thought to be difficult or when airway pathology is suspected. In patients with unilateral hemifacial microsomia, radiographic classification of the mandibular anatomy can help predict ease of intubation.[12]

Radiographic evaluation of patients with airway obstruction may be obtained in patients who present to the emergency room only if they are not in respiratory distress. Radiographs should be obtained in the upright position because obstruction may worsen in the supine position.[13] In this situation, it is mandatory that a clinician skilled in airway management and capable of managing a difficult pediatric airway accompany the patient, along with the appropriate equipment.

Radiographs have high sensitivity (>86%) for the diagnosis of airway foreign body, exudative tracheitis, and innominate artery compression. For laryngomalacia and tracheomalacia, radiography has much lower sensitivity (5% and 62%, respectively).[13] Radiologic evaluation should not take precedence over airway control in patients with a compromised airway. Other physicians, especially otolaryngologists, may be consulted and support management of a DI.

Classification of the Difficult Pediatric Airway

Difficulty with face-mask ventilation of the upper airway, laryngoscopy, ventilation using an SGA, tracheal intubation, extubation, or invasive airway is the definition of a DA according to the 2022 ASA DA management guidelines.[1] Recognition of the DA along with the circumstances that predispose to airway problems is crucial to the safe management of the pediatric airway. Classification of the difficult pediatric airway may be made according to the anatomic location affected. Major anomalies of the head, face, mouth and tongue, nasopharynx, larynx, trachea, and neck are discussed in detail later.

Pediatric Airway Equipment

To manage a DA successfully, the appropriate equipment should be immediately available. We recommend the creation of a difficult pediatric airway cart stocked with equipment for patients ranging from premature infants to small adults. The ASA has created an infographic chart that can be used as a cognitive tool during the management of a DA.[1] (Fig. 36.3). This infographic can be placed on the DA cart. In addition, the American Academy of Pediatrics section on anesthesiology recommends the creation of a DA cart for all locations anesthetizing children.[14] This cart should be dedicated only for use in a DA or a cannot intubate/cannot oxygenate (CICO) scenario (Box 36.1). At institutions where extracorporeal membrane oxygenation (ECMO) is available, clinicians should consider this as a last resort option.

Face Mask

When managing the DA, the ability to ventilate with a mask is more important than tracheal intubation. If at any point, face-mask ventilation becomes inadequate, call for help and proceed with the DA algorithm.[1] When dealing with the pediatric airway, and especially the difficult pediatric airway, have a selection of masks readily available. Disposable clear-plastic masks with an inflatable rim are typically used. These masks should extend from the chin to the bridge of the nose. A leak-free seal should be obtained with minimal pressure applied to the face or mandible. Transparent masks allow visualization of secretions or vomitus during induction. These masks can be purchased in different flavors or scented before induction to make them less intimidating.

Face masks have been modified for flexible scope intubation (FSI) in a variety of ways.[15-18] Frei and colleagues[16,17] described modifying a commercially available mask (Vital Signs) by drilling a hole into the lateral aspect of the mask and attaching a corrugated silicon tube. The center of the mask is fitted with a plastic ring covered by a silicon membrane. A hole 1 to 2 mm smaller than the outer diameter (OD) of the bronchoscope is punched

into the membrane. This airway endoscopy mask has been used to facilitate FSI in patients ranging in age from 3 days to 12 months with spontaneous ventilation and propofol sedation.[15] A commercially available face mask with a ventilation side port (MERA, Senko Ika Kogyo, Tokyo, Japan) was modified and used successfully to intubate nine patients ages 3 months to 11 years under inhalational anesthesia with a flexible scope and continuous manual ventilation.[18]

Oropharyngeal Airway

Upper airway obstruction may occur during induction of anesthesia because the infant's tongue is large in relation to the oropharynx. Appropriately sized oropharyngeal airways are necessary for air exchange. Guedel and Berman airways are the most common airways available. By holding the airway next to the child's face, the correct size can be estimated. If the airway is too short, obstruction may be worsened. If the airway is too long, the epiglottis or uvula may be damaged. Use of a tongue depressor to insert the oropharyngeal airway is recommended to avoid impaired lymphatic drainage of the tongue.[4]

Nasopharyngeal Airway

Nasopharyngeal airways are available in sizes 12- to 36-French and are used with caution in pediatric patients with hypertrophied adenoids. The modified nasal trumpet was first described by Beattie[412], followed by its use in pediatric airway management as described by Holm-Knudsen in 2005[413] (Fig. 36.3).

Endotracheal Tube

ETTs in a variety of sizes (2.5–7.0 mm) should be available for the pediatric patient. Laser-resistant, nasal/oral Ring-Adair-Elwyn (RAE) and wire-reinforced ETTs are available for use depending on the surgical requirement. Determination of correct ETT size is based on the patient's age and weight. ETTs one-half size larger and smaller than the calculated size should be available

> ## BOX 36.1 Pediatric Difficult Airway Cart
>
> Assortment of laryngoscope handles or blades
> Oxyscope
> Endotracheal tubes (ETTs): 2.0–7.0 mm
> Oral/nasopharyngeal airways
> Bite blocks
> Masks
> Stylets
> Endotracheal tube exchangers
> Laryngeal mask airways (LMAs): all sizes
> Flexible intubation scope (FIS) equipment
> Bronchoscopic swivel connector
> Retrograde intubation kit
> Percutaneous cricothyrotomy kit
> Laryngoscope
> McGill forceps
> Albuterol adapters (for metered doses)
> Intravenous (IV) catheters
> Defogger
> Yankauer: pediatric and adult sizes
> Suction catheters
> Lidocaine solution/jelly

ASA DIFFICULT AIRWAY ALGORITHM: PEDIATRIC PATIENTS

Pre-Intubation: Before attempting intubation, choose between either an awake or post-induction airway strategy. Choice of strategy and technique should be made by the clinician managing the airway.[1]

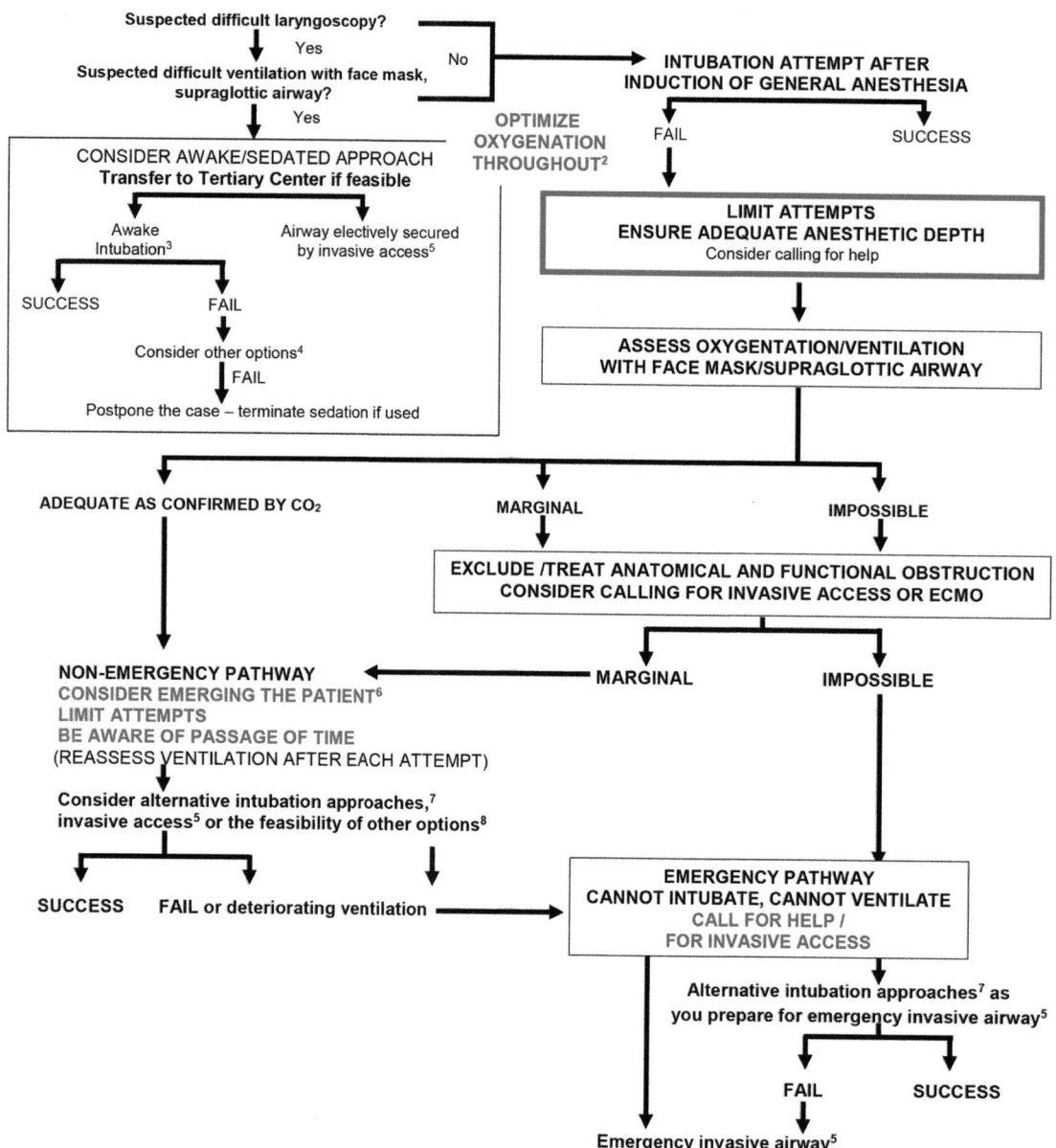

• **Fig. 36.3** Difficult airway algorithm: Pediatric patients. (1) The airway manager's assessment and choice of techniques should be based on their previous experience; available resources, including equipment, availability, and competency of help; and the context in which airway management will occur. (2) Low- or high-flow nasal cannula, head elevated position throughout procedure. Noninvasive ventilation during preoxygenation. (3) Awake intubation techniques include flexible bronchoscope, videolaryngoscopy, direct laryngoscopy, combined techniques, and retrograde wire-aided intubation. (4) Other options include, but are not limited to, alternative awake technique, awake elective invasive airway, alternative anesthetic techniques, induction of anesthesia (if unstable or cannot be postponed) with preparations for emergency invasive airway, or postponing the case without attempting the above options. (5) Invasive airway techniques include surgical cricothyroidotomy, needle cricothyroidotomy if age-appropriate with a pressure-regulated device, large-bore cannula cricothyroidotomy, or surgical tracheostomy. Elective invasive airway techniques include the above and retrograde wire–guided intubation and percutaneous tracheostomy. Also consider rigid bronchoscopy and ECMO. (6) Includes postponing the case or postponing the intubation and returning with appropriate resources (e.g., personnel, equipment, patient preparation, awake intubation). (7) Alternative difficult intubation approaches include, but are not limited to, video-assisted laryngoscopy, alternative laryngoscope blades, combined techniques, intubating supraglottic airway (with or without flexible bronchoscopic guidance), flexible bronchoscopy, introducer, and lighted stylet. Adjuncts that may be employed during intubation attempts include tracheal tube introducers, rigid stylets, intubating stylets, or tube changers and external laryngeal manipulation. (8) Other options include, but are not limited to, proceeding with procedure utilizing face-mask or supraglottic airway ventilation. Pursuit of these options usually implies that ventilation will not be problematic. (From Apfelbaum JL, Hagberg CA, Connis RT, et al. 2022 American Society of Anesthesiologists Practice Guidelines for Management of the Difficult Airway. *Anesthesiology*. 2022;136(1):31–81. doi:10.1097/ALN.0000000000004002.)

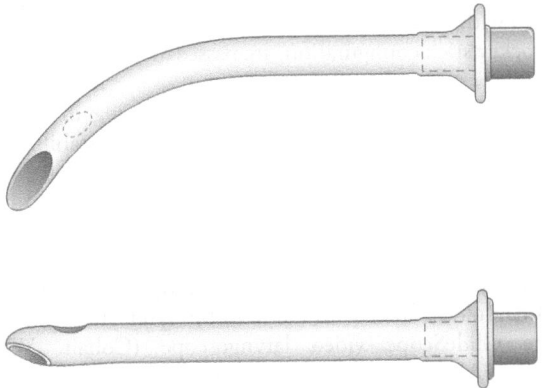

• **Fig. 36.4** Modified nasal trumpet airway by Beattie is a nasal airway with an endotracheal tube connector wedged into the flared end. The patient can be ventilated through this modified nasal trumpet. The mouth, lips, and the other naris should be closed.

TABLE 36.1	Formula for Endotracheal Tube Size and Depth of Insertion	
Type/Insertion	**Formula**	
Uncuffed ETT	(Age + 16)/4 *or* ETT >2 years, Age/4 + 4	
Cuffed ETT	Age/4 + 3.5	
Length of insertion (oral)	Age (years)/2 + 12 *or* 3 × ID (mm)	
Length of insertion (nasal)	3 × ID (mm) + 2	

ETT, Endotracheal tube; *ID*, internal diameter.

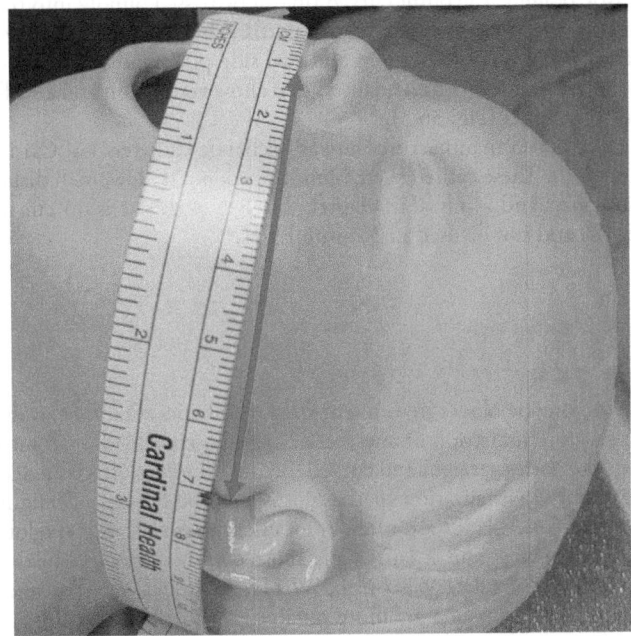

• **Fig. 36.5** Nasal-tragal length (NTL) can also be used to measure depth of insertion in neonates. A measurement is made from the center of the nasal septum to the tragus, and 1 cm is added to this number.

TABLE 36.2	Suggested Endotracheal Tube Size for Infants	
Age	**Size (mm ID)**	
Preterm (>1000 g)	2.5	
Preterm (1000–2500 g)	3.0	
Newborn to 6 months	3.0–3.5	
1–2 years	4.0–4.5	
>2 years	(Age +16)/4 = ID	

ID, Internal diameter.

(Table 36.1). Traditional teaching advocates the use of uncuffed ETTs in patients younger than 8 years of age. Pediatric ETTs with low-pressure high-volume cuffs are available for use in patients with low lung compliance or those at risk for aspiration. For cuffed ETTs, a half-size smaller tube should be used because the OD of the tube is larger with the cuff.[19]

Maintenance of air leak pressure at less than 20 cm H_2O with or without a cuff is recommended to minimize the occurrence of postintubation croup. Use of a manometer is recommended to avoid overinflation of the cuff. Koka and colleagues cite the incidence of postintubation croup as 1%.[20] In a prospective study of more than 5000 children, however, Litman and Keon found that seven patients developed croup, defined as inspiratory stridor at least 30 minutes in duration, for an incidence of 0.1%.[21] In that study, ETTs with air leak pressures greater than 40 cm H_2O were replaced with the next smaller size.[21] The presence or absence of a leak depends on the level of anesthesia and the use of muscle relaxants. Many clinicians use the degree of difficulty in passing the ETT below the vocal cords as the indicator of proper fit.

In general, there are many formulas for calculating the appropriate size of an ETT. Formulas for selecting an uncuffed ETT in children older than 2 years include (age + 16)/4 or (age/4) + 4. The use of cuffed ETTs in newborns and children under 8 years has been studied. In a group of 488 patients, patients were randomly allocated to receive a cuffed or an uncuffed ETT.[22] The formula for the cuffed tube was (age/4) + 3. This formula was appropriate for 99% of patients. In that study, three patients in each group were treated for croup symptoms. Formulas for length of insertion of an oral ETT include length (cm) + 3 times internal diameter (mm) or length (cm) = age (years)/2 + 12.[19] In the premature or newborn infant, the tip-to-lip distance in cm = 6 + weight (kg).[23] Nasal-tragal length (NTL) can also be used to measure depth of insertion in neonates. A measurement is made from the center of the nasal septum to the tragus and 1 cm is added to this number (Fig. 36.4). Whatever method is chosen, correct ETT position should be confirmed by auscultation of bilateral breath sounds (Table 36.2). Also, leaks should be checked to a permissible pressure of 20 to 25 mm Hg.

Double-lumen tubes are not available for use in pediatric patients younger than 6 to 8 years. The Arndt Endobronchial Blocker (Cook Critical Care, Bloomington, IN) has been used to provide one-lung ventilation in infants.[24] The 5.0-French blocker is available; the recommended ETT size is 4.5 mm. The Univent tube (Fuji Systems, Tokyo, Japan) is a single-lumen tube with an incorporated movable bronchial blocker inside.[25] Pediatric sizes of the Univent tube are available: 3.5-mm internal diameter (ID) and 4.5-mm ID. The 3.5-mm Univent tube does not have a lumen for suctioning or administration of oxygen to the blocked lung. A flexible intubation scope (FIS) is needed for placement. Further detail regarding one-lung ventilation is provided in Chapter 26.

Endotracheal Tube Exchangers

ETT exchangers have multiple uses; they can be used to exchange damaged ETTs and provide a conduit for reintubation, if necessary, and should be determined on a case-by-case basis. The ASA 2022 guidelines recommend minimizing the use of airway exchange catheters for extubation purposes in pediatric patients.[1]

Many different types of exchangers are available for use in adult patients. These tube exchangers are long, semirigid catheters that fit inside ETTs. The Frova Intubating Introducer (Cook Critical Care, Bloomington, IN) is available in a pediatric size (8-French) that allows placement of a 3.0-mm ETT. It is 33 cm in length with a hollow lumen and a blunt curved tip that is shaped like the gum elastic bougie. The blunt curved tip can be passed blindly into the trachea when visualization of the glottis is inadequate. The Frova catheter has a hollow lumen and two side ports and is packaged with removable Rapi-Fit adapters that allow ventilation and a stiffening cannula (Fig. 36.5).[26]

Cook also manufactures airway exchange catheters (AECs) in four sizes. These catheters are blunt tipped and hollow, with distal side ports and a Rapi-Fit adapter. The 8-French size is 45 cm in length and can be used in 3.0-mm ETTs.[26]

Laryngoscopes

Straight Versus Curved Blades

Laryngoscope blades in different sizes and shapes should be available before induction of anesthesia. Laryngoscope blades fall into two categories: straight and curved. Because the epiglottis is angled posteriorly, visualization of the glottis may be difficult. Straight laryngoscope blades are often recommended to lift the epiglottis in neonates and infants. The most common straight blades include the Miller, Wisconsin, Wis-Hipple, and Wis-Foregger blades. Curved blades are more suitable for older children.

Oxyscope

The Oxyscope is a fiberoptic Miller no. 1 blade with a port for insufflation of oxygen during intubation. Oxygen insufflation during laryngoscopy in spontaneously breathing, anesthetized infants has been shown to minimize the decrease in transcutaneous oxygen tension, thus making airway instrumentation safer.[27]

Anterior Commissure Laryngoscope

The anterior commissure laryngoscope is frequently used by otolaryngologists for visualization of the glottis. It is a rigid, tubular, straight-blade laryngoscope with a distally located, recessed light source. This design permits enhanced visualization by preventing the tongue from obscuring the field of view.[28]

Video Laryngoscopes

The angulated video-intubation laryngoscope (AVIL), invented by Dr. Marcus Weiss of Zurich, is an endoscopic intubation device. The AVIL consists of a cast-plastic Macintosh 4 laryngoscope, with the blade angulated distally, and an integrated fiberoptic endoscope (1.8 m long, OD 2.8 mm, VOLPI, Schlieren, Switzerland). The distal blade tip is angulated about 25 degrees to provide increased viewing for the fiberoptic lens. With the angulated tip, the AVIL resembles an activated McCoy blade. Flattening of the blade's vertical flange enables the device to be used in children. The fiberoptic endoscope runs from the handle to the tip of the blade. The AVIL uses conventional laryngoscopy techniques coupled with video monitoring from the blade tip. Stylleted ETTs, in a hockey stick configuration, are passed along the vertical flange of the blade under video control.[29]

The AVIL has been used in patients ranging in age from 3 months to 17 years with manual in-line neck stabilization. In infants and small children, care should be taken with insertion of the blade; initial insertion of the blade was too deep in some patients.[30] Several reports document the use of this device in pediatric patients with a DA. The video laryngoscope has been used successfully to intubate children with Morquio syndrome, as well as a 3-day-old neonate with Pierre Robin syndrome.[29,31]

The GlideScope video laryngoscope (Cobalt, Verathon; Bothell, WA) has a reusable video baton and single-use laryngoscopy blades in two sizes. The laryngoscope comes with a monitor screen, and a video recording unit is also available. The GlideScope Cobalt model features a 10-mm laryngoscope blade. The blade is inserted in the midline without displacing the tongue.[32] Two studies have been reported using the GlideScope in children with normal airways. Both studies found it suitable for intubation in pediatric patients.[33,34] In one of the studies, the time required for intubation was longer.

The Airtraq optical laryngoscope (AOL; Prodol, Vizcaya, Spain) is a single-use indirect laryngoscope for tracheal intubation. The Airtraq comes in two pediatric sizes: infant (size 0) for ETT sizes 2.5 to 3.5 and pediatric (size 1) for ETT sizes 3.5 to 5.5. Both sizes require a mouth opening of 12 to 13 mm. The rubber eyepiece may be used or a camera may be attached and used with a wireless monitor. Images from the distal tip of the blade are projected to the proximal eyepiece. The Airtraq is inserted midline, and the tip may be placed in the vallecula or used to lift the epiglottis. Once the glottis is visualized, the ETT is slowly advanced. For intubation, lubricate the ETT so that the tube advances easily. Problems with advancement of the ETT may be caused by too large diameter of the ETT, the guide channel, or incorrect angle of the ETT as it exits the channel.[32] Two case reports documented the use of the Airtraq in pediatric patients with DAs: a 9-year-old child with Treacher Collins syndrome who weighed 23 kg and an infant with Pierre Robin syndrome who weighed 4.8 kg.[33,34] Other case reports have documented difficulty with advancement of the ETT into the trachea despite a good view of the larynx.[35]

The McGRATH MAC blade is a small portable handheld device that combines direct laryngoscopy with enhanced video laryngoscopy and is produced by Medtronic (Boulder, CO). This battery-powered blade uses an LED light source and has a 2.5-inch (6.3-cm) LCD color display camera. The inline camera is anterior to provide direct and indirect views of the airway. It comes in sizes 1, 2, 3, and 4. The slim, disposable blades are packaged sterile for single use. This McGRATH MAC 1 blade has been used in neonates as small as 0.8 kg (see Video 36.1).[5]

The C MAC is a Karl Storz (Tuttlingen, Germany) video laryngoscope available in MAC sizes 2, 3, and 4, and in Miller sizes 0 and 1, as well as a pediatric D-BLADE, which can be used for DAs. This stainless steel laryngoscope blade is inserted into the airway as a MAC or Miller blade would be used and illuminates the oropharynx while producing an 80-degree diagonal field of view video image onto either a cable-linked monitor or a portable monitor. These images can be recorded. One study showed ease of use, glottic view, and successful intubation using the Storz Miller blade to be more favorable compared with other blades by residents and nurse anesthetists who had never used video laryngoscopy before in a simulated pediatric DA (see Video 36.2).[6]

The Coopdech video laryngoscope portable VPL-100 (Daiken Medical Co., Ltd, Osaka, Japan) is a handheld, battery-powered laryngoscope, similar to the McGRATH, except that the blades are reusable and can be autoclaved, and there is a zoom display option for the images. This single-unit video laryngoscope comes in pediatric sizes Miller 0 and 1 and MAC 2. The attached monitor has a 3.5-inch (8.9-cm) LCD display and uses a white LED light source to illuminate the oral cavity. There is little research at this point on this device in the pediatric population, but one study suggests the Coopdech video laryngoscope performed well in regard to successful intubation and time to effective ventilation.[8]

The Pentax airway scope (AWS; Pentax-AWS, Tokyo, Japan) is a handheld, waterproof, battery-powered video laryngoscope with an attached 2.4-inch (6-cm) color LCD screen that displays an 80-degree angle view. The screen is adjustable to allow for intubation in a variety of positions. The detachable, disposable blade has a guiding groove for the ETT, and therefore no stylet is needed. The ETT can be inserted in the groove before or after laryngoscopy. There is also a channel for inserting a suction catheter. The curve of the blade allows for intubation without neck extension. The blade is inserted along the palate, without involving the patient's tongue, inserted under the epiglottis, and then slightly elevating the epiglottis. The pediatric size will accommodate ETT with OD of 5.5 to 7.6 mm without a cuff. The neonatal size accommodates ETTs with ODs less than 5 mm. Few reports in the literature describe this video laryngoscope's efficacy in the pediatric population.[7,9]

Stylets

Various types of stylets are available as adjuncts to tracheal intubation, including the traditional malleable stylet, lighted stylets, and optical stylets. Stylets should be available for the DA. The stylet is inserted into the ETT until the distal end of the stylet is just short of the ETT tip. The ETT and stylet are bent into the desired shape, usually a hockey stick configuration. Complications associated with use of stylets include tracheal trauma, ETT obstruction, and shearing of the stylet. When removal of a stylet becomes difficult, the tip should be examined.[36]

Lighted Stylets

Several different types of lighted stylets, or light wands, are currently commercially available, including the Vital Signs light wand illuminating stylet (Vital Signs, Totawa, NJ) and the Tube Stat lighted stylet (Xomed, Jacksonville, FL). Pediatric versions are available for use with ETTs as small as 2.0 to 4.0 mm. The use of the lighted stylet to guide blind tracheal intubation relies on the principle of transillumination. The presence of a well-defined glow in the neck indicates tracheal placement. Esophageal placement is indicated by the absence of a glow in the neck. Several different reports describe successful intubation of pediatric patients with the light wand.[37,38] Successful technique includes the following principles: (1) a small shoulder roll should be used to keep the head in a neutral to slightly extended position. This is extremely important in a small infant, whose neck naturally flexes when lying on a flat surface because of the large occiput; (2) the light wand should be advanced in the midline; if the light deviates to one side, the light wand should be withdrawn and repositioned; (3) the epiglottis is elevated by lifting the jaw with the nondominant hand; (4) transillumination should be assessed before advancing the light wand too far; (5) blind nasal intubation in children is often easier with the rigid stylet left in place; and (6) the wand is bent less sharply than for an oral intubation.

Benefits of light-guided tracheal intubation include use in obstructed conditions, low acquisition costs, and disposable components that eliminate the need for disinfection of equipment. As with any new technique, experience in patients with normal anatomy should be obtained before attempts in patients with a DA.

Optical Stylets

The first optical stylet, described in 1979, was a Hopkins telescope with a fiberoptic external light source (Karl Storz, Tuttlingen, Germany).[39] The Seeing Optical Stylet (SOS) system (Clarus Medical, Minneapolis, MN) is a new, reusable, high-resolution fiberoptic endoscope with a malleable stainless-steel stylet.[32] It combines the features of an FIS and a light wand. The Shikani SOS is portable, lightweight, and available in pediatric and adult versions. The pediatric version is compatible with ETTs 3.0 to 5.0 mm in size. The SOS can be inserted directly into an ETT, allowing intubation to be performed under direct vision. Illumination is provided by a standard green-line fiberoptic laryngoscope handle or the included SITElite halogen handle. An adjustable tube stop with an oxygen port, which goes over the shaft of the stylet, allows supplemental oxygen to be delivered. Many factors do not affect the SOS, including cervical spine injury, small mouth, large tongue, and reduced jaw mobility.[32]

Pfitzner and colleagues[40] described the use of the Shikani SOS on eight occasions in seven patients with DA. There were seven successful intubations; one patient, who had previous surgery and radiotherapy for a retropharyngeal rhabdomyosarcoma, could not be intubated by any method. Two patients with limited mouth opening and one patient with a C1–C2 subluxation were intubated on the first attempt. A patient with Hunter syndrome was intubated on the second attempt. A potential difficulty mentioned with the SOS is loss of the visual field, which occurs when the lens is next to a mucosal surface. Maneuvers to increase the operating space available are use of a laryngoscope to retract the base of the tongue, lifting the mandible, and pulling the tongue forward.[41]

The Shikani Stylet is inserted into the ETT after lubrication with silicon spray. The fiberoptic cable can be connected to a video monitor. The mandible is lifted with the left hand and displaced anteriorly until the lower teeth are anterior to the upper teeth.[41] The stylet with the loaded ETT is advanced into the trachea under direct vision. Laryngoscopy may be useful in cases of DI (Fig. 36.6). The Shikani SOS (Clarus Medical, Minneapolis, MN) is a portable video stylet.

The Bonfils and Brambrink are semirigid intubation endoscopes (Karl Storz, Tuttlingen, Germany) that can also be used for

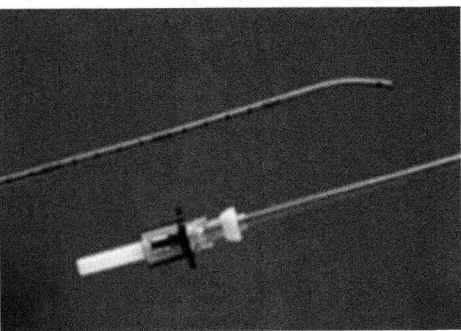

• **Fig. 36.6** Frova Intubating Introducer (Cook Critical Care, Bloomington, IN) catheter is available in a pediatric size (8-French) that allows placement of a 3-mm endotracheal tube. It is hollow with two side ports, is blunt tipped, and has a Rapi-Fit adapter.

small mouth openings in a medial or retromolar approach. They come in pediatric ODs of 2 mm and 3.5 mm with a 40-degree distal bend. There is an oxygen adaptor to allow for extended intubation time, as well as a portable LED light source. The Brambrink DCI (Karl Storz, Tuttlingen, Germany) intubation endoscope can be used with ETT sizes 2.5 to 3.5 mm. The Bonfils retromolar intubation endoscope (Karl Storz, Tuttlingen, Germany) can be used with ETT sizes 4 to 5.5 mm and uses a movable eyepiece.

Video-Optical Intubation Stylet

Another video-optical intubating stylet (Acutronic Medical Systems, Hirzel, Switzerland) consists of a flexible fiberoptic endoscope (developed by Dr. Weiss of Zurich). A sliding connector locks the video stylet onto the ETT adapter; it does not require neck extension but does require mouth opening. One report documents successful use of the video-optical intubation stylet in patients ages 6 to 16 years, with a simulated grade III laryngoscopic view; 46 of 50 patients were intubated on the first attempt; four attempts were considered failures because of prolonged intubation time (>60 seconds).[42]

Supraglottic Airways

Laryngeal Mask Airway Family

The laryngeal mask airway (LMA North America, San Diego, CA), introduced in 1983 and approved for use in 1991 by the US Food and Drug Administration (FDA), is a standard part of the ASA DA algorithm and part of a larger class of SGAs.[1,43] Pediatric versions of the LMA Classic, as well as the disposable LMA, are available for use and are part of the pediatric DA algorithm, as described by Steward and Lerman.[44] Application of the SGA requires minimum training and can be useful in neonatal resuscitation.[45] The LMA Flexible is available in sizes 2 and 2.5, and the LMA ProSeal is available in a size 2.

The size of the SGA in children is determined by the patient's weight, although a new method has been suggested. With the hand extended and palm facing up, the thumb and little finger are extended. The second, third, and fourth fingers are placed together. The fully inflated SGA is placed against the palmar side of the patient's fingers, keeping the widest part of the SGA in line with the widest part of the three fingers. In a study of 163 children at birth to 14 years old, this method was correct in 78%. In the remaining patients, a difference of only one size was observed.[46]

The SGA has been described as a conduit for blind intubation as well as a conduit for FSI.[47–51] Awake placement of the SGA has been described in an infant with Pierre Robin syndrome.[52] Anterograde intubation through the SGA with a guidewire was also described in an infant with micrognathia who could not be intubated with conventional methods. A soft-tipped guidewire was advanced through the SGA and the position confirmed by fluoroscopy. An ETT was inserted over the guidewire, followed by removal of the SGA.[53] A review of the literature demonstrates different insertion techniques.

The standard technique described with the cuff deflated for adults has also been advocated for children. In addition, a rotational or reverse technique has been described. The SGA is inserted with the cuff facing the hard palate and then rotated and advanced simultaneously. An alternative technique involves inserting the SGA with the cuff partially inflated. Reports on placement of the SGA with the different techniques are conflicting. In children, one study compared two insertion techniques. The partially inflated cuff insertion technique does not increase the incidence of downfolding of the epiglottis and is an acceptable alternative to the standard technique.[54] In another study, insertion of the partially inflated SGA required less time and was associated with a higher success rate on first attempts compared with the standard (deflated) technique.[55] Results from a study detailing the flexible scope positioning of the SGA in children with a DA show that 29.5% of patients had a grade I (full) view of the glottis, 29.5% had a grade II (partial) view, and 41% had a grade III (epiglottis only) view. Children with a mucopolysaccharide disorder had a grade III view 54% of the time and a grade I view 14% of the time.[56]

The ProSeal LMA is now available in pediatric sizes. This SGA has a second mask to isolate the upper esophagus with a second dorsal cuff to increase the seal against the glottis. Lopez-Gill and colleagues[57] found that it was easily inserted, and oropharyngeal leak pressure was greater than 40 cm H_2O (Table 36.3).

Air-Q Intubating Laryngeal Airway

The Air-Q intubating laryngeal airway (ILA; Cookgas, Mercury Medical, Clearwater, FL, USA) is an SGA used both for airway maintenance during routine anesthesia and as a conduit for tracheal intubation for patients with a DA. Unlike the LMA, the ILA was designed primarily to allow for the passage of conventional cuffed tracheal tubes when used for blind tracheal intubation, and it has the option for subsequent removal. The ILA also shares some structural features with the intubating laryngeal mask airway

TABLE 36.3 Laryngeal Mask Airway Classic Mask Size With Corresponding Cuff Volumes, Endotracheal Tube, and Flexible Bronchoscope

Mask Size	Weight (kg)	Maximum Cuff Volume (mL)	Maximum ETT Size	Maximum FIS (mm)
1	Infants up to 5	Up to 4	3.5 uncuffed	2.7
1.5	5–10	Up to 7	4.0 uncuffed	3.0
2	10–20	Up to 10	4.5 uncuffed	3.5
2.5	20–30	Up to 14	5.0 uncuffed	4.0
3	30–50	Up to 20	6.0 cuffed	5.0
4	50–70	Up to 30	6.0 cuffed	5.0
5	70–100	Up to 40	7.0 cuffed	5.0
6	>100	Up to 50	7.0 cuffed	5.0

ETT, Endotracheal tube; *FIS*, flexible intubation scope; *LMA*, laryngeal mask airway.

(ILMA). Compared with the LMA, the ILA allows for straightforward passage of a cuffed tracheal tube when used as a conduit for tracheal intubation because of three design differences. First, the airway tube of the ILA is wider, more rigid, and curved. Second, removal of the detachable 15-mm proximal connector increases the ID of the airway tube. Third, the ILA's shorter length allows for easier removal after successful tracheal intubation. The Air-Q ILA is available in six sizes (1, 1.5, 2, 2.5, 3.5, and 4.5) for single use and in four sizes (2.0, 2.5, 3.5, and 4.5) for reuse. Sizing of the pediatric Air-Q ILA is similar to the LMA, in that it is weight based (size 1 for patients <5 kg; size 1.5 for patients 5–10 kg; size 2 for patients 10–20 kg).

The self-pressurized Air-Q ILA (ILA-SP) is a new first-generation SGA for children, with a self-adjusting cuff and lack of a pilot balloon. A newer version of the ILA-SP was recently introduced into our practice for routine airway maintenance in children. The ILA is currently the only supraglottic device available in pediatric patients designed to act as a conduit for tracheal intubation with cuffed tracheal tubes.

Rigid Ventilating Bronchoscope

The rigid ventilating bronchoscope is extremely useful for ventilating patients with a DA and is included in the most recent version of the ASA DA algorithm as an alternative device in the cannot intubate/cannot ventilate (CICV) situation. In any situation of potential airway collapse, the otolaryngologist and the rigid ventilating bronchoscope should be immediately available (see Chapter 29).

Induction Technique

The principles outlined in the ASA guidelines for DA management apply to the pediatric patient. Evaluation, recognition, and preparation are key elements.[1] If a difficult airway is expected, a timeout to discuss the plan for airway management, including airway equipment and backup equipment, should be performed prior to induction. It is important to identify the primary person responsible for securing the airway, the backup or secondary person, as well as other helpers involved during this timeout, and who will be in charge of an invasive airway or ECMO, if necessary. The ASA 2022 DA guidelines infographic chart for pediatric patients can be used as a cognitive tool during management of a DA (Fig. 36.3).[1]

Preoxygenation of pediatric patients, although difficult, should be attempted if possible before any DA intervention. Studies have demonstrated that the optimal time for preoxygenation in pediatric patients is different from that in adults. Values ranging from 80 to 100 seconds have been reported for adequate preoxygenation in healthy children.[58,59] Continuous oxygenation during intubation of neonates and infants should be used to prolong the time before apneic desaturation.[60] Continuous oxygenation during intubation can be done via nasal cannula, modified nasal trumpet connected to oxygen source, blow-by-oxygen via ETT inserted in the oropharynx, or a high-flow nasal oxygenation system.[61-64] Summoning help early, using awake intubation, and preserving spontaneous ventilation during intubation attempts are also important when managing the DA. The awake or awake-sedated approach is preferred in most circumstances when managing the DA. However, in pediatric patients, the patient's cooperation may limit the usefulness of awake intubation. One well-tolerated technique is placement of a lubricated SGA in awake infants, which provides an airway for inhalational induction.[52]

The traditional approach to the difficult pediatric airway has been maintenance of spontaneous ventilation under inhalational anesthesia. Premedication with oral or intravenous atropine (0.01–0.02 mg/kg) is indicated for vagolytic and antimuscarinic effects. Inhalation induction may be performed with sevoflurane in 100% oxygen. Sevoflurane has been used in the management of the DA with success.[65,66] The low blood gas solubility of sevoflurane and consequent rapid induction and emergence are advantageous when managing the DA. When the ability to ventilate the patient by mask is demonstrated, a small dose of muscle relaxant or propofol may be given to facilitate intubation.

For patients who can tolerate an awake sedated intubation technique, a variety of sedating medications can be used. One must always keep in mind the risk-benefit ratio when sedating a patient with a DA. Sedatives may further compromise an airway. Sedatives should not be given to any patient in acute distress or with the potential for acute obstruction. Use of sedatives should be based on careful physical examination, anesthesiologist experience with agents involved, and overall patient condition. If no other options are available, slow titration of pharmacologic agents to effect, without loss of spontaneous ventilation, should be performed. Use of pharmacologic agents that are easily antagonized is recommended. For older children and adolescents, a combination of midazolam and fentanyl may be used. Remifentanil can also be used. Dexmedetomidine has been used successfully to perform an awake FSI in a morbidly obese patient with facial, cervical, and upper thoracic edema.[67] In extreme circumstances, parental presence at induction may be allowed, and careful preparation of the parent must be performed before induction. As soon as the patient separates or begins to lose consciousness, a designated member of the operating room (OR) staff should immediately escort the parent out of the OR (see Video 36.3).

Another important aspect for successful airway management is topicalization of the airway with local anesthesia. In pediatric patients, this may be obtained by nebulizing, spraying, or swabbing local anesthetic solution or by applying viscous gel to a gloved finger. FISs with suction ports can be used to spray local anesthesia on the vocal cords under direct vision. The maximum dose of local anesthetic allowed should be calculated before topicalization. The drug of choice is lidocaine because it has the best safety profile. Maximum doses of lidocaine are 5 mg/kg. Agents containing benzocaine (e.g., Cetacaine spray; Americaine ointment; Hurricaine ointment, gel, or spray) should be avoided in infants and young children because of the risk of methemoglobinemia.[7]

Airway Management Techniques

Techniques for Ventilation

Obstruction of the upper airway is a common occurrence in pediatric patients undergoing an inhalation induction. Techniques for overcoming this type of obstruction include insertion of an appropriate-size oropharyngeal airway or a nasopharyngeal airway, or both. Another common mistake is occlusion of the submandibular space with incorrect placement of the anesthesiologist's hand. Care should be taken to position the hand on the tip of the mandible and not on the submandibular space. Chin lift or jaw thrust combined with continuous positive airway pressure (CPAP) at 10 cm H_2O has been shown to improve upper airway patency.[68]

Additional techniques are available for mask ventilation. The two-person technique involves either one person holding the mask with both hands while an assistant compresses the reservoir bag or a second person assisting in jaw lift while the first person continues to compress the reservoir bag. Another option is using the anesthesia ventilator to provide ventilation so that one person can hold the face mask with both hands.[69]

Techniques for Intubation

Direct Laryngoscopy

Tips for successful visualization of the larynx include proper use of external laryngeal pressure and positioning. Direct laryngoscopy involves alignment of the oral, pharyngeal, and laryngeal axes to visualize the glottis. Because the larynx is situated in a more cephalad position and the occiput is large, the sniffing position in infants does not assist in visualization of the larynx.[4,7] The infant should be positioned with the head in a neutral position with the neck neither flexed nor extended.[70] A small shoulder or neck roll may be beneficial. Optimal external laryngeal manipulation (OELM) should also be used with a poor laryngoscopic view to improve visualization. OELM may improve the laryngoscopic view by at least one whole grade in adults. This is not cricoid pressure but rather pressing posteriorly and cephalad over the thyroid, hyoid, and cricoid cartilages. Benumof and Cooper suggest that OELM should be an instinctive and reflex response to a poor laryngoscopic view.[71] This maneuver has also proved effective in pediatric patients.[72] The main mechanism appears to be shortening of the incisor-to-glottis distance.

The two-anesthesiologist technique involves manipulating the larynx under direct vision by the laryngoscopist and intubation by a second anesthesiologist. This technique has been used successfully to intubate a 6-month-old infant with Pierre Robin syndrome and concomitant tongue-tie (ankyloglossia).[73]

The retromolar or paraglossal technique has been advocated as useful in cases of DI related to a small mandible.[74] A straight laryngoscope blade is introduced into the extreme right corner of the mouth overlying the molars, thus reducing the distance to the vocal cords. It is advanced in the space between the tongue and lateral pharyngeal wall until the epiglottis or glottis is visualized. The head is rotated to the left to improve visualization while applying external laryngeal pressure and displacing the larynx to the right. Advancement of the ETT is facilitated by retracting the corner of the mouth, to allow placement of the ETT. The styletted ETT should be shaped into the classic hockey stick configuration. An alternative approach involves placement of the ETT from the left side of the mouth.[75] Lateral placement of the laryngoscope blade reduces the soft tissue compression because the tongue is essentially bypassed. The maxillary structures are also bypassed by the lateral blade placement, thus improving the view.[4] Because there is a reduced space for displacement of the tongue in syndromes with micrognathia, this approach may be useful. The retromolar technique has been described as an alternative method for intubation of patients with Pierre Robin syndrome.[76] A pediatric version of the Bonfils Retromolar Intubation Fiberscope is the Brambrink Intubation Scope (Karl Storz, Tuttlingen, Germany). It is an optical stylet that allows a retromolar approach to the DA.[26]

In adults, the left molar approach with a Macintosh blade and OELM has been reported to improve the glottic view in cases of difficult laryngoscopy.[77] Suspension laryngoscopy is often employed by otolaryngologists as an alternative technique for visualization of the difficult larynx. Intubation of an infant with Goldenhar syndrome was accomplished by suspension laryngoscopy.[78] This method is similar to standard laryngoscopy by the retromolar technique.

With any direct laryngoscopy technique, limiting the number of attempts is recommended. Edema can rapidly occur and create a CICV scenario. The ASA 2022 guidelines for a DA state that attempts should be limited to 3 by the primary provider, and 1 attempt can be made by a secondary provider.[1] In addition to providing supplemental oxygen throughout airway management, oxygenation and ventilation should be performed between each laryngoscopy attempt.[1] After 4 attempts to secure an airway, consider waking up the patient or, if there is difficulty with ventilation, attempt to relieve any airway obstruction first and then consider waking up the patient.[1]

Flexible Scope Intubation

Aids for FSI include face masks, oropharyngeal airways, guidewires, and the SGA.[79] The Frei mask previously described or variations of commercially available masks have been used with success.[15,16,80] The Patil-Syracuse mask (Anesthesia Associates Inc, San Marcos, CA) is available in a size 2, but it is difficult to achieve a good seal with this mask. An endoscopy mask can be made by attaching a swivel FIS adapter to a pediatric face mask in one of two ways[79]: a commercially available swivel adapter (Instrumentation Industries, Bethel Park, PA) can be attached directly to the mask, or an adapter designed for attachment to the ETT (e.g., Portex bronchoscope adapter, Smiths Medical, Keene, NH) can be connected to the face mask with a 15-mm to 22-mm adapter.

Oropharyngeal airways may also be modified for use in pediatric FSI. A strip may be cut from the convex surface of a Guedel-style airway to produce an aid for oral flexible laryngoscopy, creating a channel. The flexible scope is placed in the channel, which helps maintain a midline position. The use of a smaller airway than predicted is suggested so that one may visualize the base of the tongue and epiglottis. Modified oropharyngeal airways are not effective as bite blocks, and one must be careful.[79] Also, a nipple from a baby bottle has been modified to act as a conduit for FIS in an infant with an unstable cervical spine. In this case, a hole was cut obliquely into the end of the nipple. After topicalization of the airway with 2% lidocaine, FSI was performed with a 4.0-mm uncuffed ETT.[81]

Flexible scope laryngoscopy is one of the cornerstones of DA management. Preparation for flexible laryngoscopy should include preparation of the patient (antisialogue) and checking of the FIS, light source, and suction as well as standard airway equipment. An assistant is necessary for monitoring of the patient and providing a jaw lift, which is useful because it elevates the tongue from the posterior pharynx.[7] For older children and adolescents who will be sedated for the procedure, explanation and reassurance in a calm manner are helpful. A method of delivering oxygen is necessary as well. This can be accomplished in a variety of ways, either blowby from the anesthesia circuit or by nasal cannula. For patients who are anesthetized, an SGA or an endoscopy mask may be used to ventilate the patient while the intubation is being performed. Tips for successful oral intubation include midline placement of the FIS, advancement of the FIS only when recognizable structures are visualized, and retraction of the tongue with gauze or clamps if needed.[7] If the view from the fiberscope is pink mucosa, the FIS is slowly pulled back until a recognizable structure is seen. If the nasal route is chosen, a topical vasoconstrictor may be used to reduce the chance of bleeding. In a series of 46 patients with DA, flexible nasal intubation was successful on the first attempt in 37 patients (80.4%) and on the second or third attempt in 7 patients (15.2%). Two failures occurred: one related to bleeding and the other to inability to introduce the scope nasally.[82]

FSI may be performed in a variety of ways. The standard technique involves passage of the ETT over the FIS. The ultrathin flexible laryngoscope with a directable tip allows FSI to be performed with ETTs as small as 2.5 mm. Intubation of a 3-month-old infant with Pierre Robin syndrome has been successfully performed with an ultrathin fiberscope.[83] A new 2.5-mm ultrathin FIS with a 1.2-mm suction channel has been used to intubate a newborn with a DA.[84] This FIS has a 2.5-mm OD, 1.2-mm working suction channel, angle of deflection of 160 degrees up and 130 degrees down, and working length of 450 mm.

In scenarios where the available bronchoscope is too large for the required ETT, a staged technique may be employed.[85] An FIS with a working channel, a cardiac catheter, and a guidewire are required. The guidewire is passed into the working channel of the fiberscope before intubation. The FIS guidewire assembly is then introduced into the mouth and positioned above the larynx. The guidewire is advanced into the trachea under direct visualization, followed by removal of the FIS. A cardiac catheter (used to stiffen the wire) is threaded over the guidewire. Finally, an ETT is advanced into the trachea over the guidewire-catheter assembly, which is then removed. A modification of this technique involves passage of the ETT over the guidewire without the reinforcing cardiac catheter. This has been used to intubate nasotracheally a 3-day-old infant with Pierre Robin syndrome.[86]

The flexible bronchoscope may also be used as an aid for nasal intubation either under direct vision or with a guide. In these cases, an FIS is introduced into one of the nares while the ETT is advanced into the trachea through the other naris.[34] Alternatively, if the ETT cannot be manipulated into the glottis, a guide may be placed in the opposite naris and directed into the trachea. The ETT is then removed and threaded over the guide. A urethral catheter has been used in this manner to assist in the intubation of a 2-week-old neonate with Klippel-Feil syndrome, occipital meningocele, and microretrognathia.[87] Another variation of the staged technique involves placement of a larger ETT into the larynx under flexible scope visualization, followed by removal of the FIS, leaving the larger ETT in the larynx. A bougie is placed through the larger ETT into the trachea, and the ETT is removed. An appropriate-size ETT is then advanced over the bougie into the trachea.[88]

FSI can be combined with a video laryngoscope to aid in intubation (combination technique). The video laryngoscope can first be inserted to help with jaw lift and/or partial visualization of the oropharynx. The flexible scope can then be used nasally or orally for intubation. Insertion of an FIS through an SGA has been successful.[53,54,89] Staged intubation techniques involving an SGA, FIS, guidewires, and catheters (dilators) have been reported, including the use of SGA-assisted wire-guided flexible scope tracheal intubation. In a series of 15 cases, Heard and colleagues demonstrated that this technique was safe, successful, and easy to learn.[90] After the FIS is placed through the SGA and the vocal cords are visualized, the guidewire is passed through the suction port of the bronchoscope and into the trachea. The SGA and FIS are carefully removed, and the ETT is advanced over the wire. A variation of this theme involves flexible scope visualization of the glottis through the SGA followed by passage of a guidewire through the suction port of an FIS into the trachea as before. The fiberscope is then removed and an airway catheter or a ureteral dilator passed over the wire into the trachea through the SGA. The SGA is then removed and an ETT advanced over the catheter into

the trachea.[91] This technique has been used successfully to manage the airway in children with mucopolysaccharidoses (MPS). The use of an SGA, an AEC, and a 2.2-mm-OD FIS has also been described.[92] After placement of the SGA and visualization of the vocal cords, the flexible scope is removed. The FIS is placed into the lumen of a size 11 AEC, which had been cut to 25 cm. This combination was advanced through the SGA into the trachea by a connector. The SGA and FIS are removed, and an ETT is advanced over the Cook AEC.

Przybylo and colleagues reported the performance of a retrograde FSI through a tracheocutaneous fistula in a child with Nager syndrome.[93] The ultrathin FIS was passed through the fistula in a cephalad direction past the vocal cords and exiting the nares. The ETT was then advanced over the FIS into the trachea.

Retrograde Intubation

The classic retrograde technique involves percutaneous placement of an intravenous catheter through the cricothyroid membrane into the trachea followed by placement of a guidewire. The guidewire exits the mouth or nose, and the ETT is then exchanged over the guidewire. If resistance to ETT passage occurs, counterclockwise rotation of the ETT may facilitate placement. This technique has been used for intubation of an infant with Goldenhar syndrome.[94] A 14-French retrograde intubation set is commercially available from Cook for use with ETTs of ID 5.0 mm or greater.

A combined technique using the FIS and retrograde intubation has been used successfully in management of the difficult pediatric airway as well, as previously mentioned.[95]

An FIS with a working channel is necessary for the combined technique. The guidewire is threaded into the suction port of an FIS that has a preloaded softened ETT on it. The FIS is passed along the guidewire until it is past the vocal cords. When the scope is past the vocal cords, the wire is withdrawn and the ETT correctly positioned. This technique allows passage without obstruction from the arytenoid cartilage or epiglottis. Oxygen insufflation can be performed through the suction port as well, even with the wire in place. Care must be taken to limit flow to avoid tracheobronchial injury from excessive gas velocity. Audenaert and colleagues used this technique in 20 patients with DA ages 1 day to 17 years and reported no major complications.[96] Retrograde wire-guided direct laryngoscopy has also been reported for airway management in a 1-month-old infant.[97] In that patient, attempts to pass a 2.5-mm ETT over the wire itself were unsuccessful, but tracheal intubation was achieved over the wire with direct laryngoscopy.

Emergency Access

Emergency access is divided into the emergency surgical and the emergency nonsurgical airway.[1] Emergency surgical airway access is often difficult and requires the presence of a skilled anesthesiologist. It is the last resort in the CICV = arm of the ASA DA algorithm.[98] Three procedures are referred to in this category: emergency tracheostomy, emergency cricothyroidotomy, and percutaneous needle cricothyroidotomy. In children younger than 6 years of age, emergency tracheostomy is usually the procedure of choice because the cricothyroid membrane is too small for cannulation.[96] In older children, percutaneous needle cricothyroidotomy is often preferred over a surgical approach because most anesthesiologists can perform this technique rapidly. Also, there is less risk of injury to surrounding structures.[4] Emergency cricothyroidotomy kits are available from Cook with 3.5-, 4-, and 6-mm-ID airway catheters.

The emergency nonsurgical airway access includes use of the SGA, esophageal-tracheal Combitube, and transtracheal jet ventilation (TTJV).[1] The Combitube is available in a small-adult size and is contraindicated in patients less than 4 feet (122 cm) tall.[7] The SGA is useful in the management of the difficult pediatric airway, as stated previously, as an SGA device or as a conduit for intubation; however, in the presence of glottic or subglottic obstruction, the SGA is ineffective, in which case TTJV is considered the technique of choice, as reported in two cases for laser endoscopic surgery.[99] Caution with TTJV is urged because serious complications may result from its use.[100] TTJV below a glottic or subglottic obstruction may result in barotrauma because the pathway for egress of air and oxygen is limited. Tension pneumothorax has been reported with jet ventilation through an AEC in an adult.[101]

Other Intubation Techniques

In the past, blind digital intubation has been performed.[102] The Bullard laryngoscope is no longer manufactured. The use of a dental mirror has also been described.[103]

Intubating the COVID-19 Patient

Intubation of a COVID-19 patient should be performed only by experienced personnel, and training or teaching should not be performed on an infected patient. The airway equipment should be available, and the use of video laryngoscopy is recommended to minimize proximity to the infected patient. A plan should be in place for an unanticipated DA. SGA devices are acceptable alternatives to ETTs with minimal aerosolization risk, as stated by the Pediatric Difficult Intubation Collaborative (PeDI-C),[414] a collaborative group of 35 hospitals from 6 countries including the United States and Canada. These authors suggest the use of second-generation SGA devices because they have a higher leak pressure than first-generation SGA devices. Awake FSI is not encouraged, unless it is indicated. Viral contaminant can be aerosolized during atomization. The airway equipment most familiar to the operator should be used.

Personal protective equipment (PPE) must be worn during intubation of the COVID-19 positive patient. Hand hygiene must be performed before and after donning and doffing PPE. At a minimum, an N95 respirator/mask that will fulfill the filtering efficiency criteria of the National Institute for Occupational Safety & Health (NIOSH) and eye protection must be worn. Double gloving is recommended during all airway manipulation.

During intubation and extubation, limit the number of staff in the room to reduce the risk of exposure. Prepare intubating equipment in close proximity to the patient. After intubation, place the used laryngoscope in a sealed bag and remove the outer layer of gloves. Rapid sequence intubation (RSI) is recommended to avoid positive-pressure ventilation (PPV) after adequate preoxygenation of the patient; however, this can be modified based on the patient's clinical condition. The cuff of the ETT should be inflated before PPV. Placement of a heat and moisture exhange (HME) filter is recommended between the ETT and the circuit at all times. A plastic drape or shield over the COVID-19 patient is used (Video 36.4).

Extubation often results in greater aerosol generation as compared to intubation and should be performed with the same precautions as the intubation. Once extubated, place a mask on the patient's face to minimize aerosolization in the immediate postextubation period. Once the patient is extubated and proper doffing occurs, hand hygiene must be performed. The patient should be recovered in the operating room or a negative pressure room until there is minimal risk for further airway manipulation.

Complications of Airway Management

Complications that result from intubation in adults can occur in the pediatric population as well. Airway injury accounted for 6% of claims in the ASA closed-claims database.[104] Among the airway injury claims, 4% involved pediatric patients younger than 16 years. The most frequent sites of injury reported were the larynx (33%), pharynx (19%), and esophagus (18%). Injuries to the esophagus and trachea were more frequently associated with DI. Laryngeal injuries included vocal cord paralysis, granuloma, arytenoid dislocation, and hematoma. Pharyngeal injuries included lacerations, perforation, infection, sore throat, and miscellaneous injuries (foreign body, burn, hematoma, and diminished taste).

An oropharyngeal burn related to the laryngoscope lamp occurred in a term baby weighing 3.6 kg who was easily intubated at birth.[105] The laryngoscope was switched on before intubation. Light-bulb laryngoscopes, in contrast to fiberoptic laryngoscopes, can reach temperatures that would result in burns to the oropharynx. Filaments may overlap with use, and it is common for two or more coils to touch.[105] The resistance of the lamp decreases and the current increases, thus increasing the temperature. Koh and Coleman recommend that all light-bulb laryngoscopes be switched on for less than 1 minute; if left on, the temperature of the bulb should be manually checked before intubation.[105] DI accounted for 62% of all esophageal injuries, with most involving esophageal perforation (90%). Esophageal perforation following DI has been reported in a neonate.[106]

Laryngotracheal stenosis may be classified as glottic, subglottic, or tracheal. Prolonged intubation seems to be the major etiology. The mechanism responsible seems to be ischemic necrosis caused by pressure from the ETT against the glottic and subglottic mucosa. This results in an inflammatory reaction with a secondary bacterial infection and scar formation. Risk factors include too large an ETT, prolonged intubation, repeated intubation, laryngeal trauma, sepsis, and chronic inflammatory disease.[107]

The incidence of postintubation croup varies from 0.1% to 1%.[20,21] Risk factors include age under 4 years, tight-fitting ETT, repeated intubation attempts, duration of surgery exceeding 1 hour, patient's position other than supine, and previous history of croup. Reports are conflicting concerning the risk from a concurrent upper respiratory tract infection. Classic treatment consists of humidified air, nebulized racemic epinephrine, and dexamethasone. In pediatric trauma patients, absence of an air leak at extubation was the strongest predictor of postextubation stridor requiring treatment.[108]

Airway Diseases and Implications

Head Anomalies

Airway Implications

Airway management in children with macrocephaly with abnormal anatomy, predicting a difficult airway, requires proper head and neck positioning and care of the associated airway anomalies that are a frequent finding in patients with mucopolysaccharidosis. If preoperative evaluation suggests presence of a DA, awake methods of tracheal intubation should be initially attempted.

In children, awake intubation may require careful use of sedatives in addition to topical anesthesia to the oropharynx, larynx, and nasopharynx (for nasotracheal intubation). A limited number of attempts at direct laryngoscopy may be made. If these are not successful, one of the various techniques of nonvisual or indirect laryngoscopy, as detailed previously, may be used to secure the airway. According to the Pediatric Difficult Intubation Registry (PeDI), more than two direct laryngoscopy attempts in children with difficult tracheal intubation are associated with high failure rate and increased severe complications. The PeDI data suggest quickly transitioning to an indirect laryngoscopy technique when direct laryngoscopy fails.[109]

If the patient does not comply with awake tracheal intubation without the use of sedative that risks respiratory compromise, GA may be induced if mask ventilation is possible. The patient may breathe a vapor anesthetic and/or intravenous medications may be titrated until a level of anesthesia is achieved that allows tracheal intubation. The intubation may be accomplished with or without muscle relaxation. According to a recent study using the Pediatric Difficult Intubation Registry, controlled ventilation with and without the use of muscle relaxant was associated with less hypoxemia and laryngospasm complications compared to spontaneously breathing patients.[110] Other options include flexible scope laryngoscopy in a patient breathing spontaneously through a mask or an SGA, use of a lighted stylet, use of a Bullard laryngoscope, and the retrograde technique. When mask ventilation is known to be easy, muscle relaxants may be used and have been shown to notably improve airway visualization, decrease airway trauma, and increase the chance of successful tracheal intubation.[111]

Specific Anomalies

Head Anomalies

Airway management can be adversely affected by conditions that involve enlargement of the head. Mass lesions and macrocephaly can interfere with mask ventilation direct laryngoscopy, or both. The pathologic conditions that involve enlargement of the head and affect the airway are encephalocele, hydrocephalus, and mucopolysaccharidosis, along with other, less common conditions, such as phakomatoses, cranioskeletal dysplasias, or conjoined twins with face-to-face encroachment of the heads or proximity of the chests (thoracopagus).

Encephalocele

Patients with encephalocele may have other diseases that complicate airway management. The only two syndromes associated with encephalocele in which survival past infancy is likely are Roberts-SC phocomelia syndrome (includes pseudothalidomide syndrome, hypomelia-hypertrichosis–facial hemangioma syndrome), and facioauriculovertebral spectrum (includes first and second branchial arch syndrome, oculoauricular vertebral dysplasia, hemifacial microsomia, Goldenhar syndrome). Encephaloceles, or neural tube defects of the head, usually occur in the occipital area, although they may involve the frontal and nasal regions. When large, they affect airway management by interfering with mask fit or laryngoscopy.[112]

Hydrocephalus

Hydrocephalus is associated with more than 30 malformation syndromes. Some craniosynostosis syndromes are associated with hydrocephalus and result from bone compression that prevents free flow of cerebrospinal fluid; examples include achondroplasia, Apert syndrome, and Pfeiffer syndrome. Some of these diseases may affect the airway by more than one mechanism (e.g., children with hydrocephalus who also have Arnold-Chiari malformation). Difficulties with airway management are usually associated with the underlying pathology and interference with face mask ventilation.

Mucopolysaccharidoses

The mucopolysaccharidoses are a group of seven inherited lysosomal storage disorders caused by the deficiency of specific lysosomal enzymes required for the degradation of glycosaminoglycans (GAGs), which are complex macromolecules. The inability to degrade GAGs leads to their lysosomal accumulation and the subsequent clinical features of the disorders, which can include facial coarsening, corneal clouding, valvular heart disease, hepatosplenomegaly, and dysostosis multiplex accompanied by short stature.

MPS type I, which results from the deficiency of l-iduronidase activity, can manifest as one of three different clinical phenotypes: Hurler syndrome (i.e., MPS type IH), Scheie syndrome (i.e., MPS type IS), or Hurler-Scheie syndrome (i.e., MPS type I H/S). Of these, Scheie syndrome is the mildest form of the metabolic defect. The other mucopolysaccharidoses are Hunter syndrome (type II), Sanfilippo syndrome (type III), Morquio syndrome (type IV), Maroteaux-Lamy syndrome (type VI), and Sly syndrome (type VII).

The anesthetic morbidity of the mucopolysaccharidoses is 20% to 30%.[113] Morbidity is almost always related to respiratory difficulties. Intubation and maintenance of the airway might be difficult because of a variety of upper airway abnormalities, including micrognathia, macroglossia, patulous lips, restricted motion of the temporomandibular joints (TMJs), friable tissues, and the presence of copious viscous secretions. Semenza and Pyeritz, in a retrospective study on 21 patients with the diagnosis of MPS, found that the anatomic factors affecting respiratory status included (1) upper airway narrowing by hypertrophied tongue, tonsils, adenoids, and mucous membranes; (2) lower airway narrowing by GAG deposition within the tracheobronchial mucosa; (3) decreased thoracic dimensions related to scoliosis and thoracic hyperkyphosis, and (4) decreased abdominal dimensions because of lumbar hyperlordosis, gibbus formation, and hepatosplenomegaly.[114] In addition, a short neck and an anterior and narrowed larynx may lead to an increased incidence of difficult or failed intubations.[115] In particular, patients with Hunter, Hurler, or Maroteaux-Lamy syndrome have significantly more airway difficulties as they grow older than MPS patients have with other syndromes.[116]

The incidence of DI is high. In one review of 34 patients who underwent 89 anesthetics, the overall incidence of DI was 25% and failed intubation was 8%.[115] In children with Hurler syndrome, incidence of DI was 54% and failed intubation was 23%. Herrick and Rhine administered 38 anesthetics to 9 patients with MPS (Hunter, Hurler, Sanfilippo, and Morquio syndromes) and found an overall incidence of airway-related problems of 26%, with a 53% incidence in patients with the Hurler or Hunter syndrome.[117]

Belani and colleagues reported their experience with 141 anesthetics in 30 patients with MPS.[118] Visualization of the vocal cords during laryngoscopy was easier in children with Hurler syndrome when they were younger (23 vs 41 months; $p \leq 2.01$) and smaller (12 vs 15 kg; $p \leq 2.05$). Also, children with preoperative obstructive breathing had a significantly higher incidence of postextubation obstruction. A total of 28 children underwent bone marrow transplantation; this reversed upper airway obstruction and reversed intracranial hypertension.

Failure to insert an SGA or nasopharyngeal airway and fatal outcomes have been reported.[91,119,120] Consequently, nasotracheal intubation is not recommended because of difficulties with the anatomy of nasal passages and potential hemorrhage from soft tissue trauma. Accumulation of MPS in the trachea may require a much smaller ETT than usual.[119] Tracheostomy can also be difficult technically in these patients, and in one case was impossible even postmortem.[121]

Cervical instability, potential spinal cord damage, and severe thoracic and lumbar skeletal abnormalities make positioning and intubation difficult. In their series in children with Hurler syndrome, Belani and colleagues found a 94% incidence of odontoid dysplasia, whereas 38% demonstrated anterior C1–C2 subluxation.[118] To avoid cervical cord damage in patients with cervical instability, Walker and colleagues described manual in-line stabilization during intubation and concluded that a pediatric FIS should be available for all known DIs.[115] Tzanova and colleagues reported successful anesthesia in a 23-month-old girl with Morquio syndrome and unstable neck.[122] Flexible scope nasal intubation with spontaneous ventilation has been suggested as the method of choice.

Facial Anomalies: Maxillary and Mandibular Disease

The pediatric airway may be complicated by a large number of syndromes involving the head, neck, and cervical spine. The airway and associated structures are deviated from the branchial arches. The first arch develops into the maxilla, mandible, incus, malleus, zygoma, and a portion of the temporal bone. The second arch develops into the stapes, the styloid process of the temporal bone, and a portion of the hyoid. The third arch develops into the remainder of the hyoid. The fourth and sixth arches fuse to form the laryngeal structures, including the thyroid, cricoid, and arytenoid cartilages. The pharyngeal muscle develops from the fourth arch, whereas the sixth arch gives rise to the laryngeal musculature. Failure of any of these to develop properly may lead to characteristic anomalies.

Tumors

Cystic Hygroma

Cystic hygromas are multiloculated cystic structures that are benign in nature. They form as the result of budding lymphatics and thus may occur anywhere in the body, although most frequently in the neck (75%) and axilla (20%). As the tumor grows, it may cause symptoms from pressure on the trachea, pharynx, blood vessels, tongue, and nerves and eventually may severely compromise the airway. The tongue often protrudes outside the mouth and prevents its closure, making maintenance of the airway difficult if not impossible. Airway obstruction is the most critical complication of the cystic hygroma in the neck. The safest approach in these children seems to be nasal intubation, either blind or with flexible scope assistance with the patient awake.[123] In extreme cases, tracheostomy may be necessary.

Neck Teratoma

Teratomas of the head and neck are interesting because of their obscure origin, bizarre microscopic appearance, unpredictable behavior, and often dramatic clinical presentation. The reported incidence of cervical teratomas ranges from 2.3% to 9.3% of all teratomas. A teratoma is a true neoplasm, which includes four groups: dermoid cysts, teratoid cysts, true teratomas, and epignathi (pharyngeal teratomas).

Teratomas of the head and neck frequently arise with respiratory distress or even asphyxia at delivery, and a well-established plan for early airway management should be prepared. If they are untreated, the mortality of patients with these masses is 80% to 100%.[124] Fetal ultrasonography has been used since the 1970s to aid in the prenatal diagnosis. Antenatal diagnosis is important for two reasons. First, elective cesarean section should be planned to avoid dystocia and fetal trauma. Second, because immediate establishment of a patent airway is essential for survival, a team of pediatric airway experts must be available.

The ex-utero intrapartum technique (EXIT) allows the continuance of fetoplacental circulation during cesarean section. Initially, only the infant's head and shoulders (but not the placenta) are delivered, thus maintaining uteroplacental blood flow. Intramuscular fentanyl and vecuronium are given, the infant's airway is secured, and then the umbilical cord is clamped and delivery of the infant completed. The EXIT procedure has proved useful in cases of anticipated DA instrumentation of the neonate (e.g., large fetal neck masses causing airway obstruction).[125] Once the head of the neonate is delivered, a multitude of choices are available for airway management: direct laryngoscopy, FSI, pediatric Bullard laryngoscopy,[124] or tracheostomy. The EXIT procedure has proved to be safe and efficacious, allowing establishment of an airway in a controlled manner because the placenta allows continued gas exchange during airway manipulation.[126,127] Early identification of these masses allows controlled delivery of the neonate in a setting where pediatric anesthesiologists, surgeons, and neonatologists can develop strategies to minimize the risk of a postnatal respiratory death.

Cherubism

Cherubism is a familial disease of childhood in which patients acquire mandibular and sometimes maxillary enlargement. The mandibular rami hypertrophy, limiting the submandibular space for displacement of the tongue and making visualization of the glottis during direct laryngoscopy difficult.[11]

Congenital Hypoplasia

Acrocephalosyndactyly

Maxillary hypoplasia results from premature synostosis of facial and cranial sutures and usually manifests as one of multiple abnormal features in a group of rare but complex syndromes called acrocephalosyndactylies. Acrocephalosyndactyly encompasses a number of dysostoses, not all of which can be distinguished clearly. The midface retrusion gives the appearance of prognathia, although in reality the mandible is smaller than normal. In addition, there may be associated anomalies of the central nervous system (CNS; increased intracranial pressure, absent corpus callosum), the extremities, and in a small percentage of patients the heart.[128] Both the upper and the lower airway may be compromised in these patients.[129]

Multiple pathologic conditions may be seen; maxillary regression may be associated with choanal stenosis or atresia, reduction in nasopharyngeal space,[130] and palate deformity (narrow, high arched, or cleft). These features may cause respiratory compromise or obstructive apnea early in life, although obstruction can worsen as the child grows because of continued restriction in growth of the maxillary region.[131-134] In one series, upper airway obstruction arose more frequently in Crouzon disease and Pfeiffer syndrome than in Apert syndrome.

The incidence of airway obstruction has been addressed.[135] Of a total of 40 patients with severe syndromic craniosynostosis (13 had Apert syndrome and 27 had Crouzon disease), 40% presented with airway obstruction (12.5% severe and 27.5% mild obstruction). There was no significant difference in the distribution of airway status between patients with Apert syndrome and Crouzon disease. Severe obstruction in 5 patients resulted from midface hypoplasia, lower airway obstruction, tonsillar and adenoid hypertrophy, and choanal atresia.

Lower airway disease in the acrocephalosyndactylies occurs in the form of tracheomalacia, bronchomalacia, solid cartilaginous trachea lacking tracheal rings, and tracheal stenosis. Patients with tubular cartilaginous trachea have displayed a propensity for easy tracheal injury, edema, and stenosis and a potential for lower airway infection (tracheitis and bronchitis) and mucous plugging, because tracheal ciliary activity may be deficient. Sleep apnea was described in association with tracheal cartilaginous sleeve in a patient with Pfeiffer syndrome.[136]

Airway problems can be divided into those arising from the nasal passages, nasopharynx, palate, or trachea. Nasal septal deviation is a common feature of craniosynostosis patients and is considered a principal finding in Saethre-Chotzen syndrome. Narrowing of the nasal passages arises from maxillary hypoplasia. Although choanal atresia can occur, the usual picture is generalized narrowing. The nasopharynx is shallow because of hypoplasia of the maxilla and the altered angulation of the skull base. Palatal abnormalities further impinge on the nasopharynx. These deformities may consist of arched or ridged palates or increased thickness of the soft tissue. The degree of airway obstruction varies among these patients, being among the worst in those with Apert syndrome. Complications have included cor pulmonale and even death from airway obstruction. Lower airway obstruction may result from a number of abnormalities, including subglottic stenosis and vertically fused tracheal cartilage. Subglottic stenosis is especially common in Crouzon syndrome patients. Vertically fused tracheal cartilage has been reported in patients with Apert, Crouzon, and Pfeiffer syndromes; the entire trachea is encased in a tube of nonsegmented cartilage. These children can be difficult to manage and usually present with episodes of recurrent lower respiratory tract infections, reactive airway disease, and chronically retained secretions.

Acrocephalosyndactyly disorders include Apert syndrome (type I) and Apert-Crouzon (Crouzon) disease. Acrocephalosyndactyly also occurs with other diseases, including Chotzen (Saethre-Chotzen) syndrome and Pfeiffer-type acrocephalosyndactyly.

Apert Syndrome. Apert syndrome is characterized by agenesis or premature closure of the cranial sutures, midface hypoplasia, and syndactyly of the hands and feet that is symmetrical and involves at least the second, third, and fourth digits. Prevalence is estimated at 1 in 65,000 live births (~15.5 per 1 million population). Apert syndrome accounts for 4.5% of all cases of craniostenosis. Concerning CNS abnormalities, intelligence varies from normal to mental deficiency, although a significant number of patients are mentally retarded. Malformations of the CNS may be responsible for most cases. Papilledema and optic atrophy with loss of vision may be present in cases of subtle increased intracranial pressure. Other abnormalities include cervical spine fusion, which is common and almost always involves C5 to C6; osseous fusions may also be evident in other joints of the extremities and in the spine, tracheal cartilage anomalies, and diaphragmatic hernia.[137]

Airway anomalies result from facial abnormalities, which include small nasopharynx and hypoplastic and retropositioned maxilla. DI in Apert syndrome has been reported. One of the suggested mechanisms is trismus related to temporalis muscle fibrosis.[138] Both the upper and the lower airway can be compromised by complete or partial cartilage sleeve abnormalities of the trachea and obstructive sleep apnea (OSA).[129]

Crouzon Syndrome. Crouzon syndrome (Crouzon disease, craniofacial dysostosis) is closely related to Apert syndrome. In 1912, Crouzon described the triad of skull deformities, facial anomalies, and exophthalmos.[139] Crouzon syndrome is an autosomal dominant disorder with complete penetrance and variable expressivity.[140,141] About 50% of cases represent sporadic mutations, and 40% are familial. In the United States, prevalence is 1 per 60,000 live births (~16.5 per 1 million population). Crouzon syndrome makes up approximately 4.8% of all cases of craniosynostosis at birth.[142] Crouzon disease is associated with acanthosis nigricans (5%) and CNS defects such as chronic tonsillar herniation (73%), progressive hydrocephalus (30%), and syringomyelia.[143] Multiple sutural synostoses frequently involve premature fusion of the skull base sutures, causing midfacial hypoplasia, shallow orbits, a foreshortened nasal dorsum, maxillary hypoplasia, and occasional upper airway obstruction.[144]

Crouzon syndrome is characterized by premature closure of calvarial and cranial base sutures, as well as those of the orbit and maxillary complex (craniosynostosis). Other features include beaked nose; short upper lip; mandibular prognathism; overcrowding of upper teeth; malocclusions; V-shaped maxillary dental arch; narrow, high, or cleft palate and bifid uvula; hypoplastic maxilla; and relative mandibular prognathism. Cervical fusion of C2–C3 and C5–C6 is present in 18% of cases.

Pfeiffer Syndrome (Type I). Pfeiffer (Noack) syndrome (type I) is also a close relative of Apert syndrome, although it is less severe. Pfeiffer syndrome has three clinical subtypes and is manifested by craniosynostosis, broad thumbs and toes, variable maxillary retrusion, and partial soft tissue syndactyly. Type I is classic Pfeiffer syndrome; affected patients have normal intelligence and a good prognosis. Type II is associated with cloverleaf skull, severe proptosis, and ankylosis of the elbows (Fig. 36.7). Type III is manifested by the absence of cloverleaf skull but the presence of elbow ankylosis and high morbidity in infancy. Other abnormalities are severe exorbitism that puts patients at risk for corneal exposure and damage, high-arched palate, crowded teeth, hydrocephalus, and seizures.[145]

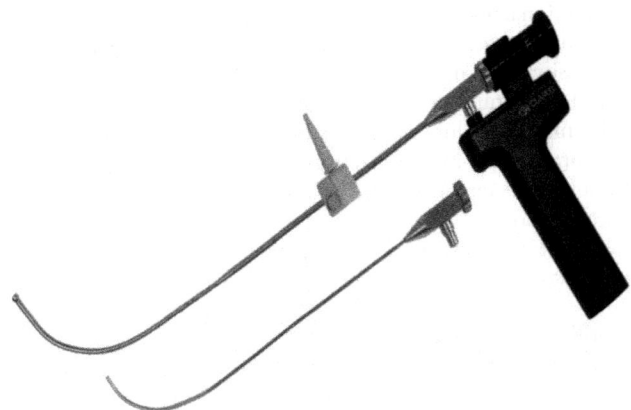

• **Fig. 36.7** Shikani Seeing Optical Stylet (Clarus Medical, Minneapolis, MN) is a reusable, high-resolution fiberoptic endoscope. The pediatric version is compatible with endotracheal tubes in the range of 3 to 5 mm. Supplemental oxygen can be delivered through the oxygen port. It can be used with the SITElite halogen handle (as shown) or a standard green line fiberoptic laryngoscope handle.

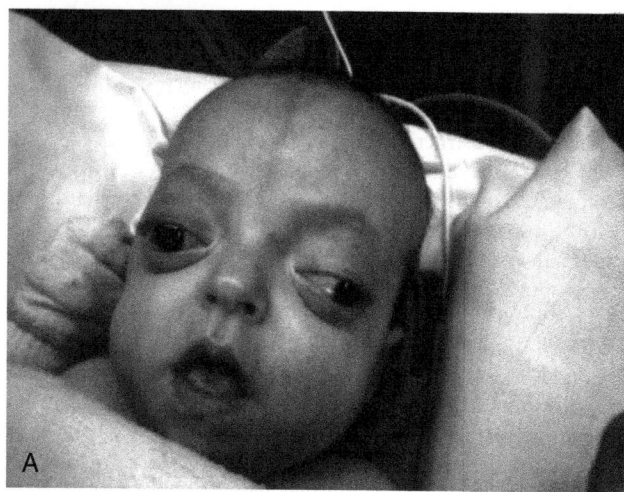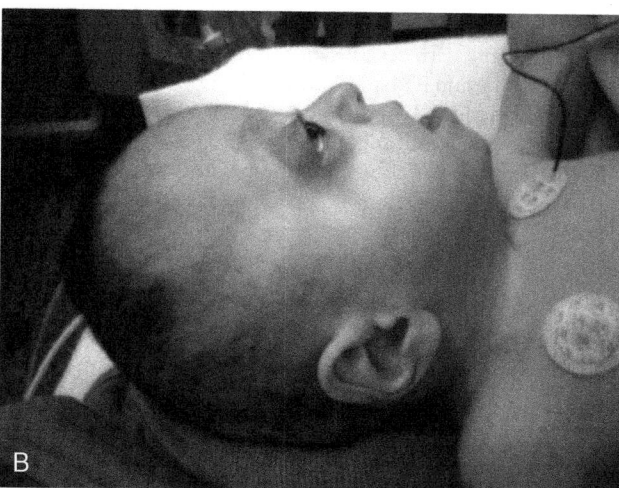

• **Fig. 36.8** (A) Pfeiffer syndrome. Craniosynostosis, marked proptosis, and maxillary retrusion are present. (B) Upper and lower airway obstruction may be present as well.

As with Apert syndrome, Pfeiffer syndrome can arise with upper and lower airway obstruction. Congenital tracheal stenosis,[146] tracheal obstruction related to congenital tracheomalacia,[147] and OSA have been reported.[148] In addition to a high incidence of vertebral fusion (73%), other radiologic abnormalities include hypoplasia of the neural arches, hemivertebrae, and a butterfly vertebra.[149] The C2–C3 level was most often involved, although fusion was noted at all levels of the cervical spine.[150]

Acrocephalopolysyndactyly

Carpenter Syndrome (Type II). Carpenter syndrome (type II) is typically evident at or shortly after birth. Because of craniosynostosis, the top of the head may appear unusually conical (acrocephaly), or the head may seem short and broad (brachycephaly). In addition, the cranial sutures often fuse unevenly, causing the head and face to appear dissimilar from one side to the other (craniofacial asymmetry). Other malformations of the skull and facial (craniofacial) region may include downslanting eyelid folds (palpebral fissures), a flat nasal bridge, small dental malformations,[151] underdeveloped (hypoplastic) upper or lower jaw (maxilla or mandible) or both, and malformed (dysplastic), low-set ears.

Additional abnormalities may include short stature, structural heart malformations (congenital heart defects), mild to moderate obesity, protrusion of portions of the intestine through an abnormal opening in the abdominal wall near the navel (umbilical hernia), or failure of the testes to descend into the scrotum (cryptorchidism) in affected males. Both normal intellect and mild mental retardation have been reported in patients with Carpenter syndrome.[152,153]

DI might be expected in Carpenter syndrome patients with hypoplastic upper or lower jaw, oral malformations, and obesity.

Mandibular Hypoplasia

Mandibular hypoplasia is one of the main anomalies of the mandible, with a profound effect on airway management. Micrognathia results in posterior regression of the tongue and a small hyomental space. The mandible develops from the first branchial arch and is a feature in many rare syndromes (e.g., Pierre Robin, Treacher Collins, Goldenhar, Nager).[154] Although micrognathia is a feature typically shared by these syndromes, they often present additional specific features with adverse effects on the airway.

The finding of periauricular skin tags or abnormally developed external ears, which also develop from the first branchial arch, may be used as a marker for a potential DA. Micrognathia may affect the airway in three ways: (1) The tongue may not be easily moved during laryngoscopy; (2) if the tongue is not pulled forward in the normal developmental manner, the laryngeal inlet appears more anterior and difficult to visualize; and (3) the oral aperture is not opened as easily or as widely.[155] Glossoptosis may further complicate the airway in micrognathic children. Glossoptosis makes displacement of the tongue to the left difficult, so the airway is difficult to visualize.

Pierre Robin Syndrome. Pierre Robin syndrome, which affects 1 in 8500 newborns,[156] was described in 1923 by Pierre Robin as airway obstruction associated with glossoptosis and hypoplasia of the mandible. This syndrome is characterized by retrognathia or micrognathia, glossoptosis, and airway obstruction. An incomplete cleft of the palate is associated with the syndrome in approximately 50% of these patients (Fig. 36.8). Pierre Robin syndrome results from failure of mandibular growth during the first several weeks of embryogenesis. This causes posterior displacement of the tongue, which prevents normal growth and closure of the palate.

The Pierre Robin syndrome represents a spectrum of anatomic anomalies whose common features include mandibular hypoplasia, glossoptosis, and cleft palate. Four types of airway obstruction have been described in patients with Pierre Robin syndrome; in only 50% is the obstruction totally related to posterior positioning of the tongue.[157] Therefore, glossopexy fails to relieve airway obstruction in approximately half of all symptomatic patients with Pierre Robin syndrome. This feature may explain why the use of an oral or nasopharyngeal airway alone may not improve an already difficult mask airway. Patients who fail to improve after glossopexy or nasopharyngeal airway placement, or both, usually require tracheostomy.[52]

A large body of literature details airway management of patients with Pierre Robin syndrome. Preoperative or postoperative airway obstruction and mask ventilation difficulties have been a frequent problem in these patients. In a 10-year retrospective study of 26 infants with Pierre Robin syndrome, Benjamin and Walker found that awake intubation without GA proved to be safer and less difficult when a special-purpose slotted laryngoscope was used.[158]

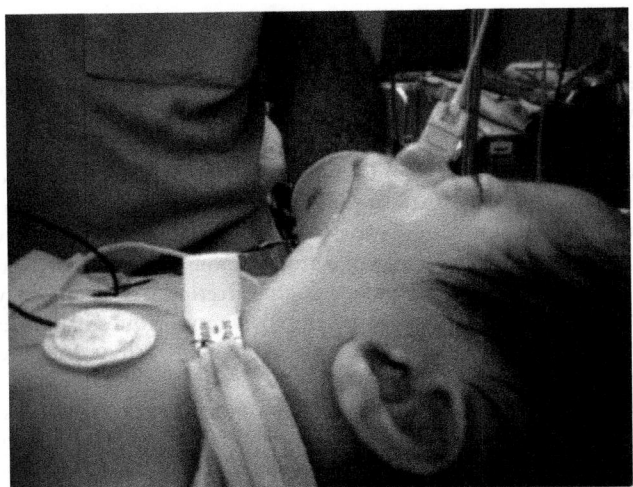

• **Fig. 36.9** Pierre Robin syndrome. Marked micrognathia, glossoptosis, and cleft palate are evident. The micrognathia causes posterior displacement of the tongue, preventing normal development of the palate. Because of the upper airway obstruction present, an elective tracheostomy was performed.

Li and colleagues reviewed the airway management in 110 children with Robin syndrome. Prone posturing was effective in the treatment of mild airway obstruction in 82 patients (90.2%) who had noisy breathing sounds.[159] Only 30% of the patients required tracheal intubation, and 6.6% required tracheostomy (all were eventually decannulated).

Alternative intubation techniques used successfully in patients with Pierre Robin syndrome include SGA,[52,160–162] FSI,[86,163,164] FSI through an SGA,[48] rigid nasoendoscope with video camera or video intubation laryngoscope,[31] Trachlight with a homemade lighted stylet,[165–167] and retrograde intubation.[168] Digitally assisted tracheal intubation and elective tracheal intubation in prone position have also been reported.[169,170]

Treacher Collins Syndrome. Treacher Collins syndrome (mandibulofacial dysostosis, Franceschetti syndrome) results from a deficient vascular supply to the first visceral arch during the initial 3 to 4 weeks of gestation and is believed to be caused by a change in the gene on chromosome 5 that affects facial development and leads to hypoplasia of the facial bones, especially the zygoma and the mandible. There is a 50% chance that the child will pass the trait on to future generations. It is often associated with DI and airway obstruction, mainly related to micrognathia.

Facial clefting causes a hypoplastic facial appearance, with deformities of the ear, orbital, midface, and lower jaw regions. The clinical appearance is a result of the zygoma (malar bone) failing to fuse with the maxilla, frontal, and temporal bones. Highly variant degrees of involvement (complete, incomplete, abortive) can be seen, but common facial features include hypoplastic cheeks, zygomatic arches, and mandible; microtia with possible hearing loss; high-arched or cleft palate; antimongoloid slant to the eyes; colobomas; increased anterior facial height; malocclusion (anterior open bite); small oral cavity and airway with a normal-size tongue; and pointed nasal prominence.

Most children with Treacher Collins syndrome have normal development and intelligence. However, additional physical findings have included a 40% hearing loss, dry eyes, cleft palate, and breathing problems. Both acute and OSAs have been described.[171,172]

An extensive array of complications can affect management. Because of the small jaw and airway, combined with the normal size of the tongue, breathing problems can occur at birth and during sleep when the base of the tongue obstructs the small hypopharynx. This can also cause serious problems during the induction of GA. Consequently, a tracheostomy may be required to control the airway adequately.

The airway of children with Treacher Collins syndrome had been successfully managed with an SGA,[173–175] the Bullard intubating laryngoscope,[176] Augustine stylet,[177] and FSI. Rasch and colleagues[178] recommend that children with obstructive symptoms have laryngoscopy before anesthetic induction. If the glottic opening is visualized, inhalational induction can proceed. If the glottic structures cannot be visualized, the anesthetist must choose between awake oral or nasal intubation, elective tracheostomy, or FSI.

Goldenhar Syndrome/Hemifacial Microsomia. Synonyms of Goldenhar syndrome (hemifacial microsomia) are first and second branchial arch syndrome, facioauricular vertebral spectrum, oculoauricular vertebral dysplasia, and oculoauriculovertebral spectrum disorder. The main feature of this condition is unilateral underdevelopment of one ear (which may not even be present) associated with underdevelopment of the jaw and cheek on the same side of the face. When this is the only problem, it is normally referred to as hemifacial microsomia, but when associated with other abnormalities, particularly of the vertebrae (hemivertebrae or underdeveloped vertebrae, usually in the neck), it is referred to as Goldenhar syndrome. However, these are likely two ends of the spectrum of the same condition.

The muscles of the affected side of the face are underdeveloped. There are often skin tags or pits in front of the ear or in a line between the ear and the corner of the mouth.

Children with the Goldenhar end of the spectrum may have some type of congenital heart disease in 5% to 58% of cases (e.g., ventricular septal defect, patent ductus arteriosus, tetralogy of Fallot, coarctation of aorta). A variety of kidney abnormalities may also be present (e.g., ectopic kidneys, renal agenesis, hydronephrosis).

Difficulties in airway management result from mandibular hypoplasia, cleft or high-arched palate, cervical vertebral anomalies, and scoliosis.[179] Suggested airway management approaches include using a lighted stylet,[180] suspension laryngoscopy,[78] or SGA under anesthesia or using awake FSI through an SGA.[181,182]

Nager Syndrome. Nager syndrome (mandibulofacial dysostosis) is a rare craniofacial disorder with fewer than 100 cases reported in the medical literature. The morphologic features of Nager syndrome include downslanted palpebral fissures, malar hypoplasia, a high nasal bridge, atretic external auditory canals, and micrognathia (severe underdevelopment of the lower jaw). Proximal limb malformations include absent or hypoplastic thumbs, hypoplasia of the radius, and shortened humeral bones.[183] Many of the characteristic facial features may be similar to those of Treacher Collins syndrome. However, patients with Treacher Collins syndrome have more severe maxillary and zygomatic hypoplasia, downslanting palpebral fissures, and lower lid coloboma.

Among the additional problems of children with Nager syndrome are stomach and kidney reflux and hearing loss. Cardiac and spine defects have also been reported.[184] Danziger and colleagues reported four patients with a cardiac defect (type unspecified),[184] and tetralogy of Fallot was reported in another patient.[154]

Difficulties with airway management and postoperative airway obstruction may occur secondary to mandibular hypoplasia with micrognathia, restricted jaw mobility, and microstomia. Associated cleft lip or cleft palate, or both, and maxillary hypoplasia with midface deformities may further complicate airway management and appropriate mask fit during mask ventilation. The airway has been successfully managed with SGA,[185] retrograde intubation,[93] and FSI.[186]

Smith-Lemli-Opitz Syndrome

Smith-Lemli-Opitz syndrome (SLOS) is an autosomal recessive syndrome characterized by congenital anomalies affecting the airway; cardiorespiratory, gastrointestinal, and genitourinary systems; and the CNS. SLOS has an incidence between 1 in 26,500 pregnancies in Canada and 1 in 50,000 pregnancies in the United States.[187,188] The syndrome results from an inborn error of cholesterol biosynthesis involving a deficiency of 3β-hydroxysterol δ7-reductase, the enzyme that catalyzes the reduction of 7-dehydrocholesterol to cholesterol.[189] Patients with SLOS can have severe growth failure, congenital anomalies affecting most organ systems, early death, developmental delay, and self-injurious and ritualistic behavior.[190–192]

Patients with SLOS can be a challenge for airway management because of the typical dysmorphic facial features, including micrognathia, prominent incisors, cleft palate, and a small and abnormally hard tongue. There are several reports of DI and abnormal laryngoscopic views in patients with SLOS.[193–195] An SGA was used successfully in managing the airway in a newborn infant with SLOS.[196]

Quezado and colleagues presented experience from a series of 20 anesthesias in 14 SLOS patients,[197] prospectively deciding to use flexible scope laryngoscopy as the initial technique of intubation in spite of the possible gastroesophageal reflux disease (GERD),[187] muscle rigidity,[195] and behavioral abnormalities in these patients.[192] In all patients, adequate spontaneous ventilation was maintained throughout the airway management. One patient had laryngospasm during induction, and one was intubated by an otolaryngologist.

Cornelia de Lange (Cryptophthalmos) Syndrome

Cornelia de Lange syndrome (CDLS) is a syndrome of multiple congenital anomalies transmitted in an autosomal dominant pattern, characterized by a distinctive facial appearance, prenatal and postnatal growth deficiency, feeding difficulties, psychomotor delay, behavioral problems, and associated malformations mainly involving the upper extremities. The incidence is 1 per 30,000 to 50,000 live births.[198] A most important feature is a striking delay in the maturation of structure and function of most organ systems, including the CNS.[199] CDLS patients are short in stature (the syndrome is also known as Amsterdam dwarfism),[200] have microcephaly (98%), and the facial features are perhaps the most diagnostic of all the physical signs. Cardiac defects occur in 15% of patients.[201]

Intubation may be difficult because of a short (86%), often webbed neck; a high-arched (66%), sometimes cleft palate; and a small mouth with micrognathia (84%). There is also a high incidence of GERD (58%) and hiatal hernia. There are a number of case reports of DI in CDLS; the airway was successfully managed by blind nasal intubation in one case.[202] Lumb and Carli reported respiratory arrest in a 3-year-old child after caudal injection of bupivacaine and hypothesized that changes in intracranial pressure secondary to caudal injection might be the cause of the cardiac arrest.[203]

Hallermann-Streiff Syndrome

Hallermann-Streiff syndrome (oculomandibulodyscephaly with hypotrichosis or oculomandibulofacial syndrome) is rare, with approximately 150 cases reported.[204] Cardinal features are dyscephaly with bird facies; frontal or parietal bossing; dehiscence of sutures with open fontanelles; hypotrichosis of scalp, eyebrows, and eyelashes; cutaneous atrophy of scalp and nose; mandibular hypoplasia; forward displacement of TMJs; high-arched palate; small mouth; multiple dental anomalies; and proportionate small stature.[205,206] Children with Hallermann-Streiff syndrome can have a multitude of cardiorespiratory problems. The incidence of cardiac anomalies is 4.8% and includes septal defects, patent ductus arteriosus, and tetralogy of Fallot. Upper airway obstruction may result from small nares and glossoptosis secondary to micrognathia, which may lead to cor pulmonale.[204]

The patients have natal teeth, which are brittle and may be easily broken or avulsed during laryngoscopy. The TMJ may be easily dislocated. At times, the TMJ is absent, making placement of the ETT by the oral route impossible. Small nostrils, deviated nasal septum, high-arched palate, and anterior larynx preclude blind nasotracheal intubation. The ascending ramus of the mandible is either underdeveloped or absent, resulting in a small mouth cavity. Intubation was achieved with difficulty in two cases with the patient under inhaled anesthesia. In both cases, mask ventilation was impossible.[206,207] Most patients with Hallermann-Streiff syndrome may require elective tracheostomy because of respiratory difficulty.[205]

Turner Syndrome

Turner syndrome (gonadal dysgenesis) is caused by the absence of a second X chromosome. Manifestations of the syndrome include primary amenorrhea, genital immaturity, and short stature; intelligence is usually normal. Additional associated features that may influence the management of anesthesia include hypertension, short neck, high palate, micrognathia, the occasional presence of aortic stenosis or coarctation of aorta, and an absent kidney.

Despite the micrognathia and the short neck, only one case of DI has been published.[208] Because of the small stature, unexpected unilateral endobronchial intubation was reported.[209]

Inflammatory Disease

Juvenile Rheumatoid Arthritis (Still Disease)

Juvenile rheumatoid arthritis (JRA) is a systemic disease of mesenchymal tissues, which may affect collagen and connective tissue of any organ and in which arthritis is one manifestation. Although it is beyond the scope of this review to describe this complex disease, the possible involvement of the heart (36% pericarditis confirmed by echocardiography) should be mentioned.

Abnormalities predisposing to DA management include temporomandibular ankylosis, mandibular hypoplasia, and cricoarytenoid arthritis. Atlantoaxial or low cervical subluxation may occur. The vertebrae may fail to grow, and ankylosis of the apophyseal joints may result.

Difficulty in maintaining the airway patency and inability to intubate the trachea are the most serious anesthetic problems in these children. Severe respiratory distress requiring tracheal intubation has been reported in children with JRA.[210–213] Vetter reported an acute exacerbation of JRA, manifesting as acute arytenoiditis and resulting in marked upper airway obstruction.[213] Symmetrical swelling of the arytenoids and moderate swelling of the epiglottis were noted at laryngoscopy. In another case, direct laryngoscopy demonstrated immobile vocal cords, which were approximated to each other in the midline secondary to arthritis of the cricoarytenoid joints.[212] In both patients, intubation was achieved with some difficulty during direct laryngoscopy, and both recovered after large doses of steroids. Nevertheless, an FIS should always be available in case of failure.

Mouth and Tongue Anomalies

Microstomia

Microstomia (a small mouth opening) is uncommon and may be congenital or acquired. Pediatric microstomia may be congenital (in Freeman-Sheldon [whistling face], Hallermann-Streiff, and otopalatodigital syndromes) but is more often acquired after accidental thermal injuries, such as biting an electrical extension cord or ingesting household lye.[95]

Congenital Microstomia

Freeman-Sheldon Syndrome. Freeman-Sheldon syndrome (whistling face syndrome, windmill-vane-hand syndrome, craniocarpotarsal dysplasia, distal arthrogryposis type 2) is a rare congenital disorder defined by facial and skeletal abnormalities. The three basic abnormalities are microstomia with pouting lips, camptodactyly with ulnar deviation of the fingers, and talipes equinovarus.

Anesthetic challenges include DA management, intravenous cannulation, and regional technique. Patients may be at increased risk for malignant hyperthermia and postoperative pulmonary complications. Oral FSI is considered the preferred airway management technique; the nasal route cannot be used because of small nostrils.[214] An SGA was used successfully in one patient after direct laryngoscopy proved to be impossible.[215,216]

Hallermann-Streiff Syndrome. As discussed previously, Hallermann-Streiff syndrome is a rare congenital disorder in which the presence of mandibular hypoplasia and microstomia makes intubation difficult.

Airway Implications. Again, these patients have brittle natal teeth that may be easily broken or avulsed during laryngoscopy. The TMJ may be easily dislocated[217] and at times is absent, making oral intubation impossible. The small nostrils, deviated nasal septum, high-arched palate, and anterior larynx preclude blind nasotracheal intubation. The ascending ramus of the mandible may either be underdeveloped or absent, resulting in a small mouth cavity. The options available to circumvent these problems are awake intubation, intubation over an FIS, retrograde intubation,[217] and intubation under inhalational anesthesia. Even tracheostomy proved to be difficult in these cases; therefore an experienced pediatric otolaryngologist should be available.[218]

Acquired Microstomia

Epidermolysis Bullosa Hereditaria Dystrophica. Postburn contractures of the neck following a burn injury may hamper cervical hyperextension and lifting of the mandible. Direct laryngoscopy may also be difficult because of rigid scar tissue, which obscures the mandibular and laryngeal anatomy, or microstomia after retraction of scar tissue in facial burns.[219] FSI is the method of choice for securing the airway,[220] but an SGA can also be used successfully. Kreulen and colleagues[219] described a quick surgical neck release of contractures to facilitate tracheal intubation in postburn patients. Bilateral commissurotomy to allow insertion of the laryngoscope into the mouth is also reported.[95] (Also see "Pharyngeal Bullae or Scarring" under "Nasal and Palatal Anomalies.")

Burns from Lye Ingestion. Microstomia from lye ingestion may be associated not only with limited mouth opening but also with such severe intraoral scarring that common landmarks

guiding either rigid or flexible scope laryngoscopy are obscured, rendering oral and nasal intubation difficult or impossible.[95,221]

Diseases of the Tongue

Increase in tongue size is known as macroglossia, defined as a resting tongue that extends beyond the teeth or alveolar ridge.[222]

Congenital Disease

Hemangioma. Hemangiomas are the most common tumor seen during infancy and affect 10% to 12% of white children.[223] Most hemangiomas (70%) are seen during the first weeks of life as an erythematous macula or a telangiectasia. All hemangiomas proliferate during the first year of life. Complications include ulceration, high-output cardiac failure, airway obstruction, and the Kasabach-Merritt syndrome, which results from platelet sequestration and destruction within the hemangioma as well as consumptive coagulopathy. It is fatal in 60% of children.

Lymphangioma. Lymphangioma is a rare congenital disease of unknown etiology.[224] Cystic hygroma of the head and neck, with large lymphatic endothelium-lined cysts, is amenable to surgical excision. Cavernous or microcystic lymphangioma, however, is composed of small lymphatic spaces and poses a therapeutic dilemma by its propensity to cause airway and feeding difficulties and by its tendency to recur despite extensive surgery. All lymphangiomas are present at birth, even though they may not become apparent until the first or second year of life. Although the lymphatic malformation affects preferentially the submandibular space and the neck, it may extend cephalad and invade the tongue and surrounding structures.[224]

Lymphangiomatous involvement of the tongue is generally diffuse and may result in dramatic macroglossia, extending the tongue outside the mouth beyond the lip margins. It is associated with airway obstruction as well as dysphagia and speech, orthodontic, and aesthetic problems. Acute enlargement of the tongue has been reported following trauma or upper respiratory tract infections.

Of the multiple therapeutic methods advocated, surgical laser resection is the mainstay. Repeat laser resection may be necessary because of the tendency for recurrence. Spontaneous resolution is uncommon. In many patients, if lymphangioma is left untreated for extended periods, pulmonary hypertension and cor pulmonale may develop.

In one series, 9 of 18 patients (50%) reviewed required tracheostomy because of the size of the lymphoma and the tendency for recurrence.[225] Nasal FSI was used successfully in these patients.[226]

Traumatic Injury

Burns of the face and mouth can affect the tongue and pharynx. Aspiration of hot liquid can occur in conjunction with upper-body scald burns, leading to thermal epiglottitis, acute compromise of the airway. Clinical features and radiologic findings are similar to those seen in patients with acute infectious epiglottitis.[227] Thermal epiglottitis can be an extremely difficult problem if subtle signs of impending airway compromise are not appreciated. The treatment should be approached with the same caution and preparedness for emergency airway management as for acute infectious epiglottitis. Immediate tracheal intubation should be performed in those with acute respiratory distress, and prompt investigation by direct laryngoscopy in the OR is appropriate in those who have not yet developed overt respiratory distress.[228] Surprisingly, only 9.2% of 1092 burn patients admitted to the Shriners Burns Institute in Galveston, Texas, over a 5-year period needed tracheal intubation or tracheostomy for more than 24 hours.[229] A similar incidence of tracheal intubation (10%) was found after accidental inhalation of caustic substances.[230]

Lymphatic or Venous Obstruction. Tongue swelling may result from prolonged surgical traction and local mechanical pressure. This may be caused by transesophageal echocardiography probe or by dentures in adults.[231,232] Angioneurotic edema or other reactions to drugs can cause marked swelling of the tongue, leading to life-threatening airway emergencies.[233–235]

Metabolic Disorders

Beckwith-Wiedemann syndrome (BWS) comprises a constellation of clinical features including the presence of omphalocele, macroglossia, hypoglycemia (related to hyperinsulinism), inguinal hernia with gigantism, organomegaly, renal medullary dysplasia, cardiac defects, and increased risk for embryonic tumors (4%–21%).[236]

The anesthetic management of children with BWS may be complicated by a potential DA related to macroglossia.[237–239] Because of the high rate of omphalocele in this syndrome, anesthetic care is frequently required during the neonatal period. The SGA has been used successfully in children with BWS.[236] Even though tracheal intubation was possible in most case reports,[237,239,240] airway obstruction presented a major concern, especially after extubation. Swelling, secretions, and blood may precipitate complete airway obstruction. Because of the size of the tongue, additional pathology (tongue hematoma and bleeding) can increase the difficulty of airway management and cause postoperative obstruction.[238]

Glycogen Storage Diseases. Glycogen storage diseases (GSDs) are a heterogeneous group of inherited disorders involving one of the several steps of glycogen synthesis or degradation. They occur in approximately 1 in 20,000 live births. Isolated deficiencies of virtually all the enzymes involved in glycogen processing have been described. The glycogen present in patients with GSD is abnormal in structure, amount, or both. Of the 10 Cori-type GSDs, only Cori type II (Pompe disease, also known as generalized glycogenosis or [lysosomal] acid maltase deficiency) is associated with glycogen infiltration of the skeletal muscle of the tongue, which can lead to macroglossia and potential airway issues.[241]

Severe macroglossia may lead to airway obstruction during anesthetic induction, emergence from anesthesia, or the postoperative period. Associated cardiomyopathy, myopathy, nervous system involvement (especially the motor neurons in the brainstem and spinal cord), and alterations in the regulation of serum glucose concentrations are part of the clinical presentation. Only a few reports address airway problems related to macroglossia in patients with GSD.[242,243]

Lipid Storage Diseases. Lipid storage diseases are characterized by abnormal lecithin-sphingomyelin metabolism, which results in an abnormal amount of lipid products being stored in the cells of the reticuloendothelial system. The lipids include cholesterol (xanthomatosis), cerebroside (Gaucher disease), and sphingomyelin (Niemann-Pick disease). In Gaucher disease, accumulation of the substrate leads to multiorgan dysfunction involving the brain, spleen, liver, lymph nodes, and bone marrow. Airway difficulties may arise because of trismus, limited neck extension, and upper airway infiltration with glucocerebroside. Kita and colleagues found it was impossible to insert an SGA in a 9-year-old child with Gaucher disease because of trismus and a narrowed oral cavity.[244] Subsequently, FSI was performed successfully.

Neurofibromatosis. Neurofibromatoses are a group of hereditary diseases transmitted in an autosomal dominant manner and characterized by a tendency to form tumors of ectodermal and mesodermal tissues. Two distinct forms recognized on clinical and genetic grounds are designated neurofibromatosis type 1 (NF1) and neurofibromatosis type 2 (NF2).[245] Von Recklinghausen NF1 is one of the most common genetic disorders related to an autosomal dominant mutation and occurs at a frequency of 1 in 3000 to 4000 live births.[246] The clinical features of NF1 include café-au-lait spots; neurofibromas involving the skin, deeper peripheral nerves, nerve roots, and blood vessels; intracranial and spinal cord tumors; kyphoscoliosis; short stature; and learning disability. One feature common to all patients is disease progression over time. NF1 is also associated with a higher incidence of malignant disease than NF2.

Possible problems in airway management of the patient with NF1 include the presence of intraoral lesions, tumors compromising the airway, and the presence of thoracic deformities or neurologic lesions. Although their presence in the upper airway is rare, neurofibromas may pose a serious problem in airway management. An estimated 5% of NF1 patients have intraoral manifestations of the disease.[247] Discrete neurofibromas may involve the tongue or the larynx.[248,249] This may cause obstruction, as well as symptoms of dyspnea, stridor, loss or change of voice, or dysphagia, and should warn the anesthetist of potential airway problems.[250] Airway obstruction after induction of anesthesia has been reported in patients with a tongue neurofibroma and a neurofibroma involving the laryngeal inlet.[247,250] Both patients required emergency tracheostomy. Even if intraoral pathology is recognized preoperatively, elective awake FSI may fail because of a grossly distorted anatomy. In addition, the presence of macroglossia, macrocephaly, mandibular abnormalities, and cervical spine involvement may contribute to difficulties of airway management.[245]

Tongue Tumors

Lingual Tonsil Hypertrophy. The lingual tonsil, a normal component of Waldeyer ring, consists of lymphoid tissue located at the base of the tongue. Acute inflammation and hypertrophy of lingual tonsils can occur and has been reported as one of the unusual causes of unexpected difficulty with both mask ventilation and tracheal intubation.[251,252] Lingual tonsil hypertrophy (LTH), or lingual tonsillar hyperplasia, has occasionally been reported in children but more often occurs in adults, particularly in atopic individuals.[253,254] The etiology is unclear. However, LTH is thought to be a compensatory mechanism following removal of the palatine tonsils or secondary to a chronic, low-grade infection of the tonsils.[254,255]

Clinically, LTH is not detectable on routine preoperative physical examination.[256] Although many patients are asymptomatic, others may complain of a globus sensation, alteration of voice, chronic cough, choking, or dyspnea.[257] The first to report a death secondary to failed airway management in a patient with unrecognized LTH were Jones and Cohle.[256] Asai and colleagues[251] reported a case of suboptimal ventilation and failed tracheal intubation using various intubation strategies, including an intubating SGA and FIS.

Enlarged lingual tonsils can impinge against the epiglottis, displacing it posteriorly. This can make mobilization of the epiglottis difficult during direct laryngoscopy. Similarly, FSI is often equally difficult because the posterior displacement of the epiglottis causes interference with the insertion of the tip of the endoscope under it. These difficulties may be compounded by the presence of redundant pharyngeal tissue interfering with flexible scope exposure and the use of muscle relaxants.[256] With the onset of neuromuscular blockade, the pharyngeal musculature relaxes, causing further posterior movement of the tongue and epiglottis.[258]

In a retrospective study of unexpected DI in 33 patients, Ovassapian and colleagues reported that the only finding common to all patients was LTH observed on flexible scope pharyngoscopy.[259] Most of the patients had normal airway measurements (Mallampati class of I or II), and 36% of patients were difficult to ventilate.

The SGA has been used in CICO situations caused by LTH with both success and partial success.[260–263] Asai and colleagues highlighted that the SGA cannot always solve a truly glottic or subglottic problem; rather, the ventilatory mechanism must get below the lesion.[251] If an airway cannot be established with an SGA, TTJV and cricothyrotomy are other options. Crosby and Skene recommended the Bullard laryngoscope (which can be fitted with a camera) as the airway device of choice for LTH patients because its robust construction permits gentle manipulation of airway tissues, allowing it to create the necessary endoscopic airspace.[261]

Other masses situated at the base of the tongue may displace the epiglottis and may distort the airway anatomy. Such masses include thyroglossal duct cysts and thyroid tumors.

Nasal and Palatal Anomalies

Nasal obstruction in pediatric patients may result from choanal atresia or stenosis, nasal masses, foreign body, trauma, or adenoidal hypertrophy, as well as choanal stenosis combined with nasal mucosal edema.[264,265] These lesions may become evident at birth or later in childhood. Nonpalatal anomalies can result in airway obstruction and feeding difficulty and can complicate airway management.

Choanal Atresia

Choanal atresia is a congenital anomaly of the nasal choana that results in lack of continuity between the nasal cavity and the pharynx. This entity is rare and results from failure of resorption of the mesiobuccal membrane at the sixth to seventh week of gestation. Congenital choanal atresia is usually bony and unilateral versus membranous and bilateral. Complete nasal obstruction in a newborn may cause death from asphyxia. During attempted inspiration, the tongue is pulled to the palate, obstructing the oral airway. Vigorous respiratory efforts produce marked chest retraction. Death may occur if appropriate treatments are not available; however, if the infant cries and takes a breath through the mouth, the airway obstruction is momentarily relieved. The crying then stops, the mouth closes, and the cycle of obstruction is repeated.

Many patients have associated narrowed nasopharynx, widened vomer, medialized lateral nasal wall, or arched hard palate. Associated malformations occur in 47% of infants without chromosomal anomalies. Such malformations include cleft palate, cleft lip, and Treacher Collins syndrome. The upper airway abnormalities are present in 56% of patients with choanal atresia.[266]

Nonrandom association of malformations can be demonstrated using the CHARGE association, which appears to be overused in clinical practice. The components of the CHARGE association are **c**oloboma, 80%; **h**eart disease, 58%; **a**tresia choanae, 100%; **r**etarded growth, 87%; development, or CNS anomalies, 97%; **g**enital hypoplasia, 75%; and **e**ar anomalies or deafness, 88%. Other airway abnormalities, as part of the CHARGE association, may be present.[267]

A high level of suspicion is required to diagnose bilateral choanal atresia. Symptoms of severe airway obstruction and cyclic cyanosis are the classic signs of neonatal bilateral atresia.

If bilateral, choanal atresia is a medical emergency that becomes evident after birth with severe respiratory distress and cyanosis. These signs resolve with crying and recur when crying stops or the infant attempts to feed. In unilateral disease, the signs and symptoms are less evident and thus may result in delayed diagnosis. These patients come to medical attention with unilateral nasal discharge and mouth breathing. Respiratory distress occurs when the second nostril becomes obstructed, as during an upper respiratory tract infection. Older children display nasal discharge, inability to blow the nose on the affected side, nasal speech, and mouth breathing.

The diagnosis is based on history and physical examination, inability to pass a nasal catheter into the nasopharynx, flexible scope examination, and radiologic studies. CT scan is useful in demonstrating the atretic area.

Treatment of the choanal atresia is directed at providing the patient with a patent airway. Infants may benefit from the placement of an oral airway. Feeding may take place in the form of gavage (tube feeding). Tracheal intubation is usually not needed unless there are associated congenital anomalies, and tracheostomy is not necessary. Surgical correction is not an emergency and uses an endonasal or a transpalatal approach to remove the bony or membranous obstruction and part of the vomer and stent the newly created path. In infants, the transpalatal approach is used less often because of the risk of injury to the palatal growth center.

Roger and colleagues evaluated the need for a tracheostomy and its timing in 45 patients during the evolution of CHARGE association.[268] They found a high percentage of associated airway abnormalities: pharyngolaryngeal anomalies leading to dyspnea (58%; discoordinate pharyngolaryngomalacia, glossoptosis, retrognathia, laryngeal paralysis, DI) and tracheobronchial anomalies (40%; tracheoesophageal fistula, esophageal atresia, tracheomalacia). Tracheostomy was necessary in 13 patients (29%) despite the posterior nasal choanae being patent in 10 patients. The authors concluded that often a tracheostomy could not be avoided in these patients, regardless of choanal patency, and that tracheostomy needs to be performed early to avoid hypoxic events.

Asher and colleagues studied the association between catastrophic airway events and developmental delay in patients with CHARGE association.[269] They found that children with CHARGE association have a propensity for airway instability and that cerebral hypoxia contributed to the developmental delay in some of the patients. They recommended early tracheostomy rather than early choanal atresia repair in these patients to protect the CNS.

If micrognathia or subglottic stenosis is present, a difficult tracheal intubation should be anticipated. Awake tracheal intubation, direct laryngoscopy, indirect visual techniques, or nonvisual intubation techniques may be tried. If the patient with choanal atresia has tracheal stenosis, a smaller-than-usual ETT must be available.

Nasal Masses

Nasal mass lesions are rare disorders in the pediatric population, with an incidence of 1 in 20,000 to 40,000 live births.[270,271] Nasal mass lesions are a diverse group of lesions that include anomalies of embryogenesis, such as encephaloceles, dermal and nasolacrimal duct cysts, tumors, and inflammatory processes.[270] Encephaloceles represent herniation of CNS tissue at the level of the cranium. Although most encephaloceles are located in the occipital area, some occur anteriorly and may contain various quantities of brain tissue. Encephaloceles may be associated with midline defects. Dermal cysts become evident as hard intranasal masses that result from herniation of dura and subsequent contact with the skin. These midline defects may manifest as a nasal obstruction without a facial mass. There is a risk of local abscess formation and intracranial infection.

Tumors located in the nasal area in children are rare and include hemangiomas, neurofibromas, angiofibromas, hamartomas, lipomas, and rhabdomyosarcomas. Radiologic studies (CT, MRI, angiography) can elucidate the size and position of the mass and display coexistence of any cranial bone defect. The mainstay of treatment is surgery.

A foreign body in the nostril is a finding in small children, usually a toy part or food substance. This typically manifests as nasal discharge, which may be purulent, foul smelling, or bloody, and obstruction of the affected side. Diagnosis is made by history, examination of the nares, and, occasionally, radiologic evaluation.

Nasal masses can affect the management of the airway by interfering with mask ventilation or with direct laryngoscopy and tracheal intubation. Nasotracheal intubation in these patients should be avoided. Extension of a cephalocele through a palatal defect interfered with tracheal intubation in one patient.[272] All the airway implications previously discussed under choanal atresia with unilateral (or even bilateral) obstruction are valid in patients with nasal airway obstruction.

Palatal Anomalies

Cleft lip and cleft palate are the most common of the craniofacial anomalies, with an incidence of approximately 1 in 800 live births; 25% of cleft lip cases are bilateral, 85% of which are associated with cleft palate. There has been a move toward earlier surgical repair of both cleft lip and palate, with cleft lip repair being performed in the neonatal period in some centers.

Anomalies of the palate include cleft and high-arched deformities and hypertrophy of the alveolar ridge area. In two studies of children undergoing palate repair, the incidence of difficult laryngoscopy (Cormack and Lehane grades III and IV) was 6.5% and 7.4%.[266,273] Of the 59 patients with difficult laryngoscopy in Gunawardana's study, 2.95% had unilateral cleft lip, 45.76% had bilateral cleft lip, and 34.61% had retrognathia.[266] Interestingly, tracheal intubation was successful in 99% of patients in whom laryngoscopy was difficult (failed intubation was 1%). There was a significant association between age and laryngoscopic view: 66.1% of patients with difficult laryngoscopies were younger than 6 months, 20.3% were 6 to 12 months, and 13.6% were 1 to 5 years old.

The presence of other associated congenital anomalies, including cardiac and renal anomalies, should always be remembered, particularly in children with isolated cleft palate. More than 150 syndromes have been described in association with cleft lip or palate, but fortunately all are rare. Some, however, have considerable anesthetic implications, and many involve potential airway problems, including the well-known Pierre Robin, Treacher Collins, and Goldenhar syndromes. Others, such as Klippel-Feil syndrome, may include abnormalities of the cervical spine.[274]

Henriksson and Skoog reviewed the records of 154 patients who underwent closure of the palate and found that 84% had isolated cleft palate, 12% had Pierre Robin syndrome, and the rest had other identified syndromes.[275] The risk of anesthetic complications was four times greater with surgery in children less than 1 year of age, with a sixfold increase when a more elaborate velopharyngoplasty technique was used.

The airway complications after palatoplasty ranged between 5.6% and 8% in two surveys.[276,277] As a rule, patients with cleft palate with the Pierre Robin syndrome or other additional congenital anomalies had an increased risk for airway problems after palatoplasty.

Palatal edema or hematoma may also develop. Swelling limited to the soft palate or uvula can cause posture-dependent airway obstruction in children.[278] Edema may result from instrumentation of the airway, burn injury, allergy, or infectious agents.

Many methods of management of DA in patients with cleft palate have been described. The use of firm pressure over the larynx (cricoid pressure) to aid laryngoscopy, with a bougie as a guide to tracheal intubation, is relatively simple to perform by any competent anesthetist and is usually successful.[266] Other techniques (e.g., SGA, FIS) have been described,[274] especially when cleft palate is associated with different syndromes.

Adenotonsillar Disease

Together, the lingual tonsils anteriorly, the palatine tonsils laterally, and the pharyngeal tonsils (adenoids) posterosuperiorly form a ring of lymphoid or adenoid tissue at the upper end of the pharynx known as the Waldeyer tonsillar ring. All the structures of the Waldeyer ring have similar histology and function and, regarding airway management, produce similar symptoms and require treatment. In response to recurrent infections, adenoids and tonsils can hypertrophy and lead to airway obstruction.[279]

Adenoidal hypertrophy peaks at 4 to 6 years of age and disappears by adolescence. Although a disease of the older child, hypertrophy can occur in the infant. One of the major complications of adenoidal hyperplasia is OSA. Signs and symptoms of airway obstruction include snoring and restless sleep, somnolence during the day, noisy breathing, mouth breathing, hyponasal speech, persistent nasal secretions, apnea, choking during feeding, respiratory distress, and behavioral disturbances.[163] If the condition is left untreated, the following may develop: failure to thrive; a characteristic, long adenoid facies with open mouth, palate, and dental malformations; and cardiovascular changes (cor pulmonale) reflective of chronic hypoxemia and hypercapnia.[280]

Airway obstruction resulting from adenoid tissue is determined not by the absolute size of the adenoids but rather by their size relative to the volume of the pharynx.[252] Patients with preexisting diseases that reduce nasopharyngeal size or alter its integrity may have airway obstruction with only mild degrees of adenoidal hyperplasia. Examples are children with craniofacial anomalies (in whom the nasopharynx may be reduced in size) and those with nasal polyps, septal or turbinate malformations, MPS, or deficient pharyngeal support (Down syndrome).

Tonsillar hyperplasia is a physiologic phenomenon of childhood that peaks at about 7 years of age. It can cause OSA with restless sleep and an irregular breathing pattern, snoring, and intermittent periods of apnea as well as daytime somnolence, irritability, and poor school performance.[281] Long-standing partial obstruction of the airway can be associated with repeated hypoxic episodes and may result in pulmonary hypertension, cor pulmonale, and right-sided heart failure. Acute exacerbation of adenotonsillar hypertrophy may necessitate emergent airway security.[282,283]

The treatment of adenoidal and tonsillar hyperplasia is adenoidectomy and tonsillectomy. These are among the most common surgical procedures in children. There are multiple indications for excision of tonsils and adenoids.[279] Upper airway obstruction is of most concern for the anesthesiologist because these patients may have airway obstruction both during induction of anesthesia and in the postoperative period.

Upper airway obstruction may occur after premedication, during induction of anesthesia, or following tracheal extubation. Visualization of the glottis during direct laryngoscopy may be difficult with tonsillar hypertrophy. Resection of tonsils and adenoids may not result in immediate relief of airway obstruction. Bleeding and edema can make the child susceptible to postoperative airway obstruction. Although it usually causes chronic upper airway obstruction, adenotonsillar hypertrophy can result in acute airway obstruction.[282–284] Airway assessment and management of patients with OSA caused by adenotonsillar hypertrophy are detailed in the next section.

Peritonsillar abscess in children manifests as a purulent mass surrounded by the tonsillar capsule. It occurs more frequently in untreated children with chronic tonsillitis or those who have been inadequately treated.[279] Signs and symptoms include fever, sore throat, tonsillar mass, dysphagia, drooling (caused by odynophagia and dysphagia), muffled voice, trismus (caused by irritation of pterygoid muscle by pus and inflammation), and variable degrees of toxic state. Peritonsillar abscess requires intravenous antibiotic therapy. If symptoms of airway obstruction develop or the patient fails to respond to medical therapy, needle aspiration, incision, and drainage with tonsillectomy are recommended.[279] In a prospective study of 50 adult patients with peritonsillar abscess, the Mallampati score did not correlate with the Cormack and Lehane glottic view during laryngoscopy because of palatopharyngeal arch distortion. There were no DIs in this study group.[285]

Peritonsillar abscess affects the airway in a manner similar to tonsillar hypertrophy, except that the patients may have trismus. There may be associated edema of the supraglottic area, uvula, and soft palate that exacerbates airway obstruction. Patients are susceptible to airway obstruction during either spontaneous breathing or manual mask ventilation. During direct laryngoscopy, care should be taken not to rupture the abscess. When large, the abscess may interfere with visualization of the vocal cords.

Obstructive Sleep Apnea

Definition
Obstructive sleep apnea syndrome (OSAS) in children is a disorder of breathing during sleep characterized by prolonged partial upper airway obstruction or intermittent complete obstruction (obstructive apnea) that disrupts normal ventilation during sleep and normal sleep patterns.[286]

Prevalence of Snoring
The prevalence of primary snoring ranges from 3.2% to 12.1%, whereas the prevalence of OSAS ranges from 0.7% to 10.3%.[35,287,288] The ability to maintain upper airway patency during the normal respiratory cycle is the result of a delicate equilibrium between various forces that promote airway closure and dilatation. This balance of pressure concept was first proposed independently by Remmers and colleagues in 1978 and Brouillette and Thach in 1979 and represents the current thought regarding the pathophysiologic mechanisms of OSAS.[289,290]

The four major predisposing factors for upper airway obstruction are as follows.
1. An anatomic narrowing of the upper airway behaves as predicted by the Sterling resistor model. The maximal inspiratory flow is determined by the pressure changes upstream (nasal) to a collapsible site of the upper airway, and flow is independent of downstream (tracheal) pressure generated by the diaphragm.

Children with OSAS close their airways at the level of the enlarged adenoids and tonsils at low positive pressures, whereas healthy children require subatmospheric pressures to induce upper airway closure.[291]
2. There is abnormal mechanical linkage between airway dilating muscles and airway walls. Control of the upper airway size and stiffness depends on the relative and rhythmic contraction of a host of paired muscles, which include palatal, pterygoid, tensor palatini, genioglossus, geniohyoid, and sternohyoid. With contraction, these muscles promote motion of the soft palate, mandible, tongue, and hyoid bone. The activity of these muscles is dependent on the brainstem respiratory network. Wakefulness conveys a supervisory function that ensures airway patency, and sedative agents that compromise genioglossal muscle activity may result in significant upper airway compromise. Roberts and colleagues demonstrated that mechanoreceptor-mediated and chemoreceptor-mediated genioglossal activity are critical for maintenance of upper airway patency in both normal and micrognathic infants.[292]
3. There is little evidence to suggest that intrinsic muscle weakness is a major contributor to upper airway dysfunction; nevertheless, in patients with neuromuscular disorders, airway obstruction is frequently observed during sleep.[293]
4. Neural regulation is abnormal. Subtle alterations in central chemoreceptor activity were found by different researchers. Gozal and colleagues reported that arousal to hypercapnia was blunted, whereas Onal and colleagues found that upper airway musculature is more stimulated than the diaphragm.[294,295]

Pathophysiology and Clinical Picture
The etiology and pathophysiology of OSAS in children are multifactorial, with anatomic and neuromuscular abnormalities playing a major role in the disorder.[296–300] Others, however, downplay the role of neuromuscular factors because the vast majority of children with OSAS can be cured by correcting anatomic obstructions. The narrowing of the airway lumen by hypertrophied lymphoid tissue, compliance, elasticity of the pharyngeal soft tissue, facial morphology, and the physiologic changes that occur in the pharyngeal dilators during sleep determine the severity of airway collapse.

Patients with dysmorphic constricted craniofacial development—such as those with Pierre Robin syndrome; Treacher Collins, Apert, or Crouzon syndrome; or neuromuscular abnormalities, as in cerebral palsy and anoxic encephalopathy—have a much higher incidence of severe OSAS.

Adenotonsillar hypertrophy plays a major role in the pathogenesis of OSAS in children. The volume of lymphoid tissue in the upper airway increases from about 6 months of age up to puberty, with the maximum proliferation occurring in the preschool years, which coincides with the peak incidence of OSAS in children. Despite this narrowing of the upper airway by lymphoid tissue, most children do not develop OSAS. A normal child's airway is less likely to collapse in sleep than the adult airway.

One of the hallmarks of sleep-disordered breathing is fragmentation and disruption of normal sleep architecture. By definition, deeper levels of sleep, especially rapid-eye-movement (REM) sleep, are less susceptible to arousal from various stimuli, including adverse ventilatory events.[301] Oxyhemoglobin desaturation therefore tends to be more frequent and more severe during REM sleep. The hypercapnia and hypoxemia with resulting arousals often lead to a reduction in REM sleep.[301,302]

While OSAS and hypertension are often associated in adults, children with OSAS also tend to have higher diastolic blood pressure. The cardiovascular changes appear to be the result of an increase in sympathetic tone that results from sleep arousals, which in turn are related to the obstructive respiratory events.[303] The clinical presentation of OSAS in children has many similarities and important differences compared with the disorder in adults (Table 36.4).[248,302,304]

Unlike findings in adults, obesity is not commonly associated in pediatric OSAS, although its role increases with the age of the child.[305] Abnormal sleep positions with preference for an upright position and hyperextension of the neck have been noted in children with sleep-related breathing disorders.[306]

Prolonged exposure to hypoxia and hypercarbia results in compensatory changes in the pulmonary vasculature. Pulmonary vascular resistance increases, causing increased right ventricular strain.[307] Severe cases may progress to pulmonary hypertension, dysrhythmias, and cor pulmonale.[308]

Laboratory Evaluation

Polysomnography (PSG) remains the gold standard for the diagnosis of OSAS in adults and children. In 1995 the American Thoracic Society adopted guidelines for performing PSG in children.[309] Use of PSG was recommended to differentiate primary snoring, which does not require any form of treatment, from OSAS, which can lead to cardiopulmonary dysfunction and functional impairment if left untreated.[310] In general, studies show that history alone does not have sufficiently high diagnostic sensitivity or specificity to be the basis for recommending therapy.[311]

In a study of 50 healthy children, Marcus and colleagues reported normal PSG values for the various respiratory events.[311] The apnea indices (number of apneas per hours of total sleep time [TST]) were 0.1 ± 0.5, with the minimum oxygen saturation being 96%, maximal drop in saturation 4%, and CO_2 greater than 55 mm Hg no more than 0.5% of TST. An abnormal study includes an apnea index greater than 1, oxygen desaturation greater than 4% more than three times an hour or associated with a greater than 25% change in heart rate, oxygen desaturation less than 92%, and elevation of end tidal CO_2 ($EtCO_2$) to more than 52 mm Hg for more than 8% of TST or 45 mm Hg for more than 60% of TST (Table 36.5).

TABLE 36.4 Adult Versus Childhood Obstructive Sleep Apnea Syndrome

Features	Adult OSAS	Childhood OSAS
Snoring	Intermittent	Continuous
Mouth breathing	Uncommon	Continuous
Obesity	Common	Uncommon
Failure to thrive	—	Common
Daytime hypersomnolence	Common	Uncommon
Gender predilection	Male	None
Most common obstructive event	Apnea	Hypopnea
Arousal	Common	Uncommon treatment
Nonsurgical	CPAP in majority	CPAP in minority
Surgery	Selected cases in majority	T&A

CPAP, continuous positive airway pressure; *OSAS*, obstructive sleep apnea syndrome; *T&A*, tonsillectomy and adenoidectomy.

TABLE 36.5 Normal Sleep Study Measurements in Children

Measurement	Normal Values
Sleep latency (minutes)	>10
TST (hours)	>5.5
REM sleep (%)	>15% TST
Stage 3 and 4 non-REM sleep (%)	>25% TST
Respiratory arousal index (no./h TST)	>5
Periodic leg movements (no./h TST)	>1
Apnea index (no./h TST)	>1
Hypopnea index (nasal/esophageal pressure catheter; no./h TST)	<3
RDI (apnea/hypopnea index)	<1
Nadir oxygen saturation (%)	<92
Mean oxygen saturation (%)	<95
Desaturation index (<4% for 5 s; no./h TST)	<5
Highest CO_2 (mm Hg)	52
CO_2 <45 mm Hg	>20% TST

no., Number; *RDI*, respiratory disturbance index; *REM*, rapid eye movement; *TST*, total sleep time.

Treatment of OSAS

Medical therapy of pediatric OSAS is not considered to be consistently effective. Systemic or topical steroids may shrink lymphoid tissue, but the long-term effectiveness is not known, and a short course of systemic corticosteroids appears to be ineffective. Topical intranasal steroids appear to reduce the severity of OSAS.[312]

Adenotonsillectomy remains the mainstay of treatment for pediatric OSAS.[313,314] The optimal age for adenotonsillectomy is 4 to 7 years, although a young age, even under 1 year, is not a contraindication for surgery for airway obstruction or OSAS. Children with Down syndrome deserve further comment because they frequently have severe OSAS.[315] Although data are conflicting on the usefulness of adenotonsillectomy in this group, it appears worthwhile if the tonsils or adenoids are obstructing the airway. If an adenotonsillectomy fails or is not considered appropriate therapy, uvulopalatopharyngoplasty may be effective.[35]

Several studies demonstrated the relative safety of adenotonsillectomy performed on an outpatient basis with a suitable period of postoperative observation and hydration. It appears that if children meet standard discharge criteria (normal respiratory parameters, no bleeding, adequate oral intake and pain control, normal mental status) at 4 to 6 hours after surgery, they can be safely discharged home regardless of age or preoperative diagnoses.

Minimal specific evidence exists for or against the use of opiates and sedatives in the perioperative period in children with OSAS. To date, there are only anecdotal reports of respiratory depression in children in response to sedatives such as chloral hydrate and in the postoperative period, including hypoxia.[316–320] Children with OSAS appear to have increased sensitivity to opioids.

Waters and colleagues found that children with OSAS develop more pronounced respiratory depression than with aged-matched control subjects when breathing spontaneously under anesthetic with the upper airway secured.[321] Addition of a small dose of opioids increased the respiratory depression in children with OSAS. The low dose of fentanyl used (0.5 µg/kg) precipitated central apnea in 46% of the OSAS group. In this study, the best predictor of opioid-induced central apnea was an increase in $EtCO_2$ to levels of 50 mm Hg or greater during spontaneous breathing after anesthetic induction. In contrast to the previous studies,[319,321–323] Wilson and colleagues found no correlation between the preoperative cardiorespiratory sleep study (PSG and home sleep studies) parameters and opioid administration and postoperative outcome.[324]

Few studies provide data pertaining to complications of surgery in children undergoing adenotonsillectomy for upper airway obstruction. All specifically address the risk of postoperative respiratory obstruction (Table 36.6).[318–320,322–327] The authors define respiratory compromise in various ways but generally consider the need for supplemental oxygen as a minimum criterion. The studies report a wide range for the incidence of postoperative respiratory complications (0%–27%), primarily because their populations include different proportions of children with neuromuscular, chromosomal, and craniofacial disorders.

Young age (<3 years) and associated medical problems were found in most studies to define the highest-risk groups. A high preoperative respiratory disturbance index (apnea/hypopnea index) also seems to be a risk factor for postoperative complications.[319,320] Time to onset of respiratory compromise after adenotonsillectomy appears to be brief, although McColley and colleagues reported that one patient required 14 hours to manifest respiratory symptoms.[319] Postobstructive pulmonary edema may develop in some children undergoing adenotonsillectomy for relief of upper airway obstruction. The incidence of this complication is unknown, and pulmonary edema often manifests immediately after tracheal intubation.

The patient's position after extubation seems to be important for the development of airway obstruction. Ishikawa and colleagues found that prone position increases upper airway collapsibility in anesthetized infants.[328] Isono and colleagues, in a study of adult patients, reported that lateral position structurally improves maintenance of the passive pharyngeal airway in OSAS patients.[329] These findings are in concordance with the current practice of extubating and transporting children in the lateral position.

In a retrospective study of 163 OSAS children, Wilson and colleagues found a 21% incidence of respiratory compromise requiring medical interventions after adenotonsillectomy.[324] Of the children with OSAS, 96% were managed in a recovery room or ward setting and 6 required postoperative admission to the intensive care unit (ICU).

Most of the polysomnographic studies done weeks after adenotonsillectomy in children with OSAS reported a cure rate between 85% and 100%.[330,331] A major concern is the effect of residual anesthetic and sedative medication as well as edema of the pharyngeal tissues on the complications related to airway obstruction in the immediate postoperative period. Helfaer and coauthors tried to respond to these concerns by comparing preoperative and first-night postoperative polysomnograms in children with mild OSAS.[318] Surprisingly, most of the children had improvements in their sleep studies on the night of surgery. Specifically, intraoperative administration of opioids was not associated with postoperative respiratory impairment. Even though this study was performed on a relatively small number of patients with mild disease, it was concluded that children with mild OSAS can be safely discharged home on the day of surgery (see Table 36.6).

In our institution, the criteria for postoperative admission are severe OSAS; age less than 3 years; associated craniofacial anomalies (including Down syndrome); associated neuromotor, cardiac, or pulmonary diseases; upper airway burn; hypotonia; morbid obesity; or recent upper respiratory tract infection. These criteria may serve as a guide to other institutions developing admission criteria for OSAS.

In conclusion, the anesthetic management of OSAS should be directed toward assessing and managing the coexisting cardiac or pulmonary diseases; managing the airway, especially in syndromic children; minimizing the amount of opioid used intraoperatively; using capnography in the postoperative period; and preventing and managing the possible postoperative complications. Preoperative sleep studies are necessary for a positive diagnosis and to guide postoperative monitoring. Therefore, anesthesiologists should review the results of the sleep study in order to devise an appropriate anesthetic plan.

Retropharyngeal and Parapharyngeal Abscesses

The various cavities and virtual spaces in the pharynx and neck are in anatomic continuity with one another. The retropharyngeal, parapharyngeal, peritonsillar, and submandibular spaces intercommunicate, and infection in one can extend to the others. The superior limit of the retropharyngeal space is the base of the skull; inferiorly, it extends into the mediastinum to the level of the tracheal bifurcation.

Retropharyngeal abscess is a rare but potentially fatal infection of the pharyngeal wall. It occurs primarily in pediatric patients; in one study, more than half of the patients were younger than 12 months.[332] In children, it usually results from suppurative involvement of lymph nodes located in the retropharyngeal space. These nodes drain lymph from the pharynx, nasopharynx, paranasal sinuses, and middle ear. The most common pathogens are *Staphylococcus aureus* (25%), *Klebsiella* species (13%), group A streptococci (8%), and a mixture of gram-negative and anaerobic organisms (38%).[332,333] Other causes of retropharyngeal abscess include spread of infection from pharyngitis or peritonsillar abscess, penetrating trauma, and foreign body ingestion.

Clinical presentation of retropharyngeal abscess varies with the patient's age. Most children have fever, some degree of toxic appearance, a hyperextended or stiff neck, dysphagia, drooling, trismus, muffled voice, and respiratory distress. Infants and young children may have stridor. Older children with mediastinal involvement may, in addition, complain of chest pain. Physical examination may reveal cervical lymphadenopathy and pharyngeal swelling. A lateral radiograph of the neck typically shows widening of the retropharyngeal prevertebral soft tissue. CT is helpful in the diagnosis of retropharyngeal abscess but is limited in differentiating cellulitis and abscess. Lateral neck radiography was found to be very specific for an abscess when the air sign was present.[334] Ultrasound imaging can also distinguish between suppurative and presuppurative stage.[335] Chest radiographs may show mediastinal involvement and tracheal deviation.[336]

Complications of retropharyngeal abscess include airway obstruction, abscess rupture, pneumonia, sepsis, and extension of the disease into the mediastinum and the carotid sheath, causing mediastinitis, jugular vein thrombosis, or penetration into the carotid artery. Treatment consists of airway support, antibiotic therapy, and early incision and drainage.

The danger of retropharyngeal abscess is related to the potential for rapid progression to airway obstruction. In one report, 5 of 65 patients required tracheostomy.[337] There is also an ever-present risk of abscess rupture and aspiration of pus into the airway. The clinical presentation of children with retropharyngeal abscess can mimic that of children with epiglottitis and croup. Deaths are

TABLE 36.6 Respiratory Compromise After Adenotonsillectomy in Children With Obstructive Sleep Apnea Syndrome

Author	Year	Methodology and Rating	Inclusion Criteria	No.	Rate of Respiratory Compromise	Comments
McGowan et al.[327]	1992	Case series, level IV	Clinical upper airway obstruction	53	25%	Risk factors for complications were prematurity, adenoidal facies, preoperative respiratory distress.
McColley et al.[320]	1992	Case series, level IV	Abnormal PSG	69	23%	Onset up to 14 hours postoperatively. Main risk factors were age and preoperative RDI.
Price et al.[321]	1993	Case series, level IV	Clinical upper airway obstruction, nap PSG	160	19%	Associations with risk factors (age, preoperative PSG) asserted but not quantitated
Rosen et al.[322]	1994	Case series, level IV	Abnormal PSG	37	27%	Postoperative obstruction occurred within hours of surgery. All patients with complications were complex and had a higher mean RDI preoperation.
Helfaer et al.[323]	1996	Case series, level IV	Mild OSAS by PSG (no severe cases)	15	0%	No postoperation desaturation or obstruction in children with mild OSAS
Geber et al.[324]	1996	Case series, level IV	Questionnaire	292	15% (38% if age <3 years)	Included complex patients. Respiratory compromise developed only in patients who snored preoperatively.
Rottschild et al.[328]	1994	Case series, level IV	Clinical diagnosis	69	7%	Specific diagnostic criteria for OSAS not specified.
Bivati et al.[323]	1997	Case series, level IV	Clinical diagnosis	355	25% (36% with abnormal PSG)	Included complex patients. No patient with normal PSA has postoperative respiratory complications.
Wilson et al.[325]	2002	Case series, retrospective	Abnormal PSG	163	21%	96% were managed in recovery room or ward setting.

OSAS, Obstructive sleep apnea syndrome; *PSG,* polysomnography; *RDI,* respiratory disturbance index.

reported with retropharyngeal abscess, but the exact incidence is not known. In a retrospective study, Ameh reported two deaths among 10 children surveyed; one child died before the abscess was drained, and the other died in the postoperative period because of laryngospasm.[338] Coulthard and Isaacs reported two deaths in 31 children with retropharyngeal abscess.[332]

All patients with the diagnosis of retropharyngeal abscess must be considered to have a DA. Case management depends on the severity of airway distress and the degree of the patient's cooperation. In most children, GA is required for airway management because few patients accept an awake technique. GA may be induced by inhalation of sevoflurane and oxygen with emergency plans for securing the airway should airway obstruction develop. If not in place, an intravenous line should be secured and atropine administered. It is advantageous to maintain spontaneous ventilation because neuromuscular blockade may relax the pharyngeal musculature and potentiate airway obstruction with an already reduced pharyngeal space.

After adequate anesthetic depth is achieved, gentle direct laryngoscopy should be attempted, taking care not to rupture the abscess. If tracheal intubation is not possible after limited attempts at direct laryngoscopy, a surgical airway should be considered for those with large lesions. In children with minimal respiratory distress and adequate mask air exchange, other intubation techniques (indirect visual or nonvisual) may be tried first. Take special precautions not to traumatize the abscess during tracheal intubation. Blind attempts at intubation, insertion of an SGA or oral airway, or overzealous direct laryngoscopy may result in rupture of the abscess.

Pharyngeal Bullae or Scarring

Epidermolysis bullosa (EB) describes a group of genetically determined mechanobullous disorders that vary in course and severity, ranging from relatively minor disability to death in early infancy.[339,340] The group is characterized by an excessive susceptibility of the skin and mucosa to separate from the underlying tissues and form bullae following minimal mechanical trauma. The affected areas can be considerable in size because the bullae enlarge by expanding and tracking along the natural tissue planes. As with all blisters, they can be extremely painful. More than 20 types of EB are described,[341] with three major subtypes: dystrophic, simplex, and junctional, with each broad category of EB containing several subtypes.

Dystrophic Epidermolysis Bullosa

Dystrophic epidermolysis bullosa (DEB), which was first described by Fox in 1879, is probably the most frequent type of EB to have surgical treatment.[342,343] The prevalence of DEB is approximately 2 in 100,000 children.[344] The majority of DEB patients have wounds that are present at birth or shortly after, with a variety of blister sizes, some even exceeding 10 cm in diameter. The blisters of DEB are usually flaccid and filled with either a clear or a blood-stained fluid. New blisters tend to develop less frequently as the child ages. Scarring is unusual after a single episode of blistering, but blistering is much more easily provoked in previously blistered areas; it is this recurrence that causes atrophic scars to form. As a result of repeated skin infection, injury, and healing, patients with the dystrophic form develop contractures, which may involve the skin of the neck and mouth.

Oral, pharyngeal, and esophageal blistering are common in DEB. The recurrent blistering leads to progressive contraction of the mouth (causing limited opening) and fixation of the tongue. The associated pain and resulting dysphagia lead to a reduction of nutritional intake because eating is a painful, slow, and exhausting experience. GER is common in patients with DEB. Esophageal scarring leads to dysmotility and the formation of strictures or webs, which contributes to the dysphagia by exacerbating oral, pharyngeal, and esophageal ulceration and by increasing dental decay.

Epidermolysis Bullosa Simplex
Almost all cases of epidermolysis bullosa simplex (EBS) are inherited in an autosomal dominant manner.[342] Although the exact prevalence of EBS is not known, it is thought to be approximately 1 or 2 in 100,000 children.[339] There are three major subtypes: Dowling-Meara, Weber-Cockayne, and Koebner.

Only the Dowling-Meara type (EBS herpetiformis) has airway implications. The onset of this type of EBS is usually in early infancy. There is a great range in the severity of Dowling-Meara, from relatively mild to exceptionally severe with death during the neonatal period. Oral involvement is usually not prominent, but a number of severely affected neonates exhibit extreme oropharyngeal involvement, which interferes with feeding. Patients may also have a tendency for GER and aspiration. Laryngeal involvement, causing a hoarse cry, is also regularly seen in Dowling-Meara EBS.

Junctional Epidermolysis Bullosa
There are three major subtypes of junctional epidermolysis bullosa (JEB): Herlitz, non-Herlitz, and JEB with pyloric atresia. Herlitz JEB is the most common form.

Formerly known as lethal JEB, Herlitz affects the larynx, producing a characteristic hoarse cry in infancy. This hoarseness is usually followed by recurrent bouts of stridor (caused by granulation tissue and not usually fresh blisters), each with the potential risk of fatal asphyxiation. The mouth and pharynx are often severely affected, causing substantial pain and feeding difficulties, which in turn lead to a profound failure to thrive. Death in the first 2 years of life is usual in Herlitz JEB, either from acute respiratory obstruction or from overwhelming sepsis related to a poor nutritional state.

Children with EB, especially DEB, are more likely to have airway management problems, with the risk of DI secondary to contracture formation. In addition to oral, pharyngeal, and laryngeal problems, head and neck skin involvement and contractures may make positioning for laryngoscopy difficult.[345] A DI should always be suspected and contingency plans made before embarking on anesthesia. To avoid prolonged facial manipulation during the procedure, airway maintenance by intubation is often preferred.[346] To reduce the risk of new laryngeal bullae formation, an ETT, one-half to one size smaller than predicted, may be necessary. If a cuffed tube is required, the cuff should be slightly inflated. The risk of bullae formation after intubation is low because the larynx and trachea are lined with ciliated columnar epithelium rather than the squamous epithelium that lines the oropharynx and esophagus.[347]

Although securing the ETT by wiring it to a tooth has been advocated,[348] a more conservative approach is to tie the tube in place with either ribbon gauze or Vaseline gauze and a collar of adhesive tape around the ETT to prevent the ties from slipping. Nasal intubation can be performed, preferably with a flexible

scope, but blind nasal intubation should be avoided. Blind techniques (e.g., blind oral intubation or lighted stylet) have been used successfully but may result in trauma to the laryngeal structures if multiple unsuccessful attempts are required and probably should be avoided.[349]

The lips should be lined with lubricated gauze at the place they touch the ET and underneath the tie to prevent chafing. An intravenous cannula should be secured with a nonadhesive dressing. Central venous and arterial cannulas, if required, should be sutured in place.

In caring for patients with EB, it is prudent to take general precautions to protect the integrity of the skin from trauma, friction injury, and adhesive products. Areas susceptible to pressure (e.g., below a face mask) should be generously lubricated.

Laryngeal Anomalies
Laryngomalacia
Laryngomalacia is the most common congenital abnormality of the larynx and is characterized by a long, narrow epiglottis and floppy aryepiglottic folds.[344] It is the most common cause of noninfective stridor in children.[344] Stridor, usually present at birth, may appear after weeks or months. It may appear only with crying or in the presence of an acute upper respiratory infection. The stridor is inspiratory, high pitched, and more obvious in the supine position.[200] In the mild form, stridor peaks at 9 months and then levels off, declines, and disappears by 2 years of age.[350] Severe laryngomalacia may cause upper airway obstruction, cyanosis, failure to thrive, and cor pulmonale. GER has been reported as well, in which case antireflux therapy is recommended.[351]

Diagnosis of laryngomalacia is by flexible endoscopy or direct laryngoscopy under anesthesia.

Patients with laryngomalacia are at risk for airway obstruction, and preparations for management of the difficult pediatric airway must be made. A gradual inhalation induction with 100% oxygen is performed, maintaining spontaneous ventilation. CPAP with 10 cm H_2O may be necessary to overcome obstruction, along with an oral airway and jaw lift. The time required for an adequate depth of anesthesia may be delayed in cases of airway obstruction. When deep levels of anesthesia are achieved, direct laryngoscopy may be performed. Topicalization of the vocal cords before laryngoscopy decreases the incidence of coughing. As stated previously, one should calculate the maximum dose before topicalization so that toxic doses are avoided.

Surgical treatment consists of either aryepiglottoplasty or laser excision of redundant supraglottic tissue.[352] Endoscopic division of the aryepiglottic folds has been suggested as the first-line therapy for severe laryngomalacia.[353]

Epiglottitis
Epiglottitis, more appropriately called supraglottitis, is a life-threatening infection of the epiglottis, aryepiglottic folds, and arytenoids. It is a true airway emergency because supraglottitis may progress rapidly to complete airway obstruction. Supraglottitis is classically described as occurring between 2 and 8 years of age, although it can occur in infants, older children, and adults.[354] *Haemophilus influenzae* type B (Hib) is the most common causative agent, although other organisms have been reported. *Pseudomonas,* group A β-hemolytic *Streptococcus,* and *Candida* have been reported in the literature as etiologies of epiglottitis as well.[354-356] The introduction of the *H. influenzae* conjugate vaccine has

dramatically reduced the incidence of supraglottitis, but vaccine failure does occur.[356] A high index of suspicion for the diagnosis of supraglottitis should be maintained because the disease has not been completely eliminated.

Children with epiglottitis often present with the four Ds of supraglottitis: drooling, dyspnea, dysphagia, and dysphonia. These children are described as anxious and appearing toxic, preferring to rest in the tripod position (upright sitting position, leaning forward with the mouth open).[355] High fevers and signs of respiratory distress evolve over a few hours. Stridor, if present, is usually inspiratory.[357]

Diagnosis is usually based on clinical findings. Radiographs are indicated only if the child has no respiratory distress and a physician capable of controlling the DA is in attendance. A lateral neck radiograph obtained with hyperextension during inspiration is the single best exposure. Classic findings include round, thick epiglottis (thumb sign), loss of the vallecular air space, and thickening of the aryepiglottic folds.[354] Definitive diagnosis is made at laryngoscopy in the OR, and should be avoided in the emergency room. Dynamic airway collapse may occur, and complete obstruction ensues.

The mainstay of therapy for supraglottitis is to obtain an airway, usually with a multidisciplinary approach in an organized and controlled manner. An otolaryngologist capable of performing an emergency tracheostomy should be present at induction. A pediatric DA cart, rigid bronchoscope, and tracheostomy set should be in the OR. When dealing with the child with epiglottitis, it is vital that the child remain calm. If separation from the parents is too stressful, parental presence at induction, after proper preparation, should be considered. Sedation is not advised in this situation. Induction should proceed with 100% oxygen in the sitting position with maintenance of spontaneous ventilation. CPAP at 10 cm H_2O may be beneficial in maintaining a patent airway. Once anesthesia is induced, an intravenous line should be placed if not already present and a volume bolus of 10 to 30 mL/kg of lactated Ringer's solution can be given for resuscitation. Atropine or glycopyrrolate can be given intravenously before laryngoscopy for antimuscarinic effect. After an adequate depth of anesthesia is obtained, direct laryngoscopy is performed, and an oral ETT is placed. Identification of a cherry-red edematous epiglottis is diagnostic. Gentle pressure applied to the chest may reveal expiratory gas bubbles to aid intubation. A styletted ETT, one or two sizes smaller than predicted, should be placed into the trachea.[357] If the patient cannot be intubated, the DA algorithm should be followed. Rigid FIS may be attempted if the condition permits, or a surgical airway may be necessary.

After the appropriate cultures are obtained, antibiotic therapy should be initiated. Some advocate changing the oral ETT to a nasotracheal tube because of its greater stability. The mean duration of intubation ranges from 30 to 72 hours. Extubation should be performed when the patient demonstrates clinical improvement and there is evidence of an air leak around the ETT. Some clinicians advocate the use of dexamethasone before extubation to reduce the incidence of postextubation stridor.[354]

Congenital Glottic Lesions

Congenital laryngeal anomalies include laryngomalacia, vocal cord paralysis, laryngeal web, and atresia. Vocal cord paralysis is the second most common cause of congenital laryngeal malformations.[358] Bilateral vocal cord paralysis is often associated with CNS abnormalities such as Arnold-Chiari malformation. Birth trauma may also induce vocal cord paralysis. The presentation of bilateral vocal cord paralysis is high-pitched inspiratory stridor and a normal or mildly hoarse cry. Severe airway obstruction may develop that requires emergency intubation or tracheostomy.[358] Occasionally, vocal cord paralysis resolves spontaneously or after a ventriculoperitoneal shunt is placed.[359] In unilateral paralysis, the left side is more frequently affected. Cardiovascular and mediastinal problems are often associated with unilateral paralysis.[358] Unilateral paralysis arises with a weak cry.[279] It seldom requires surgery.[359]

Laryngeal webs occur when there is failure of recanalization of the larynx during embryologic development. In general, webs occur at the level of the glottis, causing respiratory distress at birth. They may be thin and limited to the glottis, with minimal airway obstruction. Significant airway obstruction is usually the result of more extensive webs. These webs are thick, extending into the subglottis. Surgical treatment is endoscopic division of the web for smaller webs. Laryngotracheal reconstruction may be needed for extensive webs.

Laryngeal atresia is a rare and often fatal anomaly. Survival depends on the presence of an associated tracheoesophageal fistula or immediate tracheostomy at birth.[358]

The degree of obstruction determines the method used for airway management. Severe forms require a surgical airway; milder cases may be managed with intubation. Intubation may be performed either awake or after inhalation induction, depending on the patient and the situation. Preparations for a failed intubation should be made.

Recurrent Respiratory Papillomatosis

Laryngeal papillomatosis, or recurrent respiratory papillomatosis (RRP), is the most frequent benign tumor of the larynx, with an incidence in the United States of 4.3 per 100,000 children. It is caused by the human papillomavirus (HPV), types 6 and 11. It is also the second most common cause of hoarseness in children.[360] Laryngeal papillomas are located primarily in the larynx on the vocal cord margins and epiglottis; however, any part of the respiratory tract may be affected.[361] RRP may affect children and adults. The juvenile form is often more aggressive than the adult form of the disease. Pediatric patients with RRP often wheeze, and the diagnosis may be delayed. The primary symptom of RRP is hoarseness or a weak cry. Stridor is often the second symptom to develop, usually starting as inspiratory and progressing to biphasic with advancing disease.[360] Other symptoms may include chronic cough, paroxysms of choking, failure to thrive, and respiratory fatigue.[361] Diagnosis is made with a flexible nasopharyngoscope. If patient's cooperation limits the examination, GA may be needed. Treatment consists of CO_2 laser microlaryngoscopy, which vaporizes the lesions and causes minimal bleeding. Frequent surgical procedures may be required to control the disease. Medical management includes the use of acyclovir, interferon-α, cidofovir, and indole 3-carbinol.[361]

Airway obstruction has been reported with induction of anesthesia in patients with RRP.[362] Anesthetic evaluation should include careful preoperative assessment of the airway and the emotional status of the child.[363] Sedation is necessary because these patients require frequent surgeries, but it should be avoided in patients with respiratory compromise. In appropriate cases, parental presence in the OR may be beneficial. Anesthesia should be induced with an inhalational induction in 100% oxygen while maintaining spontaneous respirations. Patients may be apprehensive about the mask, and an alternative technique, such as cupping the hands around the circuit to increase the concentration of the inhalational agent, may be useful.[363] RRP is a recognized DA, and appropriate equipment and personnel should be in the OR before induction.

Laryngeal Granulomas

Laryngeal granulomas are frequently the result of prolonged tracheal intubation.[107] However, granuloma formation has been reported after short-term intubation as well. Other factors contributing to granuloma formation include female gender, size of the ETT, position of the ETT, traumatic intubation, and excessive cuff pressure.[80] The incidence in adults has been described as 1 in 800 to 1 in 20,000.[364] Typically, granulomas form in the posterior glottis on the medial aspect of the arytenoids.[105] Hoarseness is a common feature. Treatment consists of inhaled steroids, antireflux measures, antibiotics, and surgical removal under direct visualization.[80]

If the granulomas are large or pedunculated, airway obstruction may be seen. Awake intubation may be indicated in the adult population or, rarely, inhalation induction with intubation may be indicated in the pediatric population. ETTs smaller than predicted should be immediately available.

Congenital and Acquired Subglottic Disease

Subglottic Stenosis

Subglottic stenosis may be classified as congenital or acquired. It is defined as the presence of an abnormally small subglottic lumen (<3.5 mm in diameter in newborn).[358] Congenital subglottic stenosis is the third most common congenital anomaly.[359] Patients may present with mild or severe airway obstruction. Another common presentation is recurrent croup.[358] Patients who develop recurrent croup with upper respiratory tract infections during the first years of life should be evaluated for congenital subglottic stenosis. Acquired subglottic stenosis is usually the result of tracheal intubation. Definitive diagnosis is made with rigid endoscopy. Treatment consists of anterior or multiple cricoid splitting with cartilage graft interpositioning (mitomycin). The success rate for these procedures is approximately 90%.[359]

Croup

Croup, or laryngotracheobronchitis, is the most common cause of infectious airway obstruction in children. The incidence of croup in the United States is 18 per 1000 children annually. The peak incidence is 60 per 1000 among children 1 to 2 years of age.[354] Croup affects children between the ages of 6 months and 4 years, with peak incidence in early fall and winter. Parainfluenza type I is the most common etiologic agent responsible for croup. This is a viral infection that affects the subglottic region of the larynx, causing edema. The disease has a gradual onset, usually arising after an upper respiratory tract infection. Symptoms include inspiratory stridor; suprasternal, intercostal, and subcostal retractions; and a croupy or barking cough. Anteroposterior films of the neck show the classic church steeple sign (symmetrical narrowing of the subglottic airway).[354]

For mild cases, treatment consists of breathing humidified air or oxygen.[354] In severe cases, treatment with nebulized racemic epinephrine (0.25–0.5 mL in 2 mL of saline) is indicated. Repeated treatments, every 1 to 2 hours, may be necessary. Because the duration of action is brief (<2 hours), rebound respiratory distress may develop after treatment, and observation is necessary. Studies suggest that patients may be discharged from the emergency room after a 3-hour observation period provided that the parents are reliable and easy access to the ER is available. Racemic epinephrine should be used with caution in patients with tachycardia

or underlying cardiac abnormalities, such as tetralogy of Fallot or idiopathic hypertrophic subaortic stenosis.[365]

After years of debate, the use of steroids in the treatment of mild-to-moderate viral croup has gained acceptance.[366–368] Treatment with steroids has been associated with a reduction in admissions and length of stay.[368] Dexamethasone, 0.6 mg/kg (maximum dose, 10 mg) intravenously, is the standard dose. Dexamethasone (0.6 mg/kg) given orally was associated with more rapid resolution of symptoms than nebulized dexamethasone.[366] Heliox, a mixture of helium and oxygen, has also been used in the treatment of viral croup. Helium is an inert, nontoxic gas that has low specific gravity, low viscosity, and low density. Because of these properties, helium reduces airway resistance by decreasing turbulent flow in the airway.[369] If the preceding measures fail, intubation is necessary.

As with all cases of upper airway obstruction, preparations for management of a difficult pediatric airway must be made. The appropriate equipment and personnel must be in the OR at induction. A gradual inhalation induction is performed with 100% oxygen maintaining spontaneous respirations. Intubation is performed with an ETT, one or two sizes smaller than predicted, to decrease the risk of subglottic stenosis. Extubation is performed after an adequate air leak around the ETT is demonstrated.

Tracheobronchial Anomalies

Tracheomalacia

Tracheomalacia is characterized by weakness of the tracheal wall related to softness of the cartilaginous support. This allows the affected portion to collapse under conditions where the extraluminal pressure exceeds the intraluminal pressure.[370] Tracheomalacia may be classified as either congenital (primary) or acquired (secondary). Congenital tracheomalacia may be further subdivided into idiopathic or syndromic conditions. Tracheoesophageal fistula, CHARGE syndrome, and DiGeorge syndrome are associated with congenital tracheomalacia. Acquired tracheomalacia is typically caused by extrinsic compression of great vessels or is secondary to bronchopulmonary dysplasia. Symptoms include episodic respiratory distress, persistent dry cough, wheezing, dysphagia, and recurrent respiratory infections. Failure to wean from the ventilator or failure of extubation may also be indicative of tracheomalacia.[370]

Airway obstruction has been reported in patients with tracheomalacia during GA, even in asymptomatic patients.[371,372] Collapse of the affected segment occurs during expiration and with particularly forceful expiration or coughing. CPAP with or without intermittent positive-pressure ventilation (PPV) can alleviate the obstruction.[373] Noninvasive PPV through a face mask has been used successfully to prevent reintubation in an infant with tracheomalacia postoperatively.[374]

Bacterial Tracheitis

Bacterial tracheitis, formerly called pseudomembranous tracheitis or membranous laryngotracheobronchitis, is a potentially life-threatening disease. It is an infection of the subglottic region, and progression to full airway obstruction is possible. Bacterial tracheitis is believed to result from a bacterial superinfection preceded by a viral upper respiratory tract infection.[375] The peak incidence is in the fall and winter, affecting children 6 months to 8 years. *S. aureus*, *H. influenzae*, α-hemolytic *Streptococcus,* and group A *Streptococcus* are the usual causative agents. Patients usually present with a several-day history of viral upper respiratory symptoms, followed by rapid deterioration. The patient develops high fever, respiratory distress, and a toxic appearance. In contrast to those with supraglottitis, these patients have a substantial cough, appear comfortable when supine, and tend not to drool.[354]

In contrast to those with laryngotracheobronchitis, patients with bacterial tracheitis do not respond to racemic epinephrine or corticosteroids. Radiographs of the airway often show irregular tracheal densities and subglottic narrowing.[375] Patients with severe respiratory distress should be taken to the OR for rigid endoscopy and intubation.

Patients with bacterial tracheitis have the potential for airway obstruction. Preparations for management of the difficult pediatric airway must be made, including a rigid bronchoscope. Inhalation induction with maintenance of spontaneous respirations is preferred. Endoscopy is performed with removal of the sloughed mucosa. Intubation is performed, and specimens for culture and Gram stain are taken. Broad-spectrum antibiotics are started and continued for 10 to 14 days. Intubation is usually required for 3 to 7 days.[354]

Mediastinal Masses

Anesthesia for patients with mediastinal masses, usually anterior mediastinal masses, is associated with a high risk of airway obstruction, hemodynamic instability, or even death from extrinsic compression of three structures: the heart, great vessels (primarily superior vena cava), and the trachea and bronchi.[376] Induction of anesthesia and PPV may exacerbate the airway compression in a variety of ways. Loss of intrinsic muscle tone, reduced lung volumes, and a reduced transpleural pressure gradient combine to increase the effects of extrinsic compression. Cardiac arrest, superior vena cava syndrome, and airway occlusion are problems that can occur during induction of anesthesia.[377–379] Airway compression during induction of anesthesia can occur even in asymptomatic patients.[378] These complications may be unresponsive to position changes or open cardiac massage.

Mediastinal masses may be divided into anterosuperior, visceral, and posterior. The anatomic location of the mediastinal mass varies with age. In children, mediastinal masses are predominantly found in the posterior mediastinum. Neurogenic tumors, especially neuroblastomas, are the most common mediastinal tumor in young children. Germ cell tumors are the second most common anterior mediastinal mass in children. In adolescents, lymphomas are the most common anterior mediastinal mass.[376]

Symptoms such as orthopnea, stridor, and wheezing are ominous signs of airway obstruction.[380] Positional dyspnea, tachyarrhythmia, and syncope suggest right-sided heart and pulmonary vascular compression. Syncope during a Valsalva maneuver suggests significant vascular encroachment.[376] Children usually display symptoms earlier than adults. Small decreases in airway diameter result in increased resistance. Preoperative evaluation should focus on symptoms of respiratory compromise in the supine and standing positions. Intolerance of the supine position indicates compression by the mass on the trachea, heart, pulmonary artery, or superior vena cava. Preoperative CT scan should be obtained. Minimum criteria for safe administration of GA should be a tracheal cross-sectional area at least 50% of predicted value and a peak expiratory flow rate at least 50% of predicted value.[381]

Patients with a mediastinal mass are considered difficult to ventilate. Avoidance of GA, muscle relaxants, and PPV are the mainstay of anesthetic management for patients presenting for biopsy before irradiation or chemotherapy. Biopsies should be performed, if possible, under local anesthesia.[382] Ketamine, local anesthesia, and a 50:50 mixture of O_2 and nitrous oxide (N_2O)

while maintaining spontaneous ventilation have been used successfully for a diagnostic biopsy in a 13-year-old patient.[383] Placing the patient in reverse Trendelenburg position may help.

With pediatric patients, GA may be needed for biopsy. Recommendations have been made for a rigid pediatric bronchoscopy and femoral-to-femoral bypass standby.[378,384] If possible, irradiation of the mass before GA may reduce the risk associated with anesthesia. Peripheral shielding of the mediastinum may allow subsequent tissue biopsy.[385] For older children, an awake FSI should be performed to assess the degree of obstruction after topicalization of the airway. In small infants and children, an awake intubation is not practical. In these patients, an inhalation induction with maintenance of spontaneous ventilation is recommended. Intravenous access must be obtained in a lower extremity before induction.[384] Induction of anesthesia in the lateral semi-Fowler position has been recommended.[379] Maintenance of spontaneous ventilation is vital; however, this is not foolproof.[386] Heliox (80% helium, 20% O_2) has been used for induction with sevoflurane and an SGA for successful airway management in a 3-year-old patient with severe respiratory distress related to a massive mediastinal mass.[387]

If airway obstruction or hemodynamic collapse occurs with induction, the following steps are suggested. First, attempt to pass the ETT down the least obstructed bronchus. If passage of the ETT is not possible, rigid bronchoscopy to bypass the obstruction should be attempted. Position changes to the lateral or prone position may alleviate the obstruction by changing the weight distribution of the tumor. Finally, cardiopulmonary bypass has been recommended.[378] Airway obstruction may occur during emergence as well. Extubation should be performed with the patient awake. These patients should be monitored postoperatively in the ICU.

Vascular Malformations

Vascular malformations result from abnormal development of the arterial component of the branchial arch system, resulting in complete or incomplete encirclement of the trachea or esophagus, or both.[388] In 1945, Gross introduced the term *vascular ring* to describe this anomaly.[389] Patients with vascular rings may present with symptoms of respiratory distress or dysphagia because of tracheoesophageal compression. Patients may present with respiratory distress after birth or may be asymptomatic for life. Most children with vascular rings present with nonspecific symptoms such as stridor, dyspnea, cough, or recurrent respiratory tract infection.[390] Dysphagia is often the primary symptom in adults with vascular ring.[388] In a retrospective review of vascular rings, 74% of the malformations were symptomatic, with inspiratory stridor and wheezing as the main complaints.[390]

Various types of vascular rings have been described, including double aortic arch and right aortic arch with aberrant left subclavian artery. The double aortic arch usually arises earlier than other varieties requiring surgical correction.[388] Associated cardiac anomalies are often present with the vascular ring. Diagnosis is confirmed by radiologic studies. A chest radiograph may indicate the site of the ascending and descending aorta. A barium esophagogram may disclose extrinsic compression of the esophagus. Angiography has been considered the gold standard for identifying vascular rings. CT and MRI scans can assist in the diagnosis of vascular ring and determine the anatomy. The diagnosis of vascular ring may be delayed because of the nonspecific symptoms.[390] Patients who are symptomatic should undergo surgery. Surgical correction is by a left thoracotomy, right thoracotomy, or median sternotomy.[388]

Patients with a vascular ring are at risk of airway obstruction from compression of the trachea. Tracheomalacia may be present as well. Maintenance of spontaneous ventilation until the trachea is intubated with a reinforced ETT may be beneficial. A rigid bronchoscope should be available to serve as an airway stent in the event of airway collapse.

Foreign Body Aspiration

Foreign body aspiration is a cause of significant morbidity and mortality in the pediatric population. Young children are at increased risk for foreign body aspiration, with children less than 2 years old most often affected.[391] A second peak of aspiration occurs between 10 and 11 years of age.[392] Most of the deaths occur in children younger than 1 year. The objects most frequently aspirated are food products. There is only a slight propensity for the object to lodge on the right side because of symmetrical bronchial angles in children under 15 years old. The left mainstem bronchus is displaced by the aortic knob by age 15 years, creating a more obtuse angle at the carina.[393]

Witnessed events are easier to diagnose. A history of choking, gagging, or coughing is usually given. Patients may be asymptomatic at the time or may develop symptoms of acute distress. A persistent cough, wheezing, or recurrent pneumonia may be the initial sign if the aspiration occurred in the past. The American Academy of Pediatrics has developed guidelines for the management of choking episodes. For children under 1 year, back blows and abdominal thrusts with the child in a head-down position are recommended. The Heimlich maneuver is reserved for older children and adults.[394]

Emergency removal is indicated if the patient is in distress or if the foreign body is in a precarious location. Abnormalities of the cervical spine may decrease range of extension or flexion movement. Common conditions of limited cervical spine mobility are discussed in detail below. If the patient is stable, radiographs may be taken to assist in localizing and identifying the foreign body. Classically, peanuts should be removed promptly because of the inflammatory reaction to the peanut oil. If the foreign body is radiopaque, it is easily identified. Radiolucent foreign bodies may demonstrate soft tissue density in or narrowing of the airway.[13] Indirect signs of air trapping, mediastinal shift, or atelectasis may be present. Lateral decubitus films are helpful in infants and younger children because they cannot cooperate with expiratory films.[393] The downside lung should be deflated unless it is obstructed with a foreign body.[392]

In general, inhalation induction without cricoid pressure is the favored technique for removal of foreign bodies in the airway, regardless of the type of object, according to a postal survey of members of the Society for Pediatric Anesthesia.[391] For foreign bodies in the upper esophagus, a rapid-sequence induction *without* cricoid pressure was the preferred technique, whereas for objects in the lower esophagus and stomach, a rapid-sequence induction *with* cricoid pressure was chosen; however, cricoid pressure may cause harm if the foreign body is sharp or positioned in the larynx. If the case is not an emergency, one can wait until the appropriate nothing-by-mouth time has passed. In a retrospective review of anesthetic management for tracheobronchial foreign body removal, neither spontaneous nor controlled ventilation was associated with an increased incidence of adverse events.[395]

With an inhalation induction, a prolonged induction may occur because of airway obstruction. CPAP at 5 to 10 cm H_2O and assisted ventilation may be needed at times to maintain a patent airway. After an adequate level of anesthesia is obtained, topicalization of the airway may decrease the incidence of coughing or laryngospasm. Use of a ventilating rigid bronchoscope allows ventilation during the procedure. High oxygen flow rates may be needed to overcome the presence of an air leak around the FIS. Communication between the anesthesiologist and the endoscopist is crucial because this is a shared airway. The patient may require intermittent ventilation if desaturation occurs during the FSI. When the foreign body is grasped, the glottis should be relaxed for removal. Short-acting muscle relaxants, propofol, or deeper inhalational anesthesia may be used. The forceps and the bronchoscope are removed from the trachea as a single unit.[357] Dislodgement of foreign bodies at the glottic or subglottic area has been reported.[396] If a foreign body is dislodged and obstructs the trachea, the bronchoscope must be used to push the foreign body into a mainstem bronchus to enable ventilation of one lung. Flexible laryngoscopy with tracheotomy removal of a bronchial foreign body has been used successfully to remove an object that was too large to pass through the subglottis.[397]

When the foreign body is removed, the patient is usually intubated with an appropriate-size ETT. Depending on the amount of edema from the procedure, the patient should be able to be extubated. Postoperatively, racemic epinephrine (0.5 mL of 2.25% solution in 3 mL of saline) may be used for stridor. Dexamethasone is often given for edema.

Other Tracheal Disease

Tracheal stenosis is congenital or acquired. Congenital stenosis may be associated with congenital airway malformations such as tracheoesophageal fistula, hypoplastic lungs, and tracheomalacia. Congenital complete tracheal rings are also a cause of tracheal stenosis. In this condition, the rings are fused posteriorly, and there is no posterior membranous wall. Acquired stenosis is usually attributed to prolonged intubation, inhalational injuries, trauma, or tumors. Symptoms include stridor, wheezing, croup, tachypnea, and cough. For mild lesions, conservative therapy is warranted. Surgical treatment involves tracheal resection with primary reanastomosis for short-segment lesions. Anterotracheal split procedures may be used for longer segmental lesions. Laser excision of granulation tissue at the repair site may be needed.[279]

Tracheal stenosis may cause difficulty with ventilation or ETT advancement. Minimal trauma to the airway can lead to acute airway obstruction.[279] Use of an SGA has been described in two patients with subglottic stenosis in whom the stenotic areas were 2 mm or less.[398,399] Passage of the rigid bronchoscope should be performed only at definitive repair.

Cervical Spine Anomalies

Limited cervical spine mobility may be caused by congenital or acquired disorders. Abnormalities of the cervical spine may decrease range of extension or flexion movement. Common conditions of limited cervical spine mobility are discussed in detail below.

Klippel-Feil Syndrome

Klippel-Feil syndrome is characterized by fusion of two or more cervical vertebrae. Other features include short neck, a low posterior hairline, scoliosis, and congenital heart disease.[400] Difficulty with airway management usually arises in the latter half of the first decade of life. The degree of difficulty with airway management depends on the severity of neck fixation.

Goldenhar Syndrome

See "Mandibular Hypoplasia."

Juvenile Rheumatoid Arthritis

Juvenile rheumatoid arthritis (JRA) is a chronic arthritis with variable manifestations. Several different subgroups of disease have been identified: systemic onset (Still disease), polyarticular, and oligoarticular (see "Facial Anomalies: Maxillary and Mandibular Disease").

Careful preoperative evaluation of patients with limited cervical mobility must be done before anesthetic induction. Previous anesthetic records, if available, should be reviewed for any relevant information. Because a DA is presumed to exist, preparation for management of the difficult pediatric airway must be made. In cases of limited cervical mobility, the ability to align the oral, pharyngeal, and laryngeal axes for visualization of the glottis is impaired. The presence of TMJ involvement may limit mouth opening as well. Awake tracheal intubation is recommended in this scenario. Many techniques are available for use, including FSI, Bullard laryngoscope, retrograde wire technique, and light wand. Awake techniques may not be suitable in younger patients. For patients who will not cooperate with an awake technique, a mask induction with 100% O_2 and spontaneous ventilation is indicated. Retrograde intubation, suspension laryngoscopy, and FSI through the SGA have all been reported in pediatric patients with Goldenhar syndrome.[78,94,401] The light wand was used to intubate an 18-day-old infant with right hemifacial microsomia.[38]

Congenital Cervical Spine Instability

Cervical spine instability, if unrecognized, is a potential cause of serious morbidity and even mortality during airway management. Cervical spine instability or subluxation most often involves the atlanto-occipital joint. Congenital syndromes such as trisomy 21, Hurler syndrome, Hunter syndrome, and Morquio syndrome are associated with cervical spine instability.[402] Of these, trisomy 21 is the syndrome most often encountered by anesthesiologists.

Down Syndrome

Trisomy 21 (Down syndrome) occurs in approximately 1 of every 660 live births. Mental retardation, congenital heart disease, OSA, and congenital subglottic stenosis may be present. Approximately 20% of patients have ligamentous laxity of the atlantoaxial joint, which may allow atlantoaxial instability. This may predispose them to cervical spinal cord compression. Children are at risk for injury during hyperextension, hyperflexion, or increased rotation of the neck.[278,403] Signs of cervical spinal cord compression include loss of ambulatory function, spasticity, hyperreflexia of the lower extremities, extensor plantar reflexes, and loss of bowel and bladder control. Other signs may include increased fatigue with walking and torticollis.[403] Preoperative evaluation of the patient with Down syndrome must attempt to discover any preexisting signs or symptoms of spinal cord compression.

The issue of screening for atlantoaxial instability in patients with Down syndrome is controversial. The American Academy of Pediatrics Committee on Sports Medicine and Fitness decided that the value of cervical spine radiographs is uncertain in screening for possible catastrophic neck injury in athletes with Down syndrome.[403] However, Pueschel argued that patients should be screened for atlantoaxial instability.[404] A survey of the Society of Pediatric Anesthesia found that members obtain preoperative radiographs (18%) or subspecialty consultation (8%), or both, for asymptomatic patients. For symptomatic patients, radiographs

and preoperative consultations are obtained 64% and 74% of the time, respectively. The majority of respondents attempt to maintain the head in a neutral position for both symptomatic and asymptomatic patients.[405]

Airway management for patients with Down syndrome should consider the possibility of cervical spine instability with cord compression. In addition, the large tongue and potential for OSA can lead to upper airway obstruction. Patients who have symptoms of cord compression should have radiographic evaluation before any elective surgical procedure. Lateral extension and flexion radiographs of the upper cervical spine can reveal atlantoaxial subluxation. An odontoid process (axis) to anterior arch (atlas) distance 4.5 mm or greater indicates abnormal instability.[403]

For emergency surgery, cervical spine precautions should be used in patients who are symptomatic. In-line stabilization of the cervical spine for direct laryngoscopy should be used. Techniques for airway management that require minimal neck movement may be useful (e.g., Bullard laryngoscope, light wand, angulated video laryngoscope, SOS).

Acquired Cervical Spine Instability

Acquired cervical spine instability in pediatric patients can result from multiple trauma or head and neck trauma. Any pediatric patient with a severe head injury should be treated as though a cervical spine injury is present.[406] An estimated 1% to 2% of pediatric patients with multiple trauma have a cervical injury.[394] Pediatric patients with underlying medical conditions such as Down syndrome may be more susceptible to cervical cord injury.[394] Pediatric patients 8 years of age or younger are at increased risk for injury to the upper cervical spine and craniovertebral junction. Only 30% of cervical injuries occur below C3 in children 8 years old or younger. They also have a higher incidence of spinal cord injury without radiographic abnormality (SCIWORA).[407] Immobilization of a patient with suspected cervical injury is crucial so that further damage to the cord is prevented. A hard collar, spine board, and soft spacing devices between the head and securing straps are needed. The occiput is large, and a blanket under the torso allows the neck to rest in a neutral position.

The choice of airway management depends on the degree of urgency associated with the intubation. Techniques that minimize head extension and cervical flexion are mandatory. Trauma patients are considered at risk for aspiration, and appropriate measures must be undertaken.

For an urgent airway in a patient with a DA or facial fractures, a surgical airway may be the best option. If time allows, a limited number of attempts at direct laryngoscopy may be performed. A video laryngoscope may be useful in this situation. In an emergency, the SGA may be used to ventilate or oxygenate the patient until a formal airway is established. This does not provide protection against aspiration.

For a nonurgent intubation, further evaluation of the cervical spine is warranted. When the cervical spine has been cleared by the neurosurgeon or trauma surgeon, a rapid-sequence induction with cricoid pressure may be performed after adequate preoxygenation if the airway appears reasonable. If the cervical spine is unstable, a rapid-sequence induction with cricoid pressure may be performed with in-line stabilization. Fluoroscopy was used to assist the intubation of an 11-year-old patient with an unstable subluxation of C1–C2 after a motor vehicle crash.[408] Awake techniques such as flexible scope laryngoscopy, Bullard laryngoscope, light wand, SOS, or retrograde intubation may be indicated if the patient has an unstable cervical spine and a DA.

Pediatric Trauma

All pediatric trauma patients are considered to have a cervical spine injury until proved otherwise. In addition, these patients are at risk for aspiration. Oxygen should be administered, and ventilation assisted if needed as soon as possible. Trauma patients should be immobilized on a spine board with a rigid collar as previously described. After an evaluation of the airway, one should decide on the method of intubation. If the airway is judged to be adequate, a rapid-sequence induction with cricoid pressure and manual in-line stabilization should be employed. In children 8 years old or younger, 45% can have lateral displacement of the esophagus at the level of the cricoid cartilage. This could make cricoid pressure ineffective, especially in younger children.[408] In addition, application of cricoid pressure can compress the airway rather than the esophagus.[409] If the airway cannot be secured, the ASA DA algorithm should be followed. In a DA scenario, one of the previously described awake techniques may be used. In certain cases, awake tracheostomy or surgical cricothyrotomy may be indicated. A multidisciplinary approach to the management of the difficult pediatric trauma airway is necessary.

Extubation of the Difficult Airway

The management of the difficult pediatric airway does not end until the plan for extubation has been established. Choices include extubation over an airway catheter or guidewire or extubation when an air leak develops, as with epiglottitis. The 2022 ASA guidelines recommend minimizing use of airway exchange catheters for extubation in pediatric patients.[1] Preparations for the difficult pediatric airway must be made because extubation may fail and require reintubation. If airway edema is suspected at the end of the surgery because of either the intubation process or the surgery, dexamethasone may be of benefit. Postoperative ventilation may be indicated until the edema resolves. Extubation has been successfully performed over an airway exchange catheter in an adolescent with a DA.[410] Alternatively, a 0.018-inch (0.05-cm) guidewire has been used to maintain airway access in a 2-year-old child with severe micrognathia and tetralogy of Fallot.[411]

Conclusion

Unexpected difficulties with airway management in otherwise healthy children are rare after exclusion of predictors of DI, such as mandibular hypoplasia, limited mouth opening, and facial asymmetry, including abnormalities of the ear, syndromes, OSAS, and stridor. Difficulties that occur are probably a result of inexperience or inadequate supervision and lack of pediatric airway training. Thorough preoperative assessment and anticipation of airway difficulties, as well as education, continuous training, and regular practice in basic airway management, are necessary to reduce the incidence of pediatric airway difficulties. Besides inexperience with the pediatric airway, most morbidity and mortality in pediatric airway management are attributed to a failure to recognize and overcome functional airway problems because of insufficient depth of anesthesia or muscle paralysis and not due to a failure to intubate.

Selected References

3. Morray JP, Geiduschel JM, Ramamoorthy C, et al. Anesthesia-related cardiac arrest in children. *Anesthesiology.* 2000;93:6–14.
4. Coté CJ, Todres ID. The pediatric airway. In: Coté CJ, Todres ID, Goudsouzian NG, Ryan JF, eds. *A Practice of Anesthesia for Infants and Children.* 3rd ed. Saunders; 2001.
9. Kopp VJ, Bailey A, Valley RD, et al. Utility of the Mallampati classification for predicting difficult intubation in pediatric patients. *Anesthesiology.* 1995;83:A1147.
14. Apfelbaum JL, Hagberg CA, Connis RT, Abdelmalak BB, Agarkar M, Dutton RP, Fiadjoe JE, et al. 2022 American society of anesthesiologists practice guidelines for management of the difficult airway. *Anesthesiology.* 2021 Nov 11. Online ahead of print. PMID: 34762729.
16. Frei FJ, aWengen D, Rutishauser GE, et al. The airway endoscopy mask: useful device for fiberoptic evaluation and intubation of the paediatric airway. *Paediatr Anaesth.* 1995;5:319–324.
22. Khine HH, Corddry DH, Kettrick RG, et al. Comparison of cuffed and uncuffed endotracheal tubes in young children during general anesthesia. *Anesthesiology.* 1997;86:627–631.
47. Ellis DS, Potluri PK, O'Flaherty JE, et al. Difficult airway management in the neonate: a simple method of intubating through a laryngeal mask airway. *Paediatr Anaesth.* 1999;9:460–462.
76. Bonfils P. Schwierge Intubation bei Pierre Robin–Kindern, eine neue Methode: Der retromolare Weg. *Anaesthesist.* 1983;32:363–367.
258. Crosby ET, Cooper RM, Douglas MJ, et al. The unanticipated difficult airway with recommendations for management. *Can J Anaesth.* 1998;45:757–776.

All references can be found online at eBooks.Health.Elsevier.com.

37

Airway Management in Obstetric Patients

NAVEEN VANGA, ANA LISA RAMIREZ-CHAPMAN, AND MAYA S. SURESH

CHAPTER OUTLINE

KEY POINTS

- Anesthesia is a leading cause of maternal mortality and ranks seventh in the United States and eleventh in the United Kingdom. Airway-related complications during general anesthesia (GA) for cesarean delivery (CD) feature as a predominant cause of anesthesia-related maternal morbidity and mortality and are preventable.
- Pregnancy-related anatomic and physiologic changes are not the sole reason for difficulty with intubation, ventilation, and extubation. Other reasons include lack of preanesthesia assessment and preparedness, inadequate communication, loss of situational awareness, and lack of clinical airway management skills.
- Early preoperative assessment for patients undergoing labor and delivery must include a thorough airway history and examination and a rescue plan for potential failed tracheal intubation (TI). Appropriate airway equipment and personnel must be immediately available in labor and delivery suites to manage the difficult airway (DA).
- Although regional anesthesia (RA) is safe in most patients undergoing CD, in certain exceptional situations an awake TI is considered the safest choice in cases of anticipated or known DA in a patient undergoing nonurgent CD. Awake TI can be performed using flexible scopes or video laryngoscopes. Appropriate topical anesthesia of the airway and judicious sedation

(with minimum adverse effects on the fetus) can enable any of these techniques to be used successfully. Video laryngoscopy for awake intubation is associated with shorter intubation time; it has a success rate and safety profile comparable to flexible bronchoscopy.
- Adequate preoxygenation, left uterine displacement (LUD), head-elevated positioning and use of ramp, and supplementary high-flow oxygen via nasal cannula enhance oxygenation and prevent early desaturation.
- Video-assisted laryngoscopy should be the first line laryngoscopy.
- In a cannot intubate/cannot oxygenate (CICO) critical airway scenario, invasive airway access is a high priority. A scalpel-bougie surgical cricothyrotomy technique must be considered in the critical airway with increasing hypoxemia situation.
- Extubation airway-related problems have emerged as the most common cause of airway-related maternal mortality in recent reports from the United States and the United Kingdom.
- Simulation-based training during residency training is essential to address the declining use of GA for CD.
- High-fidelity simulation training with formal instruction in management of failed TI, difficult ventilation, and cricothyrotomy skills should be taught and practiced.

Introduction

Anesthesiologists in active obstetric anesthesia practice uniformly agree that general anesthesia (GA) for cesarean delivery (CD) should be reserved for special circumstances, such as emergent delivery for a life-threatening (mother or baby) situation, when regional anesthesia (RA) is contraindicated, or in complicated cases. Evidence-based literature from the United States and United Kingdom has demonstrated that complications of airway management, which include difficult laryngoscopy (DL), difficult or failed tracheal intubation (TI), and inability to ventilate or oxygenate following induction of GA for CD are major contributory factors leading to significant maternal morbidity and mortality.[1,2] Thus, the anesthesiologist involved in obstetric airway management respects the gravity of GA for CD. The trend in obstetric anesthesia clinical practice in industrialized countries has shifted significantly toward RA for most operative obstetric surgical procedures leading to a decline in GA for CD. Despite the decline in GA, it remains an enigma as to why the incidence of failed intubation in obstetric patients has not changed in the last four decades. Prediction of difficult airway (DA) in obstetric patients is not always reliable, yet proper airway assessment and evaluation are required. Based on published literature, the focus priorities include the following:

1. Readiness and appropriate preparation for GA in an obstetric patient;
2. Formulate strategies to manage DA and difficult intubation (DI);
3. In the event of failed intubation, outline strategies to establish ventilation;
4. In a critical airway situation with hypoxemia, the emphasis is on optimizing oxygenation to support safe outcomes for both mother and baby;

5. A strategy to manage safe extubation in a patient with known DA;
6. Availability of airway devices in an obstetric suite; and
7. Maintenance of advanced airway management (AAM) skills.

Common Obstetric Practices and Concerns

The common practice in obstetric anesthesia is to accomplish intubation using a single dose of succinylcholine when anesthetizing for CD under GA. From an obstetric anesthesia perspective, a DI is defined as when an experienced provider cannot successfully accomplish intubation within the timeframe of the initial induction.[3] The increased use of RA and the significant decline in GA for operative procedures raises three concerns: clinical, patient safety, and educational:

The clinical concerns center on the changing demographics among the obstetric patient population. As the prevalence of high-risk obstetric patients with comorbidities (particularly pregnant patients with congenital heart disease, advanced maternal age, morbidly adherent placental abnormalities requiring cesarean hysterectomy) and morbid obesity continues to increase, anesthesia providers will encounter clinical scenarios in which neuraxial anesthesia may be contraindicated or impossible, making airway instrumentation and management both necessary and challenging. Approximately one-third of obstetric general anesthetics are now administered after failed neuraxial anesthesia.[4]

Because of the declining GA experience of anesthesia trainees and the inability to acquire airway management skills in pregnant patients, the educational concern has resulted in educators opting for simulation-based training to enhance anesthesia trainees' cognitive, technical, and nontechnical skills. This includes clear communication during a simulated obstetric emergency on a high-fidelity patient simulator.[5] An emphasis on critical airway management skills and front-of-neck access cricothyrotomy techniques is essential.

Incidence of Difficult or Failed Intubation and Cannot Intubate/Cannot Oxygenate in Obstetrics

A literature review of obstetric failed intubations from 1970 to 2021 shows that the incidence of failed intubation in obstetric patients has not changed in 40 years.[4] It remains unchanged at 2.6 per 1000 anesthetics (1 in 390) for obstetric GA and 2.3 per 1000 GA (1 in 443) for CD (Table 37.1).[4] Maternal mortality from failed intubation was 2.3 per 100,000 GAs for CD (1 death per 90 failed intubations).[6] Maternal deaths were secondary to aspiration, and hypoxemia events were secondary to airway obstruction or esophageal intubation.[4]

Over the years, maternal morbidity and mortality secondary to airway-related complications have declined. However, the incidence of DI during CD has remained unchanged because of the altered anatomic and physiologic changes of pregnancy and failure to predict DI in two-thirds of the cases.[4,7] A retrospective study performed at Baylor College of Medicine in 2017 found that the incidence of failed intubation was 1:232, which is comparable to previous studies. All the failed intubations were rescued by the laryngeal mask airway (LMA).[8] As compared with the incidence of failed intubation in obstetrics, the incidence of failed intubation in surgical patients averages 1:2230. Therefore, there is a nearly eightfold increased risk for failed intubation in obstetric patients. Interestingly, in countries with a high GA usage rate during CD (i.e., South Africa), a lower failed intubation rate of 1 in 750 is reported.[9]

Cannot Intubate/Cannot Oxygenate

The incidence of simultaneous difficult mask ventilation (DMV) and DI in the obstetric population is unknown. However, the reported incidence of cannot intubate/cannot oxygenate (CICO) following intubation during GA for CD ranges from 5% to 28%.[4] A recent editorial recommends that physician focus needs to center on CICO instead of cannot intubate/cannot ventilate (CICV) to prevent poor outcomes associated with a failed obstetric airway. The focus is to improve emergency cricothyrotomy clinical skills to establish oxygenation expeditiously and prevent adverse neurologic outcomes in both mother and baby.[10] Two studies from the same institution but conducted at different periods showed that failure of mask ventilation or supraglottic airway (SGA) devices to rescue the airway in obstetric patients could result in a high incidence of CICO, with an estimated incidence ranging from 1:500 to 1:95 general anesthetics.[11,12] The current estimates include approximately 3.4 front-of-neck airway access procedures (surgical airway) per 100,000 general anesthetics for CD (1 procedure per 60 failed obstetric intubations). These procedures are usually carried out as late rescue attempts and result in poor maternal outcomes.[4,10]

Anesthesia-Related Maternal Mortality

Recent reviews on anesthesia-related maternal mortality have heightened anesthesiologists' awareness of potential airway problems in obstetric patients. Despite the increased use of RA and advances in airway management, difficult or failed intubation cases are still reported when RA is converted to GA during CD, because of either pain or hemorrhage. Concerns for rapid delivery of the fetus often lead to time pressure, which may result in poor preparation, inadequate planning, gaps in nontechnical communication, and substandard performance of technical tasks in the majority of CD under GA.[1,7]

TABLE 37.1   Incidence of Failed Intubation: 1985–2015

Data Collection	Author, Year	Incidence of Failed Intubation
1978–1983	Lyons, 1985	1 in 291
1980–1989	Glassenberg, 1990	1 in 357
1982–1985	Samsoon, 1987	1 in 281
1984–1994	Hawthorne, 1996	1 in 231
1984–2003	McKeen, 2011	CS 0
1988–2004	Saravanakumar, 2005	1 in 543
1990–1995	Tsen, 1998	1 in 536
~1991	Rocke, 1992	1 in 750
1993–1998	Barnardo, 2000	1 in 249
1993–2002	Nze, 2006	1 in 265
1997	Shibli, 2000	1 in 885
1999–2000	Bloom, 2005	1 in 1264
1999–2003	Rahman, 2005	1 in 238
2000–2005	Palanisamy, 2011	1 in 98
2000–2007	Djabetey, 2009	0
2001–2006	Tao, 2012	CS 1 in 409
2003–2004	Bullough, 2009	1 in 309
2004–2009	D'Angelo, 2014	1 in 533
2004–2011	Teoh, 2012	CS 1 in 462
2005	Pujic, 2009	1 in 399
2005–2006	McDonnell, 2008	1 in 274
2005–2008	Kessack, 2010	CS 1 in 180
2006–2011	Kirodian, 2012	1 in 118
2006–2013	Rajagopalan, 2015	1 in 232
2007–2009	Nafisi, 2014	1 in 465
2008–2010	Quinn, 2013	1 in 224
2008–2011	Madsen, 2013	1 in 164
2008–2012	Davies, 2014	1 in 391
2009	National Obstetric Anesthesia Data (NOAD)	1 in 571
2009–2010	Keen, 2011	1 in 154
2011	NOAD	1 in 564

CS, Cesarean section

Reproduced with permission, modified from Kinsella SM, Winton AL, Mushambi MC, et al. Failed tracheal intubation during obstetric general anesthesia: a literature review. *Int J Obstet Anesth.* 2015;24(3):356–374.

US Data on Anesthesia-Related Maternal Mortality

Anesthesia-related maternal mortality ranks seventh among the leading causes of maternal deaths in the United States (Fig. 37.1).[13] The first landmark study of anesthesia-related maternal mortality in the United States was reported in 1997. It revealed a 16.7 relative risk ratio increase in mortality in mothers who received GA compared with those who received RA.[14] A total of 82% of the deaths occurred during CD and mainly resulted from difficult or failed intubation, inability to ventilate and oxygenate, and pulmonary aspiration and respiratory complications. The death rates during GA for CD increased from 20 per million between 1979 and 1984 to 32.3 per million between 1985 and 1990. The relative risk ratio of GA-associated deaths was 2.3 times higher than RA-related deaths. This evidence-based data ushered in a significant change in anesthesia practice for pregnant patients who moved away from GA to predominantly RA for CD, demonstrating the death rate for RA during the same time had declined from 8.6 to 1.9 per million (Table 37.2).

In a follow-up report, a reexamination of trends in anesthesia-related maternal deaths from 1991 to 1996 compared with anesthesia-related deaths from 1997 to 2002 showed the case fatality for GA declined from 16.8 to 6.5 per million.[2] However, despite the changes in practice, 56 anesthesia-related deaths were primarily associated with complications during anesthetic induction, failure of TI (25%), respiratory failure (20%), or high spinal or epidural block (16%) followed by respiratory failure.

Maternal deaths following extubation and emergence from GA are another area of concern. A review of anesthesia-related maternal deaths during the perioperative period in Michigan (1985–2003) found that deaths occurred during emergence, extubation, or recovery from hypoventilation or airway obstruction.[15] Obesity and race (that is, African American) were considered important risk factors for anesthesia-related maternal mortality.[15] Currently, the anesthetic-related maternal death rate in the United States has stabilized to 1 out of 1 million live births.[2] Although the reasons for the reductions in anesthesia-related deaths are not fully understood, there is reason to believe that the improved outcomes are a result of (1) the changing patterns of anesthesia practice, predominantly toward RA; (2) GA in elective obstetric cases being reserved for high-risk patients with comorbidities; (3) enhanced awareness and use of protocols and DA algorithms; and (4) use of alternate airway devices, particularly SGA, in DA management.

Obstetric Anesthesia Closed Claims Studies

The American Society of Anesthesiologists (ASA) database is a structured evaluation of adverse events from the closed claims files of 35 US professional liability insurance companies. Before 1990, maternal death and newborn death/brain damage were the most common obstetric anesthesia malpractice claims in the database. Obstetric anesthesia claims for injuries from 1990 to 2003 were compared to claims before 1990, and the proportion of obstetric anesthesia claims from 1990 or later associated with CD decreased. The proportion of claims related to GA from 1990 onward decreased, and the proportion of maternal death/brain damage and newborn death/brain damage also decreased. Malpractice claims from 1990 or later related to respiratory causes of injuries decreased to 4% from the pre-1990 level of 24%. Claims pertaining to inadequate oxygenation/ventilation, pulmonary aspiration of gastric contents, and esophageal intubation have also decreased. However, the claims related to DI after 1990 in comparison with pre-1990 have not changed.[7]

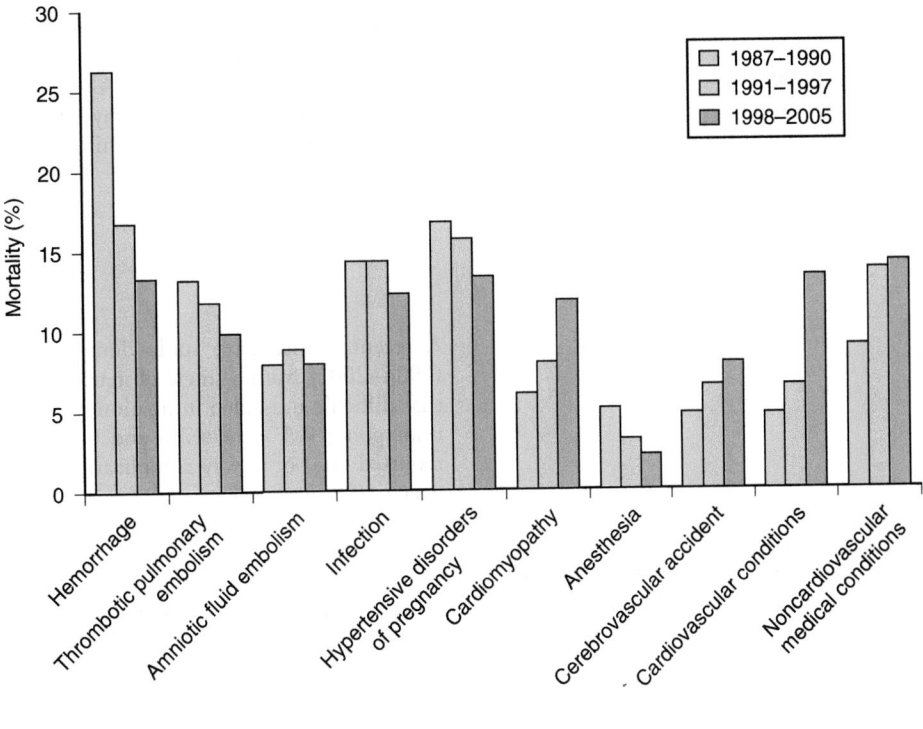

• **Fig. 37.1** Maternal mortality: United States (1998–2005). (Reproduced with permission from Berg CJ, Callaghan WM, Syverson C, Henderson Z. Pregnancy-related mortality in the United States, 1998 to 2005, *Obstet Gynecol.* 2010;116:1302–1309.)

TABLE 37.2	Case Fatality Rates and Rate Ratios of Anesthesia-Related Deaths During Cesarean Delivery by Type of Anesthesia: United States (1979–2002)		
Year of Death	CASE FATALITY RATES (DEATHS PER MILLION, GENERAL OR REGIONAL ANESTHETIC)		
	General Anesthetic	Regional Anesthetic	Rate Ratios
1979–1984	20.0	8.6	2.3 (95% CI 1.9–2.9)
1985–1990	32.3	1.9	16.7 (95% CI 12.9–21.8)
1991–1996	16.8	2.5	6.7 (95% CI 3.0–14.9)
1997–2002	6.5	3.8	1.7 (95% CI 0.6–4.6)

CI, Confidence interval
Reproduced with permission from Hawkins, JL. Anesthesia-related maternal mortality in the United States 1979–2002. *Obstet Gynecol.* 2011; 117(1):71.

• BOX 37.1 The Fourth National Audit Project (NAP4): The Most Common Recurring Themes Resulting in Adverse Airway-Related Outcomes

- Poor airway assessment
- Repeated intubation attempts
- Lack of preformulated strategy for management of the difficulty airway
- Awake fiberoptic intubation indicated but not used
- Obesity as a risk factor
- High failure rate of emergency cricothyroidotomy and other rescue techniques
- Adverse airway events during emergence and extubation
- Adverse airway-related outcomes in the intensive care unit and emergency department

Reproduced with permission from Cook TM, Woodall N, Harper J, Benger J, Fourth National Audit Project. Major complications of airway management in the UK: results of the Fourth National Audit Project of the Royal College of Anaesthetists and the Difficult Airway Society. Part 2: Intensive care and emergency departments. *Br J Anaesth.* 2011;106(5):632–642.

UK Data on Anesthesia-Related Maternal Mortality

Anesthesia-related deaths in the United Kingdom rank as the 11th leading cause of maternal death. A new consortium formed in 2014—Mothers and Babies: Reducing Risk through Audits and Confidential Enquiries across the UK (MBRRACE-UK)—initiated a collection of all medical records of all notified maternal deaths, including all maternal deaths from Ireland. The leading causes of death are listed in Fig. 37.2. The reports show that since the early 1980s, there has been a dramatic reduction in anesthesia-related maternal deaths, with the maternal mortality rate for deaths attributed to anesthesia from 1952 to 2011 having fallen dramatically (Fig. 37.3). A significant contributor to the success has been a result of a reduction in airway- and GA-related deaths. Between 2009 and 2012, 4 deaths were classified as directly because of anesthesia, a rate of 0.17 per 100,000 pregnancies. Increased use of RA, aspiration prophylaxis for CD, and improvement in airway training have likely contributed to this decrease.[16]

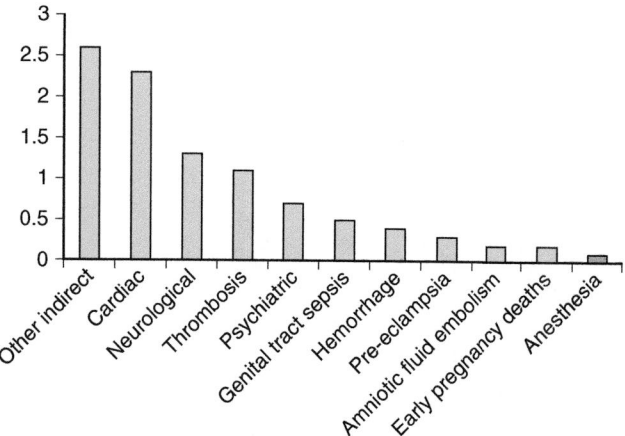

• **Fig. 37.2** Leading causes of maternal deaths in United Kingdom 2009–2012). (Reproduced with permission from Freedman RL, Lucas DN. MBRRACE-UK: saving lives, improving mothers' care – implications for anaesthetists. *Int J Obstet Anesth.* 2015;24(2):161–173.)

The current UK Obstetric Surveillance System (UKOSS) of data collection found the incidence of failed TI in obstetric anesthesia to be 1 in 224. Advanced maternal age, obesity, and a Mallampati (MP) score >1 were significant independent predictors of failure.[17] The Fourth National Audit Project (NAP4) of the Royal College of Anesthetists and the Difficult Airway Society (DAS) were designed prospectively to study the incidence of major complications of airway management in hospitals in the United Kingdom and to perform quantitative and qualitative data analysis.[18,19] In four cases, pregnant women had problems with intubation during emergency CD. These cases took place outside of regular working hours, involved complex patients, and were managed by senior anesthetists. The airway complications noted were aspiration, patient woken up followed by failed awake flexible scope intubation (FSI), a failed cricothyrotomy attempt, and a successful surgical airway. In NAP4 the most common recurring themes resulting in adverse airway-related outcomes are listed in Box 37.1. All patients were admitted to the intensive care unit (ICU) and made a full recovery.[18]

Canadian Data on Anesthesia-Related Maternal Mortality

A recent retrospective study done by McKeen and colleagues (1984–2003) from a single obstetric center in Canada indicated that difficult and failed intubation rates among obstetric patients undergoing GA were 4.7% and 0.08%, respectively.[6] Still, the reported rates of airway complications remained relatively stable over a 20-year period.

Trends in Obstetric Anesthesia

The heightened awareness among anesthesia practitioners regarding the risk for difficult and failed intubation in obstetrics along with the increased trend toward RA techniques have resulted in a marked decline in GA. The National Health Service maternity statistics show that the number of obstetric GAs for CD administered in the United Kingdom decreased from 50% to as low as 5%. Johnson and colleagues similarly found over the same period a marked decline in GA for CD, from 79% to less than 10%.[20] In the United States, Palanisamy and colleagues compared data in their large-volume,

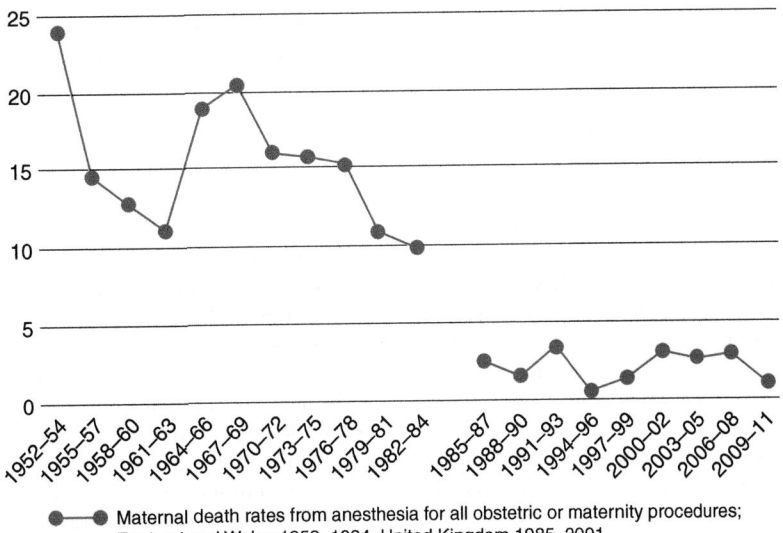

Maternal death rates from anesthesia for all obstetric or maternity procedures; England and Wales 1952–1984, United Kingdom 1985–2001.

• **Fig. 37.3** Decline in maternal deaths from anesthesia: England and Wales, United Kingdom (1952–1954 through 2009–2011). (Reproduced with permission from Freedman Rl. *Int J Obstet Anesth.* 2015;24(2):161–173. Redrawn by Deidre Tomkins, Baylor College of Medicine.)

tertiary care institutions and reported a dramatic decline in the use of GA from 4.5% (1990–1995) to 0.6% (2000–2005).[12]

The current trend in the United States and the United Kingdom is to use GA mainly for the true emergency CD, especially if there is insufficient time or a contraindication to RA. Encountering a DI in the obstetric population continues to persist; therefore, the emerging problem of declining airway skills is important, given the unchanged rate of failed TI in the past four decades.[21–23] The risk of failed TI is considerably higher for an emergency CD than for an elective CD, with 80% of airway-related fatalities occurring during an emergency CD (nights and weekends) and usually involving trainees.[21] Because of the decreased use of GA for CD, the trend in the anesthesia trainees' experience with GA in obstetric patients is also declining.[11,20,24]

Risk Assessment

Maternal, fetal, surgical, and situational factors contribute to the increased incidence and risk of failed intubation following GA for emergency CD.[1] Anatomic and physiological factors alter the airway during pregnancy. In addition, the pulmonary, gastrointestinal, and cardiovascular changes associated with pregnancy place the parturient at risk for DMV, DI, DL, hypoxemia, and cardiorespiratory arrest. The anatomic and physiologic changes during pregnancy and associated risks are highlighted in Box 37.1.

Obesity

Obesity is a significant risk factor for DI and is becoming an increasing concern in the obstetric population. In 2011–2012, the Centers for Disease Control and Prevention (CDC) reported that 34.9% of adults in the United States had a BMI above 30.32 kg/m² (BM1 >30 kg/m² is considered obese). The CDC also predicts that 50% of the population in the United States will have a BMI greater than 30 kg/m² by 2025 (Fig. 37.4). A definition of obesity specific to pregnancy does not exist, but the consensus is that a pregnant woman is considered overweight when her BMI is 25.0 to 29.9 kg/m² and to have obesity when

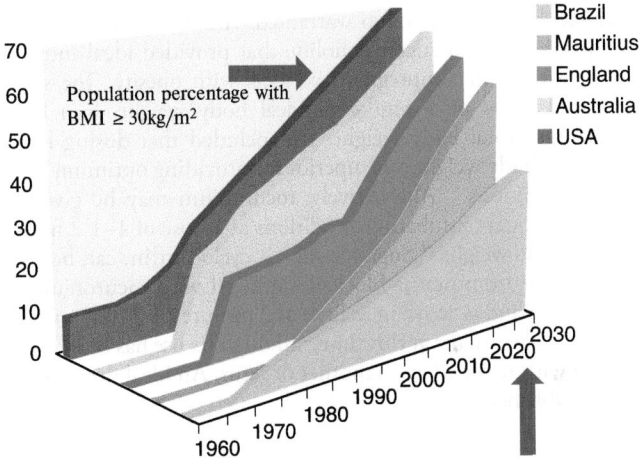

• **Fig. 37.4** Projected prevalence of obesity in adults by 2025. (Reproduced with permission from the Global Challenge of Obesity and the International Obesity Task Force. http://www.iuns.org.)

her BMI is 30 kg/m² or greater.[25] The incidence of DI in the population with obesity varies from 15.5% to a reported incidence of 33%.[26]

In 2015, the National Health and Nutrition Examination Survey showed that 36.5% of women of reproductive age (20 to 39 years) in the United States had obesity.[27] It is estimated that 15% of pregnant women in the United Kingdom have obesity, with 5% having a BMI greater than 35 kg/m².[28] The prevalence of morbid obesity (BMI >40 kg/m²) in pregnancy has increased significantly over the past decade and now represents over 10% of Western women of reproductive age.[29]

A review of anesthesia-related maternal mortality from Michigan showed that obesity was a significant risk factor for airway-related adverse events contributing to maternal mortality.[15] A 6-year review of failed intubations in obstetric patients in a region of the United Kingdom reported 36 cases of failed intubation in women whose average BMI was 33 kg/m².[22] In the confidential inquiries into maternal deaths in the United Kingdom from 2000 to 2002, 35% of all the women who died had obesity, 50% more than the general population. In the reports from 2003 to 2005, 4 of the 6 deaths directly attributable to anesthesia occurred in patients with obesity, two of whom had morbid obesity (BMI >35 kg/m²).[16] The ASA obstetric anesthesia closed claims files indicate that damaging events related to the respiratory system were significantly more common among patients with obesity (32%), than without it (7%) patients. Further, mortality was more common among patients with obesity. These data stress the importance of increased vigilance when caring for the obstetric patient with obesity and necessitates immediate availability of resources, including DA equipment in the labor and delivery suite.[30]

The American College of Obstetricians and Gynecologists (ACOG) Practice Bulletin No. 156, "Obesity in Pregnancy," recommends that an anesthesiologist should be consulted before delivery when a patient with obesity is identified. This allows adequate time for developing an anesthetic plan that addresses the availability of proper equipment for airway management, hemodynamic monitoring, appropriate venous access, and the influence of comorbid conditions such as sleep apnea.[31]

The dosing of induction agents in the parturient with obesity should be based on ideal body weight rather than actual body weight.[32] Thoughtful attention regarding the dose of neuromuscular blocking agents is also warranted. A 2006 study sought to identify the dose of succinylcholine that provided ideal intubating conditions in nonpregnant patients with obesity. The study compared doses of 1 mg/kg of ideal body weight, lean body weight, and total body weight. It concluded that dosing based upon total body weight was superior for providing optimum intubating conditions.[33] Alternatively, rocuronium may be given to provide adequate intubating conditions at a dose of 1–1.2 mg/kg of ideal body weight.[34] Sugammadex, a cyclodextrin, can be used to reverse neuromuscular blockade induced with rocuronium or vecuronium and is active in as little as 2 minutes.[35] It has not been studied in parturients at this time, although its use has been documented with no ill effect to mother or fetus. An ideal dose has yet to be established.[36]

Predictors of Difficult Mask Ventilation and Predictors of Difficult Intubation

Traditional airway assessment involves an attempt to predict the difficulty of glottic view at DL and, by inference, difficulty in intubation.[37] However, such assessment is neither sensitive nor specific and may be unreliable.[4,38] Because of this, it is essential for the anesthesia provider to take a detailed history of the patient and perform a thorough airway assessment to identify any potential risk factors for a DMV or TI. While it is imperative to prepare for a suspected DA, it is just as crucial to be prepared for the unanticipated DA to avoid potential complications. Preparedness is crucial in a parturient since, similar to patients with obesity, a gravid uterus typically leads to a decreased functional residual capacity (FRC), increased oxygen requirements, and, therefore, a tendency to more rapidly desaturate.

A retrospective audit performed on all obstetric GAs, involving a total of 3430 cases over an 8-year period, found 23 DI patients, with an incidence of 1:156. DI was anticipated in 9 patients, 3 of whom underwent an awake FSI; in the remaining 6 patients with morbid obesity, senior trainees or consultants managed the DI, and unanticipated difficulties occurred in 14 patients (61%). The

study showed a zero incidence of esophageal or failed intubation.[39] Preoperative assessment was either not recorded in 6 cases or was poorly documented in 8 cases.

Preoperative Assessment
History and Physical Examination
The ASA difficult airway algorithm (DAA) recommends a focused airway-related history to detect anesthetic, medical, and surgical factors that indicate the presence of a DA. The guidelines also recommend an airway assessment using multiple airway features before initiation of anesthetic care and airway management in all patients.[40] Additionally, the recently updated guidelines by the joint task force of the ASA and the Society for Obstetric Anesthesia and Perinatology (SOAP) recommend establishment of early and ongoing communication between the obstetric, nursing, and anesthesiology teams in a multidisciplinary setup.[38] Recognition of significant anesthetic airway or obstetric risk factors should encourage consultation between the obstetrician and the anesthesiologist.

Predictors of Difficult Airway in Obstetrics: Mallampati Classification
In obstetric patients, the MP score has been used as a single parameter to illustrate the dramatic airway changes that occur in pregnancy and to highlight the importance of preoperative assessment of the airway.

In 1995 Pilkington and coworkers evaluated the MP class at 12 weeks' and 38 weeks' gestation[41]; photographs taken at the end of each time period demonstrated the increase in MP class in the same patient, as gestation advanced. The MP score correlated with the increase in body weight, implying that oropharyngeal edema was responsible for the increase in the MP score.

Kodali and colleagues performed a two-part study to evaluate airway changes during labor and delivery.[42] In part I of the study, they used the conventional Samsoon modification of the MP airway classification. The airway was photographed at the onset of labor (prelabor) and at the end of labor (postlabor). Pregnant women with MP class IV airways were excluded from this initial part of the study. In part II, prelabor and postlabor upper airway volumes were measured by acoustic reflectometry. In part I (n = 61), a significant increase in MP class was observed between prelabor and postlabor measurements ($p < 0.0001$). The airway increased by one class in 20 patients (33%) and by two classes in 3 patients (5%). At the end of labor, there were 8 patients with MP class IV ($p < 0.01$) and 30 with MP class III or IV ($p < 0.0001$). In part II (n = 21), there were significant decreases after labor and delivery in oral volume ($p < 0.05$), pharyngeal area ($p < 0.05$), and pharyngeal volume ($p < 0.001$).

The study by Kodali and colleagues confirmed the frequent increase in MP score during pregnancy and particularly during labor.[42] These findings suggest that it is imperative to evaluate the airway in early labor and to reevaluate it immediately before anesthetic management for an operative delivery.

Sternomental Distance
Sternomental distance (SMD) is measured from the sternum to the tip of the mandible with the head fully extended and the mouth closed. The normal measurement is 13.5 cm. The SMD and the corresponding laryngoscopic view were documented in 523 parturients undergoing elective or emergency CD under GA.[43] An SMD of 13.5 cm or less had a sensitivity of 66.7%, a

specificity of 71%, and a positive predictive value of only 7.6%. Eighteen patients (3.5%) had a Cormack-Lehane grade 3 or 4 laryngoscopic view and were classified as having potentially difficult TIs. The SMD as a sole indicator of DI was not useful, and the suggestion was to incorporate it with other tests in the preoperative airway examination.

Other Bedside Predictors

Recent studies have demonstrated that bedside evaluations such as mouth opening, thyromental distance, upper lip bite test, interincisor distance, BMI, SMD, and the hyomental distance ratio (HMDR) are not useful predictors for DA in the obstetric patient, especially when utilized as an independent risk factor.[4,44-46]

Riad and colleagues were able to demonstrate that MP score and neck circumference were positive predictors for DI using univariate analysis ($p = 0.005$ and $p = 0.011$, respectively); however, this same study was unable to demonstrate that either of these two predictors can be used independently when logistic regression analysis was performed ($p = 0.53$).[47] Riad and colleagues were able to show that a neck circumference ≥33.5 cm was a sensitive predictor to detect a DI, with 100% sensitivity (95% CI 69.2–100) and 50% specificity (95% CI 38.9–61.1).[45]

Multivariate Predictors

In 1992 Rocke and colleagues were the first to use multivariate predictors to predict difficult TI.[9] They evaluated the MP classification as modified by Samsoon and Young, referring to it as the Modified Mallampati Test (MMT), along with other risk parameters in 3440 patients undergoing elective or emergency CD under GA. Data were collected on 1606 patients, representing 46.7% of the obstetric surgical patients. Of the patients studied, 1500 underwent GA. Other risk parameters for DA that they assessed included short neck, which equates with decreased anterior-occipital joint extension; receding mandible or decreased temporomandibular

joint distance (TMD [less than <6.0 cm]); and protruding maxillary incisors indicating significant overbite, which would equate to the current class C jaw protrusion or class III upper lip bite test.

Rocke's group made subjective assessments of the ease or difficulty of TI according to the following classification (Tables 37.3 and 37.4):[9]

- *Grade 1: Easy.* Intubation at first attempt with no difficulty.
- *Grade 2: Some difficulty.* Insertion of tracheal tube (TT) not achieved at first attempt; no difficulty, but successful intubation after adjustment of laryngoscope blade and/or adjustment of head position, not requiring additional equipment, removal, and reinsertion of the laryngoscope, or senior assistance.
- *Grade 3: Very difficult.* Requiring removal of the laryngoscope, further oxygenation by mask ventilation, and subsequent intubation with or without the use of airway adjuncts (e.g., Eschmann introducer, alternative laryngoscope blade) or intubation by a senior colleague.
- *Grade 4: Failed intubation.* Several attempts at intubation or unrecognized esophageal intubation by resident, followed by subsequent TI by senior anesthesiologist.

Based on these various parameters, the relative risk of experiencing difficult TI (compared with an uncomplicated MMT class I airway) was determined as follows:

3.23 for MMT class II
7.58 for MMT class III
11.3 for MMT class IV
5.01 for short neck
8.0 for protruding incisors
9.71 for receding mandible

The investigators analyzed the univariate individual risk factor (i.e., MMT class) and combinations of the various risk factors and showed that in a patient with an MMT III or IV classification plus protruding incisors, a short neck, and a receding mandible, the probability of DI was greater than 90% (Fig. 37.5).

TABLE 37.3   Ease or Difficulty of Tracheal Intubation

System	Anatomical and Physiological Changes	Risks
Airway	1. Hormonal changes: increase in estrogen, elevates ground substance of maternal airway, blood volume, and total body water. 2. Increase in hypervascularity and edema of oropharynx, nasopharynx, and respiratory tract. 3. Increase in Mallampati score during pregnancy, labor, and delivery. 4. Excessive weight gain fluid overload during pregnancy and preeclampsia.	1. Edema of the airway. 2. Increasing risk of epistaxis with manipulation of nasopharynx. 3. Difficult intubation. 4. Potential for difficult airway.
Respiratory changes	1. Gravid uterus cephalad displacement during pregnancy results in 20% decrease in FRC, which is exacerbated in the supine position. 2. O_2 consumption and CO_2 production increased by 20%–40% secondary to metabolic demands of a growing fetus, uterus, and placenta.	1. Shortens safe apnea time, resulting in rapid hypoxemia. 2. Rapid desaturation during prolonged apnea.
Cardiovascular changes	1. Compression of inferior vena cava in supine position by gravid uterus. 2. Compression of aorta by gravid uterus. 3. Decrease in cardiac output and hypoxemia during difficult ventilation and intubation.	1. Results in decrease in venous return and cardiac output. 2. Results in decrease in utero-placental perfusion. 3. Can result in development of myocardial hypoxemia and cardiac arrest.
Gastrointestinal (GI) changes	1. GI changes secondary to increased progesterone and estrogen, anatomic and physiological changes. 2. Decrease in pH; increase in intragastric pressure and incompetent gastroesophageal sphincter tone.	1. The parturient is at risk for regurgitation and aspiration. 2. Predisposes the parturient to aspiration; thus consideration for timely administration of nonparticulate antacids, H_2-receptor antagonists, and/or metoclopramide for aspiration prophylaxis.

TABLE 37.4	Association Between Oropharyngeal Structures Visualized Preoperatively and Subsequent Difficulty at Tracheal Intubation				
	OROPHARYNGEAL STRUCTURES VISUALIZED				
	Class I	Class II	Class III	Class IV	Total
Difficulty at Intubation					
Grade 1: easy	461 (96.4)	566 (90.6)	264 (82.2)	58 (76.3)	1349 (89.9)
Grade 2: some difficulty	15 (3.1)	48 (7.7)	43 (13.4)	13 (17.1)	119 (7.9)
Grade 3: very difficult	2 (0.42)	10 (1.6)	13 (4.0)	5 (6.6)	30 (2.0)
Grade 4: failed	0 (0)	1 (0.2)	1 (0.3)	0 (0)	2 (0.1)

Values are percentages ($p < 0.001$).
Reproduced with permission from Rocke DA, Murray WB, Rout CC, Gouws E. Relative risk analysis of factors associated with difficult intubation in obstetric anesthesia. *Anesthesiology.* 1992; 77(1):69.

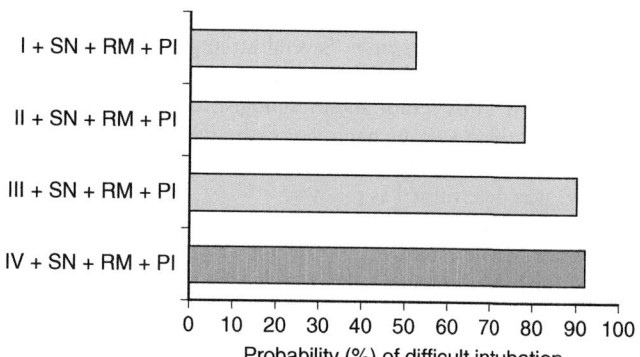

• **Fig. 37.5** Probability of experiencing difficult intubation for varying combinations of risk factors. (Reproduced with permission, modified from Rocke DA, Murray DB, Rout CC, Gouws E. Relative risk analysis of factors associated with difficult intubation in anesthesia. *Anesthesiology.* 1992;77:67–73.)

Merah and associates studied the potential of five airway measurements to predict a difficult direct laryngoscopy in 80 West African obstetric patients during CD under GA.[47,48] The five bedside tests evaluated were MMT, TMD, SMD, horizontal length of mandible, and interincisor gap. Eight patients (10%) had DL. The MMT as a sole predictor had a sensitivity, specificity, and PPV of 87.1%, 99.6%, and 70%, respectively. Increased BMI contributed to the prediction of DL. The difference between the mean weights of difficult-to-intubate patients (109 ± 12.4 kg) and easy-to-intubate patients (81 ± 12.0 kg) was statistically significant. The combination of MMT and TMD yielded values of 100%, 93.1%, and 61.5% for sensitivity, specificity, and PPV, respectively. The researchers concluded that MMT can be used as the sole predictor of difficult TI. Despite multiple sources describing MMT as an unreliable independent predictor of a DA due to its low sensitivity and specificity, Merah and associates attribute their success with MMT from ensuring they performed the test as MP described and without patient phonating or gagging.[48]

Gupta and colleagues evaluated the obstetric airway, using the MMT and the Wilson risk sum score, to assess the potential for DA in 372 patients undergoing elective or emergency CD under GA.[43] As a screening test for prediction of DI, the Wilson risk sum score was less sensitive (36%) but had almost the same specificity (98.5%) and PPV (64%) as the MMT. When both tests were combined as predictors, the sensitivity was improved to 100%, the specificity was marginally decreased to 96.2%, and the PPV (64.8%) remained almost the same, compared with the MMT score alone. Gupta and colleagues concluded that in obstetric

patients, use of the Wilson risk sum score along with the MMT score resulted in high sensitivity, specificity, and PPV.[46] This study highlighted the importance of incorporating multiple predictors rather than using single predictors of DL and intubation.

Ultrasonography

Since bedside screening tests and clinical assessment alone are not always reliable predictors of DA,[6,49] other methods have been explored for predicting DA. Ultrasonography (USG) is a quick, portable, noninvasive, inexpensive, and nonradiating means to visualize the airway; modern advancements in ultrasound technology allow for improved resolution and enhanced tissue penetration for visualization of structures such as the epiglottis, vocal cords, and ring-shaped membrane.[50] Recent studies have used USG to predict DL by measuring anterior-neck soft-tissue thickness; however, there are limited data as to whether this method could also be applied for the parturient airway.[51,52]

The use of USG is becoming popular in assessing DA management. It is a valid tool to identify critical landmarks such as the cricothyroid membrane (CTM) in a suspected or anticipated DA.[53]

Zheng and colleagues have devised a protocol in which ultrasound measurements will be taken to determine anterior cervical soft tissue thickness at five anatomical levels (hyoid bone, epiglottis, CTM, thyroid isthmus, and suprasternal notch) in the upper airway.[54] Using the Cormack-Lehane grading system, subjects will be classified as either an "easy intubation" or "difficult intubation," and these results will be compared against the ultrasound measurements. This study is currently in progress. Presently, there are no reliable methods for using the ultrasound for airway assessment.[54-56]

Metaanalysis of Bedside Screening Test Performance

Shiga and colleagues conducted a systematic review to determine the diagnostic accuracy of bedside tests for predicting difficult TI in patients with no airway pathology.[57] Thirty-five studies comprising 50,760 patients, including both surgical and obstetric patients, were selected from randomized trials (Table 37.5).

The overall incidence of difficult TI was 5.8% (95% confidence interval [CI], 4.5% to 7.5%). Screening tests included the MP oropharyngeal classification, TMD, SMD, mouth opening, and Wilson risk score.

The metaanalysis showed that in the obstetric population (2155 patients), the prevalence of difficult TI was 3.1% (95% CI 1.7–5.5). In the obstetric patients, the MP classification yielded a sensitivity of 56%, a specificity of 81%, and a likelihood ratio of 0.6%. The metaanalysis data in the obstetric patients

TABLE 37.5 Pooled Estimates of Bayesian Statistics of Six Different Bedside Tests for Difficult Intubation

Diagnostic Test	No. of Studies Included	No. of Patients	Prevalence of Difficult Intubation (95% CI), %	Pooled Sensitivity (95% CI), %	Pooled Specificity (95% CI), %	POOLED LIKELIHOOD RATIO		Pooled Log Diagnostic Odds Ratio (95% CI)
						Positive	Negative	
Overall Population								
Mallampati classification	31	41,193	5.7 (4.4–7.3)*	49 (41–57)*	86 (81–90)*	3.7 (3.0–4.6)*	0.5 (0.5–0.6)*	2.0 (1.7–2.3)*
Thyromental distance	17	29,132	6.5 (4.6–9.1)*	20 (11–29)*	94 (89–99)*	3.4 (2.3–4.9)*	0.8 (0.8–0.9)*	1.7 (1.2–2.1)*
Sternomental distance	3	1,085	5.4 (3.1–9.2)*	62 (37–86)*	82 (67–97)*	5.7 (2.1–15.1)*	0.5 (0.3–0.8)	2.7 (1.4–3.9)*
Mouth opening	3	20,614	5.6 (2.2–14.5)*	22 (9–35)*	97 (93–100)*	4.0 (2.0–8.2)*	0.8 (0.7–1.0)*	1.7 (1.2–2.3)*
Wilson risk score	5	6,076	4.0 (1.8–9.0)*	46 (36–56)	89 (85–92)	5.8 (3.9–8.6)*	0.6 (0.5–0.9)	2.3 (1.8–2.8)*
Combination of Mallampati classification and thyromental distance	5	1,498	6.6 (2.8–15.6)*	36 (14–59)*	87 (74–100)*	9.9 (3.1–31.9)*	0.6 (0.5–0.9)*	3.3 (1.5–5.0)*
Obstetric Subgroup								
Mallampati classification	3	2,155	3.1 (1.7–5.5)*	56 (41–72)	81 (67–95)*	6.4 (1.1–36.5)*	0.6 (0.4–0.8)	2.5 (0.6–4.4)*
Obese Subgroup (BMI >30)								
Mallampati classification	4	378	15.8 (14.3–17.5)	74 (51–97)*	74 (62–87)*	2.9 (1.6–5.3)*	0.4 (0.2–0.8)	2.1 (0.8–3.3)*

Posttest probability = [(pretest odds) * likelihood ratio]/[1 + (pretest odds) * likelihood ratio]; where pretest odds = pretest probability/(1 − pretest probability).
DerSimonian-Laird random-effects model was used throughout.
*Significant heterogeneity (p < 0.1) was found.
BMI, Body mass index; CI, confidence interval; Neg., negative; Pos., positive; ROC, receiver operating characteristic curve.
Reproduced with permission from Shiga T, Wajima Z, Inoue T, Sakamoto A. Predicting difficult intubation in apparently normal patients. Anesthesiology. 2005;103(2):429–437.

remained inconclusive because of the small number of studies and heterogeneity.

Management of the Difficult Airway in Obstetrical Patients in Labor

Management of the DA has emerged as one of the most important safety issues in both the surgical and obstetric populations. The ASA Task Force Practice Guidelines for Obstetric Anesthesia published in 2016 do not address the specifics of management of difficult or failed TI during GA for obstetric patients.[58] The foundation for best practices involves three important recommendations by the ASA for obstetric anesthesia: First, based on the recognition of anesthetic or obstetric risk—that is, obesity and predictors of DA—best practices should warrant consultation between the anesthesia and obstetric providers. Second, providers should consider prophylactic placement of an epidural catheter early during labor in high-risk cases such as patients with obesity, predicted DA, preeclampsia, potential obstetric complications, and trial of labor after CD. Third, providers should avoid instrumentation of the airway in patients who are at risk for DI or DMV, which requires advanced planning while the patient is

in labor, and should have the proper equipment available to deal with the management of airway emergencies.

Types of Fetal Heart Rate Tracings Affecting Anesthetic Management

The American College of Obstetricians and Gynecologists has developed a three-tiered classification of fetal heart rate (FHR) and a system for interpreting these abnormalities[59] (Box 37.2). The interpretation of the FHR and the potential for fetal acidemia, and possible neurological injury, warrant expedited operative delivery. The decision for operative delivery has significant impact on our anesthetic management. In category II FHR, despite intrauterine resuscitation, persistent late decelerations with minimum or no FHR variability warrant expedited operative delivery. Category III FHR tracings are abnormal, and these tracings have been associated with adverse neurologic abnormalities, although the predictive value is poor. When intrauterine resuscitation of these abnormalities fails, delivery should be expedient. The emergent CD under GA and airway-related morbidity are associated with high liability. Studies are lacking to demonstrate the timeframe for performance of the expeditious delivery. The traditional

Category I FHR: These are normal FHR tracings. Baseline FHR 110–160, moderate variability with fluctuations in amplitude and frequency 6 to 25 beats.

Category II FHR: Baseline FHR. Bradycardia not accompanied by recurrent decelerations; recurrent variable decelerations accompanied by minimal or moderate variability; or prolonged decelerations >2 min but <10 min.

Category III FHR: Include either no baseline variability, or the presence of recurrent late decelerations , variable decelerations, bradycardia, or sinusoidal pattern. Category III FHR tracings are abnormal and persistent category III tracings are associated with adverse neurologic outcomes and therefore require immediate intervention and expedited delivery

"decision-to-incision time" of 30 minutes to perform a cesarean section has not been validated. These situations require vigilance, anticipation, preparation, and preformulated strategies for safe anesthetic management in order to have the best outcomes for mother and baby.

Neuraxial Labor Analgesia Techniques

To ensure optimal and safe maternal and fetal outcomes, to eliminate airway-related maternal mortality, and to avoid GA, it is prudent to incorporate the best practice of early neuraxial labor epidural in the anesthetic management plan of the patient, so as to avoid instrumentation for a potential DA in the event of an operative delivery. The increased use of neuraxial techniques for providing labor analgesia and anesthesia for CD has been prompted by a number of concerns, with the most prominent being to avoid the potentially adverse outcomes with a DA and the risk of pulmonary aspiration. In the United States, implementation of best practices has been associated with a remarkable decline in airway-related morbidity and mortality.[2] The MBRRACE-UK consortium outlines the lessons learned from airway catastrophes and focuses on preventable factors, which has resulted in a decline in maternal deaths.[47] The remarkable success in reducing maternal deaths is due to reduction in airway- and GA-related complications. As noted, the combination of pregnancy and obesity poses an undue high risk for DI following induction of GA. A recent systematic review of 11 cohort studies reported that the risk of CD was increased by 50% in women with BMI of 30–35 kg/m² and was more than doubled compared to women with normal BMI (20–25 kg/m²).[60] Factors associated with higher risk for CD in parturients with obesity include medical and pregnancy-related comorbidities, as well as decreased uterine contractility, thus raising concerns for both GA and RA in an emergency. This further highlights the importance of proper planning and safe anesthetic choices with the implementation of the best practice of an early functioning neuraxial epidural while the parturient is in labor. The recommendation for prophylactic use of optimal epidural labor analgesia is based on reasonable evidence supporting a reduced risk of conversion to GA.

Another option for providing labor analgesia is the use of combined spinal epidural (CSE) labor analgesia with an intrathecal opioid and an epidural catheter in-situ. However, in a patient with a predicted or known DA, morbid obesity, or high probability of operative delivery, CSE is controversial and debatable. During the initial phase of analgesia provided by intrathecal medications, the functionality of the epidural catheter is not known,

and therefore there is no guarantee that surgical anesthesia will be achieved for an urgent or emergent CD posted during the initial CSE placement.[49] However, Bloom and colleagues reported that failed RA requiring conversion to GA occurred more commonly with an epidural than with CSE (4.3% vs 2.1% vs 1.7%, respectively).[50] Finally, as part of best practice, there should be aggressive monitoring and management of an epidural catheter that is not functioning well; it requires replacement with either a functioning continuous epidural catheter or a continuous spinal catheter.

Management of Parturient With Predicted Difficult Airway Undergoing Operative Delivery

Airway Management Is Unnecessary: Neuraxial Techniques

Predicted Difficult Airway—Operative Delivery: Category II FHR Tracing

The choice of anesthesia in patients with category II FHR tracing for operative delivery is either neuraxial or GA depending upon the clinical situation and its urgency. In modern obstetric anesthesia practice, neuraxial anesthesia is administered to some patients who would have otherwise received GA in the past—for example, patients with severe preeclampsia with decreased platelet count, placenta previa *without* active bleeding, and umbilical cord prolapse with confirmed functioning epidural catheter where surgical anesthesia can be established rapidly and without delay. In recent years, these previous contraindications have been questioned, and many such patients can now be safely managed with neuraxial anesthesia. Neuraxial techniques for CD are safe and predictable[2]; therefore in any patient undergoing elective or emergent CD, if airway intervention is not necessary, one can proceed with a neuraxial anesthetic such as single-injection spinal anesthesia, continuous epidural anesthesia, combined spinal-epidural anesthesia, or continuous spinal anesthesia.

A functioning epidural catheter in a patient allows the option of establishing surgical anesthesia by incrementally dosing the in situ functioning epidural catheter in an expeditious manner with the shortest decision to delivery intervals (DDIs). Current evidence confirms achieving surgical anesthesia with a functioning epidural, and achieving shortest DDI for emergency CD is comparable with that achieved with GA.[61,62] The investigators concluded that although GA is considered faster than either spinal or epidural anesthesia, it is well established that GA poses greater maternal risk.[4,63] Therefore, the benefits of obtaining anesthesia with GA faster versus the risk of a maternal airway-related complication must be weighed and determined by the obstetrician and anesthesiologist working in consultation together in each individual case.

The ACOG committee opinion on anesthesia for emergency deliveries endorses and advocates "Cesarean deliveries that are performed for a nonreassuring FHR pattern do not necessarily preclude the use of RA."[58]

A retrospective study confirmed that the use of GA for CD from 2000 to 2005 was low at less than 1%, and of that, 85% were emergent deliveries.[12] The majority of those performed under GA were attributed to a perceived lack of time, particularly for the emergency deliveries. Very few GA cases resulted from failure of neuraxial anesthesia techniques, with a very low incidence of

GA-related morbidity, and no cases of mortality. This study confirms several matters: First, the policy to place epidural catheters prophylactically in high-risk patients, particularly patients with obesity and potential DA, has reduced the risk of unanticipated GA. Second, the adoption of a more aggressive approach toward management of inadequate neuraxial block (by replacement of epidural catheters for suboptimal analgesia during labor) may have reduced the incidence of intraoperative conversion to GA. Third, the willingness to perform emergent spinal anesthesia, including intentional continuous spinal techniques, especially in patients with certain comorbid conditions, such as severe preeclampsia[62,64] and morbid obesity, may have been partly responsible for the reduction in GA. Although it may seem obvious, it is vital that all essential monitoring with functioning monitor alarms based on ASA basic monitoring guidelines, drugs, and equipment should be checked and ready in the OR before any major neuraxial block. Emergency airway devices and a DA cart should also be readily available in the event RA fails and a general anesthetic becomes necessary.

Airway Management Is Necessary: Awake Tracheal Intubation

Mushambi et al., in their most recent publication in 2020,[51] offer recommendations on management of obstetric high-risk patients with predicted DA who will require airway management for operative delivery. Unlike a guideline, it offers a series of practice recommendations and algorithmic decision aids based on an extensive literature review spanning more than 40 years. Lessons learned include the following:

1. Early antenatal referral to the high-risk anesthesia clinic or anesthesia service is needed for airway consultation.
2. Meticulous multidisciplinary planning takes into consideration both obstetric and anesthetic course of action.
3. Patient-centered care with patient involvement should be part of decision-making, in order for the parturient to appreciate the significant risks involved with airway management and to obtain final consent to the obstetric and anesthetic plan of action.
4. Elective CD should be planned in advance for patients with significant airway pathology and presence of other surgery specialties such as otolaryngology.
5. It is vital to have a contingency plan in case emergency CD is necessary.

Parturients with documented DA, obvious airway abnormalities, or women in whom oxygenation and manual mask ventilation or intubation is not guaranteed can present significant challenges to anesthesia teams. Further, the management of such a patient presenting for CD does not offer a straightforward decision because, following induction of anesthesia, intubation of the trachea may be impossible and a CICV situation may ensue. Conversely, regional techniques can be unsuccessful, or complications may arise that necessitate emergency intubation.[52,55,65]

Indications for Awake Tracheal Intubation in Patients Undergoing Elective or Nonurgent Cesarean Delivery

Awake TI is indicated in patients with a previously documented history of difficult/failed intubation, osteogenesis imperfecta, severe rheumatoid arthritis,[56] severe facial burn injuries, restricted mouth opening and abnormal upper airway pathology, acromegaly, lingual tonsillar hyperplasia, subglottic tracheal stenosis,

---

• BOX 37.3 Factors Associated With Difficult Airway Management and Surgical Safety Checklist

Factors Associated with Difficult Airway Management

☐ Previous history of difficult airway
☐ Morbid obesity
☐ Diabetes, acromegaly, rheumatoid arthritis, obstructive sleep apnea, osteogenesis imperfecta
☐ Trauma, facial burn injuries, swelling, head and neck infection, hematoma of the mouth, tongue, pharynx, larynx, trachea, or neck
☐ Large tongue, receding jaw, high arched palate, prominent upper incisors, short thick neck, large breasts, microstomia, fixed or "high" larynx
☐ Mouth opening, 2–3 cm jaw protrusion class C, Mallampati class III or IV, thyromental distance <6 cm, reduced head/neck mobility
☐ Voice change, shortness of breath, difficulty swallowing, choking stridor, inability to lie flat, drooling of saliva, lingular tonsillar hyperplasia

Surgical Safety Checklist: Example

Ben Taub Hospital: Obstetrical Use Only
In the event of an emergent case, do not delay proceeding in an expeditious manner in order to complete this checklist; rather, defer this checklist until the appropriate clinical time.

SIGN-IN

Surgeon Completes During Time-Out, With Attending Present
Indication and categorization (urgent, scheduled) of surgery confirmed ☐ Yes ☐ No
   Consent signed with correct attending identified and all appropriate procedures documented ☐ Yes ☐ No
   All team members have been introduced by name and role ☐ Yes ☐ No
   Patient and team members have verified her identity, surgical site, and procedure ☐ Yes ☐ No
   Known allergy? ☐ Yes ☐ No
   Antibiotic prophylaxis given within the last 60 minutes ☐ Yes ☐ No ☐ Not Indicated
   Fire safety assessment complete ☐ Yes ☐ No
   Current hemoglobin/hematocrit, platelets reviewed ☐ Yes ☐ No
   Medications currently being administered and plan for intraop and postoperative dosing discussed ☐ Yes ☐ No
   Airway and risk of aspiration evaluated and appropriate equipment available ☐ Yes ☐ No
   If risk of blood loss >1000 cc for cesarean delivery, blood products readily available ☐ Yes ☐ No (Review patient-specific risks of PPH/uterine atony and devise the plan)
   Surgeon: Review critical and unexpected steps, operative duration, anticipated complications and patient-specific concerns (e.g., arrest of descent may need a vaginal hand and/or consideration of dorsal lithotomy position)
   Anesthesia: Review patient-specific concerns (including regional versus general anesthesia plan)
   Nursing Staff: Review patient-specific concerns, equipment, supplies, sterility
   All essential imaging studies reviewed (placental location, characterization verified) ☐ Yes ☐ No
   Fetal lie verified (Leopold's maneuver sufficient) ☐ Yes ☐ No
   Discuss: Is Neonatology needed at delivery? ☐ Yes ☐ No
   Team: Discuss postoperative recovery location, duration, and anticipated postop complications.

SIGN-IN

Nurse Verbally Confirms with the Surgeon and Anesthesia Providers
Instrument, sponge, and needle counts correct ☐ Yes ☐ No
   Specimens labeled and pathology request complete ☐ Yes ☐ No
   Equipment and/or supply concerns escalated to charge nurse ☐ Yes ☐ No
   Surgeon, Anesthesia Professionals, and Nurse: Review the key concerns for recovery and management of this patient
   Team: Discusses postoperative recovery location, duration, and anticipated postop complications

morbid/super obesity with severe obstructive apnea and predicted DA (Box 37.3), or predicted impossible mask ventilation.[38,66] Other indications for awake TI include certain anatomic features which indicate that TI by conventional means is likely to be difficult or impossible, contraindications to RA, or, in a patient with predicted DA, where extensive hemorrhage is anticipated. A safe option in patients with airway challenges undergoing operative delivery is to secure the airway with the TT while the patient remains awake. In such patients, although neuraxial anesthesia may be a consideration, it may be more prudent to secure the airway awake so as to have a safe outcome for mother and baby. If RA is not an option and time is not an issue, an awake TI can be performed safely with either an FSI or a video-assisted laryngoscopy (VAL).

Incidence of Flexible Scope Intubation in Obstetrics

The incidence of awake FSI in obstetric patients performed either electively or after failed intubation is not fully known and is dependent on the institution and the skills of the anesthetists. Glassenberg evaluated data spanning more than 35 years on the liberal use of sedation and awake FSI in an attempt to decrease the incidence of failed TI within his obstetric unit.[67] Between 1974 and 1985, awake FSI was not used at all; between 1985 and 2004, it was performed in 14% of all cesarean sections; and between 2005 and 2010 it was performed in less than 15% of all cesarean sections. Glassenberg concluded that an awake FSI rate of 15% would be required to halve the failed intubation rate and then went on to suggest that a more pragmatic approach is a combination of use of video laryngoscope during rapid sequence induction (RSI) of GA and laryngeal mask after failed intubation.[67] Based on a 1-year UK obstetric unit survey conducted in 2014, failed intubations totaled 55 and awake FSI intubations totaled 24, giving an estimate rate of 1.1 per 1000 awake intubations for obstetric GA.[68] The incidence in an Australian study is similar: 1 per 1095 cases.[69]

In our retrospective study, an assessment of airway management for CD performed under GA over an 8-year period, we observed that out of 10,077 CDs, GA was used in 695 cases. Of the 695 cases, elective awake FSI was performed in 7 patients (1%) with predicted DA. The indications for awake FSI included a nonreassuring airway exam with MP scores greater than III, a short thick neck, or restricted neck movement; other indications were Noonan syndrome, severe burn contractures, nephrotic syndrome with DA, severe rheumatoid arthritis with bamboo spine, placenta previa and thrombocytopenia, twin gestation with placenta accreta, and DA.[8] Other reports document the successful use of awake FSI in parturients with DA for CD[70] and a study in 60 parturients undergoing cesarean section who underwent asleep FSI.[61]

Accomplishing Successful Awake Flexible Scope Intubation in an Obstetric Patient

The basic components for accomplishing a successful awake FSI include (1) patient counseling and psychological preparation, (2) administration of antisialagogue and judicious sedation, (3) adequate topicalization of the upper airway and elimination of the gag reflex, and (4) the AAM skills of the operator. Awake TI may be achieved by either FSI or, as recent reports suggest, the use of awake vide-assisted VAL, and preparation of the airway is similar.[62,71–73]

Patient counseling includes providing all options, discussing risks and benefits, and obtaining informed consent. It requires spending enough time with the patient and the family.

Supplemental oxygen: During airway preparation, always remember to administer supplemental oxygen via nasal cannula. Glycopyrrolate, 0.2 mg intravenously, should be administered 15 minutes before applying local anesthetic to the upper airway. Glycopyrrolate helps dry oropharyngeal secretions, thereby facilitating quick absorption of undiluted local anesthetic by the oropharyngeal mucosa and improves flexible scope visualization of the glottic opening. An additional advantage in the parturient is that glycopyrrolate, a quaternary ammonium compound, does not cross the placental barrier and, thus, has no effect on the fetus.

Sedation: Perform careful titration of sedatives such as midazolam 15–30 µg/kg intravenously to allay anxiety and fentanyl 1.5 µg/kg (ideal body weight) administered intravenously to provide analgesia, depress airway reflexes, facilitate airway instrumentation, and improve patient comfort and cooperation during the procedure without risking respiratory depression in the mother or the newborn.

Dexmedetomidine is another choice to consider for sedation as it does not cross the placenta and has been used successfully for sedation during FSI. Dexmedetomidine 1.0 µg/kg infusion over 10 minutes provides good to excellent tolerance of the procedure, allows more stable hemodynamics, and preserves a patent airway without causing respiratory depression.[74]

Topicalization: Traditionally, the oral route is used for airway access. Nasotracheal intubation is avoided in pregnant women due to the risk of initiating epistaxis from the hyperemic nasal mucosa. The aim of airway topicalization with local anesthetic such as lidocaine is to depress pharyngeal, laryngeal, and tracheobronchial reflexes and to facilitate smooth TI. A needleless approach to local anesthetic topicalization of the airway may be achieved in the following manner:

1. *Combined pharyngeal, periglottic anesthesia:* Have an assistant pull the tongue gently anterior with gauze-padded finger and thumb, then apply lidocaine gel 2% with a tongue spatula to the tip of the tongue, sides of the tongue, and base of the tongue. Place 1 inch of 5% lidocaine ointment on the tongue blade, and place it like a lollipop in the midline, posterior aspect of the tongue, as far back as the patient can tolerate.
2. *Glossopharyngeal nerve block:* (a) Employ a tongue depressor on the lateral surface to shift the tongue medially and spray 4% lidocaine on the palate, base of the tongue, uvula, posterior pharyngeal wall, and anterior/posterior tonsillar pillars. (b) The MADgic atomizer (Wolfe Tory Medical, Inc., Salt Lake City, UT) works well for the local anesthetic spray since the droplet size is very small.[75–77] The atomized particles are gently dispersed across a broad area of the mucosa for optimal coverage, and absorption of the local anesthetic is rapid. If the mucosa is dry, apply gauze balls soaked in 4% lidocaine with a curved clamp to the pyriform fossa for <5 minutes. *Eliminating the gag reflex is critical for a successful awake intubation, which means applying topical local anesthetic to the base of the tongue and the peritonsillar pillars liberally to block the* **glossopharyngeal nerve**. Use Yankauer or soft suction to clear the secretions and test for reaction (gag, cough).
3. *Superior laryngeal and recurrent laryngeal nerve blocks (The "Spray as You Go" technique):* Preload the side port of the flexible bronchoscope with a 5 mL Luer slip syringe containing 2% to 4% lidocaine. Spray 2 to 3 cc on the anterior and superior aspects of the epiglottis in order to block the **superior laryngeal nerve** and the posterior and inferior aspects of the epiglottis, the vocal cords, and the upper trachea to block the **recurrent laryngeal nerve**.[78] Because it is essential to prevent

gagging, coughing, and laryngeal spasm, adequate airway topicalization is required prior to awake TI. There has been concern that the depression of laryngeal and gag reflexes in patients at risk for regurgitation of gastric contents may place the parturient at risk for pulmonary aspiration. However, those fears have been allayed and found to have no merit in a study performed in a similar subset of patients who were at high risk for aspiration.[79] Regardless of the extent of airway topicalization with local anesthetic, lower esophageal tone seems to be preserved, provided sedation is used judiciously.

Following topicalization of the upper airway and elimination of the gag reflex, TI can be achieved with either FSI or VAL.[80,81]

Clinical Pearls to Successful Flexible Scope Intubation Technique

The following are the awake FSI strategies that have worked in enhancing our success rate in obstetric patients.

1. Before advancing the flexible scope, measure the distance from the corner of the mouth to the ear to predict intubating oral airway size (Ovassapian, Berman, Patil-Syracuse, Williams, or MAD).
2. Keep the flexible scope straight and follow the midline of the hard palate. The dominant hand performs the finer, complex movement of aiming the tip in the correct direction.
3. Advance the flexible scope to 10 cm and look at the video monitor to visualize identifiable airway structures.
4. Make small movements with the lever as you advance the bronchoscope.
5. If the beveled tip of the TT impinges on the right arytenoid cartilage, try pulling back the TT, over the flexible bronchoscope by 2 cm, and then rotating it by 90 degrees clockwise or counterclockwise so that the right beveled tip is either at the 6 o'clock or 12 o'clock position, respectively.
6. Identify the carina, advance the scope to three rings above the carina, and avoid touching the carina because it provokes coughing. Ask the patient to inhale deeply, before advancing the tube to its final position and removing the scope. If the TT meets resistance while trying to advance it into the larynx, withdraw 1 to 2 cm, rotate 90 degrees counterclockwise, and advance the TT.
7. Stabilize the TT with one hand and inflate the cuff. Confirm the tube placement with $EtCO_2$ while hand ventilating, as well as the presence of bilateral breath sounds, before inducing GA.

Training in Awake Flexible Scope Intubation

FSI is a challenging technique to learn, and even when mastered it requires regular practice to maintain skills and proficiency. The learning curve for FSI is steep, with competency achieved only after 25 successful FSI.[82] In a survey of 132 residency programs in the United States, it was determined that FSI was taught in only 64% of residency programs; however, the average FSI procedures performed before graduation were fewer than 10. Proficiency carries with it a level of mastery of the skill that is above the minimum required to gain competency. FSI is a procedure that necessitates experience with the equipment, an understanding of airway endoscope anatomy, proficiency in providing effective local anesthesia and sedation, and ongoing maintenance of FSI skills. It is likely that anesthesia providers in obstetric practice do not have proficiency and maintenance of these skills or the confidence required to perform awake FSI, especially given the preponderance of neuraxial anesthesia in obstetric practices.

Awake Video Laryngoscope-Assisted Tracheal Intubation

The majority of obstetric operating suites now have video laryngoscopes readily available. Although FSI is a gold standard technique for patients with predicted DA, video laryngoscopy is also gaining popularity as an awake technique to assess the airway or to determine the preferred airway device for the management of the DA. Video laryngoscopes have potential advantages over flexible bronchoscopes:

1. Easy to set up;
2. Wider and better glottic visualization and panoramic view of the airway;
3. No limitation on the TT diameter;
4. Easier endotracheal tube (ETT) exchange (the flexible scope must be removed to change to a different size tube); and
5. On-screen viewing by the operator creates a new dynamic interaction and enhances improvement in communication and teaching.

Further, and as noted, anesthetists need approximately 25 intubations to gain competency with FSI,[82] whereas only 1 to 6 intubations are needed to reach the same competency with video laryngoscopy.[83,84] Although there are no reports of video-assisted awake laryngoscopy in obstetric patients, one can draw from the lessons learned about general surgical patients. Alhomary et al. conducted a systematic review of 239 publications and included only 8 for a detailed metaanalysis.[80,81,85–91] The primary determination was the time needed to intubate the patient's trachea. Secondary findings included failed intubation, the rate of successful intubation at first attempt, patient satisfaction, and complications resulting from the intubation. The eight studies examining 429 patients showed awake TI time was shorter with video laryngoscopy compared to FSI. There was no significant difference between the two techniques in failure rate or the first-attempt success rate. The level of patient satisfaction was similar in both groups. The conclusion from the metaanalysis study was that video laryngoscopy for awake intubation is associated with shorter intubation time; it also seems that awake video laryngoscopy has a success rate and safety profile comparable to FSI.

In conclusion, awake TI can be performed using flexible scopes or video laryngoscopes. Appropriate topical anesthesia of the airway and judicious sedation (with minimum adverse effects on the fetus) make it possible to use either of these techniques successfully.[92] In addition, acquiring and maintaining skills with either technique are equally important.

Management of Parturient With Unanticipated Difficult Airway Undergoing Urgent/Emergent Cesarean Delivery for Maternal or Fetal Compromise

Category III FHR Tracing

CD is the most frequently performed surgical intervention. Based on the binary classification of urgent and elective, it is estimated that 800,000 urgent CDs are performed per year in the United States. In the United States, ACOG and, in United Kingdom, the Royal College of Anesthetists recommend a maximum of 30 minutes between the decision to perform an emergency CD and the incision (DDI).[93] The caveat is that certain clinical situations, such as cord prolapse or life-threatening maternal and fetal conditions, will require a much shorter DDI than 30 minutes. Several studies have shown that 10 minutes of anoxia can lead to irreversible cerebral lesions.[94] Conversely, if the infant is extracted within 30 minutes the Apgar score and pH are significantly improved.[95,96] Studies confirm that in the absence of an established and functioning epidural anesthesia or failed epidural anesthesia, the most expeditious means to meet the DDI criteria is to administer GA.[97] According to Tuffnell et al., factors related to anesthesia were implicated in 40% of prolonged DDI interval.[98] Krom et al., using an operational research model, analyzed three alternative anesthetic management approaches: (1) RSI GA with video laryngoscopy, (2) FSI, and (3) spinal anesthesia. Their results demonstrated a shorter mean time to induction of 100 seconds using rapid sequence GA compared to 9 minutes for awake FSI and 6.3 minutes for spinal anesthesia ($p < 0.0001$).[99,100] They also concluded that based on the calculated risk of ultimate failed intubation after RSI of 21 per 100,000, some mothers may accept the risk of GA in order to reduce the potential delay in fetal delivery from an extended time with other forms of anesthesia. It is an emergent life-threatening situation in an obstetric patient that presents a unique challenge to anesthesia providers, where practitioners must balance the need to deliver the fetus expeditiously despite the inherent concerns of maternal safety. The risks of GA in such a situation include difficult or failed intubation, aspiration, or inability to provide adequate rescue oxygenation, which can deteriorate into a CICO situation.

The DA is not entirely due to the anatomic and physiologic changes of pregnancy. Other important factors encountered in an obstetric operative emergency delivery also contribute to adverse outcomes, including emergent nature of delivery with compromised fetal or maternal well-being, location remote from main operating room with inadequate backup assistance, poor communication, poor training and teamwork, inadequate preparation; deficiencies in availability of proper airway equipment, and inadequate system and processes, thus predisposing to loss of situational awareness and leading to poor decision making and substandard care.

For this discussion, key recommendations for DA management strategies in the obstetric patient are based on the following guidelines:

(1) The ASA DA Practice Guidelines and Algorithm salient recommendations include (a) VAL as a primary or a rescue approach to difficult intubation, (b) the use of second-generation SGA instead of first generation, and (c) emphasis on the importance of oxygenation and making it the cornerstone of management in all situations, including emergent and nonemergent pathways.[58,101]

(2) The salient 2015 DAS guidelines emphasize (a) a more linear four-point stepwise algorithm plan, with emphasis on each step being consequent on the previous plan failing; (b) definite decision points that focus on moving forward in the algorithm; (c) use of nasal oxygen supplementation during apnea (apneic oxygenation) along with emphasis on maintenance of oxygenation during the execution of each plan; (d) use of manual breaths and gentle ventilation during rapid sequence induction (RSI) of GA; (e) recommendation that rocuronium may be more appropriate than succinylcholine with rapid reversal with sugammadex if necessary; (f) the use of second-generation SGA, particularly in patients at risk for aspiration;

(g) removal if necessary of cricoid pressure (CP) during SGA placement; and (h) seeking the best assistance available as soon as difficulty with laryngoscopy is experienced.[102]

(3) The Obstetric Anaesthetists' Association (OAA)/DAS 2015 Obstetrics Airway Guidelines emphasize (a) planning airway management, (b) acute management of failed intubation, (c) and CICO failed intubation.[1]

(4) Our previously published (2017) strategies and management of difficult and failed intubation.[16,103]

Scenario: Emergent Cesarean Delivery—Rapid Sequence General Anesthesia

Our current recommendations for emergent CD under GA include the following: the anesthesia provider must (1) be prepared with availability of airway equipment and video laryngoscope for an emergent rapid sequence GA; (2) follow an organized stepwise strategy to effectively manage an unanticipated DA encountered during GA for emergency CD; (3) limit the number of attempts at intubation to two, thus minimizing airway trauma, and move to the next step quickly contingent on the previous plan failing; and (4) emphasize maintenance of oxygenation as the cornerstone of this strategic management.

We provide a single master algorithm for management of unanticipated DA and failed TI (Fig. 37.6). Based on these principles, a logical sequential linear approach with a four-point stepwise plan is designed to address the clinical scenario of emergent CD requiring GA (Fig. 37.6), including crisis management of a critical CICO airway situation, with the ultimate goal of having safe and best outcomes for both mother and baby.

Plan A/Step 1: Optimize Preparation

The ultimate goal is safety of mother and baby, and prevention of adverse outcomes. Emphasis is on comprehensive adequate airway assessment; preparation and readiness of the operating room for GA, aspiration prophylaxis, preinduction communication and checklist, video laryngoscope, and immediate access to other adjunct airway devices and the DA cart.

Plan B/Step 2: Optimize Intubation—Best Attempt at Intubation

Rapid Sequence Induction: Ramp position, preoxygenation strategies including apneic oxygenation, CP guidance, laryngeal maneuvers during DL, and use of adjunct airway devices to aid in intubation. (Also see Box 37.4.)

Plan C/Step 3: Optimize Ventilation

Failed intubation should be declared when encountered, and strategies to optimize ventilation and oxygenation should be implemented, including two-person mask ventilation or placement of a second-generation SGA device as a definitive airway or conduit for other approaches,

Plan D/Step 4: Optimize Oxygenation in a Cannot Intubate/Cannot Ventilate Situation

Failed ventilation should be declared after failed SGA placement. Supplemental oxygen should be administered in preparation for invasive front-of-neck access

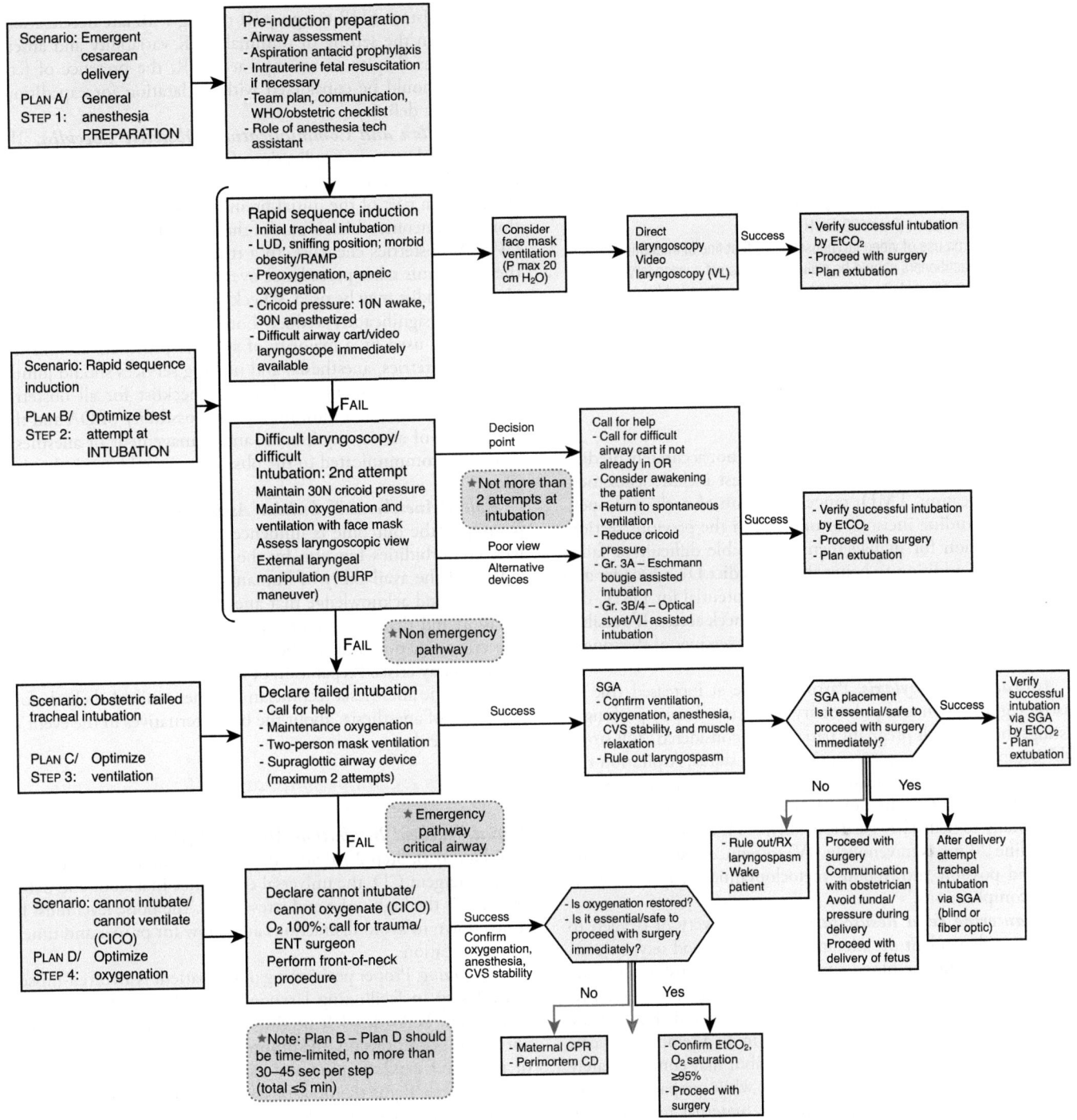

• **Fig. 37.6** Master algorithm for obstetric anesthesia: Management strategies—difficult and failed intubation. *BURP,* Backward, Upward Right Pressure; *CPR,* Cardio-Pulmonary Resuscitation; *CVS,* Cardio vascular system; *LUD,* Left uterine displacement; *SGA,* supraglottic airway.

Scenario: Emergent Cesarean Delivery Requiring General Anesthesia—Details of the Four-Step Plan

Plan A/Step 1: Optimize Preparation—Preinduction Assessment, Planning and Preparation

If the decision is made to proceed with GA, the following preparation is essential before induction of anesthesia and intubation: airway assessment, use of gastrointestinal aspiration prophylaxis, optimal positioning including the placement of a wedge under the right hip to offset aorto-caval compression, emphasis on team communication as part of preinduction briefing, and following the obstetric checklist to communicate to the team the possibility of DA (Fig. 37.6, Step 1) (Box 37.3). As part of the preparation, the obstetric emergency operating room must be in a state of readiness at all times of the day and night for the anesthesia machine check, monitors, suction, and airway equipment including video laryngoscope and adjunct airway devices (bougie and SGA). There should be immediate access and a dedicated DA cart in the obstetric operating room.

Advantages of head-up positioning and ramping are highlighted
Preoxygenation is recommended for all patients
Apneic oxygenation techniques with nasal cannula >10–15 L/min O_2 are recommended in high-risk with morbid obesity parturients.
Consider high flow nasal cannula (~30 L/min) – instruct patient to breathe through nose
The importance of neuromuscular block is emphasized
Consider mask ventilation (Pmax 20 cm H_2O)
Strong emphasis on use of video laryngoscope as first line of intubation device
All anesthesia practitioners should be skilled in the use of a video laryngoscope
A maximum of two attempts at laryngoscopy are recommended (2+1)
Cricoid pressure should be removed if intubation is difficult

Reproduced with permission from Frerk C, Mitchell VS, McNarry AF. Difficult Airway Society 2015 guidelines for management of unanticipated difficult intubation in adults. *Br J Anaesth*. 2015;115 (6):827–848.

Airway Assessment. Even though DA is not accurately predictable, airway evaluation, if time allows, must include assessment of MP classification, TMD, range of motion of neck, oral opening, and protruding incisors, as outlined in the previous section, with preparation for management of possible difficult or failed intubation. In addition to being able to predict DI, a broader aim of airway assessment is to determine the potential for DMV, difficult SGA placement, or difficult front-of-neck access. If possible, before induction of anesthesia remove oral piercings of the tongue to avoid trauma.

Aspiration Prophylaxis. Parturients are at increased risk for gastric regurgitation and pulmonary aspiration despite prolonged fasting; therefore, all pregnant patients are considered "full stomach" irrespective of the preoperative fasting status. Aspiration risk can be mitigated by administering pharmacologic prophylaxis. If time permits before induction of GA, administration of sodium citrate orally to neutralize gastric acidity,[104] H_2 receptor antagonist famotidine 20 mg intravenously (IV) to reduce gastric acid secretion, and possibly intravenous metoclopramide may reduce the risk of complications.[105]

Intrauterine Fetal Resuscitation. The delivery of oxygen to the fetus is dependent on adequate maternal blood oxygen concentration and uterine blood supply, placental transfer, and fetal gas transport. The aim of intrauterine fetal resuscitation (IUFR) while in the operating room is to increase oxygen delivery to the placenta, as well as umbilical blood flow in an attempt to reverse fetal hypoxia and acidosis, so that either labor may continue safely or the fetal condition can be improved while preparing for an urgent delivery. IUFR measures include maternal repositioning into the left lateral position (or alternatives such as right lateral or knee elbow if necessary), maternal oxygen administration at 10 L/min via nonrebreathing mask, rapid infusion of 1000 mL crystalloid (except in fluid-restricted or preeclamptic patients), decreasing uterine contractions by stopping oxytocic medications and administering tocolytic agents (terbutaline 250 μg subcutaneously or IV, glyceryl trinitrate 60–250 μg IV or sublingual spray, two puffs). A vasopressor (e.g., ephedrine or phenylephrine) may be required if there is maternal hypotension. The IUFR strategy may continue even after the patient is in the operating room. This time interval should be utilized for placement of monitors, implementation of adequate preoxygenation while drawing up induction drugs, and being prepared for GA by having airway equipment ready.

If a persistent FHR category III tracing with late decelerations continues in the setting of minimal FHR variability and absent accelerations despite an attempt at IUFR, the presence of fetal acidemia should be considered with declaration for expeditious and prompt delivery.

Team Plan and Communication: Obstetric Checklist. The goal of avoidance of complications following GA requires institutional and individual preparedness. Planning for failed intubation should form part of the initial preinduction huddle communication and timeout, which is part of the World Health Organization (WHO) obstetrics checklist. In a true stat (emergent) situation, the fetal status takes precedence over the checklist, but an abbreviated checklist may be used. Checklist implementation has been shown to significantly reduce both morbidity and mortality and is now used by a majority of surgical providers around the world. Obstetrics, anesthesia, and nursing services should jointly develop and implement an obstetric checklist for all obstetric procedures, and—at a minimum—the possibility of DA and the availability of airway equipment and management of anesthesia should be communicated to the obstetrics team before induction (Box 37.3).

Role of Anesthesia Technician Assistance. Every adverse event is unique; the outcome is influenced not only by maternal and fetal comorbidities but also by the skills of the anesthesia provider and the availability of human and technical resources. We recognize and acknowledge that anesthesiologists do not work in isolation and that the role of the anesthesia technician is crucial in a crisis situation and can be an important resource in managing an airway crisis. Preparation of GA requires brief communication with the anesthesia technician or other available help, before induction of anesthesia, about the best alternatives in the event of airway difficulty.

Plan B/Step 2: Optimize Intubation—Rapid Sequence Induction General Anesthesia

Initial Tracheal Intubation Attempt: Optimizing Intubation. (See Fig. 37.6, Step 2.) Before induction of anesthesia, especially in an emergent CD, the universal experience in a labor and delivery suite is the high noise and stress level. The noise level must be toned down to avoid distractions and allow for proper and timely communication.

Positioning. Proper positioning of the patient is an often-missed critical step in facilitating laryngoscopy, TI, and possible mask ventilation. Following left uterine displacement (LUD) to avoid aorto-caval compression, the optimal sniff position (slight flexion of the lower cervical spine and extension of the upper cervical spine), which aligns the oral, pharyngeal, and laryngeal axes into a straight line, facilitates TI when using traditional direct laryngoscopy. The neck should be flexed on a pillow and the atlanto-occipital joint extended to achieve the optimal sniffing position; however, *aligning the axes is not critical if a VL is being used.* However, in the patient with morbid obesity, one should use the head-elevated laryngoscopy position (HELP) by creating a ramp to ensure that the head and shoulders are higher than the chest.[106] The HELP position is achieved by drawing an imaginary horizontal line that connects the patient's sternal notch with the external auditory meatus, so that the head and neck are at a slightly higher elevation than the chest. The Troop Elevation Pillow (Mercury Medical, Clearwater, FL) is shaped like a ramp and is designed to optimize the HELP and sniffing positions (Fig. 37.7). Laryngeal exposure has been shown to be superior at the 25-degree elevated position; when compared with the supine position,[106] it increases

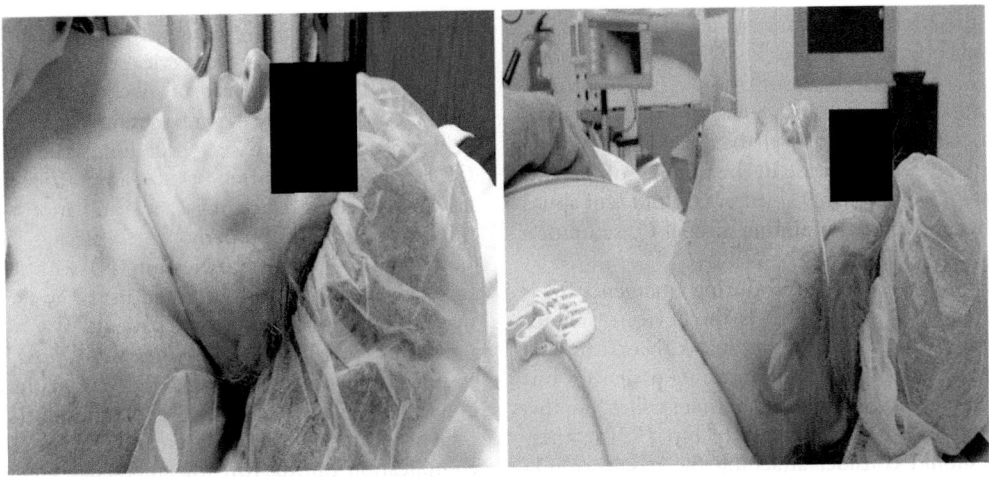

• **Fig. 37.7** Patient positioning. (Reproduced with permission from Munnur S, Suresh MS. Difficult airway management in the pregnant patient. In: Baysinger CL, Gambling D. *A Practical Approach to Obstetric Anesthesia.* Lippincott Williams and Wilkins. 2nd ed. 2016.)

the functional residual capacity (FRC) in pregnant patients and allows for prolonged apnea.[107,108]

During routine preoperative visits for nonobstetric patients, written instructions are given in the preoperative clinic to avoid hair extensions, elaborate hairstyles, and nail polish. However, for emergent CD, this is not the case. Certain hairstyles, elaborate hair braids, and large extensions with hair buns can compromise neck extension and lead to difficulty with laryngoscopy and intubation.[64,109–111]

Preoxygenation and Apneic Oxygenation: Preoxygenation is an important component of RSI, especially because term pregnant patients are at risk for rapid arterial desaturation during a period of apnea, as mentioned earlier in the physiologic changes during pregnancy. Preoxygenation is a safe, simple, and effective technique to increase apnea time. When patients desaturate below 88% to 90%, the patient's oxygenation status is on the steep portion of the oxyhemoglobin dissociation curve and can decrease to critical levels of oxygen saturation (70%) within moments,[112] thus predisposing the patient to myocardial hypoxia and anoxic brain injury. During periods of apnea associated with RSI of GA, the PaO_2 falls at more than twice the rate in pregnant than in nonpregnant women (139 mm Hg/min vs 58 mm Hg/min).[40] Effective preoxygenation with 100% oxygen increases the oxygen content of the patient's FRC from 21% toward 100%, which should produce a proportionate increase in the safe apnea time. Although in clinical practice achieving alveolar oxygen concentrations of 100% is not possible, increasing the end-tidal oxygen (EtO_2) concentration levels of 80% to 90% is usually readily achievable. Denitrogenation can be achieved with an appropriate flow of 100% oxygen through the anesthesia circuit while maintaining an effective seal until the EtO_2 is 0.87 to 0.9.

High Inspired Oxygen Concentration (FiO_2) of 100%: To maximize the safe apnea time, consideration should be given to providing oxygen and allowing tidal volume ventilation for at least 3 minutes or instructing the patient to take 8 deep breaths (DBs) in 60 seconds. The best marker of adequate lung denitrogenation[114] is to achieve a functional end-tidal oxygen ($fEtO_2$) greater than 0.9.[115] Preoxygenation of patients with obesity, in the head-up position compared with the supine position, has been shown to prolong safe apnea time after induction, and its use should be considered in obstetric anesthesia.[109] After complete denitrogenation

via inhalation of 100% oxygen, nonpregnant patients tolerate 9 minutes of apnea before oxygen saturation is less than 90%, whereas pregnant patients tolerate only 2 to 3 minutes of apnea.[40]

Technique of Preoxygenation: Replacement of nitrogen with high concentrations of oxygen being inspired during preoxygenation is a function of both the rate of alveolar ventilation and the duration of preoxygenation. Adequate preoxygenation is achieved with 3 minutes of normal tidal ventilation. Eight vital capacity breaths can achieve similar degrees of preoxygenation.[103,116] Previous clinical research and recent computer models show that a 2-minute period of preoxygenation is adequate for the term pregnant woman.[117,118] Some have argued that effective preoxygenation may be achieved by breathing an FiO_2 of 1.0 for 3 to 5 minutes or 4 DBs of FiO_2 1.0 over 30 seconds (4 DBs/30 seconds). However, the 4 DBs/30 seconds technique was later shown to predispose to rapid oxygen desaturation, especially during a period of apnea.[119] Oxygen desaturation occurs quicker and worsens faster in children, individuals with obesity, and term pregnant patients. Recent studies have shown that 8 DBs over 1 minute are comparable with 3 minutes of tidal volume breaths in patients with obesity and term pregnant patients[120] and much superior to the 4 DBs/30 seconds technique in preventing desaturation during apnea.

Apneic Oxygenation: Can Apneic Oxygenation Extend the Duration of Safe Apnea? Alveoli will continue to take up oxygen even without diaphragmatic movement or lung expansion. In an apneic patient, approximately 250 mL/min of oxygen will move from the alveoli into the bloodstream. Conversely, only 8 to 20 mL/min of carbon dioxide moves into the alveoli during apnea, with the remainder being buffered in the bloodstream.[121] The difference in oxygen and carbon dioxide movement across the alveolar membrane is attributed to the significant differences in gas solubility in the blood, as well as the affinity of hemoglobin for oxygen. This movement causes the net pressure in the alveoli to become slightly subatmospheric, generating a mass flow of gas from pharynx to alveoli.

Apneic oxygenation (AO) permits maintenance of oxygenation without spontaneous or mechanical ventilation. AO has been used for many years to provide oxygenation through the process of diffusion.[122] The use of pharyngeal oxygen insufflation has been validated by studies in healthy patients without obesity undergoing GA, who tolerated a period of 6 to 10 minutes of apnea,[123,124] without dropping their arterial O_2 saturation level below 95%. A similar study was conducted in patients with obesity, undergoing simulated DL, using oxygen insufflation via nasal prongs. Nasal oxygen administration was associated with prolongation of duration of oxygen saturation greater than 95% (5.29 minutes vs 3.49 minutes); a significant increase in the number of patients with oxygen saturation greater than 95% after 6 minutes of apnea (8 vs 1); and significantly higher minimum arterial O_2 saturation (94.3% vs 87.7%).[125]

Technique of Apneic Oxygenation: AO during emergency TI is provided with the nasal cannula, which is the device of choice in addition to preoxygenation with the face mask. Nasal cannula provides limited F_{IO_2} in a spontaneously breathing patient,[126] but the decreased oxygen demands of the apneic state will allow this device to fill the pharynx with a high level of F_{IO_2}.[127] The anesthesia practitioner should consider attaching the nasal cannula to the ancillary side port with 10 L/min O_2 flow before starting preoxygenation, to maintain bulk flow of oxygen during intubation attempts.[128] An additional benefit to the use of nasal cannula devices is that they can be left in place during the TI attempts. This has been described with an acronym, NO DESAT, which stands for **n**asal **o**xygen **d**uring **e**fforts **s**ecuring **a** **t**ube (Fig. 37.7).[129] NO DESAT allows the continued benefits of AO while TI techniques are performed.

Transnasal Humidified Rapid-Insufflation Ventilator Exchange (THRIVE): A Physiological Method of Increasing Apnea Time in Patients with DAs: A landmark study showed that the deployment of OptiFlow Transnasal Humidified Rapid-Insufflation Ventilatory Exchange, at a rate of 70 L/min in patients with DAs, extended the apnea time on an average of 17 minutes. None of the 25 patients had oxygen saturation below 90%, nor developed cardiac arrhythmias or other complications suggestive of CO_2 toxicity.[130] Two recent studies showed that high-flow nasal oxygen (HFNO), as compared to standard flow with face mask oxygen, for preoxygenation in obstetric patients did not reliably achieve end-tidal oxygen concentration >90%.[131,132] In both these studies, the investigators were not able to validate the success of HFNO for preoxygenation using end-tidal O_2 of >90% concentration as a primary outcome. There are no clinical studies that assess the role and potential benefits of HFNO in prolonging safe apnea time in obstetric patients. However, there are recent case reports highlighting the benefits of HFNO in prolonging apnea time in obstetric patients and management of DA.[133–137]

Cricoid Pressure: CP is an integral part of anesthetic management of the patient having RSI for CD. Since its first description by British anesthetist Brian Sellick in 1961, CP has become common practice for preventing the aspiration of gastric contents during RSI or modified RSI[138,139]; however, excessive or improper application of CP may displace the vocal cords anteriorly or laterally, thus preventing a good view of the larynx during direct laryngoscopy.[140]

In Sellick's original publication, the maneuver included using one's thumb and second finger to occlude the upper end of the esophagus by applying backward pressure to the cricoid cartilage against the body of the C5 vertebra. Sellick's study involved filling cadaver stomachs with water and placing the bodies in the Trendelenburg position while using the maneuver with success, noted by lack of water in the oropharynx.[138] However, what is overlooked is that Sellick historically first described the maneuver to prevent regurgitated gastric contents from entering the hypopharynx during mask ventilation and administration of GA.[138] Considering its widespread use, the evidence supporting the use of CP is of

surprisingly poor quality. Sellick described full extension of the head and neck to bring the cervical vertebrae more anteriorly.[138] In addition, full neck extension is likely to make laryngoscopy more difficult, and therefore hyperextension of the neck is not advocated. Sellick claimed that mask ventilation is safe during application of CP. However, this is often omitted in practice despite several studies demonstrating a lack of gastric insufflation while mask-ventilating with CP applied properly.[141,142] Typically, a cephalad and posteriorly pointing force of 10 Newton (N), with the thumb and index finger of the assistant, is required in the awake patient increasing up to 30 N in the unconscious patient.[143,144]

Complications and Adverse Effects of CP: As important as CP is to prevent regurgitation of gastric contents into the oropharynx, conversely excessive CP may obscure the glottic view by displacing the vocal cords anteriorly or laterally.[140] Thus, the most important complication during RSI for emergency CD is the reduced visibility on laryngoscopy and difficulty with ventilation. Palmer and colleagues examined the side effects of CP using flexible bronchoscopy through an LMA with different pressures applied (20, 30, and 44 N). They found that at 44 N, cricoid deformation was present in 90% of patients, whereas 50% had cricoid occlusion and 60% were difficult to ventilate.[145] The effect of CP on the cricoid cartilage and vocal cords was observed in an endoscopic study in anesthetized patients.[145] The advantage of VAL is that it allows the visualization of the glottic view on the monitor, thus allowing the assistant to adjust CP for external laryngeal manipulation appropriately.[146,147] The assistant is asked to transiently reduce or release CP, with suction at hand, to visualize the glottic area and vocal cords, despite the potential risk of pulmonary aspiration in the event of gastric regurgitation.

Improper CP technique can lead not only to a poor view at laryngoscopy and TI but also to prevention of proper insertion of the SGA. Thus, should an SGA be required, it is important to release the CP until the SGA is seated appropriately.[148,149]

Choice of Induction Agent and Neuromuscular Blocking Agent: The most common induction agent for CD in the United States is propofol, and the other less commonly used agents include ketamine and etomidate. Propofol suppresses airway reflexes and can be advantageous should an intubation attempt fail. Succinylcholine 1 mg/kg is the standard muscle relaxant, used for RSI in obstetric patients. It has a rapid 60-second onset and a shorter duration of action than other muscle relaxants, and the presumption is that, should intubation fail, the rapid return of spontaneous ventilation can be advantageous if the decision is to wake the patient up. However, succinylcholine-induced fasciculation can result in an increase in oxygen consumption during apnea, leading to rapid desaturation compared with rocuronium, which may prove to be disadvantageous in a failed intubation situation.[150–152] In the United Kingdom, rocuronium is currently emerging as the muscle relaxant of choice in providing better and optimum condition for intubation at the dose of 0.9–1.2 mg/kg and has been shown to provide similar intubating condition to that of intubating dose of succinylcholine. OAA/DAS guidelines suggest the use of high-dose rocuronium (1.2 mg/kg), with sugammadex backup for reversal, as a suitable alternative to succinylcholine in the surgical nonpregnant patient. The ability to antagonize and fully reverse the effect of rocuronium with sugammadex (16 mg/kg) may be advantageous.[153,154] Similarly, rocuronium is being suggested as providing an ideal condition for intubation during RSI,[150,155] having shown that reversal of rocuronium with 16 mg/kg of sugammadex is significantly faster than the spontaneous recovery from succinylcholine. In this study, the median time from TI to spontaneous ventilation was 216 seconds with a rocuronium–sugammadex combination as compared to 406 seconds with succinylcholine. The concern is with the use of high-dose rocuronium in the issue of placental transfer and its effects on the fetus. However, case series using high-dose rocuronium did not have any effect on neonatal outcomes.[156,157]

Mask Ventilation During Rapid Sequence Induction: Kinsella's review indicates that a number of dogmas exist.[4] Based on evidence, there is a paradigm change in the practice of obstetric anesthesia in North America and the United Kingdom, which is to use gentle mask ventilation after the application of CP and before TI.[1,158,159] The inherent value is that it prolongs the time to desaturation, particularly in patients with comorbidities such as sepsis or high metabolic requirements. There is no evidence that supports the once-conventional pattern of practice to refrain from bag-mask ventilation of the lungs in the interval from induction of anesthesia until laryngoscopy and TI are performed, and, in fact, there is evidence to the contrary that would encourage it.[102,160] It also provides an early indication of the ease of ventilation.[161]

Number of Attempts at Intubation: The fundamental essence of optimizing intubation and maintaining oxygenation is to maximize the likelihood of successful intubation at the first attempt or, failing that, to limit the number of intubations to two and minimize the duration of attempts (<45 seconds with each attempt) at laryngoscopy to prevent airway trauma, aspiration, and the serious progression to a CICO situation.

A suboptimal attempt at intubation is a wasted attempt, and the chance of success diminishes with each subsequent attempt. Repeated attempts at intubation also reduce the probability of successful placement of an SGA.

If the first attempt at tracheal intubation is successful, verify intubation with capnography and proceed with CD or else proceed to the next step of DL/DI (Fig. 37.6).

Scenario: Difficult Laryngoscopy/Difficult Intubation: Second Attempt at Intubation—Optimizing Best Attempt at Intubation

If DL or DI is encountered during the initial attempt at intubation, one needs to focus on ensuring adequate oxygenation and ventilation. The considerations to improve and obtain the best view at laryngoscopy and best attempt at intubation require the following steps:

1. *Call for help and the DA cart.* If it is not already in the OR, get the DA cart while quickly assessing the information gathered from the initial laryngoscopy view during the first attempt. It is prudent to call for help early in the process, either from individual(s) with expertise in DA management or a surgeon in the eventuality that surgical airway is required. Have the most experienced person available make the second attempt; use external laryngeal manipulation/BURP maneuver.
2. *Consider releasing CP transiently during the second attempt.*[162]
3. *Maintain/reinforce the head-elevated laryngoscopy position.*
4. *Perform external laryngeal manipulation.* Use the BURP maneuver with backward, upward, and right-sided pressure (Fig. 37.8).
5. *Change the laryngoscope blade type and size.* A videolaryngoscope (VL) is the preferred equipment. Use a smaller-diameter TT.

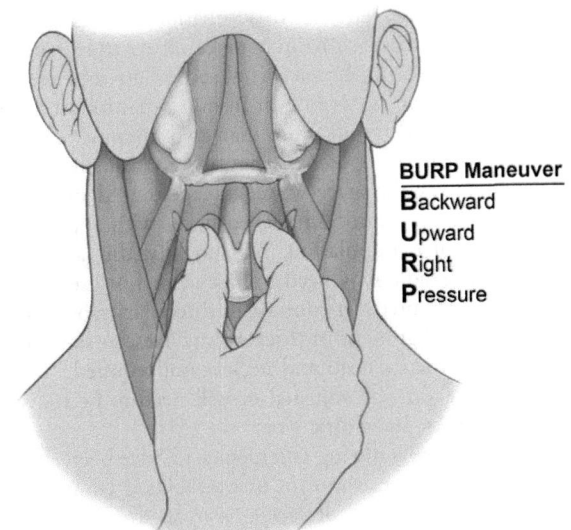

BURP Maneuver
Backward
Upward
Right
Pressure

• **Fig. 37.8** External laryngeal manipulation. (Reproduced with permission from Baylor College of Medicine, Drawn by Creative Services.)

6. *Consider using an Eschmann bougie, optical stylet with VAL.* This choice depends upon the laryngoscopic view during the initial attempt (grade 3A, 3B, 4, respectively).
7. *Attempt bag-mask ventilation and oxygenation.*
8. *Consider waking the patient.* Also consider returning to spontaneous ventilation.

External Laryngeal Manipulation: External laryngeal manipulation, referred to as the BURP maneuver, optimizes the laryngoscopic view. The use of optimal external manipulation, or backward, upward, right pressure (BURP) maneuver, involves pressure on the thyroid cartilage, which is the surface marking for the laryngeal aperture, and displacement of the larynx in three specific directions: posteriorly against the cervical vertebrae, as far superiorly as possible, and slightly laterally to the right to improve the laryngoscopic view.[163] In a study comparing glottic views with and without the use of the BURP maneuver, it has been shown that the BURP maneuver improves the glottic view by at least one whole grade and reduces the incidence of failure to view any portion of the glottis from approximately 9.2% to 1.6%.[163] The application of optimum external laryngeal manipulation to optimize the laryngoscopic view may be critical. All the preceding elements are important in managing the DI scenario and are discussed in detail later in this chapter.

The ASA DAA suggests calling for help, returning to spontaneous ventilation, and waking the patient. In all but the most urgent situations, one can consider waking the mother and reassessing the fetus before proceeding with an alternative plan. However, in urgent and emergent CD situations under GA, the goal should be balancing maternal oxygenation, prevention of pulmonary aspiration, and expeditious delivery of the fetus. Such a situation dictates addressing the management of the difficult and failed TI attempt.

Appropriate initial management and procedures following the failed initial attempt at TI can influence and ensure the final optimal and best outcome for both mother and baby. Calling for help is critical; it should be done sooner rather than later. Immediate access to the DA cart and video laryngoscope is also crucial.

Number of Maximum Attempts at Intubation: Despite optimal position and the BURP maneuver, if the first attempt at intubation fails, other alternative intubation devices should be considered such as the Eschmann bougie, optical stylet, and video laryngoscope to assist in the successful second attempt at intubation (Fig. 37.6). One needs to bear in mind that for an obstetric patient, there should be no more than two attempts at TI. The second attempt at laryngoscopy should be considered the best attempt; to increase the success rate, an experienced anesthesiologist will use the optimum/ramped position, with application of external laryngeal manipulation. Additionally, the laryngoscope blade type and handle may need to be changed or use of the VL should be implemented. In contrast to direct laryngoscopy, VAL does not require alignment of three airway axes, so specific positioning of the patient's head and neck is not required.[2] If necessary, CP may need to be adjusted or will need to be transiently released to optimize the glottic view.

Persistent attempts during emergency TI have been shown to significantly increase the rate of airway-related complications, especially as the number of laryngoscopic attempts increases from fewer than two to more than two attempts, resulting in hypoxemia (11.8% vs 70%), regurgitation of gastric contents (1.9% vs 22%), aspiration of gastric contents (0.8% vs 13%, bradycardia (1.6% vs 21%), and cardiac arrest (0.7% vs 11% ($p < 0.001$) (Fig. 37.9).[103,162,164,165]

Use of Appropriate Devices During Difficult Laryngoscopy/ Difficult Tracheal Intubation—Eschmann Introducer, Optical Stylet, Video Laryngoscope

The Eschmann Introducer: The Eschmann introducer is commonly referred to as the gum elastic bougie and is used universally to facilitate difficult TI.[166] The original Cormack and Lehane classification of laryngoscopic view[167] was recently modified by Cook, who proposed subdividing grade III into grade IIIA and grade IIIB.[167] In grade IIIA, the glottic aperture cannot be seen, but the epiglottis can be visualized and elevated, and hence the suggestion for a role and use of indirect methods, such as the Eschmann bougie. During advancement of the Eschmann bougie into the trachea, tracheal clicks are readily appreciated, as the 35-degree angulated distal coudé tip slides against the anterior tracheal rings. These tracheal clicks have been demonstrated successfully in 78% of patients with simulated and genuine grade III laryngoscopy.[168]

A second test to confirm tracheal placement is to advance the Eschmann bougie gently deeper into the trachea until it holds up at the carina.[168] With the laryngoscope blade in place in the oral cavity and the help of an assistant, the TT is railroaded over the Eschmann bougie.[168] A maneuver known as the Cossham twist has been described, where the TT is preemptively rotated 90 degrees counterclockwise on the Eschmann stylet before being advanced into the trachea to avoid delay in successful intubation.[169] The success rates between the Eschmann introducer and optical stylets in the grade IIIA airway (31 seconds vs 29.2 seconds) have been shown to be similar.[170]

Role of Optical Stylets—Grade IIIB/IV Laryngoscopic View: However, in grade III B, the epiglottis is visualized, whereas the glottic aperture cannot be visualized and cannot be elevated; in this situation, other alternative methods such as optical stylet may be useful. Optical stylets have been used successfully to facilitate rapid TI in grade IIIB laryngoscopic view[172] and help with confirmation of proper TT placement. The success rate has been shown to be higher with optical stylets than with the Eschmann introducer, and the time taken is less with optical stylets compared with the Eschmann introducer (31 seconds vs 45.6 seconds) in the grade IIIB view.[170]

Role of Video-Assisted Laryngoscopes as an Option for Initial or Rescue Tracheal Intubation—Difficult Laryngoscopic View: For almost 60 years, direct laryngoscopy was the sole method used by anesthesiologists to insert a TT into the trachea. The focus of DA algorithms has centered on difficult or failed intubation with direct laryngoscopy. Video-assisted technology has become widespread in routine anesthesia practice, and across medical/ surgical disciplines, because it enables improved visualization of anatomic detail. In 2001, GlideScope (Verathon Company, Bothell, WA) was the first VL introduced in anesthesia practice that incorporates modern video technologies. The GlideScope with a high-digital camera resolution placed at the tip of an improved Macintosh laryngoscope blade was proven to improve the Cormack-Lehane view compared to direct laryngoscopy.[172] A number of different types of VLs are currently available and have been shown to improve the laryngoscope view and are particularly useful in DAs. Besides allowing management of the DA, VAL is a useful teaching tool during both direct and indirect laryngoscopy.[173] Metaanalyses of randomized controlled trials (RCTs) in surgical patients comparing VAL with direct laryngoscopy in patients with predicted DAs report improved laryngeal views, a higher frequency of successful intubations, and fewer intubation maneuvers with VAL.[175–184] Because VLs offer improved visualization of the glottis and a higher success rate for DAs, compared with conventional direct laryngoscopy, it is now considered the first choice in many centers, including ours.[63,174,179,184-187,188] An editorial indicated that in order to increase patient safety VAL should be the new standard of care, and the conclusions include that (1) VLs should replace direct laryngoscopes, VAL be used for all intubations, and the intubation should be recorded and incorporated into the electronic health record; and (2) visualization of videos of a previous patient's TI should become standard.[188] Cook et al. demonstrated that performing a formal and prolonged trial of mandatory VAL in operating rooms led to changes in perceptions and departmental acceptance and consensus. The clinical trial resulted in their department agreeing to use C-MAC videolaryngoscopy as the default intubation technique throughout the operating rooms and intensive care units, with removal of standard Macintosh laryngoscopes from routine use.[189]

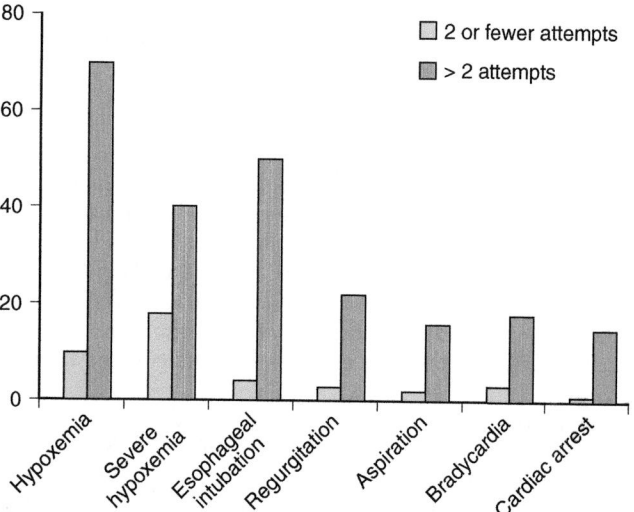

• **Fig. 37.9** Graphic display of complications by intubation attempts. (Reproduced with permission from Mort TC. Tracheal intubation: complications associated with repeated laryngoscopic attempts. *Anesth Analg.* 2004;99:607–613.)

Use of VAL in Obstetric Patients: Initially, studies on the experience and use of VAL in obstetric patients is limited.[190] In a case series comparing C-MAC VAL to direct laryngoscopy in 27 obstetric patients , the C-MAC was used after direct laryngoscopy and obtaining the glottic view. All patients were successfully intubated with the C-MAC, and in no patient did the Sao_2 decrease below 94%. However, it should be noted that 26 out of 27 patients in the study were graded as Cormack and Lehane 1 or 2 on direct laryngoscope.[191]

Arici randomized 80 women undergoing elective CD under GA and TI using McGRATH series 5 or direct laryngoscopy with the Macintosh blade.[192] Women with expected DI were excluded from the study. The results showed that intubation times were longer with VAL but that the percentage of cases with improved glottic view was higher. The authors concluded that the McGRATH Series 5 laryngoscope provided excellent glottic views in obstetric patients with normal airways.[192]

Aziz et al. did a retrospective analysis of performance of TI with either direct laryngoscopy or GlideScope in obstetric patients undergoing urgent or emergency CD.[174] During the 3-year period, they observed 180 intubations. Direct laryngoscopy resulted in 157 out of 163 first-attempt successful intubations and 1 failed intubation, whereas VAL resulted in 18 out of 18 successful intubations on first attempt. The researchers concluded that VAL might be a useful adjunct for obstetric airway management.

Initial reports confirmed the benefits of VAL in situations where initial intubation with direct laryngoscopy was unsuccessful. Later publications focused on successful intubation using VAL as the first-choice technique in patients with predicted DAs.[193–196] A case series has demonstrated the successful use of VAL for awake intubation in 2 patients, after topicalization of the airway with local anesthetic. This awake VAL was performed during an ongoing major postpartum hemorrhage situation with unstable hemodynamics.[197]

An OAA survey of all the lead obstetric anesthetists in the United Kingdom showed that 90% of the 58% respondents have video laryngoscopes. In our current practice, we have already implemented the practice of VAL as the first-choice airway device for emergent CD under GA and, in addition, for the anticipated difficult TI. Further, in the obstetric practice in several centers, VAL has been used in GA for elective and emergency CDs, including for patients with morbid obesity as well as during failed intubation.[174,190–196,198–200]

Role of Videolaryngoscopy in Obstetric Anesthesia: In determining the overall role of VAL in obstetric patients, a recent review article examined the efficacy, efficiency, and safety of VAL compared with direct laryngoscopy.[200] The review included RCTs, observational studies, case series, and case reports that reviewed the use of VAL to intubate the trachea in pregnant patients having GA. The study included four RCTs with 428 participants, nine observation studies, and 35 case series with 100 participants. The observational studies and case reports further support the role of VAL as a primary choice when difficulty with TI is expected or as a rescue modality. *The conclusion was that the evidence for the utility of VAL continues to evolve but definitely supports its increased adoption in obstetrics for use as a first-line device.* The channeled video laryngoscope (Airtraq) has been used in patients with morbid obesity undergoing emergency CD after failed TI.[193]

Given the proven fact that difficult and failed intubation is not only higher but also compounded by the unpredictably in obstetric patients, and given the efficacy of VAL in DAs both in nonobstetric and obstetric patients, it is imperative to have VLs immediately available in the obstetric operating room suite.

Role of VLs in Airway Management in COVID-19 Pregnant Patients: The COVID-19 pandemic has perhaps forever changed airway management. Current airway management guidelines from several countries have recommended that VAL be used as the first line of airway management for all patients requiring intubation.[203] Given the wealth of research highlighting the benefits of VLs, these benefits became extremely relevant where VAL eliminates the delay in changing equipment when a DI is encountered. This saves precious time when oxygenation is paramount. Because of the high risk of droplet aerosolization, the benefits of using VAL include minimization of mouth-to-mouth distance when securing the airway, as well as improved glottic visibility on the monitor, especially when wearing personal protective equipment (PPE). All of the highlighted benefits are important, relevant, and valid in obstetric patients with COVID. Given these facts, in our practice we have utilized VAL as our primary first-line management in obstetric COVID-19–positive pregnant patients requiring GA for CD and have found it to be invaluable.

Previously routine use of VAL was cost prohibitive, but the COVID-19 pandemic has catapulted the role of VAL as the first-line primary airway in mainstream anesthetic management, including obstetric patients.

In conclusion, it is essential to further improve our practice and training curriculum. Formally integrating training in VAL could play a crucial role in our preparedness to deal with challenges in airway management in the obstetric patient. However, in an obstetric emergency, in the event traditional direct laryngoscopy fails during the first attempt, the next attempt should be the use of VAL with which the operator is familiar. The use of alternative devices, such as the Eschmann introducer and optical stylets, in conjunction with VAL can enhance the intubation success rate during the second TI attempt without having to progress to the more serious critical airway with increasing hypoxemia situation.

If a second attempt at intubation is successful, verify tracheal placement with capnography and positive $EtCO_2$. If a second attempt at TI is unsuccessful, declare failed TI, pivot, and focus on optimizing ventilation and maintenance of oxygenation.

Plan C/Step 3: Declare Failed Tracheal Intubation— Optimize Ventilation and Maintenance of Oxygenation

The goals and priorities in the airway management strategies following a failed second attempt at TI, emphasis must be as follows (see Box 37.5):

1. Maintenance of maternal oxygenation;
2. Prevention of gastric regurgitation and airway protection;
3. Expeditious delivery of fetus; and
4. Avoidance of adverse respiratory, cardiac, or neurologic complications (Fig. 37.6).

Management After Failed Intubation at Cesarean Section, Decision to Wake Patient or Continue: Early acceptance of failure to intubate the trachea is paramount in arriving at the decision that maintaining oxygenation in the parturient is of utmost importance. Another change in basic assumptions is that even though the OAA guidelines advocate waking the patient after a failed intubation, there is a shift in the assumption, especially in the case of an urgent CD. The current recommendation and precedent is to use a second-generation SGA to establish adequate ventilation and oxygenation. Pregnancy-related changes can result in rapid development of hypoxemia and acidosis in the mother,[89] and the tenuous fetal status can result in a critical situation with potential

• BOX 37.5 **Key Features of Step 3: Optimize Ventilation—Role of Second-Generation SGA**

Following two optimal best attempts at yet unsuccessful intubation: Failed intubation should be declared.
The emphasis is on oxygenation via a supraglottic airway (SGA).
Second-generation SGAs are recommended.
Recommend a maximum of two attempts at SGA insertion.
During rapid sequence induction, cricoid pressure should be removed to facilitate insertion of an SGA.
Blind techniques for intubation through a SGA are not recommended.

Reproduced with permission from Frerk C, Mitchell VS, McNarry AF, et al. Difficult Airway Society 2015 guidelines for management of unanticipated difficult intubation in adults. *Br J Anaesth.* 2015;115(6):827–848. doi:10.1093/bja/aev371.

for 200% morbidity making decisions even more difficult. A review of the literature on obstetric failed TI from 1970 onward, the pooled data in a consecutive 5-year period showed a significant 1.8% per year increase in the proportion of continuing GA after failed intubation and establishment of ventilation. Before the late 1990s, most CD cases were awakened after failed intubation; however, since the 1990s, with the introduction of the LMA, GA was continued with an LMA in the majority of cases. When GA was continued, initially it was with an LMA, however the current trend has shifted toward the use of a second-generation SGA.

Face-Mask Ventilation: Because adequate oxygenation is critical, while preparing to place an SGA, face-mask ventilation with the application of CP should be attempted. If mask ventilation is difficult, an optimal or best attempt at ventilation—that is, two-person mask ventilation via a conventional face mask—is initiated while maintaining CP (30 N).[162] In the event of unsuccessful ventilation with bag and mask, then repositioning of the patient's head and chest, placement of an oropharyngeal airway, use of the airway strap around the face mask, and using a two-person technique are critical next steps (Fig. 37.10).[162] The two-person mask ventilation is performed by the primary provider holding the mask with two hands, while simultaneously providing chin elevation/jaw lift, while the assistant participates by compressing the reservoir bag and providing ventilation.

Conversely, the primary provider holds the mask in the left hand while simultaneously compressing the reservoir bag with the right hand and the assistant helps with chin elevation and jaw lift on the right side.[162] The risk with this two-person mask ventilation technique is gastric insufflation and potential risk for regurgitation/aspiration.

The emphasis with Step 3 is to maintain oxygenation, preferably with an SGA. Unsuccessful or compromised ventilation/oxygenation (CVCO) with bag and mask mandates the placement of an SGA device to maintain oxygenation in the mother and to deliver the fetus expeditiously.

Optimizing ventilation and oxygenation involves discussion of the following:
1. Role of first-generation SGA LMA as an airway rescue device;
2. Role of second-generation SGA based on DAS and OAA Failed Intubation Guidelines; and
3. Safety of second-generation SGA in obstetrical patients undergoing (a) elective CD, (b) emergency CD due to category II and III non-reassuring FHR, (c) RCTs comparing SGA versus ETT in patients undergoing CD, and (d) exchange of SGA with ETT following failed intubation in patients undergoing CD.

SGA Device Selection and Placement Following Failed Intubation: The prediction of DA is not always reliable, and given the increased incidence of failed RA, followed by failed TI,[18] every anesthesiologist practicing obstetric anesthesia should have a well-thought-out plan to deal with failed TI and a strategy for ventilation and oxygenation in an obstetric patient.

Currently, many first- and second-generation SGA devices are commercially available. The skills required for placement of an SGA compared to placement of an ETT do not have a steep learning curve, requiring less expertise and time for insertion and being associated with fewer airway-related complications.

Over the previous two decades, published obstetrical case reports and case series confirmed the role of the SGA in airway rescue following failed intubation. Internationally, there is broad general acceptance of the SGA as an alternative airway rescue device following failed intubation. The choice to use an SGA as a rescue airway device should consider protection of the airway from gastric aspiration (second-generation SGA). The SGA should also serve as a conduit for TI.

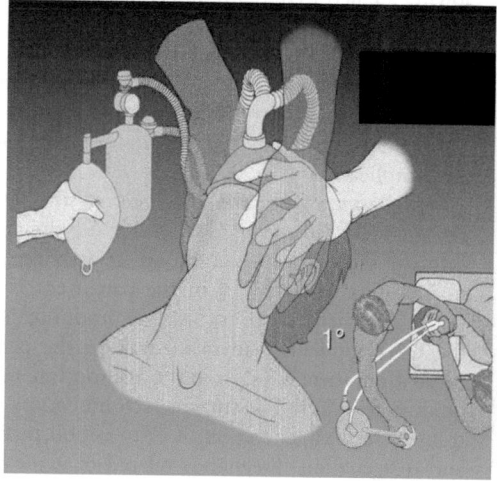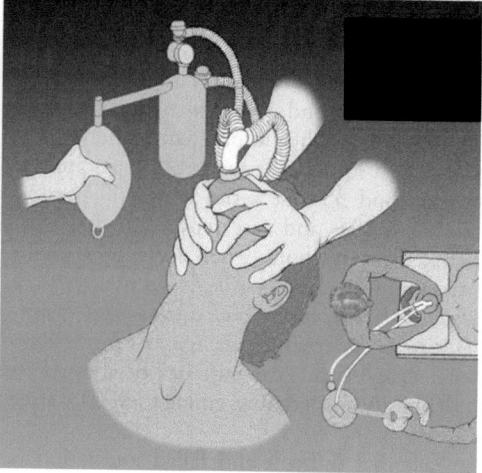

• **Fig. 37.10** Two-person mask ventilation. (Reproduced with permission from Baylor College of Medicine, Drawn by Creative Services.)

TABLE 37.6	Anesthetic Outcomes in Participants Receiving Either SLMA or ETT While Undergoing Cesarean Section Under General Anesthesia		
Characteristics	SLMA (n = 460)	ETT (n = 460)	P value
Number of Insertion Attempts			
First attempt	456	456	
Second attempt or more	4	4	1.0000
Time to effective ventilation (seconds)	16.1	39.1	<0.0001
Seal pressure (cm H₂0)	27.1	27.9	0.0014
Lowest Spo₂	99.0	98.5	0.2109
Baseline systolic blood BP (SBP)	116.8	116.8	0.9974
SBP 2 minutes after induction	114.0	133.9	<0.0001
SBP 5 minutes after induction	103.7	111.2	<0.0001
Baseline HR	84.4	85.5	0.1210
HR 2 minutes after induction	93.6	105.4	<0.0001

BP, Blood pressure; *ETT*, endotracheal tube; *HR*, heart rate; *SLMA*, Supreme laryngeal mask airway.
Reproduced with permission from Yao WY, Li SY, Yuan YJ, et al. Comparison of Supreme laryngeal mask airway versus endotracheal intubation for airway management during general anesthesia for cesarean section: a randomized controlled trial. *BMC Anesthesiol.* 2019;19(1):123. doi:10.1186/s12871-019-0792-9.

Proving the efficacy and safety of a second-generation SGA in pregnant patients first required large prospective trials in carefully selected obstetric patients undergoing *elective* CD (Table 37.6).[204] The second step was to confirm the safety of second-generation SGA in providing ventilation, oxygenation, and prevention of aspiration during *emergency* CD. This led to prospective clinical trials in select laboring patients undergoing GA for *emergency* CD.[204–208]

Since 2001, there is evolving evidence in favor of the SGA device as the primary airway during GA for CD (Table 37.6). In order to confirm the safety of second-generation SGAs as a primary airway device for pregnant patients undergoing CD, trials were conducted comparing SGA with ETT. There is now emerging data from randomized trials, comparing second-generation SGA versus ETT as a primary device in patients undergoing CD. Large observational studies on the use of different types of SGA devices in patients undergoing either elective or emergency surgery provide reassurance for the reliability of the SGA devices with minimal or no complications.[206–208] Yet, the study population cited in these studies do not match the emergency CD cohorts typically seen in everyday practice.[209–211]

Role of First-Generation SGA as a Rescue Device—Classic LMA.[213] The classic LMA has been widely used for the management of difficult obstetric airway without any episodes of gastric regurgitation or pulmonary aspiration.[21,209,213–215] There are multiple case reports on the successful use of classic LMA after failed TI in obstetrics.[213,216] Further, the utility of LMA as a rescue device has the most extensive proven successful record. In the UKOSS study of failed intubations in 57 obstetric patients spanning 2008 to 2010, the LMA Classic was used in 39 cases, Intubating LMA (ILMA) Fastrach in 4 cases, LMA ProSeal in 3 cases, and i-gel in 3 cases.[17] A national survey on failed intubation at CD conducted in the United Kingdom from 2013 to 2014 found that an LMA was used in 12 failed intubations and a second-generation SGA in 18; there was one reported failure of an SGA as a rescue device.[217]

CP and Placement of LMA SGA Device: Maintaining CP during an SGA insertion may prevent proper placement of the SGA. CP decreases the hypopharyngeal space and impedes the insertion of both first- and second-generation airway devices (Fig. 37.11).[218–221] LMA insertion has been shown to be more successful without CP (94%) versus with CP (79%).[148] Therefore it may be necessary to transiently release CP to allow proper placement of the SGA (Fig. 37.11).[162]

Classic LMA for Elective CD: Han and colleagues reported the successful use of the classic LMA as a primary ventilatory airway device in 1060 of 1067 patients.[209] There were no episodes of hypoxia, regurgitation, or aspiration reported with the use of the LMA Classic.[209] Despite the case reports on the successful use of the LMA Classic in obstetric patients after failed TI during CD, and as a primary airway device during elective CD, the current DAS RSI guideline does not recommended its use following failed TI in obstetric patients.

Intubating LMA: The Fastrach LMA or ILMA is particularly useful during failed intubation in an emergency CD because it provides ventilation and oxygenation and also because it serves as a conduit for TI and in the prevention of pulmonary aspiration. Several studies have shown the successful use of flexible bronchoscope-assisted intubation through the ILMA to assist in visually guided TI in patients who have a DA.[212,216,222] The ILMA was used successfully after failed TI during an emergency cesarean section in an eclamptic patient with morbid obesity[171] and in a second case in which RA had failed and was followed by GA, resulting in failed TI.[223] The ILMA proved to be a lifesaving device in both patients.

Role of Second-Generation SGA: Large-scale longitudinal and metaanalyses of nonobstetric patients, several DA guidelines,[1,102] and the ASA Practice Guidelines for management of DA published in 2022 all support the use of second-generation SGA

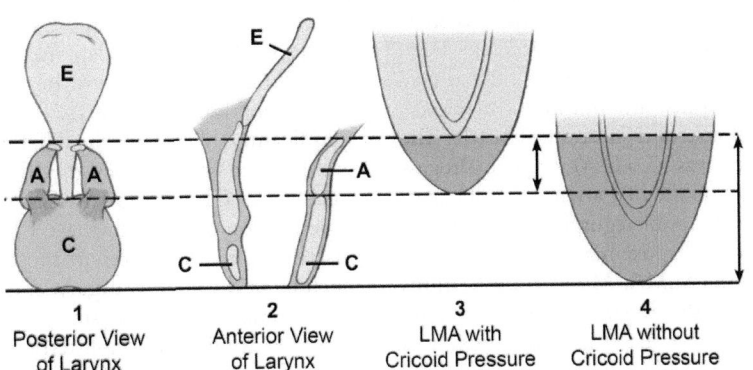

• **Fig. 37.11** LMA and cricoid pressure. *E,* Epiglottis; *A,* Arytenoid; *C,* Cricoid; *LMA,* laryngeal mask airway. (With permission from Asai T, Barclay K, Power I, Vaughan RS. Cricoid pressure impedes placement of the laryngeal mask airway and subsequent tracheal intubation through the mask. *Br J Anaesth.* 1994;72:47–51.)

following failed intubation. The proven efficacy, reliable first-time placement, high seal pressure, separation of gastrointestinal and respiratory tracts, and the increased safety and feasibility of flexible scope guided TI favor the use of the second-generation SGA. Several case studies, large cohort studies in select elective and emergency CD, and RCTs comparing SGA and ETT support the use of the second-generation SGA in obstetrical patients.

ProSeal LMA (PLMA): Reports describe the successful use of the PLMA, a reusable second-generation LMA, after failed intubation during emergency cesarean section.[224,225] Although the PLMA has been reported to be a successful rescue device for failed TI in obstetrics,[225,226] it was not until recently evaluated as a primary airway for patients undergoing elective CD. A large-scale prospective study reported experience with the PLMA in 3000 patients for elective CD from a single center using a method that involves rapid establishment of a patent airway plus gastric drainage.[210] The successful establishment of an effective airway on the first attempt was in 2992 (99.7%) patients; regurgitation and spillage of gastric contents into the mouth occurred in 1 patient (0.003%), and there was not a single case of aspiration. The conclusion from this series of 3000 patients who were considered at risk for aspiration was that the PLMA provided an effective airway in those patients undergoing elective CD, and there were no cases of aspiration.[210]

Supreme LMA (SLMA): The SLMA is a single use second-generation SGA that provides good seal for positive-pressure ventilation (PPV). It has a double aperture design that facilitates the introduction of an orogastric tube to aspirate gastric contents, thus potentially reducing gastric volume and risk of aspiration. In a large observational study, Yao and colleagues described the use of the SLMA for 700 nonemergent CDs.[211] The success rate of first-attempt insertion of the SLMA was 98% (686 patients), and time to establish effective airway was 19.5 (±3.9) seconds with maintenance of ventilation and oxygenation in all patients, and there was no evidence of aspiration. An RSI technique was performed utilizing rocuronium as the neuromuscular blocking agent. The study provides further evidence that the SLMA allows effective ventilation, despite the added risk of pregnancy-related gastrointestinal changes. The uneventful and successful use of the SLMA in 700 patients undergoing CD is reassuring. There is an important caveat: These patients were carefully selected because they were low risk, did not have obesity, had fasted for at least 4 hours, and had no gastroesophageal reflux.

Use of SLMA for Emergent CDs: Up until recently, the use and safety of the SGA has been studied in elective CDs but not in emergent CDs. Li et al. conducted a prospective clinical trial, investigating the use of SLMA for GA in parturients in active labor undergoing emergent CD.[208] This study involved the use of SLMA in 584 parturients who underwent emergent CD under GA for category II or III FHR tracing. The primary metric was first-attempt success rate, and secondary metrics included anesthetic and obstetric outcomes and maternal side effects with the airway device. The results demonstrated a first-attempt insertion success rate of 98.3%, while the overall insertion success was 100%. The mean time to effective ventilation was 15.6 (4.4) seconds. Orogastric tube insertion was successful on the first attempt in all parturients. There was no clinical evidence of regurgitation or aspiration, and there were no episodes of hypoxemia, laryngospasm, or bronchospasm associated with the SLMA. Minor complications included observation of blood on the SLMA after removal, sore throat, and hoarseness, while overall maternal satisfaction was high. Li et al. concluded that the SLMA could be an alternative effective airway in category II and III CD under GA in carefully

selected obstetric parturients. Fang et al. conducted a retrospective analysis of the use of SLMA in 1039 parturients who underwent emergency CD.[207] In this study, the first attempt was successful in all except two patients, both due to incorrect placement detected by desaturation and high airway pressure. The second attempt was successful in both cases. There was no regurgitation or aspiration and no laryngospasm or bronchospasm.

These studies demonstrate the successful use of SLMA for both elective and emergency CDs; however, there is an important caveat: Patient selection involved parturients that were low risk, did not have obesity, had fasted, and had no history of gastroesophageal reflux. These studies were conducted in hospitals that have a high rate of GA for CD, based mainly on patient preference and conducted by a small, limited number of experienced anesthesiologists where use of the SLMA is routine for CD. Therefore, its effectiveness in patients with DAs and in individuals with obesity is not known. While rapid sequence tracheal intubation remains the first line of airway management in GA for CD, the evidence from these studies shows that in a difficult or failed intubation situation, the use of a second-generation SGA should be the first primary alternative device to establish ventilation and oxygenation in obstetric patients.

Comparison of Second-Generation SLMA Versus ETT During GA for CD: In an RCT, 920 parturients who underwent GA for CD were randomized to SLMA (460) or ETT (460).[205,227] The anesthetic outcomes are shown in Table 37.6. Results showed that parturients undergoing elective CD under GA in the SLMA group had a similar first-attempt success rate as the ETT group, while potentially reducing the time taken to achieve effective ventilation with less hemodynamic change. There was limited information on the safety of SLMA use, especially pertaining to pulmonary aspiration risk, so the SLMA cannot be recommended for routine use in CD. However, given the high incidence of difficult and failed intubation in obstetrics, this study supports the current OAA/DAS guidelines recommendation on the use of second-generation SGA as a first-line ventilatory rescue device.

Comparison of Second-Generation i-gel Versus ETT During GA for CD: The i-gel, a second-generation SGA has a noninflatable soft cuff that fits well in the laryngeal inlet, creates a tight seal with minimal or no airway trauma, is easy to insert, and can be used for both spontaneous and controlled ventilation. It has been found to be an effective rescue device during failed intubation in obstetrics.[228]

Two RCTs compared i-gel to ETT for GA in elective CD.[205] In one, 80 pregnant patients posted for elective CD were randomized to the i-gel (40) or the ETT (40) group. The demographic parameters, ease of insertion, insertion times, and adequacy of ventilation were comparable between groups ($p > 0.05$). However, 8 out of 40 in the ETT group had DI. All 40 patients in the ETT group had an increase of >20% in mean arterial blood pressure (MAP) and heart rate (HR) during intubation and extubation ($p < 0.001$). Postoperative sore throat was also significantly higher in the ETT group compared to the i-gel group. In a similarly designed RCT comparing the efficacy of i-gel versus ETT for GA in CD with 80 patients, the i-gel was superior compared with the ETT in terms of ease of insertion, insertion time, first-attempt success rate, decreased incidence of bucking at the end of surgery, and complications, which include trauma and laryngeal spasm.

Other studies in nonobstetric patients have reported the efficacy of i-gel in protection of the lower airways from aspiration when there are large amounts of gastric contents.[229] In addition, the glottic view with flexible scope was better through the i-gel than the PLMA.[230]

In conclusion, studies in large series of patients and case reports have demonstrated that the first-generation SGAs—Classic and Fastrach LMAs—and, more importantly the second-generation SGAs—PLMA, SLMA, and i-gel—can be used safely in obstetric patients. The second-generation SGA should be an important part of the armamentarium as ventilatory rescue devices to establish ventilation and oxygenation, following failed intubation. There are several options for selecting the preferred type of SGA based on the experience of the practitioner, and the one best suited as a rescue device to ventilate and oxygenate the pregnant patient in an emergent situation.

Decision to Wake the Patient or Proceed With Surgery

There is a critical question to ask the obstetrician after successful SGA placement and establishment of ventilation and oxygenation: Is it essential/safe to proceed with surgery after SGA placement?

After a failed intubation, a joint decision must be made whether to wake the patient or continue GA. Kinsella's review of four decades of literature on obstetric failed from 1970 onwards shows that before late 1990 most patients were awakened after failed intubation; however, since then GA has been continued in the majority of CD cases.[4] For each successive 5 years, the rate of continuing GA without a TT has steadily increased by 1.8% per year.[4] Overall, there was a significant difference in the proportion of cases where GA was continued with SGA for emergency CD compared with elective CD (Figs. 37.12 and 37.13), When GA was continued, an LMA was usually used, with the trend shifting toward the use of a second-generation SGA.[4]

Management After Waking the Patient: The decision to wake the patient requires immediate communication with the obstetrician on the best course of action, and it is dependent on the type of emergency for which the CD is being performed. In the United Kingdom, 51 patients who were awakened after failed intubation were usually managed with either neuraxial anesthesia (spinal n = 30, epidural n = 14, CSE n = 4), local infiltration (n = 1), and sedation or GA following securing the airway awake (n = 2; flexible scope or blind nasal endoscopy).[4,226,231]

Maintaining GA After Failed Intubation: Tunstall's original algorithm recommended maintaining GA with face mask following failed intubation. Current practice shows that anesthesia is continued by face mask only if SGA/LMA placement fails.[232] A UK survey showed that GA was continued following failed intubation in 28 women with face-mask ventilation without PPV and in 10 women with PPV and administration of additional nondepolarizing neuromuscular blockers following the single dose of succinylcholine. The most commonly used inhalation anesthetics include either sevoflurane or isoflurane with a 2:1 distribution.[217,233] There were no reports of regurgitation or aspiration during or at the end of established face-mask anesthesia after experiencing failed intubation during CD.

Management of GA With SGA: Following the successful placement of the SGA and establishment of ventilation and adequate oxygenation, emphasis on communication with the obstetric team is critical (1) to avoid fundal pressure, thus preventing reflux of gastric contents, and (2) to avoid uterine exteriorization to prevent retching and vomiting. If a second-generation SGA is used, insert a 12- or 14-French gastric tube through the drainage tube and suction the gastric secretions to avoid risk of regurgitation and aspiration. Ensure that the device is positioned correctly and fixed appropriately so that gastric contents are vented through the esophageal gastric port.[212]

Selection of a Nonirritating Inhalation Anesthetic and Providing an Adequate Depth of Anesthesia: Sevoflurane provides rapid, smooth induction and adequate depth of anesthesia, it is the least irritating volatile agent,[234] while facilitating TI through the SGA in patients who have a DA and might need a definitive airway.

Decision to Intubate Through the SGA/LMA: Following delivery of the baby, one must determine that oxygenation is adequate and the maternal clinical condition is stable, following which a decision must be made whether to continue with just the SGA/LMA or to intubate. Blind intubation through the classic LMA is not recommended, except with the ILMA, which is designed for blind intubation. The LMA Fastrach has all of the ventilatory features of the classic LMA, and it is designed to provide a superior conduit for either blind or flexible scope-guided TIs. Based on the literature and data from nonobstetric patients, the overall success rate is 95.7%.[235,236]

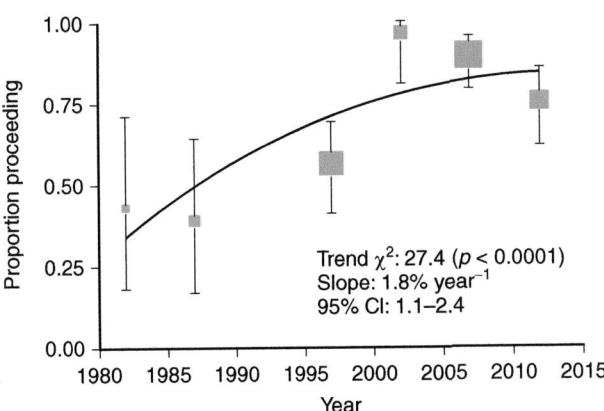

• **Fig. 37.12** The increased rate of continuation of general anesthesia after failed intubation during cesarean delivery (1980–2015). (With permission from Kinsella SM, Winton AL, Mushambi MC, et al. Failed tracheal intubation during obstetric general anesthesia: a literature review. *Int J Obstet Anesth.* 2015;24(3):356–374. Redrawn by Deidre Tomkins, Baylor College of Medicine.)

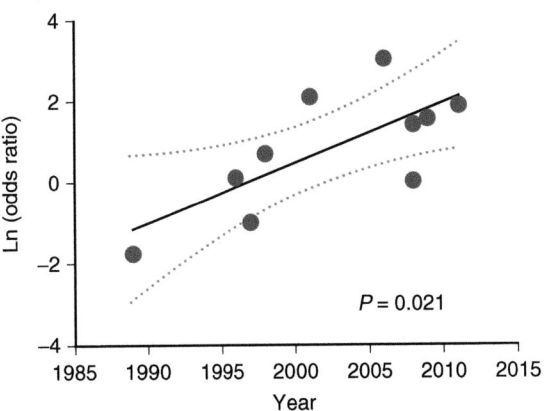

• **Fig. 37.13** Ratio proportion of general anesthesia continued after failed tracheal intubation at emergency cesarean section at elective cesarean, plotted by year of publication. *Dotted lines* = 95% confidence interval. (With permission from Kinsella SM, Winton AL, Mushambi MC, et al. Failed tracheal intubation during obstetric general anesthesia: a literature review. *Int J Obstet Anesth.* 2015;24(3):356–374. Redrawn by Deidre Tomkins, Baylor College of Medicine.)

Studies comparing insertion times and flexible scope–guided intubation show that insertion time through the i-gel was shortest (12.4 seconds) compared with the ILMA (19.3 seconds) and the C-Trach LMA (24.4 seconds).

The best flexible-scope glottic views and scores were also observed in the i-gel group. In total, 24 patients (20%) presented with DL. With the i-gel, the insertion time and FSI times were shorter than with the other two devices in this group.[237]

Flexible Scope–Guided Intubation Through an SGA Utilizing the Aintree Exchange Catheter

The seven steps of flexible scope-guided intubation through an SGA (PLMA, ILMA, or i-gel) utilizing the Aintree Exchange Catheter are illustrated in Fig. 37.14. The manufacturer recommends second-generation SGA insertion as follows:

1. Confirm capnography EtCO$_2$ for ventilation.
2. With visual guidance, introduce the flexible scope, preloaded with the Aintree catheter, via SGA into the trachea.
3. Railroad the Aintree catheter over the flexible scope into the trachea. Remove the flexible scope after visualization of the carina, leaving the Aintree catheter in the trachea, with the SGA in situ.
4. Remove the SGA over the Aintree catheter.
5. Load the TT over the Aintree catheter. Railroad and pass the ETT with an inner diameter (ID) of at least 7 mm over the Aintree catheter into the trachea.
6. Remove the Aintree catheter, and connect the ETT to the circuit and confirm ETCO$_2$.

The Aintree Exchange Catheter also has a Rapi-Fit adapter that is removable and allows for oxygen insufflation, if necessary, during the airway exchange process.[237]

Aintree Exchange Catheter–facilitated intubation has also been described with ProSeal[92,238] and i-gel SGAs.[239] However, the exchange catheter technique in a pregnant patient with confirmed DA undergoing emergency surgery is risky because of the possibility of losing the airway while the SGA is being removed over the Aintree Exchange Catheter and the potential for gastric reflux and aspiration.

Following successful intubation through the SGA, confirm proper placement with EtCO$_2$ and with the flexible scope. If SGA placement is not successful, declare failed SGA and proceed to Step 4 in the algorithm.

Plan D/Step 4: Critical Airway—Cannot Intubate/Cannot Ventilate/Cannot Oxygenate/Optimization of Oxygenation

(See Fig. 37.6 and Box 37.6.)

Emergency Cricothyrotomy

Incidence of CICO: The reported incidence of CICO in the United Kingdom and the United States following failed intubation with

---

> ### • BOX 37.6   Key Features of Step 4: Critical Airway With Hypoxemia—Cannot Intubate/Cannot Oxygenate (CICO)
>
> - CICO and Hypoxemia – Immediate necessity for front-of-neck access should be declared
> - A didactic scalpel technique has been selected to promote standardized training
> - Placement of a # 6 cuffed tube through the cricothyroid membrane facilitates normal minute ventilation with a standard breathing system
> - High-pressure oxygenation through a narrow-bore cannula is associated with serious morbidity
> - All anesthesia practitioners should be trained to perform a surgical airway
> - Training should be repeated at regular intervals to ensure skill retention
>
> Modified from Frerk C, Mitchell VS, McNarry AF. Difficult Airway Society 2015 guidelines for management of unanticipated difficult intubation in adults. *Br J Anaesth.* 2015;115(6):827–848.

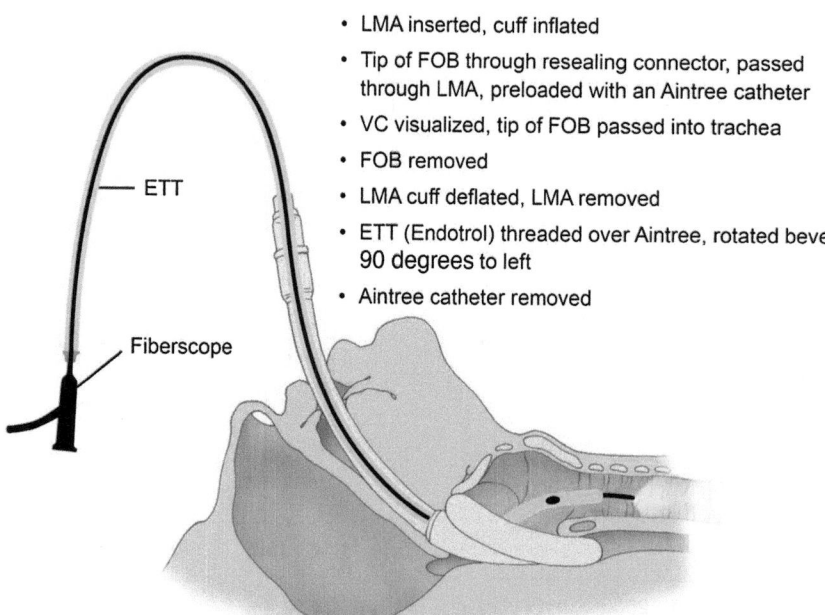

- LMA inserted, cuff inflated
- Tip of FOB through resealing connector, passed through LMA, preloaded with an Aintree catheter
- VC visualized, tip of FOB passed into trachea
- FOB removed
- LMA cuff deflated, LMA removed
- ETT (Endotrol) threaded over Aintree, rotated bevel **90 degrees to left**
- Aintree catheter removed

ETT

Fiberscope

• **Fig. 37.14** Fiberscope/Aintree guided intubation via LMA. *ETT*, Endotracheal tube; *FOB*, Fiberoptic bronchoscope; *LMA*, laryngeal mask airway; *VC*, Vocal Cords. (With permission from Suresh MS, Wali A, Crosby ET. Difficult and failed intubation: strategies, prevention and management of airway-related catastrophes in obstetrical patients. In: Suresh MS, Segal BS, Preston RL, Fernando R, Mason CL, eds. *Shnider and Levinson's Anesthesia for Obstetrics.* 5th ed. Wolters Kluwer/Lippincott Williams & Wilkins; 2013.)

GA for CD varies from 1 in 20 (5 per 100) to 5 in 18.[21,200,219,240] In the United States, among 98 general anesthetics there was one sentinel event of failed intubation and subsequent failed SGA placement that resulted in critical airway necessitating an emergency cricothyrotomy.[12] Anatomic causes of failed intubation leading to a CICO situation include high BMI,[241,242] enlarged tonsils,[171,243] and neck hematoma following carotid puncture during central access in a patient with placental abruption and coagulopathy.

Airway access can be obtained with a #14 cannula and jet ventilator as a temporizing measure, while a second attempt at intubation using a bougie.[244,245] Laryngospasm is another important cause of upper airway obstruction that must be ruled out for failure to ventilate through an SGA,[12,246] and it can be immediately relieved by the administration of a small dose of rapid-acting neuromuscular blocking agent.

Incidence of Cricothyrotomy in Obstetric Patients: There is a paucity of data with regard to cricothyrotomy after failed intubations in obstetric patients, with an incidence that is low at 1 per 60 failed intubations during cesarean section.[4] The NAP4 study provided comprehensive insight into emergency surgical airways and cannula cricothyrotomy performed when other rescue techniques to secure the airway during GA had failed, resulting in a high failure rate of 64% when performed by anesthetists.[18,247]

The recent obstetric data from the NAP4 study showed that there were four obstetric cases that developed complications associated with airway management.[18,19] All four cases took place out of hours and involved complex patients, with two cases that followed failed RA. Of the four patients, one required an invasive surgical airway that was performed successfully. Failed intubation, failed face mask, and failed SGA ventilation result in increasing hypoxemia and a CICO scenario that is often secondary to repeated unsuccessful attempts. Specifically, when a "can ventilate" situation rapidly develops into a CICV or CICO situation, it can result in significant maternal morbidity, including hypoxic brain damage, and mortality. The fetus is also at risk for severe neurologic injury. Rapid development of severe hypoxemia, particularly associated with bradycardia, is an indication for imminent intervention with an invasive airway rescue technique. In Palanisamy's study, the sentinel case of DI resulted in a critical airway incident of CICV that required an emergent surgical cricothyrotomy.[12] The researchers reported that the total time from RSI of anesthesia to surgical cricothyrotomy was less than 5 minutes, with excellent maternal and fetal outcomes.[12] Given the successful outcome, this incident has two important lessons: (1) pregnancy is associated with dynamic airway changes even in the absence of labor, particularly in the setting of preeclampsia; and (2) the early communication of an anticipated DA and the availability of expert assistance with surgical airway skills is critical in preventing management delays and subsequent adverse outcomes.[12]

Additional data from Kinsella's review on failed intubation in obstetric patients showed that 6 out of 13 cases of attempted surgical airway procedures died; the etiology could be multifactorial, including a delay in decision-making, lack of familiarity with equipment and technique, lack of appropriate skills, or decline in cognitive and motor skills because of the high stress level.[4]

Surgical airway access is rarely necessary with the acquisition of current AAM knowledge and skills. It also requires following precise DA guidelines, clear communication, and a specific threshold and criteria for performing a cricothyrotomy and, in addition, the availability of essential resources such as surgeons or anesthesiologists with FONA skills and equipment, which then immediately translates to successful outcomes.

Kristensen et al.[248] and Law et al.[249] state that the likelihood of difficulty in identifying the CTM and performance of emergency airway access must be assessed *before* induction of anesthesia; in the event that an emergency percutaneous airway access becomes necessary, it would help to optimize the success if the assessment is made before induction of anesthesia. In a category I emergent CD for life-threatening maternal or fetal condition, identifying the CTM before induction is not practical.

Failure could be attributable to patient factors affecting the identification of anatomic landmarks, such as neck positioning, obesity, equipment issues, poor insertion techniques, inadequate cannula ventilation, and inadequate training. Inexperience and psychological stress may also contribute to poor outcomes. The majority of all current guidelines recommend that practitioners involved in airway management should be proficient in surgical and cannula techniques. This requires simulation training, and the key is to transfer that knowledge and skills to actual clinical performance under any high stress situation. Howes and colleagues describe the modification of a model to replicate an obese thick neck or burnt neck to prepare the anesthesia practitioner to manage emergency cricothyroidotomy with complex anatomy so the skills can be utilized in DA clinical situations.[229,250]

The possible risks should be continually balanced against the risks of hypoxic brain damage and maternal and/or neonatal death. The decision to perform an emergent surgical airway access is a last-resort, lifesaving measure, especially in an obstetric situation to save the mother and baby. Rapid reoxygenation is critical and is best achieved with a combination of an invasive airway device and a ventilation technique that can deliver effective ventilation and high minute ventilation with an FiO_2 of 1.0.

All current airway guidelines recommend management of the CICO situation using one of the following: scalpel surgical cricothyrotomy or needle cricothyrotomy with percutaneous transtracheal jet ventilation (TTJV).[250–252]

The OAA/DAS guidelines are a proponent of standardizing the scalpel cricothyrotomy technique.[102]

Understanding CTM Anatomy: Successful outcome requires a thorough understanding of the anatomy of the CTM, the invasive airway access technique, and the nuances of the ventilation devices (Fig. 37.15).[253,254]

Any practitioner who performs intubations must know and review the structures of the neck and the structures that support the airway (thyroid cartilage, cricoid cartilage, and tracheal rings). The vocal cords are located a short distance (approximately 0.7 cm) above the thyroid notch. An attempt to place a surgical airway here would be harmful. Cricoid cartilage, a complete ring, can be felt in most individuals, except in patients with obesity. The CTM, which has a vertical height of 8 to 19 mm and a width of 9 to 19 mm, is located between the thyroid and cricoid cartilages. Branches of the thyroid arteries pierce the CTM in its upper third; it is advisable to access its lower third. Identifying the midline of the structure is important, as roughly 30% of the population have large-caliber veins within 1 cm of the midline, whereas only 10% have veins greater than 2 mm in diameter that cross the midline. In patients in whom the landmarks are difficult to identify, the CTM is usually four fingerbreadths from the sternal notch.

Role of Ultrasound: Identification of the CTM is difficult in females, whose laryngeal prominence is less obvious than in males and even more difficult in patients with obesity. Aslani and colleagues determined the accuracy of identification of the CTM by

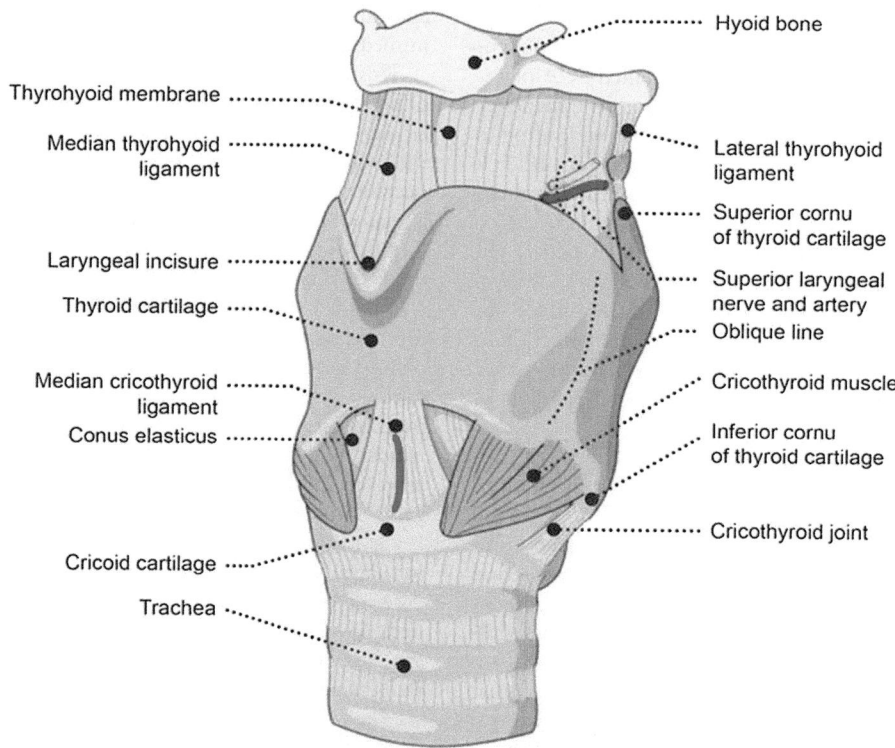

• **Fig. 37.15** Anatomy of a hyoid thyroid cartilage and cricothyroid membrane (vertical incision in obese individuals). (With permission from Baylor College of Medicine. Redrawn by Deidre Tomkins.)

palpation in females.[255] Confirmation with ultrasound showed that the accuracy of the physicians was 10 out of 41 in the patients who did not have obesity, whereas in the females with obesity the results were a dismal 0 of 15. Similarly, in two recent Canadian studies using similar methodology, Lamb and colleagues showed success rates of correct CTM identification in 72% of males without obesity versus 39% in males with obesity and 24% in females without obesity versus 35% in females with obesity.[256] Among women in labor, rates of correct CTM identification were 71% in those with obesity versus 39% in those without obesity.[257] The aforementioned studies highlight an important issue: The use of ultrasound (which is readily available in a labor and delivery suite) to identify the CTM, and the practice thereof, can be invaluable before induction of anesthesia. The role of ultrasound in actual life-threatening airway emergencies is limited. However, gaining experience in identifying the CTM with ultrasound in regular clinical practice can perhaps be beneficial in emergencies, especially if the ultrasound machine is immediately available in the obstetric suite. Caution should be exercised to prevent unnecessary delay in establishing airway access, particularly in an emergent life-threatening situation. Cricothyrotomy techniques should be taught to anesthesia trainees.

Scalpel Cricothyrotomy: Scalpel cricothyrotomy is recommended because it is the fastest and most reliable method of securing the airway in the emergency setting.[102,247,258,259] A cuffed tube in the trachea protects the airway from aspiration, provides a secure route for exhalation, allows low-pressure ventilation using standard breathing systems, and permits CO_2 monitoring.

Establishing ventilation and oxygenation can be accomplished with a rapid four-step surgical cricothyrotomy technique, which can be performed in 30 to 45 seconds:
1. Identify the CTM.

2. Perform a horizontal stab incision through skin and CTM.
3. Introduce an Eschmann bougie into the trachea through the CTM,[260] then slide the coudé tip along the blade into the trachea.
4. Railroad a 6-mm TT over the bougie into the trachea. Inflate the cuff and confirm ventilation with $EtCO_2$ capnography.

A single stab incision through the CTM is appealing in terms of its simplicity, but this approach may fail in the patient with obesity or if the anatomy is difficult, and a vertical skin incision is recommended in this situation (Fig. 37.16).

Oxygen (100%) should be applied to the upper airway throughout the procedure using an SGA, a tight-fitting face mask, or nasal insufflation. Standardization is useful in rarely encountered crises. The technique relies on the correct equipment being immediately available. Operator position and stabilization of the hands are important. Necessary equipment includes (1) a scalpel with no. 10 blade; a broad blade (with the same width as the TT) is essential; (2) a bougie with coudé (angled) tip; and (3) a cuffed 6-mm tube.

Details of Scalpel Cricothyrotomy: The optimum position involves neck extension as used in ear, nose, and throat (ENT) procedures, with shoulder support for access to the CTM. The sniffing position does not provide optimal conditions for access. In an emergency, this can be achieved by pushing a pillow under the shoulders or dropping the head of the operating table.

Details of Cricothyrotomy: A horizontal-incision technique on a palpable CTM with a scalpel and bougie[102] (Fig. 37.16) includes the following:
1. Continue attempts at rescue oxygenation via upper airway (assistant).
2. Stand on the patient's left side if you are right-handed (reverse if left-handed).

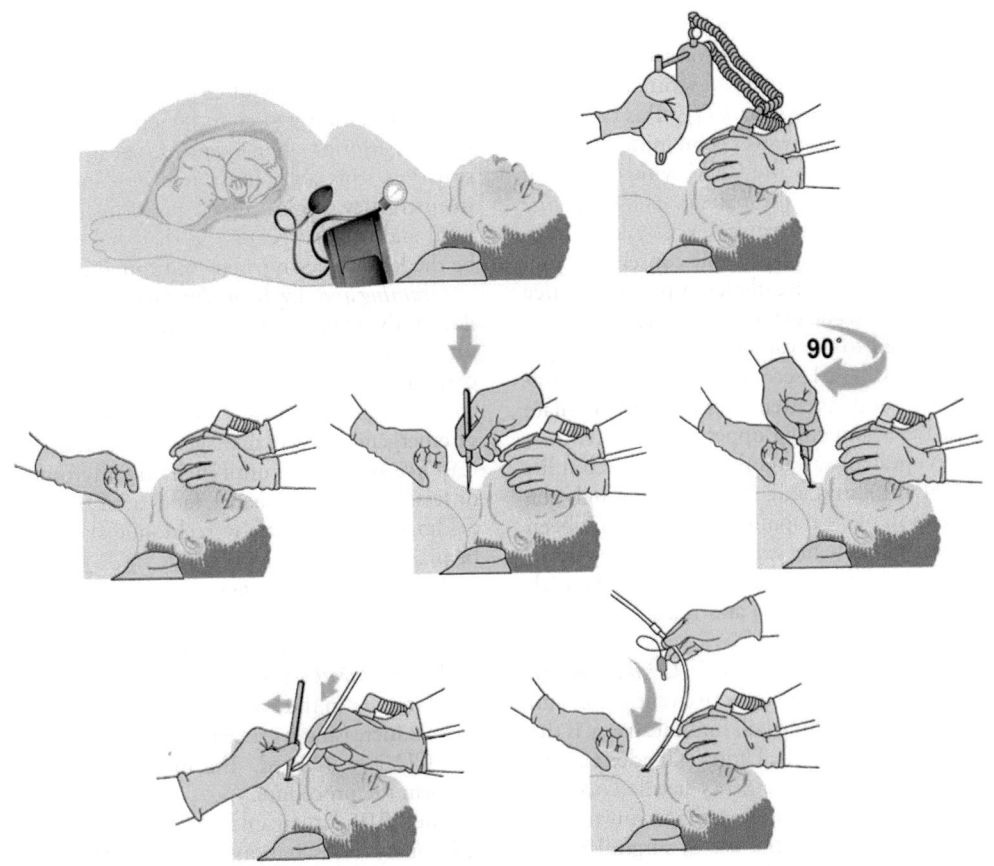

• **Fig. 37.16** Cricothyroidotomy technique. (With permission, modified from Frerk C, Mitchell VS, McNarry AF. Difficult Airway Society 2015 guidelines for management of unanticipated difficult intubation in adults. *Br J Anaesth.* 2015;115:827–848.)

3. Perform a laryngeal handshake as described by Levitan and colleagues[261] to identify the laryngeal anatomy.
4. Stabilize the larynx using the left hand.
5. Use your left index finger to identify the CTM.
6. Hold the scalpel in your right hand and make a transverse stab incision through the skin and CTM with the cutting edge of the blade facing toward you.
7. Keep the scalpel perpendicular to the skin and turn it through 90 degrees so that the sharp edge points caudally, toward the feet.
8. Swap hands to hold the scalpel with your left hand.
9. Maintain gentle traction, pulling the scalpel toward you (laterally) with your left hand, keeping the scalpel handle vertical to the skin (not slanted).
10. Pick the bougie up with your right hand; holding the bougie parallel to the floor, at a right angle to the trachea, slide the coudé tip of the bougie down the side of the scalpel blade farthest from you and into the trachea.
11. Rotate and align the bougie with the patient's trachea and advance it gently for 10 to 15 cm.
12. Remove the scalpel.
13. With your left hand, stabilize the trachea with tension on the patient's skin; railroad a lubricated size 6-mm cuffed TT over the bougie.
14. Rotate the tube over the bougie using the Cossham twist as it is advanced; remove the bougie.
15. Inflate the TT cuff, confirm ventilation with capnography and positive $EtCO_2$, then secure the tube.

If unsuccessful, proceed to the *scalpel-finger-bougie technique.*[102]
Impalpable CTM—Scalpel-Finger-Bougie Vertical Incision Technique: This approach[102] is indicated when the CTM is impalpable or if other techniques have failed. Equipment, patient, and operator position are the same as for the scalpel technique shown in Fig. 37.16:
1. Continue attempts at rescue oxygenation via upper airway (assistant).
2. Attempt to identify the laryngeal anatomy using a laryngeal handshake.
3. If an ultrasound machine is immediately available and switched on, it may help to identify the midline and major blood vessels.
4. Tension skin using the left hand.
5. Make a 2- to 3-cm midline vertical skin incision, caudad to cephalad.
6. Use blunt dissection with the fingers of both hands to separate tissues and identify and stabilize the larynx with the left hand.
7. Proceed with the scalpel technique as described above.
Needle Cricothyrotomy Using the Seldinger Technique: The needle cricothyroid technique entails using a commercial cricothyrotomy kit. Insert a no. 14 catheter (usually an intravenous catheter) through the CTM, and direct the catheter caudally at a 45-degree angle while applying negative pressure to the syringe that is attached to the catheter. Aspiration of air indicates entry into the lumen. Remove the needle and syringe while advancing the catheter to the hub. Confirm aspiration of air through the catheter. The needle through the catheter is removed and, using the Seldinger technique, a guidewire is advanced through

the catheter. The guidewire is used to advance a dilator over it, which is removed and followed by insertion of a tracheostomy tube. Attach the oxygen source to the tube and secure the airway.

Needle Cricothyrotomy With Percutaneous TTJV: This technique is similar to that described earlier. It involves combining the insertion of a large-bore catheter through the CTM with the use of a high-pressure source to oxygenate the patient. Following the insertion of the large-bore catheter, it requires a designated individual to hold the catheter firmly in place while consciously preventing dislodgment or kinking of the catheter. A pressure source (up to 50 psi) with an in-line regulator to reduce pressure to 15 to 20 psi or lower is attached to the catheter, and while using a short inspiratory time of less than 1 second and a longer expiratory time greater than 1 second, an attempt is made to ventilate and oxygenate the patient. Maintaining upper airway patency is critical; use the oropharyngeal airway and the jaw thrust/chin lift to allow for deflation of the lungs and exhalation through the upper airway and prevention of air trapping. If an SGA has been used, it can be left in situ to allow for exhalation. Jet ventilation can provide effective ventilation[262,263]; however, it is fraught with hazardous complications from barotrauma and is associated with a low success rate.[264-266]

Surgical Scalpel Cricothyrotomy Versus Needle Cricothyrotomy: When conventional approaches to obtain effective ventilation and return of effective spontaneous breathing fail, surgical airway is the last rescue option. The NAP4 audit in the United Kingdom found approximately a 60% failure rate for emergency needle cricothyrotomy, whereas surgical cricothyrotomy was almost universally successful.[18] There are data to support the use of surgical cricothyrotomy.[267,268] Most traditional surgical cricothyrotomy procedures are faster than percutaneous techniques, with the average speed of 83 ± 44 seconds (range, 28–149 seconds).[269] Conversely, Hill and colleagues found that a bougie-assisted technique is faster than standard open cricothyrotomy techniques in a sheep model (median time of 67 seconds interquartile range [IQR] = 55–82) versus 149 seconds (IQR = 111–201) for the standard technique ($p = 0.002$).[267]

Most physicians have limited lifetime experience with cricothyrotomy, and it is unclear what method should be taught for this lifesaving procedure. A prospective study was performed to compare the performance of medical personnel, naïve to surgical airway techniques, in using three commonly used cricothyrotomy techniques to establish an emergency surgical airway in cadavers.[270] The results showed that the success rates were 95%, 55%, and 50%, respectively, for surgical cricothyrotomy, QuickTrach, and Melker ($p = 0.025$). The majority of failures were attributed to cannula misplacement (15 of 20). In successful procedures, the mean procedure time was 94 ± 35 seconds in the surgical group, 77 ± 34 seconds in the QuickTrach II group, and 149± 24 seconds in the Melker group ($p < 0.001$). Few significant complications were found in successful procedures.[270] The study concluded that medical personnel naïve to surgical airway techniques establish a surgical airway more efficiently using surgical cricothyrotomy. Because the vast majority of clinicians perform emergency airway infrequently, the reluctance to use a scalpel has to be transcended. The authors in this study recommend that percutaneous cricothyrotomy sets be replaced in all airway carts by a scalpel or a set based on the surgical cricothyrotomy technique.[270] Despite regular skills-based training, anesthesia practitioners may still be unwilling to perform an emergency surgical airway. A recent study recruited 15 consultants from each specialty (n = 45): anesthetists, head and neck surgeons, and general surgeons.[271] The anesthetist

consultants completed the emergency surgical airway procedure significantly faster than general surgeons (median 50 vs 86 seconds, $p = 0.018$). Despite the strong performance, literature and survey data indicate that anesthetists still believe that surgeons are best at performing emergency surgical airway in a genuine CICO situation. This study illustrated that anesthetists regularly trained in emergency surgical airway perform at a skill level comparable to head and neck surgeons and that they should feel empowered to be the lead clinician when confronted with an emergency CICO.

Training and Acquiring Invasive Airway Technical Skills: A manikin study involving 102 anesthesiologists concluded that practice on manikins, after watching a short video, helped reduce the cricothyrotomy times and improved success rates. Although clinical correlates are unknown, some recommendations are that providers of emergency airway management be trained on manikins for at least five attempts or until their cricothyrotomy time is 40 seconds or less.[272] The performance fades after 3 months with the Melker Seldinger cricothyrotomy technique[273]; therefore, the skills must be practiced on a regular basis.

Successful Cricothyrotomy: In a critical airway situation and following successful cricothyrotomy and confirmed establishment of oxygenation, delivery of the fetus must be expedited.

Failed Cricothyrotomy—Perimortem CD and Cardiopulmonary Resuscitation: In the event airway management is unsuccessful and there is increasing hypoxemia with near cardiac arrest, a perimortem CD is warranted. The most experienced obstetrician must perform the procedure.

The 2010 American Heart Association guidelines for cardiopulmonary resuscitation recommendation of C-A-B (compressions, airway, and breathing) are also recommended by the Society for Obstetric Anesthesia and Perinatology consensus statement on the management of cardiac arrest in pregnancy.[274] The performance of a perimortem CD is a challenging aspect of maternal resuscitation. Katz and colleagues recommended a 4-minute rule from the maternal arrest to the initiation of the CD, with the fetus being delivered in 5 minutes.[275] The timing of the delivery was based on theoretical considerations such as oxygen consumption and prevention of neurologic injury. Adherence to a 4-minute rule means that the operating room and rapid response teams must rapidly assess the patient, institute appropriate resuscitation, and expedite CD.[276,277] Speed is of the essence once the decision is made to undertake delivery.

Restoration of venous return and optimal cardiac output are essential for effective maternal resuscitation. Perimortem CD results in immediate relief of inferior cava obstruction with improved venous return and cardiac output, and enhanced maternal cardiopulmonary resuscitative efforts with improved circulation.

Recommendations for Availability of Airway Devices

The DA cart should be organized to follow the sequence of clinical scenarios that one might encounter during an unanticipated DA (Box 37.7):

- *Optimizing best attempt at intubation:* The top shelf contains all the equipment and local anesthetics required for an awake intubation. This includes an Eschmann stylet as well as an optical stylet for optimizing the glottic view during a DI under GA. The flexible scope is located in a predesignated slot on the side of the DA cart. A video laryngoscope is available, on wheels, next to the DA cart.

• BOX 37.7   Difficult Airway Cart Contents

Location	Contents
Top shelf	Prep items for awake intubation Eschmann bougie Optical Stylet
Side slot	Fiberoptic bronchoscope
Drawer A	Supraglottic airway sizes 3 and 4: LMA Fastrach, LMA ProSeal, LMA Supreme
Drawer B	Specialized supraglottic airways: Second-generation SGA -, i-gel #3 and #4 , Air Q
Drawer C	Invasive airway equipment: cricothyroidotomy kit, transtracheal jet cannula with adapter, retrograde intubation kit

A videolaryngoscope is immediately available at all times in the obstetric operating suite

- *Optimizing ventilation:* SGAs of sizes 3 and 4 (LMA Excel, LMA Fastrach, LMA ProSeal, LMA Supreme, i-gel) for use in the nonemergency pathway are available in the next drawer.
- *Optimizing oxygenation:* Equipment for invasive airway access (cricothyrotomy kit, including broad blade scalpel with handle, transtracheal jet cannula with adapter) for use in the emergency pathway/critical airway situation is in the bottom drawer.

Strategies to Avoid Postoperative Airway Catastrophes

Extensive literature in international publications has focused on the topic of DA management, and a number of algorithms and recommendations have been established to safely manage patients at risk for DI. Recently, however, the focus has pivoted to complications associated following extubation and to strategies for safe extubation of the DA. The importance of developing preplanned strategies for extubation of the DA to improve patient safety and outcomes is apparent from data from both the ASA Closed Claims Analysis and the UK's recent National Audit Project of major complications of airway management.[278–280]

Similar to extubation issues with general surgery patients, an emerging problem in obstetric patients is respiratory-related complications and maternal mortality after extubation.[15] The ASA task force regarded the concept of an extubation strategy as a logical extension of the extubation process.[101] The data from the confidential inquiries into maternal death from the United Kingdom and a study from the United States on anesthesia-related deaths in Michigan indicated that airway management of the obstetric patient during induction of GA, including intubation, was without complications; however, critical airway and ventilation incidents including hypoventilation or airway obstruction occurred during emergence, extubation, or recovery.[15,26]

A review between 1985 and 2003 from Michigan identified eight anesthesia-related deaths.[15] These deaths occurred following extubation and during recovery because of airway obstruction or hypoventilation. Lapses in standard postoperative monitoring and inadequate supervision by an anesthesiologist were identified. Obesity and African American race also seemed to be important risk factors for anesthesia-related maternal mortality.

Similarly, adverse airway events were noted during emergence and extubation per the results of a NAP4 study in the United Kingdom.[18,19] Proposals to improve patient safety in obstetrics must require identification of preexisting comorbidities that can lead to postoperative respiratory complications. Standard monitoring in the postoperative period, including pulse oximetry, must be mandatory. As perioperative physicians, anesthesiologists are uniquely qualified to supervise the anesthesia care team, to manage and minimize anesthesia-related maternal risk, to provide peripartum medical diagnosis and treatment, to facilitate lifesaving airway management interventions, and to lead prompt, coordinated, and effective resuscitation efforts to prevent airway catastrophes in obstetric patients.[281] Development of a strategy to maintain continuous access to the airway with an airway exchange catheter (AEC), to facilitate potential rescue of the airway, must be considered, especially in high-risk patients such as those with obesity, an edematous airway, obstructive sleep apnea, or known or suspected airway management difficulties. An AEC is well tolerated by most patients (90%) and is, therefore, a valuable option.[281] In patients with challenging airways, experts have suggested waiting for at least 30 to 60 minutes or until the likelihood of reintubation is minimized.[16,281,282] Patients with the potential for periglottic edema may benefit either from the use of VL or from extending the duration of the indwelling AEC from 60 to 120 minutes.[281] Bhatnagar et al. highlighted the use of the video laryngoscope (King Vision, a Blade Video Laryngoscope from manufacturer AMBU, Columbia, MD) as a viable and alternative tool for safe extubation in four patients presenting with glottic and supraglottic pathology, in place of conventional laryngoscopy with the Macintosh blade.[283]

Communication, Documentation, Handoff, and Airway Alerts

The communication and documentation of information concerning patients with DAs and the associated complications with DA management are universally recognized as important components in avoiding future airway management difficulties. A range of options is available to impart this information; however, a recent survey showed there are inconsistencies and no consensus on how this information should be disseminated.[284] Options for disseminating the information include notes in the electronic or manual anesthesia and clinical record, letters to the patient and primary physician, and entries in hospital, national, and MedicAlert databases. Of the patients with an airway difficulty noted on their anesthesia record, only 14% also had a pertinent comment on their clinical record; even fewer were referred to hospital warning systems (12%) or national (6%) or MedicAlert (7%) databases.[284]

Airway-related trauma and complications have been reported with video laryngoscopes,[172] second-generation SGAs,[285] and fiber-optic intubation.[286] A recent review highlights the types and incidence of complications with SGA devices.[287] They include regurgitation and aspiration of gastric contents, compression of vascular structures, trauma, and nerve injury. Although the incidence of such complications is quite low, some carry with them a significant degree of morbidity, indicating a need to follow manufacturers' advice. The incidence of gastric content aspiration associated with the SGA devices is estimated to be as low as 0.02% with perioperative regurgitation being significantly higher but underreported. Other serious, but extremely rare, complications

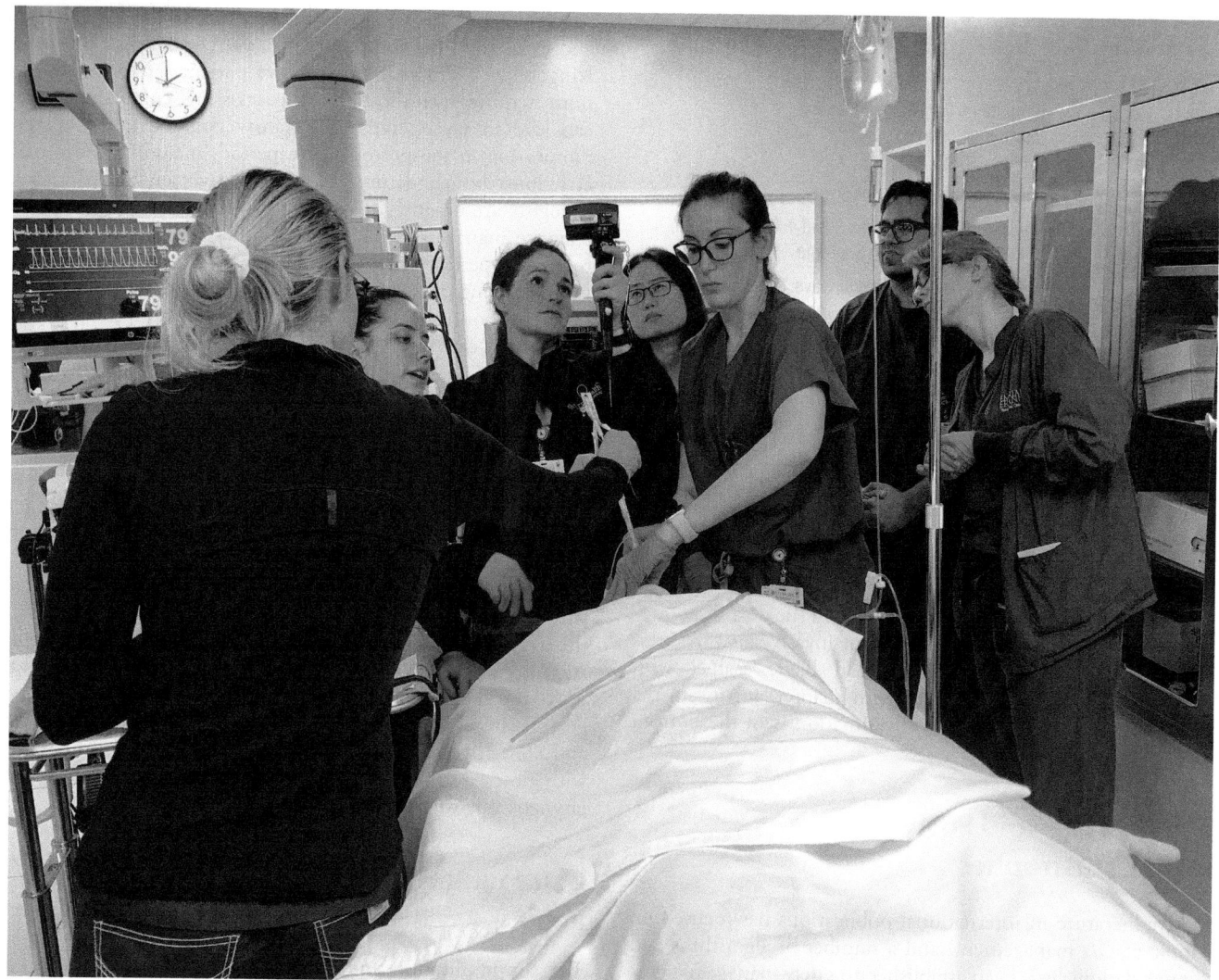

• **Fig. 37.17** Anesthesia residents practicing a difficult airway scenario in a simulation lab.

include pharyngeal rupture, pneumomediastinum, mediastinitis, or arytenoid dislocation.[287]

The ASA closed claims analysis listed pharyngeal and esophageal injuries most commonly associated with DA management[288] as possibly difficult to diagnose in the setting of pneumothorax, emphysema of the pneumomediastinum, or surgical emphysema in 50% of patients.[289] Mediastinitis secondary to airway perforation has a high mortality. Therefore, proper handoff, communication, documentation, and follow-up are required in order to enhance awareness and to promptly recognize complications secondary to airway trauma and to treat them in an expeditious manner. Patients should be observed carefully for mediastinitis and the triad of pain (severe sore throat, deep cervical pain, chest pain, and dysphagia) with painful swallowing, fever, and crepitus.[224] Postoperatively, it warrants discussion with the patient to seek immediate medical help if there is an onset of any of these signs and symptoms and consideration of giving written instructions at the time of discharge pertaining to DA.

In conclusion, documentation of DA information with the associated complications and management in the anesthetic record is widely accepted as essential[290] and is regarded as the most important form of communication. The drawback is that the records cannot be accessed if the patient seeks care in another hospital, previous notes are not readily retrievable, or prehospital airway management was conducted by first responders. Letters to the patient have been shown to be more effective, with up to 92% of patients who received a letter concerning their airway difficulty notifying a subsequent anesthesiologist about their airway when presenting for subsequent surgery.[291] In the United States, there is a MedicAlert Foundation National Difficult Airway/Intubation Registry; however, the majority of anesthesia providers are not aware of the registry and how to access the information.

The Importance of Simulation-Based Training in Obstetric Anesthesia

Anesthetic mortality related to DA management has been directly correlated to inadequate supervision, inadequate preoperative assessment, failure of communication, failure to monitor the patient, and suboptimal resuscitation.[292] These factors can be addressed in simulated settings with real-time assessment, feedback, and debriefing. Simulation training has become widely accepted as an integral part of anesthesia education and is arguably even more critical for obstetric anesthesia. Compared with trainees who do not undergo simulator-based training, trainees who do undergo such training demonstrate improved clinical performance, efficiency, and retention of cognitive, noncognitive, and performance skills in subsequent simulated anesthesia scenarios.[293] Furthermore, recent advances in simulation technology have increased realism and fidelity, translating into improved scenario accuracy.

Although guidelines for DA management have been published in the United States and the United Kingdom, there is a lack of adherence to these guidelines, and the majority of anesthesia practitioners are not prepared for a CICV/CICO situation.[294] High-fidelity simulation has been used to assess how anesthesia practitioners use the ASA DA task force guidelines to respond to an unanticipated CICV airway event.[295] The results of this study from 2009 showed that anesthesiologists had knowledge of the ASA guidelines but failed to adhere to them routinely. Instead, their approach was based on personal clinical experience, familiarity with airway devices, and selective interpretation of the guidelines.[296] Simulated training allows an organized approach to difficult or failed intubation, and strategies to establish ventilation and invasive techniques to establish oxygenation are critical in enhancing patient safety. Scavone et al. showed that anesthesiology residents participating in the simulation of GA for an emergent CD demonstrated improved performance when participating in a subsequent simulated scenario compared with residents who did not have a prior simulation experience.[293]

Over the previous decade, simulation training has incorporated several advances in technology, research, and methods. Implementing virtual reality and augmented reality modalities in conjunction with a high-fidelity manikin enhances the realism of a simulation. Obstetric environments can be more accurately created, and the dynamics of specific settings can be portrayed. Elements such as urgency, adverse events, communication challenges, treatment modalities, and such can be incorporated in real time. Simulating difficult obstetric airway scenarios can improve practitioners' technical and nontechnical skills, potentially improving clinical outcomes. Conducting routine obstetric simulations with the working clinical team members has the potential to identify factors that can impact performance and efficiency.[297] As the paradigm continues to shift in CD toward neuraxial techniques, simulation training of obstetric DA management is often referred to as an "ethical imperative," allowing for improvement in critical skills and crisis resource management without compromising patient safety.[298]

Conclusion

Management of the DA in obstetric patients has emerged as one of the most important safety issues. DL, failed TI, and inability to ventilate or oxygenate, following induction of GA for CD are major contributory factors leading to maternal morbidity and mortality. The heightened awareness of GA-related maternal mortality has led to a dramatic increase in the use of neuraxial techniques in the obstetric patient, with a consequent decrease in anesthesia-related maternal mortality. Despite the decrease in maternal mortality, in the event a GA is indicated for emergency CD, encountering a DI or inability to ventilate or oxygenate can result in a high liability for the anesthesia practitioner. Prediction of DA is not always reliable, yet there is enough evidence in the literature to suggest that performing a focused history, physical examination, and airway evaluation for predictors of DI, and/or difficult ventilation

allows the anesthesia practitioner to develop appropriate strategies for the safe airway management of the obstetric patient. Strategies must be based on standardized DA guidelines and an algorithm that is suitable and applicable to obstetric patients. GA for obstetric emergencies requires well thought-out and organized preformulated strategies for airway management *before* induction in order to have safe maternal and neonatal outcomes. Calling for help early and having important decision points is critical.

Emergency airway management strategy involves having the operating room fully prepared and in a state of readiness at all times, with immediate availability of functioning VL, adjunct airway devices, SGA, and immediate access to a DA cart. The key components of the safe anesthetic management strategy include the following:

1. Optimization of intubation, with proficiency in the use of VAL, which should be the first-line airway device used for a general anesthetic in an OB emergency. The number of intubation attempts should be restricted to no more than two. Recognition, acceptance, and declaration of a failed intubation allow the practitioner to move to the next step in emergency airway management and towards establishing oxygenation with a second-generation SGA.

2. Optimization of ventilation, with emphasis on oxygenation following failed intubation in obstetrics. Although challenging for the anesthesia practitioner, the use of a second-generation SGA is important for establishing ventilation and oxygenation.

3. Optimization of oxygenation in a critical CICO situation. If the SGA placement is not successful after two attempts, a failed SGA placement should be declared, followed by the critical and most important step in establishing oxygenation: performing a cricothyrotomy in order to save two lives and to have safe optimal outcome for both mother and baby. All anesthesia practitioners must be trained in cricothyrotomy. Crisis resource management and simulation techniques should also be an essential part of improving proficiency in obstetric emergencies.

Selected References

1. Mushambi MC, Kinsella SM. Obstetric Anaesthetists' Association/Difficult Airway Society difficult and failed tracheal intubation guidelines—the way forward for the obstetric airway. *Br J Anaesth*. 2015;115(6):815–818. doi:10.1093/bja/aev296.

2. Hawkins JL, Chang J, Palmer SK, Gibbs CP, Callaghan WM. Anesthesia-related maternal mortality in the United States: 1979-2002. *Obstet Gynecol*. 2011;117(1):69–74. doi:10.1097/AOG.0b013e31820093a9.

4. Kinsella SM, Winton AL, Mushambi MC, et al. Failed tracheal intubation during obstetric general anaesthesia: a literature review. *Int J Obstet Anesth*. 2015;24(4):356–374. doi:10.1016/j.ijoa.2015.06.008.

18. Cook TM, Woodall N, Harper J, Benger J. Fourth National Audit Project, Major complications of airway management in the UK: results of the Fourth National Audit Project of the Royal College of Anaesthetists and the Difficult Airway Society. Part 2: intensive care and emergency departments, *Br J Anaesth*. 2011;106(5):632–642. doi:10.1093/bja/aer059.

47. Freedman RL, Lucas DN. MBRRACE-UK: saving lives, improving mothers' care - implications for anaesthetists. *Int J Obstet Anesth*. 2015;24(2):161–173. doi:10.1016/j.ijoa.2015.03.004.

57. Practice Guidelines for Obstetric Anesthesia. An Updated Report by the American Society of Anesthesiologists Task Force on Obstetric Anesthesia and the Society for Obstetric Anesthesia and

Perinatology. *Anesthesiology.* 2016;124(2):270–300. doi:10.1097/ALN.0000000000000935.

61. Hodzovic I, Bedreag O. Awake videolaryngoscope - guided intubation - well worth adding to your skill-mix. *Rom J Anaesth Intensive Care.* 2019;26(1):5–7. doi:10.2478/rjaic-2019-0001.

62. Niforopoulou P, Pantazopoulos I, Demestiha T, Koudouna E, Xanthos T. Video-laryngoscopes in the adult airway management: a topical review of the literature. *Acta Anaesthesiol Scand.* 2010;54(9):1050–1061. doi:10.1111/j.1399-6576.2010.02285.x.

79. Alhomary M, Ramadan E, Curran E, Walsh SR. Videolaryngoscopy vs. fibreoptic bronchoscopy for awake tracheal intubation: a systematic review and meta-analysis. *Anaesthesia.* 2018;73(9):1151–1161. doi:10.1111/anae.14299.

94. Chauleur C, Collet F, Furtos C, Nourrissat A, Seffert P, Chauvin F. Identification of factors influencing the decision-to-delivery interval in emergency caesarean sections. *Gynecol Obstet Invest.* 2009;68(4):248–254. doi:10.1093/bja/aev29610.1159/000239783.

98. Krom AJ, Cohen Y, Miller JP, Ezri T, Halpern SH, Ginosar Y. Choice of anaesthesia for category-1 caesarean section in women with anticipated difficult tracheal intubation: the use of decision analysis. *Anaesthesia.* 2017;72(2):156–171. doi:10.1111/anae.13729.

99. Girard T, Palanisamy A. The obstetric difficult airway: if we can't predict it, can we prevent it? *Anaesthesia.* 2017;72(2):143–147. doi:10.1111/anae.13670.

113. Russell EC, Wrench I, Feast M, Mohammed F. Pre-oxygenation in pregnancy: the effect of fresh gas flow rates wixthin a circle breathing system. *Anaesthesia.* 2008;63(8):833–836. doi:10.1111/j.1365-2044.2008.05502.x.

128. Levitan RM. NO DESAT! Nasal Oxygen During Efforts Securing a Tube. *Emergency Physicians Monthly.* 2019. Available at. https://epmonthly.com/article/no-desat.

156. Williamson RM, Mallaiah S, Barclay P. Rocuronium and sugammadex for rapid sequence induction of obstetric general anaesthesia. *Acta Anaesthesiol Scand.* 2011;55:694–699.

204. Panneer M, Babu S, Murugaiyan P. Comparison of I-gel versus endotracheal tube in patients undergoing elective cesarean section: a prospective randomized control study. *Anesth Essays Res.* 2017;11(4):930–933. doi:10.4103/aer.AER_32_17.

206. Fang X, Xiao Q, Xie Q, et al. General anesthesia with the use of SUPREME laryngeal mask airway for emergency cesarean delivery: a retrospective analysis of 1039 parturients. *Sci Rep.* 2018;8(1):13098. doi:10.1038/s41598-018-31581-5.

226. Yao WY, Li SY, Yuan YJ, et al. Comparison of Supreme laryngeal mask airway versus endotracheal intubation for airway management during general anesthesia for cesarean section: a randomized controlled trial. *BMC Anesthesiol.* 2019;19(1):123. doi:10.1186/s12871-019-0792-9.

295. Borges BC, Boet S, Siu LW, et al. Incomplete adherence to the ASA difficult airway algorithm is unchanged after a high-fidelity simulation session. *Can J Anaesth.* 2010;57(7):644–649. doi:10.1007/s12630-010-9322-4.

All references can be found online at eBooks.Health.Elsevier.com.

38

Airway Management in Head and Neck Surgery

VLADIMIR NEKHENDZY AND ANIL PATEL

KEY POINTS

- Airway problems in head and neck (H&N) patients are common, and so are the airway failures. The anesthesia provider must develop and maintain excellent dexterity with a wide range of airway management devices and techniques.
- The preoperative endoscopic airway examination (PEAE) should become an integral part of the H&N anesthesia provider's armamentarium.
- In patients with compromised airway, awake or asleep flexible scope intubation (FSI) or video-assisted laryngoscopy (VAL) should substitute for direct laryngoscopy (DL) as a primary approach to tracheal intubation (TI), whenever feasible.
- High-risk H&N patients demand thorough preoperative preparation, discussion with the surgeon, and development of joint, well-thought-through airway management strategies.
- A structured and stepwise approach to a tenuous and partially obstructed airway is imperative for successful management.
- The advanced ventilation techniques, such as transnasal humidified rapid-insufflation ventilatory exchange (THRIVE), SponTaneous Respiration using IntraVEnous anaesthesia and Hi-flow nasal oxygen (STRIVE Hi), and the Tritube are being developed and are effective in selected patient populations, particularly in those with the partially obstructed airway. The use of these techniques requiring specialized expertise and teamwork in a shared airway setting.
- The principles and practice of jet ventilation (JV) must be well understood and adhered to by the anesthesia provider and the surgeon.

- For laser surgery, the fire triangle (fire triad) must be well understood and managed by all members of the team. The airway fire requires three components: fuel source, oxidant sources, and ignition source. Removal of one of these components prevents or reduces the risk. Adherence to the laser timeouts and the institutional laser safety protocols must be required.
- Close communication between the anesthesia provider and the surgeon throughout the perioperative period is critical for the success of the operation and for patient safety.

Introduction

Airway management in head and neck (H&N) surgery presents some unique challenges for the anesthesia provider (Box 38.1). The difficult airway (DA) is observed more frequently in H&N patients than in the general surgical population. In the Fourth National Audit Project (NAP4), H&N patients comprised nearly 40% of cases with airway management–related complications and almost 75% of cases where an emergent surgical airway was required for the cannot intubate/cannot oxygenate (CICO) situation.[1,2] Several large studies have demonstrated that difficult tracheal intubation (TI) (≥3 attempts on direct laryngoscopy) may be encountered in 7% to 9% of H&N cases,[3–5] which is at least two to four times higher than in the mixed surgical population.[6–9] H&N cancer patients, predominantly males, are at even higher risk: Difficult direct laryngoscopy (DL) and TI can be observed in over 12% of these patients.[1–3] Bryan and colleagues have observed that patients with oropharyngeal masses present at particularly high risk for difficult TI and associated hypoxemia: 23% of these patients required ≥3 intubation attempts, 68% were difficult to mask ventilate, and in 34% Spo_2 was below 95% during the procedure.[10] Moreover, tracheal extubation and early recovery period present increased challenges to the anesthesia provider.[1,11]

The team-centered approach to an anticipated DA in H&N surgery is paramount. Successful airway management of H&N patients requires a high degree of cooperation with the surgeon, allowing for early identification of high-risk patients, a reciprocal understanding of the potential management problems, and adequate preparation on both sides to meet the anticipated challenges that may arise.[12,13] Thorough appreciation of the complexity of the upper airway anatomy, the pathologic process involved, and all steps of the surgical procedure are necessary for devising a safe and rational perioperative airway management strategy.[14] Special expertise in H&N anesthesia and complex airway management should be encouraged because it may improve TI outcomes and result in quicker intubation times, better patient oxygenation, and fewer failures.[4]

Competent sharing of the patient's airway with the surgeon greatly contributes to safe patient management. Most of the time, not only is the patient's airway shared with the surgeon, but immediate access to the airway is also difficult or impossible, because the operating room (OR) table is turned 90 or 180 degrees away from the anesthesia provider. The endotracheal tube (ETT) must be secured diligently to prevent an accidental extubation under the surgical drapes or a withdrawal of the ETT into the larynx; a sudden air leak may negatively affect the surgical field during precision surgery

and create an airway fire hazard during intraoral procedures. Unrecognized ETT displacement out of the trachea and into the glottis carries an additional risk for the anesthesia provider to repeatedly add more air to the ETT cuff, which may lead to the compression of the anterior branch of the recurrent laryngeal nerve and vocal cord (VC) injury.[15] During oral and intranasal surgery, the patient's airway must be protected from blood, debris, and irrigation fluid, and the use of a throat pack by the surgeon may be required.

Even uncomplicated elective H&N cases require the anesthesia provider's thorough familiarity with surgery-specific airway management requirements. The spectrum of H&N surgery is broad, ranging from the most common procedures, such as tonsillectomy, to precision laryngologic and complex obstructive sleep apnea (OSA) surgery, major H&N cancer surgery with extensive reconstructive procedures, and others. The TI route, ETT size and type, and different montages of the anesthesia circuit should all be discussed with the surgeon to streamline and optimize TI and facilitate surgical access.

For example, a nasal intubation is routinely required for base-of-the-tongue (BOT) surgical work, transoral robotic surgery (TORS), orthognathic surgery, and maxillomandibular advancement for OSA surgery, and it may be requested by the surgeon for parotidectomy and some dental procedures. A nasal ETT must be appropriately sized to ensure adequate depth of tracheal placement (Fig. 38.1) and secured to prevent pressure against the alar area (Fig. 38.2). A delayed-sequence nasal intubation may be considered in patients with decreased oxygen reserve or when difficult mask ventilation is encountered or anticipated (Fig. 38.3).

For microlaryngeal surgery, the ETT is usually moved to the left corner of the patient's mouth to facilitate introduction of the surgical

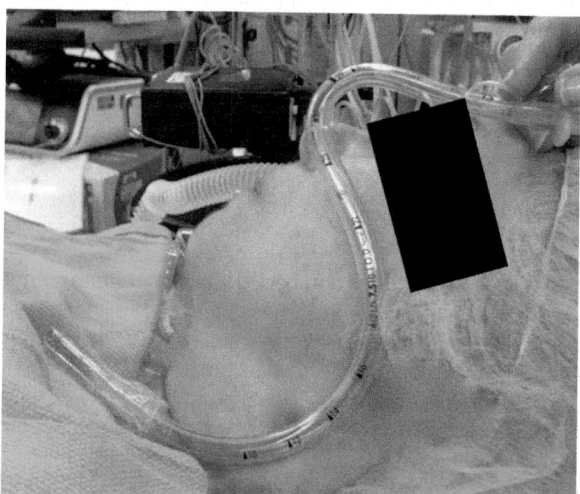

- **Fig. 38.1** Proper sizing of the preformed (nasal RAE) endotracheal tube (ETT) for nasotracheal intubation. The nasal RAE ETT is positioned along the patient's upper airway profile. With the preformed ETT bend placed against the nasal alar area, the ETT cuff should be visualized at the level of the suprasternal notch, which ensures adequate depth of ETT placement at approximately midtracheal level. (Photo courtesy Stanford Head and Neck Anesthesia and Advanced Airway Management Program, Stanford, CA.)

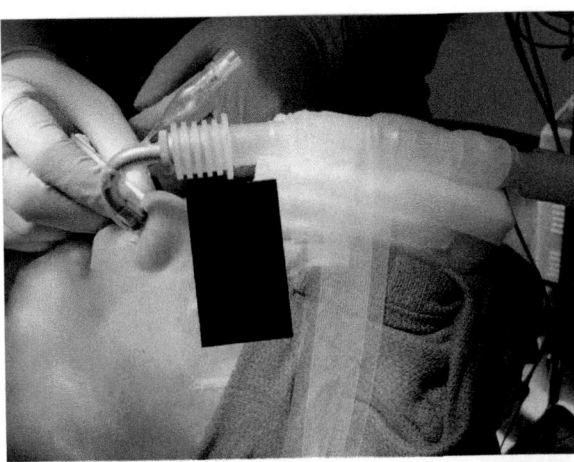

• **Fig. 38.2** Secure positioning of the nasally placed 6.0-mm-ID micro-laryngeal tube (MLT). Note the montage of the anesthesia circuit to prevent pressure of the MLT tube against the nasal alar area to avoid alar necrosis. A similar montage is frequently used for securing the positioning of the preformed nasal RAE endotracheal tubes (ETTs). The additional suturing of ETTs to the nasal septum may be required for extra ETT stability. (Photo courtesy Stanford Head and Neck Anesthesia and Advanced Airway Management Program, Stanford, CA.)

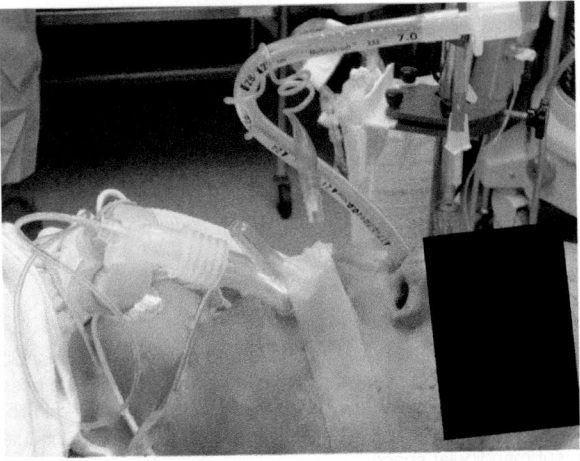

• **Fig. 38.3** A delayed sequence nasal intubation. A delayed sequence nasal intubation involves optimizing the patient's oxygenation with the supraglottic airway (SGA) device before nasal intubation. It also frees the anesthesia provider's hands to accomplish a nasal prep in an unhurried manner. The use of the SGA device with superior ventilation capabilities, such as the pictured LMA Supreme, is recommended to prolong apnea time in patients with decreased oxygen reserve (e.g., obesity), or when difficult mask ventilation is encountered or anticipated. The SGA is removed immediately before tracheal intubation. (Photo courtesy Stanford Head and Neck Anesthesia and Advanced Airway Management Program, Stanford, CA.)

instruments and must be securely taped to the lower jaw, facilitating full opening of the patient's mouth by the surgeon. The mouth opening and exaggerated full extension of the patient's neck account for ETT pullback, and a slightly deeper placement of ETT may be recommended in these patients. A small-size ETT, for example, a microlaryngeal tube (MLT) with a 5-mm inner diameter (ID) is routinely used for microlaryngeal surgery (Fig. 38.4), and a nasal intubation with a small-diameter MLT tube (5- to 6-mm ID) is frequently required to facilitate surgical access for TORS. A 6-mm-ID wire-reinforced flexible ETT is frequently preferred for many intraoral procedures.

The anesthesia provider must also become thoroughly familiar with the specialized laser and neural integrity monitor (NIM) ETTs and the techniques for their proper placement. Finally, the H&N anesthesia

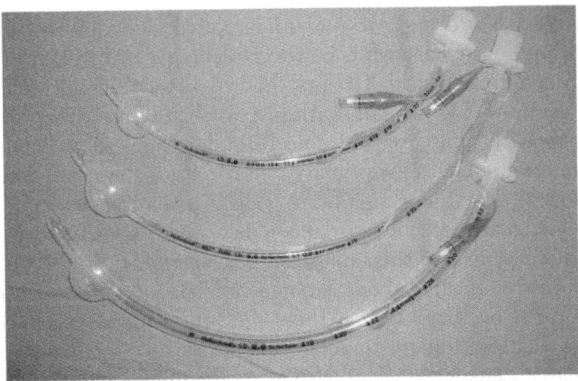

• **Fig. 38.4** Microlaryngeal tracheal (MLT) tube. A standard endotracheal tube (ETT) with an ID of 5.0 mm *(top)* is compared with a 5-mm-ID MLT tube *(center)* and an 8-mm-ID ETT *(bottom)*. A greater length and bigger cuff diameter of the MLT tube (equivalent to a standard 8.0-mm-ID ETT) allows a sufficient depth of tracheal placement, a connection to the anesthesia circuit, and an adequate seal of the trachea.

provider should be proficient with jet ventilation (JV) and other intraoperative ventilation techniques used during microlaryngeal surgery (see "Special Situations/Microlaryngeal Surgery/Jet Ventilation").

This chapter focuses on devising safe and effective airway management strategies for patients undergoing H&N surgeries based on best evidence and the authors' experience. We also discuss some specific techniques and situations deserving special attention.

Preoperative Airway Assessment and Preparation

The preoperative airway assessment must include a comprehensive general medical history, focused history related to upper airway symptoms, a directed general physical and airway examination, a thorough assessment of the previous anesthetic records, details of the surgical plan, and laboratory and imaging studies. The anesthesia provider should step outside the role of an airway proceduralist and try to conduct a joint preoperative patient evaluation with the surgical colleagues for complex H&N cases whenever possible.

History

The anatomy of H&N is largely noncompliant, and any significant pathologic processes and injuries tend to result in substantial patient suffering and functional impairment.[16] Tobacco and alcohol use are associated with most cases of H&N cancer and predispose these patients to significant comorbidities, such as chronic obstructive pulmonary disease (COPD), hypertension, coronary artery disease, and alcohol withdrawal. Appropriate diagnostic tests are indicated for these patients as part of the preoperative workup and preoperative optimization. Patients with significant lung disease and ventilation/perfusion ($\dot{V}/\dot{Q}$) mismatch may not be suitable candidates for advanced intraoperative ventilation techniques, such as spontaneous ventilation, apneic intermittent ventilation, JV, transnasal humidified rapid-insufflation ventilatory exchange (THRIVE) or SponTaneous Respiration using IntraVEnous anaesthesia and Hi-flow nasal oxygen (STRIVE Hi).[17–21] It is not uncommon for H&N cancer patients to present with chronic anemia. Appropriate laboratory studies must be obtained, and electrolyte and fluid status of these patients should be optimized preoperatively. Patients with chronic alcohol consumption require preoperative evaluation of liver function and coagulation status.

Some patients may present with increased aspiration risk, complicating DA management. Lower cranial nerve involvement (cranial nerves XI, X, and XII) may lead to airway difficulty related to aspiration or obstruction. Almost one-half of the patients presenting with laryngeal and voice disorders have silent laryngopharyngeal reflux as the primary cause or as a significant etiologic factor.[22,23] Coexistent significant glottic insufficiency (e.g., VC paralysis) may place these patients at increased risk for aspiration of gastric contents.[24,25] This can usually be diagnosed during a routine preoperative flexible scope laryngoscopy or laryngostroboscopy performed by the surgeon. Those presenting for esophagoscopy for evaluation and treatment of esophageal obstructing lesions, achalasia, Zenker diverticulum, active gastrointestinal bleeding, or esophageal foreign body removal constitute another category of patients at high risk for aspiration. Even when gastroesophageal reflux disease (GERD) is not clinically significant, adequate preoperative pharmacologic control of the symptoms is warranted: The combination of acid exposure and direct trauma from the operating procedure and TI can lead to laryngeal mucosal injury.[26]

Many patients presenting for H&N surgery are ≥60 years old and will demonstrate high incidence of undiagnosed sleep-disordered breathing and OSA.[27] The nature of many H&N diseases, the presence of craniofacial abnormalities (e.g., retrognathia, macroglossia), male sex, and a history of excessive alcohol intake must also increase the anesthesia provider's level of suspicion for OSA.[28] A variety of bedside screening tools (e.g., the snoring, tiredness, observed apnea, high blood pressure, body mass index, age, neck circumference, and male gender [STOP-Bang] questionnaire) can be used to identify patients at highest risk for OSA.[28]

Information about previous H&N surgical procedures and radiation therapy, as well as the history of anesthetic and airway management problems, must be obtained and communicated. History of previous difficult TI is one of the most important predictors of anticipated airway management difficulties,[29–31] yet it is still taken lightly in anesthesia practice.[32]

The history of prior H&N radiation therapy must be elucidated because exposure to radiation therapy frequently makes TI difficult. The radiation-induced tissue fibrosis results in loss of tissue compliance, frequently leads to long-standing glottic and epiglottic edema as a result of impaired lymphatic drainage, and may also restrict the patient's mouth opening and neck extension.[33]

Physical Examination

A systematic and comprehensive preoperative airway assessment is paramount, and the American Society of Anesthesiologists (ASA) 11-point bedside airway assessment tool is a good start.[34] However, standard airway assessment tests are poorly predictive, do not account for aspiration risk and lower airway problems, and fail to assess the severity of upper airway disease and BOT pathology (e.g., epiglottic cancer, epiglottic and vallecula cysts, lingual tonsillar hypertrophy) (Fig. 38.5).[9,35]

Postradiation changes in the neck and decreased mandibular protrusion are important factors predicting the risk of impossible mask ventilation, difficult mask ventilation, and difficult DL in patients at risk for these conditions (see Chapter 9).[36–39] The reduced submandibular compliance attributed to cancerous involvement, masses, inflammation, or previous radiation therapy (Fig. 38.6) may severely diminish pharyngeal space and restrict tongue displacement during DL, resulting in difficult or failed TI.[40]

Pharyngeal restriction can be further accentuated by a large tongue or intraoral masses, which can be exophytic and mobile.

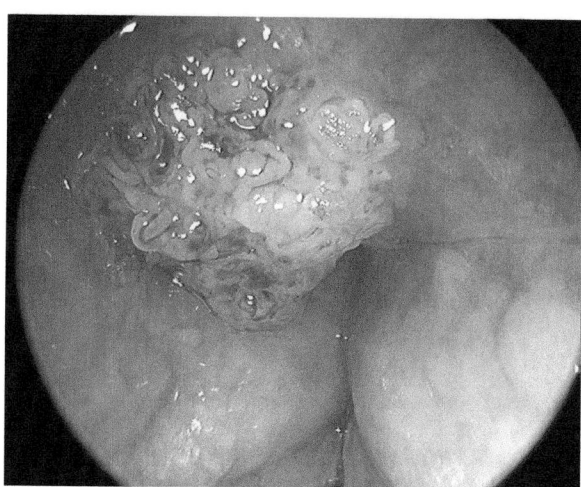

• **Fig. 38.5** Epiglottic carcinoma. (Courtesy Edward Damrose, MD, Stanford University Medical Center, Stanford, CA.)

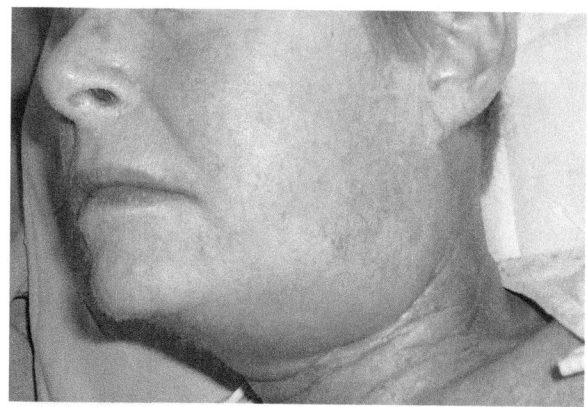

• **Fig. 38.6** Postradiation neck changes and decreased submandibular compliance in a patient presenting for panendoscopy. Note the postincisional neck scar and postradiation changes that have resulted in fibrotic changes in the skin and subcutaneous tissues of the neck and induration of the submandibular space.

Common symptoms of airway obstruction may include dyspnea at rest or on exertion, voice changes, dysphagia, stridor, and cough. Voice changes provide an early suggestion of the anatomic level, severity, and progression of the lesion. A muffled voice may indicate supraglottic disease, whereas glottic lesions often result in a coarse, scratchy voice. Physical findings may include hoarseness, agitation, and intercostal, suprasternal, and supraclavicular retraction.

Drooling, dysphagia, and expiratory snoring are the signs of marked pharyngeal restriction,[40,41] but inspiratory stridor at rest represents the most worrisome sign, suggesting a reduction in airway diameter at the supraglottic, periglottic, or glottic level of at least 50% (see "Special Considerations"/"Partially Obstructed Airway").[25,42] Airway compromise in H&N patients may also involve the lower airways. Airway narrowing at the tracheal or tracheobronchial level is typically characterized by expiratory stridor, whereas biphasic inspiratory-expiratory stridor usually points to obstructive subglottic disease.[13] In some cases, preoperative examination of the flow-volume loops may be helpful.[43]

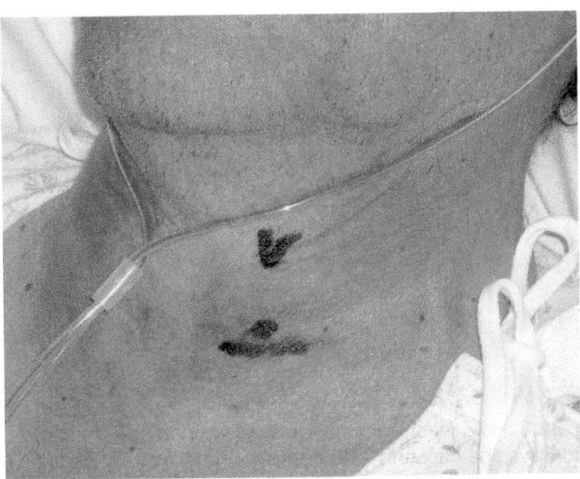

• **Fig. 38.7** A patient with a laryngeal carcinoma, fixed hemilarynx, and severe inspiratory stridor. The black check mark indicates a thyroid notch, the horizontal black line corresponds to the top of the cricoid cartilage, and the black dot represents the location of the cricothyroid membrane. Notice the inflammatory skin changes. The vocal cords were visible during preoperative nasal endoscopy.

It is prudent to assess the laryngeal mobility, the degree of tracheal deviation, and the location of the cricothyroid membrane (CTM) preoperatively.[13] Significant tracheal deviation, especially in combination with the fixed hemilarynx (Fig. 38.7) and poor or absent visualization of VC during preoperative nasal endoscopy, can be an ominous sign[42,44] and may warrant a performance of an awake tracheostomy (see "Devising Safe Airway Management Strategies for Tracheal Intubation"/ "Surgical Airway as a Primary Approach to Tracheal Intubation" and "Special Situations"/"Partially Obstructed Airway").

Endoscopy and Imaging Studies

Usually, the extent of disease in elective cases has been comprehensively evaluated preoperatively by routine chest radiography, computed tomography (CT), magnetic resonance imaging (MRI), and flexible laryngoscopy (nasal endoscopy), providing the anesthesia provider with valuable information regarding the location, size, spread, and vascularity of the obstructive lesions; the degree of obstruction; the mobility of the vocal cords; and the extent of laryngeal and tracheal deviation or compression.[13,45,46]

Patients with H&N cancer are at increased risk for CICO,[2] and if symptoms of airway obstruction are present, airway imaging and nasal endoscopy are considered a minimum necessary level of investigation for assessing airway management options.[2,14] The anesthesia provider must be thoroughly familiar with the results of these studies, and they should be reviewed and discussed jointly with the surgeon.[14]

Preoperative nasal endoscopy is usually performed by the H&N surgeon, but with sufficient practice it can be quickly and effectively executed by the anesthesia provider (preoperative endoscopic airway examination [PEAE]) as part of the preoperative assessment.[47] The PEAE (see Chapter 9) is a powerful airway assessment tool that provides precise information about upper airway and laryngeal anatomy to formulate appropriate airway management strategies.[47,48] Even in urgent situations, PEAE may help with anticipation and planning for a DA (see "Special Considerations"/"Partially Obstructed Airway").[49]

Devising Safe Airway Management Strategies for Tracheal Intubation

Determining the optimal airway management approach depends on the surgery being performed, location of the lesion, patient's symptoms, acuity of the situation, and patient's tolerance of the procedure. It may also be dictated by the anesthesia provider's skill set and equipment availability, where the need for improvement exists in both areas.[49]

The recurring theme in the NAP4 report is the need for maintaining close lines of communication with the surgical team before and during the intubation procedure.[50,51] Failure to anticipate and plan for problems and to develop safe airway strategies will contribute to failures and increase patients' morbidity.[49,52] An airway strategy can be defined as the predetermined set of sequential plans for managing failure of the previous attempts and for achieving and maintaining adequate ventilation, oxygenation, and protection against aspiration.[49]

Awake Versus Asleep Approach to Tracheal Intubation

The decision to proceed with an awake approach can be very straightforward when significant anatomic distortion is present or the patient's mouth opening is severely limited. In many cases, however, only a certain degree of difficulty can be expected, and decision-making becomes more complicated. For such patients with undefined risk, an approach to an anticipated DA should follow the framework suggested in the ASA DA algorithm,[34] with special attention directed to predictors of difficult mask ventilation, impossible mask ventilation, and their association with difficult DL and TI (see Chapter 9).[36–39]

The likelihood of difficult supraglottic airway (SGA) ventilation (see Chapter 19) and difficult surgical airway access (see Chapter 29) must also be considered and evaluated.[34] If the emergency cricothyroidotomy is contemplated as part of the airway strategy, success should not be assumed,[14] and it is best to secure the patient's airway while awake. If the patient's airway is marginal, but an awake approach is not feasible, the "airway double setup" is warranted: The CTM should be marked, the patient's neck should be prepped, and the surgical team must be present for induction as well as ready to perform an emergent cricothyroidotomy or tracheostomy. The placement of the tracheal catheter or cannula through the CTM before induction of anesthesia for passive oxygen insufflation and/or subsequent JV shall also be considered (see "Devising Safe Airway Management Strategies for Tracheal Intubation"/"Oxygenation Strategies and Special Situations"/"Partially Obstructed Airway"). Management of cases that may involve a surgical airway as a rescue technique should always be performed where the appropriate equipment is available, most commonly in the OR.[2,14]

The more complicated the patient's condition is, the more elaborate airway management strategies should become. Patients with H&N cancer, especially those with supraglottic and glottic tumors or a history of radiation therapy, require the longest intubation times and represent the highest risk for adverse TI outcomes.[1,2,4] In NAP4, airway management was considered poor in nearly 30% of these cases.[1,2] The pertinent preoperative imaging and PEAE findings for these patients must be reviewed and discussed with the surgeon to accurately estimate the degree of pathology and facilitate decision-making.

Role of Conventional and Video-Assisted Laryngoscopy

Given a high incidence of anticipated and encountered DA in H&N patients, it is prudent to reach for video-assisted laryngoscopy (VAL) as a primary TI technique in many cases. The ASA Difficult Airway Task Force recommendation to consider VAL as an initial approach to anticipated DA capitalizes on an extensive body of evidence for both steering and channeled VAL techniques (see Chapter 23).[34,53–63] The 2013 survey of the Canadian anesthesia practice also has listed VAL as the top technique to use during difficult TI.[64] For complex patients, and for patients for whom at least some degree of DL difficulty is anticipated, we therefore advocate expanding airway evaluation beyond the ASA recommendations to determine the likelihood of difficult VAL. The first-pass intubation success rate with the acute-angle VAL systems, such as the Glidescope or Storz CMac, may be expected to reach 93% to 96% in the general surgical population.[63] For patients with H&N pathology, and particularly those presenting with intraoral airway masses, inadequate glottic exposure may be observed with increased frequency, even with the use of the hyperangulated VAL blades. Hyman and colleagues have found that VAL fails to obtain an adequate view (Cormack-Lehane grade ≥3) in roughly one-third of these patients, highlighting a significantly increased risk for failed TI and oxygenation in this patient population.[65]

Difficult VAL also may be expected in patients with neck pathology (particularly a scar or a mass), abnormal neck anatomy, decreased cervical spine motion, decreased oral entry, and restricted oropharyngeal space.[55,56,61,66–69] Choosing a VAL depends on the operator's experience, but the nature and location of the lesion must be considered. For example, it may be safer to navigate around BOT tumors with a channeled VAL, such as Pentax Airway Scope, whose blade engages under the epiglottis, unlike other devices that typically require the tip of the blade to be placed in the vallecula. On the other hand, the steering technique of VAL with a styleted ETT may be more effective for maneuvering around the intraoral lesions.[70]

Difficulties with VAL notwithstanding, management of the anticipated DA with DL alone remains persistent and alarming practice. By studying over 188,000 patients in the Danish Anesthesia Database, Nørskov and colleagues have shown that half of the patients with anticipated difficult TI and over 40% of high-risk patients with anticipated combined ventilation and TI difficulty were planned to be managed by DL as a primary approach.[71]

A consistent NAP4 finding in patients with H&N pathology was the deterioration of the airway following a single or repeated attempts at DL.[1] The H&N tumors can cause considerable airway distortion and can be friable, leading to bleeding, defragmentation, airway soiling, and rapid edema formation.[1] If DL is chosen as a primary approach to TI, multiple attempts should be avoided in order to avert total airway obstruction and CICO situation.[1,2,13]

Role of Operative Laryngoscopy and Rigid Bronchoscopy

Should DL fail, the rescue with operative laryngoscopy using the anterior commissure scope or with the rigid bronchoscope by the surgeon can be successful.[34,45,72–74] The anterior commissure scopes, such as Holinger (Fig. 38.8), are very effective in handling poor laryngeal exposure or glottic obstruction and can

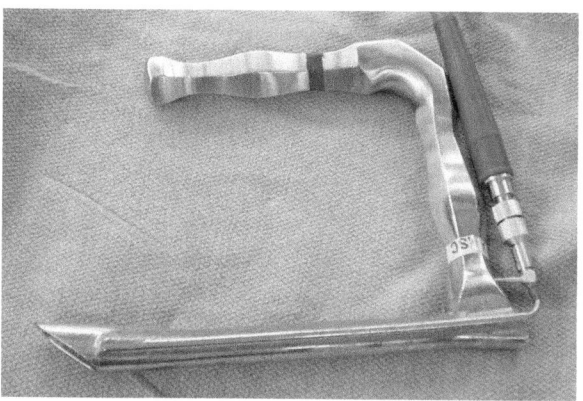

• **Fig. 38.8** Holinger anterior commissure laryngoscope. The pointed tip and the leverage capability of the laryngoscope facilitate visualization of at least part of the glottis. An anterior flare at the tip of the laryngoscope allows it to serve as a guide to endotracheal intubation.

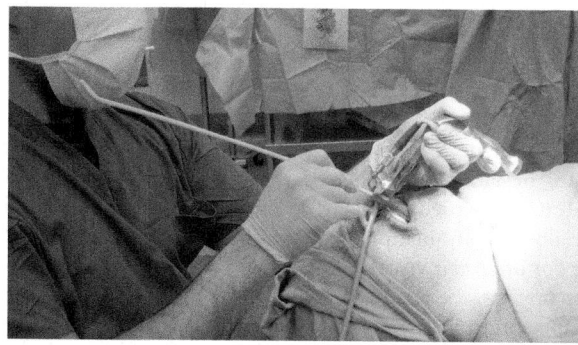

• **Fig. 38.9** Airway rescue is achieved with a bougie introducer and a Holinger laryngoscope in a patient with difficult laryngeal exposure. The endotracheal tube (ETT) cannot be directly advanced down the narrow barrel of the Holinger laryngoscope because of impaired visualization during tube advancement. The bougie introducer is used first, followed by removal of the laryngoscope and railroading the ETT over the bougie into the patient's trachea. The ETT can be directly advanced through the wider lumen of other laryngoscopes, such as the Lindholm, Dedo, or Kleinsasser.

be used as a conduit for TI when the bougie introducer or ETT is passed directly down the lumen (Fig. 38.9).[75] Hillel and colleagues have demonstrated that the use of the anterior commissure scopes by otolaryngologists, who were part of the DA response team (DART), helped secure over 35% of DAs and to decrease the number of emergent cricothyroidotomies nearly in half.[76]

In experienced hands, rigid bronchoscopy can rescue failed TI and CICO situations. It also serves as an indispensable tool for managing acute airway obstruction resulting from foreign bodies, hemoptysis, or tumors.[77,78] After the bronchoscope is placed into the patient's trachea by the surgeon, manual (Fig. 38.10) or JV can commence in a safe manner through the lumen of the bronchoscope. Subsequent airway exchange to ETT can be performed using an airway exchange catheter (AEC) or a gum elastic bougie (GEB) introducer (Fig. 38.11).[79,80]

Relying on operative laryngoscopy and rigid bronchoscopy as airway rescue assumes immediate availability of the equipment and expert surgical help. Unfortunately, even in skilled hands quick deployment of these devices can be problematic, especially when unfavorable anatomy precludes full atlanto-occipital extension and establishing the straight line of sight (Fig. 38.12).[22,73,81,82]

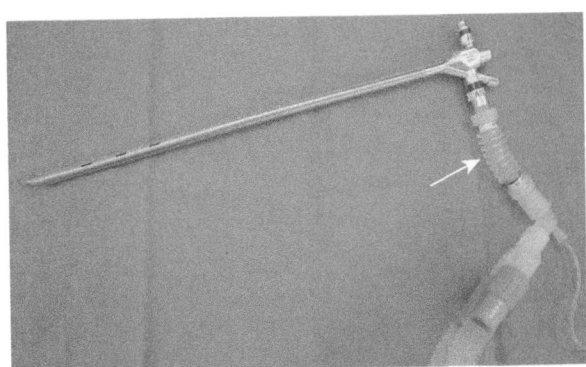

• **Fig. 38.10** A rigid bronchoscope is connected to the anesthesia circuit by a Racine adapter (arrow). A flexible diaphragm of the Racine universal adapter (SunMed, Largo, FL) connects a side arm of a rigid bronchoscope to the anesthesia breathing circuit.

Role of Inhalation Induction

Inhalation induction can be safely used in the presence of noncollapsing lesions, with anticipated failure rate of approximately 5%.[4] Difficulty in maintaining the airway during inhalation induction in patients with large pedunculated tumors, granulomas, and cysts should be anticipated, even if preoperative symptoms of airway obstruction are mild.[4,73] Early application of continuous positive airway pressure (CPAP) can help to stent the airway open, but inhalation induction should be considered highly problematic if mask ventilation difficulty is anticipated.[4] In the NAP4 study, inhalation induction failed in 12 of 16 (75%) H&N patients with the compromised airway, and in nearly all these patients (11 of 12) spontaneous ventilation became impossible.[1]

Sevoflurane is the most commonly used inhalation induction agent in adult and pediatric patients.[43,83] The minimum alveolar concentration (MAC) of sevoflurane required to provide adequate TI conditions in 50% of unpremedicated adult patients (MAC_{TI50}) is 4.5% (95% confidence interval 3.9% to 5.2%), and the 95% effective dose (ED_{95}) for TI is 8%.[84] The time for achieving this ED_{95} target in patients with normal airways is approximately 7 minutes,[85] but up to 20 minutes may be required when partial airway obstruction or the preexisting increase in minute ventilation and $\dot{V}/\dot{Q}$ mismatch are present.[41,43] The induction time can be shortened with the addition of small intravenous doses of midazolam or fentanyl[83,86] but at the expense of an increased risk of apnea and loss of the airway. Even in patients without severe airway compromise, inhalation induction frequently causes expiratory stridor (25%–40%) and breath holding (7.5%–15%), and the intubating conditions still remain inferior to the use of the neuromuscular blocking (NMB) agents.[83,85]

Overall, if inhalation induction is chosen as the primary approach to the difficult H&N airway, the possibility of failure should be anticipated, and the clear rescue strategies must be in place from the outset.[1]

Role of Flexible Scope Intubation and Optical Stylets

Recent randomized trials have demonstrated that an awake acute-angle VAL can be as effective as an awake flexible scope intubation (FSI)[87,88]; however, the latter remains the gold standard of care (see Chapter 24). It is frequently underused when indicated, probably because of a lack of confidence, skills, judgment, and equipment.[89]

Patients with H&N pathology may require awake FSI more frequently due to common occurrence and/or coexistence of H&N cancer, previous surgery, history of radiation, associated OSA, obesity, and anatomic characteristics, such as reduced mouth opening, limited neck extension, and progressive airway compromise.[90] Both awake and asleep FSI can fail frequently in H&N patients: In NAP4, such failure was observed in nearly 61% of these cases.[1] When performed by designated H&N anesthesia providers, a much lower yet still sufficiently high failure rate of 8.8% may be expected.[4] In the mixed surgical population with anticipated DA, the awake FSI may be expected to fail in 1% to 4% of cases,[87,88,90] usually without associated severe adverse effects.

The most common reasons for awake FSI failure appear to be the inability to either identify the glottis or to pass the flexible intubation scope (FIS) or ETT.[1] Additional reasons for the failure of asleep FSI include repeated TI attempts, bleeding, and airway obstruction.[1] Previous reports also documented a mere 50% success rate of FSI after repeated DL attempts,[91] and awake FSI should be chosen over an asleep approach in H&N patients whenever possible.[1,14]

The awake FSI requires a high degree of skill yet can be challenging even with proper patient preparation and cooperation. Similar to the inhalation induction strategy, the failure of either awake or asleep FSI should be anticipated in patients with advanced H&N pathology, and solid backup strategies must be in place before the start of the procedure.[1,14]

The optical intubation stylets, such as Bonfils, Shikani, Sensa-Scope, and Clarus Video System (see Chapter 22), can effectively lead within an ETT to help bypass mobile supraglottic and glottic masses. The FIS may fail in this situation, either because of the inability to displace the tumor or because the ETT simply would not pass. With optical stylets, once the glottis is entered, the ETT will follow the trajectory of the stylet into the patient's trachea. However, most of the available adult-size optical stylets require the use of an ETT with a minimum ID of 5.5 to 6 mm.

Role of the Supraglottic Airways and the Supraglottic Airway-Endotracheal Tube Exchange

The SGAs are vitally important in ventilation-centered airway management for H&N patients, who have a higher incidence of difficult and failed TI. A wide variety of SGAs are available, but their comparative performance in DA situations in general, and for H&N patients in particular, has not been vigorously investigated.[92]

By prospectively studying over 20,000 general surgical patients, Parmet and colleagues[91] documented a 94% success rate for rescue ventilation with the classic laryngeal mask airway (cLMA) in unanticipated DA.[91] The successful placement of cLMA and other types of LMA devices in patients with an abnormal airway and/or DA is probably independent of factors used to predict or score difficult TI.[93,94] However, reliable SGA ventilation in many H&N patients can be problematic because of difficulties associated with SGA insertion (e.g., restricted mouth opening), with achieving its proper positioning (e.g., space-occupying lesions, previous radiation therapy), and/or with maintaining an adequate airway seal pressure (ASP) and SGA ventilatory capability (e.g., obstructing pathology either at or below VC).

The NAP4 study has demonstrated a high failure rate of the first-generation SGAs and numerous cases of aspiration of gastric

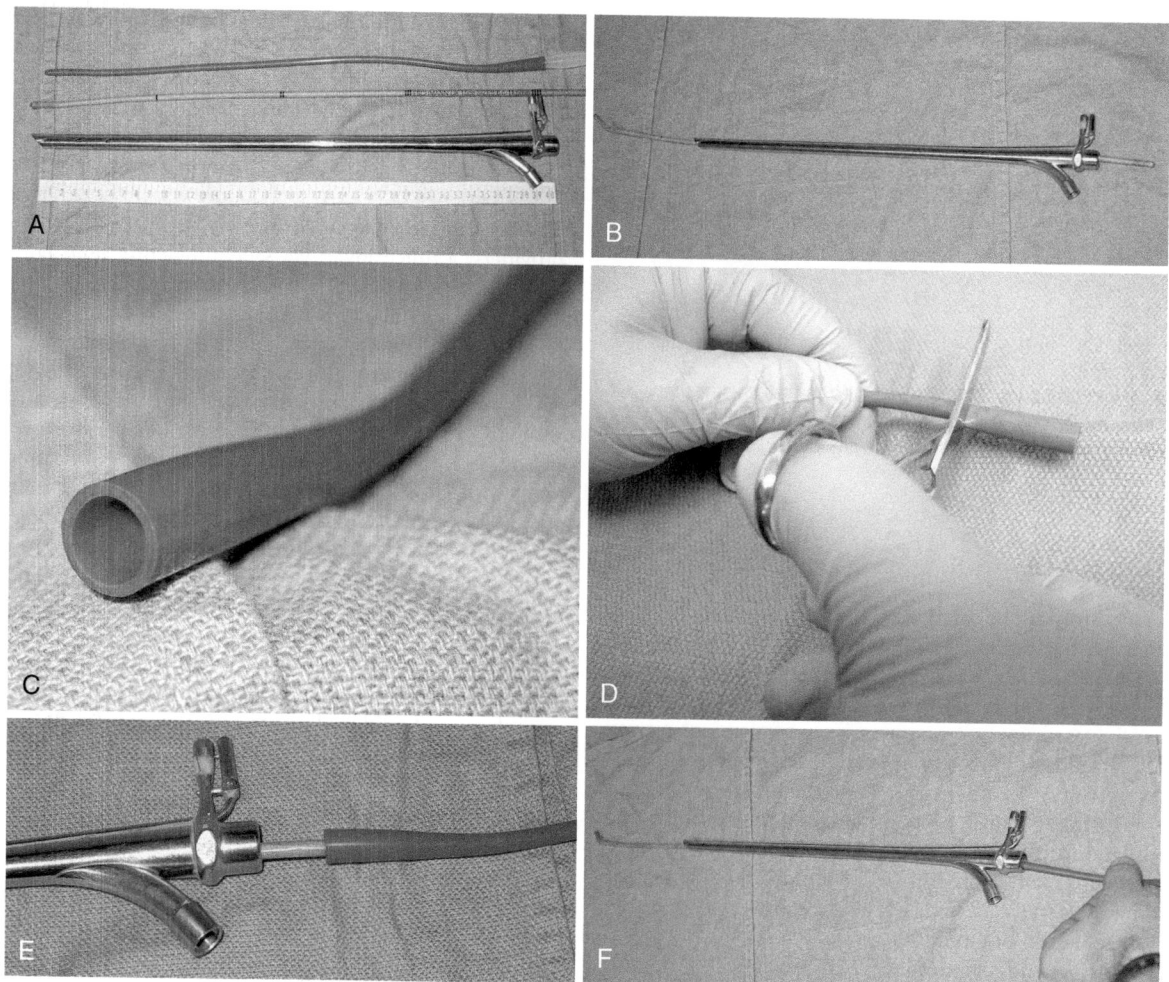

• **Fig. 38.11** Airway exchange with the bougie introducer through the rigid bronchoscope. (A) The 9-French, 40-cm-long rigid bronchoscope (CL Jackson Fiberoptic Bronchoscope, Pilling Inc., Fort Washington, PA); 15-French, 60-cm-long, multiple-use gum elastic bougie (GEB) (Eschmann Tracheal Tube Introducer, SIMS Portex Inc., Keene, NH); and 16-French, 41-cm-long, rounded, closed-tip suction catheter (Robi-Nel catheter, Kendall Dover, Mansfield, MA) are used to facilitate an airway exchange. The technique involves the following steps: deliberately passing the curved tip of the GEB through the lumen of the bronchoscope into a large-caliber bronchus, as indicated by eliciting (B) a gentle, distal hold-up; (C–E) stabilizing and extending a proximal straight tip of the GEB with a precut funnel-shaped end of the Robi-Nel suction catheter; (F) safe removal of the bronchoscope over the extended GEB-catheter assembly; and removal of the catheter and railroading the endotracheal tube over the GEB into the patient's trachea (not shown). This approach provides a better stability of the intubation guide and may be safer than the use of the airway exchange catheter (AEC). With AEC, mapping the distance to the carina during the bronchoscope withdrawal is impossible, because the AEC centimeter markings become embedded inside the bronchoscope. This predisposes the AEC to either slip below the carina, risking lung perforation, or to spring out of the trachea, risking loss of the airway. (A, B, and E from Nekhendzy V, Simmonds PK. Rigid bronchoscope-assisted tracheal intubation: yet another use of the gum elastic bougie. *Anesth Analg.* 2004;98:545–547.)

contents.[89] Should the use of SGA be required in an H&N patient, it is prudent to reach for the second-generation SGAs with greater ventilation capability and gastric access, such as the LMA Proseal or LMA Supreme. These devices will provide superior ASP and better airway protection and will allow for a quick and reliable detection of device malposition.[95]

It may be reasonable to anticipate a 3.8% to 5.2% failure rate with the second-generation SGAs.[92] To minimize failures in H&N patients, we recommend the GEB-assisted insertion technique,[96] to maximize the first-pass success (FPS) rate, and to ensure optimal esophageal and laryngeal seals.[97] The PEAE can be highly

informative in determining the feasibility of SGA placement in H&N patients after the induction of general anesthesia (see Fig. 38.13 and the illustrative case report in Box 38.2).

The LMA Fastrach (intubating laryngeal mask airway [iLMA]) represents another excellent SGA choice. It has an outstanding ventilatory capability and provides a 92% to 94% success rate of blind TI in patients with anticipated DAs.[98,99] In patients with glottic or infraglottic pathology, blind TI intubation should be superseded by FSI-guided iLMA-ETT exchange, which can be performed with or without the use of the Aintree intubation catheter (AIC) (see Chapter 19).

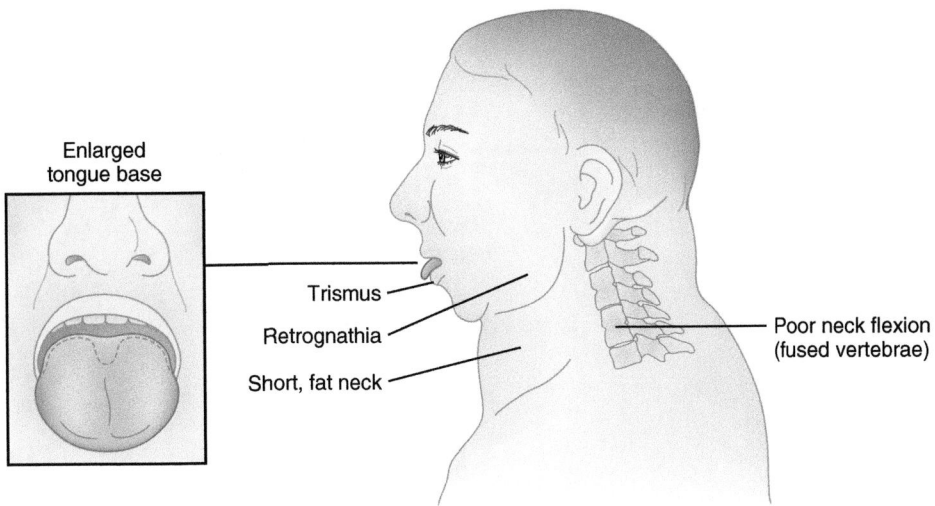

• **Fig. 38.12** Anatomic features associated with a difficult airway exposure during operative laryngoscopy and rigid bronchoscopy. Difficult laryngeal exposure may be encountered in patients with retrognathia; lingual hypertrophy or poor palatal visualization; trismus or reduced interincisor opening; short, thick neck; and limited neck extension. (From Rosen CA, Simpson CB, eds. *Operative Techniques in Laryngology*. Springer-Verlag; 2008: 56.)

The FIS-guided SGA-ETT exchange can be considered one of the core techniques in DA management. It offers the advantage of direct visualization of the laryngeal structures, carries minimal risk of intubation trauma and esophageal intubation, and allows the practitioner to ventilate the patient's lungs while performing TI. Such an exchange should be considered when DA is encountered, when SGA can easily be displaced, or when airway edema is present or anticipated.[1,14] Proceeding with the suboptimally functioning SGA as a stand-alone airway is not acceptable.[14]

The FIS-guided cLMA-AIC exchange technique may be 96% to 100% effective in patients with anticipated DA.[100,101] It worked very well in NAP4 for H&N patients with different pathology, including vertebral body fracture, hematoma, pharyngeal edema, and pharyngeal bleeding.[1] The AIC technical characteristics (4.7-mm ID, 6.5-mm OD) should be kept in mind for selecting the appropriately small FIS and ETT of 7-mm or more ID.

Despite a simple concept, the SGA-ETT exchange can fail either as a result of inability to establish the endoscopic view or the dislodgment of the AIC from the patient's trachea. It can also cause serious complications, such as perforation of the distal tracheobronchial tree because of accidental subcarinal advancement of the AIC during the exchange. The important prerequisite for success is the anesthesia provider's knowledge of the "anatomy" of the chosen SGA device and the ability to establish the landmark endoscopic view as illustrated for the LMA family of devices (Fig. 38.14). Once such a view is established, the exchange can usually proceed unhampered.

We recommend first practicing on a manikin the details of the SGA-ETT exchange for the LMAs and other mainstream SGA devices, such as i-gel, air-Q (Cookgas intubating laryngeal airway [ILA]), and laryngeal tubes (LT-D, LTS-D), in order to develop the necessary dexterity and appreciation for the important details.

The tubular SGAs, such as the Combitube and the laryngeal tubes (LT), are especially beneficial in patients with limited access to the airway and massive upper airway bleeding or regurgitation, when rapid control of the airway is necessary. Ventilation through the Combitube can be effective when other SGAs (e.g., LMA) have failed.[102] Winterhalter and colleagues have documented successful LT ventilation in 95% of patients with oropharyngeal cancer.[103] Nevertheless, the tubular SGAs cannot be considered fail-safe devices, particularly when an infraglottic obstruction is present.[104]

Combined Intubation Techniques

A combined use of VAL with FIS or optical stylet is gaining increased attention and popularity in complex airway management (see Chapter 25). The VAL facilitates FIS/optical stylet maneuvering when the anatomy is severely distorted or supraglottic/glottic tumors are present and allows for continuous observation of the intubation procedure and ETT advancement both from above and below the vocal cords, with diminished risk of tumor disturbance (see Fig. 38.15 and illustrated case report in Box 38.3.).

In the large prospective study of 140 patients with anticipated DA, Lenhardt and colleagues have shown that a combined VAL-FSI technique increases the success rate of TI in patients with cervical spine pathology who could not be intubated with VAL alone.[105] Cook and colleagues have demonstrated a 100% success rate of TI in patients with anticipated DA when a combination of a channeled VAL (Airtraq) and a flexible dynamic stylet (an introducer or FIS) was used; TI was accomplished in less than 30 seconds in 73% of these patients.[106] Mazzinari and colleagues prospectively studied a combined VAL (Glidescope)-FIS technique in 80 patients with multiple predictors of difficult TI and demonstrated 90% reduction in TI injury, 35% increase in TI FPS, and shorter intubation time.[107]

The combined techniques will likely continue to play a bigger role in complex airway management of H&N patients.[90] They demand excellent dexterity that can be achieved with prior manikin practice in the simulation lab. It should be kept in mind that the VAL-FIS technique requires the presence of two operators, with at least one of them being proficient with FIS.

Oxygenation Strategies

Oxygenation-centered airway management is critical for H&N patients, who present with the higher incidence of failed TI and

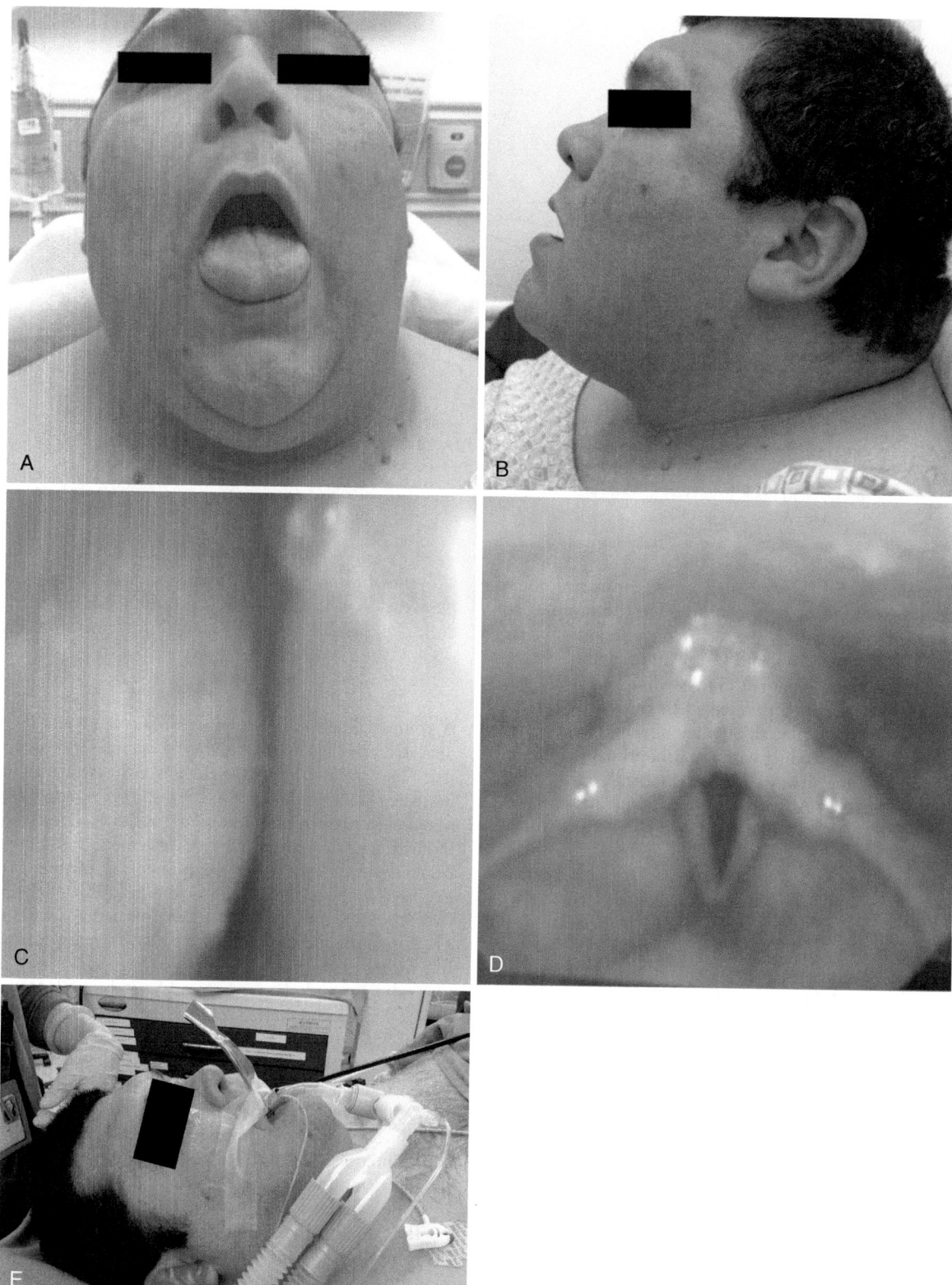

• **Fig. 38.13** (A–E) The value of the preoperative endoscopic airway examination (PEAE) in the management of an anticipated difficult airway. (A, B) Note the patient's external airway features associated with the anticipated difficult airway: morbid obesity, a Mallampati class IV airway, decreased mandibular protrusion, decreased atlanto-occipital extension, and a short, thick neck. (C) PEAE demonstrates the "kissing" tonsils, (D) a normal posterior airway, clear pyriform sinuses, and absent laryngeal pathology. (E) The PEAE negative findings were reassuring for an asleep approach to tracheal intubation, which was uneventfully accomplished via the LMA Fastrach (E). (Photos courtesy Stanford Head and Neck Anesthesia and Advanced Airway Management Program, Stanford, CA.)

A 38-year-old male with a history of severe obstructive sleep apnea (OSA; apnea-hypopnea index of 115/h, nadir nocturnal SpO_2 56%) and morbid obesity ([MO]; body mass index 63.4 kg/m², SpO_2 93% on room air) presented for elective tonsillectomy. Pertinent airway examination demonstrated multiple risk factors for both difficult and impossible mask ventilation (DMV, IMV) and difficult direct laryngoscopy (DL), such as male sex, Mallampati class IV airway, MO, OSA, a short, thick neck (neck circumference 58.4 cm), decreased atlanto-occipital extension, and reduced mandibular protrusion (Figs. 38.13A and B). The awake flexible flexible scope intubation (FSI) was strongly considered, but the patient refused.

Airway Management

With the patient's consent, preoperative endoscopic airway examination (PEAE) was performed in the operating room (OR) after application of 2 mL 4% lidocaine to the right nostril. The PEAE revealed significantly enlarged "kissing" tonsils and a greatly diminished pharyngeal space, but a clear, normal posterior airway and absent laryngeal pathology (Figs. 38.13C and D). These findings were reassuring for developing a primary strategy for using LMA Fastrach (intubating LMA, iLMA) for both ventilation and as a bridge for FOI after induction of general anesthesia.

After adequate preoxygenation and uneventful induction of general anesthesia, iLMA #5 was placed and provided adequate ventilatory control with minimal leak fraction, V_t 650 mL, SpO_2 of 98%, and $EtCO_2$ less than 40 mm Hg. Tracheal intubation (TI) with the manufacturer-supplied 7-mm-ID wire-reinforced ETT was subsequently performed using flexible scope without complications (Fig. 38.13E).

The surgery proceeded uneventfully, and TI was accomplished over the Cook Airway Exchange Catheter (CAEC). During the extubation trial, CAEC had served as a bridge for oxygenation and possible reintubation (see "Tracheal Extubation in Head and Neck Surgery"). After observing the patient for 15 min in the OR, the CAEC was removed from the patient's trachea, with the patient fully awake and able to maintain a clear airway.

Discussion

The PEAE is a minimally invasive technique that can provide highly valuable information about the upper airway in an awake patient.

The presented case illustrates the essential role of PEAE in helping to formulate optimal airway management strategies in patients with anticipated difficult airway. With awake FOI precluded by patient refusal, PEAE provided critical information about the posterior airway that was reassuring for elective supraglottic airway (SGA) placement. Therefore, we were able to proceed with SGA use as our primary strategy for ventilation and as a conduit for FOI.

In an unlikely event of iLMA failure, secondary strategies for airway management included reverting to mask ventilation (MV), placing the LMA Proseal for ventilation and as a bridge for TI using the Aintree airway catheter, and TI using video laryngoscopy.

Conclusion

The PEAE is an invaluable tool in the management of the anticipated difficult airway and can facilitate decision-making about the feasibility of the SGA placement after induction of general anesthesia. Critical anatomic information can be obtained quickly and reliably, and we encourage incorporating this minimally invasive technique into the anesthesia provider's armamentarium.

a CICO situation. The active oxygenation strategies should be in place throughout the process of DA management[34] and are described in detail in Chapter 15.

THRIVE[108] improves the patient's oxygenation during awake FSI.[109] Its use during asleep TI should be strongly considered in H&N patients, as THRIVE prolongs the apneic period, increases peri-intubation Spo_2, and improves FPS, even in patients with a severely compromised airway.[109,110] It is likely that THRIVE will continue to play an even bigger role in DA management and laryngologic surgery in the future, pending adequate validation studies.[111] Placement before induction of anesthesia of a transtracheal jet ventilation (TTJV) catheter for providing tracheal oxygen insufflation or high-frequency TTJV[112] also can be considered in complex cases; proper placement of the catheter should be confirmed by aspirating the tracheal air with the syringe and by capnography. Substituting a TTJV catheter for an Arndt cricothyroidotomy cannula offers the advantage of using its 3-mm-ID lumen with the low-pressure gas source, thus allowing for manual ventilation using the anesthesia circuit or an Ambu bag.[113]

Surgical Airway as a Primary Approach to Tracheal Intubation and Airway Rescue

An awake tracheostomy is usually undertaken in patients with significant airway compromise, where postoperatively the caliber of the airway is not expected to improve. The procedure should be performed under local anesthesia, and without sedation in advanced cases. In selected cases, judicious IV sedation may be appropriate, but it should be administered with extreme caution. The decision to proceed with the awake tracheostomy by the surgeon may also be contingent upon the lack of advanced airway skills on the part of the anesthesia provider. Data indicate that when the patient's airway is managed by dedicated H&N anesthesia providers, the awake tracheostomy can be largely avoided: In a prospective series by Iseli and coworkers, it was required in only 2 of 153 (1.3%) patients.[4]

In advanced cases, awake tracheostomy can prove technically challenging or impossible and will require general anesthesia. There is a clear preference on the part of H&N surgeons to perform a tracheostomy under controlled conditions, after induction of anesthesia, to avoid airway trauma, tumor disturbance, and tracheostomy tube displacement or obstruction.[4] An elective tracheostomy should also be considered if significant postoperative airway compromise is anticipated, if the patient may return to the OR, or after major H&N reconstructive procedures.[114]

An awake dilator cricothyroidotomy also can be safely performed and may serve as a viable alternative to tracheostomy for many H&N patients with a DA.[4,115]

For emergency airway management, surgical cricothyroidotomy is strongly preferred over transcutaneous CTM access; in the NAP4 study, the emergency transcutaneous cannula cricothyroidotomy failed in 60% of H&N patients.[1,2] The observed failure was attributed to the inability to place the cannula or to its misplacement, fracture, kinking, blockage, dislodgment, and barotrauma.[1,2] These findings highlight the need for training anesthesia providers to perform the surgical airway[89] and for the immediate availability of all the necessary equipment for surgical airway access.[49]

Tracheal Extubation in Head and Neck Surgery

A preformulated extubation strategy should constitute an integral part of DA management[34] and is especially important for H&N patients who are at high risk for extubation failure.[1,11] Within the

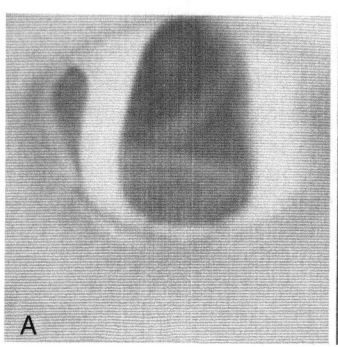
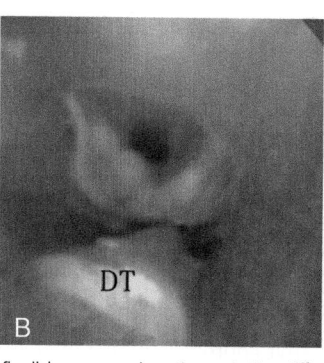
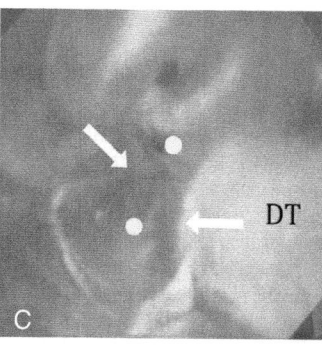
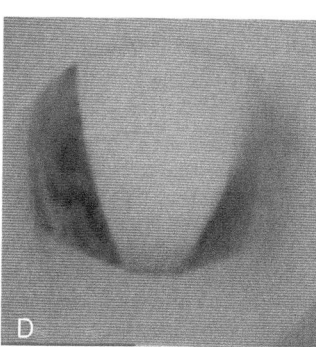

• **Fig. 38.14** A flexible scope view through the different laryngeal mask airways (LMAs) during the LMA-endotracheal tube (ETT) exchange. The important differences in the flexible intubation scope (FIS)-guided airway exchange through different types of supraglottic airway (SGA) devices. Establishing the landmark endoscopic view inside the SGA is the essential first step for such an exchange. The LMA family of devices is used commonly and was selected for this demonstration. (A) A flexible scope view of the aperture bars of the LMA Unique/Classic. The LMA-endotracheal tube exchange is commonly facilitated using the Aintree intubation catheter (AIC), which is advanced off the flexible intubating scope (FIS) through the LMA aperture bars into the patient's trachea, followed by the ETT-AIC exchange. (B) A flexible scope view of the laryngeal inlet through the airway tube of the LMA Proseal (pLMA). Note the improved access to the larynx as compared with the LMA Unique/Classic. The pLMA-ETT exchange is most easily performed using the AIC DT-drainage tube. (C) A flexible scope view on the exit from the airway tube of the LMA Supreme (sLMA). The FIS can be directed either to the left (pictured), or to the right of the sLMA drainage tube (DT). Note the SLMA fins (white arrows), creating two distinct channels (yellow dots) for the passage of the flexible fiberoptic bronchoscope (FFB). It is advisable to direct the FIS above the fins to achieve greater maneuverability with the FIS scope. The sLMA-ETT exchange is most easily performed using the AIC. (D) A flexible scope view of the epiglottic elevator bar (EEB) inside the LMA Fastrach. The space around the EEB is not sufficient to pass the FFB. As opposed to the other SGAs, the airway exchange should be led by the tip of the ETT to elevate the EEB first, thus clearing the way for the FFB advancement into the patient's trachea. The AIC can be used to facilitate this exchange but is not essential. (Photos courtesy Stanford Head and Neck Anesthesia and Advanced Airway Management Program, Stanford, CA.)

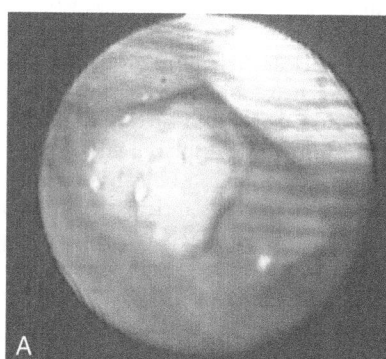
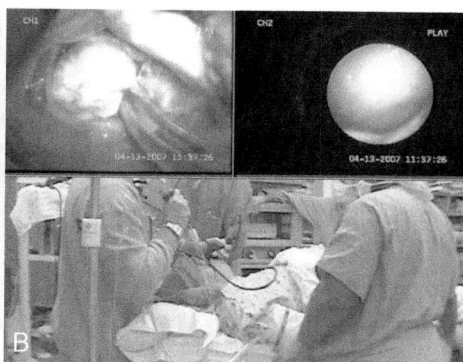

• **Fig. 38.15** A combined intubation technique using the Glidescope and the Shikani optical stylet (SOS) in a patient with a glottic tumor. (A) A ball valve laryngeal tumor seen on preoperative endoscopic airway examination (PEAE). Note a small glottic opening at the inferior-right side of the larynx (toward the 5 o'clock direction), allowing for a successful combined endoscopic approach. (B) A combined video intubation sequence with the Glidescope video laryngoscope (operator's left hand) and an SOS (operator's right hand). With the video laryngoscopy–enabled wide laryngeal exposure (left upper field), the optical stylet with the preloaded endotracheal tube is carefully maneuvered around the mass into the glottic opening (right upper field). (Images and [edited] case discussion courtesy Dr. James DuCanto, Aurora St. Luke's Medical Center, Wisconsin, and the Society for Head and Neck Anesthesia [SHANA]. http://www.shanahq.com/main/content/laryngeal-ball-valve-tumor-gvl-and-shikani-0).

NAP4 cohort, one-third of adverse airway events occurred during emergence and recovery from anesthesia, with airway obstruction being the most common cause.[89]

The comprehensive approach to the extubation of the DA is covered elsewhere (see Chapter 47), with detailed framework outlined by the Difficult Airway Society (DAS) Extubation Guidelines[116] and other high-impact publications aimed specifically at H&N patients.[11] The difficulty of the intubation procedure, the extent and duration of the surgery, the degree of postoperative swelling and anticipated airway obstruction, the possibility of postoperative bleeding, and the patient's state of consciousness on emergence, as well as the patient's preoperative

• BOX 38.3 A Combined Intubation Technique Using the Glidescope and Shikani Optical Stylet in a Patient With a Glottic Tumor

A 79-year-old male with mobile, fungating T2N0 squamous cell carcinoma of the left vocal cord involving perilaryngeal tissues presented with progressive shortness of breath and diminished exercise tolerance. The patient had minimal inspiratory stridor because he was able to self-regulate the rate and depth of breathing to reduce the degree of dynamic airway obstruction. There was no tracheal extension of the tumor, and the patient's past medical history was otherwise noncontributory.

Examination of the patient's airway revealed a Mallampati class 2 airway, normal thyromental distance, and full range of neck motion. Neck was without visible distortion or palpable masses, and the cricothyroid membrane was easily identifiable.

Preoperative discussion with the surgeon regarding airway management and surgical plan addressed the potential for an awake tracheostomy, and possible laryngectomy, should the tumor be found to deeply invade the larynx and laryngeal cartilages. Alternatively, should the tumor be removed superficially, laryngectomy could be avoided. The airway management plan was formulated to allow for avoidance of awake tracheostomy and further in-depth surgical evaluation and resection of tumor with the patient anesthetized.

Airway Management

The patient was brought to the operating room and connected to the standard monitors. Preoperative endoscopic airway examination (PEAE) revealed that the tumor was attached to the left vocal cord and pivoted anteriorly, superiorly, and leftward with spontaneous ventilation, producing a ball valve phenomenon. It was determined from this examination that the larynx and trachea could be successfully exposed and navigated with an endoscopic approach from an inferior-right approach to the larynx and tumor (toward the 5 o'clock direction, Fig. 38.15A).

Because of the size, motion, and lack of view of the larynx on PEAE, a combined intubation approach was chosen using two video-enabled endoscopes: the Glidescope video-assisted laryngoscope (GVL) and the Shikani Optical Stylet (SOS). With adequate upper airway topicalization and moderate sedation, the GVL was used to expose the epiglottis and tumor, and the SOS was introduced at the 5 o'clock position to the tumor, navigating the mass with the optical stylet positioned inside the 6-mm-ID ETT (Fig. 38.15B). Upon passing the mass, the interior of the laryngeal cartilage was visualized with the SOS video channel, and the tracheal tube was easily advanced off the stylet without resistance.

The surgery proceeded uneventfully, and the tracheostomy was avoided. A staged extubation using a Bailey maneuver (see "Tracheal Extubation in Head and Neck Surgery") was performed with an air-Q size 4.5 before emergence. Upon full emergence from anesthesia and ensuring adequate ventilation, the patient's airway was suctioned and the air-Q supraglottic airway was removed. The patient regained consciousness and awareness to such an extent that he was able to move himself over to the transport cart with minimal assistance.

Postoperatively, the patient had undergone chemotherapy and radiation therapy, with excellent results. At 4-year follow-up, he continued to be disease free, with some long-standing benign mild erythema of the left vocal cord.

Discussion

The presented case illustrates a careful, stepwise approach to airway management of a patient with the partially obstructed airway and the value of PEAE in developing optimal intubation strategy (see "Preoperative Airway Assessment and Preparation"/"Endoscopy and Imaging Studies," and "Special Situations"/"Partially Obstructed Airway"). Patients with glottic lesions present increased challenges to the anesthesia provider, and the intubation approach should maximize the laryngeal exposure.

The combined video intubation techniques can be highly effective in these patients because they allow a continuous visualization of the intubation procedure both from above and below the lesion, minimizing the chance of tumor disturbance. With video-assisted laryngoscopy–enabled wide laryngeal exposure, the optical intubation stylets can lead within ETT to help bypass mobile masses. Once the glottis is entered, the ETT will follow the trajectory of the stylet into the patient's trachea.

Maintaining spontaneous ventilation in these patients provides a superior margin of safety. An awake flexible scope intubation may fail with the obstructing glottic lesions, either because of the inability to displace the tumor or because the ETT simply would not pass. A forceful advancement of the ETT off the flexbile scope may cause tumor defragmentation, bleeding, and contamination of the lower airway.

The combined video techniques will likely continue to play a bigger role in complex airway management of H&N patients. They demand excellent dexterity, which can be achieved with manikin practice in the simulation lab.

---

status, all should play a role in the anesthesia provider's decision-making.[11,114,117] Most important, every extubation of an at-risk H&N patient should be considered a possible reintubation, and all the necessary airway equipment and professionals should be in place before the extubation trial starts.

The AEC is most commonly used to provide continuous tracheal access during the extubation trial. The AEC serves as a conduit for oxygen insufflation, JV, reintubation, and a brief suctioning. The practical points of AEC use include never advancing AEC against resistance, confirming proper AEC placement by the ability to jet ventilate before ETT removal, avoiding sucarinal placement (keep AEC at 25–26 cm on the alveolar ridge), and removing AEC only after tracheal position of the new ETT has been confirmed. Refer to Table 38.1 for the technical characteristics of Cook AECs.

Tracheal extubation of an uncomplicated H&N airway also presents a unique challenge to the anesthesia provider. Smooth emergence from anesthesia, devoid of patient straining, bucking, and coughing, is essential for avoiding the formation of hematoma, disrupting delicate surgical repairs, and minimizing undesired hyperdynamic responses. Extubating the patient's trachea at a deep plane of anesthesia is problematic in H&N surgery because of the increased risk of postextubation laryngospasm and overall

TABLE 38.1 The Characteristics of the Cook Airway Exchange Catheters Used for Extubation Trial and Tracheal Reintubation

AEC Size	AEC OD (mm)	AEC ID (mm)	AEC Length (cm)	ETT Size
8 Fr	2.7	1.6	45	≥3.0
11 Fr	3.7	2.3	83	≥4.0
14 Fr	4.7	3.0	83	≥5.0
19 Fr	6.3	3.4	83	≥7.0

AEC, Airway exchange catheters; *ETT*, endotracheal tube; *Fr*, French; *ID*, inside diameter; *OD*, outside diameter.

increased need for the airway support and protection required on the part of the anesthesia provider.

Smooth extubation strategies include the use of SGA in lieu of ETT (see "Use of the Supraglottic Airways as the Primary Ventilatory Devices in Elective Head and Neck Surgery"), the ETT-SGA exchange at the end of the case (the Bailey maneuver), and a pharmacologic approach that best relies on a low-dose remifentanil infusion to blunt the tracheal responses.

The Bailey maneuver involves, in steps, insertion of SGA (usually, the LMA) behind the existing ETT with the patient still adequately anesthetized, removal of ETT, and administration of ventilatory support through the SGA until the patient resumes spontaneous ventilation and awakens from anesthesia.[118] Remifentanil provides a predictable, rapid, and almost simultaneous recovery of consciousness and protective airway reflexes, while also blunting sympathetic responses associated with extubation.[41,119] Current data indicate that EC_{95} of effect site concentration of remifentanil for blunting tracheal reflexes after balanced desflurane and sevoflurane anesthesia is 2.3 to 2.9 ng/mL,[120–122] which corresponds to the manual infusion rate 0.08 to 0.1 µg/kg/min. This is higher than that observed with the total intravenous anesthesia (TIVA), where a target concentration of 2.1 ng/mL and a corresponding manual infusion rate of 0.07 µg/kg/min is usually sufficient.[123] The authors' experience corroborates that of others indicating that lower blood target concentrations of remifentanil (1.5–2.0 ng/mL and corresponding manual infusion rates of 0.05 to 0.06 µg/kg/min) may be equally effective, especially if TIVA was used.[119,122,124,125] A single IV bolus of lidocaine may help prevent cough at extubation in a dose-dependent manner in the range of 0.5 and 2.0 mg/kg.[126] In our experience, significant dose-response variability makes this approach less reliable compared to IV remifentanil administration. Delayed recovery of consciousness may also be observed with increased frequency with higher IV lidocaine doses given at the end of surgery.

Use of the Supraglottic Airways as the Primary Ventilatory Devices in Elective Head and Neck Surgery

This section focuses on the use of the SGAs as dedicated, stand-alone airways for elective H&N surgery. Please refer to "Devising Safe Airway Management Strategies for Tracheal Intubation"/"Role of the Supraglottic Airways and the Supraglottic Airway-Endotracheal Tube") for an overview of the role of SGAs in DA management for H&N patients.

The use of an SGA as a dedicated airway for H&N surgery may be strongly preferred over the ETT when smooth emergence from anesthesia is essential—for example, for otologic surgery, functional endoscopic sinus surgery, and facial cosmetic surgery. The SGA facilitates the resumption of spontaneous ventilation and decreases the likelihood of the airway reflex stimulation, and its placement does not require administration of a NMB. Prospective and retrospective studies have shown that the use of LMA in H&N surgery is associated with improved hemodynamic stability during airway management on induction and emergence, superior maintenance of a stable plane of anesthesia and controlled hypotension, improved quality of surgical field and faster awakening time, and decreased incidence of adverse respiratory events.[127–131]

Although both spontaneous and controlled ventilation through an SGA can be successfully employed intraoperatively, the authors usually opt for the latter (pressure control or pressure support ventilation mode) to preserve normocapnia. Continuous monitoring of the pressure-volume and flow-volume loops, the shape of the end-tidal carbon dioxide ($EtCO_2$) waveform, and total compliance on newer anesthesia machines will help to immediately detect the decreased tidal volume (V_T) and increased leak fraction associated with the lighter planes of anesthesia.[132] With SGA use,

these changes typically precede the patient's hemodynamic and motor responses, thereby facilitating hypnotic monitoring and allowing for prompt deepening of anesthesia.[132]

We agree with the opinion of others[133] that, when used appropriately in selected patients, absence of immediate access to the patient's airway should not be considered a deviation from the standard of care of SGA use in the modern era. Selection of the SGA devices that possess greater ventilating capability and provide gastric access (e.g., the LMA Proseal, the LMA Supreme) will increase the margin of safety. See Fig. 38.16 and the illustrative case report in Box 38.4 for a discussion of the principles of the safe use of SGAs with positive-pressure ventilation (PPV).

SGAs such as the i-gel and air-Q (Cookgas intubating laryngeal airway) also show promise[134–141]; however, the meta-analysis reports are conflicting,[142–144] and the ventilatory performance of these devices in H&N surgical cases awaits a formal evaluation.

The flexible laryngeal mask airway (FLMA) is of particular benefit for oral, intranasal, cosmetic, and facial plastic surgery.[127–129,145–150] The wire-reinforced shaft of the device can be freely manipulated inside the patient's mouth and bent away from the surgical field without loss of the laryngeal seal. The properly placed FLMA adequately protects the lower airway from blood, secretions, and surgical debris, thus eliminating the need for the use of the throat pack by the surgeon.

Nekhendzy and colleagues[151] have retrospectively investigated the ventilatory performance of FLMA with PPV in 685 patients who had undergone elective—mostly intranasal and facial cosmetic—H&N surgery and documented a cumulative success rate of 92.6%, which was comparable with the cLMA[152,153] and the second-generation SGAs.[92] The authors used stringent criteria for documenting adequate FLMA function and performance, such as achieving adequate ventilation (V_T ≥6 mL/kg), airway protection (ASP >12 cm H_2O in patients without preexisting GERD), and separation of the respiratory and gastrointestinal tracts (absent gastric insufflation) during PPV.[151] A 7.3% incidence of gastric insufflation was observed in this study after the initial FLMA placement despite adequate V_T and ASP, suggesting the need for routine auscultation of the epigastric as part of the confirmation tests.[151] The FLMA independent predictors of failure include male sex, advanced age, higher ASA class, higher BMI,[154] increased number (≥3) of FLMA insertion attempts, and a low airway sealing pressure (ASP),[151] which is consistent with most of the predictors for SGA failure. The low ASP highlights the need for the use of the largest FLMA size whenever possible.[155] To prevent intraoperative FLMA dislodgment, we recommend a secure taping of the FLMA shaft with a strong adhesive dressing (Fig. 38.17) and developing close cooperation with the surgeon to alert the anesthesia provider about manipulating the patient's head and airway. Maintaining a low threshold for replacing malfunctioning FLMA with TI at any time should constitute an essential part of the safety protocol.

Special Situations

Partially Obstructed Airway

Patients with an advanced airway obstruction and inspiratory stridor at rest comprise some of the most feared and complicated cases for the anesthesia provider.[41,42] The incidence of difficult mask ventilation and impossible mask ventilation among patients with severe stridor and upper airway obstruction greater than 75% of the lumen reaches 40% and 6%, respectively,[156] compared with

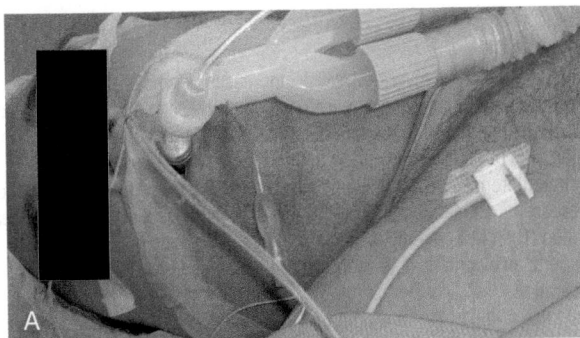

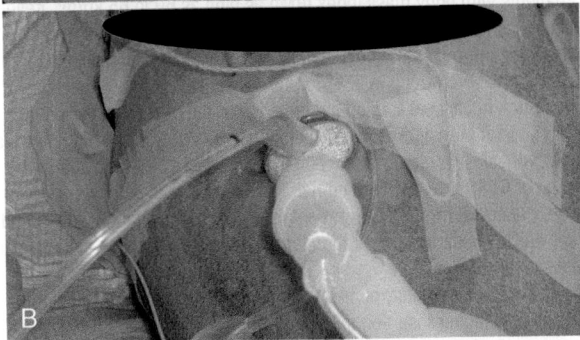

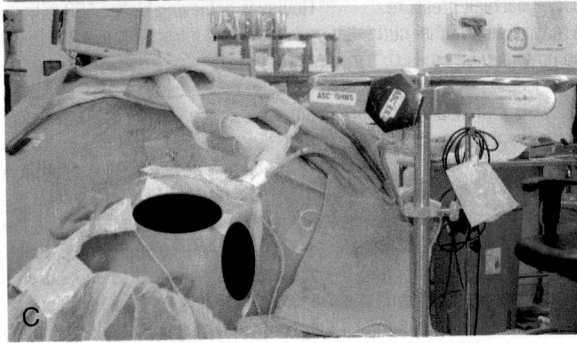

• **Fig. 38.16** The use of the supraglottic airway (SGA) as a primary ventilatory device for middle ear surgery. (A, B) Note the anatomic features associated with the difficult airway and the properly positioned SGA (LMA Supreme), which is used as a primary ventilatory device for middle ear surgery. The orogastric tube is passed through the drainage tube into the patient's stomach to facilitate safe administration of the positive-pressure ventilation. Note a proper midline fixation of the LMA Supreme over the fixation tab. See Box 38.4 for details. (C) The patient being prepped for surgery. Note the positioning of the side table on the patient's right. Such arrangement allows the anesthesia provider to reach for the patient's airway under the surgical drapes and troubleshoot the positioning of the SGA intraoperatively should the need arise. (Photos and [edited] case discussion courtesy Dr. Vladimir Nekhendzy, Stanford University Medical Center, Stanford, CA, and the Society for Head and Neck Anesthesia [SHANA]. http://www.shanahq.com/main/content/anesthesia-middle-ear-surgery-0.)

trained respiratory muscles can sustain adequate alveolar minute ventilation at rest through a 3-mm orifice, but acute deterioration occurs when a critical narrowing is reached.[157] Drooling, dysphagia, and expiratory snoring are the signs of marked pharyngeal restriction,[40,41] but inspiratory stridor at rest represents the most worrisome sign, suggesting a reduction in airway diameter at the supraglottic, periglottic, or glottic level of at least 50%.[25,42]

Preoperative assessment aims to identify the size, mobility, and site of a lesion. Very mobile lesions may cause partial airway obstruction after induction of anesthesia, but total airway obstruction is extremely uncommon. Airway obstruction is worse in a spontaneously breathing patient after induction of anesthesia because of the loss of supporting tone in the oropharynx and hypopharynx. Supraglottic lesions, if mobile, can obstruct the airway or make visualization of the laryngeal inlet difficult. Subglottic lesions may allow a good view of the laryngeal inlet but cause difficulty during the passage of an ETT. The traditional teaching of inhalational induction and maintenance of spontaneous ventilation in obstructed airways has been questioned.[157]

Airway narrowing at the tracheal or tracheobronchial level is typically characterized by expiratory stridor, whereas biphasic inspiratory-expiratory stridor usually points to obstructive subglottic disease.[13] In some cases, preoperative examination of the flow-volume loops may be helpful.[43] Tracheal compression can occur because of lesions within the trachea or compression by thyroid and mediastinal masses. The upper airway may be normal at laryngoscopy, and it may be possible to pass ETT beyond the glottis but not beyond the obstruction.[157]

The optimal technique for airway management of the stridorous patient with an advanced proximal airway obstruction (i.e., supraglottic, glottic, and subglottic levels) remains a subject of controversy. An awake FSI, inhalation induction, and intravenous induction with muscle relaxants have been used successfully, but none should be considered fail-safe.[41,42,156,158]

Modern automated jet ventilators incorporate multiple safety features, including automatic ventilator shutdown if the user preset pressure limits are exceeded (see "Special Situations"/"Microlaryngeal Surgery"/"Jet Ventilation"). This has enabled some experienced providers to successfully use transtracheal high-frequency jet ventilation (HFJV) in patients with massive supraglottic lesions and severe airway compromise, for which the use of supraglottic or infraglottic JV was not possible or surgically feasible.[156] The presence of a second anesthesia provider to facilitate monitoring and maintenance of an upper airway was required and deemed an important safety factor in preventing intraoperative pressure-related complications in all cases.[156] Although no major complications were observed in this series of 50 patients, the incidence of minor complications reached 20%, a more than threefold increase compared with the instances when transtracheal HFJV has been used in patients with less severe airway compromise.[159]

Based on our experience and review of the literature,[1,2,4,14,19,33,41,42,44,73,75,78,112,113,117,156–164] current recommendations for management of the critically obstructed airway (management of the central airway obstruction is excluded from this discussion) can be outlined as follows:

1. Preoperative nasal endoscopy (Preoperative Endoscopic Airway Examination, PEAE) should be performed in all H&N patients with symptoms of upper airway obstruction. It is the only technique that allows visualization of the lesion and degree of obstruction directly and assessment of respiratory mechanics and tumor mobility.

1.4% and 0.15% for the general surgical population.[36–38] These patients frequently present for panendoscopy and microlaryngeal surgery on an emergent or semi-emergent basis, yet they require a systematic and thoughtful approach by the anesthesia provider and the surgeon. The nature of the obstructing lesion (e.g., vascular, submucosal, pedunculated, inflammatory) and its location (e.g., supraglottic, glottic, subglottic, midtracheal, lower tracheal, and bronchial [mediastinal]) may require completely different intubation considerations and approaches.[41–43,46,73,75,78]

The slow-growing upper airway tumors can cause a high-grade airway obstruction without significant associated symptoms. Fully

The 45-year-old male patient presented for tympanomastoidectomy and ossicular chain reconstruction, scheduled in the ambulatory surgical center. Past medical history was significant for morbid obesity ([MO]; height 190 cm, weight 161.4 kg, body mass index 44.7 kg/m²), snoring, severe obstructive sleep apnea (OSA) treated by continuous positive airway pressure (CPAP), controlled systemic hypertension, and absent symptoms of gastroesophageal reflux disease (GERD).

Airway examination revealed a short, thick neck (neck circumference 54 cm), decreased oral entry (small mouth), big tongue, Mallampati (MP) class III, normal mandibular protrusion, and thyromental distance of 6 cm. Some of the airway features can be appreciated from Figs. 38.16A and B; preoperative airway pictures were not available. The rest of the airway examination was normal, and physical examination was otherwise unremarkable. Preoperative vital signs were stable, and electrocardiogram and laboratory test results were normal.

Airway and Anesthetic Management

The patient was premedicated with ranitidine 150 mg by mouth (PO) 2 hours preoperatively. After optimal preoxygenation, anesthesia was induced uneventfully with intravenous (IV) fentanyl 150 µg and IV propofol 300 mg. Once adequate depth of anesthesia was confirmed by absence of patient movement to jaw thrust,[241] the size 5 LMA Supreme (sLMA) was easily inserted using the single-handed rotational technique recommended by the manufacturer. The sLMA cuff was inflated with a total of 30 mL of air.

Correct positioning of the sLMA was confirmed by the positive suprasternal notch test, the lack of air leak from the gastric tube, the absence of gastric insufflation during positive-pressure ventilation (PPV), the presence of a square-wave EtCO₂ capnography trace, and the easy passage of a lubricated 18-French orogastric tube (OGT) through the drainage tube of the device into the patient's stomach, with subsequent aspiration of a small amount (<20 mL) of clear gastric contents.[242–245] The airway seal pressure (ASP) was recorded at 32 cm H₂O, with fresh gas flow 3 L/min and closed pressure-adjusted expiratory valve on the anesthesia machine.[246] The sLMA was taped midline over the fixation tab, with slight downward traction, to maintain deep cuff position and optimal airway seal (Figs. 38.16A and B).[245]

Intraoperatively, the patient's lungs were mechanically ventilated in a pressure-controlled mode of 28 cm H₂O. Adequacy of ventilation was confirmed by achieving an expired V_T of approximately 800 mL, minimal leak fraction (less than 5%), SpO₂ of 98%, and EtCO₂ less than 40 mm Hg. Adequacy of ventilation was further assessed continuously during the case, by monitoring V_T, EtCO₂ value, total leak fraction, and total compliance and by observing the flow-volume and pressure-volume loops and EtCO₂ waveform on the screen of the anesthesia machine.

The preventive measures aimed at reducing the risk of gastric insufflation during PPV included maintaining peak inspiratory pressure (PIP) below ASP and passively emptying gastric contents left in the drainage tube of the device into an empty IV bag through the OGT.[243,244] The in situ OGT also served as a functional guide, which would enable advancement of the sLMA back into the original position had accidental displacement of the device and loss of seal occurred intraoperatively (Fig. 38.16C).[247]

Anesthesia (total intravenous anesthesia [TIVA]) proceeded uneventfully, the emergence was smooth, and the sLMA was removed with the patient fully awake. He was admitted for overnight observation on the hospital ward and uneventfully discharged home the following morning.

Discussion

Smooth emergence from anesthesia, without associated bucking, coughing, or straining, is one of the essential requirements of the otologic surgery, and the use of SGAs may be preferred for achieving this objective.

It was anticipated that mask ventilation in this patient would be problematic because of the presence of three risk factors predictive of both difficult and impossible mask ventilation (DMV, IMV), such as obesity, MP class III airway,

snoring, male sex, and severe OSA.[248–250] Increased degree of difficulty was also expected with direct laryngoscopy (DL): full dentition and a thick/obese neck increased the number of predictors of difficult DL and associated DMV to 7, with the odds ratio of 18 (MP class V), as defined by Kheterpal et al.[251] Increased neck circumference (>40 cm), especially in combination with a high MP grade, also represents an independent risk factor for difficult DL and difficult tracheal intubation (TI) in MO patients, especially males.[252,253] Had TI been planned in this patient, an awake flexible scope intubation should have been given full consideration.

Safe use of the pLMA as a primary ventilatory device has been reported in MO patients with body mass index (BMI) as high as 60 to 65 kg/m². Keller and colleagues found that the use of the pLMA in MO patients resulted in perfect isolation of the gastrointestinal and respiratory tracts and highly effective PPV (V_T = 8 mL/kg) in 95% to 98% of patients, possibly because of improved pharyngeal seal caused by reduction of the pharyngeal volume.[254] In addition, the pLMA ventilation capabilities are independent of high MP class or poor laryngeal view during DL.[254] Whether the obese patients without the symptoms of GERD are at increased risk for aspiration of gastric contents is the subject of controversy.[255] Our patient received premedication with ranitidine for prophylaxis against acid aspiration, and the suctioned gastric volume was minimal.

The sLMA is conceptually similar to the pLMA, and its use results in the same or slightly higher insertion success rate on the first attempt but lower oropharyngeal leak pressure.[245,256,257] However, achieving higher ASP with the pLMA may require higher cuff inflation volume and intracuff pressures in excess of recommended 60 cm H₂O.[256] Timmerman et al.[245] have documented excellent performance of the sLMA in terms of the ease and speed of insertion, ASP, adequacy of controlled ventilation, and flexible scope view of the laryngeal inlet in obese patients with a BMI greater than 35 kg/m².

The use of the sLMA as a dedicated ventilatory device in this patient follows the ASA Difficult Airway Algorithm guidelines.[258] Had the PPV through the sLMA been proven suboptimal in our patient before the surgery commenced, a flexible scope exchange to the ETT was planned over the Aintree intubation catheter (Cook Medical Inc., Bloomington, IN). In the unlikely event of sLMA failure, the backup airway management plans included the use of the LMA Fastrach Airway for rescue ventilation and intubation, the tracheal intubation techniques involving the gum elastic bougie–assisted DL, and video laryngoscopy. All these strategies have been successfully used for managing anticipated and unanticipated difficult airway in obese and nonobese patients.[259–266]

A combination of TIVA with absent muscle relaxation facilitated crisp and smooth awakening and maintenance of airway patency and allowed for safe titration of opioids after emergence.

After extubation, full consideration should be given to bridging the immediate postextubation period with the Boussignac CPAP system (5–7.5 cm H₂O), if available. The traditional CPAP may be contraindicated after middle ear surgery, because middle ear pressure may increase substantially even at minimal CPAP levels, and the surgical team should be consulted before its use.

Conclusion

The use of SGAs for otologic surgery offers significant advantages, such as smooth emergence, without associated coughing, bucking, or straining; avoidance of neuromuscular blocking agents; improved cardiovascular stability; and maintenance of a stable plane of anesthesia. The use of second-generation SGAs that possess greater ventilatory capability and provide gastric access (sLMA in this case) is strongly preferred and will increase the margin of safety.

The presented case report outlines the principles of the safe use of SGAs with PPV for elective surgery. The sLMA and pLMA can be safely used in selected patients with multiple predictors of DMV and difficult DL, provided the anesthesia provider is throughly familiar with the device. The backup ventilation and TI strategies must be in place should the SGA ventilation prove suboptimal before the surgery commences. Proceeding with surgery with an inadequately functioning SGA cannot be recommended.[14]

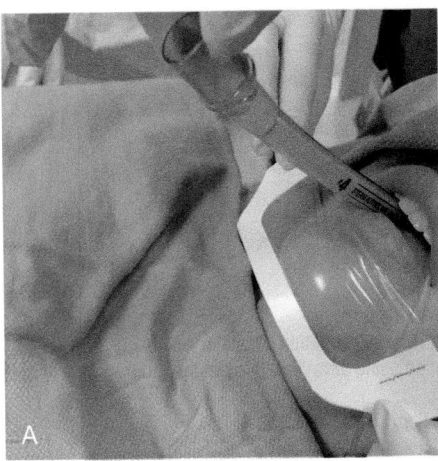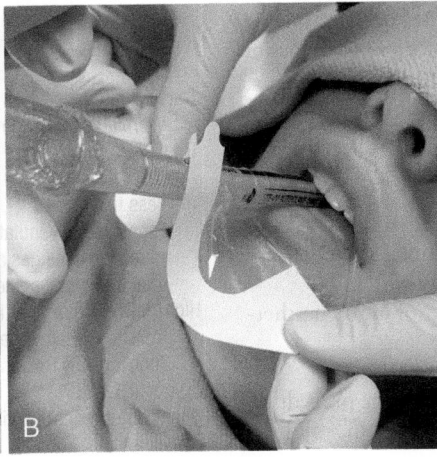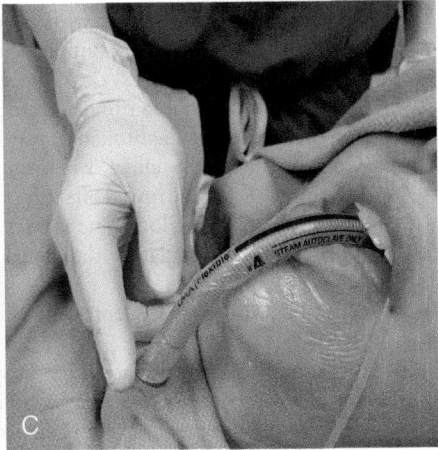

• **Fig. 38.17** The flexible laryngeal mask airway (FLMA) taping technique used by the Stanford Head and Neck Anesthesia team. (A) The first precut piece of the Tegaderm (3M Healthcare, St. Paul, MN) is placed over the patient's chin, as close to the lower lip as possible. (B) The second precut piece of the Tegaderm fully encases the FLMA shaft by creating a "mesentery." (C) The second and first pieces of the Tegaderm are connected together to secure FLMA positioning, as demonstrated by absent FLMA pullback during applied external pressure. (Photos courtesy Stanford Head and Neck Anesthesia and Advanced Airway Management Program, Stanford, CA.)

2. Management of patients with advanced airway obstruction requires a dedicated team effort. Thorough preoperative discussion of the surgical pathology and formulation of closely coordinated airway management strategies with the surgeon are essential. None of the techniques should be considered fail-safe.

3. All airway instrumentation should proceed in a careful and gentle manner. TI should be accomplished rapidly, under direct vision, and with a small ETT. The number of attempts should be limited to two, because critical airway obstruction can quickly progress to a cannot intubate/cannot ventilate (CICV) situation.

4. For patients with severe stridor (e.g., nocturnal symptoms, hypoxemia-induced agitation or panic attacks, use of accessory muscles on inspiration, a large tumor, fixed hemilarynx, gross anatomic distortion, a larynx not visible on PEAE), an awake tracheostomy under local anesthesia without sedation should be strongly considered (see "Devising Safe Airway Management Strategies for Tracheal Intubation"/"Surgical Airway as a Primary Approach to Tracheal Intubation and Airway Rescue"). If an awake approach is not feasible, the airway double setup is warranted: the patient's CTM should be marked, the neck should be prepped, and the surgical team must be present for induction, ready to deploy an anterior commissure scope or a ventilating rigid bronchoscope, or to perform an emergent surgical airway.

5. Patients with moderate stridor and a significant lesion seen on PEAE, but who are considered possible to intubate, can be managed with an awake FSI or an inhalation induction. Failure of either technique should be anticipated, and the clear rescue strategies must be in place from the outset. If TI under direct vision (DL, VAL, FSI) fails, tracheostomy can be performed, with the patient breathing spontaneously.

6. Inhalation induction is best reserved for noncollapsing lesions, when it can be rescued by mask ventilation. A sufficiently deep and stable plane of anesthesia is essential to avoid loss of the airway (e.g., cough, laryngospasm). Preparing the patient's nares with a mixture of a vasoconstrictor and a topical anesthetic before induction will allow early passage of a nasal airway to overcome early obstruction. Difficulty in maintaining the airway during inhalation induction in patients with large tumors, granulomas, and cysts should be anticipated, even if preoperative symptoms of airway obstruction are mild.

7. Oropharyngeal and hypopharyngeal obstructions due to intraoral and BOT masses, swelling, or infection usually can be effectively managed by an awake nasal FSI.

8. Supraglottic obstruction may not allow visualization of the larynx during DL or VAL. An awake nasal FSI should be considered to bypass the obstruction, but an assumption that the tumor can be simply pushed aside with ETT can prove wrong. The combined intubation techniques can be very effective (see "Devising Safe Airway Management Strategies for Tracheal Intubation"/"Combined Intubation Techniques"). If these options are not viable, an awake tracheostomy should be considered.

9. Patients with glottic or subglottic lesions present increased challenges. The approaches to these lesions are similar and should involve maximizing the laryngeal exposure. Video-assisted and operative laryngoscopy, combined intubation techniques, especially leading with the optical stylet or bypassing a lesion with the rigid bronchoscope, should be strongly considered as the primary approach (see "Devising Safe Airway Management Strategies for Tracheal Intubation"/"Role of Conventional and Video Laryngoscopy," "Role of Operative Laryngoscopy and Rigid Bronchoscopy," and "Combined Intubation Techniques"; Fig. 38.15; and the illustrated case report in Box 38.3). If these are not feasible, an awake tracheostomy should be performed.

10. In anesthetized patients, the avoidance of muscle relaxants is controversial: The improvement in ventilatory dynamics with PPV has been observed in stridorous patients with high-grade laryngotracheal stenosis after administration of NMB. If inhalation induction is used, administration of NMB should be avoided until after TI is completed to prevent sudden, complete airway obstruction, especially when the tumor is subglottic.

11. An awake FSI should be used with caution, because one or more of the following factors can precipitate a sudden loss of the airway:
    - Bleeding from a friable tumor on impaction with the FIS or seeding parts of the broken tumor into the trachea
    - "Cork in the bottle" effect, when the scope is introduced into the critically narrowed airway
    - Inhibitory effect of local anesthetics on the tongue and upper airway musculature, laryngeal muscles, and function
    - Central nervous system depressant effect of local anesthetics
    - Local anesthetic-precipitated laryngospasm
    - Patient's apprehension and agitation during the procedure, resulting in hyperventilation and "sucking in" mobile, pedunculated tumors
12. Additional fallback strategies may include the following:
    - HFJV through the SGA (e.g., LMA)
    - Placement of a TTJV catheter before induction for providing tracheal oxygen insufflation or high-frequency TTJV. Substituting a TTJV catheter for a 3-mm-ID Arndt cricothyroidotomy cannula will allow manual ventilation using the anesthesia circuit or an Ambu bag.
    - Infraglottic and transtracheal HFJV. These approaches require caution, especially in the presence of subglottic lesions, to avoid air trapping and barotrauma. If upper airway obstruction is greater than 50%, the position of the jet nozzle should be proximal to the site of the obstruction and directed toward the remaining free airway opening to prevent barotrauma. Alternatively, the obstruction must be bypassed by a rigid bronchoscope first. Total outflow obstruction with resultant barotrauma during infraglottic or transtracheal HFJV can be quickly precipitated by surgical instrumentation, glottic edema, laryngospasm, or closure of the vocal cords because of inadequate depth of anesthesia or inadequate muscle relaxation.
    - Transtracheal HFJV as a temporizing technique for high-grade upper airway obstruction, allowing time for a definitive airway to be established. A transtracheal catheter or cannula can be left in place after the surgery if the concern remains for postoperative airway patency. The use of transtracheal HFJV is best reserved for operators with significant experience and expertise.
13. Patients with inspiratory obstruction because of bilateral vocal cord paralysis or fixation of cricoarytenoid joints typically do not present ventilation or intubation problems.
14. In selected patients with high-grade obstructing lesions, THRIVE or STRIVE Hi techniques can be used successfully as the primary approach, allowing the surgeon to quickly perform suspension laryngoscopy and reduce the disease burden under general anesthesia.[21,108] Subsequently, the surgery can be concluded with the use of apneic intermittent ventilation (see "Microlaryngeal Surgery") and/or JV, if desired.
15. If tracheostomy is avoided, an extubation strategy must be decided on with the surgeon.
16. Extubation should be performed over an AEC, with the necessary reintubation equipment immediately available (see "Tracheal Extubation in Head and Neck Surgery"). Some patients should remain intubated until the airway inflammation and edema subside, at which time the patient's airway is then reevaluated.

• BOX 38.5　Ventilation Techniques for Microlaryngeal Surgery

Tracheal intubation
　Microlaryngeal endotracheal tube (MLT)
Tritube
　Laser ETT
Tubeless techniques
　Spontaneous ventilation
　Inhalation anesthesia (insufflation)
　Total intravenous anesthesia[a]
High-flow nasal oxygen insufflation
　Transnasal Humidified Rapid-Insufflation Ventilatory Exchange (THRIVE)[b]
　SponTaneous Respiration using IntraVEnous anaesthesia and Hi-flow nasal oxygen (STRIVE Hi)[c]
Apneic intermittent ventilation
Jet ventilation
　Supraglottic (operating laryngoscope)
　Infraglottic (catheter, cannula, rigid bronchoscope)
　Transtracheal (cather, cannula)
　Low frequency
　High frequency
　Superimposed high frequency

[a]Supplemental oxygen is usually administered either through traditional nasal cannula (low-flow oxygen insufflation) or through the insufflation port of the surgical suspension laryngoscope.
[b]Patient apneic.
[c]Patient breathing spontaneously.

Microlaryngeal Surgery

Overview

Demands of laryngeal surgery require the anesthesia provider to be adept with a variety of advanced airway management devices and to competently execute different intraoperative ventilation techniques and strategies. Under general anesthesia, either the patient's trachea is intubated (a "tube" technique) or "tubeless" techniques of ventilation (spontaneous ventilation, apneic intermittent ventilation, JV) are used intraoperatively (Box 38.5). The comparison of these techniques is listed in Table 38.2.

If suspension laryngoscopy fails or if the location of the laryngeal lesion is not easily accessible, some procedures can be performed with the help of an FIS inserted through an SGA.[165,166] The LMA Fastrach (intubating LMA, iLMA) offers certain advantages, such as a rigid, wide metal tube that can accommodate a large-diameter FIS, optimal alignment of iLMA aperture with the glottic opening, diminished hemodynamic responses compared with suspension laryngoscopy, and superior ventilation capability.[98,99,166]

Patients who are vocal performers or professional voice users present unique challenges, requiring the anesthesia provider to avert even the slightest trauma to the patient's vocal cords and/or cricoarytenoid joints and to protect laryngeal and vocal function at all times.[26] If TI is required, it should be smooth and atraumatic, the ETT cuff should be inflated to seal pressure only,[167] and strict adherence to smooth extubation protocol (see "Tracheal Extubation in Head and Neck Surgery") will help to avoid cough-induced vocal cord injury.[168]

Tracheal Intubation

The use of a small (5-mm-ID) MLT tube with positive-pressure ventilation remains the standard for airway management in most

TABLE 38.2	Advantages and Disadvantages of Ventilation Techniques Used for Microlaryngeal Surgery	
Technique	**Advantages**	**Disadvantages**
Tracheal intubation (microlaryngeal tube)	Adequate surgical field and surgical access to the larynx in most cases Still surgical field Adequate airway protection Control of patient immobility and vocal cord movement with NMB Stable and controlled ventilation technique Ability to continuously and reliably monitor F_{IO_2}, $EtCO_2$, Paw, and anesthetic gases Suitable for prolonged procedures	Largely unsuitable for surgery of the posterior glottic pathology (e.g., posterior glottic or subglottic stenosis, transglottic tumor) Unsuitable for laser if the need arises May not be used according to the surgeon's preference
Spontaneous ventilation (insufflation and total intravenous anesthesia)	Unobstructed surgical field and free surgical access to the larynx Ability to evaluate dynamic airway function and obstruction Suitable, but not ideal, for laser surgery	Unprotected lower airway Precision and laser surgery difficult in the moving surgical field Contamination of operating room environment with anesthetic gases with insufflation technique Difficulty controlling adequate depth of anesthesia and absence of patient movement Inability to continuously and reliably monitor F_{IO_2}, $EtCO_2$, and anesthetic gases May not be suitable for patients with significant PD or CVD or for very young pediatric patients Best reserved for short, uncomplicated cases
Apneic intermittent ventilation	Unobstructed surgical field and free access to the larynx Still surgical field Control of patient immobility and vocal cord movement with NMB Ability to intermittently control gas exchange Suitable for laser surgery	Unprotected lower airway Possible airway trauma and disruption of the surgical field because of repeated passage of the endotracheal tube Inability to continuously and reliably monitor F_{IO_2}, $EtCO_2$, and anesthetic gases Slows the pace of surgery Best reserved for short, uncomplicated cases
Jet ventilation	Unobstructed or minimally impeded surgical field and surgical access to the larynx Rather still surgical field Control of patient immobility and vocal cord movement with NMB Ability to monitor and control F_{IO_2}, $EtCO_2$ (with low-frequency JV only), driving pressure, Paw, and PEEP with automated jet ventilators Suitable for prolonged procedures Suitable for laser surgery	Sole dependence on intravenous anesthesia Association with most major (e.g., barotrauma) and minor intraoperative anesthesia-related complications Dependence on sophisticated automated jet ventilators for safe use Limitations of manual JV and transtracheal JV Significant experience required May not be suitable for patients with significant PD or CVD

CVD, Cardiovascular disease; *EtCO₂*, end-tidal carbon dioxide; *FIO₂*, fraction of inspired oxygen; *JV*, jet ventilation; *NMB*, neuromuscular blockade; *Paw*, peak airway pressure; *PD*, pulmonary disease; *PEEP*, positive end-expiratory pressure.

nonlaser microlaryngeal surgery, and it is associated with minimal or no intraoperative complications.[159,163] Adequate gas exchange can be maintained through small-ID ETTs in most adult patients,[169,170] unless the duration of surgery approaches 2 hours (which happens rarely).[169] Even then, despite a consistent trend toward progressive hypercapnia and respiratory acidosis, the pH and $EtCO_2$ values remain within physiologic range.[170]

With most glottic pathology originating in the anterior two-thirds of the larynx, consistent positioning of a small MLT tube between the arytenoid cartilages in the posterior part of the glottis leaves most of the surgical field unobstructed to the surgical view and manipulations.[12,24,25,73,171] Even with many posterior glottic disorders, it may be possible for the surgeon to gently displace the MLT tube anteriorly with the microsurgical cupped forceps or to perform the surgery using the specially designed posterior glottic laryngoscopes.[172,173]

However, if the posterior glottis is occupied by a significant surgical pathology (e.g., posterior glottic or subglottic stenosis, transglottic tumor) (Fig. 38.18), use of alternative, tubeless ventilation techniques becomes necessary.[73] Tubeless ventilation can also be requested as a primary ventilation mode from the outset of the procedure, according to the surgeon's preference.

A 2.4-mm-ID and 40-cm-long specialized cuffed ETT (Tritube, Ventinova Medical B.V., Eindhoven, The Netherlands) has been developed recently for patients undergoing upper airway surgery.[174–176] It provides airway protection, while instantly improving glottic visualization. It also facilitates TI, especially for patients with stenotic lesions in and around the airway.[174] The small lumen of the Tritube makes conventional ventilation impossible, and high inflation pressures and expiratory ventilation assistance (EVA) are required, either with the manual use of the Ventrain device (Ventinova Medical B.V.) or the Evone, an automated flow-controlled

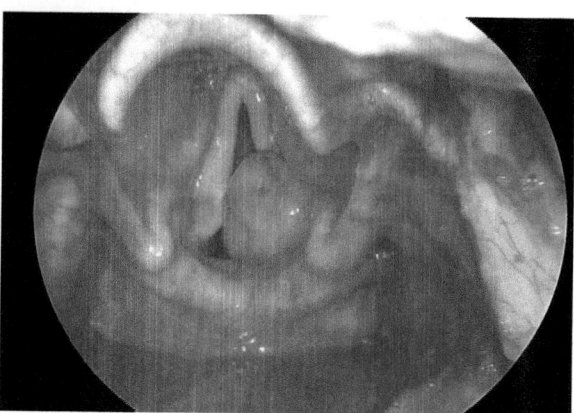

• **Fig. 38.18** A right vocal process granuloma is located in the posterior glottis. The location and the nature of the pathology preclude the use of the microlaryngeal tracheal (MLT) tube and require the use of jet ventilation. (Courtesy Edward Damrose, MD, Stanford University Medical Center, Stanford, CA.)

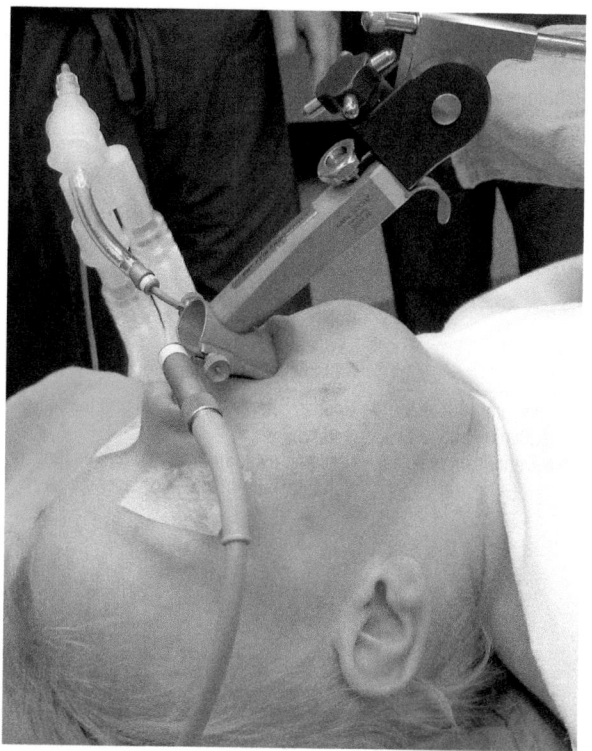

• **Fig. 38.19** A child in suspension laryngoscopy using the spontaneous ventilation (insufflation) technique. Notice the precut endotracheal tube connecting the anesthesia circuit to a metal cannula inserted into a side port of the suspension laryngoscope. (Courtesy Peter Koltai, MD, Stanford University Medical Center, Stanford, CA.)

ventilator with EVA technology (Ventinova Medical B.V.).[174–176] Small observational and randomized controlled trials have demonstrated the effectiveness of the Tritube-Evone ventilation system for laryngeal surgery in terms of oxygenation, CO_2 elimination, and airway protection,[145,176] and the future outcome-centered trials are required for wider introduction of this technology.

Spontaneous Ventilation

Spontaneous ventilation is rarely used in adult microlaryngeal surgery,[173,177–179] but it is commonly employed in the pediatric patient population, for whom it offers additional ability to evaluate dynamic airway function and level of obstruction. Anesthetic gases can be delivered (insufflated) through a nasal trumpet connected through an ETT adapter to the anesthesia circuit,[180–183] an ETT positioned in the nasopharynx,[184–186] a metal cannula, a side port of the operating laryngoscope (Fig. 38.19),[73] or a catheter placed through the vocal cords into the patient's trachea.[187–189]

Deep planes of anesthesia are usually required to blunt the laryngeal responses and to prevent patient movement, and supplementing with topical or local anesthesia of the airway facilitates maintenance of a more stable plane of anesthesia, promotes hemodynamic and respiratory stability, and decreases the incidence of intraoperative laryngospasm.[180,184,189–191]

High-Flow Nasal Oxygen Insufflation

Since its introduction to clinical anesthesia practice by Patel and Nouraei in 2015,[108] THRIVE has been rapidly gaining popularity as the sole ventilatory technique for adult laryngologic surgery. With patients anesthetized and apneic, THRIVE delivers fully conditioned oxygen through a specialized nasal cannula at or above 70 L/min, which leads to flow-dependent flushing of anatomic dead space, decreased airway resistance, generation of positive airway pressure and lung recruitment, and enhanced oxygenation and gas exchange due to interactions between the highly turbulent oxygen vortices and cardiogenic oscillations.[192,193] Intraoperatively, a combination of THRIVE-induced apneic oxygenation and apneic ventilation may eliminate or reduce the need for TI or JV and afford the surgeon with a fully unobstructed and highly stable surgical field (Fig. 38.20). A number of small observational and randomized controlled trials have documented the safe and

effective use of THRIVE for diverse laryngologic surgical procedures, including benign and malignant lesions, subglottic stenosis, and so on.[20,108,192–196] The results of some studies allow speculation that, in addition to facilitating surgical exposure, THRIVE may improve early patient recovery, suggesting its potential economic benefit for outpatient laryngologic procedures.[192]

The use of high-flow nasal oxygen insufflation in spontaneously breathing, anesthetized patients (STRIVE Hi) during microlaryngeal surgery has been advocated as an alternative to THRIVE.[21] Using STRIVE Hi, Booth and colleagues have demonstrated at least twice more effective CO_2 elimination compared to THRIVE after 30 minutes of anesthesia.[197] Relatively quick development of significant respiratory acidosis remains a major limiting factor of intraoperative THRIVE use, with the current estimate of $Paco_2$ rise ranging between 1.1 mm Hg/min and 1.8 mm Hg/min.[20,108,194] Sometimes viewed as a modern alternative to the traditional inhalation induction,[21] STRIVE Hi seems to be effective in preserving intraoperative oxygenation, CO_2 elimination, and airway patency.

Implementation of both THRIVE and STRIVE Hi techniques require close cooperation with the surgeon and may be best reserved for use by specialized teams for complex cases. The suggested protocol for THRIVE use for nonlaser laryngologic surgery[192] is listed in Box 38.6.

Apneic Intermittent Ventilation

Apneic intermittent ventilation (AIV) remains a relatively popular technique for microlaryngeal surgical procedures of short duration in some surgical centers.[159] Compared with spontaneous ventilation, it affords more stable and controlled anesthetic

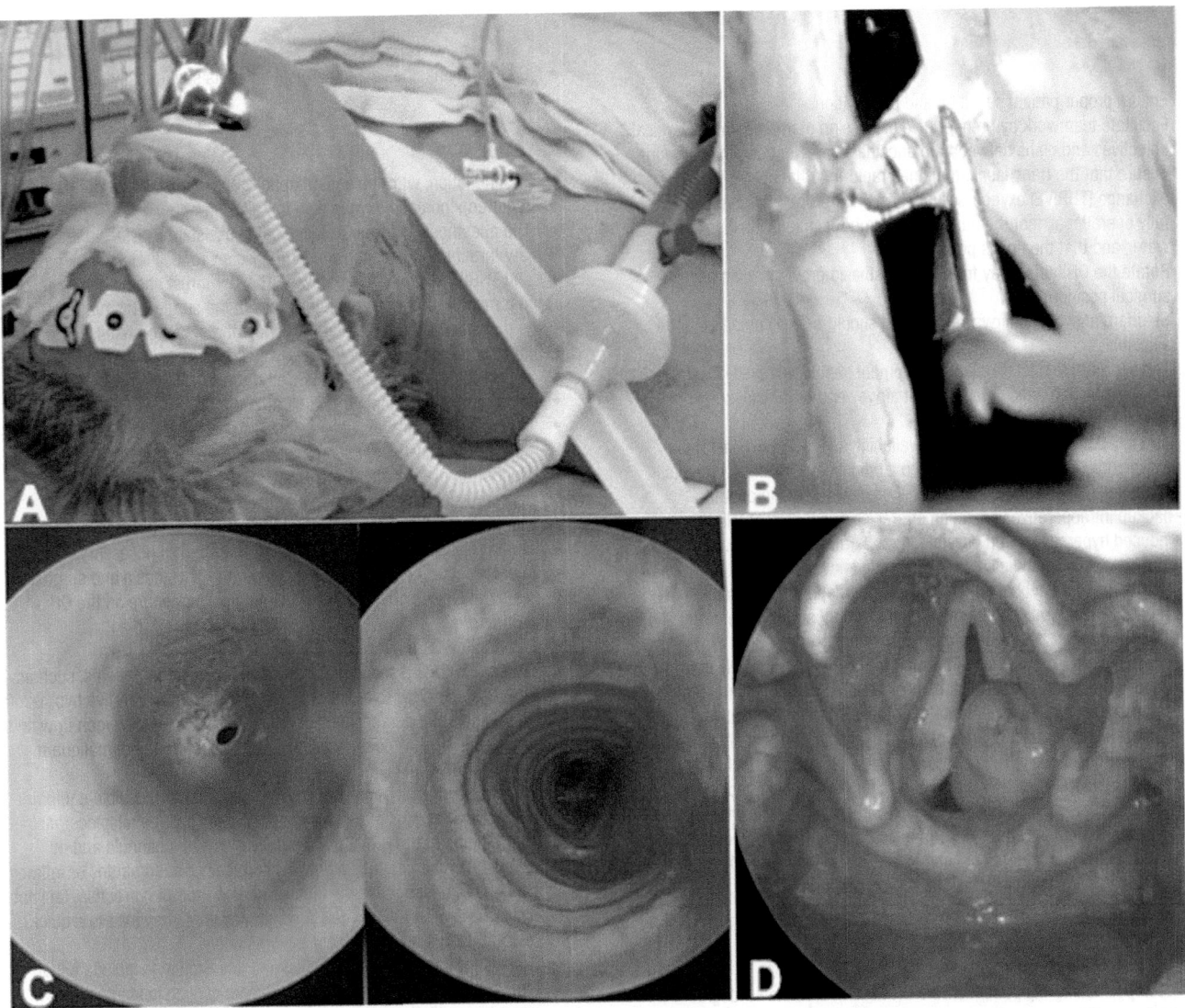

• **Fig 38.20** Intraoperative administration of transnasal humidified rapid-insufflation ventilatory exchange (THRIVE) and its effect on the surgical field. (A) Suspension laryngoscopy under general anesthesia, with the use of THRIVE as a primary ventilatory technique. THRIVE is administered using an Optiflow system (Fischer & Paykel Healthcare, Auckland, New Zealand), which delivers fully conditioned, heated, and humidified oxygen through specialized nasal cannula at or above 70 L/min. (B) Vocal cord polyp excision using THRIVE as a primary ventilatory technique. Note greatly enlarged, completely unobstructed surgical field facilitating surgical instrumentation. (C) Endoscopic treatment of Grade 3 subglottic stenosis (left image) using THRIVE as a primary ventilatory technique. THRIVE can effectively negotiate tight stenotic lesions, providing adequate intraoperative oxygenation. Right image: post dilation subglottic stenosis. (D) Excision of the right vocal process granuloma partially obstructing the glottic opening using THRIVE as a primary ventilatory technique. Note the greatly facilitated surgical access to the posterior glottic lesions. (Reproduced, with permission, from Nekhendzy V, Saxena A, Mittal B, et al. The safety and efficacy of Transnasal Humidified Rapid-Insufflation Ventilatory Exchange for laryngologic surgery. *Laryngoscope*. 2020;130:E874–E881.)

conditions, as well as full muscle relaxation. With the patient in suspension, the trachea is intubated by the surgeon with a small-diameter, preferably uncuffed ETT that is placed through the lumen of the laryngoscope,[159] and the patient's lungs are hyperventilated with an F_{IO_2} of 1.0 (Fig. 38.21). The ETT is then removed to provide a fully unobstructed and still surgical view of the larynx.

The ETT is withdrawn and reinserted as frequently as necessary to maintain an oxygen saturation by pulse oximetry (SpO_2) of 90% or greater and $EtCO_2$ between 40 and 60 mm Hg,[45,159,198] allowing periods of apnea from 5 to 10 minutes in healthy adult patients.[159,199]

Jet Ventilation

Compared with TI, supraglottic and infraglottic HFJV techniques have distinct advantages. They provide the surgeon with an enlarged and minimally distorted view of the endolarynx, facilitating surgical access and eliminating flammable material (ETT)

• BOX 38.6   Suggested Protocol for THRIVE Use During Non-laser Laryngologic Surgery

Preparation

- Ensure proper patient selection and preparation.
- Facilitate teamwork by preoperative discussion of intraoperative surgical objectives and plans between the anesthesia provider and the surgeon.
- Ensure that the transnasal humidified rapid-insufflation ventilatory exchange (THRIVE) oxygen delivery system is properly assembled, is fully operational, that the humidifier chamber is filled with distilled water, and that the unit is powered on.
- Rotate the OR table away from the anesthesia provider, to its final surgical position.
- Standard anesthesia airway equipment should be fully prepared and available.
- The appropriate difficult airway equipment should be readily available for patients with anticipated difficult airway and/or difficult surgical suspension.
- Strongly consider the immediate availability of a second-generation supraglottic airway device and video laryngoscopy for these patients.
- The anesthesia and surgical teams shall devise the appropriate backup intraoperative ventilation strategies to counteract THRIVE-induced hypercapnia and possible intraoperative hypoxemia. At the minimum, this should include the immediate availability of a 5.0-mm-ID microlaryngeal tracheal (MLT) tube (see "Intraoperative Management"). The jet ventilation (JV) equipment (automatic JV strongly preferred) shall be fully prepared and available, if deemed necessary.
- The anesthesia provider shall arrange the THRIVE oxygen delivery system and all the prepared anesthesia-related equipment in a highly ergonomic manner allowing the team to facilitate intraoperative multitasking and maintenance of situational awareness at all times.
- Strategic positioning of the anesthesia provider close to the head of the OR table may be advisable. It allows for performing effective jaw thrust during suspension laryngoscopy without interfering with surgical instrumentation; for effective communication with the surgeon and continuous observation of the surgical field and the OR monitors; and for monitoring patient's vital signs and proper functioning of the THRIVE oxygen and drug delivery systems.

Preinduction

- Upon positioning the patient on the OR table in a 30- to 45-degree backup position, immediately start oxygen at 50 L/min to promote early preoxygenation and lung recruitment. Instruct the patient to breathe slowly through the nose, with the mouth closed, to generate continuous positive airway pressure (approximately 1 cm H_2O pressure per 10 L/min of oxygen). Patient's tolerance of high oxygen flow can be facilitated with a small IV dose of midazolam (0.5–1.0 mg), as required. If the patient is unable to tolerate high-flow oxygenation, decrease oxygen flow in 5 L/min increments, but to not lower than 30 L/min.
- With the THRIVE oxygen delivery system deployed, apply the standard OR monitors and other patient monitoring equipment, as required. Intraoperative monitoring of transcutaneous CO_2 (TcP_{CO_2}) is advisable, subject to equipment availability.
- Secure the patient's comfortable position on the OR table with special attention on protecting the patient's pressure points.
- Ensure that all the surgical equipment is readily available and fully functional, and that the suspension stand is attached to the OR table in the correct position.

- Complete anesthesia and surgical timeouts sequentially prior to induction.

Intraoperative Management

- Postinduction, with the patient apneic, anesthetized, and paralyzed (as required), increase oxygen flow to 70 L/min.
- The anesthesia provider or a dedicated assistant provides a manual jaw thrust during suspension laryngoscopy to facilitate airway patency and THRIVE oxygenation pathway. The jaw thrust should be provided in a manner that does not interfere with the surgical instrumentation (e.g., while facing the patient). The jaw thrust can be released upon introduction of the suspension laryngoscope in the patient's mouth, or maintained until full suspension, as desired.
- Intraoperatively, maintain THRIVE at 70 L/min.
- Maintain total intravenous anesthesia (propofol and remifentanil are most commonly used) and adequate muscle relaxation, as required.
- Monitoring of the patient's hypnotic state and the degree of neuromuscular blockade is recommended, whenever feasible.
- Monitor the level of sterile water in the THRIVE oxygen delivery system humidification chamber, and refill the chamber, as necessary.
- Maintain close communication between the anesthesia and surgical teams and close observation of the surgical procedure on the OR monitors.
- Monitor TcP_{CO_2}, if available.
- Observe THRIVE discontinuation criteria for selected patients, such as prolonged surgical duration (>40 min), and/or intraoperative hypoxemia (Sp_{O_2} <90% and decreasing, not relieved by increased oxygen flow and/or correction of iatrogenic causes), and/or occurrence of malignant cardiac arrhythmias.
- For intraoperative hypoxemia, troubleshoot first for possible equipment-related and surgical iatrogenic causes. These include misplacement/obstruction of the THRIVE oxygen delivery system cannula and/or occlusion of the patient's airway by surgically placed patties or inflated balloon of the subglottic dilatation catheter. Prompt correction, facilitated by increasing THRIVE oxygen flows, as required, may lead to a quick restoration of a normal patient's oxygenation.
- Options for improving oxygenation and gas exchange include full or temporary (apneic intermittent ventilation) conversion to positive-pressure ventilation using a 5.0-mm-ID MLT tube (placed by the surgeon); full or temporary conversion to JV (supraglottic high-frequency jet ventilation [HFJV] is preferred as an initial maneuver to avoid surgical interruption); or withdrawing the laryngoscope and temporarily reverting to bag-mask or supraglottic airway ventilation before reinstituting THRIVE.

Emergence From Anesthesia

- Upon completion of surgery, intravenous drug delivery is discontinued, the neuromuscular blockade is reversed, as required, and the patient is allowed to emerge from anesthesia.
- Oxygenation/ventilation options during emergence include the continuation of THRIVE; placement of a supraglottic airway; bag-mask ventilation; or tracheal intubation, depending on the clinical situation and the patient's underlying medical conditions.
- The patient is transferred to the recovery room upon restoration of spontaneous ventilation and full emergence from anesthesia.

(Reproduced and modified, with permission, from Nekhendzy V, Saxena A, Mittal B, et al. The safety and efficacy of Transnasal Humidified Rapid-Insufflation Ventilatory Exchange for laryngologic surgery. *Laryngoscope.* 2020;130:E874-E881.)

---

from the patient's airway should the need for laser surgery arise intraoperatively.[19,200]

Refer to "Special Situations"/"Partially Obstructed Airway" for the discussion of the use of HFJV in patients with a partially obstructed airway.

General Principles

In contrast to conventional ventilation, where a gas volume is pushed rather slowly via an ETT into the "sealed" trachea, JV consists of rapid gas (oxygen) insufflation with high velocity via a narrow nozzle into the open airway. HFJV is most commonly used and is administered

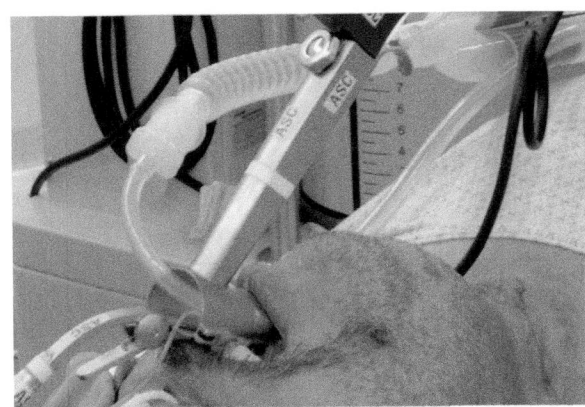

• **Fig. 38.21** Apneic intermittent ventilation during microlaryngeal surgery. The endotracheal tube is intermittently placed through the lumen of a suspension laryngoscope by the surgeon and connected to the anesthesia breathing circuit for positive-pressure ventilation.

by specialized ventilators with automatic shutdown features. The V_T generated during HFJV is small (1–3 mL/kg), and successful gas exchange predominantly occurs because of unique mechanisms, such as ambient gas entrainment, Taylor-type dispersion, molecular and facilitated diffusion, pulsatile effects of thoracic vibrations and cardiac oscillations, and collateral ventilation (pendelluft).[19,201] Both oxygenation and CO_2 elimination can be controlled in a variety of patients and a broad range of clinical situations.

In conventional ventilation, gas flow is bidirectional and happens in a sequential mode (inspiration-expiration); however, gas flow during JV is mainly coaxial and partially simultaneous in both directions (inward and outward). The exhalation happens completely outside of the JV delivery system, via a free gas exhalation pathway. If full exhalation cannot be guaranteed, JV is contraindicated.

Driving Pressure. The driving pressure (DP) is the pressure at which jets are delivered to the patient. The DP is held constant, and any change in respiratory compliance will result in a reduction of minute ventilation. Changes in DP have the greatest, but nonlinear, effect on the efficiency of gas exchange.

Ventilation Frequency. The ventilation frequency (VF) is the number of cycles generated per minute (cpm). Low-frequency JV (LFJV) is delivered at 10 to 30 cpm, and HFJV is usually initially set at 150 cpm (100–300 cpm). Higher frequencies significantly reduce laryngeal motion and afford a quiet surgical field without the need for interrupting ventilation; however, a dead space ventilation is increased with possible reduction of CO_2 elimination.[19,184,202]

Oxygenation is largely independent of the VF. The higher the VF, the more likely the auto-positive end-expiratory pressure (auto-PEEP) builds up, particularly if the inspiration duration is increased.

Inspiration Duration. The inspiration duration (ID), or inspiratory time, is usually set at 50%. Longer ID leads to a shorter pause duration, which hinders exhalation and increases the auto-PEEP.

There may be a trend toward a slight improvement of oxygenation by extending the ID, but the CO_2 elimination may become impaired. Prolonged ID may also shift the thoracic excursions into a deeper inspiratory position, with increase in airway pressures and worsened gas exchange.[19] Because of the variable effects, it may be recommended to keep ID at or near 50%.

Oxygen Concentration. The oxygen fraction of the gas at the jet nozzle ($Fjeto_2$) is set by the operator, but the FiO_2 that is delivered to the patient will always be lower because of air entrainment.

Administration of infraglottic or transtracheal HFJV will result in higher FiO_2, because entrainment of air is reduced deep inside the airway.

Gas Volumes. The pressure-driven nature of JV and the multiple mechanisms responsible for gas exchange produce more variability in V_T and minute ventilation compared with conventional positive-pressure ventilation. The V_T is directly influenced by changes in DP and ID, but this relationship is not linear.

Airway Pressure. The airway pressure (Paw) is influenced by various factors, mainly by DP. As long as the exhalation remains unimpeded, Paw remains very low in the magnitude of a few millibar (1 mbar = 1 cm H_2O). The VF and ID usually have little direct impact on the Paw.

If a double-lumen HFJV catheter is used, Paw can be continuously monitored through the smaller lumen and displayed as a pressure curve with numerical values indicating peak inspiratory pressure (PIP), mean airway pressure (mPaw), and end-expiratory pressure (EEP). The Paw in the trachea may be accepted as a good approximation of the distal airway pressure, and therefore elevated Paw carries the risk of lung distention and lung injury.[19,201]

The pause airway pressure (PP) is intermittently measured between JV cycles through the main jet line. The PP must be undercut before the next insufflation can be released.

The automatic ventilator shutdown occurs if the user-determined pressure limits are exceeded.

Jet Gas Conditioning. Prolonged ventilation with unconditioned (dry and cold) ventilation gas may cause severe damage to the tracheobronchial mucosa and produce a heat loss resulting in intraoperative hypothermia. The optimal conditioning is provided by a combination of moisture supply and heating of the jet gas and should be used whenever possible, even for short cases.

Supraglottic Jet Ventilation

With supraglottic JV, the jet nozzle is positioned above the glottic opening. Supraglottic JV can be performed through the side port

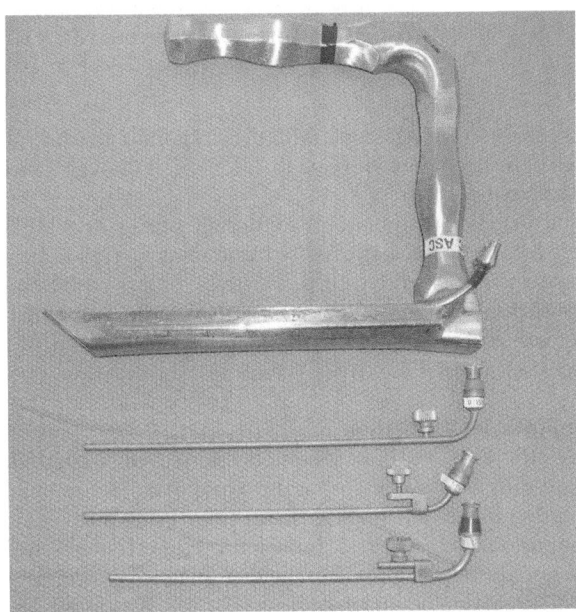

• **Fig. 38.22** A Dedo operating laryngoscope with the integrated side port *(top)* that can be used for supraglottic jet ventilation. Jetting metal cannulas *(bottom)* also can be inserted directly through the laryngoscope lumen.

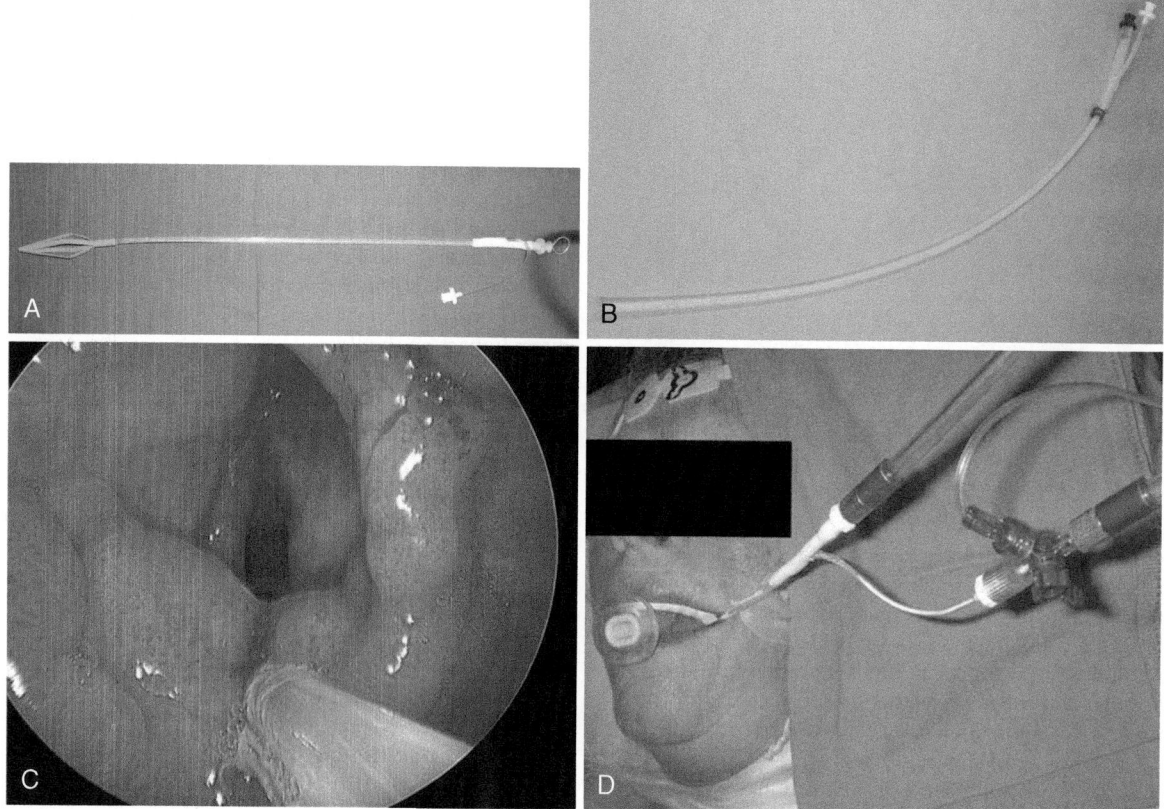

• **Fig. 38.23** (A) The Hunsaker Mon-Jet Ventilation Tube (Medtronic Xomed Inc., Jacksonville, FL) and (B) a double-lumen catheter (LaserJet, Acutronic Medical Systems AG, Hirzel, Switzerland) are laser resistant, come with the metal stylet to facilitate tracheal placement, and have a large port that is used for jet ventilation (JV) and a smaller port that is used for monitoring the distal airway pressure and respiratory gases. The green, basket-shaped distal end of the Hunsaker Mon-Jet tube facilitates self-centering of the tube within the trachea, preventing the catheter "whip" that may lead to submucosal gas injection and possible occlusion of the distal end of the jet tube by tracheal mucosa. (C) The small-diameter Hunsaker Mon-Jet tube is placed through the glottis to facilitate a clear surgical view and surgical access. (D) The Hunsaker Mon-Jet tube is taped in place during JV, with the monitoring port connected to the ventilator through a three-way stopcock. The jet ventilator tubing is suspended to prevent kinking, and an oral airway is inserted to facilitate full egress of air during JV. (B, Courtesy Acutronic Medical Systems AG, Hirzel, Switzerland; C and D, from Davies JM, Hillel AD, Maronian NC, et al. The Hunsaker Mon-Jet tube with jet ventilation is effective for microlaryngeal surgery. *Can J Anaesth.* 2009;56:284–290.)

of a suspension laryngoscope, with the jet cannula attached to the lumen of the laryngoscope (Fig. 38.22)[19,82,203] or through a specialized jet laryngoscope.[204,205]

The inability to monitor Paw during supraglottic HFJV is largely inconsequential; the risk of barotrauma is very low because the system is not tightly sealed. However, proper positioning of the suspension laryngoscope against the glottis is essential for safety and effectiveness of the technique, and misalignment may cause barotrauma.

Infraglottic Jet Ventilation

Infraglottic HFJV is most commonly employed: a continuous, upward-directed flow of gas creates a positive-pressure buildup, preventing blood and surgical debris from being directed down an unprotected airway.[206–208] Infraglottic HFJV is established by bypassing the larynx from above with a small (3- to 4-mm-OD), laser-resistant double-lumen catheter (Fig. 38.23), a metal jet cannula, or a rigid bronchoscope.

The use of the rigid bronchoscope provides a wide margin of safety: The airway is constantly kept open for exhalation, the

danger of intraoperative laryngospasm is eliminated, and Paw monitoring during HFJV is not required.

With an HFJV catheter, strategies for minimizing the risk of barotrauma on initiation of infraglottic HFJV may include starting ventilation with low driving pressures at or below 1.0 bar (1.0 bar is approximately 15 psi); promoting sufficient exhalation time by using LFJV first; and maintaining the patient's airway patency with the assistance of an oral airway or providing a jaw lift.[156,159,163,202,209] Alternatively, initiation of the infraglottic HFJV can be held off until the suspension laryngoscope is deployed, and ventilation is supported conventionally through a face mask or SGA. It may be prudent to confirm absence of the infraglottic catheter obstruction by the $EtCO_2$ return and to check the catheter or cannula position endoscopically before HFJV commences.[163,202]

On emergence from anesthesia, small V_T and low peak and mean airway pressures associated with infraglottic HFJV facilitate a transition to spontaneous ventilation.[19,43,163,210,211] If the conversion to spontaneous ventilation through a small subglottic catheter proves difficult, the patient's airway can be supported through a face mask, SGA, or ETT.

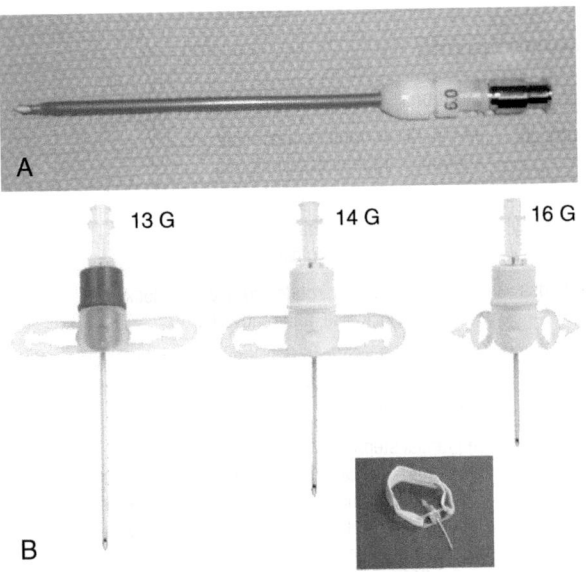

13 G   14 G   16 G

- **Fig. 38.24** Devices for transtracheal jet ventilation (TTJV). (A) The 7.5-cm-long, 2-mm-ID TTJV catheter (Cook Medical Inc., Bloomington, IN) is mounted on a 14-gauge (G) needle. The catheter is wire reinforced to prevent kinking. (B) Different sizes of the Ravussin-type cricothyrotomy catheter (VBM Medizintechnik GmbH, Sulz, Germany) for TTJV. The 13-gauge, 1.3-mm-outer-diameter catheter with the fixation flange and foam Velcro neck tape is most frequently used in adults. (Courtesy Acutronic Medical Systems, GmbH, Salzburg, Austria.)

Transtracheal Jet Ventilation

With transtracheal JV, the larynx is bypassed from below by a long catheter or Ravussin-type cannula (Fig. 38.24) placed through the CTM.[156,163,212] The routine use of FIS or a rigid bronchoscope is advocated by some to monitor the procedure in anesthetized patients and to minimize the risk of posterior tracheal wall laceration, which may lead to submucosal gas injection and barotrauma.[159,206,213]

The ability to monitor PP during transtracheal HFJV is helpful, but the overall level of safety is decreased compared with infraglottic and supraglottic JV. The automatic cut-off features may not be able to remedy all possible causes of barotrauma associated with transtracheal HFJV: complications may be related to the TTJV catheter insertion problems, laryngospasm, and high-pressure episodes (e.g., coughing, active expiration) during the recovery period.[112,163]

Notwithstanding the attractive features of high-frequency TTJV, such as a motionless surgical field and a particularly easy transition to spontaneous respiration,[163] it may be advisable to reserve the elective use of this technique for the most complicated patients[156] and to designate operators with significant clinical experience and expertise.[112,156,163,206]

Clinical monitoring of the patient to prevent barotrauma should remain the standard of care for all JV techniques.[159,163] Essential for the patient's safety are ensuring an adequate level of anesthesia, analgesia, and muscle relaxation; painstaking attention to maintaining unobstructed exhalation; and diligent monitoring of vital signs and chest excursions.[82,159,163,214] Close cooperation between the surgeon and the anesthesia provider is essential; if the operating laryngoscope moves or is removed without warning to the anesthesia team, major barotrauma may result.

Jet Ventilation Problems

The risk of barotrauma remains one of the major limiting factors of JV techniques. An overall incidence of major barotrauma complications (e.g., cervicomediastinal emphysema, pneumothorax, tension pneumothorax) is small (0.2% to 0.5%),[159,206,215] and these complications are most frequently observed during TTJV (1%).[159,163]

The higher ASA physical status correlates with the higher incidence of complications with infraglottic and TTJV techniques,[159] and these patients should be given special attention. Patients with previous neck radiation therapy are at higher risk for multiple attempts at TTJV catheter placement and subsequent risk of developing intraoperative barotrauma.[163] The anesthesia provider should also be thoroughly familiar with the other problems in JV management that may arise intraoperatively (Table 38.3).

Laser Laryngeal Surgery

Good communication, cooperation, and the development of a team approach are essential requirements for successful laser airway surgery. The surgeon and anesthesia provider should be familiar with the principles of a laser, the types of laser available, hazards of laser use, the management of an airway fire, and the advantages and disadvantages of the various anesthetic techniques available.

For an airway fire, three components of the fire triad are needed: fuel source, oxidant sources, and ignition source. Removal of one of these components prevents or reduces the risk of an airway fire, which in practice means removing or protecting the fuel sources, minimizing the oxidant sources, and not using an ignition source. To avoid an airway fire, all safety checks (e.g., laser timeout) shall be instituted and observed during the laser airway surgery.

For laser airway surgery, the CO_2, argon, neodymium:yttrium-aluminum-garnet (Nd:YAG), potassium titanyl phosphate (KTP), and diode lasers are the most commonly used (Table 38.4).

Carbon Dioxide Laser

The CO_2 laser is particularly suited for laryngeal and H&N surgical procedures and is used for the treatment of benign laryngeal pathology, such as nodules, polyps, papillomas, granulomas, Reinke edema, webs, hemangiomas, subglottic stenosis, arytenoidectomy, as well as for phonosurgical procedures. CO_2 lasers allow precise cutting and shallow penetration of tissues (Fig. 38.25).

Most commonly, the CO_2 laser can be directed into the patient through a micromanipulator. It emits invisible infrared light at a wavelength of 10,600 nm in the infrared range of the electromagnetic spectrum, and the light cannot be seen by the human eye. To allow the CO_2 laser to be seen, a second, low-intensity (0.8-mW) coaxial helium-neon (He-Ne) laser is incorporated into the CO_2 laser and acts as a red-light pointer.

The CO_2 laser can be used in a continuous, pulsed, or superpulsed mode. The superpulsed mode reduces the exposure time to a few nanoseconds while delivering high energies of 400 to 500 W with each peak (Fig. 38.26). The rest time between each peak allows the tissues to cool and reduces thermal injury to adjacent tissues.

Flexible-fiber CO_2 lasers (Omniguide, Cambridge, MA; Fiberlase CO_2 Fiber, Lumenis, CA) have been developed for use in airway procedures, including BOT tumors, laryngeal tumors, tracheal tumors, laryngeal papillomas, tracheal stenosis, and laryngeal lesions.[216–221] The flexible laser fiber can be passed through a rigid bronchoscope or flexible bronchoscope or can be used with a handpiece.

TABLE 38.3   High-Frequency Jet Ventilation Troubleshooting and Problem Solving

Problem	Causes	Solutions
Difficult insertion of the suspension laryngoscope by surgeon	Unfavorable upper airway anatomy for creation of a straight line of sight	Infraglottic or transtracheal HFJV Alternative intubation techniques
Impossible insertion of infraglottic jet catheter	Unfavorable or distorted upper and/or lower airway anatomy	Supraglottic or transtracheal HFJV Alternative intubation techniques
Difficulty advancing infraglottic jet catheter into the trachea	The tip of JV catheter abutting against the tracheal mucosa	Retract JV catheter, rotate180 degrees clock- or counterclockwise, and readvance
Advanced airway stenosis (≥50% of lumen)	Scars, tumors	Position JV nozzle (catheter tip) proximal to stenotic lesion, or bypass stenosis with the rigid bronchoscope first. Transtracheal HFJV
Activated pause pressure (PP) alarm	JV frequency too high: insufficient time for PP to decrease below the set alarm limit Possible airway obstruction if Paw not monitored concomitantly	Sequential steps: Check for adequate egress of air, as indicated by absent concomitant increase in peak airway pressure, and a detectable air leak out of the patient's mouth Decrease inspiratory time Lower JV frequency Set higher PP limit
Activated peak airway pressure (Paw) alarm	Impaired gas egress Kinking of JV line or catheter Displacement of JV catheter, with catheter tip abutting against the mucosa Dissipating neuromuscular blockade (infraglottic JV)	Sequential steps: Check for adequate egress of air, as indicated by absent concomitant increase in PP pressure, and a detectable air leak out of the patient's mouth Check for JV line/catheter kinking Retract JV catheter 0.5–1 cm and/or rotate axially Reestablish neuromuscular blockade
Decreased SpO$_2$	Various degrees of restrictive, obstructive, and combined lung diseases	Sequential steps: Increase FiO$_2$ Increase JV driving pressure Increase inspiratory time, up to a maximum of 60% Increase JV frequency Switch from supraglottic to infraglottic JV Add an O$_2$ bias flow in the vicinity of the jet nozzle If the above measures fail, revert to conventional ventilation
Decreased CO$_2$ elimination	Various degrees of restrictive, obstructive, and combined lung diseases Noncompliant chest wall	Sequential steps: Increase JV driving pressure Decrease inspiratory time to prolong alveolar emptying Increase entrainment of ambient air by decreasing JV frequency in steps of 50 cycles per minute. Convert to low frequency JV If the above measures fail, revert to conventional ventilation
Hypotension	Anesthetic overdose Hemodynamic instability Barotrauma	Check anesthetic plane, volume status Exclude cardiovascular problems If tension pneumothorax, urgent insertion of chest tube(s)

FiO$_2$, Fraction of inspired oxygen; *HFJV,* high-frequency jet ventilation; *JV,* jet ventilation; *Paw,* peak airway pressure; *PP,* pause pressure; *SpO$_2$,* oxygen saturation by pulse oximetry.

The pressurized gas exiting the fiber tip during the laser procedure may cause gas emboli, and the fiber tip should not be brought into direct contact with blood vessels or vascular tissues. Pressurized gas exiting the fiber tip during the laser procedure also may cause separation of submucosal flaps or mild emphysema under superficial layers of tissue, and the CO$_2$ fibers should not be used for lesions below the carina.

Potassium Titanyl Phosphate Laser
The KTP laser is strongly absorbed by hemoglobin and melanin, and it is used for otolaryngologic lesions, vascular diseases, and hemorrhages.[222] It is used in vascular lesions within the airway,

and because it can be transmitted through clear substances and can pass through a flexible scope channel, it can be used in areas where a direct line-of-site laser cannot. Most commonly, the KTP laser is directed into the larynx using a metal laryngeal suction adapted as the carrier for the fiber.

General Laser Hazards

Eye Damage

Lasers can easily damage the eyes by direct or indirect exposure, causing serious corneal and retinal injuries that may be irreversible.

TABLE 38.4	Characteristics of Commonly Used Medical Lasers			
Type of Laser	Laser Wavelength (nm)	Color	Fiberoptic Transmission	
Gas				
Helium-neon	633	Red	Yes	
Argon	500	Blue-green	Yes	
Carbon dioxide	10,600	Invisible	No	
Solid				
Ruby	695	Red	Yes	
Nd:YAG	1,060	Invisible	Yes	
KTP	532	Green	Yes	

KTP, Potassium titanyl phosphate; *Nd:YAG*, neodymium:yttrium-aluminum-garnet. Modified from Sosis MB. Anesthesia for laser surgery. *Probl Anesth.* 1993;7:160.

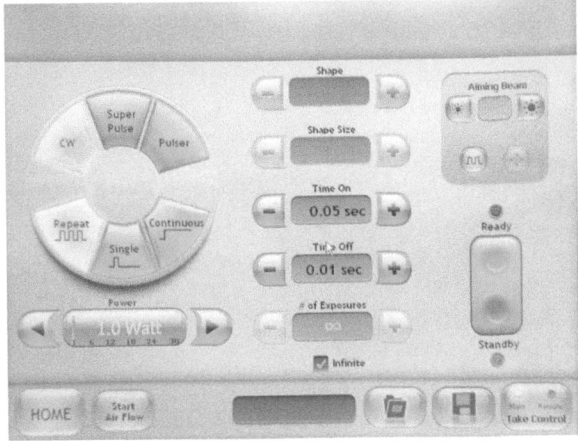

• **Fig. 38.26** CO_2 laser parameters include continuous, pulsed, and superpulsed modes.

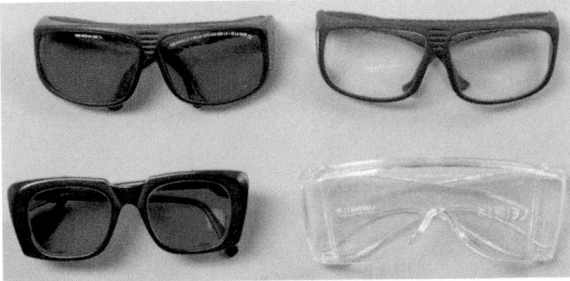

• **Fig. 38.27** In the selection of laser glasses, notice the protection offered by the sides of the glasses, which wrap around the eye.

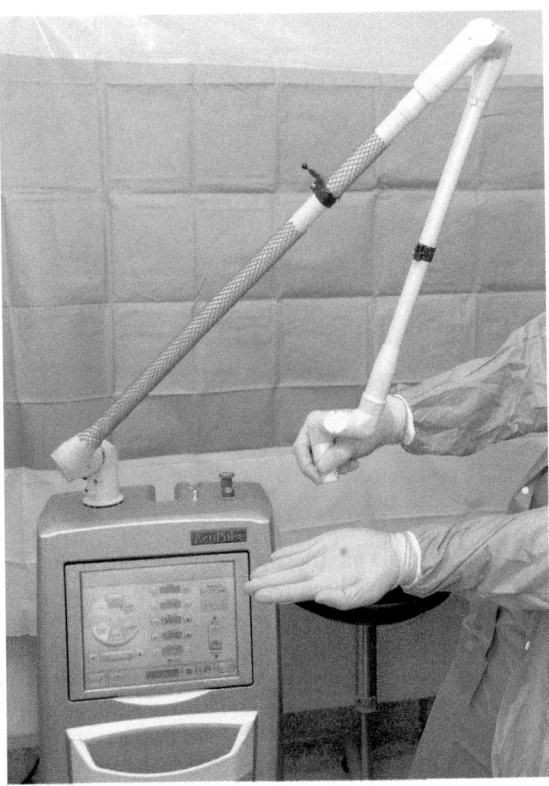

• **Fig. 38.25** The CO_2 laser (AcuPulse, Lumenis, Yokneam, Israel) has an articulating arm for attachment to a surgical microscope or handheld device. The coaxial helium-neon, low-intensity laser can be seen as a continuous, visible red light.

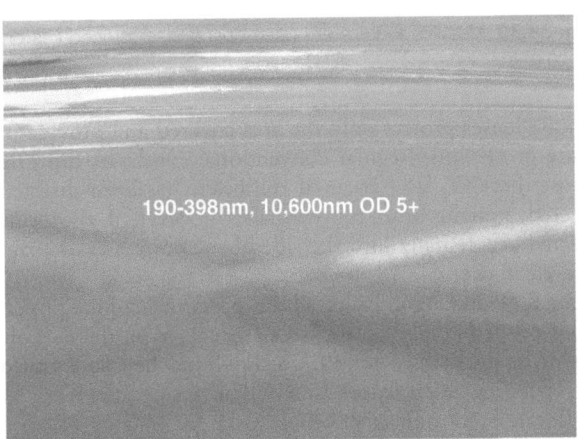

190-398nm, 10,600nm OD 5+

• **Fig. 38.28** Eyes must be protected from laser energy. Laser glasses are labeled with the optical density value, the wavelengths against which protection is afforded, and maximum radiant exposure or irradiance to which eyewear is exposed.

Eye protection is essential for anyone within the OR, including the patient, auxiliary staff, nursing staff, surgeon, and anesthesia provider (Fig. 38.27). General precautions for the patient include taping the eyes closed and avoiding the use of petroleum-based eye lubricants. Further protection includes saline-soaked eye pads, protective eyeglasses, or metal eye goggles, depending on the wavelength and type of laser used.

All laser glasses should be labeled clearly with the optical density value, the wavelengths against which protection is afforded, and maximum radiant exposure, or irradiance, to which the eyewear can be exposed (Figs. 38.28 and 38.29).[223] The correct protective eyeglasses must be used for the type of laser used for the procedure; failure to do so provides no protection for the eyes. In hospitals where only one type of laser is in use, this is less of a problem, but meticulous care must be taken in hospitals with many types of lasers and protective eye goggles.

For CO_2 lasers, the damage to the eye is limited to the cornea because its radiation is largely absorbed by water, and the cornea is more than 75% water.[224] There is no risk to the retina.

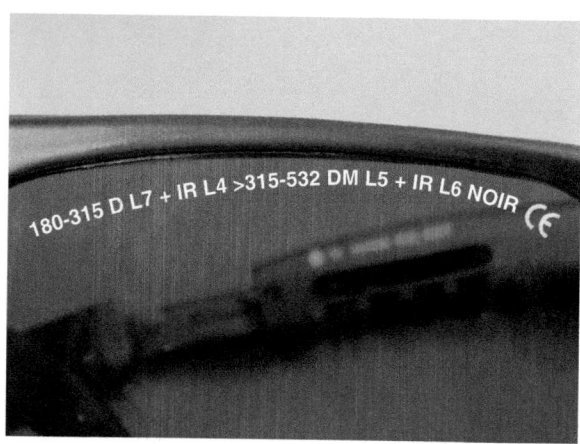

• **Fig. 38.29** The correct protective eyeglasses must be used with any given laser. The optical density value, the wavelengths against which protection is afforded, and maximum radiant exposure or irradiance to which eyewear is exposed are part of the design of laser glasses.

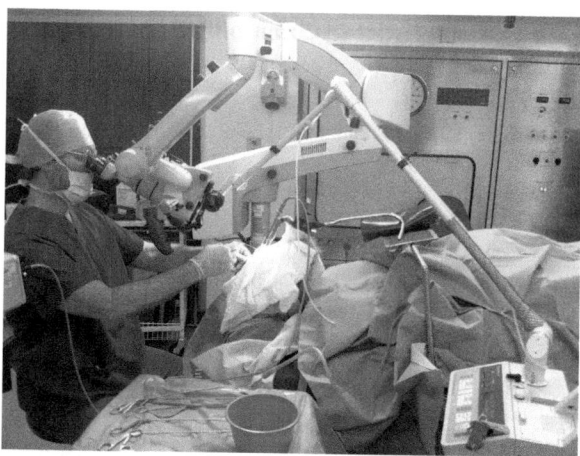

• **Fig. 38.31** Care should be taken with wet towels to ensure complete coverage of the face and area around the surgical laryngoscope. A CO_2 laser is attached to the operating microscope by an articulating arm.

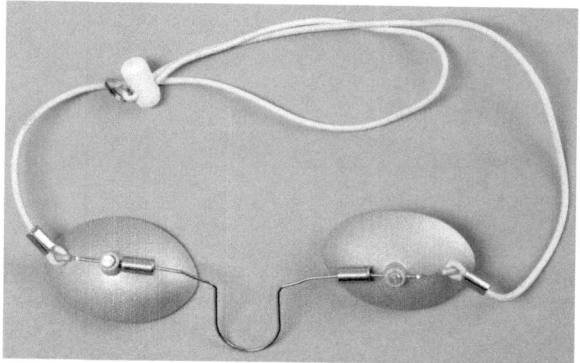

• **Fig. 38.30** Metallic goggles are used during laser procedures on the surface of the skin.

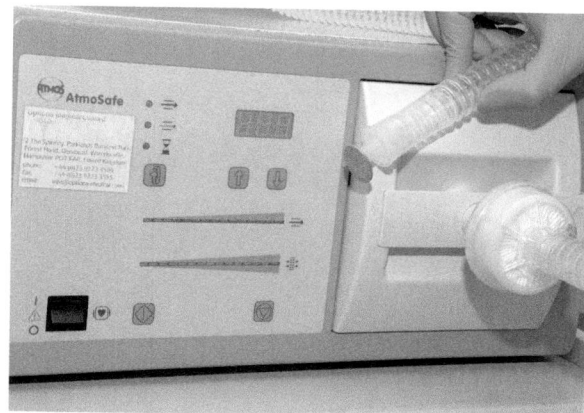

• **Fig. 38.32** The AtmoSafe smoke evacuator (Atmos Medical Limited, Hampshire, UK) holds a metal coin by its suction.

Contact lenses protect only the area covered and provide inadequate protection. Regular conventional eyeglasses can protect against the CO_2 laser beam if the beam has been directed or reflected straight onto the eyeglass; however, if the beam is reflected accidentally into the side of the eyeglasses, damage to the eye can occur.

For KTP and argon lasers, all OR personnel require protective amber-colored eyeglasses; for laser procedures on the face, metal goggles are used (Fig. 38.30). For rigid and flexible endoscopes and operating microscopes, filters that absorb the KTP wavelength can be introduced.

Skin and Drape Damage

The aberrant laser hit may cause skin burns, and the face or exposed areas should be protected with wet towels and drapes. For laser airway procedures involving a suspension laryngoscope, all the area around the surgical laryngoscope and face should be completely covered with wet towels, which must be kept wet throughout the procedure. Care should be taken, particularly around the draping of the proximal portion of the surgical laryngoscope, to ensure that the lips and nose are fully protected because this region is more likely to be struck by a reflected laser beam from the proximal rim of the surgical laryngoscope (Fig. 38.31).

Preparation solution should not contain alcohol. Disposable surgical drapes are a potential fire hazard. Although they are treated with flame-retardant chemicals and are water resistant, all types of surgical drapes are potentially flammable. Many cases of drapes catching fire have been reported. When drapes catch fire, it is difficult to extinguish them because the drapes are water resistant and water rolls off them. A CO_2 fire extinguisher should be available. Drapes, once ignited, go up in flames immediately, causing the OR to be inundated with smoke and making it difficult for everyone to see and breathe.[225–227] It is important to keep the towels moist because they also can catch fire.

Laser Plume

The plume of smoke produced by vaporization of tissues in electrocautery or laser surgery may be hazardous. The smoke contains fine particles (mean size, 0.31 μm; range, 0.1 to 0.8 μm) that can be efficiently transported and deposited in the alveoli.[228] Viral DNA has been detected in plumes from condylomas and skin warts but not from laryngeal papillomas.[229–232] CO_2 lasers seem to produce the most smoke from vaporization of tissue. OR personnel can be protected by using an efficient smoke evacuator at the surgical site (Fig. 38.32).[233,234]

Gas Embolism

Gas embolism has been reported with Nd:YAG laser resection of tracheal and bronchial tumors, and it may be a risk factor for flexible-fiber CO_2 lasers introduced into the bronchial tree.[235,236]

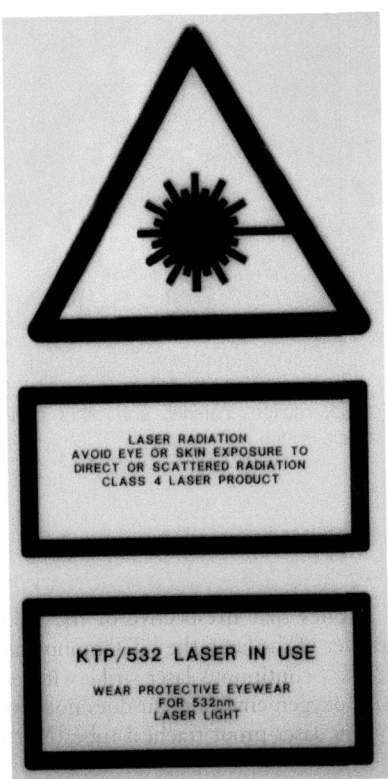

• **Fig. 38.33** The sign warns personnel entering the operating room that a potassium titanyl phosphate (KTP) laser is being used.

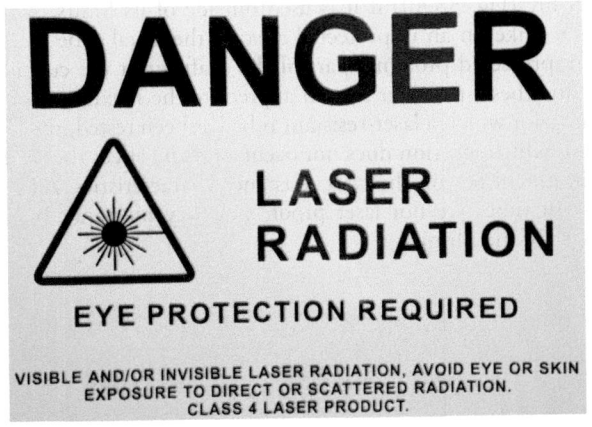

• **Fig. 38.34** A warning sign should be placed on the operating room door to prevent personnel from inadvertently entering during laser surgery.

Misdirected Laser and Laser Protocol

A misdirected laser may result from equipment failure or inadequate knowledge of that equipment. Close communication between the laser operator and surgical team must ensure that any laser is put in standby mode when not in use.

A warning sign should be placed on the OR door so that anyone entering is informed that the laser is in use (Figs. 38.33 and 38.34). To prevent personnel inadvertently entering the OR during laser surgery, the doors may be automatically locked when the OR is in laser mode (Fig. 38.35). Extra goggles should be available for personnel entering the OR.

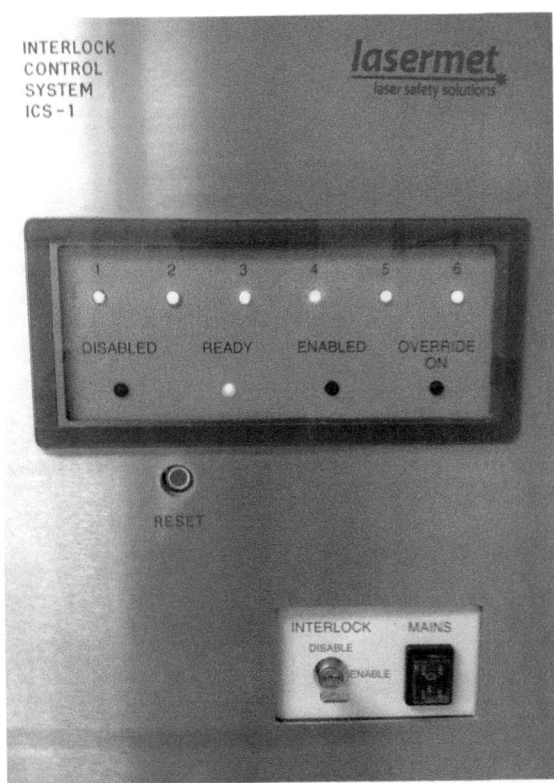

• **Fig. 38.35** An Interlock Control System in the operating room prevents entry during laser use. When these systems are engaged, operating room doors are locked automatically.

Fire Triad

Fires require three components (i.e., fire triad): a fuel source, an oxidant source, and an ignition source. A fuel source includes flammable material, such as ETTs, gauze, sponges, drapes, towels, volatile anesthetics, masks, nasal cannulas, suction catheters, gloves, gowns, endoscopes, and any material that may burn in the presence of an oxidant-rich atmosphere. The only exception is stainless steel. An oxidant-rich atmosphere exists within closed breathing circuits when high concentrations of oxygen or nitrous oxide are present, and this increases the chances of an airway fire. An oxidant-rich atmosphere also can occur under drapes or masks and can increase the likelihood of a fire. Any high-energy source has the potential to ignite a fire.

During laser airway surgery, the laser is the ignition source. Other ignition sources include electrocautery devices, scope cables, light cables, defibrillator pads, heated probes, and drills.

The high energy of the laser and its potential for combustion can cause an airway fire when the surgical field is near to the airway (Fig. 38.36). When a laser strikes the unprotected external surface of a tracheal tube during laser airway surgery, the surface starts to disintegrate and can catch fire. If the fire is not recognized and the laser continues to be applied, it can produce a hole in the tracheal tube and expose the burning surface to the oxidant-rich gas within the anesthesia system. At this stage, an explosive blowtorch-like fire may occur and rapidly spread in a distal and proximal manner. Any airway fire is a life-threatening complication, but the blowtorch fire is especially feared (Fig. 38.37).

If the cuff of an ETT is punctured, the oxidant-rich gas within the circuit becomes exposed to the external surface of the ETT, and the risk of an airway fire, including a blowtorch fire, is increased significantly. Examination of an ETT after a

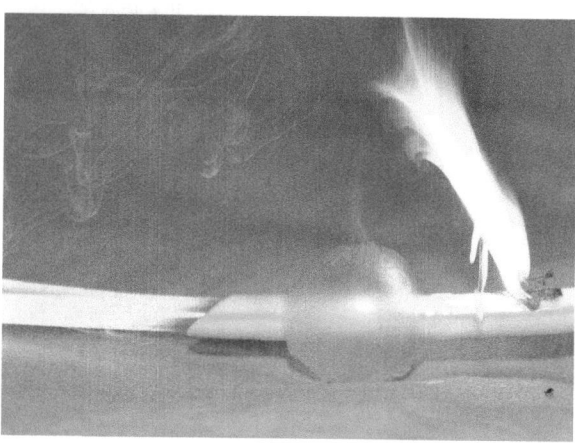

• **Fig. 38.36** An airway fire results when a laser strikes the polyvinyl chloride endotracheal tube (ETT).

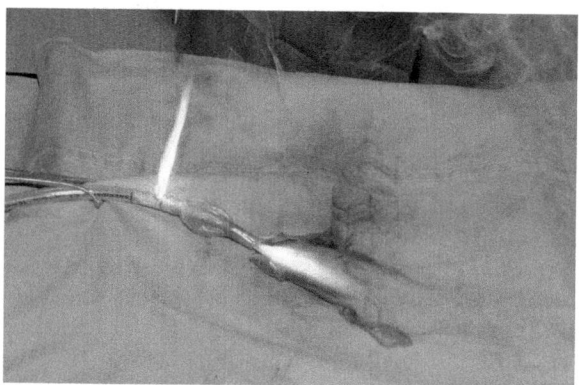

• **Fig. 38.37** Continued laser application can produce a hole in the tracheal tube and expose the burning surface to the oxidant-rich gas within the anesthesia system, producing a blowtorch airway fire.

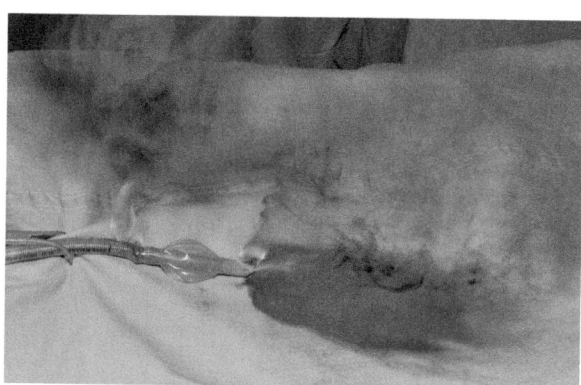

• **Fig. 38.38** Smoke, molten material, and other particulate material spread out after an airway fire.

blowtorch laser fire reveals total or near-total destruction of the ETT, with molten material, smoke, and other particulate material spreading out from the distal end of the tube (Figs. 38.38 and 38.39).

It is thought that OR fires are underreported and that 100 to 200 OR fires probably occur in the United States each year. Of the reported fires, 20% result in serious injury to the patient. One or two deaths per year are caused by airway fires.[237]

Preventing Airway Fires

The risk of an airway fire during laser airway surgery depends on the many factors that affect the three components of the fire triad. The first component is the fuel source, and the most common fuel source is the ETT. Attempts have been made to reduce the risks of a fire by covering the tube shaft with metal foil or with laser-protective coatings to protect it, adding saline to the tube cuff, and developing specially manufactured laser tubes suitable for laser airway surgery.

The second component is the oxidant source. An understanding of the effect of anesthetic gases on tracheal tube flammability is required, as well as an appreciation of the flammability limits of potent inhaled anesthetics.

The third component is the ignition source. The type of laser used, the laser operation mode (continuous vs pulsed), the power settings and the lasing time should all be taken into consideration in assessing and mitigating the risk of airway fire.

Fuel Source Considerations

Special Endotracheal Tubes for Laser Airway Surgery

"Laser proof" implies that irrespective of the oxidant environment and the power of the laser, the ETT cannot catch fire. With a laser-proof ETT, a continuous laser strike with extremely high power in a 100% oxygen environment does not produce a fire of the tube. Only one laser-proof tracheal tube (Norton) has been designed.[238]

All other manufactured ETTs for laser airway surgery are "laser resistant." Laser-resistant tubes provide some degree of protection against a laser strike, but these tubes vary in their materials, protective coating, relative size, and number of cuffs used. Any laser-resistant tube can result in an airway fire or blowtorch fire (Fig. 38.40) if it is used outside of its limits, such as a laser strike on an unprotected area on the distal tube shaft, at the unprotected proximal part of the shaft, or at the cuff itself. The anesthesia provider should appreciate the maximum power settings for which a laser-resistant tube has been tested, the range within which ignition does not occur, and the effect the oxidant environment has on the laser resistance characteristics. All laser-resistant tubes are not laser proof, and they must not be used outside of their limits.

Oxidant Source Considerations

Effect of Anesthetic Gases on Endotracheal Tube Flammability

The anesthetic gases used during airway laser surgery can profoundly influence combustibility. Oxygen and nitrous oxide support combustion very well. Helium and nitrogen are inert gases, and when added to oxygen, they can delay ETT flammability.[239] In clinical practice, administration of air and oxygen is most frequently used during laser airway surgery, and nitrous oxide should be avoided.

The oxygen concentration should be kept as low as clinically feasible while the laser is in proximity to the tube.

Management of an Airway Fire

Many factors must be considered when an airway fire occurs. All OR personnel must be prepared for the possibility of an airway fire during laser endoscopic surgery. If an airway fire occurs, sterile isotonic saline or water should be immediately available

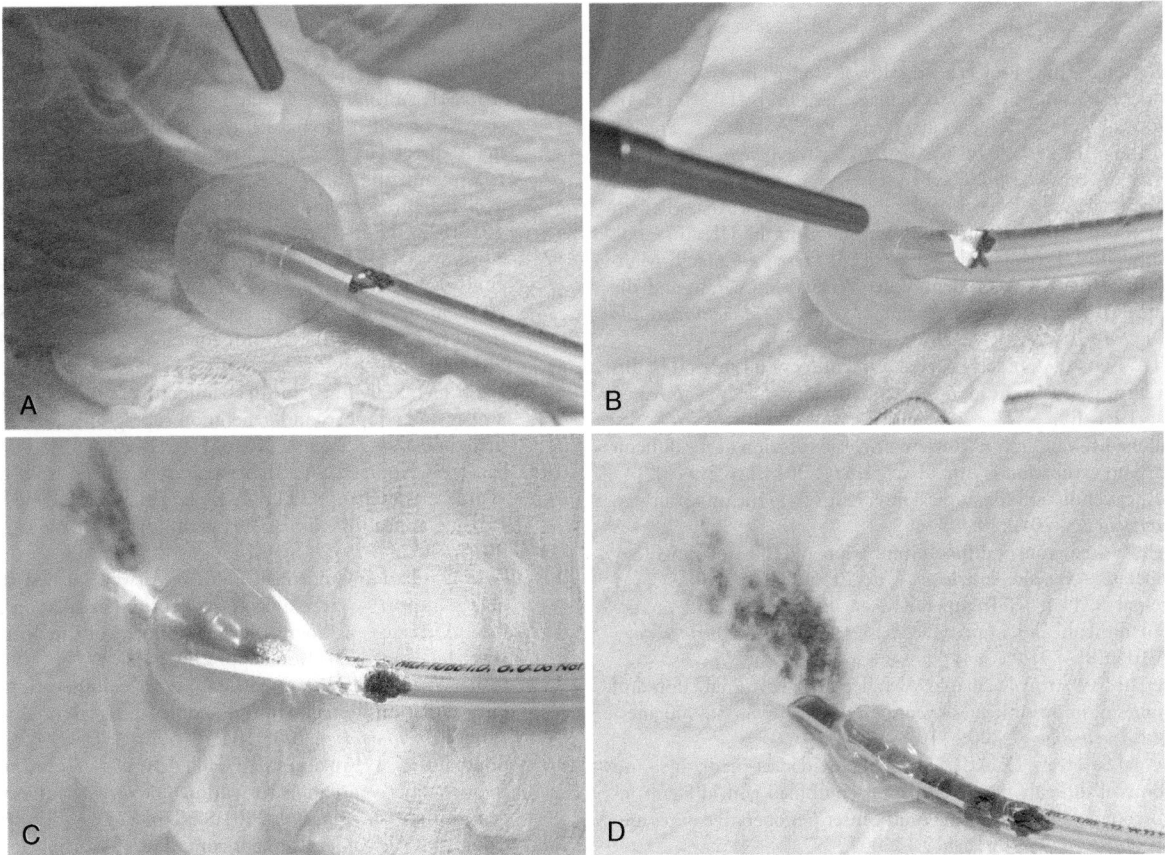

• **Fig. 38.39** A laser striking the polyvinyl chloride endotracheal tube (ETT) created an airway fire. (A) Smoke emerges from the outer shaft of the ETT after a continuous laser strike. (B) The outer surface glows orange. (C) After perforation into the inner aspect of the ETT in the presence of 100% oxygen flow, flames emerge from the puncture site and distal ETT. (D) After the fire is extinguished, damage to the ETT and material spreading out from its distal end can be seen.

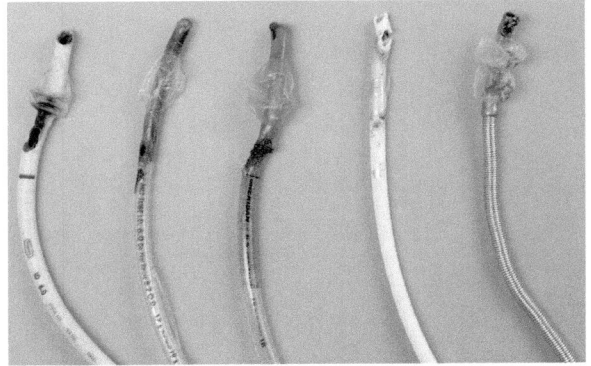

• **Fig. 38.40** Laser-induced fire damage to endotracheal tubes (ETTs). Left to right, the first three are standard nonlaser polyvinyl chloride ETTs, and all three have been damaged by an airway fire. The two ETTs on the right are designed for laser use. Both tubes have sustained fire damage in their unprotected areas distal to the cuff by high-energy, sustained CO_2 laser strikes to the ETTs with 100% oxygen passing through them.

in a 30- or 60-mL syringe. Another laser and polyvinyl chloride (PVC) ETT should be available. A plan of action should be rehearsed by OR personnel so that rapid action can be taken. (See the American Society of Anesthesia Providers Practice Advisory for the Prevention and Management of Operating Room Fires.[240])

An understanding of the fire triad and the steps that can be taken to avoid a fire is an essential requirement before undertaking laser airway surgery. General laser hazards include eye and skin injury, drape fires, and laser plumes. Airway fires occur when a laser strikes the unprotected surface of a tracheal tube or any other material within the airway that acts as a fuel source. Any high-energy source, such as diathermy, can act as an ignition source and can result in an explosive blowtorch fire.

Conclusion

The airway challenges in H&N anesthesia will continue to grow because of increasing complexity of the surgical procedures and improved patient survival. Airway management in H&N surgery demands a truly comprehensive approach. It should suit the patient and clinical situation, involve good understanding of the disease process, and require sound clinical judgment and a wide range of advanced airway skills.

Achieving favorable patient outcomes frequently depends on the close working relationship between the anesthesia provider and H&N surgeon. A lack of mutual collaboration and planning can turn even a routine case into a chaotic, life-threatening airway crisis. As anesthetic challenges continue to grow, so will the demand for a wide range of unique skills and expertise from the anesthesia provider to ensure patient safety and favorable surgical outcomes.

Selected References

1. 4th National Audit Project of the Royal College of Anaesthetists. Major complications of airway management in the UK. In: Cook T, Woodall N, Frerk C, eds. Chapter 18. Patel A, Pearce A, Pracy P. Head and Neck Pathology. *The Royal College of Anaesthetists and the Difficult Airway Society.* 2011;143–154.

2. 4th National Audit Project of the Royal College of Anaesthetists. Major complications of airway management in the UK. In: Cook T, Woodall N, Frerk C, eds. Chapter 13. Frerk C, Cook T. Management of the 'Can't Intubate Can't Ventilate' Situation and the Emergency Surgical Airway. *The Royal College of Anaesthetists and the Difficult Airway Society.* 2011;105–113.

4. Iseli TA, Iseli CE, Golden JB, et al. Outcomes of intubation in difficult airways due to head and neck pathology. *Ear Nose Throat J.* 2012;91:E1–E5.

11. Cavallone LF, Vannucci A. Review article: extubation of the difficult airway and extubation failure. *Anesth Analg.* 2013;116:368–383.

19. Biro P. Jet ventilation for surgical interventions in the upper airway. *Anesthesiol Clin.* 2010;28:397–409.

33. O'Dell K. Predictors of difficult intubation and the otolaryngology perioperative consult. *Anesthesiol Clin.* 2015;33:279–290.

37. Kheterpal S, Han R, Tremper KK, et al. Incidence and predictors of difficult and impossible mask ventilation. *Anesthesiology.* 2006;105:885–891.

38. Kheterpal S, Martin L, Shanks AM, Tremper KK. Prediction and outcomes of impossible mask ventilation: a review of 50,000 anesthetics. *Anesthesiology.* 2009;110:891–897.

39. Kheterpal S, Healy D, Aziz MF, et al. Incidence, predictors, and outcome of difficult mask ventilation combined with difficult laryngoscopy: a report from the multicenter perioperative outcomes group. *Anesthesiology.* 2013;119:1360–1369.

42. Mason RA, Fielder CP. The obstructed airway in head and neck surgery. *Anaesthesia.* 1999;54:625–628.

45. Xiao P, Zhang XS. Adult laryngotracheal surgery. *Anesthesiol Clin.* 2010;28:529–540.

49. Woodall N, Frerk C, Cook TM. Can we make airway management (even) safer? - lessons from national audit. *Anaesthesia.* 2011;66(suppl 2):27–33.

62. Aziz MF, Abrons RO, Cattano D, et al. First-attempt intubation success of video laryngoscopy in patients with anticipated difficult direct laryngoscopy: a multicenter randomized controlled trial comparing the C-MAC D-Blade versus the GlideScope in a mixed provider and diverse patient population. *Anesth Analg.* 2016;122(3):740–750.

71. Nørskov AK, Rosenstock CV, Wetterslev J, et al. Diagnostic accuracy of anaesthesiologists' prediction of difficult airway management in daily clinical practice: a cohort study of 188,064 patients registered in the Danish Anaesthesia Database. *Anaesthesia.* 2015;70:272–281.

95. Cook TM, Kelly FE. Time to abandon the "vintage" laryngeal mask airway and adopt second-generation supraglottic airway devices as first choice. *Br J Anaesth.* 2015;115:497–499.

108. Patel A, Nouraei SA. Transnasal humidified rapid-insufflation ventilatory exchange (THRIVE): a physiological method of increasing apnea time in patients with difficult airways. *Anaesthesia.* 2015;70:323–329.

116. DAS Extubation Guidelines. Difficult Airway Society; 2018. Available at https://www.das.uk.com/content/das-extubation-guidelines.

157. Patel A, Pearce A. Progress in management of the obstructed airway. *Anaesthesia.* 2011;66(suppl 2):93–100.

159. Jaquet Y, Monnier P, Van Melle G, et al. Complications of different ventilation strategies in endoscopic laryngeal surgery: a 10-year review. *Anesthesiology.* 2006;104:52–59.

163. Bourgain JL, Desruennes E, Fischler M, et al. Transtracheal high frequency jet ventilation for endoscopic airway surgery: a multicentre study. *Br J Anaesth.* 2001;87:870–875.

206. Cook TM, Alexander R. Major complications during anesthesia for elective laryngeal surgery in the UK: a national survey of the use of high-pressure source ventilation. *Br J Anaesth.* 2008;101:266–272.

All references can be found online at eBooks.Health.Elsevier.com.

39

Airway Management in Neurosurgical Patients

IRENE P. OSBORN, ROBERT NARUSE, AND HAITHAM IBRAHIM

KEY POINTS

- In addition to airway assessment, neurologic examination and communication with the surgeon is invaluable before the induction of anesthesia for neurosurgical procedures.
- Patients with an unstable cervical spine may be unable to cooperate with an awake flexible scope intubation (FSI) because of intoxication, hypoxia, or head injury. The need for a cervical spine injury (CSI) patient's airway to be secured is often urgent because of the CSI or associated head or facial injury.
- A rigid cervical collar may make airway management difficult, impeding mouth opening and application of cricoid pressure. Therefore with manual in-line immobilization in place, the front part of the collar should be removed or opened before attempted intubation.
- Patients with acromegaly frequently have obstructive sleep apnea and should be induced and ventilated with caution.

- Direct laryngoscopy and video-assisted laryngoscopy (VAL) are the most effective intubation techniques.
- Elective patients who demonstrate neurologic symptoms of the extremities with neck flexion or extension should have awake, topicalized tracheal intubation.
- Become familiar with alternative airway devices and practice in normal airways before treating patients with difficult airways.
- Be attentive and inspect the degree of neck flexion in patients positioned prone, lateral, or in any head fixation device.
- A cuff leak test may be helpful before extubation after prolonged surgery in the prone position; always have reintubation strategies and plans. Consider trial extubation over an airway exchange catheter.

Introduction

Airway management in the neurosurgical patient can be a challenging endeavor. In achieving and maintaining a patent airway it is important to consider its impact on the central nervous system (CNS) and the well-being of the patient. The variety of neurosurgical procedures, anesthetic techniques, and airway devices has increased dramatically over the past decade. The evolution of neurosurgical practice and the growth of complex spine surgery provide a myriad of clinical challenges.

The goal of this chapter is to address issues specific to the dedicated neuroanesthesiologist, as well as those related to the neurosurgical patient that might be encountered by the generalist anesthesia provider. This discussion reflects the ever-changing considerations in the airway management of neurosurgical patients and offers solutions to common clinical problems that may occur.

The Neurosurgical Patient

The American Academy of Neurological Surgeons (AANS) estimates that almost 1 million neurosurgical procedures are performed annually in the United States. Spine procedures are performed at three times the rate of cranial surgeries.[1] When considering the range of potential neurosurgical procedures, the variety of patient pathophysiology is substantial. A patient presenting for neurosurgery may appear to be completely normal or can present with clinical symptoms of intracranial hypertension. The airway might be assessed as "normal," but the patient's head is fixed in a frame. Also, the patient may present with acromegaly for pituitary surgery or may have a previous history of difficult intubation (DI). Additionally, the unanticipated difficult airway becomes an even greater challenge in patients at risk for cerebral aneurysm rupture. Other challenges include the spine surgery patient in the prone position and considerations for extubation after prolonged surgery. Patients with CNS disease can be sensitive to the effects of hypnotic agents, rendering them susceptible to apnea when premedication is given. These are just a few examples of challenges that will be further addressed in this chapter.

Although neurosurgical procedures comprise only 7% of cases in the American Society of Anesthesiologists (ASA) closed-claims database, they are associated with settlements that are 1.6 to 4 times more than general surgical procedures.[2] Understanding the patient's physiologic requirements, in addition to the surgeon's plan, is extremely important in these patients. It is wise to have a number of techniques for achieving, maintaining, and rescuing the neurosurgical airway.

Intracranial Dynamics and the Airway

Intracranial pressure (ICP) is the pressure within the rigid skull. Airway management in the face of intracranial hypertension is a frequent challenge for the neuroanesthesiologist, neurointensivist, and emergency physician. The patient who does not require immediate airway control may benefit from the simple maneuver of elevating the head. The head-up position may have beneficial effects on ICP through changes in airway pressure, central venous pressure, and cerebrospinal fluid displacement.[3] Cerebral perfusion pressure (CPP) is the effective perfusion pressure driving blood through the brain, defined as the difference between mean arterial pressure (MAP) and ICPs (CPP = MAP – ICP). A frequent consideration in the neurosurgical patient is the need to balance and maintain intracranial dynamics, avoiding increases in ICP, yet maintaining cerebral perfusion.

Laryngoscopy and intubation, if performed with difficulty or improperly, can severely compromise intracranial dynamics and increase morbidity. Both the sympathetic and the parasympathetic nervous systems mediate cardiovascular responses to tracheal intubation.[4] Acute increases in ICP and MAP during laryngoscopy and tracheal intubation have been well documented.[5] In 1975 Burney and Winn[6] measured ICP in 12 patients undergoing craniotomy and 2 patients for carotid arteriography. ICP did not change in response to the injection of contrast medium but increased significantly and dramatically in response to laryngoscopy and intubation. The increase appeared related to the initial ICP of these patients, possibly representing exhaustion of compensatory mechanisms. Special attention must be given to this factor during manipulation of the larynx in neurosurgical patients with initially increased ICP or space-occupying intracranial lesions.

Techniques to blunt this sympathetic response include (1) an additional dose of opioids or propofol; (2) the use of beta-blockers or other antihypertensive agents; and (3) the use of intravenous (IV) lidocaine. Esmolol or lidocaine as an IV bolus of 1.5 mg/kg before laryngoscopy and intubation does not completely prevent the increase in MAP and ICP.[7,8] Etomidate has been shown to cause an early "burst suppression" pattern on the electroencephalogram (EEG), minimal changes in CPP, and a marked reduction in ICP. This decrease in ICP is maintained during the first 30 seconds and the following 60 seconds after intubation, as MAP and heart rate remain unchanged.[9] Although not practical, this approach demonstrates the extent of efforts often made to obtund this response. Numerous methods have been advocated to prevent undesirable cardiovascular disturbances at intubation.[10] Whereas the cardiovascular response can be dramatic and substantial, the ICP response may lag and persist longer. Once the patient is intubated, ventilation parameters may be adjusted to the clinical situation.

Clinical Strategies for the Neurosurgical Patient

Airway assessment of the neurosurgical patient requires similar considerations, as described in other chapters of this textbook. The patient who has undergone previous surgery and has a history of DI warrants particular attention. A review of the anesthetic record should reveal which techniques produced success or failure. Difficult mask ventilation is of particular concern because of the potential for causing hypercarbia and the detrimental changes previously described.

Patient for Craniotomy

Patients who are neurologically intact may demonstrate no evidence of intracranial pathology or alteration. In addition to the history and physical examination, preoperative computed tomography (CT) or magnetic resonance imaging (MRI) scans of the head may give valuable information, because lesions associated with greater than 10 mm in midline shift or cerebral edema usually indicate intracranial hypertension.[11] These patients should be appropriately managed to avoid undue increases in ICP and cerebral blood flow (CBF). Such measures include proper head positioning, preoxygenation, and appropriate dosing of induction agents and relaxants to achieve a smooth intubation. The primary challenge in anesthetizing a patient with a supratentorial mass lesion is to avoid further increases in ICP when one has limited intracranial compliance. There is no "ideal anesthetic" for this group of patients, and the perioperative management should be individualized. However, the practitioner should be aware of the effects of anesthetic agents on intracranial dynamics.

The preoperative use of midazolam for anxiety in these patients should not cause harm if they are carefully observed. A 1- to 2-mg dose of IV midazolam in adult patients may facilitate the induction of anesthesia without altering intracranial dynamics.[12] Opioids, on the other hand, should be restricted to very small amounts and given preoperatively under constant supervision because of possible hypercarbia and resultant effects. The efficacy was recognized early on as a technique for avoiding intracranial hypertension.[13] In the 1980s deep inhalation anesthesia was replaced by a combination of IV induction agents, notably thiopental, in combination with fentanyl. Barbiturates, methohexital and pentobarbital, produce a dose-dependent reduction in CBF and cerebral metabolic rate of oxygen ($CMRo_2$) consumption. ICP is reduced by barbiturates, likely because of the reduction in CBF and cerebral blood volume (CBV). Propofol has replaced thiopental (no longer manufactured in the United States) as the induction agent of choice for neuroanesthesia. Despite initial concerns about decreasing MAP and CPP, propofol provides a smooth transition to unconsciousness without an increase in heart rate, as observed with thiopental. This often produces less hypertension with laryngoscopy and intubation.[14]

Clinical doses of most opioids have minimal to modest depressive effects on CBF and $CMRo_2$. Early studies demonstrate that ICP is either not elevated or slightly decreased with fentanyl alone or in combination with droperidol. Reported ICP increases in patients with space-occupying lesions have been attributed to hypercapnia. The variability in response to opioids appears to be caused by the background anesthetic. When vasodilating drugs are used as part of the anesthetic management, the effect of the opioid is consistently that of a vasoconstrictor. Sufentanil was thought to produce an increase in ICP in patients with intracranial mass effect, but this was later attributed to a decrease in MAP.[15] Alfentanil produces little change or a slight decrease in CBF.[16] The beneficial effect of synthetic opioids is their ability to blunt the hemodynamic response to laryngoscopy and intubation without affecting intracranial dynamics. Remifentanil produces the most profound and consistent response, with a lack of hypertension, tachycardia, or an increase in ICP.[17] A continuous infusion throughout induction may provide the most effective hemodynamic control, while adequate ventilation is maintained.

The volatile agents, including nitrous oxide, can be considered dose-dependent cerebral vasodilators.[18] As a component of neuroanesthesia, volatile agents are typically used in moderate doses, in combination. Their effects on cerebral circulation and metabolism of sevoflurane and desflurane are largely comparable to isoflurane. Both induce a direct vasodilation of the cerebral vessels, resulting in a less pronounced increase in CBF, compared with the decrease in cerebral metabolism.

Induction may be followed by ventilation with a volatile agent to deepen the anesthetic, decrease $CMRo_2$ (and CBF), and provide bronchodilation in patients with asthma or chronic obstructive pulmonary disease (COPD). Sevoflurane is useful in both pediatric and adult patients by allowing inhalation induction without the adverse effects of coughing or breath-holding.[19] A frequently employed technique in the cooperative patient is the use of active hyperventilation before induction to initiate hypocapnia and decrease CBF as the patient loses consciousness. The use of topical anesthesia applied to the larynx and trachea can also prevent further response to laryngoscopy and intubation.[20] The large number of techniques recommended to suppress cardiovascular responses indicates that no single method has gained widespread acceptance (Table 39.1).

The obtunded patient with symptoms of intracranial hypertension requires additional attention to detail, avoiding premedication and maneuvers that increase coughing. If a rapid sequence induction is not indicated and the patient's airway anatomy is adequate for laryngoscopy, anesthetic induction may proceed with voluntary hyperventilation with 100% oxygen by mask, if possible. After loss of consciousness, manual hyperventilation should occur both before and after the administration of muscle relaxant. Opioid administration may begin at this time to prevent the sympathetic response to laryngoscopy. IV lidocaine (1 mg/kg) may be administered to blunt the hemodynamic and ICP response to laryngoscopy. Alternatively, a beta-blocker or an additional dose of propofol may be given. Esmolol or lidocaine, 1.5 mg/kg as an IV bolus before laryngoscopy and intubation, does not completely prevent the increase in MAP and ICP.[21] Complete neuromuscular blockade should be verified before laryngoscopy to prevent cough and associated increases in ICP. Proper airway management is

TABLE 39.1	Anesthetic Techniques to Avoid Increased Intracranial Pressure	
Technique	**Precaution(s)**
Avoid hypercapnia	Be vigilant of patient's respiratory status. Avoid undue sedation.
Avoid hypoxia	Supplemental oxygen use is mandatory. Be vigilant of patient's respiratory status. Take precautions to avoid aspiration. Use preoxygenation before induction of anesthesia or tracheal intubation.
Avoid marked hypertension	Be vigilant to changes in degree of painful stimulation. Ensure adequate depth of anesthesia before intubation attempts or surgical/procedural attempts.
Avoid severe neck rotation	Attempt to maintain neck in neutral position. Be vigilant to head positioning of patient during surgery.
Avoid compression of jugular veins	Consider avoiding internal jugular neck lines when possible.
Elevate head	If backup position is not possible, use reverse Trendelenburg (avoid hypotension).
Decrease blood viscosity and intracerebral vascular volume	Avoid rapid infusion of mannitol, which may paradoxically increase intracranial pressure.
Avoid sustained increases in intrathoracic pressure	Use maneuvers or pharmacologic agents to avoid bucking, movement, and vomiting. Avoid high ventilatory pressures when possible. Avoid excessive PEEP when possible.
Avoid cerebral venodilators	Consider beta-blocker use to treat hypertension. Consider calcium channel blockers. Avoid nitroglycerine and nitroprusside, if possible.

PEEP, Positive end-expiratory pressure.

essential to avoid the dual threat of hypoxia and hypercarbia. An obstructed airway may also lead to a rise in intrathoracic pressure. This may produce an elevated venous pressure, increased intracranial blood volume, and elevated ICP. If the patient can be mask ventilated but intubation is difficult, one may choose to proceed with video-assisted laryngoscopy (VAL) or another alternative device to facilitate intubation.

The intubating laryngeal mask airway (ILMA) is particularly useful in the failed intubation sequence, and the ability to ventilate is extremely important in neurosurgical patients. The success of the ILMA as a ventilatory device has been well established, as demonstrated in several of the early evaluation studies.[22,23] While it is used less often with the availability of VAL, it remains very useful in the setting of a failed flexible scope intubation (FSI).[24]

The patient for aneurysm surgery who presents with a difficult airway is particularly problematic. If the airway is anticipated or known to be difficult, FSI is often the method of choice. This is assuming that one is skillful in using the flexible intubation scope (FIS) and is prepared to perform this technique in the awake, cooperative patient (see Chapter 25). IV fentanyl and midazolam may be carefully administered if the patient does not exhibit signs of intracranial hypertension. An arterial line is sometimes placed before induction for careful monitoring. Additional techniques include remifentanil infusion (0.05 μg/kg/min) or dexmedetomidine infusion.[25,26] Both techniques require careful patient monitoring and may be useful. Once the glottis is viewed, a dose of lidocaine may be given via the FIS to prevent coughing and "bucking" with intubation.

Alternative techniques for failed sedation or topicalization include awake placement of the ILMA or other techniques that do not produce excessive hemodynamic responses. The concomitant administration of beta-blockers or vasodilators may be necessary for blood pressure control. Essentially, the ASA Difficult Airway Management Algorithm should be followed with close monitoring of blood pressure and heart rate at all times until the airway is secured.

Head-Injured Patient

Traumatic brain injury (TBI) remains a prevalent problem in the United States and the world. The incidence of TBI is 175 to 300 per 100,000 population and accounts for 56,000 deaths per year in the United States.[27] With the increased use of seatbelts, motor vehicle accidents are now secondary to gunshot wounds as the leading cause of TBI. Early intubation of the head-injured patient is critical and is often established in the field if providers are so trained. It is essential for the optimal management of the patient, providing for efficient ventilation and oxygenation, helping to prevent aspiration of gastric contents, and allowing for suction of the lungs and pulmonary toilet. However, patients who are unconscious and breathing adequately may be transported with oxygen by mask throughout their initial assessment. This is intuitive in the apneic and unresponsive patient with a Glasgow Coma Scale (GCS) score of 8 or less.

The provider caring for the patient with TBI must understand that although primary mechanisms of injury (primary insults) are a large determinant of patient outcome, attention to secondary insults, such as hypoxia, hypotension, intracranial hypertension, and decreased CPP, can impact morbidity, mortality, and quality of life of the TBI patient.[28] Evidence supports the impact of secondary harm, with mortality from TBI nationally decreasing over the decades.[29] Hypoxia in TBI patients is a frequent occurrence, particularly in the prehospital setting. Interestingly, hypoxia was

identified in 44% of patients with TBI on arrival in the emergency department.[30] Similarly, Jeremitsky and colleagues[31] report that hypoxia is one of three predictors of mortality in adult brain-injured patients (with hypothermia and hypoperfusion). Hypoxia dramatically impacts morbidity and mortality in TBI, and hypercapnia further increases mortality.

Hypotension is the secondary insult that has been most frequently cited as contributing to poor outcome after TBI. Hypotension is independently related to mortality in multivariate analysis.[32] Information from the Traumatic Coma Data Bank demonstrates that a systolic blood pressure of less than 80 mm Hg was one of five factors that worsened patient outcome at 6 months. Hypotension during any phase in the brain trauma patient's hospital course is associated with a greater likelihood of severe disability and vegetative state. However, early in the course of brain trauma, especially when combined with hypoxia, hypotension is devastating. When hypotension and hypoxia occur together, mortality is 75%.[33]

Techniques minimizing head movement should be used in TBI patients and by the most skilled clinicians. However, concern about a cervical fracture should never take precedence over relieving hypoxemia. It is of critical importance to ensure that appropriate monitoring is present throughout airway maneuvers. Nasal intubation should be avoided in head-injured patients, particularly in those with known or suspected basilar skull fractures and sinus injuries. Alternative airway devices, such as video laryngoscopes, any of the indirect rigid laryngoscopes, ILMA, or optical stylets, may be useful when the head must remain immobilized.[34] Most emergency patients are assumed to have a full stomach, so it is important to weigh the risk of aspiration, which is a potential problem during laryngoscopy and intubation. If the situation warrants, surgeons should be prepared to perform a rapid cricothyrotomy, if intubation attempts fail and ventilation becomes impossible.

Patient With Cervical Spine Disease

Management of Acute Injury and the Unstable Spine

Spinal injuries occur in approximately 13% to 30% of polytrauma patients, and cervical spine injury (CSI) represents about 0.9% to 3% of all polytrauma patients.[35,36] The relative risk of CSI is increased in the presence of severe head injury by a factor greater than 8.[37] In the United States cervical trauma has an incidence of approximately 5 per 10,000 population annually, making up 4% of all blunt trauma. In trauma victims with a GCS score of 13 to 15 the incidence of CSI is 1.4%, but this rises dramatically to 10.2% if the GCS score is less than 8. It is of vital importance to capture all injuries in the unconscious polytrauma patient within an emergent time frame. If a CSI is missed or its detection delayed, the incidence of secondary neurologic deficit increases from 1.4% to 10.5%. For this reason, the Advanced Trauma Life Support (ATLS) protocol was created and is updated and broadly followed in most trauma centers. When a diagnosis of CSI is delayed, almost one-third of patients may develop permanent neurologic deficit.[38] One of the areas of controversy is how to best "clear" the cervical spine in the trauma patient. The detection of CSI requires a variety of modalities that vary in sensitivity, including clinical evaluation, plain radiography, CT, MRI, and dynamic fluoroscopy.

Clinical Evaluation

To clear the cervical spine clinically, the following criteria must be met:

1. GCS score of 15, with the patient alert and oriented
2. Absence of injuries that may draw attention away from a CSI
3. Absence of drugs or intoxicants that may interfere with the patient's sensorium
4. Absence of signs or symptoms on examining the neck, specifically:
    a. No midline pain or tenderness
    b. Full range of active movement
    c. No neurologic deficit attributable to the cervical spine

Clearly, there will be only a small number of trauma patients who fulfill these criteria.

Plain Radiography

The cross-table lateral view alone, even if technically adequate and interpreted by an expert, will still miss 15% of cervical injuries. Of cross-table lateral films taken in emergency rooms, approximately a quarter of the films are anatomically inadequate, necessitating further imaging modalities for evaluation, usually of the cervicothoracic junction. A three-view cervical series includes the cross-table lateral view, open-mouth odontoid view, and anteroposterior (AP) view (Figs. 39.1–39.3). Using these views, the sensitivity increases to detect 90% of those with an actual injury. Again, anywhere from 25% to 50% of these series may be inadequate anatomically. In low-risk patients plain radiography is an efficient diagnostic examination with a specificity of 100%. In high-risk patients plain radiography is a good adjunctive screening test in conjunction with a CT scan, with a sensitivity of 93.3% and specificity of 95%.

Computed Tomography

CT scanning, either of the entire cervical spine or directed at areas missed by plain radiographs, provides a complementary approach

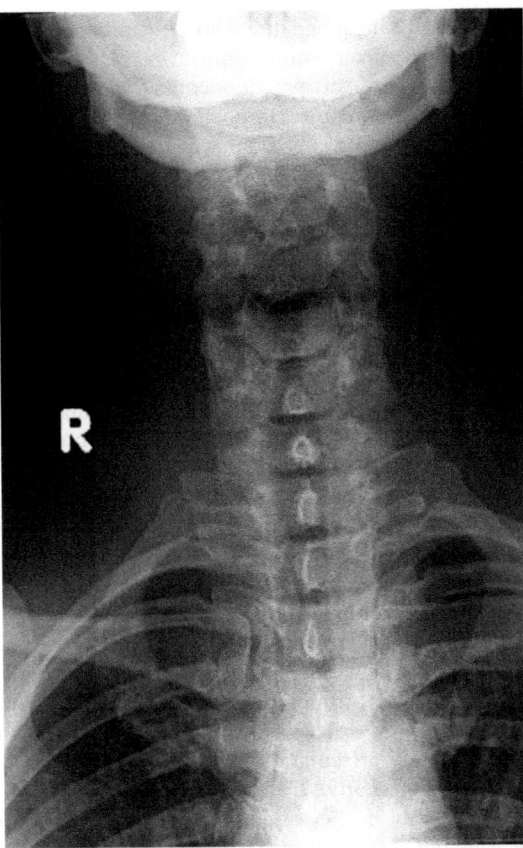

• **Fig. 39.2** Normal anteroposterior cervical spine x-ray view. (Courtesy Prasanna Vibhute, MD, USA, Department of Radiology, Mount Sinai Medical Center.)

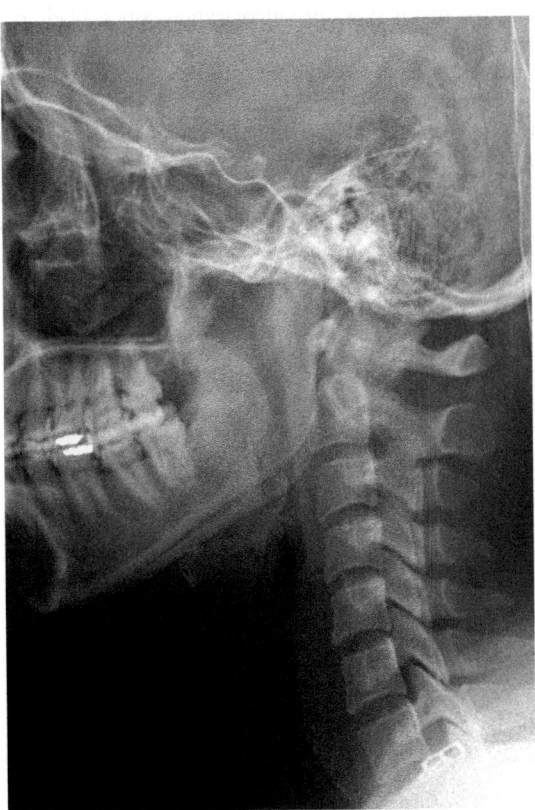

• **Fig. 39.1** Normal lateral cervical x-ray view. (Courtesy Prasanna Vibhute, MD, USA, Department of Radiology, Mount Sinai Medical Center.)

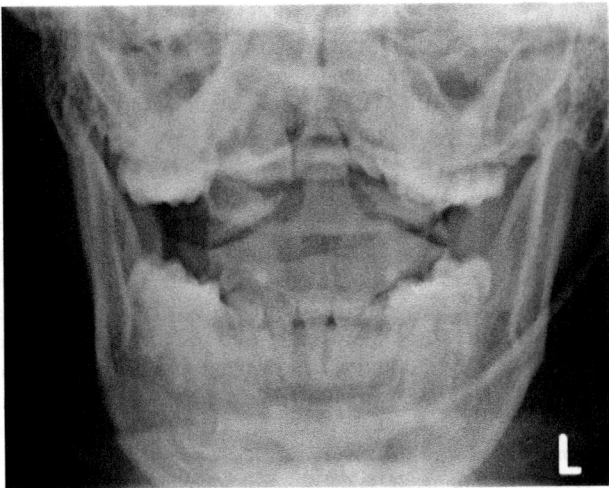

• **Fig. 39.3** Normal odontoid cervical spine x-ray view. (Courtesy Prasanna Vibhute, MD, USA, Department of Radiology, Mount Sinai Medical Center.)

when used in addition to the three-view cervical series, reducing the risk of missing a CSI to less than 1%. In the evaluation of the cervical spine a helical CT scan has higher sensitivity and specificity than plain radiographs in the moderate-risk and high-risk trauma population, but it is more costly. In fact, a helical CT scan is the preferred initial screening test for the detection of cervical spine fractures among moderate-risk to high-risk patients seen in urban trauma centers, reducing the incidence of paralysis resulting from false-negative imaging studies and institutional costs when settlement costs are taken into account.[39]

Intubation. The airway practitioner may be confronted with a patient with CSI who requires intubation. In one case series 26% of patients admitted to a large trauma center required intubation over the first day of admission. Furthermore, a growing body of literature indicates that any patient with a CSI above C5 should be intubated electively, early during the presentation.[40] Because all maneuvers that are typically performed to facilitate airway management produce some degree of cervical motion, the major concern during the acute care of patients with potential CSI is the avoidance of further deterioration of the neurologic function. Therefore independent of the technique chosen to secure the airway, it is crucial to preserve spinal stability by maintaining physiologic spinal alignment and establishing early immobilization of the spine. Techniques to provide cervical spine immobilization include sandbag-tape immobilization and cervical collars of various consistency.[41] The same rationale is applied when the management of the airway is required in the patient with suspicious CSI. The goal is to achieve tracheal intubation with the least amount of cervical motion. Although thorough evaluation for respiratory failure is necessary, the current consensus is that early intubation is mandatory in patients with complete CSI, and evidence of respiratory failure should prompt immediate airway intervention.[42] The following survey reviews airway devices and assigns utility based on the clinical presentation of cervical injury (Box 39.1).

Direct Laryngoscopy. If performed appropriately, direct laryngoscopy is safe in the patient with CSI.[43–45] No neurologic sequelae were noted in a review of 73 patients with known cervical spine fractures intubated after rapid sequence induction with the application of cricoid pressure and manual in-line stabilization (MILS) of the head and neck and direct laryngoscopy.[46] When intubating the patient with direct laryngoscopy, the anterior portion of the hard cervical collar can be removed to facilitate the opening of the mouth at intubation.

As currently recommended by the ATLS protocol, direct laryngoscopy and VAL with MILS are most often performed and have been extensively investigated.[47]

The effects of direct laryngoscopy have been studied in a range of patients, including those with normal neck anatomy under anesthesia, as well as in cadavers with cervical lesions caused to simulate fractures at a variety of levels. In the anesthetized patient with normal cervical anatomy, using neuromuscular blockade and a 3 Macintosh blade, a variety of movements occur. On the elevation of the blade to obtain a view of the larynx, there is superior rotation of the occiput and C1 in the sagittal plane, C2 remains near neutral, and there is mild inferior rotation of C3–C5.[48] The most significant movement is produced at the atlantooccipital and atlantoaxial joints (Video 39.1).[49] In cadaveric models of unstable cervical segments (C1–C2) the movements associated with maneuvers such as chin lift and jaw thrust are greater than those produced by the intubation itself. The application of cricoid pressure produced no significant movement at the site of injury in these patients; however, this maneuver is performed less due to its potential to obstruct the laryngeal view.

Stabilization. In view of the risk of secondary neurologic injury, unstable cervical spine, to the acutely injured, it is widely viewed as the standard of care to stabilize the cervical spine when this is suspected. The most common measures include MILS, immobilization of the head between two sandbags, and placement of a rigid cervical collar and a spinal board. This management is itself associated with significant morbidity and mortality. It may

increase the difficulty of intubation or increase the likelihood of airway compromise and risk of aspiration. Nonetheless, the use of MILS is the best means to minimize the movement of the cervical spine during airway manipulations and should always be practiced. It should be recognized, however, that the presence of a cervical collar does not necessarily protect against movement at the occipitocervical and cervicothoracic junctions.

Significantly less movement was reported when the Miller straight blade was used compared with the Macintosh and the McCoy blades.[50] The worsening of the glottic view caused by MILS has been shown to increase the pressure applied by all direct laryngoscopy blades, potentially aggravating the pathologic craniocervical motion.[51]

The laryngoscopic pressure, which reflects a degree of difficulty in glottic visualization, can be significantly diminished by using video laryngoscopes, such as the Airtraq and the Pentax Airway Scope.[52,53] These channeled video laryngoscopes allow for indirect laryngoscopy and provide an optimal view of the glottis without the alignment of the oropharyngeal and orotracheal axes (Video 39.2). For these reasons, they have been successful in allowing tracheal intubation in the presence of cervical collars. The GlideScope is a widely used video laryngoscope with a record of success in cervical spine immobilization.[54,55] Using cinefluoroscopy, Robitaille and colleagues[56] found that the GlideScope did not produce less cervical spine movement than the Macintosh blade but did provide an improved laryngoscopic view and successful intubation (Fig. 39.4).

Video Asssisted Laryngoscopy. The most significant development in the last 20 years has been the introduction of VAL for intubation. The specifics and techniques for practice are described elsewhere in this book but its impact on airway management for cervical spine pathology is immense and reassuring. Currently, there are two major types of videolaryngoscopes: blade type and channel type. The blade-type scopes are more frequently used since the technique is more similar to direct laryngoscopy. Subsequent studies using the McGRATH MAC VL have yielded similar results with improved ability and success of intubation, particularly with MILS.[57]

Awake Intubation. In a cooperative patient awake FSI can be performed. One of the benefits of this technique is that it allows for the patient to be intubated without the movement of the cervical spine. It may be performed with a hard collar in place.

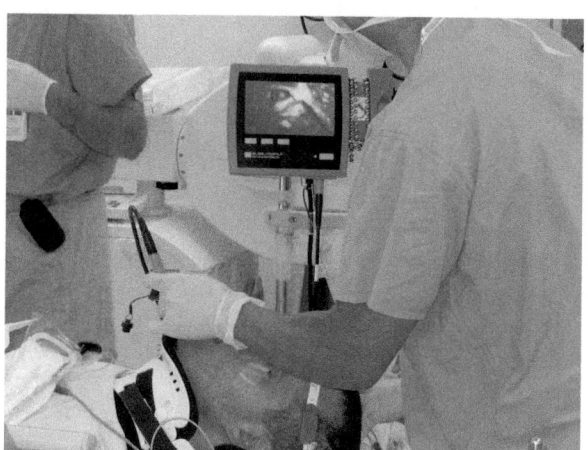

• **Fig. 39.4** Intubation using the GlideScope in a cervical collar. (Reproduced with permission from © Verathon Inc., Bothell, WA)

The patient's airway may be topicalized, but this may, in theory, increase the potential for aspiration in patients at risk for regurgitation and aspiration. However, Ovassapian and others found no evidence of aspiration in 105 patients at risk.[58] Awake FSI may prove to be time consuming and requires expert topicalization and operator skills for success. Because of the lack of assurance of expedient intubation and the risk of aspiration, we advocate that the FIS be used in the cooperative patient in an urgent situation and in the nonurgent patient who is not at risk of aspiration. This recommendation is a general guideline, and expertise with any given airway device must be considered when using an airway technique in a specific clinical situation.

Supplemental oxygen is recommended during FSI and high-flow nasal oxygen (Optiflow) during FSI may be useful in maintaining oxygenation in the sedated or obtunded patient and preventing arterial hypoxemia during intubation.[59]

Laryngeal Mask Airway. Another alternative to direct or videolaryngoscopy is the ILMA. Waltl and colleagues[60] reported that the ILMA produced less extension of the upper cervical spine than direct laryngoscopy.[61] Ferson and colleagues, in 254 difficult-to-manage airways, reported that 70 patients with acutely unstable necks were all successfully intubated with the ILMA, 92.6% on the first attempt and 7.4% on the second attempt.[62] There was no report of worsening neurologic outcome or aspiration because of this intervention. The authors were skilled users of the device and practicing anesthetists who had vast clinical experience with the ILMA. Other studies were not as successful. Bilgin and Bozkurt reported that optimum conditions for ventilation through the ILMA could be achieved at the first attempt only in 59% of the patients wearing a semirigid neck collar and that two to four attempts were necessary for 42% of the patients.[63] Successful blind intubation could be performed in all patients but only 53% at the first attempt. On the contrary, first-attempt and overall success rates were reported to be higher than with blind techniques using an FIS or Lightwand-guided tracheal intubation under vision through the ILMA. The clear disadvantage of this approach was the prolonged intubation time.

However, this information must be viewed in light of cadaveric experiments in which the ILMA has been demonstrated to create posterior pressure on the midportion of the cervical spine.[64] This may be particularly relevant in cervical flexion injuries. If the ILMA is to be used in a patient in a hard cervical collar with cricoid pressure, one should be aware of the difficulties described in this scenario. Wong and colleagues[65] presented two cases where the ILMA was used in awake topicalized patients with an unstable cervical spine without difficulty. In light of these studies indicating that the ILMA may produce cervical motion and excessive pressure on the cervical spine and that it is difficult to place with the application of cricoid pressure and the presence of a hard cervical collar, the ILMA cannot be recommended as a primary device in the patient with acute cervical injury. It should be viewed as a rescue device if direct or FSI fails. In the current era of videolaryngoscopy this device and technique are less frequently used. It may be helpful in the soiled airway and for maintaining oxygenation in patients with limited reserve.

Cricothyrotomy. Although suggested as an alternative to direct laryngoscopy in patients with cervical neck trauma,[66] cricothyrotomy may produce a small but significant movement of the cervical spine.[67] Although often suggested as a primary mode of intubation of the unstable patient with CSI, the procedure is associated with a high complication rate.[68] In one study of long-term complications in emergency departments in the United

Kingdom only 41.5% survived till hospital discharge. A mere 25.9% of these patients who survived experienced no long-term complications (10.9% of all patients receiving emergency cricothyrotomy).[69] This high incidence of complications may be related to the decreasing number of cricothyrotomies performed and the unfamiliarity of many physicians with the procedure. The incidence of an emergency surgical airway in the setting of trauma has decreased over the past several decades. Therefore emergency cricothyrotomy should be reserved as a rescue procedure in the management of the airway in patients with acute CSIs.

Summary

As can be appreciated from the previous discussion, the problem with airway management in patients with CSI is that the techniques normally employed to secure the airway have the potential to cause spine movement and thereby risk causing secondary neurologic injury. Although a strategy for "clearing" the cervical spine is previously outlined, the emergent nature of the management of these frequently multiply injured patients may mean that time does not permit this to be performed. Therefore a group of patients remain whose cervical spinal integrity is uncertain and who must be managed as if their cervical spine is injured. It is essential to proceed in the most expedient manner with the techniques that have been carefully practiced.

Chronic Spine Disease With Myelopathy

In the same manner as patients with ischemic heart disease present for noncardiac surgery patients with cervical spine disease present for surgery for non-neurosurgical procedures. As such, their airway management is of interest to all, not solely those providing anesthesia for complex spinal surgery. One of the problems for this patient group is predicting difficulty with intubation, both by direct laryngoscopy and fiberoptic intubation.[70,71]

Regarding FSI, the traditional bedside tests used to predict difficult direct laryngoscopy may not necessarily be predictive of difficulty in FSI. Difficulty with visualizing the vocal cords in FSI has been extensively documented and is most often caused by secretions and blood in the airway, distortion of the upper airway, and of particular relevance, resistance to the passage of the endotracheal tube (ETT) in a high proportion of cases. This ETT problem has been linked to the size of the FIS in relation to the ETT and, indeed, the design of the ETT itself. Patients with rheumatoid arthritis (RA) may pose additional difficulty because of alteration in the plane of their vocal cords. Efforts at establishing which patient features influence difficulty in the passage of the ETT or impingement have been directed at examining radiologically common features. Neither the Mallampati grade nor the thyromental distance correlated with the degree of impingement on passage of the tube. There was, however, a positive correlation between the size of the epiglottis and the size of the tongue. In particular, the thickness was more important than the length of the tongue, an issue of relevance in patients with acromegaly.

DI is well recognized as more common in patients with cervical spine disease. In particular, ankylosing spondylitis, RA, and Klippel-Feil abnormality present additional difficulty.[72] One of the problems with predicting DI is its incidence, and the sensitivity and specificity of the tests used to detect it.[73] DI in the undifferentiated anesthesia community has an incidence of approximately 1%. The positive predictive value (PPV; proportion of difficult cases predicted to be difficult) of the common tests such as Mallampati or Wilson Risk Sum is about 8%, and the PPV of the tests used in combination is approximately 30%.[74] Tests predicting DI with a sensitivity of 95% and specificity of 99% will have a 51% false-positive rate. However, if the prevalence of DI is theoretically 10%, the problem of false-positive cases would decrease to 8.7% (with a sensitivity of 95% and specificity of 99%). One might therefore expect the prediction of DI to be more rewarding in a patient subgroup with a high incidence of DI, such as those with cervical spine disease.

A number of important correlates have emerged from this examination. As previously discussed, when performing direct laryngoscopy, the most significant movement is produced at the atlantooccipital and atlantoaxial joints.[75] Not surprisingly, patients with reduced mobility at this level present increased difficulty of intubation.[76] However, a highly significant association exists between disease of the occipitoatlantoaxial complex and impaired mandibular protrusion. This is mainly, but not uniquely, caused by rheumatoid disease. Also, extension at the craniocervical junction is needed to open the mouth fully, another limiting factor with direct laryngoscopy.

Rheumatoid Arthritis

Three especially relevant areas in which RA affects the airway and cervical spine are cricoarytenoid arthritis, temporomandibular arthritis, and atlantoaxial instability.[77] Laryngeal involvement in RA has a prevalence of 45% to 88%. Depending on the investigation, 59% of patients with RA have laryngeal involvement on physical examination, 14% show extrathoracic airway obstruction on spirometry, and 69% have one or more signs of laryngeal involvement. Of the latter, 75% have symptoms of breathing difficulty. For these RA patients, the greater airway management risk may be after extubation. Intubation, even if of brief duration, can lead to sufficient mucosal edema to cause postextubation stridor and airway obstruction. Interestingly, the incidence of postextubation stridor is much lower after FSI (1%) than after direct laryngoscopy (14%).[78]

Up to two-thirds of patients with long-standing RA may have limited temporomandibular joint (TMJ) mobility with consequent limited mouth opening. Of those with severe TMJ destruction, up to 70% may suffer episodes of airway obstruction similar to that seen in patients with micrognathia or obstructive sleep apnea syndrome.

Atlantoaxial instability is present in about 25% of all patients with RA and is more likely in those with severe peripheral rheumatoid involvement. Symptoms correlate poorly with radiologic findings, and a serious concern is that some series have found atlantoaxial instability in approximately 5% of RA patients presenting for elective orthopedic surgery. The direction of the instability is variable, and a significant percentage will exhibit vertical subluxation, or cranial "settling." This can also result in the impingement of the odontoid peg on the brainstem.[79]

Summary

The patient who presents for elective surgery with symptoms of cervical myelopathy deserves careful airway management to avoid further injury. Intubation techniques described for the CSI patient are appropriate and best performed by experienced practitioners. When possible, awake intubation, followed by the demonstration of extremity movement, is ideal and recommended. When this is not possible, a technique that produces minimal head movement and airway maintenance is acceptable. A thoughtful approach is based on patient anatomy, risk of intubation difficulty, and a rescue plan for intubation or ventilation failure.

• **BOX 39.1** Airway Techniques for Patients With Unstable Cervical Spine

Awake flexible scope intubation
Nasal intubation
Indirect rigid laryngoscopy
Bullard, Wu, and Upsher laryngoscopes
    Video laryngoscope (GlideScope, McGRATH, and C-MAC systems)
    Airtraq and Pentax AWS laryngoscopes
Direct laryngoscopy with manual in-line stabilization
Flexible scope intubation using SGA as conduit
    LMA Classic
    LMA Fastrach
Lightwand or optical lighted stylets
    Trachlight
    Shikani Optical Stylet and Bonfils Retromolar Intubation Fiberscope
    Clarus video system
Retrograde intubation
Surgical airway
    Cricothyrotomy
    Tracheostomy
Supraglottic airways

Failed Intubation or Anticipated Difficult Airway

Patient in a Halo Frame or Stereotactic Headframe

Early halo immobilization is common practice in patients with potentially unstable cervical injuries and may facilitate the diagnostic work-up and treatment of trauma patients with multiple injuries.[80] The halo device provides the most rigid form of external cervical immobilization. Although the halo frame is an effective form of cervical immobilization, complications can occur. This cumbersome device prevents easy access to the patient's airway and also prevents extension of the head.

Patients treated with halo fixation present unique challenges in terms of airway control. The halo frame prevents proper positioning for laryngoscopy by restricting atlantooccipital extension. Oral intubation is often possible, but it is dependent on other variables, such as mouth opening, tongue size, upper dentition, and the ability to protrude the lower jaw forward. In the nonemergency setting FSI can overcome the difficulties in intubating these patients,[81] but in an emergency setting these intubations can be extremely difficult. Sims and Berger[82] reported a retrospective survey of 105 patients managed with halo fixation at a level 1 trauma center. In this series 14 of the patients (13%) required emergent or semiemergent airway control, with almost half the patients dying in the attempts or shortly after. Based on their findings, the authors suggest that early tracheostomy be considered in hospitalized trauma patients requiring halo fixation who present with a high injury severity score (ISS), history of cardiac disease, or a condition requiring intubation on arrival. Patients who are intubated on arrival may be more likely to require emergent reintubation during their hospital stay. Older patients and those with a history of cardiac disease are more at risk for arrest-related death (Box 39.2).

Respiratory failure or airway obstruction in the patient wearing a halo frame becomes a serious emergency. If the airway needs to be secured and tracheal intubation has failed, the use of adjuncts

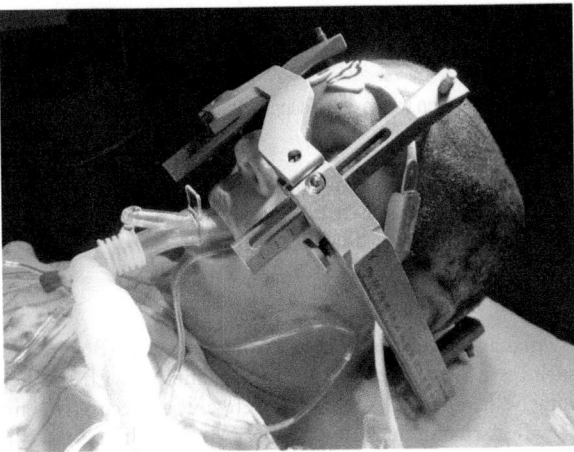

• **Fig. 39.5** Leksell frame allows the placement of a supraglottic airway. (Courtesy LMA Supreme; Teleflex Incorporated, Wayne, PA.)

may be lifesaving. The halo frame immobilizes the head and neck and prevents the use of the "sniffing position" for laryngoscopy or assisted ventilation. Case reports have described a variety of techniques for airway rescue in the patient wearing halo fixation. The Bullard laryngoscope has been used after failed laryngoscopy in a patient who additionally had a difficult airway.[83] The ILMA was successfully used in an awake patient when an FIS was unavailable.[84] This device was also used by one of the authors after a failed intubation attempt following a respiratory arrest. A Combitube was used in a 78-year-old patient with respiratory deterioration after extubation when LMA insertion proved impossible.[85] In recent reports 15 patients in halo-vest fixation were electively intubated for surgery under general anesthesia using the GlideScope, and a 14-year-old patient unable to tolerate awake FSI was successfully intubated with the Pentax AWS.[86,87]

Patients who present for elective surgery in halo fixation should be approached carefully with a plan for intubation. The techniques described earlier for the anticipated difficult airway should be employed. It is imperative that (1) clinicians involved have the skills and equipment for alternative intubation techniques; (2) a neurosurgeon or professional can safely remove the halo if necessary; and (3) a rescue plan is prepared in case of failed ventilation in these challenging patients.

Stereotactic Headframes

Stereotactic localization is widely used in neurosurgery and has revolutionized practice over the past 30 years. The term *stereotactic* originated from the Greek words *stereo,* meaning "three-dimensional," and *tactos,* meaning "touched." Lars Leksell is best known as the neurosurgeon who brought stereotaxis into clinical use, although it was originally described by Horsley and Clarke in 1908.[88] In 1949 Leksell designed the first instrument to be based on the arc-center principle, a system that provided precise mechanical three-dimensional control in the intracranial space. It served to identify the target and to calculate the angles and distances to be used with the frame. The stereotactic system has undergone many refinements over the years. The early stereotactic frames produced by Leksell provided head fixation but significantly interfered with airway access. The later frames have a crossbar that may be directed cephalad for easier access to the nose and mouth. The crossbar can be removed by unscrewing two screws with an Allen wrench (which should always be available). Newer designs feature a movable front piece (Fig. 39.5). Despite moderate access to the airway, head positioning and fixation to the table can make proper positioning for airway management extremely challenging.

Applications of stereotaxis are presently used for biopsy, craniotomy, and procedures for movement disorders. Neuronavigational techniques require the acquisition of radiologic studies, such as CT or MRI, while the patient is wearing the stereotactic frame. Stereotactic neurosurgery may require general anesthesia or conscious sedation. Cooperative patients who are neurologically intact may easily tolerate frame placement under sedation with local anesthetic applied at the pin sites. Conscious sedation is sometimes required when patients must be transported for diagnostic radiologic procedures in the headframe. This is the anesthetic technique appropriate for intracranial biopsies and the surgical treatment of movement disorders and Parkinson disease. The use of IV sedation must be carefully monitored, and the agents chosen should provide analgesia, sedation, and cardiovascular stability.[89] Supplemental oxygen should be administered and the monitoring of capnography is extremely useful. It is essential to monitor head positioning during frame fixation to the operating table. Excessive head flexion may lead to airway obstruction when sedative agents are given.[90]

Potential complications of the surgical procedure include bleeding and the potential for air entrainment. Air entrainment may occur from the surgical site if near the venous sinuses or from the pin sites if placed near diploic veins.[91] This is usually noted by the development of coughing, dyspnea, and decreased oxygen saturation. It is important to make the diagnosis and inform the surgeon, who should immediately flood the operative field to prevent further air entry. Another and more serious risk is internal bleeding. Postoperatively, patients usually undergo a CT scan to check for signs of hemorrhage or hematoma formation.

Patient cooperation is an important factor in these procedures; pediatric patients, obtunded patients, and those at risk for seizures present increased management challenges. The obese patient or the patient prone to airway obstruction requires careful consideration for the stereotactic headframe technique, perhaps performed under general anesthesia. When this decision is made, the patient is anesthetized and intubated before frame placement and must be ventilated, sedated, and monitored for transport to and from a diagnostic radiologic area. Alternatively, a cooperative patient may tolerate the placement of the headframe and diagnostic radiology, although if the lesion is in the occipital region, it may require prone positioning. This problem may be solved by awake intubation in the headframe, followed by positioning after anesthesia is induced. If awake intubation fails, an alternative technique may be used. Supraglottic airways (SGAs) are extremely useful in this scenario and may be used as the sole airway in smaller patients having the procedure in the supine position. Be familiar with a number of airway techniques and have a plan for alternative methods of

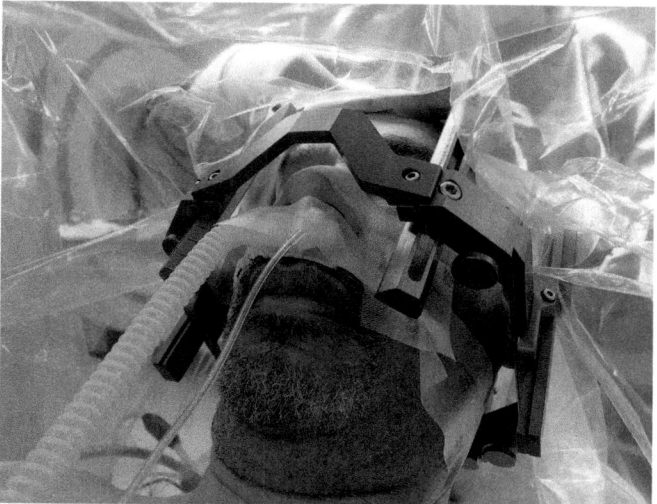

• **Fig. 39.6** Patient receiving high-flow oxygenation during stereotactic surgery. (Courtesy Optiflow THRIVE; Fisher & Paykel Healthcare, Aukland, New Zealand.)

airway management should these challenges occur (Box 39.3).[92] A reassuring study was performed using manikins with the Leksell stereotactic headframe. Clinicians were able to secure the airway using various techniques, including VAL, but the fastest way to manage the airway was using a laryngeal mask.[93]

Patient for Awake Craniotomy or Embolization Procedures

Craniotomy in the awake state has been performed since ancient times. Current indications include the resection of a lesion in the eloquent or speech center of the brain. Surgical procedures for the treatment of epilepsy, tumors, or arteriovenous malformation (AVM) are also sometimes performed in the awake patient. With the refinement of neurophysiologic monitoring techniques, awake craniotomies are necessary in only a small percentage of patients. However, surgery for movement disorders has again increased the use of this technique. Intraoperative complications of awake craniotomy include restlessness and agitation.[94] This may occur when the patient is oversedated but experiences discomfort. More serious complications are hypoventilation, nausea, and seizures. [95] Changing the level of sedation will often resolve these problems. It is important to maintain a good rapport with the patient. Comfortable positioning of the patient to avoid discomfort, allowing surgical access and avoiding a claustrophobic atmosphere, is essential and requires the cooperation of the entire operating room (OR) staff.

The evolution of the anesthetic technique has progressed from the use of fentanyl/droperidol to the current use of propofol infusion with alfentanil or remifentanil or dexmedetomidine.[96,97] Intraoperative nausea is rare with the use of propofol infusions. *Dexmedetomidine* (Precedex) is a selective α_2-adrenergic agonist used for continuous IV sedation. Dexmedetomidine has been shown to produce sedation and analgesia without respiratory depression. The onset is slower than with propofol, and dexmedetomidine must be administered by infusion. This may be beneficial for the older patient, pediatric patient, or potentially debilitated patient and has been used throughout intraoperative testing. Seizure control is sometimes necessary; methohexital (1 mg/kg) or a benzodiazepine (midazolam) is effective. Terminating the seizure requires careful titration of sedatives to avoid apnea.

Oxygenation may be provided using high flow nasal oxygen, which is easily tolerated and may provide humidity and warmth for the patient (Fig. 39.6). If necessary, general anesthesia may be required for the uncooperative or very young patient.[98] The "asleep–awake–asleep" technique has been used by some centers in an effort to minimize patient discomfort and provide better operating conditions for the surgeon. The patient undergoes a "light general anesthetic" with additional local anesthesia and is awakened intraoperatively for testing at the appropriate time.

Airway management can be challenging, and several maneuvers have been reported. Huncke and colleagues used awake FSI, which was accomplished in 10 patients.[99] This effective but arduous technique required significant skill and a special catheter to deliver local airway anesthetic. Some clinicians have also used nasal airways and blind nasal intubation, assuming that bleeding or significant discomfort is avoided. The most useful technique in recent years has been the laryngeal mask airway for the control of the airway.[100] The LMA has been described in several reports and can be placed (with skill) without having to remove drapes or change patient position.[101] In our experience using the LMA Classic and the LMA Supreme, patients could be induced and reanesthetized for the resection after intraoperative testing. This allows the surgeon a "quiet field," because many patients become hypercarbic while awake and sedated. The LMA Supreme or any second-generation device is particularly advantageous for the ability to provide positive-pressure ventilation and access to the gastric tract. A recent cadaver study demonstrated the ease and utility of this technique for patients in the lateral position.[102]

Embolization Procedures

The endovascular treatment of intracranial aneurysm and AVM is now an option for many patients. This new therapy offers significantly reduced morbidity, mortality, and hospital stay compared with craniotomy.[1] In patients with acute subarachnoid hemorrhage (SAH) considerations must be made for the likelihood of increased ICP, changes in transmural pressure, and cerebral ischemia. During endovascular treatment, the two most serious potential complications are cerebral infarction and hemorrhage. Endovascular coiling may be safely applied within hours of the aneurysm rupture with a low probability of aneurysm perforation. General anesthesia is preferred for patients with acute SAH. Despite concern for neurologic evaluation, most neuroradiologists now prefer general anesthesia for the optimal imaging of studies and techniques. Airway control through an ETT or LMA allows for improved oxygenation, anesthetic administration, and a motionless patient. Radiologic imaging methods include high-resolution fluoroscopy and high-speed digital subtraction angiography (DSA) with a "roadmapping" function. The computer superimposes images onto live fluoroscopy so that the progress of the radiopaque catheter tip can be seen. Any motion during this stage of the procedure profoundly degrades the image. The anesthesiologist is typically situated off to the side of the patient and must negotiate around the myriad of monitors and equipment, which are part of this terrain. One benefit of this environment is the ability to obtain fluoroscopic confirmation of ETT positioning, confirm proper central line location, if placed, or make the diagnosis of atelectasis.

Although the radiology suite may be in a remote location, the patient with an anticipated difficult airway should be approached in the same manner as in the OR. A potential limiting factor is the flat table, which does not allow the patient's head to be raised. Supporting blankets should be used to produce the optimal position for laryngoscopy or awake intubation, if necessary. The techniques described earlier apply in this setting, and we have also used the FIS, ILMA, and VAL in the radiology suite. Emergence from anesthesia should be smooth, avoiding excessive coughing and bucking. Hypertension should be controlled to prevent potential cerebral edema and bleeding at the femoral cannulation site. There is minimal pain, but patients are required to remain supine for a time.

Patient With Acromegaly

Acromegaly is a rare condition afflicting 3 to 4 per 1 million people.[103] After Marie's 1882 description of the disease,[104] Chappel[105] reported the death of an acromegalic patient secondary to airway obstruction in 1886. Airway obstruction is one of several mechanisms associated with DI in these patients. The association between difficult airway management and acromegaly has long been recognized in the anesthesiology community. Compared with the nonacromegalic population, acromegalic patients have a higher incidence of DI, unpredictable difficult airway, and problematic mask ventilation.

The occurrence of the difficult airway in acromegaly is well described, and the incidence of difficult laryngoscopy in these patients ranges from 9% to 33%.[106] The hypersecretion of growth hormone characterizing acromegaly results in a number of alterations in airway anatomy. Patients develop hypertrophy of the facial bones with coarsening of the features. The hypertrophy of the mandibular bone leads to prognathism. In addition to significant macroglossia, hypertrophy of laryngeal and pharyngeal soft tissues and structures (e.g., vocal cords, arytenoepiglottic and ventricular folds) is well documented. Schmitt and colleagues[107] found a 26% incidence of Cormack and Lehane grade III views on direct laryngoscopy in acromegalic patients.

Airway management in the acromegalic patient remains problematic, particularly because face-mask ventilation may also be challenging. Various explanations have been described as the reason for the difficulty in ventilating these patients. The prognathic jaw may impede proper mask placement; the large tongue or redundancy of soft tissue may lead to airway obstruction with recumbency and use of muscle relaxants; and the decreased range of neck motion secondary to cervical osteophyte formation may impede the attainment of proper sniffing position. There is a 16% to 30% incidence of upper airway obstruction diagnosed by spirometry in patients with acromegaly.[108] Additionally, the incidence of sleep apnea is increased in these patients.[109] A history of obstructive sleep apnea, hoarseness, or stridor should alert the anesthesiologist to possible glottic and infraglottic involvement and the potential for difficulty with intubation and face-mask ventilation. Although the use of asleep oral FSI may prove difficult or fail in patients with acromegaly,[110] some advocate the use of awake FSI in patients with acromegaly to avoid the creation of a surgical airway.[111,112] Indeed, the awake FSI remains the present standard of care for expected difficult airways, particularly if difficult ventilation is expected. When considering awake FSI, the increased incidence of coronary artery disease in patients with acromegaly should also be considered.[113] An anesthetic plan must be formulated to balance the risks of losing the airway and precipitating myocardial ischemia. The plan should include (1) a second skilled laryngoscopist if a difficult airway is anticipated; (2) a difficult airway cart; and (3) a surgeon skilled in performing a surgical airway.

This propensity for airway obstruction must also be considered in the immediate postoperative period, especially in the patient with bilateral nasal packing.[114,115] Postoperative negative-pressure pulmonary edema has been described in acromegalic patients from partial obstruction after extubation (Box 39.4).

The use of VAL is generally found to be beneficial in acromegalic patients. Prospective studies are lacking, but we continue to have excellent results at our institutions using the GlideScope, C-MAC, and the McGRATH video-assisted laryngoscopes as primary or secondary instruments for intubating patients with acromegaly. The construction of most blade-type video laryngoscopes allows easy navigation around the large tongue and redundant soft tissue and usually provides excellent visualization of the glottic opening.[116] Experience with VAL is recommended in normal airways before attempting its use in a potentially difficult airway.[117]

Role of Supraglottic Airway in Neurosurgery

Although the use of both the LMA and the ILMA for neurosurgical procedures has been previously described, this section addresses additional issues and further details regarding their use in the neurosurgical patient population. Although the SGA cannot substitute for the ETT, it can be used in a number of situations where an ETT would be difficult or impossible to insert. In addition, the beneficial effects on cardiovascular and intracranial reflexes make the SGA a wise choice in certain neurosurgical procedures. This assumes that the clinician is skilled in SGA placement and manages the anesthetic appropriately. Several case reports describe LMA use in craniotomy, but these were scenarios of failed intubation and the necessity for an airway in fasted patients.[118,119] Although the intubating LMA has been discussed extensively as a device for airway management in patients with limited neck movement, Combes and colleagues[120] demonstrated its role in the failed-intubation scenario. In their prospective study of unanticipated DI they concluded that the ILMA and the gum

---

• BOX 39.4 Airway Considerations in Patients With Acromegaly

Prognathic jaw
Macroglossia
Osteophyte formation of the cervical spine; decreased range of motion of the neck
Thickening of pharyngeal and laryngeal soft tissue
Thickening of the vocal cords
Recurrent laryngeal nerve paralysis
Decrease in the width of the cricoid arch
Hypertrophy of arytenoepiglottic folds
Hypertrophy of ventricular folds
Central sleep apnea

elastic bougie effectively solve most problems occurring during unexpected difficult airway management. This is particularly important for the neurosurgical patient, who may not easily tolerate repeated laryngoscopy attempts, inadequate ventilation, and excessive hypertension and tachycardia.

The LMA can also be used as a conduit for FSI and as a rescue airway technique that is preferred by some clinicians rather than the ILMA.[121] The LMA, as well as the ILMA, can be inserted in a variety of patient positions. This becomes useful in the dreaded situation of extubation in the prone position, as well as loss of the airway in a sedated patient fixed in a headframe.[122] Assuming the mouth opening is adequate, the device can be easily placed by facing the patient and using the thumb to insert along the hard palate. A case report describes anesthetic induction and management in the prone position for a penetrating spine injury at C1–C2 using an LMA.[123,124] Elective use in the prone position, although considered controversial by some, can be safely performed in appropriate patients with proper positioning. There is a growing body of experience and literature on the utility of this technique with the LMA Supreme. Studies have shown the ease of insertion with the patient positioned prone for surgery. This obviates the need for turning an anesthetized patient and allows for efficient use of OR time.

Hypertension, coughing, and bucking are preferably avoided in the neurosurgical patient. When these are a particular consideration or the patient has severe asthma or COPD, extubation may be facilitated by exchanging the ETT for an SGA (using SGA as a "bridge to extubation").[125] This is performed while the patient is still deeply anesthetized, without airway reflexes. The exchange technique is also useful when an elaborate head draping is required, and excessive neck movement will likely provoke coughing and bucking. The technique is also known as the "Bailey maneuver," used at the Royal Throat, Nose and Ear Hospital in London.[126] An SGA provides a number of airway options for the neurosurgical patient and should always be readily available.

Postoperative Considerations

Airway Injury and Function After Neurosurgery

A range of airway problems is possible in the patient who has undergone neurosurgery. Potential risks include an intraoperative seizure, hypoxia, and hypoperfusion of an ischemic penumbral area, which may produce an obtunded postoperative state. These factors, along with the residual effects of anesthetic drugs, may render the patient unable to maintain the airway safely. Patients undergo neurosurgery in a variety of positions other than supine, and the effects of gravity, venous pressure, and fluid administration may alter the integrity of the airway structures. Thus although the airway itself may not be considered a difficult airway, there are reasons why airway function may not automatically return immediately after neurosurgery. In addition to this global effect on the ability to maintain the airway, there are specific risks of alteration in airway function after neurosurgery.

After Supratentorial Craniotomy

In addition to general issues regarding the impaired level of consciousness, patients who have previously undergone temporoparietal or pterional craniotomy may present with airway problems. When these patients subsequently present for surgery, they may now have a difficult airway because of limited mouth opening not evident at the original craniotomy. This is a consequence of scar formation in the region of the temporalis muscle.[127] This is

much more likely to occur in those who have had a period of sedation and ventilation in the intensive care unit following their original craniotomy, because they do not resume normal eating and talking activities. Even patients extubated immediately after craniotomy and who do resume normal eating and talking are at risk of developing restricted mouth opening if they themselves limit jaw movement and subsequently develop restrictive scarring. Kawaguchi and colleagues were able to characterize postcraniotomy changes in mouth opening that occurred in 92 patients after surgery.[128] The postoperative reduction in maximal mouth opening was greater in the group who underwent frontotemporal craniotomy (vs parietal or occipital regions). Limited mouth opening resolved after 3 months in most patients. Supratentorial craniotomies separated by short intervals can increase the risk of limited mouth opening, which may result in a DI.

There is a risk that the anesthesia provider may be lulled into a false sense of security in this setting if they limit their assessment of the airway to reviewing the previous anesthesia chart. This will only describe the grade of laryngoscopy at that time, and if they do not perform a new postcraniotomy assessment of the airway with particular reference to mouth opening, they may find a critical reduction in ease of laryngoscopy.

After Cervical Spine Surgery

The intraoperative management of the patient scheduled for cervical spinal surgery was discussed in detail earlier. A significant number of problems, however, present themselves only on completion of the surgery. Although the surgical goals included alleviating spinal cord compression, reduction of dislocation, or fixation of instability, almost invariably, these procedures result in a reduced range of cervical movement. Consequently, on emergence, it may be difficult to maintain the airway in the presence of residual anesthesia because airway maneuvers possible after the induction of anesthesia are no longer viable.

Anterior cervical spinal surgery may result in recurrent laryngeal nerve injury or hematoma, causing airway obstruction after extubation. The most common cause of vocal cord paralysis is compression of the recurrent laryngeal nerve within the endolarynx. Monitoring of ETT cuff pressure and release after retractor placement may prevent injury to the recurrent laryngeal nerve.[129] A subgroup of patients with chronic myelopathy are those undergoing anterior cervical discectomy and fusion (ACDF). These patients are at increased risk of recurrent laryngeal nerve injury, which is related mainly to surgical dissection and retraction. A neural integrity monitoring (NIM) ETT is a commonly used tool to help with the intraoperative monitoring of the integrity of the recurrent laryngeal nerve. It has become a gold standard for use in many thyroid surgeries[130] (Fig. 39.7).

Tracheoesophageal edema or perforation may also develop in the tissues of the neck because the esophagus and trachea are retracted during these procedures to obtain access to the cervical spine.[131] In contrast to problems associated with recurrent laryngeal nerve injury that occur early, such as angioedema or hematoma, this edema may not develop for 2 to 3 days postoperatively. Patients requiring reintubation often exhibit the following: greater number of levels manipulated, higher the operated levels, duration of surgery, and intraoperative blood loss. When these patients require reintubation, it is often difficult to perform, with significant rates of mortality and hypoxic sequelae. Consequently, attempts have been made to identify the risks previously described and the strategies to predict at-risk groups and plan alternative management.

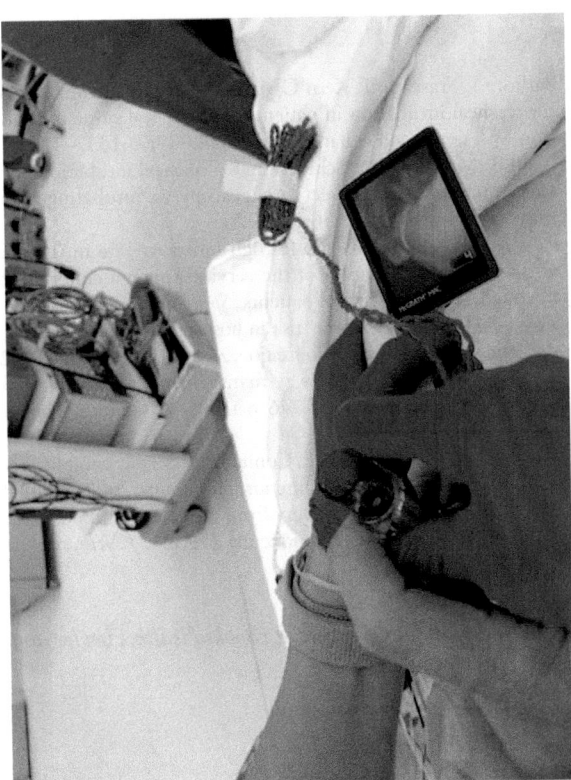

• **Fig. 39.7** Placement of a neural integrity monitoring (NIM) tube using videolaryngoscope.

Sagi and colleagues demonstrated that 19 patients (6.1%) had an airway complication, 6 patients (1.9%) required reintubation, and 1 patient died. Symptoms developed on average 36 hours postoperatively.[132] All complications except for two were attributable to pharyngeal edema. Variables found to be statistically associated with an airway complication were exposing more than three vertebral bodies; intraoperative blood loss greater than 300 mL; exposures involving C2, C3, or C4; and surgery longer than 5 hours. A history of myelopathy, spinal cord injury, pulmonary problems, smoking, anesthetic risk factors, and the absence of a drain did not correlate with an airway complication. Thus patients with prolonged procedures (5 hours), exposing more than three vertebral levels that include C2, C3, or C4 and with more than 300-mL blood loss, should remain intubated or should be extubated over an airway exchange catheter and watched carefully for respiratory insufficiency. Neurophysiologic monitoring, especially transcortical motor-evoked potentials, has been noted to result in tongue, dental, and other oral injuries. The use of bite blocks with periodic inspection may minimize the risk of bite injuries.[133]

Swallowing difficulties and dysphonia may occur in patients undergoing anterior cervical discectomy and fusion. The etiology and incidence of these abnormalities are not well defined. Once again, there is a tendency for patients undergoing multilevel surgery to demonstrate an increased incidence of swallowing abnormalities on postoperative radiographic studies.[134] Patients undergoing multilevel procedures are at an increased risk for these complications, in part because of soft tissue swelling in the neck. Although rarer, the risk of migration of the bone, synthetic graft, or plate into the airway or compressing the airway with resultant obstruction may also be present. In addition to necessitating reintubation, this has the added hazards of intubation being required in a patient with a potentially unstable cervical spine and the need for further surgery.[135,136]

The issues surrounding airway complications of posterior cervical spinal surgery, which are in addition to those of anterior cervical spinal surgery, relate mainly to anesthesia conducted with the patient in the prone position.

After Posterior Fossa Surgery

Because of the position of the lower cranial nerves in relation to the posterior fossa, the patient's ability to maintain the airway may be compromised postoperatively. The performance of a careful history preoperatively may unmask subtle impairment of the gag reflex with increased episodes of choking on food, and family members may have noticed changes in the character of speech. The duration of surgery, proximity of the surgical site to the lower cranial nerves, and presence of either edema or hematoma in relation to these nerves may result in both the loss of gag reflex and loss of the ability to maintain and protect the airway after posterior fossa surgery. Because of the proximity to the brainstem, further hazards are presented postoperatively because central control of respiration may be jeopardized, and these factors will dictate the safety of the timing of extubation.[137,138]

Potential postoperative airway problems can be divided into those of the prone and sitting positions and those related to surgery on the structures in the posterior fossa. Patients are at risk of ETT dislodgement because securing the ETT is hampered by secretions and skin preparation solutions. Even if securely fastened to the skin, facial edema may result in ETT migrating out of the trachea, especially in children in whom the distance between endobronchial intubation and extubation is small. Facial edema itself is not necessarily hazardous to the airway, but macroglossia and oropharyngeal edema clearly are problematic.[139]

A variety of mechanisms have been proposed to account for the macroglossia seen after posterior cervical spinal and posterior fossa surgery.[140] Clearly, if the tongue becomes inadvertently trapped between the teeth, lingual edema will result. The venous drainage of the tongue may be obstructed by the presence of an oropharyngeal airway, and if an esophageal stethoscope is used along with an oral ETT, these further risk impairing the venous and lymphatic drainage of the tongue in the prone position. Other factors that may contribute to the formation of edema are lateral rotation of the head and neck and flexion of the neck, because these two maneuvers may impair the venous drainage of the head and neck.[141] The duration of surgery, as well as blood loss and fluid replacement, should also be taken into account to predict the likelihood of developing macroglossia.[142]

In all these settings, although macroglossia may be immediately apparent and may preclude extubation, the oropharyngeal airway and the ETT may be the only elements maintaining the airway, and only upon their removal does the edema become apparent, risking airway compromise. A rarer neurologic complication impacting airway function after surgery in this position is quadriplegia. This may be caused by a combination of prolonged hyperflexion, overstretching of the spinal cord, and compromised blood supply to the cord.[143] The devastating complication of quadriplegia has been reported as another risk of surgery in the seated position. Clearly, extubation of the neurosurgical patient after prolonged surgery requires careful consideration, including a review of the patient's intraoperative course and assessment of airway and neurologic responses. Patients who appear to have obvious facial or airway swelling with minimal response to the ETT are best left intubated until the edema is fully recovered and they meet all criteria for extubation.

Conclusion

The scope of airway considerations in the neurosurgical patient is vast. General and specific concerns for patient management include airway assessment and emergency airway algorithms. These patients often present with a number of disease processes, which must be considered in relation to the anesthetic as well as to airway management. This task becomes more challenging as patients become older, live longer, and present with multiple medical problems. Additionally, neurosurgical procedures are becoming more complex with time. Some procedures will be done with the neurosurgical patient in prone, lateral, or sitting positions. Others will require the patient to be awake temporarily and then anesthetized. The approach to airway control is a decision made by the anesthesia provider, often in collaboration with the surgeon. It is important for the practitioner to explore new airway devices and techniques and to gain skill in those that will benefit the neurosurgical patient population. Many problems may occur in the patient after neurosurgery, and thus vigilance both intraoperatively and postoperatively is essential. Anesthesiologists' role as perioperative physicians requires that they provide close observation of the patient throughout the perioperative period and render the safest care possible.

Selected References

54. Bathory I, Frascarlo P, Kern C, et al. Evaluation of the GlideScope for tracheal intubation in patients with cervical spine immobilization by a semi-rigid collar. *Anaesthesia.* 2009;64:1337–1341.

60. Waltl B, Melischek M, Schuschnig C. Tracheal intubation and cervical spine excursion: direct laryngoscopy vs. intubating laryngeal mask. *Anaesthesia.* 2001;56:221–226.

79. Paus AC, Steen H, Røislien J. High mortality rate in rheumatoid arthritis with subluxation of the cervical spine: a cohort study of operated and nonoperated patients. *Spine.* 2008;33:2278.

82. Sims CA, Berger DL. Airway risk in hospitalized trauma patients with cervical injuries requiring halo fixation. *Ann Surg.* 2002;225:280–284.

106. Nemergut EC, Zuo Z. Airway management in patients with pituitary disease: a review of 746 patients. *J Neurosurg Anesthesiol.* 2006;18:73–77.

132. Sagi HC, Beutler W, Carroll E, Connolly PJ. Airway complications associated with surgery on the anterior spine. *Spine.* 2002;27:949–953.

136. Bruder N, Ravussin P. Recovery from anesthesia and postoperative extubation of neurosurgical patients: a review. *J Neurosurg Anesth.* 1999;11:282–293.

All references can be found online at eBooks.Health.Elsevier.com.

40

Obesity, Sleep Apnea, the Airway, and Anesthesia

MATTHEW W. OH, BABATUNDE OGUNNAIKE, AND TIFFANY SUN MOON

CHAPTER OUTLINE

KEY POINTS

- A high body mass index (BMI) is a weak but statistically significant predictor of difficult intubation (DI) and difficult mask ventilation (DMV). Body fat distribution, rather than the BMI value, may be a better predictor of difficult laryngoscopy. Measuring the neck circumference at the thyroid cartilage level is a useful addition to the normal daily practice of measuring weight or BMI during preoperative airway evaluation.
- For those suspected of having obstructive sleep apnea (OSA) based on clinical criteria, anesthesiologists may elect to proceed with a presumptive OSA diagnosis unless the patient has significant comorbidities.
- General anesthesia with a secure airway is preferable to deep sedation without an airway for superficial procedures and patients with OSA undergoing procedures involving the upper airway. Intraoperative positive airway pressure (PAP) or high-flow nasal cannula (HFNC) can be used in the patient with morbid obesity and OSA to augment spontaneous ventilation and provide good sedation for surgery.
- Intubation under general anesthesia should be carried out with the patient fully preoxygenated to prevent hypoxia. The relatively low functional residual capacity (FRC) found in patients with obesity causes them to desaturate more rapidly. Extension of apnea time during laryngoscopy through apneic oxygenation

- can prolong the safe apnea time and increase first-pass intubation success.
- The head-elevated laryngoscopy position (HELP) significantly elevates the head, upper body, and shoulders above the chest so that an imaginary horizontal line connects the sternal notch with the external auditory meatus to create a better alignment among the three axes to improve laryngoscopy conditions.
- Rapid sequence intubation (RSI) is often recommended in patients with obesity because of the high prevalence of lower esophageal sphincter hypotonia, which increases the prevalence of gastroesophageal reflux disease. Still, the benefits should be weighed against the risks of DMV or DI.
- Pressure-controlled ventilation volume-guaranteed (PCV-VG) may be advantageous in the patient with obesity because it ensures a minimum tidal volume with lower peak inspiratory pressures.
- The endotracheal tube (ETT) should be left in place, or extubation should be carried out over an airway exchange catheter if any doubt exists about the patient's ability to breathe spontaneously or the practitioner's ability to reintubate in an emergency.
- Tracheal extubation should occur in the semi-upright or head-up position only after the patient with obesity and OSA regains

full consciousness after general anesthesia and after confirming airway patency and verification of complete reversal of neuro-muscular blockade.

- Patients with obesity and OSA may need a higher level of monitoring postoperatively due to an increased risk of opioid-induced postoperative upper airway obstruction.

Introduction

The prevalence of obstructive sleep apnea (OSA) among patients with obesity ranges from 35% up to as high as 94%, with a majority of studies reporting a prevalence of at least 60%.[1] With obesity at epidemic proportions worldwide, OSA remains a major contributing factor to airway management difficulties. Surgical patients with OSA have been found to have a higher incidence of pulmonary and airway complications,[2,3] and numerous studies have reported major respiratory complications, including brain damage and death.[4-8] These devastating outcomes can result from failure to secure the airway during the induction of anesthesia, airway obstruction immediately following tracheal extubation, and respiratory arrest after the administration of opioids or sedation in the postoperative period.

The prevalence of OSA globally is estimated to be 18.6% in adults (age 30–69).[9] In the US adult population (age 30–70), its prevalence is estimated to be 26%, and it is the most common type of sleep-disordered breathing (SDB).[10] It occurs due to partial or complete airway obstruction during sleep,[11] and it is associated with episodic hypoxemia and hypercarbia.[12-14] However, with the US population aging and becoming more obese, the prevalence of OSA is expected to increase significantly. Among the surgical population, patients with morbid obesity and OSA tend to be overrepresented because of the higher rates of obesity and OSA-related complications requiring surgical therapy. However, a significant proportion of these patients are often undiagnosed or untreated for OSA.[15]

Definitions of Obesity and Obstructive Sleep Apnea

In 2013, the American Medical Association and several other organizations officially recognized obesity as a disease requiring treatment and prevention efforts. The Obesity Medical Association defines obesity as a "chronic, relapsing, and treatable multifactorial, neurobehavioral disease, wherein an increase in body fat promotes adipose tissue dysfunction and abnormal fat mass physical forces, resulting in adverse metabolic, biomechanical, and psychosocial health consequences."[16] When utilized as a tool to categorize individuals based on relative weight and assess population-level measurements of risk factors, obesity is defined as a body mass index (BMI) or weight in kilograms (kg) divided by height in meters (m^2) >29.9, and overweight is defined as a BMI of 25 to 29.9 kg/m².[17,18] Morbid obesity is classified as a BMI of ≥40 and a BMI of ≥50 kg/m² designates super morbid obesity. Obesity and morbid obesity are associated with increased risk for several chronic medical comorbidities, including cardiovascular disease, diabetes, and chronic kidney disease,[17,19] which may influence perioperative morbidity and mortality.[20,21]

OSA is a sleep disorder characterized by repetitive upper airway collapse during which airflow ceases for more than 10 seconds, five or more times per hour, despite continuing ventilatory effort. It is usually associated with decreased arterial oxygen saturation (Sao_2) of more than 4%.[22] Obstructive sleep hypopnea is defined as a decrease in airflow, ranging from ≥30 to 50%, associated with a decrease in arterial saturation ≥3% to 4% for ≥10 seconds occurring five times or more per hour of sleep.[23,24]

Pathophysiology of Obstructive Sleep Apnea

Pharyngeal Muscle Activity and Airway Patency

Three pharyngeal segments—the nasopharynx (i.e., retropalatal pharynx), oropharynx (i.e., retroglossal pharynx), and laryngopharynx (i.e., retroepiglottic pharynx)—form the upper airway, which is a long, soft-walled tube that lacks bony support on the anterior and lateral walls, making it collapsible (Fig. 40.1).[24] The transmural pressures across the pharyngeal walls (i.e., the difference between extraluminal and intraluminal pressure) determine the upper airway's patency. Activation of pharyngeal dilator muscles, the tensor veli palatini, the genioglossus, and the hyoid bone's muscles (geniohyoid, sternohyoid, and thyrohyoid) during inspiration counteracts the narrowing effects of reduced intraluminal pressure associated with inspiration. In addition to this inspiration-associated activation, the tonic activity of these muscles during wakefulness helps stabilize the pharyngeal walls.

The cause of upper airway collapse is multifactorial and can be attributed to several factors. A reduction in pharyngeal dilator muscle activation, which likely results from the loss of the stimulatory effect of wakefulness (i.e., during sleep), reduction in respiratory drive, depression of negative pressure reflexes, loss of lung volume, and overaction of the respiratory pump muscles, decreases longitudinal traction on the pharyngeal walls and increases the likelihood of upper airway collapse.[25,26] *Loop gain* is a term utilized to describe the stability of a feedback control system, and patients with severe OSA have been shown to have high loop gain, rapidly and aggressively responding to minimal changes in CO_2, which leads to a higher tendency of periodic breathing.[25,27]

Patients with OSA also tend to have a reduced respiratory-tract diameter. The pharynx has a round shape, compared to an oval shape, attributing to a larger anteroposterior diameter rather than a larger transversal diameter. This ultimately generates a hindrance in the mechanics of the dilator muscles of the pharynx.[25]

Sleep Pattern, Airway Obstruction, and Arousal

Normal sleep consists of four to six cycles of non-rapid-eye-movement (NREM) sleep, followed by rapid-eye-movement (REM) sleep. The four stages of NREM sleep and one stage of REM sleep represent a progressive slowing of the electroencephalographic waves. Rhythmic activity of the upper airway muscles decreases during deeper sleep stages, which accompanies a significant increase in upper airway resistance and consequent upper airway collapse.[28] Patients with OSA have a decreased or even absent airway reflex during non-REM sleep. REM sleep is associated with impaired respiratory arousal and an increase in nocturnal hypoxemia episodes.[26,29]

Contraction of the diaphragm during inspiration creates a subatmospheric pressure within the airway that may narrow the collapsible segments of the pharynx.[30] As pharyngeal pressure

UPPER AIRWAY ANATOMY

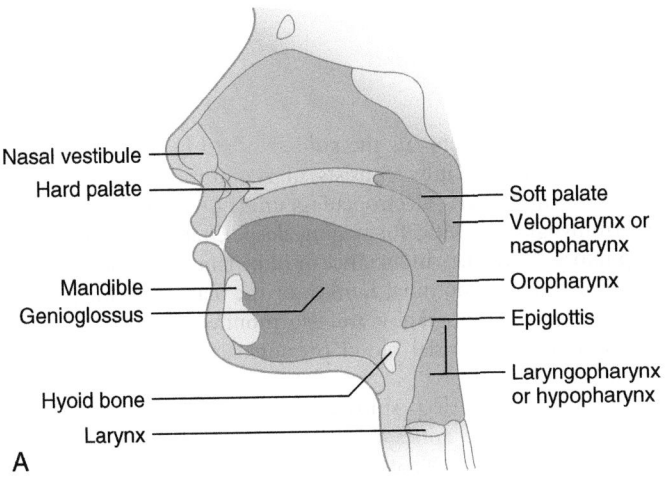

A

ACTION OF THE UPPER AIRWAY DILATOR MUSCLES

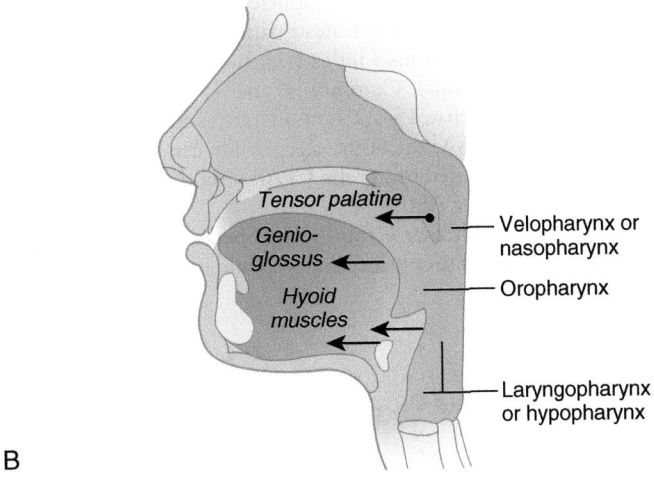

B

SITES OF OBSTRUCTION DURING SLEEP APNEA

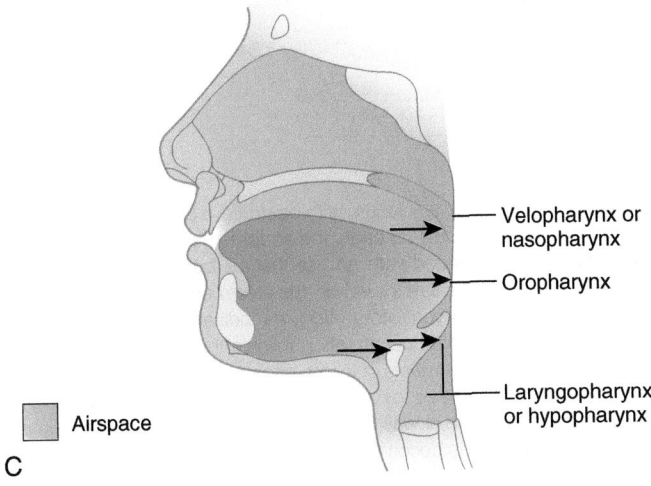

C

• **Fig. 40.1** Airway obstruction during sleep apnea. (A) The schematic drawing shows the important upper airway anatomy. The nasopharynx ends at the tip of the uvula; the oropharynx extends from the tip of the uvula to the epiglottis; and the laryngopharynx extends from the tip of the epiglottis to the posterior cricoid cartilage. (B) The drawing shows the action of the most important dilator muscles of the upper airway. The tensor palatine, genioglossus, and hyoid muscles enlarge the nasopharynx, oropharynx, and laryngopharynx, respectively. (C) The drawing shows collapse of the nasopharynx at the palatal level, the oropharynx at the glottic level, and the laryngopharynx at the epiglottic level. (From Benumof JL. Obstructive sleep apnea in the adult obese patient: implications for airway management. *J Clin Anesth.* 2001;13:144–156.)

becomes more negative, pharyngeal collapse increases progressively. The most compliant and common pharyngeal collapse site is the lateral pharyngeal walls, a significant pharyngeal adipose tissue deposition site.[31] In patients with obesity, deposition of fat around the pharyngeal walls narrows the upper airway and increases the extraluminal pressure and risk of collapse.[25,32,33] Increased fat deposits, in addition to the gravitational effects of being in the supine position, also lead to increased compression to the retropalatal airway and retroglossal airway, which tend to be smaller in this patient population.[25] For a given degree of loss of pharyngeal muscle tone and pharyngeal muscle collapse, a greater degree of pharyngeal obstruction is observed in patients with a posteriorly set tongue (caused by micrognathia and retrognathia or a receding mandible), displacement of the hyoid bone often associated with obesity, a large tongue, large tonsils, and nasal obstruction. Other factors that contribute to upper airway narrowing and subsequent collapse during sleep include large neck circumference, anatomic or craniofacial abnormalities affecting the airway, gender, and age.[25,26,34,35]

Airway collapse leads to obstructive apnea and consequently causes a decrease in arterial oxygen tension (Pao_2) and an increase in arterial carbon dioxide tension ($Paco_2$), which increases neural traffic in the reticular activating system, progressively increasing ventilatory efforts[36,37] and causing arousal from sleep. Arousal, expressed as extremity twitching, gasping or snorting, vocalization, and increased electroencephalographic activity, reactivates the pharyngeal muscles and opens the upper airway. As the upper airway opens, an increase in diaphragm activity leads to hyperventilation, reversing the blood gas disturbance, correcting hypoxia and hypercarbia,[38] and decreasing the central drive.[25] The cycle repeats itself when the patient falls asleep again (Fig. 40.2).

Frequent arousals and the subsequent cycle of wake and sleep prevent deep restorative sleep phases and lead to excessive daytime somnolence,[25] which has been shown to exist in up to 32% of highly compliant patients with continuous positive airway pressure (CPAP) during the night.[39] Oxygen desaturation, sympathetic hyperactivity, and a systemic inflammatory response may contribute to cardiovascular comorbidities such as systemic hypertension, cardiac arrhythmias, myocardial ischemia, pulmonary hypertension, and heart failure.[40]

Diagnosis of Obstructive Sleep Apnea

Because OSA is undiagnosed in up to 80% of patients at the time of surgery[41] and failure to recognize OSA preoperatively is one of the major causes of perioperative complications,[14] all perioperative patients should be screened for OSA. Obtaining a thorough history and physical examination helps to determine a presumptive

PATHOPHYSIOLOGY OF OBSTRUCTIVE SLEEP APNEA

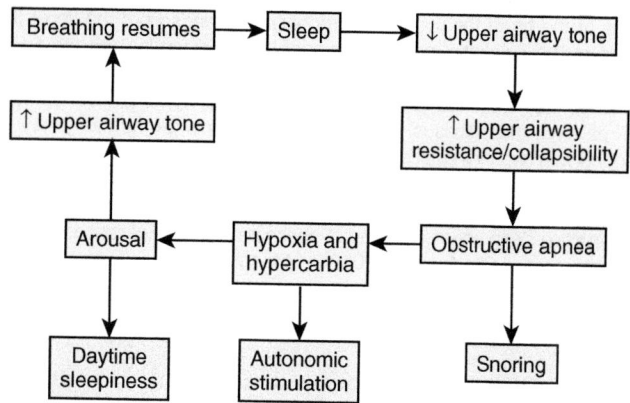

• **Fig. 40.2** Pathophysiology of obstructive sleep apnea.

diagnosis of OSA. However, only polysomnography can confirm the diagnosis and severity of OSA and determine the need for and level of CPAP needed.

Clinical Diagnosis

A presumptive clinical diagnosis of OSA may be made from the observation of components that make up the classic triad of sleep-disordered breathing (i.e., history or observation of apnea or snoring with hypopnea during sleep), arousal from sleep (i.e., extremity movement, turning, vocalization, or snoring), and daytime sleepiness (i.e., easily falling asleep during quiet times of the day) or fatigue. Because arousals may not be readily apparent, the diagnosis of OSA is commonly based on two of the three components: sleep-disordered breathing and daytime somnolence.

A systematic review and meta-analysis of clinical screening tests for OSA reported that the STOP-Bang screening tool was easy to use and a good predictor of severe OSA (i.e., apnea-hypopnea index [AHI, described below] >30) (Box 40.1).[42,43] The STOP-Bang questionnaire has a sensitivity of 93% and specificity of 43% at an AHI >15 and a sensitivity of 100% and specificity of 37% at an AHI >30.[43] Other questionnaires, including the Berlin questionnaire and the American Society of Anesthesiologists (ASA) checklist, are also in clinical use and have similar predictive

• BOX 40.1   STOP-Bang Scoring System

S = Snoring. Do you snore loudly (louder than talking or loud enough to be heard through closed doors)?
    T = Tiredness. Do you often feel tired, fatigued, or sleepy during daytime?
    O = Observed apnea. Has anyone seen you stop breathing during your sleep?
    P = Pressure. Do you have or are you being treated for high blood pressure?
    B = Body mass index >35 kg/m²
    A = Age >50 years
    N = Neck circumference >40 cm
    G = Male gender
    Risk of Obstructive Sleep Apnea
High risk: ≥3 questions answered yes
Low risk: <3 questions answered yes

(From Chung F, Yegneswaran B, Liao P, et al. STOP questionnaire: a tool to screen patients for obstructive sleep apnea. *Anesthesiology.* 2008;108:812–821.)

accuracy for OSA.[44–46] However the STOP-Bang questionnaire is the most accurate screening tool for detecting mild, moderate, and severe OSA.[47]

Polysomnography

Polysomnography remains the gold standard in the diagnosis of OSA. Polysomnography consists of monitoring the electroencephalogram (EEG), electrooculogram (EOG), and submental electromyogram (EMG) for staging sleep. Oral and nasal airflow, respiratory efforts (i.e., inductance or impedance pneumography to monitor thoracoabdominal motion or the diaphragmatic EMG), oximetry, and capnography are also monitored as well as body position, sound, arterial blood pressure, and the electrocardiogram (Fig. 40.3).[48]

The results of a sleep study are reported as events and indices. Events include apnea (no airflow ≥10 seconds), hypopnea (tidal volume [V_t] ≤50% of the control awake value ≥10 seconds), desaturation (>4% decrease in Sao_2), and arousal, which may be detected clinically (i.e., vocalization, turning, or extremity movement) or by an electroencephalographic burst.[49] Indices are measured as events per hour, which include the AHI (i.e., number of times a patient was apneic or hypopneic per hour), oxygen desaturation index (i.e., number of times a patient had a ≥4% decrease in Sao_2 per hour), and arousal index (i.e., number of times a patient was aroused per hour). Commonly, an AHI value 5–14 is considered mild severity, 15–29 is moderate, and ≥30 is severe. If the patient has OSA, the entire sleep study can be repeated with CPAP titration to determine the CPAP level that causes a significant decrease in the AHI.

It is unclear whether a routine preoperative sleep study (i.e., polysomnogram or home sleep study) could improve perioperative

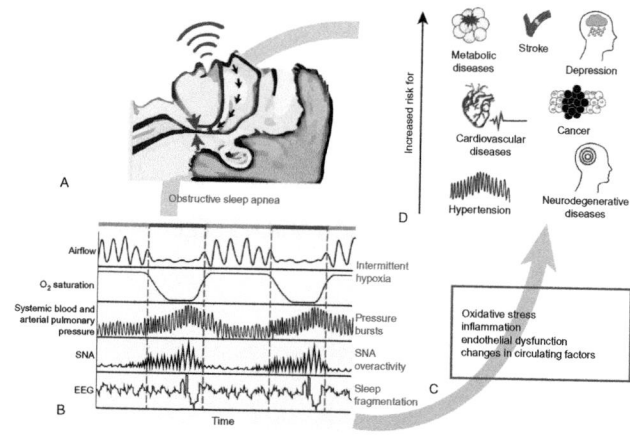

• **Fig. 40.3** Upper airway closure with obstructive apnea. Increasing ventilatory effort is seen in the rib cage, the abdomen, and the level of esophageal pressure (measured with an esophageal balloon), despite lack of oronasal airflow. Arousal recorded on the electroencephalogram is associated with increasing ventilatory effort, as indicated by the esophageal pressure. Oxyhemoglobin desaturation follows the termination of apnea. During apnea, the movements of the rib cage and the abdomen (effort) are in opposite directions (*arrows*) as a result of attempts to breathe against a closed airway. After the airway opens in response to arousal, rib cage and abdominal movements become synchronous. (From Gaspar, L.S., Alvaro, A.R., Moita, J., Cavadas, C. 2017. Obstructive sleep apnea and Hallmarks of aging. *Trends Mol. Med.* 23 [8], 675–692. https://doi.org/10.1016/j.molmed.2017.06.006. Copyright © 2017 Elsevier Ltd.)

outcomes. The optimal duration of preoperative CPAP therapy before proceeding with elective surgical procedures is unknown, and CPAP compliance varies. For those suspected of having OSA based on clinical criteria, anesthesiologists may elect to proceed with a presumptive diagnosis of OSA and provide an anesthetic appropriate for patients with OSA.[14]

Obesity, Obstructive Sleep Apnea, and the Airway

Patients with morbid obesity have excess adipose tissue deposits in the neck, breast, thoracic wall, and in the mouth and pharynx that may impede patency of and access to the upper airway.[50] Magnetic resonance imaging (MRI) studies of patients with obesity found greater amounts of fat in areas surrounding the collapsible segments of the pharynx in those with OSA,[51,52] which may explain a higher incidence of airway management difficulty in patients with obesity and OSA. In a retrospective study evaluating the influence of morbid obesity on intubation and mask ventilation, the overall incidence of difficult intubation (DI) was similar when comparing patients with morbid obesity (4.3%) to patients without morbid obesity (4.2%), and DI was related more to anatomic features than BMI.[53] Evidence suggests that obesity may not be an independent risk factor for difficult airway.[54–57] The distribution pattern of body fat may be a more relevant factor contributing to difficult airway management than BMI itself.[58]

Patients with severe OSA (AHI >30) are at a significantly higher risk for difficult mask ventilation (DMV) and DI, leading to speculation that these patients may have different anatomic characteristics compared with patients who have less severe OSA.[59] A recent study showed that patients with obesity with undiagnosed OSA and any patients with STOP-Bang scores of 3 or more have a significantly higher risk of DI.[60] Patients with obesity and OSA have larger neck circumferences than patients with equal obesity (i.e., similar BMI) and without OSA.[32,61] This neck "mass loading" (up to 28% increase in neck soft tissue) may be responsible for a more collapsible airway, leading to DMV and DI.[32] Men have a higher percentage of soft tissue and fat in the neck compared with women,[62,63] which may explain greater airway difficulties in male patients with OSA compared with female patients with OSA, such as more DMV.[64] A logistic regression model identified neck circumference at the thyroid cartilage level as the sole significant predictor of DI.[65] Probability of a DI increases significantly with a neck circumference of 40 cm or more.[65] Neck circumference corrected for height (i.e., neck circumference/height) is sensitive and specific for detecting OSA compared with neck circumference alone.[66]

Effects of Anesthesia and Surgery on Postoperative Sleep

Sedatives, hypnotics, and opioids impair neural input to the upper airway muscles and therefore may worsen or even induce obstruction. These drugs also decrease the ventilatory response to hypoxemia and hypercarbia, further exaggerating the negative impact of obstruction. In contrast to natural sleep, in which patients with OSA are aroused in response to asphyxia, drug-induced airway obstruction and apnea are associated with a lack of ability to arouse and respond adequately to asphyxia. These drug-induced events may have life-threatening consequences.

Other factors that influence sleep patterns and exacerbate sleep disorders include the stress response to surgical insult and postoperative anxiety, pain, and opioids.[67] These factors lead to reduced REM sleep in the immediate postoperative period, followed by a rebound REM sleep. REM sleep returns acutely and can last for several days after surgery.[68] Since increased REM sleep is associated with more frequent apneic events, rebound REM sleep makes patients with OSA even more vulnerable to airway obstruction.[26,68]

Perioperative Risks of Obesity and Obstructive Sleep Apnea

Factors that augment perioperative risks for patients with obesity and OSA include the degree of obesity (BMI), severity of OSA, invasiveness of anesthesia and surgery, and postoperative opioid requirements.[45] The ASA practice guidelines propose a scoring system that may be used to estimate whether a patient with OSA is at increased risk for perioperative complications and to determine perioperative management (Box 40.2).[45] However, this scoring system is not yet validated, and thus its clinical utility is questionable. When comparing the STOP-Bang questionnaire to both the Berlin questionnaire and the ASA-OSA checklist, only the STOP questionnaire and the ASA-OSA checklist could identify patients who are likely to develop postoperative complications.[46]

> **• BOX 40.2 American Society of Anesthesiologists Scoring System for Estimating Perioperative Complications**
>
> A. Severity of sleep apnea is based on sleep study (i.e., AHI) results or clinical indicators if a sleep study is not available:
> None = 0
> Mild OSA = 1
> Moderate OSA = 2
> Severe OSA = 3
> Subtract a point for patients using CPAP or BiPAP preoperatively and postoperatively.
> Add a point for a patient with a $Paco_2$ greater than 50 mm Hg.
> B. Invasiveness of surgery and anesthesia:
> Superficial surgery under local or peripheral nerve block anesthesia without sedation = 0
> Superficial surgery with moderate sedation or general anesthesia or peripheral surgery under spinal or epidural anesthesia (with no more than moderate sedation) = 1
> Peripheral surgery with general anesthesia or airway surgery with moderate sedation = 2
> Major surgery or airway surgery under general anesthesia = 3
> C. Requirement for postoperative opioid:
> None = 0
> Low-dose oral opioids = 1
> High-dose oral opioids or parenteral or neuraxial opioids = 3
> D. Estimation of perioperative risk:
> Overall score = score of A plus larger score of B or C
> Patients with an overall score of 4 or greater may be at increased perioperative risk from OSA.
> Patients with an overall score of 5 or greater may be at significantly increased perioperative risk from OSA.
>
> *AHI*, Apnea-hypopnea index; *BiPAP*, bi-level positive airway pressure; *CPAP*, continuous positive airway pressure; *OSA*, obstructive sleep apnea; *Paco₂*, arterial partial pressure of carbon dioxide. Adapted from Gross JB, Bachenberg KL, Benumof JL, et al. Practice guidelines for the perioperative management of patients with obstructive sleep apnea: A report by the Task Force on Perioperative Management of patients with obstructive sleep apnea. *Anesthesiology.* 2006;104:1081–1093.

There is a higher incidence of airway-related complications with ambulatory anesthesia in those with obesity, including hypoxemia, airway obstruction, laryngospasm, and broncho-spasm. These complications have not been found to greatly influence the incidence of an unplanned admission or other serious complications.[69] However, there have been reported incidents of patients with morbid obesity and patients with OSA undergoing ambulatory surgery and suffering perioperative anoxic brain injury death. Thus, when considering suitability for ambulatory surgery, surgical factors should also ensure minimized risk for blood transfusion and no need for specialized postoperative care.[70]

Preoperative Evaluation

During the preoperative evaluation, a thorough review of past medical records should include a history of a difficult airway during previous anesthetics plus other congenital or acquired medical conditions that may impact airway management, such as naso-pharyngeal characteristics, neck circumference, tongue size, and available sleep studies.

Patients with obesity do not necessarily have increased gastric volumes when appropriately fasted. However, bedside point-of-care ultrasound (POCUS) is a noninvasive bedside tool that can help ascertain gastric contents in patients with obesity. POCUS is utilized by measuring the antrum cross-sectional area, optimally when the patient is in the right lateral decubitus (RLD) position, and this value is used in a validated model to estimate liquid gastric volume[71]: Volume (mL) = $27.0 + 14.6 \times$ right lateral CSA $- 128 \times$ age.[72] Although the antrum is typically identifiable in patients with obesity, it tends to be deeper and more difficult to visualize than patients without obesity. Further, baseline absolute gastric volumes are significantly higher in patients with obesity. However, the fasting volume per unit of weight remained comparable between patients with obesity and without obesity.[73] Fasting volumes up to 1.5 mL/kg are normal and do not increase the risk for aspiration.[74,75]

It is recommended that preoperative use of positive airway pressure (PAP) should be considered before surgery. However, the data suggesting improved outcomes with preoperative PAP use are limited.[76] Nevertheless, patients receiving preoperative CPAP should be encouraged to use the device before surgery and possibly bring it to surgery to use as a bridge after extubation. The scientific literature regarding ambulatory surgery safety in patients with OSA is sparse, and of limited quality,[7] and the suitability of these procedures remains controversial. With a trend of increasing ambulatory surgeries compared to inpatient surgeries, it is important to be cognizant of the risk for adverse outcomes in high-risk patients and patients with OSA.[77] Patients who are at significantly increased risk for perioperative complications utilizing the ASA practice guidelines scoring system (score ≥5) are not good candidates for ambulatory surgery.[45] Other risk factors to consider include BMI ≥50, male sex, hypertension, the risk for thromboembolic disease, and age ≥45, as patients who had four or more of these risk factors had an increased rate of mortality.[78]

However, the consensus statement from the Society of Ambulatory Surgery (SAMBA) recommends that patients with a presumed diagnosis of OSA based on a screening tool, such as the STOP-Bang questionnaire, may be suitable for ambulatory surgery if their comorbidities are optimized and there is minimal need for opioids postoperatively and, for those patients with known OSA, that PAP devices are utilized postoperatively.[79–81]

Intraoperative Considerations

The primary concerns during anesthesia induction in patients with obesity and OSA include DMV, DI, and possible hemodynamic perturbations.[79,82] General anesthesia with a secure airway is considered preferable to deep sedation without an airway.[45] In patients with morbid obesity and OSA undergoing a procedure using sedation-analgesia technique, intraoperative positive airway pressure devices or high-flow nasal cannula (HFNC) can be considered to improve oxygenation and ventilation.[83]

Finding the correct dose of opioids for patients with obesity can be difficult as there is a large degree of individual variation in opioid requirements. These patients are typically more sensitive to opioids than patients without obesity, requiring reduced opioid dosing for comparable analgesia levels.[84] A multimodal approach is recommended, utilizing regional anesthetics, local anesthetics, and nonsteroidal antiinflammatory drugs (NSAIDs) over systemic opioids, which has shown beneficial postoperative outcomes.[83,84]

Preinduction Considerations

Alterations in pulmonary function (e.g., reduced functional residual capacity [FRC]) in patients with obesity increase the risk of severe hypoxemia, even after short periods of apnea or hypoventilation, such as during intubation (Fig. 40.4).[85] Thus, certain precautions should be taken, including positioning the patient in the head-elevated laryngoscopy position (HELP), which can be achieved by stacking blankets or using specially designed foam pillows. This maneuver aims to elevate the head, upper body, and shoulders above the chest so that an imaginary horizontal line connects the sternal notch with the external auditory meatus to create a better alignment among the oral pharyngeal and laryngeal axes (Fig. 40.5).[86] This position structurally improves maintenance of the passive pharyngeal airway, facilitates bag-mask ventilation, and improves mean arterial oxygen tension and the success of tracheal intubation.[87]

Other techniques used to avoid postinduction hypoxemia include preoxygenation with 100% O_2 until the end-tidal oxygen value is at least 90% and use of 10 cm H_2O of CPAP or bilevel positive airway pressure (BiPAP) ventilation (i.e., intermittent positive-pressure ventilation [PPV] with positive end-expiratory pressure [PEEP]) with the patient in a 25-degree head-up position.[87–90] Preinduction techniques followed by 10 cm H_2O of PEEP during bag-mask ventilation and after intubation can reduce postintubation atelectasis and improve arterial oxygenation.[91]

The principle of apneic oxygenation has also been proven to decrease the incidence of desaturation during airway management in patients with obesity.[92,93] The safe apnea time is defined as the time from the beginning of laryngoscopy until the saturation reaches 92%; this time is much shorter for patients with obesity.[85,93] However, it can be extended through continuous delivery of oxygen through a nasal cannula during attempts at laryngoscopy.[85,93] Transnasal humidified rapid-insufflation ventilatory exchange (THRIVE) combines the benefits of apneic oxygenation with CPAP and gas exchange through flow-dependent dead space flushing to help bridge the oxygenation gap between induction and ventilation via intubation. In one study,[94] an OptiFlow nasal cannula was used to preoxygenate patients (at 40-degree head-up inclination and 70 L/min) before intravenous induction of anesthesia and resulted in extended apnea time by an average of 17 minutes without significant desaturation (<90%) or carbon dioxide toxicity (e.g., cardiac arrhythmias).[94]

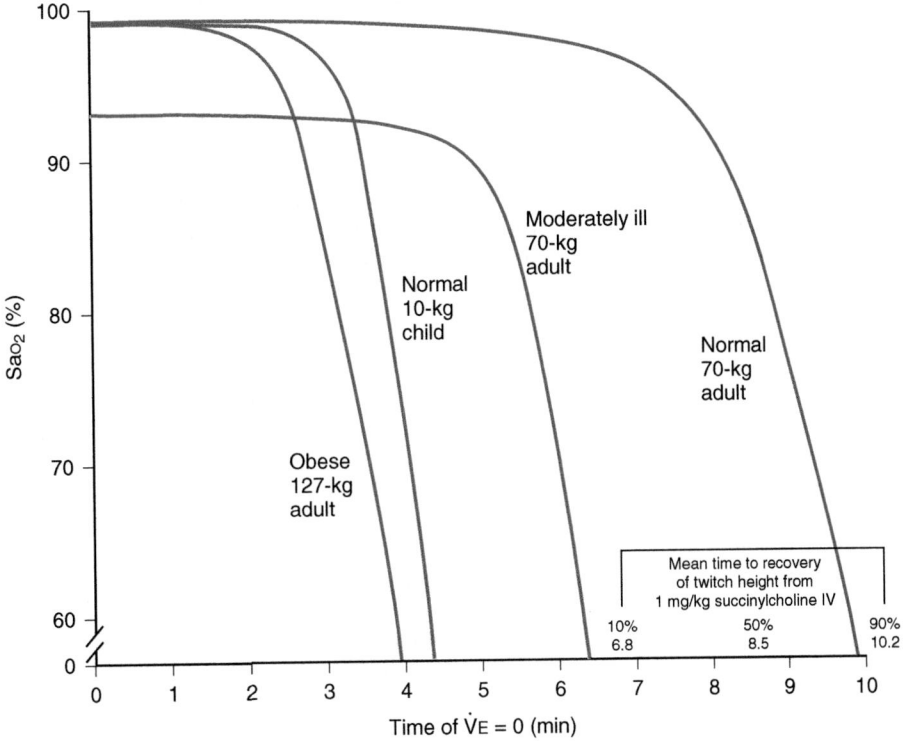

TIME TO HEMOGLOBIN DESATURATION WITH INITIAL $F_{AO_2} = 0.87$

• **Fig. 40.4** Arterial oxygen saturation (Sao_2) versus time of apnea for various types of patients. Mean times to recovery from 1 mg/kg of intravenous succinylcholine *(lower right corner)*. Critical hemoglobin desaturation occurs before return to an unparalyzed state after 1 mg/kg of intravenous succinylcholine. (From Benumof JL, Dagg R, Benumof R. Critical hemoglobin desaturation will occur before return to unparalyzed state following 1 mg/kg intravenous succinylcholine. *Anesthesiology.* 1997;87:979–982.)

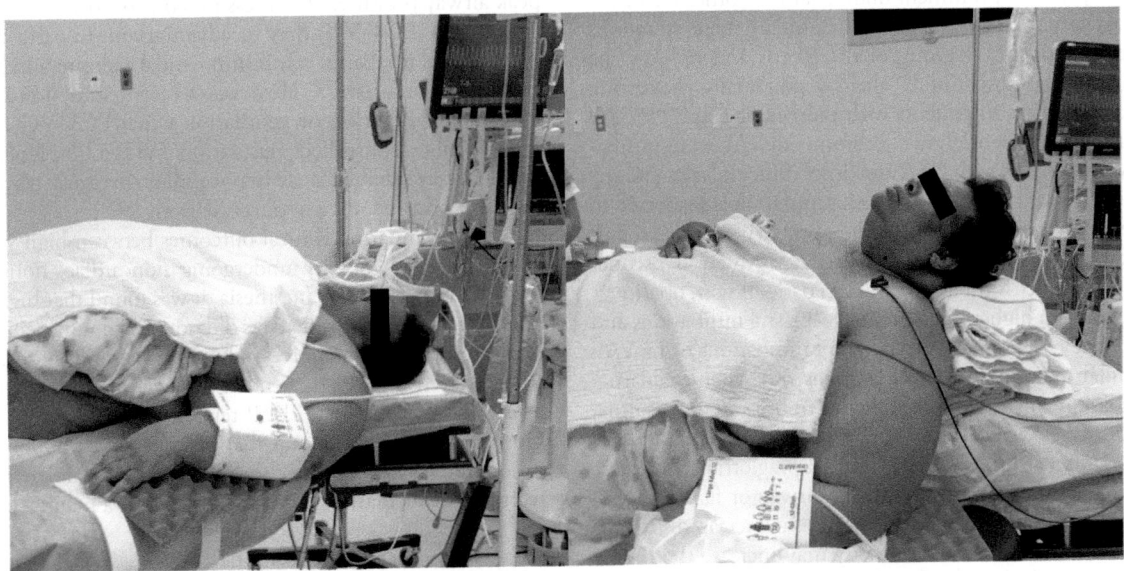

• **Fig. 40.5** Incorrect versus correct patient positioning. *(Left)* The patient is positioned incorrectly in the supine position. *(Right)* The patient is placed in the head-elevated laryngoscopy position achieved through the use of stacked blankets, allowing for alignment of the oral, pharyngeal, and laryngeal axes.

Awake Tracheal Intubation

One of the critical decisions regarding the induction of general anesthesia in patients with obesity and OSA is to determine whether awake intubation should be performed. Awake intubation may be considered when any triple maneuver component (i.e., mandible advancement, neck extension, and mouth opening) is unattainable.[95] Patients with OSA and obesity typically are more difficult to intubate than those without OSA, but obesity by itself is not necessarily associated with difficult laryngoscopy or DI.[53,57,62,96] A retrospective analysis performed to identify patient characteristics that influence the choice of awake flexible scope intubation (FSI) or intubation after general anesthesia in patients with obesity revealed that awake intubation patients were more likely to be male, have a BMI of 60 kg/m² or more, and be assigned to a Mallampati class of III or IV.[97] Because no single factor predicts DMV or DI, it may be prudent to combine multiple predictors, such as Mallampati class III or IV,[98] neck circumference of 40 cm or more, limited mandibular protrusion,[56] and severe OSA (AHI ≥40), to determine the need for awake intubation.

It is important to provide adequate topicalization for awake FSI with local anesthetics. Sedatives and opioids should be avoided because of the high risk of airway obstruction when these agents are administered.[10] Dexmedetomidine is a highly selective α₂-adrenergic agonist with sedative, amnestic, analgesic, and sympatholytic properties that do not cause respiratory depression.[99] It reduces salivary secretions through sympatholytic and vagomimetic effects, which should help facilitate and improve visualization during awake FSI. Compared with fentanyl and placebo group patients, patients who received IV dexmedetomidine had significantly decreased postoperative pain scores, increased opioid-free time intervals in the postanesthesia care unit (PACU), and opioid-sparing effects for up to 24 hours.[100] However, dexmedetomidine-treated patients experienced longer times in the PACU and increased time to emergence from anesthesia.[100]

Tracheal Intubation After Induction of Anesthesia

Emergency airway equipment (e.g., video laryngoscopes, supraglottic airways, flexible intubation scopes) and additional help should be immediately available. Combined DMV and DI infrequently occur in the same patient (0.4%).[101] In patients with both DMV and DI, sleep apnea is a prominent finding, among other factors.[101] Video-assisted laryngoscopy (VAL) is helpful in these situations because it offers superior viewing of the glottis and reduces the duration of tracheal intubation,[102] thereby potentially preventing significant desaturation in patients with morbid obesity.[103–105] The ASA Difficult Airway Algorighm[106] recommends VAL as an intubation strategy for patients with OSA and other difficult laryngoscopy predictors as a primary technique if mask ventilation is suspected to be adequate or as a rescue technique when primary intubation fails in the maskable pathway. Others believe that video laryngoscopes should be a first-choice intubation device in patients with obesity.[107] Studies have found a higher frequency of successful intubations and a higher frequency of success at first-attempt intubations using VAL but with similar outcomes to direct laryngoscopy when evaluating time to intubation, airway trauma, lip/gum trauma, dental trauma, or sore throat.[108–110] Awake intubation by VAL has been highly successful in patients with morbid obesity.[111] Supraglottic airways are an effective rescue device for the difficult airway or failed airway, even in patients with obesity.[112,113] However, the increased intraabdominal pressures associated with obesity may increase the risk of gastric aspiration with the use of an SGA because it does not completely seal the airway. Restrictive pulmonary disease in patients with obesity can increase the peak inspiratory pressures and cause leaks around an SGA cuff, leading to hypoventilation and gastric insufflation.[114,115]

Because of concerns about aspiration and a difficult airway, rapid sequence induction of general anesthesia with propofol and succinylcholine or rocuronium is frequently performed for patients with morbid obesity. A short-acting muscle relaxant (e.g., succinylcholine) is recommended because it allows a rapid recovery, which may allow the rapid return of spontaneous breathing. However, even with low-dose succinylcholine, recovery of breathing and pharyngeal patency may not occur before the development of severe hypoxemia because patients with morbid obesity can desaturate rapidly.[24] The dose of succinylcholine should be based on total body weight (TBW), which results in more optimal intubating conditions in patients with morbid obesity.[116] Use of high-dose rocuronium may allow rapid intubating conditions, but its longer duration of action may be detrimental during a DI or DMV. Sugammadex can rapidly reverse rocuronium-induced muscle relaxation in case of impossible or difficult bag-mask ventilation or tracheal intubation.[117]

Mechanical Ventilation

Mechanical ventilation in patients with obesity aims to prevent progressive atelectasis, hypoxemia, and volutrauma, commonly seen in this patient population.[118] Although the optimal settings for mechanical ventilation in patients with obesity remain uncertain,[119,120] low tidal volume ventilation has been shown to reduce postoperative complications.[92,120] Proposed ventilatory strategies for patients with obesity include the use of lower inspired oxygen concentrations (Fio_2), ideally less than 0.8, to maintain physiologic oxygenation,[121] low V_t (6–8 mL/kg of ideal body weight),[122] application of PEEP (5–10 cm H_2O), and inclusion of recruitment maneuvers (i.e., large manual or automatic lung inflations).[119,123–126] Recruitment maneuvers to adequately open up the collapsed alveoli may require up to 55 cm H_2O of airway pressures, which may have deleterious effects on hemodynamic consequences and therefore should be performed only after hemodynamic stabilization and be maintained for only a short period.[127] Use of pressure-controlled ventilation may allow improved distribution of gases and lower peak airway pressure.[128,129] Pressure-controlled ventilation volume-guaranteed (PCV-VG) may be advantageous in patients with obesity because it ensures a minimum tidal volume with lower peak inspiratory pressures.[130] However, a recent study found no differences in oxygenation or ventilation when PCV-VG is compared with volume controlled ventilation (VCV).[131] Hyperventilation should be avoided because hypocapnia may cause metabolic alkalosis and postoperative hypoventilation.[118]

When comparing clinical outcomes between high vs low PEEP in patients with obesity undergoing noncardiac, nonneurological surgeries under general anesthesia, it was found that high PEEP and alveolar recruitment maneuvers did not provide any benefits in terms of decreasing postoperative pulmonary complications.[132] Patients who received high PEEP tended to have more hypotension, while those who received low PEEP tended to have more hypoxemia.[132] However, it has been found that postoperative pulmonary complications are associated with the use of high peak airway pressure and recruitment maneuvers performed by giving a manual breath.[119]

Postoperative Considerations

The ASA has published Practice Guidelines for Management of the Difficult Airway since 1993, including preformulated extubation strategies for the difficult airway. Recently updated in 2013, this Guideline recommends (1) comparing the benefits and drawbacks between extubating while awake or while unconscious, (2) considering the clinical factors that may lead to adverse outcomes in ventilation postextubation, (3) and if adequate ventilation cannot be maintained postextubation, having a proper airway management plan in place.[133]

There is a high risk of postextubation airway obstruction in patients with obesity and OSA. In patients with morbid obesity and OSA emerging from anesthesia after nonnasal surgery, Camacho et al recommend utilizing the Double Barrel Technique, placing one longer nasal trumpet (extending to the base of the tongue or hypopharynx) and one shorter nasal trumpet (extending beyond the soft palate) allowing for a stented upper airway pathway.[134] Carefully inserting these lubricated nasal trumpets can help mitigate some of the potential risks of obstruction and allow for safe emergence from anesthesia in patients predisposed to upper airway obstruction.[71,134] A nasopharyngeal or oropharyngeal airway may prevent postextubation airway obstruction.[135]

According to the Fourth National Audit Project (NAP4), 1 in 22,000 serious airway complications occurred during general anesthesia, and patients with obesity (BMI 30–35) and with morbid obesity (BMI >35) had, respectively, two and four times as many airway problems compared to patients without obesity. Of the recorded primary airway problems, extubation problems had the third-highest frequency behind the aspiration of gastric contents and failed intubation.[136]

Factors to consider when determining whether to leave the patient intubated after surgery include BMI, the severity of OSA, associated cardiopulmonary disease, ease of bag-mask ventilation and intubation at the induction of anesthesia, type and duration of surgical procedure, and other nuances of the intraoperative course. As the pathophysiology likely remains the same during extubation as intubation, patients with OSA should be extubated in a semi-recumbent position, allowing for a better diaphragmatic excursion, improved FRC, and the displacement of the abdominal contents caudally,[71] after they are fully awake. As these patients are extremely sensitive to residual neuromuscular blockade, verifying adequate reversal of neuromuscular blockade is critical before extubation.[71]

Postoperative Noninvasive Positive-Pressure Ventilation

CPAP and BiPAP are the most commonly used positive airway pressure devices. CPAP is the most commonly used form of noninvasive PPV in patients with OSA. It works by acting as a pneumatic splint to prevent airway collapse, thereby reducing the work of breathing to reduce respiratory muscle load, thus improving lung function and improving gas exchange.[137,138]

CPAP or BiPAP should be applied as soon as possible after surgery to patients who may need it postoperatively. Contraindications to the use of CPAP include nausea, vomiting, facial surgery, and patient intolerance.[45] The use of CPAP or BiPAP immediately after tracheal extubation may improve postoperative pulmonary function.[139] It has been shown to improve oxygenation and ventilation-perfusion matching, reduce respiratory failure and atelectasis, and decrease the need for reintubation.[71] Extubating to HFNC is another option to consider. HFNC is better tolerated by patients and provides additional benefits, including reduced air trapping, better airway function, and decreased airway resistance due to improved mucociliary clearance.[71] A retrospective study of patients with OSA undergoing bariatric surgeries found that patients with known OSA who used CPAP both pre- and postoperatively had a shorter length of stay than patients with presumed OSA who did not use CPAP.[140]

Postoperative Disposition

Requirements for postoperative monitoring depend on patient-specific factors (e.g., high BMI, severe OSA, associated cardiopulmonary disease), invasiveness of the anesthetic technique, the type and duration of surgery, and the intraoperative course.[141] The majority of adverse events occur within the first 24 hours postoperatively, and better outcomes are associated with higher levels of monitoring.[77] It is important to risk-stratify patients with obesity and OSA to allow for patients who are at a high risk of postoperative adverse events to receive the highest level of monitoring. Patients with severe OSA undergoing an extensive surgical procedure that requires significant opioid analgesia may require close monitoring in a monitored environment (e.g., intensive care unit, step-down unit, or remote surveillance monitoring). The creation of intermediate care (observational) units with higher nursing ratios has been suggested as the most rational solution for postoperative care of patients with morbid obesity and OSA who have moderate disease and whose conditions are not severe enough to qualify for an intensive care unit.

A review of 60 patients with death or near-death complications revealed that 83% of these patients had been diagnosed with OSA. The remaining 17% were later diagnosed with OSA, with 81% of the adverse events occurring within the first 24 hours.[142] Factors associated with these critical events include suboptimal use of postoperative CPAP, co-administration of opioids and sedatives, undiagnosed OSA, morbid obesity, and lack of medical personnel appropriately monitoring patients.[77,142]

Expert opinion suggests that patients with OSA should be monitored for a median of 3 hours longer than their counterparts without OSA before discharge from the facility.[45] Similarly, experts suggest that monitoring should continue for a median of 7 hours after the last episode of airway obstruction or hypoxemia while breathing room air in an unstimulated environment.

COVID-19 Considerations

With the increasing prevalence of COVID-19, healthcare providers need to be cognizant of the risks associated with airway management in these at-risk patients. Although CPAP is typically recommended for patients with OSA, the decision to use noninvasive ventilation (NIV), such as CPAP, BiPAP, and HFNC, needs to be carefully considered as there is a high risk of viral transmission by aerosol generation.[143] It is recommended that for surgical patients, regional anesthesia should be utilized to avoid aerosol-generating procedures, and patients at increased risk, primarily those with moderate to severe OSA who receive opioids, should be monitored with pulse oximetry, and ideally with capnography.[143]

Conclusion

As the incidence of obesity and OSA continue to increase, anesthesiologists must be cognizant of the pathophysiology caused by these diseases and the associated anesthetic techniques that can be used to facilitate care for this physiologically vulnerable group of patients. Since the prevalence of OSA among patients with obesity is so high, all patients should be thoroughly screened for OSA and undergo preoperative polysomnography, if possible. It is necessary to develop multimodal anesthetic techniques that are opioid sparing and maximize the use of adjuncts such as neuraxial anesthesia and NSAIDs. Postoperatively, patients with OSA and obesity are more susceptible to airway obstruction, especially with opioid use. Thus, anesthesiologists must consider various techniques and strategies, including postoperative monitoring and extubating directly to positive airway pressure devices, among other recommendations.

Selected References

3. Opperer M, Cozowicz C, Bugada D, et al. Does obstructive sleep apnea influence perioperative outcome? a qualitative systematic review for the Society of Anesthesia and Sleep Medicine Task Force on Preoperative Preparation of Patients with Sleep-Disordered Breathing. *Anesth Analg.* 2016;122(5):1321–1334.

5. Kaw R, Chung F, Pasupuleti V, Mehta J, Gay PC, Hernandez AV. Meta-analysis of the association between obstructive sleep apnoea and postoperative outcome. *Br J Anaesth.* 2012;109(6):897–906.

8. Chan MTV, Wang CY, Seet E, et al. Association of unrecognized obstructive sleep apnea with postoperative cardiovascular events in patients undergoing major noncardiac surgery. *JAMA.* 2019;321(18):1788–1798.

42. Memtsoudis SG, Besculides MC, Mazumdar M. A rude awakening—the perioperative sleep apnea epidemic. *N Engl J Med.* 2013;368(25):2352–2353.

46. American Society of Anesthesiologists Task Force on Perioperative Management of Patients with Obstructive SleepApnea. Practice guidelines for the perioperative management of patients with obstructive sleep apnea: an updated report by the American Society of Anesthesiologists Task Force on Perioperative Management of Patients with Obstructive Sleep Apnea. *Anesthesiology.* 2014;120(2):268–286.

54. Moon TS, Fox PE, Somasundaram A, et al. The influence of morbid obesity on difficult intubation and difficult mask ventilation. *J Anesth.* 2019;33(1):96–102.

57. Kheterpal S, Martin L, Shanks AM, Tremper KK. Prediction and outcomes of impossible mask ventilation: a review of 50,000 anesthetics. *Anesthesiology.* 2009;110(4):891–897.

72. Moon TS, Van de Putte P, De Baerdemaeker L, Schumann R. The obese patient: facts, fables, and best practices. *Anesth Analg.* 2021;132(1):53–64.

76. Van de Putte P, Perlas A. The link between gastric volume and aspiration risk. In search of the Holy Grail? *Anaesthesia.* 2018;73(3):274–279.

81. Nagappa M, Mokhlesi B, Wong J, Wong DT, Kaw R, Chung F. The effects of continuous positive airway pressure on postoperative outcomes in obstructive sleep apnea patients undergoing surgery: a systematic review and meta-analysis. *Anesth Analg.* 2015;120(5):1013–1023.

137. Cook TM, Woodall N, Harper J, Benger J. Major complications of airway management in the UK: results of the Fourth National Audit Project of the Royal College of Anaesthetists and the Difficult Airway Society. Part 2: intensive care and emergency departments. *Br J Anaesth.* 2011;106(5):632–642.

All references can be found online at eBooks.Health.Elsevier.com.

41

Regional Anesthesia and the Difficult Airway

BETTINA U. SCHMITZ AND SARA GUZMAN-REYES

CHAPTER OUTLINE

KEY POINTS

- Regional anesthesia can provide an alternative to general anesthesia for certain surgical procedures; these includes surgeries to the thoracic and abdominal cavities and wall, and surgery to the extremities. The surgeries should be of limited duration (i.e., not more than 90 to 120 minutes) with only minor blood loss and, preferably, with the patient in the supine position.
- Ultrasound assessment of the regional target area and the airway can be included in the preoperative assessment.
- Regional anesthesia, especially using catheter techniques, provides better postoperative pain control, opioid sparing, and subsequent reduction in postoperative respiratory depression risk.
- Adequate anesthesia must be confirmed before the start of surgery. Incomplete blocks or patchy blocks can often be

- supplemented with more peripheral single nerve blocks or infiltration of local anesthesia in the surgical field.
- Acute emergencies related to complications or side effects of regional anesthesia are rare.
- An airway plan for emergent and nonemergent airway management, including fallback strategies for both plans, must be formulated before starting anesthesia.
- Oxygenation should be optimized throughout the perioperative period and can include high-flow nasal cannula oxygen and continuous positive airway pressure (CPAP).
- Communication is key: All team members need to know about the plan to manage the airway if necessary. This communication is best achieved during a team prebrief.

Introduction

The American Society of Anesthesiologists (ASA) guidelines, the Canadian Airway Focus Group (CAFG) guidelines, and the Difficult Airway Society (DAS) guidelines recommend regional anesthesia as an alternative to general anesthesia in patients with a difficult airway (DA).[1-4] In obstetrics, for a patient population that is generally presumed to have a higher incidence of DA, neuroaxial anesthesia became the preferred method for elective cesarean sections, resulting in significant reduction of maternal mortality.[5]

Techniques to achieve surgical anesthesia include neuroaxial blocks, plexus blocks, thoracic and abdominal wall blocks, peripheral nerve blocks, and infiltration of local anesthetic (LA).[6-13]

Beyond the avoidance of managing a DA, reasons to perform regional anesthesia include the preferences of the surgeon and patient, improved surgical outcomes in certain procedures, patient conditions with a high risk for general anesthesia, and reduction of postoperative nausea and vomiting due to lower opioid require-ments.[14–16]

Regional anesthesia can be a safe alternative to general anesthesia in the patient with a DA; however, the decision to proceed with regional anesthesia instead of general anesthesia and management of the airway should be made individually for every patient by taking multiple factors into account.

Preparation and Communication

Patient

Not all patients are good candidates for regional anesthesia. The use of regional anesthesia for anesthetic management, rather than securing the airway, may be considered in adult patients who are calm, motivated, possess adequate communication skills, and understand and accept the risks and benefits of a regional technique over general anesthesia.

In a patient with a known or anticipated DA, this condition and its implications must be discussed in detail with the patient. The benefits of regional anesthesia in general and specifically for the individual patient should be explained. The regional anesthesia procedure itself, effects, side effects, and complications, as well as general anesthesia, including the plan for airway management, must be discussed comprehensively because the need to manage the airway can arise at any time during the procedure.[17,18] Therefore, the anesthesia consent should include the perioperative management of the airway.

Contraindications for regional anesthesia include physical and psychological conditions of the patient, such as the inability to lie flat on a hard operation room table for a long period of time; back pain; restless leg syndrome; other movement disorders; anxiety; panic disorder; claustrophobia; or posttraumatic stress disorder. These factors can limit the patient's tolerance for undergoing a surgical procedure under regional anesthesia and the feasibility of this approach. In addition, an increased requirement for sedation may represent a contraindication for the use of regional anesthesia.

Patients with morbid obesity are especially challenging, as these patients may be difficult to mask-ventilate and intubate. Additionally, neuroaxial and peripheral regional blocks may be taxing for this patient population, as surface landmarks are difficult to palpate and the target structures are deep and harder to identify with ultrasound (US). Furthermore, sedation is problematic as these patients often have obstructive sleep apnea. Nonetheless, regional anesthesia techniques are beneficial for this population as they are at higher risk for pulmonary complications and side effects of opioid medications with alternate techniques.[19–22]

An appropriate assessment of the patient's airway is the first step, irrespective of any initial thoughts. Although the ability to accurately predict a DA preoperatively would be of great value, it is evident from the literature that no single airway assessment nor any composite score can reliably do this.[23,24] Nevertheless, a preoperative airway history and physical examination should be performed to facilitate the choice and management of the DA, as well as to reduce the likelihood of adverse outcomes.[23] Findings that are not reassuring should prompt a reconsideration of the primary airway management plan and exit strategies.[23,24]

The physical assessment of the airway should include assessments for indicators of difficult intubation (DI) and potentially difficult alternative or fallback strategies, such as face-mask ventilation, supraglottic airway (SGA) placement, and front-of-neck access.[2–4,23] Both face-mask ventilation and SGA are recommended

fallback techniques or alternatives in the ASA's DA algorithm, the recommendation of the CAFG, and the British DAS guidelines, and a front-of-neck approach to the airway is the recommended step in the "cannot intubate/cannot oxygenate" (CICO) situation.[1–4]

Surprisingly, routine airway assessment is not performed reliably by all anesthesiologists in every patient undergoing general anesthesia, and even less so in patients undergoing regional anesthesia. In 2012 McPherson and colleagues took a survey in the United Kingdom and Europe of anesthesiologists' practices for predicting DI. They found that 33% of the European and 44% of the UK anesthesiologists did not assess the airway in all patients undergoing general anesthesia, and 62% of the UK anesthesiologists and 52% of the European anesthesiologists did not always assess the airway in patients undergoing surgery under regional anesthesia.[25]

The information that patients can provide about a previous DI differs widely. If available, review of a DA letter, previous anesthesia records, or imaging of the airway can provide further information; however, gaining timely access to such records can be challenging.

Notwithstanding the depth of information available regarding a previous intubation, any changes in the patient's body habits and airway since that event must be explored because they can further complicate airway management. Information such as additional weight gain, radiation treatment, and scar formation also needs to be evaluated. Previously successful techniques might not be feasible when additional conditions further alter the airway.

A preoperative endoscopic airway examination (PEAE), done at the bedside, can provide further information about the current status of the airway and potential problems.[26]

In a review of 50,000 anesthetics, Kheterpal and colleagues reported an incidence of impossible mask ventilation in 0.15% of the patients; 25% of these patients were difficult to intubate, but only 1 patient required surgical airway access.[27] A history of radiation, male gender, Mallampati score of III or IV, and a beard were identified as risk factors for difficult mask ventilation. Ramachandran and colleagues reviewed 15,795 patients undergoing anesthesia with the Laryngeal Mask Airway Unique (LMA Unique) and reported a failure to achieve an airway in 1.1% of the patients; more than 60% of these patients developed hypoxia, hypercapnia, and airway obstruction.[28] The risk for difficult mask ventilation was three times higher in patients with failed LMA Unique placement compared with successful placements. Independent risks for LMA Unique failures reported were male gender, poor dentition, elevated body mass index (BMI), and surgical table rotation.

Ultrasound Assessment: Area of Interest for Regional Anesthesia

A brief US preassessment of the body area where the regional anesthesia will be performed can provide valuable information about the feasibility of regional anesthesia during the preoperative assessment and can support the provider and patient in their decision to choose a specific regional anesthesia technique for the surgical procedure. This includes the assessment of the spinal column, as studies have shown that preprocedural US of the spine can facilitate a neuroaxial approach.[29–33]

Airway

A US assessment of the airway with identification of the cricothyroid membrane can also be performed during the preoperative visit. This examination does not require more than a couple of minutes and can be especially helpful in patients with ambiguous neck anatomy.[34–36]

Portable handheld ultrasound probes are now widely available and simplify a screening assessment of both the airway and regional anesthesia target.[37]

Airway Management Plans

Poorly planned airway management strategies in patients with potential DA and delays in changing unsuccessful strategies were identified as problems in the Fourth National Audit Project (NAP4) study.[38] Joffe and colleagues identified lack of adequate planning as a contributing factor for airway-related morbidity in an analysis of closed claims.[39] Because routine airway management techniques might not secure the airway in a patient with a DA, a safe plan specific for the individual patient needs to be delineated.[6,27,40] This plan should include strategies for an emergency/urgent access and a nonurgent/nonemergent access. A stepwise approach for both situations should be outlined, as well as alternative strategies in case the primary plan fails to successfully secure the airway. A flexible intubation scope, video laryngoscope, and SGA should be readily available for the patient during the entire time in the perioperative area.

Any plan is only as good as the anesthesia provider who executes the plan. Competence with the techniques and familiarity with the equipment are critical aspects for choosing a specific plan.[39]

Surgery

Surgical Procedures Suitable for Regional Anesthesia

Surgeries of the extremities, the abdominal and thoracic wall, and selected procedures of the thoracic and abdominal cavity can possibly be performed under regional anesthesia (Table 41.1, Fig. 41.1).

Surgical Considerations Under Regional Anesthesia

Even though a surgical procedure can be performed under regional anesthesia, other factors can limit the feasibility of this approach (Box 41.1):

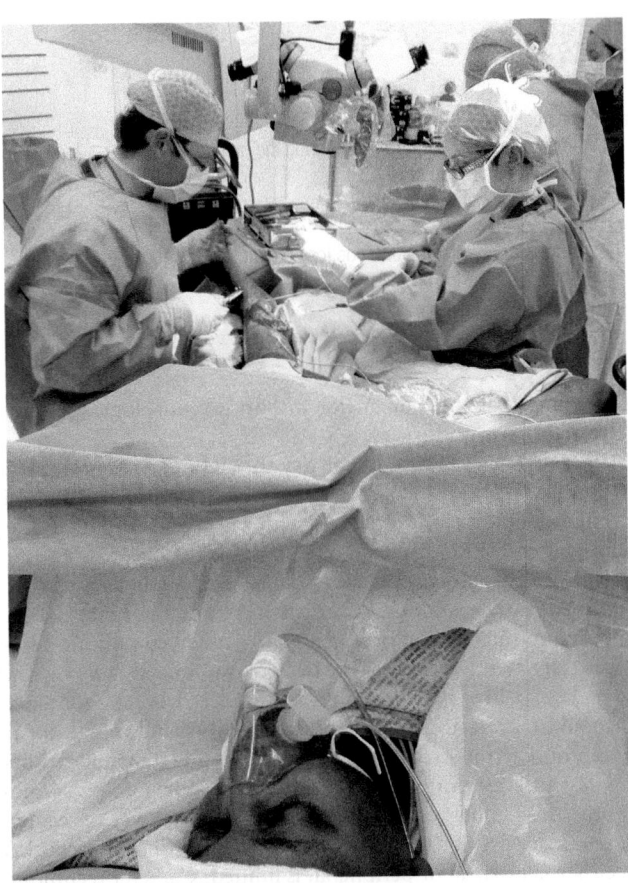

• **Fig. 41.1** Lower-extremity surgery performed under epidural anaesthesia. (From Galatzine S, Wilson K, Edington M, Burumdayal A, McNally M. Patients' reported experiences and outcomes following surgical excision of lower limb osteomyelitis and microvascular free tissue reconstruction under 'awake' epidural anaesthesia and sedation. *The Surgeon,* Copyright © 2020 Royal College of Surgeons of Edinburgh [Scottish charity number SC005317] and Royal College of Surgeons in Ireland.)

Blood loss: Because major blood loss can result in hemodynamic instability, preemptive management of the airway is advisable for surgery where major blood loss is expected or very likely;

TABLE 41.1	Examples of Surgeries That Can Be Performed Under Regional Anesthesia	
Body Area	**Surgery**	**Regional Anesthesia Method**
Upper extremity: shoulder, arm, forearm wrist, hand	Arthroscopy, fractures repair, tendon repairs, carpal tunnel release, arteriovenous fistula creation, joint replacements	Brachial plexus block: interscalene, supraclavicular, infraclavicular, axillary; intravenous regional, local infiltration
Chest wall	Lipoma excision, lumpectomy, mastectomy	Thoracic epidural, paravertebral block, erector spinae, serratus plane, pectoralis I and II block
Abdominal wall	Herniorrhaphy, lipoma excision	Epidural, paravertebral block, erector spinae block, transverse abdominis plain block, quadratus lumborum block, ilioinguinal block, LA
Thoracic cavity		Segmental epidural
Abdominal cavity	Cholecystectomy, urological procedures, gynecological procedure	Spinal, combined spinal esspidural, epidural anesthesia
Lower extremity: hip, knee, ankle, foot	Arthroscopy: *hip*, knee, ankle; joint replacement: hip, knee, ankle; fractures, tendon repair, foot surgery	Spinal, epidural, lumbar plexus block, femoral, adductor canal, sciatic block

examples can include major orthopedic oncological surgery and hip revision surgery.

Patient position: Access to the airway throughout a surgical procedure is preferred for any anesthesia under regional anesthesia but even more so in the patient with a DA. Surgeries performed in prone position (Achilles tendon repair), lateral position (hip replacement), or beach chair position (some shoulder arthroscopies) do not permit this immediate and continuous access. These positions might result in a delay and/or might complicate necessary airway intervention. The decision to proceed with regional anesthesia in a patient with a DA under these circumstances should take all these concerns into account and might not be appropriate for some. The supine position is the preferred and safest position for a patient with a DA undergoing a surgical procedure under regional anesthesia with the airway unsecured.

Duration of surgery: The duration of action of a single dose of LA, either neuroaxial or peripheral, is limited. Catheter techniques can be used for both neuroaxial and peripheral regional anesthesia and can provide extended periods of surgical anesthesia. However, patient comfort is also a limiting factor and may require increasing levels of sedation to tolerate an uncomfortable operating room (OR) table for a longer period. Lengthy sedation may not be a safe option for a patient with a DA. Total OR time longer than 120 minutes might be tolerated by some patients, but for other patients general anesthesia is the better choice under these circumstances.

Tourniquet pain: Pain related to a tourniquet can be a significant problem for surgeries performed under peripheral regional anesthesia. Tourniquet pain can be present immediately after inflation of the cuff but usually develops slowly with increasing duration of the tourniquet. Systemic analgesia and sedation are typically used to mitigate this pain, but again this option is limited in the patient with a DA. Instead, a regional anesthesia approach that not only covers the surgical area but additionally the area of the tourniquet should be chosen. An infraclavicular approach to the brachial plexus covers the tourniquet on the distal humerus better than an axillary approach.[41] Likewise, spinal anesthesia will provide better coverage of the pain resulting from the tourniquet in knee surgery than would a femoral/sciatic nerve block (Box 41.2).

Surgeon and Team Members

The decision to proceed with regional anesthesia in a patient with a DA should include the surgeon. In some instances, the surgeon is already aware of the DA, but more often they are not. It is advisable before any in-depth discussion with the patient to discuss the DA and the option to perform the procedure under regional anesthesia with the surgeon in order to avoid the impression of

less than optimal team communication that could result in patient concerns and anxiety. Part of the discussion should be the feasibility of performing the planned procedure under regional anesthesia in the specific patient. Even if a procedure can be performed under regional anesthesia, specific patient conditions could make this approach less suitable. Other aspects to discuss are expected duration of the surgery, the need for a tourniquet in extremity surgery, patient position, and expected blood loss. Furthermore, a plan and solution for potential problems should be discussed at this point. These include possible supplementation of an incomplete block with local anesthesia in the field by the surgeon, limiting the duration of tourniquet inflation, and possible interruption of the surgery to manage the airway if necessary. An existing collegial and trustful relationship between anesthesiologist and surgeon provides a good base for managing these patients, as continuous cooperation between both is necessary throughout the procedure.

It is preferred that the anesthesiologist responsible for providing the anesthesia care is comfortable with managing a DA, as well as with the regional anesthesia procedure. However, the latter could be managed in close cooperation with a regional anesthesia specialist.

Other anesthesia team members (i.e., anesthesia technicians) must be familiar with the various pieces of equipment used for managing a DA and with their setup.

Effective communication is a key element in crisis situations, and communication failure was recognized as a contributing factor for adverse outcomes in DAs in the NAP4 study.[38] The entire team, including circulating registered nurse, OR technician, and anesthesia technician, need to know the concerns regarding the particular patient, the regional anesthesia plan, the airway management action plan, their roles, and the equipment that will be needed to secure the airway to facilitate effective intervention when problems arise. This information sharing should occur during the time-out or prebrief before anesthesia starts.[1]

Environment

Environmental considerations include procedure location and available resources to assist in an emergency or during times when personnel and support for a procedure are more limited.

In a review of the closed claims database, there was significantly higher incidence of respiratory damaging events, specifically inadequate oxygenation/ventilation in a remote location compared with the OR area,[42] and the number of claims occurring outside of the operating room grew in a more recent analysis.[39] Nonoperating room anesthesia (NORA) environments present the anesthesiologist with multiple challenges: patients may have a higher ASA status score, access might be limited during the procedure, and many of these cases are urgent/emergent and performed after normal working hours. The locations are often not originally designed as anesthesia locations and often provide very limited space for anesthesia equipment and personnel. Anesthesia providers are not as familiar with the location and the personnel in those areas as they are with the OR and with OR personnel. Similarly, healthcare providers in areas with limited or rare contact with anesthesia may not be comfortable with anesthesia-related problems and less able to assist in an emergency because of lack of exposure and experience. Last, but not least, equipment, drugs, and blood components that are readily accessible in the OR suite will often not be immediately available in nonoperating room anesthesia locations. Providing anesthesia care in these locations can be challenging even in patients with uncomplicated airways but more so in patients with a DA.[43–45] The decision to manage a DA in these environments versus avoiding the airway management and pursuing the procedure under local or regional anesthesia must take all aforementioned factors into account. If there is more than little concern about the possibility to perform the procedure successfully under local/regional anesthesia, preemptive airway management either in the remote area itself or in the OR before transferring the patient to the respective area should be considered.

Sedation and Other Patient Comfort Strategies

Patient satisfaction with regional anesthesia was higher in patients who received sedation during regional anesthesia, according to a 2014 study by Ironfield and colleagues.[46] However, sedating a patient with a DA can be challenging. Strategies used for sedation during awake airway management are suitable for sedation procedures under regional anesthesia.

Benzodiazepines, opioids, propofol, ketamine, and dexmedetomidine have all been used alone or in combination to obtain analgesia, amnesia, and anxiolysis while maintaining adequate ventilation, hemodynamic stability, and minimal or no respiratory depression. A Cochrane review of four randomized trials with a total of 211 patients with anticipated DA requiring awake flexible scope intubation (FSI) concluded that the α-2 agonist dexmedetomidine was a good sedative alternative to the use of opioids and benzodiazepines because it produced less cardiovascular and respiratory depression.[47,48] A literature review by Johnston and Rai related to sedation for FSI from 1996 to 2012 concluded that remifentanil and dexmedetomidine provided the best intubating conditions and hemodynamic stability with less airway events and more patient satisfaction.[49]

Dexmedetomidine, a potent selective α-2 agonist, is increasingly used for sedation as well as an adjunct to peripheral nerve blocks. It exhibits sedative and analgesic properties without significant respiratory depressive action.[50–52] However, when used in combination with opioids and other sedatives, respiratory depression is possible.[53] If face-mask ventilation is known or presumed to be difficult, further caution should guide the practitioner.

Meticulous attention to patient comfort should be provided as feasible and possible; knee pillows, head position, warm blankets, noise control in the OR, and even headphones with the patient's choice of music can reduce the need for sedation.

Oxygenation

Oxygenation via a nasal cannula or through a face-mask is standard for most procedures performed under regional anesthesia and

sedation. For patients with a known or assumed DA, high-flow oxygen and/or continuous positive airway pressure (CPAP) can widen the margin of safety when sedation is required. The latter is especially valuable in patients with obstructive sleep apnea (OSA).[54,55]

Strategies for Successful Management of a Patient With a Difficult Airway Under Regional Anesthesia

Benefits of Regional Anesthesia

Regional anesthesia is an essential part of opioid-free or sparing anesthesia techniques, multimodal pain management protocols, and Enhanced Recovery after Surgery (ERAS) protocols as it provides excellent postoperative pain control as well as reductions in systemic opioid requirements, postoperative nausea and vomiting, and respiratory complications.[11–16,21,56–68]

In the context of a DA, a lower need for systemic opioids decreases the risk for opioid-related side effects and complications, such as respiratory depression, that could be catastrophic in these patients. Continuous nerve block catheter techniques extend the aforementioned benefits well into the postoperative period.

Patient satisfaction with regional anesthesia is high. An analysis by Ironfield and colleagues of 600 satisfaction questionnaires of patients who underwent surgery either with regional anesthesia as the sole anesthetic or in combination with general anesthesia demonstrated that 94.6% (confidence interval [CI]: 94%–95.1%) were willing to have regional anesthesia again in the future. Factors that reduced the willingness to have a peripheral nerve block performed again were reported as block failure (only 4%), severe or moderate postoperative pain, and lower scores for patient-anesthesiologist interaction.[47]

Contraindications for Regional Anesthesia

Neuroaxial blocks are contraindicated in patients with coagulopathies, concurrent antifibrinolytics, or high-dose anticoagulation therapy. Regional anesthesia procedures that can result in accidental hematoma could jeopardize the airway (i.e., interscalene approach to the brachial plexus) and are, therefore, not advisable in patients with altered coagulation. Peripheral regional anesthesia and neuroaxial anesthesia can be safely performed in a number of neurologic conditions, but for certain conditions a risk-benefit assessment should guide the decision because deterioration of the neurologic situation can develop independently from the anesthesia method.[69,70] Specific guidelines for both conditions have been published by the American Society of Regional Anesthesia (ASRA).[69,70] The interscalene approach to the brachial plexus, and less often the supraclavicular approach, can result in paralysis of the ipsilateral diaphragm and should not be performed in patients with severe chronic obstructive pulmonary disease (COPD) or other conditions that reduce significantly the pulmonary function.

Side Effects and Complications of Regional Anesthesia

Severe side effects and complications related to regional anesthesia are rare. In a prospective study in France from August 1998 to May 1999, Auroy and colleagues reported 4 deaths, 11 cardiac arrests, 7 respiratory failures, and 7 seizures in 158,083 neuroaxial and peripheral regional anesthesia procedures.[71]

In a prospective audit of 7156 peripheral regional anesthetics by the Australian Regional Anesthesia Collaboration from January 2006 to May 2008, LA systemic toxicity (LAST) presenting with neurologic symptoms was reported in 8 patients: 0.98 per 1000 (CI: 0.42–1.9:1000) blocks. No cardiac arrest resulted from that LA toxicity.[72] In the Third National Audit Project in the United Kingdom, Cook and colleagues recorded major complications of central neuraxial blocks over a 1-year period.[73] A total of 707,455 neuraxial blocks were performed during this period with 84 major complications recorded. In an analysis of a prospective clinical registry in 2012, 4 out of the total of 6 reported deaths were attributed to LA. Sites and colleagues reported an incidence of 0.08 (CI: 0.0–0.3) of seizures and no cardiac arrests in 12,668 US-guided peripheral regional anesthetics.[74]

Acute and severe complications requiring urgent or emergent control of the airway include respiratory failure resulting from a high spinal block after neuraxial block or lumbar plexus block and LAST presenting as seizure or cardiac arrest. Preventive measures include close monitoring of the developing block level in spinal and epidural anesthesia and the use of a test dose and titration of the local anesthesia in epidural anesthesia. US-guided technique with continuous visualization of the needle tip and LA spread, slow injection of small increments of LAs, and lower volumes of LA are recommended for peripheral regional anesthesia.[75]

Failure of regional anesthesia is a far more common concern than severe side effects. Over the last few decades, US guidance for regional anesthesia has become widespread because it provides visualization of the neural structures and surrounding structures, the passage of the needle through the tissue planes and the position of the needle tip, and, when applicable, the catheter tip in relation to the neural or other structures of interest. The spread of the LA can be observed in real time. These advantages over the anatomic (landmark) and functional (nerve stimulation) techniques can explain the better success rate of US-guided regional anesthesia as well as other observed benefits such as shorter procedure time, faster onset, and successful block with lower amounts of LA.[76–81]

Regional Anesthesia Procedure

Timely planning of the regional anesthesia procedure is critical, as enough time for the block to take effect is necessary. However, the duration of a single injection block is limited, and the patient should undergo the procedure as soon as possible once the block is adequate. Catheter insertion with continuous infusion of LA can prolong the duration of regional anesthesia, and supplemental single nerve blocks can complement a patchy block distribution. It is paramount to verify appropriate surgical anesthesia before patient care is released to the surgeon.

The regional anesthesia procedure can be performed in the OR, but a dedicated regional anesthesia area is preferred because

TABLE 41.2	Strategies for Regional Anesthesia in a Patient With a Difficult Airway
Regional Anesthesia	Timely, Verify Completeness and Supplement When Necessary Before Surgery Start
Airway management plan	Emergent and nonemergent plan to manage airway, fall-back strategies for both plans
Ultrasound airway	Skin mark at the level of cricoid membrane
Patient	Information, explanation, and assurance
Surgeon and team	Preoperative briefing about anesthesia plan, airway management plan, role assignment
Sedation and comfort strategies	Careful titration of sedation, optimizing patient comfort, support oxygenation

it allows time for the block to take effect and makes for a more comfortable patient care environment.

Along with standard equipment for cardiovascular collapse, airway equipment should always be available in areas where regional anesthesia is performed (Table 41.2).

Conversion from Regional Anesthesia to General Anesthesia

Certain situations require conversion from regional anesthesia to general anesthesia, and these can arise at any time during the performance of regional anesthesia and surgical procedures. The need for conversion might develop slowly, allowing for some time to secure the airway, or emergently, demanding immediate intervention.[17] Probable causes can be related to the regional anesthesia procedure itself, the surgery, sedation, or the patient (Table 41.3).

Airway Management Strategies

Airway patency and presence or absence of respiratory drive are determining factors for the strategy to use to manage the airway. In an awake and sufficiently breathing patient who is reasonably hemodynamically stable, any technique expected to secure the airway successfully can be chosen, including awake techniques. When pursuing an awake intubation, one should take into account

TABLE 41.3	Reasons for Conversion from Regional Anesthesia to General Anesthesia			
Cause/Time Available	Regional Anesthesia	Surgical Procedure	Sedation	Patient
Emergent	LAST: seizure, cardiovascular collapse	Extensive blood loss	Respiratory depression	Uncooperative, combative
Nonemergent	Initial or subsequent failure to provide appropriate anesthesia	Need to extend surgery beyond area covered by regional anesthesia Longer duration of surgery	Increasing sedation requirements not safe without a protected airway	Discomfort with position Inability to remain immobile

the amount of local anesthesia already given during the regional anesthesia procedure to avoid LAST. By contrast, choices are more limited in a patient with airway obstruction, a patient with insufficient or absent respiratory drive, or a patient who is combative. Options in these scenarios include video laryngoscopes alone or in combination with a flexible intubation scope, optical stylet, or SGA placement with subsequent endotracheal intubation through the SGA. Irrespective of the strategy chosen, supplemental oxygen should be delivered throughout the procedure.[82-84]

The use of algorithms, such as the ASA DA algorithm, cognitive aids such as the Vortex approach, specialized airway guidelines such as the DAS Awake Tracheal Intubation guidelines, and or checklists are strongly recommended. [4,39,51,85]

The surgical team and anesthesia support team need to be informed about the necessity to manage the airway, including whether the situation is urgent or emergent. The procedure should be stopped, if feasible, until the airway is secured and confirmed. Requesting additional help should be considered.

Conclusion

Regional anesthesia represents an acceptable alternative to general anesthesia with airway management under certain conditions. Several factors, including patient, surgeon, surgery, and the regional anesthesia technique, must be considered. Strategies for emergent and nonemergent management of the airway during the procedure should be delineated and communicated to the entire team.

Selected References

1. Frerk C, Mitchell VS, McNarry AF, et al. Difficult Airway Society 2015 guidelines for management of unanticipated difficult intubation in adults. *Br J Anaesth.* 2015;115(6):827–848.

31. Li M, Ni X, Xu Z, et al. Ultrasound-assisted technology versus the conventional landmark location method in spinal anesthesia for cesarean delivery in obese parturients: a randomized controlled trial. *Anesth Analg.* 2019;129(1):155–161.

34. Kristensen MS, Teoh WH, Rudolph SS. Ultrasonographic identification of the cricothyroid membrane: best evidence, techniques, and clinical impact. *Br J Anaesth.* 2016;117(suppl 1):i39–i48.

39. Joffe AM, Aziz MF, Posner KL, Duggan LV, Mincer SL, Domino KB. Management of difficult tracheal intubation: a closed claims analysis. *Anesthesiology.* 2019;131(4):818–829.

43. American Society of Anesthesiologists. Standards and Guidelines: Statement on Nonoperating Room Anesthetizing Locations, Committee on Standards and Practice Parameters (CSPP), Reaffirmed October 2018 [Internet]. Available at https://www.asahq.org/standards-and-guidelines.

73. Cook TM, Counsell D, Wildsmith JAW. Major complications of central neuraxial block: report on the Third National Audit Project of the Royal College of Anaesthetists. *Br J Anaesth.* 2009;102:179–190.

75. Neal JM, Barrington MJ, Fettiplace MR, et al. The Third American Society of Regional Anesthesia and Pain Medicine Practice Advisory on Local Anesthetic Systemic Toxicity: Executive Summary 2017. *Reg Anesth Pain Med.* 2018;43(2):113–123. doi:10.1097/AAP.0000000000000720. PMID: 29356773

82. Patel A, Nouraei SAR. Transnasal Humidified Rapid-Insufflation Ventilatory Exchange (THRIVE): a physiological method of increasing apnoea time in patients with DAs. *Anaesthesia.* 2015;70(3):323–329.

All references can be found online at eBooks.Health.Elsevier.com.

42

Airway Management in Non-Operating Room Locations

LOUISE ELLARD AND DAVID T. WONG

KEY POINTS

- Specific training for non-operating room anesthesia (NORA) should be incorporated into anesthesia residency programs.
- Monitoring for both oxygenation and ventilation is required during sedation, including the use of capnography.
- Intubation of the patient with an anticipated difficult airway (DA) may be best managed in the operating suite with optimal equipment and familiar anesthesia staffing before transporting the patient to the NORA location.
- An anesthesia machine offers convenient means of providing oxygenation, ventilation, volatile anesthesia, suction, and ease of conversion to general anesthesia, if required.

- Sedation can be safely used for many NORA procedures, but the precautionary principle should be applied for complex, lengthy procedures or where the need for immobility or risk of hemodynamic instability is present.
- Management of the unanticipated DA in a NORA location should be the same as in the OR, utilizing DA algorithms and calling for assistance early.
- Long anesthesia circuits are especially useful in many NORA locations.

Introduction

In recent years, the coverage responsibilities of anesthesiologists have evolved from traditional operating room (OR) locations to encompass more remote areas in the hospital. Non-operating room anesthesia (NORA) refers to administration of anesthetic care outside of the OR for patients undergoing procedures.[1] Under the umbrella of NORA fits a diverse range of procedures with unique procedural requirements, equipment, and risks that are united in their out-of-OR location. NORA locations and specialties include endoscopy, cardiology, pulmonology, and radiology and are detailed in Table 42.1. As expert providers of sedation and general anesthesia both inside and outside of the OR,

anesthesiologists should take the lead in ensuring that safety is maintained in this growing specialty.

A rapidly increasing proportion of cases are being performed in remote locations due to advances in diagnostic and interventional techniques and greater patient expectations for amnesia and sedation. From 2005 to 2007, approximately 12% to 15% of the total anesthesia workload was outside of the OR.[2,3] Data from the National Anesthesia Clinical Outcomes Registry (NACOR) for the period 2010 to 2014 showed that NORA as a proportion of all anesthesia cases increased from 28.3% in 2010 to 35.9% in 2014.[4] In other countries, NORA composes a much smaller percentage of all cases, accounting for only 8.2% of all cases in a large Korean study of 199,764 cases between 2013

TABLE 42.1	Some of the Most Common Procedures in NORA Locations
NORA Location	**Procedures**
Neuroradiology	Diagnostic angiography Embolization of cerebral aneurysm or arteriovenous malformation Mechanical thrombectomy (i.e., emergency clot retrieval) Carotid or vertebral artery angioplasty/stenting
Diagnostic radiology	Computed tomography (CT) Magnetic resonance imaging (MRI) Positron emission tomography (PET)
Interventional radiology	Chemoembolization and radiofrequency ablation Endovascular stents Transjugular intrahepatic portosystemic shunt (TIPS) Percutaneous transhepatic cholangiography (PTC) CT-guided abscess drainage and biopsies Insertion of vascular lines Kyphoplasty/vertebroplasty
Gastrointestinal endoscopy suites	Upper gastrointestinal endoscopy Endoscopic retrograde cholangiopancreatography (ERCP) Percutaneous endoscopic gastrostomy (PEG) tube placement Colonoscopy Endoscopic submucosal resection
Cardiovascular	Transesophageal echocardiography (TEE) Electrophysiology studies and treatment Pacemaker/defibrillator insertion or extraction Cardioversion Percutaneous coronary intervention Percutaneous valve replacement or repair[a]
Pulmonology	Diagnostic bronchoscopy Endobronchial ultrasound (EBUS) with biopsy Endobronchial lung volume reduction for chronic obstructive pulmonary disease (COPD) using endobronchial valves Airway stents Bronchoalveolar lavage
Psychiatry	Electroconvulsive therapy (ECT)
Oncology	Radiation oncology Bone marrow biopsy Therapeutic lumbar puncture and chemotherapy

[a]In some centers with hybrid theaters, these procedures are done within the OR complex.

and 2017.[5] There are estimates that, within the next decade, the proportion of NORA will approach or even exceed traditional OR cases.[6,7]

Safety Profile and Risks of NORA

Safety data for non-OR locations are not reassuring, performing poorly compared with OR locations. Certain NORA locations feature prominently in closed claims analyses and observational studies, including the endoscopy suite, radiology, and cardiac catheterization suites.[8–11] These closed claims analyses showed that injuries in NORA locations were more severe and more likely to result in death when compared to OR closed claims.[8–10] Most adverse events in NORA locations are respiratory in origin, which is often attributed to oversedation resulting in inadequate ventilation and oxygenation during monitored anesthesia care (MAC).[8,12]

A prospective multicenter observational study in 2132 patients undergoing gastrointestinal endoscopy with propofol sedation confirmed the risks of NORA, reporting unplanned events in 23% of patients, significant hypotension in 11.8%, and a 30-day mortality of 1.2%.[13] A large database study found that the incidence of cardiac arrest and death was 3.92 per 10,000 in patients undergoing gastrointestinal endoscopy, with most arrests attributed to hypoventilation and hypoxemia.[14] Studies in the pulmonology suite and cardiac electrophysiology laboratory both report high rates of adverse events that are often respiratory in origin.[15,16]

Although some studies, especially those with a large proportion of pediatric patients, show that complications in the NORA setting are rare,[5,17,18] other studies point to concerning rates of complications when compared with OR locations. An understanding of the nature of these complications, including the overrepresentation of respiratory causes, is needed to improve the safety of NORA.

NORA locations are generally found at a distance from the main ORs; therefore, access to skilled anesthesia personnel and equipment may not be immediately available. Unlike the standardized layout of most ORs, NORA locations are highly differentiated, resulting in an unfamiliar working environment for the anesthesia provider. These suites are designed for the specific procedure being undertaken, incorporating bulky imaging and procedural equipment, resulting in limited available workspace for anesthesia personnel and equipment. Access to the patient, specifically the airway, may be limited as the anesthesia provider is often more physically distant from the patient during the procedure. The procedure table may lack the degree of adjustability of an OR table. The environment can be noisy and dimly lit, interfering with observation of the patient and monitors. Lower ambient temperatures are typical to avoid overheating of equipment, which can result in patient hypothermia. Radiation safety must be considered for both patients and staff, requiring the use of lead aprons, thyroid shields, and glass lead screens.[19] Equipment that is taken for granted in OR locations may not be readily available, including scavenging and suction systems; piped wall air, oxygen, and inhalational anesthesia; an anesthesia machine; or difficult airway (DA) carts, cardiac arrest carts, and malignant hyperthermia carts.

Staff in NORA locations are generally less familiar with anesthesia procedures, their unique requirements and equipment, emergencies, and airway management. A growing number of emergency procedures and procedures are being performed outside of normal working hours when reduced staff familiarity and resource limitations are likely to be amplified.[4] Because many procedures occurring in NORA locations are minimally invasive, they may be offered to patients who are otherwise too frail or unfit for open surgical procedures; thus NORA patients tend to be older and sicker than those in OR locations.[4,17,20]

In addition to the general risks of NORA, specific risks according to the procedure and patient cohort are outlined in Table 42.2. Prior to anesthetizing a patient in a NORA location, the anesthesia provider should understand the planned procedure, duration, patient positioning, need for immobility and sedation, expected level of discomfort, and other specific requirements.

Monitoring Requirements of NORA

To ensure NORA locations meet the same safety profile as the OR, patient assessment and optimization should be equally

TABLE 42.2   Risks in NORA Locations

Procedure	Procedure-Specific Risks	Risk Due to Patient's Condition
Neuroradiology	General requirement for immobility Restricted access to the patient's airway is likely Control of intracranial pressure may be required Risk of thromboembolic complications Risk of vascular rupture (sudden onset of elevated intracranial pressure resulting in hypertension and bradycardia)	Presenting neurological condition may result in confusion, lack of cooperation, or reduced level of consciousness[19]
MRI	Unique physical environment Darkened room High level of noise Interference with equipment caused by magnetic fields Potential for heat generation within monitoring wires (e.g., pulse oximeter, electrocardiogram) causing burns Equipment in room limited to nonferrous items	Often extremes of age Claustrophobia/extreme anxiety Cognitive impairment/intellectual disability
Upper gastrointestinal endoscopy	Shared airway Endoscope may obstruct the airway Deep sedation often required to suppress gag and cough reflexes	Aspiration risk if gastric bleeding
PEG tube insertion	Same as for upper gastrointestinal endoscopy	Patient generally unwell, with end-stage neuromuscular disorders common
Endoscopic retrograde cholangiopancreatography	Semi-prone position Uncomfortable procedure requiring deep sedation or general anesthesia	Aspiration risk due to underlying pathology, including pancreatic pseudocyst, biliary obstruction, or liver disease
Colonoscopy	Manual abdominal pressure to overcome technical difficulties may increase the risk of aspiration[46]	
Percutaneous aortic valve replacement	Risk of aortic rupture, tamponade, or valve maldeployment	Aortic stenosis Patient may be medically unfit for open aortic valve replacement
Bronchoscopy	Constant stimulation of the airway and coughing Preference for akinesia Risk of hemoptysis	Severe lung disease is common Lung cancer and associated paraneoplastic syndromes High proportion of smokers
Radiotherapy	Fiberglass immobilization mask is used to direct the position of the radiation beam for intracranial lesions, which precludes the use of an oral airway or supraglottic airway once in place[51]	

thorough. Organizational policies should address minimum facility and equipment requirements. The use of a smaller pool of dedicated anesthesia providers for NORA locations[21] who have undergone specific NORA training[6,22] can further assist with risk mitigation.

In closed claims analyses, inadequate oxygenation and ventilation feature highly in NORA claims, with anesthesia care often judged to be substandard and preventable by better monitoring.[8–10] Patient monitoring in remote locations should be equivalent to OR standards and should adhere to guidance provided by the major national anesthesiology societies, including those published by the American Society of Anesthesiologists (ASA) (Box 42.1),[23] the Canadian Anesthesiologists' Society,[24] the Australian and New Zealand College of Anaesthetists,[25] and the Association of Anaesthetists of Great Britain and Ireland.[26]

Pulse oximetry should be used for all patients undergoing general anesthesia or procedural sedation,[24,25,27,28] although it must be recognized that this is a useful indicator of oxygenation but not ventilation, as a fall in oxygen saturation may be delayed relative to the onset of apnea.[29,30] The oxygen reserve index is a novel noninvasive measure of oxygen reserve detecting Pao_2

levels <150 mm Hg,[31] giving an early warning of impending desaturation.[32,33]

When capnography is used during procedural sedation, respiratory depression is more likely to be detected prior to the onset of hypoxia.[20,34] Monitoring for presence of exhaled carbon dioxide (CO_2) became an ASA standard for general anesthesia in 1991[28] and was extended to moderate or deep sedation in 2011.[28,35] International guidelines endorse the use of exhaled CO_2 monitoring for sedation, in addition to general anesthesia.[25–27] Closed claims data support that monitoring requirements for oxygenation and ventilation should be independent of the depth of sedation,[21,36] and the findings in the Fourth National Audit Project of the Royal College of Anaesthestists (NAP4) were another major factor in encouraging widespread adoption of end-tidal CO_2 monitoring outside of the OR.[37]

CO_2 monitoring during sedation can be achieved using capnography from a sampling line incorporated into nasal prongs or attached to a face mask or bite block. When used in this manner, air entrainment and dilution by high fresh gas flows will result in lower end-tidal CO_2 levels and underestimation of arterial CO_2.[38] However, there is value in detecting qualitative changes including

1. A reliable source of oxygen adequate for the length of the procedure as well as a backup supply (a central oxygen source is preferred, and a backup source should include at least a full E-cylinder)
2. A reliable suction source
3. An adequate system for scavenging waste anesthetic gases
4. A self-inflating resuscitator bag capable of administering at least 90% oxygen as a means to deliver positive-pressure ventilation
5. Adequate anesthetic drugs, supplies, and equipment for the intended anesthetic care
6. Adequate monitoring equipment that adheres to the ASA Standards for Basic Anesthetic Monitoring,[28] which should be applied to all cases involving general anesthesia, regional anesthesia, and monitored anesthesia care
7. In any location where inhaled anesthetics are used, there should be an anesthesia machine equivalent in function to that used in the operating room and maintained to current operating room standards
8. Sufficient electrical outlets that adhere to facility standards
9. Adequate illumination of the patient and equipment
10. Sufficient space to accommodate necessary equipment and personnel to allow rapid access to the patient and equipment when needed
11. Immediate access to an emergency cart with a defibrillator, emergency drugs, and other equipment to provide cardiopulmonary resuscitation
12. Adequate anesthesia support staff readily available at each location
13. Appropriate postanesthesia management and recovery with adequately trained staff and monitoring equipment

Modified with permission from American Society of Anesthesiologists (ASA). Statement on nonoperating room anesthetizing locations. Available at https://www.asahq.org/standards-and-guidelines/statement-on-nonoperating-room-anesthetizing-locations. Reaffirmed October 17, 2018.

waveform shape, respiratory rate, evidence of airway obstruction, or apnea.[31,39]

Other methods of monitoring ventilation are described in Table 42.3, including acoustic respiratory monitoring, impedance monitoring, respiratory volume monitoring, and transcutaneous CO_2 monitoring, with potential advantages over traditional capnography.

Choice of Anesthesia and Sedation

Many NORA cases can be performed using procedural sedation, especially brief procedures in relatively healthy patients. For complex procedures, medically unwell patients, or patients with an identified DA, general anesthesia with preemptive control of the airway may be preferred.

The purpose of sedation is to control pain or anxiety, improve patient cooperation,[40] and/or provide amnesia and decreased awareness.[29] The ASA defines four distinct levels of sedation on a continuum: minimal, moderate, deep, and general anesthesia.[41] The commonly used term *conscious sedation* refers to mild or moderate sedation.[41] Deep sedation is frequently chosen in NORA locations and is generally accomplished without a definitive airway. A 2015 survey of 409 Australian anesthesiologists of individual sedation practice for endoscopy patients revealed that a deep level of sedation, where the patient was unresponsive to painful stimulation, was targeted by 54% of respondents.[42] In a study of 87 patients undergoing colonoscopy, the measured depth of anesthesia in the 43 patients who received propofol-based sedation was consistent with general anesthesia for a significant part of the procedure.[43] MAC is commonly employed in NORA locations and featured highly in closed claims analysis.[8,9,12] MAC involves an anesthesia provider participating in the care of a patient undergoing a diagnostic or therapeutic procedure and includes all aspects of anesthesia care, including sedation and treatment of complications and coexisting medical problems.[44,45] A key requirement is that the qualified anesthesia provider must be prepared to convert to general anesthesia if necessary.[45]

Risks of Sedation

Patients undergoing sedation are at risk of airway obstruction and/or respiratory depression, which can result in hypoxia, hypercarbia, or both.[30,38] Independent risk factors for sedation-induced hypoxemia include high body mass index (BMI), hypertension, diabetes, heart disease, and procedures that include upper gastrointestinal endoscopy and colonoscopy.[29] Sedation-induced oxyhemoglobin desaturation is accelerated in patients with a reduced functional residual capacity (FRC), including infants and obese patients.[36]

TABLE 42.3 Other Methods of Monitoring Ventilation During Procedural Sedation

Category	Examples	Description	Potential Advantages Over Capnography
Acoustic respiratory monitoring	Massimo Rad-87[80–81]	Detects sound of airflow in the pharynx using a piezoelectric sticker applied to the neck	Greater specificity to detect apneic events during procedural sedation compared to end-tidal CO_2 monitoring[81] Single monitor provides both pulse oximetry and respiratory rate[80] Sticker applied to the neck does not require close proximity to the airway and avoids interference by supplemental oxygen or movement of the endoscope
Respiratory volume monitoring	Respiratory Motion ExSpirion	Uses electrical impedance changes to derive a signal that strongly correlates with minute ventilation[38]	Useful during longer sedation cases Detects decreases in minute ventilation Higher sensitivity and specificity for determining hypoventilation compared to capnography for procedural sedation[82,83]
Transcutaneous CO_2 monitoring	SenTec digital monitoring system	Controlled heating of the skin to arterialize the capillary bed allowing CO_2 to diffuse into a chamber containing a Clarke-Severinghaus electrode[38]	Useful during longer sedation cases Able to provide a more accurate estimate of arterial CO_2 during procedural sedation[38] Does not require monitor proximity to the airway and is not interfered with by supplemental oxygen (however, does not detect apnea)

Management of respiratory depression, apnea, or airway obstruction includes verbal or physical stimulation to breathe, reversal of sedation, insertion of an oral or nasopharyngeal airway, or mechanical ventilatory support using bag-mask ventilation, insertion of a supraglottic airway (SGA), or tracheal intubation. Another respiratory complication of sedation is aspiration, which is more likely in patients with symptomatic gastroesophageal reflux, gastric outlet obstruction, gastric stasis, gastrointestinal bleeding, and inadequate fasting times.

Medication Choices

Many different medications can be used for sedation in NORA locations, including propofol, opioids, benzodiazepines, ketamine, and dexmedetomidine, without firm evidence for a preferred option with superior outcomes. Propofol is easily titratable, providing rapid onset and short duration of action. Addition of a short-acting opioid (fentanyl or remifentanil) suppresses coughing but can increase the risk of apnea.[46] When comparing propofol and remifentanil with propofol alone in patients undergoing colonoscopy, the addition of remifentanil reduced the dose of propofol but was associated with more respiratory depression.[47] Ketamine and propofol can be mixed together as "ketofol" for procedural sedation.[22] Remimazolam, a novel benzodiazepine with quicker onset and offset compared to midazolam, may be increasingly useful for procedural sedation.[48]

Dexmedetomidine can also be used for sedation, and its benefits include lack of a respiratory depressant effect, patient cooperation when roused, and an analgesic effect.[49] This may be a particularly useful drug in patients with obesity and sleep apnea. A typical dose is 1 µg/kg over 10 minutes followed by an infusion of 0.6 µg/kg/h titrated to required effect.[22] The efficacy and safety of high-dose dexmedetomidine (2 µg/kg bolus followed by 1 µg/kg/h) was investigated as a sole sedative agent in 544 children undergoing MRI. In 78.5% of cases, no additional medication was required.[50] Side effects of dexmedetomidine include bradycardia and hypotension.

Airway Considerations in NORA

Routine Airway Management

Anesthesia and airway equipment in NORA locations should mimic that in the OR as much as possible. A system should be in place to ensure that restocking of off-site locations occurs with the same frequency and degree of certainty as for the OR[51]; a suggested list of essential airway equipment is outlined in Box 42.2. One convenient option is a mobile anesthesia cart, or a fleet of carts, to hold all required equipment; these can be housed in the main operating theater complex and checked and restocked daily.[36] As needed, these carts can then accompany the anesthesia provider to the NORA location.

An anesthesia machine is a familiar and convenient device for the anesthesia provider and provides the ability to oxygenate and ventilate the patient, administer volatile anesthesia, and provide suction. The drawers in an anesthesia machine can house additional airway supplies to prevent possible oversights when trying to assemble all necessary equipment.[44] Long anesthesia circuits should be considered in various NORA locations, as it may be impossible to have the anesthesia machine immediately adjacent to the airway. Given the potential for progression to general anesthesia due to patient deterioration or procedural complications, the presence of an anesthesia machine or its component parts should be immediately available.[44]

• BOX 42.2 **Suggested Airway Equipment in NORA Locations**

Airway devices
Oral and nasopharyngeal airways[a]
Nasal prongs[a]
Face masks[a]
Supraglottic airways[a]
Endotracheal tubes[a]
Stylets for endotracheal tubes[a]
Bougies[a]
Laryngoscope handle and blades[a]
Oxygen
Self-inflating resuscitation bag with a positive end-expiratory pressure (PEEP) valve or portable breathing system capable of delivering high oxygen concentrations (Mapleson C breathing system) with an oxygen supply that is independent of the anesthesia machine
Wall gas
Backup oxygen supplies (cylinders)
Other
Suction and Yankauer catheters (for exclusive use of the anesthetist at all times)
Scavenging system if inhalational anesthesia is planned
Syringes
Stethoscopes
Tape
McGill forceps

[a]Various sizes according to patient population.

Anticipated Difficult Airway

When considering the challenges associated with NORA locations and the overrepresentation of respiratory morbidity, management of the patient with a known DA must be carefully considered. The DA is exacerbated by the difficult environment in which the airway is being managed. Situational difficulties may arise, which must be anticipated, including lack of skilled personnel, missing equipment including airway tools, and poor patient access.

DA algorithms apply equally to OR and NORA settings.[52,53] For many NORA procedures, there is no initial plan to intubate, making the Vortex approach particularly suited to NORA locations. The Vortex approach is based on the principle that there are only three nonsurgical ways to manage the airway. These three "lifelines" (face mask, SGA, and endotracheal tube [ETT]) are arranged in a circle, meaning that airway management could commence with any method and proceed to the remaining two in any sequence, regardless of the initial airway choice.[54]

In an anticipated difficult intubation, awake intubation should be considered, ideally in the controlled environment of the operating suite, where a full complement of familiar advanced airway equipment and personnel are located. Next, the intubated patient can be transferred to the NORA location.[51,55,56] The benefits of this approach need to be considered against the inherent risks of transporting an intubated patient with potential for ETT displacement. Similar consideration should be given to managing extubation in patients with a DA back in the OR, in case advanced techniques (e.g., extubation over an airway exchange catheter) or reintubation are required.

If the anticipated risk of difficulty is relatively low, the patient can be induced in the NORA location and a clearly delineated intubation plan followed. This could include video-assisted laryngoscopy (VAL), a hybrid approach combining intubation through a SGA, or a combined VAL and bronchoscopic intubation technique. If airway difficulties are encountered in a NORA location, the practitioner should call for help early.

If intubation is not planned, sedation must be extremely judicious to ensure that oversedation does not lead to respiratory depression or apnea, resulting in the need to emergently manage a DA in a challenging environment.

Unanticipated Difficult Airway

The approach to an unanticipated DA in a NORA location should be identical to management within the OR, incorporating DA algorithms and agreed hospital protocols.[52–54] An "out-of-area" DA cart must be readily available, with suggested contents shown in Box 42.3. The management of airway and other emergencies will be aided by using standardized code carts throughout an organization and poster displays of agreed-upon DA protocols, so that nonanesthesia personnel can rapidly and reliably assist and retrieve critical items.[51]

Procedure Specific Airway Management

Neuroradiology and Other Interventional Radiology

Many interventional radiology procedures are prolonged, with challenging access to the patient once the procedure is underway. General anesthesia and tracheal intubation are often required to permit absolute immobility, breath holds,[7] accurate stent deployment, and management of complications. This is especially true for interventional neuroradiology procedures to minimize the risk of vessel perforation or malpositioning of embolic material, controlled ventilation for optimal imaging, and rapid management of vascular complications should they arise. The need to attend to airway issues while simultaneously managing catastrophic intraprocedural complications, such as intracerebral hemorrhage, is avoided with preemptive intubation.[19]

Multiple trials have sought to answer the question whether emergency clot retrieval for acute ischemic stroke should be performed under general or local anesthesia with sedation. Recent randomized controlled trials have shown no difference in outcomes between conscious sedation or general anesthesia.[57–59] The anesthesiologist should consider the patient's state of consciousness and level of cooperation, severity of the stroke, anticipated technical difficulties of the procedure, and challenges with airway management, if required, when deciding on the anesthesia and airway management plan in such patients.

Magnetic Resonance Imaging

Many patients who require anesthesia for MRI can be safely managed with an SGA. For more complex patients or those in whom airway difficulty is anticipated, preemptive tracheal intubation is desirable. During an MRI scan, access to the patient's airway is limited and difficulties with visual and auditory assessment of the patient can occur.[56] If the need to manage the patient's airway arises midprocedure, the scan would need to be interrupted and personnel brought in from outside of the room.

A comprehensive guide to promote staff and patient safety in the MRI environment is published in the ASA's Practice Advisory on Anesthetic Care for MRI, including details of the four zones that correlate with the intensity of the magnetic field and the personnel and equipment permitted in each zone.[51,56]

> **• BOX 42.3   Suggested Contents of a Difficult Airway Cart in NORA Locations**
>
> *Rescue bag-mask ventilation*
> Oropharyngeal airways[a]
> Nasopharyngeal airways[a]
> Masks[a]
> Self-inflating bag with PEEP valve
> *Rescue supraglottic airway*
> Classic (first-generation) supraglottic airways[a]
> Second-generation supraglottic airways[a]
> Intubating supraglottic airway (e.g., Ambu AuraGain)[a]
> *Rescue intubation*
> Endotracheal tubes[a]
> Videolaryngoscope
> Range of laryngoscope blades[a] (straight, short handle, McCoy, Kessel)
> Tracheal tube introducer (bougie)[a]
> Stylet
> Airway exchange catheter[a]
> Aintree Intubation Catheter (Cook Medical, Bloomington, IN)
> *Awake flexible scope intubation equipment*
> Flexible bronchoscope and screen
> Atomizer device
> Ovassapian (or similar) airway
> Airway topicalization drug box
> Endoscopy masks[a]
> *Rescue emergency invasive airway*
> Scalpel size 10 blade
> Bougie
> Endotracheal tube size 6 cuffed
> 14G IV catheter
> Rapid-O_2 oxygen cricothyroidotomy insufflation device (Meditech Systems Ltd, Shaftesbury, UK) (jet ventilation via cannula) or Enk Oxygen flow modulator (Cook Medical, Bloomington, IN) or Ventrain (Ventinova, Eindhoven, The Netherlands)
> Emergency cricothyrotomy catheter set (e.g., Melker [Cook Medical, Bloomington, IN])
> *Miscellaneous*
> Magill forceps
> Qualitative CO_2 measurement device (e.g., colorimetric CO_2 detector)
> Sugammadex
> Suction catheters[a]
> Cuff manometer
>
> [a]Various sizes according to patient population.

Within the MRI room (zone IV), any anesthesia and airway equipment must be MRI compatible. It is worth noting that the only component of a laryngoscope that is not usually MRI safe is the battery, which can be replaced with a lithium battery.[51] Most videolaryngoscopes, flexible intubation scopes, and their respective towers are not MRI compatible.[51] Most SGAs are MRI compatible, although those with reinforced metal coils can interfere with image quality and the pilot balloon must be taped out of the imaging field for scans of the head and neck.[51,60] Complex airway management (i.e., flexible scope-guided intubation) should be performed in a controlled environment outside zone IV, and MRI-safe airway devices should be immediately available in the MRI suite, including suction equipment.[56]

Upper and Lower Gastrointestinal Endoscopy

Most upper gastrointestinal endoscopy can be performed under sedation without an airway device. In the event of respiratory depression, apnea, or airway obstruction, many rescue airway

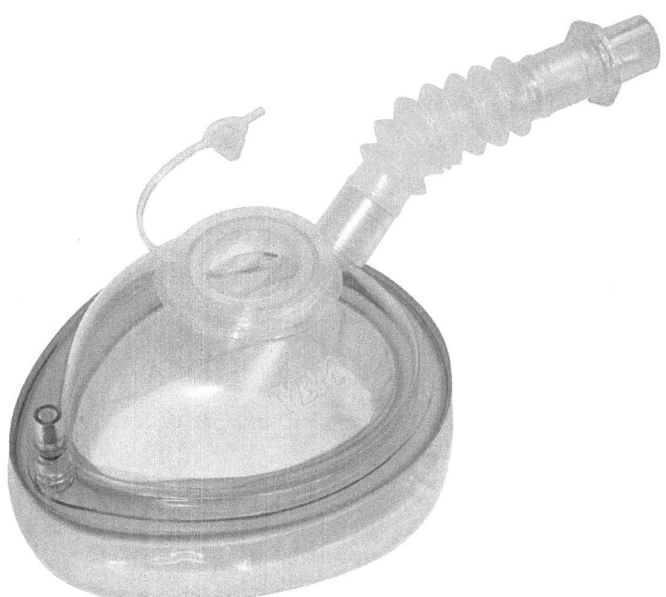

• **Fig. 42.1** The endoscopy mask. (Courtesy VNM, Medizitchnik, Sulz am Neckar, Germany).

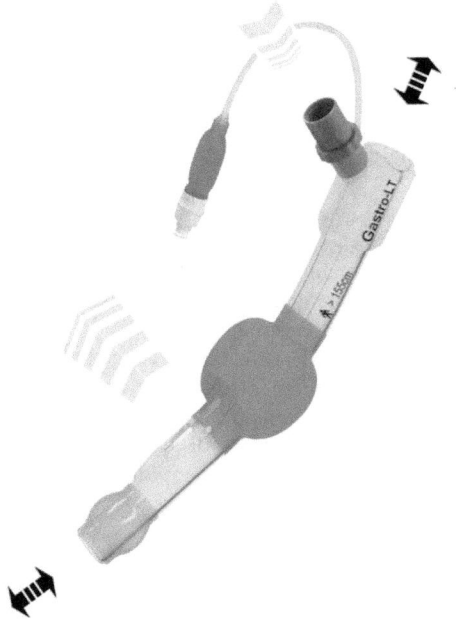

• **Fig. 42.2** The Gastro-Laryngeal Tube. (Courtesy VNM, Medizitchnik, Sulz am Neckar, Germany.)

maneuvers (insertion of an oropharyngeal or nasopharyngeal airway, bag-mask ventilation, SGA insertion, or tracheal intubation) can only be applied after withdrawal of the endoscope.

Supplemental oxygen during sedation is considered standard of care, which can be challenging to deliver through a standard face mask during endoscopy procedures. Several specifically designed bite blocks permit endoscopy access and include features for oxygen delivery, capnography monitoring, and a suction port to clear secretions.[31,61] The Goudra ventilating bite block incorporates a port for cuff inflation and an air-tight self-sealing diaphragm for insertion of the endoscope; when used in combination with the supplied nasal occlusion device, the closed system permits CO_2 monitoring.[62] The Endoscopy Mask (VBM Medizintechnik, Sulz am Neckar, Germany) has a leakproof cushioned seal that allows positive-pressure ventilation and delivery of almost 100% oxygen (Fig. 42.1).[31] The DEAS (DEAS, Castel Bolognese, Italy) cannula is a modified nasopharyngeal cannula allowing oxygen delivery, medication administration through a dedicated channel, and end-tidal CO_2 sampling.[63]

The LMA Gastro (Teleflex, Morrisville, NC) is a modified, disposable SGA that was developed to improve airway management during upper gastrointestinal endoscopy. It has a dedicated large-bore channel for passage of an endoscope and a separate airway channel for ventilation and end-tidal CO_2 (EtCO$_2$) sampling (Fig. 42.2).[63] The Gastro-Laryngeal Tube (VBM Medizintechnik, Sulz am Neckar, Germany) has two cuffs: the distal one inflates in the esophagus to prevent regurgitation of gastric contents, and the second cuff lies proximally to block air leak via the naso/oropharynx.[31] Between these two cuffs, multiple perforations in the tube lie adjacent to the larynx to allow positive-pressure ventilation if required. The gastroscope is inserted via a separate channel built within the tube, and there is a connection for capnography (Fig. 42.3).[31] Safety and efficacy have been demonstrated for both the Gastro-Laryngeal Tube[64–67] and LMA Gastro in clinical practice.[68–70]

Tracheal intubation should be considered for complex, lengthy procedures such as double-balloon enteroscopy and endoscopic

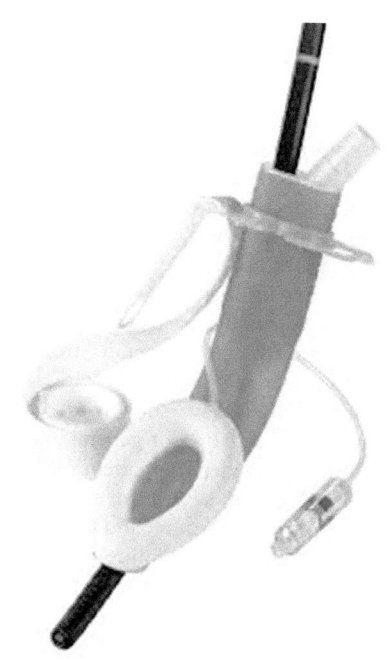

• **Fig. 42.3** The LMA Gastro. (Courtesy Teleflex, Morrisville, NC)

mucosal resection[71] or for procedures that result in an increased aspiration risk, including upper gastrointestinal bleed or pancreatic pseudocyst drainage where fluid is drained into the stomach.

A cohort study of 91 patients undergoing submucosal resection of gastric tumor compared propofol-based sedation (54 patients) to volatile-based general anesthesia with an ETT (37 patients). The general anesthesia group had faster dissection speed and lower incidence of desaturation, coughing, and nausea.[72] In a retrospective cohort study of 119 morbidly obese patients (BMI >40 kg/m²) presenting for outpatient upper gastrointestinal endoscopy, low rates of hypoxia were attributed to a technique involving a nasopharyngeal airway connected to a Mapleson circuit, and supine head-up positioning to preserve FRC. Only two patients recorded oxygen saturation <90% (89% and 82% were the lowest recorded saturations for brief periods).[73]

Endoscopic Retrograde Cholangiopancreatography

Optimal airway management for patients undergoing endoscopic retrograde cholangiopancreatography (ERCP) remains a contentious area without agreed consensus. Semi-prone positioning makes rapid airway securement challenging, if required during the procedure. In a survey of Australian anesthetists, 22% routinely intubate elective ERCP patients, and 64% routinely intubate emergency ERCP patients.[72] A randomized controlled trial compared general endotracheal anesthesia vs propofol-based MAC in 200 patients at high risk of sedation-related adverse events undergoing ERCP. Patients considered to be at risk of sedation-related adverse events had a STOP-BANG score ≥3, ascites, BMI >35 kg/m², chronic lung disease, ASA score >3, Mallampati class 4 airway, or moderate-heavy alcohol abuse.[74] Composite respiratory adverse events were higher in the sedation group (51.5% vs 9.9%), and there was a 10.1% rate of conversion to general anesthesia. There was no difference in procedure duration, success, recovery, or time in the endoscopy suite. These authors argue for elective tracheal intubation in ERCP with patients at risk of adverse respiratory events, given the superior safety profile and lack of impact on efficiency.[74]

Cardiac and Cardiovascular Interventional Units

Many interventional cardiology procedures are lengthy and present a risk of hemodynamic instability (e.g., resulting from tamponade or significant arrythmia) and may require the use of transesophageal echocardiography. For this reason, tracheal intubation is often chosen. Transcatheter aortic valve replacement (TAVR) has been performed since 2002 for management of aortic stenosis.[75] When performed via the transapical or transsubclavian routes, general anesthesia is typically chosen. However, the transfemoral route, increasingly being performed without the need for transesophageal echocardiography, lends itself to MAC in many centers.[76]

Pulmonology

The three main options for airway management during diagnostic or therapeutic bronchoscopy include local anesthetic topicalization with or without sedation, general anesthesia using an SGA, or general anesthesia with muscle paralysis and an ETT. The choice of airway management primarily depends on procedural requirements including the need for spontaneous ventilation (e.g., to diagnose tracheomalacia), visualization of the vocal cords, access to proximal mediastinal lymph nodes (excluding use of an ETT), the expected duration of the procedure, need for immobility, use of laser, and choice between flexible and rigid bronchoscopy.

Flexible bronchoscopy can be performed using local anesthetic topicalization with minimal sedation. Airway topicalization can be achieved in a number of ways, but the use of a DeVilbiss or another atomizer allows this to be rapidly and easily achieved. Supplemental local anesthetic to the distal bronchial tree can be given by the proceduralist. As diagnostic and therapeutic procedures are

becoming more complex and there is a greater desire for patient immobility, techniques involving general anesthesia and an SGA are increasingly preferred.[77–79]

Endobronchial ultrasound (EBUS) and transbronchial needle aspiration represent a complex diagnostic technique allowing sampling of mediastinal and hilar lymph nodes for lung cancer staging and diagnosis. Although EBUS can be performed using topicalization and sedation, the duration of the procedure, desire for immobility, and precision required to sample lymph nodes adjacent to blood vessels mean that general anesthesia with an SGA is often chosen.[78,79] The choice of an SGA rather than an ETT provides access to proximal mediastinal lymph nodes higher in the trachea. Muscle relaxation is often used to prevent cough and movement during biopsy.[78]

Conclusion

Demand is increasing for anesthesia services in locations outside of the OR, involving older and sicker patients. The most common NORA locations include interventional and diagnostic neuroradiology, the cardiac catheterization laboratory, and the gastrointestinal and pulmonology suites. Safety data on NORA locations have not been reassuring, with particular concern surrounding respiratory complications and inadequate monitoring. Emphasis must be on ensuring that NORA locations are just as safe as the OR, with attention to organizational safety standards, equipment, monitoring requirements, personnel training, and emergency drills. The anesthesia provider should understand the procedural requirements, risks, and patient comorbidities prior to embarking on a given case and deciding on airway management.

Many diagnostic and brief procedures can be safely managed using procedural sedation. Complex procedures with higher risk of complications, or involving patients with greater risk of airway difficulties, should be managed with general anesthesia and tracheal intubation. If uncertain, the precautionary principle should be applied. For both planning of and execution of anticipated and unanticipated airway difficulties, published airway guidelines apply equally to NORA and OR locations. Anesthesiologists are ideally positioned to take the lead in this quest to optimize safety for patients undergoing procedures in NORA locations.

Selected References

4. Nagrebetsky A, Gabriel RA, Dutton RP, Urman RD. Growth of nonoperating room anesthesia care in the United States: a contemporary trends analysis. *Anesth Analg.* 2017;124(4):1261–1267.

8. Metzner J, Posner KL, Domino KB. The risk and safety of anesthesia at remote locations: the US closed claims analysis. *Curr Opin Anaesthesiol.* 2009;22(4):502–508.

13. Leslie K, Allen ML, Hessian E, et al. Safety of sedation for gastrointestinal endoscopy in a group of university-affiliated hospitals: a prospective cohort study. *Br J Anaesth.* 2017;118(1):90–99.

31. Goudra B, Singh PM. Airway management during upper GI endoscopic procedures: state of the art review. *Dig Dis Sci.* 2017;62(1):45–53.

35. Apfelbaum JL, Gross JB, Connis RT, et al. Practice Guidelines for Moderate Procedural Sedation and Analgesia 2018: A Report by the American Society of Anesthesiologists Task Force on Moderate Procedural Sedation and Analgesia, the American Association of Oral and Maxillofacial Surgeons, American College of Radiology, American Dental Association, American Society of Dentist Anesthesiologists, and Society of Interventional Radiology. *Anesthesiology.* 2018;128(3):437–479.

37. Cook TM, Woodall N, Frerk C, Fourth National Audit Project. Major complications of airway management in the UK: results of the Fourth National Audit Project of the Royal College of Anaesthetists and the Difficult Airway Society. Part 1: anaesthesia. *Br J Anaesth.* 2011;106(5):617–631.

54. Chrimes N. The Vortex: a universal 'high-acuity implementation tool' for emergency airway management. *Br J Anaesth.* 2016;117:i20–i27.

56. Apfelbaum JL, Singleton MA, Ehrenwerth J, et al. Practice advisory on anesthetic care for magnetic resonance imaging. An updated report by the American Society of Anesthesiologists Task Froce on Anesthetic Care for Magnetic Resonance Imaging. *Anesthesiology.* 2015;122(3):495–520.

63. Sorbello M, Pulvirenti GS, Pluchino D, Skinner M. State of the art in airway management during GI endoscopy: the missing pieces. *Dig Dis Sci.* 2017;62(5):1385–1387.

76. Lee DW, Wasowicz M. Recent advances in nonoperating room anesthesia for cardiac procedures. *Curr Opin Anaesthesiol.* 2020;33:601–607.

78. Galway U, Zura A, Khanna S, Wang M, Turan A, Ruetzler K. Anesthetic considerations for bronchoscopic procedures: a narrative review based on the Cleveland Clinic experience. *J Thorac Dis.* 2019;11(7):3156–3170.

All references can be found online at eBooks.Health.Elsevier.com.

43

Airway Management in Intensive Care Medicine

ANDY HIGGS AND JARROD M. MOSIER

CHAPTER OUTLINE

KEY POINTS

- Intensive care unit (ICU) patients' airways are extremely demanding; airway-related mortality and severe morbidity may be orders of magnitude higher than in general OR practice. Difficult airway (DI) is at least twice as common. Airway intervention must be prompt and smooth: The critically ill simply do not tolerate poor airway management.
- The ICU must have immediate access to a flexible intubation scope (at least a disposable one).
- Head-of-the-bed signage detailing the known features of a patient's airway is invaluable in a crisis. It should indicate whether a stoma is a tracheostomy or a laryngectomy.
- If a patient with a neck stoma suffers respiratory deterioration, oxygen should be applied to the nose, mouth, and stoma.

- All ventilator-dependent patients should have waveform capnography in constant use.
- Before airway interventions, the patients should be properly preoxygenated with positive end-expiratory pressure (PEEP).
- All cuff leaks are partial displacement or tube herniation until proven otherwise.
- If any respiratory deterioration occurs in an intubated/tracheostomy patient, the breathing circuit should be made as simple as possible, such as a Mapleson C circuit directly to the artificial airway. Capnography should be checked.
- Tube exchange is fraught with danger. The use of an airway exchange catheter (AEC) should always be considered.
- Reintubation in the ICU is associated with more complex management and higher complication rates.

Introduction

Airway management has always been central to the provision of intensive care. Intensive care medicine first developed when Danish anesthesiologist Bjørn Ibsen applied his advanced airway skills and understanding of positive-pressure ventilation to the care of victims of the 1952 Copenhagen polio epidemic. His revolutionary insight was to understand that protecting the airway and ventilating patients' lungs with positive pressure would improve outcomes.[1] Patients were intubated, tracheostomized, and, famously, manually ventilated by medical students. Mortality plummeted from 87% to 11%, and the medical profession was delivered a new specialty, with expertise in managing the airway, its *sine qua non*.[2,3]

Nearly 70 years later, airway management in intensive care medicine is again front-and-center of cutting-edge medical practice during the global COVID-19 pandemic. Leading the discussion is when and how to secure the airway of patients with acute respiratory failure to improve mortality while minimizing viral transmission to healthcare workers. It is a timely reminder that expertise in securing access to the airway is fundamental to the provision of modern advanced respiratory support.

Defining the Problem

Tracheal intubation is the most commonly performed procedure in the intensive care unit (ICU) and is associated with significant mortality and morbidity,[4,5] the incidence of which is higher in the ICU than in the operating room (OR).[5–10] Nonetheless, some ICUs still manage tracheal intubation in a relatively primitive manner.[4,11] Few studies address how many ICU patients have a difficult airway (DA) and caseloads vary, but Astin and colleagues provided useful context for the intensivist: in general ICUs 4.1% of patients had been admitted to the unit for a primarily airway-related reason, and overall 6.3% were judged to have a DA.[12] Studies quantifying airway difficulties in the ICU are also rare. Martin and colleagues reported 3423 emergency tracheal intubations performed by anesthesia residents with 60% occurring in the ICU. Difficult intubation (DI) (Cormack and Lehane [CL] grade 3 or 4, or >2 attempts) occurred in 10%, and complications were observed in 4.2% of intubations.[9] This is approximately twice the incidence of DI seen in the OR (5.8%)[13] and is consistent with other ICU studies reporting DI rates of 7% to 13%.[3,5,7,8,14] Mort reported a failed intubation rate of 1 in 10 to 20 attempts outside the OR,[14]

and Jaber and colleagues reported death as a complication in 0.8% of intubation attempts in the ICU.[8] Thus, the DA in the ICU is potentially lethal and dramatically increases the risk of life-threatening complications (51% vs 36% with non-DAs).[15]

The Fourth National Audit Project (NAP4) of the Royal College of Anaesthetists was a nationwide, prospective observational audit conducted over 1 year in the United Kingdom (UK).[6,16] It included data from the OR, emergency department (ED), and ICU. Inclusion criteria were airway-related mortality, brain damage, emergent surgical access, ICU admission, or prolongation of ICU stay. There were 38 airway-related deaths: 16 in the OR, 4 in the ED, and 18 in the ICU. Considering the denominator values were 2.9 million anesthetics in the OR, 20,000 tracheal intubations in the ED, and 58,000 episodes of advanced respiratory support in ICU, airway-related death is approximately 58 times more common per patient in the ICU than in the OR.[6] The rates of death or brain damage seen when DAs are encountered in the ICU were 61%, compared with 14% in the OR. This suggests airway-related mortality rate of 1 in 2700 ICU patients versus 1 in 180,000 in the OR. NAP4 assessors stated that many of these ICU deaths were avoidable and found a higher incidence of poor and mixed-quality airway care than in the OR. One crucial difference is when ICU-related airway problems occur: The UK National Reporting and Learning System ICU airway incidents database documents 18% occurring at tracheal intubation but 82% after the airway had been secured, and 25% of these contributed to mortality.[17] Other studies and closed claims analyses are consistent, and all suggest that many of these incidents are preventable. An updated analysis from 2019 of the Anesthesia Closed Claims Project demonstrated that 76% of cases had at least one predictor of DI, and 41% had at least two.[18]

Why Is ICU Airway Management So Hazardous?

Common to all reports that evaluate ICU airway management is failed tracheal intubation, delayed recognition of esophageal intubation, training deficiencies, poor communication, and poor judgment (late recognition of evolving crises and slow escalation strategies). Institutional preparedness is often poor (e.g., inconsistent equipment provision, meager supervision of residents, or few local algorithms). The commonalities can be distilled into failure to evaluate and plan for the DA and failure to recognize and rescue the failed airway. There are repeated problems relating to displaced airways, particularly in obese patients and on patient movement or transfer. Often, patients with a DA are not recognized, and even when potential problems are identified early, coherent plans to manage crises are not formulated, including proper equipment and expertise being immediately available in the ICU. When difficulty arises, rescue techniques fail more frequently in the ICU than in other clinical settings.[6,16]

There are several reasons why the ICU is associated with such high risks. ICU patients are physiologically compromised, having significant ventilation/perfusion ($\dot{V}/\dot{Q}$) abnormalities and lower functional residual capacities (FRCs), which renders preoxygenation less effective and leads to reduced or nonexistent tolerance of apnea.[19–21] Patients are frequently not fasted or have delayed gastric emptying. Patients are hemodynamically compromised, with exaggerated physiological responses to vasodilation from induction agents and the hemodynamic consequences of the transition to positive-pressure ventilation, especially in the setting of right ventricular strain.[21] Severe metabolic acidosis means apnea and rising carbon dioxide (CO_2) levels are poorly tolerated. Intubation in the ICU is often urgent, with little time for assessment or preparation, and minimally conscious or unconscious patients prohibit intubation options that are available in awake and cooperative patients. Apnea and hypercarbia are detrimental in patients with raised intracranial pressure (ICP). Airway assessment in the critically ill is problematic,[22–24] so difficulty is often unanticipated. These issues are collectively referred to as "the physiologically difficult airway."[19]

Furthermore, ICU patients may have artificial airways in situ for days or months and are cared for by staff whose expertise is not primarily airway management. Patients' airways are manipulated by these staff during oral hygiene and insertion of feeding tubes or other devices. They are positioned prone and transferred to remote areas of the hospital, during which artificial airways are extremely vulnerable to displacement. Often, critically ill patients are agitated and liable to self-extubate. Although sedation holds are vital to optimal ventilation,[25,26] they may lead to self-extubation. The fluid status of critically ill patients is problematic as well; patients can be hemodynamically compromised and may poorly tolerate sedatives and raised intrathoracic pressure, or may have significantly positive fluid balances with generalized edema, including of the airway, especially if prone ventilation is used. Even normal patients become difficult in such circumstances.[22,27]

In the ICU, access to the patient is challenging. Beds rather than operating tables, poor lighting, and lack of space make intervention difficult.[6,28] A commonly used approach during failed management in the OR is simply to allow the patient to awaken, but when intubation is indicated for respiratory, cardiovascular, or neurologic failure, this is not an option. Airway rescue with supraglottic airway devices (SGAs) and invasive access, especially needle cricothyrotomy, fails more commonly in the ICU.[6] ICU equipment is often different from that in other areas of the hospital and deficient in important ways. The most striking of the NAP4 practice deficiencies, and one also seen around the world, is the poor use and understanding of capnography in the ICU.[6,29–31] Although the availability of life-saving airway devices is crucial, this should be team appropriate. Simply providing a plethora of devices reveals that unit leaders have failed to agree on how airways should be managed and have no clear strategies developed. Additionally, this paradox of choice hampers team performance because expertise can only be achieved in a relatively small number of techniques. Airway equipment should be purchased with the least experienced user in mind.[32,33]

Airway-related problems in the ICU occur after hours more commonly than in the OR (46% vs 31%).[6] When difficulty with airway

management arises, senior medical help or experienced airway surgeons are not available to help residents; some of the residents interviewed following NAP4 incidents did not recognize terms such as *backward, upward, rightward pressure* (BURP) or *Combitube*, revealing a lack of basic airway knowledge.[6] The expertise of the doctors is important.[34,35] Joffe and colleagues conducted a national survey of airway training in US internal medicine ICU fellowships, and only 58% had a designated program. Actual experience varied markedly: Before graduation, 67% of fellows reported performing less than 50 direct laryngoscopies (DLs), 73% had used an SGA fewer than 10 times, 60% had used an intubating stylet fewer than 25 times, and 73% had used video-assisted laryngoscopy (VAL) fewer than 30 times.[36] An SGA learning curve is more than 15 uses. Minimal competence in many other techniques is achieved with perhaps 30 to 60 uses, and expertise with more than 100 uses.[37,38] This problem is global.[6,12,39] Only two-thirds of ICUs in the UK have a resident in possession of the initial assessments of airway competency, equivalent to 3 months of dedicated airway training, and in only 27% of ICUs had the resident received specific training in how to manage a displaced airway.[12] In 72% of Australian ICUs, the night doctor is not required to have prior anesthetic or airway training; in 97% of them, the senior airway doctor at night is either not stationed in the unit or may have duties elsewhere. Only 15% of the Australian units have a doctor who is present in the hospital overnight, who does not have other clinical commitments, and always has formal airway training.[30] The skill set of ICU doctors is rarely specified: For instance, the US Accreditation Council for Graduate Medical Education simply states that a fellow in an internal medicine critical care fellowship "must demonstrate competence in airway management" but does not define this, specify a target number of procedures, or describe methods for formal competency assessment.[40]

Evidence-Based Improvements

Evidence suggests that training and experience in airway management are likely the most important factors for improving airway-related outcomes in the ICU.[41] A study with data from 22 of the 24 ICUs in Scotland suggested that airway care led by experienced practitioners can result in higher first-attempt tracheal intubation success rates (90% vs 63%–75%) and lower complication rates than in many other studies.[7,8,14,34,42] In this study,[34] 74% of ICU physicians had more than 24 months of anesthesia training, and only 10% had fewer than 6 months of such training (all but one of the novice tracheal intubations were supervised by a senior). Success rate in tracheal intubation was related to duration of anesthesia training ($p < 0.001$). In contrast, Griesdale did not demonstrate improved outcomes with experts rather than nonexperts, but in this study, 92% of nonexperts were immediately supervised by experts: The impact of a lack of expertise was therefore unclear, other than to confirm that nonexperts need significantly more attempts to achieve tracheal intubation, and more than two attempts is associated with more severe complications.[7] Tellingly, Jaber and colleagues found that the presence of two operators (a junior and a senior) was protective against tracheal intubation complications in the ICU.[7,8] De Jong and colleagues reported that most studies are inadequately powered to analyze the effect of operator experience and that 24 months of anesthesia training was significantly associated with a lower incidence of DI.[43] However, experience is not always protective. A 2018 study of patients intubated in the ICU within 30 days of an elective operation found that, despite being intubated by the same anesthesiologists, there was worsened glottic visualization, an 8% lower first-attempt success, a 7% increase in moderate or difficult intubation (16% overall), and a 31% increase in complications when intubated in the ICU.[35]

Nontechnical factors are extremely important for DA-related outcomes. Pathologic thought processes occur during airway crises—practitioners overanalyze the situation, become task-fixated on tube placement, and neglect rescue oxygenation. An idealized, as opposed to pragmatic, solution is sought by the practitioner, which leads to delay and perseveration; the operator's appreciation of how urgently they must deal with the situation fails. A loss of situational awareness means timely progression through airway algorithms slows or stops.[32] This is especially true in the ICU, where high-risk physiologic derangements and the emergent need to secure an airway simply overload even experienced practitioners' cognitive strategies. Crisis management can be taught and improved.[43] Although there are similarities between OR and ICU airway management, there are sufficiently important differences to justify ICU-specific guidelines, as there are in obstetric and pediatric anesthesia practices.

There is no single innovation that can mitigate these risks. Like all demanding areas of human activity, performance is improved by the aggregation of marginal gains—achieving small improvements in every element of the task, whether relating to individuals, teams, or institutions. Quality improvement initiatives incorporating many of the following components discernibly improve performance metrics[41,44]: the use of intubation bundles to minimize procedural difficulty (e.g., checklists, standards of practice), optimizing human factors, adequate training and supervision, continuous waveform capnography, sound assessment and backup planning, using appropriate equipment with which the team is familiar and practiced, immediate availability of appropriate rescue devices, deploying the most appropriate rescue techniques when faced with difficulty, attention to detail once the airway has been secured, and carefully planned extubation.

Noninvasive Ventilation

Noninvasive positive-pressure ventilation (NIPPV) includes continuous positive airway pressure (CPAP) and bi-level positive airway pressure (BiPAP) applied via full face mask, nasal mask, or helmet. It is used to manage various types of respiratory failure, manage obstructive sleep apnea (OSA), and preoxygenate patients before tracheal intubation. A full description of NIPPV is beyond the scope of this chapter (see Chapter 18), but intensivists must be familiar with the implications NIPPV has for upper airway management. Important contraindications to NIPPV are listed in Box 43.1.

High-flow nasal oxygen (HFNO) has evolved as an alternative noninvasive oxygen therapy for acute respiratory failure.[45] High-flow nasal cannula (HFNC) provide a flow-dependent increase in end-expiratory lung volume, which reduces atelectasis and increases oxygenation through this positive end-expiratory pressure (PEEP)-like effect.[46–48] HFNO also reduces arterial carbon dioxide tension ($Paco_2$) through dead space clearance, which decreases inspiratory effort and reduces work of breathing (WOB).[46,48]

Indication-Specific Points Relevant to Airway Management

Noninvasive Strategies Used to Avoid Tracheal Intubation

Avoiding tracheal intubation is associated with reduced mortality rates in hypercarbic and hypoxemic respiratory failure.[49–53] Invasive

• **BOX 43.1**   Important Contraindications to Noninvasive Positive-Pressure Ventilation

Airway-Related Contraindications	Nonairway-Related Contraindications
Upper airway obstruction	Respiratory arrest
Low level of consciousness (CO_2 narcosis)	Agitated or uncooperative patient
Excessive secretions	Untrained staff
Unacceptable seal/leak with mask	Hemodynamic instability (shock)
Inability to protect airway	Uncontrolled cardiac ischemia/arrhythmia
Impaired swallow	Upper GI bleeding
Recent upper GI or airway surgery	Significant metabolic acidosis
Trauma: epistaxis, facial/skull fracture, pneumothorax/ pneumomediastinum	Multiorgan failure

GI, Gastrointestinal.

ventilation is associated with myopathy, as a result of continuous intravenous (IV) sedation, and nosocomial pneumonia.[54–56] NIPPV reduces the risk of these adverse outcomes. NIPPV with a full-face mask is usually preferable to a nasal interface because of the oral leak,[57] and NIPPV by helmet interface may yield the best outcomes.[49]

For patients with acute hypoxemic respiratory failure, both HFNO and NIPPV may be beneficial for avoiding intubation. A recent systematic review and meta-analysis showed that noninvasive respiratory strategies reduce the need for intubation and mortality, but the benefits are skewed heavily by helmet NIPPV, and comparisons show no difference between NIPPV by face mask and by HFNC.[49] Two other systematic reviews and meta-analyses have recently compared HFNO and NIPPV, and both found that HFNO was associated with a significant reduction in intubation rate compared to conventional oxygen, but not compared to NIPPV.[58,59] However, a subgroup analysis showed that HFNO was associated with a lower intubation rate than NIPPV in patients with an arterial oxygen tension to fraction of inspired oxygen (Pao_2/Fio_2 [P/F]) ratio <150, but not in patients with higher P/F ratios.[60]

Noninvasive Strategies Following Extubation

Prophylactic NIPPV or HFNO may help prevent postextubation respiratory failure and may decrease ICU mortality.[61–70] There is no clear evidence to support one strategy over the other, but there are logistical and patient comfort advantages to extubation to HFNO. However, extubation failure leads to worse outcomes and early reintubation should not be delayed.[71,72]

Patients Who Fail Noninvasive Strategies: Implications for Intubation

In patients with respiratory failure, NIPPV reduces the risk of requiring intubation, but when NIPPV fails, the risk of death is increased. The source of this increased mortality is the delay in tracheal intubation, cardiorespiratory stress, patient self-inflicted lung injury, as well as the complications associated with emergent tracheal intubation.[8,53,73,74] The increased risk of mortality with failure of HFNO does not appear to be the same, suggesting that NIPPV may be intrinsically injurious through patient self-inflicted lung injury.[75,76] The physiologic ramifications of delayed intubation may make complications of tracheal intubation more likely or more severe. Mosier and colleagues studied patients intubated after failed NIPPV and compared composite airway outcomes (hypoxemia, hypotension, and aspiration) with patients who were similarly intubated but had no prior NIPPV. A propensity-adjusted model for factors affecting the decision to use NIPPV showed an adjusted odds ratio for a complication of intubation in patients failing NIPPV of 2.20 (95% confidence interval [CI]: 1.14–4.25). Furthermore, when one of these complications occurred, the odds ratio of death in the ICU was 1.79 (1.03–3.12). There was no difference in the incidence of DI or number of attempts, and all tracheal intubations were supervised by an experienced senior.[53] Certainly, the decision regarding timing of intubation when NIPPV fails is of vital importance. As patients receiving a trial of NIPPV fail, tachypnea, tachycardia, hypoxemia, acidosis, agitation, poor mask tolerance, loss of consciousness, and hemodynamic instability develop. If these become apparent by 1 to 2 hours after NIPPV is initiated, then even worse deterioration should be avoided by prompt intubation. This is especially true when the indication for NIPPV was weak in the first place: for instance, pneumonia or hypoxemic respiratory failure. For patients on HFNO, a ROX index (ratio of oxygen saturation [SpO_2]/FiO_2 to respiratory rate) <4.88 at 2, 6, and 12 hours is an accurate predictor of patients who will likely fail and require intubation.[77]

Tracheal Intubation

Assessment

It is advantageous to identify DA patients to avoid prolonged, complicated, unanticipated DA management and to facilitate better planning. Within the anesthetic literature, prediction of difficulty is credited with a reduction in mortality and morbidity, but this is not certain.[78–81] Standard airway assessments all suffer from variably poor sensitivity and poor-to-moderate specificity and translate only partially to the critical care arena.[23,82] Emergent ICU intubation usually precludes detailed imaging investigation. A common approach in emergency patients is the LEMON (look, evaluate, Mallampati, obstruction, neck mobility) mnemonic.[83,84] Of the "look" criteria, Reed and colleagues found that only large incisors, reduced inter-incisor gap, and reduced thyrohyoid distance were associated with DI. Reduced thyromental distance, obstruction, and Mallampati score trended to significance. Only 57% of subjects in this study were suitable for Mallampati scoring. Similarly, Levitan found that only 32% of ED patients could follow simple commands (needed to perform Mallampati) while also not having cervical spine protection in place (permitting a cervical spine mobility assessment).[82] However, Levitan and colleagues used the classic Mallampati assessment with the patient sitting up, opening the mouth fully, and maximally protruding the tongue, although it can be scored in the supine position in cooperative patients.[85] They questioned LEMON's utility because, even if it was able to better guide practitioners, few options for management other than rapid sequence intubation (RSI) or primary surgical airway exist in the ED. They stated that awake intubation has almost no role in uncooperative patients, those needing immediate intubation, or those with secretions, blood, or vomit in the airway.[82]

Importantly, De Jong and colleagues developed the only ICU-specific assessment tool:[43] The MACOCHA score (Table 43.1). It is a seven-item assessment with ICU-specific risk factors for

TABLE 43.1 MACOCHA Score

Factors	Points
Factors related to patient	
Mallampati score III or IV	5
Obstructive sleep apnea syndrome	2
Reduced mobility of cervical spine	1
Limited mouth opening <3 cm	
Factors related to pathology	1
Coma	1
Severe hypoxemia (<80%)	
Factor related to operator	1
Non-anesthesiologist	1
Total	12

MOCOCHA, Mallampati score III or IV, apnea syndrome (obstructive), cervical spine limitation, opening mouth smaller than 3 cm, coma, hypoxia, anesthesiologist nontrained. Coded from 0 to 12: 0 = easy; 12 = very difficult.

DI. A score of 3 or greater is recommended as the cutoff value. Its discriminant value is high. The MACOCHA predictive score includes two ICU-specific criteria: hypoxemia and coma before intervention. These are important because hypoxia permits less time for preparation, leads to quicker desaturation, and may increase operator stress; coma makes assessment more difficult and is associated with greater laryngeal contamination. Uniquely, MACOCHA scores operator experience: specifically, anesthesia training of at least 24 months. MACOCHA makes it explicit that OSA, rather than obesity per se, causes DAs.[86,87] The Mallampati score in this study was determined in the recumbent position and obtained in 77% of subjects. The best predictor of a DA is documentary evidence of previous difficulty, but documentation is typically poor.[88–90] If a history is suggestive of upper airway obstruction, flexible nasal endoscopy is a valuable tool. Even when a DI is not predicted, unanticipated difficulty is still possible. Predictors of difficult mask ventilation (DVM) and SGA ventilation have been described but not validated in the ICU setting.[91–97]

Awake Intubation

Awake intubation is regarded as the gold standard for management of the DA, and there is certainly a place for it in the ICU. Advantages include maintaining airway patency and spontaneous ventilation. Awake intubation includes flexible scope intubation (FSI), VAL, tracheostomy, cricothyrotomy, retrograde intubation, and intubation via an SGA. Combined upper and lower respiratory tract pathology renders ICU patients with DAs particularly challenging.[5,19,21,98,99] Contraindications to awake intubation in the ICU include noncooperative patient, inexperienced operator, need for immediate intubation, absolute refusal by patient, raised ICP, and dependency on NIPPV (although HFNO may significantly mitigate this contraindication).

Some patients have physiologic abnormalities that make RSI risky because of limited or no safe apnea time. These patients, usually suffering refractory hypoxemia, have reduced FRC, as well as high shunt fractions that create conditions unsuitable for maintaining hemoglobin saturation during apnea. In these patients, awake intubation can sometimes be advantageous to maintain spontaneous breathing if oxygen saturation is adequate using HFNO until they can be immediately transitioned to positive pressure ventilation.[5,19] No definitive studies favor awake intubation or RSI. Some authorities believe PEEP dependency prior to intubation favors RSI, especially if postinduction bag-mask ventilation eliminates the apneic phase. Significant hemodynamic compromise before intubation may lead to cardiovascular collapse with adequate doses of induction agents: Awake techniques should be considered.

Awake Intubation: Technique

Several airway management techniques can be used for awake intubation; practitioners should use the technique with which they are most familiar (see Chapter 13). Some tips that are particularly useful in the ICU setting include (1) HFNO (e.g., Optiflow, Vapotherm) is useful to maintain Spo_2 during awake intubation and pneumatically splint the airway open to some extent; (2) performing awake intubation in a sitting, upright position optimizes FRC, tidal volume, and patient comfort and reduces the risk of aspiration; and (3) sedation should be just sufficient to ensure cooperation—amnesia is not required. Opioid sedation is commonplace; remifentanil is easily titratable and fully reversible with naloxone. Dexmedetomidine, propofol, midazolam, and ketamine are also widely used.

Awake intubation in the ICU should always have a backup plan in place. If the intubation fails, it can be rescued by a more experienced operator or an alternative technique. Occasionally in the ICU, time pressure, lack of immediate assistance, and lack of patient cooperation mean that one must proceed with intubation after induction of anesthesia. However, preparations should be made for rescue oxygenation and immediate surgical airway if this fails.

Routine Awake Intubation for ICU Patients

Some authorities recommend that awake intubation should be used for all ICU patients, especially when airway management is performed by novices. This does not refer solely to FSI for a predicted DA but rather to simply topicalizing the airway and using standard laryngoscopy. Some ICU patients will accept this procedure under topical anesthesia alone, relying on the sedative effects of critical illness, sepsis, hypotension, hypoxemia, and hypercarbia.[11] However, critically ill patients should be intubated well before they reach the perilous physiologic state whereby they can be intubated under rapidly applied (incomplete) topicalization alone. In addition, borderline respiratory status can easily deteriorate even with gentle intubation attempts (because of laryngospasm, vomiting, trauma, and/or complete loss of the airway) or with small amounts of sedation. The hypertension and tachycardia associated with awake intubation can cause cardiac ischemia. Indeed, in the ICU, the frequency of RSI is inversely related to the incidence of DIs.[100,101] Adoption of RSI by anesthesiologists and ED practitioners has improved success rates and reduced complications for emergency intubation and therefore is recommended in the ICU, where it has also shown an increase in first-pass success and a reduction in complications.[5,102,103]

Intubation Care Bundle

No single intervention can improve airway safety in the ICU, and so care bundles are required. Jaber and colleagues demonstrated that implementation of a 10-component bundle reduced life-threatening complications compared with controls.[104] The incidence of Spo_2 less than 80% reduced from 25% to 10% using

the bundle, as did hypotension (defined as systolic blood pressure [SBP] <65 mm Hg) from 26% to 15%. The incidence of esophageal intubation did not decrease, but the incidence of esophageal intubation with hypoxia reduced from 50% to 0%. The protocol, specifically aimed at reducing airway-related complications, included five evidence-based elements: the use of NIPPV,[105,106] the presence of two operators,[107] RSI,[101] capnography,[108] and protective ventilation;[109] plus five elements that were regarded as good practice based on experience: fluid loading in absence of cardiogenic pulmonary edema, preparation of long-term sedation, use of the Sellick maneuver, norepinephrine for diastolic hypotension, and prompt initiation long-term sedation. Which individual components resulted in improvement is open to question. Marshall and Mehra demonstrated that cognitive aids and checklists improve team performance and help clinicians complete tasks without freezing or panicking.[67] Importantly, the checklist should cover all the areas that must be addressed prior to induction—namely, preparation of the patient, preparation of all equipment/medications that might be required, and preparation of the whole intubation team rather than just the operator. In addition, the checklist guides the team in how to verbalize preparation for DI, if it arises.[68] A recent pragmatic trial by Janz and colleagues showed that a checklist prior to intubation did not improve outcomes.[110] We advocate for using a bundle, which is proposed in Box 43.2 and borrows from Jaber's work.[104] This approach is amenable to simulation training and checklist-style deployment, which should be embedded into ongoing training.[41,44,111]

Rapid Sequence Induction and Intubation

ICU patients are rarely fasted and often have intraabdominal pathology or functional ileus; as a result, they are at high risk of regurgitation of gastric contents and pulmonary aspiration. The definition of RSI varies, but it is a technique to reduce the risk of pulmonary aspiration during intubation by minimizing the time interval between drug-induced loss of intrinsic airway reflexes and restoration of airway protection using an endotracheal tube (ETT) with its cuff inflated. The adoption of RSI by anesthesiologists and emergency physicians has improved success rates for the emergency tracheal intubation and has decreased complications, with similar results in the ICU.[102,103] Critical care physicians should learn to perform and become comfortable with all aspects of RSI.

Cricoid Pressure

In the classic RSI, cricoid pressure (CP) is applied and no face-mask ventilation occurs between induction and tracheal intubation; however, gentle face-mask ventilation during CP application is acceptable and is often necessary in patients with borderline or failing pulmonary function to prolong the time to desaturation.[5,112–116] One recent trial showed a significant reduction in desaturation rates when mask ventilation was applied between induction and laryngoscopy.[112] There is great controversy about whether or not CP prevents regurgitation. CP has variable, but mostly unfavorable, effects on laryngoscopic view,[117] and prevents proper insertion of SGAs.[118–120] Outcomes data with CP are lacking. A recent Cochrane review concluded that more evidence is needed,[121] and a clinical trial in 2019 failed to show noninferiority of sham CP versus CP.[122] However, CP is recommended by the 2018 Difficult Airway Society guidelines.[123] If used, CP must be applied by trained staff, and if mask ventilation, laryngoscopy, or intubation is difficult (or active vomiting occurs), it should be released.

• BOX 43.2 Intensive Care Unit Rapid Sequence Intubation Care Bundle

	Who?
1. Preintubation: assemble airway team	
Lead nurse (runs preprocedure checklist): team coordinator	N1
1st operator (physician)	O1
2nd operator (senior physician who may administer initial drugs)	O2
Cricoid operator (staff nurse; also monitors vital signs on monitor)	N2
Intubator's assistant (second staff nurse)	N3
Manual in-line stabilization operator (additional team member, as appropriate)	M1
2. Preintubation preparation	
Checklist commences (lead by N1 with all team present)	N1/O2
This must be read aloud to entire team	
2.1 Reliable intravenous access; time for arterial line?	O1/O2
2.2 Turn on capnography (EtCO$_2$); ensure self-check has completed before induction	N1/O1
2.3 Apply full monitoring, if not already	N2/N3
2.4 Sit patient to 20- to 25-degree head up or ramp as appropriate (unless contraindicated)	N2/N3
2.5 Chart/bedhead signage/handover communication reviewed: DA or allergy?	O1/TEAM
2.6 Assess airway	O1/O2
2.7 Aspirate gastric tube	N2/N3
2.8 Administer oxygen via nasal cannula	N2/N3
2.9 Start preoxygenation with NIPPV (F$_{IO_2}$ = 1.0; PEEP = 5–8 cm H$_2$O; PS to V$_T$ of 6–8 mL/kg; good mask fit)	N1/N2/N3
2.10 Commence 500-mL fluid bolus (unless contraindicated); optimize inotropes	O1/O2
2.11 Confirm Waters circuit or Ambu bag available for bag-valve-mask ventilation	N1
2.12 Yankauer suction working	N1
2.13 Ensure intubation cart with difficult airway equipment is at bedside If flexible bronchoscope is not on cart, is it immediately available?	N1/O1
2.14 Prepare intubation drugs: hypnotic, relaxant, atropine, bolus pressor/inotrope	O2/O1
2.15 Prepare continuous sedation drugs	N2/N3
2.16 Confirm sugammadex 16 mg/kg immediately available, if appropriate	N1/TEAM
2.17 DECISION: If intubation fails, can patient be woken up?	O2

	Who?
3. Verbal confirmations	
Team coordinator asks:	
3.1 Operator 2 states intubation plan	O2
3.2 Does anyone have any concerns? Opportunity for team to clarify plan	TEAM
3.3 Has patient been preoxygenated for 3 minutes?	O1
3.4 EtCO$_2$ working?	O1
3.5 EtO$_2$ >0.9	O2
3.6 Can patient be optimized further before induction?	O2
Team coordinator states checklist complete	**N1**
4. Intubation attempt	
4.1 Optimize head neck: sniffing position with face parallel to ceiling if possible	O1/O2
4.2 Push induction drugs Ketamine 2 mg/kg, rocuronium 1.2 mg/kg No contraindication to succinylcholine, if used	O2
4.3 Cricoid pressure	N2
4.4 As face mask removed, ensure nasal cannula flow 15 L per minute	N3
4.5 Bag ventilation	O1
4.6 Intubation	O1
4.7 Confirm intubation with waveform EtCO$_2$	O1/O2
4.8 Auscultate both lungs	O1/O2
4.9 Cuff pressure 20 to 25 cm H$_2$O	N2
5. Postintubation care	
5.1 Pressor for MAP <70 mm Hg	O1/O2
5.2 Initiate sedation	N2
5.3 Initiate invasive ventilation: V$_T$ 6–8 mL/kg ideal body weight; PEEP 5 cm H$_2$O; RR 10–20; F$_{IO_2}$ 1.0; Plateau pressure <30 cm H$_2$O, as appropriate	N2
5.4 Recruitment maneuver if stable (CPAP 30 to 40 cm H$_2$O for 30 to 40 seconds)	O2
5.5 Chest radiograph and annotate intubation details in medical record	O1/O2
5.6 Note tube depth on chart	N2
5.7 Arterial blood gas	N2
5.8 Titrate F$_{IO_2}$ down to target Pao$_2$ and V$_E$ to target Paco$_2$	N2
5.9 Complete intubation audit documentation	N1/O2

CPAP, Continuous positive airway pressure; *DA*, difficult airway; *EtCO$_2$*, end-tidal carbon dioxide; *EtO$_2$*, end-tidal oxygen; *MAP*, mean arterial blood pressure; *NIPPV*, noninvasive positive-pressure ventilation; *PEEP*, positive end-expiratory pressure; *PS*, pressure support; *RR*, respiratory rate; *V$_E$*, minute ventilation; *V$_T$*, tidal volume.

Use of Neuromuscular Blockade

RSI is part of the only intubation bundle seen to reduce complications of ICU intubation.[104] Recent guidelines for the management of unanticipated DA are unequivocal in stating that if airway management or tracheal intubation is difficult, further attempts should not proceed without full relaxation to abolish laryngeal reflexes, increase chest compliance, and facilitate mask ventilation.[113,123] Studies of DI in the ICU have shown a high incidence of DI and low use of neuromuscular blockade. Le Tacon and colleagues also reported low levels of neuromuscular blocking drug (NMBD) use and high levels of DI; subgroup analysis of this work showed that RSI was associated with a much lower incidence of DI.[124] NMBD use has been shown to be associated with fewer complications at emergent tracheal intubation.[5,98,102,103] Levitan[82] states that, after deciding awake intubation is impractical in the uncooperative ED patient, "if difficult laryngoscopy is anticipated, it

is counterintuitive to expect that attempting laryngoscopy under suboptimal conditions (without neuromuscular blockade) will succeed." A study looking at failed intubation in the ED identified RSI as the most common way that failed awake intubation was rescued.[125] In 1665 patients, Langeron and colleagues found that failure to use NMBDs was significantly associated with DI.[126] Walls reviewed 8937 ED tracheal intubations and reported improved success with relaxants (97% vs 91%); complication rates were 1.7 times higher without neuromuscular blockade.[127] The key to intubation in the ICU is the avoidance of hypotension, hypoxemia, and minimizing the number of intubation attempts. The best way to accomplish these goals is to use neuromuscular blockade. Patel reports that during the NAP4 expert case reviews, delay/avoidance in using NMBDs led to adverse outcomes.[128] Patel opines that NMBDs usually improve mask ventilation and never worsen it, which has been corroborated in recent studies.[5] NMBDs facilitate chin-lift, head-tilt, jaw-thrust, and mouth opening required to safely manage the airway. The risk-critical step is inducing anesthesia in the first place and not the administration of NMBDs. When apnea occurs and face-mask ventilation is difficult or fails, the point of no return has already been passed (the administration of sedatives). The solution is to rapidly optimize face-mask ventilation, SGA insertion, or tracheal intubation, all of which are improved by NMBDs.[91,129–132] The major risk of ICU airway management is apnea-inducing sedatives; what makes that safer and more successful is the concomitant use of NMBDs. NAP4 is unequivocal in stating that "obstruction and hypoxia should never be allowed to progress to the stage of needing emergent surgical airway access without giving a muscle relaxant".[128]

Facilitated Intubation: Sedation Without Relaxants

The alternative to RSI is facilitated intubation using sedation only. The strength of this technique is said to be maintenance of spontaneous respiration, and its proponents claim excellent results.[133] Proponents argue that using NMBDs risks the ability to perform face-mask ventilation following a failed intubation and lethal hyperkalemia secondary to succinylcholine; however, the literature supports NMBDs improving mask ventilation, and modern RSI uses high-dose rocuronium. Facilitated intubation requires that spontaneous respiration is maintained; however, this technique often results in incrementally increasing doses of drugs, such as propofol, to allow tracheal intubation. This often results in hypotension and apnea/obstruction in a patient at risk of aspiration. The worst possible scenario is an unconscious, ineffectively breathing patient who is not optimized for laryngoscopy and intubation. ICU patients are usually intubated for respiratory impairment, so failed tracheal intubation results in a patient in end-stage respiratory failure who is now under the influence of powerful respiratory depressants and whose larynx has been traumatized by multiple failed tracheal intubation attempts. The patient often cannot return to a stable state; this is extremely hazardous. Gagging associated with laryngoscopy during light sedation leads to aspiration; concomitant use of topical anesthesia to the airway heightens this risk. Mayo and colleagues describe a series of ICU tracheal intubations following an extremely well-devised training scheme with 15 simulation crew resource sessions and the avoidance of relaxants. This is an exacting and rigorous regimen, yet the DI rate in this paper was still perhaps twice as high (20%) as in other ICU studies and had an 11% esophageal intubation rate and a low (62%) first-pass intubation rate.[133]

Preintubation and Periintubation Oxygenation

Critically ill patients tolerate upper airway intervention and apnea poorly. Mort found that all ICU patients who needed three or more tracheal intubations developed hypoxemia with an SpO_2 of less than 70%.[10] Saturation this low risks arrhythmias, cardiovascular collapse, brain damage, cardiac arrest, and death.[134] Severe hypoxemia complicated 26% of ICU intubation attempts in Jaber's study, and 1.6% sustained cardiac arrest.[8] The underlying reasons for the profound drop in SpO_2 are a combination of intrapulmonary shunt, low mixed venous saturation (as a result of low cardiac output, anemia, and hypermetabolic states), and apnea/hypoventilation. The oxygenation maneuvers described here address these issues.

Preintubation: Preoxygenation and Positioning

Preoxygenation prolongs the safe apnea time (i.e., the time from the onset of apnea until SpO_2 reaches 88%–90%).[20,116] Preoxygenation

denitrogenates the FRC, filling it with oxygen to act as a reservoir to draw upon during apnea.[20] The efficacy of denitrogenation can be assessed by measuring the end-tidal oxygen concentration (EtO_2), which represents alveolar gas. SpO_2 and blood gas tensions are composites of cardiorespiratory interactions and cannot be used. Adequate preoxygenation is achieved at an EtO_2 more than 90%, which can be achieved with high-flow oxygen or positive-pressure ventilation through a closed circuit.[135,136]

Desaturation to an SpO_2 less than 85% in a typical ICU patient may occur in as little as 23 seconds. This is 25 times faster than healthy patients.[134,137–139] Basic preoxygenation techniques (without added PEEP) have been shown to be only marginally effective in the ICU.[140] However, the patients in this study who were intubated for airway protection (with normal lungs) did respond to this basic preoxygenation technique, whereas the patients with advanced pulmonary disease hardly improved at all.

A tight-fitting anesthetic-type full face mask must be used for preoxygenation. Leak around the face mask is the most common source of failure of preoxygenation and is identified by loss of the EtO_2 tracing.[20,136,141,142] Correct mask sizing and the use of two hands reduce leaks. Anesthesia circuits are useful and can provide high flow and a good seal (although it is difficult to control PEEP levels). The combination of a high-flow rate of oxygen and a reservoir bag means that the high peak inspiratory flow rates of dyspneic patients are met without entrainment of room air and the FIO_2 approaches 1. If there is unavoidable leak, the efficacy of mask preoxygenation can be improved by applying high-flow oxygen by nasal cannula at 15 L per minute during preoxygenation.[143] Standard nonrebreather face masks only achieve FIO_2 of 70% and should not be used if possible; increasing the oxygen flow rate through the nonrebreather mask to "flush rate" has been shown to be as effective as preoxygenation with a face mask.[144,145] If the SpO_2 remains low after 4 minutes of preoxygenation, this is diagnostic of intrapulmonary shunt, which can be highly refractory to simple preoxygenation when the shunt fraction is >30%.[19,20,146]

More advanced methods of preoxygenation are required in these patients with moderate to severe hypoxemia.[5,19] HFNO and positive pressure using either CPAP or NIPPV are both effective options. Alveoli can be recruited using positive pressure; PEEP of 5 to 10 cm H_2O is used. Computed tomography studies show that PEEP of 10 cm H_2O during preoxygenation reduces atelectasis from 10% to 2%.[147] NIPPV and CPAP can help prevent the absorption atelectasis that results from breathing 100% oxygen.[148] Ensuring that peak inspiratory pressure remains below that which would overcome the esophageal sphincter pressure (20 to 25 cm H_2O) avoids gastric distension.[149] Baillard's preoxygenation regimen includes PEEP of 5 cm H_2O and pressure support adjusted to a tidal volume of 7 to 10 mL/kg for 3 minutes.[105] In volume replete patients, there are few cardiovascular or gastric distension side effects, although these can occur. HFNO provides a flow-dependent increase in end-expiratory volume, which provides a PEEP-like effect, can recruit alveoli, and can be left in place for apneic oxygenation during laryngoscopy.

The literature on HFNO vs NIPPV is mixed; however, heterogeneity across the studies and arbitrary saturation cutoffs make an overall assessment difficult. HFNO prevents or limits the incidence and depth of desaturation and prolongs safe apnea time compared to simple face-mask preoxygenation in most studies.[150,151] However, in patients with more severe hypoxemia, NIPPV for preoxygenation has shown the best outcomes in preventing desaturation,[152,153] although HFNO can be left in place for apneic oxygenation and perhaps can limit the depth of desaturation.[154]

The supine position facilitates dorsal lung collapse, which is more pronounced in ICU patients but is ameliorated when sitting head up.[155] Baillard used the semi-sitting position, which makes laryngoscopy easier,[105,156] consistent with ramping.[157] In spinal trauma, 20-degree reverse Trendelenburg can alternatively be used if the patient is hemodynamically stable.[158]

In patients with refractory hypoxemia, some experts support that maintaining spontaneous breathing with HFNO during intubation may be the safest option to prevent rapid increase in V̇/Q̇ mismatch, rapid desaturation, and cardiac arrest.[19] However, in the absence of definitive evidence, others maintain that if significant PEEP-dependency has already been established, replacing it with only HFNO prior to intubation may precipitate abrupt desaturation and RSI is indicated.

Apneic Period: Intermittent Face-Mask Ventilation

Intermittent face-mask ventilation with PEEP can be used while waiting for onset of neuromuscular blockade to stabilize open lung units and prolong the safe apnea time.[118,159] It also helps control $Paco_2$ in patients with brain injury and elevated ICP. Peak inflation pressures should be kept low, and an oropharyngeal airway should be used to minimize gastric insufflation. Aggressive face-mask ventilation with high rates and tidal volumes can lead to gastric regurgitation; it also causes hypotension in patients with shock, COPD, or asthma because of an abrupt drop in venous return. A gentle approach using low-rate, low-volume, and low peak-inspiratory pressure, but with PEEP, is well tolerated.[160] A recent clinical trial demonstrated a significant reduction in desaturation rates with mask ventilation between induction and laryngoscopy in critically ill patients at low risk of aspiration.[112] If mask ventilation is not used, it is important to keep the source of oxygen used for preoxygenation in place until the patient is fully apneic, as any spontaneous breaths in the absence of oxygen results in rapid loss of the oxygen reserve.[161]

Apneic Period: Apneic Oxygenation Using Nasal Cannula

The standard nasal cannula provides limited supplemental oxygen to a spontaneously breathing patient, but apnea permits the pharynx to fill with a high Fio_2; at 15 L per minute, the Fio_2 in the hypopharynx of an apneic patient can reach close to 100%, allowing for apneic oxygenation during airway management.[160,162–165] The nasal cannula can be placed under the face mask during preoxygenation and remains on during tracheal intubation. Apneic oxygenation requires a patent airway for tracheal entrainment to occur. In obese patients, Ramachandran and colleagues found that using HFNC led to a longer time to desaturation, from 3.5 to 5.3 minutes.[165] Patel and Nouraei described conducting entire surgical procedures using 70 L per minute flows from commercially available devices in healthy patients.[166] The only clinical trial of apneic oxygenation in critically ill patients failed to show a benefit[167]; however, there are significant limitations to the available studies. The balance of evidence suggests that HFNO, when left in place for apneic oxygenation, prevents the incidence and depth of desaturation. In critically ill patients with high degrees of shunting (>40% shunt fraction), apneic oxygenation alone is unlikely to be sufficient, although it is still useful in animal models at shunt fractions of 25%,.[168] Apneic oxygenation is not a recruitment technique; if desaturation occurs, bag-mask ventilation is required. If the face-mask seal is impaired by the cannula, the HFNC may need to be removed.

Adjuvant Techniques

The following techniques are additional strategies to improve oxygenation during airway management in the ICU:
- When indicated, the lower airways can be cleared by physiotherapy before induction, rendering preoxygenation more efficient.
- Low venous oxygen saturation (caused by low cardiac output, anemia, or a hypermetabolic state) can contribute to hypoxemia in the ICU; it is worsened with concomitant intrapulmonary shunt. If the patient with shunt is in hemodynamic shock, improving the cardiac output improves arterial oxygenation[169,170]; therefore, the anesthetic agents chosen for induction should preserve cardiac output.
- High-dose rocuronium (1.2 mg/kg) is associated with longer safe apnea times than is succinylcholine; this is attributed to succinylcholine's fasciculation-induced increase in oxygen consumption.[171,172]
- Delayed sequence intubation is a technique used in patients who cannot tolerate face-mask preoxygenation, usually because of agitation.[173] It is essentially procedural sedation using dissociative doses of ketamine (1–2 mg/kg in 0.5 mg/kg divided doses) to achieve sedation with preserved spontaneous ventilation and intact airway reflexes. The patient is then preoxygenated as earlier. After 3 minutes, additional induction agent and an NMBD are given, and intubation is performed.
- A recruitment maneuver is a sustained increase in inspiratory pressure (to 40 cm H_2O) for 30 to 40 seconds to reestablish FRC immediately postintubation. It increases Pao_2 for 30 minutes after tracheal intubation. Hemodynamic stability is required to administer a recruitment maneuver because of the associated decrease in venous return.[174]

Pharmacology of ICU Airway Management

Induction Agents

ICU patients are often hypovolemic, septic, and/or in hemodynamic shock. Approximately half of all severe complications of ICU tracheal intubation are hemodynamic,[8] and there is a 2% to 4% rate of cardiac arrest.[15,175] Predictors of postintubation hypotension often include the induction agents administered.[176,177] The induction agents most commonly used in patients in shock are etomidate or ketamine.[5,28,178–181] Generally, the dose of sedative agents can be decreased up to 30% to 50% in ICU patients. Using NMBDs allows further reductions in induction dose.

Etomidate is well tolerated in hemodynamically compromised patients. Historically, there has been significant concern over etomidate use in critically ill patients because of its suppression of 11β-hydroxylase,[182–184] and concern over etomidate-associated adrenal insufficiency and mortality.[183–187] This concern has not been validated by clinical trials, and there is no definitive data showing that etomidate increases mortality. Both Jabre et al. and Price et al. compared etomidate and ketamine in combination with succinylcholine and found no difference in airway parameters or other outcomes; despite altered cortisol metabolism, mortality was not affected.[179,188] Hinkewich and Green noted a trend to increased mortality using etomidate in trauma patients and questioned its use.[189]

The primary concern regarding the use of ketamine is elevation of ICP; however, its effect on arterial blood pressure usually results in an increase in cerebral perfusion pressure, and so this agent is increasingly used in trauma and can be used in head injury if the patient is adequately ventilated.[190,191] Recent observational studies comparing ketamine and etomidate show that ketamine has higher odds of postintubation hypotension[192,193]; however, it is increasingly used around the globe. No induction agents demonstrate definitive superiority.[123]

Propofol is often avoided in the ICU because of concerns over hypotension. However, a Scottish group achieved excellent outcomes using mainly propofol, illustrating the overriding importance of experience in using a particular drug, rather than rigid prescriptions.[34]

Neuromuscular Blocking Drugs

Succinylcholine is the NMBD traditionally used in the ICU[194]; however, the intubating conditions achieved with rocuronium and succinylcholine have been shown to be clinically equivalent in this setting.[195–198] Of relevance in hemodynamically unstable ICU patients, the speed of onset of rocuronium is dependent on cardiac output.[199] Succinylcholine fasciculations can be problematic in the ICU as such muscle activity raises oxygen consumption and precipitates earlier desaturation—116 seconds earlier with succinylcholine than with rocuronium.[171] The most dangerous concern with the use of succinylcholine in the ICU is hyperkalemia attributed to the development of extrajunctional acetylcholine receptors with prolonged immobility. There is no clear guidance as to the duration of immobilization that puts patients at highest risk, though many clinicians use 10 to 14 days as a cutoff.[200] The incidence of anaphylaxis seen with succinylcholine and rocuronium is similar[201]; however, a recent report demonstrated succinylcholine was far more likely to lead to anaphylaxis compared to the other NMBDs.[202]

Neuromuscular Blockade in Failed Intubation

The concept of waiting for succinylcholine to wear off in failed airway management is an old one, but the residual effects of sedation, laryngeal trauma from failed intubation attempts, and the underlying cardiorespiratory failure in ICU patients make this unreliable. During the interval of incomplete blockade, the patient will try to move and is at risk of active regurgitation. Full recovery of neuromuscular function in healthy patients takes up to 10 minutes, after administration of succinylcholine, but patients desaturate before this.[137] The NAP4 study makes the point that if emergent surgical access is required, neuromuscular blockade

must be assured, so the effects of succinylcholine wearing off are problematic.[16] In ICU patients, there is wide variability in plasma cholinesterase levels and duration of succinylcholine's action.[203,204] Some recommend that it should be removed from the ICU. Booij comments that it is unlikely authorities would approve succinylcholine if it were presented today as a new drug.[200] It has lethal side effects with no apparent benefit over nondepolarizing alternatives.

An RSI dose of rocuronium can be reversed by sugammadex (16 mg/kg) in less than 10 minutes.[205] However, the same rationale applies for rocuronium in a failed airway. Reversing rocuronium with sugammadex will result in an incompletely paralyzed, incompletely breathing, critically ill patient who still requires intubation. For these reasons, reversing rocuronium or waiting for succinylcholine to metabolize have no role in a failed airway, and the operator should proceed with rescue oxygenation and emergency invasive airway access.

Laryngoscopy

Difficult laryngoscopy is more common in the ICU, regardless of who performs the procedure, and an increased number of intubation attempts is associated with critical hypoxemia, hemodynamic collapse, and cardiac arrest.[10,14,35,206,207] Maximizing first-pass success is intuitively advantageous and is consistent with current airway philosophy, which advocates limiting laryngoscopic attempts.[123,207–209] VAL is becoming a standard of care in the ICU because it definitely improves laryngeal view (Fig. 43.1).[5] VAL may reduce movement of the cervical spine during intubation,[210,211] and awake VAL is possible, if uncommon.[212] The evidence supporting VAL as a primary technique is incomplete and contradictory, however.[5] It has been demonstrated to both improve and worsen tracheal intubation in the ICU.

The purported advantages of VAL are relevant to the ICU and include allowing all members of the team to see the laryngeal view and facilitating teaching, assistance (by optimizing BURP maneuvers without relying on verbal directions from a task-fixated operator), and communication. De Jong's meta-analysis of nine trials of VAL in the ICU showed that VAL reduced the risk of DI; reduced

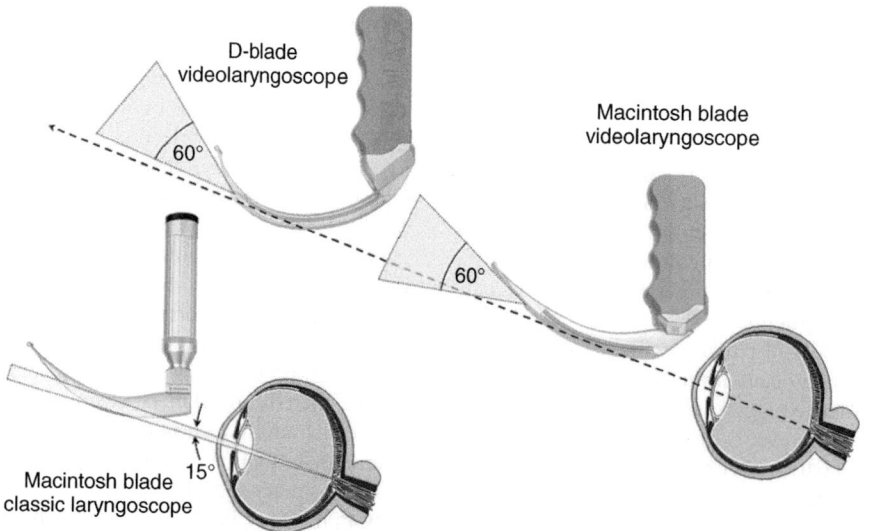

• **Fig. 43.1** Vertical visible angle of view (60 degrees) with a C-MAC Mac blade and D-blade, compared with the 15-degree angle of view of a classic Macintosh laryngoscope. (From van Zundert A, Pieters B, Doerges V, Gatt S. Videolaryngoscopy allows a better view of the pharynx and larynx than classic laryngoscopy. *Br J Anaesth.* 2012;109:1014–1015.)

the incidence of CL grade 3 and 4 views and of esophageal intubation; and increased first-pass success.[213] There was no reduction in the frequency of hypoxemia, hypotension, or airway trauma. This study, however, included only three randomized controlled trials,[214–216] and when only these are considered, there is merely a trend toward less DI and better first-pass success. The apparent contradiction of fewer attempts but no fewer major complications is perhaps explained by underpowering and uncontrolled confounding variables such as sedation, NMBDs, preoxygenation, and device-specific training. The studies describing VAL in the ICU use different devices, training programs, operator experience, and use of NMBDs. Control group performance is poor: a mean intubation time of almost 4 minutes, a first-pass success rate of about 40%, and an incidence of severe hypoxia greater than 50%.

There are potential pitfalls of VAL in ICU practice—blood, secretions, and vomitus in the airway can undermine their use, although recent evidence still supports the superiority of VAL over DL.[217,218] VAL, specifically hyperangulated VAL, can require more time than DL,[215,219,220] which is a concern in patients with significant V̇/Q̇ mismatch. VAL failure is often rescued by DL; however, VAL is still more likely than DL to succeed after a failed first attempt.[221] Any technique requires training, and simply introducing a new videolaryngoscope (VL) to the ICU with no corresponding training is problematic. Some ICUs may lack sufficiently experienced trainers to provide this because even experienced doctors cannot be assumed to have expertise in VAL.[222] VLs themselves are different, and proficiency gained with one is not wholly transferable to others (a concern for rotational ICU trainees). Channeled and nonchanneled VLs are clearly different, but in-group variation is still significant. Novices may fail to appreciate that highly angulated VAL requires specifically shaped stylets or bougies to facilitate passage of the ETT, even when the laryngeal view is good. VAL technology reduces the performance gap between novices and experts,[223] and all intensivists should be trained in VAL techniques, preferably with a screen visible to all members of the team.

Confirmation of Tracheal Intubation

Confirmation of tracheal intubation is one aspect of airway management in the ICU that has traditionally differed from OR practice, where capnography is ubiquitous. Unrecognized ETT misplacement is potentially catastrophic and avoidable in a majority of cases. However, in the UK in 2003, only 15% of ICU intubations were formally confirmed with capnography, despite the technology being available to some extent in 80% of units.[31] Two of the most revelatory findings from NAP4 were mainly related to ICU practice—capnography was not used in 75% to 100% of unrecognized esophageal intubations, and most of these patients died; lack of capnography materially contributed to 77% of all ICU deaths, including ETT displacements. In some cases, when waveform capnography was used, the tracing was misinterpreted, resulting in death[6]; specifically, physicians wrongly interpreted flat capnography waveforms to imply no cardiac output during cardiac arrest, when, in fact, cardiopulmonary resuscitation (CPR) provides sufficient pulmonary blood flow to generate a capnographic signal (Fig. 43.2). Clinical signs, such as chest wall excursion, auscultation, ETT condensation, SpO$_2$, and radiography are unreliable and cannot be used without confirmation by an advanced technique.[209] Advanced techniques include waveform capnography, DL or VAL confirming transglottic tube insertion, or flexible scope visualization of the tracheal lumen. Nevertheless, none of these are wholly without false positives/negatives. The gold standard remains continuous waveform capnography (see Chapter 30).

A flat capnography tracing should immediately trigger assessment of ETT position; such a tracing implies esophageal intubation, complete absence of cardiac output (cardiac arrest without CPR), complete obstruction of the airway, severe bronchospasm, or ventilator circuit disconnection. Immediate inspection should be performed using DL or VAL; flexible scope examination through the ETT is more reliable if it is immediately available. In cases of delay or uncertainty, the maxim "If in doubt, take it out" applies. Capnography does not identify endobronchial intubation.

In response to the NAP4 audit, recommendations for the use of continuous waveform capnography in ventilator-dependent patients were reissued.[224] This has resulted in almost universal use in UK ICUs (T. Cook, NAP4 author, personal communication, 2016). This was also part of the intubation bundle used by Jaber that resulted in lower complication rates in ICU tracheal intubation.[104] Central to this is adequate training of physicians and nurses in the ICU.[225] Ultrasonography (USG) has become popular, but transtracheal USG at the suprasternal notch has a high failure rate for confirmation of tracheal intubation.[226] Intensivists who routinely use thoracic USG can simply confirm bilateral pleural lung sliding with ventilation to confirm tracheal intubation. This cannot be used in the presence of surgical emphysema or pneumothoraces.[227,228]

Failed Initial Intubation Plan

When the initial intubation plan has failed, focus must turn to oxygenation. The risk of a failed intubation is critical hypoxemia, further (largely iatrogenic) deterioration of the airway, aspiration, and progression to a cannot intubate/cannot oxygenate (CICO)

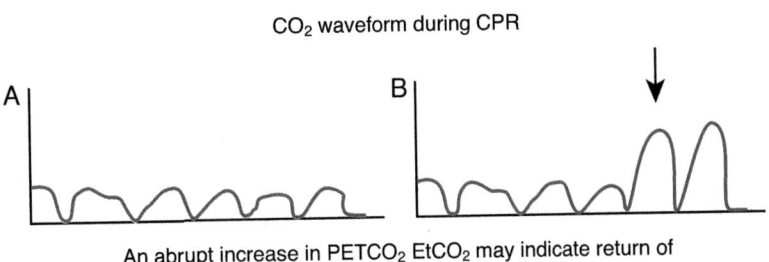

CO$_2$ waveform during CPR

An abrupt increase in PETCO$_2$ EtCO$_2$ may indicate return of spontaneous circulation (ROSC). Increase in pulmonary circulation brings more CO$_2$ into the lungs for elimination.

• **Fig. 43.2** Capnography tracing during cardiopulmonary resuscitation. Note the recognizable waveform. Return of spontaneous circulation is indicated by an abrupt and sustained increase in the height of the capnogram (*arrow*). (Modified from Kodali BS, Urman RD. Capnography during cardiopulmonary resuscitation: current evidence and future directions. *J Emerg Trauma Shock.* 2014;7:332–340.)

situation. It is critical that this phase is recognized and accepted by the team. Declaring a failed intubation helps focus the entire intubation team's efforts on what is most appropriate and how the operators can best be assisted. Nasal high-flow oxygen should continue, and ventilation using a face mask or SGA should be attempted in keeping with published airway algorithms including guidelines specific for the critically ill.[123] SGAs may be more effective at oxygenation than face masks.[229–231] The use of an SGA in place of a face mask not only leads to less hand fatigue but frees the operator's hands to prepare the backup device. To avoid airway trauma, bleeding, and swelling, the number of SGA insertion attempts should be limited to no more than three. Persistent attempts at SGA placement also delay recognition of failure of this Plan B stage, which can lead to critical hypoxia. Second-generation SGAs are recommended for reasons that are highly salient in the ICU (see Chapter 19). They are designed to enhance safety by (1) having 50% higher seal pressures, allowing for positive-pressure ventilation and application of PEEP,[232–237] which is vital in the ICU; (2) providing an improved esophageal seal so that regurgitation of gastric contents is less likely; (3) having a drainage tube to vent regurgitated material away from the airway, decreasing the risk of aspiration; and (4) in some cases, providing a conduit for intubation of the trachea. CP impedes SGA placement and should have already been removed during failed laryngoscopy. In a majority of cases, oxygenation via an SGA after failed intubation is possible[238]; the exact incidence of failed SGA oxygenation in the ICU is not known.

If oxygenation via an SGA is achieved, there are three options at this point: allow the patient to wake up and breathe spontaneously, though this is rarely applicable in ICU; intubate via the SGA; or surgical tracheal access.

The Intubating Laryngeal Mask Airway (ILMA; LMA North America, San Diego, CA), known as the LMA Fastrach, is an SGA specifically designed to facilitate intubation, although many second-generation SGAs provide a conduit for tracheal intubation. If an SGA that cannot facilitate tracheal intubation is used for rescue of oxygenation, an extremely useful technique is to mount an Aintree Intubation Catheter (AIC; Cook Medical, Bloomington, IN) on a flexible intubating scope (FIS) and to pass these through the SGA. The trachea is entered under visualization (minimizing trauma), and the AIC is placed in the trachea. The FIS and SGA are then removed, leaving only the AIC in the trachea. An ETT is then advanced over the AIC. Using a Bodai connector permits ventilation with PEEP throughout most of this sequence. This technique has been described in emergency failed tracheal intubation and was used in 128 patients with a 93% success rate.[239–241] Most of these patients had CL grade 3 or 4 views, and some could not be ventilated via face mask. It has been used with most SGAs.[239,242,243] If intubation proves impossible and critical hypoxia develops, emergency invasive airway access should be performed.

Endotracheal Tube Choice

Endotracheal Tube Size

The choice of ETT size is always a compromise between the short-term advantages and long-term sequelae of larger tubes, and therefore is different from OR practice. In the ICU, ETTs have ancillary purposes in addition to ventilation—they must accommodate adult-size therapeutic bronchoscopes as well as suction catheters large enough to cope with thick secretions and blood. Rosen and Hillard showed that if the ratio of the outer diameter (OD) of the suction catheter to the internal diameter (ID) of the ETT is >0.5, then the negative pressure generated during suctioning

causes atelectasis and cardiovascular compromise.[244] A standard bronchoscope is 5.7 mm in diameter with a 2-mm suction channel and must be inserted into at least a 7.5-mm ID ETT. Ongoing ventilation during bronchoscopy via an 8.0-mm ID ETT means 42% of the lumen is occluded, which can cause intrinsic PEEP, 80% reduction in tidal volume, and peak airway pressures as high as 70 cm H_2O with resultant hypoxia and hypercarbia.

Spontaneous breathing trials during weaning are performed using the ETT. WOB increases by as much as 490% as the ETT size drops from 9.0 mm to 6.0 mm ID.[245,246] Respiratory secretions accumulate inside the ETT, which reduces the effective diameter significantly; after 3 days, the average biofilm depth is 2 mm (range 0–5 mm) and increases with time.[247,248] Small ETTs become blocked and must often be replaced with larger ones, which is extremely hazardous. Although larger tubes mitigate short-term problems, they certainly make long-term complications worse.[249] Laryngeal trauma is more common with larger ETTs, especially at the posterior glottis.[250]

Ventilator-Associated Pneumonia Prophylaxis

ETTs play a central role in the development of ventilator-associated pneumonia (VAP) in that VAP incidence is influenced by ETT choice.[251–253] The pathogenesis of VAP is microaspiration of bacteria past the ETT cuff into the lower trachea. The ETT breaches the natural defense of the glottis, and sedation impairs the cough reflex, providing an opportunity for bacteria to enter the lungs. ETTs impregnated with silver reduce VAP rates by decreasing the rate of ETT bacterial colonization.[254]

The ETT cuff is pivotal: standard high-volume/low-pressure cuffs are only partially inflated in vivo, and the resultant folds permit secretions to channel caudally. Newer, low-volume/low-pressure cuffs, such as the Microcuff (Kimberly-Clark, Irving, TX), reduce cuff folds and minimize leakage of secretions past the cuff.[255] Thinner polyurethane cuffs form narrower folds than traditional polyvinyl chloride (PVC) cuffs and are associated with lower VAP rates.[256,257] ETTs designed with ports that allow for subglottic drainage reduce the incidence of microaspiration by up to 50%.[258,259] They are stiffer and more traumatic than usual tubes, however, and repeated subglottic suctioning may cause mucosal injury leading to laryngeal edema and a higher incidence of reintubation.[260] The OD of these ETTs is larger to accommodate the suction channel. If ventilation is expected to last 48 hours or more, these newer ETTs should be considered, although concerns remain regarding their cost, efficacy, and safety.[261]

Human Factors

It is increasingly recognized that nontechnical skill factors play a central role in adverse outcomes. Human factors are more important than which particular device is chosen, and the deciding factor in performance is the ability of the practitioner to maintain the presence of mind to change the plan when situations change. It is not necessary for the ICU airway manager to be proficient in all available techniques, but one must be proficient in managing oneself and the team. NAP4 concluded that 40% of major complications were caused in part by human factors.[262] However, subsequently conducted in-depth interviews with a sample drawn from the NAP4 using a human factors investigation tool concluded that human factors were relevant in all the incidents. There was a mean of 4.5 (range: 1–10) human factors per incident.[262] A recent closed claim analysis reported that human factors judgment errors are unfortunately not improving over time.[18]

The ICU scores highly in all domains for potential human factor contribution to critical incidents. Recent guidelines for unanticipated DI include explicit instructions to stop and think at key stages of evolving crises. ICU airway managers typically use guidelines designed for OR practice that are not wholly applicable in the ICU setting.[123] For these reasons, NAP4 describes the ICU as an environment that is hostile to airway management, and efforts have been made to improve this. Training and simulation optimize performance in the ICU, and cognitive aids such as the Vortex approach are useful.[41,263,264] Safe and effective airway management in the ICU should focus on human performance rather than adoption of the latest gadget (see Chapter 12).

Emergency Invasive Airway Access

Emergency invasive airway access is indicated in a CICO crisis and is a necessary skill for all doctors who practice in the ICU, where patients are far more likely to require emergency invasive tracheal access as critical hypoxemia occurs more rapidly and waking the patient is rarely possible. The term *CICO* itself is particularly important in the ICU; the traditional phrase *cannot intubate/cannot ventilate* implies that if the patient's lungs can be ventilated, then adequate oxygenation is achieved; however, ICU patients have $\dot{V}/\dot{Q}$ abnormalities such that borderline face-mask or SGA ventilation may not improve profound hypoxemia. If dangerous hypoxemia cannot be reversed and tracheal intubation is impossible, emergency invasive airway access is required. The American Society of Anesthesiologists (ASA) Closed Claims Project describes how most CICO crises are to some extent iatrogenic, in that the natural history of an airway crisis often proceeds in stages through difficulty, trauma, swelling, bleeding/aspiration, and complete obstruction.[18,265] Underappreciated is how imperative a prompt decision to perform emergency invasive airway access is in determining outcomes and the importance of the operator avoiding task fixation. There is a dearth of high-quality evidence regarding emergency airway access in the ICU.

The default approach for emergency invasive airway access is through the cricothyroid membrane (CTM). This is preferred over open tracheotomy because the CTM is relatively superficial, usually palpable, and less likely to be covered by overlying vessels or the thyroid isthmus. As a result, cricothyrotomy is quicker to perform. The cricoid cartilage is a complete ring, and the posterior lamina protects the esophagus from damage during the potentially injurious procedure. Although open tracheostomy performed by surgeons was used in several of the NAP4 emergency invasive airway access cases, in many of these situations CICO was not ongoing, and some (minimal) oxygenation was occurring while the formal tracheotomy was created. Airway access via the CTM is more rapid in the true CICO scenario, and surgeons are often inexperienced in fast-moving crisis management.[266–268]

Percutaneous dilatational tracheotomy is well described and has been suggested as a viable method for emergency invasive airway access that can be practiced and perfected in elective ICU circumstances.[269,270] It cannot, however, be recommended as a first-line technique.[123] Considerable skill and specific equipment are required, and intensivists performing percutaneous tracheostomy usually use flexible bronchoscopy to confirm access to the trachea; this significant safety feature is not possible in emergent situations. The benefits of percutaneous tracheostomy include the fact that it is a definitive airway, whereas cricothyrotomy requires conversion to formal tracheostomy; percutaneous tracheostomy is quicker than open tracheotomy and can be performed within 3 minutes. Emergent percutaneous tracheostomy should be reserved for

three situations: when the CTM cannot be located, when an ICU patient has had a previous percutaneous tracheostomy that was recently decannulated, and when access via the CTM has failed. In an emergency, when percutaneous tracheostomy is performed without a bronchoscopy, it is key to understand the importance of smooth tactile passage of the guidewire. This relies on the operator: It is successful in experienced hands, but novices should avoid it. It has been suggested that the sternal notch in the morbidly obese is more palpable than the CTM, favoring percutaneous tracheostomy over cricothyrotomy. However, in these circumstances, a vertical incision over the presumed site of the CTM, deep palpation to identify it and subsequent cricothyrotomy are preferable.

Three basic techniques are described to access the airway via the CTM: surgical cricothyrotomy, percutaneous dilatational cricothyrotomy (PDC), and transtracheal jet ventilation (TTJV) via a needle cricothyrotomy. The evidence supporting one technique over the others is not definitive, but some general observations are useful.

As many as 14% of CICO patients are obstructed in both the inspiratory and expiratory phase of ventilation. This means that TTJV, which relies on passive expiration through the native airway, is doomed to fail and risks barotrauma. Achieving adequate oxygenation of ICU patients requiring high F_{IO_2} and high PEEP with TTJV is unlikely to be successful, and poor lung compliance reduces the efficacy of devices like the Ventrain (see Chapters 28 and 38).[271] Most intensivists have little experience with TTJV, and high-frequency jet ventilators are rarely available in ICUs. The fine motor control required to perform needle cricothyrotomy or PDC is lost amid the stress of an emergent CICO scenario. The ASA Closed Claims analysis identified 26 patients in whom needle cricothyrotomy was attempted, and all had a poor outcome; 89% of cases where TTJV was used resulted in barotrauma. Failed needle cricothyrotomy was often managed by open cricothyrotomy, which was successful.[265] NAP4 showed similar results with needle cricothyrotomy: 12 out of 19 attempts failed (63%) attributed to misplacement, misuse, device failure, or catheter kinking; 7 were rescued by tracheotomy and 1 each by open cricothyrotomy, tracheal intubation, and SGA insertion. Open techniques were consistently successful in accessing the airway. There is no case series in which needle cricothyrotomy has a high success rate[272]; only practitioners who are specifically trained in needle cricothyrotomy should attempt it.

There are few reports of commercial PDC kit usage in the ICU. New devices appear regularly on the market, with slightly different characteristics, and often consist of multiple steps. The number and variation of the devices mean that adequate training is difficult, and there is no good evidence that they are advantageous. Failure can occur, even when the wire is in the trachea. Most literature suggests that open cricothyrotomy is more successful than PDC.[17] Open cricothyrotomy is a reliable technique with good success rates and requires only equipment readily available in any ICU (see Chapter 29).

Airway Care in the Mechanically Ventilated Patient

The time when an ICU patient is at highest risk for airway-related complications is after his or her airway has been secured. This is not surprising because patients are often intubated for days or weeks. In the UK between 2005 and 2007, 1085 ICU airway-related events were reported: 77% occurred after the airway had been satisfactorily secured; most of these complications involved some degree of dislodgement or obstruction. Avoidable death is mainly associated with partial dislodgements of tubes rather than complete removal because it is more difficult to diagnose. This was attributed to the low incidence of capnography use in UK ICUs at this time.[17,273] NAP4 made repeated references to failure to identify patients with high-risk airways and failure of planning to prevent adverse airway events. The goal must be prevention, early identification, and prompt management of complications. The approach must be systematic and lend itself to a care bundle approach (see Chapter 44).

Confirmation of Initial Tube Position

Waveform capnography confirms that the ETT is in the trachea and should be routine. The distal tip should be at the mid-trachea, then secured and insertion depth documented. Confirmation of position involves clinical assessment, usual insertion depth (21 cm for females, 23 cm for males), and radiography. Used alone, none of these individual elements is sensitive, but the combination is useful (see Chapter 30).[274] The practice of daily chest radiographs should be abandoned and performed only when indicated; the process of obtaining a chest radiograph risks dislodging the ETT, and daily films do not reduce complications. Chest radiographs should be taken in the neutral position; flexing the neck causes migration of the ETT toward the carina, and extending the neck withdraws it. The ETT tip should be between the clavicular heads, about 5 cm above the carina.

Tube Stabilization

Many different methods are used to secure an ETT in the ICU, including adhesive tape, knotted cotton twill, and commercially available products. This variety is testament to a lack of a universally applicable method. All methods are affected differently by perspiration, saliva, vomitus, blood, skin temperature, and facial hair. Commercial devices have more reproducible, if not more successful, outcomes than tape or twill.[275] Audited quality outcome measures often include avoidance of dermal injuries, but it has been suggested that unplanned extubation should be regarded as a quality indicator in ICU as well.

Documentation: Communication and Hand-Over

The depth of the ETT and the relevant landmark should be annotated on the observations chart every day and checked each shift or in the event of any change in the patient's respiratory status. Pertinent details of the intubation should be recorded, including the device used, laryngoscopic view, airway manipulations required (e.g., external laryngeal manipulation, ramping), and the identity of the operator. Many units now display signs at the head of the ICU bed with airway-related information regarding patients with a tracheostomy or a DA. Signs should record the same information as described previously, together with a preemptively agreed-upon management plan for reintubation. Hand-over forms should identify patients with DAs. The senior physician each shift should ensure that an airway plan is in place and that it remains appropriate considering each shift's available personnel and their expertise with the available equipment.

Minimization of Airway Swelling

Positioning a patient's head up 30 degrees reduces upper airway edema.[27,199] Likewise, avoiding positive fluid balances reduces swelling and reintubation rates.[27,199,276] ETT ties and fixation

devices can impede venous drainage. If surgery has sacrificed jugular vessels bilaterally, airway swelling should be expected. Treatment with corticosteroids is discussed in the section Extubation in the Intensive Care Unit.

Cuff Pressure

ETT cuff pressure should be maintained at 20 to 25 cm H_2O. This minimizes leaks, aspiration, and VAP.[277] Pressures less than 20 cm H_2O are associated with VAP, whereas pressures greater than 30 cm H_2O are associated with mucosal necrosis. At high peak-airway pressures, cuff pressures may need to be increased, but this is not without risk.[278] Automatic cuff control results in lower pressures than usual but does not reduce complications.[279,280]

Pulmonary Toilet and Gas Humidification

Patients should be suctioned using sterile technique with closed suction systems to minimize nosocomial contamination.[281] Heat-moisture exchangers can be used for at least 48 hours without complication. Suction frequency depends on the quantity of secretions.

Intubated Patient: Airway Red Flags

Airway red flags are warning signs caused by evolving life-threatening conditions, which, if acted upon promptly, can help prevent significant complications (Box 43.3). Experienced clinicians involved with airway management develop a very low threshold for investigating the airway if any of these occur. All medical, nursing, and respiratory therapy staff should be trained to appreciate the importance of these events. If these are associated with clinical deterioration, the breathing circuit should be immediately simplified by attaching a Waters (Mapleson C) circuit to the ETT, removing any extraneous devices from the proximal end of the ETT such as filters, closed suction attachments, and so on. This narrows the focus of investigation to the ETT and the patient.

> **• BOX 43.3**   **Intubated Patient Red Flags**

- No CO_2 detected on waveform capnography tracing
- Obvious respiratory distress; accessory muscles, tracheal tug, subcostal retractions
- Audible air leak at the mouth, nose, or tracheostomy stoma
- Bubbles of saliva at the mouth
- Vocalization; means the ETT is above the glottis
- Any noisy breathing (grunting, snoring, or stridor); ETT tip is above the glottis
- ETT is not at the depth that the chart/intubation note says it should be
- Deflated pilot balloon or need to repeatedly reinflate it
- No chest wall movement on inspiration
- Rising airway pressure and/or decreasing tidal volume
- Subcutaneous emphysema
- Inability to pass a suction catheter
- Gastric contents on ETT suction
- Significant bleeding from ETT
- Visual evidence of ETT damage
- Any respiratory deterioration after patient is turned or after gastric tube insertion
- Increasing oxygen requirements
- Anxiety, agitation in a conscious patient

ETT, Endotracheal tube.

Often, this solves the problem, but if not, a useful drill is to auscultate the chest, deflate the cuff (stops cuff herniation), and pass a suction catheter to check ETT patency. Help should be called for as early as possible. The glottis should be inspected with DL or VAL, and a flexible scope should be passed through the ETT. This underlines the importance of having a flexible bronchoscope immediately available in the ICU.[123] Cuff leaks in ICU patients are common, and ETT displacement, which occurs more commonly, may mimic a cuff leak. All cuff leaks should be assumed to be a displaced airway until proven otherwise.

Difficult Tube Exchange

Changing an ETT in a critically ill patient can be extremely hazardous and should never be embarked upon lightly. Tube exchange is required urgently in conditions such as cuff failure, luminal obstruction, or kinking. Similarly, semielective tube change may be required to alter its size or type to facilitate flexible bronchoscopy or weaning from mechanical ventilation. Importantly, patients with DAs often undergo awake nasal intubation, usually with narrow nasal tubes. Such ETTs are not well suited to prolonged ICU ventilation. Minute ventilation is reduced, and $Paco_2$ rises. This permissive hypercapnia is well tolerated and in the context of a DA, it is often best to accept this usually benign condition (pH >7.2 is almost always safe in the absence of metabolic acidosis or elevated ICP). Tube exchange is safest when continuity with the airway is not lost, but although the concept of tube exchange over some form of airway catheter is simple, performing it requires skill, experience, and attention to detail.[282] Patients are sometimes transferred to the OR to change an ETT; such transfers risk fatal tube dislodgement. It is almost always safest to perform ETT exchange in the ICU.

Preexchange Laryngoscopy

Before ETT exchange, it is crucial to determine the exact position of the existing tube. For instance, out of 655 exchanges, in 171 cases the presumed cuff leak was actually partial displacement.[283] This not only makes tube exchange unnecessary, but passing an airway exchange catheter (AEC) through a malpositioned tube may result in an esophageal intubation and loss of the airway. DL in intubated ICU patients often reveals a poor view because of the ETT, secretions, feeding tubes, and swelling. VAL is superior for this adjunct laryngoscopy: Mort discovered the best DL view in over 80% of ICU patients was CL grade 3; this improved to 87.9% having a CL grade 1 or 2 view with VAL. First-pass success rates for ETT exchange were significantly improved using VAL. The much higher DL complication rates (Spo_2 <80%, bradycardia, esophageal intubation, and cardiac arrest) and a need for rescue techniques were attributed to the poorer DL view. Poor glottic view leads to multiple attempts, a factor universally associated with higher complication rates.

Laryngoscopy helps to open a pathway for reintubation by displacing the tongue. Laryngoscopy should be performed throughout the exchange sequence to assess the glottis, to confirm the position of the AEC, to recognize bowing or coiling of the AEC advancing the ETT, to diagnose and manage tube hold-up, to confirm that the ETT enters the glottis, to check the depth of insertion of the ETT, and to facilitate immediate rescue for reintubation failure. If VAL fails to reveal the glottis, then a flexible scope should be passed through the existing ETT to ensure it is well inside the trachea and the tip is mid-trachea; this avoids passing an AEC through a herniated tube.

Selection of the Airway Exchange Conduit

In general, the largest airway exchange conduit that will easily pass through the existing ETT should be chosen as larger conduits are stiffer and bend less. This also minimizes the gap between the ID of the new ETT and the external diameter of the conduit, facilitating advancement of the ETT. It is prudent to use a catheter that allows insufflation of oxygen if necessary (see later discussion). The AIC allows insertion of a standard 4-mm FIS, which facilitates direct visual confirmation of its position and correct tube deployment; however, the smallest replacement tube an AIC will accommodate is 7.0 mm ID. An alternative is to use a standard AEC.

Advancement of an ETT over an airway conduit is facilitated by a 90-degree counterclockwise rotation, lubrication, and use of flexible ETTs; the use of smaller tubes or the Parker Flex-Tip tube (Parker Medical, Highlands Ranch, CO) is also beneficial.[283–285] Some advocate using FISs as the airway conduit.[286] The replacement ETT is premounted onto the FIS, which is then advanced into the trachea alongside the existing ETT; the new ETT is advanced over the FIS as the existing ETT is withdrawn. In such circumstances, if the new ETT will not pass, the FIS must be fully withdrawn, potentially resulting in loss of the airway. Smaller AECs (11-French) can pass through the Murphy's eye of indwelling tubes. This has resulted in esophageal intubation when this occurs in conjunction with a slightly herniated ETT at the glottis. Ensure that the ETT and the AEC can move independently of each other; if they do not, then this complication may have occurred. Another problem with smaller AECs is their flexibility, resulting in coiling at the glottis as the replacement ETT is advanced with inadvertent esophageal intubation. If a smaller AEC has been inserted and there is concern it may bend or flick out of the trachea during advancement of the new ETT, then an AIC can be slid over a size 8-French, 11-French, or 14-French AEC; this increases the width of the conduit and makes it stiffer (Fig. 43.3).

Oxygenation via an Airway Catheter

The primary role of AECs is to act as a placeholder to maintain tracheal access while one ETT is exchanged for another. However,

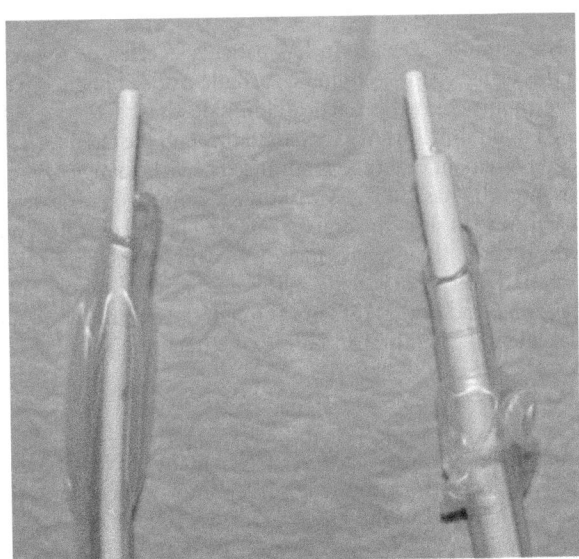

• **Fig. 43.3** Advancing a 7.0-mm internal diameter (ID) endotracheal tube (ETT) over an 11-French airway exchange catheter (AEC) can result in impingement on laryngeal structures due to the sizable gap between the two devices (left). Placing an Aintree intubation catheter between the AEC and ETT reduces the gap and facilitates advancement through the larynx (right).

oxygenation via the device is possible, although controversial. It can cause barotrauma secondary to oxygen insufflation or jet ventilation; the latter is particularly associated with barotrauma and is not recommended. The authors recommend that oxygen should only be administered when the AEC tip is 3 cm or more above the carina and when egress of gas from the glottis is confirmed, but this is extremely difficult. If an AEC is in situ and a patient's Spo$_2$ deteriorates to critical levels, then oxygenation to safe (not maximal) levels can be attempted by insufflation of oxygen at 1 to 3 L per minute, provided the clinician is certain the tip is above the carina and gas egress is confirmed; there should be a low index of suspicion for barotrauma. The primary solution for this problem, however, is reintubation.

Other Considerations

Occasionally, an AEC cannot be passed through the existing ETT. This may be because the original tube is too small but may also be associated with ETT kinking, as PVC becomes more malleable at body temperature. With oral ETTs, this usually occurs at the posterior oropharynx; palpating the tube in the back of the mouth will facilitate diagnosis and can straighten it out sufficiently to pass an AEC, although it rarely cures the problem because kinking recurs. If the inability to pass an AEC or FIS is caused by endoluminal accretion, this may be removed by using a device such as the complete airway management (CAM) Rescue Cath (Omneotech, Tavernier, FL).

Endotracheal Tube Exchange Procedure

An algorithm for exchanging ETTs in the ICU can be seen in Fig. 43.4. Some additional tips are as follows: (1) assemble staff and equipment before starting (including smaller ETTs, FIS, a full range of AEC sizes, SGAs, and bougies); (2) ensure functioning of capnography; (3) preoxygenate using 100% O$_2$ and PEEP (even with apparent cuff leak); (4) apply high-flow nasal O$_2$; (4) empty the stomach if there is an indwelling gastric tube; (5) optimize patient position—consider ramping; and (6) use adequate sedation with or without neuromuscular blockade.

Nasal to Oral Endotracheal Tube Exchange

This is a common scenario in DA patients. A safe way to accomplish this using VAL is as follows: A coudé-tipped bougie is passed via the mouth into the trachea alongside the ETT (the cuff is deflated to do this). An AEC is passed through the nasal ETT. The larger replacement oral tube is advanced over the bougie up to the glottis, and the nasal ETT is withdrawn from the glottis, leaving the nasal AEC in situ. The oral ETT is then passed over the bougie into the trachea. If the replacement ETT will not pass, the original is reinserted over the nasal AEC. The alternative of simply pulling the proximal end of the AEC out through the mouth can result in displacement of the distal end out of the trachea.

Tracheostomy Complications

Approximately 10% to 15% of ICU patients have a tracheostomy.[287] A detailed, nationwide survey into tracheostomy practice was conducted in the UK over 11 weeks in 2014. Of 2546 tracheostomies placed, 69.6% were percutaneous procedures performed by intensivists; the remainder were surgical. The most common major complications were inadvertent decannulation/displacement, obstruction, bleeding, and pneumothorax.[288] This corroborated evidence from NAP4, which highlighted that displacement incidents were frequently fatal; 14 displacement

episodes causing serious complications were described (7 were fatal, and 4 caused serious brain damage). Two-thirds were displaced when the patient was turned or moved by staff. Half of these patients had BMI greater than 30, and none of the displacements resulting in serious complications used capnography. Half occurred in units without a preformulated standard operating procedure (SOP) to manage tracheostomy displacement (Fig. 43.5). Tracheostomies reported in NAP4 became displaced when secured with surgical sutures, Velcro straps, or both, and the value of stay sutures in the lower part of the stoma, which when pulled help identify the tracheal edge, was unclear. Partial displacement (tracheostomy tube is in the stoma, but the tracheostomy tube tip lies either outside the trachea or abutting the posterior tracheal wall) led to more fatal complications than complete decannulation.[289] This can be ascribed to the delay before a partial displacement is recognized and uncertainty in how to manage this. Blind replacement of a displaced tracheostomy tube is often problematic and may lead to pretracheal placement (creation of a false lumen). The true incidence of tracheostomy tube complications is unknown, as few displacement or obstruction episodes not resulting in harm are recorded on hospital clinical incident databases.

Sixty-two percent of tracheostomies are inserted into overweight patients,[288] which increases the risk of tube displacement and obstruction. Mallick and colleagues showed that even in nonobese patients, standard-length tracheostomy tubes are too short and that the lengths of the stomal and tracheal limbs varied widely between different manufacturers and models, as did the angle between them (90 to 140 degrees).[290] These authors called for manufacturers to develop more anatomically faithful tracheostomy tubes with limbs at least 1 cm longer and an angle of 110 to 120 degrees. Obese patients benefit from adjustable, flanged, flexible tracheostomy tubes. These are available for use at the point of insertion, but only 17% of obese patients had such tracheostomy tubes inserted initially in the UK.[288]

That these problems occur in all healthcare systems is evidenced by the development of the Global Tracheostomy Collaborative, which is a powerful resource for raising standards in tracheostomy care. The NAP4 authors opine that "it is likely that tracheostomy tube displacement in the ICU is unavoidable" and then proceed to make several recommendations. The greatest protection is offered by early recognition of partial displacement. Similar to most critical incidents, there are warning signs akin to the red flags listed in Box 43.3. Continuous waveform capnography and increased staff awareness of the dangers of displacement during turns, movement, and instrumentation are critical. This complication is eminently predictable, and training in SOPs for tracheostomy emergencies should be mandated (see Fig. 43.5).

When faced with a deteriorating patient in the setting of a displaced tracheostomy tube, a sensible approach is to attach a Waters (Mapleson C) circuit with capnography to the tracheostomy and administer 100% oxygen via it and a nonrebreather face mask (unless it is certain the patient has a laryngectomy rather than a tracheostomy—if in doubt, oxygen should be administered to the nose and mouth anyway). The collapsible bag of the Waters circuit demonstrates spontaneous breathing and allows for tactile feedback during manual ventilation. The circuit should be made as simple as possible by removing speaking valves, caps, or humidifiers; this reduces the risk of extraneous causes for breathing difficulties. The neck should be inspected for emphysema (especially seen with fenestrated tracheostomy tubes), and it should be confirmed that the cuff is not herniated over the tracheostomy tube

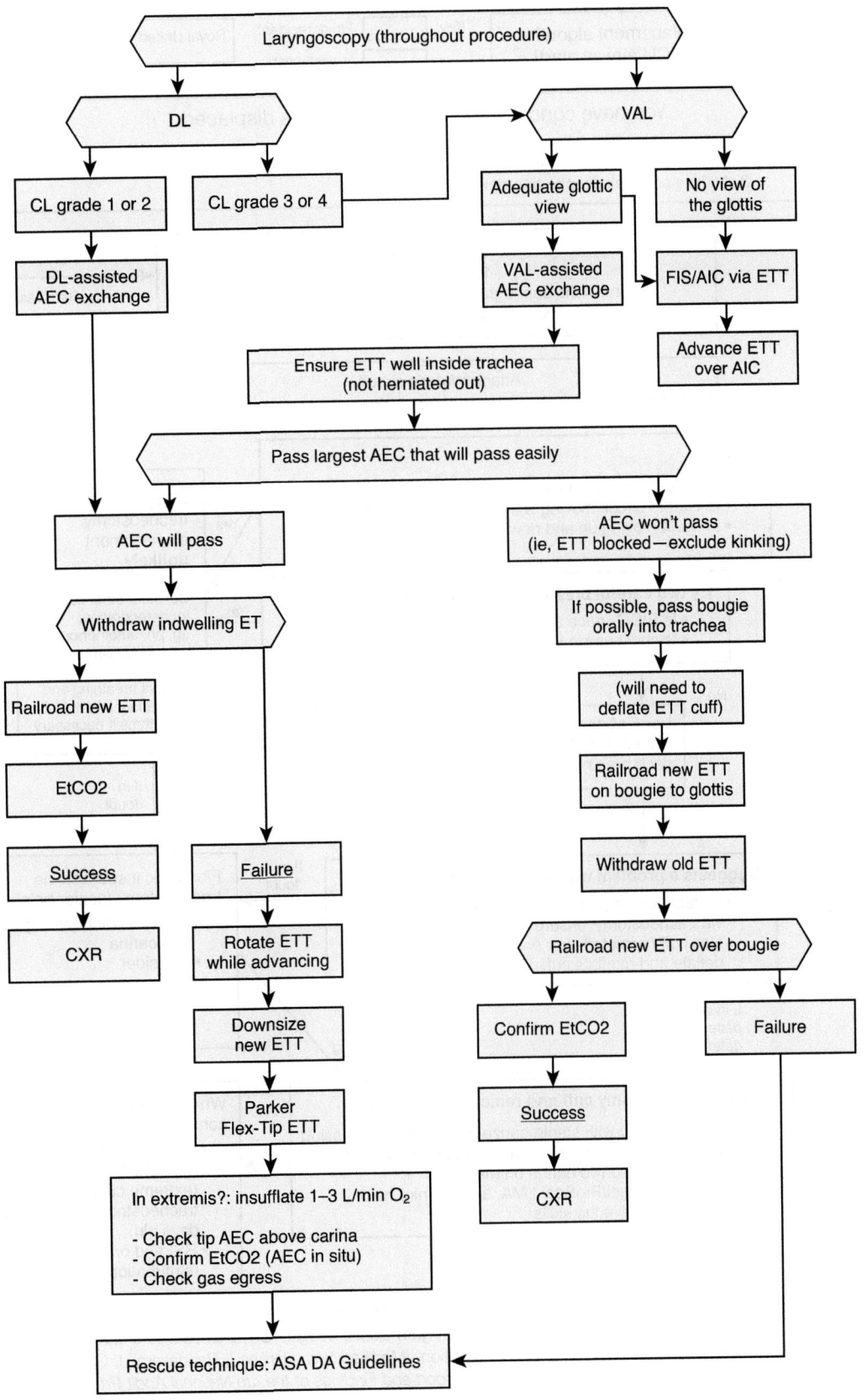

• **Fig. 43.4** Endotracheal tube exchange algorithm. *AEC*, Airway exchange catheter; *AIC*, Aintree intubation catheter; *ASA*, American Society of Anesthesiologists; *CL*, Cormack-Lehane; *CXR*, chest x-ray; *DA*, difficult airway; *DL*, direct laryngoscopy; *EtCO₂*, end-tidal CO_2, *ETT*, endotracheal tube; *FIS*, flexible intubation scope; *VAL*, video-assisted laryngoscopy.

NB: If no view with VAL and neither AEC nor FIS will pass, prepare for extremely difficult exchange with likely failure & need for airway rescue including surgical airway.

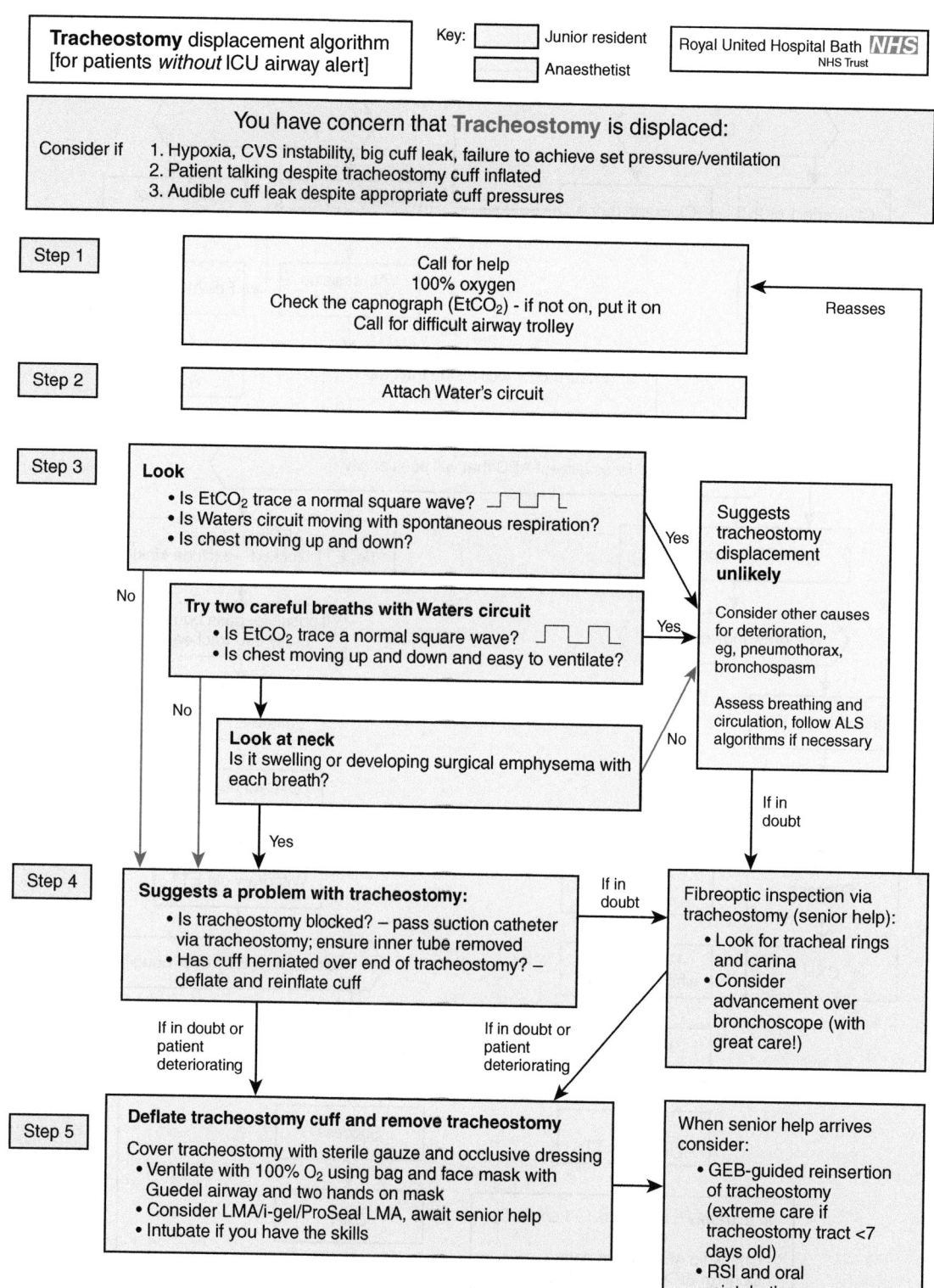

Fig. 43.5 Example algorithm for tracheostomy displacement in the intensive care unit. *CVS,* Cardiovascular system; *EtCO₂,* end-tidal carbon dioxide; *GEB,* gum-elastic bougie; *ICU,* intensive care unit; *LMA,* laryngeal mask airway; *RSI,* rapid sequence intubation. (Modified from Harper J, Rangasami J, Cook T. Major events in patients with a tracheostomy. In: *Report and Findings of the 4th National Audit Project of the Royal College of Anaesthetists and the Difficult Airway Society.* 2011:121–128.)

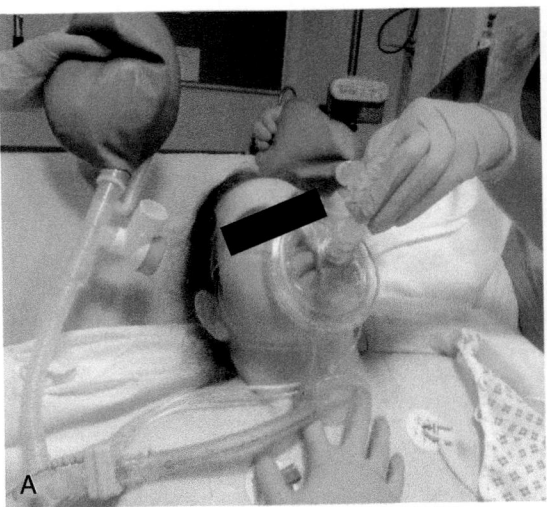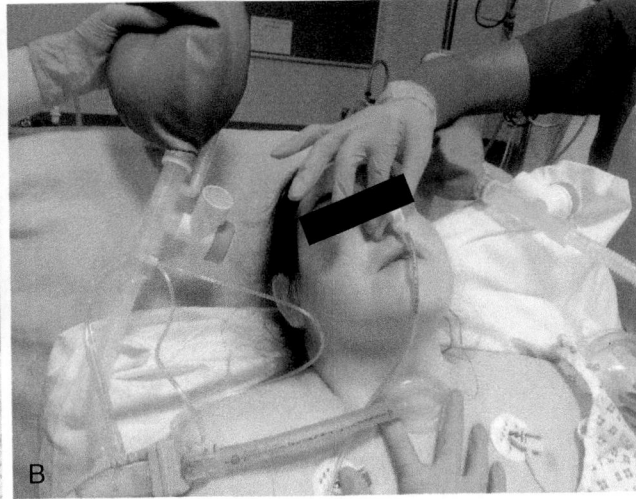

• **Fig. 43.6** Ventilation via a tracheostomy stoma using a laryngeal mask airway (LMA). (A) Dual ventilation via the upper airway by face mask and the tracheal stoma by LMA. (B) LMA ventilation of the tracheal stoma while minimizing leak by closing the mouth and nose.

tip by deflating it. Patency can be checked by passing a suction catheter down the tracheostomy tube.

If a situation is reached in which the cuff is deflated, a suction catheter will not pass, and ventilation is difficult, the tracheostomy tube is nonfunctioning. If staff with advanced airway skills capable of flexible scope inspection of the airway via the tracheostomy tube are not immediately available, the tracheostomy tube should be removed, and the airway managed with bag-valve-mask ventilation. An innovative means of oxygenation via the stoma itself is to hold an inflated size 3 LMA over the stoma and ventilate the lungs using this. Closing the mouth and occluding the nose minimize leak. This is an excellent temporizing technique while awaiting help (Fig. 43.6).

The tracheostomy tube can be directly inspected with an FIS; an evolution of this technique is to mount an AIC on the scope. Fig. 43.7 demonstrates this technique, which works equally well for obstruction, partial displacement, or even complete displacement when the AIC-loaded FIS is simply passed into the stoma. The advantages of this technique over other methods of tracheostomy tube replacement are (1) direct visualization of the trachea confirms that the AIC always remains in the airway, (2) directional control of the FIS helps to avoid traumatic insertion, (3) the AIC fits tightly into the tracheostomy tube, avoiding a large step at the leading edge that may impede insertion, (4) the AIC is flexible but firm enough to resist kinking, which can lead to creation of a false passage, (5) the AIC is disposable, (6) if ventilation through the original tracheostomy tube is possible, then by using a Bodai connector, the AIC/FIS can be inserted through the self-sealing port such that the lungs can be ventilated throughout the procedure until the moment the tracheostomy tube is removed, (7) the procedure is easily learned/practiced during routine tracheostomy tube changes or on manikins, and (8) if insertion of the tracheostomy tube is impossible, AICs can be used as ventilating bougies (see the section Oxygenation via an Airway Catheter).

Hemorrhage at the tracheostomy insertion site can occur, as can later erosion of the tracheostomy tube into neighboring blood vessels (e.g., tracheo-innominate fistula). One preventative strategy is to use ultrasound scanning of the tissues overlying the planned insertion site. It is not known what caliber vessels preclude percutaneous techniques; arterial vessels are easily identified using USG, and surgical approaches should then be used (Fig. 43.8).

The Obstructed Airway in the Intensive Care Unit

General ICU practice mandates familiarity with the natural history, clinical assessment, investigation, and management of patients with acute upper airway obstruction, such as patients with Ludwig's angina, epiglottitis, and angioedema, who have a high incidence of mortality and morbidity. Such patients often present acutely in extremis or at least in danger of sudden deterioration to nonspecialist centers and to relatively inexperienced physicians. Optimal management is controversial. Oral and oropharyngeal upper airway obstruction (angioedema) can lead to difficult mask ventilation and DL or difficult VAL. The aim must be to bypass the obstructed airway without traumatizing it. If the glottis and lower airway are normal, awake FSI is the method of choice; if this is not possible, awake tracheostomy is needed. Regarding lesions of the tongue base or supraglottis (Ludwig's angina or acute epiglottitis), induction of general anesthesia can be dangerous. It may precipitate total airway obstruction as tone diminishes, DL or VAL may cause trauma with swelling/bleeding, and techniques requiring placing a blade tip in the vallecula are unreliable; awake FSI or awake tracheostomy is indicated. NAP4 noted several points related to the management of acute upper airway obstruction: a high failure rate of FSI performed after induction of anesthesia, a dearth of opportunities for junior surgeons to learn open tracheostomy since the advent of percutaneous techniques, and that most (two-thirds) of emergency cannula cricothyrotomies in upper airway obstruction fail. The paper suggests that the best plan depends on the circumstances, considering the experience of the anesthesiologist, surgeon, overall team, and available equipment. No plan is always successful, and the hallmarks of good practice are early senior involvement and thorough assessment, including imaging if available. A plan using techniques and equipment with which the team is familiar should be made; prompt recognition that an initial plan may fail and moving to plan B before loss of the airway are essential. If the airway strategy includes possible tracheostomy, an experienced surgeon should be present from the beginning.

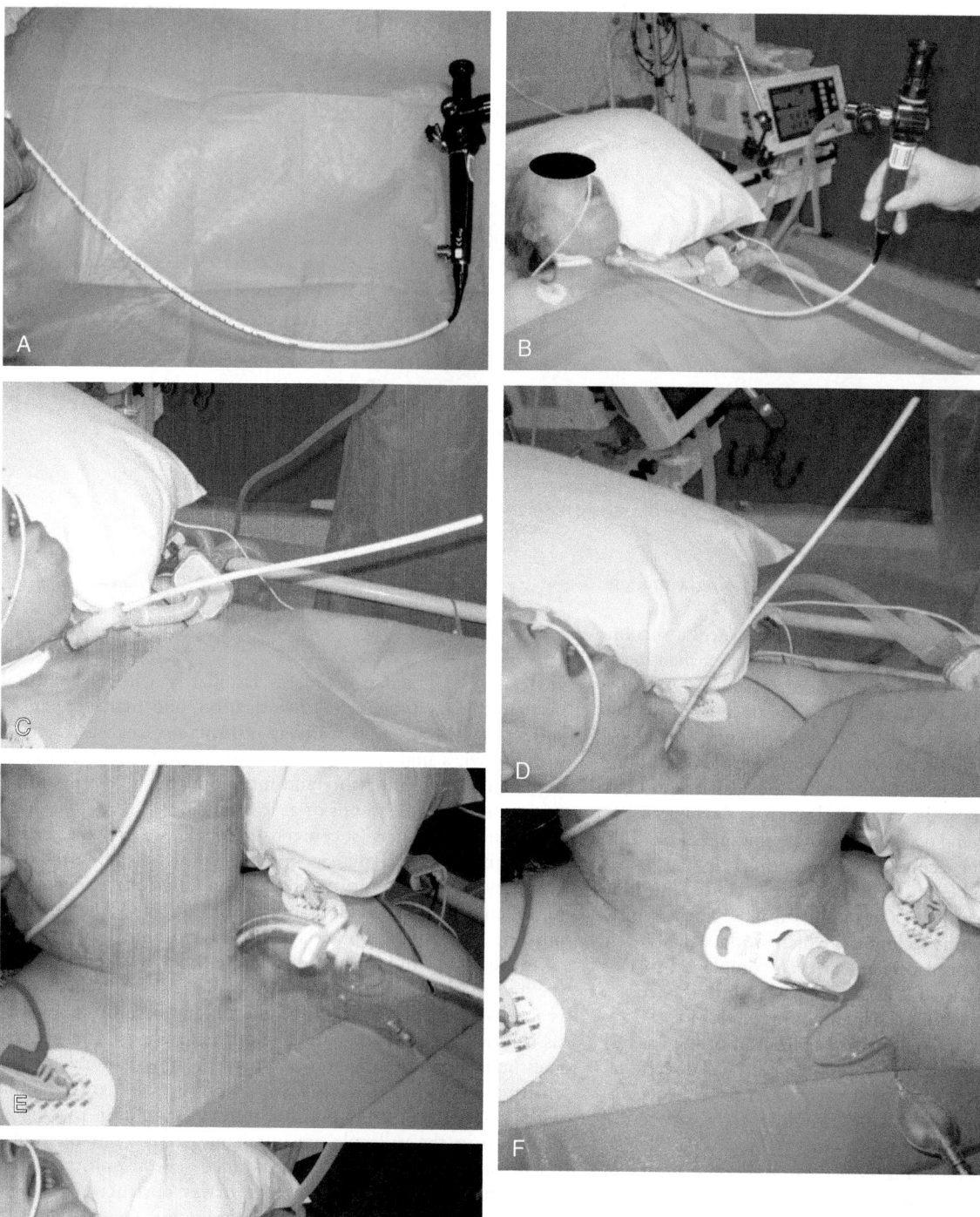

• **Fig. 43.7** Tracheostomy tube replacement using the Aintree intubation catheter (AIC) technique. (A) An AIC is mounted onto a flexible intubation scope (FIS). (B) The FIS/AIC is inserted into a partially occluded tracheostomy tube. (C) The FIS is removed, leaving the AIC through the stoma in the trachea. (D) The existing tracheostomy tube is removed over the AIC; at this point, there is no ventilation. (E) A new tracheostomy tube is placed over the AIC. (F) A new tracheostomy tube in situ. (G) Positioning of the replacement tracheostomy tubes performed using the FIS; ventilation has resumed.

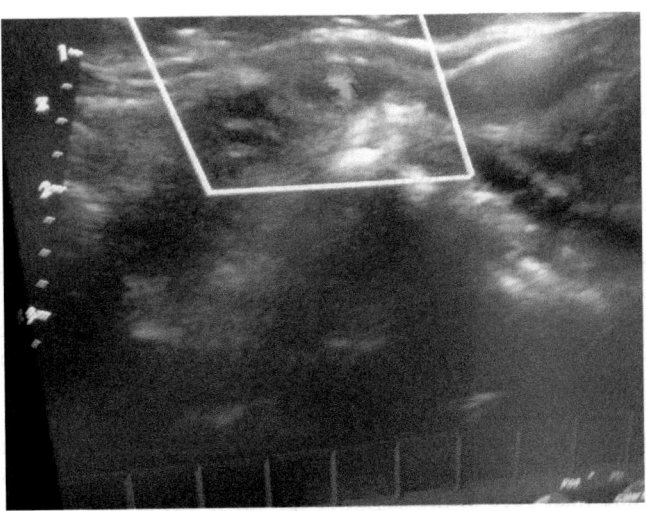

• **Fig. 43.8** Ultrasound image with color Doppler showing a large vein overlying the trachea before insertion of a percutaneous tracheostomy, subsequently deferred for a surgical approach.

Ludwig's Angina

Ludwig's angina illustrates many of the subtleties involved in managing upper airway obstruction in the ICU. The resulting upper airway obstruction develops insidiously until virtually complete, when abrupt asphyxiation can occur. Conservative management (not protecting the airway in all cases) is increasingly popular and comprises antibiotics, humidified oxygen, positioning head-upward

30 degrees, fasting, judicious administration of IV fluids, steroids, and extremely close observation in a monitored environment such as the ICU. Despite the success of medical management, however, it can fail with disastrous results.[291,292] The risk of a conservative approach is that the signs of early and retrievable upper airway obstruction are subtle, and loss of the airway can be sudden. Classic signs such as stridor, retractions, and cyanosis are clinically obvious but occur late so cannot be relied upon to prompt timely intervention.[293] The experience of ICU residents who are first responders to airway deterioration varies enormously.[294]

Signs of Airway Deterioration

Greenland and colleagues reported a novel approach on how to identify clinical deterioration in a review of deaths from Ludwig's angina reported to Australian coroners over 8 years to 2008.[295] This report looked primarily at patients who died of upper airway obstruction after extubation following surgical decompression of Ludwig's angina. The authors noted a premorbid sequence in which the voice changes and then poor cough caused by edema of the glottis and difficult cord adduction develop. Drooling (poor control of oral secretions) implies the oral and/or pharyngeal phases of swallowing are impaired because Ludwig's angina displaces the tongue and reduces its mobility. Stridor, respiratory distress, and orthopnea indicate impending complete airway obstruction, potentially too late for controlled tracheal intubation. Desaturation is an extremely late sign.[296] Greenland and colleagues constructed a table of signs, what these imply, and recommended actions (Fig. 43.9). Senior physicians should instruct ICU residents and nurses in what signs to report. The precise order

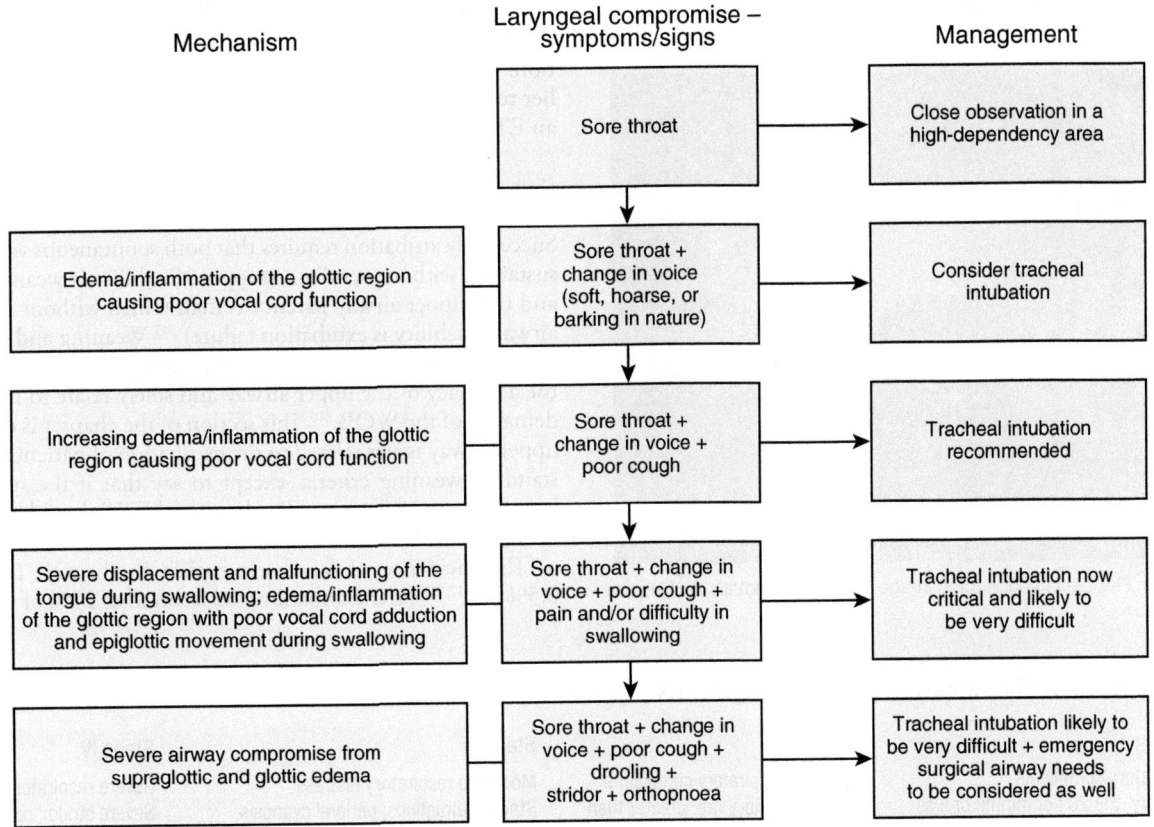

• **Fig. 43.9** Signs and symptoms of laryngeal compromise in Ludwig's angina with subsequent clinical management. (Modified from Greenland KB, Acott C, Segal R, Riley RH, Merry AF. Delayed airway compromise following extubation of adult patients who required surgical drainage of Ludwig's angina: comment on three coronial cases. *Anaesth Intensive Care.* 2011;39(3):506–508.)

can vary, but loss of voice, effective cough, or effective swallow mandates senior review. These signs should always prompt airway endoscopy, and if there is laryngeal swelling, or an obstructed view of the larynx, the airway should be secured immediately.

Securing the Airway

If, after flexible endoscopy, the larynx is deemed able to accommodate an ETT, awake FSI performed in the sitting position is recommended. Ovassapian and colleagues reported 26 such attempts with only one failure (because of narrow nasal passages).[297] During awake intubation, it is important to avoid irritation of the airway as laryngospasm and loss of the airway may occur.[298,299] Opioids are useful to depress airway reflexes before topical spray as you place a patient under anesthesia; some patients will not need any topicalization, especially with remifentanil titration. Real-time preintubation USG is useful to gauge the dimensions of the airway and identify the anterior neck anatomy in case this is needed for airway access.[300] Awake tracheostomy has been described as the gold standard and is certainly the default technique when awake tracheal intubation is unavailable, unfeasible, or fails.[301] Awake tracheostomy may be extremely challenging and risks spreading infection to the mediastinum, bleeding, and loss of the airway. Extreme caution is needed in positioning the patient for awake tracheostomy: semirecumbent is preferable to supine, which can cause total airway obstruction.

Acute Epiglottis

Acute epiglottitis in adults is more accurately described as supraglottitis with variable spread (Fig. 43.10).[302,303] Management is controversial; most adults' airways are not jeopardized, and

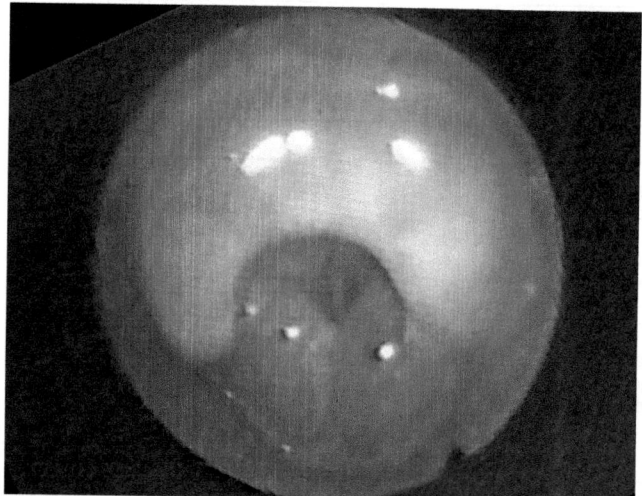

• **Fig. 43.10** Flexible laryngoscopic image of acute epiglottitis and supraglottitis.

intervention is becoming more conservative[304]; however, medical management must be selective and only used in the context of vigilant clinical observation because sudden death can occur.[305] Mortality has been reduced dramatically from 32% to 1%.[304–308]

Friedman and colleagues classified four stages of acute epiglottitis progression and asserted that respiratory arrest does not occur with no prior evidence of airway compromise (Table 43.2).[309] Stage IV requires immediate intervention,[302] often awake tracheostomy. Stage I and most stage II and III patients do not need airway intervention, but stridor or respiratory distress within a day of developing symptoms indicates a need for control of the airway.[304] Simple clinical indices, however, are insufficient for airway intervention decision making.

Airway endoscopy is well tolerated in adults with acute epiglottitis.[310] Katori and Tsukuda used endoscopic criteria such that intervention is needed when severe swelling narrows or obscures more than 50% of the larynx or spreads to the arytenoids; this was also associated with stridor and a recent onset of symptoms.[311] As many as 20% of adults with acute epiglottitis require intubation.[312] Awake tracheostomy is indicated for those with no airway visible on endoscopy or if the larynx will not accommodate an ETT.[313] Steroids may reduce length of stay in the ICU.[304,307,313]

Angioedema

All patients with angioedema will benefit from endoscopic examination. These patients should have their airway secured if they exhibit dyspnea, voice changes, difficulty controlling secretions, altered mental status, respiratory distress, or stridor, unless they demonstrate an adequate response to treatment with nebulized racemic epinephrine and IV steroids (Fig. 43.11). Angioedema can recur during the same admission without specific provocation. Significant laryngeal involvement akin to that described earlier requires awake FSI. Again, if the larynx cannot accommodate an ETT, awake tracheostomy is indicated.[314]

Extubation in the Intensive Care Unit

Successful extubation requires that both spontaneous ventilation is sustained without ventilator support (inability is weaning failure) and that upper airway patency is maintained without an artificial airway (inability is extubation failure).[315] Weaning and extubation failure can overlap. Standard extubation criteria do not address the adequacy of the upper airway and solely relate to meeting the demands of the WOB.[316] This section of the chapter is confined to upper airway issues related to the extubation of patients who meet standard weaning criteria, except to say that if the spontaneous breathing tests fail, a partially obstructed ETT should be ruled out using flexible bronchoscopy.

The incidence of failed extubation in the OR is less than 0.5%;[276,317,318] ICU extubations fail as often as 25% of the time.[319]

TABLE 43.2	**Friedman Classification of Acute Epiglottitis**		
Stage I	**Stage II**	**Stage III**	**Stage IV**
No respiratory complaints Respiratory rate 20 per minute or less (average)	Subjective respiratory complaints and/or respiratory rate greater than 20 per minute (average)	Moderate respiratory distress Stridor, retractions, perioral cyanosis PCO_2 greater than 45 mm Hg Respiratory rate greater than 30 per minute (average)	Severe respiratory distress Severe stridor, retractions Cyanosis, delirium, loss of consciousness, hypoxia Respiratory arrest

form, accounts for most extubation failures. The most significant exception in the ICU is poor control of secretions.

Assessment

ICU extubation decisions involve many difficult-to-quantify elements and are, by nature, imprecise. The elements related to the decision to extubate are identification of upper airway obstruction before the ETT is removed, determination of ease of reintubation should this be needed, assessment of the ability of the patient to control secretions, assessment of level of consciousness, and ensuring that reintubation is not needed for predictable, nonphysiologic reasons (e.g., surgery or radiologic imaging). The DAS extubation guidelines use a sequential approach to identifying an at-risk extubation (one in which reintubation or oxygenation after extubation may be difficult).[321] The airway assessment before extubation comprises:

1. **Externally observed risk factors** visible by bedside clinical examination that will restrict access to the airway if reintubation is necessary (e.g., halo fixation, maxillomandibular fixation, cervical collar, or facial swelling).

2. **Assessment of the supraglottis,** including the tongue, oropharynx, and hypopharynx using DL or VAL. This will identify restricted mouth opening or neck extension, obvious edema, airway trauma/bleeding, and surgical complications such as retropharyngeal hematoma. The utility of this assessment has been questioned because ETTs often obscure the supraglottic structures, and there is no evidence that it impacts morbidity. Concerns regarding this visual inspection include the ETT causing a poor view,[322–324] difficult quantification of swelling,[325] and edema that molds around the ETT such that, even in the absence of worsening of edema, this existing edema redistributes, causing obstruction after extubation. Redistribution of airway edema may be responsible for deterioration soon after extubation (within 2 hours). If an adequate view of the supraglottis cannot be obtained with DL or VAL, inspection with a flexible scope can be performed. Although the assessment remains subjective, if the glottis can be easily visualized, it will, when performed by an experienced airway clinician, form an important element in the decision to extubate and may allow extubation when it may otherwise be delayed.

3. **Visual assessment of the glottis and subglottis** is impossible with an ETT in place; however, the functional cuff leak test can provide valuable information regarding the caliber of the glottic and subglottic airway.[326] If the airway lumen narrows by more than 50%, inspiratory stridor results. Postextubation laryngeal edema is seen in 5% to 54.4%, and postextubation stridor is seen in 1.5% to 26.3% of ICU extubations. The reported incidence of reintubation attributed to postextubation laryngeal edema is 1.1% to 10.5%; risk factors include female gender, ETT diameter greater than 45% of tracheal diameter, cuff pressure greater than 25 to 30 cm H_2O, difficult or traumatic tracheal intubation, prolonged intubation more than 3 days, attempted phonation while intubated, and gastroesophageal reflux. The primary utility of the cuff leak test is in identifying patients not at risk of postextubation laryngeal edema or stridor: the negative predictive value is more than 90%. The corollary is that a positive cuff leak test (no or minimal leak) does not mean that a patient will develop postextubation laryngeal edema or stridor. The predictive values of the cuff leak test are improved using quantitative means. The cuff leak test is performed after thorough glottic suctioning and using

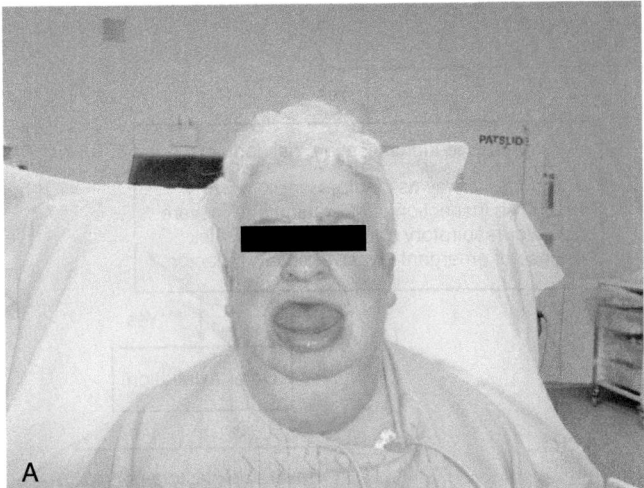
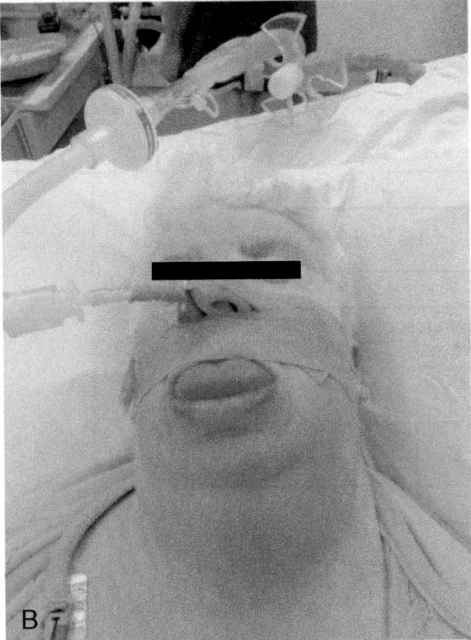

• **Fig. 43.11** Angioedema. (A) This patient had a virtually inaudible voice, no cough, and mild drooling. At initial endoscopic assessment in the emergency department, the larynx was said to be uninvolved. (B) Thirty minutes later, the patient began to deteriorate clinically. Such severe glottic involvement was seen during awake flexible scope intubation that a 5-mm internal-diameter endotracheal tube was required.

Patients with a DA are at high risk during reintubation. The ASA Closed Claims analyses have confirmed that the rates of death and brain damage are higher for adverse events at extubation than at other times during airway management.[320] Likewise, the NAP4 audit confirmed that extubation is extremely risky in that one-third of all major complications occurred at extubation, and these had a combined incidence of death and brain damage rate of 13%; the NAP4 authors identified inadequate risk assessment and poor planning as root causes. As intended extubation is an elective process and ICU patients are very vulnerable during reintubation, extubation should be well planned, and the Difficult Airway Society (DAS) extubation guidelines are applicable in the ICU.[321] An example of an extubation algorithm for the ICU is shown in Fig. 43.12. The risk factors for failed extubation are not specific enough to predict failed extubation. Airway obstruction, in some

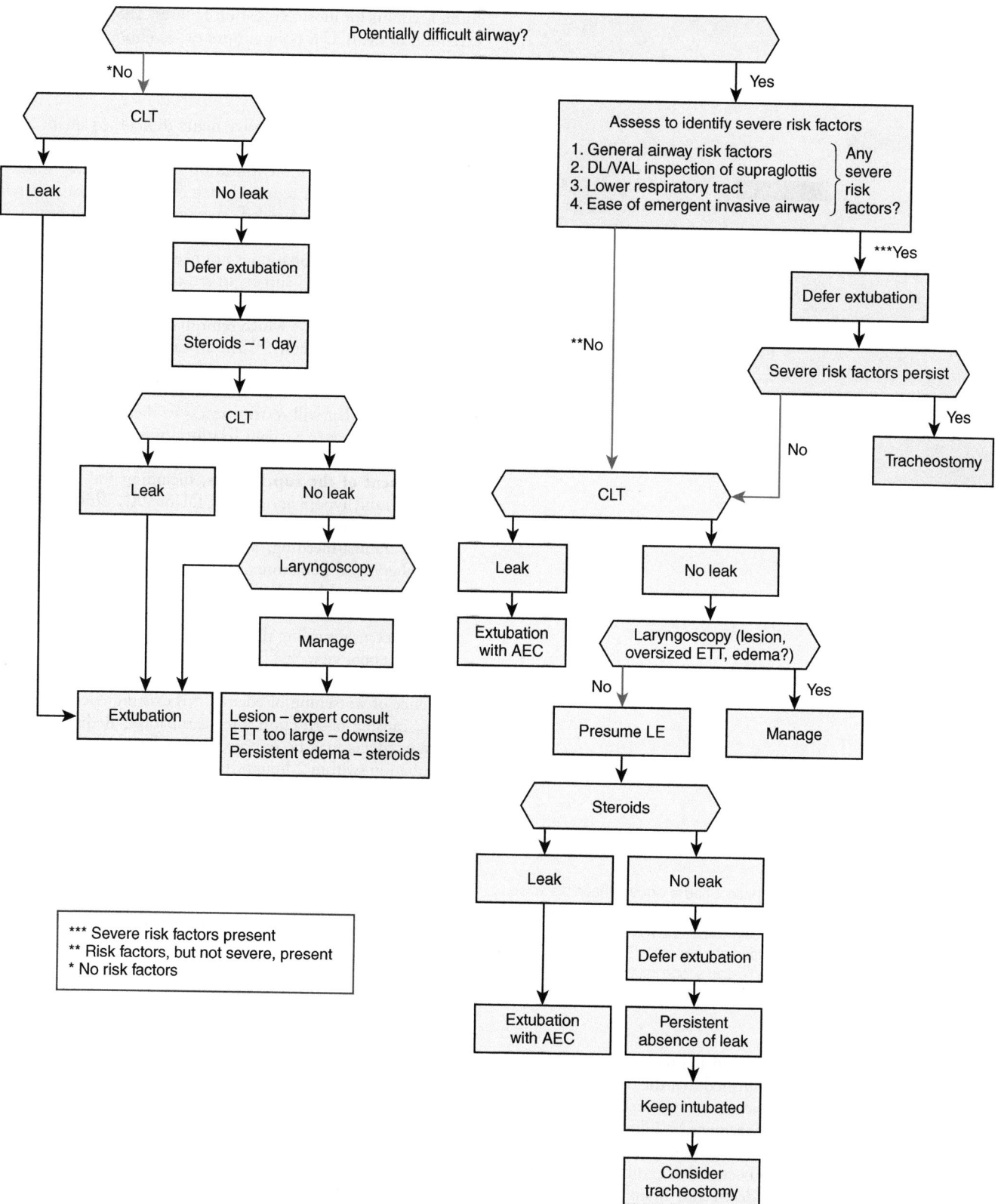

• **Fig. 43.12** Algorithm for extubation in the ICU. *AEC,* Airway exchange catheter; *CLT,* cuff leak test; *DL,* direct laryngoscopy; *ETT,* endotracheal tube; *LE,* laryngeal edema; *PEEP,* positive end-expiratory pressure; *SBT,* spontaneous breathing trial; *VAL,* video-assisted laryngoscopy.

volume-controlled ventilation. An acceptable cuff leak volume is 12% to 24% of the tidal volume with the cuff inflated or 110 to 130 cc in an adult.[323,326,327] Do not persist with cuff leak tests during spontaneous ventilation if there is no leak at all. Forced inspiration against a closed airway can result in postobstructive (negative pressure) pulmonary edema. If there is a poor or absent cuff leak, the glottis should be examined to exclude a laryngeal lesion, an oversized ETT, or the presence of excessive secretions. Overall, the cuff leak test is useful as part of a comprehensive extubation assessment such that, on the precautionary principle, the absence of an acceptable leak in patients at high risk for extubation and/or with predictors of a DA should usually lead to deferment of extubation.

4. **Assessment of the lower airway** for the complications of DA management: bronchial intubation, gastric distension with diaphragmatic splinting from aggressive mask ventilation, or pneumothorax. Chest x-ray helps exclude these.

5. **Assessment of secretion control.** In the ICU, the balance between production and clearance of respiratory secretions is essential. Suction frequency is a useful composite measure of this balance: a requirement for tracheal suctioning more than twice hourly precludes extubation.[328] An adequate level of consciousness is crucial and requires eye opening, hand grip, tongue protrusion, and cough to command.[329]

6. **Assessment of the feasibility of emergency invasive access should extubation fail.** If emergency invasive access looks problematic, extubation success should be confidently expected before the ETT is removed.

Preparation: Optimizing Conditions for Extubation

The general condition of the patient and ventilation requirements must be suitable for extubation. Airways with any evidence of laryngeal edema, previous trauma, or surgery should be treated with steroids. Methylprednisolone 20 mg IV every 6 hours for four doses is commonly used.[319,330,331] In high-risk patients, steroids reduce the incidence of postextubation stridor and reintubation significantly. Note that steroids do not reduce noninflammatory edema caused by venous obstruction. ETT fixation devices should be ensured to not impede venous drainage, and the patient should be positioned head up as much as possible. Excessive fluid administration should be avoided.

Classifying Risk and Extubation

At the conclusion of the preextubation assessment, an experienced airway operator must form an opinion. The question to be answered is this: "Are there any risk factors identified which suggest that if extubation should fail, I would not be able to secure the airway?" These severe risk factors absolutely preclude extubation. Paucity of evidence means it is not currently possible to quantify these severe risk factors; asking an experienced airway specialist to perform the examination described previously is the current best practice.

A preextubation assessment allows classification patients into three groups: (1) no anticipated difficulty; (2) there may be some difficulty, but extubation is reasonable; features suggest that a DA potentially exists but are not so severe that extubation is precluded (no severe risk factors); and (3) patients with severe risk factors suggest that, if extubation fails, reintubation would be extremely difficult (see Fig. 43.12).

If there is no expected difficulty, the clinician can proceed with an awake extubation after a cuff leak test confirms there is a leak. With an inadequate cuff leak, the precautionary principle should apply: defer extubation, introduce/continue steroids, and repeat the assessment in 24 hours. If the clinical picture suggests extubation is reasonable, but that reintubation or postextubation oxygenation is potentially complicated (e.g., nonswollen, good cuff leak, but known DA), it is reasonable for this at-risk extubation to proceed. The risk is mitigated using an airway conduit such as an AEC.[332,333] This is group 2 as outlined previously.

The AEC tip should be positioned in the mid-trachea. To achieve this, the DAS guidelines recommend measuring the distance between a facial landmark (e.g., nostrils or lips) and the mid-trachea with a flexible bronchoscope via the ETT before the AEC is inserted. The AEC is then inserted, secured, and labeled, and the depth is annotated on the chart. Its position in the airway is confirmed using waveform capnography (Fig. 43.13). AECs

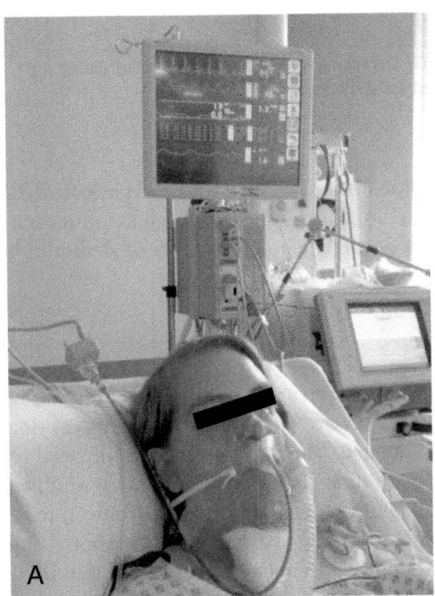

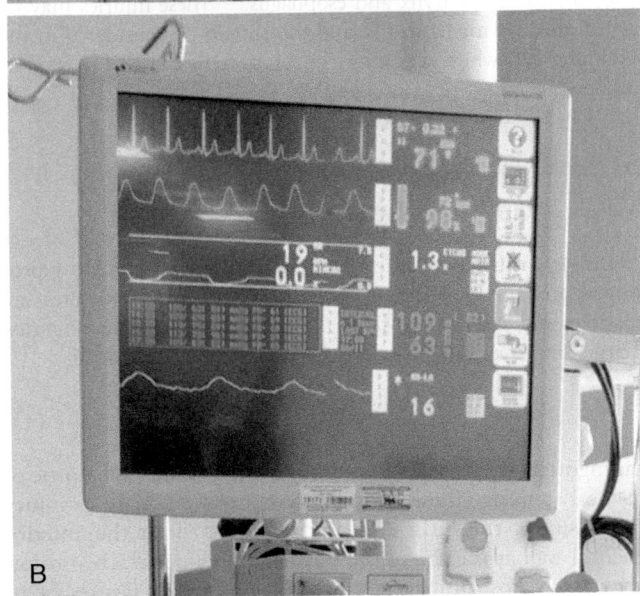

• **Fig. 43.13** (A) Patient with an airway exchange catheter (AEC) in situ. (B) Close-up of the capnograph tracing, confirming intratracheal placement of the AEC.

- If respiratory insufficiency occurs, reintubation should proceed without delay. Stridor can be temporized with nebulized epinephrine and intravenous or nebulized steroids. These do not usually alter the natural history of extubation failure but can be used to buy time to prepare for reintubation.
- Call for help experienced in emergent invasive airway access.
- Sit patient upright and administer 100% oxygen via face mask/nasal cannula.
- Assemble all necessary intubation equipment.
- Check $EtCO_2$ tracing from AEC, and check that there is a leak (in absence of leak, never administer oxygen via an AEC).
- Oxygenation via AEC only if life-threatening hypoxia (maximum 2 to 3 L per minute).
- Sedation and neuromuscular blockade, if needed (usually is).
- VAL to displace tongue to facilitate reintubation (DL is acceptable but inferior).
- Advance the smallest suitable ETT over the AEC.
- Confirm $EtCO_2$.

AEC, Airway exchange catheter; *DL,* direct laryngoscopy; *$EtCO_2$,* end-tidal carbon dioxide; *ETT,* endotracheal tube; *VAL,* video-assisted laryngoscopy.

reduce reintubation-related morbidity.[332–334] If a patient deteriorates with an AEC in situ, medical causes such as pulmonary edema should be excluded, and the process in Box 43.4 should be followed.

Postextubation Care

It is crucial that the recently extubated DA patient be monitored closely, with regular medical review and an experienced airway doctor being immediately available. Measures to mitigate the need for reintubation include positioning the patient upright, humidified oxygen, fasting, avoidance of excessive fluid administration, respiratory care, and analgesia. Noninvasive respiratory support using HFNO or NIPPV is useful.[61–66] DA management can be traumatic, especially to the pharynx and esophagus.[335] These injuries may be complicated by mediastinitis, and this should be considered in the ICU after DI, where it is a rare but important cause of pyrexia of unknown origin.

Delayed Complications of Intensive Care Unit Airway Management

Intensivists must be aware of important complications of prolonged airway management because preventative measures are possible, and early diagnosis in the ICU, as well as following discharge, improves outcomes (see Chapter 48 for more detail).

Laryngotracheal Stenosis

Laryngotracheal stenosis commonly refers to either subglottic or tracheal stenosis. These pathologies most often relate to injury at the site of the ETT cuff postintubation or at the anterior tracheal wall at the site of the tracheal stoma posttracheostomy, respectively. Postintubation subglottic stenosis and posttracheostomy tracheal stenosis should be regarded as separate entities.[336] Postintubation subglottic stenosis usually occurs at the ETT cuff site as a weblike, fibrous growth. Its etiology is mucosal ischemia

leading to circumferential injury and contracture.[337] Ischemia begins within a few hours of tracheal intubation and can result in weblike fibrosis within 3 to 6 weeks. To prevent ischemia, ETT cuff pressures greater than the mean capillary perfusion pressure of the tracheal mucosa (27 cm H_2O) must be avoided. Cuff inflation pressure should ideally be less than 25 cm H_2O and not exceed 30 cm H_2O.[338] Other risk factors include incorrect ETT size (too small, which necessitates high cuff pressures, or too large), ETT movement in agitated patients, gastric reflux, vascular disease, intubation greater than 10 days,[339] traumatic intubation, hypotension, female gender, and infection. Conversely, posttracheostomy tracheal stenosis results from abnormal wound healing with excess granulation tissue at the stoma site. This can also develop over fractured cartilage, which can occur during the tracheostomy procedure.[336,340] Wound infection is said to be causative in 42% of stenoses following open tracheostomy (Figs. 43.14 and 43.15).

The incidence of late laryngotracheal stenosis resulting in more than 50% luminal obstruction is 3.1% for 6 to 12 months

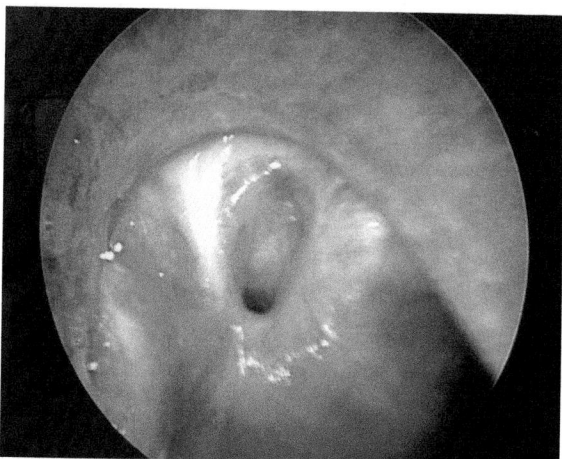

• **Fig. 43.14** Myer-Cotton Grade 1 subglottic stenosis.

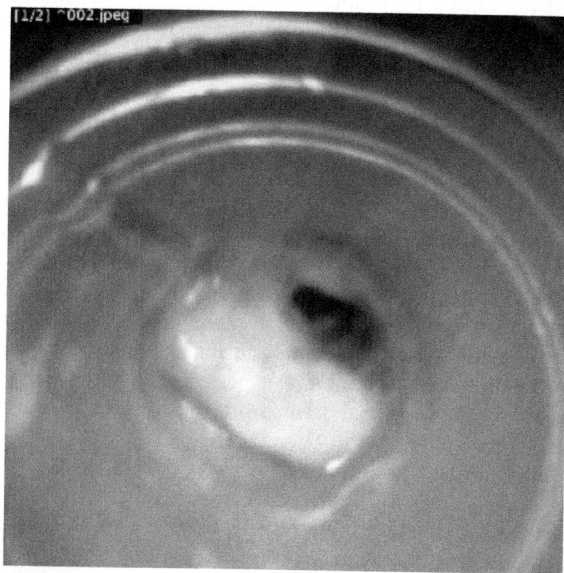

• **Fig. 43.15** Early granuloma at 6 weeks after insertion of a tracheostomy tube causing approximately 50% occlusion with failure to wean from the ventilator.

postdecannulation. If lesser degrees of subglottic/tracheal stenosis are considered, the incidence rises to 4.6%.[339] Extrapolating this to UK ICU survivors and the known number of laryngotracheal therapeutic interventions carried out,[341] Nouraei and colleagues have estimated that as many as four out of five patients with severe stenosis do not receive treatment. This is because patients are lost to follow-up after ICU discharge, the evolving respiratory compromise is misdiagnosed, and even severe luminal obstruction is only revealed clinically when the patient attempts a certain level of physical activity. Many convalescing ICU patients remain so debilitated that this functional limitation is never revealed. Stenosis is often asymptomatic until the tracheal lumen is reduced by 75%, and stridor does not occur in some cases until the tracheal diameter is 5 mm or less. In the ICU, a high index of suspicion and prompt endoscopy to rule out stenosis should be considered in patients who fail decannulation.

Diagnosis

There are various diagnostic modalities for investigation of laryngotracheal stenosis:

- Flexible endoscopy: the single best investigation because it identifies type, site, and severity of the stenosis and whether there is cartilage involvement, and it can be performed in the ICU. In patients requiring reintubation after failed extubation, flexible endoscopic examination should be considered to exclude airway stenosis as the culprit. Early lesions, including edema, ulceration, granulation, and vocal cord dysfunction, are commonly seen. It is also easily performed in the ICU follow-up clinic where minor abnormalities of the tracheal lumen are common (<10% stenosis).
- High-resolution computed tomography: requires thin (1 mm) cuts with sagittal and/or coronal reconstruction to ensure the full extent of the stenosis is identified.
- Spirometry: flow-volume loops can be used as a screening tool in cooperative patients in post-ICU follow-up clinics and are also useful to monitor for restenosis after therapeutic intervention.

Prevention and Management

To mitigate the risk of development of laryngotracheal stenosis, the risk factors listed above should be avoided when possible and translaryngeal intubation should be limited to 10 days; prolonged intubation followed by tracheostomy should especially be avoided. If it is clear early in the hospital course that tracheostomy will be required, this should be ideally performed by day 5 to 6. Cartilage fracture during percutaneous tracheostomy can be avoided by using bronchoscopy during the procedure. Fenestrated tracheostomy tubes are more likely to cause granulation tissue. Early diagnosis within a few weeks of extubation is beneficial as inflammatory conditions in the airway respond to intralesional steroids followed by laser reduction of the granulation tissue and balloon dilatation.[342,343] Patients receiving this early treatment require significantly fewer surgical interventions than with later diagnosis. The possibility of stenotic disease should be considered when previous ICU patients are readmitted for intubation; smaller ETTs should be available.

Glottic Stenosis

A third form of laryngotracheal stenosis is fixation of the arytenoids caused by postintubation interarytenoid scarring. This causes hoarseness and dysphagia with persistent aspiration after extubation and may evolve to dyspnea and upper airway obstruction.[344,345] Early tracheostomy minimizes the risk of glottic stenosis and impaired vocal cord mobility.[339]

Other Lesions

Vocal cord paralysis occurs as a result of compression of the internal branch of the recurrent laryngeal nerve as it enters the larynx between the cricoid and thyroid cartilages by a high-lying cuff when the cuff pressure exceeds 30 cm H_2O. Tracheomalacia results from cuff pressure necrosis, mechanical erosion attributed to ETT movement, inflammation, and infection destroying tracheal cartilage. Tracheo-innominate fistula arises when pressure necrosis at the anterior tracheal wall causes local erosion; it classically presents with a sentinel bleed followed by massive hemoptysis 3 to 24 days after a low tracheostomy.[346] Management centers on emergent surgical repair or embolization, temporized by hyperinflation of the cuff to tamponade bleeding. If the latter maneuver fails, the tracheostomy tube should be removed and replaced with an ETT inserted into the stoma so that the cuff is below the bleeding point. A finger is then inserted through the stoma to compress the anterior tracheal wall and vessel against the sternum to allow time for emergent transport to the OR. Survival is poor (14%).[347,348] Tracheoesophageal fistula is caused by a similar mechanism with posterior cuff pressure causing mucosal necrosis and erosion into the esophagus. It presents with food suctioned from the airway, coughing at feeding, and recurrent aspiration pneumonitis.[349] Early referral is required. Impaired swallowing is common postintubation,[350] but significant aspiration is much less frequent.

Conclusion

ICU patients' airways are extremely demanding; airway-related mortality and severe morbidity may be orders of magnitude higher than in general OR practice. DI is at least twice as common. Airway intervention must be prompt and smooth: The critically ill simply do not tolerate poor airway management.

Thorough preoxygenation, competent use of VAL, and an intubation checklist incorporating RSI are key management strategies. However, the hazards of airway management in the ICU only begin once the tube is inserted. An intubated patient care bundle including capnography should be followed. Partially displaced tubes present diagnostic uncertainty, and the accompanying delay is harmful. The key to successful management is training and having a well-formulated airway plan that is shared with the entire team and that uses equipment with which team members are proficient. Difficult extubation is increasingly part of ICU practice. Tracheostomy insertion is unique to ICU airway management, but more challenging still is to ensure that tracheostomy patients remain safe after the stoma is created.

Confidence in dealing with tracheostomy emergencies is a core ICU skill. Another essential element of intensivists' airway repertoire is the management of patients with acutely inflamed airways. Intensivists must be able to recognize the patterns of airway deterioration to which these patients are susceptible. Timely intervention requires constant vigilance, experience, and shrewd judgment, not to mention exacting technical skill.

It is incumbent on those who train intensivists to ensure that their fellows are equipped to provide these singularly vulnerable patients with the best possible care, remembering that the emphasis is no longer on devices but on training, good planning, and teamwork.

Selected References

2. Higgs A, Cook TM, McGrath BA. Airway management in the critically ill: the same, but different. *Br J Anaesth.* 2016;117(suppl 1):i5–i9. doi:10.1093/bja/aew055.

5. Mosier JM, Sakles JC, Law JA, et al. Tracheal intubation in the critically ill. Where we came from and where we should go. *Am J Respir Crit Care Med.* 2020;201:775–788. doi:10.1164/rccm.201908-1636CI

6. Cook TM, Woodall N, Harper J, et al. Major complications of airway management in the UK: results of the Fourth National Audit Project of the Royal College of Anaesthetists and the Difficult Airway Society. Part 2: intensive care and emergency departments. *Br J Anaesth.* 2011;106:632–642. doi:10.1093/bja/aer059

7. Griesdale DEG, Bosma TL, Kurth T, et al. Complications of endotracheal intubation in the critically ill. *Intensive Care Med.* 2008;34:1835–1842. doi:10.1007/s00134-008-1205-6

15. De Jong A, Rolle A, Molinari N, et al. Cardiac arrest and mortality related to intubation procedure in critically ill adult patients: a multicenter cohort study. *Crit Care Med.* 2018;46:532–539. doi:10.1097/CCM.0000000000002925

21. Mosier JM, Joshi R, Hypes C, et al. The physiologically difficult airway. *West J Emerg Med.* 2015;16:1109–1117. doi:10.5811/westjem.2015.8.27467

34. Simpson GD, Ross MJ, McKeown DW, et al. Tracheal intubation in the critically ill: a multi-centre national study of practice and complications. *Br J Anaesth.* 2012;108:792–799. doi:10.1093/bja/aer504

All references can be found online at eBooks.Health.Elsevier.com.

PART 6

Postintubation Procedures

44

The Endotracheal Tube and Respiratory Care

THOMAS C. MORT, JEFFREY P. KECK JR., SRIHARSHA SUBRAMANYA, DHAMODARAN PALANIAPPAN, AND SAIMIR SHAROFI

CHAPTER OUTLINE

KEY POINTS

- Polyurethane endotracheal tube (ETT) cuffs that have high-volume/low-pressure (HVLP) cuffs can conform to the irregular borders of the tracheal lumen and, therefore, are more effective at preventing microaspiration.
- ETT placement has mechanical and physiologic consequences. Vigilant surveillance of skin hygiene, airway patency, cuff integrity, and ventilatory support is necessary to minimize injury and maximize support.
- Evaluation of a cuff/air leak is a multifaceted endeavor requiring vigilance, diligence, and skill. An analysis of the potential causes

by patient evaluation and airway assessment should provide the needed clinical information to determine the cause and direct a therapeutic intervention.
- Once an ETT is in place, efforts must be aggressive and perpetual to decrease the risk of ventilator-associated pneumonia (VAP); deploying a multi-dimensional VAP bundle incorporating the use of specially designed ETTs and advanced nursing care regimens appears warranted. VAP appears to be more multifaceted than previously believed. Subglottic suctioning and biofilm management are just the beginning steps.

- It is better to investigate any perceived ETT problem electively than to deal with its consequences after it becomes an acute emergency.
- The landscape of ETT design, construction, and maintenance has changed and will continue to evolve over the next decade.

Not all variations will prove effective, but improved patient care will take place.

Introduction

The role of the endotracheal tube (ETT) in medicine is as invaluable as that of any other medical device created to date. The establishment of a definitive airway via the ETT in both elective and emergency situations has allowed for the delivery of immediate life-sustaining therapies during resuscitation, the maintenance of oxygenation and ventilation in prolonged illness, and the (temporary) delivery of inhaled anesthesia.[1] This chapter begins with a brief history of the development of the ETT. It describes the various types of ETTs available along with their indications for use and respective limitations. It reviews basic airway anatomy with regard to ETT placement, proper positioning and stabilization of the ETT, and complications attributed to its use. Finally, it addresses respiratory care of the intubated and mechanically ventilated patient.

Properties of the Endotracheal Tube

Anatomy of the Endotracheal Tube

When ether was introduced in the 1840s, the performance of surgical procedures accelerated in number. General anesthesia was administered using devices that covered the patient's mouth and nose. Aspiration as a complication of anesthesia administration was not well appreciated, and postoperative pneumonia was a common problem. Trendelenburg was credited with having designed the first inflatable cuff in 1869. It consisted of a thin rubber bag fitted over the end of a tracheostomy tube with the goal of providing a tight seal of the tracheal lumen to prevent aspiration under anesthesia.

In 1893, Eisenmenger first described the use of a cuffed tube coupled with the concept of a pilot balloon to monitor intracuff pressure.[2-6] The precursor for the modern ETT was developed in 1917 by Magill and Rowbotham, who manufactured them from rubber for the purpose of administering anesthesia.[7] In 1928, when Guedel and Waters added a protective cuff to prevent aspiration, the modern ETT was born. During the polio epidemic in the 1960s, the potential value of cuffed tubes for application of positive-pressure ventilation in respiratory failure was appreciated.[8] Early ETTs made of red rubber had limitations in this application, however, such as increased stiffness with rising temperature and limited adhesive properties with different polymers, requiring the cuffs to be manufactured from the same polymer as the tube.[9] These shortcomings led to the search for alternative materials.

In 1967, polyvinyl chloride (PVC) was popularized by Dr. S. A. Leader, and it has since been the material most used. One property that makes PVC attractive is that it provides stiffness to an ETT at room temperature to assist with intubation yet becomes more malleable as its temperature increases in vivo. Other beneficial properties include the ability to embed radiopaque stripes in the material to assist with positioning and recognition on a radiograph. The low cost of PVC and its compatibility with many different materials provides distinct advantages. It affords manufacturers the opportunity to exteriorize the inflation line and pilot balloon assembly to the PVC ETT with a variety of cuff materials.[10]

The simple yet clever design of the 15-mm adapter allows for universality between ventilating devices such as a bag-mask ventilation system, anesthesia circuit, or ventilator circuit. The adapter fits ETTs as large as 12-mm internal diameter (ID) and as small as 3 mm ID, thereby providing further commonality among multiple ETTs and ventilating devices. Having one standard size also allows for interchange between devices made for tracheostomies or ETTs. The adapter is removable to allow for passage of intraluminal devices (e.g., a bronchoscope or suction catheter) or to allow passage of the ETT via a supraglottic airway (SGA). Adapter removal may facilitate the extraction of extensive biofilm accumulation or mucous plugs. Additionally, removal and reattachment of the adapter allows the clinician to resize (shorten) the ETT.[11]

The Murphy eye, an elliptically shaped opening in the distal end of the ETT, is designed to provide an extra (secondary) portal for ventilation should the most distal lumen become blocked by bodily fluids, foreign bodies, or soft tissue. The most typical manifestations of this phenomenon occur when the distal lumen abuts the soft tissue of the tracheal tree or when secretion buildup occludes the distal opening. Despite its advantages and useful design features, its presence may allow an airway exchange catheter or bronchial blocker to travel astray with the potential for patient harm.

The cuffs on early ETTs were, like the tubes themselves, composed of rubber. Rubber ETT cuffs had limitations, such as the need for elevated inflation pressures (high-pressure, low-volume [HPLV]) to fill the cuff and occlude the airway surrounding the ETT. The cartilaginous U- or D-shaped trachea with a softer, flattened posterior wall is not properly shaped to be completely sealed with a round or ovoid cuff. HPLV cuffs inflate in a circular manner, thereby altering the structure of the trachea; the high pressure exerted on the tracheal wall, typically greater than 30 cm H_2O, impairs capillary perfusion pressure and, thus, blood flow, which may result in mucosal ischemia.[12] The use of HPLV cuffs has diminished significantly. The ETTs with HPLV cuffs used in current practice are primarily the silicone ETTs used with intubating laryngeal mask airways (LMAs). Caution should be exercised when using these ETTs for prolonged periods; given their inherent risk of tracheal mucosal damage, strong consideration should be given to exchanging the HPLV ETT, unless the time of intubation is projected to be brief.

The introduction of PVC-based cuffs has reduced this problem because of a thinner and more supple cuff wall, allowing the cuff to accommodate high volume under low pressure (HVLP), and thus providing an adequate seal with lower lateral wall pressures (Fig. 44.1).[9,12,13] The main value of the HVLP cuff is its ability to better conform to the irregular borders of the trachea.[14-16] Polyurethane is thinner (10 μm vs 50 μm for PVC tubes) and more pliable with increased tensile strength, allowing for higher volumes, larger contact areas, and minimal mucosal pressures.[17] Foam-based cuffs provide maximal conformation to the tracheal walls, but, unfortunately, they do little for the prevention of microaspiration.[16]

Remodeling of the cuff has been particularly driven by the desire to improve prevention of ventilator-associated pneumonia

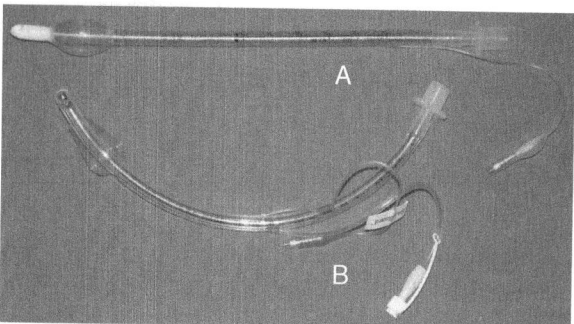

• **Fig. 44.1** Structural comparison of (A) a high-pressure, low-volume (HPLV) cuff and (B) a high-volume, low-pressure (HVLP) cuff. (Courtesy LMA North America, San Diego, CA.)

(VAP), and, as such, the shape of the cuff has also been altered. The Mallinckrodt TaperGuard Evac ETT (Medtronic, Minneapolis, MN) has a conical-shaped (tapered) cuff and has been demonstrated in randomized, controlled trials to reduce microaspiration by as much as 83% compared with traditional HVLP barrel-shaped cuffs (Fig. 44.2).[15] It is postulated that a barrel-shaped cuff tends to wrinkle and fold in an attempt to conform to the tracheal wall, creating small channels that allow for potential microaspiration of nasooropharyngeal secretions, debris, or gastroesophageal reflux-mediated aspiration, whereas the bulbous, conical shape of the TaperGuard Evac ETT may reduce wrinkling and thus decrease the incidence of microaspiration. A recent meta-analysis revealed that the use of tapered ETT cuffs alone did not reduce the incidence of VAP.[18] Continued work in this area may lead to improved tracheal wall sealing capabilities at safe levels of pressure while minimizing potential pathways for the translocation of nasooral and gastroesophageal secretions, which is thought to be the primary etiologic pathway for VAP.[19] An additional feature of the TaperGuard Evac ETT is subglottic drainage of secretions. This is accomplished by applying low wall suction to the separate dorsal suction lumen located just above the cuff via a separate suction line assembly. Utilization of this type of ETT is associated with a lowering of VAP incidence but does not clearly provide benefit regarding a reduced duration of mechanical ventilation,

length of stay, antibiotic usage, or mortality in the intensive care unit (ICU).[18]

The pilot balloon of an ETT functions as an indirect volume gauge for the ETT cuff, relative to the amount of air located in the cuff (inflated or deflated). Manual assessment of the pilot balloon does not provide accurate information about the absolute volume insufflated or the pressure exerted on the tracheal mucosa except when the pilot balloon is firm (high pressure, e.g., >60 cm H_2O) or when underpressurized or nearly collapsed (low pressure, e.g., <10 cm H_2O). Use of a manometer is recommended for accurate cuff pressure assessment. When a pilot balloon assembly fails (balloon and/or tubing), options are generally limited to ETT exchange or bedside repair.[20–22] Pilot balloon assembly failures have multiple causes: shearing along the ETT connection (usually because of contact with dentition), cracked inflation valves (from syringe manipulation or trauma), material aging, or pilot tubing laceration attributed to biting, among others.[23–26] Simple techniques have been described to replace a pilot balloon in a variety of clinical situations using equipment readily available in the operating room (OR) or ICU setting. Needles or intravenous catheters with stopcocks or Luer connectors, epidural clamp connectors, and commercially available repair kits (Fig. 44.3) provide reliable substitutions for an incompetent pilot balloon assembly.[27,28] The procedure for replacing an incompetent valve if a commercially available repair kit is not available is as follows: cut the inflation tube; insert a needle or intravenous catheter into the cut end (or affix the hub of an epidural catheter to the cut end); use a stopcock or Luer adaptor on the needle or catheter after insufflation; and evaluate the cuff pressure with a manometer. This option is best for the weaning patient in anticipation of extubation; otherwise, formal ETT exchange is recommended.

Development and Properties of the Endotracheal Tube

The purpose of the ETT has always been the same, and it has always had the same inherent problems. Technology continues to advance the standard ETT for improved function and decreased physiologic insult. Rather than compensate for the resistance produced by a rubber or PVC ETT, an ultra-thin polyurethane ETT that is reinforced with wire to resist collapsing and kinking is available. The

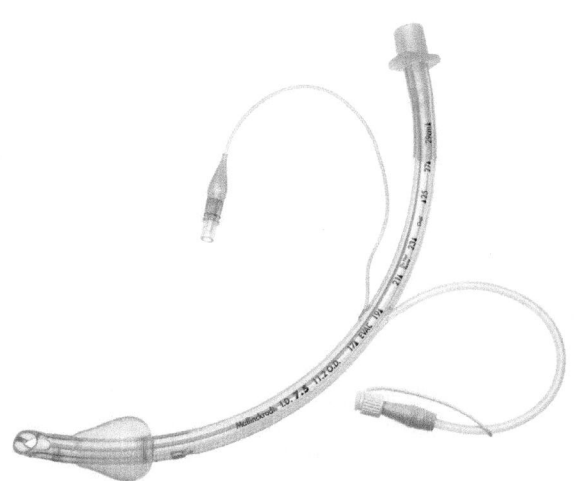

• **Fig. 44.2** TaperGuard endotracheal tube cuff. (Courtesy Covidien, Boulder, CO.)

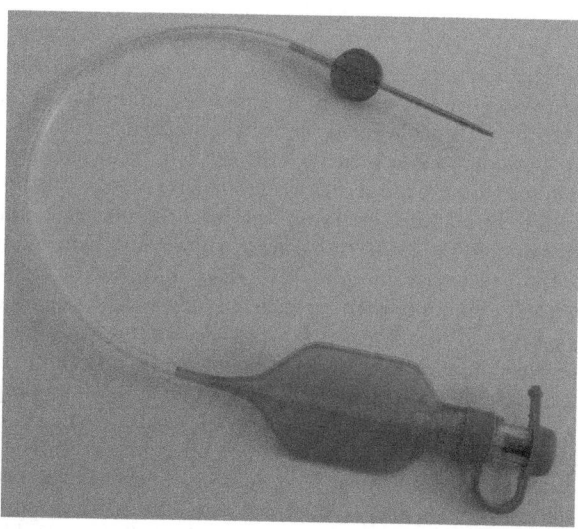

• **Fig. 44.3** Pilot balloon repair device. (Courtesy Instrumentation Industries, Bethel Park, PA.)

wire reinforcement is unique in that it has an elastic shape memory to prevent deformation. The ID is increased without compromising the rigid shape of the ETT. The result is a tube with a resistance similar to that of the upper airway that is lighter, offers less airflow resistance, and, when compressed, forms an egg shape rather than an oval.[29] Experimentally, this new design has been shown to decrease inspiratory and expiratory resistance by 60% each and the inspiratory, expiratory, and total work of breathing (WOB) by 70%, 47%, and 45%, respectively.[30,31] Unfortunately, the wire-reinforced ETT may undergo crimping or kinking due to acute bending or patient biting. Such extreme damage will not recoil, and the luminal diameter will not return toward its original caliber.

Use of the ETT continues to expand—no longer is it expected to be simply a conduit for ventilation. As the technology has advanced, the original ETT has steadily been outfitted with a host of successful innovations to improve patient care, whether for convenience or necessity. For example, modifications to the cuff to improve occlusion of the trachea in an effort to prevent microaspiration, coupled with an extra subglottic suctioning port (and other patient care maneuvers), have served to vastly reduce the incidence of VAP.[14–16,18] Another example is the modification of the surfaces of the ETT to minimize bacterial adhesion and thereby minimize biofilm accumulation.[32] As for bells and whistles, there are ETTs with fiberoptic cameras at the distal tip, allowing for ease of placement and the possibility of continued intratracheal surveillance. Another example is the addition of multiple sensors, for so-called bioimpedance cardiography, that are capable of monitoring stroke volume variation, cardiac output (CO), systemic vascular resistance, and arterial pressures (because of the proximity of the ETT and the aorta) and thereby, at least theoretically, preventing the need for additional invasive technologies. Continued study of these modifications may provide justification to adapt these technologies to patient care, with the potential of limiting physiologic insult and reducing iatrogenic complications (e.g., from central line placement or radial arterial catheterization in the example of an ETT equipped for bioimpedance cardiography).

Physiologic Effects of Endotracheal Tube Placement

The placement of an ETT, whether oral, nasal, or translaryngeal, is unnatural. Certain physiologic changes occur that must be addressed, including those created by the ETT itself and those modified by its presence. The properties inherent to the ETT are relatively obvious: It causes a partial obstruction, resulting in a decrease in the normal airway circumference, and creates the potential for turbulent air flow patterns. Additionally, the narrowed conduit leads to higher pressures concurrent with lower flows because of the reduced airway diameter; higher pressures may lead to mucosal damage distally, particularly at points of turbulence or obstruction. The presence of an ETT is a trigger for the inflammatory cascade; despite its relatively hypoallergenic profile, it is still a recognizable foreign body and, as such, triggers well-defined host responses. Placement of the device, regardless of the care used in placing it, may result in mechanical trauma and therefore decreases the ability of the respiratory mucosa to protect itself. Finally, the ETT may cause airway alterations secondary to pressure injury, either caused by ETT translational pressures from resting against the mucosa or by turbulent flow patterns. Ventilatory strategies employed because of ETT placement may also lead to a triggered inflammatory response.

The body's response to the ETT is also multifaceted, affecting mechanics, structure, and physiologic function. Loss of humidity and heat is the most obvious effect of replacing the regular mucosa with a foreign conduit. Bypassing the patient's natural ability to warm and humidify the incoming air may lead to problems in the distal tracheobronchial tree. The delivery of dehumidified and cool gases may reduce ciliary function, thicken secretions, and increase mucous plugging. The normally motile respiratory cilia are essentially paralyzed and rendered dormant, leading to impaired secretion management. The body lacks its normal ability to move debris in a proximal (cranial) direction, and collection sites develop within the tracheobronchial tree, leading to multiple potential areas for infection. Additionally, these partially or completely occluded areas may result in lobar collapse and, consequently, a ventilation-perfusion mismatch. Obstructions caused by mucous plugging can also create an inability to completely exhale, leading to breath stacking and auto-positive end expiratory pressure (auto-PEEP) and possibly resultant barotrauma.

Complications of Endotracheal Tube Placement

Complications associated with ETT placement can be grouped into three major subcategories: those that occur at intubation, those that occur with the ETT in situ, and postextubation sequelae.[33] The problems associated with ETT placement are numerous and can be worsened because of emergency situations, inherent physiologic or anatomic complications leading to multiple attempts, the use of a variety of devices, operator inexperience, and patient-related anatomic factors.[34] Problems at placement include dental and oral injury, maxillofacial damage, displacement of the arytenoid cartilages, vocal cord ulceration or dysfunction, airway perforation (Fig. 44.4), autonomic hyperactivity, and,

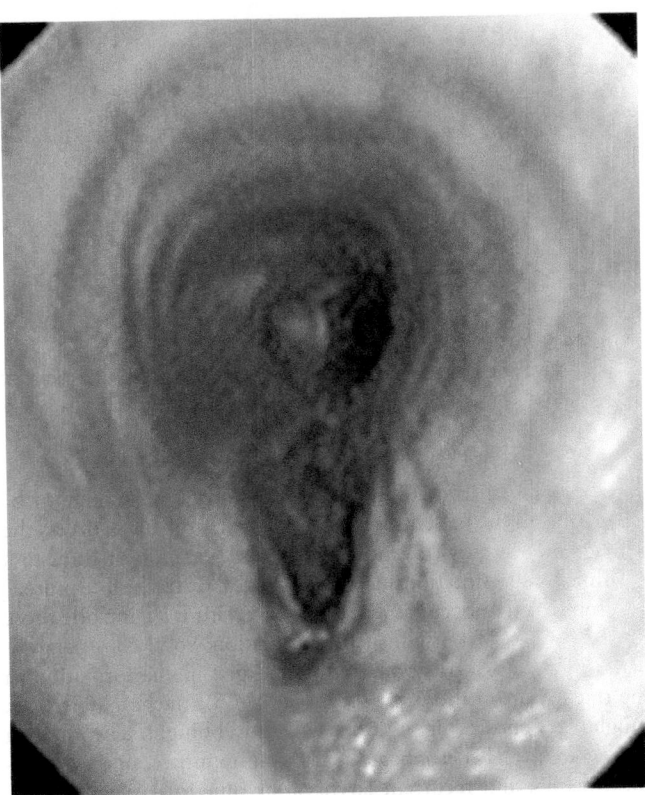

• **Fig. 44.4** Trauma along the posterior tracheal wall from intubation with a styletted endotracheal tube.

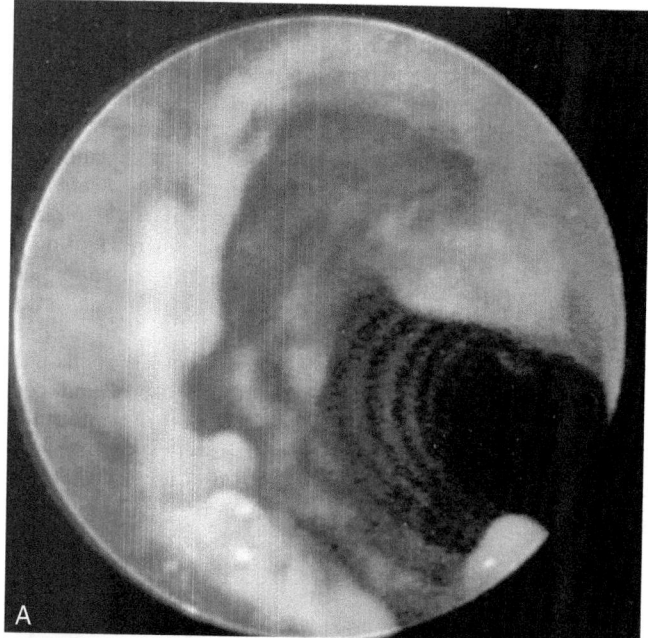

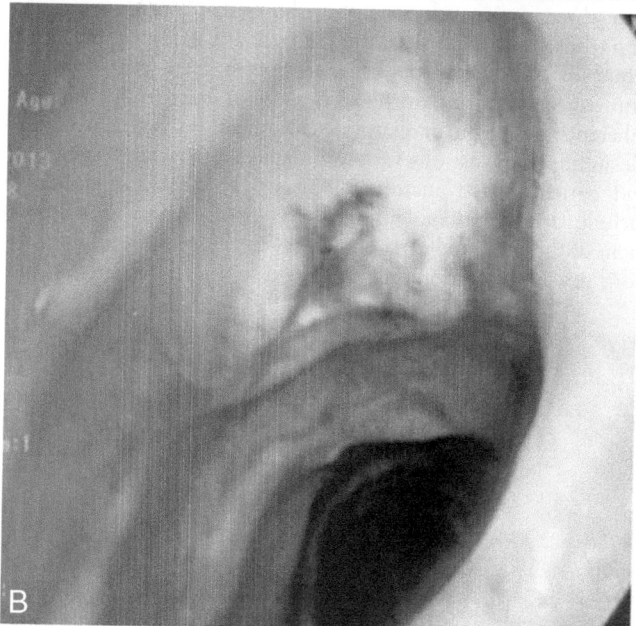

• **Fig. 44.5** (A) Tracheal wall denudation and cartilaginous exposure following 7 days and (B) a combined 15 days (two intubations). Both injuries were noted during bronchoscopic exam.

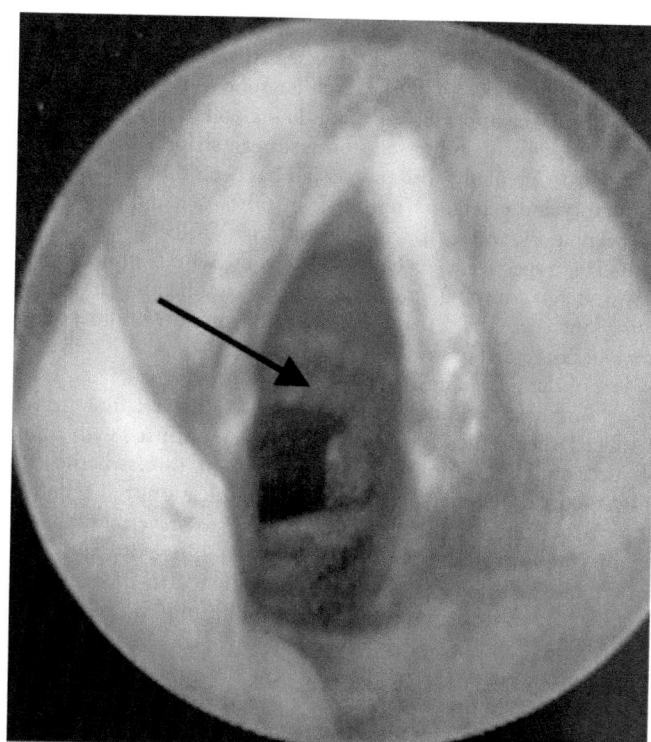

• **Fig. 44.6** Laryngoscopic view of subglottic stenosis (*arrow*) from prolonged, multiple intubations. The patient was stridorous and short of breath after extubation on multiple occasions prompting reintubation.

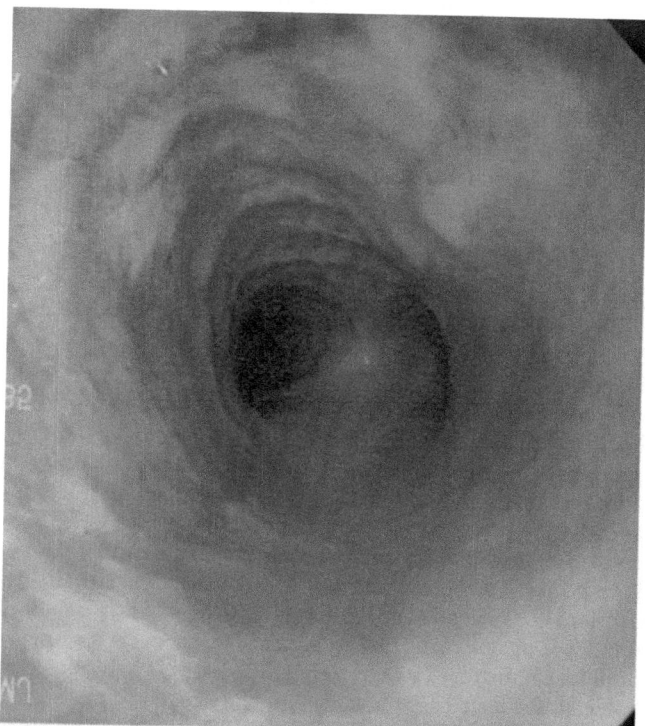

• **Fig. 44.7** Bronchoscopic exam prompted by continuous air leak revealing widening of the distal trachea (tracheomalacia).

of course, failed intubation. Structural damage is unlikely to be repaired until the patient no longer requires intubation, unless the damage interferes with ventilation and oxygenation or leads to a life-threatening situation such as esophageal or tracheal rupture.

Problems that occur as a result of an in situ ETT include those caused by the ETT itself, such as aspiration; vocal cord paralysis or transient nerve palsy; ulceration and granuloma formation in the trachea or on the vocal cords (Fig. 44.5); tracheal synechiae; subglottic stenosis (Fig. 44.6); laryngeal webbing; tracheomalacia (Fig. 44.7); tracheoesophageal, tracheoinnominate, or tracheocarotid fistula; and recurrent laryngeal or superior laryngeal nerve damage.[35] Overpressurization of the ETT cuff contributes to these maladies, as can head and neck position and movement or forces from the ventilation circuit causing ETT angulation. Other complications are related to mechanical ventilation facilitated by the ETT and include aspiration, barotrauma (e.g., pneumothorax or pneumomediastinum), VAP, and ETT dislodgment.[36]

Finally, postextubation complications can lead to long-term morbidity or the urgent need for reintubation. Many of the postextubation culprits have already been encountered as complications of ETT placement or presence, particularly subglottic stenosis, vocal cord injury, and hoarseness.[36,37] Without a doubt, the most common postextubation issue is acute respiratory failure and the subsequent need for reintroducing invasive airway access.

Postextubation dysphagia is a common but often unrecognized issue in the critically ill patient requiring intubation for greater than 48 hours. Dysphagia associated with speech and swallow discoordination is linked to aspiration risk.[38] Periglottic edema, ulceration, granulation tissue formation, scarring and vocal cord dysfunction may accompany intubation, particularly if extended in duration. Autopsy evaluation supports the nearly ubiquitous presence of laryngotracheal injury, to various degrees, in the majority of patients who experience prolonged tracheal intubation.[39]

Tracheal stenosis, an abnormal narrowing of the tracheal lumen, is related to both tracheal intubation and creation of a surgical airway. Narrowing typically occurs at the site of the ETT cuff (or malpositioned ETT tip). Following mucosal denudation and injury, local inflammation and infection may lead to chondritis of the anterior and lateral tracheal walls.[39–41] Vascular granulation tissue may develop at the injury site and impede airflow or contribute to hemorrhage during reintubation or ETT manipulation. Granulation tissue undergoes fibrosis and epithelialization followed by stenosis of the cartilaginous walls. Common risk factors include prolonged intubation, traumatic intubation, hypotension, sepsis, gastroesophageal reflux, advanced age, malnutrition, debility, inappropriately sized ETTs (too large or small), and excessive tracheal wall irritation from ETT motion.[39–41]

Excessive cuff pressure, even for as short as 15 minutes, may initiate a cascade of compromised tracheal mucosal blood flow leading to ischemia or necrosis. Left unchecked, as in the ICU setting, webbed fibrotic changes, cartilaginous wall injury, and contracture may occur within 3 to 6 weeks. However, an even shorter duration overpressurization (e.g., in the OR) may contribute to dysphagia, altered phonation, coughing, blood-tinged sputum, and stridor. This may be worsened when accompanied by anterior tracheal wall damage from aggressive advancement of a styletted ETT with a hyperangled configuration. The basis of the ischemia is overpressurization of the cuff (>25–30 cm H_2O) as it relates to the average mucosal capillary perfusion pressure ($\approx$27 cm H_2O). Ideally, cuff pressure should be maintained <25 cm H_2O. HVLP cuff designs for both ETT and tracheostomy tubes have improved this undesirable consequence of airway control but not eliminated it. Head position and positive-pressure ventilation will alter the intracuff pressure as will N_2O administration in the OR. Shearing forces from the ETT or its cuff may further aggravate injury. ETT cuff pressure is also directly related to peak inspiratory pressure during mechanical ventilation support. Even if cuff pressures are initially within recommended limits, increases in peak inspiratory pressure may result in an increase in cuff pressure.[42–45]

The degree of local or circumferential contracture leading to tracheal luminal reduction varies widely and may remain clinically underappreciated and underreported in many patients. Dyspnea at rest or stridor may not be noted until the tracheal narrowing is <5 mm. Therapy for symptomatic tracheal narrowing is typically provided in a stepwise fashion based on the degree of narrowing and its response to one of many therapies.[39,40] Often, evaluation and diagnosis are performed with flexible scope assessment in the ICU, clinic, or office, and operative intervention may be indicated. Diagnostic and therapeutic rigid bronchoscopy alone

or combined with serial tracheal dilatation may be successful. Moreover, stenting of the narrowed tracheal segment may be performed as a temporary intervention. If successful, the stent may be upsized or removed. If narrowing recurs, a permanent stent may be the best option. For patients with an acceptable medical/surgical history, surgical resection of the stenotic segment and tracheal reconstruction are considered the ideal management of postintubation tracheal stenosis since the development of safe surgical techniques.[39,40] As an alternative, the higher-risk, frail, or debilitated patient may be better candidate for serial dilatation with or without stenting.[39–41]

Tracheomalacia, a weakening of the tracheal wall often accompanied by dilatation or compression, results from ischemic injury to the trachea following intubation or tracheostomy (see Fig. 44.7). Tracheal wall injury leading to chondritis may enhance destruction and necrosis of the supporting tracheal cartilage. Respiratory symptoms result from tracheal wall weakening and its collapse during expiration. Clinically, air trapping, failure to tolerate weaning of PEEP, limitation of expiratory airflow, and retained secretions may complicate patient care. FB may allow visualization of the expiratory collapse of the trachea.[39,40]

Intolerance of the extubated state has many confounding factors and etiologies. Marginal cardiopulmonary reserves or preexisting medical/surgical conditions combined with acute and chronic disease are prominent causes of extubation/decannulation failure. However, the presence of tracheal wall injury can be a hidden contributing factor to such intolerance that may not be appreciated until the patient undergoes reintubation or the tracheal stoma is recannulated. Even then, the formation of granulation tissue, luminal narrowing, scarring, tracheomalacia, or tracheal stenosis may not be appreciated until several extubation/decannulation failures prompt more detailed scrutiny of the airway. HVLP cuff designs have led to significant reduction, but not elimination, of tracheal wall injuries. Moreover, maintaining the cuff pressure in a safe zone (<25 cm H_2O) has a prime role in decreasing the rate of ischemic injuries and postextubation stenosis. Unfortunately, the ETT itself acts as a foreign body exerting variable but persistent pressure on sensitive tissues. This contributes to periglottic edema and additional sites of laryngeal injury (e.g., true and false vocal cords, arytenoid cartilages, aryepiglottic folds, and posterior commissure) (Fig. 44.8).[39,40] These, too, may contribute to postextubation respiratory distress, stridor, dysphagia, phonation difficulties, hoarseness, vocal cord dysfunction, and laryngeal incompetence. Laryngeal maladies include edema, ulceration, granulation tissue, and abnormal vocal cord mobility, paresis, or paralysis. Risk factors appear to be prolonged intubation duration, female gender, emergency intubation, difficulty with airway management, multiple attempts at intubation, self-extubation, and a smaller height:ETT diameter ratio.[39,40]

Unilateral or bilateral glottic scarring may lead to glottic stenosis. Arytenoid immobility due to scarring or dislocation may complicate prolonged or difficult intubation. Phonation difficulties, hoarseness, and impaired swallowing with an increase in aspiration risk postextubation may be rooted in such laryngeal injury. Air hunger and airway obstruction may be present in severe cases. If postextubation phonation difficulties or hoarseness persist, evaluation is encouraged. A delay in assessment may allow further scar tissue formation that could endanger or limit future therapy.

Indirect injury to the branches of the recurrent laryngeal nerve from a high-lying (subglottic), overpressurized ETT cuff compressing the internal nerve branch as it traverses the larynx at the level of the thyroid and cricoid cartilages is, fortunately,

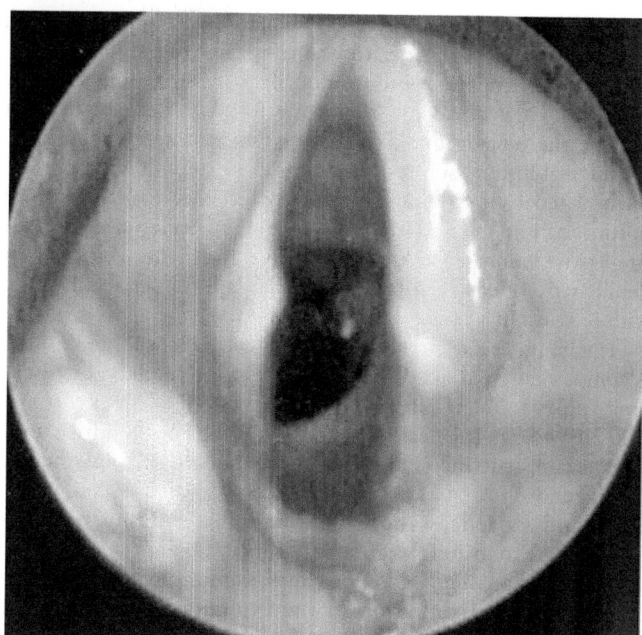

• **Fig. 44.8** Scarring of the arytenoids and a posterior glottic "chink" with subglottic injury and subsequent stenotic narrowing.

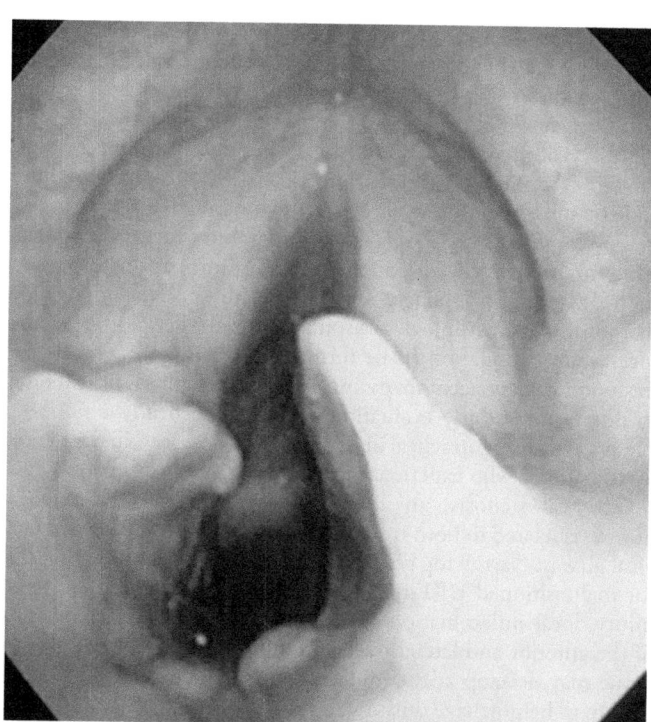

• **Fig. 44.9** Image captured during fiberoptic endoscopic evaluation of swallowing at bedside in the intensive care unit revealing significant true and false vocal cord edema, arytenoid edema, and a large posterior gap where the previous endotracheal tube was positioned for 6 days before extubation was achieved.

uncommon. Vocal cord paresis or paralysis may be based on similar factors that increase the risk for other laryngotracheal injuries (e.g., duration of intubation, cuff location and pressure, ETT size and curvature), as well as advancing age, vascular disease, hypotension, sepsis, and other potential low-perfusion states. Separating out individual causative factors may be difficult.

Diagnosis of Laryngotracheal Injuries

Given the variety of airway-related maladies that may afflict patients who have required tracheal intubation or placement of a surgical airway, careful evaluation with an elevated index of suspicion is warranted. Employing bronchoscopy, tracheoscopy, nasopharyngoscopy, or VAL at the bedside or the OR may be helpful. Defining and documenting any periglottic or tracheal pathology may shed light on weaning intolerance, failed decannulation, swallowing disorders, phonation difficulties, and tracheal pathology. Bedside video-assisted swallowing evaluations may provide valuable insight. Bedside flexible endoscopy may offer empiric evidence that the patient may benefit from a more thorough evaluation in the OR (e.g., rigid bronchoscopy or suspension laryngoscopy) with the opportunity for biopsy, excision, electrocautery, cryoablation, glottic injections, stenting, or dilatation of uncovered airway abnormalities. Ultra-high resolution computed tomography imaging or swallowing studies may render useful information. Spirometry, while limited in its application in the ICU setting, may provide evidence of obstruction and restriction of air flow.

Assessment and Therapy for Postextubation Disorders

It is imperative that patients receive assessment and therapy for postextubation disorders. Speech-language pathologists (SLPs) deliver clinical services for a broad range of disorders, including swallowing, speech, and voice disorders so prevalent in postintubation and tracheostomy patients. Moreover, stroke, traumatic

brain injury, Parkinson disease, dementia, or instrumentation or trauma of the oropharynx, esophagus, and/or trachea may lead to brief, intermediate, and long-term consequences related to swallowing, speech, and voice integrity. The muscles and nerves that regulate speech, voice, and swallowing via the lips, tongue, pharynx, and larynx are intimately interlinked, thus providing coordinated choreography for swallowing, breathing, and phonation. Postintubation and posttracheostomy alterations deserve individualized screening tools, bedside swallowing evaluations, and assessment of hyolaryngeal movement and swallow coordination by hands-on midline palpation of the larynx. Intubation and tracheostomy placement may disrupt the essential biomechanical constructs of the three-way glottic closure mechanism directing foods and liquids to the esophageal portal (i.e., true and false vocal cord adduction and a downfolding epiglottis). Advanced diagnostic testing beyond a modified barium-swallow study is termed "instrumental studies" and is now the gold standard for assessment of such disorders. Instrumental testing may include pH manometry, ultrasonography, and fiberoptic endoscopic evaluation of swallowing (FEES) (Fig. 44.9). Box 44.1 presents excerpts from SLP evaluations demonstrating their broad scope of practice in the postextubation and tracheostomy patient.

Endotracheal Tubes and Other Airway Adjuncts

Choice of Endotracheal Tube Size

In selecting an ETT, consideration must be given to the functional reason for placement, as well as patient-specific factors,

• BOX 44.1　Speech-Language Pathology Evaluations

Patient A: 70-year-old female with diabetes mellitus, multiple hospitalizations and intubations for hypoxic respiratory failure (most recently discharged 5 days ago after intubation for pneumonia), on 2 to 3 L/min of nasal cannula oxygen at baseline. The patient presented to emergency department for right-sided back pain and hypoxia. Speech/language pathologist recommended an MBS to formally rule out silent aspiration vs. evaluate for reflux aspiration given history of gastroesophageal reflux disease. MBS revealed functional oropharyngeal swallow mechanism with no aspiration across consistencies. Oral phase characterized by intact bolus manipulation, cohesion, and transit across trials with no oral residue postswallow. Good bolus coordination observed across consistencies. Pharyngeal motor response was timely, consistently initiating at the level of the ramus. Intact hyolaryngeal elevation/excursion resulted in complete epiglottic inversion and laryngeal closure. The patient maintained adequate airway protection across trials with no airway compromise across consistencies. Functional base of tongue retraction and pharyngeal stripping wave present, with complete pharyngeal clearance and no stasis postswallow. Adequate bolus flow from the pharynx into proximal esophagus. Of note, upon transferring patient back to her bed, she had significant coughing with expectoration of thick secretions and barium-tinged contrast likely indicative of esophageal dysphagia and concern for reflux aspiration.

Patient B: The patient evaluated 4 hours postextubation (two emergency intubations, total of 7 days intubated). Seated upright in bed on 3 L/min of nasal cannula oxygen. Alert and oriented to person, place, and time. The patient was severely dysphonic and displayed a weak volitional cough. Clinical swallow evaluation was concerning for pharyngeal dysphagia (weak reflexive coughing observed with trials of ice chips and mildly thick liquids). Recommend continued NPO status except crushed meds and ice chips. Plan for FEES. FEES completed with patient alert and seated upright in bed. On 4 L/min of nasal cannula oxygen, pulse oximetry was 92% to 93% at baseline. Study demonstrated a functional oropharyngeal swallow. Adequate labial seal, bolus control, and mastication/manipulation with complete oral clearance. Timely swallow initiation with clear liquids only. Functional epiglottic inversion with normal-appearing whiteout. Functional pharyngeal stripping with minimal postswallow vallecular residue. Moderate amount of thin secretions pooled in pyriform sinuses. Significant glottic posterior gap from prolonged endotracheal tube presence (see Fig. 44.9). True vocal cords showed reduced movement bilaterally with posterior glottic gap visualized during phonation. High risk for aspiration due to periglottic edema and residual gap opening in posterior glottis. Abnormal airway protection with penetration and aspiration visualized. Of note, intermittent coughing was observed throughout the exam. The patient desaturated to 72% on pulse oximetry during consumption of ice chips and clears. Recommended initiation of a limited diet (ice chips only) and implementation of aspiration precautions. Consider otorhinolaryngologic consult to evaluate vocal cord dysfunction, glottic edema, and the glottic gap.

FEES, Fiberoptic endoscopic evaluation of swallowing; *MBS,* modified barium swallow; *NPO,* nothing by mouth (*nil per os*)

---

such as body height, gender, airway integrity, airway pathology, and previous airway manipulation or instrumentation. Theoretically, short-term placement for anesthesia should be different from placement for prolonged support with mechanical ventilation or for fiberoptic bronchoscopy to aid therapy. Generally, the trachea of an adult female accepts a tube of 7.5- to 8.0-mm ID and that of a male accepts one of 8.5- to 9.0-mm ID, but typically a 7.0-mm ID ETT is used for females and an 8.0-mm ID tube is used for males, at least in the United States. It is also generally accepted that an ETT of at least 8.0-mm ID is needed for an adequate adult bronchoscopic investigation.

Small Tubes and Airway Resistance

The physics of laminar gas flow through a conduit is described by the Hagen-Poiseuille equation, which reflects the relationship of resistance varying inversely with the fourth power of tube radius. Air flow through an ETT is often turbulent, which leads to increased airway resistance. The net effect on the increase in airway resistance with each millimeter decrease in ETT diameter is considerable, ranging from 25% to 100%.[46] Airway resistance is affected by more than tube diameter; the presence of secretions within the tube, ETT kinking, and positioning of the head and neck may also increase the tendency for turbulent flow.[47] The fundamental principle to be mindful of is that airway resistance induced by an ETT is inversely proportional to the tube size.[48]

Airway resistance increases with decreasing ETT diameter whether because of internal occlusion, smaller size, or external compression. As airway resistance increases, WOB also increases.[46] The increase in WOB associated with a 1-mm reduction in ETT diameter varies in accordance with tidal volume and respiratory rate at a given minute ventilation and can range from 34% to 154%.[46] When ventilation is controlled, the increase in WOB related to ETT resistance is seldom of any consequence because it is overcome by ventilator adjustments. However, small-diameter tubes create greater difficulty for patients in weaning from ventilatory support because of the higher levels of resistance encountered when attempting to breathe spontaneously.[49,50] It has been suggested that an inability to spontaneously ventilate because of the increased WOB imposed by a 7.0-mm ETT might indicate that extubation will fail regardless of tube size.[51,52]

Increased airway resistance associated with a smaller-diameter ETT may also be associated with inadvertent PEEP. Patients with high oxygen consumption, increased carbon dioxide production, or ventilation/perfusion relationships that produce high dead space ventilation ($\dot{V}_D$) often require higher minute ventilations to achieve appropriate ventilation and oxygenation. The gas flows necessary to maintain such minute ventilation are also quite high, and the resistance imposed by a smaller-diameter ETT further prohibits the completion of expiration before initiation of the subsequent inspiration. This breath stacking results in air trapping and unwanted PEEP, magnifying the risk of mechanical ventilation as barotrauma and subsequent intrathoracic overpressure could result in circulatory compromise.[53]

The restriction to gas flow through any ETT increases dramatically when devices, such as a suction catheter or bronchoscope, are placed in the lumen. The cross-sectional area of the tube is effectively reduced by an amount equal to the cross-sectional area of the device inserted into the tube. This limitation of gas flow has consequences for both the inspiratory and expiratory phases: inspiratory flow may be inadequate to maintain oxygenation and ventilation during the procedure, and obstructed expiratory flow may lead to overdistention of the lungs, resulting in barotrauma or circulatory compromise because of reduced venous return, particularly in the hypovolemic or hemodynamically compromised patient.[54]

Large Tubes and Trauma

Whereas smaller diameter ETTs have disadvantages related to gas flow and airway resistance, larger tubes are more frequently associated with traumatic placement and damage to both the laryngeal structures and the tracheal mucosa.[51,52,55] Larger ETTs are associated with a higher incidence of sore throat after general anesthesia compared with smaller diameter tubes, but this difference is relatively negligible with long-term intubation.[56] With prolonged intubation, laryngeal trauma is more likely. Women and those of shorter stature, because of the inherently smaller size of their airway, are more susceptible to injury than men.[57,58]

Laryngeal structures at particular risk for trauma are the arytenoid cartilages and the cricoid cartilage. Trauma results not only from the shape discrepancy between the round ETT and the angular, wedge-shaped glottic opening but also from direct contact and pressure on these structures and from repetitive tube movement, which leads to ulceration or erosion of the protective mucosa.[58-60] Tracheal mucosal injury can also occur because of the irregular surfaces created by wrinkling and folding of the ETT cuff or the externalized pilot tube used to fill the ETT cuff. If the tracheal lumen is "overcrowded," airway injury is more likely to occur when large tubes are used, and little cuff volume is required to seal the airway.[61]

Potentially Beneficial Alternatives to the Standard Endotracheal Tube

Preformed and Reinforced Tubes

Modifications to the ETT that are made in the OR setting to accomplish specific surgeries are often developed in response to interference and access issues. The ability to work without disturbing the ETT has led to several variations of the ETT that can be placed safely and remove the risk of inadvertent advancement, dislodgment, kinking, or obstruction. ETTs used in remote locations also have airway access issues associated with tube kinking and partial occlusion, which typically are related to positioning problems and associated comorbidities. In part because of less stringent vigilance, unintended consequences of ETT use outside the OR may result in more drastic outcomes. In response to these dilemmas, a variety of tubes have been developed to maintain their shape and patency in locations where distortion might cause kinking and occlusion.

Rigid, preformed tubes such as those developed for long-term use in tracheostomy were known to maintain their patency despite the need for angulation. Preformed tubes have been developed for specific application in anesthesia practice as well. The Mallinckrodt Ring-Adair-Elwyn (RAE) tubes (Medtronic, Minneapolis, MN), both oral and nasal models (Fig. 44.10), maintain a fixed contour similar to the average facial profile, allowing for head and neck surgery while minimizing surgical field interference. Their contour also reduces the risk of pressure injury to the posterior pharynx when repositioning is desired. The intraairway length is tied to the size of the ETT, with a relatively appropriate depth based on the average size of a patient for whom the tube might be selected.[62,63]

Wire-reinforced ETTs (also referred to as anode or armored tubes) have an embedded wire coil designed to minimize kinking even with exaggerated position-induced angulation. Wire-reinforced tubes are popular for use in head and neck surgery where remote airway access and the potential for kinking of the ETT are concerns. Placement of a wire-reinforced tube through a tracheostomy for procedures such as a laryngectomy is a common practice; it allows placement during surgical procedures such that the tube can be mobilized, or the circuit draped away from the field without a high risk of tube kinking. The other common use of a

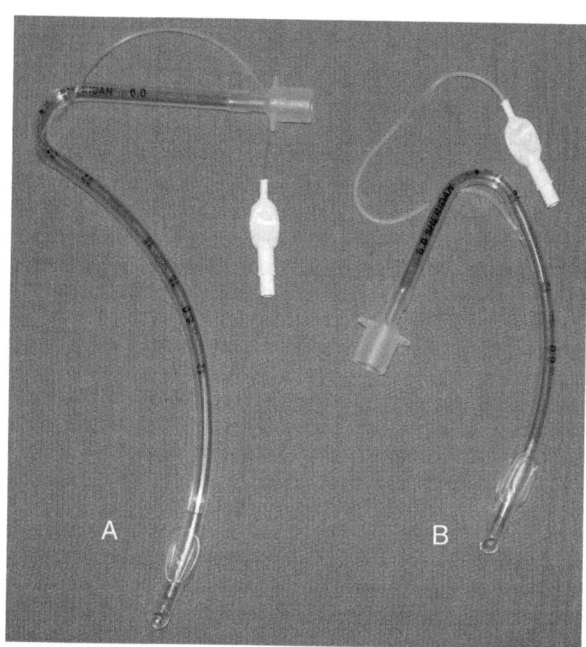

• **Fig. 44.10** (A) Nasal and (B) oral Ring-Adair-Elwyn (RAE) preformed endotracheal tubes. (Courtesy Covidien, Mansfield, MA.)

wire-reinforced tube is with the intubating laryngeal mask airway (ILMA). These tubes are designed to facilitate placement through the device and to be used for short periods of time. The HPLV cuff and the theoretical possibility of kinking and resultant airway obstruction make the long-term use of ILMA silicone ETTs risky.

The embedded wire concept of the reinforced ETT has also been developed for long-term tracheostomy use. Although the reinforced tracheostomy tube is not free of risks, one advantage is that its flexibility allows its length and intratracheal depth to be adjusted, which may be beneficial if tracheomalacia at the level of the cuff develops.[64] These tracheostomy tubes are also popular for use in morbidly obese patients, in whom, because of the depth of tissue, preformed tracheostomy tubes may not have the shape required to fit an individual patient.

One major consequence of this type of reinforced ETT may occur when external pressure is applied to the wire-reinforced component (e.g., by patient biting). Once a compression threshold is reached, the luminal support provided by the wire may be compromised, and a permanent, irreparable indentation remains that can significantly impair ventilation and suctioning capabilities.

Laser Tubes

Progress in laser technology has advanced surgical capabilities, particularly for airway surgery. To protect patients and healthcare providers from laser-induced injury to eyes and airways, special precautions are required. Fire is the most serious danger associated with the use of lasers in the OR, especially when a laser is used in airway surgery.[65-67] A major complication related to the use of lasers for laryngeal surgery is ignition of the ETT.[68] The laser beam may ignite the tube by direct penetration or indirectly if burning tissue is inhaled into the tube.[65,66,69] The ease of ignition is related to the ETT material, the concentration of oxygen in use, and any other adjunctive materials or gases that could support combustion.[66,69] Most ETTs are constructed of PVC, which is highly flammable. Ideally, PVC tubes should not be used for airways when a laser is employed.[65,69,70]

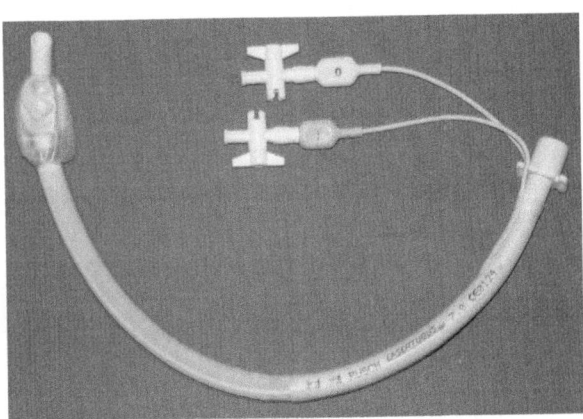

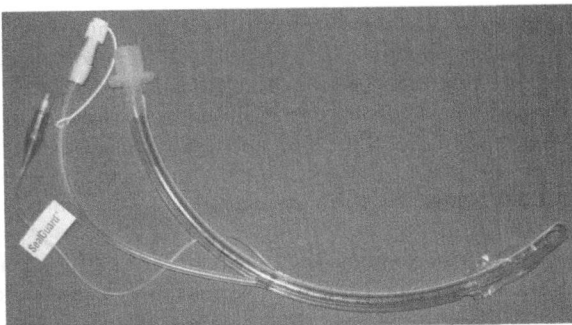

• **Fig. 44.12** Mallinckrodt SealGuard Evac endotracheal tube. (Courtesy Covidien, Mansfield, MA.)

• **Fig. 44.11** Rüsch Lasertubus laser-safe endotracheal tube. (Courtesy Teleflex Medical, Durham, NC.)

ETTs can be laser proofed or protected from the laser beam by wrapping them with reflective metal tape. Ideally, they should be constructed from noncombustible materials. In particular, the ETT cuff is vulnerable to puncture by the laser beam and should be filled with saline or water, which allows more energy to be absorbed before disruption.[66,69] A technique to enhance detection of a penetrated cuff is to place a dye indicator, such as methylene blue, into the solution that is instilled into the cuff. Any leakage will clearly mark the airway and alert the provider to the potential dangers.[71] Protecting the tube from the laser beam by wrapping it with foil tape has proved effective (commercial devices are available) (Fig. 44.11).[72] Tubes made of materials, such as metal and silicone, and those with special double cuffs also reduce the risk of airway fires and injury during laser airway surgery.[65,72] (See Chapter 38.)

Subglottic Suctioning "Evac" Endotracheal Tubes

Hospitalized patients who require mechanical ventilation are susceptible to the development of aspiration pneumonia. VAP is known to increase hospital length of stay, healthcare costs, and mortality.[73] Organisms that grow in pooled subglottic secretions above the inflated cuff of the ETT, but beneath the glottis, have previously been immeasurable with any reliability but now have been demonstrated to be a major source of VAP.[18] Several medical and nursing care measures may be taken to reduce the incidence of VAP caused by this route, including personnel handwashing, improved and frequent oral care, elevating the head of the bed past 30 degrees, frequent suctioning, and ensuring postpyloric tube feedings; however, none of these measures will completely eliminate the collection of secretions.[18,74]

The presence of these pooled collections has led to the development of specific ETTs that possess a dedicated suction system capable of emptying this area of debris. Drainage of subglottic secretions has been shown to prevent VAP.[18,75–77] The currently available subglottic drainage ETTs have a suction lumen that opens on the external (posterolateral) surface of the ETT immediately above the cuff (Fig. 44.12). The lumen is attached to constant or intermittent suction for active drainage of the space. Although these ETTs are beneficial, their efficacy is not 100%, and therefore all the aforementioned nursing care actions remain vital to good hygiene and prevention of VAP.[18] Subglottic drainage tubes continue to be refined in cuff construction (materials, shapes, volumes, locations) and suction capabilities that help to reduce aspiration of the subglottic debris.

Subglottic secretions are not the only recognized cause for VAP. Biofilm is an accumulation of debris adhered to the internal circumference of the ETT that is composed of tissue, secretions, mucus, and an undetermined bacteria load. Biofilm can be aspirated, resulting in a source of infection or causing an area of obstruction to airflow. Biofilm may also contribute to luminal narrowing of the ETT with resultant increases in airway resistance. Biofilm removal and reduction through oral hygiene and routine ETT care are demonstrated improvements to minimize these complications.[78] Although mechanical options for treatment are available and discussed later in this chapter, no better method exists than prevention. As such, there is growing interest in the reduction of biofilm through construction of ETTs impregnated with antimicrobial agents.[79–81] The ability of such developments to affect the incidence of VAP has not yet been proven.

Double-Lumen Endotracheal Tubes

The uses of a double-lumen endotracheal tube (DLT) can be separated into relative and absolute indications (Fig. 44.13). The absolute indications are lung isolation to avoid soilage or contamination of the contralateral lung when dealing with infections or frank hemoptysis from a unilateral location, bronchoalveolar lavage, and one-lung ventilation (OLV). The most common reason for placement is OLV for surgical exposure, but OLV can also be important in cases of bronchopleural or bronchocutaneous fistula, unilateral pulmonary hemorrhage, giant unilateral bulla or

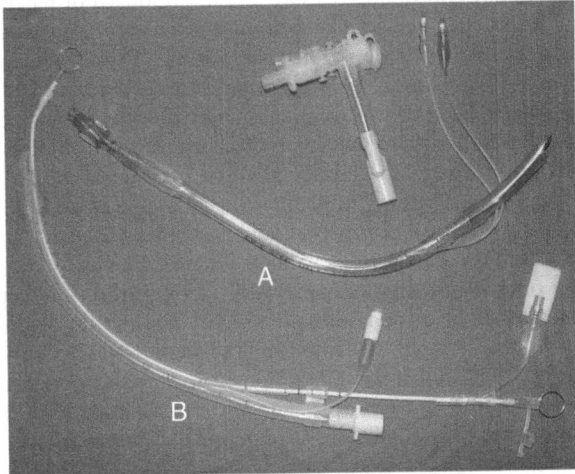

• **Fig. 44.13** Endobronchial blocking devices for lung isolation. (A) Mallinckrodt Endobronchial Tube (Covidien, Mansfield, MA); (B) Fuji TCB Univent Tube (Phycon Products, Tokyo, Japan).

cyst, and severe unilateral ventilation/perfusion mismatch. The relative indications all deal with surgical exposure. Complementing the DLT as another option for lung isolation, particularly if a DLT cannot be placed, are bronchial blocking devices. However, the primary advantage of the DLT is the ability to pass suctioning catheters or fiberoptic devices into the area of concern without dramatically jeopardizing OLV or contaminating the contralateral side. (See Chapter 26.)

Relative contraindications to the placement of a DLT are fairly minimal. They include patient refusal (likely because of risk of trauma secondary to the large size), a known difficult airway, and the speed with which an isolated airway must be established. In patients with difficult airways, specially designed airway exchange catheters (AECs) can be used after placement of a conventional single-lumen tube (SLT) to facilitate DLT placement. The time required for placement is usually the biggest detractor to the use of DLTs. Situations such as frank hemoptysis or a patient with limited cardiopulmonary reserve may benefit from initial placement of an SLT for stabilization.

Using a DLT in the ICU setting (>24 to 48 hours) must be approached with caution because the larger overall tube size can lead to mucosal damage, and the two smaller-diameter lumens are at significantly increased risk for partial or complete occlusion. Consideration should be given to close monitoring of luminal patency with fiberoptic evaluation on a regular basis and optimization of luminal hygiene to reduce mucus or biofilm accumulation. It is important to recognize that maintenance of a DLT requires specialized equipment because of the smaller-airway lumens; a standard adult-size therapeutic bronchoscope will not fit in a DLT. To that end, if a DLT is in use, a difficult airway cart with the appropriately sized bronchoscopic equipment should be readily available.

Proper Safeguarding of the Airway

Cuff Pressure Monitoring

Probably the most overlooked parameter in daily airway care is cuff pressure.[43–45,82,83] Almost universally, this measurement is neglected in OR intubations, particularly in the adult population. However, it is well documented that excessive pressure applied to the tracheal mucosa, even for a short time, leads to mucosal ischemia and may contribute to a sore throat. Prolonged or repetitive mucosal ischemia can lead to erosion, tracheoesophageal fistula, cartilage necrosis, scarring, synechiae, vocal cord paralysis, nerve damage, or ulceration.[43,44,83–85] Cuff pressures of 30 cm H_2O for 4 hours have been shown to impair ciliary motility for at least 3 days.[44,85–87] In addition, animal studies have revealed diminished circulation in the tracheal mucosa with a pressure of just 20 cm H_2O, exaggerated greatly in the presence of hypotension.[88]

Normal occlusive pressures should be between 20 and 25 cm H_2O to avoid complications while maintaining an adequate seal in the tracheal lumen circumferentially around the cuff to prevent microaspiration and, ultimately, VAP.[85–88] This pressure range seems to be effective at accomplishing this task both in vitro and during in vivo animal studies, although efficacy is dependent on the type of cuff. For example, standard HVLP cuffs have been demonstrated to be ineffective at preventing microaspiration with pressures as high as 60 cm H_2O,[14] whereas polyurethane cuffs seem to be effective down to 15 cm H_2O.[14,17,88]

Much of the morbidity associated with ETTs is related to either inappropriate inflation of an ETT cuff or a defective cuff.[83–85]

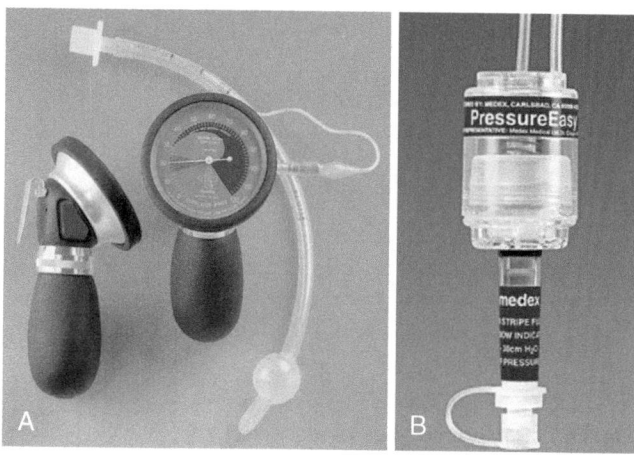

• **Fig. 44.14** (A) Posey Cufflator aneroid manometer and (B) PressureEasy Pressure Controller Device for monitoring endotracheal tube cuff pressure. (Courtesy Posey Company, Arcadia, CA, and Smiths Medical, Minneapolis, MN.)

One scenario that leads to increased morbidity is frequent ETT exchanges for suspected cuff leaks; trended values for cuff pressure could help to minimize some of these unnecessary procedures. Importantly, it has been demonstrated that manual palpation of the cuff or inflation with a standardized volume of air often leads to higher cuff pressures than desired, resulting in unrecognized complications.[82–85] Therefore, it is recommended that frequent examination of the cuff pressure be documented and trended using manometry.

Reusable aneroid manometers can be tedious to calibrate and are often difficult to locate; in addition, they pose a recurring risk of cross-contamination for each patient. The manometers currently in use in most ICUs provide only a single data point at the time of collection. Commercially available, disposable, precalibrated devices that constantly measure airway cuff pressures are available. One such device, the PressureEasy Cuff Pressure Controller (Smiths Medical, St. Paul, MN), attaches to the pilot balloon and visually indicates when the measured cuff pressure is in the optimal range of 20 to 30 cm H_2O (Fig. 44.14).[82–85] Current technology allows variable cuff pressures to fluctuate according to a baseline pressure and the pressure required to maintain tracheal wall occlusion during the delivery of a relatively high-pressure mechanical breath.

Measurement of ETT cuff pressure in the ICU setting is imperative. Conversely, adapting this habit in the OR for both the ETT and inflatable SGAs should be equally stressed as a prudent maneuver to optimize cuff pressures, even for brief cases of 1 to 2 hours duration.

Evaluation of a Cuff Leak

An ETT "cuff leak" or an "air leak" in mechanically ventilated patients poses unique challenges. Although ETT cuff leaks pertain most often to longer-duration intubations in the ICU, short-term tracheal intubation in the OR may also present with an apparent leak. The most relevant question is "When is a cuff leak really a cuff leak?" An audible leak implies that air is escaping from the presumably closed ETT system. The characteristics of the leak are variable and may be continuous or intermittent and may vary with the posture of the patient. The leak may compromise oxygenation and ventilation in addition to increasing the risk of aspiration.

TABLE 44.1	Differential Diagnosis of a Cuff/Air Leak

ETT Cuff Above Trachea

ETT cuff–tip complex dislocation (partial/complete extubation)

- Cuff within glottis (Grade I)
- Cuff above glottis, ETT tip within glottis (Grade II)
- Cuff and tip above glottis (complete extubation, Grade III)

ETT Cuff Within Trachea

- Cuff perforation, tear
- Incompetent or broken pilot balloon assembly
- Subglottic suction ETT (port on suction mimics leak)
- Tracheal wall–ETT cuff gap
  - Tracheomalacia
  - Anatomic distortion (tracheal)
  - ETT cuff design
  - ETT size
  - ETT cuff located immediately below glottis
  - Inadequate cuff inflation volume/pressure
  - ETT cuff at tracheocarinal junction
  - Device/foreign body between cuff and tracheal wall[a]
- Respiratory-digestive tract communication[b]

[a]For example, nasogastric tube, orogastric tube, temperature probe, tooth
[b]Tracheoesophageal, gastrotracheal, gastrobronchial, bronchoesophageal fistula

ETT, Endotracheal tube

Simply assuming that a cuff leak is strictly related to the cuff itself is a common mistake. A systematic approach to evaluate the varied etiology is a must for appropriate corrective action to prevent harm. Cuff leak may be caused by a structural defect in the cuff or a dysfunctional pilot balloon and inflation valve system. However, as outlined by El-Orbany and Salem, the etiology of a cuff leak is much more varied and extensive (Table 44.1).[89] Air leakage may be caused by cuff underinflation, cephalad migration of the ETT (supraglottic extubation), a misplaced orogastric or nasogastric tube or temperature probe, a discrepancy between the ETT cuff and tracheal wall dimensions (tracheomalacia, cuff positioned at the carina/mainstem bronchus junction, or a cuff abutted against the subglottic opening), or increased peak airway pressure causing a leak around an intact cuff (Fig. 44.15). Cephalad migration of the ETT leading to unrecognized partial or complete extubation may be the most common cause of cuff leak not related to the cuff itself.[90] For better understanding, a grading system has been described to define the various ETT tip-cuff positions (Table 44.2). An "air leak" is often managed by repeated inflation of the pilot balloon by the provider thinking there is a cuff leak (Figs. 44.16 and 44.17). This may temporarily resolve the "leak" but result in further ETT displacement (Grade I/II → Grade III) (Figs. 44.18 and 44.19). It is imperative to investigate a leak rather than assume that the ETT cuff is leaking or dysfunctional. Determining the cause of the leak will assist in planning corrective

measures, if indicated. Thus, an airway assessment combined with a brief review of the patient's history and recent bedside activities (e.g., recent chest radiograph or feeding tube placement) may offer valuable clues. For example, the airway team may be asked to "change the ETT" due to a "cuff leak." If the team assumes

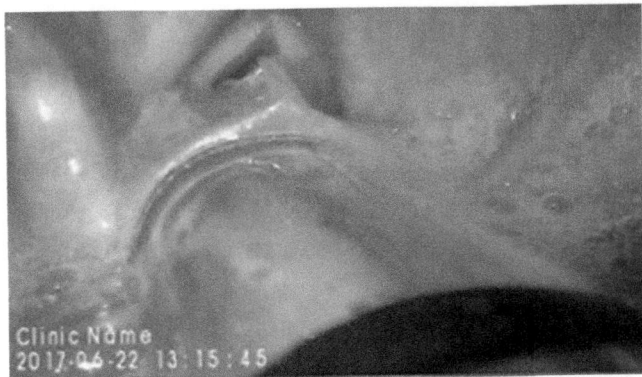

• **Fig. 44.16** Grade I partial extubation. Endotracheal tube cuff lies between the vocal cords.

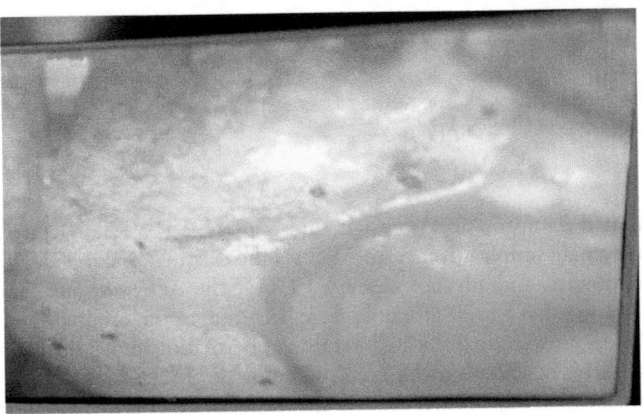

• **Fig. 44.17** Grade II partial extubation. Video-assisted laryngoscopic view of complete cuff herniation above glottis with the endotracheal tube tip at the glottic inlet.

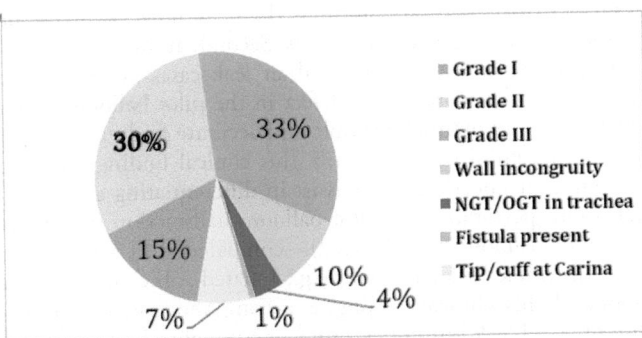

Legend (pie chart):
- Grade I — 33%
- Grade II — 30%
- Grade III — 15%
- Wall incongruity — 7%
- NGT/OGT in trachea — 1%
- Fistula present — 10%
- Tip/cuff at Carina — 4%

• **Fig. 44.15** Etiology of cuff/air leak in 935 intensive care unit patients.

TABLE 44.2	Partial/Complete Extubation Grading System		
Grade I		**Grade II**	**Grade III**
Partial extubation: ETT cuff between the vocal cords		Partial extubation: ETT tip at the level of vocal cords	Complete extubation: ETT tip above the vocal cords

ETT, Endotracheal tube.

Illustrations by Anna J. Mort and Thomas C. Mort.

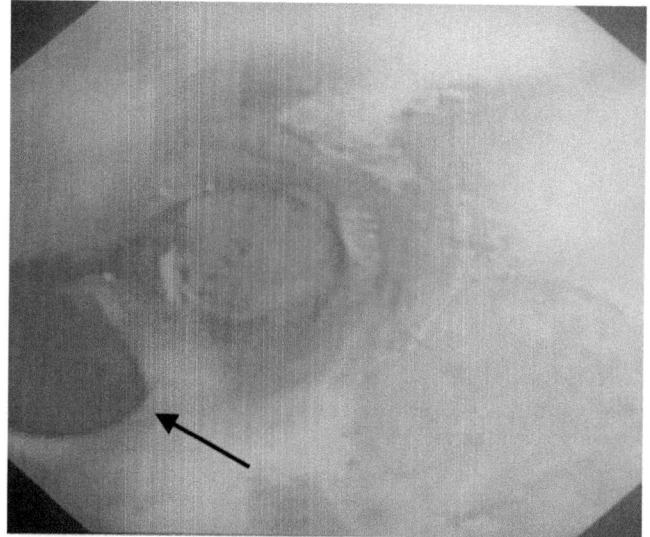

• **Fig. 44.18** Grade III complete extubation. Endotracheal tube tip impingement against supraglottic tissues with air exchange via the laterally positioned Murphy eye (*arrow*).

that the information is correct and that there is a leaking ETT, they may simply advance an AEC via the existing "leaking" ETT, remove it, and advance a new ETT over the AEC without considering that the "leak" could have been due to the original ETT being proximally dislocated because of herniation above the glottis. The newly advanced ETT may now be located outside the tracheal airway. This illustrates the importance of a preexchange or preprocedural airway assessment. Table 44.3 presents a streamlined "problem/solution" outline. Each etiology of the "cuff leak"

may have a differing corrective measure that could endanger the patient if implemented erroneously. Performing an external airway assessment complimented by flexible bronchoscopy (FB) and/or laryngoscopy (conventional direct laryngoscopy or, preferably, VAL) will allow the team to better define the problem and then develop a management plan. Both FB and VAL are excellent for diagnostic and therapeutic correction. However, preparation for management of a difficult airway is justified. Forward advancement of a thermally softened, nonstyletted Grade III ETT toward the glottic opening combined with a hyperangulated videolaryngoscope (VL) blade may lead to difficulty with reintubation of the trachea. Such cases are best managed with the advancement of a new, styletted ETT. Extreme caution should be exhibited on the use of VAL together with an AEC in managing complete extubation (Grade III), as maneuvering the straight-tipped AEC into the trachea can be challenging and may delay securing the airway.[91]

Two important clinical points are worthy of mention, as they pose valuable diagnostic clues regarding the evaluation of a "cuff/air leak." First, the depth markings on the ETT have little correlation to the actual depth of the ETT cuff and tip in partial/complete extubation (Fig. 44.20). Therefore, assuming a depth of greater than 24 to 26 cm infers the ETT must be in a good position could be grossly erroneous. Second, an intact pilot balloon, present in 97% of the cuff/air leak cases not related to an actual cuff perforation or defect in the pilot balloon assembly, presents a potentially simple and accurate finding that may serve as a helpful clinical sign.[92] This clinical finding offers an intriguing diagnostic clue to assist in differentiating a true cuff leak—cuff perforation or pilot balloon malfunction (incompetent pilot balloon, e.g., deflated)—compared with a dislocated ETT tip (intact pilot balloon, e.g., inflated). The authors have embraced this clinical finding as a component in the evaluation of a cuff leak but not as a sole determinant of unrecognized

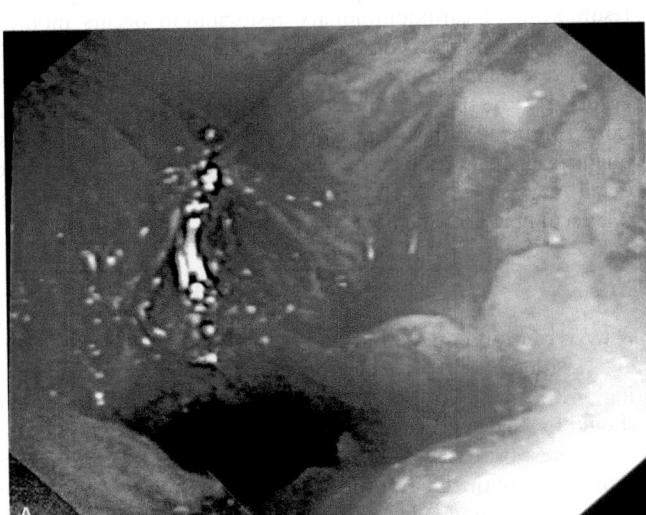
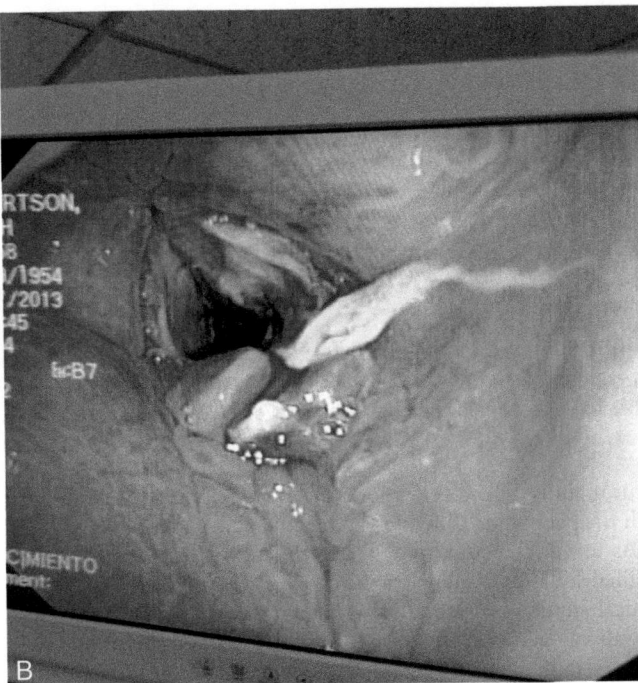

• **Fig. 44.19** (A and B) Grade III complete extubation. Bronchoscopic views from inside the indwelling endotracheal tube that were noted to be well above the glottic opening.

TABLE 44.3	Simplified Problem-Solution Approach for a Cuff Leak	
Problem	**Solution**	**Risk Level**
Cuff perforation	Exchange ETT (only feasible choice)	High
Incompetent pilot valve/pilot balloon line	Exchange ETT	High
	Clamp line (Kelly, Hemostat)—short-term solution	Low
	Place stopcock or cap on valve	Low
	Replace pilot balloon–line assembly	Low
Displaced ETT (intact pilot balloon)	Perform flexible endoscopic evaluation—diagnostic	Low–moderate
	Blindly advance ETT	Very high
	Video-assisted laryngoscopy evaluation	Low–moderate
	Blindly pass airway exchange catheter	High
	Perform direct laryngoscopy	Low–moderate
Tracheocarinal/mainstem intubation	Retract ETT	Low–moderate
Respiratory-digestive tract communication (tracheo/broncho-esophago/gastro fistula)	Surgical consult, reposition ETT, radiographic evaluation	Moderate–high
Foreign body between tracheal wall and cuff	Advance/retract/change/remove NGT/OGT/temperature probe	Low–high

ETT, Endotracheal tube; *NGT*, nasogastric tube; *OGT*, orogastric tube.

tracheal extubation. Also, ready access to other airway device adjuncts is central to providing safe rescue airway management that frequently accompanies critically ill patients outside the OR environment. To summarize, evaluation of the pilot balloon assembly may render useful diagnostic information regarding the origin of the cuff leak, and, despite a seemingly adequate depth at the dentition line, the ETT should be evaluated for potential displacement.

Documentation of Placement

Clinicians who care for patients who are intubated for long periods in the ICU may find it difficult to obtain pertinent airway management details. This situation could result for many reasons: lack of relevance (routine intubation before the patient's surgery), lack of continuity (the intubator is no longer involved in the patient's care), or an incomplete or total lack of documentation. This information, however, is essential when airway emergencies

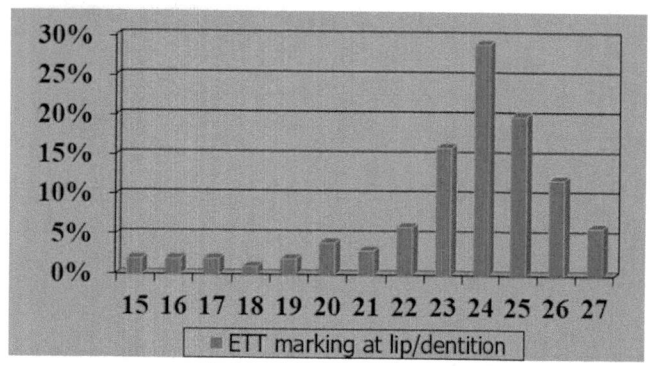

• **Fig. 44.20** Depth of the endotracheal tube (*ETT*) at the lips/gingival line in 729 intensive care unit patients with partial/complete extubation.

occur in an ICU and practitioners who are potentially unfamiliar with the patient are called to emergently manage the airway.

As an ICU course progresses, the details surrounding the original ETT placement may prove less relevant as the patient's clinical status and airway are dynamic, not static. A previously easy airway may remain so, but difficulty often increases as airway edema, trauma, and secretions accumulate. These changes, combined with acute and chronic physiologic deterioration of the patient, provide a challenge to future attempts at airway management. Anatomic abnormalities may be hidden or exaggerated by excessive fluid administration or a capillary leakage phenomenon in the critically ill patient, and examination of the airway may become impossible.

When airway management is necessary on a previously intubated patient, knowledge of the techniques and airway adjuncts that have been previously attempted is imperative. Immediate availability of pertinent historical airway management details may prove helpful in delivering better care. A summary of airway interventions, medical/surgical history, allergies, medications, recent lab work, and procedures can be computer generated, printed, and provided to practitioners in a timely manner (Fig. 44.21). In an emergency, this may improve communication and decrease the incidence of adverse events during airway management in a typically chaotic environment. The advent of the electronic medical record (EMR) has presented benefits, as well as pitfalls. A quick, computer-based review of previous airway interventions at the bedside is a welcome advantage. However, if the notes are poorly written or lacking in detail, they may not provide useful clinical information that may be applied to the airway intervention. The EMR invites the quick checking of boxes to construct a note. This may lead to a cookie-cutter product that lacks insight, description, or details of the patient's clinical situation or their response to the airway intervention. The addition of a standardized template or "phase" outlining what was done or encountered may offer improved communication, as long as the template does not simply add to the box-checking problem.

If the EMR-based airway management note includes a selection of complications, this too may present data-mining issues. The definition of what constitutes a complication is variable. A common finding observed with EMR-based airway notes is that "no complications" is highlighted, yet a memo box with free-text details about the airway intervention offers documentation of details. If data-mining reports are generated by focusing on checked complication boxes, many complications will elude detection, which could lead to the underreporting of complications unless the memo section is specifically reviewed.

Describing the clinical situation surrounding the airway intervention may reap substantial benefits. For example, responding to a cardiac arrest call, the airway team arrives to see the return of spontaneous circulation with chest compressions halted. Intubation takes place for airway protection. Deterioration necessitating resumption of cardiopulmonary resuscitation occurs moments later. Due to poor documentation of the clinical setting by the airway team, another provider notes in their documentation of the events that the patient suffered a cardiac arrest following intubation. This detail is then copied and pasted multiple times in subsequent progress notes by other care providers. This lack of clinical detail may not serve well for official review of the case and does not accurately describe the acute event.

Stabilization of the Endotracheal Tube

After verification and confirmation of proper tracheal placement and position have been achieved, care should be focused on securing the ETT in its proper position, and frequent assessments should be made to recognize malpositioning.[92,93]

At the most basic level, recording and confirming the depth in centimeters of the ETT at the patient's teeth or lips should be routine. This measurement should be documented on the respiratory care flow sheet. In patients requiring prolonged mechanical ventilation, the depth should be assessed and documented frequently (e.g., every shift or every 4 hours), along with clinical assessments of ETT patency and hygiene, chest expansion, and auscultation findings.

Securing and surveillance of the ETT are important not only to ensure proper depth and positioning but also to reduce the incidence of inadvertent extubation.[92] Unplanned extubation is primarily a problem in the ICU, with a reported incidence ranging from 2% to 16%. As many as 80% of unplanned extubations require reintubation, and unplanned extubation leads to a higher rate of airway-related complications, hemodynamic alterations, patient morbidity, and mortality.[62,94–96] The most frequently identified cause is inadequate sedation of a mechanically ventilated patient.

Few studies have specifically addressed techniques used to secure ETTs. In a study comparing four such techniques, Levy and Griego concluded that the use of simple adhesive tape split at both ends and secured to both the ETT and the patient's face was more effective than proprietary methods and allowed more effective nursing care, improved oral hygiene, and greater comfort for the patient.[93] However, Barnason and colleagues found no statistical difference between two methods studied in preventing unplanned extubation, allowing oral hygiene, or maintaining facial skin integrity.[97] Because there have been no definitive studies on the topic, no consensus exists on the best method of securing the ETT.

One important caveat should be understood regarding proper ETT position at the gum line or lips in all intubated patients: The ETT marking at these locations does not guarantee the depth and location of the distal ETT tip. Although this problem pertains most often to the ventilated ICU patient, an ETT located at 25 cm at the gum line and seemingly secured by tape or a commercial device does not guarantee tracheal intubation (with or without a cuff leak). Typically, a continuous or intermittent apparent cuff leak leads to further insufflation of the pilot balloon in an attempt to reduce the leak. An intact (inflated) pilot balloon in this clinical situation should arouse suspicion that the cuff-tip complex may lie at or above the glottis. Proper assessment of ETT

Department of Anesthesiology Airway Management Note

Airway Management Procedure:
[ ] Elective   [ ] Urgent   [ ] Emergent
[ ] Cardiac or Respiratory Arrest
[ ] Intubation   [ ] ETT Exchange   [ ] Extubation   [ ] Other: _____

Date: _____ Call Time: _____ Arrival Time: _____
Location: _____ Staff: _____

Height: _____ Weight: _____ NPO Status: _____
BP: _____ HR: _____ Oxy Sat: _____ on _____%
[ ] Room Air   [ ] Nasal   [ ] Face mask   [ ] NRB   [ ] NIPPV

Isolation Precautions: [ ] Contact   [ ] Droplet   [ ] Airborne
                                [ ] Vector   [ ] Common Vehicle

Condition Upon Arrival (check all that apply):
[ ] Awake   [ ] Hypoxemic   [ ] Dyspnea   [ ] Secretions
[ ] Sedated   [ ] Hypercarbic   [ ] Tachypnea   [ ] Vomitus
[ ] Agitated   [ ] Stridorous   [ ] Bradypnea   [ ] Blood
[ ] Unconscious   [ ] Wheezing   [ ] Apnea   [ ] Foreign Matter...
[ ] Other/Comments: _____

Underlying Pathologies/Co-Morbidities (if known, mark all that apply):
Neurologic: [ ] CVA   [ ] Increased ICP   [ ] ICH/SDH   [ ] Seizure
                 [ ] SCI   [ ] Δ Mental Status   [ ] Drug Overdose

Pulmonary: [ ] Asthma   [ ] COPD   [ ] ARDS   [ ] OSA   [ ] PE
                 [ ] PNA...   [ ] CAP   [ ] VAP   [ ] Pulm. Contusion
                 [ ] Pneumo/Hemothorax   [ ] Upper Airway Issue...
                 [ ] Post-operative Respiratory Failure   [ ] NPPE

Cardiac: [ ] AMI   [ ] CHF   [ ] Dysrhythmia...   [ ] Tamponade
Metabolic: [ ] Acidosis...   [ ] Electrolyte...   [ ] Alcohol Withdrawal
                 [ ] UGIB or LGIB   [ ] SBO   [ ] Mesenteric Ischemia

Infectious: [ ] Immune compromised   [ ] Sepsis   [ ] PTA
                 [ ] Tonsil/Epiglottitis   [ ] Tracheitis/Bronchitis

Trauma: [ ] Cranial/Spinal...   [ ] Thoracic...   [ ] Abdominal...
                 [ ] Orthopedic...

Other/Comments: _____

Airway Management Procedural Documentation:
Preoxygenation: [ ] Room Air   [ ] Face mask/NRB   [ ] 100%, Bag-Mask
Ventilation: [ ] Assisted   [ ] Controlled   [ ] Easy   [ ] Difficult
                     [ ] Oral Airway   [ ] Nasal Airway   [ ] Two-person
Positioning: [ ] Supine   [ ] Ramped   [ ] Elevated HOB
                     [ ] Sitting   [ ] Other: _____
Induction: [ ] Awake   [ ] Sedated   [ ] General Anesthesia   [ ] None
                     [ ] Topical Anesthesia   [ ] Airway Block...   [ ] Paralysis...
                     [ ] Rapid Sequence Induction   [ ] Cricoid Pressure
                     [ ] Other: _____
Medications: [ ] Etomidate _____ mg   [ ] Propofol _____ mg
                     [ ] Ketamine _____ mg   [ ] Other: _____
                     [ ] Succinylcholine _____ mg   [ ] Rocuronium _____ mg
1st Attempt: [ ] DL: MAC _____ MILLER_____   [ ] Glidescope/VL   [ ] FOB
                     Other: _____
                     C-L View: [ ] 1   [ ] 2a   [ ] 2b   [ ] 3a   [ ] 3b   [ ] 4
                                  [ ] Secretions   [ ] Blood   [ ] Edema
                     AirwayAdjuncts: [ ] Bougie   [ ] ILMA   [ ] LMA
                     Other/Comments: _____

• **Fig. 44.21** Example of a detailed airway record for emergency intubations.

2nd Attempt: [ ] DL: MAC_____ MILLER_____   [ ] Glidescope/VL   [ ] FOB
              Other:_____

              C-L View: [ ] 1   [ ] 2a   [ ] 2b   [ ] 3a   [ ] 3b   [ ] 4
                            [ ] Secretions   [ ] Blood   [ ] Edema
              AirwayAdjuncts: [ ] Bougie   [ ] ILMA   [ ] LMA
              Other/Comments: _____

_____
_____

3rd Attempt: [ ] DL: MAC_____ MILLER_____   [ ] Glidescope/VL   [ ] FOB
              Other:_____

              C-L View: [ ] 1   [ ] 2a   [ ] 2b   [ ] 3a   [ ] 3b   [ ] 4
                            [ ] Secretions   [ ] Blood   [ ] Edema
              AirwayAdjuncts: [ ] Bougie   [ ] ILMA   [ ] LMA
              Other/Comments: _____

_____
_____

Airway Device Ultimately Placed: [ ] ETT...   [ ] LMA...   [ ] Combitube
        Size:_____ Type: [ ] Standard   [ ] ORAE   [ ] NRAE
                                    [ ] Subglottic EVAC   [ ] ECOM
        Placement Location:_____ cm @ lip
Confirmation: [ ] Esophageal bulb device   [ ] ETCO$_2$ [ ] Direct Visual
                  [ ] Bilateral BS   [ ] Bronchoscopy   [ ] Chest X-ray

Post-Procedure Vital Signs:

BP: _____   HR: _____   Oxy Sat:_____ on_____%

Other/Comments: _____
_____
_____
_____
_____
_____
_____
_____
_____
_____
_____
_____

Signature:_____   Date/Time:_____

• **Fig. 44.21, cont'd**

position, preferably with flexible optical laryngoscopy or VAL for diagnostic and therapeutic maneuvers, is indicated. Detection of the ETT tip-cuff complex using ultrasound technology can allow serial monitoring of ETT position to combat ETT tip migration leading to partial or complete tracheal extubation.

Taping

The classically described methods for taping the ETT are a "barber's pole" technique for OR intubations, a simple split tape technique (Fig. 44.22), and a more secure "four-point" technique for intubations anticipated to last for 24 hours or longer. In each of these methods, tape is used to anchor the ETT to the face. Moisture (in the form of sweat, skin oils, secretions, or vomitus) and facial hair can jeopardize the integrity of the bond between adhesive and skin, putting the security of the ETT at risk.[92,98] Additionally, patient comfort is an issue when tape is used for this purpose. Skin breakdown because of allergic reactions, pressure necrosis, or repetitive trauma has been documented as a potential problem resulting from taping the ETT for prolonged periods.

The four-point method is more secure than the barber's pole technique because the tape encircles the patient's head and is not as susceptible to moisture because it is anchored to itself as well as to the patient's skin. Razor stubble, facial hair of any amount, makeup, and the buildup of oil/sebum on facial skin reduce tape adherence. Cleansing of the skin to enhance adhesiveness is a valuable adjunct for improving ETT stabilization. Additionally, liquid adhesives (e.g., Mastisol or benzoin) can increase the tackiness of skin and help to improve adherence of tape and dressings.

Commercially Available Devices

Although several options are available, a proprietary device has been developed to help secure the ETT and provide increased patient comfort while facilitating airway care. This device, the AnchorFast Guard (Hollister Inc., Libertyville, IL), incorporates an ergonomically designed frame to minimize well-known pressure points, a latex-free adhesive on a pad, and a padded Velcro-style retaining strap that encircles the head (Fig. 44.23). Preliminary studies comparing this device against classic adhesive tapes

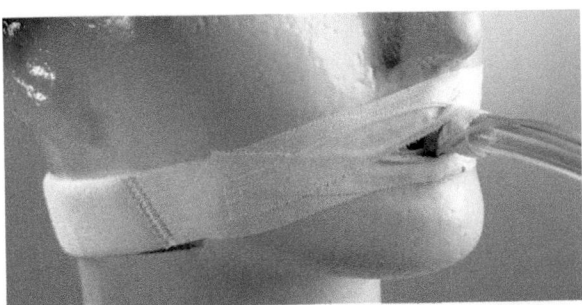

• **Fig. 44.22** The split-tape method of taping the endotracheal tube.

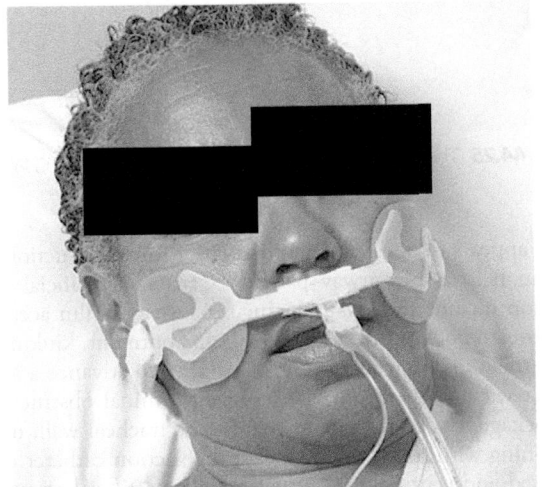

• **Fig. 44.23** The AnchorFast system for endotracheal tube stabilization. (Courtesy Hollister Inc., Libertyville, IL.)

showed reduced skin breakdown, fewer lip ulcers, and improved patient comfort.[93,98] The AnchorFast Guard incorporates a tube protection sleeve that serves as a bite block.

Stapling for Facial Burns

The overall incidence of burn patients in most practices is very small, and this creates an unfamiliarity with their care, particularly as it relates to airway management. In addition to difficulties with tracheal intubation initially, replacement of an ETT after a burn resuscitation is far more challenging because of a multitude of unique injuries. The two major problems with securing an ETT for the patient with a facial burn are the worsening edema of the airway and facial tissue because of ongoing inflammatory processes and continued resuscitation, and the burned skin, which weeps constantly and is often debrided or sloughing. It should be obvious that adhesive devices, both simple tape and proprietary devices, are ineffective in this situation. A well-documented and accepted method in these patients is to secure the ETT with tape and subsequently anchor the tape to the skin by stapling it to the burned areas. This is surprisingly well tolerated, but more important, it is very reliable for maintaining the airway. (See Chapter 35.)

Maintenance of the Endotracheal Tube

There is currently no alternative to the placement of an oral, nasal, or transtracheal ETT, whether to maintain airway patency, perform ventilation, improve oxygenation, remove secretions, or deliver necessary therapies. However, the ETT is only as good as its most pristine state. Despite the unavoidable decision, some still look on the placement of an ETT as a necessary evil. The conundrum arises in preserving or remastering the physiologic function of the host tissues while combating their inherent defenses aimed at reacting to the new artificial airway and protecting the new foreign device to maintain its optimized function as in its original condition.

The presence of an ETT bypasses the host defenses of the upper airway, prevents the humidification of inspired gases, increases the WOB, limits the administration of medications, and restricts prophylactic oral hygiene. All these changes promote bacterial colonization, inflammation, and sputum production. Inability to actively clear secretions because of a poor cough or increased difficulty of passive removal by healthcare personnel can lead to plugging of proximal and distal airways as well as the ETT. These retained secretions may result in the formation of atelectasis, ventilation/perfusion mismatching in the form of shunt or dead space, hypoxemia, and increased respiratory load, thereby prolonging the duration of mechanical ventilation.[99,100] Therefore, aggressive respiratory care must be provided for the intubated patient to avoid these complications and further morbidity.

Heat and Humidity of Inspired Gas

During normal breathing, air is delivered to the carina at a temperature of 32°C and an absolute humidity of 30.4 mg H_2O/L.[101] The insertion of an ETT via the nose, mouth, or trachea bypasses the upper airway and causes the body's natural ability to heat and humidify inspired gas to be lost. The American Association for Respiratory Care states that devices should provide a minimum of 30 mg of H_2O/L of delivered gas at 30°C.[102] If inspired air is not warmed and humidified, the result is a dry, cool gas that is damaging to the respiratory tract and impedes mucociliary function. Secretions may become dry and inspissated, possibly leading to partial or complete occlusion of the ETT lumen. If left unrecognized, this occlusion may lead to barotrauma and other life-threatening crises. The most common method to protect against this situation is the use of an active heated humidifier or a passive heat and moisture exchanger (HME) (Fig. 44.24).[103]

HMEs are typically cylindrical devices that are fitted to the ventilator circuit, usually just proximal to the ETT connector and the Y-piece, with limited changes on airway mechanics.[104,105] This is the most effective site for HME placement for maximizing humidity and temperature retention in the patient circuit.[103,106] HMEs provide heat, humidification, and filtering properties, earning the device the nickname "artificial nose."[107] They are

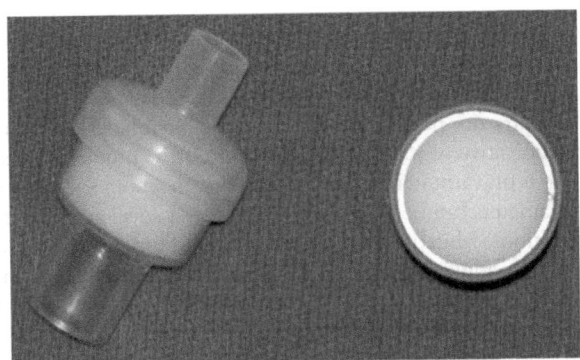

• **Fig. 44.24** A heat and moisture exchanger.

lightweight and inexpensive, require no power source, and reduce circuit condensation, making them attractive alternatives to the more expensive heated humidifiers.

Use of heated humidifiers is associated with the production of almost 100% humidity in the inspiratory gas and is thus more effective than use of HMEs. These units require an external power source and additional circuitry, increasing cost. Accidental overheating can occur and may create additional damage to the airway if temperatures are not frequently monitored. There is no consensus about the proper duration of use of these implements. Multiple studies have failed to show a correlation of increased incidence of pneumonia with heated humidifiers versus HMEs or with frequent changes of HMEs or heated humidifiers. Therefore, frequent changes of ventilator circuits (i.e., more often than every 7 days), unless they are visually soiled, are neither cost-effective nor medically efficacious.[108–111]

Suctioning

Airway suctioning is commonly used in respiratory care to promote optimal tracheobronchial toilet and airway patency in critically ill patients. Because of the perceived simplicity and limited complications, airway suctioning is frequently employed. However, both its overuse and underutilization present patient care problems. If proper indications and technique are not appreciated, the potential for significant complications exists.

The principal goals of suctioning include keeping the lungs free of active infiltrate while causing the least possible impairment of cardiopulmonary function and damage to tracheal mucosa, maintaining patency of the artificial airway, and decreasing the incidence of atelectasis due to mucous plugging of airway.

When suctioning is performed carelessly, complications may occur, including soft tissue or airway trauma, aspiration, laryngospasm, increased intracranial pressure, bronchospasm, hypoxemia, and cardiac dysrhythmias.[112] Hypoxemia can be minimized with preoxygenation using a 100% fraction of inspired oxygen (F_{IO_2}). In patients with intracranial hypertension, mild hyperventilation or blunting of the cough reflex with intravenous lidocaine just before suctioning may reduce the risks of additional increases in intracranial pressure. The evacuation procedure should be brief and intermittent. The vacuum should be applied only after the suction catheter has been advanced to its distal position. After each pass of the catheter, lung reexpansion with a few gentle, manual recruitment breaths should be administered. Suctioning can be applied by a single-use open system in which the catheter is unprotected and open to the environment or by a closed system that sheathes the catheter in a sterile protective covering (Fig. 44.25).

Indications

Suctioning of the airway should not be done without appropriate clinical indications. The audible (auscultatory) or visible presence of airway secretions is the most common indication. Increasing peak inspiratory pressures in mechanically ventilated patients are often indicative of retained secretions. Routine prophylactic suctioning is unwarranted except in neonates, in whom the small airway diameters can be acutely obstructed by a small accumulation of secretions. Moreover, the presence of DLT or a smaller-caliber ETT in an adult may benefit from a more aggressive suctioning schedule to reduce the risk of compromising the patency of the smaller cross-sectional lumen.

In addition to removal of secretions, suction catheters are employed as aids in evaluating airway patency. If an artificial

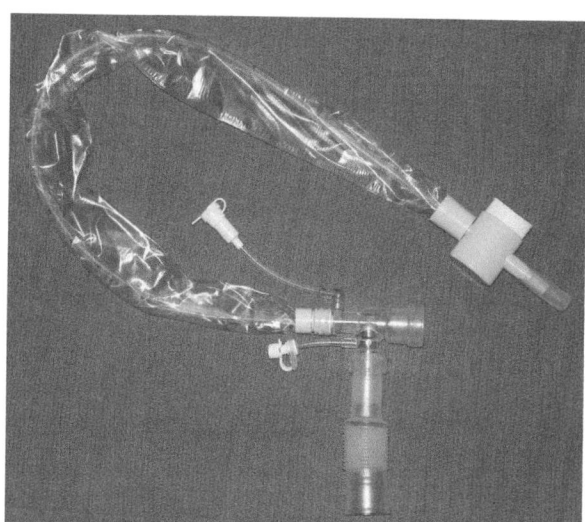

• **Fig. 44.25** The Ballard closed endotracheal tube suctioning system.

airway appears to be occluded, an attempt to pass a suction catheter can help assess airway patency. Causes of artificial airway occlusion include mucous plugging, excessive biofilm accumulation, foreign body obstructions, ETT tip abutment, kinking, and cuff herniations. Furthermore, the inability to advance a suction catheter via a tracheostomy may suggest luminal obstruction or tip blockage, tip impingement against the tracheal wall, or malpositioning within a false passage. If the suction catheter cannot be passed and ventilation is obstructed, the artificial airway may require a simple remedy such as removal of the inner cannula or it may require complete replacement, as this could be life-threatening. Bronchoscopic evaluation may assist the clinician in the evaluation of the airway. Provision of airway suctioning depends on an appreciation of the available equipment, the appropriate techniques, and the potential complications.

Equipment

Numerous commercial suction catheters exist.[113,114] The ideal catheter is one that optimizes secretion removal and minimizes tissue trauma. Specific features of the catheters include the material of construction, frictional resistance, size (length and diameter), shape, and position of the aspirating holes. A reasonable clinical recommendation would be to use a suction catheter that occludes less than 50% of the lumen of the ETT in children and adults and less than 70% in infants. Additionally, an opening at the proximal end of the catheter to allow the entrainment of room air, neutralizing the vacuum without disconnecting the vacuum apparatus, is ideal. The proximal hole should be larger than the catheter lumen. Tracheal suctioning can occur only with occlusion of this proximal opening. The conventional ETT suction catheter has side holes and end holes to lessen the maximum suction action at the tip, thus reducing mucosal trauma (Fig. 44.26). This concept applies to both airway suction catheters and those used to suction the oropharyngeal cavity (e.g., the Yankauer suction catheter).

The length of the typical suction catheter should allow it to pass beyond the distal tip of the artificial airway. The diameter of the suction catheter is very important; the optimal catheter diameter should not exceed one-half of the ID of the artificial airway. A catheter that is too large can produce an excessive vacuum and evacuation of gases distal to the tip of the airway, promoting atelectasis because of inadequate space for entrainment of air around the

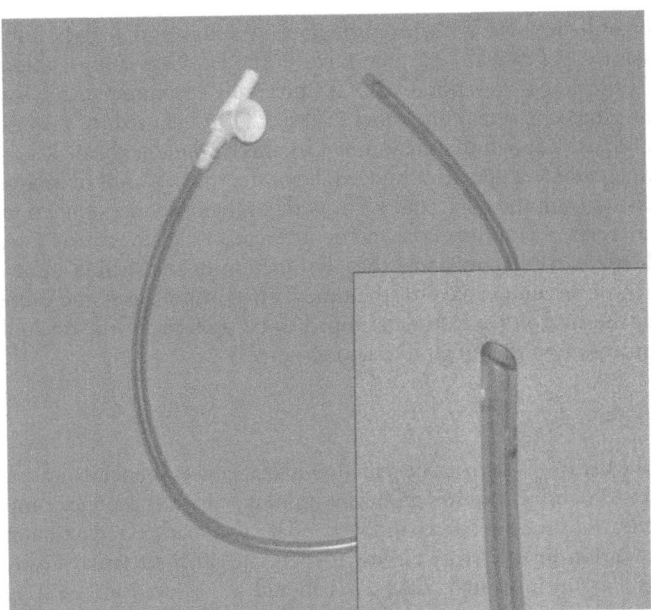

• **Fig. 44.26** A conventional suction catheter has side and end holes. (*Inset*) Enlarged view of the beveled tip and dual side holes.

suction catheter. If the catheter is too small, the efficacy of removal of secretions, depending on their viscosity and volume, can be compromised. Closed suctioning systems are usually incorporated into the ventilator breathing circuit at the junction of the Y-piece and the ETT or tracheostomy tube, allowing continued ventilation during suctioning with no need to disconnect the circuit. The advantage of not having to disconnect is important for patients who require aggressive ventilator management (e.g., high PEEP therapy), making them less susceptible to alveolar derecruitment compared with open suctioning. The retractable catheter does not add any additional restriction to airflow (when not deployed). There are concerns that colonization of these devices with aspiration of bacterial particles and cross-contamination may predispose to VAP.[113] Such concerns have led to differing opinions on the appropriate timing of any system changes. Kollef and colleagues randomly assigned patients to scheduled circuit changes every 24 hours or to no change except when there was a malfunction or visible soiling.[114] In both groups, 15% of patients developed VAP. The only difference was in total cost: There was a 13-fold increase in equipment cost in the group with scheduled changes versus the group with no scheduled changes.[115]

Technique

Suctioning technique is important for the optimal removal of secretions and limitation of complications. This should be a sterile procedure necessitating appropriate care in the handling of the catheter. Gloves and handwashing are necessary unless a closed system is employed. Other necessary equipment includes a vacuum source, sterile rinsing solution, self-inflating bag-valve mask, and lavage solution. The optimal vacuum pressure should be adjusted for the patient's age.

Before suctioning, the patient should be preoxygenated by increasing the FIO_2 to 100% or by manual ventilatory assistance. Preoxygenation minimizes the hypoxemia induced by circuit disconnection and application of the suction vacuum. After preoxygenation, the sterile catheter is advanced past the distal tip of the artificial airway without the vacuum. When the catheter can no

longer easily advance, it should be slightly withdrawn, and intermittent vacuum pressure should be applied while the catheter is removed in a rotating fashion. This technique reportedly reduces mucosal trauma and enhances secretion clearance. The vacuum (suction) time should be limited to 10 to 15 seconds, and discontinuation of ventilation and oxygenation should not exceed 20 seconds. After removal of the catheter, reoxygenation and ventilation are essential. Throughout the procedure, the patient's stability and tolerance should be monitored. If signs of distress or dysrhythmias develop, the procedure should be immediately discontinued, and oxygenation and ventilation reestablished. Suctioning is repeated until secretions have been adequately removed. After airway suctioning, oropharyngeal secretions should be suctioned, and the catheter should be disposed of and replaced with a new catheter, unless it is a closed system.

Optimization of secretion removal necessitates adequate hydration and humidification of delivered gases. Occasionally, secretions can become quite viscous. Instillation of 5 to 10 mL of sterile normal saline can aid removal. In critically ill patients, using a closed system or swivel adapter to allow simultaneous suctioning and ventilation limits the consequences of airway disconnection, minimizes the loss of PEEP, and enhances sterility. These disposable systems are usually more costly but are used for up to 72 hours.

When an artificial airway is absent, nasotracheal suctioning techniques are employed. These techniques are technically less effective and more difficult than oral suctioning without an artificial airway and have the potential for additional complications. After appropriate lubrication, the catheter is inserted into a patient's nasal passage (often through a previously placed nasopharyngeal airway). The catheter is advanced distally toward and possibly into the larynx. Breath sounds from the proximal end of the catheter are often used as an audible guide. On the catheter's entry into the larynx, the patient often coughs. The vacuum is connected and suctioning of the trachea is accomplished, as previously described. The stimulated cough may serve as an impetus for the patient to expel otherwise retained secretions buoyed by a weakened cough.

Complications

Complications of suctioning can be significant.[113] Factors influencing complications include the suctioning technique, suction frequency, and higher levels of PEEP. The incidence of complications can be reduced by the implementation of suctioning guidelines. Although the suction vacuum is used to remove secretions, it also removes oxygen-enriched gases from the airway. If inappropriately applied and monitored, suctioning can produce significant hypoxemia. The use of arterial oxygen monitors (e.g., pulse oximetry)—a standard of care in the ICU and intermediate/step-down setting—can often help detect alterations in SaO_2, heart rate, and the presence of dysrhythmias. Hypoxemia, particularly in the significantly debilitated or compromised patient, may lead to tachycardia, arrhythmias, and even cardiac arrest. For this reason, the patient must be oxygenated manually or with 100% FIO_2 via ventilator before, during, and following the procedure. Neonates are the exception to this rule because of a higher risk of adverse effects from hyperoxia; when suctioning a newborn, the FIO_2 should be increased by an absolute 10%.

Cardiovascular alterations during suctioning are common. Hypertension and tachycardia are common in response to vigorous suctioning; however, dysrhythmias and hypotension can also occur. Arterial hypoxemia (and eventually myocardial hypoxia) and vagal stimulation from tracheal suctioning are recognized precipitating causes of cardiovascular complications. Coughing induced by stimulation of the airway can reduce venous return and ventricular preload. Avoidance of hypoxemia, prolonged suctioning (>10 seconds), appropriate monitoring, and adequate sedation and analgesia help to reduce the incidence and significance of these complications.

Inappropriate suction catheter size can produce excessive evacuation of gas distal to the artificial airway because of inadequate space for proximal air entrainment. This leads to hypoxemia and atelectasis. It is best avoided by reducing the catheter size to less than one-half of the ID of the airway. Auscultation of the lungs before and after suctioning can help detect significant atelectasis. After suctioning, several hyperinflation or recruitment breaths may assist with reinflating atelectatic lung segments.

The concern for intracerebral hemodynamic alteration in at-risk patients (e.g., patients with intracranial hypertension) is a major concern. Limiting the frequency and intensity (duration) of suctioning may be needed in high-risk patients. Pretreatment with lidocaine (intravenous or instilled into the airway) or sedative-hypnotic or opioid medication may assist in subduing the intracranial response. A prolonged coughing episode is capable of causing a significant increase in intracranial pressure and deleterious effects for patients. Hypotension may occur due to bradycardia resulting from vagal stimulation or prolonged coughing, bucking, or straining during suctioning.

Mucosal irritations and trauma are common with frequent suctioning. The incidence and severity of trauma depend on the frequency of suctioning, technique, catheter design, absence of secretions, degree of direct mucosal contact, and amount of vacuum pressure applied. This may be exaggerated in the presence of anticoagulation, antiplatelet therapy, coagulopathy, thrombocytopenia, others. Significant bleeding may require bronchoscopic evaluation and possibly correction of coagulopathy or the changing of medication regimens. Another consideration in patients who have undergone lobectomy or pneumonectomy is the possibility of passing the suction catheter through the bronchial stump anastomosis. Catheter length and the depth of its passage are important consideration; close attention to the length of catheter passed is recommended. Blood in the secretions is usually the first sign of tissue trauma. Meticulous technique is essential to limit this complication. Airway reflexes can be irritated by direct mechanical stimulation.

Extremely vigorous cough, patient agitation, or a poorly secured ETT may result in accidental extubation. Extreme head turning side to side or hyperextension of the neck may also result in inadvertent extubation, particularly in younger patients. Wheezing resulting from bronchoconstriction can necessitate bronchodilator therapy.

Subglottic Care

Secretion management has, by necessity, moved beyond the ETT lumen. Suctioning of secretions that are pooled above the ETT cuff, in the subglottic space, is a crucial step in good tracheal care and is important for the prevention of VAP.[114-118] Subglottic suctioning has been shown to decrease the incidence of VAP in the ICU from 16% to 4%.[116] Specialized ETTs with dedicated subglottic suctioning ports are commercially available but are more expensive than a standard ETT (a 5- to15-fold difference in cost).[119] Despite this increased cost, the estimated cost benefit

of utilizing an ETT with a subglottic suction port may be substantial per case of VAP prevented.[119] The US Centers for Disease Control and Prevention (CDC) universally recommends the use of subglottic suctioning tubes in the ICU to help reduce the rate of VAP.[120] Subglottic suctioning can also be done with small suction catheters that are advanced down the trachea until resistance is met from the ETT cuff. ETTs with a subglottic suctioning port are certainly not infallible and do not replace vigilant airway care. It has been demonstrated that dysfunction of the suction lumen can occur almost 50% of the time.[121] In 43% of cases, the cause of the suction loss was determined to be prolapse of the tracheal mucosa into the subglottic suction port.[121]

Bronchoscopy

The use of FB for routine secretion management is not advocated. It is expensive, requires proficient training, and may produce complications such as barotrauma secondary to a marked reduction or cessation in expiratory airflow (depending on the relative airway caliber) in intubated patients. It should be reserved for assisting with lobar collapse caused by mucous plugging or inspissated secretions not amenable to conventional mucolysis, to perform so-called pulmonary toilet bronchoscopy that may be needed after an inhalation injury, to evaluate for tracheobronchial injury, to aid in the diagnosis of significant hemoptysis, or to assist with specimen procurement when clinical suspicion merits sampling. Again, patient care involving a DLT in the ICU must be meticulously approached with periodic surveillance bronchoscopy because of the smaller-caliber lumens combined with the underlying indication for the DLT (blood, secretions, etc.). Acute luminal obstruction can be catastrophic, in general, but particularly in the patient with limited cardiopulmonary reserve or one with difficult airway characteristics.

Biofilm Management

Biofilm and adherence of secretions (Fig. 44.27) within the ETT have been implicated in the development of VAP, increased WOB, delays in extubation, and other complications.[122-125] Biofilm can easily be identified by bronchoscopy, yet newer technologies using acoustic reflectometry have also been developed to help with monitoring the accumulation of biofilm and evaluating the integrity of the intubated airway. The SonarMed airway monitoring device (SonarMed, Indianapolis, IN) employs this technology to assess ETT positioning and movement as well as ETT patency.

Traditional methods used to manage biofilm include catheter suctioning, bronchoscopic lavage, and ETT exchange. Catheter suctioning is often ineffective for biofilm removal. Biofilm frequently evades detection because the suction catheter navigates the patent luminal channel formed by a single or multiple concretions, thereby leaving the impression that the lumen is patent. Bronchoscopic lavage and ETT exchange are hampered by significant costs, extended time employed during retrieval attempts, and hazards for both practitioners and patients. Another option is a device similar to a Fogarty catheter (which employs an inflatable cuff to remove a vascular thrombus) that essentially "scrapes" the biofilm from the luminal surface. The CAM (complete airway management) Rescue Cath (Omneotech, Tavernier, FL), among other products, has an inflatable balloon at the distal end of a catheter that is encased in a latticed netting to provide traction and atraumatic scraping of the ETT lumen (Fig. 44.28). It is introduced into the ETT and advanced to the distal end (based

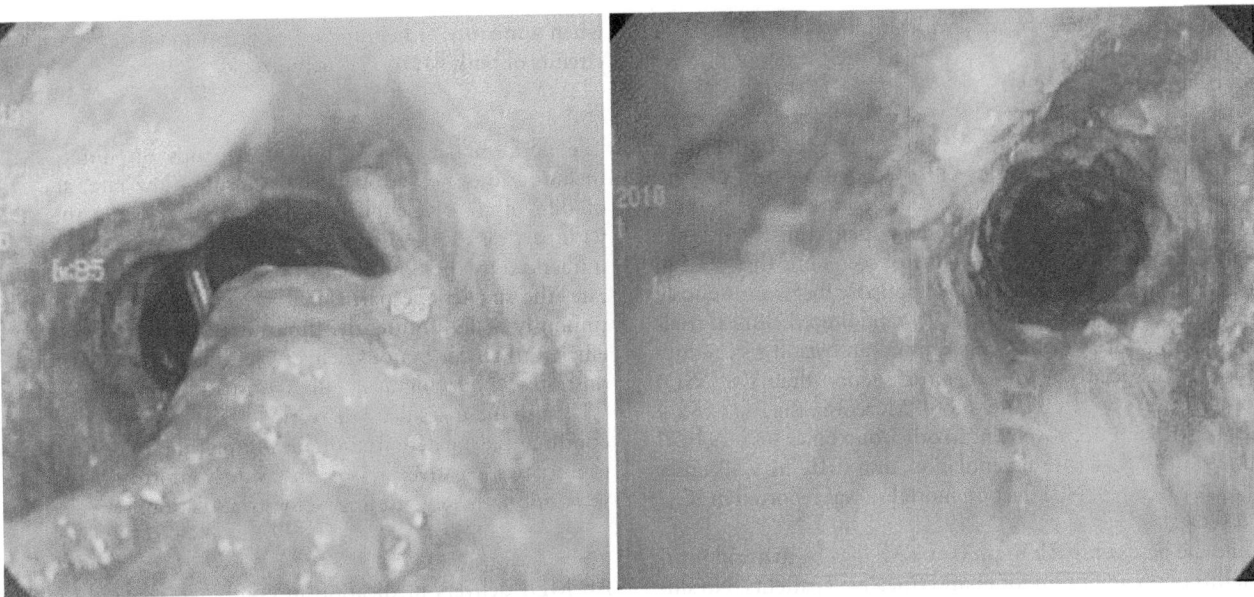

• **Fig. 44.27** Examples of biofilm accumulation inside the lumen of an endotracheal tube.

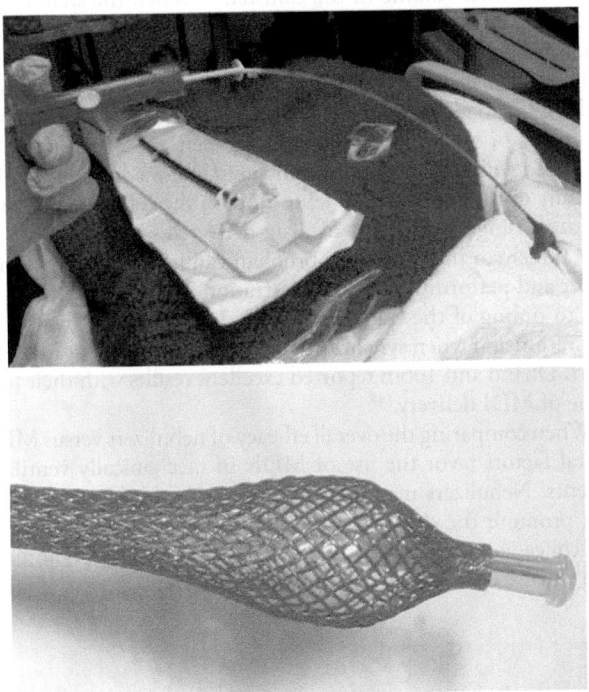

• **Fig. 44.28** The Omneotech CAM (Complete Airway Management) Rescue Cath. (Courtesy Omneotech, Tavernier, FL.)

on ETT and CAM depth markings); the balloon is then inflated, and the catheter is fully withdrawn from the ETT, bringing any luminal biofilm with it. This device and procedure may prove to be a useful option in already hypoxic or PEEP-dependent patients in whom time-consuming bronchoscopies could be hazardous. The CAM Rescue Cath is also a good option for patients with a potentially difficult airway, in whom ETT exchange can pose a considerable risk.[126]

Conflicting information exists on the prevention of biofilm formation. One study showed no difference in the rate of *Pseudomonas aeruginosa* and *Staphylococcus epidermidis* biofilm formation among different ETT materials including PVC, silicone, stainless steel, and sterling silver.[127] ETTs and tracheostomy tubes coated with various chemical or pharmaceutical substances (e.g., silver or chlorhexidine) may help reduce the rate of biofilm accumulation and its subsequent colonization.[128] The preventive management of biofilm may not be far in the future, but chlorhexidine-coated ETTs are currently not commercially available. For now, the best strategy to manage biofilm is increased vigilance, fastidious respiratory care, and new technologies that may alert the patient care team to its accumulation with the aim of biofilm minimization and safe clearance.

Prevention of Ventilator-Associated Pneumonia

VAP is categorized and defined as a pneumonia that develops more than 48 hours after tracheal intubation.[129] VAP is known to increase hospital length of stay and healthcare costs and is associated with significant morbidity and mortality. The pathogenesis of VAP is related to the numbers and virulence of microorganisms entering the lower respiratory tract and the response of the host. VAP may be caused by a wide variety of pathogens, can be polymicrobial, and may be due to multidrug-resistant pathogens. The main risk factor for VAP is the presence of an ETT, which bypasses the natural defense mechanisms of the upper respiratory tract by impairing mucociliary clearance and cough.[130–132] The diagnosis of VAP should be suspected in patients with new onset of fever, purulent sputum, leukocytosis, and worsening oxygenation. The primary route of infection of the lungs is through microaspiration of organisms that have colonized the oropharyngeal tract (or to a lesser extent the gastrointestinal tract). Even though the ETT cuff prevents gross aspiration of supra- and subglottic secretions, it cannot prevent microaspiration around the microfolds of the ETT cuff, a phenomenon that has been reproduced in studies using dye.[133]

The development of biofilm inside the ETT is another pathophysiological process that is known to cause VAP. This leads to microbial colonization and is protected against host defenses. Biofilm has formed as early as 48 hours after intubation.[131,134,135] As such, there is growing interest in the reduction of biofilm through construction of ETTs impregnated with antimicrobial agents.[136,137] The ability of such developments to affect the incidence of VAP has not been proven.[130]

Several ETT tube designs have been investigated to achieve reduction in the incidence of VAP, but none have been shown to provide a complete seal inside the tracheal lumen to prevent microaspiration.[138] One of the modified ETT designs includes a subglottic suction channel (EVAC tubes) placed just above the tracheal cuff that helps with suctioning of secretions that pool in the subglottic space. Suction can be applied either continuously or intermittently. A meta-analysis of 13 randomized clinical trials including a total of 2442 patients showed an overall risk reduction for VAP associated with subglottic suction drainage (SSD) (relative risk 0.50, 95% CI 0.46–0.66). Moreover, the use of SSD was associated with improvement in other outcomes such as ICU stay, duration of mechanical ventilation, and delay in VAP onset (2.7 days on average). No effect on mortality was reported in ICU and hospital stay.[18,139]

While the best approach to prevent VAP may be to avoid intubation, this is not an option for many critically ill patients. No single intervention by itself is known to reduce the incidence of VAP. Current evidence suggests a care bundle approach—a group of interventions that, when applied together, lead to better outcomes in prevention.[4] Some of these preventive strategies include maintenance of hygiene by healthcare personnel with frequent handwashing during patient care, elevation of head of the bed more than 15 degrees, daily spontaneous breathing trials to assess readiness for extubation, chlorhexidine oral wash to reduce colonization of microorganisms, the preferential use of postpyloric tube feeds, and the use of EVAC tubes if a patient requires mechanical ventilation for longer than 48 hours.

Respiratory Therapies for the Intubated Patient

Inhalation Therapy

The presence of an ETT does not limit drug delivery to the lungs and may enhance it. Many clinicians take advantage of this route of administration. The two predominant methods used to deliver agents are metered-dose inhalers (MDIs) and nebulizers. The drugs delivered by these devices are most commonly bronchodilators, mucolytics, corticosteroids, and antibiotics. For pulmonary conditions, inhaled drugs achieve efficacy comparable with or exceeding that of systemically delivered drugs with a smaller dose.[140–142] Tracheal administration of some traditionally systemic drugs often requires much higher doses to ensure absorption.

Inhalation drug delivery has other advantages over systemic administration. Because systemic absorption is markedly decreased, side effects can be reduced. Variable reports regarding penetration and distribution of an aerosol to the lower respiratory tract range from 0% to 42% with nebulizers and 0.3% to 98% with MDIs. However, when the delivery method was standardized, the amount delivered in either method was similar, about 15%.[143–145]

Particle size also plays an important role in delivery. The larger the particle, the less likely it is to be delivered down the tracheobronchial tree to the alveoli. Aerosol particles ranging between 1 and 5 μm are optimal for proper deposition.[140,141,144,146] The density of the gas carrying the aerosol also influences the delivery in an inverse relationship. Improvement in delivery has been reported

when a mixture of helium and oxygen was used in the ventilator circuits of both MDIs and nebulizers.[142,147]

Nebulizers

The performance of a nebulizer depends on multiple factors including the model, operating pressure, flow rate, and volume of diluent used. Nebulizers are capable of generating aerosols with particle sizes of 1 to 3 μm, and the size produced is inversely influenced by the flow rate or pressure used: The greater the flow rate, the smaller the particle.[140,141] Nebulizers may be used continuously or intermittently. Intermittent use appears to be more efficient than continuous delivery, with less waste of aerosol demonstrated.[148] Placing a nebulizer upstream from the Y-piece and ETT also increases drug delivery.[146,148,149] Interestingly, the use of continuous drug nebulization may impair the ability of the patient to initiate a negative-pressure inspiratory effort in the PS mode of ventilation, thereby leading to hypoventilation.[150]

Metered-Dose Inhalers

An MDI delivers medication in combination with a mixture of pressurized propellants, preservatives, flavoring agents, and surfactants. The final concentration of active drug constitutes about 1% of the total volume in the canister.[140] When the stem on the MDI canister is depressed, a fixed amount of drug is released at a certain velocity, and a spray cloud develops. Various adapters are available that fit in line with the ventilator circuit or on the end of the ETT to aid in the administration of inhalational therapies. Chambers or spacers appear to provide better delivery of aerosol compared with the more commonly used elbow adapters.[151] MDIs typically cause more aerosol deposition on the ETT than nebulizers, decreasing the amount of drug delivered. These particles, in turn, adhere to the ETT. This problem can be reduced by using a spacer and performing the administration with meticulous attention to timing of the ventilatory cycle: It is most effective during inspiration and when synchronized with the patient's spontaneous effort. Dhand and Tobin reported excellent results with their technique of MDI delivery.[148]

When comparing the overall efficacy of nebulizers versus MDIs, several factors favor the use of MDIs in mechanically ventilated patients. Nebulizers may become colonized with bacteria, which may promote the delivery of an aerosolized inoculum. Bowton and colleagues reported a potential saving of $300,000 annually with the use of MDIs compared with nebulizers.[152]

Chest Physiotherapy

Chest physiotherapy encompasses a variety of techniques for reducing the buildup of secretions that include position changes, percussion and vibration of the chest wall, and stimulation of a cough response. These are relatively dogmatic approaches that have historically provided poor results. They also tend to be burdensome to both the respiratory therapist and the patient. Newer, alternative techniques show promising results.

Percussion and Postural Drainage

Used extensively in patients with cystic fibrosis, the technique of percussion with postural drainage uses external percussion of the chest wall overlying the affected lung region. Percussion can be applied manually with a cupped hand or by an automated, usually pneumatic, device. The application of percussion, vibration, or both to the chest wall functions to loosen secretions in the bronchi and facilitate their mobilization.[153,154] A steep Trendelenburg position of 25 degrees or more may be employed (depending on patient tolerance) to facilitate the gravitational effects on mucus clearance.[155,156]

Relative contraindications to the postural component of this therapy include the presence of increased intracranial pressure; the possibility of an unprotected airway and the potential for aspiration; recent esophageal, ophthalmic, or intracranial surgery; congestive heart failure; and uncontrolled hypertension.[157] As for the application of percussion or vibration, placement of the technique over recent surgical sites or sites of injury (e.g., split-thickness skin grafts, rib fractures or chest trauma, pulmonary contusions, burns, unstable spine fractures) or in the presence of coagulopathies, subcutaneous emphysema, or bronchospasm are reasonable to be considered relative contraindications. Hazards include hypoxemia and accidental extubation.

Clinically and experimentally, the use of percussion with postural drainage in patients with cystic fibrosis is well supported.[158-161] However, patients' compliance remains a concern, because the technique is burdensome for patients and caregivers. Optional features for newer model ICU beds include positioning and percussive therapy.

Positive End-Expiratory Pressure Therapy

PEEP therapy, as a secretion-clearance technique, creates a restriction to expiratory flow by means of a face mask or mouthpiece. The resistance is adjusted to 10 to 20 cm H_2O of back pressure during expiration, which allows airflow to move into distal airways and associated lung units, forcing past secretions and causing them to move toward the larger airways, where suctioning is more feasible. The maneuver is used with gentle and forceful coughs lasting up to 20 minutes and aerosolized medications that can be administered concurrently. Patients with increased WOB or severe dyspnea may have difficulty performing this technique because of temporary lapses in ventilation. PEEP therapy is at least as effective for secretion clearance as percussion with postural drainage, if not more effective, and patient satisfaction is markedly more favorable.[107,162,163]

Intrapulmonary Percussive Ventilation

Intrapulmonary percussive ventilation (IPV) can be delivered through a mouthpiece or to the end of the ETT. Its high-frequency, percussive oscillations function to loosen retained secretions, expand airways and lungs, and reduce atelectasis. Conceptualized and designed by Dr. Forrest Bird, IPV uses a Phasitron—a sliding Venturi device capable of providing 5 to 35 cm H_2O pressure during oscillations of 2 to 5 Hz.[164] Aerosolized medications may also be delivered during IPV treatments. Favorable results have been reported for secretion clearance and lung expansion in patients with cystic fibrosis, as well as in other disorders with an increased incidence of thickened secretions.[165,166] IPV offers an advantage to patients who lack the ability to tolerate percussion with postural drainage or high PEEP therapies.

High-Frequency Chest Wall Compression

Therapy with high-frequency chest wall compression entails the wearing of an inflatable vest around the chest. Air is instilled into the vest bladder and then rapidly withdrawn in a cyclic manner, essentially creating an artificial cough. The high-frequency oscillations that are produced range from 5 to 25 Hz and can generate pressures as high as 50 cm H_2O. These oscillations create a gentle "squeezing" of the patient's chest that mimics small coughs. The frequency of the oscillations may be adjusted, and sensors in the vest can reduce the pressure delivered when the patient's chest expands (as with a sigh breath or a deep cough).[167] Secretion clearance and improvement in mucus rheology have also been reported, yet a key hurdle is the high investment cost for each unit.[168,169]

Conclusion

The establishment and maintenance of a secure and dependable airway are paramount in the care of the critically ill patient. From the very onset of admission to the ICU, care of the airway should begin with surveillance and a determination of which airways will be difficult to secure or difficult to maintain. The proper choice of an artificial airway not only facilitates ventilatory requirements for improved oxygenation but protects the patient from untoward iatrogenic problems encountered with instrumentation. Regardless of the intervention, unfettered vigilance is the key to improved outcomes. Proper ETT care, early performance of a tracheostomy (when indicated), frequent pulmonary hygiene, and the use of established protocols and proven preventive measures should help to ensure safe and successful outcomes in critically ill patients.

Selected References

16. Spiegel JE. Endotracheal tube cuffs: design and function. In: *Anesthesiology News Guide to Airway Management*. McMahon Publishing; 2010:51-58.
18. Muscedere J, Rewa O, McKechnie K, Jiang X, Laporta D, Heyland DK. Subglottic secretion drainage for the prevention of ventilator associated pneumonia: a systematic review and meta-analysis. *Crit Care Med*. 2011;39(8):1985-1991.
31. Chastre J, Fagon JY. Ventilator-associated pneumonia. *Am J Respir Crit Care Med*. 2002;165:867-903.
34. Mort TC. Emergency tracheal intubation: complications associated with repeated laryngoscopic attempts. *Anesth Analg*. 2004;99:607-613.
38. Altman KW, Yu G, Schaefer SD. Consequence of dysphagia in the hospitalized patient: impact on prognosis and hospital resources. *Arch Otolaryngol Head Neck Surg*. 2010;136(8):784–789.
39. Epstein SK. Late complications of tracheostomy. *Resp Care*. 2005;50:542-529.
40. Durbin CG. Early complications of tracheostomy. *Resp Care*. 2005;50 (4):511-515.
42. Vyas D, Inweregbu K, Pittard A. Measurement of tracheal tube cuff pressure in critical care. *Anaesthesia*. 2002;57(3):275-277.
76. Berra L, De Marchi L, Panigada M, et al. Evaluation of continuous aspiration of subglottic secretion in an in vivo study. *Crit Care Med*. 2004;32:2071-2078.
77. Dezfulian C, Shojania K, Collard HR, et al. Subglottic secretion drainage for preventing ventilator-associated pneumonia: a meta-analysis. *Am J Med*. 2005;118:11-18.
84. Hoffman RJ, Parwani V, Hahn IH. Experienced emergency medicine physicians cannot inflate or estimate endotracheal tube cuff pressure using standard techniques. *Am J Emerg Med*. 2006;24:139-143.
85. Sengupta P, Sessler DI, Maglinger P, et al. Endotracheal tube cuff pressure in three hospitals and the volume required to produce appropriate cuff pressure. *BMC Anesthesiol*. 2004;4(1):8.

All references can be found online at eBooks.Health.Elsevier.com.

45

Mechanical Ventilation

REEBA MATHEW, MARK T. WARNER, AND BELA PATEL

CHAPTER OUTLINE

KEY POINTS

- The indications for mechanical ventilation include hypoxemic and hypercapnic respiratory failure, altered mentation with patient inability to protect the airway, hemodynamic instability, and maintenance of adequate oxygenation and ventilation during deep sedation, general anesthesia, or neuromuscular blockade.
- Positive end-expiratory pressure (PEEP) improves oxygenation in patients with hypoxemic respiratory failure, optimizes alveolar recruitment, and decreases cycles of recruitment and derecruitment of alveolar lung units.
- Assist-control ventilation (ACV) can be volume-targeted upon initiation of mechanical ventilation or pressure-targeted when increased oxygenation is required and there is concern about increasing airway pressures.
- A lung protective strategy should be employed in all patients with acute respiratory distress syndrome (ARDS). Using low tidal volumes of 6 mL/kg predicted body weight with plateau pressures of 30 cm H_2O or less has become the standard of care for patients with ARDS.
- Synchronized intermittent mandatory ventilation (SIMV) incorporates some characteristics of ACV and pressure support ventilation (PSV). The purpose of the two types of breaths (mandatory and spontaneous) is to allow increased diaphragmatic activity and increased work of breathing with patient-triggered spontaneous breaths.
- Airway pressure release ventilation (APRV) uses high and low pressures to aid in recruitment of atelectatic lung units and allows spontaneous breathing. It can decrease airway pressures and improve alveolar recruitment oxygenation, and cardiac output.
- High-frequency ventilation improves oxygenation by providing oxygen-rich and CO_2-poor gas that rapidly mixes with sinusoidal flow at stroke volumes that approximate anatomic dead space. Each type of high-frequency ventilation—high-frequency jet ventilation (HFJV), high-frequency oscillatory ventilation (HFOV), and high-frequency percussive ventilation (HFPV)—has its subtleties and specific indications.
- Noninvasive positive-pressure ventilation (NIPPV) is useful in many situations, including exacerbations of chronic obstructive pulmonary disease (COPD), cardiogenic pulmonary edema, and in other select patient groups.
- During weaning from mechanical ventilation, daily interruption of sedation (unless contraindicated by severe hypoxemia or the need for neuromuscular blockade) and daily trials of spontaneous breathing should be employed for all patients.

Introduction

Breathing is normally an automatic process during which inspiration is active and expiration is passive. The typical normal human undergoes negative pressure breathing wherein elevation of the rib cage and flattening of the diaphragm create a negative intrathoracic pressure, and this facilitates movement of air into the lungs. Following this, relaxation of the diaphragm and other respiratory muscles allow for exhalation. The lung performs two principal functions: oxygenation of the blood through diffusion of oxygen across the alveolar-capillary membrane and exhalation of CO_2 that has diffused out of the serum and into the lungs. When either or both of these functions are decompensated relative to a patient's physiologic needs, the patient is considered to be in respiratory failure. The primary means of supporting a patient in respiratory failure is with a mechanical ventilator. This chapter will discuss the use of both invasive and noninvasive mechanical ventilation. Mechanical ventilation is frequently used to provide respiratory support in times of critical illness or in patients undergoing general anesthesia. The main goals of mechanical ventilation include (1) augmentation of oxygenation utilizing the ability to increase the fraction of inspired oxygen (Fio_2) that is delivered, adding positive end-expiratory pressure (PEEP), and changing inspiratory time, and (2) CO_2 elimination, which is ensured by maintaining an adequate minute ventilation. Minute ventilation is the product of tidal volume and respiratory rate.

Significant advances in positive-pressure ventilation have occurred since Fell and O'Dwyer designed the foot-pump ventilation apparatus in 1888. Although mechanical ventilation can be lifesaving, it can injure the lungs. Therefore, safe application of mechanical ventilation to limit ventilator-induced lung injury (VILI) and negative interactions with other organ systems is fundamental in managing patients who require mechanical ventilatory support. This chapter reviews different modes of mechanical ventilation and describes their characteristics, attributes, and shortcomings.

Esteban and colleagues reviewed the use of mechanical ventilation in intensive care units (ICUs) in North America, South America, Spain, and Portugal. Among the indications for mechanical ventilation, acute respiratory failure was the most common (66%), followed by coma (15%), exacerbation of chronic obstructive pulmonary disease (COPD) (13%), and neuromuscular weakness (5%). The principal causes of acute respiratory failure across all centers were pneumonia (16%), sepsis (16%), postoperative infection (15%), heart failure (12%), acute respiratory distress syndrome (ARDS) (12%), trauma (12%), unspecified causes (13%), and aspiration (3%). Endotracheal tubes (ETTs) were used three times more often than tracheostomies to provide artificial airways. There was some variability in the modes of ventilation used in the different countries participating in the study. Assist-control ventilation (ACV) was the most common worldwide, followed by synchronized intermittent mandatory ventilation (SIMV) and pressure support ventilation (PSV). However, in North American ICUs, ACV and SIMV were used equally.[1]

Prior to a discussion on noninvasive and invasive mechanical ventilation, which by convention implies positive-pressure ventilation (PPV), a basic understanding of negative-pressure ventilation is essential, especially in view of the interest in negative-pressure ventilators in the context of resource utilization in a pandemic. Negative-pressure ventilators were the first form of ventilation used in the early to mid-20th century with the first

clinical application by Drinker and McKhann in 1928 in a child with poliomyelitis.[2] The apparatus, essentially a tank around the patient's body with the head protruding out, subsequently came to be known as the "iron lung." Use of the iron lung became more prevalent during the polio epidemic in the 1950s. Negative-pressure ventilators work by applying subatmospheric pressure to the chest wall, causing lung expansion and air entry into lungs—hence simulating normal physiologic negative pressure with inspiration. It can be used in continuous negative, intermittent negative, or biphasic modes. Patients are able to breathe spontaneously, and an endotracheal or oronasal interface is not needed. A physiotherapy mode can be used that adds oscillation and secretion clearance functions. Despite the theoretic benefit of simulating natural respiration by virtue of negative pressure, use of the iron lung was limited due to size and weight considerations and impaired access to the patient, leading to a pivotal change in the 1960s with development of PPV. There have, however, been advances over the years with development of smaller negative-pressure ventilators such as the cuirass. Current use of negative-pressure ventilation with the chest cuirass is infrequent, with use limited to pediatric patients and the outpatient management of neuromuscular disease, chest-wall disorders, and central hypoventilation syndrome.[3–5]

Noninvasive Ventilation

Mechanical ventilation can be delivered to the patient by invasive or noninvasive methods. Noninvasive positive-pressure ventilation (NIPPV) is delivered by an external nasal or oronasal interface such as a face mask. The decision to use invasive or noninvasive mechanical ventilation depends on the severity and the anticipated timing of the reversibility of the underlying condition and the mental status of the patient. Using NIPPV in the setting of respiratory failure, either hypoxemic or hypercapnic, is generally considered for patients who have a condition in which there is the potential to rapidly improve the decompensated physiologic variables. (The use of NIPPV in the ambulatory setting for obstructive and central sleep apnea will be discussed separately.) The mechanics of NIPPV involve the application of positive pressure to the nasopharynx or oropharynx, which splints open the airway, and its transmission downstream to the lungs, where it increases lung volume. Several cardiovascular effects are seen with NIPPV, including increased intrathoracic pressure, decreased venous return, and decreased left ventricular afterload, which in combination have varying effects on cardiac output depending on the patient's underlying physiology. Fig. 45.1 details the interaction of the effects of NIPPV on the cardiopulmonary system.

Patient selection is paramount in the decision to initiate NIPPV. NIPPV is not recommended for patients with upper airway obstruction, cardiac arrest, hemodynamic instability, respiratory arrest, injury to the face, massive gastrointestinal bleeding, a high risk of aspiration, significantly depressed mentation, or an inability to clear secretions (Table 45.1).[6–8] Proper patient selection includes ensuring that the goals of using mechanical ventilation are being accomplished with the application of NIPPV—namely, improvement in the patient's level of consciousness, improvement or maintenance of hemodynamic stability, and objective evidence of improved gas exchange. NIPPV can be delivered using a standard ventilator through a face mask, nasal mask, or nasal plugs. Heated humidification of the delivered gas may improve the patient's comfort.[9] Common modes of ventilation used to deliver NIPPV are continuous positive airway pressure (CPAP), bi-level

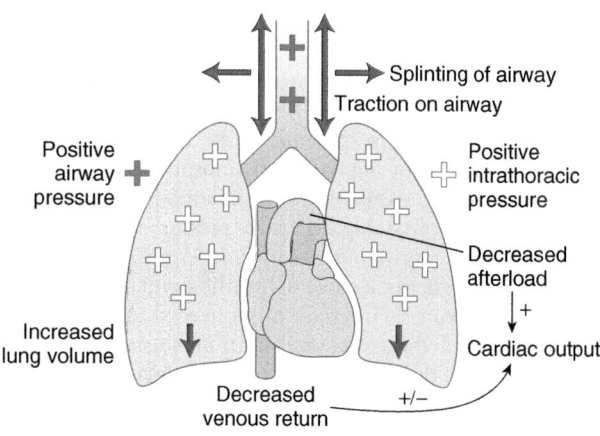

• **Fig. 45.1** Physiologic effects of positive airway pressure. (Adapted from Antonescu-Turcu A, Parthasarathy S. CPAP and bi-level PAP therapy: new and established roles. *Respir Care*. 2010;55:1216–1228.)

TABLE 45.1	Factors for Success or Failure of Noninvasive Positive-Pressure Ventilation	
Success	**Failure**	
High Paco₂ with low A-a gradient	High APACHE score	
Improvement in pH, Paco₂, and decreased respiratory rate after 1 hour of NIPPV	Pneumonia on chest radiograph	
	Copious secretions	
	Edentulousness	
Good level of consciousness	Poor nutrition status	
	Confusion or delirium	

A-a, Alveolar to arterial; *APACHE*, Acute Physiology and Chronic Health Evaluation; *PaCO₂*, arterial partial pressure of carbon dioxide; *NIPPV*, noninvasive positive-pressure ventilation.

positive airway pressure (BPAP), PSV, proportional assist ventilation (PAV), and ACV. Differences in airway pressures, flow, and tidal volume among different modes of NIPPV are illustrated in Fig. 45.2. Modes of NIPPV are selected based on patient characteristics. For example, patients who require greater support in reducing the work of breathing should be placed on ACV mode, whereas patient-ventilator dyssynchrony may be improved with PSV.[10] No difference in mortality rates among these modalities for various disease states has been demonstrated.[11–14] The patient

should be monitored very closely after initiation of NIPPV. If prompt improvement is not evident within 1 or 2 hours, the clinician should proceed to intubation and invasive mechanical ventilation.[15] In a prospective multicenter cohort study, NIPPV failed in 30% of patients, requiring intubation. The highest intubation rates occurred in patients with ARDS or community-acquired pneumonia (50%), and the lowest rates were for those with pulmonary contusion (18%) or cardiogenic pulmonary edema (10%).[16]

NIPPV improves mortality rates and length of stay for patients with severe COPD exacerbations.[17] A meta-analysis of patients with severe and mild COPD exacerbations demonstrated no mortality benefit for the patients with mild COPD exacerbations.[18] In cases of cardiogenic pulmonary edema, NIPPV decreases the rate of intubation, but the mortality benefit is uncertain because of conflicting study results.[19,20] NIPPV use in postextubation failure has been studied; if used immediately on extubation in patients with hypercapnia during a spontaneous breathing trial, NIPPV may prevent reintubation and is associated with a reduction in mortality rates.[21] NIPPV use in patients after the development of postextubation failure did not reduce reintubation rates and increased mortality rates, with a longer median time from extubation failure to reintubation in the NIPPV group.[22] The American Thoracic Society/European Respiratory Society (ATS/ERS) practice guidelines on NIPPV use in acute respiratory failure are as follows: NIPPV is strongly recommended in exacerbations of COPD with hypercapnia[18, 23–25] and cardiogenic pulmonary edema[26–28] and may be considered in acute respiratory failure in the postoperative setting and in chest trauma patients. Other recommendations with some evidence for NIPPV use include acute respiratory failure in immunocompromised patients, weaning from invasive mechanical ventilation in hypercapnic respiratory failure, and to prevent postextubation respiratory failure in high-risk patients. NIPPV should not be used to treat established postextubation respiratory failure. Hence in patients with severe COPD exacerbations and cardiogenic pulmonary edema, NIPPV should be attempted if no contraindications exist. In other causes of respiratory failure, NIPPV may be considered if the patient does not meet the criteria for intubation and invasive mechanical ventilation. However, if the patient does not stabilize in the first 2 hours, management should rapidly progress to intubation and invasive mechanical ventilation.

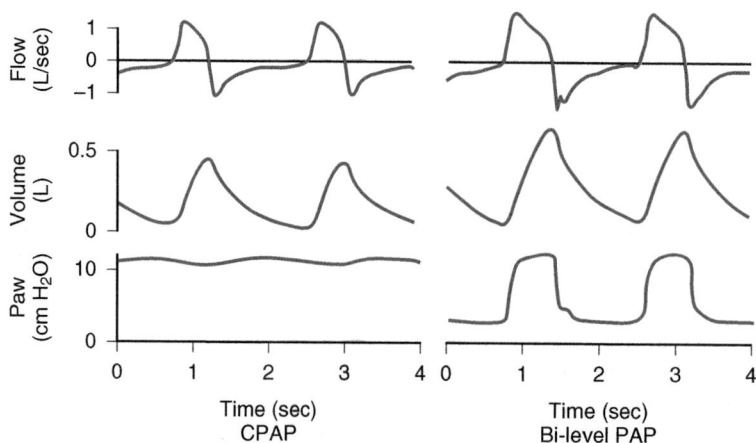

• **Fig. 45.2** Airflow, volume, and airway pressure (Paw) versus time tracings for continuous positive airway pressure (CPAP) and bi-level positive airway pressure (Bi-level PAP). (From Antonescu-Turcu A, Parthasarathy S. CPAP and bi-level PAP therapy: new and established roles. *Respir Care*. 2010;55:1216–1228.)

NIPPV is used in ambulatory and inpatient settings for obstructive and central sleep apnea. Positive airway pressure (PAP) therapy has been well-established in the treatment of sleep-disordered breathing.[29] CPAP is used for obstructive sleep apnea, whereas BPAP is frequently used for obstructive sleep apnea with alveolar hypoventilation.[30] Other modes used in the ambulatory setting include auto-titrating positive airway pressure (APAP), adaptive servo-ventilation (ASV), average volume-assured pressure support (AVAPS), and neurally adjusted ventilator assist (NAVA).[31,32] All of these modes seek to both improve patient-ventilator synchrony and ensure adequate minute ventilation in times of sleep to reverse physiologic abnormalities.

Invasive Mechanical Ventilation

To initiate invasive mechanical ventilation, the patient must have in place an artificial airway to interface with the mechanical ventilator. Various types of airway devices are discussed in other chapters of this textbook. Patients are most frequently connected to a mechanical ventilator with an ETT (orotracheal or nasotracheal) or a tracheostomy.

Common reasons for insertion of an artificial airway are to maintain airway patency, to prevent aspiration, to facilitate clearance of secretions, and to allow mechanical ventilatory support.[33] There are several indications for mechanical ventilation: hypoxemic respiratory failure, hypercapnic respiratory failure, mixed respiratory failure, altered mentation with inability by the patient to protect the airway, hemodynamic instability, and maintenance of adequate oxygenation and ventilation during deep sedation, general anesthesia, or neuromuscular blockade. Hypoxemic respiratory failure, defined as a failure to maintain a arterial oxygen tension (Pa_{O_2}) greater than 60 mm Hg with a Fi_{O_2} of 60% or more, can generally be treated with application of high-flow oxygen by nasal cannula. However, if the disease process causing hypoxemia is severe pneumonia, acute pneumothorax, progressive noncardiogenic pulmonary edema, or other situations where NIPPV would be contraindicated, the patient would meet criteria for invasive mechanical ventilation. In hypercapnic respiratory failure, defined as an arterial carbon dioxide tension (Pa_{CO_2}) greater than 50 mm Hg with a concomitant pH less than 7.30, lack of improvement in mental status or Pa_{CO_2} levels with application of NIPPV would be indication for invasive mechanical ventilation. Other situations that are relative contraindications for NIPPV include recent upper gastrointestinal surgery, a high risk for aspiration, facial trauma, burns or surgery to upper airway and face, or fixed airway obstruction. Patients with these conditions who require mechanical ventilatory support will usually require invasive mechanical ventilation.[34,35]

The choice of airway device depends on the anatomic considerations of the patient as well as the urgency of the situation. NIPPV can be applied through a nasal or oronasal mask and may be appropriate in some settings. ETTs and tracheostomies are more secure airways and are employed with invasive mechanical ventilation. Nasotracheal tubes may be used in airway emergencies, including trauma, burns, and angioedema, or for specific surgeries. Laryngeal mask airways (LMAs) and other supraglottic airways (SGAs) should be considered unsecure airways and are not used in an ICU setting.

Characteristics of Mechanical Ventilation

After the decision to initiate invasive positive-pressure mechanical ventilation, several variables must be considered for effective implementation. They include tidal volume, respiratory rate, PEEP, Fi_{O_2}, peak pressure, plateau pressure, driving pressure, trigger sensitivity, flow rate, and flow pattern.

Tidal Volume

Tidal volume is the volume of air delivered to the lungs with each breath by the mechanical ventilator. Historically, initial tidal volumes were set at 10 to 15 mL/kg actual body weight and delivered to patients with neuromuscular diseases receiving mechanical ventilation. Over the past two decades, studies have shown that excessive tidal volumes can lead to VILI as a result of alveolar overdistention.[36,37] The mechanism of lung injury includes regional overinflation, stress of repeated opening and closing of lung units, and sheer stress between adjacent structures with differing mechanical properties.[38–41]

A low tidal volume strategy, which uses 6 mL/kg predicted body weight, has become the standard of care for patients with ARDS, following the Acute Respiratory Distress Syndrome Network (ARDS Network) publication in 2000.[42] The ARDS Network prospectively studied intubated patients with acute lung injury (ALI) or ARDS to determine whether a low tidal volume strategy, using a tidal volume of 6 mL/kg predicted body weight and plateau pressures of 30 cm H_2O or less, compared with a traditional tidal volume strategy, using a tidal volume of 12 mL/kg predicted body weight and plateau pressures of 50 cm H_2O or less, could improve mortality and decrease ventilator days. The final analysis showed a 23% reduction in all-cause mortality and a 9% absolute decrease in mortality with the use of a low tidal volume strategy. Low tidal volume ventilation, also known as lung protective ventilation, is now recommended for all patients with ARDS. In patients without ARDS, a retrospective review demonstrated an association between ALI and the use of tidal volumes greater than 10 mL/kg predicted body weight.[43] Considering the current evidence, tidal volumes greater than 10 mL/kg predicted body weight should not be routinely used in the care of the mechanically ventilated patient.

Respiratory Rate

The respiratory rate during mechanical ventilation depends on the desired minute ventilation. Minute ventilation is a product of the respiratory rate and the tidal volume and is expressed in liters per minute. After a patient is intubated and placed on a mechanical ventilator, adequate minute ventilation must be ensured because the underlying pathophysiology or pharmacologic interventions can suppress a patient's ability to compensate for metabolic demands. In many scenarios, the rate is determined by observing the patient's native respiratory rate before intubation. A normal minute ventilation is 5 to 7 L/min. In patients with sepsis or diabetic ketoacidosis, the native minute ventilation may be as high as 12 to 15 L/min, requiring a higher respiratory rate. To adequately compensate for the acid-base derangements and ensure adequate minute ventilation, it is necessary to titrate the set respiratory rate until the desired pH and Pa_{CO_2} goals are met. Permissive hypercapnia (i.e., allowing the Pa_{CO_2} to increase intentionally to achieve other goals) may be appropriate in certain clinical conditions, such as in ARDS. Auto-PEEP (intrinsic PEEP) must be measured to ensure it remains less than 5 cm H_2O. After the goal is achieved, it is safe practice to set the respiratory rate at 4 breaths per minute below the spontaneous breathing rate in the event that intrinsic or extrinsic factors suppress respiration. In patients on SIMV, the respiratory rate is initially set to meet up to 80% of the minute ventilation demands.

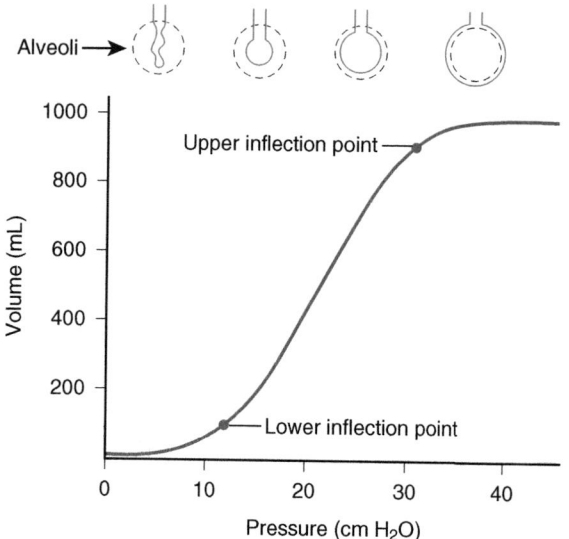

• **Fig. 45.3** Calculation of optimal positive end-expiratory pressure (PEEP). Mechanical ventilation delivers low levels of PEEP to keep unstable alveoli from collapse at end expiration. The volume-pressure curve can be used to assess changes in lung compliance and to determine a ventilation strategy by identifying the lower inflection point, which is the critical opening pressure of collapsed alveoli, and the upper inflection point, which indicates a state of lung overinflation. (From Haitsma JJ. Physiology of mechanical ventilation. *Crit Care Clin.* 2007;23:117–134.)

Initial respiratory rates are usually 12 to 16 breaths per minute, but respiratory rates in the high 20s to low 30s may be required in patients with ARDS. In those with obstructive lung disease (e.g., asthma), a lower respiratory rate is desired because of the significant risk of auto-PEEP. (Assessment and management of auto-PEEP are discussed later). In general, respiratory rates up to 35 breaths per minute may be safely delivered as long as one is diligent to observe for development of auto-PEEP, but rates higher than this should not routinely be used. It is prudent to use the lowest respiratory rate that is effective for the patient.

Positive End-Expiratory Pressure

PEEP is the alveolar pressure above atmospheric pressure at end-expiration. PEEP applied using a mechanical ventilator is known as applied PEEP or extrinsic PEEP and maintains positive pressure at the end of expiration to keep unstable lung units from collapsing.[44] PEEP increases the peak inspiratory pressure, which directly overcomes the opening pressure of the unstable lung units. Low levels of PEEP (3 to 5 cm H_2O) are routinely used in patients on mechanical ventilation. It can decrease alveolar collapse at end-expiration and may reduce the incidence of ventilator-associated pneumonia (VAP).[45] Higher levels of PEEP are employed to improve oxygenation in patients with hypoxemic respiratory failure. Goals in managing ARDS are to optimize alveolar recruitment and decrease cycles of recruitment and derecruitment of alveolar lung units. Several strategies are used to determine optimal PEEP, but there are limited data to support their routine use. Determining the lower inflection point of the pressure-volume curve (P_{flex}), which reflects the transition from low to higher compliance, and applying PEEP of 2 cm H_2O greater than this point may be used to estimate the appropriate level of applied PEEP (Fig. 45.3).[46]

As it is often impractical to routinely obtain pressure-volume curves, algorithms have been developed (e.g., in ARDS Network trials) with FiO_2 and PEEP combinations to achieve adequate oxygenation (Pao$_2$ 55- to 80 mm Hg or SpO$_2$ 88%- to 95%) (Table 45.2).[42,47] Measuring esophageal pressure to estimate transpulmonary pressure has been studied as a method to determine the appropriate applied PEEP in patients with ARDS, and this approach has demonstrated improvement in oxygenation and pulmonary compliance.[48] Trials of increasing or decreasing PEEP can also be used.[49,50] Higher levels of PEEP in postoperative patients have been shown to confer no additional benefit.[51]

The etiology of VILI in patients with hypoxemic respiratory failure is heterogeneous. Because the collapse and repeated opening and closing of unstable lung units leads to further injury, its prevention would be the optimal ventilator strategy. High PEEP have been used to mitigate alveolar collapse and cyclic alveolar stress. Several trials demonstrated that high PEEP increases

TABLE 45.2	Combinations of Positive End-Expiratory Pressure and FiO_2 Used in the Acute Respiratory Distress Syndrome Network Trials												
Component	**Allowable Combinations of PEEP and FiO_2[a]**												
Lower-PEEP Group													
FiO_2	0.3	0.4	0.4	0.5	0.5	0.6	0.7	0.7	0.7	0.8	0.9	0.9	0.9	1.0
PEEP	5	5	8	8	10	10	10	12	14	14	14	16	18	18–24
Higher-PEEP Group[b]													
FiO_2	0.3	0.3	0.3	0.3	0.3	0.4	0.4	0.5	0.5	0.5–0.8	0.8	0.9	1.0
PEEP	5	8	10	12	14	14	16	16	18	20	22	22	22–24
Higher-PEEP Group[c]													
FiO_2	0.3	0.3	0.4	0.4	0.5	0.5	0.5–0.8	0.8	0.9	1.0			
PEEP	12	14	14	16	16	18	20	22	22	22–24			

[a]Combinations of positive end-expiratory pressure (PEEP in cm H_2O) and fraction of inspired oxygen (FiO_2) used in the acute respiratory distress syndrome (ARDS) network trials.
[b]Before the protocol changed to use higher levels of PEEP.
[c]After the protocol changed to use higher levels of PEEP.

(Adapted from National Heart, Lung, and Blood Institute ARDS Clinical Trials Network. Higher versus lower positive end-expiratory pressures in patients with the acute respiratory distress syndrome. *N Engl J Med.* 2004;351:327–336.)

oxygenation but does not improve mortality rates.[47,52] However, a meta-analysis of high PEEP trials indicated a mortality benefit for patients with a PaO_2/FiO_2 ratio of less than 200.[53] The ideal method for determining optimal PEEP has not been established.[44] Trials in ARDS patients have demonstrated that PEEP requirements in this cohort are usually between 12 and 20 cm H_2O.

Fraction of Inspired Oxygen

On initiation of mechanical ventilation, the FiO_2 is usually set at 1.0. The goal is to rapidly reduce the FiO_2 to the target PaO_2 and SpO_2 to limit the consequences of excessive supplemental oxygen. In most patients, a target PaO_2 of 60 mm Hg and SpO_2 of 90% meets oxygenation requirements. However, some patients may have higher PaO_2 or SpO_2 targets based on their underlying cardiopulmonary status (e.g., myocardial ischemia or pulmonary hypertension) and in conditions such as acute stroke, cluster headaches, pregnancy, sickle cell crisis, carbon monoxide toxicity, air embolism, and pneumothorax. In patients with ARDS, targeting a PaO_2 as low as 50 mm Hg may be appropriate to limit alveolar injury.[54] A prolonged high level of FiO_2 has been associated with airway and parenchymal injury, atelectasis from nitrogen washout (absorption atelectasis), and an increased risk of diffuse alveolar damage, which is even higher in patients receiving bleomycin therapy.[55,56] If the need for supplemental FiO_2 remains greater than 0.6, FiO_2 should be reduced with strategies such as applied PEEP, prone positioning, and alternative ventilator modes.

Peak Pressure

Peak airway pressure is a measurement of the maximum pressure subjected to the airway during inspiration. In the anesthetized or calm patient, peak airway pressure depends on the respiratory rate, tidal volume, and inspiratory flow rate in volume-targeted modes of mechanical ventilation. When awake and active, a patient's effort contributes to the peak airway pressure. In pressure-targeted ventilator modes, the peak pressure is directly related to the inspiratory pressure that is set and the inspiratory flow rate.[57] Studies have not consistently shown barotrauma to be an adverse consequence of increased peak pressures.[58,59] Peak airway pressure typically is higher than the plateau pressure, and the difference indicates airway resistance.

Plateau Pressure

Plateau pressure is the pressure applied by the mechanical ventilator to the small airways and alveoli. The plateau pressure is measured at end-inspiration with an inspiratory hold maneuver on the mechanical ventilator of 0.5 to 1 second in duration. A meta-analysis demonstrated a significant correlation between plateau pressures greater than 35 cm H_2O and the risk of barotrauma.[60] In the ARDS Network trial, lower tidal volume ventilation with plateau pressures less than 30 cm H_2O was associated with a lower mortality rate than that for conventional tidal volumes using plateau pressures less than 50 cm H_2O.[42]

Common reasons for increased plateau pressures are the use of high PEEP, high inspiratory flow, and high tidal volumes. Adverse consequences of high plateau pressures are barotrauma resulting in VILI, pneumothorax, pneumomediastinum, and subcutaneous emphysema. If barotrauma develops, it may be beneficial to reduce plateau pressures further by decreasing the tidal volume, PEEP, or inspiratory flow or by deepening the patient's level of sedation.

Driving Pressure

Driving pressure is calculated as the difference between plateau pressure and applied PEEP. Described differently, it is the ratio of tidal volume to the compliance of the respiratory system; this is used to determine functional lung size, which can be more individualized to the patient than adjusted body weight. Driving pressure has been described as a potential marker of recruitable lung and also as a factor that could predict increased ventilator-associated mortality in ARDS. In a study by Amato and colleagues, driving pressure was derived from data pooled from previous studies and was a variable shown to independently be associated with survival; an increase in driving pressure of as little as 7 cm H_2O was associated with a 1.41 relative risk for increased mortality.[61] Higher driving pressure has also been shown to be associated with increased mortality in other studies, and a maximum driving pressure of 20 cm H_2O has been suggested.[62–64] Despite evidence of driving pressure being a marker of mortality, current guidelines are still cautious about accepting it independently from PEEP and tidal volume.[65]

Trigger Sensitivity

Sensors on the ventilator detect a patient's effort in terms of negative inspiratory pressure applied to the circuit or inspiratory flow of air generated by the patient. This is referred to as triggering the ventilator or triggering a breath. Pressure trigger sensitivity typically is set between –1 and –3 cm H_2O, and a breath is triggered when a negative inspiratory effort is greater than the set sensitivity. A flow-triggered breath is delivered when the ventilator senses the patient's effort by detection of a change in the flow through the ventilator circuit; flow-trigger sensitivity is typically set at 2 L/min. When the patient does not provide adequate negative inspiratory pressure or flow rate to trigger breaths, the ventilator provides mandatory breaths to the patient at the set parameters. The breaths are initiated by the ventilator at the set time, as determined by the set respiratory rate, and it delivers the breath at the prescribed flow rate until the desired tidal volume has been achieved, after which the ventilator cycles off for passive exhalation.

Flow Rate

Flow rate, or peak inspiratory flow rate, is the maximum flow at which a set tidal volume breath is delivered by the ventilator. Most modern ventilators can deliver flow rates between 60 and 120 L/min. Flow rates should be titrated to meet the patient's inspiratory demands.[66] If the peak flow rate is too low for the patient, dyspnea, patient-ventilator dyssynchrony, and increased work of breathing may result. High peak flow rates increase peak airway pressures and lower mean airway pressures, which may decrease oxygenation.[57] In most patients, peak flow rates of 60 L/min are adequate. Higher flow rates are required in patients with higher ventilator demands. Higher peak flow rates may also be necessary in patients with obstructive lung disease to decrease inspiratory time, thereby increasing the expiratory time and reducing the risk of development of auto-PEEP.[66–68]

Flow Pattern

Modern mechanical ventilators can deliver various inspiratory flow patterns. A constant (or square wave) flow pattern represents inspiratory flow delivered by the mechanical ventilator during volume-cycled modes of ventilation. In this pattern, inspiratory flow remains constant until the desired tidal volume is delivered, which is held until expiration. In this pattern of inspiratory flow, the airway pressure varies and depends on the patient's effort and compliance of the lung. A sinusoidal wave pattern is characterized by gradually increasing and decreasing inspiratory flow throughout the respiratory cycle. In a decelerating ramp wave pattern, the flow rate begins maximally and decreases until the end of inspiration. It parallels the normal inspiratory pattern most closely. The ramp wave yields the most homogeneous distribution of ventilation in most conditions, decreases peak airway pressures, improves work of breathing, and decreases dead-space ventilation.[69] For patients who are triggering the ventilator, this strategy of ventilation is recommended (Fig. 45.4).

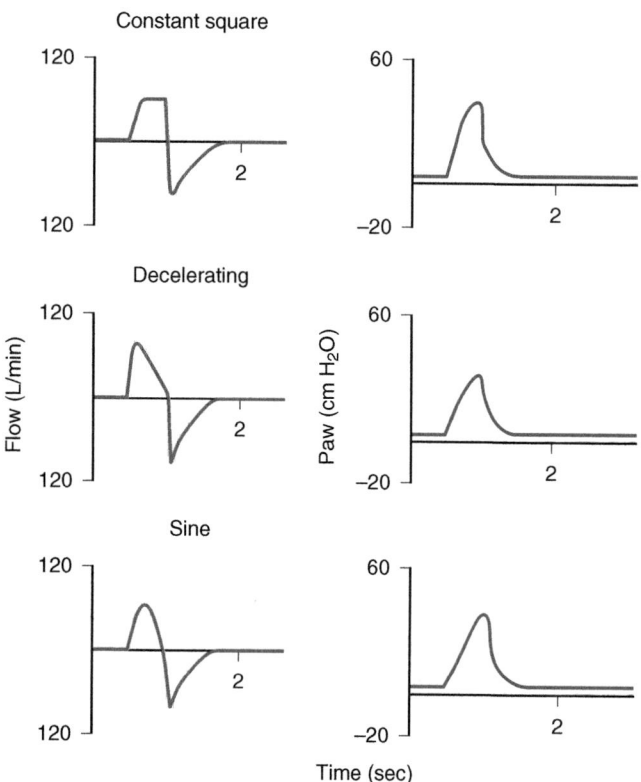

• **Fig. 45.4** The three most common inspiratory flow patterns for mechanical ventilation *(left)* are compared with their corresponding pressure versus time curves *(right)*. (From Yang SC, Yang SP. Effects of inspiratory flow waveforms on lung mechanics, gas exchange and respiratory metabolism in COPD patients during mechanical ventilation. *Chest.* 2002;122:2096–2104.)

Common Modes of Mechanical Ventilation

The three most commonly used modes of mechanical ventilation are ACV, SIMV, and PSV. Each mode determines whether breaths are volume constant or pressure constant, which breaths are mandatory or spontaneous or both, and which variables determine a change in function. All three modes have uses throughout the spectrum of stabilization of ventilation, maintenance of ventilation, and weaning from mechanical support.

The choice of mode of mechanical ventilation is most often determined by whether resting of the respiratory muscles is indicated, such as in patients who are hemodynamically compromised, patients with severe oxygenation or ventilation derangements, or those undergoing general anesthesia. In these cases, it is prudent to choose a mode of ventilation that accomplishes ventilation without the need for spontaneous respirations; ACV is most often used. However, if use of muscles of respiration is desired, SIMV or PSV should be considered. Patients in whom the use of respiratory muscles is desired are usually those being weaned from mechanical ventilation or undergoing assessment of muscle strength and adequacy of spontaneous work of breathing. PSV is the only mode of the three that relies entirely on the patient spontaneously breathing. Table 45.3 shows the set and variable parameters in each common mode of ventilation.

The earliest mechanical ventilators utilized controlled mechanical ventilation (CMV) or control mode ventilation, although these are now outdated terms and the current preferred term is *continuous mandatory ventilation*. In this mode, the patient receives positive-pressure breaths at a set rate without the ability to influence how it is delivered. Current ACV modes function as CMV in patients who are unable to influence the ventilator, such as patients under deep sedation and neuromuscular blockade or patients without a neural respiratory drive.

Assist-Control Ventilation

Volume assist-control ventilation (VACV) is the most frequently used initial mode of ventilation and has several advantages in stabilization and maintenance of adequate ventilation. Using VACV allows adequate oxygenation and ventilation and decreases the work of breathing. It is commonly used in patients expected to be passive, such as in the operating room for general anesthesia and for comatose patients.

VACV is a combination mode of ventilation in which a preset tidal volume is delivered either in response to inspiratory effort or if no patient effort occurs within a set period. The period is determined by the backup respiratory rate set on the ventilator. A patient-triggered breath is sensed by a change in airway flow

TABLE 45.3	Set and Variable Parameters for Common Modes of Mechanical Ventilation				
Ventilation Mode	**Respiratory Rate**	**Tidal Volume**	**Peak Inspiratory Pressure**	**PEEP**	**Fio₂**
ACV	Set	Set (VACV)/Variable (PACV)	Set (PACV)/Variable (VACV)	Set	Set
SIMV	Set	Set	Variable	Set	Set
PSV	Variable	Variable	Set	Set	Set

ACV, Assist-control ventilation; *FiO₂,* fraction of inspired oxygen; *PACV,* pressure assist-control ventilation; *PEEP,* positive end-expiratory pressure; *PSV,* pressure-support ventilation; *SIMV,* synchronized intermittent mandatory ventilation; *VACV,* volume assist-control ventilation.

or pressure. When the change reaches the trigger threshold, the ventilator delivers the predetermined tidal volume. In VACV, the limit variable that increases to the set threshold before inspiration ends is volume or flow or both. The cycle variable that ends inspiration is volume or time. Peak inspiratory airway pressure and plateau pressure are variable in this setting. As discussed, in patients under deep sedation and neuromuscular blockade, the ACV mode functions like CMV. The advantage of ACV is that it substantially decreases both work of breathing and myocardial oxygen demand. The disadvantages of ACV in the active patient are that it is less comfortable than spontaneous breathing and, in a hyperventilating patient, it can induce respiratory alkalosis and breath-stacking (Table 45.4).

When ACV is used in a volume-targeted mode, airway pressures vary. When patients with severe hypoxemia (e.g., ARDS) require high PEEP and Fio_2 settings to maintain adequate oxygenation, the airway pressures that are generated to deliver the desired tidal volume increase. This increasing pressure can be measured as the peak inspiratory pressure, the mean airway pressure, or the plateau pressure, all of which attempt to describe the pressures that are transmitted through the airways at different levels and at different points in the respiratory cycle. As the plateau pressures increase, reflecting increasing alveolar pressure, it may be prudent to use a pressure-control or pressure-targeted variant of the ACV mode.

Similar to VACV, the pressure-targeted ACV (PACV) mode requires an input of the desired frequency (i.e., respiratory rate), PEEP, and Fio_2, but instead of a preset tidal volume, the upper limit of the inspiratory pressure that is allowable is set. As the ventilator delivers a breath, the inspiratory flow continues until the maximum pressure or allotted time is reached, and the flow then ceases. In PACV, the tidal volume varies, and consistency is sacrificed to prevent barotrauma by high pressures (Table 45.5).[70] Fig. 45.5 depicts the differences in VACV and PACV in graphs of pressure versus time and airflow versus time.

Synchronized Intermittent Mandatory Ventilation

SIMV is a frequently used mode of ventilation in medical and surgical units that incorporates characteristics of ACV and PSV. SIMV requires the same settings as ACV: frequency, tidal volume, PEEP, and Fio_2; however, it also includes a setting for a prescribed pressure support for spontaneous breaths. The purpose of the two types of breaths (i.e., mandatory and spontaneous) is to allow increased diaphragmatic activity and increased work of breathing by the patient when triggering spontaneous breaths. SIMV is sometimes used as a weaning mode, but it can prolong mechanical ventilation and is therefore not routinely recommended for weaning.[71]

When a patient is deeply sedated or paralyzed, SIMV functions in the same manner as ACV. The patient receives a fixed number of mandatory breaths as determined by the set respiratory rate with set tidal volume, PEEP, and Fio_2. However, in patients with spontaneous ventilatory effort, SIMV assists the patient when a mandatory breath is triggered and supports spontaneous breaths above the set number of mandatory breaths with the prescribed pressure support and PEEP. The advantage of this mode is that it allows the patient to receive a fixed number of mandatory breaths by controlling the breaths (if the patient is not initiating inspiration) or assisting breaths (if the patient is triggering the start of inspiration), and the patient is allowed to breathe spontaneously at a higher frequency than the set respiratory rate SIMV can also be used in a pressure-targeted mode, where a preset inspiratory pressure is used instead of a tidal volume. The use of SIMV may reduce sedation requirements (see Table 45.4).[72]

Pressure Support Ventilation

PSV is used for patients who are capable of spontaneous breathing. PSV was initially developed to reduce work of breathing in SIMV but evolved into a stand-alone mode of ventilation.

TABLE 45.5	Comparison of Volume-Targeted and Pressure-Targeted Assist-Control Ventilation	
Parameter	Volume-Targeted Ventilation	Pressure-Targeted Ventilation
Frequency (rate)	Set	Set
Tidal volume	Set	Variable
Inspiratory flow	Set	Set
Peak inspiratory pressure	Variable	Set
PEEP	Set	Set
Fio_2	Set	Set

PEEP, Positive end-expiratory pressure; *Fio_2*, fraction of inspired oxygen.

TABLE 45.4	Advantages and Disadvantages of Conventional Modes of Ventilation	
Ventilation Mode	Advantages	Disadvantages
ACV	Predictable tidal volumes (VACV) Mandatory respiratory rate Useful for reliable ventilation Good for stabilization of hypoxemia Decreases work of breathing	Uncomfortable for the awake patient Respiratory alkalosis possible Breath-stacking, auto-PEEP Not a weaning mode Usually requires sedation
SIMV	More comfortable Allows respiratory muscle work	Spontaneous breaths vary Increases weaning time
PSV	More comfortable Allows for evaluation of spontaneous work of breathing Weaning mode	No guaranteed respiratory rate No guaranteed tidal volume Apnea can be disastrous

ACV, Assist-control ventilation; *PEEP*, positive end-expiratory pressure; *PSV*, pressure-support ventilation; *SIMV*, synchronized intermittent mandatory ventilation; *VACV*, volume assist-control ventilation.

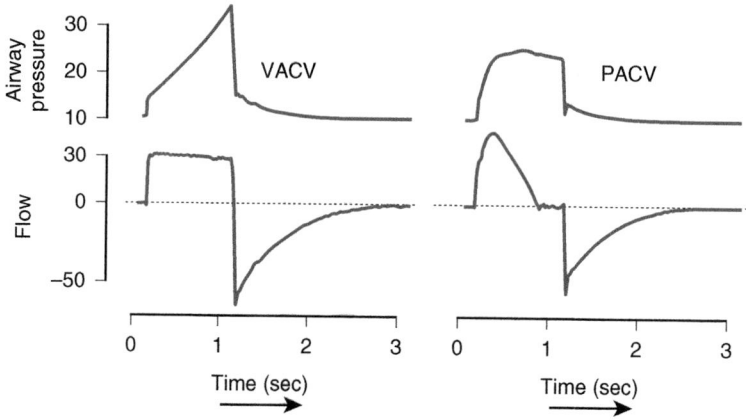

• **Fig. 45.5** Graphs of airway pressure versus time and airflow versus time compare volume assist-control ventilation (VACV) and pressure assist-control ventilation (PACV). (From Marini JJ. Point: Is pressure assist-control preferred over volume assist-control mode for lung protective ventilation in patients with ARDS? Yes. *Chest.* 2011;140:286–290.)

PSV augments a patient's spontaneous inspiratory efforts with a selected level of pressure support. The inspiratory pressure is delivered until the flow decreases to a predetermined level (usually 25% of peak flow). In PSV mode, pressure support, PEEP, and Fio_2 are set parameters. This mode relies entirely on spontaneous breaths by the patient, who must have an intact ventilatory drive. The work of breathing in PSV is inversely proportional to the level of pressure support and the flow rate.[73] Because no tidal volume is guaranteed by this mode of ventilation, pressure support must be titrated to allow the patient to achieve an adequate tidal volume. However, any change in lung compliance or airway impedance results in a change in tidal volume. A certain level of pressure support is needed to overcome the resistance of the ventilator circuit and ETT. This typically is less than 10 cm H_2O, although it can be higher with narrower ETTs.[74] Pressure support above that needed to overcome the artificial airway resistance supplements the achieved tidal volumes. Typical pressure support settings are between 5 and 25 cm H_2O. When full ventilatory support is needed for a patient, PSV may not be the ideal mode because it requires a higher work of breathing and minute ventilation is not guaranteed (see Table 45.4).

Pressure-Regulated Volume Control

Pressure-regulated volume control (PRVC), also known as volume control plus (VC+), is a controlled mode of ventilation that combines features of pressure-controlled and volume-controlled ventilation; it can be employed with ACV or SIMV. This dual mode of ventilation introduced in recent years utilizes adaptive control of inspiratory pressure with the goal of targeting a desired tidal volume. A target tidal volume is set as in volume-controlled ventilation (VCV), but breaths are delivered with a decelerating ramp flow pattern, as in PCV. The ventilator provides a breath at a low pressure and then calculates the peak pressure necessary to deliver the set tidal volume; that pressure level is delivered during the next breath. If the target is not attained, the peak pressure is adjusted by 1 to 3 cm H_2O for the next breath. This allows breath-to-breath correction and enables increased airway pressure control. Because the inspiratory flow is autoregulated, PRVC results in a lower peak airway pressure for a given tidal volume. PRVC can be useful even

when the patient is not breathing spontaneously because it delivers guaranteed tidal volumes with a decelerating ramp inspiratory flow pattern, minimizing peak inspiratory pressures. Many modern anesthesia machines incorporate similar ventilation modes for this reason (e.g., volume AutoFlow [AF] on Dräger machines and volume-guarantee pressure support [VG-PS] on GE machines). A potential drawback to the mode can be seen in conditions where there is increased ventilatory effort such as anxiety, pain, and acidosis. Because the ventilator responds to the patient's effort in PRVC, as the patient's respiratory effort increases, inspiratory pressure decreases, thereby increasing the patient's work of breathing and causing patient-ventilator dyssynchrony.[75,76]

Uncommon Modes of Ventilation

Inverse Ratio Ventilation

Inverse ratio ventilation (IRV) is positive-pressure ventilation with an inspiratory-to-expiratory (I:E) ratio greater than 1. It has been used in the management of severe ARDS to improve oxygenation when PEEP has been optimized.[77] I:E ratios usually range from 1:2 to 1:5, whereas in IRV they may be 1:1, 2:1, or higher. Increasing the inspiratory time increases mean airway pressure without increasing the inspiratory plateau pressure, which may improve oxygenation.[78,79] This application is most commonly used with time-cycled pressure-controlled ventilation (PCV), but it can also be used with VCV. The improvements in oxygenation are modest, and CO_2 elimination is preserved[79,80]; however, not all studies have shown benefit.[81] Development of auto-PEEP is common in IRV and may be responsible for some of the improvements in oxygenation; however, this also increases the risk of barotrauma. Because the benefits of IRV are controversial, it should be limited to use in patients with severe ARDS with refractory hypoxemia.[82]

Airway Pressure Release Ventilation

Airway pressure release ventilation (APRV) can be seen as a blend of inverse ratio PCV and PSV. APRV offers two levels of CPAP ventilation, in which it uses high and low pressures to aid in recruitment of atelectatic lung units and allows for spontaneous breathing.[83,84] A continuous high positive pressure (P_{high}) is delivered by the ventilator for a prolonged duration (T_{high}) and then drops to a lower pressure (P_{low}) for a short duration (T_{low}). Spontaneous breathing can occur during high and low pressures. Overall, increasing P_{high} or T_{high} or both improves hypoxemia; ventilation is improved by increasing P_{high} while simultaneously decreasing T_{high} or by increasing T_{low} alone.[85] When the patient cannot initiate breaths, the mode is identical to inverse ratio PCV.[86] One study of 24 patients with ARDS showed that when APRV was compared with PSV, APRV improved oxygenation and cardiac parameters, along with improvements in ventilation-perfusion matching in the lung.[87]

APRV can decrease peak airway pressures, improve oxygenation, improve alveolar recruitment, and improve cardiac output; however, findings have been inconsistent, and there has been no evidence of a mortality benefit.[88–91] During periods of transition between low and high pressures, patient-ventilator dyssynchrony can occur. APRV is not recommended for patients with obstructive lung disease or in patients that require high minute ventilation (Figs. 45.6 and 45.7).

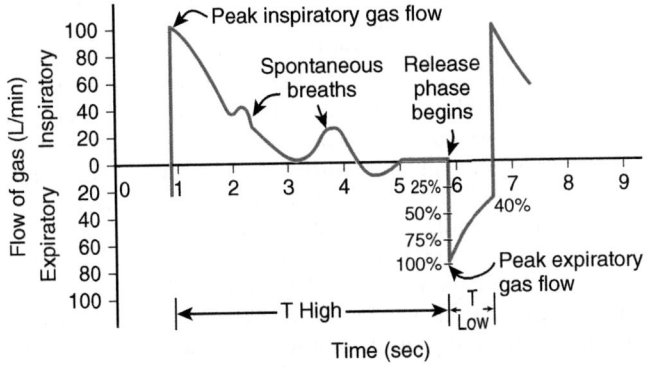

• **Fig. 45.6** Inspiratory and expiratory flow of gas in airway pressure release ventilation. *T High,* Number of seconds spent at the higher pressure; *T Low,* number of seconds spent at the lower pressure. (From Frawley PM, Habashi NM. Airway pressure release ventilation: theory and practice. *AACN Clinical Issues.* 2001;12:234–246.)

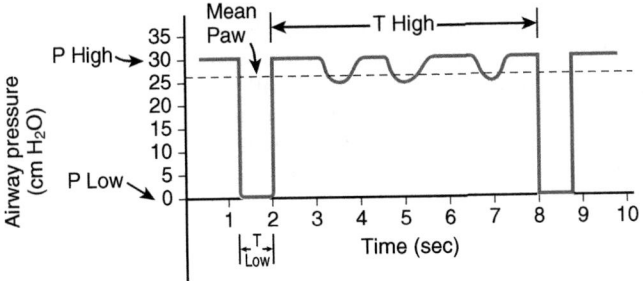

• **Fig. 45.7** Pressure-time curve for airway pressure release ventilation. *Paw,* Airway pressure; *P High,* higher pressure used for respiration on bi-level (e.g., 30 cm H_2O); *P Low,* lower pressure used on bi-level (e.g., 0 cm H_2O); *T High,* number of seconds in the respiratory cycle spent at the higher pressure; *T Low,* number of seconds spent at the lower pressure. (From Frawley PM, Habashi NM. Airway pressure release ventilation: theory and practice. *AACN Clinical Issues.* 2001;12:234–246.)

Bi-level ventilation is similar to APRV but has additional features.[92] The cycling of the ventilator between low and high pressures is coordinated with the patient's effort to reduce dyssynchrony. T_{low} is usually longer in bi-level ventilation, which allows more spontaneous breaths to occur at this pressure level. As in APRV, bi-level ventilation has been used primarily in patients with ARDS, and it should be avoided in patients with obstructive lung disease because of the risk of auto-PEEP from shortened expiratory times.

High-Frequency Ventilation

There are many types of high-frequency mechanical ventilation. High-frequency ventilation is positive-pressure ventilation with tidal volumes near the anatomic dead space and respiratory rates greater than 60 breaths per minute. The theoretical advantages over conventional ventilation are that the tidal volumes of 1 to 3 mL/kg and the higher levels of PEEP reduce the risk of cyclical alveolar injury and limit alveolar overdistention. The ability to maintain high mean airway pressures can improve oxygenation.

High-frequency oscillatory ventilation (HFOV), sometimes called the oscillator, is a means of improving oxygenation by providing an oxygen-rich and CO_2-poor gas at high respiratory rates that rapidly mixes with sinusoidal flow at stroke volumes that approximate anatomic dead space. HFOV is the most commonly used high-frequency ventilator in adults. HFOV uses a pump to generate a respiratory frequency of 3 to 6 Hz or 180 to 360 breaths per minute. In a 1984 publication, Chang described five mechanisms of oxygen delivery by high-frequency oscillation: direct alveolar ventilation of lung units adjacent to proximal airways, bulk convective gas mixing in conductive airways by recirculation of air among neighboring airways in different cycles of opening and closing of the alveolus, convective transport of gases, longitudinal dispersion by airway turbulence, and molecular diffusion.[93]

Selection guidelines for HFOV do not exist, but patients with ARDS who develop refractory hypoxemia on conventional ventilation were historically considered.[94–96] HFOV uses high airway pressures during very short time intervals to help recruit and oxygenate atelectatic lungs. The mean airway pressure is set by manipulation of the inspiratory flow rate and an expiratory back-pressure valve. HFOV in patients with obstructive lung disease (e.g., COPD, asthma) may lead to significant auto-PEEP. The oscillator requires vigilance on the part of the physician and respiratory therapist because patients are usually severely hypoxemic at the initiation of HFOV. Because the oscillator is uncomfortable for patients, increased sedation and often neuromuscular blockade is required. Careful titration of inspiratory pressure and frequency are needed to obtain optimal settings. During HFOV, ventilation is a passive process, and the patient must have the ETT cuff deflated to allow for passive exhalation of CO_2. In initial studies, HFOV appeared to be equivalent to conventional ventilation in ARDS patients and useful in the management of refractory hypoxemia and severe air leaks (Fig. 45.8).[97]

A multicenter trial of 148 patients with ARDS compared conventional ventilation to HFOV. Patients were randomized to receive conventional mechanical ventilation or HFOV and were followed to compare 30-day ventilator-free survival. The results demonstrated improved 30-day mortality rates in the HFOV group, but statistical significance was not achieved in this primary outcome, nor in various secondary endpoints, including 6-month

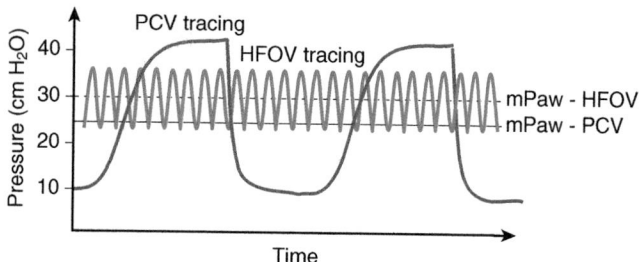

• **Fig. 45.8** The pressure-time curve for high-frequency oscillatory ventilation (HFOV) is superimposed on the tracing for pressure-controlled ventilation (PCV) for comparison. (From Chang KP, Stewart TE, Mehta S. High-frequency oscillatory ventilation for adult patients with ARDS. *Chest.* 2007;131:1907–1916.)

mortality rates and duration of mechanical ventilation.[95] A systematic review and meta-analysis in 2010 noted that patients had a higher Pao_2/Fio_2 ratio on HFOV than on conventional mechanical ventilation but noted higher mean airway pressures in the HFOV group.[98] This review of eight randomized trials, which included 419 patients in total, concluded that HFOV might improve survival and was unlikely to cause harm. Subsequently, two multicenter trials of HFOV for ARDS failed to show benefit in HFOV and showed a trend toward potential harm, compared with conventional mechanical ventilation.[99,100] The OSCAR trial randomized 795 patients with a Pao_2/Fio_2 ratio less than 200 mm Hg to receive either conventional mechanical ventilation or HFOV and showed no difference in 30-day mortality between the two modes of ventilation.[99] The second trial, OSCILLATE, was terminated early after randomizing 548 patients with moderate to severe ARDS to either HFOV or conventional mechanical ventilation.[100] This trial showed a higher mortality in the HFOV group (47%) versus conventional mechanical ventilation (35%), signaling that HFOV may not decrease and may actually increase mortality when compared with conventional ventilation. Based on the results of these two large trials, HFOV has fallen out of favor for treating ARDS in many ICUs.

In high-frequency jet ventilation (HFJV), a pressurized gas is introduced by inserting a cannula from the HFJV device into the ETT. An initial pressure of 35 pounds per square inch (psi) is set with a rate of 100 to 150 breaths per minute and an inspiratory fraction (inspiratory time divided by the sum of inspiratory and expiratory times) of 30%.[101] HFJV is more commonly employed in pediatric patients, but it has some use in interventional pulmonary procedures and in upper airway surgeries including laryngeal and tracheal surgery (see Chapter 38).[102,103] The drawback of conventional jet ventilators is that there is not an adequate measure of intrapulmonary pressure in the circuit, and the patient may be at risk for volutrauma from alveolar overdistention.

High-frequency percussive ventilation (HFPV) is a time-cycled, pressure-limited mode of ventilation that delivers subphysiologic tidal volumes at rates as high as 500 breaths per minute.[104] HFPV has been used in burn units, specifically for patients with inhalation lung injury, and for salvage therapy in patients with severe ARDS.[105] The basic tenets are the same as for HFOV, but it oscillates at two different pressure levels. A Phasitron valve (Percussionaire Corp., Sagle, ID) at the end of the ETT delivers small tidal volumes at frequencies of 200 to 900 breaths per minute

superimposed on PCV. Whereas the HFOV uses rapid oscillations of small volumes at high frequencies that transiently reach high airway pressures, HFPV prolongs the application of high airway pressure at high frequencies to assist in clearance of mucus and sloughing airway secretions. A single-center, prospective, randomized trial comparing HFPV with low tidal volume ventilation in burn patients with ARDS demonstrated no difference in mortality rates or ventilator-free days.[106]

Proportional Modes

Proportional modes are more novel modes of ventilation in which ventilator-delivered breaths are adjusted during inspiration in proportion to the patient's respiratory effort. The two proportional modes are proportional assist ventilation (PAV) and neurally adjusted ventilator assist (NAVA).

PAV is a form of synchronized partial ventilatory assistance in which the ventilator monitors the flow and volume that the patient's effort generates, calculates the total pressure that is required to be delivered, and delivers the pressure proportional to the patient's needs. There are no preset variables such as flow, pressure, volume or time, which are all under the patient's control; however, the provider is able to set the percentage of the assist from the ventilator and does it adaptively. PAV can be used in invasive mechanical ventilation as a weaning mode and also as noninvasive mechanical ventilation in acute and chronic respiratory failure. A recent trial compared PAV with PSV in patients who met criteria for spontaneous breathing but had not yet passed a spontaneous breathing trial (SBT) to be safely extubated.[107] The trial was based, in part, on a previous study showing that PAV had benefits of increasing patient-ventilator synchrony, adapting to changes in ventilator demand, and improving sleep in ICU patients undergoing mechanical ventilation.[108] PAV was associated with decreased time to extubation and decreased ICU length of stay as compared with PSV. Although PAV was developed to improve patient-ventilator interaction, specifically in weaning from mechanical ventilation with the goal of improving synchrony and comfort, implementation of this mode in ICUs has been slow and may be due to providers' lack of familiarity with the mode and lack of demonstration of superiority over more conventional weaning modes such as PSV.

NAVA is a mode similar to PAV; it differs in that the proportional assistance of the ventilatory effort is determined based on the patient's diaphragmatic activity. Specifically designed nasogastric tubes with electromyographic (EMG) electrodes at the distal end are used to acquire signals of diaphragmatic activity. Similar to PAV, the ventilator pressure is delivered in proportion to the patient's effort (i.e., the EMG signal) with improved patient-ventilatory synchrony. Although a promising tool, studies thus far have not clearly demonstrated improvement in clinically relevant outcomes. Current use is mostly in the neonatal and pediatric ICU population.[109–111]

Volume Guarantee Ventilation

Volume guarantee (VG) ventilation is a volume-targeted modality that can be applied to ACV, SIMV, or PSV. VG is a pressure-limited, volume-targeted, time-cycled or flow-cycled mode of ventilation.[112] It adjusts inspiratory pressure to changes in exhaled tidal volumes, therefore compensating for air leak around uncuffed ETTs. VG has been used primarily in neonates and has been shown to be both feasible and effective. In a Cochrane review, SIMV with VG was shown to have a lower mortality than SIMV with PSV.[113]

Management of Acute Respiratory Distress Syndrome

ARDS, commonly seen in medical and surgical patients, is synonymous with noncardiogenic pulmonary edema and presents dilemmas in treatment.[114,115] ARDS has many direct and indirect causes. Examples of direct injury are pneumonia, gastric fluid aspiration, and inhalation injury; indirect causes of injury include severe sepsis, shock, pancreatitis, blood product transfusion, and narcotic overdose.[116] Historically, according to the 1994 American-European Consensus Conference (AECC) definition, ARDS was recognized as a spectrum including ALI (defined as Pao_2/Fio_2 ratio ≤300 mm Hg) and ARDS (defined as Pao_2/Fio_2 ratio ≤200 mm Hg). Other characteristics of ARDS per the AECC definition were the acute onset of bilateral pulmonary infiltrates in the setting of a pulmonary capillary wedge pressure less than 18 mm Hg (i.e., no evidence of elevated left atrial pressure). In 2012, the ARDS definition task force developed the Berlin definition of ARDS because of shortcomings in the AECC definition.[117] A lack of explicit criteria in defining acute onset of the process, the sensitivity of the Pao_2/Fio_2 ratio to different ventilator settings, poor reliability of chest radiograph criteria, and difficulties in distinguishing purely noncardiogenic pulmonary edema from hydrostatic edema were some of the limitations of the AECC definition.

The Berlin definition first states that the occurrence of ARDS must be within 1 week of a known clinical insult or new or worsening respiratory symptoms must have developed in the past week. Second, the chest imaging findings must depict bilateral opacities that are not fully explained by pleural effusions, pulmonary nodules, or lobar or lung collapse. Third, the Berlin definition recognizes that noncardiogenic pulmonary edema may coexist with development of a component of cardiogenic pulmonary edema in the ICU patient because of fluid and medication administration intravenously, so the definition suggests that, in the opinion of the treating physician, the respiratory failure may not be fully explained by cardiac failure or fluid overload. Last and possibly most important, the Berlin definition does away with the notion of ALI as a separate entity to ARDS and describes the process as a continuum that is reclassified into mild, moderate, and severe ARDS. These distinctions correlate with differences in mortality as well as interventions that are delineated between levels of severity. For mild ARDS, the Pao_2/Fio_2 ratio for inclusion is 201 to 300 mm Hg and PEEP or CPAP ≥ 5 cm H_2O. Patients with mild ARDS may be managed with invasive or noninvasive mechanical ventilation. Moderate ARDS is defined as Pao_2/Fio_2 ratio of 101 to 200 mm Hg with PEEP ≥ 5 cm H_2O. Most patients with moderate ARDS will be managed with invasive mechanical ventilation and may require increased PEEP. Lastly, severe ARDS is defined as Pao_2/Fio_2 ratio ≤100 mm Hg with PEEP ≥5 cm H_2O. All patients with severe ARDS are managed with invasive mechanical ventilation, and additional therapies may be applicable in this group of patients, including higher PEEP, prone positioning, neuromuscular blockade, inhaled nitric oxide, extracorporeal CO_2 elimination, or extracorporeal membrane oxygenation. Additionally, the Berlin definition noted increased mortality with increasing

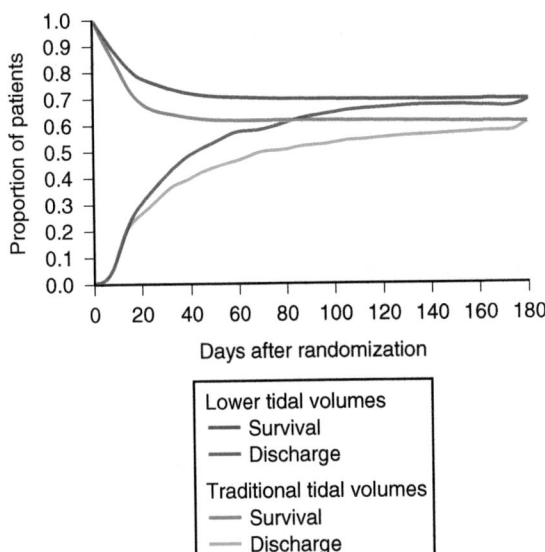

• **Fig. 45.9** The Kaplan-Meier curve from the ARDS Network study compares survival to 180 days and discharge to home without breathing assistance in the lower tidal volume group and the traditional tidal volume group. (From Acute Respiratory Distress Syndrome Network. Ventilation with lower tidal volumes as compared with traditional tidal volumes for acute lung injury and the acute respiratory distress syndrome. *N Engl J Med.* 2000;342:1301–1308.)

severity: 27% in mild ARDS, 32% in moderate ARDS, and 45% in severe ARDS.

Ventilatory strategies for the management of ARDS are based on the results of the ARDS Network studies, which demonstrated that patients given tidal volumes of 6 mL/kg predicted body weight had improved mortality rates compared with patients with tidal volumes of 12 mL/kg predicted body weight. Another finding was that plateau pressures less than 30 cm H_2O protect the lung from injury (Fig. 45.9 and Table 45.6).[42] In 1998, Amato and colleagues demonstrated the mortality benefit of lower tidal volumes and a lower rate of barotrauma (Fig. 45.10).[46] Two meta-analyses demonstrated decreased mortality rates with the use of low tidal volume ventilation (i.e., lung protective ventilation).[118,119] In ARDS management, plateau pressures should be less than or equal to 30 cm H_2O or at the lowest possible level. A high-PEEP strategy decreased the mortality rate in patients with Pao_2/Fio_2 ratio of less than 200 mm Hg in a meta-analysis of 2299 ARDS patients.[53] Randomized trials of ventilation strategies in ARDS patients are summarized in Table 45.7.

Weaning From Mechanical Ventilation

The process of weaning from mechanical ventilation is a continuum from decreasing support provided by the ventilator to assessment of readiness using multiple variables and eventual discontinuation of mechanical ventilation.

In 2001, a collective task force from the American College of Chest Physicians, the American Association of Respiratory Care, and the American College of Critical Care Medicine examined the issue of discontinuation of mechanical ventilation and defined patients who required prolonged mechanical ventilation and strategies to liberate them from the mechanical ventilator. They found

TABLE 45.6 Main Outcome Variables in the Acute Respiratory Distress Syndrome Network Trial of Low Tidal Volumes Versus Traditional Tidal Volumes in Patients With Acute Respiratory Distress Syndrome

Outcome Variable	Group Receiving Lower Tidal Volumes	Group Receiving Traditional Tidal Volumes	p Value
Death before discharge home and breathing without assistance (%)	31.0	39.8	0.007
Breathing without assistance by day 28 (%)	65.7	55.0	<0.001
Number of ventilator-free days, days 1 to 28 (%)[b]	12 ± 11[a]	10 ± 11[a]	0.007
Barotrauma, days 1 to 28 (%)[c]	10	11	0.43
Number of days without failure of nonpulmonary organs or systems, days 1 to 28[d]	15 ± 11[a]	12 ± 11[a]	0

[a]Mean ± standard deviation.

[b]The number of ventilator-free days is the mean number of days from day 1 to day 28 during which the patient had been breathing without assistance for at least 48 consecutive hours.

[c]Barotrauma was defined as any new pneumothorax, pneumomediastinum, subcutaneous emphysema, or a pneumatocele greater than 2 cm in diameter.

[d]Circulatory failure was defined as a systolic blood pressure of 90 mm Hg or less or the need for treatment with any vasopressor; coagulation failure as a platelet count less than or equal to 80,000/mm³; hepatic failure as a serum bilirubin concentration 2 mg/dL (34 μmol/L) or more; and renal failure as a serum creatinine concentration 2 mg/dL (177 μmol/L) or more.

From the Acute Respiratory Distress Syndrome Network. Ventilation with lower tidal volumes as compared with traditional tidal volumes for acute lung injury and the acute respiratory distress syndrome. *N Engl J Med.* 2000;342:1301–1308.)

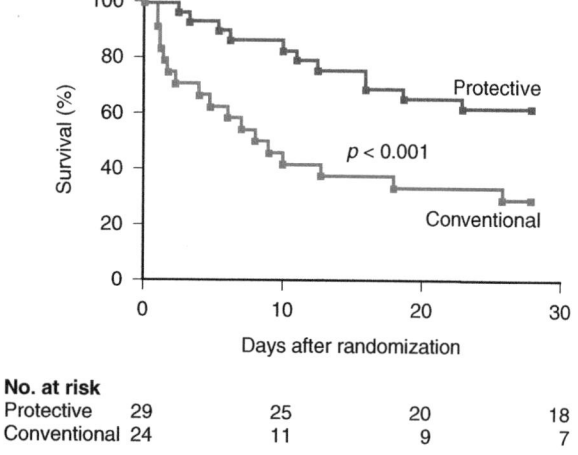

No. at risk

Protective	29	25	20	18
Conventional	24	11	9	7

• **Fig. 45.10** Comparison of the 28-day survival of patients with acute respiratory distress syndrome (ARDS) assigned to protective or conventional mechanical ventilation. (From Amato MB, Barbas CS et al. Effect of a protective-ventilation strategy on mortality in the acute respiratory distress syndrome. *N Engl J Med.* 1998;338(6):347–354.)

that mechanically ventilated patients spend approximately 42% of their ventilator time undergoing the weaning process. The task force offered 12 recommendations to standardize practice for discontinuing mechanical ventilation. These include searching for causes of respiratory failure; early discontinuation of sedation of postoperative patients; ensuring daily SBTs for patients who meet the criteria for hemodynamic, pulmonary, and mental stability; outlining criteria for evaluation of patients on an SBT; strategies for prolonged weaning and daily SBTs assisted by nonphysician practitioners within the healthcare organization. The clinical criteria outlined by the task force include clinically improving cause of respiratory failure, adequate oxygenation (defined as Pao_2/Fio_2 >150 mm Hg or oxyhemoglobin saturation greater than ≥90%

while receiving Fio_2 ≤0.4 and a PEEP ≤5 cm H_2O), hemodynamic stability (absent or low-dose vasopressors and no signs of myocardial ischemia), arterial pH 7.25 or more; and a patient who is able to initiate a spontaneous inspiratory effort.[120]

A study of 300 patients published in 1996 demonstrated the value of daily screening of patients followed by trials of spontaneous breathing. In the study, the nurse, respiratory therapist, and physician screened patients daily, and if preset guidelines were met, patients underwent a 2-hour SBT. If the patient passed the trial, the physician was notified and the patient was extubated. The study demonstrated a decrease in ventilator days, a decrease in the number of complications including reintubation, and lower hospital costs.[121] Another study showed a decrease in the number of ventilator days and ICU days with daily interruption of sedation.[122]

In 2007 a second task force produced the Statement of the 6th International Consensus Conference on Intensive Care Medicine, which identified the characteristics that predicted favorable and unfavorable weaning outcomes and determined which modes of ventilation should be used when a patient fails an SBT. The task force also addressed the use of noninvasive ventilation and prolonged ventilator dependence. The task force's recommendations were as follows: wean as early as possible; use SBTs to determine if the patient can be extubated; SBTs should last 30 minutes and consist of either T-tube breathing or low levels of pressure support; avoid SIMV as a weaning mode; use PSV or ACV after a failed weaning attempt; and NIPPV should not routinely be used after failed extubation—rather, it should be used only in select patients with hypercapnia, although CPAP may be useful in preventing hypoxemia in postoperative patients. Successful weaning was defined as 48 hours free of the ventilator after extubation (Table 45.8).[123]

In 1995 the Spanish Lung Failure Collaborative Group prospectively compared the use of SIMV, PSV, intermittent trials of spontaneous breathing, and once-daily SBTs. The study showed that SBTs in either form were superior to SIMV or PSV in terms

TABLE 45.7	Summary of Randomized, Controlled Trials of Ventilatory Strategies Used for Adult Patients Who Have or Are at Risk for Acute Respiratory Distress Syndrome to Prevent Ventilator-Associated Lung Injury				
Study Component	Amato et al.[46] (n = 53)	Brochard et al.[125] (n = 108)	Brower et al.[126] (n = 52)	Stewart et al.[127] (n = 120)	NIH[a] (n = 861)
Population					
Entry criteria	LIS > 2.5 PAWP < 16 mm Hg MV < 7 days	LIS > 2.5 MV < 3 days	Pao_2/FIO_2 < 200 MV < 1 day	Pao_2/FiO_2 < 250 MV < 1 day	Pao_2/FiO_2 < 300 MV <36 hours
Exclusion criteria	Coronary insufficiency, prior lung disease, barotrauma, uncontrolled acidosis, intracranial hypertension, terminal disease	Left heart failure, acute or chronic organ failure, chest wall abnormality, intracranial hypertension, head injury, terminal disease	Age < 18, left heart failure, acute neurologic disease, chronic lung disease, thoracic surgery	Age < 18, left heart failure, myocardial ischemia, acute or chronic neurologic disease, PIP > 30 for 2 hours, terminal disease	Age < 18, left heart failure, acute neurologic disease, life expectancy < 6 months, hepatic failure
Characteristics at Inclusion					
APACHE II	28 vs 27	18 vs 17	90 vs 85 (APACHE III)	22 vs 21	
Pao_2/Fio_2	112 vs 134	144 vs 155	129 vs 150	123 vs 145	
LIS	3.4 vs 3.2	3.0 vs 3.0	2.7 vs 2.8		
Targeted Settings					
Intervention	VT < 6 mL/kg PIP < 40 cm H_2O $P_{driving}$ < cm H_2O CPAP recruiting	$P_{plateau}$ ≤ 25–30 cm H_2O VT = 6–10 mL/kg	$P_{plateau}$ ≤ 30 cm H_2O VT ≤ 8 mL/kg IBW	PIP < 30 cm H_2O VT ≤ 8 mL/kg IBW	VT ≤ 6 mL/kg IBW Reduce VT if $P_{plateau}$ > 30 cm H_2O
Control	VT = 12 mL/kg $Paco_2$, 35–38 mm Hg PIP unlimited	VT = 10–15 mL/kg, PIP < 60 cm H_2O	$P_{plateau}$ ≤ 45–55 cm H_2O VT = 10–12 mL/kg IBW	PIP ≤ 50 cm H_2O VT = 10–15 mL/kg IBW	VT = 12 mL/kg IBW Reduce VT if $P_{plateau}$ > 50 cm H_2O
PEEP (cm H_2O)					
Intervention	2 above P_{flex}	0–15, titrated to best P/F ratio	5–20 titrated to best P/F ratio	5–20 titrated to best P/F ratio	Titrated to gas exchange
Control	Titrated to P/F ratio	Titrated to P/F ratio	Titrated to P/F ratio	Titrated to P/F ratio	Titrated to gas exchange
Resulting Settings[b]					
$P_{plateau}$ (cm H_2O)	30 vs 37	26 vs 32	25 vs 32	22 vs 28	25 vs 32–34
PEEP (cm H_2O)	16 vs 7	11 vs 11	10 vs 9	9 vs 7	8–9, both groups
VT (mL or mL/kg)	350 vs 770 mL	7 vs 10 mL/kg	7 vs 10 mL/kg	7 vs 11 mL/kg	6.2 vs 11.8 mL/kg
Pao_2 (mm Hg)	55 vs 32	60 vs 41	50 vs 40	54 vs 46	
Outcomes					
Mortality	13/29 (45%) vs 17/24 (71%)	47% vs 38%	13/26 (50%) vs 12/26 (46%)	30/60 (50%) vs 28/60 (47%)	31 vs 39%
Barotrauma[c]	2 (7%) vs 10 (42%)	8 (14%) vs 7 (12%)	1 (4%) vs 2 (8%)	6 (10%) vs 4 (7%)	No difference

APACHE II, Acute Physiology and Chronic Health Evaluation II; *CPAP*, continuous positive airway pressure; *FiO₂*, fraction of inspired oxygen; *IBW*, ideal body weight (formulas used for calculation were not uniform across studies; Brochard and coworkers used dry weight to determine tidal volume); *LIS*, lung injury score; *MV*, mechanical ventilation; *Pao₂*, partial pressure of arterial oxygen; *P_driving*, driving pressure; *PEEP*, positive end-expiratory pressure; *P/F*, Pao₂/FiO₂, fraction of inspired oxygen; *P_flex*, pressure at the lower inflection point of the pressure-volume curve; *PIP*, peak inspiratory pressure; *PAWP*, pulmonary artery wedge pressure; *P_plateau*, plateau pressure; *VT*, tidal volume.

[a]National Institutes of Health (NIH) Acute Respiratory Distress Syndrome (ARDS) Network Trials, as reported on the NIH Web site (www.nih.gov).

[b]Precise comparison of resulting settings across the studies is difficult, because there is variation in the schedule of reporting; we attempted to compare mean values on days 1 through 3.

[c]Barotrauma was defined by Amato et al. as clinical barotrauma; by Brower et al. as pneumothorax; by Stewart et al. as pneumothorax, pneumomediastinum, subcutaneous emphysema, and lung cysts on a chest radiograph; and by Brochard et al. as pneumothorax requiring a chest tube.

Adapted from American Thoracic Society, European Society of Intensive Care Medicine, and Societé de Réanimation de Langue Française. International Consensus Conference in intensive care medicine: ventilator-associated lung injury in ARDS. *Am J Respir Crit Care Med.* 1999;160:2118–2124.)

TABLE 45.8	Time From Initiation of Weaning to Successful Extubation With Various Ventilation Modes		
Weaning Technique	Median (days)	First Quartile (days)	Third Quartile (days)
Intermittent mandatory ventilation	5	3	11
Pressure-support ventilation	4	2	12
Intermittent trials of spontaneous breathing	3	2	6
Once-daily trial of spontaneous breathing	3	1	6

From Esteban A, Frutos F, Tobin MJ, et al: A comparison of four methods of weaning patients from mechanical ventilation. Spanish Lung Failure Collaborative Group. *N Engl J Med.* 1995;332:345–350.

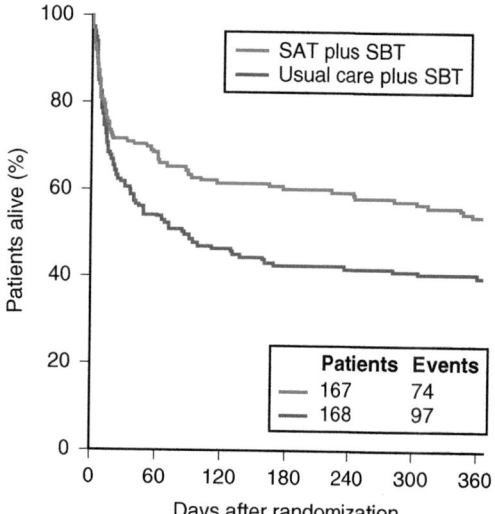

Patients at risk

SAT plus SBT	167	110	96	92	91	86	76
Usual care plus SBT	167	85	73	67	66	65	59

• **Fig. 45.11** Survival at 1 year after randomization to usual care with trials of spontaneous breathing (SBT) or to trials of spontaneous awakening (SAT) with SBT. (From Girard TD, Kress JP, Fuchs BD, et al. Efficacy and safety of a paired sedation and ventilator weaning protocol for mechanically ventilated patients in intensive care [Awakening and Breathing Controlled trial]: a randomised controlled trial. *Lancet.* 2008;371:126–134.)

of time from initiation of weaning to successful extubation and probability of successful weaning.[71]

The interaction of SBTs with daily interruption of sedation was illustrated by the Awakening and Breathing Trial in 2008. The trial showed that after randomizing 336 patients to the standard protocol or to daily discontinuation of sedation and daily SBTs, the intervention group had 3 fewer days on the mechanical ventilator, fewer ICU days, shorter hospital days, and improved survival rates compared with the standard protocol (Fig. 45.11 and 45.12).[124] Numerous weaning parameters have been studied to hasten liberation from mechanical ventilation, but none has been shown to be superior to using clinical criteria combined with an algorithmic approach to discontinuation of sedation and ventilation.

Complications of Mechanical Ventilation

Mechanical Complications

Mechanical ventilation may produce complications from the use of an artificial airway and from positive-pressure ventilation. Common complications of artificial airways are laryngeal edema and irritation, tracheal stenosis, sinusitis, vocal cord damage, and vocal cord paralysis. Mechanical complications of positive-pressure ventilation include barotrauma from high airway pressures, volutrauma from large distending volumes, and atelectrauma from ventilation at low volumes. Barotrauma can lead to alveolar rupture and a continuum of pneumothorax, pneumomediastinum, and subcutaneous emphysema. The lungs are susceptible to alveolar hyperinflation because of high tidal volumes delivered by the ventilator resulting in volutrauma. Due to the heterogeneous nature of the lung, even lower volumes may be disproportionally delivered to open alveoli.[125–127] Atelectrauma, or cyclic atelectasis, is sheer-force trauma resulting from repeated opening and collapsing of the alveolus in response to positive-pressure ventilation (Fig. 45.13). Biotrauma is VILI caused by local and systemic effects of cell mediator release and activation of cell signaling in the lung resulting from mechanical ventilation.[128]

Volutrauma and atelectrauma are within the spectrum of the ill-defined entity of VILI, which appears to be more common in patients with ARDS or other conditions that cause injury to the lung parenchyma or chest wall, creating the phenomenon of the stiff lung. VILI is an entity well described in animal models. It is a syndrome of diffuse alveolar damage that is morphologically identical to ARDS with formation of hyaline membranes caused by mechanical ventilation.[129] Alveolar injury results in increased permeability, loss of functional surfactant, release of cytokines, and alveolar collapse (Fig. 45.14). Other factors that may be associated with an increased risk for VILI include immunosuppression,[130] high ventilator rates,[131] supine body position, and hyperthermia.[132]

Auto-Positive End-Expiratory Pressure

Intrinsic PEEP, or auto-PEEP, results from incomplete alveolar emptying before the initiation of the next breath.[133] The alveolar pressures remain positive relative to atmospheric pressures at end-expiration. High minute ventilation from high tidal volumes or high respiratory rates is a common cause. When high respiratory

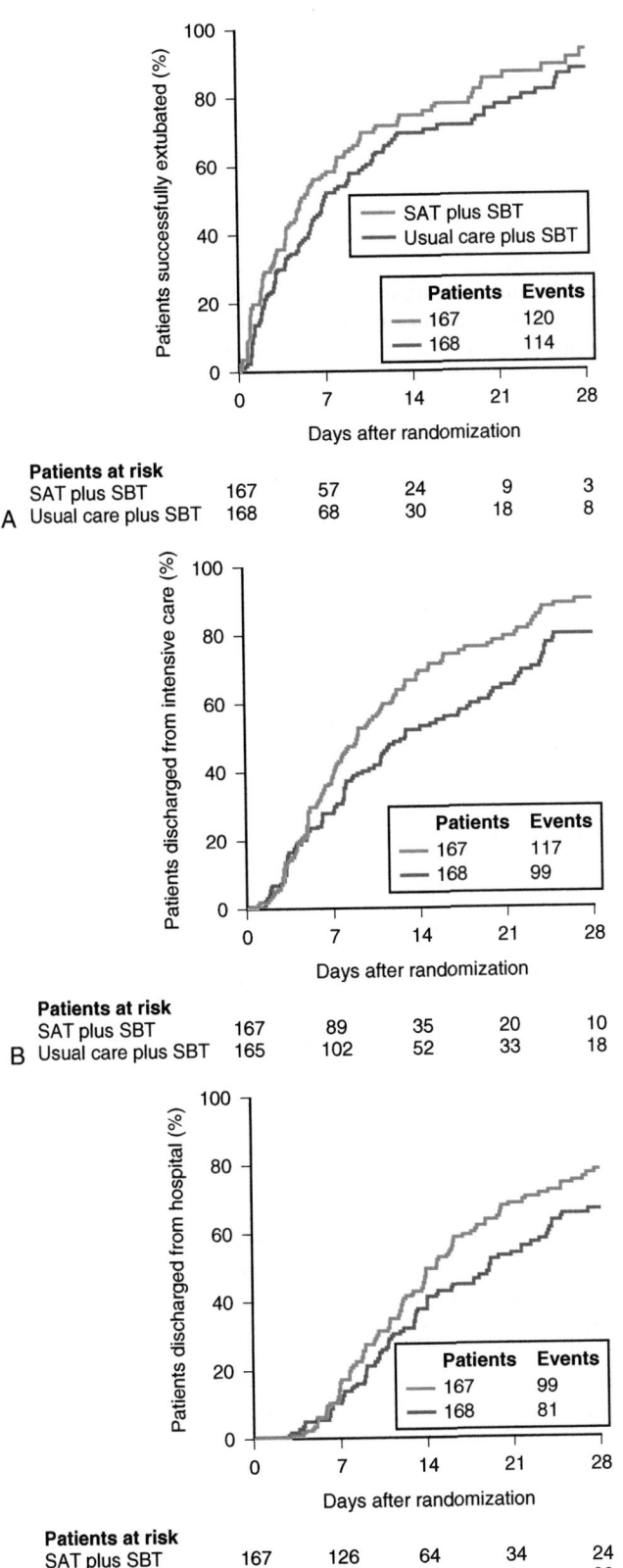

• **Fig. 45.12** Probability of successful extubation (A), discharge from intensive care (B), or discharge from hospital (C) within the first 28 days after randomization. *SAT*, Spontaneous awakening trials; *SBT*, spontaneous breathing trials. (From Girard TD, Kress JP, Fuchs BD, et al. Efficacy and safety of a paired sedation and ventilator weaning protocol for mechanically ventilated patients in intensive care [Awakening and Breathing Controlled trial]: a randomised controlled trial. *Lancet.* 2008;371:126–134.)

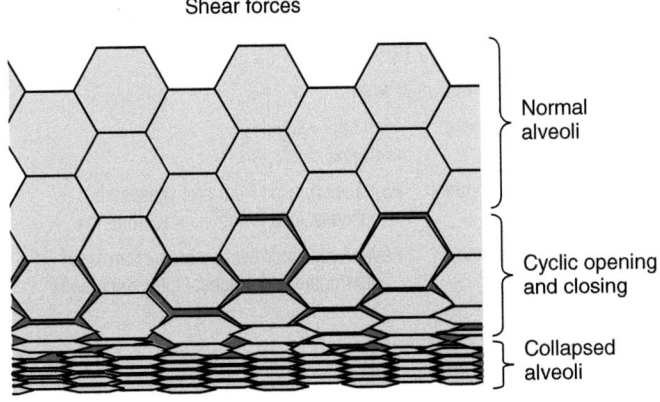

• **Fig. 45.13** Atelectrauma (i.e., cyclic atelectasis) results from the sheer forces generated by repeated opening and collapsing of the alveoli in response to positive-pressure ventilation. (From Papadokos PJ, Lachmann B. The open lung concept of mechanical ventilation: the role of recruitment and stabilization. *Crit Care Clin.* 2007;23:241–250.)

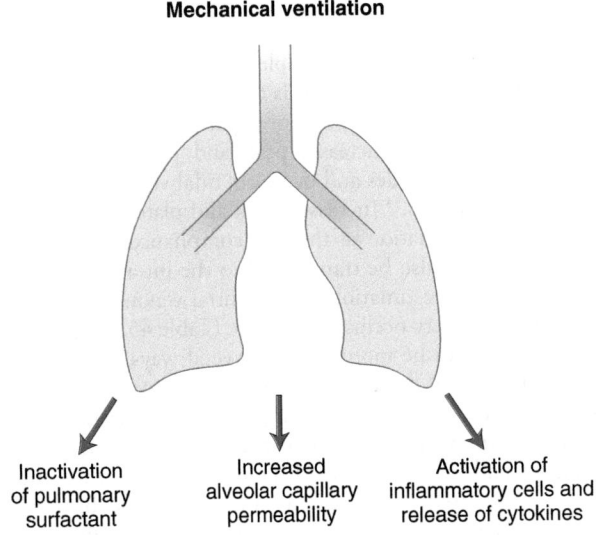

• **Fig. 45.14** Downstream effects of lung injury from mechanical ventilation. (From Papadokos PJ, Lachmann B. The open lung concept of mechanical ventilation: the role of recruitment and stabilization. *Crit Care Clin.* 2007;23:241–250.)

rates exist, expiratory time may be decreased to a point at which the full tidal volume is not exhaled before the next breath. High tidal volumes are less likely to be exhaled entirely before the next breath. Patients with obstructive lung diseases such as COPD and asthma often develop auto-PEEP while on mechanical ventilation because of disease-related limitations in expiratory flow.[134] Expiratory resistance from any obstruction of the ETT (e.g., kinks, secretions) or patient-ventilator dyssynchrony can also lead to auto-PEEP. Auto-PEEP can hence result from high tidal volumes, a high respiratory rate, or a decreased expiratory time relative to inspiratory time in any disease state (Table 45.9).

TABLE 45.9	Intrinsic Positive End-Expiratory Pressure (Auto-PEEP) Factors	
Causes of Auto-PEEP	**Factors**	
High minute ventilation	High tidal volume High respiratory rate	
Expiratory flow limitation	Airway narrowing from bronchospasm, collapse, inflammation, or remodeling	
Expiratory resistance	Patient-ventilator dyssynchrony, Narrow or obstructed endotracheal tube, Secretions	

PEEP, Positive end-expiratory pressure.

Consequences of Auto-Positive End-Expiratory Pressure

Auto-PEEP can decrease venous return, reduce cardiac output, reduce ventricular compliance, and induce hypotension.[135] Hypovolemic patients are at increased risk for PEEP-related hypotension. Alveolar distention from auto-PEEP can lead to barotrauma, worsening oxygenation from ventilation-perfusion ($\dot{V}/\dot{Q}$) mismatch, and VILI. Auto-PEEP increases the work of breathing by raising the pressure differential the patient must generate to trigger a ventilator breath. For example, if the breath is triggered at -2 cm H_2O and the auto-PEEP is 6 cm H_2O, the patient needs to overcome both (-8 cm H_2O of negative pressure) to initiate a breath. Auto-PEEP increases peak and plateau pressures in volume-controlled modes and decreases tidal volume in pressure-controlled ventilation.[54] Increased peak and plateau pressures can lead to an overestimation of thoracic compliance. Increased plateau pressures can also be transmitted to the intrathoracic vessels and lead to an overestimation of the central venous pressures and the pulmonary artery occlusion pressure (Table 45.10).

Auto-PEEP can be monitored in several ways but can sometimes be difficult to detect. Graphs of flow versus time will demonstrate initiation of a new breath before the expiration reaches zero flow. End-expiratory alveolar pressure, measured by introducing an end-expiratory breath-hold and subtracting applied PEEP, can be used to quantitate auto-PEEP. The breath-hold allows the pressure in the proximal airways to equilibrate with alveolar pressure. Auscultation for airflow at the end of expiration is also useful.[136]

TABLE 45.10	Consequences of Intrinsic Positive End-Expiratory Pressure (Auto-PEEP)	
Affected System	**Consequences**	
Cardiac	Decreased venous return Hypotension Overestimation of CVP and PCWP	
Pulmonary	Alveolar overdistention Barotrauma or pneumothorax Increased peak and plateau in pressure ventilation Increased work of breathing Underestimation of thoracic compliance	

CVP, Central venous pressure; *PCWP,* pulmonary capillary wedge pressure; *PEEP,* positive end-expiratory pressure.

Management of auto-PEEP is targeted at promoting alveolar emptying and increasing expiratory time. Reducing minute ventilation by targeting tidal volume or the respiratory rate, or both, and increasing inspiratory flow can be effective measures in reducing auto-PEEP. Management of the underlying condition is important, especially for patients with obstructive lung diseases treated with bronchodilators, steroids, and antimicrobial therapies. In patients with COPD or asthma, the limited expiratory flow can be counterbalanced by application of extrinsic PEEP.[137] Small amounts of applied PEEP can decrease intrinsic PEEP by keeping the small airways open at end-expiration. However, the applied PEEP should be less than intrinsic PEEP to prevent an increase in alveolar pressures.[138]

Infectious Complications

VAP, a type of hospital-acquired pneumonia, is defined as pneumonia that develops more than 48 hours after tracheal intubation. Studies of management with noninvasive ventilation show a decreased incidence of pneumonia when tracheal intubation is avoided.[21] The sooner pneumonia is diagnosed after onset of mechanical ventilation, the better the prognosis. Pneumonia diagnosed later during mechanical ventilation is likely caused by a drug-resistant organism and carries a worse prognosis. Several practices can help minimize the occurrence of pneumonia on the ventilator. These include elevation of the head of the bed to the semirecumbent position of 30 to 45 degrees, aggressive weaning of sedation, use of orotracheal and orogastric tubes to decrease the potential for sinusitis, daily assessments to liberate from mechanical ventilation, avoidance of gastric overdistention, avoidance of unplanned extubation, oral care with antiseptic solution, and limiting contamination of ventilator tubing.[139,140] Once a VAP occurs, there is no difference in mechanical ventilation–free days, the length of ICU stay, the number of organ failure–free days, or mortality rates on day 60 between groups receiving 8 versus 15 days of treatment with appropriate antibiotics.[141]

Conclusion

Various modes of mechanical ventilation can be used to provide respiratory support in critical illness or in patients undergoing general anesthesia. Safe application to limit VILI and negative interactions with other organ systems is fundamental in managing patients receiving mechanical ventilation. NIPPV can be safely and effectively applied to patients with acute respiratory failure from COPD, pulmonary edema, or other conditions. Mechanical ventilation selection using common or uncommon modes is determined by several factors, including hemodynamic instability, severe oxygenation or ventilation derangements, administration of general anesthesia, and patient comfort. A lung-protective strategy incorporating tidal volumes of 6 mL/kg predicted body weight and plateau pressures below 30 cm H_2O improves outcomes in ARDS. Tidal volumes greater than 10 mL/kg predicted body weight should not be routinely used with mechanical ventilation. PEEP can be applied to improve oxygenation and to limit collapse and repeated opening and closing of unstable lung units, which can lead to lung injury. Plateau pressures greater than 35 cm H_2O have been associated with increased risk of barotrauma and VILI. Auto-PEEP should be monitored to avoid related complications. Measures to reduce the risk of VAP should be instituted on initiation of mechanical ventilation.

Daily interruption of sedation and daily trials of spontaneous breathing expedite weaning and liberation from mechanical ventilation. Ventilator-weaning algorithms that allow for nonphysician providers to assess the readiness of patients for extubation when they meet certain preset criteria are often useful.

Selected References

16. Antonelli M, Conti G, Moro ML, et al. Predictors of failure of non-invasive positive pressure ventilation in patients with acute hypoxemic respiratory failure: a multi-center study. *Intensive Care Med.* 2001;27:1718–1728.

43. Gajic O, Dara SI, Mendez JL, et al. Ventilator associated lung injury in patients without acute lung injury at the onset of mechanical ventilation. *Crit Care Med.* 2004;32:1817–1824.

46. Amato MB, Barbas CS, Medeiros DM, et al. Effect of protective-ventilation strategy on mortality in the acute respiratory distress syndrome. *N Engl J Med.* 1998;338:347–354.

47. Brower RG, Lanken PN, MacIntyre N, et al. National Heart, Lung, and Blood Institute ARDS clinical trials network. Higher versus lower positive end-expiratory pressures in patients with the acute respiratory distress syndrome. *N Engl J Med.* 2004;351:327–336.

53. Briel M, Meade M, Mercat A, et al. Higher vs lower positive end-expiratory pressure in patients with acute lung injury and acute respiratory distress syndrome: systematic review and meta-analysis. *JAMA.* 2010;303:865–873.

71. Esteban A, Frutos F, Tobin MJ, et al. A comparison of four methods of weaning patients from mechanical ventilation. Spanish Lung Failure Collaborative Group. *N Engl J Med.* 1995;332:345–350.

124. Girard TD, Kress JP, Fuchs BD, et al. Efficacy and safety of a paired sedation and ventilator weaning protocol for mechanically ventilated patients in intensive care (Awakening and Breathing Controlled trial): a randomized controlled trial. *Lancet.* 2008;371:126–134.

128. Slutsky AS, Ranieri VM. Ventilator-induced lung injury. *N Engl J Med.* 2013;369:2126–2136.

All references can be found online at eBooks.Health.Elsevier.com.

46

Monitoring the Airway and Pulmonary Function

NEAL H. COHEN

CHAPTER OUTLINE

KEY POINTS

- The most reliable method for determining the intratracheal location of an endotracheal tube (ETT) is direct visualization of the tube passing through the vocal cords; flexible scope assessment can define the specific location of the ETT in the airways.
- When using CO_2 detection in exhaled gas from an ETT to document whether it is within the trachea, CO_2 should be present for four or five breaths.
- Paradoxical abdominal wall motion (i.e., abdominal expansion during inspiration without chest excursion) in a patient without upper airway obstruction is an early and critical indicator of respiratory muscle fatigue and impending respiratory failure.
- Bedside thoracic ultrasonography (USG) is a useful way to assess respiratory function and determine response to clinical interventions in selected clinical situations.
- The pulse oximeter is a valuable monitor of oxygenation, but its limitations must be recognized. The accuracy of pulse oximetry is altered by several factors, including external light sources, motion, poor perfusion, and dyshemoglobinemias.
- Analysis of the plethysmographic waveform from a pulse oximeter has clinical utility in the hemodynamic assessment of patients and can be helpful in assessing intravascular volume status in selected patients.
- Although measurement of end-tidal CO_2 tension (P_{ETCO_2}) is a valuable monitor of ventilation during adjustments of ventilatory parameters, it may be an insufficiently accurate measure of ventilation in patients with traumatic brain injury.
- The dead space volume (V_{DS}) to tidal volume (V_T) ratio (V_{DS}/V_T) can be used as a marker of disease severity in patients with acute lung injury.
- When adjusting ventilatory parameters or transitioning a patient from mandatory to spontaneously initiated modes of ventilation, ongoing assessment of gas exchange, work of breathing (WOB), and respiratory mechanics is essential.

Introduction

Monitoring of the airway and respiratory function is critically important for any patient undergoing anesthesia and surgery. It is also an important part of the management of acutely ill patients receiving analgesics or other medications that affect ventilation, as well as patients with obstructive sleep apnea or other abnormalities of the airway. Although several monitoring techniques and clinical assessment tools are available to assess the airway, oxygenation, ventilation, and respiratory function in many clinical situations, the assessment can be challenging, requiring both an understanding of the value and limitations of each monitoring technique, as well as interpretation of the data based on the underlying physiologic considerations. As a parallel example, although there are well-designed algorithms for management of the airway during elective or emergency intubation,[1] even with this evidence-based approach, the clinical situation, goals of therapy, and clinical skills of the provider must be considered in determining the best approach to securing the airway. For each patient, there is rarely a single or best monitoring technique for each clinical situation. The underlying clinical problem for which airway management and/or ventilator support is required will influence the selection and interpretation of each monitoring technique. As a result, the clinician should have a broad understanding of the available monitors, the information each provides, and their limitations.

This chapter describes techniques for monitoring and evaluating the airway, gas exchange, and respiratory function in a variety of clinical situations. It provides an overview of the monitors used to assess each patient and describes specific monitors that are most useful in selected settings. Because the options for securing the airway and providing for ventilatory support have expanded considerably, it is critical for the clinician to know how to interpret the information provided, correlate the data with the clinical situation, and, in some cases, reconcile differences (or contradictions) in information about the patient being provided by the monitors and clinical assessment to make appropriate clinical decisions. In addition, when using these devices for clinical decision making, it is crucial to understand the limitations of each monitoring technique.

Although this chapter will concentrate on identifying specific monitors and monitoring techniques used to assess the airway and pulmonary function, it will also describe the importance and value of the history and physical examination, as an integral part of the assessment and its significance in determining how to optimize clinical management.

Monitoring the Airway

A wide variety of monitors are available to assess the airway in both intubated and nonintubated patients. Although this discussion will emphasize monitoring techniques for the patient requiring tracheal intubation, it is also important to understand what monitors are available to monitor the nonintubated patient. Ensuring that every patient maintains a patent airway, particularly those patients whose underlying clinical conditions place them at risk for obstruction or who are receiving respiratory depressants or medications that compromise either the airway or ventilation, is paramount. Over the past decade, the expanding use of opioid analgesics to ensure that every patient's pain is well managed has, in some cases, contributed to unintended consequences, including hypoventilation and airway obstruction. Newer techniques for monitoring airway patency in the nonintubated patient, although

not perfect, have improved our ability to determine if a patient has obstruction during sleep or with changes in position,[2,3] if the patient is at risk for aspiration,[4] as well as if there is obstruction or reduced cross-sectional area of a tracheal tube.

Monitoring the Native (Nonintubated) Airway

Assessing a patient's airway is critically important to ensure that it is patent, to assess any limitation to gas flow, and to evaluate vocal cord function and ability of the patient to protect his or her airway. This assessment is a routine part of perioperative care. However, although anesthesiologists are aware of the importance of airway assessment before tracheal intubation and use a variety of approaches to evaluate the airway itself and ease of intubation,[5] assessment is equally important for patients who may require analgesics or sedatives, each of which has the potential to affect airway patency or gas exchange. Outside of the operating room (OR) environment, most clinicians assume that the patient can maintain a normal airway, so in most cases the assessment is cursory. For selected patient populations, however, whether scheduled to undergo a procedure or not, it is important to obtain a more detailed history to assess for evidence of upper airway obstruction, particularly during sleep. To do so requires specific questioning of patients (and/or their family members) about sleeping patterns, snoring, daytime somnolence, or sleep deprivation. In addition, patients should be asked about their use of continuous positive airway pressure (CPAP) or bi-level positive airway pressure (BiPAP) and, if used, whether the use has improved their sleep pattern.

For most patients without a history of upper airway obstruction during sleep, assessment of the airway is relatively straightforward. If a patient is breathing comfortably, has a normal voice, and is handling oral secretions without difficulty, then the upper airway is generally intact. However, in some situations, the clinical assessment can be challenging and may underestimate the degree of airway compromise and its implications. For example, if a patient is breathing with low inspiratory flow and low respiratory rate, an assessment may not capture the magnitude of change in airway diameter or vocal cord function that might be present because of a mass or other abnormality. As a patient's respiratory rate or flows increase (e.g., with exercise, fever, or agitation), airway resistance increases markedly, causing stridor or obstruction. As a result, if there is any concern about vocal cord function or large airway narrowing based on history or comorbidities, the patient should be assessed during rapid breathing or while performing mild exercise (e.g., during brisk walking).[6]

Evaluation of the patient who is scheduled for anesthesia and surgery or who may require tracheal intubation in other settings requires a more thorough assessment of the airway, including evaluation of mouth and neck mobility, ease of visualization of the airway, and identification of airway abnormalities that could influence the approach to securing the airway.[1,5] In addition, for patients who are being intubated because they have respiratory failure requiring ventilatory support, assessment of the upper airway before instrumentation helps not only to define how best to access the airway but also to clarify the extent to which upper airway compromise might be contributing to respiratory failure.

Under elective circumstances, assessment of the airway should include a review of the patient's medical history and comorbidities that might influence airway management decisions, a review of past experiences with airway management (if available), and any previous episodes of respiratory failure for which the patient required supplemental oxygen or ventilatory support. As previously noted, the patient (or family) should be questioned about snoring or episodes of airway obstruction during sleep; use of CPAP or BiPAP; previous experiences with tracheal intubation, including difficult intubation; hoarseness after airway manipulation or with exercise; history of neck radiation; and known airway or tracheal abnormalities, including stenosis, tracheomalacia, or neck masses (e.g., goiter).[1] Patients with rheumatoid arthritis should be questioned about upper airway problems, particularly those related to potential arthritic changes in the cricoarytenoid joints, as well as any history of associated pulmonary disease.[7] Patients who have had previous neck or mediastinal surgery should be carefully evaluated for evidence of unilateral or bilateral vocal cord dysfunction. In emergency situations, the assessment may not be as thorough as in elective situations but should include some focused elements of the history and a rapid physical assessment, which can be very useful in identifying potential problems with airway management or tracheal intubation. For patients unable to provide a history, discussion with family members or the nurse caring for the patient, a review of the medical record, and direct observation of the airway and ventilatory pattern while preparing equipment for airway intervention will also provide useful information to guide management decisions.

Clinical examination should include a thorough assessment of the upper airway, including evaluation of dentition; mobility of the jaw, chin, and neck; and assessment of the anticipated ease or difficulty of tracheal intubation based on the size of the mandible and visualization of the airway (i.e., Mallampati classification).[8,9] Most often, this evaluation can be completed expeditiously, at least to assess anticipated relative ease or difficulty of intubation. For patients with obvious signs of upper airway compromise or obstruction, the evaluation may be limited by the emergent need for intervention. Although a lateral neck radiograph can provide useful information about the upper airway, presence of masses in the airway, or epiglottic edema, for most patients a radiologic evaluation is of limited value[10,11] or cannot be completed without putting the patient at significant risk by delaying access to the airway. However, evaluation of the airway can often be performed while managing the airway with bag-mask ventilation, assuming the airway is not completely obstructed. In all cases, if a patient is not ventilating adequately or has significant hypoxemia, the patient should be provided with supplemental oxygen or positive airway pressure by mask, while preparing for the tracheal intubation. For patients with abnormalities of the upper airway that may make routine laryngoscopy difficult, alternative methods to secure the airway must be considered and the appropriate equipment brought to the patient's bedside to allow rapid control of the airway. Most hospitals have developed "difficult airway carts" that provide the needed equipment to facilitate tracheal intubation or other access to the airway, including supraglottic airways (SGAs) of varying styles and sizes, standard laryngoscope, a videolaryngoscope, a flexible intubation scope (FIS), intubating stylets, and cricothyroidotomy kits. For patients whose airways are anticipated to be difficult to manage, a surgeon who can perform emergency tracheostomy should be notified and be available at the bedside to gain control of the airway if noninvasive techniques fail.

Monitoring the Airway During Tracheal Instrumentation

For the patient who requires tracheal intubation, although several monitors are available and useful, the clinical judgment of the clinician provides the most important assessment of the airway and respiratory status. An evaluation of a patient's pattern of ventilation, chest wall and diaphragmatic movement, and mental status can help guide decision-making. Monitoring of oxygenation is also critically important before and during manipulation of the airway because of the risk of hypoxemia, particularly in patients with reduced functional residual capacity (FRC) or high oxygen consumption. During airway management, administration of supplemental oxygen is important, even if the delivery system is not optimal or the delivery of supplemental oxygen is only intermittent, as the airway is being secured. Pulse oximetry is a useful noninvasive monitor for ensuring that the oxygen saturation remains satisfactory during airway manipulation and for guiding delivery of supplemental oxygen and bag-mask ventilation, as clinically appropriate. Although oxygen saturation by pulse oximetry (SpO_2) is an important monitor during tracheal intubation, it is also important to emphasize that pulse oximetry is not a monitor of ventilation. During delivery of supplemental oxygen, even the apneic patient may maintain a satisfactory SpO_2 despite progressively rising arterial carbon dioxide tension ($PaCO_2$) and respiratory acidosis.[12,13]

Monitoring ventilation and carbon dioxide (CO_2) levels based on clinical assessment is challenging. Using the electrocardiogram (ECG) leads to monitor chest wall movement (impedance pneumography) is not reliable in upper airway obstruction because there may be chest wall movement despite inadequate ventilation. Other techniques for monitoring air movement are more useful for monitoring ventilation when upper airway obstruction is of concern, such as nasal cannulae that allow monitoring of CO_2 in expired gas or thermistors in the airway to document changes in temperature of inspiratory and expiratory gases. When using a noninvasive monitor of expired CO_2, the measured CO_2 may not accurately reflect the end-tidal CO_2 ($EtCO_2$) or adequacy of ventilation but will confirm air flow if CO_2 is present during exhalation.

SGAs may provide a satisfactory airway, either for short-term airway management or to facilitate tracheal intubation. For patients undergoing a surgical procedure for which positive-pressure ventilation is not required, an SGA may be used to secure the airway and allows initiation of positive-pressure ventilation using low airway pressures if clinically required. For any patient who has an SGA inserted, proper positioning of the airway must be verified. Direct visualization of SGA placement is usually not required; positioning can be confirmed using clinical signs. If the patient is breathing comfortably without evidence of obstruction, the SGA is usually in a good position. For the spontaneously breathing patient, this clinical assessment is usually sufficient. In selected clinical cases, when positive-pressure ventilation may be required, better confirmation of the correct position is desirable because of the potential risks associated with improper positioning of the SGA. If the SGA is not correctly positioned, positive-pressure ventilation may cause a leak around the SGA, compromising the ability to provide an adequate tidal volume (V_T). In addition, ventilation through an SGA does not prevent entrainment of gas into the stomach, and the risk of regurgitation and aspiration must be considered. In this situation, correct positioning of the SGA must be confirmed, and if there is any question about the appropriate placement, its position must be verified by direct visualization or must be repositioned.

Although a variety of masks and other devices are available to facilitate ventilatory support without the need for tracheal instrumentation, many patients require tracheal intubation for both airway protection and to ensure ventilation either using an endotracheal tube (ETT) inserted through the mouth or nose or with a tracheotomy. When tracheal intubation is required, confirmation of correct placement of the ETT is essential. The most reliable method to assess endotracheal placement is direct visualization of the tube passing through the vocal cords at the time of intubation.

Physical examination is also important to ensure that both lungs are being ventilated after placement of the airway. Auscultation over both lung fields (particularly the apices of the lungs) and stomach should routinely be performed to assess ETT placement. When the ETT is within the trachea, equal breath sounds should be heard over both lung fields while listening over the apices. Auscultation over the upper lung fields minimizes the likelihood of hearing sounds transmitted from the stomach. For most adult patients, if the ETT is located within the trachea, no breath sounds should be heard over the stomach. Unfortunately, auscultation can be misleading. Occasionally, particularly in children, breath sounds are transmitted to the stomach even when the ETT is properly positioned. For patients with extensive parenchymal lung disease, effusions, or endobronchial lesions, breath sounds may not be heard equally over both lung fields even when the ETT is properly positioned within the trachea.

Other clinical signs can be useful for confirming tracheal intubation. They include identifying condensation within the lumen of the ETT during exhalation, palpation of the cuff of the ETT in the suprasternal notch, and the normal feel of a reservoir bag during manual ventilation. Despite the clinical usefulness of these methods, none is infallible, and false-positive and false-negative evaluations have been reported.[14]

A more reliable monitor for confirming tracheal intubation is identification of CO_2 in exhaled gas. If the airway is within the trachea and the patient is ventilating spontaneously or receiving positive-pressure ventilation, CO_2 should be eliminated by the lungs. The presence of CO_2 in exhaled gas or direct measurement of CO_2 concentration can be used to determine the location of the ETT. Several devices are available to monitor CO_2 in expired gases. In the OR, CO_2 can be measured using an infrared device,[15] Raman effect scattering, or mass spectrometry. In the intensive care unit (ICU), emergency department (ED), or other settings including out-of-hospital locations, colorimetric techniques are often used to qualitatively estimate the CO_2 concentration. More commonly, however, infrared capnography is used to directly measure the CO_2 concentration in expired gases.[16,17] As a result of the ease of use and widespread availability of this modality, the documentation of the presence of CO_2 in exhaled gas after placement of an airway device (i.e., capnography) has become a standard of care in anesthesia practice and is routinely used during emergency airway management in many hospitals and emergency settings. A detailed description of capnography is provided in Chapter 30.

CO_2 detection can provide misleading information, however, and is not foolproof.[18–20] For example, when a patient has been ventilated by mask before intubation, CO_2-containing gas may remain in the stomach; a capnogram may then indicate the presence of CO_2 in expired gas that does not reflect CO_2 from the lungs. This problem can also occur when capnography is used to monitor the patient who has recently received bicarbonate-containing solutions or has been drinking beverages containing CO_2 before placement of the airway device. In these situations, CO_2 is eliminated from the stomach during the first few breaths provided through a misplaced ETT in the esophagus. The presence of CO_2 from exhaled gas should, therefore, be monitored for several breaths. If CO_2 continues to be eliminated through the ETT after 4 or 5 breaths, endotracheal placement of the tube can be ensured.[19] Another limitation of capnography is that CO_2 elimination occurs only if a patient has sufficient cardiac output to deliver CO_2 to the lungs. If the patient has suffered a cardiac arrest and cardiac output is very low or absent, no CO_2 is delivered to the lung, leading to no detection of CO_2, even when the ETT is within the trachea.[21–24] During cardiopulmonary resuscitation, chest compressions may be effective at eliminating enough CO_2 from the lungs to confirm ETT placement, even when cardiac output is inadequate. In addition, the presence of CO_2 in exhaled gas provides confirmation that the cardiac output has improved and CO_2 is being eliminated from the lungs.

Other techniques can be used to confirm tracheal intubation. The use of a self-inflating bulb has been advocated as a simple way to confirm the proper positioning of an ETT in out-of-hospital intubations. The technique uses a bulb that is applied to the ETT; self-inflation of the bulb within 4 seconds confirms that the ETT is in the proper position. Although the technique has some proponents, most studies are unable to demonstrate that this is a reliable method to verify ETT placement.[25] More recently, the use of ultrasound has been demonstrated to be helpful for confirming tracheal intubation.[24,26]

Once tracheal intubation has been confirmed, assess the exact location of the ETT within the trachea to avoid placement that is too proximal (increasing the risk of accidental extubation) or too distal (endobronchial). Incorrect positioning of the ETT has been associated with several complications, including pneumothorax and death.[27] The position of the ETT should be confirmed at the time of placement and should be regularly assessed while it remains in place because the position can change even after it is secured. Flexion of the neck moves the ETT toward the carina, whereas extension moves the tube up toward the vocal cords. In adult patients, flexion and extension of the head change the position of the ETT tip by as much as 2 cm.[27,28] Additionally, ETT position can change because of softening of the plastic as it warms or as a result of the patient manipulating the ETT with the tongue. These changes in ETT position place patients at risk for self-extubation, even when the ETT is properly secured and the extremities are restrained.

Several techniques can be used to assess proper positioning of the ETT within the trachea. For example, securing the ETT at a predetermined depth has been advocated as a way to minimize the likelihood of endobronchial intubation. At least one study has suggested that endobronchial placement of the ETT could be avoided if the tube was at a depth of 21 cm in women and 23 cm in men when referenced to the anterior alveolar ridge or the front teeth.[29] However, subsequent studies have not confirmed that this technique prevents endobronchial intubation in critically ill adults or that it is predictive of the relationship between the position of the ETT at the teeth and the tube's position relative to the carina (see Chapter 30).[30–32]

Flexible laryngoscopy/bronchoscopy is now commonly used to confirm ETT placement if there are clinical concerns about the location of the tip of the ETT.[33] This technique is useful, although not without some risk. Insertion of an FIS reduces the effective cross-sectional area of the ETT, potentially compromising ventilation and oxygenation.[34] Peak inspiratory pressure increases during the visualization. Partial obstruction of the ETT results in an increase in airway resistance, which may lead to the unrecognized development of elevated end-expiratory pressure, increasing the risk of pneumothorax or hemodynamic compromise.[35] Despite these limitations, in experienced hands the assessment can be completed rapidly and without complications. It is a particularly useful way of documenting the location of the ETT within the trachea in the patient for whom the specific location of the tube is critically important, such as one with abnormal tracheal anatomy, the patient at risk for obstruction of the right upper lobe bronchus, or one with specific needs related to the planned surgical procedure.

Capnography can also be a useful tool for identifying endobronchial migration of an ETT in some patients.[36] With distal migration of the ETT, the EtCO$_2$ falls; this is usually associated with an increase in peak inspiratory pressure. These changes, although not always reliable, can provide early evidence of ETT migration because the EtCO$_2$ changes precede a change in arterial blood gases (ABGs) or other signs of displacement.

Probably the most used method to assess the positioning of the ETT within the trachea is the routine postintubation chest radiograph. The distance of the ETT from the carina can be measured from a portable anteroposterior radiograph obtained at the bedside. Although many clinicians have questioned whether the cost of chest radiography warrants its routine use for documentation of ETT placement, it remains the most useful and reliable method to determine the appropriate depth of the ETT within the trachea.[30,32] Alternative methods, such as ultrasonography (USG), are becoming more commonly used to assess positioning of the ETT,[24,26] although the chest x-ray continues to be used, not only for assessment of the ETT but also to confirm placement of catheters, to assess lung fields, and to identify potential complications of mechanical ventilatory support.

One special clinical situation warrants additional monitoring of the airway. Some patients require placement of a double-lumen tube (DLT) to facilitate a unilateral surgical procedure on the lung, to provide differential lung ventilation, or to protect one lung from contamination with blood or infected secretions from the other lung. In these cases, proper placement of the DLT must be ensured. Physical examination alone and other monitoring techniques are usually insufficient to confirm proper positioning. Flexible bronchoscopic evaluation is required to confirm DLT position after initial placement and to reevaluate placement after the patient is repositioned for a surgical procedure or while requiring differential lung ventilation in the ICU.[37] Direct visualization of the tip of the DLT and the relationship between the tracheal and bronchial lumens ensures that the tube is in the proper position and that the two lungs are isolated. Other techniques can be used to diagnose malpositioning of DLTs, although few studies confirm their value. Capnography, which can be useful in identifying endobronchial migration of a single-lumen ETT,[36] may provide information about the position of a DLT, particularly if only one lung is being ventilated at the time of evaluation. Spirometry, which can be obtained from in-line monitoring devices added to the anesthesia circuit or monitoring modalities provided by critical care ventilators, can also provide early detection of DLT malpositioning.[38,39] As an ETT migrates, expiratory flow obstruction can be detected as a change in the shape of the expiratory limb of the flow-volume loop; inspiratory obstruction is best diagnosed by a change in the pressure-volume loop.

Monitoring the Airway in the Mechanically Ventilated Patient

As noted, confirmation of the placement of an airway device in the patient receiving mechanical ventilatory support should be done routinely. Most often, the assessment is performed by a respiratory therapist who assesses the position of the ETT at the lip or incisor

level to ensure that it has not migrated. Although this assessment can be reassuring, the position of the ETT within the trachea cannot be confirmed by documenting the location of the tube within the mouth. After intubation, the ETT becomes soft and more pliable, allowing it to migrate. In addition, some patients will use the tongue or teeth to manipulate the ETT, occasionally causing the cuff of the ETT to migrate above the vocal cords. ETTs that remain in place for longer periods of time can malfunction, including tearing of the cuff or leaking of the pilot balloon, leading to malpositioning. As a result, every intubated patient should have the ETT assessed regularly and should have the pressure within the ETT cuff assessed to ensure that it is neither over- nor underinflated. A variety of techniques have been recommended to assess ETT cuff pressure, although no foolproof methods for confirming either its location nor the appropriate cuff pressure have been identified.[40]

When a patient is clinically stable and ready for removal of the ETT, a careful evaluation of the patient's airway should be performed before tracheal extubation and immediately after the ETT is removed. After the patient is weaned from ventilatory support and is being prepared for extubation, the patient's ability to protect and maintain the airway after tracheal extubation must be assessed. Unfortunately, despite efforts to assess the airway and its patency before extubation, it is not possible to completely assess the airway with an ETT in place. Various clinical criteria have been used to determine whether an intubated patient can protect his or her airway. The most common criteria are to determine if the patient has a normal gag response and a strong cough. Neither of these can be completely assessed with an ETT in place. A patient cannot have a normal cough with a tube inserted into the airway. Most often the cough is elicited when the patient's airway is suctioned and reflects stimulation/irritation of the carina, rather than an assessment of the ability to cough and clear secretions from the airway. Despite these limitations, if a patient gags when the back of the throat is stimulated and coughs during suctioning, most clinicians feel confident that the patient will be able to prevent aspiration after extubation. These criteria, however, have never been subjected to scientific evaluation. Some patients who have a poor gag or cough with the ETT in place can handle secretions and cough effectively after tracheal extubation. Others who seem to have a satisfactory cough or gag before extubation are still unable to protect the airway when extubated. The inability of a patient to adequately protect the airway may become clinically apparent only when the patient begins to eat, because pharyngeal function may remain abnormal for several hours to days after tracheal intubation.[41-43] Nonetheless, these criteria continue to be the most used to determine whether the patient can be extubated safely, but they should be interpreted with caution.

In addition to assessing a patient's gag and cough, the airway should be assessed to ensure there is no edema or other abnormality, such as vocal cord dysfunction, that might compromise ventilation before ETT removal. For patients electively intubated for a straightforward surgical procedure, routine clinical evaluation is usually sufficient; no formal assessment of airway size is required before extubation. However, if the patient develops significant edema of the head and neck during surgery, as might occur during a procedure performed in the prone position, or for a patient undergoing a head or neck procedure that may compromise the airway, a more thorough assessment is required. A common technique used to assess airway size is to determine whether the patient can breathe around the ETT when the cuff is deflated and the ETT is occluded (cuff leak test); if the patient is able to breathe around the ETT, the patient can be successfully extubated. Some patients, however, become agitated during this maneuver or cannot tolerate breathing around the uninflated cuff of the ETT. As a result, the technique, although useful in some situations, is not a reliable method for assessing tracheal diameter in all intubated patients.

Many patients cannot breathe adequately around the occluded ETT because of the increased resistance with the ETT in place; therefore alternative methods have been suggested. The cuff leak test has been used to assess the airway pressure required for a leak to develop around the cuff when positive-pressure ventilation is applied through the ETT with the cuff deflated.[44] Although the specific pressure at which the leak develops has not been well correlated with successful extubation, some clinicians require that a leak occur when the airway pressure is low (usually <15 cm H_2O) before extubation. Unfortunately, some studies, including a systematic review of the literature, have been unable to confirm the diagnostic value of the test or a specific leak pressure or volume above which extubation is contraindicated.[45] If the airway pressure required to identify a leak during positive-pressure inspiration is high (20 to 25 cm H_2O), the patient may have sufficient upper airway edema to warrant leaving the ETT in place until the edema resolves. If, however, the leak occurs at a low airway pressure, the likelihood of successful extubation is reassuring. A patient who has significant head, neck, facial, or conjunctival edema postoperatively because of large fluid requirements may not be ready for extubation. As the edema in the face, head, and neck resolve, the edema of the airway is also most often reduced as well.

Monitoring the Airway After Tracheal Extubation

After tracheal extubation, the airway must be closely monitored. For most surgical patients, the risk of airway compromise after successful extubation of the trachea is small. Occasionally, airway edema can become a problem after removal of the ETT. Less commonly, vocal cord dysfunction or cricoarytenoid dislocation, which was not obvious while the ETT was in place, can cause hoarseness or airway obstruction.

As noted, patients who have extensive edema after surgery or a critical illness can have the ETT safely removed when the clinical signs of edema resolve. However, in some cases, the airway is stented open when the ETT is in place; after removal, the airway diameter may be reduced. In this situation, the airway narrowing becomes evident as the patient's inspiratory flow increases, resulting in stridor and increased airway resistance. If stridor develops and edema of the airway is the likely cause, aerosolized vasoconstrictors, such as nebulized racemic epinephrine, can be administered to reduce airway swelling. The vasoconstrictive effects of the epinephrine reduce the edema and improve the cross-sectional area of the airway. When epinephrine is required, it must be administered with caution. After discontinuation of the epinephrine, rebound hyperemia can occur. If repeated epinephrine treatments are required, the epinephrine dose and frequency of treatment should be tapered (in frequency or dose) rather than abruptly withdrawn. Systemic steroids can also be administered either before or immediately after extubation to reduce upper airway edema. Because the onset of action of steroids is prolonged, it is often most appropriate to administer them 6 to 8 hours before the time of anticipated extubation. When edema, stridor, or other unanticipated complications occur after extubation, emergent reintubation may be required. In patients for whom the clinical assessment is not entirely clear but the risks of extubation are outweighed by the benefits, specialized intubation equipment,

including an FIS and a cricothyroidotomy kit, should be readily available to facilitate emergent intubation, if needed.

Assessment of vocal cord function should also be considered before extubation. After some surgical procedures involving the neck or upper airway, such as thyroidectomy or parathyroidectomy, vocal cord function may be compromised because of transection of or trauma to the recurrent laryngeal nerve. Recurrent laryngeal nerve dysfunction can also occur because of high tracheal mucosal pressure transmitted from an overinflated ETT cuff or as a result of direct trauma at the time of tracheal intubation.[46,47] Unfortunately, assessment of vocal cord function is very difficult while the ETT is in place. If vocal cord dysfunction is suspected, the airway can be assessed by inserting an FIS through the ETT and, with the patient sedated or anesthetized, slowly removing the ETT while evaluating vocal cord motion through the scope. If vocal cord function is compromised, the ETT can be advanced back into the airway, using the flexible bronchoscope as a stylet. In most cases, however, assessment of vocal cord function requires that the ETT be removed. After extubation, evaluation of laryngeal and vocal cord function can be assessed with an FIS based on clinical findings, such as stridor or voice hoarseness. In those patients for whom there is concern about vocal cord function or upper airway patency, the assessment should be performed in the OR or in an ICU setting. When performed in the ICU, a surgeon or other physician who can perform a tracheotomy should be at the bedside at the time of the evaluation. Alternatively, the assessment and ETT removal can be performed in the OR under more controlled conditions, where emergency airway and surgical equipment is immediately available. In this case, the evaluation and trial extubation can be performed while the patient is anesthetized with a volatile anesthetic agent or topical anesthesia and is breathing spontaneously. If severe stridor or airway obstruction develops with removal of the ETT, the patient can be reintubated or have a tracheostomy performed for long-term airway maintenance. In most cases, even in the setting of unilateral recurrent laryngeal nerve or vocal cord injury, the patient will be able to breathe normally without stridor, unless inspiratory flows are excessive. The greater risk exists for the patient who suffers bilateral vocal cord palsies. While still sedated, the patient may not have stridor or evidence of airway obstruction. However, as the patient awakens and inspiratory flows increase, the stridor becomes obvious and usually requires emergent tracheal intubation or, more commonly, tracheostomy.

Stridor can alternatively occur as a result of dislocation of the cricoarytenoid joint. The risk of cricoarytenoid dislocation is greatest in patients with rheumatoid arthritis, in whom the joint may be affected. However, dislocation of the arytenoid should be considered for any stridorous patient for whom intubation was difficult, requiring multiple attempts and extensive manipulation of the airway. When present, the arytenoid may require surgical manipulation to reposition and prevent persistent upper airway compromise.

Monitoring the Airway in the Patient With a Tracheostomy

For patients with a tracheostomy, the patency and positioning of the tracheostomy tube should be assessed regularly. As part of the monitoring and assessment of the airway, it is essential to understand the reason for tracheostomy and the consequences of the tracheostomy tube becoming occluded or dislodged. For the patient who has a permanent tracheotomy tube in place, the management options depend on whether the patient has a patent upper airway or has undergone a laryngectomy. If the latter, the patient cannot be intubated from above under any circumstance, and, in this case, the patient may or may not require a cuffed tube because the risk of aspiration is minimal. For most of these patients, the tracheal stoma is well healed and risk of loss of the stoma is low. Many of these patients can remove the tracheostomy tube for cleaning and replace it without difficulty. On the other hand, for patients with a fresh tracheostomy, monitoring of the airway is critically important. If a freshly placed tracheotomy tube becomes dislodged, replacing the tube can be very difficult, because the stoma may be difficult to cannulate, and the risk of misplacement is high.[48] To minimize the likelihood of loss of the airway, the physician who performed the procedure will usually place stay sutures into the tracheal wall to facilitate replacement of the tube in case of dislodgement. Even when care has been taken to allow easier access to the airway, if a fresh tracheotomy tube becomes dislodged, reinsertion carries significant risk. As a result, whenever caring for a patient with a new tracheotomy tube in place, the clinician should review the patient records to determine whether oral intubation was difficult and, if so, what was done to ensure proper placement and to identify the reason that the tracheostomy was performed. At all times, additional backup airway equipment, including replacement tracheotomy tubes, should be readily available.

Most tracheotomy tubes used to facilitate mechanical ventilation or provide airway protection are disposable, although for those patients with a permanent tracheostomy, an uncuffed metal tube may be used to access the airway. For most other applications, a disposable tracheostomy tube is used; most have inner cannulas, which can be replaced or removed for cleaning. In every case, the clinician caring for the patient should be knowledgeable about the device used to secure the airway and backup equipment should be available. Alternative approaches to the airway may be necessary if the patient develops upper airway obstruction or other clinical complications, such as occlusion of the inner cannula. It is useful to have a clearly defined algorithm for addressing these clinical challenges.[49] Many hospitals have developed signage to clarify the reason for the tracheostomy, the patient's underlying anatomy, and the options for securing the airway, should it become dislodged. This approach can be very helpful in addressing emergent situations, particularly when those involved in the placement of the original airway are not available to assess the patient and guide clinical decision-making.

Monitoring Respiratory Function

Clinical Assessment

Clinical examination remains one of the most important and valuable methods to monitor a patient's respiratory status. Too often, attention is placed on technologically sophisticated monitoring devices, and the physical examination is cursory, or the clinical findings are undervalued. Nonetheless, much information about actual or potential airway problems and abnormalities in pulmonary mechanical function or gas exchange can be obtained from a carefully performed and thorough examination. Many of the early signs of respiratory failure are apparent on physical assessment before the abnormalities are apparent by other means. For example, the respiratory rate provides important information about respiratory reserve, dead space, and respiratory drive,

particularly when interpreted in conjunction with $Paco_2$. Tachypnea is frequently the earliest sign of impending respiratory failure. The patient's pattern of breathing should be evaluated. Subtle changes in the respiratory rate, V_T, and pattern of breathing may provide an early indication of increased work of breathing (WOB) (as may occur with reduced lung compliance, increased airway resistance, or phrenic nerve dysfunction) or altered ventilatory drive. Although inspiratory flow and minute ventilation ($\dot{V}E$) are difficult to quantify by clinical examination alone, respiratory distress often manifests as the patient attempts to increase alveolar ventilation by taking larger, more rapid inspirations.

Upper airway obstruction, as may occur after manipulation of the airway or in association with epiglottitis or a mass in or around the airway, can be assessed by careful clinical evaluation. Nasal flaring, stridor, and chest wall movement in the absence of airflow suggest upper airway obstruction. If the patient is making respiratory efforts and has abdominal expansion during inspiration without chest excursions, he or she has upper airway obstruction and may require manipulation of the upper airway, including a jaw thrust, initiation of noninvasive positive-pressure ventilation (NIPPV), or tracheal intubation. When the patient presents with stridor, the physical evaluation is also useful in identifying the location of airway compromise. When the stridor occurs primarily during inspiration, it is caused by extrathoracic obstruction; when it occurs during exhalation, it reflects an intrathoracic obstruction. If the stridor occurs during both inspiration and exhalation, the obstruction is fixed, such as may occur with tracheal stenosis. A fixed obstruction is rarely amenable to conservative treatment, and tracheal intubation is most often required until a more definitive therapy can be provided. In selected patients, helium therapy can be used as a temporizing intervention until a more definitive treatment can be provided.[50]

Respiratory dyssynchrony (when the patient has no evidence of upper airway obstruction) is an early and critical indicator of respiratory muscle fatigue and impending respiratory failure.[51,52] Respiratory dyssynchrony is identified by assessing chest wall and abdominal movement during normal tidal breathing. A paradoxical respiratory pattern suggests that the patient may have inadequate muscle strength to sustain spontaneous respiration and that positive-pressure ventilation support may be required. Tobin and colleagues found that respiratory muscle dyssynchrony could occur before the development of fatigue, although fatigue of the respiratory muscles does not always result in the development of dyssynchrony.[53–55]

Clinical observation of the patient should include careful assessment of the respiratory muscles to assess the patient's respiratory reserve. Use of accessory muscles, including the sternocleidomastoid and scalene muscles, is commonly seen in patients with long-standing respiratory failure associated with chronic obstructive pulmonary disease (COPD).[56] The position of the diaphragm and diaphragmatic motion are also affected in patients with severe COPD. The patient who relies on accessory muscles and has minimal diaphragmatic excursion does not have any respiratory reserve and is at risk for recurrent respiratory failure; these patients present a significant challenge during weaning when mechanical ventilatory support is required.

A routine physical examination of the lungs should be performed as part of the assessment for every patient. The examination can provide evidence of parenchymal lung abnormalities and cardiopulmonary pathology. Auscultation of the lungs can provide useful information about the presence of pleural effusions, pneumothorax, or other extrapulmonary air and can assess the location of the diaphragms. The examination can provide information about potential physiologic abnormalities and guide the selection of other monitoring techniques, including ABGs and chest radiography.

Although the physical examination is useful and should be performed routinely, some of the physical signs and symptoms of respiratory failure are not diagnostic but instead reflect the physiologic manifestations of the underlying problem. The greatest value of the physical examination is that it provides an initial baseline assessment of the patient, and subsequent examinations can clarify the response to clinical interventions. The physical examination combined with other monitoring modalities remains an important monitor of respiratory status.

Imaging

The chest radiograph is another important monitor of pulmonary status, although it represents a static picture of the clinical situation. The chest radiograph can confirm proper placement of central venous and other catheters, the ETT,[32] and implantable cardiac devices. Routine portable chest radiography usually provides evidence of pulmonary infiltrates and pulmonary edema, if present. Radiographic findings that suggest pulmonary edema include bronchial cuffing, perihilar pulmonary infiltrates, and Kerley B lines. Although these findings are helpful, in many critically ill patients, diffuse bilateral infiltrates caused by infection can be difficult to differentiate from pulmonary edema. When underlying pulmonary diseases such as COPD coexist with acute pulmonary edema, the classic bilateral, fluffy pulmonary infiltrates may not be present. In these circumstances, the x-ray findings must be correlated with other clinical data to explain the radiographic findings.

The chest radiograph can occasionally identify abnormalities in the larger airways, including tracheal stenosis and dilatation (as may occur when the ETT cuff is overinflated), although confirmation of the suspected findings usually requires computed tomography (CT) or magnetic resonance imaging (MRI). The presence of tracheomalacia is more difficult to identify because the airway may look normal on a routine chest radiograph. The tracheal abnormality is more evident on clinical examination (i.e., stridor with forced exhalation) or on a dynamic radiographic study, such as a cine-CT scan.

The routine chest radiograph has limitations when used as a monitor of respiratory status. Radiographic findings do not always correlate with other clinical and physiologic monitors because the radiologic changes can be delayed in onset and resolution. The radiologic technique also influences the value of the chest radiograph as a monitor. Most commonly, for intubated and mechanically ventilated patients, a portable anteroposterior radiograph is obtained with the patient in the supine position. In most cases, the chest radiograph is obtained during maximal inspiration. The timing of the film to the respiratory cycle can be difficult in patients who are tachypneic or require a high minute ventilation. As a result, interpretation of changes in heart size, the presence or absence of atelectasis and pleural effusions, or detection of pneumothoraces can be challenging. When trying to identify any of these abnormalities, other views, including upright or lateral decubitus x-ray films, may be obtained, depending on the suspected pathology and the ability to obtain good images in these different positions. Occasionally, an ultrasound or CT scan of the chest may be a more useful way of confirming the presence of pleural effusions, pulmonary abscesses, or other abnormalities.

Other imaging evaluations can be useful to assess abnormalities observed on the chest radiograph or physical examination. Ventilation/perfusion ($\dot{V}/\dot{Q}$) scans have been used to detect pulmonary emboli, although they are often inadequate or impossible to obtain in the mechanically ventilated critically ill patient. For the ICU patient with suspected pulmonary emboli, pulmonary arteriograms or more commonly CT angiograms are performed because they can be completed quickly and provide better diagnostic information than the $\dot{V}/\dot{Q}$ scan alone.

CT and MRI can also be obtained to assess the airways and pulmonary parenchyma. These scans can identify the location, extent, and character of upper airway abnormalities, including mass lesions, pulmonary intraparenchymal lesions, pleural effusions, and other pulmonary and extrapulmonary abnormalities (see Chapter 2).

Ultrasound examination of the lung is increasingly being used as a diagnostic aid in the clinical evaluation and management of critically ill patients, not only to assess presence of pleural effusions but for a variety of other reasons.[57-59] In recent guidelines on the use of bedside USG in the critically ill, thoracic USG has been recommended to complement or replace the routine use of chest radiography in the diagnosis of pneumothorax and to be the primary diagnostic modality used for interstitial and parenchymal disease in patients with respiratory failure.[59] Lung USG can also be used to evaluate lung aeration both before and after a trial of spontaneous breathing, during changes in the level of positive end-expiratory pressure, and to quantify and characterize the burden and etiology of pulmonary edema.[58] Bedside USG has also been demonstrated to have clinical value in the assessment of both the lungs and heart in the hemodynamically unstable patient. It has been shown to reduce diagnostic uncertainty and guide clinical interventions.[60] A standardized hypotension protocol examination includes a focused cardiac examination, abdominal scan, and transthoracic scan.[60] The use of USG in emergency clinical situations has been described as a visual stethoscope allowing rapid assessment of both hemodynamic and respiratory status in some unstable patients.[57,61]

Assessment of Gas Exchange

One of the most important goals in monitoring pulmonary function is to determine whether the lungs can maintain satisfactory oxygenation and ventilation. For these purposes, both invasive and noninvasive monitors of gas exchange are used routinely. Although noninvasive devices are useful and provide important information about oxygenation and ventilation, the ABG remains the most reliable monitor of oxygenation, ventilation, and acid-base abnormalities.[62]

Blood Gas Monitoring

ABG measurement is an essential component of respiratory monitoring. It provides direct measurement of arterial oxygen tension (Pao_2), $Paco_2$, and pH. From these measured parameters, bicarbonate concentration (HCO_3^-), oxygen saturation (Spo_2), and base excess or base deficit are calculated. The measured and calculated parameters define adequacy of gas exchange, acid-base balance, and overall cardiorespiratory status.

ABGs including Pao_2, $Paco_2$, and pH are used routinely in the OR, ICU, ED, and occasionally in other clinical settings to evaluate gas exchange and respiratory reserve. Direct measurement of Pao_2 from a sample of arterial blood obtained from a direct arterial puncture or from an indwelling arterial catheter has been the traditional method for assessing oxygenation. To interpret Pa_{O_2} accurately requires an understanding of normal pulmonary physiology and the influences of alterations in ventilation and perfusion on the predicted value of Pa_{O_2}. Normal values of Pa_{O_2} can vary over time by as much as 10%, as can the measurement error by the blood gas machine. In addition to these technical and physiologic determinants of the Pa_{O_2}, "normal" Pa_{O_2} declines with age. Hypoxemia can result from several factors, including inadequate inspired oxygen (i.e., low alveolar oxygen tension [Pa_{O_2}], $\dot{V}/\dot{Q}$ mismatch, shunt, or inadequate cardiac output (i.e., low mixed venous oxygen tension [Pv_{O_2}]). Documentation of an acceptable Pa_{O_2} is reassuring, although it is important to put the Pa_{O_2} value into context. It alone does not ensure that a patient's O_2 delivery is sufficient. To assess the adequacy of oxygen delivery, additional studies are necessary, including evaluation of acid-base status, measurement of serum lactate and mixed venous oxygen content, and cardiac output measurement.

The Pa_{CO_2} is used to assess adequacy of ventilation, differentiating whether ventilation is normal or abnormal (too high or too low). The normal Pa_{CO_2} is 40 mm Hg. If the Pa_{CO_2} is 40 mm Hg or less, the patient is hyperventilating; if the Pa_{CO_2} is 40 mm Hg or more, the patient is hypoventilating. However, the Pa_{CO_2} alone is only one measure of the adequacy of ventilation. It must be interpreted in relation to the pH. In response to changes in pH, ventilatory drive changes. When a patient develops a metabolic alkalosis, as might occur after a bicarbonate infusion or the transfusion of large quantities of citrated blood, the ventilatory drive is decreased. The Pa_{CO_2} rises, but the decrease in minute ventilation, $\dot{V}E$, is appropriate and is not an indication of respiratory failure. Similarly, the patient who has a significant metabolic acidosis should increase $\dot{V}E$ to normalize the pH. In interpreting whether the patient is ventilating appropriately and has a normal ventilatory drive, the Pa_{CO_2} and pH must be evaluated concurrently. For example, if a patient has a normal Pa_{CO_2} of 40 mm Hg, but the pH is below normal (e.g., 7.25), the ventilatory effort is inadequate, suggesting inadequate respiratory compensation because of medications that are suppressing ventilatory drive or underlying respiratory failure.

When arterial blood cannot be obtained, venous blood sampling (peripheral or central) can be used to estimate arterial Pa_{CO_2}. In some clinical situations, the difference between Pa_{CO_2} and venous CO_2 tension (Pv_{CO_2}) is small, and Pv_{CO_2} can be used as an estimate of Pa_{CO_2}. However, the exact relationship between arterial and venous Pa_{CO_2} is not consistent from patient to patient or within a single patient as clinical conditions change; therefore, Pv_{CO_2} cannot be used as a simple substitute for Pa_{CO_2}. Although venous blood can be helpful in assessing ventilation, it does not provide meaningful information about arterial oxygenation.

Although monitoring gas exchange using blood gas measurements has clinical use, the technique has limitations. Blood gas monitoring is invasive, and samples must be drawn from an indwelling arterial catheter, an arterial puncture, or, in some cases, venous access sites. Frequent blood gas sampling can result in significant blood loss, which may pose problems for any unstable patient, particularly the pediatric patient or anemic adult. In addition, arterial catheters placed to allow frequent sampling and for blood pressure monitoring carry the potential risk of complications, including hemorrhage, hand ischemia, arterial thrombosis and embolism, development of arterial aneurysms,[63] and infection.[64,65] Arterial catheters are an underrecognized source of catheter-related bloodstream infection in critically ill patients.[66]

Unfortunately, the use of barrier precautions during placement of arterial lines, as recommended by the Centers for Disease Control guidelines on prevention of catheter-related infections, is not a routine practice in many critical care units.[67]

Another limitation of blood gas monitoring is its intermittent nature. When a patient's respiratory status is unstable or rapidly evolving, or when frequent adjustments in ventilatory support are required, intermittent monitoring may be insufficient. In these clinical situations, continuous monitoring is preferable. Continuous intraarterial blood gas monitors can provide useful real-time data regarding gas exchange and acid-base status,[68,69] although the clinical use of these monitors has not been validated and the technology is not widely available.[70,71] These monitors use fluorescence-based probes placed through an arterial catheter to provide a continuous assessment of Pa_{O_2}, Pa_{CO_2}, and pH. The information obtained from these instruments should provide more immediate information about changes in gas exchange or acid-base balance. However, the probes and monitors are more expensive than intermittent blood gas analysis, their reliability has not yet been validated, and, as a result, these continuous monitoring devices have not become routine monitors.

Noninvasive Monitoring

Assessment of gas exchange using noninvasive techniques has revolutionized clinical care, particularly for anesthesiologists and intensive care providers. Because clinical assessment of gas exchange is unreliable and often a late sign of deterioration,[72] noninvasive devices that continuously monitor oxygenation and ventilation have become valuable tools when caring for patients in the OR, ICU, and, increasingly, in other clinical settings. Several noninvasive methods are available for evaluating oxygenation and ventilation. The most commonly used devices include pulse oximetry for monitoring oxygenation and the capnogram for evaluating ventilation.

Pulse Oximetry

Pulse oximetry provides a rapid, continuous, and noninvasive estimation of the oxygen saturation of hemoglobin in arterial blood, and it is used routinely to monitor clinical care involving airway management in the OR, ED, and ICU.[73-76] It has become the standard monitor of oxygenation during administration of sedation for procedures and during general medical care.[77-80] With routine use of this monitor, a high prevalence of clinically undetected hypoxemia in adults and children has been demonstrated.[73,80-82] These episodes of desaturation may affect morbidity and mortality.[83,84] With severe and sustained hypoxemia (i.e., Sp_{O_2} <85% for more than 5 minutes), patients with known cardiac disease were shown to be twice as likely to have perioperative ischemia after noncardiac surgery.[84] Among medical patients, those who experienced episodes of hypoxemia within the first 24 hours of hospitalization were three times more likely to die 4 to 7 months after discharge.[83]

It is logical to assume that the routine use of pulse oximetry has made caring for patients safer by increasing the detection of hypoxemia, better understanding its causes, and allowing more rapid and effective interventions to correct the pathophysiologic causes. It has been suggested that the early detection of arterial oxygen desaturation with the use of pulse oximetry may improve outcomes.[84-87] Although clinical studies have not confirmed this, they do not negate the presumed benefit of this monitoring tool.[88-91] A systematic review of the Cochrane database found no evidence of an outcome benefit with the use of pulse oximetry in anesthesia practice.[92] Despite the lack of good outcome data to document the value of pulse oximetry, its use is considered standard of care for critically ill patients and patients receiving general anesthesia or moderate to deep sedation. When using pulse oximetry, however, interpretation of the information provided requires an understanding of the measurement technique and its limitations—including a recognition that it is not a monitor of ventilation.

To measure the oxygen saturation of hemoglobin in arterial blood, pulse oximetry uses two fundamental principles: the differential light absorption of oxyhemoglobin (O_2Hb) and reduced (deoxygenated) hemoglobin (HHb) and the increase in light absorption produced by pulsatile blood flow compared with that of background connective tissue, skin, bone, and venous blood.[79,93] The spectrophotometric principle that forms the basis for oximetry is the Lambert-Beer law (Eq. 1), which allows determination of the concentration of an unknown solute in a solvent by light absorption.

$$I_1 I_0 = e^{-alc} \tag{1}$$

where
I_1 = intensity of the light out of the sample
I_0 = intensity of the incident light
a = absorption coefficient of the substance
l = distance the light travels through the material (i.e., path length)
c = concentration of the absorbing species
e = base of the natural logarithm

Use of the Lambert-Beer law allows the determination of the concentration of a solute in a solvent if the extinction coefficient is known. It also follows that for a solution with multiple solutes, a separate wavelength of light is needed for differentiation of the solutes. For a solution with four solutes, four wavelengths of light are required.

Commercially available pulse oximeters use light-emitting diodes (LEDs) that transmit light at specific wavelengths: 660 nm (red) and 940 nm (infrared). These wavelengths were selected because the absorption characteristics of O_2Hb and HHb are sufficiently different at these wavelengths to allow differentiation of O_2Hb and HHb (Fig. 46.1). The pulse oximeter determines arterial saturation by timing the measurement to pulsations in the arterial system. During pulsatile flow, the vascular bed expands and contracts, creating a change in the light path length.[74] These pulsations alter the quantity of light transmitted to the sensor and provide a plethysmographic waveform.[94] This timing of the signal allows the pulse oximeter to differentiate arterial oxygen saturation from venous saturation based on the ratio of pulsatile and baseline absorption of red and infrared light (Fig. 46.2).

The pulse oximeter displays the SpO_2 based on a ratio (R) of pulsatile and baseline absorption at the two wavelengths transmitted (i.e., 660 and 940 nm) in the tissue bed. The relationship is shown in Eq. 2:

$$R = \frac{\text{Pulsatile absorbance at 660 nm/}}{\text{nonpulsatile absorbance at 660 nm}} \Big/ \frac{\text{Pulsatile absorbance at 940 nm/}}{\text{nonpulsatile absorbance at 940 nm}} \tag{2}$$

The SpO_2 displayed by the pulse oximeter is empirically related to this calculated value based on calibration curves derived for healthy, nonsmoking adult men breathing oxygen at various concentrations. Most commercially available pulse oximeters are calibrated over the range of 70% to 100%. The accuracy of pulse

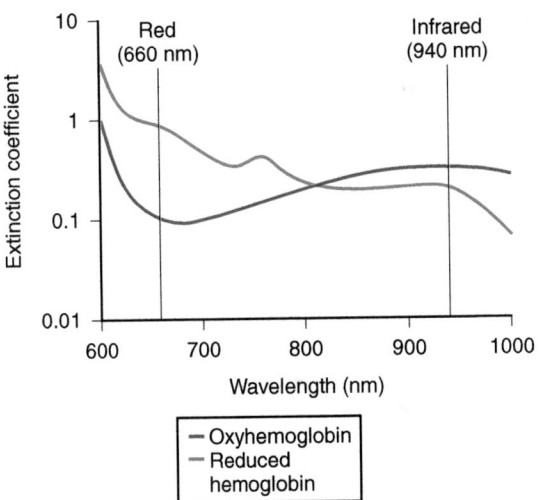

• **Fig. 46.1** Absorption (extinction) characteristics of oxyhemoglobin and reduced hemoglobin are shown. There are marked differences between the two at light wavelengths of 660 nm (red) and 940 nm (infrared). (From Tobin MJ. Respiratory monitoring. *JAMA.* 1990;264:244–251.)

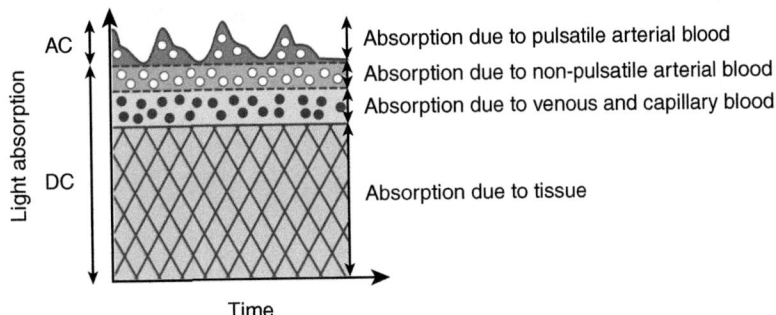

• **Fig. 46.2** Schematic representation of light absorption through living tissue. Notice that the alternating current *(AC)* signal results from the pulsatile component of arterial blood and that the direct current *(DC)* signal comprises all the nonpulsatile absorbers of light in the tissue, including nonpulsatile blood in the veins and capillaries, and nonpulsatile blood in all other tissues. (From Tremper KK, Barker SJ. Pulse oximetry. *Anesthesiology.* 1989;70:98–108.)

oximetry in determining the SaO$_2$ has been excellent over this range,[74] with an error of ±3% to ±4%.[80]

Modern pulse oximeters visually display the measured SpO$_2$, and they also produce an auditory tone whose pitch changes with the SpO$_2$ level. This sonification of the signal allows clinicians to hear changes in the oxygen saturation of their patient; as the SpO$_2$ falls, so does the pitch of the signal produced by the device. This design advance in pulse oximeters was first introduced by Nellcor in 1983. Unfortunately, among the various manufacturers of these devices, there is no standardization in the tone frequency (pitch) used for various levels of SpO$_2$. In most commercially available devices, the relationship between SpO$_2$ and tone frequency is linear. This creates a problem in the processing of the information provided by the tone, in that pitch perception by humans (the physiologic equivalent of frequency) is not linear but is, rather, logarithmic.[95] Clinicians are able to discriminate between high and low SpO$_2$ measurements by tone but have limited ability to estimate the actual saturation based on the perceived pitch. Brown et al. tested the ability of 40 anesthesiologists to judge absolute SpO$_2$ levels and the direction and magnitude of change in SpO$_2$ using pulse oximeters that used either a linear or logarithmic pitch scale. The use of the logarithmic scale resulted in a significant increase in the accuracy of the physicians' ability to identify the absolute value of the SpO$_2$ as well as that of the change between two values.[95] The investigators suggest that the development of standardized logarithmic scales for tones of pulse oximetry data could improve patient management and safety.

Although pulse oximetry has become a ubiquitous monitoring device, particularly to confirm adequacy of oxygenation during airway management, it has certain limitations. First, the measurement of SpO$_2$ does not provide a direct assessment of oxygen tension. Because of the shape of the oxygen-hemoglobin dissociation curve, at higher levels of oxygenation, measurements of SpO$_2$ are insensitive in detecting significant changes in PaO$_2$ (Fig. 46.3). Second, the pulse oximeter is not accurate when oxygen saturation is less than 70%. The inaccuracy results from the limited range of oxygen saturations used in the calibration process and the difficulty in obtaining reliable human data at these low oxygen saturations.[94,96]

The accuracy of pulse oximeters during hypoxemia has been extensively studied and reviewed.[53,97-100] Most of these studies have been performed on healthy volunteers who had hemoglobin desaturation induced by breathing hypoxic gas mixtures for short periods. Pulse oximeters from different manufacturers varied in their accuracy during hypoxemia; the direction of error differs among these devices, with some overestimating and some underestimating true arterial oxygen saturation. Some study results discovered problems with the calibration curves, which led to revision of the algorithms by the manufacturers.[96-101] These modifications to the algorithms have improved performance of the oximeters.[80]

Other factors affect the performance of pulse oximeters. The response characteristics of pulse oximeters are clinically important, particularly in situations in which the saturation may be changing rapidly, as can occur during management of the difficult airway. Several investigators have studied the response characteristics of pulse oximetry in clinical practice.[96-101] West and colleagues studied five obese, nonsmoking men with sleep apnea syndrome.[102] During rapid changes in saturation, the pulse oximeter readings did not reflect real-time changes in oxygenation. During episodes of spontaneous desaturation, the pulse oximeter underestimated the minimum SpO$_2$, and during spontaneous recovery of oxygen saturation, there was an overshoot of the maximum SpO$_2$.

The location of the pulse oximeter probe also influences the response time for the device. Probes placed on the ear respond more quickly to a sudden decrease in SaO$_2$ than do probes placed on a digit.[99] The response time to changes in SaO$_2$ also depends on heart rate. For fingertip sensors, as heart rate increases, the response to an acute change in saturation is faster; for ear or nasal probes, the relationship is reversed, and the response to changes in SaO$_2$ is slower as heart rate increases.[102] The specific digit on which

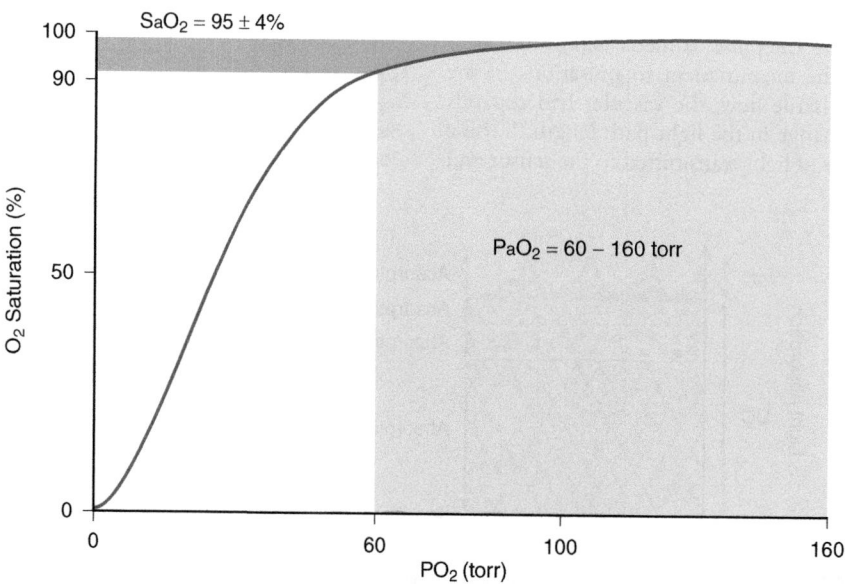

• **Fig. 46.3** Oxygen-hemoglobin dissociation curve. Because pulse oximeters have 95% confidence limits for SaO$_2$ of ± 3% to 4%, an oximeter reading of 95% can represent a PaO$_2$ of 60 mm Hg (saturation of 91%) or 160 mm Hg (saturation of 99%). (From Tobin MJ. Respiratory monitoring in the intensive care unit. *Am Rev Respir Dis*. 1988;138:1625–1642.)

the pulse oximeter probe is placed may affect the accuracy of measurement. In 27 healthy volunteers, Basaranoglu and colleagues found that in right-handed individuals, the right middle finger gave the most accurate results, followed by the right thumb.[103] Likewise, in left-handed subjects, the left middle finger and left thumb produced the most accurate SpO_2 reading.

Accuracy of the pulse oximeter is influenced by several other factors (Box 46.1). Excessive light, such as fluorescent or xenon arc surgical lights, bilirubin lights, and heating lamps, can cause falsely low or high SpO_2 values.[80,96,104] Covering the probe with an opaque material that absorbs red and infrared light (blue, green, or black in color) helps to eliminate this problem. Electrocautery devices can produce significant electrical interference that results in improper functioning of the pulse oximeter.[79] The infrared pulse waves used by neurosurgical image guidance systems interfere with the signal quality and SpO_2 detection by pulse oximetry[105]; the use of aluminum foil as a shield was effective in restoring the accuracy of six brands of pulse oximeters when exposed to the infrared signal generated by a neurosurgical navigation device.[106] Misalignment of disposable pulse oximeter probes may cause falsely low SpO_2 measurements despite a high-quality plethysmographic tracing; this can have important implications in anesthetic management.[107] In 100 patients entering the postanesthesia care unit (PACU) at Massachusetts General Hospital, only 6 had perfect placement of the probes, and for the remaining 94, the average misalignment distance was 5.4 mm (range, 0 to 23 mm).[107] In a single case report, a pulse oximeter displayed an uninterrupted waveform and normal SpO_2 during asystole in a patient undergoing abdominal surgery.[108]

Motion of the pulse oximeter probe, such as when a patient or caregiver moves the digit on which the probe is placed, can cause artifactual readings. Vibration of the sensor delays the detection time for hypoxemia and causes spurious decreases in SpO_2.[109] Movement can result in errors of as much as 20%.[110] In a large, prospective study, patient motion was the major reason for abandoning the use of a pulse oximeter in the PACU.[111] In pediatric patients, 71% of all alarms were false.[112] Attempts have been made to minimize the effect of motion by linking the measurement of SpO_2 to the timing of the heart rate on the ECG; pulse oximeters that use this technology have performed better during vibration than those without this feature.[109] Although this ECG interface is helpful, it has not completely eliminated motion artifact, particularly in very active or agitated patients. Another approach to decreasing the effect of patient motion on the accuracy of pulse oximetry has been to reject motion artifact, retrospectively using changes in the plethysmographic waveform that immediately preceded the questionable event.[110] This results in fewer detected episodes of false oxygen desaturation, although at the price of missing true events.[113]

Several manufacturers have incorporated additional technology designed to minimize motion artifact and to extract a more accurate pulse oximetry signal. The Masimo SET (Irvine, CA) uses unique sensor designs and software algorithms to reduce the incidence of false alarms. When the performance of oximeters using this technology was compared in volunteers with that of the Nellcor N-3000 Symphony (Medtronic, Minneapolis, MN) with improved low-signal performance (Oxismart) and the older Nellcor N-200, the oximeters using Masimo SET were superior in error and signal dropout rate.[114] Baker and colleagues compared the functioning and accuracy of 20 pulse oximeter models in volunteers with hypoxemia during motion and found that the Masimo SET had the best overall performance.[115] When used in the neonatal ICU, Masimo SET resulted in dramatically fewer false alarms and captured more true events than the Nellcor N-200.[116] Oximeters using Masimo SET were more reliable than the N-3000 in detecting bradycardia and hypoxemic episodes in patients in the neonatal ICU.[117] This is evidence that more reliable data from oximetry can improve the process of care in a cost-effective manner. In adults after cardiac surgery, the use of more reliable oximeters (those with Masimo SET) compared with conventional oximeters resulted in a more rapid reduction in fraction of inspired oxygen (FiO_2) and the need for fewer ABG determinations during mechanical ventilation.[118] Petterson and colleagues have reviewed the various technologies used to prevent the effects of motion artifacts on the accuracy of pulse oximeters.[119]

An oximeter can differentiate only as many substances as the number of wavelengths of light it emits.[79,101] Standard commercially available oximeters can detect only two types of hemoglobin, reduced (deoxygenated) and oxygenated (HHb and O_2Hb). Pulse oximeters derive a functional saturation of hemoglobin, which is defined in Eq. 3:

$$\text{Functional saturation} = \frac{O_2Hb \times 100\%}{O_2Hb + HHb} \qquad (3)$$

This functional saturation does not account for other hemoglobin derivatives, such as methemoglobin (MetHb) or carboxyhemoglobin (COHb). When COHb or MetHb is present, the pulse oximeter does not provide a true measurement of oxygen saturation.[120,121] The presence of COHb causes a false elevation in the SpO_2 measurement.[120] As shown in Fig. 46.4, COHb has minimal light absorption at 940 nm, and at 660 nm its absorption coefficient is almost identical to that of O_2Hb. Because the pulse oximeter cannot differentiate COHb from O_2Hb, it overestimates the SpO_2.[120] The SpO_2 displayed by the pulse oximeter approximates the sums of COHb and O_2Hb. This problem is important to consider when assessing oxygenation in patients who have sustained smoke inhalation or patients who have smoked tobacco immediately before airway management. COHb can also be present in long-term ICU patients because carbon monoxide (CO) is a metabolic product of heme metabolism.[122,123] The influence of this potential endogenous source of CO on the accuracy of SpO_2 in the critically ill patient requires further evaluation. In any case, when high CO levels are suspected, oxygen saturation should be measured using a CO-oximeter rather than a pulse oximeter (see below).

> ● **BOX 46.1** Conditions Affecting the Accuracy of Pulse Oximetry
>
> External light sources
> Electrocautery
> Motion of the probe
> Dyshemoglobinemias: carboxyhemoglobin, methemoglobin
> Dyes and pigments: indocyanine green, methylene blue, indigo carmine
> Nail polish
> Severe anemia
> Low perfusion
> Excessive venous pulsations

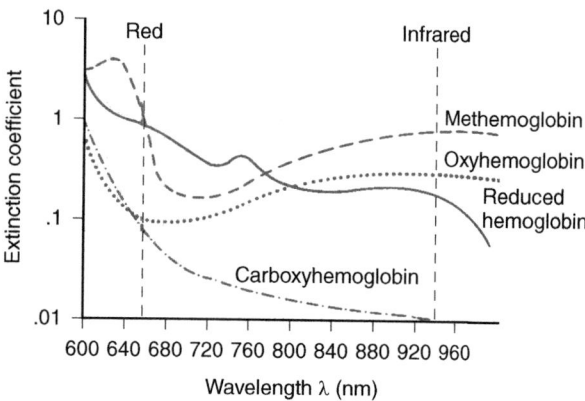

HEMOGLOBIN EXTINCTION CURVES

• **Fig. 46.4** Transmitted light absorbance spectra of four hemoglobin species: oxyhemoglobin, reduced hemoglobin, carboxyhemoglobin, and methemoglobin. (From Tremper KK, Barker SJ. Pulse oximetry. *Anesthesiology.* 1989;70:98–108.)

MetHb also interferes with pulse oximeter measurements.[121,124] As MetHb levels exceed 30% to 35%, Spo_2 becomes independent of the MetHb level, approaching 85% to 90%. This inaccuracy occurs because the MetHb absorption coefficient at 660 nm is almost identical to that of HHb, whereas at 940 nm, it is greater than that of other hemoglobin derivatives (see Fig. 46.4). The pulse oximeter therefore overestimates or underestimates the true Sao_2, depending on the level of MetHb.[101] Some causes of high MetHb levels include administration of nitrates, local anesthetics (e.g., lidocaine, benzocaine), metoclopramide, sulfa-containing drugs, ethylenediaminetetraacetic acid (EDTA), diaminodiphenyl sulfone (dapsone), and primaquine. Some patients can also have congenitally high MetHb levels. Fetal Hb does not affect the accuracy of the pulse oximeter.[79,80,104] The effect of other dyshemoglobinemias, such as sulfhemoglobin, on the accuracy of pulse oximetry has not been investigated.[104]

To assess for the presence of COHb and MetHb, two additional wavelengths of light must be incorporated into the measuring device. Spectrophotometric heme oximeters (CO-oximeters) that use four or more wavelengths of light can measure other hemoglobin species and calculate the fractional saturation using Eq. 4:

$$\text{Fractional saturation} = \frac{O_2Hb \times 100\%}{O_2Hb + HHb + MetHb + COHb} \quad (4)$$

Modern CO-oximeters use 8 to 12 wavelengths of light. Devices developed by Masimo, the Rainbow SET Radical-7 and the Rad-57 pulse CO-oximeters, can detect and accurately measure the concentrations of COHb and MetHb.[125] An advantage of these devices is the ability to continuously monitor the level of dyshemoglobinemia and monitor the response to treatment.[126–130] The clinical value of this technology has been documented in numerous case reports of detection of carboxyhemoglobinemia and methemoglobinemia. However, the specific algorithms used to detect these hemoglobin derivatives impact the accuracy of these devices. For example, the accuracy of the Masimo Radical-7 pulse CO-oximeter in measuring MetHb during coincident hypoxemia (Sao_2 <95%) was poor in 14 healthy adults with overestimation of MetHb levels by 10% to 40%.[131] After the company made modifications to the software and separated the optical sensors for MetHb and COHb, the accuracy for measuring MetHb concentrations improved considerably.[132]

Pulse CO-oximetry can also be used to continuously determine the hemoglobin concentration in arterial blood (SpHb).[133] Macknet and colleagues used a Masimo Radical-7 with a spectrophotometric adhesive sensor using 12 wavelengths of light to measure SpHb in 20 healthy volunteers undergoing hemodilution (with removal of 500 mL of whole blood) compared with the standard total hemoglobin (tHb) measurement using a laboratory CO-oximeter.[134] The investigators found the average difference between SpHb and tHb to be –0.15 g/dL, with a standard deviation of 0.92 g/dL, and they concluded that SpHb is accurate to within 1.0 g/dL. Park and colleagues studied 26 patients having surgical procedures and found that the use of sevoflurane during induction of anesthesia improved the accuracy of SpHb measurements.[135] In 20 patients undergoing spinal surgery, Miller and colleagues compared SpHb with tHb measured with a point-of-care device, the HemoCue.[136] There was an overall tendency for the SpHb to overestimate the corresponding tHb, especially when the perfusion index (PI) was higher than 1.4, the manufacturer's threshold value for accuracy of SpHb. This study also calls into question the utility of using SpHb in making clinical decisions, because 22% of the pulse CO-oximeter tests determined hemoglobin values were more than 2.0 g/dL different from the tHb values.[136] In an evaluation of pulse CO-oximetry in patients undergoing abdominal and pelvic surgery, investigators found that the average difference between time-matched samples of SpHb and laboratory-measured tHb (bias) was significantly larger than that in normal volunteers when blood loss was more than 1000 mL, the measured tHb was less than 9 g/dL, an intraoperative transfusion had been administered, or there had been a decrease in tHb of 2 g/dL or more during the procedure.[137]

Some investigators, however, have found clinical use for SpHb in the OR.[138–140] In a prospective study of 327 patients undergoing orthopedic surgery, noninvasive continuous SpHb measurement resulted in a 4% absolute reduction in the risk of having a blood transfusion when compared with standard care and monitoring.[138] Likewise, Awad and colleagues found that SpHb monitoring reduced transfusions of red blood cells during high-blood-loss neurosurgical procedures[139]; in this study, the difference between SpHb measurements using a Masimo CO-oximeter and laboratory determination of tHb was 0.0 ± 0.8 g/dL. They also found that the trend accuracy of SpHb measurements yielded a coefficient of determination (R^2) of 0.96 with time-matched laboratory determination of tHb. This ability to accurately trend tHb over time may allow clinicians to more rapidly respond to anemia and better manage transfusion therapy.[139] Berkow and colleagues used SpHb in 29 patients during complex spine surgery and found that pulse CO-oximetry had clinically acceptable accuracy compared with laboratory values, that it may provide more timely information on hemoglobin status than intermittent blood sample analysis, and thus that it has the potential to improve blood management during surgery.[140]

The use of SpHb monitoring in ICUs has also been studied.[141,142] Frasca and colleagues compared SpHb to that obtained invasively with either a point-of-care device (HemoCue Hb 301, Ängelholm, Sweden) or a laboratory CO-oximeter in 62 patients in a French ICU. They found that the hemoglobin measurement by pulse CO-oximetry had both absolute accuracy and trending accuracy similar to that of the invasive methods used at bedside with the added benefits of being continuous and noninvasive.[141]

In a study of hemoglobin measurement by pulse CO-oximetry in ICU patients with severe gastrointestinal bleeding, investigators found that 19% of SpHb measurements were unavailable from the CO-oximeter.[142] In patients receiving norepinephrine infusions in the study, SpHb could not be determined in 42% of attempted measurements, a significant limitation of the technology.[142]

These disparate findings on the reliability of SpHb measurements speak to the need for clarity on the goal of measuring a parameter such as hemoglobin and how to compare the accuracy of different technologies over the clinically important range of physiologic variables. SpHb measurement is not intended as a replacement for the laboratory determination of hemoglobin but, rather, is a supplement that allows trending of the hemoglobin to determine if it is changing during clinical care.[143] Rice and colleagues make the point that using SpHb would be advantageous in helping guide red blood cell transfusion only if the accuracy of the device is verified to be within 1 g/dL when the measured hemoglobin is within the range when a transfusion may be clinically indicated (i.e., 6 to 10 g/dL).[144] The data comparing SpHb with laboratory-measured tHb in this clinically important range are not available. It is worth emphasizing that decisions to transfuse should not be based solely on a hemoglobin value but on the patient's physiologic state, the estimated blood loss, and an estimate of the likelihood of ongoing hemorrhage. Perhaps it is the trend in the measured SpHb value over time that may be of most value in determining the need for blood replacement, taking into account the clinical scenario and course.[145] In addition to having clinical use, the device must remain accurate during low perfusion states, hypothermia, and the administration of vasopressors.[146] The differences in the findings may also be related to variability in populations studied, to the different technologies used for comparison, and the accuracy and variability of these "gold standard" devices.[145]

Substances that absorb light at 660- and 940-nm wavelengths can interfere with pulse oximetry. Intravenous dyes that interfere with the accuracy of pulse oximeter measurements include indocyanine green, methylene blue, and indigo carmine.[104] These dyes cause transient artifactual falls in saturation; the extent of the problem depends on the absorption characteristics of the dye. Skin pigmentation has minimal effect on pulse oximeter readings, although very dark pigmentation can result in a slight decrease in accuracy.[147,148] During hypoxemia, however, darker skin pigments can produce falsely high SpO_2 readings. The positive bias in patients with dark skin may be as much as 8% when SaO_2 is 80% or less; it is less pronounced in patients with intermediate pigmentation and smallest in those with the lightest skin.[149] This may be explained by the use of light-skinned individuals for the testing and calibration of pulse oximeters; however, not all oximeters produce this result. Jaundice can cause artificially low and artificially high pulse oximeter readings.[119] In most studies, however, even very high bilirubin levels had no effect on the accuracy of the SpO_2.[128,150] Certain shades of nail polish can alter significantly the accuracy of pulse oximetry when the sensor is placed directly over the fingernail. The extent to which accuracy is affected depends on the absorption characteristics of the nail polish at 660 and 940 nm. Black, blue, and green polishes can falsely lower the measured SpO_2 by up to 6%; red nail polish has little effect on pulse oximeter measurements.[104,151,152] If a patient has a darkly pigmented polish, it should be removed from the finger that is going to receive the probe, or the probe should be placed over the sides of the digit, thereby avoiding transmission of the signal through the fingernail.[104,152] The Masimo Radical-7

oximeter with an adhesive, disposable probe was found to underestimate oxygen saturation in hypoxic subjects.[153]

Severe anemia can affect the accuracy of the pulse oximeter. Lee and colleagues demonstrated that the pulse oximeter was inaccurate when the hematocrit was 10% or less.[154] Vegfors and colleagues also found that the pulse oximeter is inaccurate when the hematocrit is very low,[155] but they suggested that the problem was caused by poor perfusion rather than the hematocrit level alone. Of more importance in the management of the severely anemic patient is the assessment of oxygen delivery, rather than oxygen saturation, even when the pulse oximeter is accurate. SpO_2 reflects only oxygen saturation and does not provide a guide to adequacy of the oxygen-carrying capacity of the blood or oxygen delivery. In patients with sickle cell anemia, pulse oximetry correlates well with SaO_2 measured by CO-oximeter, although with a clinically insignificant bias toward underestimation.[156]

When patients become hypotensive, hypovolemic, or markedly vasoconstricted, the peripheral pulse diminishes. This results in an additional problem with the performance of the pulse oximeter because the monitor works only when the patient has adequate and detectable arterial pulsations. When the patient's peripheral perfusion is poor, the pulse oximeter may be unable to measure SpO_2. In one study of patients with poor perfusion after cardiopulmonary bypass, only 2 of 20 brands of pulse oximeters could give SpO_2 values within 4% of that obtained using a CO-oximeter.[157] Attempts to improve the accuracy of pulse oximeters in hypoperfused conditions have not adequately solved the problem. Alternative probe locations, such as the nose or ear, and reflectance, rather than transmittance, techniques have been tried with various degrees of success.[158,159] The feasibility and accuracy of nasal alar pulse oximetry has recently been assessed by Morey and colleagues. The nasal alar is perfused by branches of the external and internal carotid arteries, and thus perfusion may be preserved better than in other tissue beds during periods of altered blood flow or with movement. The investigators found that nasal alar SpO_2 was accurate over the range of 70% to 100% and was in fact more precise than values obtained from the patients' digits when compared with arterial samples.[160]

Investigators have evaluated pulse oximetry using probes placed in the esophagus.[161–163] When placed in the esophagus or other internal tissue sites, the measurement of SpO_2 depends on reflectance and not on detection of the transmitted signal on the side opposite the emitter, as in standard transmission pulse oximetry.[164,165] Esophageal pulse oximetry in critically ill surgical patients results in more consistent SaO_2 readings than with standard surface probes, and the function of the probes was not affected by changes in perfusion or temperature.[163] Esophageal pulse oximetry has also been used successfully in neonatal and older pediatric patients.[166] Fetal pulse oximetry uses reflectance technology.[167] Unfortunately, although this technique was thought to provide better evidence of fetal perfusion and viability, it has not reduced the rate of cesarean delivery.[168] On the other hand, the use of other approaches to document oxygenation has influenced clinical management.

In patients with severe peripheral vascular disease, the use of a forehead reflectance probe has been shown to be an acceptable alternative to the standard transmission probe place on the earlobe.[164] Even with the use of alternative sites for placement of probes in such patients, pulse oximetry may not be an effective monitor because the pulse amplitude is too low (or absent) for there to be an acceptable signal. In addition, for patients who have a continuous flow left ventricular assist device (LVAD) in situ, the absence of a pulse limits the value of most pulse oximeters. Aldrich and colleagues recently reported the development of pulseless oximetry.[169] The technique described uses diodes emitting light at 660 nm (red) and 905 nm (infrared) to transilluminate a digit. The radial and ulnar arteries on that hand are occluded for 5 to 10 seconds and then released. The changing attenuation of each of the two wavelengths is then measured 1 second after release of the occluded arteries to calculate the red/infrared attenuance ratio. Preliminary results in 5 normal patients and 7 pulseless patients with an LVAD demonstrated that pulseless oximetry estimates SaO_2 with acceptable accuracy. This technique, if commercialized, would obviate the need to obtain ABGs in patients with LVADs to determine their oxygenation—currently the only method available if measuring SpO_2 is not possible.

The accuracy of SpO_2 measurements in hypothermic patients has also been a limitation of the pulse oximeter. Although limited studies report the accuracy of the pulse oximeter in the hypothermic patient, the accuracy seems to depend primarily on the presence or absence of an adequate pulse signal rather than temperature itself.[170] In one study, active warming of patients improved the ability of pulse oximeters to detect a signal and decreased the incidence of false alarms.[171]

Pulsations other than arterial pulsations interfere with the performance of the pulse oximeter. When venous pulsations are pronounced, for example, the pulse oximeter may underestimate the true arterial oxygen saturation of hemoglobin.[172] In a group of patients with severe tricuspid insufficiency, pulse oximetry underestimated the oxygen saturation by up to 11%. Other clinical situations in which venous pulsations may be important include patients with severe congestive heart failure and patients who require very high venous pressure, such as after a Fontan procedure performed as treatment for tricuspid atresia.

Although rare, severe burns and injury to the digits have been reported from the application of pulse oximeter probes.[173–175] Frequently rotating the site of application and increasing vigilance can minimize these events. Burns of the skin have occurred with the application of pulse oximeters to patients after photodynamic therapy with porfimer sodium, a photosensitizer.[176] During intraoperative photochemotherapy with verteporfin, frequent rotation of the site of the pulse oximeter at intervals of 7 to 15 minutes during the 6-hour procedure prevented cutaneous injury.[177]

Pulse oximeters have other potential value in monitoring patients in the OR or ICU. The plethysmographic waveform produced by many pulse oximeters has been evaluated as a noninvasive method to determine blood pressure, intravascular volume, and perfusion.[151,178–184] Respiratory-induced changes in photoplethysmography as a predictor for volume responsiveness in mechanically ventilated patients are similar to that seen in the arterial pressure waveform, and these dynamic measurements are superior to the static measurements obtained from intravascular catheters.[185–187]

Some patient conditions may limit the use of these dynamic indicators of volume responsiveness, including dysrhythmias, a requirement for positive-pressure ventilation with a V_T greater than 8 mL/kg, and low levels of positive end-expiratory pressure (PEEP).[188] Plethysmographic variations induced by the use of positive-pressure ventilation were more reliable in predicting fluid responsiveness than central venous pressure or pulmonary artery occlusion pressure in mechanically ventilated cardiac surgery patients postoperatively.[189] Photoplethysmographic pulse variation of more than 9% produced by mechanical ventilation identified patients who were likely to respond to fluid administration with an increase in cardiac output.[185] In this study, there was

no relationship between directly measured arterial pressure and the amplitude of the photoplethysmogram. Respiratory changes in the amplitude of the plethysmographic pulse were found to be as accurate as changes in pulse pressure from an arterial catheter produced by mechanical ventilation in septic patients for the prediction of fluid responsiveness.[190] The use of respiratory variations in photoplethysmography has been as reliable and as accurate an indicator of mild hypovolemia (up to a 20% decrease in estimated circulating blood volume) as the use of arterial waveform analysis in hemodynamically stable, mechanically ventilated patients undergoing autologous hemodilution.[191] Conversely, Landsverk and colleagues found that there exists larger intraindividual and interindividual variability in critically ill patients in indices derived from pulse oximeter technology than from those using arterial waveforms. Based on this information, the value of pulse oximetry in predicting volume responsiveness must be interpreted with caution.[192]

The use of the respiratory-induced waveform variation (RIWV) in photoplethysmography may also be useful in detecting hypovolemia in spontaneously breathing patients.[193,194] In a study of trauma patients in the prehospital setting, Chen and colleagues found that RIWV in photoplethysmography was independently correlated with major hemorrhage and that it may enhance detection of hypovolemia beyond the use of standard vital signs.[193] In a study of volunteers, McGrath and colleagues progressively reduced central blood volume using lower body negative pressure up to −100 mm Hg and investigated the pulse shape features of the photoplethysmographic pattern obtained from sensors placed on the finger, forehead, and ear to determine which might serve as an indicator of hypovolemia.[194] The investigators found that reductions in pulse amplitude, width, and area under the curve of the pulse oximeter waveform from the ear and forehead were strongly correlated with reductions in stroke volume, with the forehead sensor demonstrating the best performance. These waveform changes were seen before reductions in arterial blood pressure. The increased sympathetic activity that accompanies hypovolemia and the concomitant peripheral vasoconstriction were thought by the investigators to reduce the ability of the photoplethysmogram obtained from the finger probe to function, as well as the probes in other locations for detecting hypovolemia.

The Masimo Corporation developed a proprietary algorithm—the pleth variability index (PVI)—which allows continuous and automated calculation of respiratory-induced variations of the photoplethysmographic waveform. PVI is a dynamic measure of the changes in the perfusion index (PI) that occur over a complete respiratory cycle. The PI is the ratio of pulsatile absorption of the pulse oximeter signal (AC) to that obtained during the baseline nonpulsatile signal (DC) and reflects the amplitude of the plethysmographic waveform (see Fig. 46.2).[151] To calculate PI, the pulsatile signal is indexed to the nonpulsatile blood flow and expressed as a percentage: $PI = (AC/DC) \times 100$. The PVI calculation uses the maximal (PI_{max}) and minimal (PI_{min}) PI values over the respiratory cycle: $PVI = [(PI_{max} - PI_{min})/PI_{max}] \times 100$, expressed as a percentage.[195] Studies have investigated the usefulness of the PVI to predict fluid responsiveness in patients and guide clinical management.[196–198] In patients after cardiac surgery, PVI was able to predict the reduction in cardiac output produced by the application of PEEP of 10 cm H_2O when patients were mechanically ventilated with a V_T greater than 8 mL/kg.[195] When patients were ventilated with a V_T of 6 mL/kg, the PVI and the change in pulse pressure variability (PPV) were unable to accurately assess the hemodynamic effects of PEEP. In a study of goal-directed fluid management, PVI was used to assess volume responsiveness in 82 patients undergoing abdominal surgery. The use of PVI resulted in a decrease in the volume of fluid administered in the OR and reduced lactate levels in the intraoperative and postoperative periods.[197] Zimmermann and colleagues found that PVI is comparable with stroke volume variation as an indicator of volume responsiveness.[199] PVI can also predict fluid responsiveness in mechanically ventilated critically ill patients with circulatory insufficiency after a 500-mL colloid bolus.[198] In this study, a higher PVI at baseline was associated with a larger change in cardiac output after fluid administration.

The peripheral perfusion index (PPI), which is derived from the photoelectric plethysmographic signal of the pulse oximeter, may be a useful noninvasive tool for measuring peripheral vasomotor tone.[200] The index is derived from the ratio between the arterial component (pulsatile) and the nonpulsatile component (venous) of the light detected by the pulse oximeter.[200] In healthy volunteers subjected to progressive reductions in central blood volume by the stepwise application of lower-body negative pressure (LBNP), van Genderen and colleagues found that the use of PPI detects early central hypovolemia before the onset of cardiovascular decompensation.[201] More recently, a novel machine-learning model—the compensatory reserve index (CRI)—has been developed as a measure of the physiologic reserve available to compensate for reduced central blood volume and was found to identify central hypovolemia better than estimates of stroke volume or traditional vital signs[202,203] a CRI of 1 indicates supine euvolemia, and 0 represents the onset of hemodynamic decompensation. Janak and colleagues compared the discriminative ability of PPI, PPV, and CRI (all determined by the photoplethysmographic arterial waveform obtained from a Masimo pulse oximeter) to predict the occurrence of hemodynamic collapse in 51 healthy volunteers subjected to stepwise LBNP from –15 to –100 mm Hg.[204] Compared with both PPI and PPV, CRI had statistically superior discriminative ability to predict the onset of hemodynamic decompensation induced by central hypovolemia at all levels of simulated hemorrhage. This technology may allow the early recognition and treatment of hypovolemia, which has been long sought after in the management of both medical and surgical patients.

In the postoperative period, continuous pulse oximetry can be a useful surveillance monitor and can reduce respiratory complications. One commercially available system uses a paging system to alert the nursing staff when preset physiologic alarm limits are breached. In one study that evaluated the clinical benefits of the Masimo Patient SafetyNet System, careful selection of the alarm limits reduced the number of false alarms but provided notification to the nurse of changes in physiologic parameters, including SpO_2. The investigators demonstrated a decrease in ICU transfers and a reduced need for rescue events (i.e., activation of a rapid response team, cardiac arrest team, or stat airway team) compared with the number of events noted before the implementation of the system.[205] Further investigation of the clinical value of these systems is needed to justify widespread use.

The use of pulse oximetry as a novel marker for the quality of chest compressions during cardiopulmonary resuscitation has been studied by Xu and colleagues in a porcine model of cardiac arrest.[206] The investigators found that both the area under the curve and absolute amplitude of the pulse oximetry plethysmographic waveform correlated well with both the cerebral perfusion pressure and the $EtCO_2$ levels in the animals. Thus, it may be advantageous to use these parameters from the

pulse oximeter to monitor the effectiveness of compressions during CPR.

Pulse oximetry has also been investigated in combination with lung ultrasound as a tool to screen for acute respiratory distress syndrome (ARDS) in clinical situations where access to chest radiography and blood gas analysis may be limited.[207] This use of the pulse oximeter as an adjunct to the information obtained from other noninvasive monitors should be considered in selected clinical settings.

Capnography

Capnography provides a noninvasive method to assess ventilation and ventilation/perfusion relationships.[208–210] A capnograph provides a continuous display of the CO_2 concentration of gases from the airways. The CO_2 concentration at the end of normal exhalation ($EtCO_2$) reflects gas from the distal alveoli; it therefore represents an estimate of the alveolar CO_2 concentration ($Paco_2$). When ventilation and perfusion are well matched, the $Paco_2$ closely approximates the $Paco_2$, and $Paco_2 \cong Paco_2 \cong Petco_2$. The normal gradient between $Paco_2$ and $Petco_2$ ($P[a–et]co_2$) is about 5 to 6 mm Hg. The gradient between $Paco_2$ and $Petco_2$ increases when pulmonary perfusion is reduced or ventilation is maldistributed.

Various methods of gas analysis are commercially available, including mass spectrometry, Raman scattering, and infrared absorption spectrometry. The most commonly used method is infrared spectrophotometry. It is based on the principle that CO_2 absorbs infrared light. As the infrared light is passed through a sample of gas, the amount of infrared light absorbed is proportional to the concentration of CO_2 in the sample.

Two different sampling techniques are used for capnography: mainstream and sidestream devices. The mainstream (in-line) capnograph has a transducer that is connected to the patient's ETT. The transducer contains the infrared light source and a photodetector. The mainstream capnograph has a faster response time because no gas is withdrawn from the patient's airway. Secretions usually do not prevent accurate measurement because they are easily removed from the sensor site. The mainstream device does have some limitations, including the weight of the connectors, the increased equipment dead space (as much as 20 mL), and the inability to use mainstream devices in extubated patients. The sidestream (diverting) capnograph aspirates gas from the patient's airway to the capnograph through a sampling tube. Analysis of the CO_2 concentration is performed in the monitor rather than at the airway adapter. Because the analysis is not done at the airway, the airway connector is smaller and adds no significant dead space or weight to the Y-connection between the ETT and ventilator circuit. The sidestream device can also be used with a modified nasal cannula to monitor CO_2 concentrations in the airway of nonintubated patients. The response time of the sidestream capnograph is slower because it aspirates gas from the airway. The sampling can be compromised by significant water condensation in the catheter and pulmonary secretions.

Capnography has important applications during airway management and mechanical ventilatory support. It is a useful monitor during tracheal intubation and to confirm placement of the ETT within the trachea. It can document adequacy of ventilation during mechanical ventilatory support, spontaneous ventilation in intubated and nonintubated patients, and adequacy of cardiopulmonary resuscitation. Capnography is useful when evaluating the patient with a tenuous airway or gas exchange who may require urgent or emergent tracheal intubation and mechanical ventilatory support.

The capnogram is a waveform that graphically represents the CO_2 concentration over time. The capnogram provides information about adequacy of ventilation, potential airflow obstruction, and, in conjunction with other monitors, $\dot{V}/\dot{Q}$ relationships. A normal capnogram has four components: the ascending limb, alveolar plateau, descending limb, and baseline (Fig. 46.5). The ascending limb represents the CO_2 concentration of the gas in rapidly emptying alveoli. The alveolar plateau occurs because the CO_2 concentration from uniformly ventilated alveoli is relatively constant. The $EtCO_2$ is the point at which the CO_2 concentration is highest, representing the CO_2 concentration approximating true alveolar gas. The rapid, descending limb of the capnogram signals inspiration. The baseline represents the CO_2 concentration of inspired gas. The capnogram can be used to identify significant inspiratory or expiratory airway obstruction, including intrinsic airway obstruction or a kinked ETT (Fig. 46.6). With expiratory obstruction, the waveform does not have a normal alveolar plateau. By continuously monitoring the capnogram waveform, the response to bronchodilator therapy can be visually confirmed. The capnogram waveform can also be used to diagnose rebreathing of CO_2; with rebreathing, as can occur when fresh gas flow is inadequate, the baseline (inspired) CO_2 concentration increases.

Despite its clinical use, capnography has significant limitations as a monitor of ventilation for patients with impaired pulmonary function or hemodynamic instability. The biggest problem is that the correlation between $Paco_2$ and $Petco_2$ varies and is sometimes poor in patients with low cardiac output or altered $\dot{V}/\dot{Q}$ relationships. The correlation varies as the patient's clinical condition changes, making interpretations of ventilation from $Petco_2$ measurements alone unreliable. This has been documented in patients suffering severe traumatic injury, particularly those with traumatic brain injury for whom hypocapnia and hypercapnia should be

avoided.[211,212] In a study of 180 trauma patients presenting to an ED, the correlation between $Petco_2$ and $Paco_2$ was poor.[213] Following common recommendations for ventilation in these patients to maintain $Petco_2$ values between 35 and 39 mm Hg resulted in significant hypoventilation. The $Paco_2$ was more than 40 mm Hg in 80% of cases and more than 50 mm Hg in 30% of cases. The correlation between $Petco_2$ and $Paco_2$ was best for patients with traumatic brain injury and poor for those with chest injuries or decreased perfusion. An increased difference between $Paco_2$ and $Petco_2$ in patients with traumatic brain injury was observed for those with coexistent severe chest trauma, hypotension, and metabolic acidosis. For patients without significant extracranial trauma, the $Paco_2$ and $Petco_2$ were 100% concordant.[214] Capnography may be used to guide ventilatory therapy in patients with traumatic brain injury, but only if there is limited injury to other organ systems. It can provide useful noninvasive information in patients undergoing apnea testing to confirm brain death,[215] although most clinicians perform confirmatory ABG analysis to document the $Paco_2$ before declaring brain death.

Monitoring Pulmonary Function During Mechanical Ventilatory Support

Assessment of pulmonary mechanical function can be performed using a variety of monitoring techniques for the patient who is breathing spontaneously and for the mechanically ventilated patient.[216–219] The techniques are useful for optimizing ventilatory support in the critically ill patient, determining the extent to which the patient can initiate spontaneous ventilation, guiding the use of supportive modes of ventilation (e.g., pressure support ventilation [PSV]) and determining when and how to initiate weaning from mechanical ventilatory support. With several new modes of ventilation and supportive techniques to augment patient-initiated breaths, these monitoring techniques have become an essential component of respiratory management.

Assessment of Ventilation

Most clinicians measure $Paco_2$ to determine whether the patient has adequate ventilation, defined as effective removal of CO_2 by the lungs. $Paco_2$ is an essential measure of respiratory function and cardiorespiratory relationships, although interpretation of $Paco_2$ requires an understanding of respiratory function, acid-base status, and compensatory mechanisms by which the patient may adjust to decreased alveolar ventilation ($\dot{V}A$). Evaluating the adequacy of ventilation requires an understanding of $\dot{V}A$ and dead space ventilation ($\dot{V}Ds$). The determinants of $Paco_2$ are represented in Eq. 5:

$$Paco_2 = k\dot{V}co_2 / \dot{V}A \qquad (5)$$

where
k = 0.863
$\dot{V}co_2$ = CO_2 production (mL/min)
$\dot{V}A$ = alveolar ventilation (L/min)

The equation assumes that inspired CO_2 is zero. CO_2 elimination through the lung depends solely on the $\dot{V}A$, the area within the lung where gas exchange occurs.[219] The remainder of the lung and large airways represent dead space, the volume of gas that

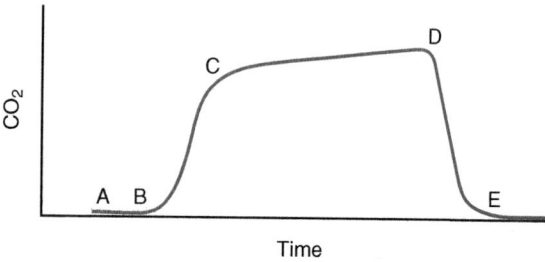

• **Fig. 46.5** Normal capnogram. Exhalation begins at point *A* and continues to point *D*. Segment *C–D* is the alveolar plateau. Point *D* represents the end-tidal carbon dioxide. Inspiration is represented by rapid, descending limb of segment *D–E*, which reaches the zero baseline.

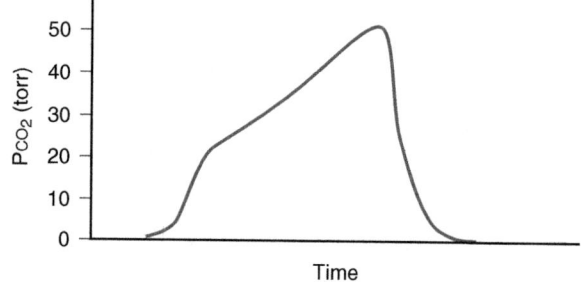

• **Fig. 46.6** Capnograph waveform in a patient with airflow obstruction demonstrates lack of an alveolar plateau.

does not participate in gas exchange; $\dot{V}_{DS}$ has no effect on CO_2 elimination.

The required $\dot{V}_E$ to maintain CO_2 homeostasis, however, depends on the relationship between $\dot{V}_A$ and $\dot{V}_{DS}$. As dead space increases, the WOB (respiratory rate or V_T) must increase to compensate for the inefficient ventilation and maintain a normal $Paco_2$. $\dot{V}_E$ is the sum of $\dot{V}_A$ and $\dot{V}_{DS}$, as shown in Eq. 6:

$$\dot{V}_E = \dot{V}_A + \dot{V}_{DS} \tag{6}$$

Assessment of $\dot{V}_{DS}$ is critical to understanding the nature of a patient's respiratory dysfunction and defining the ventilator needs of the patient. The $\dot{V}_{DS}$ represents inefficient ventilation in that it increases the WOB without contributing to gas exchange. Dead space is composed of anatomic dead space, alveolar dead space, and dead space imposed by equipment used to maintain the airway and ensure ventilation. The anatomic dead space is the volume of gas within the conducting airways; in a normal, 70-kg man, it averages about 156 mL (about 1 mL/lb).[220] The volume of the anatomic dead space increases with higher lung volumes and decreases when the patient is in the supine position.[221-224] Intubation of the airway with an ETT decreases the anatomic dead space by about 50% because of the elimination of the extrathoracic airway (i.e., the nose and mouth), which does not contribute to gas exchange.[223,225] Depending on the intraluminal volume of the ETT and any additional apparatus dead space, the actual reduction of the anatomic dead space that occurs after tracheal intubation is most often inconsequential. Alveolar dead space is defined as the amount of gas that penetrates to the alveolar level but does not participate in gas exchange. In healthy individuals, this volume is minimal; however, alveolar dead space is increased in patients with $\dot{V}/\dot{Q}$ mismatch, such as those with pulmonary emboli or severe lung injury (e.g., emphysema). The physiologic dead space is the sum of the anatomic and alveolar dead spaces and is represented by the total volume of gas in each breath that does not participate in gas exchange.

The portion of each breath that is dead space can be determined by calculating the ratio of dead space volume ($\dot{V}_{DS}$) to tidal volume (V_T) ($\dot{V}_{DS}/V_T$). The $\dot{V}_{DS}/V_T$ is a useful clinical monitor of the overall WOB. It can be estimated using the Bohr equation:

$$\dot{V}_{DS}/V_T = \frac{Paco_2 - P\bar{E}co_2}{Paco_2 - Pico_2} \tag{7}$$

where

$Paco_2$ = alveolar CO_2 tension
$P\bar{E}co_2$ = CO_2 tension in mixed expired gas
$Pico_2$ = inspired CO_2 tension

The $\dot{V}_{DS}/V_T$ can be estimated more easily by assuming that $Pico_2$ is zero and estimating alveolar CO_2 as arterial CO_2. This simplified formula represents the Enghoff modification of the Bohr equation:[93,96,225]

$$\dot{V}_{DS}/V_T = \frac{Paco_2 - P\bar{E}co_2}{Paco_2} \tag{8}$$

$P\bar{E}co_2$ can be measured by collecting expired gas in a large-volume reservoir (e.g., Douglas bag, meteorologic balloon) for 3 to 5 minutes (depending on the $\dot{V}_E$) and measuring the CO_2 tension of a sample of this gas.[225,226] $Paco_2$ is measured from blood gas obtained simultaneously during the collection of the expired gas.

The normal $\dot{V}_{DS}/V_T$ is 0.3 at rest; it decreases during exercise, primarily as a result of an increase in V_T—a more efficient way to increase alveolar ventilation with increasing oxygen consumption and CO_2 production.[223,225] Patients with severe respiratory failure may have a $\dot{V}_{DS}/V_T$ value as high as 0.75, even with an ETT in place. In this situation, the patient's WOB is so high that discontinuation of some level of ventilatory support is not possible,[227] although modes of ventilation that increase V_T without an accompanying increase in WOB, such as PSV, may facilitate spontaneous ventilatory work.

Some technical factors must be considered when measuring $\dot{V}_{DS}/V_T$ in mechanically ventilated patients. A correction must be made for gas compression within the ventilator, connecting tubing, and any additional dead space from the apparatus.[228] If the compression volume is ignored, the true physiologic dead space is underestimated by as much as 16%. Newer ventilators adjust the V_T to account for the compression volume of the ventilator circuit. Several ventilator parameters can influence the accuracy of the measurement of $\dot{V}_{DS}$. For example, physiologic dead space was found to increase markedly when the duration of inspiration during mechanical ventilation was decreased from 1 to 0.5 seconds in paralyzed patients.[229] A nomogram of the relationship between $\dot{V}_E$, $\dot{V}_{DS}/V_T$, and $Paco_2$ in mechanically ventilated patients was developed to aid in the titration of ventilatory support, assess the response to medical therapy, and increase the precision of the therapeutic management of critically ill patients.[230]

A simpler method for estimating $\dot{V}_{DS}/V_T$ has been described. Measurement of the CO_2 tension (Pco_2) in the condensate of expired gas in the collection bottle from the expiratory limb of the mechanical ventilator is equivalent to the cumbersome technique of collecting the mixed expired gas.[226] This Pco_2 value can be substituted for $P\bar{E}co_2$, greatly simplifying the measurement of physiologic dead space in mechanically ventilated patients.

Another approach to the noninvasive assessment of the physiologic $\dot{V}_{DS}/V_T$ ratio substitutes $Petco_2$ for $Paco_2$. For normal subjects, the relationship between $Petco_2$ and $Paco_2$ is well established.[231,232] At rest, $Petco_2$ underestimates $Paco_2$ by 2 to 3 mm Hg. However, with exercise, $Petco_2$ can overestimate $Paco_2$. The difference between $Petco_2$ and $Paco_2$ varies directly with V_T and cardiac output and inversely with respiratory rate. For patients undergoing general anesthesia or with respiratory failure, the gradient between arterial and $Petco_2$ increases.[223,233] This increase reflects more ventilation to lung units with high $\dot{V}/\dot{Q}$ relationships. For patients with normal pulmonary function who are mechanically ventilated during general anesthesia, the arterial to end-tidal partial pressure gradient of carbon dioxide ($P[a-et]co_2$) averages 5 mm Hg; the $P[a-et]co_2$ can be as high as 15 mm Hg in the supine position. The average $P[a-et]co_2$ increases to 8 mm Hg when these patients are placed in the lateral decubitus position.[234] In patients with respiratory failure, the $P[a-et]co_2$ can be even greater. In patients with respiratory failure, there is a close correlation between $P[a-et]co_2$ and $\dot{V}_{DS}/V_T$.[233] The $P[a-et]co_2$ can therefore be used as an indicator of the efficiency of ventilation.

In patients with acute lung injury, an increase in $\dot{V}_{DS}/V_T$ correlates with increased mortality and with a decrease in ventilator-free days. As a result, the $\dot{V}_{DS}/V_T$ can be used as a marker of severity of disease.[235,236] Frankenfield and colleagues developed and validated an equation that uses clinically available data to estimate $\dot{V}_{DS}/V_T$: $\dot{V}_{DS}/V_T = 0.32 + 0.0106 \ (Pa_{CO_2} - Et_{CO_2}) + 0.003$ (respiratory rate) $+ 0.0015$ (age in years).[237] The equation was constructed from data obtained from 135 patients and validated on an additional 50 patients ($r^2 = 0.67$). Recently Bhalla and colleagues found that increased dead space is also associated with increased mortality in critically ill children.[238] Others have also suggested that dead space should be measured in clinical trials of ARDS to enable secondary analysis and show that if $\dot{V}_{DS}/V_T$ is not directly measured, the Harris-Benedict equation may be a useful way to estimate the dead space fraction.[239]

Volumetric capnography, also called the single-breath test for CO_2, can be used to estimate physiologic dead space.[233] Volumetric capnography enlists a plot of the expired CO_2 against the exhaled volume of a single breath. Volumetric capnography in combination with D-dimer testing has been used in the ED to help evaluate patients with suspected pulmonary emboli and to select the optimal level of PEEP in anesthetized, morbidly obese patients.[240,241]

Assessment of Tidal Volume and Airflow

V_T and airflow can be valuable information when monitoring patients on mechanical ventilation. V_T assessment is important in situations such as ARDS, when low V_T ventilation is needed.[242] V_T is directly related to other parameters and indices. In volume-targeted ventilation, after getting volumetric parameters on mechanical ventilators, information about airway pressures, compliance, resistance, WOB, and dead space (Table 46.1) can be obtained.[243–245] During low V_T ventilation, other parameters must be monitored to effectively ventilate and prevent harm in a patient with respiratory failure. The principles of low V_T ventilation encourage low V_T and reduced plateau pressures with optimal PEEP and F_{IO_2}. If higher PEEP is necessary, driving pressures become an important factor. In patients who are not making any respiratory effort, driving pressure can be calculated as plateau pressure minus PEEP. This measure may better predict cyclic strain in ARDS compared with V_T alone during low V_T ventilation with increased levels of PEEP.[246]

With respect to pressure-targeted modes of mechanical ventilation, V_T becomes the dependent parameter. Transpulmonary pressure can vary depending on the patient's WOB and compliance. If the patient is generating a breath, the combination of the negative intrapleural pressure and the pressure-regulated breath can create a situation where excessive V_T and alveolar distention occur without an increase in measured airway pressures.[247] Therefore, for patients receiving a pressure-targeted mode of ventilation, monitoring V_T is critically important.

Inspiratory flow during mechanical ventilation can affect the overall delivery of gas. Depending on the patient's $\dot{V}_E$ requirement and other patient-specific issues, the set inspiratory flow rate and pattern (decelerating ramp versus square wave) can influence the patient's comfort level, volume delivered, and transpulmonary pressure changes. If flows are not sufficient to match the patient's flow requirements, air hunger may develop early in the ventilated breath. Inspiratory flow is particularly important in patients with high $\dot{V}_E$. When provided a decelerating flow pattern, the inspiratory flow at mid-inspiration may be too low to meet the patient's need. This can be overcome by changing modes from a volume-targeted to a pressure-targeted mode or, in some cases, by adjusting the peak flow or flow pattern of the delivered breath.[247] Different clinical situations and patients may necessitate changes to the mode of ventilation, volume, time constants, pressures, or inspiratory flow and therefore require ongoing monitoring and adjusting of ventilatory parameters (see Chapter 45).

Assessment of Work of Breathing

WOB is another important monitor of a patient's respiratory status, respiratory reserve, and likelihood of being successfully weaned from mechanical ventilatory support. The patient's WOB can be qualitatively assessed by clinical evaluation at the bedside or calculated using data obtained from an esophageal balloon and flow transducer at the airway.[221,248] Clinical evaluation of WOB, although useful, can be misleading. Some patients who appear to have excessive WOB indicate that they are comfortable. Others with a low $\dot{V}_E$ and slow respiratory rate are already working maximally, and although they appear comfortable at the current level of ventilatory support, they cannot tolerate any further increase in their WOB.

WOB can be measured directly using bedside monitors. These monitors require placement of an esophageal balloon to measure esophageal pressure as an estimate of intrapleural pressure. The WOB is calculated by integrating the area under the pressure-volume loop. With an understanding of each of the components of WOB, modifications can be made in ventilator parameters to minimize the patient's WOB. This monitoring technique has

TABLE 46.1 Monitored Ventilatory Parameters

Volume-Related Assessment	Pressure-Related Assessment	Non-volume, Non-pressure Assessment	Waveforms and Loops	Additional Parameters Specific to Ventilator Brand and Mode
Expired tidal volume	Peak circuit pressure	Delivered oxygen concentration	Pressure vs. Time	Work of breathing parameters
Expired minute volume	Mean circuit pressure	Inspiratory time	Flow vs time	CO_2 parameters
Inspired tidal volume	Plateau pressure	Expiratory time	Volume vs time	Dead space parameters
Spontaneous minute volume	Positive end-expiratory pressure (PEEP)	Inspiratory to expiratory ratio (I : E)	Pressure-volume loop	Electrical activity of the diaphragm
Leak volume	Intrinsic PEEP (iPEEP)	Respiratory rate	Flow-volume loop	
Rapid shallow breathing index		Compliance parameters		
		Resistance parameters		

been recommended to adjust PSV to optimize gas exchange while minimizing WOB. Although the additional information about the patient-ventilator interface has resulted in modifications of methods for ventilating critically ill patients, no studies have documented which parameters are most useful to monitor and which modifications to ventilator management result in the best outcomes.

Ventilatory Waveform Analysis

Ventilatory waveform analysis is a useful method for assessing airway patency, pulmonary function, and the patient-ventilator interface. Most critical care ventilators have a variety of waveform monitoring capabilities; for ventilators that do not have integrated waveform monitoring capability, separate monitors are available to assess the waveform, WOB, capnography, and other useful monitoring parameters, such as oxygen consumption, CO_2 production, and calculated energy expenditure. Although all these measures can help a clinician optimize the overall care of critically ill patients, ventilatory waveforms are particularly useful in assessing the patient's air movement, identifying the presence of air trapping, and, for many patients, providing critically important information about the adequacy of the ventilatory parameters in addressing patient needs. Evaluating the flow-time and pressure-time curves can provide information about whether or not a patient is able to trigger the ventilator to initiate supported breaths (e.g., pressure support) and to determine whether the peak inspiratory flow and flow pattern are adequate to meet the patient's needs.[249–251] When a patient appears agitated or dyssynchronous with the ventilator, the ventilatory waveforms can be useful in giving direct feedback about whether the problem is related to inappropriately low inspiratory flow, other ventilator-dependent parameters, or inadequate analgesia or sedation.[252–254]

In many cases, modifications to the ventilator can improve the clinical situation and minimize the need for excessive sedation. In addition to displaying inspiratory and expiratory flow patterns, the ventilator displays pressure-volume and flow-volume loops, both of which can be useful in assessing whether the peak inspiratory flow is too high or too low or the VT is too high, putting the patient at risk for pulmonary volutrauma.[255] For patients with ARDS, in whom the deleterious effects of high VT and airway pressures are well recognized, analysis of ventilatory waveforms can aid in adjusting ventilator parameters to optimize gas exchange without increasing the risk of lung injury.[256] Fig. 46.7 illustrates a waveform that identifies excessive WOB during a patient-initiated breath.

Airway Resistance and Lung-Thorax Compliance

In the intubated, ventilated patient, airway resistance and lung-thorax compliance can be differentiated by evaluating peak and plateau pressures and the difference between them (Fig. 46.8). The peak airway pressure generated by the ventilator reflects the pressure necessary to overcome airway resistance and compliance of the lung and chest wall. The peak pressure is elevated when airway resistance is increased, as may occur with increased pulmonary secretions, a kinked ETT, or when lung-thorax compliance is reduced.[257] The peak pressure is influenced by other factors, including ventilator parameters such as inspiratory flow rate and pattern, VT, and ETT size. The ratio of the VT delivered divided by the difference between the peak inspiratory pressure and PEEP is the dynamic compliance. Dynamic compliance is reduced when airway resistance is increased or lung-thorax compliance is reduced.

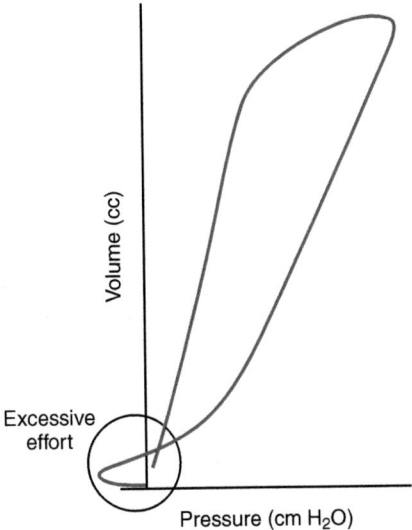

• **Fig. 46.7** Pressure-volume curve identifying excessive effort by the patient to initiate a patient-triggered breath for assist-control ventilation or pressure-support ventilation. (From Novametrix Medical Systems. *Bedside Respiratory Mechanics Monitoring.* Novametrix Medical Systems; 1998.)

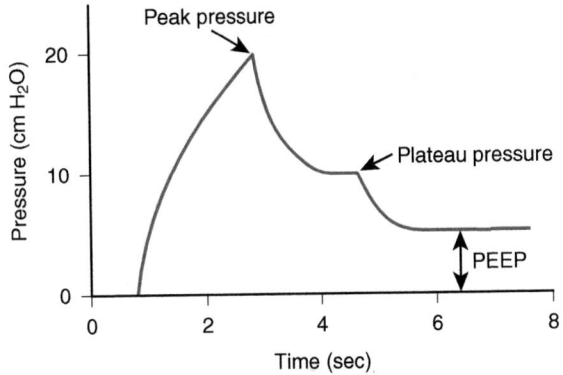

• **Fig. 46.8** Graphic display of airway pressure in a mechanically ventilated patient. Peak inspiratory pressure is achieved during gas flow into the lung. Plateau pressure is achieved by temporary occlusion of expiratory tubing. From these pressures, dynamic and static compliance can be calculated. *PEEP,* Positive end-expiratory pressure.

To distinguish the cause of reduced dynamic compliance and increased peak airway pressure, the static compliance must be calculated. Static compliance can be assessed by determining the plateau pressure, which is the pressure achieved in the airways when the lung is inflated to a specific VT under conditions of zero gas flow. Static compliance is measured when inspiration is complete and the lung remains inflated with no further gas flow. Most mechanical ventilators have the capability to provide an inspiratory pause (hold) that allows measurement of the plateau pressure. The pressure generated in the lung during the inspiratory pause is the pressure required to overcome lung and chest wall compliance. Because there is no gas flow at the time of measurement, airway resistance does not contribute to the measured pressure. The static compliance can be estimated by dividing the VT by the difference between the plateau pressure and PEEP. The normal static compliance measured using this method is 60 to 100 mL/cm H_2O. The static compliance is reduced in patients with an extensive pulmonary infiltrate, pulmonary edema, atelectasis, endobronchial intubation, pneumothorax, or any decrease in chest wall compliance, as may occur with chest wall edema or subcutaneous emphysema.

Intrinsic Positive End-Expiratory Pressure

Hyperinflation (overdistention) of the lung occurs in some mechanically ventilated patients because of air trapping. Gas can be trapped within the lung during the expiratory phase because of dynamic airflow limitation (e.g., associated with asthma) or inadequate expiratory time, as may occur when the inspiratory flow is so low that it causes a high inspiratory-to-expiratory (I:E) ratio. The hyperinflation that results is referred to as auto-PEEP, intrinsic PEEP (iPEEP), or occult PEEP.[258,259] The presence of iPEEP increases the risk of barotrauma, compromises hemodynamics by reducing venous return, increases the patient's WOB, and can result in unilateral lung hyperinflation.[228,258,259]

Identification of iPEEP is challenging in critically ill patients. iPEEP is not reflected in the pressure measured on the manometer of the ventilator at the end of exhalation, because at end expiration the exhalation valve is open to atmospheric pressure (PEEP = 0 cm H_2O) or reflects the level of PEEP provided by the ventilator. iPEEP can be quantified by occluding the expiratory port of the ventilator circuit at the end of exhalation immediately before the next breath is delivered and allowing the pressure in the lungs and ventilator circuit to equilibrate; the level of iPEEP is then displayed on the manometer. Although this approach provides an estimate of the magnitude of gas trapping, it is technically difficult and hard to reproduce. Another method to qualitatively determine whether iPEEP is present involves evaluation of the expiratory flow waveform. If expiratory flow does not fall to zero before the next inspiration, gas is trapped within the lung, creating iPEEP (Fig. 46.9). When iPEEP is identified using this method, the flow waveform can be monitored while adjusting ventilator parameters to minimize iPEEP. Still another method to estimate iPEEP in a passive patient is to perform an expiratory hold maneuver, which allows the airway and circuit to equilibrate to estimate the presence of iPEEP.

Special Considerations During Noninvasive Ventilation

NIPPV refers to mechanical ventilation via a nasal or oronasal mask, without the use of invasive airways such as ETTs, tracheostomy tubes, and SGAs. For purposes of this discussion, NIPPV will include CPAP and BiPAP. The clinical situations for which NIPPV are most appropriate include patients with underlying COPD who have acute worsening hypercapnic respiratory failure and patients with hypoxemic respiratory failure associated with acute cardiogenic pulmonary edema.[260–262] In each of these situations, a trial of NIPPV can be attempted while optimizing other therapeutic interventions to reverse the acute cause for the respiratory failure.

Monitoring of patients receiving NIPPV should focus on the effects of the positive pressure on reducing WOB and improving overall gas exchange. When initiating NIPPV, the patient should be closely observed and monitored to ensure that the ventilator support is appropriately applied and that there is clinical evidence to demonstrate that it is in fact reducing respiratory distress. When properly implemented, the patient should have evidence of a decreased respiratory rate, decreased use of accessory muscles, and reduced paradoxical abdominal wall motion.[263] Placement of the mask is critically important when implementing NIPPV in the nonintubated patient. Special attention should be given to the mask fit to ensure that there is no significant air leak when using either CPAP or BiPAP. Ventilator parameters that are important to monitor include air leak, V_T, and patient-ventilator synchrony.[263] V_T measured during expiration is the preferred way to document the level of ventilatory support. If there is a significant leak during inspiration, the V_T delivered to the patient may be less than the inspired V_T delivered by the ventilator. Other monitors of gas exchange can also be used to document the clinical value of NIPPV in improving ventilatory status. For example, gas exchange can be monitored noninvasively using continuous pulse oximetry, capnography, or, in selected cases, transcutaneous P_{CO_2} measurement, which has been successfully used to monitor ventilatory (Pa_{CO_2}) trends in patients with COPD exacerbations.[264] Based on the assessment, adjustments in V_T, $\dot{V}_E$, PEEP, and F_{IO_2} can be made to address persistent hypercapnia and hypoxemia, respectively.[265] Although NIPPV is generally used for short-term support, it has been helpful in optimizing gas exchange in selected other situations. When used for longer-term support, the mask application and site must be monitored closely. With prolonged use, complications include skin irritation or abrasion, mucosal dryness, mucous plugging, and nasal congestion.[265]

Assessment During Weaning From Mechanical Ventilatory Support

Several measures of pulmonary mechanical function are used to evaluate the likelihood of weaning success in the mechanically ventilated ICU patient.[227] Vital capacity (VC) and maximum

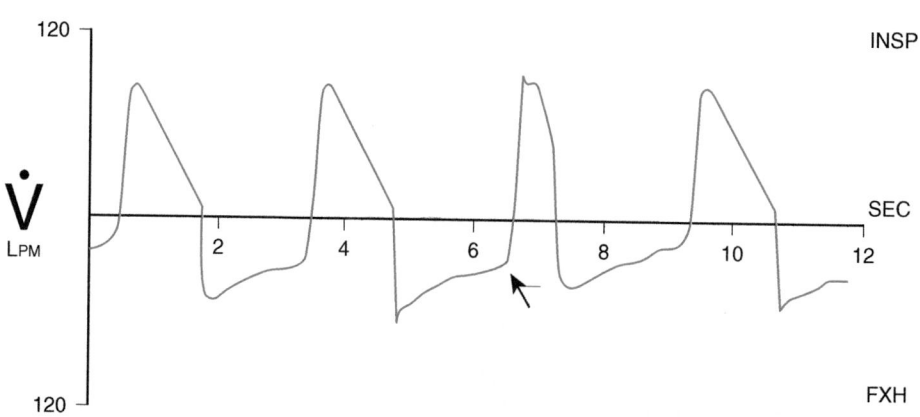

• **Fig. 46.9** Flow-time curve demonstrates expiratory flow continuing until initiation of inspiration *(arrow)*. In a normal patient, expiratory flow falls to zero, indicating complete emptying to functional residual capacity. Continued expiratory flow indicates air trapping.

inspiratory pressure (MIP or PI_{max}) are commonly employed to evaluate pulmonary mechanical function. A VC of 10 mL/kg and PI_{max} more negative than –20 cm H_2O are useful predictors of weaning success in some patients. Other measures of mechanical function that have been used to predict weaning success include maximum voluntary ventilation (MVV) greater than two times the resting level and $\dot{V}E$ less than 10 L/min. A $\dot{V}DS/VT$ greater than 0.6 has consistently predicted weaning failure, particularly if a patient with such a high dead space develops a fever, mucous plugging, or any minimal reduction in VT. Unfortunately, although each of these parameters can be used to assess pulmonary mechanical function, several studies have demonstrated that none accurately predicts weaning success.

Other monitoring techniques have been employed to predict weaning success, including continuous measurement of oxygen consumption.[266] Although many studies have attempted to define key factors in predicting weaning success, changes in mechanical ventilatory capabilities and our understanding of the risks and benefits of mechanical ventilatory support have had a major impact on methods for assessment and monitoring of patients. The use of PSV and noninvasive modes of ventilatory support have made interpretation of the studies and recommendations difficult. One of the key components in the decision-making process concerning weaning and discontinuation of mechanical ventilatory support is related to the patient's ability to protect the airway and the need for intensive respiratory care rather than specific respiratory mechanical parameters. Many patients previously thought to be unable to wean can now be provided with ventilatory assistance using pressure-support ventilation through an ETT or using NIPPV; therefore, traditional methods for assessing weaning may no longer apply. Nevertheless, an understanding of the various methods that have been used to assess weaning potential is critical to defining the most effective way to transition a patient from positive-pressure ventilation to spontaneous ventilation.

Indices to Predict Weaning From Mechanical Ventilator Support

Several indices have been developed to predict when a patient can be successfully weaned from mechanical ventilatory support. These indices combine multiple individual parameters to predict weaning success; some incorporate indices of gas exchange. One study evaluated multiparameter indices, including the rapid shallow breathing index (RSBI), which is the ratio of respiratory frequency divided by VT in liters, and the CROP index (thoracic compliance, respiratory rate, arterial oxygenation, PI_{max}), which incorporates measures of dynamic lung compliance, respiratory rate, gas exchange, and inspiratory pressure.[267] An RSBI of 105 or less was shown to have a high predictive value for weaning success, whereas the CROP index and more traditional indices had poor predictive values. A study could not confirm these findings and demonstrated that an RSBI of 105 or less did not consistently predict weaning failure.[268]

Breathing Pattern Analysis

Respiratory impedance plethysmography (RIP) can be used to assess the breathing pattern by measuring VT, respiratory frequency, inspiratory time, and the contribution of the rib cage and abdomen to lung volume changes.[53,54] Using RIP, the relationship between rib cage and abdominal contributions to VT (i.e., respiratory muscle dyssynchrony) has been quantitated. RIP is useful for evaluating changes in FRC and level of auto-PEEP as ventilator parameters are adjusted. As a method for predicting weaning success, the technique has had variable success.

Airway Occlusion Pressure

The airway occlusion pressure has been used as an index of respiratory drive, although it is rarely used as a routine monitor of ventilatory drive. Airway occlusion pressure ($P_{0.1}$) is the pressure generated 0.1 second after initiating an inspiratory effort against an occluded airway. The $P_{0.1}$ in normal subjects usually is less than 2 cm H_2O. Some studies suggest that a $P_{0.1}$ value greater than 6 cm H_2O is incompatible with successful weaning for patients with COPD.[269] Few studies have confirmed the value of airway occlusion pressure as a predictor of successful weaning success,[270,271] and its clinical utility remains unclear.

Assessment of Respiratory Function With Spontaneously Initiated Modes of Mechanical Ventilation

During mechanical ventilation, spontaneously initiated breaths are used during spontaneous breathing trials, spontaneous modes of ventilation (e.g., PSV), and sometimes in conjunction with controlled modes of ventilation (e.g., intermittent mechanical ventilation). When spontaneously initiated modes are used, the patient's breathing efforts can be variable with partial to full ventilator support. By observing ventilatory parameters and patients' physiologic signs and assessing gas exchange, the provider can determine if more, less, or no mechanical ventilation is needed. The parameters or indices most often used to determine performance during a spontaneous breathing trial are respiratory rate and pattern, gas exchange, hemodynamic stability, and patient comfort.[272] The theoretical advantage of decreased WOB from overcoming the resistance of the ETT and circuit is apparent in spontaneously initiated modes of ventilation. In addition, it may allow patient control of inspiratory time, frequency, and VT. Oftentimes this enhances patient comfort and possibly prevents respiratory muscle atrophy. Given these advantages, the patient must also be consistently breathing spontaneously. Any prolonged period of apnea would trigger a backup machine-controlled mode of ventilation. Providers must also be aware of variables in the patient's condition that may cause inadequate support, such as worsening lung compliance or increasing WOB. Inadequate support may lead to patient fatigue and continued respiratory failure.

During PSV, the ventilator augments a patient's spontaneous inspiratory effort with a set positive pressure. PSV improves patient comfort and WOB and has become a frequently used mode for assisted ventilation. The pressure that is produced for PSV increases inspiratory flow and VT as the pressure reaches a plateau.[273] Because the level of pressure augmentation is set, it is important to assess the volume delivered proper gas exchange, and the breathing pattern. A higher level of support than necessary can deliver larger volumes, causing overdistention and lung injury. A less than adequate level of support can result in higher respiratory rates and increased WOB. Although synchrony of the supported breath is timed with a flow or pressure gradient, a small lag can exist.

Another form of spontaneously initiated ventilation is proportional assist ventilation (PAV). PAV uses instantaneous feedback of flow rate and volume from the ventilator to the patient. The total applied pressure is based on the relationship between flow rate and resistance plus volume and elastance.[274] The elastance (or the inverse of compliance) and resistance can be measured or estimated by the ventilator. The percentage of the total applied pressure is set based on the amount of support desired for each breath. In addition to parameters that are usually assessed during conventional modes, other parameters that are assessed may include resistance, compliance, auto-PEEP, and WOB.

Finally, neutrally adjusted ventilator assist (NAVA) is a unique mode that monitors the electrical activity of the diaphragm (EA_{di}) by processed signals from electrode arrays placed in the esophagus. The amount of support is set depending on the amount of electrical activity.[275] The clinician should be aware of different parameters for NAVA, such as the amount of pressure support per microvolt of EA_{di} and electrical activity peaks and minimums. These newer spontaneously initiated modes may become more useful for weaning along with other treatment options as patient physiologic cues regulate the amount of support the ventilator provides, but they have not been widely adopted as significant benefits have yet to be determined.[276]

When utilizing spontaneously initiated modes of ventilation, monitoring of the patient and the patient-ventilator interface is critically important. In some cases, only minimal support using one of these modes of ventilation may be required; however, without this support, the patient may not have adequate gas exchange or may have excessive WOB that is not sustainable. As a result, the amount of support required can be difficult to determine, and the line between success and failure can be thin. When using any of these spontaneously initiated modes of ventilation, careful ongoing assessment of V_T, respiratory rate, and other parameters of respiratory function must be performed to prevent premature extubation or weaning failure. The specific monitors of readiness to wean and extubation will vary from one patient to the next, depending on the underlying clinical condition, the relationship between ventilation and hemodynamics, as well as associated comorbidities. Recently, USG has been found to be an effective way to assess diaphragmatic function by measuring the thickening fraction of the diaphragm during assisted spontaneous breathing in postoperative patients.[277] Although USG and other methods have been used to monitor patients during weaning from positive-pressure ventilation to assess weaning success, further clinical trials will be required to determine which technique has the greatest value in predicting successful transitions from ventilator support, particularly in deconditioned, critically ill patients who have suffered from prolonged respiratory failure.

Conclusion

Several modalities are available to monitor the airway and pulmonary function in the patient who requires tracheal intubation and mechanical ventilatory support. Monitoring techniques include clinical assessment, monitoring of gas exchange, and a variety of methods to evaluate pulmonary mechanical function. Selection of the most appropriate monitors for each patient depends on an understanding of the clinical situation, the availability of specific monitoring techniques, the information each monitor provides, and the monitors' limitations. The challenge for the clinician is to identify and appropriately use techniques that optimize clinical management and reduce morbidity and mortality, rather than using any monitor simply because it is available.

Acknowledgments

This chapter provides an updated version of Chapter 46: Monitoring the Airway and Pulmonary Function. The author and editors acknowledge the work of Hokuto Nishioka, MD and David E. Schwartz, MD for their contributions to the chapter included in the previous edition of the book.

Selected References

33. Salem MR. Verification of endotracheal tube position. *Anesthesiol Clin North Am.* 2001;19:813–839.
59. Frankel HL, Kirkpatrick AW, Elbarbary M, et al. Guidelines for appropriate use of bedside general and cardiac ultrasonography in the evaluation of critically ill patients – part 1: general ultrasonography. *Crit Care Med.* 2015;43:2479–2502.
79. Schnapp LM, Cohen NH. Pulse oximetry: uses and abuses. *Chest.* 1990;98:1244–1250.
210. Szaflarski NL, Cohen NH. Use of capnography in critically ill adults. *Heart Lung.* 1991;20:363–372.
225. Lumb AB, Nunn JF. *Nunn's Applied Respiratory Physiology.* 7th ed. Churchill Livingstone 2010.
237. Frankenfield DC, Alam S, Bekteshi E, et al. Predicting dead space ventilation in critically ill patients using clinically available data. *Crit Care Med.* 2010;38:288–291.
247. Rittayamai N, Katsios CM, Beloncle F, et al. Pressure-controlled vs volume-controlled ventilation in acute respiratory failure: a physiology-based narrative and systematic review. *Chest.* 2015; 148:340–355.
250. Hess DR. Ventilator waveforms and the physiology of pressure support ventilation. *Respir Care.* 2005;50:166–186.
251. Fernandez-Perez ER, Hubmayr RD. Interpretation of airway pressure waveforms. *Intensive Care Med.* 2006;32:658–659.
254. Nilsestuen O, Hargett KD. Using ventilator graphics to identify patient-ventilator asynchrony. *Respir Care.* 2005;50:202–234.

All references can be found online at eBooks.Health.Elsevier.com.

47

Extubation and Reintubation of the Difficult Airway

RICHARD M. COOPER AND MATTEO PAROTTO

CHAPTER OUTLINE

KEY POINTS

- Careful planning of tracheal extubation or tube exchange is as vital as the planning required for intubation. Airway complications are as common after tube removal as during insertion.
- Anticipating a successful extubation is an inexact science. Any emergent reintubation is likely to be more complex because of physiologic instability and contextual challenges.

- Reintubation may fail because of inadequate access to the airway (e.g., halo fixation, maxillomandibular fixation), anatomic features (e.g., retrognathism, prominent incisors, macroglossia), inadequate preparation, lack of expertise or insufficient information (e.g., emergencies), a rapidly deteriorating clinical state, or blood, secretions, or swelling obscuring the visual field.

- The primary objective of airway management is the maintenance of oxygenation. If this can be achieved, the necessary
  resources can be summoned if reintubation initially fails.
  Repeated attempts to reintubate may worsen an already precarious situation.
- Many life-threatening circumstances can be anticipated and
  managed preemptively with a preplanned extubation strategy.
- Extubation strategies include deep extubation, bronchoscopic
  examination under anesthesia through a supgraglottic airway
  (SGA), substitution of an endotracheal tube (ETT) with an SGA,
  and extubation over an airway exchange catheter (AEC).

- The safest extubation strategy may be a preemptive surgical
  airway.
- An SGA or AEC should be left in place (off-label recommendation) until it is likely that reintubation will not be required.
  Premature removal is a common mistake.
- A reintubation strategy may include the judicious administration of oxygen by insufflation or jet ventilation; advancement
  of an ETT over an AEC, preferably with tongue retraction; or
  indirect laryngoscopy.
- Clear communication among those providing care is essential to
  mitigate adverse secondary outcomes.

Introduction

Anesthesia and airway management are often compared with flying an airplane. No one would dispute that its landing is any less
important that its takeoff. Similarly, tracheal intubation and extubation are of equal importance to patient safety. Although there
is a growing appreciation of the frequency and severity of airway
difficulties following tracheal extubation, it remains insufficiently
studied. Indeed, it was recently reported that for every published
article concerning extubation, there are 36 regarding intubation
despite the frequency and severity of the problem.[1] Clinical surveys,[2] closed claims analysis,[1,3] and the Fourth National Audit
Project (NAP4) in the United Kingdom highlight the importance of adverse events following extubation.[4] This has led to several reviews,[5–8] the inclusion of an extubation component within
comprehensive airway management guidelines,[9–11] and standalone
documents on tracheal extubation.[12,13] Complications at extubation range from the relatively minor ones, such as coughing and
transient breath-holding that have little impact on outcome, to
those that are life-threatening. The American Society of Anesthesiologists (ASA) Closed Claims Project analyzed adverse respiratory events and found that 16% and 4% of brain injuries and
deaths occurred after extubation in the operating room (OR) and
postanesthesia care unit (PACU), respectively.[1] Furthermore, the
Closed Claims Project showed that while a significant reduction
in airway claims relating to intubation occurred in the decade
following the 1993 ASA Practice Guidelines on Management of
the Difficult Airway,[14] there was no such improvement in those
relating to extubation. The Closed Claims Project also noted that
brain injury and death were the more likely outcomes in extubation claims compared with intubation claims.[3] The NAP4 audit
found that major airway complications during emergence or
following extubation that led to death, brain injury, unplanned
emergency surgical airway, or airway-related intensive care unit
(ICU) admission were only slightly less frequent than those resulting from failure to intubate or the aspiration of gastric contents.[15]
Because extubation should be regarded as an elective procedure,
this offers the opportunity to anticipate, prepare, and provide safer
management. This chapter discusses the complications associated
with routine and more complex tracheal extubation or reintubation, emphasizing the importance of anticipating and preparing
for higher-risk extubations (and reintubation).

Low-risk or routine extubations have been reviewed elsewhere
and are not the focus of this chapter.[5,13,16] The primary concerns
with routine extubation include ensuring recovery from neuromuscular blockade, opioids, and volatile and intravenous (IV)
sedatives; hemodynamic stability; the adequacy of ventilation and

oxygenation; normothermia; freedom from noxious stimulation;
and airway patency.[17–19] This chapter deals almost exclusively with
adults because there is limited literature relating to the pediatric population.[20] The controversy surrounding deep versus awake
extubation has been addressed elsewhere.[21,22]

Extubation Failures and Challenges

Two dimensions contribute to the risk of extubation: (1) the
patient's tolerance of extubation and (2) the likelihood that reintubation, if required, succeeds free of complications.

Clearly, when extubating a patient with limited physiologic
reserve, the risk of extubation failure is increased. If the patient
also has an anatomically difficult airway (DA), the consequences
of a failed extubation may also be greater. It is probably inaccurate
to think of risk as binary: easy versus difficult. Rather, risk exists
along a continuum that demands clinical judgment. Extubation
should be planned, deliberate, and elective. When necessary, it can
be postponed until conditions are optimal. *When* it is performed
may mitigate the risk of reintubation being required; *how* it is performed may determine whether reintubation can be accomplished
safely. In short, intubation is a skill; extubation is an art.

Extubation failure occurs when a patient is unable to maintain
oxygenation, adequate ventilation, clearance of respiratory secretions, or airway patency. *Reintubation failure* occurs when extubation is followed by an immediate or delayed but unsuccessful
attempt to reintubate the trachea. There is no agreement concerning the time frame for failure; thus, the reported incidences vary.
Furthermore, effective rescue interventions such as noninvasive
ventilation,[23] high-flow nasal oxygen, or helium-oxygen delivery
that obviate the need for reintubation may blur the definition
of extubation failure. Reintubation may ultimately succeed, but
multiple or prolonged attempts have been associated with serious
complications, particularly in the ICU[24] and emergency department (ED).[25] Complications such as desaturation, esophageal
intubation, aspiration, and hemodynamic instability may be overlooked by studies focusing on success or failure per se.

Compared with routine postoperative patients, ICU patients
pose a greater risk of extubation failure due to neurologic obtundation, airway edema, debilitation, impaired clearance of secretions,
altered pulmonary mechanics, increased dead space, and venous
admixture. In the ICU, failed extubation is relatively common,
occurring in 10% to 20% of patients despite the use of numerous
criteria to identify independence from ventilatory support.[3,26,27]
Such criteria are imperfect[28] and may not focus enough attention
on aspects such as airway obstruction, cough strength, airway
protection, and nonrespiratory factors. Also, the consequences of

extubation failure are likely proportional to the patient's clinical acuity. Even when reintubation is uneventful, extubation failure is associated with a significant prolongation of ICU stay and an increase in mortality.[28–30] Given that extubation failure among ICU patients is both common and consequential, the prudent clinician should be prepared with the appropriate supportive interventions and the equipment and expertise to facilitate reintubation if required.[31]

Minor complications associated with the extubation of postoperative patients are common and often transient, rarely requiring reintubation. Studies involving a wide case mix of postoperative patients show a high degree of concordance. In four large studies enrolling more than 150,000 patients, the incidence of required postoperative reintubation ranged from 0.06% to 0.19%.[32–36] The reintubation rate appears to be significantly higher (1%–3%) after selected surgical procedures such as panendoscopy[29,32] and a variety of head and neck procedures.[37–40]

Postoperative reintubation, although uncommon, may offer some unanticipated challenges, including anatomic distortion, physiologic instability, incomplete information, lack of essential equipment, severe time constraints, ergonomics, and inexperienced personnel. An airway that would be easily managed electively may become a life-threatening emergent event.

Extubation Risk Stratification

The overall risk of any extubation relates to the interaction between the risk of extubation not being tolerated and, if required, the success and safety of reintubation. Both aspects have some level of uncertainty. Most extubations are planned and turn out to be uneventful, but even routine extubations may be associated with complications (Box 47.1).

The causes of a failed extubation can be classified as a failure of oxygenation or ventilation, inadequate clearance of pulmonary secretions, or loss of airway patency. One cannot always predict which patients will require reintubation, but if reintubation is likely to be difficult, it is prudent to employ strategies expected to maximize the likelihood of success.

Rates, Causes, and Complications of Routine Extubation Failure

Unplanned Extubation

Unplanned extubation, either the deliberate removal of the ETT by the patient or the inadvertent displacement during maneuvers, results in significant harm and death. The incidence of this event

---

> **• BOX 47.1** Complications of Routine Extubations

Unintended extubation
Fixation of endotracheal tube
Hypertension, tachycardia
Increased intracranial pressure
Increased intraocular pressure
Coughing, breath-holding
Laryngeal injury
Laryngospasm or vocal cord paralysis
Stridor, airway obstruction
Postobstructive pulmonary edema
Laryngeal incompetence
Aspiration

---

in the ICU population has been reported as 0.1 to 3.6 per 100 intubation days.[41,42] In the OR, and more recently in the ICU and ED as a result of COVID-19, placement of the patient in the prone position increases the risk of accidental extubation.[43] Often these are patients experiencing critical failure of oxygenation, demanding the return of the patient to a supine (head-up) position and replacement of the ETT. In the ICU, unplanned extubation can occur during repositioning for radiographs or during routine nursing care, more commonly in delirious or insufficiently sedated patients.[44,45] The majority of these patients require reintubation, and when this occurs in the ICU, ICU and hospital length of stay are significantly prolonged and associated with an increase in mortality. Fastidious attention to securing the ETT and supporting the breathing circuit is essential. Unplanned extubation is a quality indicator; the risks, consequences, and strategies for its prevention have been reviewed elsewhere.[41]

Planned Postoperative Extubations

A retrospective database review from the University of Michigan analyzed 107,317 general anesthetics administered between 1994 and 1999.[35] Of the 191 (0.1%) that required reintubation in the OR or PACU, 59% were for respiratory causes, mostly hypercapnia or hypoxemia. Upper airway obstruction including laryngospasm accounted for most of the balance. Incomplete neuromuscular reversal was responsible for approximately 6% of the reintubations. Reintubation more commonly occurred in the OR versus the PACU. This study was retrospective and should be interpreted with caution.

A prospective study from Thailand found a higher reintubation rate of 27 per 10,000 patients occurring within 24 hours.[46] The precipitating factor in this study was thought to be residual neuromuscular blockade in almost three-quarters of cases requiring reintubation. A Taiwanese database surveyed 138,000 patients undergoing general anesthesia between 2005 and 2007, finding that 83 reintubations (0.06%) were performed after planned extubation.[36] Comparing these patients with a matched cohort not requiring reintubation, the investigators identified the following factors as most predictive of a need for reintubation: chronic obstructive pulmonary disease (COPD; odds ratio = 7.17; 95% confidence interval [CI], 1.98–26.00), pneumonia (odds ratio = 7.94; 95% CI, 1.03–32.78), ascites (odds ratio = 13.86; 95% CI, 1.08–174.74), and systemic inflammatory response syndrome (odds ratio = 11.90; 95% CI, 2.63–53.86).

Hypoventilation

The ASA Closed Claims Project found that 4% of 1175 closed claims resulted from critical respiratory events in the PACU. The highest proportion was attributed to inadequate ventilation, and many of these patients died or suffered brain damage.[47] Pulmonary complications may be the most common postoperative complication with respiratory failure being the most frequent within this group.[48] A multicenter, prospective survey in France examining almost 200,000 general anesthetics administered between 1978 and 1982 found that postoperative respiratory depression accounted for 27 of 85 life-threatening or fatal respiratory complications.[49] A respiratory rate of <8 breaths per minute was observed by PACU nurses among 0.2% of 24,000 adult patients after general anesthesia.[34] These studies were conducted at a time when longer-acting neuromuscular blocking agents (NMBAs) were widely used, monitoring blockade reversal was subjective or not done at all, and oximetry was rarely available. A more recent prospective, multicenter study assessed residual neuromuscular blockade among adult patients following abdominal surgery; almost all of these patients had received rocuronium, and most had been reversed with neostigmine. The incidence of incomplete reversal observed at the time of extubation and on arrival to PACU, defined as a train-of-four (TOF) ratio less than 0.9, was 63.5% (95% CI, 57.4%–69.6%) and 56.5% (95% CI, 49.8%–63.3%), respectively.[50] Although the literature is somewhat conflicting, it appears that even a TOF ratio of 0.9, compared to 0.95, is associated with increased postoperative pulmonary complications.[51] These include aspiration, airway obstruction, hypoxia, and pharyngeal/esophageal complications. Sugammadex appears to reduce the incidence of residual neuromuscular blockade compared to neostigmine and, among some patient groups, is associated with fewer postoperative pulmonary complications.[51] Miskovic and Lumb summarized the major factors contributing to postoperative ventilatory failure as continued sedation from residual anesthetic drugs and opioids, residual neuromuscular blockade, and impaired ventilatory responses to hypercapnia and hypoxia.[48]

The residual effects of trace levels of volatile anesthetic drugs may also contribute to inadequate postoperative ventilation; however, it appears that the ventilatory response to hypercapnia is less affected than the response to hypoxia.[52] It may be aggravated by incomplete reversal of neuromuscular blockers,[53,54] hypocalcemia or hypermagnesemia, or the administration of other drugs that potentiate neuromuscular blockade.

Hypoxemic Respiratory Failure

A comprehensive review of the many causes of postoperative hypoxemia is beyond the scope of this chapter but include hypoventilation, a low inspired-oxygen concentration, ventilation/perfusion mismatch, right-to-left shunting, increased oxygen consumption, diminished oxygen transport, and impairment of oxygen diffusion. The effect of residual volatile anesthetic agents on the ventilatory response to hypoxia is variable and dependent on the agent as well as a number of prevailing circumstances, such as patient stimulation.[53] Hypoxemia is more common in some clinical situations due to preexisting medical conditions, surgical interventions, persistent anesthetic influences, atelectasis, or splinting. If sufficiently severe, there may be a requirement for noninvasive positive-pressure ventilation (NIPPV) or reintubation. Hypoxemia (Spo_2 <90%) was the most common cause of a critical postoperative respiratory event in a study of over 24,000 adult patients.[34]

Inability to Protect the Airway

The inability of patients to protect their airway may be a consequence of soft tissue collapse resulting in obstruction or the loss of the reflexes that would guard against aspiration of gastric contents. This may be the result of persistent anesthetic influence including residual neuromuscular blockade, opioids and other analgesics, or sedatives, or it may be due to a preexisting medical condition such as obtundation or neurologic injury. It may be possible to temporize by repositioning patients to reduce regurgitation risk (head up), aspiration risk (head down), obstruction (on their side), or placement of an airway obturator (e.g., an oral, nasopharyngeal, or supraglottic airway [SGA]). The use of reversal agents (e.g., naloxone, flumazenil, or sugammadex) may also be helpful, if indicated. When such measures are inappropriate or ineffective, NIPPV or reintubation may be required.

Failure to Clear Pulmonary Secretions

Inadequate clearance of pulmonary secretions may result from a depressed level of consciousness with impaired airway reflexes,

overproduction of secretions, alteration of sputum consistency leading to inspissation and plugging, impaired mucociliary clearance, or inadequate neuromuscular reserve. These problems may lead to aspiration, atelectasis, or pneumonia with resultant hypoxemic respiratory failure. Alterations in pulmonary mechanics may also lead to hypercapnia, necessitating reintubation.

Airway Obstruction

Postextubation stridor

Several of the complications of tracheal intubation may not be apparent while the patient remains intubated. Although anatomic or functional laryngeal problems are more likely to develop as a consequence of multiple, prolonged, or blind intubation attempts, glottic or tracheal injury may also occur despite a good laryngoscopic view or during awake bronchoscopic intubation.[55–57] Airway injuries may range from those that are subtle and reversible to the more extreme that necessitate reintubation. They include laryngeal edema, ulceration, laceration, hematoma, granuloma formation, vocal fold immobility, tracheal and esophageal perforation, and subluxation or dislocation of the arytenoid cartilages.[58–60] Reports often omit details regarding the ETT size, cuff type, methods of cuff inflation, laryngoscopist, or clinical context. A recent systematic review detailed the findings of 21 publications involving over 6000 patients restricted to prospective studies involving adults undergoing elective surgical procedures with postoperative laryngeal examination. The incidence of edema ranged from 9% to 84% and was identified in the following locations in decreasing prevalence: arytenoid, interarytenoid, vocal folds, Reinke's space, postcricoid, and unspecified locations. The study did not specify whether any patients required reintubation despite identifying some with arytenoid subluxation and vocal cord paralysis. Most of the injuries were short lived, resolving without intervention; however, 4% to 5% of the injuries were classified as moderate to severe.[60] Presumably, patients requiring emergent or prolonged intubation are more susceptible to laryngeal injury.

Upper airway edema is a pathologic diagnosis, suggested by postextubation stridor resulting in turbulent flow due to decreased caliber of the airway lumen. The resultant increased work of breathing (WOB) may culminate in respiratory failure. The reported incidence of postextubation respiratory failure associated with stridor in ICU populations ranges from 1.8% to 31%.[61] Recognition of patients at risk of failing extubation due to airway edema is challenging and has involved inspection, the cuff leak test, and ultrasonography (USG). Management of airway edema depends on its severity. This may involve the use of a lower-density helium/oxygen blend (heliox), aerosolized epinephrine, or reintubation.

The cuff leak test has been advocated as a tool to predict postextubation stridor. The test can be performed in a variety of ways with results of variable predictive value. Essentially, the test determines the adequacy of airflow around an occluded ETT after the cuff is deflated. It can be performed qualitatively by simply listening during exhalation,[62] or quantitatively[63] by comparing the difference between inspiratory tidal volume and the average expiratory volume. The sensitivity and specificity of this test will depend upon the cutoff value chosen, but other factors undoubtedly come into play, such as compliance of the respiratory system and the mechanical forces the patient is able to generate.[61] The presence of a leak reduces the likelihood of postextubation stridor and subsequent need for reintubation.[61,63] Patients with postextubation stridor required reintubation in 18% of cases compared with 7.9% of patients without stridor. Reintubation was usually required within a median of 2 hours (range 1–6) in those with stridor, compared with 20 hours in those without (3–43 hours). Although the cuff leak test is recommended in higher-risk patients,[64] it has "limited diagnostic power"[63] with moderate sensitivity and excellent specificity.[65] A quantitative test is more discriminating, but performance depends upon the selected cutoff value (leak volume) and the population being studied. If no cuff leak is identified, deferral of extubation might be prudent until conditions improve, especially if the airway is anatomically challenging or the patient is physiologically marginal.

USG can be used to better define the amount of space between the vocal cords and the ETT. This space was found to be significantly less in patients who subsequently develop postextubation stridor, though the sensitivity and specificity of this diagnostic application vary widely across studies. Several studies have compared USG with the cuff leak test[65]; however, the findings must be interpreted cautiously since so few patients with stridor were included. A large study involving 400 ventilated children, 44 of whom exhibited postextubation stridor, observed significant decreases in the quantitative cuff leak and the ultrasound-measured air column around the ETT in those who subsequently exhibited stridor. The ultrasonographic assessment demonstrated higher sensitivity and specificity.[46,66] Video-assisted laryngoscopy (VAL) can be used as a tool to record the laryngeal anatomy and clinical progress,[67] but one must be very cautious in using this as a predictive tool of postextubation stridor, as the ability to accurately assess the anatomy is limited while the ETT remains in situ.

It is unlikely that laryngeal edema can be eliminated, but it may be possible to minimize it by attempting to achieve a visually controlled, atraumatic intubation with an appropriately sized ETT, a compliant cuff inflated just sufficiently to achieve a seal (with cuff-pressure manometry), minimizing the duration of intubation, optimizing patient positioning, and timely administration of IV corticosteroids. The benefits of corticosteroids with respect to postextubation stridor and the reintubation rate have been variable and likely depend upon patient selection, the steroid used, the dose, its timing, and when and if the dose is repeated. A meta-analysis of three randomized controlled trials involving patients with no cuff leak found that corticosteroids were associated with a reduced rate of reintubation and postextubation stridor.[64] To be effective, these must be given in adequate doses, sufficiently before and, often enough, following extubation.[68–71]

As mentioned, in the face of airway swelling or postextubation stridor, temporizing measures, such as head-up positioning, nebulized epinephrine, and heliox may be of some value. The efficacy of NIPPV in the symptomatic patient following extubation will depend upon the severity of the respiratory difficulty and the pre-existing factors. Large-scale studies have not looked specifically at patients who fail as a consequence of laryngeal edema. One meta-analysis found that NIPPV had a greater effect on reducing reintubation rates in postoperative patients compared with ICU patients (odds ratio 0.24 [95% CI, 0.12–0.50] vs 0.72 [0.51–1.02]).[72] Another meta-analysis concluded that, compared with standard medical therapy, the risk of reintubation was not significantly reduced by the use of NIPPV.[73] A prospective study comparing NIPPV with standard medical therapy, involving 37 centers in 8 countries, failed to demonstrate benefit with respect to reducing reintubation; in fact, the study was stopped prematurely because of an increased mortality rate in the NIPPV group.[74]

Laryngospasm

Laryngospasm involves bilateral adduction of the true vocal cords, vestibular folds, and/or aryepiglottic folds.[75] This is protective to the extent that it prevents aspiration of solids and liquids; it becomes maladaptive when sustained or restrictive of ventilation and oxygenation. The intrinsic laryngeal muscles are the main mediators of laryngospasm, and they include the cricothyroid, lateral cricoarytenoid, and thyroarytenoid muscles. The cricothyroid muscles are the vocal cord tensors, an action mediated by the superior laryngeal nerve (SLN).

The diagnosis of laryngospasm is based upon visualization of laryngeal and supraglottic closure with inspiratory stridor, paradoxical breathing, and suprasternal retraction. Laryngospasm is believed to be a common cause of postextubation airway obstruction, particularly in children.[76] Even in adults, Rose and colleagues stated that it accounted for 23.3% of critical postoperative respiratory events, although the diagnosis was presumptive.[34] Emergency surgery, nasogastric tubes, and surgery for tonsillectomy, cervical dilation, hypospadias correction, oral endoscopy, or excision of skin lesions appear to be risk factors.[76] The triggers are generally noxious but nonspecific, including vagal, trigeminal, auditory, phrenic, sciatic, and splanchnic nerve stimulation; cervical flexion or extension with an in situ ETT; or vocal cord irritation from blood, vomitus, or oral secretions.[77] A risk assessment questionnaire was used to prospectively study over 9000 children undergoing general anesthesia. A positive history of nocturnal dry cough, exertional wheezing, or more than three wheezing episodes in the prior 12 months was associated with a 4-fold increase in the risk of laryngospasm in the PACU and a 2.7-fold increased risk of airway obstruction during surgery or in the PACU.[78] In this study, twice as many children were managed with a laryngeal mask airway (LMA) than with an ETT, and an equal number had their devices removed awake and asleep. The depth of anesthesia at the time of device removal did not influence the incidence of laryngospasm, although this contradicts conventional teaching.[75]

Nevertheless, it is widely believed that prevention of laryngospasm is best achieved by extubating at a sufficiently deep plane of anesthesia or awaiting recovery of consciousness.[79] Potential airway irritants should be removed, and painful stimulation should be discontinued. If laryngospasm occurs, oxygen by sustained positive pressure may be helpful, although this may push the aryepiglottic folds together more tightly.[80] Larson described a technique of applying firm digital pressure to the "laryngospasm notch" between the ascending mandibular ramus and the mastoid process, stating that this technique is rapid and highly effective.[81] Very small doses of a short-acting neuromuscular blocking drug (NMBD) with or without reintubation may be necessary.[82,83] Recently, a case report described the successful use of transnasal humidified rapid-insufflation ventilatory exchange (THRIVE) in a patient with refractory laryngospasm, circumventing the need for reintubation.[84]

Macroglossia

Macroglossia, or severe enlargement of the tongue, can result in airway obstruction and increase the risk of extubation failure. One cause is angioedema, which may be caused by a hereditary or acquired deficiency of C1-esterase inhibitor. These cases are usually recurrent with varying severity; oropharyngeal involvement is less common but can be life-threatening when encountered.[85] Most other cases of angioedema are mediated by mast cells, which release histamine, heparin, leukotriene, and prostaglandin, enhancing capillary permeability and producing tissue edema. It may be triggered by exercise or an allergic reaction to food, latex, or drugs, most commonly to angiotensin-converting enzyme inhibitors or angiotensin receptor blockers, aspirin, or nonsteroidal anti-inflammatory drugs (NSAIDs).[86,87] Although involvement of the tongue is the most obvious manifestation, the uvula, soft tissues, and larynx may also be affected.

Massive tongue swelling also can complicate prolonged posterior fossa surgery performed with the patient in the sitting, prone, or park bench position[88] and steep or prolonged Trendelenburg positioning. Robotic surgery, coupling extreme Trendelenburg positioning with peritoneal insufflation, can also give rise to facial and airway swelling. Likewise, transoral placement of robotic instrumentation into a confined space may result in compressive injuries to the tongue and other oral structures. Other causes of macroglossia include hypothyroidism, acromegaly, lymphangioma, idiopathic hyperplasia, metabolic disorders, amyloidosis, cystic hygroma, neurofibromatosis, rhabdomyosarcoma, sublingual or submandibular infections, and chromosomal abnormalities such as Beckwith-Wiedemann syndrome.[89]

In the ICU setting, macroglossia may be seen as a complication of extreme volume overloading or tongue trauma, particularly when it is further complicated by a coagulopathic state. If this occurs or progresses after extubation, it can lead to partial or complete airway obstruction, making reintubation necessary but difficult or impossible.[90] Macroglossia may result from venous or lymphatic compression leading to immediate swelling or arterial insufficiency and subsequent reperfusion injury.[91]

Laryngeal or Tracheal Injury

Airway injuries from the lips to the distal trachea can include lacerations, edema, arytenoid dislocation, and vocal fold damage. The lip or tongue may be compressed between the laryngoscope blade and the maxillary teeth, resulting in swelling or bleeding, although this is unlikely to be severe enough to delay or complicate extubation. The glottis may be injured as a result of the blind advancement of the ETT. This probably results in universal swelling or mucosal erosion of varying degrees to the posteromedial larynx that is largely unrecognized. The trachea can be lacerated or penetrated by the ETT or its introducer or by ischemic compression of the tracheal mucosa by the cuff. Arytenoids may become dislocated during difficult intubation efforts.[59] Palatopharyngeal injuries have been described as a consequence of blind insertion of an ETT during VAL.[92,93] The epiglottis can be downfolded during placement of an ETT, the consequences of which are unknown.[94,95] Although these injuries are not often apparent at the time of intubation or SGA placement, they are typically managed conservatively and should not complicate extubation.

Laryngeal injuries accounted for 33% of all airway injury claims and 6% of all claims in the ASA Closed Claims Project database.[96] These range from transient hoarseness to vocal fold paralysis. Even when direct laryngoscopy (DL) provides a satisfactory glottic view or intubation is facilitated by flexible bronchoscopy,[55,57] airway injury can occur and go unsuspected until after the ETT is removed or only when symptoms prompt further investigation. Airway injuries are presumed to be less likely if intubation is easy, but analysis of the ASA Closed Claims Project revealed that 58% of airway trauma and 80% of laryngeal injuries were associated with intubations that were not described as difficult.[96,97] The Closed Claims Project observed that difficult intubations were more likely to result in injuries to the pharynx and esophagus than to the trachea.

Vocal fold immobility can result from injury to the recurrent laryngeal nerve or the arytenoid cartilages.[59,98,99] Arytenoid immobility has resulted from seemingly uneventful DL,[100] double-lumen tube (DLT) insertion,[101] and lighted stylet intubation.[102] In

a prospective study involving over 3000 intubations, postoperative hoarseness was observed in approximately half of intubated patients on the day of surgery, persisting to days 3 and 7 in 11% and 0.8% of patients, respectively.[103,104] Three patients (<0.1%) had arytenoid dislocation, and four had vocal cord paralysis.[103,104] Arytenoid dislocation is confirmed by endoscopic visualization of an immobile vocal cord associated with a rotated arytenoid cartilage.[59,99] If the diagnosis is made prior to the onset of ankylosis, it may be possible to manipulate the arytenoid back into position.

Vocal fold paralysis results from injury to the vagus nerve or one of its branches (i.e., the recurrent laryngeal nerve [RLN] or external division of the SLN [ex-SLN]) and may resemble arytenoid dislocation or ankylosis. Differentiation may require palpation of the cricoarytenoid joints under anesthesia or laryngeal electromyography.[99] When vocal fold paralysis occurs as a surgical complication, it is usually associated with neck, thyroid, or thoracic surgery. The left RLN can also be compressed by thoracic tumors, aortic aneurysmal dilatation, left atrial enlargement, or during closure of a patent ductus arteriosus. Occasionally, a surgical cause cannot be implicated. Cavo postulated that an overinflated ETT cuff might result in injury to the anterior divisions of the RLN.[105,106]

The RLN supplies all the intrinsic laryngeal muscles except the cricothyroid, the true vocal cord tensor, which is innervated by the ex-SLNs. Unilateral ex-SLN injury results in a shortened, adducted vocal fold with a shift of the epiglottis and the anterior larynx toward the affected side. This produces a weak, breathy voice but no obstruction and usually resolves within days to months. Bilateral ex-SLN injury causes the epiglottis to overhang, and the vocal cords may appear bowed and lacking in tension. This does not produce obstruction. The vocal quality is hoarse with a reduction in volume and range. Unilateral RLN injury causes the affected vocal fold to assume a fixed paramedian position and may produce a hoarse voice or weak cough, though many patients with unilateral vocal cord paralysis are asymptomatic. Bilateral RLN injury results in both vocal folds being fixed in the paramedian position and inspiratory stridor, often necessitating a surgical airway.[105,107]

Prolonged or stressful contact between the ETT and the posteromedial aspects of the vocal cords, arytenoids, or posterior commissure may result in ulceration of the perichondrium, which can heal with fibrous adhesions leading to vocal cord fixation. An otolaryngologist should assess a patient with persistent postextubation hoarseness, a breathy voice, or an ineffective cough.

Pharyngeal, nasopharyngeal, and esophageal injuries include perforation, lacerations, contusions, and infections. These injuries may be associated with difficult laryngoscopy or intubation, but they may also result from passage of a gum elastic bougie,[108] nasogastric tube,[109] nasotracheal tube,[110] orotracheal tube,[92] suction catheter, esophageal stethoscope, esophageal temperature probe, or transesophageal echocardiogram probe.[111] Penetrating injuries can communicate with the esophagus, resulting in a tracheoesophageal fistula, or with the mediastinum, resulting in mediastinitis, retropharyngeal abscess, or death.[98]

After a brief intubation, soft tissue injuries resulting in airway obstruction are more likely to result from edema or hematoma than infection. Most of the described injuries do not significantly complicate extubation. Laryngeal and tracheal stenoses are serious complications, but they are rarely evident at the time of extubation.

Postobstructive Pulmonary Edema

Severe airway obstruction from any cause and at any anatomic level may complicate extubation by leading to postobstructive pulmonary edema (POPE), also called negative-pressure pulmonary edema.[112,113] This occurs when a forceful inspiratory effort is made against an obstructed airway (also known as the Mueller maneuver). The most common causes include a closed glottis, occlusive biting on an SGA or ETT, laryngospasm, bilateral vocal cord paralysis, croup, or epiglottitis. A strong inspiratory effort results in large negative intrapleural pressures, promoting venous return.[114,115] Type I POPE can occur with the onset of obstruction (e.g., laryngospasm, croup, epiglottitis, foreign body aspiration, hanging, biting, or neck hematoma). Type II POPE (reexpansion pulmonary edema) is seen following relief of the obstruction (e.g., chronic partial obstruction from enlarged tonsils, adenoids, or a laryngeal mass).[116] The consequences of the Mueller maneuver include increased venous return, leftward shift of the interatrial and interventricular septa, decreased left ventricular compliance, and elevated pulmonary pressures and flow. The increased negative intrapleural pressure coupled with the increased hydrostatic pressure promotes transudation of fluid, resulting in pulmonary interstitial and alveolar edema.

Perioperatively, Type I POPE most commonly occurs in healthy patients capable of generating large negative intrathoracic pressures when inhaling against airway obstruction caused by occlusive biting on an ETT or SGA. Fortunately, this can be prevented by the routine placement of a bite block prior to awakening. Care must be taken not to place this as the patient is emerging from anesthesia as it may provoke more biting, dental damage, a gag reflex, or regurgitation. An effective bite block might be fashioned from a roll of gauze wrapped by tape with a "tail" to prevent its aspiration.

Type II POPE follows relief of the obstruction and occurs as follows: An expiratory effort opposed by an obstructed airway (i.e., a Valsalva maneuver) reduces venous return and raises intrapleural and alveolar pressures. With relief of the obstruction, the sudden increase in preload elevates the hydrostatic pressures leading to pulmonary edema. This state is exacerbated by circumstances promoting pulmonary vasoconstriction, such as hypothermia, hypercapnia, hypoxia, and adrenergic stimulation.[116]

POPE typically has a rapid onset. The diagnosis should be suspected when tachypnea, crackles, rhonchi, frothy sputum, hypoxemia, and diffuse pulmonary infiltrates are observed following the relief of upper airway obstruction. The diagnosis is supported by the clinical context, exclusion of other more common causes, and more rapid resolution than that typically seen with other causes of pulmonary edema. Other than ensuring airway patency, treatment primarily consists of positive pressure ventilation (including NIPPV); diuresis is only appropriate when there is associated volume overload.[116,117]

Hypertension and Tachycardia

Transient hemodynamic disturbances accompany the extubation of most adults. These responses may be prevented by deep extubation,[118] exchange of an ETT for an SGA before emergence,[12,119,120] or attenuated with the administration of medication. Healthy patients not on antihypertensive agents exhibit increases in heart rate and systolic blood pressure at extubation of 20% or more.[121] The consequences of such alterations, though generally transient, may be of clinical importance in susceptible patients. The attenuation of these responses may be part of an extubation strategy aimed at minimizing the hemodynamic changes without unduly extending awakening. Strategies may include ETT cuff inflation with alkalinized lidocaine,[122] topical lidocaine,[123] IV lidocaine,[124,125] β-blockers,[126,127] calcium channel blockers,[124,128] dexmedetomidine,[125] opioids,[129] and nitrates. The efficacy undoubtedly depends upon patient selection, dosage, and timing, making comparisons difficult.

Intracranial Hypertension

Tracheal intubation and suctioning are associated with a rise in intracranial pressure (ICP). Extubation is probably associated with comparable or even greater increases in ICP. There is evidence, albeit contradictory, that IV and endotracheal lidocaine attenuate ICP responses to various noxious stimuli in different clinical settings.[130]

Intraocular Pressure

Madan and colleagues compared the intraocular pressure (IOP) changes of tracheal intubation and extubation in children with and without glaucoma.[131] In both groups, they observed significantly greater increases 30 seconds and 2 minutes after deep extubation compared with the corresponding times after uncomplicated intubations. It is likely that significant increases in IOP observed after deep extubation would have been even higher had extubation occurred after recovery of consciousness, but this was not studied. Lamb and colleagues observed similar effects of extubation on IOP in adults, finding that the increase in IOP was greater at 2 minutes after extubation than following intubation. The authors compared the changes observed in patients managed with an ETT or LMA. The IOP measured at 1 minute after removal of the ETT was higher than at any other point; values did not increase in the LMA group. Although the IOP findings achieved statistical significance, the study had only 10 patients in each limb, measurements were not taken beyond 1 minute postextubation, actual values were not presented, and the level of consciousness at extubation was not described. The authors commented that IOP levels measured after ETT removal were high enough "to cause concern" in those patients with critical glaucoma and concluded that steps should be taken to control IOP at extubation.[132]

Coughing

Coughing on emergence from general anesthesia is common, particularly when an ETT is used.[133] Although it is a protective reflex, it can be particularly troublesome in the setting of ophthalmologic, neurologic, oronasopharyngeal, or neck surgery.

Several strategies have been proposed to minimize coughing, including deep endotracheal extubation, primary use or conversion to an LMA (the Bailey maneuver),[120,134,135] dexmedetomidine,[136] opioids, IV local anesthetic, topical application of local anesthetic to the vocal folds, and the use of intracuff lidocaine.[122,123] However, coughing on emergence is relatively benign and generally a helpful protective reflex for most patients.

Tracheal Tube Entrapment

Rarely, an ETT can become entrapped due to a defective cuff, crimped pilot tube, or fixation by hardware. Partial surgical transection of the ETT during a maxillary osteotomy has resulted in the partially cut tube forming a barb that caught on the posterior aspect of the hard palate.[137] Mechanical obstruction of an entrapped tube is a life-threatening complication. One report of a fatality involved entrapment of a DLT sutured to the pulmonary artery.[138]

Higher-Risk Extubations

Although the previously described complications can follow a routine or lower-risk extubation, two additional groups of patients may be affected: those with a higher risk of requiring reintubation and those in whom successful airway management after extubation might be challenging or impossible.

Patients with higher-risk airways may be physiologically challenged[139,140] or anatomically difficult. These difficulties operate along a risk continuum. Examples of very difficult or impossible situations are described later and may include patients in whom mask or supraglottic ventilation, intubation, or emergency invasive airway access is more likely to fail (see Table 47.1).[141,142]

TABLE 47.1   Complications of Higher Risk Extubations

Complication	Surgical and Medical Setting
Inability to Tolerate Extubation and Required Reintubation	
Airway obstruction	Laryngeal edema
	Postextubation stridor
	Laryngospasm
	Macroglossia
	Laryngeal or tracheal injury
	Paradoxical vocal cord motion
	Postobstructive pulmonary edema (negative pressure pulmonary edema)
	After thyroidectomy, anterior cervical surgery, or carotid artery surgery:
	Wound swelling, hematoma
	Vocal cord dysfunction (e.g., recurrent laryngeal nerve injury)
	Hypoglossal nerve injury
	Maxillofacial or nasopharyngeal trauma
	Obesity, morbid obesity, and obstructive sleep apnea
	Rheumatoid arthritis
	Parkinson disease
	Prolonged intubation
Inadequate ventilation	Increased work of breathing (decreased compliance/increased resistance)
	Diaphragmatic splinting
	Central hypoventilation syndrome or obstructive sleep apnea
	Severe chronic obstructive pulmonary disease
	Residual sedation or neuromuscular blockade
	Preexisting neuromuscular disorder
	Relative hypoventilation (e.g., increased CO_2 production)
Inadequate oxygenation	Inadequate inspired oxygen concentration
	Ventilation-perfusion mismatch
	Right-to-left shunt
	Increased oxygen consumption
	Decreased oxygen delivery (mixed venous desaturation)
	Impaired pulmonary diffusion
Failure of pulmonary toilet	Obtundation
	Pulmonary secretions
	Increased volume of secretions
	Inspissated secretions
	Impaired mucociliary clearance
	Neuromuscular impairment
Inability to protect airway	Obtundation
	Neuromuscular disorder
Difficulty Reestablishing the Airway	
Airway injury	Thermal injury, smoke inhalation
	Blood or trauma obscuring the view
	Blood or trauma obstructing the airway
Previous airway difficulties	Anatomically difficult airway (prior difficulties; multiple attempts, devices, or operators)
	Cormack-Lehane class ≥3 for laryngeal view
Limited airway access	Maxillomandibular fixation
	Intraoral or mandibular resection
	Cervical immobilization, unstable cervical spine, or halo fixation
	Tracheal resection (e.g., guardian suture)
	Major head and neck surgery, head and neck free flap reconstruction
Emergent setting	Lack of knowledge regarding prior or potential difficulties
	Lack of expertise
	Insufficient time to prepare personnel, equipment, and medications

Reintubation is likely to occur in an urgent or emergent setting where limited information, personnel, and equipment may be available. These contextual challenges compound the anatomic and physiologic difficulties. The patient is more likely to be hypoxic, acidotic, agitated, or hemodynamically unstable. The procedure may be done in haste by whomever is immediately available, unaware of prior difficulties or successful measures. Thus, a reintubation is fundamentally different from a controlled elective intubation. A preemptive extubation strategy is critical for managing patients at higher risk of extubation failure.

Perioperative Settings

The following section identifies some perioperative settings associated with extubation difficulties. This is undoubtedly a partial list, but it may be useful in identifying the issues that pertain to other clinical settings and for which there is a body of literature.

Ear, Nose, and Throat Surgery

Mathew and colleagues looked at 13,593 consecutive PACU admissions from 1986 through 1989.[33] Of these patients, 26 (0.2%) required reintubation while in the PACU; 7 of them had undergone ear, nose, and throat procedures. Of the seven patients, three had laryngeal edema, one was obstructed from a large thyroid, two bled at the operative site, and one developed POPE following a tonsillectomy.

Patients undergoing laryngoscopy and panendoscopy (i.e., laryngoscopy, bronchoscopy, and esophagoscopy) are at an increased postoperative risk for airway obstruction and are approximately 20 times more likely to require reintubation compared with patients undergoing a wide variety of other surgical procedures.[32] Reviewing the records of 324 diagnostic laryngoscopies and 302 panendoscopies, Hill and colleagues found that patients who had undergone laryngeal biopsy were at the greatest postoperative airway risk. Of 252 patients, 13 (5%) required reintubation, most within 1 hour of extubation. Of the 13 who required intubation, 12 had undergone laryngeal biopsy. Most of these patients had COPD, and their need for reintubation was attributed largely to this.

Robinson prospectively studied 183 patients who had 204 endoscopic laryngeal procedures.[143] Because of their high-risk airways, seven patients had tracheostomies before or after their surgery. Of the remaining patients, two developed postoperative stridor, one requiring reintubation and the other a delayed tracheostomy. Indirect laryngoscopy carried out 4 to 6 hours after surgery revealed mucosal hemorrhage or laryngopharyngeal swelling in 32% of cases. Because the patients undergoing tracheostomy were not detailed, it is possible that the low incidence of reintubation resulted from an aggressive approach to preemptive tracheostomy. Some patients undergoing endoscopies may have received head and neck radiation, making their tissues more susceptible to injury and altering tissue compliance, leading to challenges with airway management.

Thyroid Surgery

A variety of airway-related injuries can be associated with thyroidectomies, including SLN and RLN injuries, wound hematoma, and tracheomalacia. Patients at greater risk of transient or permanent RLN injury include those undergoing reoperation, those with scarring or nerve encasement, patients in whom the RLN was not or could not be identified, those with thyroid cancer rather than benign goiter, more extensive surgery, and operations performed by surgeons with less thyroidectomy experience.[144] The actual rate of injury is unknown, although RLN is reported to be the leading major complication of thyroid surgery.[145] The published rates are generally reported by surgeons with a higher volume of thyroid operations and thus may not be representative of the overall frequency and severity.[145,146] RLN injury more often results from traction or compression than transection, particularly in patients with anatomic variants.[147] A recent Cochrane systematic review and meta-analysis looked at five randomized controlled trials involving 1558 patients undergoing thyroid surgery. It compared the value of intraoperative visualization and neurophysiologic monitoring of the RLN with visual identification only. The studies excluded patients undergoing repeat thyroid or parathyroid procedures. Looking for permanent or transient nerve injury, the investigators were unable to demonstrate evidence of an advantage or disadvantage to routine intraoperative monitoring of the RLN.[148] Identification of patients with RLN injury is dependent upon how and when such an assessment is made: preoperative assessment may reveal asymptomatic unilateral disease. One study reported preoperative vocal cord dysfunction in 70% and 0.3% of 365 patients with invasive and benign thyroid disease, respectively.[149] Postoperative laryngoscopy is necessary to differentiate between hoarseness resulting from nerve injury and intubation; delayed postoperative evaluation may miss transient injury.

SLN injury is more challenging to diagnose. It produces dysphonia and vocal fatigue, particularly in the higher registers. In a 5-year multicenter study involving 42 centers and nearly 15,000 thyroid operations, the diagnosis was suspected in 3.7% and confirmed in 0.4% of patients.[150]

Local hemorrhage or hematoma occurs postoperatively in 0.1% to 1.6% of patients undergoing thyroid surgery.[39,150-153] These complications can occur from 5 minutes to 7 days postoperatively. Airway obstruction may result from bleeding or significant laryngeal and pharyngeal edema. When swelling at the wound site is acute, the emergent release of sutures and wound evacuation may facilitate airway management; this is less likely to be effective when the swelling is of slower onset. A hematoma may result from or be aggravated by coagulopathies, NSAIDs, ligature slippage, coughing, vomiting, or reoperation.

Tracheomalacia is rarely diagnosed after thyroidectomy, even in patients with significant retrosternal tracheal compression, although it may exist subclinically.[154-157] Although symptoms, computed tomography (CT), and pulmonary function test results make it easy to recognize airway compression preoperatively, tracheomalacia may be difficult to predict or even detect from the surgical field and does not become apparent until after the resumption of spontaneous ventilation and extubation.[158,159]

Carotid Artery Surgery

Neck swelling or hematoma formation after carotid endarterectomy may be relatively common. The New York Carotid Artery Surgery (NYCAS) study analyzed 9308 procedures performed between 1998 and 1999 at 167 hospitals.[160] A hematoma was identified in 5% of patients, substantially increasing the risk of death (odds ratio = 4.30; 95% CI, 2.72–5.00) and stroke (odds ratio = 3.89; 95% CI, 2.82–5.38). Hematoma occurrence reported in the literature ranges from 1.2% to 12%, depending on the definition used.[160] The overall rate of wound hematomas in the North American Symptomatic Carotid Endarterectomy Trial (NASCET), involving 1415 patients, was 7.1%; the severity was considered mild with no delay in discharge, moderate delaying discharge, or severe resulting in permanent disability or death in 3.9%, 3.0%, and 0.3%, respectively. The moderate and severe cases required reexploration or wound evacuation. Hematoma contributed to the death of four patients.[161] When wound hematomas are identified by a comparison of preoperative and postoperative CT scans, it occurs far more frequently (26%).[162] The postoperative reintubation or exploration rate is 1% to 3.3%.[161,163]

Kunkel and colleagues described 15 patients who developed wound hematomas after carotid endarterectomy.[164] Eight of these were evacuated under local anesthesia. In six of seven cases where general anesthesia was induced before opening the wound, difficulties arose with airway management, resulting in two deaths and one patient with severe neurologic impairment. O'Sullivan and colleagues reported a similar experience for six patients with airway obstruction after carotid endarterectomy not relieved by preoperative wound evacuation.[165] Cyanosis and extreme bradycardia or asystole occurred in four patients, leading the authors to endorse Kunkel's recommendation for wound evacuation prior to induction. They emphasized that the external appearance may lead to an underestimation of the situation's gravity. Voice change may be a harbinger of danger, with subsequent stridor and rapid clinical deterioration.[166]

A 10-year retrospective review of 3224 carotid endarterectomies performed at the Mayo Clinic revealed that 44 patients (1.4%) required wound exploration within 72 hours of surgery, despite the nonreversal of heparin.[167] In two patients, reexploration occurred before the initial extubation. The decision to reexplore was made in the PACU for 7 patients; the remaining 35 were identified in the ICU or ward. Only one patient required a surgical airway when DL failed in the ICU. Various intubation techniques were initially employed: awake flexible scope intubation (15 of 20 were successful), DL after induction (13 of 15 were successful), and awake DL (5 of 7 were successful). When awake flexible scope intubation failed, DL was successful whether the patient was awake (3 of 3) or asleep (2 of 2). When DL initially failed after induction in two patients, it succeeded after opening the incision. When awake DL failed, one patient required a surgical airway; in the other, DL succeeded after opening the incision. Despite the size of this series, it is not possible to draw conclusions about which technique is best. Success likely depends on the skill and judgment of the airway manager. It is also possible that this study differed from the other studies in that the decision to reexplore was made earlier in patients with less airway distortion.

Several nerve injuries can result from carotid artery surgery or the associated anesthetic technique. The range reported in the literature is 3% to 23%, although most of these resolve within 4 months of surgery.[168] In the NYCAS study, cranial nerve palsies occurred in 514 (5.5%) of 9308 patients and involved the hypoglossal nerve, a branch of the facial nerve; the glossopharyngeal nerve, a branch of the vagus nerve (which may involve the RLN); the trigeminal nerve, a branch of the cervical plexus; or more than one nerve group.[160]

Bilateral vocal cord paralysis and bilateral hypoglossal nerve palsies have been described after staged, bilateral carotid endarterectomies.[37,38] In the latter case, the first procedure, performed under regional anesthesia, had been complicated by a wound hematoma, resulting in numbness over the anterior neck and diminished sensation in the C2 and C3 distribution. The subsequent endarterectomy, performed 4 weeks later under deep cervical plexus block with subcutaneous infiltration, caused intraoperative airway obstruction and asystole. The airway was secured, but repeated attempts at extubation resulted in persistent obstruction caused by bilateral hypoglossal nerve palsy. In another case, performed under

cervical plexus block, the patient developed bilateral vocal cord paralysis that required intubation and subsequent tracheotomy. It is suspected that she had a previously unrecognized contralateral vocal cord palsy from a prior thyroidectomy, identifying the importance of the preoperative assessment of patients who have had prior head and neck surgery.[169]

Cervical Spine Surgery

Cervical spine procedures may lead to airway-related complications, including vocal cord paralysis and airway obstruction. Vocal cord dysfunction was present in 5% of 411 patients undergoing anterior cervical discectomy and fusion, one of whom had stridor requiring a tracheostomy. Of the 17 patients, 16 had recovered by 15 months, and 1 was lost to follow-up.[170]

Sagi and colleagues conducted a retrospective chart review of 311 anterior cervical procedures in an effort to identify the factors associated with airway complications.[171] In this series, 19 patients (6.1%) had airway complications, but only 6 (1.9%) required reintubation. Most of these complications were attributed to pharyngeal edema. Risk factors included increased intraoperative bleeding, prolonged surgery (>5 hours), and exposure of more than three vertebral bodies, particularly when they included C2, C3, or C4. Reviewing the literature, these investigators identified an airway complication rate of 2.4% (among 1615 cases), 35 of whom required reintubation or tracheostomy. On average, those requiring reintubation did so by 24 hours. Suk and colleagues prospectively evaluated 87 patients by radiography and found that swelling caused by prevertebral edema peaked on the second and third postoperative day. The swelling was more severe in procedures involving the upper cervical discs. Reintubation was necessary in one patient (1.1%).[172]

Epstein and colleagues developed a collaborative protocol involving the neurosurgeon and anesthesiologist. Their objective was avoidance of reintubation.[173] Their study enrolled 58 high-risk patients undergoing lengthy, multilevel procedures with significant blood loss. All patients remained electively intubated overnight and underwent flexible endoscopic airway examination before considering extubation. Most patients were extubated the day after surgery, but three remained intubated until day 7. Only one patient required reintubation, a rate that was essentially the same as that observed by others.[172,174]

Patients undergoing posterior cervical surgery face the risk of macroglossia and significant retropharyngeal and hypopharyngeal swelling, which may be aggravated by fixation of the cervical spine, making intubation more challenging.[175] There is a low probability (1.1%–1.7%) that reintubation will be required, but accomplishing this may be very difficult.

Maxillofacial Surgery and Trauma

Maxillary and mandibular surgery produces conspicuous and often worrisome swelling. Anxiety regarding postoperative care may be heightened by limited airway access, fear that airway intervention may disrupt the surgical repair, and anecdotal reports of near misses or actual fatalities.[176]

Although these concerns demand special attention, deaths rarely occur. In a review of 461 perioperative deaths reported to the Ontario, Canada, coroner between 1986 and 1995, investigators found only one death associated with orthognathic surgery, although they were unable to determine how many such cases had been performed.[177] They were unable to identify nonlethal complications. Our group performed magnetic resonance imaging (MRI) approximately 24 hours after orthognathic surgery in

40 patients.[178] Despite the significant facial swelling seen in almost all the patients, none exhibited soft tissue swelling from the base of the tongue to the glottis.

Complete airway obstruction after elective orthognathic surgery has been reported. Dark and colleagues described a case involving a young woman who underwent seemingly uneventful mandibular and maxillary osteotomies with submental liposuction.[179] Immediately after extubation, she developed airway obstruction requiring reintubation. Repeated endoscopic examination and CT scanning showed severe and extensive edema from the tongue to the trachea, which was maximal at the level of the hyoid. By the fourth postoperative day, a cuff leak was detected, and the patient was successfully extubated over an airway exchange catheter (AEC). Hogan and Argalious described a patient in whom maxillo-mandibular advancement was performed for obstructive sleep apnea (OSA).[180] The procedure lasted 9 hours, during which he received 7200 mL of crystalloid and 500 mL of 6% hetastarch. The patient remained intubated overnight, and after demonstrating adequate spontaneous ventilation and a cuff leak, he was extubated over a 19-French AEC. Extubation was immediately followed by clinical evidence of airway obstruction, and he was reintubated over the AEC. The obstruction was attributed to fractured hardware and a hematoma in the piriform fossa that caused extrinsic compression. The investigators concluded that patients undergoing this type of surgery face a high risk of airway complications and recommended nasopharyngolaryngoscopy before extubation.

Clinical assessment of airway edema can be misleading,[178] and the cuff leak test is neither sufficiently sensitive nor specific. Endoscopic assessment may or may not identify occult clots (i.e., coroner's clot) in the nasopharynx or hypopharynx; it may also give rise to troublesome bleeding. Whenever possible and appropriate, the nasopharynx should be inspected and suctioned at the time of nasotracheal extubation. It might also be helpful to apply gentle suction to the nasotracheal tube upon its withdrawal.

Maxillofacial injuries may result from unrestrained occupants of motor vehicles encountering an unyielding dashboard, windshield, or steering wheel. Gunshot wounds or physical altercations also cause maxillofacial injury. Airway obstruction is a primary cause of morbidity and mortality in these patients, and many die before they reach the hospital.[181] Those with less life-threatening injuries are likely to present with a full stomach, and many have associated head and neck injuries, lacerations, loose or avulsed teeth, intraoral fractures, and fractures extending into the paranasal sinuses, into the orbit, or through the cribriform plate. They may also have an unstable cervical spine or damage to the neural axis. Injuries to the lower face raise the possibility of a laryngeal fracture. Intermaxillary fixation may be part of the surgical plan, necessitating a nasal intubation or a surgical airway. Timing of tracheal extubation is complex and must take into consideration factors such as the patient's level of consciousness, ability to maintain satisfactory gas exchange, coagulation status, and integrity of protective airway reflexes. Attention must be paid to the difficulties originally encountered in securing the airway and an evaluation of whether reintubation would be easier or more difficult after surgery and resuscitation. Most of the trauma literature about airway management addresses intubation and offers little help with extubation, making cooperation among the anesthesiologist, surgeon, and critical care physician essential.[182,183] Intermaxillary fixation requires that wire cutters be at the bedside and that personnel who know how to use them are available. A flexible intubation scope (FIS), provisions for an emergency invasive airway access, and the required expertise should

be immediately available at the time of extubation. Alternatives include prophylactic tracheotomy, submental intubation,[184-186] nasal intubation, and bronchoscopic airway evaluation performed before extubation,[187] although assessment may be limited to supraglottic structures and exclusion of tube entrapment. Ideally, extubation should be accomplished in a reversible manner, permitting supplemental oxygenation, ventilation, and reintubation, if needed (see section Extubation Strategies).

Major intraoral surgery, composite mandibular resections that include extensive neck dissections, and free flap reconstructions make for awkward airway access. This may be further exacerbated by prior radiation to the area, indurated or taut tissue, bulky flaps, or a marginal blood supply giving rise to further postoperative swelling. Many patients undergoing these procedures have comorbidities associated with postoperative complications that may necessitate urgent airway management. The decision when and how to extubate and when to perform an elective tracheostomy should involve a discussion between those responsible for subsequent care, including the surgeon, anesthesiologist, and ICU or PACU physicians, as appropriate. Several scoring systems have been advocated but have not been widely used.[188]

Nasal and Nasopharyngeal Trauma

Passage of any device through the nasopharynx can result in occult bleeding. This includes temperature probes, nasogastric tubes, or nasotracheal tubes. Significant bleeding will generally declare itself upon oropharyngeal inspection; minor bleeding, however, tends to pool in the dependent nasopharynx where it may clot, concealed above and behind the soft palate. Following extubation, the patient may take a deep breath, aspirating the clot and obstructing their airway. Ventilation may fail without prompt recognition and correction of the problem. After adenoid surgery, there is generally a high index of suspicion of nasopharyngeal bleeding, which gives rise to a careful inspection. In other contexts, the potential for a "coroner's clot" is less obvious. Related injuries resulting from nasal cannulation include submucosal dissection (which can lead to mediastinitis), turbinectomy, unintended adenoidectomy, and retropharyngeal cannulation. In the authors' opinion, even after a seemingly atraumatic nasal intubation, the nasopharynx should be carefully examined prior to waking the patient. This can be performed with slight retraction of the nasotracheal tube near the uvula using Magill forceps and applying gentle suction with a Yankauer suction catheter.

Thermal Airway Injury

Burn patients can have intrinsic and extrinsic airway injuries. Circumferential neck involvement is an example of an extrinsic injury. Smoke inhalation or thermal injuries are examples of intrinsic injuries. Burn patients are at particular risk of requiring reintubation. They can have bronchorrhea, impaired mucociliary clearance and local defenses, laryngeal and supraglottic edema, increased carbon dioxide production, impaired consciousness from carbon monoxide intoxication, and progressive acute respiratory distress syndrome. It may be difficult to secure an ETT because of involvement of the adjacent skin, and burn victims may be agitated or uncooperative, increasing the risk of unintended extubation.[189] Kemper and colleagues reported their management of extubation in 25 pediatric trauma patients. Treatment for postextubation stridor was required in 7 out of 11 patients with burns, 5 of whom required reintubation, and in only 1 out of 19 without burns. Postextubation stridor among children with facial burns was best predicted by the absence of a cuff leak.[190] See also Chapter 35.

Deep Neck Infections

Infections involving the submandibular, sublingual, submental, prevertebral, parapharyngeal, and retropharyngeal spaces are significant airway management challenges, whether intubation is achieved for surgical drainage or for protection during medical management. In expert hands, flexible scope intubation can often be achieved.[191] When this is unsuccessful or poses a significant risk of rupturing the abscess, a surgical airway before incision and drainage may be indicated.[192] Potter and colleagues retrospectively compared the outcomes of 34 patients in whom a tracheotomy was performed with 51 patients who remained intubated after surgical drainage.[193] All patients had undergone surgical drainage for impending airway compromise and required airway support postoperatively. The investigators could often not determine why a particular strategy was chosen, and these groups were likely not identical. Airway loss occurred more commonly in the intubated patients, but this characteristic was not statistically significant. Two deaths occurred, one resulting from an unintended extubation and the other from postextubation laryngeal edema and an inability to reestablish the airway. The latter patient had a cuff leak prior to extubation, but obstruction developed within 30 minutes of extubation. Surgical drainage rarely results in immediate airway improvement, and reintubation or emergent placement of a surgical airway, if required, may be complicated by edema, tissue distortion, and urgency.

Posterior Fossa Surgery

Posterior fossa surgery can cause a variety of injuries that increase the risk of extubation failure, including cranial nerve palsies, vocal cord paralysis, brainstem or respiratory control center injury, and macroglossia.[29,90,91,115,149,194] Because the nerve roots may be very close to the operative site, the resultant injuries may be bilateral, extensive, and either transient or permanent. Gorski and colleagues suggested that tolerance of the ETT and the absence of a gag reflex on oral suctioning should arouse suspicion of injury.[195] Howard and colleagues described a patient with a recurrent choroid plexus papilloma involving the fourth ventricle. Preoperatively, the patient displayed bulbar dysfunction. Extubation on the first postoperative day was complicated by complete airway obstruction, hypoxia, and a seizure. Laryngoscopy performed after neuromuscular blockade revealed mildly edematous vocal cords. After reintubation and elective tracheostomy, endoscopic examination showed adducted vocal cords, consistent with bilateral paralysis. Nocturnal positive-pressure ventilation and tracheostomy were still required at 3 months. This patient demonstrated central apnea and bulbar dysfunction with hypoglossal and vocal cord paralysis.[196]

Artru and colleagues described a patient with a cerebellar mass, severe papilledema, and bulbar signs. Despite recovery of consciousness and strength, the patient remained apneic and required ventilatory support for 7 days. The investigators cautioned that the dorsal pons and medulla are the sites of the cardiovascular and respiratory centers that control hemodynamics and ventilation. The area is also host to several cranial nerve nuclei. Damage to these areas can result from edema, disruption, ischemia, or compression and may cause a loss of respiratory drive or airway obstruction.[194] Dohi and colleagues described a patient who developed bulbar signs, including bilateral vocal cord paralysis after excision of a recurrent cerebellopontine angle tumor. POPE developed as a consequence of a bilateral, presumably central, RLN injury, and a tracheostomy was required until recovery 3 months later.[115]

Early vocal cord evaluation after extubation has been advocated along with the involvement of a neurosurgeon, otolaryngologist, speech therapist, and intensivist to manage patients who have developed laryngeal dysfunction.[197] A tracheostomy and an enteral feeding tube may be needed. A preemptive approach, the Bailey maneuver (described later), involves flexible laryngoscopic assessment through an SGA after removal of the ETT.

Stereotactic Surgery and Cervical Immobilization

Stereotactic neurosurgical and neuroradiologic procedures are finding increasing applications. Head frames and cervical immobilization devices may impede access for SGA placement or laryngoscopy. Planning for extubation in these circumstances is critical because reintubation may be difficult and rapid surgical access may be virtually impossible. The usual considerations, such as recovery of strength and consciousness, may have been compromised by the preoperative state or the surgical procedure. It is important to demonstrate the persistence of the respiratory drive, the presence of a cuff leak, preservation of protective reflexes, and absence of significant tongue swelling. Postoperative seizures, vomiting, elevated ICP, and neurologic obtundation may make extubation particularly hazardous. Higher-risk extubation strategies should be considered in managing such patients.

Tracheal Resection

Patients with moderate or severe airway narrowing may present for surgical repair. Management of their airways is demanding during all phases of care. These patients may have laryngeal, subglottic, or tracheal stenosis that may be rigid or dynamic, extrathoracic or intrathoracic. Tracheomalacia or bronchomalacia will only be apparent with spontaneous ventilation. Patients may undergo laser resections, rigid dilatations, or tracheal resection. In the latter case, significant shortening may be temporarily managed with a guardian suture from the chin to the chest to reduce tension on the anastomoses. This leaves the patient in a position of cervical flexion and could make reintubation challenging (Fig. 47.1).[198,199]

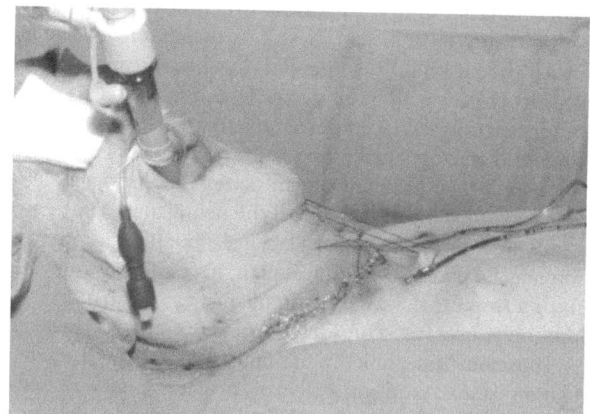

• **Fig. 47.1** This patient has undergone a cricotracheal resection. Cervical extension is restricted by placement of a chin-to-chest guardian suture. The patient has been extubated, and a laryngeal mask airway was introduced before reversal of neuromuscular blockade or awakening. This reduces coughing on emergence, allowing gradual recovery and assessment of spontaneous respiratory function while minimizing the potential distraction of the surgical anastomosis. It also provides the optimal means of performing flexible laryngobronchial examination under controlled conditions. (Courtesy Patrick Gullane, MD, University Health Network, Toronto, ON, Canada)

Efforts to minimize coughing or retching following extubation are also important.

Palatoplasty

A variety of surgical procedures have been employed to treat OSA, including uvulopalatopharyngoplasty (UPPP), midline glossectomy, mandibular advancement, limited mandibular osteotomies with genioglossal advancement, and hyoid bone suspension.[200] These procedures offer benefits but also carry significant risks, including death, since many patients with OSA have relevant comorbidities.[201,202] A multicenter cohort review of 3130 UPPPs performed at Veterans Health Administration institutions between 1991 and 2001 found that the risk of defined serious complications (0.6%–8.9%), including death (0.0%–1.6%), varied widely among institutions. Respiratory complications were the most common (1.1%). The reintubation and emergent tracheostomy rates were 0.5% and 0.2%, respectively.[202]

Preexisting Medical Conditions

The following section describes several medical conditions associated with postextubation airway complications, some of which are widely recognized and others that may be less well known to airway practitioners. Some of these conditions are very common, but the airway implications are not widely recognized, such as Parkinson disease and rheumatoid arthritis. Morbid obesity and OSA are pervasive but frequently undiagnosed, and guidelines offer limited assistance. Other conditions described in the literature may be less likely to be familiar to airway practitioners. Paradoxical vocal cord motion (PVCM) epitomizes this discussion, as patients suffering with this disorder are easily intubated but can be very difficult to extubate.

Obesity, Morbid Obesity, and Obstructive Sleep Apnea Syndrome

According to the World Health Organization (WHO), obesity—defined as a body mass index >30—has nearly tripled since 1975 and is the fifth leading risk of global deaths.[1] Many patients presenting for surgery, particularly the obese, are at risk of having undiagnosed OSA. The perioperative complications suffered by patients with diagnosed OSA undergoing nonbariatric surgery have been reviewed.[203,204] For patients with undiagnosed OSA, complications are often worse, as they are less likely to have been managed with continuous positive airway pressure (CPAP) pre- or postoperatively and less likely to be managed by a team with a specific expertise in managing such patients.[205] Obese and morbidly obese patients are more likely to have a diminished ventilatory drive and to experience rapid oxygen desaturation, difficult mask ventilation, and gastric reflux; be difficult to properly position for (re)intubation; experience airway obstruction following extubation; and present a challenge for intubation or an emergent surgical airway if required.[206] NAP4 reported that 76 out of 171 adults (44%) with serious adverse airway outcomes were obese, despite representing only 25% of patients overall. The dicrepancy was even more stark for those with BMI ≥40; they accounted for 8% of the events but only 2% of the population.[4] In the ASA Closed Claims Project analysis of adverse respiratory events, 65 of the 156 perioperative events (42%) involved obese patients; for claims specifically related to extubation, 12 of the 18 were obese, and 5 of these patients had been diagnosed with OSA.[3] A recent

review of the legal literature between 1991 and 2010 identified 24 adult cases in the United States wherein OSA was determined to be responsible for adverse outcomes, resulting in tried malpractice suits. Eight of these cases related to extubation, which was generally premature, resulting in airway obstruction further complicated by the inability to reintubate: two resulted in immediate death, five resulted in anoxic brain injury, and one sustained damage to the upper airway. The authors further observed that, whereas the number of medical malpractice suits in the United States between 2001 and 2010 has annually declined by 35%, the number of suits related to OSA appears to be increasing.[207] An accompanying editorial highlights the limited medical data contained in the legal reports and the potential bias of a database that excludes out-of-court settlements. The authors draw attention to the fact that 55% of cases were settled prior to trial and 22% of cases were dropped, all of which were excluded from review.[208]

Although not all obese patients have OSA and not all OSA patients are obese, OSA does correlate positively with age and increased body weight. OSA is present in a significant proportion of the general population; obesity predisposes such individuals to conditions requiring surgical care, and most cases of OSA remain undiagnosed when patients present for care.[209] The pathophysiology and perioperative airway management of OSA in obese patients has been reviewed.[210-212] A report of over 530,000 patients undergoing total hip or knee arthroplasties found that the risk of emergent reintubation among patients with diagnosed OSA was significantly increased (odds ratio 10.26; 95% CI, 9.0–11.7).[213] A meta-analysis that included 13 studies involving nearly 4000 adults diagnosed with OSA by screening questionnaires, oximetry, or polysomnography found that those with OSA were significantly more likely than a matched cohort without OSA to have postoperative respiratory failure (odds ratio 2.43; 95% CI, 1.34–4.39), postoperative desaturation (2.27; 1.20–4.26), and require reintubation (2.05; 0.92–4.55).[204]

The ASA Practice Guidelines for the Perioperative Management of Patients with OSA provide limited guidance regarding extubation beyond a strong recommendation that patients be fully awake and full reversal of neuromuscular blockade be confirmed before extubation. If possible, extubation and recovery should be carried out in the lateral or semiupright position,[214] nasal CPAP should be available or routinely implemented, and consideration should be given to extubation over a tube exchanger. Individually, these strategies have been associated with better outcomes, but they have not been subjected to randomized controlled trials and were not addressed by the ASA task force. The NAP4 study reminds us that obese patients, particularly those with OSA, are at significant risk of experiencing respiratory complications requiring careful planning and monitoring prior to extubation. They are especially susceptible to oxygen desaturation, hypoventilation, and airway obstruction. Mask ventilation, placement of an SGA, tracheal intubation, and emergency invasive airway access may all be particularly challenging.[4]

Paradoxical Vocal Cord Motion

Although obesity, morbid obesity, and OSA are common, frequently undiagnosed, and challenging with respect to both extubation and (re)intubation, PVCM is almost always misdiagnosed. It is the quintessential example of an easy intubation but very difficult extubation. PVCM is frequently mistaken for refractory asthma or recurrent laryngospasm.[215-220] It has been referred to as vocal cord dysfunction, Munchausen stridor, psychogenic stridor, factitious asthma, pseudoasthma, and irritable larynx

---

[1]https://www.who.int/news-room/fact-sheets/detail/obesity-and-overweight (dated April 2020; accessed Dec 14, 2020)

syndrome.[220] The pathogenesis is thought to be multifactorial, including psychogenic components, laryngeal hyperresponsiveness, altered autonomic balance, and direct stimulation of local nerve endings resulting in adduction of the true vocal cords and supraglottic structures on inspiration. It is likely exacerbated by stress, exercise, gastroesophageal reflux, irritant exposure, and/or airway manipulation. The diagnosis is dependent upon high-level clinical suspicion, with a history of refractory asthma and sudden-onset, often recurrent, respiratory difficulty primarily on inspiration. Confirmation of the diagnosis is made by endoscopic visualization of vocal cord adduction on inspiration, usually with a small posterior glottic chink. Although this is most marked while the patient is symptomatic, it may be possible to elicit these signs and symptoms with panting and deep breathing. Topical and IV lidocaine, as well as benzodiazepines, may mask these findings. Pulmonary function tests show normal expiratory but flattened inspiratory flow loops while the patient is symptomatic. Color Doppler ultrasound of the vocal cords has recently been described as a diagnostic modality and may be as useful as endoscopy without the stimulation. It is important to differentiate this condition from asthma, laryngospasm, laryngeal or tracheal stenosis, anaphylaxis, angioedema, gastroesophageal reflux, and vocal cord paralysis. The incidence of PVCM is unknown.

Hammer and colleagues described a 32-year-old woman with recurrent episodes of stridor, sometimes associated with cyanosis, despite normal flow-volume loops and pulmonary function tests. The diagnosis of PVCM was made endoscopically and managed with relaxation techniques. After preoperative sedation, topical lidocaine, and bilateral SLN blocks, she underwent awake bronchoscopic intubation. After surgery, extubation was performed after she was fully awake, but sustained inspiratory stridor ensued, resulting in reintubation. A subsequent attempt the next day confirmed inspiratory vocal fold adduction, and a tracheostomy was required for 58 days.[221] In the absence of features predicting a challenging intubation, there seems little justification for awake intubation, and it may contribute unnecessarily to an anxiety disorder.

PVCM per se poses no particular challenge for intubation. The abnormality is functional rather than anatomic. Appropriate management depends upon making the correct diagnosis. Oxygenation by CPAP, heliox, calm reassurance, diversion of attention, instructing the patient to pant, low-dose benzodiazepines, and ketamine have all been recommended. Speech therapy, psychotherapy, hypnosis, and reassurance may be helpful in long-term management.[219,222] The optimal extubation strategy of a patient with PVCM may be deep extubation, assuming there are no contraindications, but this has not been investigated (nor has the use of IV lidocaine or remifentanil). One of the authors (RMC) has successfully managed such a patient using a Bailey maneuver (see later discussion) followed by a titrated propofol infusion monitored by flexible endoscopy.

Parkinson Disease and Multiple System Atrophy

The estimated global burden of Parkinson disease more than doubled between 1990 and 2016 to over 6 million people. Aging of the population increases not only the incidence but also the duration of illness.[223] It is the second most common neurodegenerative disease after Alzheimer disease. Susceptibility to aspiration is common among patients with Parkinson disease and is the most common cause of death. Dysphonia, most frequently hypophonia, occurs in approximately 70% to 90% of patients with Parkinson disease.[224,225] Video stroboscopic findings include laryngeal

tremor, vocal fold bowing, and abnormal glottic opening and closing.[225]

Several neurodegenerative diseases, including multiple system atrophy (MSA), have some features in common with Parkinson disease, including dysphonia, and these patients may exhibit bilateral abductor vocal fold paresis. They may also exhibit nocturnal stridor and may benefit from CPAP or bi-level positive airway pressure.[224] Patients with MSA, which is frequently misdiagnosed as Parkinson disease in its early manifestations, have daytime hypoxemia associated with abnormal laryngopharyngeal movements, including airway obstruction at the arytenoids, epiglottis, base of the tongue, and soft palate.[224] The significance of these problems is unclear, but they may contribute to complications after extubation.[226]

Vincken and colleagues studied 27 patients with extrapyramidal disorders.[227] Pulmonary flow-volume loops were observed in 24 patients. Many of the loops demonstrated 4- to 8-Hz saw-toothed oscillations, reminiscent of cogwheel rigidity, even in the absence of respiratory symptoms. These were associated with irregular movements of the glottis and supraglottic structures. Among the patients, 10 exhibited intermittent upper airway obstruction, whereas 4 patients had stridor or dyspnea. The investigators believed that the upper airway was the primary site of involvement. In a subsequent report, they observed symptomatic improvement and increased inspiratory and expiratory flow with levodopa treatment, despite persistence of the oscillatory pattern on flow-volume loops.[228] Bronchodilators provided no additional benefit. This may have important implications for the perioperative management of patients with Parkinson disease.

Easdown and colleagues described a patient with Parkinson disease who had a respiratory arrest 60 hours after surgery.[229] Before that event, the patient had episodic desaturation, labored breathing, and progressive hypercapnia in the absence of tremor or rigidity. Treatment with bronchodilators provided no benefit, and his condition improved immediately after intubation. With the ETT in place, pulmonary compliance and resistance appeared normal. This patient's levodopa-carbidopa had not been resumed postoperatively, and the investigators speculated that this caused or contributed to upper airway obstruction. Because most patients with Parkinson disease are elderly and may have comorbidities that can make the diagnosis uncertain, consider involvement of the upper airway and the dramatic effect that withdrawal and reinstatement of medications can have on their clinical course. This concern is reinforced by a case report describing a patient who developed airway obstruction and acute respiratory acidosis requiring intubation preoperatively after five doses of his antiparkinson medications were withheld during preoperative fasting.[230] The reports draw attention to the need for continuation of these medications and the avoidance of dopamine antagonists throughout the perioperative period.

Liu and colleagues described airway obstruction during induction of anesthesia in a patient with Parkinson disease.[231] The obstruction resolved with intubation but recurred 24 hours later following extubation. Endoscopic examination showed inspiratory vocal fold adduction necessitating reintubation. It is unclear whether they were observing manifestations of Parkinson disease, PVCM, or simple laryngospasm, but extubation was uneventful 24 hours later after increasing the dosage of levodopa-carbidopa.

Parkinson disease is a common disorder, yet associated stridor is quite rare. It may be an imprecisely tuned protective mechanism against aspiration. The pathogenesis of upper airway obstruction is unknown. It may be mediated by the basal ganglia and nucleus ambiguus. A similar phenomenon involving esophageal spasm has been associated with Parkinson disease.[225]

Rheumatoid Arthritis

Rheumatoid arthritis (RA) is a common chronic disease capable of producing widespread articular and extraarticular destruction. In addition to the cervical spine, practitioners involved in airway management should be concerned about three additional areas: the temporomandibular (TMJ), cricoarytenoid (CAJ), and cricothyroid (CTJ) joints. The incidence of laryngeal involvement ranges between 13% and 75% of RA patients, depending on the criteria and whether the assessment is made by indirect laryngoscopy, CT imaging, or at autopsy.[232] The symptoms of laryngeal involvement may include fullness in the throat, hoarseness and difficulty speaking, odynophagia, dysphagia, and stridor. Depending upon the structures involved, RA patients may have an unstable cervical spine, narrowed glottic aperture, limited mouth opening as a result of involvement of the TMJs, laryngeal deviation, and CAJ, CTJ, or vocal cord involvement.

The incidence of cervical instability in RA patients presenting for joint replacement can be as high as 61%, with associated atlantoaxial subluxation, atlantoaxial impaction, and subaxial subluxation. Age, disease activity, and disease duration are associated with higher rates of subluxation, but symptoms do not reliably predict severity.[233]

Kohjitani and colleagues retrospectively described four RA patients undergoing bilateral TMJ replacement; three had glottic erythema and swelling on endoscopy, three had OSA, and three experienced laryngospasm during awake intubation and after extubation.[234] TMJ involvement resulting in loss of height of the mandibular ramus may contribute to or be causative of OSA.

Laryngeal involvement in patients with RA is nearly universal at autopsy and may include CAJ fixation, recurrent laryngeal nerve involvement, myositis, and nodules.[235] Symptoms may include odynophagia, dysphagia, a change in voice quality or strength, and croup. The nature of CAJ involvement may be unilateral or bilateral swelling or joint destruction resulting in unilateral vocal cord impairment or bilateral vocal cord fixation. The pathologic findings include hyperemia, edema, pannus formation, joint destruction, and ankylosis. It is helpful to have an appreciation of the extent of laryngeal involvement before embarking on elective airway management, particularly in the symptomatic RA patient. Severe CAJ involvement to the point of complete airway obstruction may even precede the articular manifestations of RA.[235-237] When vocal fatigue is described, CTJ involvement should be considered. Laryngoscopy may reveal varying degrees of edema, hyperemia, deformation, and submucosal vocal cord nodules ("bamboo nodes").[235,238]

Keenan and colleagues described tracheal scoliosis in a patient with RA, which consisted of tracheal deviation, rotation and anterior angulation of the larynx, and vocal fold adduction seen endoscopically and on CT imaging.[239] It was presumed to result from the loss of vertical height and asymmetric bony erosions.

Wattenmaker and colleagues studied patients with RA undergoing posterior cervical spine procedures.[240] Their primary objective was to compare the perioperative airway complications seen in RA patients when intubation was performed by DL or flexible bronchoscopy. Retrospectively reviewing 128 consecutive posterior cervical procedures, upper airway obstruction characterized by stridor occurred in 9 of 128 patients, 1 of 70 patients intubated with a flexible bronchoscope, and 8 of 58 patients intubated by direct laryngoscopy or a blind nasal technique. In the nonbronchoscopic group, five required emergency reintubation that proved to be very difficult, with two near fatalities and one death. Although the two groups were similar with regard to age, gender, American Rheumatology Association classification, ASA physical status, duration of surgery and anesthesia, fluid balance, and postoperative immobilization, there were significant differences in time to extubation. Among the patients, seven could not be intubated by flexible bronchoscopy and were therefore intubated by other methods. The patients were not randomized to the different methods; criteria for the method of intubation and techniques were not described; all patients were intubated awake; and the study was carried out over an 11-year period.[241] Although it is not possible to draw firm conclusions from this study, there was a high incidence (7%) of postextubation stridor and difficult or failed reintubation, regardless of the intubation technique.

Patients with RA are generally at higher risk of extubation because of anatomic challenges (such as a fixed or unstable cervical spine, TMJ ankylosis, known difficulty with intubation) and are also at increased risk of postextubation airway obstruction. Several investigators have recommended postponing extubation until the patient is wide awake. The prevailing wisdom is that patients with limited mouth opening and a potentially unstable cervical spine should be intubated with an FIS. However, this method involves blind passage of the ETT through the cords, which can be traumatic,[55,241] particularly in the face of preexisting CAJ or CTJ arthritis. Regional anesthesia should be considered as an alternative to general anesthesia when appropriate. When intubation cannot be avoided, proposed extubation strategies include a method that facilitates reintubation or, rarely, a preemptive tracheostomy. Neither strategy has been prospectively evaluated in this population.

Tracheomalacia

Tracheomalacia is a dynamic airway obstruction resulting from partial or complete loss of the cartilaginous tracheal support. Symptoms of tracheomalacia are nonspecific, but the diagnosis should be considered when the patient has dyspnea on exertion with difficulty clearing secretions and a seal-like, incessant cough.[242,243]

Patients with tracheomalacia are frequently misdiagnosed with asthma and fail to respond to escalating therapy. Pulmonary function tests (i.e., forced expiratory volume at 1 second, forced vital capacity, and peak expiratory flow) show severely diminished expiratory flow with relative preservation of the inspiratory flow; however, the findings correlate poorly with clinical severity.[244] The diagnosis can be confirmed and the severity estimated endoscopically during spontaneous quiet breathing and provocative maneuvers, such as coughing and Valsalva; dynamic helical CT scans also can establish the diagnosis and severity. The extent of the airway affected can range from localized to widespread involvement of the tracheobronchial tree as might be seen with severe COPD or relapsing polychondritis. Collapse less than 50% is generally within normal limits; 50% to 75% is considered mild, whereas collapse greater than 91% is regarded as severe.[244] Acquired tracheomalacia can result from extrinsic compression, such as from an intrathoracic goiter or arterial compression or chronic air trapping (e.g., COPD), cartilaginous destruction (e.g., relapsing polychondritis), or a combination of factors (e.g., prolonged intubation). The latter can be caused by ETT cuff–induced erosion of the tracheal cartilage with or without extension to the membranous trachea.

The severity of the dynamic obstruction is proportional to the expiratory force. It may not be apparent during quiet breathing but is disabling when the same patient is distressed. Positive-pressure ventilation or bypassing the lesion with an ETT provides temporary relief while further management options are considered, such as medical management, surgical resection, or placement of a stent.[243,244] Suggestions for the extubation of a patient with suspected tracheomalacia are described later.

Laryngeal Incompetence

Laryngeal function can be depressed after tracheal extubation despite recovery of consciousness. In one study, 8 of 24 patients intubated for 8 to 28 hours aspirated swallowed radiopaque dye 4 hours following extubation; 5 showed radiologic evidence of massive aspiration; the number diminished to 1 of 24 by 24 hours. None of the patients who aspirated coughed when challenged with the dye.[245] Tanaka and colleagues found that there is depression of laryngeal reflexes following even brief surgical procedures regardless of whether an SGA or ETT had been used to manage the airway. This study was performed on patients breathing sevoflurane at 1 MAC (minimum alveolar concentration), making it difficult to know whether the observations are applicable in the fully recovered patient.[246] When patients randomized to an SGA or ETT were deemed fit for discharge from the PACU, they were requested to swallow barium, which was detected in the trachea of 1 out of 40 patients.[247]

The results of these studies are inconclusive concerning the circumstances that put patients at greater risk of laryngeal incompetence and its prevalence. It is worrisome that the patients who did aspirate did not cough, thereby indicating their predisposition to aspiration or atelectasis.[245,247,248] This problem can be compounded by incomplete reversal of neuromuscular blockade, the antitussive effects of opioids, the increasing use of IV lidocaine as an analgesic adjunct, and the proemetic effects of many of the agents to which patients are exposed during general anesthesia. Residual neuromuscular blockade is a common problem in postoperative patients and can result in hypoventilation, hypoxemia, pharyngeal and laryngeal dysfunction, or increased pulmonary aspiration.[249]

Pulmonary Aspiration of Gastric Contents

Although more patients are being diagnosed with gastroesophageal reflux, the diagnosis of perioperative pulmonary aspiration has not increased.[250,251] Despite this, in the NAP4 study of nearly 3 million general anesthetics, aspiration was the single greatest contributor to anesthetic mortality and equal to failed intubation as the primary airway problem.[4] Aspiration was also responsible for 23 of the 29 patients admitted to the ICU following an airway event.[252] Factors predisposing a surgical patient to aspiration include emergency surgery, pain, obesity, opioids, nausea, ileus, bowel obstruction, pregnancy, some surgical positions, a depressed level of consciousness, inadequate depth of anesthesia, postoperative drowsiness, and residual neuromuscular blockade. Despite the ubiquity of these conditions, perioperative aspiration is not commonly identified. Indeed, in the review by the ASA Closed Claims Project, it was responsible for only 3 of 156 perioperative events.[3,251,253] Before intubation, difficult bag-mask ventilation can result in gastric distention, which can be further complicated if laryngoscopy proves difficult. This not only delays securing the airway, but forceful laryngoscopy often opens the esophagus and may promote regurgitation. Repeated laryngoscopic attempts can cause edema, thereby increasing glottic resistance. Aspiration can also result from obtundation or conditions that impair vocal cord apposition (e.g., vocal cord paralysis, laryngeal incompetence, residual neuromuscular blockade, or granulomas).

Although most incidents of aspiration seem to occur at induction, this can occur at any point in the perioperative period, including after extubation.[254] Numerous strategies have been described to reduce the risk at induction, but relatively little information is available on how best to prevent aspiration from occurring subsequently. Premature extubation, postoperative nausea, residual neuromuscular blockade, induced gagging with oral suctioning, supine recovery, and impaired laryngeal competence can make emergence from anesthesia and tracheal extubation as problematic as induction.

Anatomical, Physiological, and Contextual Factors Affecting Extubation and Reintubation

An extubation strategy optimizing reintubation should be considered for patients in whom management had been or might have become problematic. Examples include patients requiring multiple attempts at laryngoscopy, the use of specialized equipment or techniques, or management by more experienced personnel. In addition, patients with known or presumed difficulty in establishing or maintaining ventilation and oxygenation (by face mask or SGA) warrant such consideration.

In urgent or emergent circumstances, the methods, devices, or personnel that had previously achieved success may not be available. These contribute to contextual challenges.[255] Patients may be encountered lying on the floor or in a PACU or ICU bed where headboards, infusion pumps, or monitors create barriers. Uncertainty regarding the ease of ventilation or intubation may lead to reluctance to administer paralytic and sedating drugs, making both ventilation and laryngoscopy more difficult.

The patient with a physiologically difficult airway due to hypoxia, acidosis, hypotension, or risk of regurgitation poses additional challenges.[256] Repeated attempts at laryngoscopy may exacerbate preexisting physiologic abnormalities and are associated with a significant increase in the risk of hypoxemia, esophageal intubation, regurgitation, aspiration, bradycardia, and cardiac arrest.[24,25,257]

Anatomic considerations include limitations to airway access by maxillomandibular fixation, temporomandibular ankylosis, cervical restriction or instability, macroglossia, neck swelling, and the chin-to-chest guardian suture used following cricotracheal resection to minimize tension on the anastomosis (see Fig. 47.1). Although these examples may be extreme, situations where access to the patient's airway is awkward or worse are not uncommon.

Risk Stratification

As stated, risk stratification is best understood as a risk continuum. Higher-risk extubations imply that either extubation or reintubation (or both) has a greater likelihood of failing; if extubation fails but the airway can be easily managed, the consequences may not be severe. If, on the other hand, the extubation fails and the airway cannot be easily managed, the results may be devastating. Where that patient is on the risk continuum is dependent upon the clinical context and the resources available to manage the problems. For example, the risk is less when well-informed and highly experienced personnel with the necessary equipment and expertise are readily available; the risk is increased if the patient is more susceptible to regurgitation or oxygen desaturation, regardless of the personnel present.

Ultimately, *how* oxygenation is achieved is less important than *how quickly* it can be achieved. Multiple attempts at reintubation may be more damaging than successful face-mask ventilation, SGA ventilation, or high-flow nasal oxygenation. Extubation failure is often unanticipated and must be dealt with as it occurs in a manner most likely to succeed given the clinical setting, the equipment available, and the skills of the care team. The previous section identified circumstances in which the stakes are raised because of clinical conditions, such as morbid obesity, OSA, PVCM, unstable or restricted cervical spine, RA, and others. Certain surgical procedures associated with increased risk were also discussed, such as airway endoscopy, surgery involving the airway or neck, and extreme positioning.

The clinical playing field may not be level at all hours of the day or in all locations. The immediate availability of highly trained primary and support personnel, equipment, and the necessary clinical information may be problematic at night or during periods of intense activity. The ASA Task Force on Management of the Difficult Airway, the Canadian Airway Focus Group (CAFG), and the Difficult Airway Society (DAS), among others, have recommended a preformulated strategy for extubation of the DA. Patients at risk for hypoventilation, hypoxemia, and loss of airway patency have been discussed. The remainder of this chapter addresses specific extubation strategies.

Extubation Strategies

When traveling by air, a pilot ultimately wants to ensure that passengers safely arrive at their destination. If conditions are not suitable for a safe landing, this may require delays or an alternative airport. Likewise, when conditions do not favor a safe extubation, it is prudent to postpone or consider an alternative strategy, one that maximizes the likelihood of successful oxygenation by face mask, SGA, noninvasive ventilation, reintubation, or surgical airway access. Ideally, the strategy should permit the continuous, effective administration of oxygen with little discomfort or risk of patient harm.

Respiratory Droplet Concerns

As this text is being written, the world is being confronted by the COVID-19 pandemic, which is exhausting our healthcare resources and challenging the safety of healthcare workers, particularly those involved in aerosol- and droplet-generating procedures. The risk to healthcare workers and optimal airway management of patients with viral respiratory infections is still uncertain. It is likely that the risk to the patient is greatest at intubation when critical hypoxemia exemplifies the physiologically challenged patient. These patients are very likely to be intolerant of even brief periods of apnea, although neuromuscular relaxation significantly reduces the risk of aerosol generation. At extubation, a vigorous cough potentially threatens the health of those providing care, particularly if personal protective equipment (PPE) are in short supply or imperfectly deployed. Brown and colleagues found that the magnitude of detectable aerosols was 15 times greater at extubation compared with intubation; however, they also found that the amount of aerosols generated at extubation was considerably less than that produced by a "volitional cough."[258] It is important to point out that the comparison at extubation involved only four patients (without quantitative evidence of recovery from the NMBA) with one nonanesthetized, healthy subject who performed the volitional cough (personal communication, Jules Brown, November 3, 2020). Several strategies have been proposed, including the use of barrier devices, to contain droplets.[43,259–261]

Deep Versus Awake Extubation

Extubation can be performed before or after recovery of consciousness. Extubation before the recovery of consciousness—deep extubation—has long been practiced in pediatric anesthesia to reduce coughing, bucking, and laryngospasm. It is less commonly performed in adults and has been regarded as an advanced technique reserved for patients with anatomically normal airways who are not at risk of aspiration.[12]

Deep extubation ordinarily occurs after full recovery of neuromuscular function and the resumption of spontaneous ventilation. Its purported advantage is the avoidance of the adverse reflexes associated with extubation, such as hypertension, dysrhythmias, coughing, laryngospasm, and increased IOP or ICP. The fundamental disadvantage of deep extubation is the patient's inability to protect his or her airway against obstruction and aspiration. When deep extubation is improperly executed, laryngospasm and its subsequent complications are more likely to occur. In the perioperative setting, not having to wait for the recovery of consciousness may accelerate OR turnover, although this approach is difficult to justify with anesthetic agents that are eliminated relatively quickly. When patients are transferred to a PACU while still exhaling volatile anesthetic agents, unscavenged agents pollute the OR environment and may represent an occupational health hazard.

A recent prospective, observational study of deep extubation in 300 adults following ophthalmologic or head and neck surgery found that 13% experienced at least one respiratory complication such as persistent coughing, SpO_2 <90% for more than 10 seconds, laryngospasm, bronchospasm, or necessitated reintubation. The anesthetic management and suitability for deep extubation were at the discretion of the attending anesthesiologist. There were no specified exclusion criteria, nor was there an extubation protocol. Patients who experienced respiratory complications were more likely to have a higher BMI and to have lower SpO_2 prior to extubation.[22] The incidence of respiratory complications associated with deep extubation likely depends on patient selection, anesthetic agents used, and the extubation protocol.

One small study included 62 adults who were extubated while breathing desflurane at ≥1.5 MAC or desflurane at 1 MAC with a remifentanil infusion at a target 1 ng/mL effect-site concentration. The recovery time and respiratory complications were significantly lower (3.8% vs 48%) in the desflurane and remifentanil group. The respiratory complications observed were primarily breath-holding and coughing. The authors cautioned that because of the "delayed awakening and difficulty securing the airway, this approach should be performed by experienced anesthesiologists after careful judgment" regarding the risks and benefits.[262] Deep extubation is ill advised when the risk of maintaining or restoring oxygenation or the risk of aspiration is increased.

Extubation With a Supraglottic Airway

On emergence from general anesthesia, most patients tolerate a well-placed SGA better than an ETT with less coughing and fewer changes in IOP, ICP, and arterial blood pressure (see Fig. 47.1).[132,134,263–266] The substitution of an ETT for an SGA prior to emergence from anesthesia is referred to as the Bailey maneuver. Silva and Brimacombe described exchanging an ETT for an LMA Classic in a small series of patients while still under general anesthesia and paralyzed at the end of neurosurgical procedures.[266] Muscle relaxation was subsequently reversed, and the anesthetic was discontinued. The LMA was removed after the patients resumed spontaneous ventilation and obeyed commands. None of the 10 patients coughed, and changes in the heart rate–blood pressure product (indicating cardiac oxygen requirements) were minimal. The investigators suggested that the technique might prove useful in patients undergoing other types of surgical procedures. They stressed that this substitution should be performed only by those skilled in LMA insertion, a point emphasized in the DAS extubation guidelines wherein it was described as an advanced maneuver.[12] Patients must be at a sufficient depth of anesthesia, or coughing, breath-holding, laryngospasm, and the very pressor responses this substitution is intended to avoid may occur. Bailey and colleagues recommended that the LMA Classic be inserted before removal of the ETT to prevent losing the airway after tracheal extubation.[134,267] Compared with deep tracheal extubation followed by Guedel oral airway insertion, there was a lower incidence of coughing and requirement for airway manipulation.[267] Koga and colleagues compared this technique with deep and awake tracheal extubation.[263] They observed no difference in recovery conditions among patients in whom the ETT was removed by deep or awake methods; however, they noticed a significant improvement in recovery conditions when the LMA substitution was performed. This technique is useful but demands meticulous execution and should be practiced on routine airways before use in higher-risk extubations.[11,234] The Bailey maneuver has been performed with other SGAs, such as the ProSeal LMA and the i-gel, with similar findings.[268,269]

When a failed extubation is rescued by placement of an SGA, techniques for safely exchanging the SGA to an ETT are useful. Many SGAs are now designed to allow trans-SGA intubation with a standard-size ETT. For those that are not, such as the LMA Classic, an Aintree catheter can be used to facilitate the exchange (see Chapter 25).[270–272] Matioc and Arndt described a technique to substitute an ETT for a ProSeal LMA.[273] Using an Arndt AEC Set (Cook Critical Care, Bloomington, IN) (Fig. 47.2), they introduced an FIS through the ProSeal LMA into the trachea and, through its working channel, inserted the 144-cm guidewire included with the set. The FIS was removed, an 11-French, 70-cm AEC was advanced over the guidewire, and the ProSeal LMA was removed. The replacement ETT was then advanced over the AEC.

Extubation or Reintubation With a Flexible Intubation Scope

When tube entrapment is a possibility, insertion of an FIS can identify the potential problem that prevents or complicates extubation. Extubation over an FIS also provides the opportunity for visually assessing the trachea and laryngeal anatomy. If the patient is breathing spontaneously, vocal cord movement and tracheal integrity can also be assessed. This is useful if supraglottic or laryngeal injury, tracheomalacia, or PVCM are concerns. This can be facilitated by judicious sedation, an antisialagogue, and suction of oral secretions. We recommend two suction devices: one attached to the FIS and a second to a Yankauer or flexible suction catheter. The pharynx is suctioned, taking care to avoid inducing a gag reflex. The FIS is introduced through the ETT and advanced to a position proximal to the carina. The cuff is deflated slowly to minimize coughing. The ETT is carefully withdrawn into the oropharynx, followed by very gradual withdrawal of the FIS to the

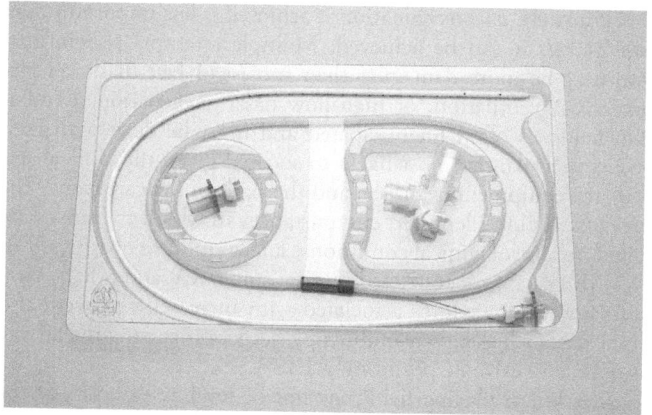

• **Fig. 47.2** The Arndt airway exchange catheter set consists of a bronchoscopic adapter, a stiff Amplatz guidewire, a tapered airway exchange catheter (AEC), and a Rapi-Fit adapter. The bronchoscopic adapter permits continuation of positive-pressure ventilation, while a bronchoscope is introduced through the original endotracheal tube (ETT). The guidewire is inserted through the bronchoscope's working channel, and the original ETT and bronchoscope are withdrawn. The tapered AEC is advanced over the guidewire, and it may be connected with a 15-mm Rapi-Fit adapter to provide ventilation. The replacement ETT is then advanced over the AEC. (Reproduced with permission from Cook Medical, Bloomington, IN.)

supraglottic region. At this point, many patients swallow, cough, or have difficulty tolerating the gradual withdrawal of the FIS, thereby hindering the assessment.

It is far easier to accomplish this procedure by replacing the ETT with an SGA as previously described (the Bailey maneuver). If properly seated, the SGA sequesters oropharyngeal secretions; permits regulation of supplemental oxygen, assisted ventilation, and IV or volatile sedation; and, importantly, provides unimpeded laryngeal exposure.

If an ETT exchange is required, this can be accomplished with an FIS. The FIS can be preloaded with a replacement ETT and passed alongside the existing tube.[274] This approach can be used to convert nasal to oral intubation and vice versa (see later discussion in "Techniques for Airway Exchange").[275]

Use of a Tracheal Introducer

Finucane and Kupshik described an awake blind nasal intubation in a patient with cervical instability complicated by damage to the ETT cuff, requiring a tube exchange.[276] They used the 4-mm outer diameter (OD) plastic sleeve from a brachial central venous catheter as a tube exchanger. Others have used a tracheal introducer (also known as a gum elastic bougie) to achieve similar objectives. Cook Critical Care designed the Mizus ETT replacement obturator (METTRO) for the replacement of endotracheal and tracheostomy tubes, but this product has been discontinued. Other devices such as nasogastric tubes have been used as exchange devices. Generally, they are too flexible and become more so as they are warmed after insertion. They are not reliable as exchange devices.

Commercial Airway Exchange Devices

Bedger and Chang coined the term *jet stylet* to refer to a self-fashioned, 65-cm-long, plastic catheter with a removable 15-mm adapter at the proximal end. It could be connected to an anesthesia machine or jet injector.[277] They created three side ports cut into the distal 5 cm to reduce catheter whip during jet ventilation. They used their stylet for the extubation or reintubation of 59 patients. It also functioned adequately in six patients when used for jet ventilation and oxygen insufflation. Although no complications were described in this series, an earlier report by these authors described tension pneumothoraces in 3 of 600 patients ventilated through a 3.5-mm OD pediatric chest tube at 15 psi.[278] This device had been used to provide airway access and ventilation during DL. They speculated that the pneumothoraces might have resulted from endobronchial migration of the catheter.

Several commercial products feature long hollow catheters with connectors that are intended for manual or jet ventilation. Most have length and radiopaque markers. Many have end and distal side holes. They can be introduced through an existing ETT, permitting the latter's withdrawal. Oxygen insufflation or jet ventilation can be provided through the tube exchanger. The advisability of insufflation and jet ventilation will be discussed in "Insufflation and Ventilation Through Catheters." High-fidelity capnography can be achieved since placement in the distal third of the trachea virtually eliminates dead space. Spontaneous breathing takes place around the device. In most reports, these catheters have been tolerated without the need for sedation or topical anesthesia and can be left in situ until the need for reintubation is deemed unlikely. They must be properly secured to ensure that they are not dislodged prematurely (Fig. 47.3). Even with the catheter in place, most patients will be able to talk or cough.

If reintubation or a tube exchange is required, gentle laryngoscopy, by retracting the tongue, makes tube exchange easier even if the larynx cannot be visualized. In a patient with an anatomically difficult airway, VAL not only displaces the tongue; it also permits visualization of ETT advancement. Correction can be made if the

ETT impinges on the arytenoids, and confirmation of successful placement is immediate.[279]

Like intubation over an FIS, the greater the difference in diameters between the tube exchanger and the advancing ETT, the more likely the ETT is to impinge upon the epiglottis, arytenoids, posterior commissure, or the vocal cords. If a tube exchange is required, it is best to choose an exchange catheter whose OD closely matches the ID of the replacement ETT. An assistant should be delegated to ensure that the exchange catheter does not migrate deeper into or out of the airway during reintubation. If resistance is encountered, counterclockwise rotation of the ETT may successfully release the tube. Visualized tube exchange makes this easier. Another useful technique is to lower the exchange catheter so that is in the same plane as the trachea. If these measures are unsuccessful and VAL is unavailable, an Aintree intubation catheter (Cook Critical Care, Bloomington, IN) can be advanced over the airway exchange device to bridge the gap between a small tube exchanger and a larger ETT.[280]

These techniques are consistent with practice guidelines from the ASA Task Force on Management of the Difficult Airway, CAFG, and DAS recommendations regarding the extubation of the DA[9,10,12]; however, it is important to note that these are "off-label" applications for the most commonly used device (Cook Airway Exchange Catheter [C-AEC]), running counter to the approval granted by regulatory bodies such as the Food and Drug Administration (FDA) in the United States.[281] Although the C-AEC was designed as an "exchange device," it is widely used to provide continuous access to the airway following the extubation of a higher-risk airway, and under such circumstances its use is off label. Maintaining airway access increases the probability of success should reintubation of the patient with a DA become necessary.[282] If difficulty is encountered and hypoxemia becomes life-threatening, the device can be used to provide oxygen by low-flow insufflation or short-term jet ventilation until alternative strategies can be implemented (see the section Insufflation and Ventilation Through Catheters).

The differences among various commercial exchange devices are less important than the concept of a reversible extubation. Because the prediction of successful extubation is imperfect, an extubation strategy that maximizes the probability of both a successful extubation and reintubation is strongly encouraged in the patient with a DA. The C-AEC will be described in the most detail because it is the most widely used.

Cook Airway Exchange Catheters

Cook Critical Care has developed a family of hollow stylets known as C-AECs (Fig. 47.4A). They are available in 8-, 11-, 14-, and 19-French sizes, appropriate for ETTs with IDs of greater than 3, 4, 5, and 7 mm, respectively. A C-AEC intended for the exchange of double-lumen tubes is described later (see "Exchange of Double-Lumen Tubes"). The 8-French C-AEC is 45-cm long, while the others are 83-cm long. To permit the exchange of an ETT, the AEC must be at least twice the length of the tracheal tube being replaced. They are radiopaque with distance markings between 15 and 30 cm from the distal end, two distal side holes, and an end hole. Proximally, two types of Rapi-Fit connectors are provided: a 15-mm connection and a Luer-Lok jet ventilation attachment that are secured and released by a patented crimping collar (Fig. 47.4B). These were designed for rapid removal and reattachment while the ETT is being offloaded and replaced. The length and IDs (1.6–3.4 mm) make manual ventilation with a resuscitation bag possible but useful only for short periods because

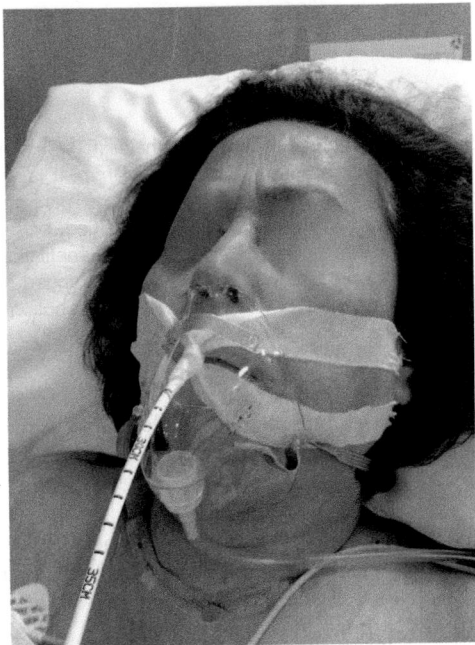

• **Fig. 47.3** A Cook AEC has been properly secured with four-point fixation in the center of the patient's mouth. Alternatively, the catheter can be secured to the mandible in the midline, permitting the patient to open his or her mouth more easily. This minimizes lateral displacement and tongue-thrusting to dislodge the device. A hole has been cut in the bridge of a face mask, and the AEC has been passed through. In this case, supplemental oxygen is being administered by face mask. (Courtesy of Dr. Richard Cooper.)

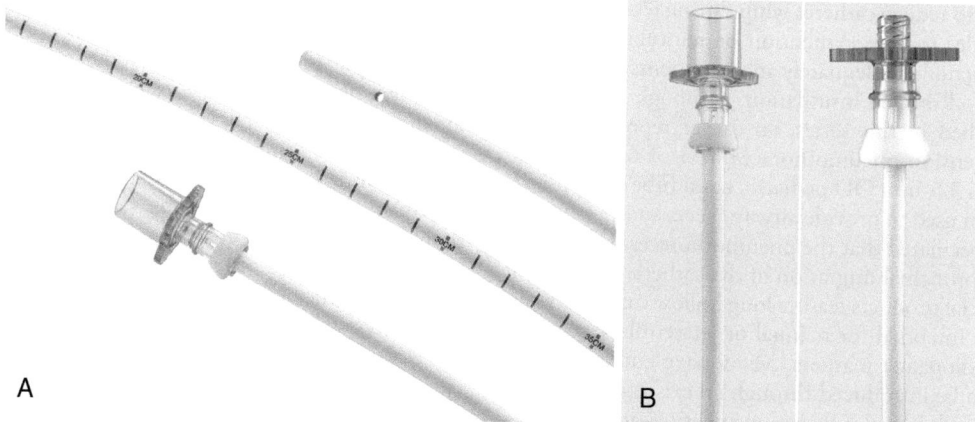

• **Fig. 47.4** The Cook airway exchange catheters (AECs) are available in four diameters and two lengths. They are radiopaque and have distance markings at each centimeter throughout the working length. (A) The proximal Rapi-Fit adapter, the middle section, and the distal end of a Cook AEC. Notice that there are two distal side holes and one end hole. (B) Two Rapi-Fit adapters: a 15-mm connector *(left)* and a Luer-Lok jet adapter *(right)*. (Reproduced with permission from Cook Medical, Bloomington, IN.)

resistance is very high. The Luer-Lok jet Rapi-Fit adapter allows jet ventilation, but the paucity of distal side holes potentially increases catheter whip and the risk of barotrauma.[283]

Mort evaluated the concept of reversible extubation in patients with DAs.[282] From an institutional database, he identified patients who were extubated in the OR, PACU, or ICU with a C-AEC. The tube exchanger was left in place until the need for reintubation was considered unlikely. Over a 9-year period, 354 patients with difficult airways qualified. Two groups emerged: those who required reintubation while the AEC was still in place and those requiring reintubation after the AEC had been removed. Airway-related complications were compared for the two groups. The AEC dwell time was a mean of 3.9 hours (range: 5 minutes to 72 hours). Of 354 patients, 288 were extubated in the ICU and had previously required three or more laryngoscopic attempts or alternative devices to achieve intubation. These patients exemplified the concept of a higher-risk extubation. Comparing the overall success rate in the two groups, 47 of 51 patients in the AEC group were successfully reintubated, 87% on the first attempt. The four failures in this group resulted from inadvertent withdrawal of the AEC in three patients during the exchange; one patient could not be reintubated despite progressive downsizing of the ETT. Mild (SpO$_2$ <90%) and severe hypoxia (<70%) was experienced by 8% and 6% in the AEC group but 50% and 19% in the non-AEC group. Three or more intubation attempts were required in 10% versus 77%, and esophageal intubations occurred in none of the AEC group but in 18% of the non-AEC group. In all cases, reintubation was attempted by an attending anesthesiologist or an anesthesiology resident under supervision. Although reintubation over an AEC does not guarantee first-pass success, this strategy was strikingly more effective (87% vs 14% first-pass success) and had far fewer life-threatening complications. Another important lesson from this report is that only 41% of these ICU reintubations occurred within the first 2 hours of extubation, meaning that 59% occurred more than 2 hours following extubation, most between 2 and 10 hours. This is long after the time many practitioners might consider removing an exchange device. Mort generally performed the reintubation using gentle laryngoscopy with sedation in most of the patients but generally without neuromuscular blockade. The authors of

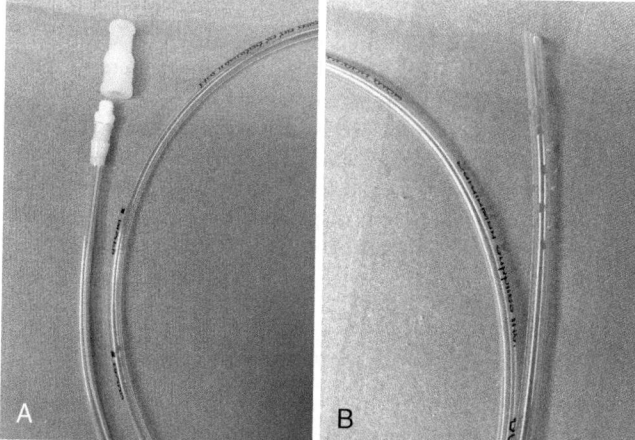

• **Fig. 47.5** The endotracheal ventilation catheter (ETVC) is available in one length (85 cm) with an outer diameter of 4 mm. It is nonthermoplastic and has a radiopaque stripe along its length. There are distance markings every 4 cm. (A) Proximally, there is a welded, barbed, plastic connector with a threaded Luer-Lok adapter for jet ventilation. (B) Distally, there is a blunt end hole with eight helically arranged side holes, which minimize catheter whip and reduce the jet injection pressure. (Courtesy of Dr. Richard Cooper.)

this chapter use neuromuscular blockade almost universally to facilitate reintubation.

Other Airway Exchange Devices

The CardioMed Endotracheal Ventilation Catheter (ETVC; Lindsay, ON, Canada) was the first hollow exchange device (Fig. 47.5). It is made of a hybrid plastic and is 85-cm long with a 4-mm OD (12-French) and 3-mm ID. It has a radiopaque stripe along its entire length and distance markings at 4-cm intervals. Proximally, it has a male hose barb with a threaded adapter welded into the catheter that connects to a removable Luer-Lock adapter. Distally, it has a blunt end with one end hole and eight helically arranged side holes. If jet ventilation is used, the multiple side holes are intended to minimize catheter whip and reduce jet injection pressures. Designed for a reversible extubation, one of the authors has used this in over 600 patients, the first 202 of which were published.[284] Although the ETVC had been used to facilitate reintubation, this was required in only 22 (11%) of 202 cases, a rate that was very similar to that reported by others.[285] Reintubation was successful in 20 out of 22 patients.

Potential complications of airway exchange devices include intolerance, unintended dislodgment, tracheal perforation, barotrauma, and failure to successfully facilitate reintubation. Intolerance should prompt reassessment of the depth of insertion. If the depth is clinically and radiographically appropriate, and the exchange device continues to be required, tolerance usually can be achieved by instilling lidocaine through the device. Dislodgment may occur if the device is inadequately secured. This allows the patient to push the catheter out with his tongue. The authors recommend midline, four-point fixation if used orally (see Fig. 47.3). A secure fixation is more easily achieved if the catheter is nasally situated, but care must be taken to avoid pressure on the nasal ala.

The Arndt AEC set (Cook Critical Care, Bloomington, IN) consists of an Amplatz extra-stiff guidewire with position markings, a Rapi-Fit adapter, a bronchoscopic port, and a distally tapered 14-French (4.7-mm OD), 70-cm-long radiopaque AEC. It was designed for the exchange of SGAs, DLTs, and ETTs (see Fig. 47.2). Bronchoscopy is performed through the bronchoscopy port adapter attached to the existing airway device. The flexible end of the guidewire is introduced through the working channel of the bronchoscope under visual control and is advanced to a position approaching the carina. The bronchoscope is removed over the wire, taking care that the wire is neither advanced nor withdrawn. The original airway is carefully removed, and its replacement is advanced over the AEC such that the distance markings on the ETT are aligned with those of the AEC. The exchange catheter is then removed, and the position of the new tube is confirmed.[270] This device may be particularly advantageous when exchanging the LMA Supreme to an ETT due to the challenges posed for navigating through the oval-shaped airway.[286] If the device is being used for staged extubation rather than reintubation, only the guidewire is left in place; the AEC is advanced if reintubation is required.

As of this writing, the Cook Staged Extubation Set (Cook Critical Care, Bloomington, IN) has not been approved for use in North America. It is conceptually similar to the AEC; however, rather than leaving a catheter in the airway, a guidewire is positioned by its distance marking within the existing ETT (Fig. 47.6). The guidewire has a 0.035-inch OD with a nickel titanium core and polymeric coating. It was designed for greater patient comfort following extubation. If reintubation is required, a 14-French exchange catheter (83 cm long) with a blunted tip and multiple side ports is advanced over the guidewire and advanced to the appropriate depth. The guidewire is removed, and the new ETT is introduced over the exchange catheter. There is limited clinical experience with this device, and it is unclear whether this adds value or simply cost and complexity.[287–289]

Techniques for Airway Exchange

Exchange of Double-Lumen Tubes

For patients who may be difficult to initially intubate with a DLT, it may be preferable to initially place a single-lumen tube and subsequently exchange this with a DLT. It may also be necessary to replace a DLT because of inappropriate sizing or a defective tube.

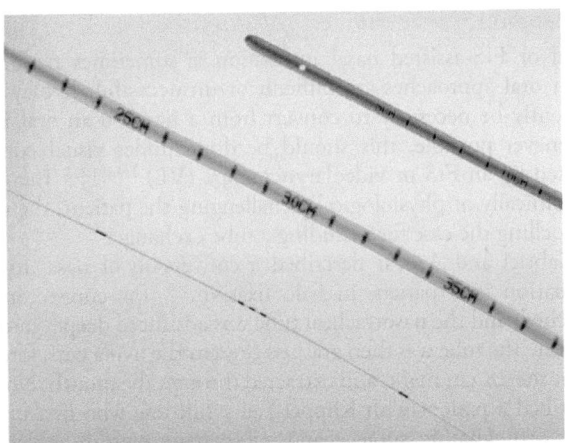

• **Fig. 47.6** The Staged Extubation Set consists of a polymeric-coated 0.035-inch (145-cm long) nickel titanium guidewire with depth markings, a soft, blunt-tipped 14-French airway exchange catheter and a 15-mm Rapi-Fit adapter. (Reproduced with permission from Cook Medical, Bloomington, IN.)

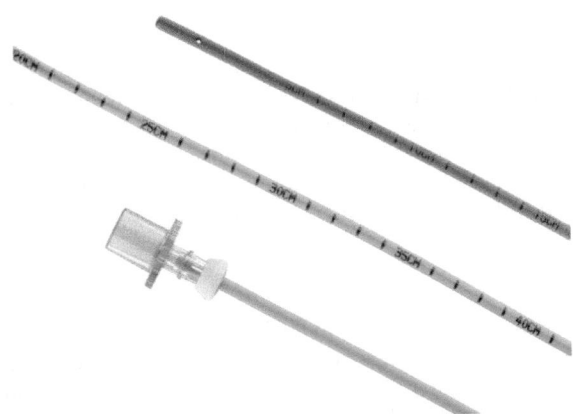

• **Fig. 47.7** The Cook Airway Exchange Catheter—Double-Lumen Tube with Soft Tip is available in two sizes: 11 and 14-French. Each is 100 cm long to enable proximal control when passed through the longer double-lumen tubes. The green part of the catheter is extra firm, whereas the purple distal 7-cm segment is soft tipped. (Reproduced with permission from Cook Medical, Bloomington, IN.)

Alternatively, it may be preferred to exchange a DLT for a single-lumen tube for postoperative management. These substitutions can be achieved or facilitated by DL or VAL.[290] If the larynx can be visualized, the DLT is withdrawn and immediately replaced with a single-lumen ETT or a replacement DLT. Occasionally, this is not easily accomplished[291] or may be deemed too risky, and the use of an AEC may facilitate the tube conversion.

Whether the substitution is a single-lumen tube to DLT, DLT to single-lumen tube, or DLT to DLT, the requirements are similar, and the previously described tube exchangers may not be sufficiently long or stiff.[292,293] Cook AECs for DLT conversion are "Extra Firm with a Soft Tip" and are available in 11- and 14-French sizes. They are 100 cm long and designed specifically for the exchange of DLTs. The 11-French device is suitable for a 35- or 37-French DLT (ID ≥4 mm); the 14-French device can be used with a 39- or 41-French DLT (ID ≥5 mm). The soft tip refers to the distal 7-cm segment of the catheter (Fig. 47.7).

Conversion From Nasal to Oral Intubation

Blind or FIS-assisted nasal intubation is sometimes performed when oral approaches are difficult or unsuccessful. It may subsequently be necessary to convert from a nasal to an oral ETT. Whenever possible, this should be done under visual control, assisted by an FIS or videolaryngoscope (VL).[279,294,295] The more anatomically or physiologically challenging the patient, the more compelling the case for including a tube exchanger.

Gabriel and Azocar described a conversion of nasal to oral intubation in a patient in halo fixation.[296] The connector was detached, and the nasotracheal tube was advanced deeper into the trachea. The tube was then grasped close to the uvula with forceps, cut at the 28-cm mark, and extracted through the mouth. Novella described a patient with Klippel-Feil syndrome who first underwent orthognathic surgery and subsequent septorhinoplasty.[297] After completion of orthognathic surgery, an AEC was inserted into the nasal ETT and the latter was withdrawn. The AEC was then grasped with two Magill forceps; the caudal one was used to stabilize the catheter, and the cephalad one was used to withdraw the proximal end out of the mouth. An oral tube was then advanced over the AEC.

Conversion From Oral to Nasal Intubation

Smith and Fenner performed an oral to nasal ETT conversion using an FIS preloaded with an ETT inserted nasally and advanced through the glottis, anterior to an oral ETT.[298] The oral ETT was withdrawn, and a nasal ETT was advanced over the endoscope. Many of the difficulties in performing a tube exchange can be avoided with the use of indirect laryngoscopy, ideally in combination with AECs.

Conversion From a Supraglottic Airway to a Tracheal Tube

Conversion of various SGAs to ETTs was mentioned briefly above (Arndt Airway Exchange Set). A fuller discussion is beyond the scope of this chapter. Whenever possible, this conversion should be facilitated by visual guidance, using direct or indirect laryngoscopy. These techniques include the use of a flexible endoscope and Aintree catheter or a video laryngoscope (see Chapters 19, 24, and 25).[299,300]

Insufflation and Jet Ventilation Through Stylets

The preceding sections stressed the importance of being able to provide supplemental oxygen during a tube exchange. Recent publications have raised concerns about the safety of high-pressure ventilation and insufflation through AECs. A chilling case was described involving misuse of an AEC that resulted in dramatic and fatal barotrauma.[301] The operators were using an AEC in the appropriate setting but in a completely inappropriate manner. As the patient became more hypoxemic, they increased the oxygen flow through a catheter that was almost certainly endobronchial. This emphasizes the importance of being familiar with the devices used and how the manufacturers intended them to be used.

Perhaps more disturbing is a case in which an AEC was reportedly used in an appropriate patient, as the manufacturer had directed, with low-flow oxygen insufflation. Nonetheless, the result was fatal barotrauma. This prompted a review by the Chief Coroner of Ontario, Canada, and a thoughtful publication by Duggan and colleagues.[176] They reviewed oxygen supplementation through AECs and concluded that jet ventilation through such a device carries a significant risk of barotrauma, whereas oxygen insufflation has a lower risk. They recommend that supplemental oxygen be delivered by means of a face mask. The authors of this chapter agree with these recommendations except in circumstances where hypoxemia becomes life-threatening despite supplemental oxygen. If insufflation or jet ventilation is deemed necessary, the practitioner must pay careful attention to details and be vigilant for complications. The objective is to avert life-threatening hypoxemia, not normalize ventilation or maximize oxygenation. Significant airway obstruction is a contraindication to the use of an exchange device as a conduit for either insufflation or jet ventilation. The depth of placement and security of the device are critical. When required, insufflation should involve low flows (1–2 L/min). Jet ventilation should only be used if life-threatening oxygenation cannot be achieved by other means, such as high-flow nasal oxygen, face mask, or insufflation. The catheter's location above the carina should be reconfirmed. The driving pressure should be the lowest possible that results in chest expansion, and the expiratory time should be sufficient to permit chest recoil. If ventilation is manual, the driving pressure can be controlled with an in-line pressure-reducing valve.[293,302]

The Ventrain device (Ventinova Medical, Eindhoven, Netherlands) appears to permit safe and effective ventilation through small-bore catheters using the Bernoulli principle to achieve active exhalation. This has been tested on a lung simulator,[303] in two desperate situations involving near totally obstructed neonates intubated with a 1.66-mm ID (2.66-mm OD) Frova intubation catheter (Cook Critical Care, Bloomington, IN),[304] and in hypoxic pigs using a 2-mm cricothyrotomy catheter with complete upper airway obstruction.[305] In the latter experiment, the SpO_2 improved from a median of 45% to 100% within 20 seconds, and although hyperemia of the posterior tracheal wall was noted, there was no evidence of barotrauma at postmortem examination.[306] Fearnley and colleagues described a patient scheduled for laser excision of laryngeal fibrosis producing critical obstruction. A cricothyrotomy (2-mm ID) was performed and ventilation was provided using the Ventrain over a 60-minute period during which the SpO_2 remained at 100%.[307] The Ventrain appears to produce active flow-dependent inspiration and expiration, significantly reducing the risk of barotrauma (Fig. 47.8). Hopefully it will extend the safety of airway exchange devices when oxygenation and ventilation are in jeopardy.[306]

Communication

As previously stated, extubation should always be performed at the optimal time and place. If delayed, it may be performed by different individuals or in a different location than the initial airway management. It is essential that clear documentation and communication occur to minimize adverse outcomes. There is no universally agreed upon way of achieving this; however, it is best to ensure that details of the problems encountered and the effective (and ineffective) measures employed be indicated on the record and verbally communicated with those responsible for ongoing care. It is advisable that this be as conspicuous as possible using a sign over the patient's bed, a highly visible bracelet, and/or a flag on the patient's chart. It would be tragic to successfully manage a DA and transfer the patient's ongoing care to another individual incompletely informed of the difficulties, only to have them recur with an adverse outcome (see Chapter 50).

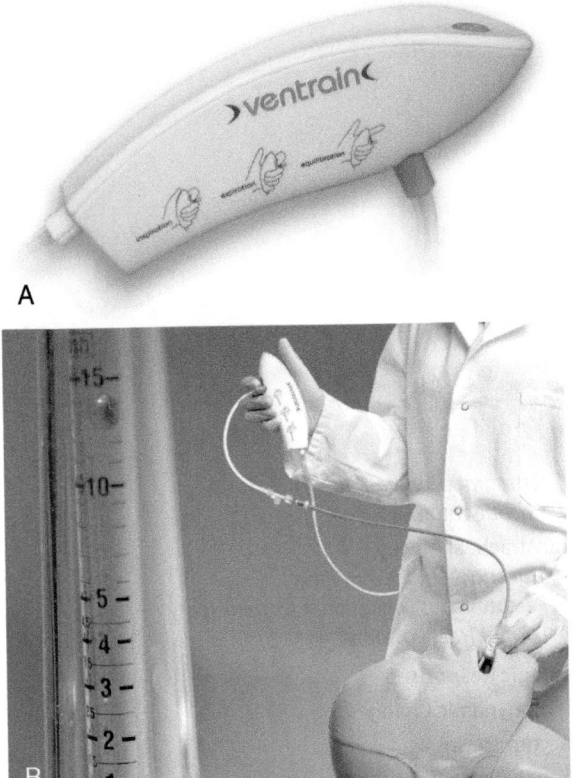

• **Fig. 47.8** The Ventrain device (Ventinova, Eindhoven, Netherlands). (A) A close-up image of the device, which provides active expiration by employing the Bernoulli principle. (B) This is accomplished by connecting the device to an oxygen flow meter and intermittently applying and releasing the thumb from the port, producing inspiration and expiration, respectively. (Reproduced with permission from Ventinova.)

Conclusion

Successful airway management does not end with tracheal intubation any more than a safe flight is only concerned with the takeoff. Although respiratory complications are more common at extubation than during intubation, most are relatively minor and do not require reintubation. However, the need for reintubation should always be anticipated. Some patients are at increased risk of requiring reintubation, which may prove to be difficult and dangerous in a variety of circumstances. The ASA Task Force for Management of the Difficult Airway, the CAFG, and the DAS, among others, have recommended that every anesthesiologist have a preformulated extubation strategy for higher-risk

patients. A risk stratification scheme has been proposed to identify patients for whom special extubation precautions seem warranted. Although many strategies are available, their benefits have not been subjected to rigorous evaluation. A reversible extubation can be performed with an AEC. The use of such a device does not guarantee that reintubation will succeed. The probability of a successful reintubation or tube exchange may be further enhanced if it can be performed under visual control using DL or indirect laryngoscopy. Oxygen insufflation and jet ventilation through an AEC risks barotrauma; however, the Ventrain device shows promise of greater safety, even in the face of critical upper airway obstruction.

Selected References

4. Cook TM, Woodall N, Frerk C. Fourth National Audit Project of the Royal College of Anaesthetists and Difficult Airway Society. Major complications of airway management in the United Kingdom. Report and Findings, Royal College of Anaesthetists London 2011. Available at http://www.rcoa.ac.uk/nap4.

8. Cavallone LF, Vannucci A. Extubation of the difficult airway and extubation failure. *Anesth Analg.* 2013;116:368-383.

10. Apfelbaum JL, Hagberg CA, Caplan RA, et al. Practice guidelines for management of the difficult airway: an updated report by the American Society of Anesthesiologists Task Force on Management of the Difficult Airway. *Anesthesiology.* 2013;118:251-270.

12. Popat M, Mitchell V, Dravid R, Patel A, Swampillai C, Higgs A. Difficult Airway Society Guidelines for the management of tracheal extubation. *Anaesthesia.* 2012;67:318-340.

33. Mathew JP, Rosenbaum SH, O'Connor T, Barash PG. Emergency tracheal intubation in the postanesthesia care unit: physician error or patient disease? *Anesth Analg.* 1990;71:691-697.

34. Rose DK, Cohen MM, Wigglesworth DF, DeBoer DP. Critical respiratory events in the postanesthesia care unit. Patient, surgical, and anesthetic factors. *Anesthesiology.* 1994;81:410-418.

35. Lee PJ, MacLennan A, Naughton NN, O'Reilly M. An analysis of reintubations from a quality assurance database of 152,000 cases. *J Clin Anesth.* 2003;15:575-581.

176. Duggan LV, Law JA, Murphy MF. Brief review: supplementing oxygen through an airway exchange catheter: efficacy, complications, and recommendations. *Can J Anaesthesia.* 2011;58:560-568.

279. Mort TC. Tracheal tube exchange. Feasibility of continuous glottic viewing with advanced laryngoscopy assistance. *Anesth Analg.* 2009;108:1228-1231.

282. Mort TC. Continuous airway access for the difficult extubation. The efficacy of the airway exchange catheter. *Anesth Analg.* 2007;105:1357-1362.

301. Ruxton LM. Inquiry Under the Fatal Accidents and Inquiries (Scotland) Act 1976 into the Sudden Death of Gordon Ewing. Scottish Courts and Tribunals. Available at https://www.scotcourts.gov.uk/search-judgments/judgment?id=328e86a6-8980-69d2-b500-ff0000d74aa7.

All references can be found online at eBooks.Health.Elsevier.com.

48

Complications of Managing the Airway

JAN-HENRIK SCHIFF, ANDREAS WALTHER, CLAUDE KRIER, AND CARIN A. HAGBERG

CHAPTER OUTLINE

KEY POINTS

- Serious complications of airway management result from not recognizing the degree of airway difficulty.
- To minimize injury to the patient, the airway practitioner should examine the patient's airway carefully, identify potential problems, devise a plan that involves the least risk for injury, and have a backup plan immediately available. Common sense should prevail at all times.
- In the practice of airway management, errors of omission are more common than errors of commission. Errors of omission include failure to recognize the magnitude of a problem, make appropriate observations, and act in a timely manner. Errors of commission include actions such as trauma to the lips, nose, or laryngotracheal mucosa; forcing sharp instruments into areas in which they do not belong; or introducing air or secretions into regions of the body that will lead to further complications.
- Many complications in airway management result from insufficient communication among the members of the medical team and improper coordination of the patients on the daily

- operating room schedule. A patient with known difficult airway (DA) problems should be scheduled at a time when the most experienced anesthesiologists and surgeons are available.
- Delayed recognition of complications leads to delayed therapy. Inadequate monitoring, nonfunctional equipment, and untrained staff can contribute to airway catastrophes.
- The overall risk of aspiration and regurgitation using the laryngeal mask airway (LMA) is about the same as for tracheal intubation when the indications and contraindications for the LMA are respected. The risk of aspiration, which is a consequence of the airway device's design, should be weighed against the advantages of the LMA in cases of difficult intubation and ventilation.

- Because of the increased risk associated with multiple attempts to perform any airway technique, a maximum of three attempts is recommended to minimize trauma to the airway.
- Any airway device technique may cause movement and subsequent injury to the patient with an injured cervical spine.
- A patent airway is an absolute requirement for safe anesthesia. Airway obstruction can occur at any time during administration of general anesthesia, particularly in prolonged operations or in patients with predisposing anatomic abnormalities. The most serious complication after extubation is the occurrence of acute airway obstruction.

Introduction

Airway management in anesthesia practice is often uncomplicated; however, complications, when they do occur, can have serious and long-lasting consequences. The Fourth National Audit Project (NAP4) of the Royal College of Anaesthetists and the Difficult Airway Society was established to estimate the incidence of major to disastrous complications of airway management and provide detailed information about the factors contributing to poor outcomes. In general, difficult airway and "cannot intubate, cannot oxygenate" (CICO) scenarios accounted for 39% of all serious events, followed by aspiration and extubation problems.

In the latest analysis of the American Society of Anesthesiologists (ASA) Closed Claims Project, 10% of recent claims concerning difficult intubation resulted in airway injury as compared to earlier claims, where airway injury was more common (34% of claims).[1,2] In general, most airway injuries are temporary, and death is a very rare outcome in routine practice (Table 48.1).[1] However, patients in more recent difficult tracheal intubation claims were significantly more likely to suffer death than patients in earlier difficult intubation claims (73% vs 42%).[2]

International studies exploring the incidence of complications during general anesthesia have been published in several countries, including the United Kingdom,[3,4] Australia,[5] France,[6]

and Germany.[7] The procedural problems and airway complications found in these studies are summarized in Table 48.2. The rates of anesthesia-related death attributed to airway management problems cover a wide range: Biboulet and colleagues reported 25%,[8] Braz and colleagues 55.5%,[9] Charuluxananan and colleagues 21.3%,[10,11] Gibbs 15%,[12] Kawashima and colleagues 7.9%,[13] Newland and colleagues 20%,[14] and Sprung and colleagues 80%.[15]

The inability to secure the airway and subsequent failure of oxygenation constitute a life-threatening complication. In the absence of major oxygen reserves, failure of oxygenation leads to hypoxia, followed by brain damage, cardiovascular breakdown, and death. As soon as oxygenation is no longer achievable, tissue damage is initiated, and irreversible injury occurs in a few minutes. The ultimate goal of airway management is oxygenation of the patient, not placement of an endotracheal tube (ETT).

Some complications are dramatic and immediately life-threatening (e.g., unrecognized esophageal intubation, tracheal rupture); some are severe and long-lasting (e.g., nerve injuries), and some are painful for the patient (e.g., sore throat). Good clinical practice aims to avoid all these complications.

In anesthesia practice, errors of omission are more common than errors of commission. Errors of omission include failure to recognize the magnitude of a problem, make appropriate observations, or act in a timely manner. Errors of commission include trauma to the lips, nose, or airway mucosa; forcing sharp instruments into areas where they do not belong; and introducing air or secretions into regions of the body that will lead to further complications. The primary goal of anesthesiologists is to ensure the safety and well-being of their patients, and they are usually careful in performing the technical aspects of their jobs. The most frequent cause of fatal errors in medical practice, especially in the field of airway management, is to ignore inadequate experience and skills and not call for help.

Complications With Mask Ventilation

Difficult mask ventilation is an underestimated aspect of managing a difficult airway (DA). Ventilation using a bag-mask breathing system is an essential skill for airway practitioners and may be life-saving for the patient. The CICO scenario represents the most severe form of airway difficulty.[2,16] Mask ventilation is used at the beginning of most cases of general anesthesia. Although the mask itself and the technique may seem benign, each can potentially cause problems.

TABLE 48.1   Severity of Injury and Standard of Care

Site of Injury (n)	SEVERITY OF INJURY		STANDARD OF CARE	
	Nonfatal n (%)	Fatal n (%)	Standard n (%)	Substandard n (%)
Larynx (87)	86 (99)	1 (1)	74 (96)	3 (4)
Pharynx (51)	46 (90)	5 (10)	29 (71)	12 (29)
Esophagus (48)	39 (81)	9 (19)	25 (60)	17 (40)
Trachea (39)	33 (85)	6 (15)	20 (63)	12 (38)
TMJ (27)	27 (100)	0	21 (100)	0
Nose (13)	13 (100)	0	11 (85)	2 (15)

TMJ, Temporomandibular joint.
Modified from Domino KB, Posner KL, Caplan RA, Cheney FW. Airway injury during anesthesia: a closed claims analysis. *Anesthesiology.* 1999;91:1703.

TABLE 48.2 Procedural Problems and Airway Complications Encountered During General Anesthesia

Respiration	Equipment	Drugs	Management
Difficult intubation	Substandard monitoring	Missing drugs	Insufficient training
Difficult ventilation	Defective apparatus	Mix-up of drugs	No specialist on call
Failed intubation	Equipment not available	Drug overdose	Inadequate assistance
Aspiration		Drug hangover	Insufficient diagnosis
Laryngospasm			Nonfasted patient
Bronchospasm			
Pneumothorax			
Airway trauma			
Airway obstruction			
Respiratory depression			

The Sterilization Process

Many of the devices used to ventilate the patient and secure the airway are disposable, although some equipment is still reusable. All devices should be checked before use, and reusable items should be free of residual cleaning agents. Masks may have pinhole defects in their air-filled bladders, allowing air leaks or extravasation of cleaning fluid, which can cause severe irritation to the patient's eyes or mucous membranes.[17,18] In one reported case, residual glutaraldehyde on an improperly rinsed laryngoscope blade caused life-threatening allergic glossitis resulting in massive tongue swelling.[19] Care must be taken to thoroughly rinse the working channel of a flexible intubation scope (FIS) after cleaning; residual agents may drip from the working channel into the larynx or trachea, causing severe chemical burns.

Mechanical Difficulties

A mask is typically applied to a patient's face before induction of general anesthesia. Preoxygenation of the patient is the first step in securing the airway. The mask should be applied during spontaneous breathing, before induction drugs are administered. During placement, direct contact of the rigid parts of the mask with the bridge of the nose or mandible should be avoided because they are at particular risk for compromised blood flow.[20] Bruising and soft tissue damage may occur in these regions with excessive pressure, and pressure damage to the mental nerves as they exit the mental foramina has been implicated in lower lip numbness in two patients.[21] Care must be taken to avoid contact with the eyes to prevent corneal abrasions, retinal artery occlusions, and blindness. As induction proceeds, firmer mask pressure and stronger lifting pressure on the angle of the mandible become necessary to maintain a tight mask fit and secure the airway. Pressure on the soft tissue of the submandibular region may obstruct the airway, especially in small children, or can damage the mandibular branch of the facial nerve, resulting in transient facial nerve paralysis.[22]

During induction, the base of the tongue may fall back into the oropharynx and obstruct the airway. Oropharyngeal airways must be gently inserted into the mouth to avoid injury, such as broken teeth or mucosal tears. Improper placement may worsen airway obstruction by forcing the tongue backward. Equal care should be given to the placement of nasopharyngeal airways to avoid bleeding and epistaxis.

Before insertion of an oropharyngeal or nasopharyngeal airway, the oropharyngeal space should be enlarged. During conventional mask ventilation, the mandible is pressed against the maxilla, blocking condylar motion and hindering sufficient mouth opening and maximal extension of the base of the tongue. The mouth is opened and the mandible gently drawn forward and upward to displace the base of the tongue to a ventral position and increase the oropharyngeal space.

The lifting pressure applied to the angle of the mandible is sometimes sufficient to subluxate the temporomandibular joint (TMJ). Patients may experience persistent pain or bruising at these points or may have chronic dislocation of the jaw, which can cause severe discomfort. Positive airway pressure can force air into the stomach instead of the trachea, producing gastric distention, difficult ventilation, and an increased risk for regurgitation. The ability to achieve adequate mask ventilation should be assessed preoperatively.

The incidence of difficult mask ventilation is about 2 to 6 in 300.[23] Independent risk factors for difficult mask ventilation are the presence of a beard, increased body mass index (BMI), edentulousness, age older than 55 years, history of snoring, sleep apnea or a high STOP-Bang score,[24] limited mandibular protrusion, male gender, Mallampati class III or IV (used to predict ease of intubation), and airway masses or tumors.[25,26]

Other factors may make mask ventilation difficult or impossible, such as a large tongue, facial burns or deformities, stridor, or nasal polyposis. In these cases, it may be best to avoid mask ventilation and perform a rapid sequence induction or an awake intubation. Patients with trauma to the pharyngeal mucosa who are mask ventilated may be at risk for subcutaneous emphysema.

Laryngoceles may manifest as or cause upper airway obstruction during induction of anesthesia. Congenital factors contribute to development of laryngoceles, and persons who play wind instruments also may be at risk because high intrapharyngeal pressures can weaken soft tissue and cause laryngoceles in the lateral pharynx.[27,28]

Prolonged Mask Ventilation

Because mask ventilation offers no protection against regurgitation, the anesthesiologist should be vigilant for questionable airway noise, coughing, or bucking. Transparent masks allow visualization of the mouth and early identification of vomitus. Extra care should be taken to avoid undue pressure on vulnerable parts of the face. When continuous positive airway pressure (CPAP) is applied to patients with basilar skull fractures, pneumocephalus may occur.[29-31] At least one case report identified positive airway pressure as the cause of bilateral otorrhagia.[32]

Mask ventilation is relatively contraindicated in nonfasting patients, intestinal obstruction, Trendelenburg position, extreme obesity, tracheoesophageal fistula, and massive nasooropharyngeal bleeding, although it may be life-saving when other airway devices fail. Especially in pediatric cases, it may be necessary to avoid hypoxia.[33]

Adequate monitoring during mask ventilation includes observation of chest movement, pulse oximetry, measurement of end-tidal carbon dioxide ($EtCO_2$), and control of inspiratory pressure. In infants, a precordially placed stethoscope is recommended.

Complications With Supraglottic Airways

Laryngeal Mask Airway

Placing a laryngeal mask airway (LMA) and similar supraglottic airways (SGAs) correctly can be difficult in some patients. The mask may fold on itself, or the epiglottis may become entrapped in the laryngeal inlet of the mask. The epiglottis may be pushed down into the glottis, increasing work of breathing and producing coughing, laryngospasm, or complete airway obstruction.[34,35] Excess lubricant can leak into the trachea, promoting coughing or laryngospasm.[36] Regardless of the problems encountered in placing the LMA, airway patency is usually maintained. An inadequate mouth opening (<1.5 cm), inadequate depth of anesthesia, insertion with an underdeflated cuff, inappropriate size of the LMA, inappropriate force during insertion, and inadequate volumes for cuff inflation can cause malpositioning of the LMA.

Numerous complications are associated with the LMA. Perhaps the greatest limitation is the inability of the LMA to protect against regurgitation of gastric contents and pulmonary aspiration. Because the LMA does not isolate the trachea from the esophagus, its use is risky when the patient has a full stomach or when high airway pressures are necessary for positive-pressure ventilation. The overall risk of aspiration and regurgitation using the LMA seems to be in the same low range as for tracheal intubation when the indications and contraindications for the LMA are respected.[37] The risk of aspiration, which is a consequence of the design of the device, should be weighed against the advantages of the LMA in cases of difficult intubation and ventilation. Other complications have been reported with the use of the LMA. Their incidence and severity depend on the user's skills and experience, depth of anesthesia, and anatomic or pathologic factors.[38]

Failure to correctly place the LMA results from inadequate depth of anesthesia, suboptimal head and neck position, incorrect mask deflation, failure to follow the palatopharyngeal curve during insertion, inadequate depth of insertion, application of cricoid pressure (CP), or oral anatomic variations such as large tonsils. Laryngospasm and coughing result from inadequate depth of anesthesia, tip impaction against the glottis, or aspiration of gastric contents. A mask leak or the inability to ventilate the lungs results from inadequate depth of anesthesia, a malpositioned mask, inadequate mask size, or high airway pressure. Displacement of the LMA after insertion is caused by inadequate anesthesia depth, a pulled or twisted tube, or inadequate mask size.

Problems during recovery are removal of the LMA at an inappropriate anesthesia depth, laryngospasm, and coughing when oral secretions enter the larynx after cuff deflation, tube occlusion caused by biting, and regurgitation. Effects on pharyngolaryngeal reflexes such as laryngospasm, coughing, gagging, bronchospasm, breath-holding, and retching may be associated with LMA use.

The incidence of sore throat with the LMA is between 17% and 26%.[38] The incidence of failed placement is 1% to 5%, although this rate tends to decrease with increasing operator experience.[39] The LMA cuff is permeable to nitrous oxide and carbon dioxide, which can result in substantial increases in cuff pressure and volume during prolonged procedures.[40,41]

Several case reports cite edema of the epiglottis, uvula, posterior pharyngeal wall, and vocal cords; in the worst cases, these conditions have led to airway obstruction.[42-44] Nerve paralysis (e.g., lingual, recurrent, hypoglossal, and glossopharyngeal), postobstructive pulmonary edema, tongue cyanosis, and transient dysarthria have been reported. Control of cuff pressure can reduce at least some of these complications.[38,45-48] Respiratory morbidity is reduced by up to 70% by using a cuff control device, and respiratory morbidity decreases even further if the cuff pressure does not exceed 25 cm H_2O.[49] Other problems with the LMA include dislodgment, kinking, and foreign bodies in the tube, leading to airway obstruction.[50]

Newer designs of the LMA were developed to increase comfort, handling, or safety in various situations. Second-generation LMAs combine the option of inserting a gastric tube through a separate drainage tube with an improved seal by design, which enables positive airway pressure ventilation at higher inspiratory pressures.[34] Nonetheless, cases of gastric insufflation with malpositioned second-generation LMAs have been reported.[50,51]

The intubating laryngeal mask airway (ILMA) was designed to overcome unexpected difficult laryngoscopic intubation. Use of the ILMA has been successful in patients with DAs.[52,53] Tracheal intubation through the ILMA using specialized ETTs is easier than with the standard LMA, and the success rate for blind insertion of an ETT through the ILMA is greater than 90%.[54-57] Branthwaite reported a case of esophageal perforation secondary to attempts at intubation using the ILMA in a patient with an undiagnosed high esophageal pouch leading to mediastinitis and the patient's eventual death.[58] Flexible scope-guided insertion of an ETT through an LMA has had the highest success rate for intubation and the lowest rate for damage of laryngeal structures. Modifications of the LMA have overall rates of complications similar to those already described.[59,60]

Classic contraindications to using an LMA include nonfasted patients, extreme obesity, necessity of high inspiratory pressures (>20 cm H_2O) in the presence of low pulmonary compliance or chronic obstructive pulmonary disease (COPD), acute abdomen, hiatal hernia, Zenker's diverticulum, trauma, intoxication, airway problems at the glottic or infraglottic level, and thoracic trauma. Nevertheless, the LMA's successors, particularly those with a channel for the insertion of a gastric tube, have led to more liberal use of LMA devices.[61-63] Specifically, second-generation LMAs seem useful and safe for prolonged periods of use and for use in minor laparoscopic procedures, in the obese, in cesarean section, and in the prone position, provided the contraindications are heeded and there is adequate clinical expertise.[34]

Other Supraglottic Airway Devices

Many devices are available for managing the airway at the supraglottic level: the cuffed oropharyngeal airway (COPA), the laryngeal tube (LT), the LaryVent (MedExNet, Amsterdam, the Netherlands), the glottic aperture seal airway (GO2 airway), the Cobra perilaryngeal airway (CobraPLA), and the King laryngeal tube suction (LTS).[64–66] Overall, they seem to cause complications and physiologic alterations similar to those found with the LMA.[67,68] The devices were designed for separating the airway from the esophagus but do not efficiently protect the airway from regurgitation and aspiration. They share several advantages and disadvantages. Contraindications include nonfasted patients, gastroesophageal reflux, hiatal hernia, pregnancy, obesity, reduced pulmonary compliance, glottic or infraglottic stenosis, and mechanical obstruction of the oropharynx. Most complications arise from dislodgment, overinflating the cuff, or insufficient depth of anesthesia. Most of the devices were developed over the past few years, and acceptance in routine practice has varied. It should be emphasized again that in clinical and preclinical settings, cuff pressure control for any of these devices is paramount in reducing adverse sequelae.[69]

Another concern is the wide range of available supraglottic devices. In addition to the limited storage space provided on the airway management cart, it seems impossible to maintain regular and sufficient training with all devices for all practitioners. Many complications in airway management are caused by operator inexperience and by inadequate or nonfunctional equipment. The recommendation for all anesthesiologists is to select a few devices that are used routinely or for which practitioners are well trained.

Esophageal-Tracheal Combitube and EasyTube

The esophageal-tracheal Combitube (Medtronic GmbH, Meerbusch, Germany) is an esophagotracheal, double-lumen airway designed for emergency use when standard airway management measures have failed.[70,71] Its use in elective surgery has also been reported.[72–75] The Rüsch EasyTube (Teleflex Inc., Wayne, PA) is a dual-lumen airway with a similar design to the Combitube.

The Combitube is inserted blindly into the mouth and advanced to preset markings. The distal tube is usually positioned within the esophagus at this point. A distal cuff is inflated within the esophagus, and a large-volume proximal cuff is inflated inside the pharynx. Ventilation is then attempted through the proximal lumen because esophageal intubation occurs in approximately 96% of insertions. If ventilation through this lumen fails, ventilation is attempted through the distal lumen. The device is designed for single use, but a study of multiple uses of the Combitube found no problems arising from reprocessing.[76] Another study warned against reuse because insufficient cleaning may lead to transmission of iatrogenic infections.[77]

The 37-French (small adult) Combitube is not recommended for patients shorter than 120 cm, and the 41-French Combitube is not recommended for patients shorter than 150 cm. Disregarding these recommendations may cause serious esophageal injury. Further contraindications to using a Combitube are intact gag reflexes, ingestion of caustic substances, known esophageal disease, airway problems at the glottic or infraglottic level, and latex allergy.[78]

The Combitube has major disadvantages because of its design. It can be used for a maximum of 8 hours (because tracheobronchial care is difficult through the Combitube), suctioning of the trachea is not possible with the device in the esophageal position (which may be problematic in the case of copious tracheal secretions), it may injure pharyngeal and esophageal soft tissues, and no pediatric sizes are available.

Various complications have been reported with use of the Combitube. In two patients, the device was inserted too far,

causing the large pharyngeal cuff to lie directly over the glottis and obstruct the upper airway.[79] This was easily resolved by partially withdrawing the Combitube until breath sounds were auscultated. Tongue discoloration has been reported while the pharyngeal cuff was inflated, although this usually resolves immediately without further adverse sequelae after the cuff is deflated. The Combitube has also been linked to glossopharyngeal and hypoglossal nerve dysfunction, esophageal rupture, subcutaneous emphysema, pneumomediastinum, pneumoperitoneum, and tracheal and esophageal injury and bleeding.[80–82] Esophageal lacerations are most likely caused by incorrect use; in both referenced cases, the distal cuff was overinflated, and the larger Combitube (41 French) was used in a small patient. When compared with intubation with a standard ETT, the EasyTube and Combitube show a higher incidence of minor trauma.[82] Despite their disadvantages, the Combitube and the EasyTube are widely accepted as devices for managing the DA.

Complications With Intubation

Tracheal Intubation

Laryngoscope Modifications and Rigid Optical Instruments

Laryngoscopes are designed for visualization of the vocal cords and for placement of the ETT into the trachea under direct vision. The two main types are the curved Macintosh blade and the straight blade (e.g., the curve-tipped Miller blade or the straight-tipped Wisconsin or Foregger blades). All blades are available in different sizes for patients of every age. The main injury caused by using laryngoscopes is damage to the teeth. In cases of inadequate visualization of the glottis, a change of the patient's head position may lead to success. In some cases, a blade of inadequate size is responsible for intubation failure. Backward-upward-rightward pressure (BURP) on the thyroid cartilage or optimal external laryngeal manipulation (OELM) may move the glottis into the line of vision and facilitate intubation (see Chapter 20).[83,84]

Obtaining a view of the glottis with a conventional laryngoscope requires optimal positioning of the patient. With flexible scope intubation (FSI), positioning is not an issue, and damage to the teeth is less likely. Similarly, with video-assisted laryngoscopy (VAL), a video image of the oropharynx and the laryngeal inlet is transmitted from the camera in the tip of the blade and allows laryngoscopy and intubation in positions other than the sniffing position. The advantages of these instruments help to reduce the number of difficult or failed intubations and the incidence of dental damage. In studies on manikins or patients with normal airways, these devices have been demonstrated to perform better than or equal to the Macintosh laryngoscope, and other studies have demonstrated successful intubation of patients with known or suspected DAs.[85,86]

Although visualization of the glottis is easier with VAL, insertion of the ETT can be difficult. The monitor view reveals only the laryngeal inlet, and advancing the tube into the larynx may require an introducer or a built-in guiding channel, which can make the instrument bulky and the technique more complicated than with a conventional laryngoscope. Several cases of pharyngeal injuries have been reported with the rigid GlideRite stylet of the GlideScope, and palatal perforation has been reported with the McGrath video laryngoscope.[87–89] Increased awareness of potential complications, better training and supervision, and appropriate equipment and patient selection can reduce the incidence of complications. In addition, choosing a tube with a flexible anterior tip (such as the Parker Flex-Tip) may reduce complications.[90]

Laryngoscopy requires deep anesthesia because it causes strong stimulation of physiologic reflexes, and respiratory, cardiovascular, and neurologic adverse effects are possible.[91] Hypertensive patients, pregnant patients with hypertension, and patients with ischemic heart disease are particularly at risk. Deep anesthesia, application of topical anesthetics, prevention of the sympathoadrenal response with drugs such as opioids or intravenous (IV) lidocaine, and minimizing mechanical stimulation can attenuate the adverse effects. Multiple case reports exist for awake intubations using VAL under topical anesthesia.[92–101]

Rigid optical instruments such as the Bonfils retromolar intubation fiberscope and its modifications,[102] the Bullard laryngoscope, and the intubation tracheoscope[103] are not as commonly used in anesthesiology. They require skilled handling, and experience should be gained in routine cases to apply to DA situations. The rigid intubation tracheoscope, a familiar device in otorhinolaryngologic surgery, has special indications and may be useful in the hands of anesthesiologists.

The disadvantages of these instruments are a relatively closed view through the tube, a high risk of damage to the teeth and laryngeal structures, possible perforation of the hypopharynx, and risk of aspiration. High-flow oxygen insufflation through a port can induce subcutaneous cervical and facial emphysema.[104]

Traumatic Intubation

Despite optimal positioning of the head and neck, the glottis is sometimes impossible to visualize, even in patients without obvious predisposing features.[105–107] Difficult intubations, particularly unexpected ones, are often traumatic. In a case of difficult intubation, the practitioner tends to increase the lifting forces of the laryngoscope blade, which may damage the intraoral tissues and osseous structures. Continuing attempts to intubate the patient many times without changing the approach or technique leads to traumatic intubation. Use of increasing force may cause swelling, bleeding, or perforation, resulting in a more difficult intubation and possibly leading to a CICO situation. A maximum of three attempts to achieve intubation using a laryngoscope is recommended. If intubation fails after three attempts, another airway-securing technique should be used following a DA algorithm.

Lip Injury

Lip injuries, which typically occur on the upper lip, include lacerations, hematomas, edema, and teeth marks. They are usually caused by inattentive laryngoscopy performed by inexperienced practitioners, the laryngoscope blade, and the teeth. Although these injuries are annoying to the patient, they are usually self-limited.

Dental Injury

The incidence of dental injury associated with anesthesia is greater than 1 case in 4500 procedures.[108] A prospective observational study reported the rate of any dental damage, including enamel fracture, to be 25%.[109] Maxillary central incisors are most at risk; 50% of these injuries happen during laryngoscopy, 23% after extubation, 8% during extubation, and 5% in the context of regional anesthesia. With the use of an SGA, the incidence of dental injuries is up to six times lower than with laryngoscopy.[110] However, the use of SGAs and oropharyngeal airways can result in dental injury. With insufficient anesthetic depth, biting against the device is possible, causing injury. Dental injuries are most

common in small children; in patients with periodontal disease (in which structural support is poor), fixed dental work (e.g., bridges or caps), protrusion of the upper incisors (i.e., an overbite), or carious teeth (poor preexisting dental status); and in cases of difficult intubation. Preexisting dental pathology, the most significant preexisting risk factor,[111] should be explored, and all loose, diseased, chipped, or capped teeth must be documented in the chart before anesthesia induction and intubation.[112,113]

The patient must be advised of the risk of dental damage and should be consented for removal of very loose teeth. Tooth guards may be used, but they can be awkward and obstruct visualization of the glottis,[114] although they do not seem to significantly prolong time to intubation.[115]

Fragments of chipped or partially broken teeth and completely avulsed teeth should be located and retrieved. Care should be taken to ensure that no foreign bodies slip into the pharynx to later become lodged in the esophagus or the respiratory tract. Tooth aspiration may cause serious complications requiring rigid or flexible bronchoscopy for removal. Avulsed teeth should be saved in moist gauze or in normal saline without cleaning them. With a rapid response from an oral surgeon or a dentist, an intact tooth can often be reimplanted and saved. The optimal time is within the first hour; thereafter, reimplantation success diminishes with increasing time.[116]

Tongue Injury

Massive tongue swelling, or macroglossia, has been reported in adult and pediatric patients.[117,118] Macroglossia can occur with a bite block or oral airway in place, with soft tissue compression of the chin, or with no protective device. A risk factor is substantial neck flexion during prolonged surgery. Macroglossia results from obstructed venous and lymphatic drainage of the tongue, and it has been associated with angiotensin-converting enzyme inhibitors.[119] The ETT may severely compromise the circulation on one side of the tongue, causing hemimacroglossia. One report described the sudden onset of tongue swelling after prolonged surgery to repair a cleft palate, during which the tongue was retracted extensively.[120] Obstruction of the submandibular duct by an ETT may lead to massive tongue swelling.[121] Reduced sense of taste, tongue cyanosis, or loss of tongue sensation is possible after compression of the lingual nerve or lingual artery during forced intubation or because of an oversized, malpositioned, or overinflated SGA.[69]

Injury to the Uvula

Injury to the uvula is usually associated with the use of ETTs, oropharyngeal and nasopharyngeal airways, or SGAs,[122] and with overzealous blind use of a suction catheter.[123] The results of damaging the uvula are edema and necrosis.[124] Sore throat, odynophagia, painful swallowing, coughing, foreign body sensation, and serious life-threatening airway obstruction have been reported.[125]

Pharyngeal Mucosal Injury

A postoperative sore throat (POST) likely represents a broad constellation of signs and symptoms. The incidence of POST after intubation (34.3%) is higher than after SGA use (21.5%) and after face-mask ventilation.[126,127] The incidence of POST associated with the use of the Combitube was 48%.[128] Aggressive suctioning is probably a contributing factor. The incidence is substantially higher in women and in patients undergoing thyroid surgery. No correlation is seen with factors such as age, use of muscle relaxants, type of narcotic used, number of intubation attempts, or duration of intubation. Smaller ETTs, lower cuff inflation pressures, topical treatment with local anesthetics, and inhalation of steroids have a beneficial impact on POST.[129] Pain on swallowing usually lasts no more than 24 to 48 hours and can be relieved in part by having the patient breathe humidified air.

Laryngeal Trauma and Injury to the Vocal Cords

Trauma to the larynx may occur after tracheal intubation, depending on the skill of the practitioner and the degree of difficulty. In one large study, 6.2% of patients sustained severe lesions, 4.5% had hematoma of the vocal cords, 1% had hematoma of the supraglottic region, and 1% sustained lacerations and scars of the vocal cord mucosa.[130] Recovery is typically prompt with conservative therapy.[131] Hoarseness may appear as late as 2 weeks postoperatively.[132]

Granulomas usually occur as a complication of long-term intubation (Fig. 48.1); however, a small but significant number of patients sustain laryngeal injuries during short-term intubation.[133] Intubation can cause various degrees of laryngeal trauma, including thickening, edema, erythema, hematoma, and granuloma of the vocal folds.[134,135] Injuries of the laryngeal muscles and suspensory ligaments are possible (Fig. 48.2). The larynx should be inspected for injury before insertion of the ETT to document

and treat preexisting lesions. Anesthesiologists should be vigilant in all cases of hoarseness, and patients with sustained postoperative hoarseness should be examined by an otorhinolaryngologist.

Arytenoid dislocation and subluxation have been reported as a rare complication of intubation.[136] Associated factors include traumatic and difficult intubations, repeated attempts at intubation, extubation with an inflated cuff (e.g., self-extubation), intubation using blind techniques (e.g., light-guided intubation or retrograde intubation),[137] or use of the McCoy laryngoscope.[138] Early diagnosis and conservative or operative treatment are necessary,[139] because fibrosis with subsequent malpositioning and ankylosis may occur after 48 hours (Fig. 48.3).

The vocal process of the arytenoid is the most common site of injury by the ETT because it is positioned between the vocal cords. Granuloma formation most commonly occurs at this site. The degree of injury worsens with increasing tube size and duration of intubation.[140]

There have been numerous case reports of unilateral or bilateral vocal cord paralysis after intubation, which is usually temporary.[141-144] One report associated vocal cord paralysis with use of ethylene oxide to sterilize ETTs.[145] Hoarseness occurs with unilateral paralysis, whereas respiratory obstruction may occur with bilateral paralysis. The most likely source of injury is an ETT cuff malpositioned in the subglottic larynx with pressure on the recurrent laryngeal nerve.[146,147] Permanent voice change after intubation because of external laryngeal nerve trauma has been reported in up to 3% of patients undergoing surgery at sites other than the head or neck. The incidence may be decreased by avoiding overinflation of the ETT cuff and by placing the ETT cuff at least 15 mm below the vocal cords.[146]

Eroded vocal cords may adhere to one another, eventually forming synechiae. This is a potential problem when airflow between the vocal cords has been compromised as a result of tracheostomy.[146] Surgical correction is usually necessary.

Tracheobronchial Injury

Tracheal injury has many causes, including an overinflated ETT cuff, inappropriate ETT size, or malpositioning of the ETT tip, laryngoscope, stylet, tube exchanger, or related equipment.[147] Predisposing factors include anatomic abnormalities, blind or hurried intubation, inadequate positioning, poor visualization,

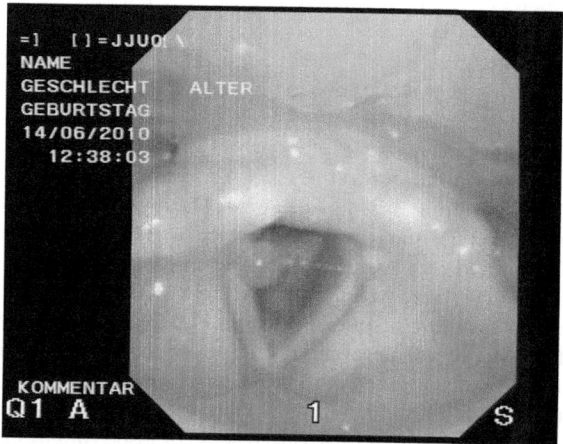

• **Fig. 48.1** Granuloma on the anterior aspect of the left vocal cord after endotracheal intubation. (Courtesy Prof. Christian Sittel, MD, Head of Department, Otorhinolaryngology/Head and Neck Surgery, Klinikum Stuttgart, Germany.)

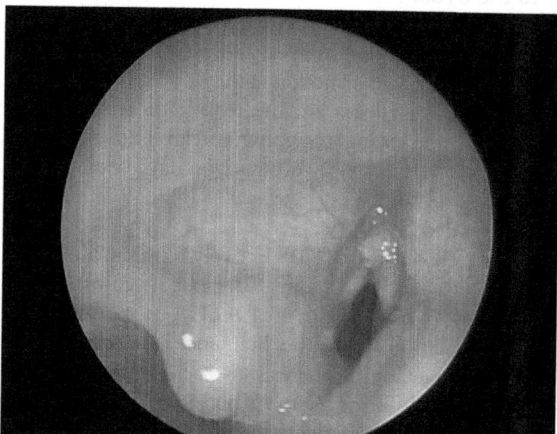

• **Fig. 48.2** Injury to the anterior commissure of the vocal cords in a child. (Courtesy Prof. Christian Sittel, MD, Head of Department, Otorhinolaryngology/Head and Neck Surgery, Klinikum Stuttgart, Germany.)

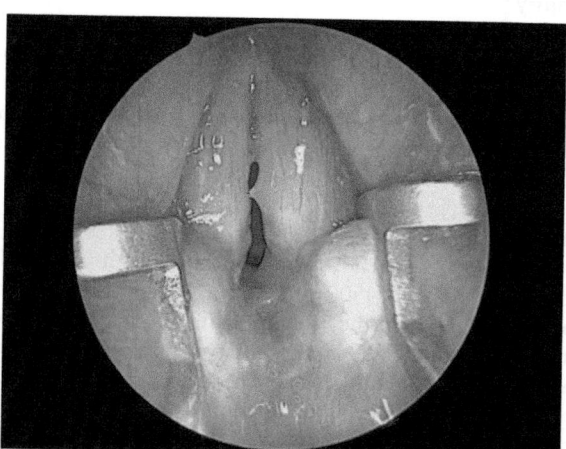

• **Fig. 48.3** Interarytenoid fibrosis after intubation. A fibrotic lesion has developed between the arytenoid cartilages after prolonged intubation. (Courtesy Prof. Christian Sittel, MD, Head of Department, Otorhinolaryngology/Head and Neck Surgery, Klinikum Stuttgart, Germany.)

and, most commonly, inexperience of the practitioner. The presence of an ETT in the trachea may lead to edema, desquamation, inflammation, and ulceration of the airway (Figs. 48.4 and 48.5).[148] The severity of the injury may be related to the duration of intubation, although this relationship is not well established.[149] Any irritating stimulus, such as pressure from an oversized ETT, dry inhaled gases, allergic reactions to inhaled sprays, or chemical irritation from residual cleaning solutions, can initiate an inflammatory response and cause mucosal edema in the larynx or trachea. Edema after extubation decreases the lumen diameter and increases airway resistance. Small children are most susceptible to this problem, with the sudden increase in airway resistance leading to postintubation croup; almost 4% of children 1 to 3 years old develop croup after tracheal intubation.[150,151] Microcuff pediatric ETTs (Kimberly Clark, Atlanta, GA) have improved tracheal sealing characteristics, providing an adequate seal with cuff pressures greater than 10 cm H_2O in children; their use will likely decrease the incidence of some of the previously mentioned problems.[152,153]

Mechanical trauma may result from sharp objects within the trachea, such as a stylet tip that extends beyond the length of the ETT. Tracheal ruptures, especially after emergency intubation, have been reported.[154] Bronchial rupture caused by an airway exchange catheter (AEC) has also been described.[155]

ETT cuffs inflated to a pressure greater than that of the capillary perfusion may devitalize the tracheal mucosa, leading to ulceration, necrosis, and loss of structural integrity.[156] Ulceration can occur at even lower cuff pressures in hypotensive patients. The need for increasing cuff volumes to maintain a seal is an ominous sign that heralds tracheomalacia.[157] Massive gastric distention in an intubated patient may signal the presence of a tracheoesophageal fistula as the cuff progressively erodes into the esophagus.[158] Any patient with more than 10 mL of blood in the ETT without a known cause should be assessed for a tracheocarotid fistula.[159] The various nerves in this region of the neck are also at risk. Erosion of the ETT into the paratracheal nerves may result in dysphonia, hoarseness, and laryngeal incompetence. Tracheomalacia results from erosion confined to the tracheal cartilages. The ETT cuff should only be inflated as much as necessary to ensure an adequate airway seal. When nitrous oxide is used during a lengthy surgical procedure, pressure in the cuff should at least be periodically checked by a manometer or using a cuff pressure control device. In the presence of 70% nitrous oxide, intracuff pressures increase to levels that are potentially high enough to cause tracheal ischemia in only 12 minutes on average.[160] ETT cuff pressure should not exceed 25 cm H_2O. Increasing cuff pressure caused by surgical manipulations can also be observed and prevented by using a manometer or cuff pressure control device.

Tracheal intubation may erode the tracheal mucosa, leading to scar tissue, which ultimately retracts and leads to tracheal stenosis. The reported incidence of granulomas is 1 case in every 800 to 20,000 intubations.[161,162] They are more common in women than in men and occur rarely in children. Avulsion of mucous membranes may also result from electrodes wrapped around the ETT for laryngeal nerve stimulation because these provide sharp edges (Fig. 48.6). The most common site of erosion is along the posterior laryngeal wall, where granulation tissue easily overgrows. Side effects of granulomas include cough, hoarseness, and throat pain. The growths may be prevented by minimizing the trauma associated with laryngoscopy and intubation. When granulomas occur, surgical excision is usually required.

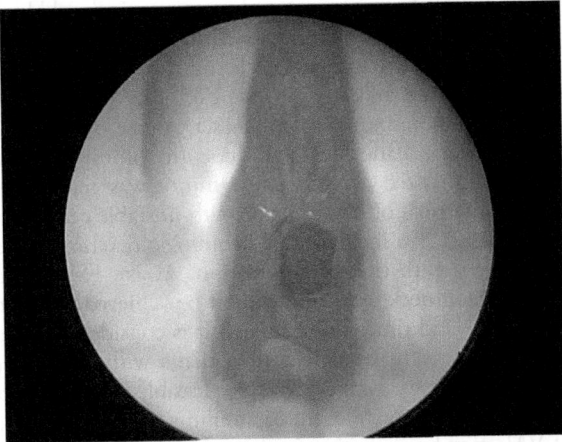

• **Fig. 48.4** Subglottic stenosis. An endotracheal view through the vocal cords shows subglottic stenosis after long-term intubation. (Courtesy Prof. Christian Sittel, MD, Head of Department, Otorhinolaryngology/Head and Neck Surgery, Klinikum Stuttgart, Germany.)

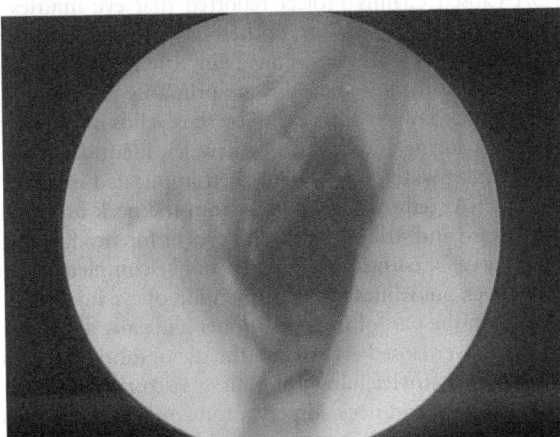

• **Fig. 48.5** Ulcerative lesion in the area of the left vocal cord after long-term intubation. (Courtesy Prof. Christian Sittel, MD, Head of Department, Otorhinolaryngology/Head and Neck Surgery, Klinikum Stuttgart, Germany.)

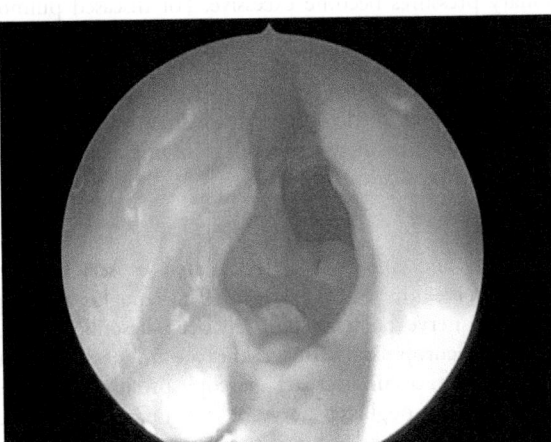

• **Fig. 48.6** An endotracheal view shows avulsion of the mucous membranes caused by wrapping of the endotracheal tube with stimulation electrodes for neurosurgery in a 2-year-old child. (Courtesy Prof. Christian Sittel, MD, Head of Department, Otorhinolaryngology/Head and Neck Surgery, Klinikum Stuttgart, Germany.)

Membranes and webs may eventually replace tracheal and laryngeal ulcers. These growths are commonly thick and gray. Care should be taken while intubating patients with these lesions because inadvertent detachment may result in respiratory obstruction or bleeding into the airway. With time, the inflammatory process associated with laryngeal ulcers may extend to the laryngeal cartilage. If this occurs, the cartilage may become inflamed (i.e., chondritis) or softened (i.e., chondromalacia).

Several months after prolonged tracheal intubation, tracheal stenosis and fibrosis may occur. This usually represents the end stage of a progression from tracheal wall erosion to cartilaginous weakening to healing with fibrosis.[148] Stenosis typically occurs at the site of an inflated cuff, although it may occur at the location of the ETT tip. Symptoms include a nonproductive cough, dyspnea, and signs of respiratory obstruction. Dilation of the stenosis is curative in its early stages. However, surgical correction may be necessary after the tracheal lumen has been reduced to 4 to 5 mm in adults.[162,163]

Supraglottic complications induced by long-term intubation may be prevented by early tracheostomy. There is no evidence supporting an ideal time for tracheostomy in long-term ventilated patients.

Barotrauma

Barotrauma results from high-pressure distention of intrapulmonary structures. High-flow insufflation techniques in which small catheters are used distal to the larynx are most often associated with barotrauma. These problems are common in microlaryngeal surgery when jet ventilation is used.[164-168] Direct impingement of the catheter tip on the tracheal mucosa may also cause barotrauma.[166] Edema or hematoma may occur if the jet of air strikes the mucosa of the larynx or the vocal cords, leading to laryngospasm. When air leaks into the peribronchial tissues, it can traverse into the subcutaneous space, the lung interstitium, or the pleural and pericardial cavities. Pneumomediastinum or tension pneumothorax and possibly cardiac tamponade are the results, and chest tubes may be necessary. Progressive accumulation of air may cause loss of pulmonary compliance and loss of ventilatory volume; if the accumulation is large enough, cardiopulmonary compromise and impossible ventilation may result. Safety mechanisms should be in place to prevent high-pressure airflow in the event that intrapulmonary pressures become excessive. For diseased pulmonary tissue, the lowest possible airway pressure should be used to prevent parenchymal blowout. This advice also applies to patients with blunt thoracic trauma who have subcutaneous emphysema; they should be presumed to have a bronchial leak unless proved otherwise. Barotrauma may also result from upper airway obstruction during jet ventilation.[169]

Nerve Injuries

Laryngoscopy and cuffed SGA devices may cause temporary or permanent nerve injury. Lingual, recurrent, hypoglossal, and glossopharyngeal nerve paralysis have all been described for LMA devices, and neuropraxia with weakness, numbness, or paralysis of the tongue can occur after laryngoscopy, presumably caused by pressure on the hypoglossal nerve.[45,170] Damage to the internal branch of the superior laryngeal nerve resulting in supraglottic anesthesia may occur during a difficult intubation and may lead to aspiration.[171] Malposition of the cuff or tube may be one reason for nerve injury. Ahmad and Yentis postulated that lingual nerve injury may occur where the nerve distal to its gingival branch is compressed by the LMA tubing against the side of the tongue.[172]

Spinal Cord and Vertebral Column Injury

Airway management techniques such as chin lift, jaw thrust, and direct laryngoscopy (DL) transmit movement to the cervical spine. When a patient's neck is fused, adequate neck extension may be impossible to obtain. Attempting to hyperextend the neck of these patients may result in cervical fractures and quadriplegia.[173] A head that is fixed in a cervical collar or halo does not allow neck extension and limits the successful use of DL. Using an FIS to assist intubation should be considered in these cases. If immediate intubation is necessary, patients with acute cervical spine fractures may be carefully intubated with manual in-line stabilization, whereby the head is protected against excessive movement by a second person.[174] C1 and C2 fractures seem to be particularly vulnerable because any degree of extension or flexion may compromise spinal cord function. Between 10% and 25% of spinal cord injuries occur because of improper immobilization of the vertebral column after trauma, and neurologic deterioration has been associated with DL in patients with cervical spine injury.[175-178]

Several conditions, such as Down syndrome and rheumatoid arthritis, are associated with atlantoaxial instability.[179-182] Excessive neck extension in a patient with an undiagnosed Arnold-Chiari malformation may cause worsening of cerebellar tonsil herniation.[183] Patients with underlying diseases such as connective tissue disorders, lytic bone tumors, and osteoporosis should be intubated carefully, and extreme neck extension should be avoided in every patient because of loss of muscle tone by curarizing drugs. A range-of-motion test and an assessment of neck extension should be performed before inducing anesthesia. A case of quadriplegia after bag-mask ventilation, DL, and cricothyrotomy in a patient with an unrecognized cervical spine injury was reported.[178] A review of the records of 150 patients with unstable cervical spine injury found a 1.3% incidence of neurologic deterioration after elective surgery with tracheal intubation. Awake FSI should be considered when neck extension cannot be achieved without the risk of damage and time is not crucial. It is considered the safest method for airway management in patients with cervical spine injury. In cases where awake FSI is not feasible (e.g., uncooperative patients and small children) or attempts are unsuccessful, the use of VAL may be an option as these devices minimize cervical spine movement during intubation.[179,184-188] Alternatively, an SGA may be used to manage the airway.[174]

Eye Injuries

The ASA Closed Claims Project reported that eye injuries were responsible for 3% of all claims; of these, 35% were related to corneal injuries, with corneal abrasions being the most common eye complication.[189] Corneal abrasions are primarily caused by a face mask being placed on an open eye or by the eyelids not being completely closed during anesthesia.[190,191] Jewelry, identification cards, and loose-fitting watch bands have been implicated in scratching the cornea.[192] A stethoscope hanging from the neck of a clinician can fall forward and strike the patient's eyes or forehead. Other factors that may cause cornea abrasion may not be completely controllable. However, guidelines for the prevention of eye injuries consist of vigilance on the part of the practitioner and early application of adhesive tape over closed eyelids and the use of lubricants containing an aqueous methylcellulose solution or viscous gel for high-risk surgery (e.g., head and neck surgery, prone or lateral positioning). The incidence of corneal injury varies widely between studies and ranges between 1 in 1000 to 1 in 10,000.[193-195]

Although most corneal injuries typically heal within 24 hours, they are usually painful and can lead to corneal ulceration. An immediate ophthalmologic consultation is recommended. Local anesthetics should not be applied because they can delay regeneration of the epithelium and may promote keratitis. Treatment consists of allowing the injured eye to rest by using an eye patch and applying an antibiotic ointment.

Temporomandibular Joint Injuries

TMJ anatomy is special in that one side cannot be moved without the other side. Both joints represent a functional unit, and injuries to one TMJ affect the other side. Opening the mouth is a combination of rotary and translational movement in the joint. The rotary movement allows only a mouth opening of about 25 mm; maximal opening is achieved by the translational movement. Pathologic changes such as bone cysts, rheumatoid arthritis, and atrophy of the mandible as a result of age can reduce joint mobility and may lead to fractures. Rupture of the lateral ligament is possible. TMJ injuries are caused by increasing forces during laryngoscopy to optimize the view of the vocal cords. Limited mouth opening, pain in the joint, lateral deviation of the mandible (i.e., unilateral luxation), protrusion of the mandible (i.e., bilateral luxation), and lockjaw (i.e., fixation after joint luxation) may occur. Most reported cases of TMJ injury were not associated with a DA.[196]

Nasotracheal Passage

Cranial Intubation

Nasotracheal intubations are potentially hazardous. In patients with basilar skull fractures or certain facial fractures (e.g., Le Fort II or III fractures), the ETT may be inadvertently introduced into the cranial vault (Fig. 48.7).[197] Fractures of the frontal part of the skull base with cerebrospinal fluid rhinorrhea, intranasal abscesses or abscesses with intranasal expansion, choanal atresia, hyperplastic tonsils, a tendency for uncontrollable nasal bleeding, and coagulopathies are considered contraindications to nasotracheal intubation. In one case of nasotracheal intubation, asystole occurred after the ETT was introduced into the orbit.[198] In another instance, cranial base injury after transnasal tracheal intubation was reported, resulting in a defect to the left skull base with bifrontal pneumocephalus.[199] However, if care is taken, the complication rates of oral and nasal intubation are not different.[200]

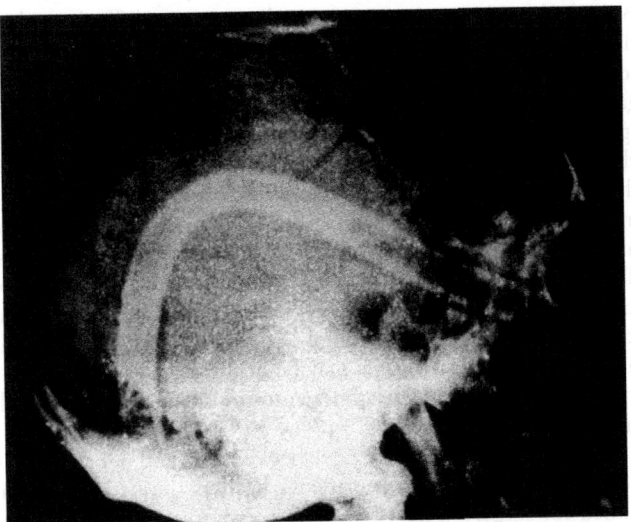

• **Fig. 48.7** Intracranial nasotracheal tube (computer enhanced). (From Horellou MF, Mathe D, Feiss P. A hazard of naso-tracheal intubation. *Anaesthesia*. 1978;33:73.)

Nasal intubation in a patient with a known or suspected skull fracture should be performed only with extreme caution by using flexible bronchoscopy via the inferior nasal meatus. In midface fractures with intact dura mater, it is possible to open the dura by manipulation during nasotracheal intubation.

Nasal Injury

Nasotracheal intubation may be problematic in the presence of hypertrophic turbinates, extreme deviation of the nasal septum, prominences on the nasal septum, chronic infections in the nasal cavity, and nasal polyposis. Minor bruising occurs in 54% of nasal intubations and most commonly involves the mucosa overlying the inferior turbinate and the adjacent septum.[201] If epistaxis occurs, the ETT cuff can be inflated and left to remain in the nasal cavity to tamponade the bleeding.

The nasal mucosa must be treated with a vasoconstrictor before instrumentation.[202] Some agents used for this purpose are 0.5% phenylephrine, 0.01% epinephrine, or 0.05% oxymetazoline.[203] The risk of nasal injury can be minimized with the use of a small, well-lubricated ETT with a flexible tip that has been soaked in warm water.[204]

Possible complications of nasotracheal intubation include dislodgment of nasal polyps, avulsion of nasal turbinates,[205,206] adenoidectomy, injury to the nasal septum, and perforation of the pyriform sinus or the vallecula. In case of injury to the pyriform sinus, the internal branch of the superior laryngeal nerve, the soft tissue of the pharynx, the larynx, and the superior laryngeal vessels may be damaged. Nasotracheal tubes may dissect and run behind the posterior pharyngeal wall. Patients with an obstructed nasal passage caused by convoluted turbinates are at increased risk for this complication. Tears in the pharyngeal mucosa can mature into retropharyngeal abscesses.[207] One case of external compression of the nasotracheal tube caused by the displaced bony fragments of multiple Le Fort fractures was reported.[208]

Delayed complications of nasotracheal intubation include pharyngitis, rhinitis, and adhesion of the nasal septum and inferior turbinate bone. After the ETT is secured in the trachea, ensure that it is also secured properly at the level of the nostril. Distortion of the nasal alar can lead to ischemia or nasal adhesions. Using anatomically preformed nasal tubes for head and neck surgery or compression of the nasal alar may lead to necrosis in the worst cases (Fig. 48.8). Wrapping the tube with foam material at the level of the nasal alar and careful attention in cases of long-term intubation may reduce or avoid this complication.

Even in the absence of gross trauma, mechanical damage to the superficial epithelial layers caused by nasal intubation results in mucociliary slowing and bacteremia.[209–212] The most common organisms introduced into the blood are nasopharyngeal commensal organisms (e.g., *Streptococcus viridans*), which can cause endocarditis and systemic infection. Even short-term intubation has caused nasal septal and retropharyngeal abscesses. Acute otitis media has occurred in 13% of nasally intubated neonates.[213] Paranasal sinusitis has been reported, most commonly occurring with nasal intubation for more than 5 days.[214,215] Infection may be related to sustained edema and occlusion of the sinus drainage pathways. Prompt diagnosis is critical, and paranasal sinusitis should be suspected in any patient with facial tenderness, pain, or purulent nasal discharge or in any nasally intubated patient who develops sepsis with no other obvious source. The nasal structures must be checked again postoperatively. The use of a nasogastric tube as a guide to facilitate tracheal tube passage was found to reduce the incidence and severity of epistaxis, to improve

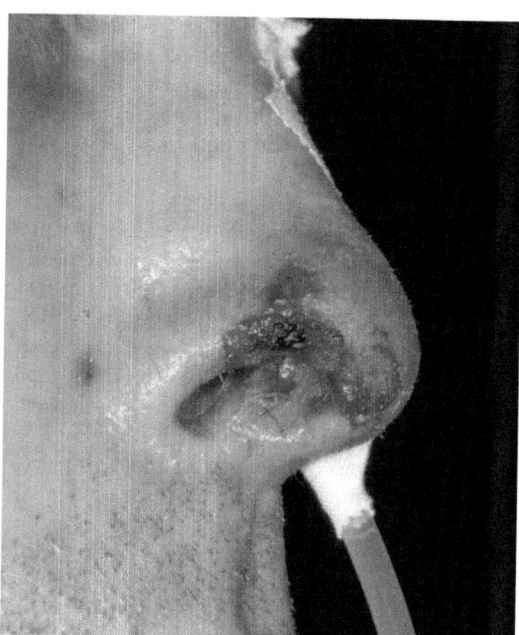

• **Fig. 48.8** Necrosis of right nasal wing after 3 days of intubation with an anatomic, preformed tube.

navigability, and to require fewer manipulations than the conventional technique.[216]

Hyposmia and anosmia following uncomplicated nasotracheal intubation for head and neck surgery have been reported. Most cases resolve in 3 to 6 months, though some may be permanent.

Foreign Bodies

The nostrils are common sites for entry of foreign bodies. Small children, known for placing small objects into their orifices, find the nostrils one of the most accessible sites. More than 80% of patients who aspirated a foreign body were children, and most were between 1 and 3 years old.[217–219] Foreign body aspiration is the cause of death of 7% of children younger than 4 years of age.

Smith and colleagues reported a rhinolith that was dislodged during nasotracheal intubation; the mass had formed around the rubber tire of a toy car that the patient had placed in his nose 30 years earlier.[220] Nasotracheal intubation can dislodge similar foreign bodies that may obstruct the ETT, pharynx, or trachea. If a nasal foreign body is known or suspected, it should be gently dislodged, advanced into the oropharynx, and retrieved before intubation. Mask ventilation may also dislodge foreign bodies to lower parts of the airway.

Esophageal Intubation

Endotracheal Tube Placement

When visualization of the glottis is difficult, the ETT may inadvertently be introduced into the esophagus. Esophageal intubation is more common among inexperienced practitioners, but it also may occur in the hands of experienced clinicians. As a proportion of anesthesia malpractice claims, delayed detection of esophageal intubation declined from approximately 3% to 8% before 1990 and to 1% to 2% per year in 1990 and later.[221]

Although intubating the esophagus is not disastrous, failing to detect and correct the condition is. Recognition of this error must be rapid to avoid the adverse effects of prolonged hypoxia. Preoxygenation can ameliorate this problem by allowing a longer apneic period for tracheal intubation and by delaying the onset

of hypoxemia. End-tidal capnography is essential in confirming endotracheal placement of the tube. Capnography should be available wherever intubation is performed. In out-of-hospital practice and emergency medicine, where capnography may not be available, calorimetric single-use CO_2 detectors or an esophageal detector device can help to identify failed intubation in 94.6% of cases.[222] Esophageal intubation can briefly produce a positive end-tidal capnogram (e.g., in the presence of CO_2-containing drinks in the stomach), but the waveform diminishes rapidly after three to five breaths.[223,224] Flexible bronchoscopy is another safe way to confirm the correct position of the ETT. Other signs, such as equal bilateral breath sounds, symmetric bilateral chest wall movement, epigastric auscultation and observation, and tube condensation, are potentially misleading.[225] A misplaced tube should remain in place while the trachea is properly intubated. This helps to identify the correct orifice for intubation and protects the trachea from regurgitated stomach contents. Once tracheal intubation is achieved after an esophageal intubation, the stomach should be suctioned to minimize vomiting, gastric perforation, or compromise of ventilation.

Esophageal Perforation and Retropharyngeal Abscess

Perforation of the esophagus has been reported on several occasions.[226–234] It seems most likely to occur when inexperienced clinicians handle emergency situations, when intubation is difficult, or in the presence of esophageal pathology. Perforation occurs most commonly over the cricopharyngeus muscle on the posterior esophageal wall, where the esophagus is narrow and thin. Subcutaneous emphysema, pneumothorax, fever, cellulitis, cyanosis, throat pain, mediastinitis, empyema, pericarditis, and death can occur. Early detection and treatment of the condition are critical because the mortality rate of mediastinitis is high. An esophageal perforation should be suspected in any patient with a fever, sore throat, and subcutaneous emphysema after a difficult intubation. One case report identified a traumatic tracheal perforation through the esophagus in a patient with a difficult intubation.[235] Cases of esophageal perforation have been associated with the use of the Combitube.[80,81]

Bronchial Intubation

Use of an Endotracheal Tube

Bronchial intubation is common and sometimes difficult to identify. Asymmetric chest expansion, unilateral absence of breath sounds (especially on the left side), and eventual arterial blood gas abnormalities are diagnostic features. Bronchial intubation (preferentially right-sided) is more common in newborns and children, because of the small distance between the carina and the glottis. The position of the tip of the tube should be carefully monitored in children. If bronchial intubation goes undetected, it may lead to atelectasis, hypoxia, and pulmonary edema.[236] Transillumination of the neck with a lighted stylet can assist in tube location,[237] although not in cases of obesity or large goiter. Flexible bronchoscopy is the best tool to detect proper position of the tube. Alternatively, the ETT may be deliberately advanced into a mainstem bronchus and withdrawn until bilateral breath sounds are auscultated.

The tip of the ETT may move between 3.8 and 6.4 cm during flexion or extension of the patient's head as the patient is positioned for surgery (Fig. 48.9).[238] It is easy to remember that the tip of the ETT moves in the same direction as the patient's nose. If the patient's neck is flexed, the nose is pointed downward, and the ETT advances farther into the trachea. The tube moves away

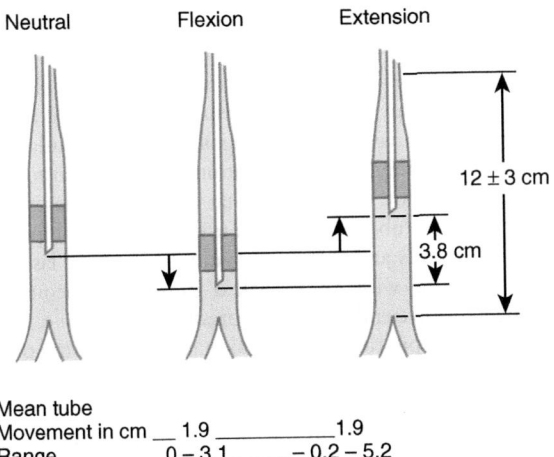

Neutral   Flexion   Extension

12 ± 3 cm

3.8 cm

Mean tube
Movement in cm __ 1.9 _____ 1.9
Range _____ 0 – 3.1 _____ – 0.2 – 5.2

• **Fig. 48.9** The mean movement of an endotracheal tube with flexion and extension of the neck from a neutral position. The mean tube movement between flexion and extension is one-third to one-fourth of the length of a normal adult trachea (12 ± 3 cm). (From Conrardy PA, Goodman LR, Lainge F, et al. Alteration of endotracheal tube position: flexion and extension of the neck. *Crit Care Med.* 1976;4:8.)

from the carina an average of 0.7 cm during lateral rotation of the head. Care should be taken in case of cleft palate surgery or tonsillectomy. Special blades used by the surgeon to achieve a direct view may move the ETT forward during positioning of the blade. A stethoscope placed on the left chest helps to identify an ETT tube that is being displaced into the right main bronchus.

When inadvertent bronchial intubation is discovered, the tube should be withdrawn several centimeters (smaller distances in children) and the lungs inflated sufficiently to expand any atelectatic areas. In cases of chronic atelectasis, bronchoscopy may be required to remove mucous plugs. This problem can be avoided by measuring the length of the ETT alongside the patient before intubation. The tip of the tube should ideally be at least 2 cm above the carina, which may be approximated at the sternal angle (of Louis) adjacent to the junction of the sternum with the second rib. Appropriate orotracheal tube depths are approximately 21 cm from the teeth in adult women and 23 cm in adult men, and nasotracheal tube depths are approximately 25 cm in women and 27 cm in men from the naris.[239]

Use of a Double-Lumen Tube

Safe limits for the placement of a double-lumen tube (DLT) have been outlined by Benumof and colleagues.[240] Modern flexible bronchoscopes have removed the guesswork surrounding DLT tip location. A DLT may be inserted blindly into the appropriate bronchus, followed by bronchoscopic confirmation of its position, or the bronchoscope may be inserted initially and used as a stylet over which the DLT is advanced.[241] Flexible bronchoscopy significantly reduces malposition of the DLT, and its routine use is recommended after intubation, changing of the patient's position, increasing ventilation pressure, and irregular auscultation sounds.

Even in the best of hands, however, tracheobronchial injuries can occur with DLT placement.[242,243] Bronchial rupture is a serious complication that requires immediate attention. Using DLTs that are too large may be the cause of bronchial trauma. Thermal softening of a double-lumen endobronchial tube may help to reduce sore throat, hoarseness, and vocal cord injuries, as does the use of VAL for tube placement.[244] The recommended DLT size is 37- to 39-French for women and 39- to 41-French for men. It is

noteworthy that the DLTs of different manufacturers vary substantially in diameter and length.[245]

Maintenance of the Endotracheal Tube

Airway Obstruction

A patent airway is an absolute requirement for safe anesthesia. Airway obstruction can occur at any time during administration of general anesthesia, particularly in prolonged operations or in patients with predisposing anatomic abnormalities. Airway obstruction should be considered when an intubated patient has diminished breath sounds associated with increasing peak inspiratory pressures. Many clinicians mistakenly treat the patient for bronchospasm when the increased airway resistance originates from the ETT, not from the patient.

Obstruction can result from various sources,[246] including a sharp bend or kink in the ETT; a tube that has been bitten closed; or a tube that is obstructed with mucus, blood, foreign bodies, or lubricant.[246,247] As the ETT warms with continued use during prolonged procedures, it becomes more malleable; under these circumstances, the tube may kink and become obstructed. The ETT and connecting hoses should be supported and, if necessary, taped to prevent kinking caused by their own weight. Inspiratory gases should be humidified during long anesthetics to prevent tube obstruction from dried secretions. At least two cases have been reported in which the plastic coating on a stylet sheared off and occluded the lumen of an ETT.[248,249] In another case, an ETT was obstructed by the prominent knuckle of an aortic arch.[250] Nitrous oxide can cause expansion of gas bubbles trapped in the walls of an ETT, leading to airway obstruction.[251] The cuff of an ETT can cause airway obstruction. An overinflated cuff may compress the bevel of the ETT against the tracheal wall, occluding its tip[252]; the cuff may also herniate over the tip of the tube and cause an obstruction.[253]

When faced with any of these problems, the best solution is to pass a suction catheter or a fiberoptic bronchoscope down the lumen of the ETT and attempt to clear it. If the tube is totally obstructed, passage of a stylet may be attempted. Complete obstruction that cannot be remedied quickly requires removal of the ETT and reintubation as rapidly as possible.

Unusual causes of airway obstruction have been reported. In two patients, complete airway obstruction occurred secondary to achalasia and esophageal dilation.[254,255] At least two cases of tension hydrothorax that caused airway obstruction during laparoscopic surgery have been reported. One patient had malignant ascites that, when combined with a pneumoperitoneum, led to a rapid accumulation of pleural fluid with respiratory and cardiovascular compromise.[256] A second case occurred during operative hysteroscopy when a large volume of glycine was absorbed through opened myometrial vessels under high intraabdominal pressure.[257] In each case, more than 1.5 L of clear fluid were drained once chest tubes were placed.

Disconnection and Dislodgment

A common and serious complication of tracheal intubation is disconnection of the ETT from the remainder of the anesthesia circuit. This was identified as the most common critical incident in a study of anesthesia-related human errors and equipment failures.[258] A trained anesthesiologist usually identifies this problem immediately. The low-pressure alarm sounds first, and the patient's breath sounds become absent. However, if the ventilator continues to function normally, the physician may be unaware of the nature of the problem. Disconnections are most likely to occur if the connections are made of dissimilar materials, if the patient's head is turned away from the anesthesiologist, or if the airway connections are hidden beneath the surgical drapes. Alarms to signal airway disconnection are included on all modern anesthesia machines, and their signals should be taken seriously.

Connections between the ETT and the breathing circuit should be checked and reinforced at the outset, before the anesthesiologist loses visual control of the airway. There should be no tension on the connections from the weight of the corrugated tubing or the drapes on the tubing. Members of the surgical team should be discouraged from inadvertently leaning on any portion of the breathing circuit. The exact site of disconnection should be ascertained rapidly by checking each connection, beginning at the patient's airway and moving proximally back to the machine.[259] Nevertheless, the anesthesiologist must have a prearranged plan in mind in the event that an airway is inadvertently disconnected or dislodged during surgery.

Circuit Leaks

Leaks in an air delivery circuit can cause hypoventilation and the dilution of inspired gases by entry of room air into the system. With an ascending bellows system, such as that found in newer models of anesthesia machines, the bellows do not rise completely during exhalation if there is a leak. This situation indicates that the circuit leak exceeds the inflow of fresh gas. Older machines with a descending bellows system do not provide such a visual cue and typically appear to function normally. The anesthesiologist should be vigilant at all times for signs of a circuit leak. The inspired oxygen concentration measured at the gas sampling port is reduced because of dilution with room air, and the partial pressure of end-tidal CO_2 increases. Cyanosis, decreased oxygen saturation (SpO_2), or hypertension and tachycardia associated with hypercapnia may be the presenting signs, although each of these is typically a late finding.

The useful mnemonic DOPE addresses the aforementioned common causes of problems maintaining the airway such as displacement or obstruction of the ETT, pneumothorax, and equipment (ventilator) failure.[260]

Laser Fires

Lasers are frequently used in the operating room to ablate benign and neoplastic tissues in the airway. The use of special laser-guarded or metal tubes is recommended, and all flammable materials such as prosthetic teeth and nasogastric tubes should be removed. One of the most catastrophic events associated with the use of lasers is an airway fire, which occurs when the laser ignites an ETT.[261-263] The risk that a laser beam will contact the wall of an ETT is 1 in 2.[264] Perforation of the tube may occur and produce a blowtorch-like flame. Oxygen-rich inspired gas concentrations fuel brisk ignition of the plastic in the ETT and can fuel a fire in both directions. The ETT acts as a blowtorch; the fire is fed by the combustible walls of the tube and is intensified by the high rate of oxygen flow. The heat and fumes of the burning plastic may cause severe damage to the airway. Treatment consists of immediately disconnecting the circuit from the ETT and removing the burning tube from the airway. If the tube is not burning or if complete loss of the airway may occur with removal of the tube, leaving the tube in situ may be considered. The fire should be extinguished with saline solution, and the patient should be supported by face-mask ventilation. The airway should be evaluated for damage with

bronchoscopy, and appropriate supportive respiratory care should be given.

Many precautions can reduce the risk of an airway fire. If possible, placement of an ETT may be avoided altogether if air can be delivered through a ventilating laryngoscope, a jet ventilation system, or by intermittent apneic ventilation.[265] If a tracheostomy tube is in place, ventilation may occur distal to the site of laser surgery. The choice of laser tubes should be consistent with the type of laser used. Blocking cuffs are particularly vulnerable to the laser beam. Covering the tube with saline-soaked gauze or noncombustible tape, using a positive end-expiratory pressure (PEEP) of 5 to 10 cm H_2O to prevent aspiration of material in case of cuff puncture, and filling the cuff with saline to act as an extinguisher in the event of puncture are measures that can protect the patient's airway.[266,267] Placing a dye, such as methylene blue, in the saline can further alert the anesthesiologist in the event of cuff rupture. Nitrous oxide should be avoided because it supports combustion. Oxygen concentrations should not exceed 40% for the same reason.[268,269]

Special Techniques

Flexible Scope Intubation

FSI is the technique of choice in most cases of an anticipated DA. Use of an FIS is not an expedient technique and should probably not be considered when speed is required. Although the device can be used in many different situations involving airway management and the preoperative evaluation of critical patients, it also has several limitations and potential complications.

Operator experience with the technique and proper preparation are essential. Connecting the device to a video system can help with guidance by a more experienced bystander, particularly in training situations.[270]

Potential complications associated with FSI include bleeding, epistaxis (when a nasal intubation is attempted), laryngotracheal trauma, laryngospasm, bronchospasm, and aspiration of blood, saliva, or gastric contents. Another possible hazard is associated with the practice of insufflating oxygen through the suction channel. Although this technique can help to keep the tip of the scope clean and provide supplemental oxygen,[271] it can also cause high-pressure submucosal injection of oxygen if the tip cuts into the pharyngeal mucosa. If this occurs, the result may be pronounced subcutaneous emphysema of the pharynx, face, and periorbital regions.[272]

Lighted Stylets

Lighted stylets may be used to facilitate intubation under local or general anesthesia. A light at the tip of a malleable stylet is used to transilluminate the soft tissues of the pharynx. The device can be used blindly or as an aid when DL is difficult. It may also confirm that the tip of an ETT is still within the cervical trachea and establish that the tube has not been advanced too far.[273,274]

Because use of the lighted stylet in the DA setting is often a blind procedure, pharyngeal pathologic conditions cannot be visualized or avoided. This technique should not be used in patients with suspected abnormalities of the upper airway, such as tumors, polyps, infections (e.g., epiglottitis or retropharyngeal abscess), trauma, or foreign bodies. The lighted stylet should be used with caution in patients in whom transillumination of the anterior neck is limited, such as those with dark skin pigmentation, morbid obesity, limited neck mobility, a large tongue, or a long epiglottis. If placement of the stylet is difficult, the anesthesiologist should consider abandoning the technique to avoid worsening a pathologic process.

Several real and potential complications have been reported with the use of lighted stylets. Sore throat, hoarseness, mucosal damage, and arytenoid subluxation are possible. Several cases have been reported in which the light fell off the end of the stylet. In another instance, the protective tubing was not removed from the stylet and had the potential to become dislodged within the trachea. Heat damage to the tracheal mucosa during a prolonged intubation procedure is a potential risk with inappropriate handling.

Lighted stylets are not recommended for use in emergency cases because the risk of regurgitation is high, CP may affect the ease of intubation, and, in some cases, more than one attempt is necessary. The transillumination technique is not suitable for verification of ETT position because of the potential for misinterpretation.

Submandibular and Submental Approach for Tracheal Intubation

The oral route for tracheal intubation can interfere with some maxillofacial surgical procedures, and the nasal route can be contraindicated or impossible. Nasotracheal intubation is contraindicated in patients with fractures in the cribriform plate of the ethmoid, which frequently accompany Le Fort II and III maxillary fractures, because of the potential complication of infection and the possibility of cranial intubation. Tracheostomy is the usual solution in these circumstances, but it also carries complications. An alternative method is to introduce the tracheal tube through a submental or a submandibular incision, bypassing the surgical area and avoiding the complications of tracheostomy. Damage to adjacent structures with bleeding, tube displacement, aspiration, infection, and hypoxia when passing the tube through the submental incision have been reported.[275,276]

Complications With Infraglottic Procedures

Infraglottic airway access is the last step in the ASA airway management algorithm. When tracheal intubation is impossible, a patient's airway is compromised, and the patient's condition deteriorates into a CICO situation threatening brain damage or death, life-saving steps must be undertaken immediately. There are no contraindications for infraglottic procedures in these critical situations. The most severe complication is failure to establish an airway before brain damage or death occurs. Complications arise because the decision to progress to a surgical airway is not made soon enough or because the procedure is performed too slowly. In all cases of DA, the practitioner should evaluate the possibility of an infraglottic airway access. Difficult anatomic situations, scars, abscesses, and morbid obesity may limit infraglottic access techniques.

Infraglottic airway techniques are suitable for emergency situations, and are also indicated for oxygenation and ventilation of anesthetized patients. Surgical procedures of the upper airway, laryngeal surgery, and diagnostic procedures have been successfully managed with this technique.

Translaryngeal Airway

Retrograde Intubation

Retrograde intubation is an excellent technique for securing a DA. It can be used when anatomic limitations obscure the glottic opening. Because the technique is blind, it is important to exercise caution and not to worsen any preexisting conditions. The technique has variations, such as using an FIS by passing the wire through the working channel or using an AEC (see Chapter 21).[277]

Although simple in concept, the basic technique has numerous potential complications. The procedure takes some time to perform and should not be considered under emergency circumstances unless the practitioner is very experienced. The tip of the ETT may get caught on the glottic structures during advancement over the wire. The problem may be alleviated somewhat by using a tapered AEC inside the ETT. Bleeding may occur at the site of the tracheal puncture in sufficient quantities to cause a tracheal clot or airway obstruction. Cases of severe hemoptysis with resultant hypoxia, cardiopulmonary arrest, arrhythmias, and death after retrograde wire intubation have been reported.[278–280] Subcutaneous emphysema localized to the area of the transtracheal needle puncture is common but usually self-limited. In severe cases, the air may track back through the fascial planes of the neck, leading to tracheal compression with resultant airway compromise, pneumomediastinum, and pneumothorax.[281,282] Laryngospasm may result from irritation by the retrograde wire unless the vocal cords are anesthetized or relaxed. Other less common complications include esophageal perforations, tracheal hematoma, laryngeal edema, infections, tracheitis, tracheal fistulas, trigeminal nerve injury, and vocal cord damage.[283,284] The complications reported with retrograde wire intubation were most often associated with multiple attempts, large-gauge needles, and untrained staff members in emergency settings.[285]

Cricothyrotomy

Two methods are described here: the surgical cricothyrotomy (using a scalpel) and the percutaneous cricothyrotomy (using a Seldinger technique). In both procedures, the cricothyroid membrane (CTM) must be perforated. Acute complications include bleeding (especially during surgical cricothyrotomy), misplacement of the tube (especially after needle cricothyrotomy), failure of airway access, wound infection, displaced cartilage fractures, and laryngotracheal separation.[286,287] Other complications include breaking and bending of the needle, subcutaneous emphysema, pneumothorax, pneumomediastinum, and pneumopericardium. When cricothyrotomy is performed in the case of total upper airway obstruction, barotrauma may occur because of expiratory blockade.

Granulation tissue around the tracheostomy site, subglottic stenosis, laryngeal mucosal trauma, endolaryngeal hematoma and laceration, vocal cord paralysis, hoarseness, and thyroid cartilage fracture with dysphasia are direct long-term complications. Every emergency translaryngeal airway should be changed to a formal tracheostomy as soon as possible to avoid the development of subglottic stenosis as a delayed complication.

Transtracheal Airway

Transtracheal Jet Ventilation

One emergency technique for oxygenation in a CICO situation is transtracheal jet ventilation (TTJV), which is accomplished by introducing a small, percutaneous catheter into the trachea through the CTM and insufflating the respiratory tract with high-pressure oxygen using a jet ventilator or a hand jet-ventilation device (e.g., the VBM Manujet). Although this technique may be helpful in critical situations, life-threatening problems can be associated with it.

To accomplish TTJV, a long large-bore catheter is advanced through the CTM into the trachea. If this catheter is displaced from the trachea, subcutaneous emphysema, hypoventilation, pneumomediastinum, pneumothorax, severe abdominal distention, or death may result.[166] The hub of the TTJV catheter must be continuously pressed firmly against the skin to prevent migration into the subcutaneous tissues.

Barotrauma is another potential complication of TTJV.[288,289] Oxygen delivered through a transtracheal catheter must be able to escape the lungs freely, or overdistention and pulmonary rupture may occur.[290,291] Any changes in breath sounds, chest wall expansion, or hemodynamics should be considered to result from pneumothorax. In cases of total airway obstruction, the risk for pneumothorax is greatly increased because gas cannot escape from the lungs in a normal manner. Strong consideration should be given to placing a second transtracheal egress catheter in these circumstances. Laryngospasm can impede the outward flow of oxygen from the trachea. It should be prevented by providing adequate local anesthesia to the neighboring structures or by relaxing the patient.[288] If the larynx is obstructed by a foreign body, only low-flow oxygen should be delivered until safe egress of gas is established. These problems may be minimized by using the Ventrain, a manually operated ventilation device that allows expiratory ventilation assistance.[292–295] Inadvertent placement of a gas delivery line into the gastrointestinal tract may result in complications including gastric rupture, esophageal perforation, bleeding, hematoma, and hemoptysis.[296,297]

Damage to the tracheal mucosa may occur in patients who are managed with long-term TTJV, especially if the gas is not humidified.[298] The possibility of tracheal mucosal ulceration should be considered in any patient if nonhumidified TTJV is attempted through single-orifice catheters for a prolonged period.

Percutaneous Dilatational Tracheostomy

Percutaneous dilatational tracheostomy is not primarily recommended for emergency use. With further development, these insertion techniques have become faster and appear to be suitable for some emergency situations in skilled hands. Several different commercial sets are available.[299–303]

Bleeding, subcutaneous and mediastinal emphysema, pneumothorax, airway obstruction, aspiration, infection, and death are early complications. Accidental extubation is a serious complication, because replacement of the cannula may be impossible. In this situation, orotracheal intubation or translaryngeal oxygenation is required.[304] Bacteremia also has been reported.[305]

Delayed complications include tracheal stenosis, scars, hoarseness, and tracheoesophageal or tracheocutaneous fistulas. The incidence of injury for percutaneous dilatational tracheostomy is 2%, which is lower than for formal tracheostomy.

Formal Tracheostomy

A formal tracheostomy is rarely recommended in emergency situations. Various types of instruments, assistance, and sterile conditions are required, and the tracheostomy should be performed only by a trained surgeon. In NAP4, emergency surgical airway was attempted in 58 (43%) of the 133 anesthesia-related reports. In 29 of these, surgical tracheostomy was the first choice for emergency surgical airway over cricothyrotomy, although is it unclear how many of these were formal tracheostomies versus percutaneous dilatational tracheostomies. Of the 25 cases where an emergency surgical airway was attempted by an anesthesiologist, 11 failures were rescued by a surgeon-performed formal tracheostomy, and 1 was rescued by percutaneous tracheostomy placed by a colleague.[306]

Bleeding is a complication of all surgical procedures, including airway access procedures. The inflated cuff used in formal tracheostomy prevents pulmonary aspiration of blood. In rare cases, the innominate artery can rupture into the trachea because of excessive pressure from the tracheostomy tube, with resultant massive hemorrhage into the airway. Air embolism during the operative procedure is possible.

If an air leak occurs and the cervical skin has healed around the tracheostomy tube, air can escape into the subcutaneous spaces of the neck, resulting in subcutaneous emphysema. If the condition goes unrecognized and the patient is maintained on high-pressure mechanical ventilation, the air may track to other locations. Air escaping into the paratracheal spaces can result in a pneumomediastinum. Air released into the pleural cavity can result in a tension pneumothorax.

Tracheal stenosis is a complication of long-term tracheostomy. A tracheostomy tube can cause tracheal erosion, particularly into the esophagus (i.e., tracheoesophageal fistula) or the brachiocephalic artery. These tubes typically sit low in the trachea and are designed with a fixed curve. Tube pressure can damage the skin at the insertion site.

Accidental extubation and dislodgment of the cannula occur occasionally, most often in the early postoperative period. If the cannula is inadvertently removed from a fresh tracheostomy, it should be replaced as quickly as possible. Infection, mediastinal sepsis, tracheal stenosis, and tracheomalacia are rare late complications.

Physiologic Responses

The larynx has the greatest afferent nerve supply of the airway. Airway reflexes are important in protection of the airway. They must be suppressed for seamless airway management, especially for tracheal intubation. Intensive autonomic responses may occur during placement, maintenance, and removal of all airway management devices.

Hemodynamic Changes

DL and tracheal intubation are potent stimuli that may instigate an intense autonomic response, regardless of the instrument used.[307–309] Tachycardia, hypertension, arrhythmias, bronchospasm, and bronchorrhea are common; hypotension and bradycardia occur less often. Patients with preexisting hypertension are even more at risk when they are under stress.

Oczenski and colleagues showed that the insertion of a Combitube was associated with a significantly higher and longer-lasting increase in systolic, diastolic, and mean arterial pressure; heart rate; and plasma catecholamine concentration compared with insertion of an LMA and laryngoscopic tracheal intubation (Fig. 48.10).[310] Hemodynamic and catecholamine responses to insertion of an LMA are minimal.[311,312] The magnitude of a stimulus to the upper airway depends on the number of attempts and the duration of intubation. In DA situations, a greater hemodynamic response should be anticipated. The sympathetically mediated responses to mechanical stimulation of the larynx, trachea, carina, and bronchi may be completely or partially blocked by topical or IV lidocaine.[313] The hemodynamic response may also be blunted by the administration of opioids or short-acting selective β$_1$-blockers before laryngoscopy and intubation.[314] In

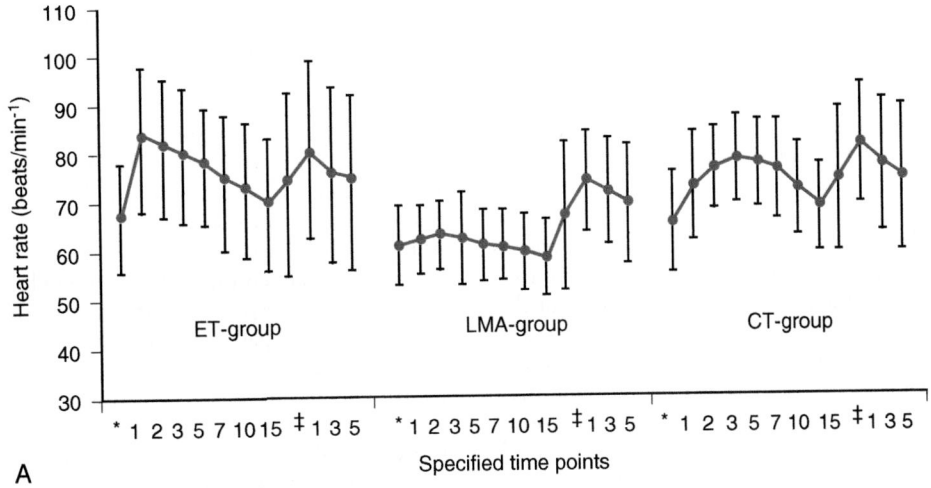

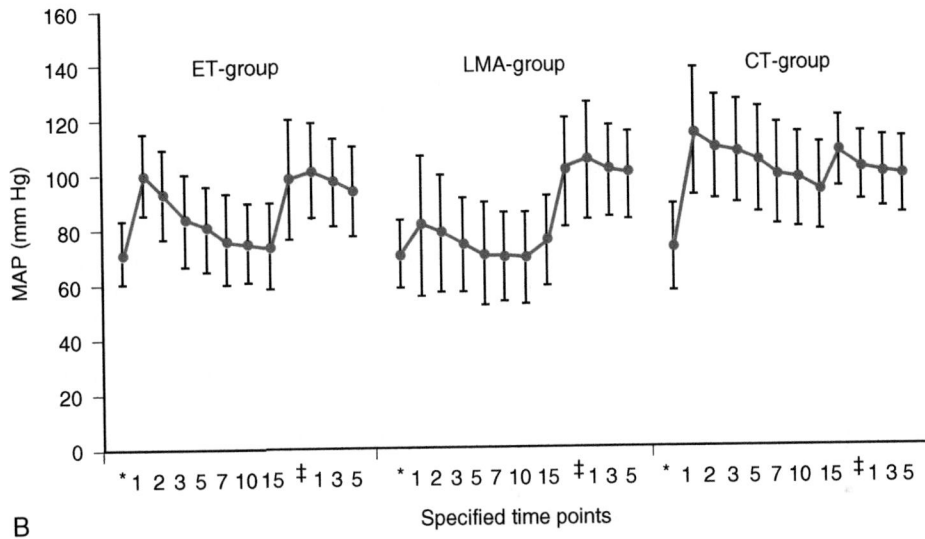

*(Baseline): immediately before intubation/insertion of the airway
‡Immediately before extubation/removal of the airway

• **Fig. 48.10** Heart rate (A) and mean arterial blood pressure (MAP) (B) at specified times (mean ± SD, n = 73) during insertion of an endotracheal tube (ET), laryngeal mask airway (LMA), and Combitube (CT). *SD*, Standard deviation. (From Oczenski W, Krenn H, Dahaba AA, et al. Hemodynamic and catecholamine stress responses to insertion of the Combitube, laryngeal mask airway or tracheal intubation. *Anesth Analg.* 1999;88:1389.)

patients with cardiovascular disease who cannot meet increased myocardial oxygen demands, large hemodynamic responses must be prevented. Over 10% of patients with myocardial disease develop some degree of myocardial ischemia during intubation.[315] The key is to provide an adequate depth of anesthesia with IV or inhalational agents before instrumentation of the airway.

Awake FSI performed under sufficient local anesthesia and conscious sedation is an appropriate technique to prevent major hemodynamic changes during intubation, although minor hemodynamic changes and minor increases in plasma catecholamine concentrations may occur. In one study, FSI resulted in fewer hemodynamic changes than DL after induction of anesthesia; the lowest cardiovascular responses were seen with LMA insertion.[316]

Laryngospasm

Laryngospasm is a vagally mediated protective reflex to prevent aspiration of foreign bodies into the trachea. It may be provoked by movement of the cervical spine, pain, vocal cord irritation by secretions, or sudden stimulation while the patient is still in a light plane of anesthesia.[317]

In some cases of laryngospasm, the patient makes respiratory efforts but cannot move air in or out of the lungs; if DL was performed, the vocal cords would be completely adducted. However, laryngospasm involves more than just spastic closure of the vocal cords. An infolding of the arytenoids and the aryepiglottic folds occurs. These structures are subsequently covered by the epiglottis.[318] Malpositioning, incorrect insertion of an

LMA, secretions or blood in the airway, and inadequate depth of anesthesia during intubation or extubation may induce laryngospasm. It may also occur during FSI performed in a patient with an unanesthetized or underanesthetized larynx. A firm jaw thrust can sometimes break laryngospasm; the hyoid is elevated, thereby stretching the epiglottis and aryepiglottic folds to open the forced closure.

When managing laryngospasm, the stimulus should be removed, a change of airway should be considered, and secretions should be suctioned. Positive pressure by mask with 100% oxygen may help by distending the pharynx or vocal cords, but this technique is not always successful. Gentle chest compression in children or a Larson maneuver (firm inward pressure in the notch situated slightly cephalad to the earlobe and between the mastoid process [posteriorly] and mandibular condyle [anteriorly]) may also help.[319] Deepening the plane of anesthesia with small doses of IV propofol (0.25–0.8 mg/kg) has been shown to successfully treat laryngospasm. Alternatively, laryngospasm can be treated with a short-acting muscle relaxant, such as succinylcholine (0.1–0.3 mg/kg).[319] Topical or IV administration of lidocaine is effective in preventing laryngospasm in children.[320]

Bronchospasm

Tracheal irritation from the ETT can cause bronchospasm that is sufficiently severe to prevent air movement throughout the lungs.[321] Approximately 80% of the measurable resistance to airflow occurs in the large central airways; the remaining 20% occurs in the smaller peripheral bronchioles.[322] The incidence of intraoperative bronchospasm is nearly 9% with tracheal intubation, 0.13% with an LMA, but almost 0% with mask ventilation.[323,324] Poor correlation is seen with age, sex, duration or severity of reactive airway disease, duration of anesthesia, or the FEV_1 (forced expiratory volume in 1 second).[325] Other factors that may contribute to bronchospasm include release of allergic mediators, viral infections, or pharmacologic factors (including β-blockers, prostaglandin inhibitors, and anticholinesterases). Bronchospasm may occur during fiberoptic intubation if parts of the subglottic airway are insufficiently anesthetized. Bronchospasm can be treated with inhalation of epinephrine, isoproterenol, or a $β_2$-agonist (e.g., albuterol or terbutaline) or by deepening the level of a volatile anesthetic.

Coughing and Bucking

Two additional adverse responses to intubation are coughing and bucking on the ETT.[325,326] These responses are potentially hazardous in cases of increased intracranial pressure,[326] intracranial vascular anomalies, open-globe injury or ophthalmologic surgery, or in cases where increased intraabdominal pressure may rupture an abdominal incision.[327] Intubating a patient only when an adequate depth of anesthesia has been achieved helps to prevent this reflex.

Coughing and bucking occur less frequently with the LMA; however, they can occur as a result of light anesthesia, malpositioning, or excess lubricant falling into the airway.

Vomiting, Regurgitation, and Aspiration

The overall incidence of aspiration during general anesthesia has been reported to range from 1 in 2131 procedures (in Sweden) to 1 in 14,150 procedures (in France). The incidence in the United States was 1 in 3216 procedures with an associated mortality rate of 1 in 71,829 cases.[328] A meta-analysis of 547 publications

regarding use of the LMA suggested that the overall incidence of pulmonary aspiration was about 2 in 10,000 cases.[329] Tracheal intubation and devices with an esophageal cuff, such as the Combitube, are the most effective airway management strategies for preventing pulmonary aspiration. To reduce the risk of pulmonary aspiration, SGAs such as the LMA ProSeal, the LMA Supreme, and the King LT-S were designed. An analysis of 700 patients for elective and urgent cesarean section found no cases of aspiration using an LMA Supreme Airway.[330]

In any patient considered to have a full stomach, the likelihood of vomiting in response to irritation of the airway is increased, and aspiration of gastric contents is a concern. Aspiration leads to coughing, laryngospasm, and bronchospasm, assuming that protective reflexes are intact. Hypertonia, bradycardia, asystole, and hypoxia may occur. The eventual effect of pulmonary aspiration is a chemical pneumonitis, which can be mild to fatally severe, depending on the type and quantity of the aspirated material (see Chapter 14).[331]

The use of CP, also known as the Sellick maneuver, is controversial. Although some strongly endorse the technique and trust its effectiveness, others think that CP should be abandoned because it may add to the risk of aspiration (as a result of increased difficulty with airway management and a decrease in lower esophageal sphincter tone) with no evidence of gained benefit. Other practitioners apply CP because they believe it is a low-risk technique that may work in some patients. The future of CP use lies in the answer to the question of whether it is effective in preventing regurgitation or an unnecessary hazard.[332]

It is possible to completely obstruct the airway with CP. CP has resulted in airway obstruction in patients with lingual tonsillar hypertrophy, lingual thyroid glands,[333] and undiagnosed laryngeal trauma.[334] If any doubt exists about the success of an oral intubation in a patient at high risk for aspiration, awake intubation techniques should be considered.[335]

Intraocular Pressure Changes

Intraocular pressure increases during DL and extubation but not during LMA insertion.[336,337] Decreased intraocular pressure was observed during tracheal intubation under general anesthesia with both propofol and sevoflurane combined with remifentanil.[338]

Sufentanil is effective in preventing intraocular pressure increases caused by rapid sequence induction (RSI) with succinylcholine; alternatively, rocuronium can be used.[339] More recently, dexmedetomidine was found to attenuate IOP during routine and RSI of anesthesia.[340,341] Increased intraocular pressure should be strictly avoided in patients with penetrating eye injuries.

Intracranial Pressure Changes

Intracranial pressure markedly and transiently rises during laryngoscopy and tracheal intubation. Patients with head injury are at risk from this increase because it reduces cerebral perfusion and may increase the likelihood of secondary brain damage.[342] Flexible bronchoscopy produces a substantial but transient increase in intracranial pressure.[343] Deep anesthesia during induction can prevent these adverse effects.

Latex Allergy

In the 1980s, a striking increase in natural rubber latex allergy was seen. Since then, many measures have been taken to prevent latex allergy, and a significant decline in the number of patients sensitized/clinically allergic to latex has been reported.[344] In the late 1990s, 16.6% of all anaphylactic events occurring during surgical procedures were related to latex allergies.[345] Latex rubber is thought to be the second most common trigger for anaphylactic reactions during anesthesia in many studies, whereas other investigations have found latex-induced anaphylaxis to be less common.[346,347] Although the reasons for this are not known, a possible explanation is that hospitals have adopted latex-free measures in many clinical areas, which may have reduced exposure rates and sensitization.

To prevent anaphylaxis during anesthesia and surgery, the patient's history should be evaluated preoperatively. There is no therapy for latex allergy, and avoidance of latex-containing products is mandatory for predisposed individuals.[348] Latex allergy affects 8% of the US general population and has a prevalence of 30% among healthcare workers.[349,350] The prevalence of latex sensitivity among anesthesiologists is about 12.5%, and the prevalence of allergy is 2.4%.[351]

Patients with spina bifida, rubber industry workers, atopic patients, and patients with a history of multiple previous surgeries are most at risk.[352] Patients with certain fruit allergies (e.g., banana, kiwi, or strawberry) may also have a coexisting latex allergy[353]; in one study, the rate was 86%.[354]

Patients with type I hypersensitivity are at risk for anaphylaxis with hypotension, rash, and bronchospasm. Type I hypersensitivity symptoms are localized contact urticaria with pruritus and edema. Generalized reactions include rash or hives, tearing, rhinitis, hoarseness, dyspnea, nausea, vomiting, bronchospasm, abdominal cramping, and diarrhea.

Exposure to latex during anesthesia is possible through direct contact from face masks, endotracheal and gastric tubes, gloves, syringes, and electrodes; through inhalation from contaminated circuits and room air; and through the parenteral path with latex-containing IV administration sets.

Most airway management devices are available as latex-free products. The oropharyngeal cuff of the Combitube contains latex; therefore, it is contraindicated in patients with known latex allergy. All anesthesiology departments should have a special latex-safe cart with all medical supplies and devices.

Complications With Extubation

Several complications are associated with extubation, including local and systemic responses (Box 48.1). The same responses after intubation may be observed at extubation. During intubation, the patient is more protected by the induction of anesthesia induction, so hemodynamic responses may be even more exaggerated during extubation. The most serious complication after extubation is acute airway obstruction. Decreased consciousness with central respiratory depression, decreased muscle tone, and tongue collapse to the posterior pharyngeal wall may lead to inspiratory or expiratory stridor, dyspnea, cyanosis, tachycardia, hypertension, agitation, and sweating. Laryngospasm is also possible, and urgent treatment is necessary to prevent hypoxia, brain damage, and death. Other complications after extubation are not caused by the removal of the tube itself; they are consequences of the previous intubation efforts and the duration of tube placement, such as laryngitis, edema, ulcerations, granuloma, or synechiae of the vocal cords. The quality of tracheal intubation contributes to laryngeal morbidity, and excellent intubating conditions are less frequently associated with postoperative hoarseness and vocal cord sequelae.

• BOX 48.1 Pathophysiologic Effects of Tracheal Extubation

Primary Local Effects

Airway
Obstruction
Coughing
Breath-holding
Damage to the vocal cords
Arytenoid dislocation/subluxation

Primary Systemic Effects

Cardiovascular System
Tachycardia
Increased systemic arterial pressure
Increased pulmonary arterial pressure

Secondary Effects

Central Nervous System
Increased intracranial pressure

Eyes
Increased intraocular pressure

Modified from Hartley M. Difficulties in tracheal extubation. In Latto IP, Vaughan RS, eds. *Difficulties in Tracheal Intubation.* Saunders; 1997.

Hemodynamic Changes

Hemodynamic changes, including a 20% increase in heart rate and blood pressure, occur in most patients at the time of extubation,[355,356] and symptoms that are associated with sympathoadrenal activity should be expected. These changes are usually transient and rarely require treatment. Although most patients tolerate these hemodynamic responses well, patients with cardiac disease, pregnancy-induced hypertension,[357] and increased intracranial pressure may be at particular risk for life-threatening ischemic myocardial episodes.[358] Cerebral hemorrhage is possible. Patients with cardiac disease have had decreased ejection fractions at the time of extubation.[358] Management consists of extubation under deep anesthesia or pharmacologic therapy. Deep extubation is inappropriate for patients with a DA, those at high risk for aspiration, and those with compromised airway access. Pharmacologic strategies emphasize the importance of decreasing the heart rate, such as with short-acting β-blockers.[359] Topical local anesthetics or IV lidocaine can effectively reduce hemodynamic responses and coughing during extubation of the trachea.[360,361] Using an SGA may significantly reduce local and cardiovascular responses at removal if the cuff pressure is minimized to avoid overstimulation of the patient.[37]

Laryngospasm

A recent study found a higher incidence of severe and critical respiratory events at extubation (i.e., laryngospasm, bronchospasm, or postoperative stridor) of 3.9% in children undergoing ENT surgery, as compared to 2.6% in children undergoing non-ENT surgery. Risk factors include younger age, history of snoring, recent upper respiratory tract infection, and recent wheezing.[362]

The optimal course for treating laryngospasm is to avoid it in the first place. (Treatment was described above.) When laryngospasm is anticipated, the patient may undergo a deep extubation.

A patient undergoing deep extubation should be placed in the lateral position with the head down to keep the vocal cords clear of secretions during emergence. It is best to extubate patients during a positive-pressure breath to remove residual secretions. A study showed that children could be safely extubated under deep anesthesia with 1.5 MAC (minimum alveolar concentration) of sevoflurane or desflurane.[363] Koga and colleagues showed that the rate of airway obstruction in patients extubated during deep anesthesia (17 of 20) was not higher than in patients extubated after they regained consciousness (18 of 20).[364]

Laryngeal Edema

Laryngeal edema is an important cause of postextubation obstruction, especially in neonates and infants. This condition has various causes and can be classified as supraglottic, retroarytenoidal, or subglottic.[365] Supraglottic edema most commonly results from surgical manipulation, positioning, hematoma formation, overaggressive fluid management, impaired venous drainage, or coexisting conditions (e.g., preeclampsia or angioedema). Retroarytenoidal edema typically results from local trauma or irritation. Subglottic edema occurs most often in children, particularly neonates and infants. Factors associated with the development of subglottic edema include traumatic intubation, intubation lasting longer than 1 hour, bucking on the ETT, changes in head position, or tight-fitting tubes. Laryngeal edema usually manifests as stridor within 30 to 60 minutes after extubation, although it may start as late as 6 hours after extubation. Regardless of the cause of laryngeal edema, management depends on the severity of the condition. Therapy consists of humidified oxygen, nebulized epinephrine, head-up positioning, and occasionally reintubation with a smaller ETT. The practice of administering parenteral steroids with the goal of preventing or reducing edema after long-term (>36 hours) ventilation may prove beneficial for adult patients, but routine administration for anesthesia is controversial.[366]

Laryngotracheal Trauma

Unlike trauma during intubation, airway trauma at the time of extubation is not well described. Arytenoid cartilage dislocation has been reported after difficult and routine intubations.[136,367] Symptoms become apparent soon after extubation and may be mild (e.g., difficulty swallowing, voice changes) or major (e.g., complete airway obstruction). Management depends on the severity of the condition. Options include reintubation, arytenoid reduction, and tracheostomy. If laryngotracheal trauma is suspected, an otolaryngology consultation is warranted.

Bronchospasm

In patients at risk for bronchospasm, the timing of extubation is important. These patients may be extubated during deep anesthesia (if this approach can be used safely) or when they are fully awake and airway reflexes have recovered. Although the degree of spasm in this condition may be severe, it is usually self-limited and short-lived.

Negative-Pressure Pulmonary Edema

When airway obstruction occurs after extubation in the case of laryngospasm, negative-pressure pulmonary edema may occur in a spontaneously breathing patient. As a result of inspiratory effort against a closed glottis, patients can generate a negative intrapleural pressure of more than 100 cm H_2O. Rib retraction with poor air movement, laryngospasm, and stridor may lead to the rare diagnosis. Increased left ventricular preload and afterload, altered pulmonary vascular resistance, increased adrenergic state, right ventricle dilation, intraventricular septum shift to the left, left ventricular diastolic dysfunction, increased left heart loading conditions, enhanced microvascular intramural hydrostatic pressure, negative pleural pressure, and transmission to the lung interstitium may result in a marked increase in transmural pressure, fluid filtration into the lung, and development of pulmonary edema.[368]

Negative-pressure pulmonary edema is seen within minutes after extubation. Hemoptysis and alveolar hemorrhage are rare symptoms. Management involves removing the obstruction, supporting the patient with oxygen, monitoring the patient closely, and reducing the afterload. CPAP therapy is useful, and reintubation is occasionally necessary. Most cases resolve spontaneously without further complications.

Aspiration

Pulmonary aspiration of gastric contents is a constant threat for any patient who has a full stomach or is at risk for postoperative vomiting. Laryngeal function is altered after tracheal extubation.[369] Coughing is a physiologic response to protect the airway from aspiration. Depression of reflexes, along with the presence of residual anesthetic agents, places most recently extubated patients at risk. Aspiration is probably more prevalent than is appreciated; most cases are so minor that they do not affect the patient's postoperative course. Reducing gastric contents by suctioning through a gastric tube and extubation with the patient placed in the lateral position with a head-down tilt are the safest protections against aspiration. Perioperative problems in minor cases, if they do occur, are usually attributed to factors such as atelectasis. Management consists of supportive measures. Depending on the extent of aspiration, measures include supportive care, ranging from administration of oxygen through a nasal cannula to reintubation with mechanical ventilation, bronchoscopy, and PEEP.

Airway Compression

External compression of the airway after extubation may lead to obstruction. An excessively tight postoperative neck dressing is a cause of external compression that is easily resolved. A more ominous situation is a rapidly expanding hematoma close to the airway. This may occur after certain operations, such as carotid endarterectomy, and must be quickly diagnosed and treated before total airway obstruction occurs.[370] Immediate surgical reexploration is indicated, although the airway concerns for these patients should be approached with extreme caution. To minimize airway distortion, general anesthesia should be avoided until the wound is evacuated under local anesthesia. However, even after surgical drainage, airway obstruction may occur as a result of venous or lymphatic congestion. The use of neuromuscular blockade during anesthetic induction in these patients may result in catastrophe, regardless of whether the wound was previously drained. Conservative options for managing the airway in this situation include awake FSI, surgical airways, or inhalational induction. Strong consideration should be given to avoidance of neuromuscular blockade until the airway is secured.

External compression of the neck, such as from chronic compression from a goiter, may also lead to tracheomalacia.[371] This condition is usually seen after the goiter has been removed, although cases were reported in which the airway collapsed with induction or after extubation.[372,373] Airway obstruction in these patients becomes apparent soon after extubation. Management includes reintubation, surgical tracheal support (i.e., stenting), or tracheostomy below the level of obstruction.

Difficult Extubation

Occasionally, ETTs are difficult to remove. Possible causes are failure to deflate the cuff, use of an oversized tube,[374] adhesion of the tube to the tracheal wall,[375] or fixation of the tube by an inadvertent suture to a nearby organ, a wire, a screw placed in an oromaxillofacial operation, or a broken drill.[376–380] Possible sequelae of these complications include airway leak, aspiration, tube obstruction, and trauma from attempts at forceful extubation. One case was reported in which a nasogastric tube made a loop around the ETT.[381] In most cases, the problem arises from an inability to deflate the cuff, commonly as a result of failure in the cuff-deflating mechanism. If this problem occurs, the cuff should be punctured with a transtracheal needle. If tube fixation is suspected, the lumen of the tube should be checked with a suction catheter or an FIS. Forceful removal of an ETT with the cuff inflated may result in damage to the vocal cords or arytenoid dislocation.

Accidental Extubation

Accidental extubation during anesthesia has been reported with disposable tonsillectomy instruments,[382] change of the patient's head position, and in neurosurgery with the patient in the knee-elbow position.[383] Most accidental extubations were reported from intensive care unit patients, for whom self-extubation was the most common incident at 77% to 85%. The rate of reintubation was 37% to 57%.[384–386] The requirement for reintubation is higher for patients with full ventilatory support than for patients during the weaning phase.

Patients at risk for accidental extubation are characterized by the absence of physical restraints, a high nurse-to-patient ratio, trips out of the intensive care unit (59%), light sedation (43%), use of bedside portable radiography, accidental removal of the nasogastric tube or tugging on the ETT, oral intubation, and insufficient sedation.[387] Complications after accidental extubation may be hypoxia, hypercarbic respiratory failure, aspiration, retention of pulmonary secretions, arrhythmias, and tachycardia. To avoid unplanned extubation, ETTs can be secured with special tube holders,[388,389] with waterproof tape, and with fixation using a knot or a bow.[390,391]

Reintubation may be very difficult, especially after a difficult intubation. The use of a Combitube or an SGA is required in some cases of inadequate access to the patient's head in the intensive care setting.[392]

Conclusion

Anesthesiologists face many challenges and complications when managing airways. Errors may be technical or judgmental. By learning from the mistakes of the past, we can avoid or minimize them by anticipating problems, devising safe primary and backup plans for every patient, maintaining vigilance throughout all operative procedures, and using common sense at all times.

Selected References

25. El-Orbany M, Woehlck HJ. Difficult mask ventilation. *Anesth Analg.* 2009;109:1870.
38. Seet E, Yousaf F, Gupta S, et al. Use of manometry for laryngeal mask airway reduces postoperative pharyngolaryngeal adverse events: a prospective, randomized trial. *Anesthesiology.* 2010;112:652.
45. Brimacombe J, Clarke G, Keller C. Lingual nerve injury associated with the ProSeal laryngeal mask airway: a case report and review of the literature. *Br J Anaesth.* 2005;95:420.
55. Benumof JL. Laryngeal mask airway and the ASA difficult airway algorithm. *Anesthesiology.* 1996;84:686.
63. López AM, Valero R, Brimacombe J. Insertion and use of the LMA Supreme in the prone position. *Anaesthesia.* 2010;65:154.
84. Benumof JL, Cooper SD. Quantitative improvement in laryngoscopic view by optimal external laryngeal manipulation. *J Clin Anesth.* 1996;8:136.
86. Mihai R, Blair E, Kay H, Cook TM. A quantitative review and meta-analysis of performance of non-standard laryngoscopes and rigid fibreoptic intubation aids. *Anaesthesia.* 2008;63:745.
174. Ghafoor AU, Martin TW, Gopalakrishnan S, Viswamitra S. Caring for the patients with cervical spine injuries: What have we learned? *J Clin Anesth.* 2005;17:640.
193. Martin DP, Weingarten TN, Gunn PW, et al. Performance improvement system and postoperative corneal injuries: incidence and risk factors. *Anesthesiology.* 2009;111:320.
335. El-Orbany M, Connolly LA. Rapid sequence induction and intubation: current controversy. *Anesth Analg.* 2010;110:1318.
386. Tanios MA, Epstein SK, Livelo J, Teres D. Can we identify patients at high risk for unplanned extubation? A large-scale multidisciplinary survey. *Respir Care.* 2010;55:561.

All references can be found online at eBooks.Health.Elsevier.com.

PART 7

Societal Considerations

49

Airway Management Education

PAUL ANDREW BAKER, SABINE NABECKER, AND ROBERT GREIF

CHAPTER OUTLINE

KEY POINTS

- Maintaining expertise in airway management is the responsibility of every airway practitioner. This responsibility extends throughout one's professional career and reaches far beyond the formative years of medical training into lifelong learning to stay competent.
- The essential ingredients of expertise are the willingness to become an expert, deliberate practice, immediate feedback, problem solving, and evaluation with an opportunity to modify or repeat performance.
- Traditional in situ education in the operating room can be optimized and structured to minimize any adverse effect on patient care. Background knowledge and skill can be assessed before entering the operating room, educational goals can be clarified, and supervision is provided during the case with immediate feedback.
- The features of a good clinical teacher include good content knowledge combined with an ability to provide a positive learning environment, excellent listening skills, constructive feedback even in difficult situations, and enthusiasm for education and the learners.
  - Simulation-based medical education (SBME) provides valuable opportunities to supplement or even supplant traditional clinical training. Procedural and nontechnical skills can be developed and assessed in an environment that is safe for the patient, the learner, and the instructor. Training is conducted without patient involvement where mistakes can be safely repeated, procedures can be interrupted for feedback, difficult scenarios can be rehearsed, and trainees can learn at their own rate. Short, structured briefing before the case and debriefing after can be rehearsed and this habit can be integrated into daily clinical practice.
- Assessment provides a vital link between airway management education and improved patient care. Learning should be measured and performance assessed to meet defined levels of expertise. Ideally, these standards of performance should be associated with patient audits to ensure improved patient care. Signing off for independent practice is based on a new educational concept: entrusted professional activities.
- There are many opportunities to improve education in airway management. Research is required to expand the opportunities offered by SBME. Assessment techniques should be implemented and refined, and training options should be evaluated to establish the value of new opportunities provided by remote learning.

Introduction

Education, along with research and clinical patient care, is one of the three pillars of academic medicine. For any practitioner engaged in airway management, education is an essential requirement for their own development and as a teacher imparting knowledge and skill to junior or senior colleagues. Generally, those "airway teachers" are expected to display a high standard of knowledge, procedural skill, and professionalism throughout their careers. Sadly, these standards sometimes fall short and, consequently, that can lead to patient harm. This was reported in the Fourth National Audit Project (NAP4) of the Royal College of Anaesthetists and the Difficult Airway Society. In that audit 184 patients with severe airway morbidity or mortality were reviewed by an expert panel looking for causal or contributory factors. Poor judgment (59%) and inadequate education or training (49%) were the second and third most common contributory factors of risk, respectively, after patient factors (77%). Deficiencies in airway assessment, failure to follow an airway plan, inappropriate use of supraglottic airways, and underutilization of awake intubation were found. Difficult, delayed, and failed tracheal intubation accounted for 39% of adverse events identified in this UK survey. That was a kind of "wake-up call," and suddenly, airway management was in the middle of the debate to improve the anesthetist's performance and patient safety. Over the last decade, new concepts from education research have been developed and new opportunities for teaching are now available, which are being applied to develop a safer approach to airway management.

Before embarking on a detailed discussion of education for airway management, it would be helpful to understand where the deficiencies remain. An international survey conducted in 61 countries, including 4948 individual questionnaires, found deficiencies in accessing practice guidelines and key airway equipment, particularly in low-income countries (LIC).[1] For example, in low-resource settings emergency front-of-the-neck equipment was available in less than 60% and videolaryngoscopes in less than 50% of locations. In total, 91% of the respondents agreed that airway management skills should be assessed, and 60% of respondents thought training should be mandatory for trainees, but only 34% felt it should be mandatory for continuing medical education. Lack of confidence performing a number of skills was reported, including emergency invasive airway access, awake intubation with a flexible intubation scope (FIS), intubation via a supraglottic airway (SGA), asleep FIS, and retrograde intubation.[1] Similar findings were reported in a Danish survey, where most anesthesiologists rated their competence as high or very high for basic airway management. Conversely, confidence dropped for advanced airway management techniques, where low procedural volume was a problem.[2]

In this chapter we will review the strengths and weaknesses of current education practice in airway management and identify areas for improvement. We will examine the role of simulation-based medical education (SBME) and review other opportunities to expand airway management competencies. Undergraduate and postgraduate airway management education and the importance of lifelong learning for all persons dealing with airway management will be considered, along with the importance of training the airway trainers and faculty development. Consideration of human factor training, leadership development, and current concepts in airway management research will conclude the chapter. The reader will not be surprised that very little specific evidence exists about education in airway management. Very often, approaches and results from studies in other fields of medicine need to be translated for their use in the teaching and learning of airway procedures. That again leads to a call for high-impact research in airway management education.

Clinical Teaching

Most airway practitioners have learned airway management at work, by acquiring practical skills and maybe learning from a mentor while attending to patients. This apprenticeship model of medical education can be traced back over a hundred years and is still a widely applied form of medical education for airway management. At the turn of the 20th century, Dr. William Osler and Dr. William Halsted from Johns Hopkins Hospital were the first to formalize and structure medical training and are credited with laying the foundations for our current residency training programs. Emphasis was placed on mentors, behavioral modeling, rotations, and evidence-based medicine.[3] Halsted characterized surgical teaching in three phases: "See one, do one and teach one." This stepwise learning was a good idea at the time. Medical trainees first observed someone performing a procedure, then after understanding the procedure, they performed it, mostly under supervision, and after mastering a skill, the final aim was to teach the procedure.[4] Halsted's idea about resident education revolutionized medical education as it meant not "learning by doing" and is not that far away from currently applied teaching practice. Exposure to cases to gain experience and competence is still widely discussed with very diverse opinions.[5-7] The current question is how can we train young doctors without jeopardizing safety or harming patients when performing procedures for the first time, as well as in subsequent practice?[8]

1. In many anesthesia teaching institutions this traditional apprenticeship model of medical education is still regarded as the standard for teaching. Learning airway management during patient care has obvious advantages of involving real anatomy, physiology, and pathology with a wide range of patient presentations. Despite these positive features, there are many difficulties and inadequacies associated with the apprenticeship model. It is becoming increasingly difficult for trainees to find sufficient time in their rotations to gain expertise in managing a challenging or difficult airway. Skill development takes time, and that time varies between individuals. In the interest of patient safety and the well-being of doctors at their workplace, limitations have recently been imposed on trainee working hours. In Europe that limit is between 40 and 56 hours per week, and 80 in the United States. Restrictions have also been imposed on the duration of on-call time and a requirement for time off after being on-call. These initiatives are designed to reduce fatigue and burnout, but inevitably they impact education and training time, as well as case load. The apprenticeship model relies on exposure to patients with normal and abnormal airways and the availability of a dedicated airway teacher for supervision and guidance. Due to the low incidence of many complex airway problems, it can take a long time to gain the required experience necessary to be considered trustworthy at managing a difficult airway (Table 49.1).

New concepts were introduced, defining not only competencies but also skilled performance that enable supervisors to trust a learner in their performance.[9] These Entrustable Professional Activities (EPAs) are a further development of the

TABLE 49.1	Incidence of Various Types of Difficult Airways in Adults
Difficult intubation	6.2%[155]
Difficult bag-mask ventilation	1.4%[156]
Difficult bag-mask ventilation, difficult laryngoscopy	0.4%[155]
Impossible bag-mask ventilation	0.15%[157]
Impossible laryngeal mask	1.1%[158]
Impossible intubation, difficult bag-mask ventilation	0.3%[155]
Impossible intubation, impossible ventilation	0.0019%[157]

From Baker P. Assessment before airway management. *Anesthesiol Clin.* 2015;33:257–278; with permission.

apprenticeship model as still the "master" defines the EPA and the learner needs to reach these aims with all the limitations described before.[10]

2. During the formative stage of skill development, patients are exposed to novices with an increased risk of side effects and complications. For example, paramedics intubating in an emergency prehospital situation had a 36% failed intubation rate and 11% unrecognized esophageal intubation rate. All of these patients were subsequently successfully intubated by prehospital physicians.[11] Failed intubation and esophageal intubation are associated with a high incidence of morbidity and mortality, demanding close supervision of novices during their skill development.[12] Similar results were seen with emergency physicians engaged in out-of-hospital retrieval medicine, where high rates of esophageal and endobronchial intubation were reported.[13]

3. Teaching in the operating room can increase the workload of the tutor and may cause distraction by diverting attention away from the patient.[14] The often noisy environment with a lot of people in the room does not create a learning-suitable climate for both the learner and the airway teacher.[15]

4. Training in the operating room has financial implications. Clinical bronchoscopy takes 50% longer when a trainee is involved and 18 minutes can be added to procedure time. There is also a threefold increase in complication rates.[16] Operating room efficiency often takes precedence over teaching, and therefore trainees can be neglected during rapid turnover operating sessions.[17]

5. Ethical issues arise concerning patient safety when unorthodox techniques or unnecessary procedures are used for clinical training. Selecting an SGA for teaching when a tracheal intubation might have been a safer option or distorting the larynx to create a difficult intubation are examples where patient safety could have been compromised.[18–21] Ideally, patients should be informed and give consent for trainee care, particularly when that trainee is performing a complex procedure such as flexible bronchoscopy for the first time.

6. Trainees find it confusing when they are exposed to a range of different tutors and a lack of standardization.[22] A very disturbing downside of the apprenticeship model is when instructors each have "their own way."

These issues have prompted a reassessment of the apprenticeship model for airway management training. Alternative training methods have the potential to supplement or even replace traditional clinical teaching with the aim to educate more efficiently and overcome the deficiencies of the apprenticeship model by dealing with a limited clinical case load.

The Features of a Good Clinical Teacher

Effective education in airway management is far easier with a mentor who is interested in the learners and wants to facilitate the development of cognitive and practical skill, as well as personal and professional growth, to an expert level. Most clinicians have not received any formal education as a clinical teacher, but teach-the-teacher courses are becoming more common and certain characteristics have been identified as worthy attributes for this task. Many of the attributes of a good clinical teacher relate to their personality.[23,24] The features of a good clinical teacher include good content knowledge and clinical skills, combined with an ability to create a positive learning environment, have excellent listening skills, provide feedback (even in distressing and embarrassing situations), and show general enthusiasm[25] for teaching. These attributes apply particularly to medical teaching but also are required of clinical teachers who serve as a specialty role model for the learners and their situation. Senior faculty often act as a coach in short-term rotations, achieving previously established educational goals, but can act as mentors to junior faculty and reinforce positive attributes in long-term relationships over residencies and beyond.[24,26–29]

Providing feedback is viewed increasingly as a normal component of the teacher–learner relationship in both directions, to the learner but also from the residents to the teaching staff.[30] Feedback extends into debriefing competencies, which are components of excellence in teaching.[31] Such teaching excellence needs to be recognized and rewarded by the corresponding institutions and educational bodies as it improves the performance of faculty and prevents burnout.[32,33] Bould et al. identified techniques to improve clinical teaching, which emphasize the importance of constructive and supportive feedback[34] (Table 49.2).

Creating a Learning Experience

Effective learning experiences can be created before and after clinical contact. This also minimizes the impact of some of the problems already discussed, including distraction from patient care during teaching and the creation of a proper learning climate.[35] It is important before the case for the learner to establish familiarity with the level of knowledge, competence, and understanding of the airway problem of the patient. In learner-centered education the specific educational goals can be discussed and defined and the teacher might seek agreement with the learner on the teaching plan that describes how the learner is going to achieve their objective with the help of the teacher. An educational goal to achieve competency in a particular task is intimately linked to the level of knowledge and prevailing skill of the learner. A novice achieving competency at holding a face mask on a patient with normal morphology is quite a different educational goal from that demanded of an advanced trainee who is required to hold a face mask on a patient with a difficult airway due to a beard. Theoretical concepts can be acquired beforehand by reading or video-assisted instruction appropriate for the learner. The concrete techniques can be discussed and rehearsed on a manikin outside the operating room prior to patient contact. The concept of the "flipped classroom" to engage the learners with the theoretical background before

TABLE 49.2	Techniques to Improve Clinical Teaching in the Operating Room

Before the Case
- Identify the learner's basic level of knowledge[23]
- Identify learning goals[159]

During the Case
- Help the learner develop an anesthetic action/organization plan for each patient[23]
- Use an open-ended questioning approach to challenge understanding[23]
- Challenge the learner to be prepared for the unexpected[23]
- Provide supervision appropriate to the case[23]

After the Case
- Find time for feedback[23,160]
- Feedback should focus on the task, not the individual's personality[161]
- Feedback should focus on one or two items to prevent overwhelming the learner[161]
- Feedback should not undermine self-esteem but should not simply consist of praise[160,161]
- Feedback can be delayed, but the information that informs the feedback should not be recorded retrospectively.[160] Feedback is most effective if given at the time of an event or shortly afterward
- Motivation to recipients benefit from authentic feedback that facilitates the learner's own reflections[160]
- Feedback should include a discussion of what the learner can practically do to improve future performance[161]
- Constructive feedback includes reflection on and understanding of items to be corrected, including an action plan of change developed by the recipient of the feedback

From Bould MD, Naik VN, Hamstra SJ. Review article: new directions in medical education related to anesthesiology and perioperative medicine. *Can J Anaesth.* 2012;59:136–150; with permission. From references 19, 28–30.

being involved with a patient in the OR or in the classroom setting is highly effective and accommodates the busy clinical environment by allowing the learner to enter directly into the clinical education of the airway skill.[36–39] After the case, debriefing provides constructive and corrective feedback, which will further enhance the learning experience (Table 49.2).

Miller's Learning Pyramid

A useful concept that relates clinical skills, competence, performance, and assessment is Miller's learning pyramid[9,40] (Fig. 49.1). Four stages are described: knows, knows how, shows how, and does. This concept can apply to the development of a procedural skill with an airway device such as an SGA. Equally, nontechnical skills can develop with this model. These stages can be conducted outside the operating room using simulation with assessment and feedback provided at each level. The final stage of "does" leads to the transfer of the newly developed skill into the clinical environment.

The base of Miller's learning pyramid is the cognitive knowledge level, which forms the foundation upon which all other

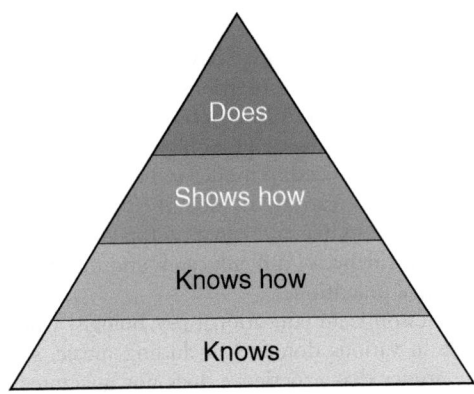

Fig. 49.1 Miller's pyramid. This diagram illustrates hierarchical levels of performance that can be used to assess learning. The bottom two levels refer to cognition: "knows" refers to the retention of factual information, and "knows how" refers to the interpretation and integration of this knowledge into a management plan. The top two levels describe behavior: "shows how" refers to a demonstration of learning, and "does" refers to an assessment of actual clinical practice. (Modified from Bould MD, Naik VN, Hamstra SJ. Review article: new directions in medical education related to anesthesiology and perioperative medicine. *Can J Anaesth.* 2012;59:136–150; with permission.)

aspects of learning rest. This "knows" level is commonly assessed by using written objective tests. The "knows how" level requires the ability of the learner to manipulate and apply knowledge and the understanding of relationships between concepts in an appropriate way to suit the environment. This would require the learner to explain the context of use, the technical details of ancillary equipment. This "knows how" level usually is assessed by written and online (gaming) tests with problem solving or oral examinations. The "shows how" level may require a standardized simulation exercise on manikins, incorporating learners' communication skills and a demonstration of the appropriate use of devices or techniques in a safe nonclinical environment. This demonstration is assessed mostly in standardized observations or measurements, like objective structured clinical exams (OSCE) in a simulation environment or with simulated patients, and often accompanied by feedback. The "does" level may occur under supervision at the workplace with assessment by the direct clinical observation of procedural skills (DOPS) or clinical encounters (Mini-CEX) in the clinical environment, including multisource feedback.[41] Recently, a fifth top level has been proposed,[9] namely, trust of clinical responsibilities in learners working without supervision or assistance. That means the readiness to cope and the capability to adapt to familiar and unfamiliar challenges in clinical practice as needed. That might be assessed during observation of clinical practice and risk assessment.

Developing Expertise in Airway Management

An expert airway practitioner needs to be able to manage a broad range of challenging and difficult airways. How can that expertise be acquired? Traditionally it has been assumed that with experience, expertise will follow. Similarly, training has been based on the volume of practice to reach a satisfactory level of competence. A study found that it took 200 tracheal intubations under supervision to achieve 95% success in the operating room.[42] Based on the figures from Table 49.1, it could take a very long time for a trainee or a young specialist to gain significant exposure to managing rare events such as difficult or failed intubation. Another study examined the learning curve for SGA and found that supervision was required for the first 40 insertions.[43] This number might not include any impossible SGA insertions because of the 1.1% incidence of that problem. These figures highlight the problems associated with the apprenticeship model and experiential learning of airway management (learning by doing) in the operating room, where experience is ad hoc and based on the volume of cases seen by chance, the incidence of difficult cases, and the rate of learning by the individual practitioner.

Anders Ericsson is an educational psychologist who has studied expertise in various domains, including music, science, and sport.[44] He argues that experience does not guarantee expertise. An individual may perform an activity poorly over a long period of time without ever developing expertise. In a systematic review of the relationship between clinical experience and quality of health care Choudhry et al. found decreasing performance with increasing years of practice.[45] A systematic review of the effect of experience and exposure on expertise showed that exposure to cases is the driving factor to maintain competency[46] that relates to better patient outcome.

Ericsson has identified the key behaviors of experts who excel in their field. Besides their positive attitude, these behaviors include deliberate practice, immediate feedback, problem solving, and evaluation with an opportunity to modify or repeat their performance,[47] which means voluntary engagement in constant challenges to master beyond daily clinical practice: ideally, to have others provide formative feedback on the performance aiming for small but constant improvements and finally to rehearse and redo the professional and manual skills, if the clinical context permits. The development of airway management expertise can evolve with these same behaviors.

Learning how to use an airway device can initially show rapid improvement. This early formative period is associated with cognitive and associative phases where feedback from mentors, repeated performance, and problem solving are associated with the rapid advancement of ability. Eventually, this advancement tends to plateau, and the learner enters a phase of automaticity. At this stage, the practitioner can perform with little effort, but the development of behavior can stall with little further improvement toward expertise (Fig. 49.2). Experience gained at this stage may decrease the *effort* of performance by producing automaticity, but this does not necessarily improve the *quality* of performance. This can be a problem encountered by senior practitioners who mostly compensate by experience, if gained from case load. To break away from automated behavior, the learner should embark on Ericsson's described "deliberate practice," where they take on challenges and difficult cases that provide new exposure and push the learner beyond their comfort zone. This process is further enhanced by distributed learning, where new challenging experiences are spread out and occur at regular intervals.[48]

Even with a concerted effort by the learner to engage in deliberate practice, the development of expertise takes time (the so-called 10,000 hours of training or 10 years of clinical practice). Hampered by the constraints of clinical practice, some airway practitioners struggle to achieve the requirements of deliberate practice and distributed learning. Under these circumstances, simulation can play a role in rapidly accelerating the learning experience by providing multiple procedures of varying difficulty in a short time. A study with the AccuTouch bronchoscopy simulator (CAE Montreal, Canada) found that novice residents

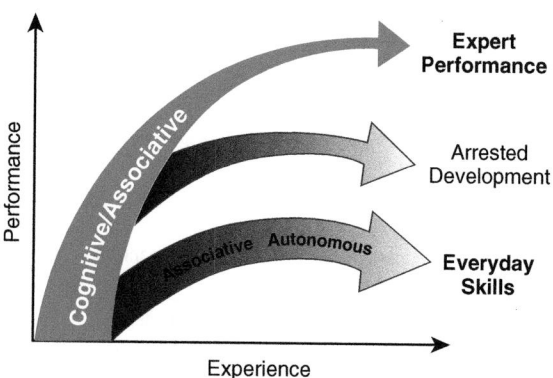

• **Fig. 49.2** Illustration of the qualitative difference between the course of improvement of expert performance and of everyday activities. The goal for everyday activities is to reach as rapidly as possible a satisfactory level that is stable and "autonomous." After individuals pass through the "cognitive" and "associative" phases, they can generate their performances virtually automatically with a minimal amount of effort (see the *gray/white plateau* at the *bottom* of the graph). By contrast, expert performers counteract automaticity by developing increasingly complex mental representations to attain higher levels of control of their performance and will therefore remain within the cognitive and associative phases. Some experts will, at some point in their career, give up their commitment to seeking excellence and thus terminate regular engagement in deliberate practice to further improve performance, which results in premature automation of their performance. (Based on Ten Cate O, Carraccio C, Damodaran A, et al. Entrustment Decision Making: Extending Miller's Pyramid. *Acad Med.* 2021 Feb 1;96(2):199-204. doi:10.1097/ACM.0000000000003800.)

performed an average of 17 oral virtual flexible bronchoscopy intubations in 39 minutes. These residents were able to increase their dexterity with the flexible bronchoscope after this short exposure.[49]

Competency-Based Medical Education Curriculum

Internationally, there has been a shift away from the time-based apprenticeship model to competency-based medical education (CBME). Defined quite simply, the words competence and competency can be used as they are defined in the Oxford Dictionary of English, meaning *the ability to do something successfully.* An example of a CBME curriculum is that adopted by the Australian and New Zealand College of Anaesthetists (ANZCA) or the Anaesthesiology European Training Requirements by the Anaesthesiology Section of the European Union Medical Specialities (EBA UEMS).[50] These curricula define clinical fundamentals and competencies, including airway management. Airway management competencies, including tracheal intubation, SGA use, bag-mask ventilation, flexible scope intubation and flexible bronchoscopy, awake intubation, and emergency airway management (or cannot intubate, cannot oxygenate [CICO]), are part of that clinical fundamental. A series of assessments are used throughout a trainee's progress to ensure that they have met the criteria to proceed to the next level of training. In order for this system to function there is a requirement for teachers to engage in direct observation, coaching, feedback, and reliable valid assessment.[51] Attendance by specialist anesthesiologists at CICO courses is also encouraged by ANZCA.

CBME has not escaped criticism. Critics suggest that CBME applies primarily to trainees and focuses too much on the development of competencies that some regard as a minimum standard of ability.[52] In airway management our goal should be to educate practitioners to be experts at managing difficult airways. This requires a lifelong commitment to keeping up to date with new knowledge, skills, and techniques. Basic competence may not be enough to reach the standard required of an airway expert in anesthesiology. With the constant barrage of new concepts and devices, trainees and specialists need to be fully versed in the recommendations of current airway management practice guidelines.

Airway Education Backed up by Practice Guidelines, Algorithms, and Other Cognitive Aids

Practice guidelines for airway management are usually the result of a detailed analysis of medical literature and a summary of current opinion. The development should follow recognized methodological standards and, wherever possible, be evidence based from reputable sources. They are usually a good resource for teaching content and teaching strategies, provided they are kept up to date with regular reviews.[53]

Airway management guidelines often contain algorithms as a form of graphically distilled information derived from the practice guideline and serve as a cognitive aid. The algorithms are not only a useful source of information during didactic teaching sessions, but they are also a great tool during the debriefing of airway simulations, where critical steps and decisions can be discussed and changes in approaches to difficult airways can be rehearsed. In the same manner an algorithm can guide a morbidity and mortality conference on difficult airway management. Due to the complexity of some algorithms, there has been a trend toward simpler cognitive aids, which are used as resources for group simulation sessions as well as applied during clinical cases.

Cognitive aids are prompts, mnemonics, charts, and graphics designed to improve performance, especially during emergencies.[54] An example of an airway management cognitive aid is the Vortex Approach,[55] which prompts the user to progress through each nonsurgical airway technique using a limited number of attempts at each step before improvement or an emergency surgical airway[56] (Fig. 49.3).

Mastery Learning

Mastery learning is a strict form of CBME where the learner is required to meet predetermined goals before progressing to the next instructional objective. The aim of mastery learning is for learners to achieve a consistent standard and complete all educational goals, irrespective of the time required to reach those goals.[57] At least seven complementary features have been described for mastery learning: (1) baseline or diagnostic assessment; (2) clear learning objectives sequenced as units in increasing difficulty; (3) engagement in powerful and sustained educational activities (e.g., deliberate skills practice, data interpretation, reading) focused on reaching objectives; (4) a fixed minimum passing standard (e.g., test score, checklist percentage); (5) formative assessment with feedback to determine the unit's completion at the minimum passing standard for mastery; (6) advancement to the next educational unit, given measured achievement, at or above the mastery standard (summative assessment); and (7) continued practice or study on an educational unit until the mastery standard is reached.[58]

A meta-analysis and systematic review was published by Cook et al. on mastery learning for health professionals using

The Vortex

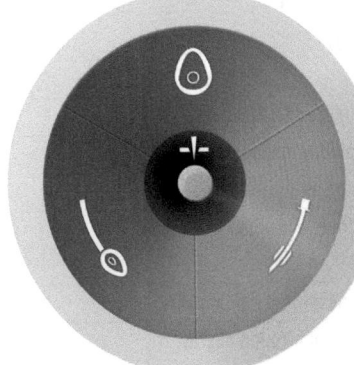

For each lifeline consider:
1. Manipulations:
   - Head & neck
   - Larynx
   - Device

2. Adjuncts
3. Size/type
4. Suction/O$_2$ flow
5. Muscle tone

Maximum three attempts at each lifeline
At least one attempt should be had by most experienced available clinician
Cico status escalates if best effort at any lifeline fails

• **Fig. 49.3** The Vortex Approach. A cognitive aid for airway management. (Courtesy Nicholas Chrimes, MBChB, FANZCA and Peter Fritz, MBChB, FACEM, Melbourne, Australia.)

technology-enhanced simulation.[59] Results showed that mastery in SBME was associated with large effects on skills but moderate effects on patient outcomes.

A Staged Approach to Developing Airway Expertise

Residency and Fellowship Training

The CBME changes introduced by ANZCA and similar colleges and certification boards will inevitably demand more training programs. This increase in airway residency programs or airway fellowships has already occurred within the United States and Canada with associated changes in content and teaching techniques.[60,61] These changes place an increased demand for teachers required to instruct trainees and senior practitioners.

The training program should follow a graduated system where training builds on existing knowledge and skills in a stepwise manner, following an agreed syllabus. An example of an airway management syllabus is presented in Table 49.3. The components of an airway management syllabus might be derived from airway practice guidelines.[62]

TABLE 49.3	An Example of a Minimal Skill Set to Be Acquired by a Trainee During an Airway Rotation

- Optimal bag-mask ventilation technique
- Optimal direct laryngoscopy and intubation with a range of laryngoscopes and intubation aids
- The use of supraglottic airways
- The use of rigid optical devices including videolaryngoscopes and optical stylets
- The use of flexible bronchoscopes
- Cricothyroidotomy

From Baker PA, Weller JM, Greenland KM, Riley RH, Merry AF. Education in airway management. *Anaesthesia* 2011;66:101–111; with permission.

TABLE 49.4	Items That Might Be Included in an Airway Management Program

- Airway anatomy and physiology
- Assessment of the airway
- The maintenance of oxygenation and ventilation
- Avoidance of trauma during airway management
- Utilization of preplanned strategies
- The importance of calling for help and when to do this
- Airway algorithms
- Management of known and unexpected difficult airways
- Establishment and confirmation of an open airway
- Awake intubation
- Rapid sequence induction
- Intubation via a supraglottic airway
- Retrograde intubation
- Emergency techniques for cannot ventilate, cannot oxygenate situations
- Extubation strategies
- Dissemination of information concerning the critical airway
- Human factor training in relation to airway management

From Baker PA, Weller JM, Greenland KM, Riley RH, Merry AF. Education in airway management. *Anaesthesia* 2011;66:101–111; with permission.

Airway training programs typically include a combination of written material, didactic and practical instruction, simulation and clinical training, and assessment of competencies reached. The content of the training program should comply with best practices and ideally correspond with operating procedures and equipment held within the trainee's hospital (Table 49.4). It is ideal to standardize training and equipment throughout a hospital to focus airway education not only on a variety of devices but much more on the team performance and patient safety issues during training.

Airway Fellowships

Airway fellowships are becoming increasingly popular and widespread as the importance of airway management becomes recognized. These fellowships extend airway management training beyond the CBME curriculum and provide advanced trainees the opportunity to engage in research and airway audits, airway management education, and advanced clinical skills. The graduates of airway fellowships often become champions for the advancement of airway management education in their region.[60]

Senior Practitioners

Education in airway management should not cease after graduation from an airway fellowship or residency program. Lifelong learning of airway management–related issues should occur throughout a specialist's career. This learning is driven by constant changes in the approach to the difficult airway and new devices that are being developed and that often demand acquiring new skills. There are currently many opportunities for senior practitioners to maintain

their knowledge and procedural skill, but these options are usually optional and rarely associated with assessment. More and more evidence in education points out that short but often repeated educational sessions result in longer-lasting learning rather than rare "big-bang" sessions[63,64] like workshops in conferences. These smaller and shorter airway education sessions might be easier to organize at the departmental level.

As described before, advancing age and experience does not guarantee the development of expertise.[45] Decline in psychomotor skill after the age of 45 to 50 years has been noted as a cause of decreased performance at cricothyroidotomy.[65] Unfortunately, there is a lack of insight on the part of some practitioners who tend to overrate their own level of expertise based on their self-assessment.[66] This is another reason why continuous assessment of individual competence with constructive feedback is needed.

There is another argument for mandatory airway education throughout a practitioner's career, associated with assessment and audit of patient outcome.[67] This level of continuing education is commonplace in the airline industry, where commercial airline pilots are required to pass regular assessments in flight simulators in order to retain their license to fly. Assessment is followed by intensive retraining if a suitable standard is not met, and return to work is allowed once competency has been established. This system is designed to maintain safety standards and ensure consistent levels of performance.[68] Such programs for anesthesia competence recertification are mandatory in the United States and are assessed by the American Board of Anesthesiology's Maintenance of Certification in Anesthesiology Program (MOCA), where airway management is part of the simulation education courses.[69]

Procedural Skill Education

Airway Equipment

It is known that many practitioners are self-taught in the use of airway devices.[70] An example of that is transtracheal jet ventilation (TTJV), where device knowledge is poor. There are currently no evidence-based or consensus guidelines for best practice to use high-pressure source ventilation. Cook et al. point out that TTJV is rarely performed and therefore it should be avoided if possible. TTJV is associated with serious complications and should be used with extreme care while adhering to best practice.[71] Other clinical problems have resulted from inadequate knowledge and training with equipment, notably oropharyngeal trauma from videolaryngoscopes and their stylets and barotrauma from airway exchange catheters with TTJV.

Understanding the function and limitations of airway equipment is fundamental to safe airway management. The tendency to pick up new devices and work out how to use them directly on a patient from first principles can lead to patient harm. Coroner's cases have been reported where anesthetists were unable to assemble emergency equipment.[59] The use of improvised emergency equipment without proper preparation or time to use them can lead to delays in patient care or poor outcomes.[72–74] Suggestions have been made to "sign off" practitioners to use new equipment only after they have demonstrated competence in its use.[75] Parallels can be found in other clinical areas, for example, approval to perform percutaneous carotid artery stenting is now dependent on relevant simulation-based training by physicians.[76] It is an ethical obligation on the part of all airway practitioners to keep up to date through lifelong learning. First use on manikins might be wise to gain familiarity with the function of a device before it is applied clinically.

Airway Workshops

Airway workshops have a long history and provide a varied syllabus for airway practitioners from different specialties, including anesthesiology, emergency medicine, and intensive care. Content can be focused on basic and advanced airway techniques; others address specific areas of interest, like the ANZCA CICO module, which is a 90-minute hands-on tutorial with procedural skill and human factor content designed for specialist anesthesiologists.[77] Workshops designed specifically for flexible bronchoscopy and awake intubation use participants as volunteer subjects for awake intubation.[78] Other workshops are more comprehensive, providing a broader range of content.[79] A survey has reported improved accuracy and confidence with airway evaluation, adoption of unfamiliar airway devices, and changes in practice when managing patients with difficult airways after attending airway workshops.[80] The decay of learned skills is an issue if skills are not practiced regularly. Research is warranted to establish skill decay following the initial improvement of workshop attendance and the time for retraining. The maintenance of skill is likely to be enhanced by distributed learning in the workplace over time or regular simulation training on task trainers, which are easily accessible. Small airway laboratories are being provided in many centers near the workplace to encourage regular training.[81] This is particularly important for those tasks that benefit from team participation and for procedures that are rarely performed clinically, such as cricothyroidotomy.

Choosing the Appropriate Training Method

The educational goal of an airway management learning session should reflect the existing competencies of the learner. This starting point of learner-directed teaching will also determine the educational methods and type of training devices used to assist with teaching. Novices tend to learn rapidly during the early stage of skill development, but their skill development soon plateaus if they are learning on a low fidelity simulator.[82] An example could be training flexible bronchoscopy. A novice can learn basic dexterity skill on a simple model consisting of slabs of wood with holes drilled asymmetrically to create a tortuous pathway.[83] These basic dexterity skills have proven to be adequate to navigate a flexible bronchoscope through a patient with a normal airway. Conversely, an advanced trainee or experienced practitioner benefits from more sophisticated training adjuncts such as a virtual reality simulator or a human volunteer.[78,82,84] There are numerous examples of simple models and training devices that have been used for airway management training purposes. Some of these devices and techniques were reviewed several years ago by Stringer et al., who recommend the presence of a training block in each hospital to help trainees learn airway skills and decision-making. Unfortunately, some areas lack an organized training program.[85] To help with this problem, the Difficult Airway Society and other organizations have recommended the appointment of airway coordinators or "Departmental Airway Leads" to promote training programs, as suggested in previous reviews.[86,87]

Other options for training include cadavers, anesthetized animals, or animal tissue.[88–92] The use of animals for training

is prohibited by law in some countries including the United Kingdom, and some doubt exists about the specific gained competences and expertise by the use of live animals for training, particularly when cadavers or well-designed simulators are considered equivalent or superior.[93] The logistics of animal anesthesia, including properly trained veterinarians and the ethics approval for the use of animals for teaching purposes, also needs to be considered.

Video recordings of airway management for teaching purposes can be a very useful tool.[94] This applies not only to the recordings of direct and videolaryngoscopy but also to other forms of optical intubation, including optical stylets and flexible bronchoscopy. These images of airway management of the trainee or instructor can be projected and easily viewed during training sessions.[95]

Videos of expert hands-on instruction have been recorded for training.[79,94] Local legislation regarding informed consent about such recordings for teaching purposes needs to be respected. Video can also facilitate assessment with global rating scores.[96] A number of studies describe the benefit of imaging the larynx with videolaryngoscopes to assist instruction during training in laryngoscopy.[97–100] Teaching neonatal tracheal intubation to inexperienced neonatal trainees has also been demonstrated with the assistance of videolaryngoscopy.[101]

Video recording of the entire airway management for teaching purposes is easily achieved with the ubiquitous smartphone that produces high-quality videos. By discussing recordings in a debriefing, after securing the airway, learners have the chance to review immediately what happened and can reflect directly not only on their abilities with the airway devices but also on how they interacted with the team. This teaching technique creates the opportunity to make immediate improvements that can be followed up in the next case. Provided these videos are used only for training purposes and have to be deleted after the debriefing, little concern exists about the personal rights of patients and team members.

At each stage of learning development, a trainee should be provided with constructive but also corrective feedback and a global assessment of their performance. Graduation to patient care occurs once the trainee has proven competence at an appropriate task. For a trainee or colleague to be trustworthy to manage a patient with a difficult airway, they need to demonstrate that they possess a number of competencies required to be trusted to perform a particular task up to an acceptable standard.[102] This relatively new concept of EPAs establishes recorded evidence of satisfactory performance to complete a procedure such as a rapid sequence intubation without supervision. The use of EPAs reflects a transition that is being integrated into curricula. Once this is established, it is planned to audit EPAs as a means to plot a practitioner's lifelong learning.

Simulation-Based Medical Education

Full-scale high-fidelity simulation, in contrast to airway simulation with low-fidelity part-task trainers, offers a number of advantages, particularly given the problems associated with traditional airway management training in the operating room (Table 49.5).

Issenberg et al. have listed desirable features that make such simulation preferable to traditional educational models: validity, feedback, repetitive practice, curriculum integration, varying levels of difficulty, multiple learning strategies, capturing clinical variation, controlled environment, individualized learning, no patient risk, and defined outcomes or benchmarks.[103] Unfortunately, this comprehensive list of features is not incorporated in many forms of low fidelity skills training.

Simulation provides the learner opportunities to improve knowledge, skill, and behavior in a safe, controlled environment. According to Gaba, "Simulation is a technique – not a technology – to replace or amplify real experiences with guided experiences that evoke or replicate substantial aspects of the real world in a fully interactive manner."[104] SBME uses "devices, trained persons, lifelike virtual environments and contrived social situations that mimic problems, events, or conditions that arise in professional encounters."[103] Extensive research, including meta-analyses, studying the efficacy of this form of education confirms the benefits of SBME in comparison with no treatment and traditional clinical education.[105,106]

There is a wide range of models, manikins, full-body simulators, and virtual reality simulators that have been used in airway management education. It is important to choose a training device that is fit for the purpose. That underlines the importance of having an educational strategy for the use of simulation in airway teaching before exploring how to use expensive manikins or simulation equipment. That choice depends on the trainee's basal level of knowledge and the educational goal of the training exercise.

Simulator Fidelity

The fidelity of a simulator plays an important role in the outcome of the training exercise. The word fidelity in the context of medical simulation has many interpretations and definitions, and there is disagreement and confusion about the meaning of various definitions.[107] As a simple definition, fidelity means faithfulness, and the level of fidelity becomes more important when considering the relationship between simulation-based learning and clinical performance.[108] The degree of the faithfulness of a simulator becomes important when defining the educational goal. Also, fidelity becomes relevant to the training exercise. A simulator that provides high-fidelity cardiovascular simulation may have poor airway fidelity. It is known that the overlap in fidelity between two sets of conditions will determine the transfer of learning between those two conditions.[108] If the educational goal is to learn how to apply a face mask and use a ventilation bag on a patient with a normal airway, an appropriate simulator could be a simple airway manikin. If the educational goal is to learn how to manipulate a bougie under a displaced epiglottis and advance a tracheal tube during direct laryngoscopy, the attainment of skill by the trainee and transfer of that skill to a patient is likely to improve if an

anatomically correct manikin is chosen with distorted epiglottis anatomy.

There are many different airway manikins available with varying fidelity. A radiological study compared human anatomy from computerized tomograms to four high-fidelity patient simulators and two airway trainers. The upper airway dimensions of the manikins were significantly different from those of humans.[109] Another study examined the SimBaby (Laerdal Medical, Stavanger, Norway) high-fidelity simulator and found similar results, where the SimBaby airway dimensions did not correlate with pediatric human airway anatomy.[110] In a study of eight neonatal airway simulators a panel of neonatal healthcare professionals found significant differences between the simulators.[111] The AirSim simulators (Trucorp, Belfast, Northern Ireland) are based on human computerized tomography (CT) scans and they were not included in the study by Schebesta et al. In a follow-up study the AirSim compared favorably with human CT data.[112]

Issenberg et al. defined positive features of simulators and included the ability to simulate varying levels of difficulty and multiple learning strategies and capture clinical variation.[103] There are a few examples of these features commercially available. Trucorp have designed pediatric airway manikins with Pierre Robin sequence. There is also a set of four difficult AirSim airway manikins with different airway anatomy, including various epiglottic shapes and the ability to enlarge the base of the tongue (Trucorp, Belfast, Northern Ireland). There are also virtual reality simulators that reproduce airway difficulty.[49,84]

Simulation for Assessment

Simulation-based airway training and assessment is already in use to teach technical and nontechnical skill. Accurately measuring time and other metrics on computer-based simulators can provide an objective assessment of performance to guide feedback. Using a simulator, assessment can occur without involving a patient, and therefore measurement can be safely applied more often in a standardized manner. High-stakes assessment using simulation for the certification of trainees and senior clinicians has been investigated in pilot studies using validated simulated patients; however, recommendations for certification under these conditions do not accurately reflect surgical skills. The development of validated and reliable scores for multiple surgical procedures has already been achieved. Major advances have already been reported in the surgical literature.[113] This is an important area of research for education in airway management that needs to be actively pursued.[114]

Preprocedural Warm-Up

The maintenance of procedural skill is a problem for some practitioners who rarely have an opportunity to perform certain procedures. An example is flexible bronchoscopy, which is a complex skill requiring regular practice. Flexible scope intubation is usually utilized to manage patients with difficult airways. This may be used electively during an awake intubation or acutely following a failed direct or videolaryngoscopy technique. A study from New Zealand found that the average anesthesiologist performed flexible scope intubation only three times per year, which creates a lack of confidence and reluctance to perform this procedure.[70] A useful technique, particularly for the occasional user, is warm-up, which means using simulation immediately before a rarely performed procedure. This technique can rapidly improve clinical performance. In a study of 33 anesthesia residents who performed a flexible bronchoscopy on patients with normal airways global skill scores and time to completion were significantly better in those residents who spent 5 minutes preoperatively performing a guided warm-up on a bronchoscopy simulator versus a second group of residents who did not warm up.[115] Warm-up is well known in sport and music, and this technique has also been applied in surgery, where simulators have been used for warm-up prior to laparoscopic cholecystectomy with significant improvement in surgical trainees.

Translational Outcomes

Translational outcomes concern the implications of education beyond the teaching environment. These include cost savings, skill retention, and improved patient outcomes. The face value of some simulators can be high, but global cost savings may be significant. Expensive repairs for flexible bronchoscopes can be reduced by up to 84% by training on simulators.[116] Skill retention, technical ability, and compliance with an algorithm for cricothyroidotomy for up to 1 year were enhanced by using simulation training.[117] A systematic review of the literature suggests that simulation-based training is equally as effective as traditional patient-based training for colonoscopy, endoscopic sinus surgery, and laparoscopic camera navigation.[118]

Other Sources of Airway Management Education

Airway Societies

Several airway societies now exist worldwide that share a common goal of promoting the science, education, and practice of airway management. In 1995 the UK-based Difficult Airway Society (DAS) and the North American Society for Airway Management (SAM) were formed. The 20th anniversary of these two societies was marked by a combined scientific meeting at the first World Airway Management Meeting (WAMM) in 2015. The European Airway Management Society was formed in 2003 with the aim of spreading high-stakes airway education throughout Europe. Now we can find such airway management societies in South America, Asia, Australia, and New Zealand.

Airway societies are a valuable resource for airway management education through their publications, online discussions, and annual meetings, which include lectures, workshops, problem-based learning, poster presentations, and expert sessions. All these societies actively promote and support the conduct and publication of airway management research.

E-Learning

E-learning is the use of internet technology to enhance learning. A wide range of applications for web-based information, including online libraries for research, internet repositories for course notes, interactive learning with feedback and assessment, case-based learning, hypermedia, and simulations, exists and is growing on a daily basis. Content can be delivered using real-time, instructor-led e-learning techniques (teleconferencing, webinars, internet chat forums, and instant written or visual messaging). Alternatively, content can be delivered asynchronously, where the delivery and receipt of information are not simultaneous. The instructor and learner can communicate by email, bulletin boards, or weblogs, but not in real time. Using e-learning can potentially free the educator from the role of a resource of information to a facilitator of learning and assessment. Research concerning the effectiveness of e-learning suggests that results are equivalent to traditional lecture-based learning.[119]

An adaptive e-learning program has been used to evaluate the knowledge of core topics in a Danish adult airway management curriculum. This study identified important knowledge gaps in three key areas, namely, preoperative planning, optimization of basic techniques, and advanced techniques, highlighting the benefit of objective assessment to guide continuing medical education.

Social Media Medical Education

The volume of new literature appearing daily is increasing exponentially. It is almost impossible to keep up with current knowledge through publication. Using free open access medical education (FOAM), which includes blogs, podcasts, microblogs (such as Twitter®), and smartphone apps, readers can rely on feeds about relevant articles and join chat groups to share ideas. Using this medium, information is disseminated and discussed instantly and globally, long before conventional journal publications. FOAM aims to be informative and entertaining and attracts large audiences, both online through learning platforms (lifeinthefastlane.com, intensivecarenetwork.com, and emcrit.org) and at scientific meetings.

The significant downside of this form of medical education is the lack of robust review processes. FOAM is heavily based on opinion, which sits at the lowest level of medical evidence on the five-point scale designed by the Oxford Centre for evidence-based medicine.[120] A common ground has been suggested where journals could operate their own blog sites moderated by clinicians and publications could be discussed, reviewed, and corrected online.[121] A critical review of internet-based material used for teaching purposes is recommended prior to use. This is to ensure firm scientific evidence of the proposed educational material.

Assessment, Feedback, and Debriefing

Assessment is the process by which learning is validated based on predefined learning outcomes. In contrast, evaluation validates the process, like an airway curriculum or airway teaching program. Airway teachers initially establish "where their learner stands" by trying to understand the existing competencies of the learner. This guides assessment of how effective the previous teaching was and gives insights into how best they can help learners improve performance. Teachers then gain insights into how they can assist learners to improve their performance. To do so, feedback provides learners with information about their performance with the aim of developing a realistic plan for improvements.

The learners are basically interested in three questions as a result of the assessment:
1. Where am I going?
2. How am I going?
3. Where to next?[122]

The assessor needs to "Feed Up" for the first question ("What are the learning outcomes to be achieved"), "Feed Back" for the second ("How was the performance"), and "Feed Forward" for the third ("What am I going to change to become better?")[123] Obviously all three questions should work together and should address how well the airway task was understood or performed. Was the framework understood? Was self-monitoring regulating the action? Finally, was there personal self-assessment and feedback about the self as a person?[122]

In airway teaching mostly formative feedback is used to help learners develop a plan of action or new learning goals. Sometimes summative assessments are used to grade airway skills or to assess whether residents are ready to perform procedures on their own. The latter concept is occurring more often with the introduction of EPAs into airway management curricula, as discussed above.[124,125]

Assessment and feedback is a framework aiming to improve the learner's progress and ideally to determine how the airway learner's own perception of their performance compares to the external view of the learner.[126] The integration of self-assessment by the learner into the feedback allows an assessor to judge if the discussed points have been noted. This may prompt a change in behavior or performance.

Workplace-based assessment (WBA) refers directly to the skill or performance of the learner. It is of utmost importance to provide corrective and constructive reasons for agreement or disagreement with a correct or incorrect execution of a skill. In other words, it is desirable to strengthen strengths and weaken weaknesses by assisting learners in their development of ideas and plans and how they can improve their skill performance. The task of the airway teacher is to provide safe opportunities in the clinical environment to train and rehearse these skills up to the expected level of competence. A meta-analysis of assessment in educational research concluded that "formative assessment does improve learning" and that gains in achievement appear to be quite considerable.[127]

Assessment and feedback during clinical airway management is usually associated with a one-to-one exchange between the learner and teacher. It is important for the learner to announce this special learning situation to reduce the stress of "being examined" and to have at least some minutes for the feedback conversation after the airway procedure. It is best not to interrupt during the assessment observation; otherwise, the assessor will never get a picture of the performance of the learner. Patient safety is paramount and should always take precedence over teaching and assessment. To minimize patient safety concerns during assessment, it is important to carefully select appropriate clinical situations and also be mindful of the correct assessed skill and level of expectation for the learner.

A variety of assessment tools or feedback forms have been developed to standardize the process and provide structured feedback during the development of new learning goals to improve airway management performance. Most studied are WBA, including "direct observation of procedural skills" (DOPS), "Mini-Clinical Evaluation Exercise" (Mini-CEX), case-based discussion, and multisource feedback.[128] These tools are helpful in the busy clinical environment of airway management teaching and can be applied during the few minutes in which an airway procedure happens. These standardized WBA tools are easy to apply and make it easy to focus on feedback to the learner to improve their clinical performance while at the same time directing their learning to the desired competencies of airway performance.[129] This type of WBA of airway management in the operating room does require assessor training.[130]

WBAs are now used internationally in training programs with the stated aim to "provide regular structured formative feedback to trainees, to facilitate teaching and learning, and to inform the in-training assessment process." It is also stated that "failure to meet the minimum WBA requirements at each core unit review will result in failure to progress to the next core unit and hence the trainee will enter into a period of extended training." Trainees tend to regard all WBAs as high-stakes, but a distinction needs to be made between assessment during the formative stage and assessment during the summative stage of training. Formative assessments apply during teaching, learning, and feedback. Assessment for promotion is summative. When skills and concepts are being developed, the stakes are low and the standard of feedback and assessment can afford to be less reliable. Summative assessment is high-stakes and may determine whether a trainee progresses in their training.[114] Trainees at this stage need to be examined more rigorously. Under these circumstances, assessment should be based on multiple observations by experienced observers and reliability is critical.[131] WBA, including DOPS, has been associated with poor interrater reliability.[132] Practical solutions to improve observational assessment have been described by Williams et al. in a series of recommendations.[133] These solutions were summarized by McGaghie et al.[134] (Table 49.6).

Using smartphone technology with very high-quality video recording capability is a possible solution to provide direct visible material for feedback discussion. Very short clips of airway procedures can be recorded to show learners how well they performed and allow them to understand areas for improvement. This technique is highly instructive and provides visible evidence for the learner and instructor to plan an airway management strategy for the next patient in real time. Because these recordings can

TABLE 49.6	Recommendations for Observational Assessment
1.	Rating instruments should be kept short and focused
2.	Apply immediate feedback to benefit teaching and learning
3.	Keep a record of performance rates in case ratings are delayed
4.	Use a wide range of clinical situations for assessments
5.	Use unobtrusive observations to supplement formal observations
6.	Separate summative from formative assessment
7.	Provide adequate time for assessments to allow thoughtfulness
8.	Train the raters
9.	Provide raters with feedback about their relative ratings (hawk vs. dove)
10.	Use multiple raters for observational assessments
11.	Apply only a maximum of seven quality rating categories
12.	Use structured, objective clinical examination and workplace-based assessment to supplement traditional clinical observations
13.	Use a group of reviewers or raters rather than a single rater for promotional or grading requirements
14.	Consider continuous (visual analog) rather than categorical measurement (global rating scale) to increase score accuracy
15.	Promote ratings of specific performance rather than global ratings
16.	Use standardized clinical encounters, skill training, and assessment protocols to supplement clinical performance
17.	Aim to clarify ratings by establishing clear limits or ranges applicable to the rating
18.	Regularly use and revise ratings to establish their meaning
19.	Review assessment from other professions
20.	Realize that observational assessment has limitations and aim to improve it

Data from Williams RG, Klamen DA, McGaghie WC. Cognitive, social and environmental sources of bias in clinical performance ratings. *Teach Learn Med.* 2003;15:270–292.

and must be deleted directly after such a short WBA, there is no need for patient or coworker consent. Standards of patient confidentiality for the viewed video are essentially the same as those for all other exchanges in such a feedback learning conversation. Video-assisted feedback on airway management provides an excellent way to reflect on the skill performance in the real clinical world. The benefit of providing feedback as soon as possible after the procedure enhances discussion with a larger group about the interprofessional or interdisciplinary interactions, which is rarely possible in the clinical environment.

Examination of team interaction can be aided by video-assisted feedback during simulation-based assessment. Safe and fast front-of-the-neck procedures can be trained and rehearsed until the expected level of performance can be observed and seen from the trainee. This type of training is compatible with high-fidelity airway simulation training, which can include reflection and debriefing of team interaction, procedural skill, leadership properties, handling of situation awareness, and decision-making under stressful conditions. Feedback is particularly relevant for the individual development of airway skills. Debriefing after simulation training is particularly helpful for the analysis and modification of group behavior during the entire process of airway management. Debriefing intends to go a step further back than simply analyzing an action and what happened to an outcome. During such debriefings, "reflective practice" aims to identify an individual's own assumptions or professional beliefs and may uncover internal images of external realities. Understanding why certain actions resulted in a particular outcome might be the first step to understanding a trainee's behavior. This method leads to a pairing of advocacy with inquiry.[135]

Successful debriefing can be performed quite simply without video recording.[136] The most important variable for successful debriefing is a properly trained airway teacher who provides feedback.[137] Obviously, a high standard of airway knowledge and technical airway skills are essential requirements for the airway instructor, but the teaching and learning of briefing and debriefing are very important for education in airway management.[138–141] It is assumed and hoped that by teaching the key points of airway management procedures using checklists and standard operating procedures, the adherence to standards and guidelines will result in increased patient safety.

Simulation is an excellent way to train and rehearse these airway briefings, as there is a tendency to cut corners over time, especially if the teams are well known to each other with little change in personnel. Debriefing has been shown to improve patient survival in the emergency setting of a cardiac arrest, but this has not been shown in airway management.[142,143] Similarly, performance-driven direct debriefing after airway procedures, as well as weekly or monthly debriefings of airway management incidents, might improve the long-term performance of the entire anesthesia staff. The key to success seems to be if the institution holds regular training events with mandatory participation. This involves reflection based on evidence with the intention to improve performance and not to blame the involved participants.

Faculty members need to be involved in strategies to implement feedback and debriefing in their clinical environment and departments. The purpose and process of assessment followed by feedback needs to be taught. Faculty need to understand the theoretical background of how feedback and debriefing can help learners improve performance. Assessment requires training to ensure that the quality of observations is valid and represents reliable reflections of trainee performances. The proper use of checklists

might help standardize the scoring in assessment.[144] Giving effective feedback needs to be trained. In roleplay participants can assume different roles. This enables the teacher to convey their own response to challenging situations during the debrief.

Under- and Postgraduate Airway Management Education

Teaching Airway Teachers

As mentioned above, very few clinicians have formal training as clinical teachers. Despite this, it is assumed that being a specialist includes the ability to teach. To facilitate this, short formal faculty development programs enable clinicians to improve their teaching ability. Interestingly, most clinicians like to teach but often find that time pressure in the OR and increasing case loads interfere with their ability to teach. Many clinicians believe that teaching airway management takes too much time in the OR. Clinical teaching in the busy OR does not necessarily require cutting out time or looking for slots of protected time to teach airway management. Teach-the-airway-trainer programs intend to show how to productively use these short periods of time for learning. Obviously, all the theoretical background and handling of equipment have to be trained beforehand, but to get experience and to become an expert in airway management needs direct patient contact and constant challenges covered by proper feedback. These competencies can be trained in airway trainer courses. Topics could cover:

1. How to create a learning climate in the OR
2. Communication of the learning goals for the given session or airway procedure
3. Short insights about the methods of simulation
4. Skill training on real patients
5. How to focus on nontechnical skills for the more advanced learners

Assessment followed by feedback, either based on direct observation and structured assessment forms or an introduction to video debriefing, needs to be part of such faculty development. To improve on-site teaching, such courses can use the same approach as real OR education (e.g., the flipped classroom concept, on-site training, roleplay, simulation and train-the-trainer courses with immediate feedback and video debriefing).

In 2013 the European Airway Management Society created the "EAMS Teach the Airway Teacher" (TAT) course, focusing primarily on the best way to teach airway management rather than on teaching specific airway devices or procedures. The TAT course is geared toward clinicians who deal with learners on a daily basis. This is where formative airway management education happens and where large numbers of teachers need support to provide quality airway management education. It has been planned to roll this course out across Europe. Competencies learned in such courses also serve to improve the teaching of airway experts at conference workshops.

Skills Training: Hands-On and Didactic Teaching

Airway management is a practical haptic competence based on specific skills. Skill is defined as ability, a specific behavior, or an adaptively carried out complex activity acquired through deliberate, systematic, and sustained effort. For airway education, we need cognitive skills dealing with the theoretical background and functions, technical skills to perform airway procedures and apply devices, and interpersonal skills to do the job properly together for the benefit of the patient. Having that in mind, hands-on and didactic teachings are complimentary for airway education.

We need to facilitate the understanding and retention of theoretical concepts, functions, and principles on which hands-on training is based. The transition of knowledge to the practical aspects of airway management starts with basic and advanced airway procedures on low-fidelity manikins. When skills are mastered on manikins, they can be applied to patients under direct supervision. This is followed by deliberate practice under immediate supervision up to an expert level. Finally, fulfilling predefined EPAs might be a point when skills teaching develops further to a level where airway experts start to instruct others.

Distance Learning

Distant learning refers to the use of multimedia methods, including a variety of web-based instruction. Learning occurs simultaneously and can be interactive (webinars) or recorded. Face-to-face teaching with podcasts, streaming conferencing through television or video, and combinations of electronic and traditional education can all be used. Distant learning also includes a separation of geographical locations and has a strong focus on learner-to-learner/instructor interaction. For airway management education, it might be helpful to flip the classroom for preparation for upcoming airway workshops or conferences, as well as for supervision and rehearsal and most probably also for recertification in very remote areas. Modern video technology not only allows us to watch new procedures or the application of new devices in airway management, but it also allows the remote observation and feedback of learners by tutors.

In 2020 during the COVID-19 pandemic, some experts expressed concern about a threat to airway management education caused by the demand for clinical duty and restriction on travel, both of which resulted in decreased allocated time for training. Efforts have been made to counteract this trend by increasing the use of distance learning.

Human Factors and Leadership Education

Human factor science is a multidisciplinary field devoted to optimizing performance and reducing human error as a result of human interactions. Human factor issues can relate to human abilities, behaviors, and limitations at work. It can apply at a system level or individual level. These human factors were considered to have contributed to an adverse outcome in over 40% (75/184) of cases reported to the NAP4. Important nontechnical skills include, besides communication issues, situation awareness, task management, decision making, and teamwork. These skills and proper leadership skills need to become part of safety training for all airway practitioners.

Effective teamwork is important in airway management, so is the ability to make appropriate decisions in good time; there is evidence that even experienced practitioners may feel considerable reluctance to progress to a surgical airway in an emergency, and more work is needed to find effective ways to address this reluctance.[145,146] Specific leadership training may have a place in airway management education. In recognition of the importance of human factors in the management of anesthetic crises the ANZCA commissioned the development of a course, the Effective Management of Anaesthetic Crises (EMAC). This 2 ½-day,

simulation-based course includes a strong theme of human factors and teamwork training. A half-day of this course is dedicated to the management of airway crises and includes skills stations, airway drills, and instruction on human error and decision making. This is reinforced in the immersion simulations of critical events, using a whole-body computerized manikin, followed by debriefing and facilitated reflective learning.[147] The aim is to ensure anesthetists are ready, willing, and able to intervene effectively in airway crises and, in fact, to recognize potential problems to avoid adverse events. While EMAC is now a compulsory component of training and recognized for continuing professional development, consideration could be given to regular, compulsory training for anesthetists in airway management, similar to the requirements of aviation pilots.

One of the key steps in managing a difficult airway is to call for help early. Trained anesthetic assistants have been shown to improve the safe management of simulated anesthesia crises,[148] and their help may be particularly useful provided they understand their role in the management of a difficult airway. Anesthetists and their assistants need to be familiar with their environment and particularly with the required equipment and its whereabouts in their own institution. It is therefore worrying that an audit of airway management equipment in a metropolitan region in New Zealand found that 20% of anesthetic and nonmedical staff had never been orientated to the difficult airway container and did not know the contents.[149] It is likely that such deficiencies exist in many other countries. In situ simulation means simulation at the workplace, including the operating room or the intervention area. This might not only reveal such deficits but offer a way to stimulate reflection and improvements at the organizational level.

It is useful to consider techniques used by the airline and other industries to mitigate the risk of human error. The use of cognitive aids, such as standard operating procedures and checklists, is an integral part of safe practice in many high-reliability organizations internationally.[150] Relevant checklists for anesthesia and surgery include the "Crisis Management Manual" from the Australian Patient Safety Foundation,[151] a new crisis checklist from Gawande's group at the Harvard School of Public Health,[152] and the World Health Organization's Safe Surgery Checklist, which includes an airway component.[153] NAP4 also recommended the use of checklists and standard operating procedures for a number of circumstances, such as intubation outside the operating room and rescue of the inadvertently dislodged airway in the ICU.[12]

Human factors and leadership education focuses on interprofessional and interdisciplinary approaches to team training and simulation.[154] It is most valuable to include all personnel from the clinical area when simulating an airway crisis. Implementing short briefings before a case focusing on the key aspects of airway management and after a case conducting a debriefing as to how it worked out and what might be improved in the future impacts the long-run collaboration of different persons during airway management. Proper education of airway managers in doing such short, structured briefings and debriefings is needed and ideally should be implemented into the daily workflow.

Research for Airway Management Education

Unfortunately, there is very little published research that addresses the best way to teach airway management. Simulation offers many potential opportunities through accelerating learning, creating rare and difficult situations, and augmenting clinical training. A domain of simulation includes team training on human factors and behavioral aspects of crisis management. Many benefits of simulation training have been proven, but unanswered questions still remain. The assessment of individuals and teamwork skills in surgical simulation is now well described, but optimum feedback and debrief techniques have yet to be elucidated.[113]

As with any intervention in medicine, such as drugs or devices, we need to investigate the effect of educational intervention to discover how large the effect size of the desired outcome will be. For many of our teaching methods, whether traditional or technology-enhanced learning, we lack this rigorous research data needed to show what techniques would give the desired educational outcome and finally improve patient safety.

For some research questions, the classic medical randomized controlled trial design might be appropriate. Blinding is problematic, however, because the learner is always aware of the teaching methods. More appropriate options in these circumstances would be questionnaires, surveys, or qualitative studies. Researchers who are in the field of airway teaching and research need to open their "tool box" of research methodology in that direction and need to get acquainted with these methods.

There is a long list of questions that remain unanswered in airway management, but priorities in airway education should include translational research showing that educational effort and resources result in improved physician performance and reduced patient morbidity and mortality. Another important topic is the decay of competencies after initial training: How do we maintain skills after workshops, particularly in the case of rarely used devices or procedures such as front-of-the-neck access? How often do we need retraining? What is an appropriate case load to stay clinically competent for a standard airway management procedure? What is the best teaching method to establish, maintain, and retrain procedural skill? Is it better to attend an airway workshop at a conference or should we use departmental skills labs for low-dose but high-frequency training at our institutions? Does e-learning offer better results or is the concept of "warm-up," "mental imagining," or low- and high-fidelity training much better in keeping the clinician up to date? When and for which purpose is a manikin or an animal tissue model best to learn?

There is an obvious need for more research concerning SBME, procedural skill development, and the impact of human behavior and nontechnical skill on airway management. The optimum methods to acquire and maintain expertise in airway management have yet to be defined. The effort and cost involved in this research should be justifiable.

Conclusion

Education in airway management is undergoing rapid change. Existing training programs are adopting teaching techniques originating from education research. CBME curriculum and moves toward mandatory airway education with assessment are likely to create more formalization of airway training. We can anticipate improvements in training techniques as a result of research into medical education. Trainees can expect the assessment of their competence in airway management to become much more rigorous in the near future. Regular reassessment of this competence is likely to become the norm for both trainees and qualified practitioners. These changes will affect all anesthesiologists. A career-long commitment to relevant education and maintenance of skills is clearly integral to the credibility of anesthesiologists' claim of being experts in airway management.

Selected References

1. Armstrong L, Harding F, Critchley J, et al. An international survey of airway management education in 61 countries. *Br J Anaesth*. 2020;125(1):e54–e60.
2. Bessmann EL, Rasmussen LS, Konge L, et al. Anesthesiologists' airway management expertise: identifying subjective and objective knowledge gaps. *Acta Anaesthesiol Scand*. 2021;65:58–67.
9. Ten Cate O, Carraccio C, Damodaran A, et al. Entrustment decision making: extending Miller's pyramid. *Acad Med*. 2020;13:13.
24. Sutkin G, Wagner E, Harris I, Schiffer R. What makes a good clinical teacher in medicine? A review of the literature. *Acad Med*. 2008;83(5):452–466.
31. Coggins A, Zaklama R, Szabo RA, et al. Twelve tips for facilitating and implementing clinical debriefing programmes. *Med Teach*. 2021;43(5):509–517.
34. Bould MD, Naik VN, Hamstra SJ. Review article: new directions in medical education related to anesthesiology and perioperative medicine. *Can J Anaesth*. 2012;59(2):136–150.
36. McLean S, Attardi SM, Faden L, Goldszmidt M. Flipped classrooms and student learning: not just surface gains. *Adv Physiol Educ*. 2016;40(1):47–55.
44. Ericsson KA. Deliberate practice and the acquisition and maintenance of expert performance in medicine and related domains. *Acad Med*. 2004;79(10 Suppl):S70–S81.
45. Choudhry NK, Fletcher RH, Soumerai SB. Systematic review: the relationship between clinical experience and quality of health care. *Ann Intern Med*. 2005;142(4):260–273.
58. McGaghie WC, Issenberg SB, Barsuk JH, Wayne DB. A critical review of simulation-based mastery learning with translational outcomes. *Med Educ*. 2014;48(4):375–385.
103. Issenberg SB, McGaghie WC, Petrusa ER, Lee Gordon D, Scalese RJ. Features and uses of high-fidelity medical simulations that lead to effective learning: a BEME systematic review. *Med Teach*. 2005;27(1):10–28.
106. McGaghie WC, Issenberg SB, Cohen ER, Barsuk JH, Wayne DB. Does simulation-based medical education with deliberate practice yield better results than traditional clinical education? A meta-analytic comparative review of the evidence. *Acad Med*. 2011;86(6):706–711.

All references can be found online at eBooks.Health.Elsevier.com.

50

Dissemination of Critical Airway Information

JESSICA L. FEINLEIB, LAURA V. DUGGAN, LYNETTE J. MARK, AND
LORRAINE J. FOLEY

CHAPTER OUTLINE

KEY POINTS

- The consequences of a difficult airway (DA) may include minor or major adverse medical events or death, professional liability to the practitioner, and direct and indirect costs to the patient and healthcare system. DA still accounts for the highest percentage of closed claims in anesthesia.
- The American Society of Anesthesiologists (ASA) Practice Guidelines for the DA recommend the following components for dissemination of critical airway information: (1) a written report or letter to the patient, (2) a report in the medical record, (3) a chart flag, (4) communication with the patient's surgeon or primary caregiver, and (5) a notification bracelet or equivalent identification device. MedicAlert is currently the only organization that can readily provide this service.
- The MedicAlert Foundation, founded in 1965 and endorsed by the ASA in 1979, is the only 501(c)(3) nonprofit organization

that provides a comprehensive medical service to members, in the form of visible medical ID, a separate wallet card, a Web-accessible personal health record, and a 24/7 live emergency response service. It is accessible at http://www.medicalert.org/difficult-airwayintubation-registry.
- The Airway APP and international Airway Collaboration is data collection for Emergence Surgical Airway:Front of Neck Access. One is able to follow results on www.airwaycollaboration.org.
- The foundation has an updated National DA/Intubation Registry form available on both its website and that of the Society for Airway Management (www.samhq.org).
- Development of an Airway Lead or Airway Team within each individual hospital can serve to guide the alert process and subsequent patient action plan.

Introduction

All airway practitioners encounter a difficult airway (DA), and likely encounter a failed airway, during their career. The consequences of

failed airway maintenance and endotracheal intubation are devastating to the patient, the practitioner, and the healthcare system.[1] Complex airway management is a multifaceted problem involving healthcare providers in a variety of clinical settings. Although a large percentage of difficult intubations can be predicted via a careful review of history and airway examination, unanticipated DAs are still reported at a rate of 1% to 3% among hospitalized operative patients.[2-5] Since Cooper's classic 1978 paper on human errors, anesthesiology has made great strides to reduce preventable harm.[6] A history of a DA and its recognition as a risk factor for future airway management have been helpful in the mitigation of risk in the clinical management of the DA patient.[7,8] Additionally, technology and new devices have improved anesthesiologists' ability to secure airways. Remaining difficulties include the cryptic anatomy encounter or other anatomic barriers to airway maintenance that were not communicated. Thus, a new "human error" of airway safety is poor forward information transmission. The critical data lacking often include identification of such patients along with the complete documentation of airway management techniques that failed and those that were successful. The effective and efficient dissemination of this critical airway information to healthcare providers and patients is the current task set to our interdisciplinary professions.

Although a patient's DA was most likely first made evident in the setting of an operating room, subsequent events could occur in a variety of settings (even in the home or in public places) and could involve physician or nonphysician providers, such as paramedics, emergency room physicians, physicians of other specialties (e.g., otolaryngology), certified registered nurse anesthetists, and/or anesthesiologists. Therefore, it is incumbent on airway practitioners to make every effort to identify DA patients in and out of the operating room and transmit this knowledge in widely accessible forms using terminology that is directed toward other airway specialists, healthcare providers, and patients or laypersons. The fundamental differences between the successful management of known versus unanticipated DAs are clearly seen in the enhanced patient outcomes observed in the former scenario.[2,9,10]

Currently, numerous DA communication reporting mechanisms exist, including airway databases and registries, although the field is migrating from a nascent stage toward a more nationally and internationally integrated stage. This transition is nonetheless still characterized by many competing elements, fractured systems, and diverse goals. We present a taxonomy of DA databases, registries, and clinical practices that have been successfully implemented.

Current Difficult Airway Databases

Systems in Place

There are two major goals of DA databases: (1) to identify specific patients for their protection and future care and (2) to collect data to study the epidemiology and cause of DAs to improve systems of care and clinical practice. Based on these goals, there are three types of DA databases: (1) patient protective DA database; (2) epidemiologic and etiologic DA database; and (3) combined patient protective, epidemiologic, and etiologic DA database. The first two accomplish one, but not both, of the aforementioned goals as would be the ideal. Other important features include the time frame (either time limited or perpetual) and accessibility for data reporting and retrieval. Data reporting can be restricted to predetermined institutions and patients or may be broadened to include global data reporting and retrieval. The data elements that are collected obviously determine the use of that databank. For incidence and

prevalence calculations, the denominator of the total number of airway management occurrences is needed, along with the numerator of untoward airway events. To illustrate this taxonomy of DA databases, we have reviewed and analyzed multiple examples, highlighting their strengths and weaknesses. The databases are grouped according to the criteria, and at the end of each synopsis any additional factors defining that airway database are encapsulated. This discussion is not an exhaustive listing of all DA databases but covers the most substantial ones. This analysis also provides a framework for the evaluation of such databases and guidance for future discussions about DA database goals and their future use.

Type I: Patient Protective Difficult Airway Database

These databases are organized to identify and protect individual patients during their hospitalization and for their future care. It has long been the practice of many anesthesiology groups to keep an informal record of patients with DAs. Over time, many groups formalized this collective knowledge into more comprehensive databases, patient record flags, and patient notification systems. These databases are usually limited to a specific location or anesthesiology practice, and access to this information is usually confined to that group.

Single In-Hospital Difficult Airway Registry

In 2005, the Johns Hopkins Hospital in Baltimore, Maryland, developed an emergent call system to notify and engage a multidisciplinary difficult airway response team (DART). A DA registry note and local EMR registry were also developed with the DART, and additional notifications were employed to ensure that all hospital personal are aware of the patient DA status.[11] Over the ensuing years, this system has been fully or partially replicated by many other healthcare systems.[12]

Database factors: Access, limited; Timeframe, ongoing; Denominator, not included.

Veterans Affairs Healthcare System

In 2012, the Veterans Affairs (VA) Healthcare System (approximately 150 hospitals) set forth a comprehensive series of airway management standards through the Out of Operating Room Airway Management Directive (VHA Directive 1157). Included in this series of standards were guidelines stating that all VA hospitals had to have "a plan for managing the known or emergently identified difficult airway" and "a process for notifying such patients." The implementation method of these guidelines was left to the individual VA hospitals to determine. Most VA hospitals now have a DA patient electronic flag; however, these flags are only local VA flags and do not attach to the patient's national electronic record. The establishment of a national patient record flag requires congressional assent. Additionally, the airway information collected by each VA hospital is not standardized, nor is there a searchable database of the information collected across the VA system. Although this directive sought to improve patient safety at local VA hospitals, it failed to create a nationally integrated system, which has impeded the ability to ascertain the issues of DAs within the VA system through data collection and analysis.

Database Factors: Access, limited; Timeframe, ongoing; Denominator, none.

Type II: Epidemiologic and Etiologic Difficult Airway Database

These databases are organized to determine the epidemiology of DAs or to catalog DA events to identify etiologic factors. The selection of patient characteristics, airway management techniques, and providers that are included in these databases determines their use for analyzing airway events. Further differentiation between these types of databases can be made in reference to their temporal framework and their accessibility.

American Society of Anesthesiologists Closed Claims Project

The American Society of Anesthesiologists (ASA) Closed Claims Project is the most widely recognized and fully established database of this type. Since its inception in 1984, this group has analyzed anesthesia-related events resulting in completed legal claims in the United States.[9] The results of these multiple rounds of analysis have had a profound and positive impact on the practice of anesthesiology worldwide.[9,13] However, the usefulness of these data in the context of airway management is somewhat limited. The only airway management data included in this sample is that of failed airways that resulted in patient harm, and that by definition resulted in a legal contest. Such bias to the most extreme airway events lacks the inclusion of a total number of airway management attempts needed to determine an event incidence. Moreover, because these data are based on insurance claims, rich clinical detail may be lacking.

Database Factors: Access, limited; Timeframe, ongoing; Denominator, none.

Airway Continuous Quality Improvement Program and Airway Registry

An Airway Continuous Quality Improvement Program and Airway Registry was started in 2007 at an Urban Academic Level 1 Trauma center in Tuscon, Arizona. With the ongoing monitoring, it allowed improvement of airway performance in the ED with increased first past success and decreased adverse events.[14]

Database Factors: Access linked, Timeframe: ongoing, Denominator: included.

The Airway App

The Airway App using smartphone technology was established in 2016 as an anonymous data-gathering app regarding the emergency front-of-neck access (eFONA) technique and first-pass success. eFONA is a rare event. This tool gathers firsthand experience of health care provided worldwide. This app collects data on the type of eFONA procedure: Seldinger technique vs scalpel and bougie-assisted cricothyrotomy. At this time, data showed the highest first-pass success rate to be scalpel and bougie-assisted cricothyrotomy.[15]

Database Factors: Access: easy; Timeframe, ongoing; Denominator, none.

National Emergency Airway Registry and National Emergency Airway Registry for Children

The National Emergency Airway Registry (NEAR) is an ongoing project established in 2003. It prospectively collects emergency department intubation data from more than 30 international institutions (http://www.nearstudy.net). This World Wide Web–based database includes more than 16,000 emergency department intubations defined by a standardized data collection form. The data are only accessible to the participating institutions for analysis and publication of findings and are de-identified. As such, this registry is incapable of providing providers and patients with airway information for future airway management. However, this database collects information on all intubations, regardless of difficulty, allowing for the calculation of incidence and prevalence of airway factors within the population of participating institutions.

NEAR for children (NEAR4KIDS) was established subsequently to NEAR and further focuses on pediatric intensive care unit intubation data. (https://www.research.chop.edu/near4kids). It was originally comprised of a handful of institutions and has now grown to include 22 children's hospitals.

Database Factors: Access, limited; Timeframe, ongoing; Denominator, included.

National Audit Project 4

The National Audit Project 4 (NAP4) was a time-limited joint effort of the Difficult Airway Society and the Royal College of Anaesthetists. Over a 1-year period (September 2008–September 2009) all participating UK hospitals documented every airway management event that resulted in an unanticipated intensive care unit admission, death, brain damage, or an emergency surgical airway (http://www.das.uk.com/natauditproject).[10] These data were then carefully analyzed for patient and provider factors that precipitated these events. In addition, the event rates could be calculated because of the inclusion of all airway management occurrences in the database system. This audit resulted in a profound reexamination of airway management outside of the operating room and during extubation. However, the data collection time frame was limited and therefore only provides a snapshot view of airway events. Determination of any change in airway management event rate subsequent to this period requires an additional audit.

Database Factors: Access, limited; Timeframe, proscribed; Denominator, calculated.

Australia and New Zealand Emergency Department Airway Registry

In response to the results of the NAP4 effort, the Australia and New Zealand Emergency Department Airway Registry was established by emergency physicians in 2011 (https://aci.health.nsw.gov.au/networks/eci/research/current-research-and-quality-activities/airway-project). It prospectively collects data from all intubations preformed in approximately 20 emergency departments in Australia and New Zealand. This registry's data are submitted by a clinical champion at each site via a standardized and patient de-identified form. The inclusion of all airway management occurrences in the database system allows for the calculation of airway morbidity and mortality rates. Since NAP4, multiple national databases, similar to this one, have been enacted (e.g., Danish system: https://clinicaltrials.gov/show/NCT01718561).

Database Factors: Access, limited; Timeframe, ongoing; Denominator, included.

Anesthesia Quality Institute: Anesthesia Incident Reporting System

The Anesthesia Incident Reporting System collects data on all anesthesia incidents, including those relating to airway management events. These data are then incorporated into the National Anesthesia Clinical Outcomes Registry, which includes more than 22 million cases from individual practitioners, hospitals, and anesthesia practices (http://www.aqihq.org/airs/airsintro.aspx). This system has gained wide acceptance and participation; as of 2014, 25% of all anesthesia cases in the United States were captured by this system. This system collects data on adverse airway events and the total number of anesthesia cases in an ongoing database, allowing for the calculation of the incidence of airway events, and these rates can be followed over time. In 2014, the Anesthesia Quality Institute and the Society of Airway Management established a formalized relationship through a letter of understanding. This provides for an analysis of this substantial database by airway specialists. However, this database is not of use for maintaining individual patient data.

Database Factors: Access, limited; Timeframe, ongoing; Denominator, included.

Type III: Combined Patient Protective, Epidemiologic, and Etiologic Difficult Airway Databases

These databases are organized to identify and protect individual patients while also cataloging DA events for epidemiologic and etiologic analysis. This requires recording and storing patient identifiers associated with the airway event information and management data. Additionally, this type of system facilitates data access by future airway providers and should ideally provide patients with airway information.

MedicAlert Foundation: Difficult Airway/Intubation Registry

Founded in 1956, the MedicAlert Foundation is a 501(c)3 nonprofit organization that innovated a national and international emergency medical identification emblem and 24/7 emergency response system. The MedicAlert Foundation was endorsed by the ASA in 1979, the World Federation of Societies of Anaesthesiologists in 1992, and the American Academy of Otolaryngology-Head and Neck Surgeons in 1993.

In 1992, an Anesthesia Advisory Council comprised of anesthesiologists, otolaryngologists, and experts in safety and risk management joined with the nonprofit MedicAlert Foundation to establish the MedicAlert National Registry for Difficult Airway/Intubation (Andrew Wigglesworth, personal communication, 2010). The major objectives of the MedicAlert Anesthesia Advisory Council were to (1) develop mechanisms for uniform documentation and dissemination of critical airway information, (2) establish a database to store and transmit protected patient information between the MedicAlert Foundation and healthcare facilities (nationally and internationally), and (3) determine through clinical practice if dissemination of clinical airway information could prevent future adverse outcomes and lower healthcare costs. A specialty enrollment form for the MedicAlert National Registry for Difficult Airway/Intubation was designed

that included a "Dear Patient" panel, "Dear Practitioner" panel, airway database, legal statement, and information for patient enrollment.

Between 1992 and 2014, there were nearly 12,000 patient enrollments in the Difficult Airway/Intubation Registry. In a preliminary survey of these patient enrollments, more than 150 healthcare institutions from all 50 states are represented. Institutions include freestanding clinics, community hospitals, tertiary care centers, teaching institutions, and military institutions. Approximately 12% of these enrollments included "Dear Patient" letters from their healthcare providers. Review of these letters identified three broad categories of patient information: (1) generic "difficult airway/intubation alert" only, (2) generic "difficult airway/intubation alert" supplemented with database elements further describing the nature of the DA, and (3) either category 1 or 2 with scanned original documentation from the patient's medical record (e.g., anesthesia operating room records, surgical operative notes).

In response to this comprehensive review, in 2014 the SAM MedicAlert Task Force updated the National Difficult Airway/Intubation brochure and registry form (20140515-Difficult_Airway_Intubation_form.pdf (medicalert.org)). Healthcare providers from any background or location can document specified patient airway factors, management techniques, and airway outcomes via a World Wide Web–based system. The providers can either download the registry form and complete it and give it to the patient along with a "Dear Patient" letter (see example) or assist patients with online registration. This information is securely stored for patients to access, and patients can avail themselves of official MedicAlert medical identification notifying healthcare providers of their airway status. This information can then be used to provide the appropriate airway management for that patient, without having to locate and contact the prior healthcare provider.

Both the SAM and the Canadian Airway Focus Group recommend the use of a national registry, such as MedicAlert, in addition to documentation of a patient's DA.[16,17]

Database Factors: Access, global; Timeframe, o; Denominator, none.

Clinical Practices and Patient Identification

The 2003, ASA Practice Guidelines for Management of the Difficult Airway contained a DA algorithm that described in great detail the choices and techniques available and the pathways for the management of the unanticipated or anticipated DA/intubation.[18] Subsequent ASA editorials suggested that successful airway techniques and devices would vary, depending on the clinical setting, the skill and experience of the practitioner, and unique characteristics of the patient.[19] How then can these many variations, successful and unsuccessful, be communicated to the next healthcare provider?

It is also known that repeated attempts at intubation cause swelling and bleeding, with each attempt increasing the likelihood of failed intubation and the possibility of brain damage or even death.[20-22] Prolonged and multiple attempts at intubation can increase the rate of complications up to 70%.[23,24] Given the serious patient safety and liability implications of repeated attempts at intubating the DA patient, how can repeated attempts at intubation be avoided during future events?

The answer to these questions lies in implementing a well-defined, uniform, reliable, and nationally accessible mechanism to document and disseminate critical information about a patient's

DA/intubation. The communication of successful and unsuccessful airway management techniques consists of two parts: (1) documentation in the electronic medical record (EMR) at the time of the event for concurrent providers during that episode of care and (2) dissemination of that information to the patient and future care providers during subsequent episodes of care.[1]

The ASA Practice Guidelines recommend that "the anesthesiologist should document the presence and nature of the airway difficulty" at the time of the event. This should include "a description of the airway difficulties that were encountered. The description should distinguish between difficulties encountered in face mask or laryngeal mask airway ventilation and difficulties encountered in tracheal intubation." It should also include "a description of the various airway management techniques that were employed. The description itself should indicate the extent to which each of these techniques served a beneficial or detrimental role in management of the difficult airway."[18] The ASA endorses preanesthesia, anesthesia, and postanesthesia documentation, ideally within a special airway management section of the EMR. This section would contain required fields and a comment section for free text.

Many practitioners have put great thought into airway documentation. Combining elements from all of these systems leads to the following list of what to document:
1. Date and institution where DA was identified
2. Provider contact information
3. Patient characteristics on airway examination, body mass index, and other significant comorbidities
4. Type of difficulty encountered with each technique, such as mask ventilation, supraglottic devices, intubation, and extubation
5. Unsuccessful techniques
6. Successful techniques with best view
7. Implications for future
8. Recommendation for registration with MedicAlert[20]

Documentation in the Anesthesia Record

DA documentation should be evident to all care providers. The preceding list encompasses the most complete system of DA documentation. Traditionally this was a cover sheet of the patient's paper chart. With the advent of the EMR and the electronic anesthesia record, many systems are now being used. One shortcoming of current systems is the inability to transfer DA data automatically from the electronic anesthesia record to the main EMR. Additionally, many electronic systems require that the provider know where to look for DA data, thus hindering many healthcare providers from obtaining this information. Many systems provide the ability to "flag" a patient's chart for a few select conditions. When activated, the DA flag appears each time the patient's EMR is accessed and must be acknowledged before progressing through the rest of the record.

Patient Consultation

The 2003 ASA practice guidelines and the Veterans Health Administration (VHA) recommend that the anesthesiologist notify the patient (or family/responsible party) of the patient's DA/intubation (VHA Directive 2012-032).[18]

Effective notification has usually been interpreted to include verbal and written notification, typically a discussion between the anesthesiologist and the patient delineating the nature of the DA. Anesthesiologists comply with this recommendation and speak with the patient in the postanesthesia care unit. However, this verbal communication to the patient and/or family may be invalidated because of the patient's postoperative pain, anxiety, or sedation and the family's more immediate concerns about the patient's surgery and recovery as communicated by the surgeon.[25] One study found that 50% of patients informed verbally did not recall or were unsure that they had a postoperative conversation with their anesthesiologist.[26] The additional burden of unfamiliar medical words further complicates successful verbal communication of a DA or intubation event. Given all of these factors, a patient reentering a facility may not remember this verbal information and may deny having a history of DA during subsequent preoperative evaluations. The limitations of verbal notification should thus be recognized, particularly with respect to the patient having "a role in guiding and facilitating future care" or being able to accurately disseminate critical information to future healthcare providers.[18] Thus, the component of verbal communication to the patient is best completed when the patient is alert and oriented or just before being discharged home. The addition of written notification at the time of verbal communication completes the classic patient teaching methods that are used for postoperative instructions.

This process has been formalized in some VA hospitals, as well as many others, into a "Difficult Airway Consult" package, including patient record flag, patient record note, patient notification letter, and verbal communication with the patient or patient designee (VHA Directive 2012-032).

Patient and Physician Letters

A letter, as in the previous example, should be given to the patient during the time of verbal communication. Also, a copy of the letter should remain in the patient's chart and a copy should be sent to the primary care physician if possible. The following letter is an example of a letter for the patient: www.medicalert.org/difficultairway.

In-Hospital Bracelet

The use of bracelets to promote patient identification and safety is now standard of care and endorsed by the World Health Organization and the International Joint Commission (http://www.who.int/patientsafety/solutions/patientsafety/PS-Solution2.pdf). The extension of this highly successful patient safety initiative to denote critical patient comorbidities with color-coded bands is often used. However, there is only marginal standardization as to what the colors indicate (http://endurid.com/blog/2013/06/the). This leads to confusion when staff or patients move between healthcare systems with different color codes.

The use of an identification bracelet for DA could increase patient safety but is more effective if the patient's condition is stated in text form. This is often seen as a potential Health Insurance Portability and Accounting Act (HIPAA) violation, and therefore it is often not incorporated into a DA patient bracelet system. The use of MedicAlert bracelets to inform healthcare providers of patient comorbidities has a long history and is well accepted by patients.

The use of in-hospital DA bracelets can safeguard patients but must be implemented at the hospital level while practitioners remain aware of the potential pitfalls. An in-hospital DA bracelet system would never be effective as the only part of a notification system—only as an additional measure combined with the other elements discussed in this chapter.

Nonoperative Patient Screening

Most hospitalized patients do not enter the operating room. In this population, most patients with DAs go undiagnosed. Therefore, efforts should also be made to increase identification of these patients. To this end, nonairway physicians and providers should be educated regarding the negative impact that an unidentified DA can have on a patient's outcomes. All healthcare providers should be encouraged and educated to assess their patients' airways. They could then obtain airway consultations from airway physicians. These efforts could decrease the discovery of a DA in an emergent scenario and avoid harm to these patients. Additionally, these services could be incorporated into a billing system to further encourage this type of screening.

Hospital Policies for Patients With Known Difficult Airways

After a patient has been diagnosed with a known or likely DA, hospital policies should be in place to support care in the safest manner. For example, a multidisciplinary group or airway lead should establish hospital policies regarding the out-of-operating room postoperative estuation, elective intubation, and emergent intubation of these patients. Additionally, procedural sedation of DA patients can place them in jeopardy. These scenarios should be anticipated and systems put in place to safeguard patients.

Future Directions

Although recommendations for DA documentation and data dissemination have existed since the early 1990s, several surveys and studies have shown that such recommendations have not been widely implemented.[27-29] One study found that only 20% of anesthesiologists consistently wrote a DA letter to the patient's general practitioner. Of those practitioners who received a DA letter, 98% thought airway information was important, but only half of them forwarded the information to other care providers.[30] A DA letter follow-up survey found that only 50% of patients remembered having a conversation with an anesthesiologist postoperatively, 80% remember getting a letter, 41% of primary providers were aware of the condition, and 23% of patients registered with MedicAlert.[31]

In-hospital DA registries have been shown to decrease emergency surgical airways and empower providers without advanced airway skills to call for assistance earlier in an event.[11,31] Cook and MacDougall-Davis[32] state that "human factors" including communication, judgment, and training are common factors resulting in airway complications.

In addition to effective DA documentation and communication of this critical information to all relevant healthcare providers, other measures can further safeguard patient security. These measures include broadening airway screening systems and implementing care policies for patient with documented DAs. These are evolving areas, and, as such, little research has been done evaluating their effectiveness in supporting patient care.

Conclusion

The need for a universal, ongoing, fully accessible, and comprehensive patient protective DA database is obvious to all active airway practitioners. In this age of the Internet and "big data," lack of critical information should no longer plague patients and healthcare practitioners. The ideal database would satisfy all of these requirements while also allowing for the statistical analysis of epidemiologic and etiologic factors that produce unrecognized DAs.

Selected References

2. American Society of Anesthesiologists Task Force on Guidelines for Management of the Difficult Airway. Practice guidelines for management of the difficult airway. *Anesthesiology.* 1993;78:597–602.

10. Pearce A, Shaw J. Airway assessment and planning. In: Cook T, ed. *NAP4 Major Complications of Airway Management in the United Kingdom.* The Royal College of Anaesthestists and the Difficult Airway Society; 2011: 135–142.

12. Sheeran P, Walsh B, Finley AM, et al. Management of difficult airway patients and the use of a difficult airway registry at a tertiary care pediatric hospital. *Paediatr Anaesth.* 2014;24:819–824.

13. Joffee A, Aziz M, Posner K, et al. Management of difficult tracheal intubation: a closed claims analysis. *Anesthesiology.* 2019;131:818–829.

14. Sakles J, Augustinovich C, Patawoola A, et al. Improvement in the safety of rapid sequence intubation in emergency department with use of an airway continuous quality improvement program. *West J Emerg Med.* 2019;20:610–618.

15. Duggan LV, Lockhart SI, Cook TM, et al. The Airway App: exploring the role of smartphone technology to capture emergency front-of-neck airway experiences internationally. *Anesthesia.* 2018;73:703–710.

25. Koenig HM. No more difficult airway, again! Time for consistent standardized written patient notification of a difficult airway. *APSF Newsletter.* 2010;-6.

32. Cook T, MacDougall-Davis S. Complications and failure of airway management. *Br J Anaesth.* 2012;109:i68–i85.

All references can be found online at eBooks.Health.Elsevier.com.

51

Airway Research

ALISTAIR F. MᶜNARRY AND NARASIMHAN JAGANNATHAN

CHAPTER OUTLINE

KEY POINTS

- Conducting airway research is difficult, partly because of the low incidence of truly difficult airways and the ethics of exposing patients to unnecessary risk (e.g., a randomized controlled trial [RCT] in front-of-neck access).
- Although a meta-analysis of RCTs may be regarded as the epitome of research (level 1a), there may not be enough RDTs in a certain field to provide meaningful answers.
- Surrogates for airway management outcomes are commonly used (time to intubation or percentage of glottic view obtained), and although these are useful scientific tools, they may not tell you if a technique or a device is appropriate for your clinical practice.
- Many similar devices are available, from supraglottic airways (SGAs) to video laryngoscopes, but similarities in form and function do not necessarily equal similarities in clinical effectiveness, and each device must be evaluated carefully.
- When managing the difficult airway, the performance of any airway device must be considered along with the performance of the individual and the entire team under stress (so-called human factors).

- No matter how effective a device has been demonstrated to be in a study, it can only be effective if the user has been trained to use it.
- Many national societies have generated guidelines for the management of difficult airways; these have been constructed using different methodologies and must be considered in the way they were constructed.
- There is much to be learned from the analysis of near misses, critical incidents, or closed claims even though these may not be hypothesis-driven research in their own right.
- Although pediatric research can be difficult practically and ethically, good research in the field of pediatric airway management can be conducted and is important in informing best practice. Just as studies among devices must be extrapolated with care, so must device or procedure efficacy between adults and children and vice versa.
- Novel pathogens may force researchers to extrapolate from preexisting knowledge until necessary research can be carried out, as happened with COVID-19 disease.

Introduction

Airway research is a broad topic, from the physiology of why airways tend to obstruct when consciousness is lost to evaluation of the many different devices available for airway management today.[1] The COVID-19 pandemic brought strategies in airway management to the fore and forced clinicians to combine various strands of research to deliver coordinated patient care. This was not always the case. The paper describing the Macintosh laryngoscope occupied less than one printed page and, although it included a description and picture of the device, it did not include any patients.[2] Similarly, Archie Brain's initial report of the (classic) Laryngeal Mask Airway (cLMA) in the *British Journal of Anaesthesia* reported its use in just 23 patients.[3] New devices have spawned new terminology, such as oropharyngeal leak pressure (OLP) and percentage of glottic opening (POGO), and ways to measure them.[4] New devices have also given rise to new strategies for dealing with intubation difficulties.[5] However, while this problem-based or reactionary approach to airway research is appealing, a structured approach is better. There is a graded hierarchy when assessing the evidence provided in a study (Table 51.1). This is separate to the grade assigned to recommendations based on evidence (Table 51.2), as used in some airway guidelines.[6]

Systematic Reviews, Meta-Analysis, Randomized Controlled Trials

Randomized controlled trials (RCTs) are regarded as the best way to determine whether a given outcome is a result of a specific treatment (cause-effect relationship) or whether it is a random effect.[7] RCTs can be combined to improve the evidence base. A systematic review is an attempt to answer a specific research question by gathering all evidence that meets clearly predefined criteria.[8] Part of that process is an explicit methodology, which would produce the same results if it was reapplied by other researchers. Thus, bias is minimized but it can *never* be eliminated entirely. Findings of included studies should then be presented. This further reduces the risk of bias or the influence of the authors' opinions as may be unintentionally present in a narrative review.[9] An ability to adequately assess the methodology of a study is a vital component of deciding how and when to apply results to clinical practice.

Meta-analysis is a statistical procedure that integrates the results of several independent studies deemed combinable to provide a more objective assessment of the available evidence.[10] It reports an effect between two groups (e.g., intervention and control), which will have both magnitude and direction. Poorly conducted meta-analyses will produce misleading results, particularly if study designs, within-study biases, variation across studies, and reporting biases are not considered.[11]

Once eligible studies have been identified, a measure of the treatment effect with its 95% confidence intervals (CI) of each individual study is made (odds ratios [ORs] or relative risks [RRs] are usually included), then an overall effect as a weighted average is calculated. Greater emphasis is given to more informative studies by using a weighting factor (inverse of the variance).[12] This means larger studies, with smaller standard errors, have a greater impact on the overall results than smaller studies.[11]

Results of a meta-analysis are presented in a forest plot[13] (Fig 51.1[14]). The squares on the horizontal lines are the component studies, with their confidence intervals, plotted on either side of a line of no effect depending on the individual study result. The overall estimate is presented at the bottom of the plot in the

TABLE 51.1	Evidence-Based Medicine Hierarchies of Evidence
Level of Evidence	**Type of Study**
1a	Systematic review of RCTs
1b	Single RCT
1c	All-or-none study (i.e., when all patients died before the therapy became available, but some now survive on it; or when some patients died before the therapy became available, but none now die on it)
2a	Systematic review of level 2b cohort studies
2b	Single cohort study or low-quality RCT
2c	Outcomes studies that investigate outcomes of healthcare practices using epidemiology to link outcomes (e.g., quality of care, quality of life) with independent variables such as geography, income, lifestyle, etc.
3a	Systematic review of level 3b studies
3b	Single case-control or historical-control study
4	Case report or case series
5	Expert opinion or ideas based on theory, on bench studies, or first principles alone

The strongest is level 1a; the weakest is level 5. *RCT*, Randomized controlled trial. (Modified from Pandit JJ, Popat MT, Cook TM, et al. The Difficult Airway Society 'ADEPT' guidance on selecting airway devices: the basis of a strategy for equipment evaluation. Anaesthesia. 2011;66:726–737.)

TABLE 51.2	Grading of Recommendations Based on the Level of Evidence Available
Grade	**Level of Evidence Available**
A	• Consistent systematic reviews of RCTs, single RCTs or all-or-none studies
B	• Consistent systematic reviews of low-quality RCTs or cohort studies, individual cohort study, or epidemiological outcome studies
	• Consistent systematic reviews of case-control studies, individual case-control studies
	• Extrapolations from systematic reviews of RCTs, single RCTs or all-or-none studies
C	• Case series, case reports
	• Extrapolations from systematic reviews of low-quality RCTs, cohort studies or case-control studies, individual cohort study, epidemiological outcome studies, individual case-control studies
	• Extrapolations from systematic reviews of case-control studies
D	• Expert opinion or ideas based on theory, bench studies, or first principles alone
	• Troublingly inconsistent or inconclusive studies of any level

RCT, Randomized controlled trial. From Ahmad I, El-Boghdadly K, Bhagrath R, et al. Difficult Airway Society guidelines for awake tracheal intubation (ATI) in adults. *Anaesthesia.* 2020;75:509–528.

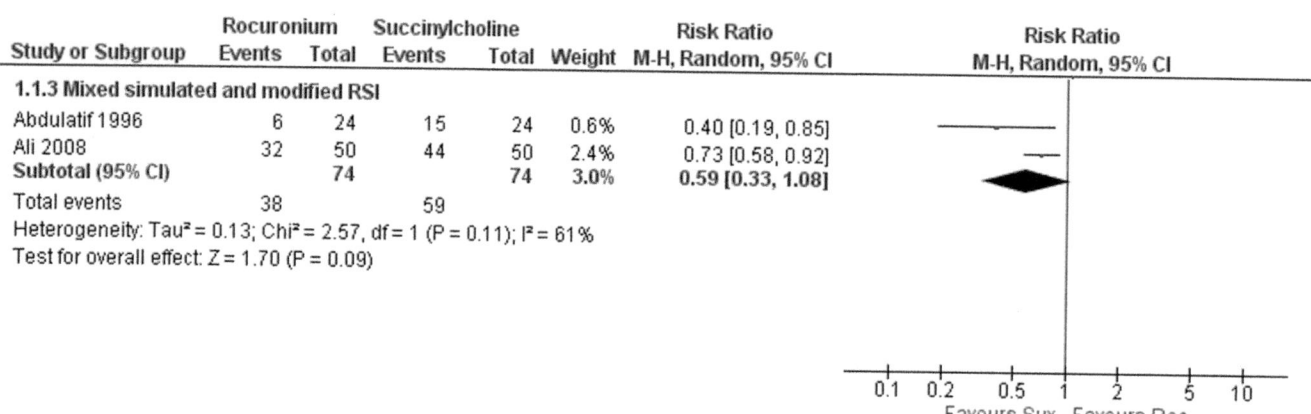

• **Fig. 51.1** An example of a forest plot comparing rocuronium versus succinylcholine for rapid sequence induction intubation. (Modified from Fig. 5 published in Tran DTT, Newton EK, Mount VAH, Lee JS, Wells GA, Perry JJ. Rocuronium versus succinylcholine for rapid sequence induction intubation. *Cochrane Database Syst Rev.* 2015;2015(10):CD002788.)

shape of a diamond. The center of the diamond represents the pooled point estimate, and the horizontal extremes represent the confidence interval. A long, thin diamond represents a wide confidence interval with the potential for a great deal of uncertainty, whereas a broad, short diamond shows that the evidence for effect is strong.[15] Regardless of shape, if the diamond crosses the line of equality/no effect, then there is good evidence that there is no observed difference (absence of effect).[16]

Meta-analyses should also include an assessment of heterogeneity, which asks whether it is reasonable to pool the data from separate studies. If the CI for the results of individual studies (the horizontal lines) have poor overlap, this generally indicates the presence of statistical heterogeneity. This is a clinical judgment, and although it is possible to report a statistical test for heterogeneity ($p < 0.05$ may indicate a problem), most meta-analyses are not sufficiently powered to allow its detection.[12] Meta-analyses are not perfect, and misleading conclusions can be generated.[17] Various tools exist to help readers assess systematic reviews in a methodical way.[18]

Systematic reviews sit at the top of the evidence-based hierarchy but are not guaranteed to provide clear answers. For example, the meta-analysis of the Pentax AWS[19] showed no clinical benefit when using this video laryngoscope despite including over 1800 patients. This is contrary to the demonstration of its effectiveness in 293 patients with previously recorded or likely-to-be difficult airways.[20]

Similarly, a meta-analysis can only be conducted if there is more than one sufficiently sized RCT randomized controlled trial to allow meaningful conclusions to be drawn. One review assessing "the safety and effectiveness of a flexible intubation scope (FIS) used for tracheal intubation in obese patients (body mass index [BMI] >30) with other methods of intubation" concluded that "More primary research is needed."[21] Another Cochrane Review sought to establish whether succinylcholine or rocuronium provided better intubating conditions.[14] It "found no statistical difference in intubation conditions when succinylcholine was compared with 1.2 mg/kg rocuronium; however, succinylcholine was clinically superior, as it has a shorter duration of action." The review clearly stated that it did not consider sugammadex, giving it a clear methodology but making it more difficult to apply to clinical practice and studies comparing the intubating conditions provided by the two agents continue.[22]

Cochrane Reviews are systematic reviews, made available in the Cochrane Library (www.cochranelibrary.com). The Cochrane Library is the world's largest independent provider of systematic reviews. Searching the library with the Medical Subject Headings (MeSH) keywords "Airway Management" revealed 199 reviews (date of search: March 21, 2021). Cochrane produces a variety of resources, including a workbook that acts as the official guide for the preparation of a Cochrane Review.[11]

Literature Review

A comprehensive literature review is a common place to start any research investigation; however, all of the available databases, some of which are outlined here, are subtly different and the benefit of expert advice from a qualified medical librarian cannot be underestimated.

Conventional Databases

Medline is the National Library of Medicine journal citation database started in the 1960s, with records going back to 1946. It currently indexes over 5200 journal titles. PubMed (https://pubmed.ncbi.nlm.nih.gov) has been available since 1996. It contains over 31 million references and includes the Medline database with additional entries.[23] EMBASE is a database maintained by Elsevier, which indexes over 8500 journals from over 95 countries, including all Medline titles.[24] There are other databases—for example, EBSCO (Elton B. Stephens Company) and Continuing Education Module Tutorial (CINAHL; cumulative index to nursing and allied health literature). Different institutions and libraries will have permissions to access different databases. PubMed is freely accessible through the Internet, complete with a variety of online tutorials and videos to improve search results.[25] The TRIP database (originally *Turning Research Into Practice*, https://www.tripdatabase.com) claims to be a clinical search engine delivering research evidence to support practice and care. However, to derive most benefit from these search engines, users must understand how the algorithm scores and weights articles as this will influence the order in which search findings are presented.

Other free academic search engines (e.g., Google Scholar at http://scholar.google.com) offer a wide variety of features to both researcher and author, including citation alerts and export options to bibliography management software. A study into the ranking algorithm suggested that the citation count was the most important feature, meaning that highly cited articles appear earlier in search results than those cited less frequently.[26]

Open-Access Journals

Open-access journals are separate from individual articles, which are made open access by a specific journal. Authors may be required to pay an article processing charge, which covers the cost of the review and editing process, and the article is then free to download for all users. These journals may or may not be listed in all bibliographic databases, but there is now a directory of open-access journals (http://doaj.org), which had indexed 3599 journals under its Medicine heading as of March 2021. Readers should always check how open-access articles are selected for publication by different journal titles because the quality of peer review can vary.

Observational Studies

Observational or longitudinal studies that look at the incidence of infrequent events can be conducted, either by looking at the incidence of device failures (e.g., a supraglottic airway [SGA] or video-assisted laryngoscope [VAL][27-31]) or the incidence of a rare condition in its own right. These types of investigations have advantages and disadvantages. De Jong's study looked at 11,035 patients in the operating room and 1400 in critical care.[32] In patients with obesity, the incidence of difficult intubation (DI) was twice as frequent in the intensive care unit (ICU) as in the operating room (16.3% vs 8.2%). However, the study defined obesity as being a BMI >30 (giving an incidence of 20%), and difficulty was defined as three or more laryngoscopic attempts to place the endotracheal tube, as lasting longer than 10 minutes using conventional laryngoscopy, or both. Other cohort studies report different findings based on their inclusion criteria. The incidence of anticipated airway difficulty was 2.2% in the Fourth National Audit Project (NAP4) of the Royal College of Anaesthetists and the Difficult Airway Society study.[33] Nørskov's study suggested an incidence of difficult tracheal intubation of 1.86%.[34] The vast majority of these were unanticipated, whereas there were a high number of false-positive DIs. Again, without considering the methodology, results can be confusing.

With a relatively low incidence of absolute difficulty, studies must include very large numbers of people to ensure the inclusion of enough patients with genuinely difficult airways. This problem is compounded when considering patients with predicted difficult airways. Most patients anticipated to be difficult were not (75%, 700/929).[34] Therefore, when using airway assessment as an indicator of difficulty, a large number of patients who are not difficult to intubate will also be included; this naturally skews the results of any investigation.

Difficulty in intubation may be overcome (VAL or flexible scope intubation [FSI]) or circumvented (waking the patient up). Difficult face mask ventilation (FMV) presents an anesthetist with a much more immediate problem. Kheterpal's group looked at factors predicting difficult mask ventilation and difficult laryngoscopy.[35] They found several factors (age ≥46, BMI >30, male sex, Mallampati III or IV, neck mass or radiation, limited thyromental distance, sleep apnea, presence of teeth or beard, thick neck, limited cervical spine mobility, limited jaw protrusion) to be independent risk factors for difficult FMV and difficult laryngoscopy

(actual incidence 0.4%). This is a useful finding in and of itself, but it is featured here because to achieve this the group considered 492,239 cases across four institutions, taking 6 years. Such effort is a salutary warning to anyone who wishes to conduct meaningful airway research.

Many observational studies of SGAs (including Brain's in 1983) included relatively small numbers of patients.[3,36,37] Pandit, however, recently reiterated the risks of concluding that a device was effective based on a small study, suggesting that when considering an SGA, we should accept an upper 95% CI for failure of around 2.5% (based on the failure rate of the cLMA of <1%).[31,38] He described how to see at least one failure of a device using these parameters a trial must include around 250 observations/device insertions. Requiring this many observations of a device to define its likely success makes any such observational trial more difficult to perform, but it must be considered when reviewing the available evidence for a device.

This does not mean that small studies are not of value. Any preliminary investigation should feature small numbers so that larger studies can be developed, effectiveness and safety ascertained. This small initial study approach can also be seen in the development of the videolaryngoscope, where the use of the GlideScope was reported in just one case,[39] or in apneic oxygenation using high-flow nasal oxygen (HFNO) where the initial cohort study considered its use in 25 patients.[40]

Ideal Trial

Although the ideal design for any trial is an RCT, the fundamental tenets of such a study, including a clearly defined question, two nearly identical groups, control of everything except the variable under investigation, and researchers blinded to the intervention, can be virtually impossible to create in the field of airway management. Blinding operators in equipment trials is virtually impossible. That knowledge may (subconsciously) influence their behavior with it. Similarly, many studies of equipment are, at least in some way, funded by the equipment manufacturers (e.g., the provision of cheap or at-cost airway devices). This again may (unintentionally) influence an investigator's opinions and induce reporting bias. Even the absolute benefit of an RCT given its cost versus the benefit derived has been questioned.[41]

The Difficult Airway Society (DAS, United Kingdom) devised the ADEPT process (airway device evaluation project team). The authors sought to address the key questions regarding the purchasing of an airway device based on evidence. The group concluded that "All airway-related equipment under consideration must fulfil the minimum criterion, that there exists for it at least one source of level 3b trial evidence concerning its use, published in peer-reviewed scientific literature."[42] This is completely different standard than that required by regulatory bodies to approve the sale of airway devices.

European devices are governed by European Union (EU) law and, as such, must all carry a Conformité Européenne (CE) mark. For medical devices this means that it meets the standards of EU Directive 93/42/ EEC.

In the United States, this governing role falls to the US Food and Drug Administration's Center for Devices and Radiological Health (CDRH), and in Australia it is within the remit of the Therapeutic Goods Administration within the Department of Health.

Despite the ADEPT recommendations for level 3b evidence, many clinicians have found observational studies of both SGAs and VALs beneficial in terms of determining whether or not a device should be used in clinical practice.[27–30] Noble as the ADEPT standards are, at the time of writing there have been no published studies using this methodology.

Pitfalls With Airway Research

A well-crafted research question does not however lead to an easy-to-conduct airway study. Considering the technique of an FSI illustrates the problems that can be faced when conducting airway research. An FSI is a recognized way of facilitating tracheal intubation in a patient known or anticipated to be a DI, and guidelines about its conduct have recently been released.[6] However very few of the recommendations were derived from the highest levels of evidence (see Table 51.2); most were recommendations at Grade D (Expert opinion, inconclusive studies). However, constructing the study as to how FSI might be most effectively conducted or even taught is difficult. Fig. 51.2 shows the various aspects that must be considered when performing an awake FSI. In an ideal study, all parameters in Fig. 51.2 would be standardized, barring the one under investigation. However, the number of features to be standardized is high, making the perfect study difficult to design and conduct.

The number of awake FSIs that should be performed to make an individual competent varies among investigators.[43–46] However, skilled FIS manipulation requires many more FSIs than those required to make the laryngoscopist just competent. The immediate assistance available to the laryngoscopist will also have a role in the success of the procedure, and although this can be standardized (e.g., the same assistant used in every case or a standardized operating procedure for the assistant), it is almost impossible to

control for all such external factors that will potentially impact the study findings.

The BMI or lean body mass of the patient will determine the total safe dose of local anesthetic that can be used,[47] but this may limit the topicalization techniques available to use for some patients. Does this mean that study protocols must accommodate these different techniques? If so, are all the investigators equally trained in each technique? Even the scope chosen may have some bearing on the success of the procedure. The nature of the tube used will impact the success of an awake FSI,[48–50] but at least some part of tube selection may be influenced by the intended surgical procedure. The underlying pathology will also determine both route chosen and difficulty of the procedure. A new technique for topicalizing the airway will fail if all the patients in the intervention group have complex airway lesions that take time and skill to negotiate. Given that it is unlikely that anyone's practice will be able to standardize for the nature of the airway lesion, it is easy to see how the study of an awake flexible technique will be compromised by the impossibility of a controlled study design. One option might be to investigate its use in an anesthetized patient; however, the practicalities of FSI in anesthetized patients are different than that in awake subjects. This makes extrapolating findings from a study on asleep patients directly to an effective awake technique very difficult.

It is also worth considering the effective outcome measures. In terms of adequacy of topicalization, outcome measures such as success of the procedure (ETT through the cords) must be coupled with measures of outcome such as patient tolerance and compliance. This means a standardized premedication/sedation regimen must be employed; however, this may be influenced by the underlying pathologic condition. Similarly, to give unbiased assessment of the technique studied, awake patients' anxiety levels

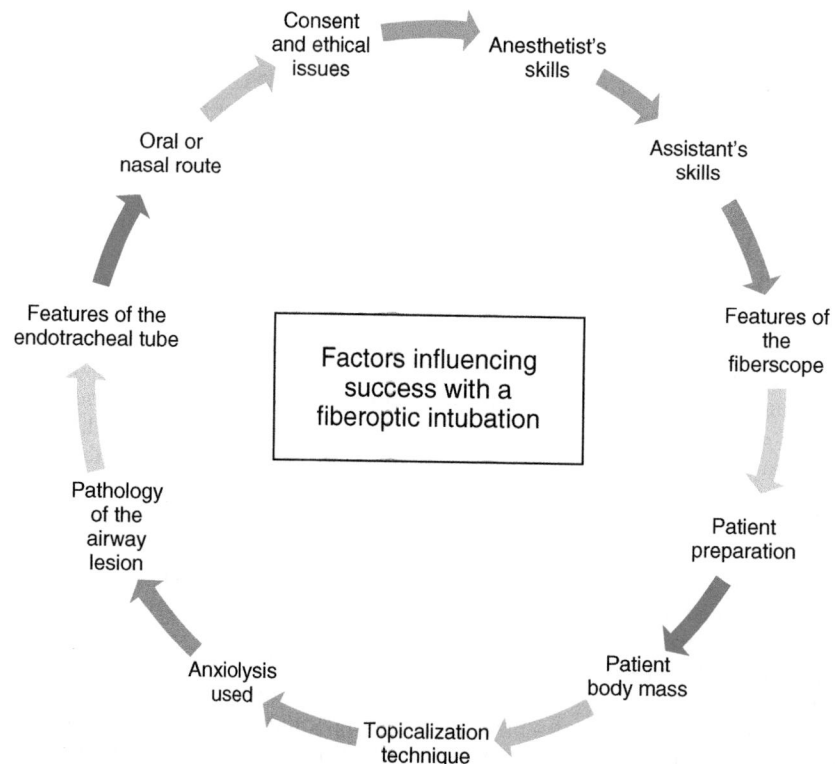

• **Fig. 51.2** Eleven steps that can influence the outcome of a fiberoptic intubation and thus affect the outcome of a study looking at the success of the technique. Standardizing 10 components to study 1 in isolation would be very difficult.

also must be recorded and included in any study analysis. One option might be to test and assess these factors in patients with known normal airways. Although this has been done on medically qualified subjects wishing to learn the technique,[47,51] there are complications associated with it,[52] making ethical approval and subject recruitment more difficult.

The perfect airway study is, therefore, immensely difficult to design. Given the actual low incidence of difficult airways, many studies rely initially on making extrapolations from patients with normal airways or the use of surrogate endpoints for procedure effectiveness.

Airway Research: Questions or Answers

Airway management is not a single topic area but one that involves a complex interplay among a wide variety of factors and features, all of which could be studied in detail. The simplest question is how can patients be effectively oxygenated (and ventilated) while they are anesthetized, given the propensity of the airway to obstruct after induction.[1] This opens up a wide range of topics from effective oxygenation techniques, to equipment used to avoid airway obstruction, and the human factors involved in performing airway management maneuvers, particularly when oxygenation may be compromised. Apneic oxygenation using HFNO has recently been described in a variety of settings.[40,53-56] While mechanisms have been postulated,[57] the most important question: How can a clinician predict when a patient is not going to be effectively oxygenated by HFNO? (i.e., when should this technique of oxygenation not be used?) remains unanswered; although there is some evidence that obesity may play a part.[56] An RCT has demonstrated that this technique does not seem to be as effective in preventing desaturation in patients with a critical illness in the ICU.[58] This variety of evidence has prompted others to try to summarize the available known effects and necessary cautions.[59] Clinicians must decide, based on limited evidence and their own analysis of the quality of that evidence, whether they should adopt the technique. This must be done in the absence of any reported major harm from the technique, but also in the absence of an RCT or a large case series describing its efficacy. The arrival of COVID-19 disease has made many of these assessments of efficacy and safety more pressing (see below).

The original work on desaturation involved modeling,[60,61] which suggested that we should be investigating techniques of oxygenation and also considering methods to avoid desaturation (e.g., that which might be induced by the fasciculation caused by succinylcholine). The availability of rocuronium and sugammadex may reduce the incidence of desaturation from succinylcholine, but sugammadex is a relatively new drug and there may be other complications from its use, not least in the difficult airway setting.[62]

Studying devices to manage the airway generates further questions. Which device or which phase of airway management? For example, devices to manage the airway can include simple bag-valve-mask ventilation, the use of an SGA, or tracheal intubation with a laryngoscope and ETT. Each of these devices can be studied in its own right, but none of them can completely manage the airway in every situation. Therefore, the results of any study involving them must be considered in conjunction with their impact on clinical practice.

The impact of a device in clinical practice usually depends on how it performs in the so-called difficult situation, but even difficulty must be defined to allow meaningful use of study findings.

- Which grade of laryngoscopic view defines difficulty?
- Should the view obtained with a videolaryngoscope be classified using the Cormack and Lehane grading system, or is a new separate system required?[63,64]
- What do studies that use patients with potentially difficult (as predicted by various airway scoring systems) airways actually mean in clinical practice, given that they will contain mostly patients with airways that are not difficult?
- Is it ethical to try new techniques of airway management on patients with known difficult airways before we record their effectiveness in patients with normal airways?

These last two points create a circular argument that usually leads to a pragmatic approach being taken regarding the potential benefits of a device, based on the *available* evidence.

Some suggest that the question which needs to be addressed is not "Which device should be used?" but "When should the airway be secured in relationship to induction of anesthesia?"[65] This then raises questions about how the airway might be secured before induction. Should this be done with awake FSI, awake tracheostomy, or awake VAL? All are possible, but choosing the best technique for a given clinical situation is complex and unlikely to be addressed by the answers from one single study or meta-analysis. Instead, airway practitioners must collate the information available to them from a wide number of sources to apply the best procedure for that patient. An awake FSI may be deemed the most appropriate means of securing a difficult airway. However, if the airway practitioner involved lacks the skills to perform the procedure, it becomes inappropriate. No airway management device tool or strategy can ever be 100% effective. Investigations must be adequately powered not just to achieve statistical significance but also to allow the reader to derive some idea of clinical relevance.

Studies in Airway Assessment

The idea that "prevention is better than cure" is attributed to Dutch philosopher Desiderius Erasmus in around 1500. The ability to identify patients who may be difficult to intubate or to ventilate with a face mask has spawned many scores and airway assessment tools. Airway assessment prior to induction of anesthesia was a recommendation of the NAP4 report.[33] However, constructing a reliable scoring system is difficult. The original Mallampati test defined only three classes and looked at only 210 patients.[66] This was then modified and had its positive predictive value redefined in the light of current practice and definitions and even its use questioned.[67-69]

Yentis described the characteristics of the ideal screening test, which should include a measurable feature that divides the population, have a test that is 100% sensitive (correctly identifies patients with a difficult airway), and 100% specific (patients graded as difficult will be difficult).

This goal is unachievable; Frerk commented that no test could be 100% sensitive.[70] This means that (1) the positive predictive value (PPV, a positive test's likelihood of identifying a difficult airway) of prediction tests will become dependent on the low incidence of a truly difficult airway in the general population (vide supra), (2) unanticipated difficulty will still be encountered and is an entire area of airway research in its own right, and (3) the search for the perfect test will continue.

Several studies have investigated the risk of difficult intubation in the patient with obesity. Brodsky's study in 2002 looked at the relationship between obesity and difficulty in tracheal intubation.[71] In patients with a BMI >40, with a neck circumference of 40 cm, the probability of a problematic intubation was approximately 5%, and at 60 cm this probability rose to 35%. However, only 100 patients were in the study, and in all but 1 patient tracheal intubation by direct laryngoscopy was successful. The study of 180 patients by Neligan et al. in 2009 suggested that neck circumference predicted difficulty in laryngoscopy but not difficulty in intubation.[72] Although they reported no failed intubations, six patients required three or more intubation attempts (DI rate of 3.3%), and they reported an 8.3% incidence of Cormack and Lehane grades III or IV. Riad's study of 104 patients with morbid obesity reported that a neck circumference of greater than 42 cm or a BMI of greater than 50 were independent predictors of DI, but intubation difficulty was defined using the Intubation Difficulty Scale, and all patients were placed in the ramped position before the induction of anesthesia.[73,74] Conversely, Ozdilek's study of 120 patients reported no link between neck circumference and difficult mask ventilation.[75] A meta-analysis by Shiga and colleagues in 2005 suggested that the incidence of DI was three times higher in patients with morbid obesity.[76] However, the meta-analysis was done in 2005, before the widespread availability of VAL, and its principal purpose was to assess the effectiveness of bedside airway assessment tests to predict difficult direct laryngoscopy.

Making sense of well-conducted studies from eminent authors in the field of airway research that are not directly comparable to one's clinical practice is challenging, more so when the results are potentially conflicting. Clinically and practically, an awareness of the results is what is important. If a morbidly obese male with a history of sleep apnea and a neck circumference of 60 cm presents requiring airway management, then the sensible distillation of the literature is to assume the airway might be difficult. If it turns out not to be, it is impossible to say whether that was because of preparedness or because it would always have been straightforward.

Box 51.1 lists 12 questions to help a reader make sense of any article by assessing the quality of evidence it provides.

> • **BOX 51.1** Evidence-Based Medicine Questions to Ask When Reviewing Any Study
>
> 1. Do the study methods accurately allow for testing of the hypothesis?
> 2. Do the statistical tests correctly test the results to allow differentiation of statistically significant results?
> 3. Are the conclusions valid, considering the results?
> 4. Did any results get omitted, and if so, why?
> 5. Did the authors suggest areas for further research?
> 6. Did the authors make any recommendations based on the results and were they appropriate?
> 7. Is this study relevant to my clinical practice?
> 8. What level of evidence does this study represent?
> 9. What grade of recommendation can I make based on this result alone?
> 10. What grade of recommendation can I make when this study is considered alongside other available evidence?
> 11. Should I change my practice based upon these results?
> 12. Should I audit my own practice based upon these results?
>
> Modified from the questions which were first used in 2003 by the Evidence Based Medicine Group of the Scottish Intensive Care Society. They are now used in the *Journal of the Intensive Care Society* as part of a Critical Appraisal Tool.

Facilitating Airway Research

Role of Manikins in Airway Research

Manikins have been advocated in airway research.[77] They have (at least) three potential roles: (1) early evaluation of new equipment, (2) training of staff in the technical skills required to do a procedure, and (3) use in a simulation setting to teach the nontechnical skills required to manage an anesthetic or, more specifically, an airway crisis.[78]

Manikins have limitations—for example, low-fidelity manikins are inexpensive but potentially unrealistic, a recent study reporting that three assessed manakins were potentially anatomically unrealistic, leading to imprecise airway device development, negatively affecting training, and causing overconfidence in users.[79] One study investigating second-generation SGAs suggested that, to optimize performance during training, the airway manikin should be chosen depending on the SGA in use.[80] Similarly, a study of a flexible bronchoscope in two manikins concluded (regardless of its findings) that "This manikin study does not predict performance in humans and a clinical study is required."[81] High-fidelity scenarios are resource intensive and can only deliver an educational or assessment opportunity for a few people at any one time. However, a meta-analysis found that simulation for airway management training was associated with improved outcomes compared with no intervention,[82] and a nonsimulation intervention and low-fidelity training has been recommended in teaching or reinforcing airway skills.[83] Computer modeling can be used to determine what might happen in various clinical situations, although this is entirely dependent on the parameters used to inform the model in the first place.[61]

Surrogates of Effective Airway Management

The size of the study required to effectively compare two airway devices may be large, depending on the primary outcome. Studies have sought to avoid this challenge by using surrogate outcomes of efficacy, such as time to insertion or glottic view achieved, but these do not actually tell clinicians whether the device will be useful in their clinical practice. The time to insert or use a device is often seen as an indicator of ease of use. For the investigator, this is a continuous variable and likely to require smaller sample sizes to demonstrate a statistically significant p value. Whether a difference in intubation time that can be measured in terms of a few seconds genuinely matters in a group of patients in whom no desaturation occurs is a point for academic discussion and requires clinical consideration.

Understanding and Training of the Investigator

Any investigation of equipment is dependent on the investigating team having achieved a minimum level of confidence with a device. However, some studies suggest that the learning curve for device use may be large. Brimacombe suggested that the learning curve for the cLMA was somewhere between 75 and 750 uses, a difficult standard to attain when assessing a new device.[84,85] Similarly, when making assessments, a grade I Cormack and Lehane view may be defined, but reporting on this score is variable.[86] How can studies be compared if even their basic definitions cannot be reliably replicated?

Comparing Different Laryngoscopes

Identifying the best tool to facilitate tracheal intubation is an obvious area for which detailed airway research should be conducted.

Rose and Cohen suggested that the incidence of difficult or awkward intubation (based on the number of laryngoscopies) was 4.3%.[87] The failure rate of actual tracheal intubation, however, was only 0.3%. Shiga's meta-analysis of 35 studies involving almost 51,000 patients suggested that the incidence of DI was 5.8%.[76] Aziz's longitudinal study of the performance of the GlideScope found the success rate at tracheal intubation was at least 97%.[30] In Asai's study[20] of 293 patients, the Pentax-AWS was successful at achieving tracheal intubation in 268 cases of 270 (99.3%), known to be Cormack and Lehane grades II, III and IV. Of the 256 patients with a conventional view of grade III or IV, the Pentax-AWS view was grade I or II.

VAL achieves a better view of the larynx than conventional laryngoscopy, but that is not the same as a difficult tracheal intubation. Early data with the McGrath Series 5 laryngoscope suggested an excellent view of the glottis did not necessarily equate with an easy tracheal intubation, but the study could not report whether this was a failure of the device or a failure of training with the device.[88]

Based on a comparison between Shiga's study and Asai's study it would appear reasonable to look at the incidence of good glottic view between video and conventional laryngoscopy. One could presume a good glottic view is obtained with a VAL in approximately 98% of patients, whereas it is approximately 94% with conventional laryngoscopy (using Cormack and Lehane grade I or II as the definition of good glottic view). Using these assumptions, a study to demonstrate a statistically significant difference would be demonstrable with 300 patients in each group. A study of 600 patients is possible to achieve but relies on the assumption that all patients who are Cormack and Lehane grade III will be difficult to intubate and that anyone with a "good" video laryngoscopic view will be easy to intubate. If the same analysis were applied to two video laryngoscopes to try to determine which one was most effective (taking as an example a success rate of 98% vs 99%), then each group size would have to be around 1500. Data could be gathered on patients with known difficult airways, but it may then prove more difficult to recruit enough participants. The Cochrane review of VAL in 2016 looked at 64 studies and 7044 patients.[89] It concluded that statistically significantly fewer failed intubations were reported when a videolaryngoscope was used. While this clearly demonstrates the benefit of videolaryngoscopy to facilitate successful tracheal intubation, it does not help individual clinicians choose the device best suited to their specific clinical situation, for which factors such as budgets, cleaning protocols, space, user experience, and training programs all must be considered.

Reliance on Only One Feature

We have described how airway management is a complex interplay of many factors; however, even individual devices can be described and defined by several different features, all of which may have a separate impact on device performance and should be considered when choosing one device over another. Laryngeal mask airway (LMA or SGA) outcomes can be defined and described by OLP, the ability to insert an orogastric tube, ability to intubate through the device, or ease of device insertion. Some devices may have very good outcomes in one area (e.g., the OLP with the Baska mask) but may be less effective in others (they have a low first-time insertion success rate).[37,90] Similarly, the Supreme LMA has a high first-time insertion success rate, but because it might be difficult to use for an airway exchange technique, it has been specifically not advocated in certain guidelines.[29,91] To confuse matters

further, van Zundert and colleagues have now suggested that an exchange technique with this device is possible.[92] How should this then apply to an individual's clinical practice? It may be that one device is better suited to the elective situation, whereas another might be best for an airway emergency where tracheal intubation has failed. Cook and Kelly have suggested scoring all the features of an SGA to arrive at the optimal device,[93] but this sort of conclusion depends on many other studies of SGAs being available.

Guidelines for Airway Management

Many national societies or colleges have produced guidelines for airway management regarding assessment, intubation, and extubation with the German Society of Anesthesiology and Intensive Care Medicine and the Difficult Airway Society on their second iteration and the American Society of Anesthesiologists on their third.[91,94–98] The Difficult Airway Society has produced and co-authored guidelines that extend to obstetric airway management, airway management on critical care, awake tracheal intubation, obstetrics, pediatrics, and extubation.[6,99–102] The guidelines are meant to summarize practice and provide clinicians with a rational airway management strategy to use in their daily practice without the need to interpret large quantities of research in airway management with every case.

However, the wide variety of guidelines available are, in themselves, testament to the fact that none of the guidelines contains all the answers. The Project for the Universal Management of the Airway (www.universalairway.org) has started to publish its guidelines[103]; however, it remains to be seen whether this ambitious project to unify airway guidelines will gain traction at a local level.

Guidelines take time to prepare, and it is likely that after publication new evidence will be published that could not have been considered. It then becomes the responsibility of the anesthesia practitioner to interpret the new research in the context of the guidelines. How this is done is especially important as guidelines tend to dictate the practice of those assisting the anesthesiologist or responding in an airway emergency. Failure is more likely if participants are working from different mental models.

Surgical Airway/Emergency Invasive Airway Access

Emergency invasive airway access or airway rescue is the final step for oxygenation when alternative techniques in the anesthetized patient have failed. Various methods for achieving this are described, but none of the techniques can carry a grade A recommendation. The techniques have all been established by reviews of events, simulation in models, from the animal wet-lab experience, or are based on effective techniques in the elective setting.[33,104,105–107] There are some longitudinal studies from prehospital investigations.[108] However, although convincing arguments and examples can be made for both the "cannula-first" and "scalpel-only" techniques,[109–112] decisions as to which technique to employ and teach at a local level are much more nuanced and will depend on local or even national practice alongside teaching and training strategies and available equipment. Sheep are not human patients, and the out-of-hospital trauma scenario is different from the in-hospital elective orthopedic or general surgical list. Even if the general approach is agreed, the specifics of the technique may vary.[113–115]

There will never be an effective clinical study into the best method to create a surgical airway in patients where all other attempts at airway management have failed and who are now critically hypoxic. Not only are these factors impossible to recreate, but also the environment where the rescue technique is to be performed will also influence performance, as will the grade and training of staff members involved.

In the NAP4 report, the 95% confidence intervals for each of the surgical airway access techniques considered were remarkably similar (Table 51.3), making it impossible to draw a meaningful conclusion from the evidence collated, despite the initial impression that ths cannula cricothyrotomy failure rate was much higher than that for surgical cricothyrotomy.

NAP4 correctly identified prediction and prevention of cannot intubate/cannot oxygenate (CICO) as an important area for research, and although some suggested that the failures may be educationally related,[116] this is a multifactorial problem with two difficulties: (1) it is unlikely that any project of sufficient size will be conducted in the near future to measure the impact of any changes, and (2) there is not enough evidence at present to suggest what that change should be. Despite the deficiencies of observational cohort studies, it is likely that this will have to be the source of information in this area. In silico studies, physiological parameters predicted based on a validated model may be a useful tool[117,118]; however, it remains to be established whether these studies will be regarded as adequate evidence to inform and influence practice.

Pediatric Research

Research in children is a potentially complex area both ethically and practically. In recent years, several impactful multicenter studies in children have potentially heightened awareness of complications and offered best practices suggestions during pediatric airway management. Engelhardt and colleagues published a secondary subgroup analysis on difficult airway and ventilation management in children from multiple European centers that participated in the Anaesthesia Practice in Children Observational Trial (APRICOT).[119] Their results provide better insight into the current management of the pediatric difficult airway throughout Europe. These findings highlight several areas where new evidence may be applied to improve airway management outcomes in children.

APRICOT was designed as a European, multicenter observational cohort to study critical events in pediatric anesthesia,

	TABLE 51.3	**Success or Failure of Various Front-of-Neck Airway Strategies as Reported in Fourth National Audit Project of the Royal College of Anaesthetists and the Difficult Airway Society**

	Headline Failure Rate	95% CI for Failure
Narrow-bore cannula	12/19	38.3–83.7
Wide-bore cannula	3/7	0–81.6
Surgical	0/3	0–70.7

CI, Confidence interval.
From Fourth National Audit Project of the Royal College of Anaesthetists and Difficult Airway Society. *Major Complications of Airway Management in the United Kingdom. Report and Findings.* Cook TM, Woodall N, Frerk C, eds. Royal College of Anaesthetists; 2011.

includes over 30,000 children, and is perhaps the best available snapshot of current pediatric anesthesia practices. The initial analysis revealed a relatively high incidence of critical events in pediatric anesthesia at 5.2%.[120] Particularly common were respiratory events, including laryngospasm, bronchospasm, and stridor, with an overall incidence of 3.1%.

A subgroup analysis on difficult airway management in children reveals that difficult or failed intubation is rare, occurring in only 131 of 31,024 patients (0.42%).[119] However, failed intubation was associated with a twofold increase in risk for respiratory critical events. Difficult or failed SGA placement was found to be similarly rare, occurring in just 49 patients, but resulted in a fourfold increase in critical respiratory events.

The Pediatric Difficult Airway Registry (PeDIR)[121] collaborative was collecting data on more than 2000 difficult airway events in the United States. Similar outcomes are revealed in their analyses. Both APRICOT and PeDIR found an increased likelihood of airway difficulty in younger children, particularly infants. These findings regarding incidence of difficult airway are like other single center reports of difficult laryngoscopy in infants.[122,123] Both the APRICOT and PeDIR studies also noted significantly increased respiratory events in patients with three or more attempts at intubation, suggesting the possibility that morbidity may be decreased by reducing the total number of tracheal intubation attempts.

Observations from PeDIR publications offer clues for reducing critical events associated with difficult airway management. It has been shown that tracheal intubation success is abysmally poor with use of direct laryngoscopy, with success rates of 4% of initial attempts and an eventual success rate of 21%.[124] In comparison, both VAL and FSI via SGA offer much higher rates of initial and eventual success.[124,125] In infants, FSI through an SGA was particularly successful and had the added benefit of allowing continuous ventilation during attempts, a practice which may reduce hypoxemic events (oxygen desaturations) that eventually lead to more serious critical events.[125] Clinicians should consider devices and approaches to minimize complications during tracheal intubation attempts. The use of passive oxygenation may prolong the margin of safety during intubation attempts and should be implemented in patients where a high risk of oxygen desaturations would likely occur.[126–130]

Another multicenter analysis of difficult tracheal intubation in neonates and infants, from a European observational cohort study of critical events in pediatric anesthesia (the NEonate-Children Study of Anaesthesia Practice in Europe [NECTARINE] study)[131] included neonates and infants up to 60 weeks postconceptual age undergoing anesthesia. In this cohort, difficult tracheal intubation, defined as two failed attempts of direct laryngoscopy, occurred at an incidence of 5.8% (95% CI 5.1% to 6.5%). In two-thirds of those patients, difficult intubation was unexpected. The most frequent intervention used to achieve a successful tracheal intubation consisted in changing the laryngoscope blade as well as calling for experienced help. Advanced alternative indirect techniques such as use of a videolaryngoscope or flexible bronchoscope were only utilized in a limited number of cases where difficult intubation was expected. Successful intubation was achieved in 98% of cases within an average of three attempts, with no patients requiring surgical airway access. Bradycardia occurred in 8% of the cases with difficult intubation, and a significant decrease in oxygen saturation (Spo$_2$ <90% for 60 seconds or longer) occurred in 40%. Difficult tracheal intubation did not lead to a significant increase in 30-day and 90-day morbidity or mortality.

Considering the recent evidence, it is now time to develop formal recommendations to help guide clinicians with best practice strategies for children during airway management. Clinicians must also familiarize themselves with advanced airway techniques to gain the skills and confidence needed to manage these challenging airways.

The Role of Audits, Surveys of Practice, and Case Reports

Although audits and surveys of practice are not accorded the same level of evidence as RCTs, systematic reviews, and meta-analysis, they can provide a great deal of information about clinical practice and should not be disregarded. Similarly, they are frequently a starting point for researchers with an interest in airway management and consideration should be given as to how to conduct them effectively.

Audits

The most significant audit project to have been conducted in airway management was the NAP4, which was published in 2011.[33] This study was UK wide and had specific entry criteria including death, brain damage, and unanticipated critical care admission secondary to the complications of airway management or emergency surgical airway. A team of experts then reviewed each of the cases included in the data set and generated a series of recommendations for patient management, for anesthetists' behavior, and for institutional preparedness to reduce the incidence of adverse events. Unlike a conventional study, the NAP4 audit was designed to record episodes of airway management with an adverse outcome. It did not record cases of good or excellent airway management and did not record any details of those cases, which may have included an adverse event but were managed well and thus did not meet the inclusion criteria of the report.

Adverse event reporting is used to improve practice in other countries. J.B. Cooper is regarded as the pioneer of incident reporting in anesthesia following his work published in 1978.[132,133] The Australian Incident Monitoring Study followed. The American Society of Anesthesiologists closed claims database was started in 1985, and although it looks at claims rather than incidents, it is a useful source of information, not least in relation to airway injury. Sadly, the most recent report looking at difficult tracheal intubation found that inadequate airway planning and judgment errors were contributors to patient harm.[134] Not only are these similar to the themes identified in NAP4, but they are not solved by the study of a single device or technique and will require a multifactorial approach. Smith and Mahajan report the development of such systems in several countries,[135] and there are obvious benefits in improving patient safety, even though they are not a study with a specific null hypothesis.

Surveys

Surveys of practice in airway management are common, and although they do not answer a specific clinical question, they inform opinion around a particular topic and can be useful for assimilating knowledge on a particular technique or facet of airway management. The advent of online survey tools has made gathering data easier for the researcher as surveys can be distributed around the globe, although it is important to realize the limitations and benefits of surveys.[136] Bruce and Chambers suggested

a variety of features to improve the information that might be gleaned from survey-based research: (1) careful choice of the question to be answered, (2) identifying the correct group who should answer the question (not necessarily the group easiest to target), (3) questionnaire piloting, and (4) aiming for a response rate of 70% to 80% to allow inferences to be drawn.[137]

A question on training opportunities should be addressed to trainees. It can be answered by senior members of the staff, but the results may not be as meaningful, and it is possible to draw the wrong conclusions.

The most obvious failing of a questionnaire, regardless of careful selection of the question and group, is the problem of response rate. Would absent responses greatly influence a survey's findings? The short but honest answer is that no one can know, but a high response rate helps mitigate the effect of the nonresponder group. Although online tools have made distribution of surveys much easier, privacy issues arise in having access to participants' email addresses, which are necessary to allow follow-up.

The use of incentives has been shown to improve response rates, as in postal returns doubling when monetary incentives were used,[138] but this strategy raises ethical concerns.

Despite their drawbacks, surveys remain a useful way of collecting views and opinions and raising awareness of certain issues. However, to be most effective they probably need to be part of research and/or education strategy (i.e., followed up by a method of dealing with the issues identified), rather than being treated as a stand-alone research tool.

Case Reports

Case reports or case series are regarded as level 4 evidence, and journals vary as to whether they accept them. They can be useful sources of information for the management of a rare condition or as an example of a rare or less common complication of the management of an otherwise straightforward incident. When writing a case report the authors must consider the learning points for the reader, whereas when reading a case report the reader must consider carefully how the limited amount of evidence presented applies to their clinical scenario.

COVID-19

Pneumonia of unknown etiology was first reported to the Centers for Disease Control and Prevention (CDC) and the World Health Organization (WHO) on December 31, 2019.[139] The WHO declared a pandemic on March 11, 2020.[140]

While well-constructed RCTs were developed rapidly (e.g., RECOVERY[141]) and allowed for the swift publication of actionable results[142] for drug treatments and vaccine development,[143,144] resolution of airway management dilemmas was even more urgent, as patients presented with life-threatening hypoxia requiring emergent airway management.

Reports published even before a pandemic had been declared suggested that 2.3% of COVID-19 patients required tracheal intubation.[145] By the end of February 2020, almost 100,000 cases had been reported.[146]

Several countries, colleges and universities, and airway interest groups produced guidelines to address these issues, based on prior experience (of SARS-CoV-1) and their understanding of the modes of transmission.[147-155]

Although all these guidelines and cohort reports were produced using the best available evidence, not all the recommendations have borne the scrutiny of ongoing clinical experience. Working out how to ensure the safety of healthcare workers had to be extrapolated from the lessons learned during the first SARS outbreak in 2003,[156–158] and correspondingly, many early guidelines suggested that "Transmission is thought to be predominantly by droplet spread."[147] This assumption was revised as better evidence emerged, and guidance was updated to clearly state the risk of airborne transmission.[159] This has led to several studies of aerosol-generating procedures, but to date these do not include patient-based studies.[160,161]

HFNO has been recognized as beneficial in the treatment of the hypoxia of acute respiratory failure.[162] However, in the setting of COVID-19 disease, concerns were raised about the risk of aerosol generation and the possibility of exhausting hospitals' finite supplies of oxygen during an overwhelming pandemic. This led to HFNO being "not currently recommended" or advice that its prolonged use should be avoided in the earliest editions of some COVID airway management guidelines.[145,154]

On the other hand, a multicenter prospective cohort study of 122 patients showed that HFNO led to an increase in ventilator-free days and a reduction in ICU length of stay, but that further studies were required.[163] The applicability of HFNO is marginal for apneic oxygenation in patients with severe shunting.

The most recent publications suggest that "There is currently no convincing evidence that HFNO increases the levels of nosocomially transmitted COVID-19 in healthcare workers."[164,165]

The concept of intubation boxes or drapes to minimize the risk of exposing the intubator to infected aerosols or droplets (check) was discussed early in the pandemic, with some early studies claiming to show benefit but this was questioned.[166,167] A literature review and simulation study followed while other authors promoted not a box but a drape to prevent aerosol transmission without inhibiting intubator function.[168–170] This practice is highly controversial, and there remains a pressing need for RCTs to guide barrier precautions during COVID-19 airway management.

What can we learn from the responses to the COVID-19 pandemic? A great deal of this chapter has been spent outlining how well-constructed research can be used to answer a specific research question. Literature reviews and meta-analyses of RCTs are meant to be the best means of defining valid answers. However, in the field of airway management, we are often confronted by situations where well-constructed randomized clinical trials are virtually impossible—for example, the best technique for awake tracheal intubation. An A randomized controlled trial in patients may even be considered unethical, as would be the case when investigating the best technique for creation of an emergency surgical airway.

Patients presenting with acute hypoxia from COVID-19 disease compelled clinicians to use the information they had to produce management principles and deliver patient care. This entailed unavoidable extrapolation from what was understood historically, while accepting that these approaches would be refined and improved as the pandemic developed.

The controversies related to HFNO highlight the need to devise a suite of robust clinical questions, as there are several issues that will have to be addressed:

1. Does HFNO delay or prevent intubation, and in what circumstances is it superior to CPAP?
2. Does HFNO actually contribute to improved survival for patients?
3. Is HFNO an aerosol-generating procedure, and if so, what are the safety precautions required to mitigate the risks to attending staff?
4. Might HFNO actually reduce aerosol production in patients with respiratory distress?
5. What criteria indicate that a trial of HFNO should be abandoned to avoid unnecessarily delaying intubation?

Clearly several research questions still need to be addressed, even as vaccines start to bring the pandemic under control. Carefully designed RCTs are still required to confirm or refute the invocations of rapidly formulated early clinical guidelines, which leaned heavily on expert opinion in the absence of objectively derived evidence.

Conclusion

Airway research is a necessary part of our understanding of difficult airway management, and although this chapter does not attempt to describe how to conduct a study in absolute detail, it provides the reader with some of the considerations necessary to design (or interpret) a study that will have statistical significance while being clinically relevant to allow necessary changes in clinical practice.

Selected References

3. Brain AIJ. The laryngeal mask—a new concept in airway management. *Br J Anaesth.* 1983;55:801–806.
8. Uman LS. Information management for the busy practitioner: systematic reviews and meta-analyses. *J Am Acad Child Adolesc Psychiatry.* 2011;20:57–59.
11. Higgins J, Thomas J, Chandler J, et al. *Cochrane Handbook for Systematic Reviews of Interventions.* 2nd ed. John Wiley & Sons; 2019. Available at https://training.cochrane.org/handbook.
33. Fourth National Audit Project of the Royal College of Anaesthetists and Difficult Airway Society. *Major Complications of Airway Management in the United Kingdom. Report and Findings.* Cook TM, Woodall N, Frerk C, eds. Royal College of Anaesthetists; 2011.
35. Kheterpal S, Healy D, Aziz MF, et al. Incidence, predictors, and outcome of difficult mask ventilation combined with difficult laryngoscopy: a report from the multicenter perioperative outcomes group. *Anesthesiology.* 2013;119:1360–1369.
63. Cormack RS, Lehane J. Difficult tracheal intubation in obstetrics. *Anaesthesia.* 1984;39:1105–1111.
89. Lewis SR, Butler AR, Parker J, Cook TM, Schofield-Robinson OJ, Smith AF. Videolaryngoscopy versus direct laryngoscopy for adult patients requiring tracheal intubation: a Cochrane Systematic Review. *Br J Anaesth.* 2017;119:369–383.
121. Fiadjoe JE, Nishisaki A, Jagannathan N, et al. Airway management complications in children with difficult tracheal intubation from the Pediatric Difficult Intubation (PeDI) registry: a prospective cohort analysis. *Lancet Respir Med.* 2016;4:37–48.
134. Joffe AM, Aziz MF, Posner KL, Duggan LV, Mincer SL, Domino KB. Management of difficult tracheal intubation: a closed claims analysis. *Anesthesiology.* 2020;131:818–829.
147. Cook TM, El-Boghdadly K, McGuire B, McNarry AF, Patel A, Higgs A. Consensus guidelines for managing the airway in patients with COVID-19: Guidelines from the Difficult Airway Society, the Association of Anaesthetists the Intensive Care Society, the Faculty of Intensive Care Medicine and the Royal College of Anaesthetists. *Anaesthesia.* 2020;75:785–799.
161. Wilson NM, Marks GB, Eckhardt A, et al. The effect of respiratory activity, non-invasive respiratory support and facemasks on aerosol generation and its relevance to COVID-19. *Anaesthesia.* 2021;76(11)1465–1474. doi:10.1111/anae.15475.

All references can be found online at eBooks.Health.Elsevier.com.

52

Airway Management and Outcomes Reporting

ALEXANDER NAGREBETSKY AND RICHARD P. DUTTON

CHAPTER OUTLINE

KEY POINTS

- Adequate documentation of airway management outcomes supports the goal of never having an unanticipated difficult airway.
- Parallel documentation of data in different sections of an electronic medical record allows for cross-checking of information, potentially increasing its reliability, but also increasing methodologic confounding if the sources do not agree.
- Automatization of clinical documentation is a particularly important function of an anesthesia information management system (AIMS)—the AIMS can be used to record objective physiologic data during periods when the anesthesiologist's attention is focused on the patient and procedure.

- The AIMS should seek to create discrete data (i.e., a menu of options for recording laryngoscope type is better than a free-text field, because the resulting data will be easier to analyze).
- Whenever possible, difficult airway management should be defined in terms of highly objective data such as video recording and automatically captured vital signs.
- Implementation of objective and standardized definitions of airway management outcomes will increase the validity of results obtained in quality improvement projects and academic research.

Introduction

Airway management is a core skill of anesthesia professionals and something we take justifiable pride in doing well. This textbook illustrates the importance of airway management in clinical practice, and the many papers cited provide ample evidence of the growth of scientific understanding in this domain. This chapter will focus on the methodology behind clinical research in airway management, summarizing the data elements and metrics used to evaluate success and presenting options for future research in the era of electronic healthcare records, national registries, and comparative effectiveness research fueled by big data.

Documentation of Airway Management Outcomes

Documentation of airway management outcomes and the techniques used to achieve them serve two important purposes. First is the traditional role of medical documentation in supporting continuity of care. Future providers can learn from the experience of those who have gone before. While past returns of the stock market do not predict future performance, a past history of easy intubation is the best predictor that a future intubation attempt will be straightforward. And the situations where this might not be true—say when there is an expanding mass in the airway or active bleeding—are usually obvious to the clinician.

Even more important than evidence supporting easy airway management is the opposite: documentation of previous difficulties. Because airway management outcomes are likely to be better when the clinician can plan ahead, foreknowledge of anatomic abnormalities can be crucial in supporting the patient safety goal of never having an unanticipated difficult airway.

The second role of documentation is to support clinical research, with the goal of continuously improving patient care. Published studies of airway management techniques number in the thousands and extend back in time for decades. Historically, data have been captured from clinical records (in retrospective studies) or by direct observation and contemporaneous documentation. While some of the outcomes and metrics observed are "structured" (i.e., objectively defined in a digital format), a frustrating number of key elements are subjective in definition or documentation. "Laryngoscope blade used" is an objective data element, often structured in electronic records by inclusion in a list of menu options. "Mallampati score" is a structured element (a common, numeric definition exists), but it is subjectively measured (different providers may score the same patient differently), whereas "Difficult intubation" lacks both a common definition and interrater reliability. Difficulty can vary based on the skills and experience of the providers, as well as on the initial approach; a patient who is difficult to intubate via direct laryngoscopy (DL) might be easy when a video-assisted laryngoscope (VAL) is used. A practitioner using VAL as the initial plan would never know that airway management with DL would be difficult.

The history of airway management outcomes documentation is, thus, a quest for better and more objective methods of defining the patient and clinical experience. The purpose is to develop performance data that can be used to assess different techniques and devices in an evidence-based fashion. These data enable design of instruments, development of protocols and algorithms, and continuous quality improvement of both institutions and individuals. In the modern era of electronic record-keeping, the potential for passive, automatic uptake of large quantities of structured data is enormous but still largely unrealized. We can see the potentials but not yet grasp the prize.

The most important element of airway management documentation remains the clinical narrative, the story of what happened. Paradoxically, it is becoming harder to reconstruct a clinical narrative in the Information Age, because the electronic medical record (EMR) fragments information across multiple forms and screens or hides ad hoc comments in out-of-the-way places. Yet the ability to retrospectively understand the course of airway management in a given patient—especially if difficulties are encountered—remains critical to our ability to improve. This is why initiatives, such as the Anesthesia Incident Reporting System (AIRS) and the Anesthesia Closed Claims Project (CCP), remain so important to ongoing quality improvement. Each of these programs captures narrative detail about unusual cases. AIRS is an online system (http://www.aqiairs.org) that enables immediate reporting of adverse events, near misses, and interesting cases. The narratives are captured in a deidentified registry maintained by the Anesthesia Quality Institute, secure from legal discovery, and are used to generate illustrative case reports and teaching exercises. Now in its 30th year, CCP is a retrospective review of malpractice activity involving anesthesiologists, powered by expert review of detailed clinical and insurance company records. Airway cases captured in CCP are, thus, the worst of the worst, almost always resulting in death or serious injury. Neither system can accurately estimate the *rate* of problems in airway management, but each provides important information about what *can* happen. For rare events, such as patient injury from airway management, these narratives are an important source of learning and have been used to design and promulgate clinical countermeasures against identified risks. The goal of incident-report collection systems is to never make the same mistake twice.

Quality Improvement in Anesthesia

The medical specialty of anesthesiology has a laudable record of continuous process improvement based on self-examination of outcomes and development and application of evidence-based guidelines and protocols. Anesthesia is arguably safer than ever, enabling complex procedures on very sick patients. Advances have been achieved dating back to at least 1954 and the work of Henry Beecher in defining perioperative mortality in a coalition of major teaching hospitals.[1] There have been numerous subsequent studies of anesthesia patient safety, ranging from descriptions of serious adverse events (e.g., the many reports from the Closed Claims Project) to prospective randomized trials of new medications, monitors, and devices. All are based on the collection of clinical data, systematic analysis, and academic reporting to the professional community.

Collecting Data

Assessing the outcomes of airway management is one facet of this overall quality improvement effort, now accelerating in the Information Age. Registries of clinical information create the capability to simultaneously link patient and procedural risk factors with anesthesia interventions, then examine the outcomes achieved. This process of using available medical documentation rather than painstakingly abstracted research data to compare interventions is known as administrative database research. While in theory it is straightforward and inexpensive, the results are subject to a number of methodologic issues:

- Data points must be commonly defined across all records.
- Definitions must be applied in a uniform way by all observers.
- Outcomes must be observed at similar times in all locations.
- Sufficient information must be gathered to understand differences in patient, procedure, and facility variables, and then used to provide valid risk adjustment of the outcomes.

For airway management, the ultimate outcomes of interest include survival, avoidance of major complications (e.g., hypoxic brain injury), avoidance of cricothyroidotomy, and patient satisfaction. Intermediate outcomes include the time taken to achieve a stable airway, the number of attempts, the need to change technique or operator, and the stability of vital signs. Variables that influence risk include patient age, sex, BMI, anatomic presentation, and comorbidities, as well as other elements such as emergent status, facility type, and type of surgery being performed.

Systematic Analysis and Reporting

Once data collection is underway, decisions must be made on how to present the results. Reporting must be purpose specific. Considerations include who will see the report (e.g., the public, federal government, hospital administration, department leadership, or individual practitioner), how frequently reports are delivered (daily, monthly, quarterly, yearly), and whether to report raw numbers, rates, or risk-adjusted metrics. In general, raw numbers and rates will be most appropriate for internal quality reporting, because variable risk factors such as patient population, operations performed, surgeons, anesthesiologists, and facility type will not change from month to month. Risk adjustment is important—and necessary—when making external comparisons and when reporting to federal regulatory programs designed for public transparency.

Change Management

Once data are collected, analyzed, and reported, the role of the quality program is to facilitate improvements in patient care—to put the data to work. This can include new policies or procedures, introduction of new devices, or even prohibitions on activities found to be too dangerous. Whenever possible, the clinicians affected should be the ones reacting to the data and suggesting options for improvement. "Solutions" imposed from on high are often impractical in the real world and suffer from a lack of buy-in. Discussion of adverse airway events in the monthly Morbidity and Mortality (M&M) conference is an excellent way to heighten awareness of potential problems and to solicit countermeasures from the clinical staff—for example, "We should bring a video laryngoscope to every intubation outside the operating room."

Anesthesia Information Management Systems

Overview

An anesthesia information management system (AIMS) is a subtype of EMRs used to collect, store, and facilitate retrieval and analysis of clinical data. Unlike in most settings, data management for anesthesia care involves multiple data streams and a high volume of data transmitted via each stream (e.g., pulse oximetry values every second). For this reason, automatization of clinical documentation is a particularly important function of the AIMS.

The AIMS has significant potential for clinical decision support. There is evidence that relatively simple prompts from the AIMS improve adherence to standard monitoring practices and can influence anesthesia provider behavior.[2,3] The next step in clinical decision support may be to combine data obtained during the case with other data recorded in the electronic health record (EHR) in near real-time. For example, the AIMS could compare the patient's current cardiac rhythm to that on several previous electrocardiograms stored in the EHR and notify the provider of significant changes. Some monitoring solutions, such as Alert-Watch (www.alertwatch.com), can be used as a secondary monitoring system in the perioperative setting, provide an intuitive high-level overview of patient physiology, and highlight potential problems.[4]

Apart from a strictly clinical application, the AIMS can play a key role during all stages of systematic quality control and improvement, from data collection to change monitoring. This is especially true for the dynamic process of airway management; the AIMS can record objective physiologic data during periods when the anesthesiologist's attention is focused on the patient and procedure.

Build and Scripting

Different AIMS applications are available from different vendors. The dynamics of software updates and development make it impractical to review specific products or software versions. What is important is that each application has these features:

- Meets the safety standards of the industry
- Can be integrated into an existing system of EHRs
- Is customizable
- Is regularly upgraded
- Has cross-platform support (desirable)
- Has maintenance and troubleshooting systems in place
- Offers ways to provide user feedback (desirable)
- Is customized to the workflow of the anesthesia practice (this requires the active participation of one or more subject matter experts)

Automatic data collection and storage by the AIMS is fast and reduces the likelihood of random errors. However, incorrect configuration of the software may lead to systematic errors in the collected data. The volume of data generated from each clinical case can be controlled by adjusting the number of data streams and the temporal resolution of collected data (i.e., vital signs every 30 seconds vs every 3 minutes).

User Interface

The user interface of the AIMS should be as intuitive as possible and should prioritize easy recording and display of the most critical data. Vital signs should be captured automatically and displayed continuously. Episodic events, such as administration of medications, should require as few "clicks" as possible. Common procedures—such as induction of general anesthesia followed by endotracheal intubation—should be templated to make routine entry as easy as possible. Good interface design will increase user acceptance and diminish the burden of documentation. Increasingly, this includes the use of multipane displays, with vital signs streaming on one screen while documentation is recorded on another. Colored text or backgrounds and dynamic displays (e.g., blinking figures) can be used to provide various levels of alerts and warnings as part of an electronic decision support system.

Whenever possible, the AIMS should seek to create discrete data, (e.g., a menu of options for recording laryngoscope type is better than a free-text field, because the resulting data will be easier to analyze in the future). These elements should be as standardized as possible, for instance following the recommendations of the International Organization for Terminology in Anesthesia, a committee of the International Health Terminology Standards Development Organization. Quality improvement organizations, such as the US Anesthesia Quality Institute, and expert members of the Society for Airway Management will play an important role in creating and promulgating standards for domain-specific data elements in airway management.

Airway Management Outcomes Reported in the Literature

The evolution of individual physicians' and institutional approaches to airway management is greatly influenced by the availability and quality of scientific evidence. The increasing number of publications related to airway management (Fig. 52.1) and improved access to the literature with portable and handheld

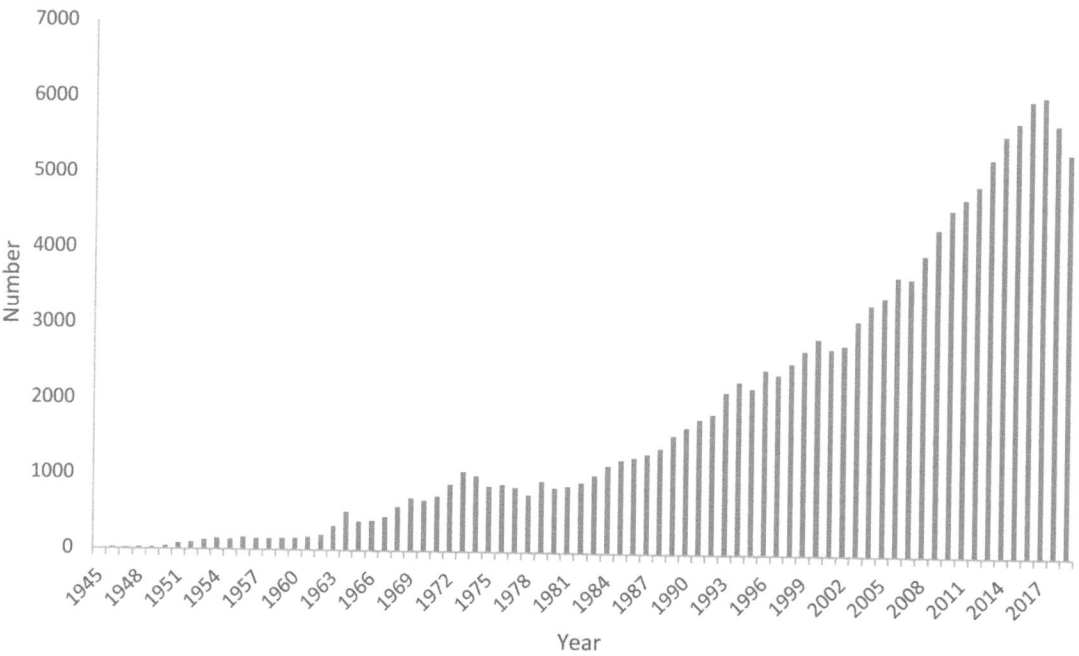

• **Fig. 52.1** Numbers of year-specific PubMed results for "airway management" from 1945 to 2019.

devices make clinical evidence readily available in most developed countries. In this section we will explore the metrics and outcomes commonly reported in the airway management literature.

The potential for rapid clinical deterioration and death during airway management distinguishes it from other routine procedures and determines the key performance outcomes: severe morbidity and mortality. Although serious, such outcomes are rare and therefore remain within the domain of large studies or individual case reports. Smaller studies explore technical aspects of airway management, including the setting, technique, equipment, and provider, but they usually lack the statistical power to comment on major safety outcomes. The more recent literature is notable for relatively complex quality measures, designed to assess the relationship between patient characteristics, clinical management, and outcome. These more complex measures may be difficult to interpret outside of the country- and institution-specific context, but their value lies in targeting the performance of a system of managing the airway-related health risk, rather than focusing on the success of its individual components. Ongoing standardization and universal collection of outcomes data will further strengthen the role of such complex metrics. However, even the simplest metrics in the hierarchy of airway management outcome, such as patient characteristics and the study setting, may be critical to understanding and applying scientific evidence.

Patient Characteristics

In a European nationwide prospective survey, patient characteristics were deemed to contribute to three-quarters of airway events.[5] Among patient characteristics, airway assessment is a critical determinant of airway-related risk. Studies that focus on airway management outcomes commonly report preprocedure airway assessment that ranges from a binary outcome of anticipated difficult airway and widely used numeric scores to novel approaches such as facial image analysis.[6-8] These metrics can be used to estimate the accuracy of clinical assessment and to derive conclusions such as the fact that most cases of difficult airway are unanticipated.[9,10]

Patient health status is typically reported using the American Society of Anesthesiologists Physical Status Classification System,[5,11] although further details, especially in patients with severe or emergent health conditions, are also frequently included.[12]

Setting

The spectrum of reported settings ranges from the prehospital trauma scene to specialized inpatient units.[6,12] The physical setting in which the airway is managed generally reflects the available resources and expertise. However, there is considerable regional variability. For example, in some European countries, physician-led specialized teams are available even at the prehospital level. The more specific inpatient settings reported in the literature typically include hospital units that account for most airway interventions: the operating room area, the intensive care units, and the emergency department.[13-15] Airway management in a specialized trauma unit has been extensively described in the literature.[9,16] In addition to the environment at the prehospital level and location within the hospital, timing with regard to normal working hours can contribute to availability of resources and expertise.[5] Recent studies and large-scale outcome registries such as NACOR and the Multicenter Perioperative Outcomes Group (MPOG, https://mpog.org) emphasize collection of precise time data.[6,17,18]

Physiologic Changes

Vital signs and oxygenation are typically monitored even during the most basic airway management in the field. Thus, in theory, such basic data can be documented and reported for every case of airway management. These metrics have been included in the recommended template for prehospital advanced airway management.[19] In more advanced settings, sophisticated physiologic data are frequently available and documented. For example, each case of anesthesia, in addition to the minimum monitoring standards, may include measurements of end-tidal concentration of anesthetic gases, electroencephalography, and tissue oxygen saturation. With increasing use of EMRs, reporting of continuously monitored physiologic measurements is likely to become routine. In fact, some records in NACOR contain detailed physiologic metrics imported from AIMS. Recent publications also include samples of continuously recorded oxygen saturation and end-tidal CO_2 and average peak airway pressure.[13,16] In addition to cardiopulmonary function, the function of virtually any other body system could be monitored and reported. For example, one research group reported the force applied via a laryngoscope during manipulation of potentially compromised cervical skeleton.[20] In the latter study, spectral entropy monitoring served as a descriptor of intubating conditions. However, basic qualitative reports such as the occurrence of hypotension or hypoxemia have been more common.[21,22]

Induction and Neuromuscular Blocking Agents

The clinical effects of pharmacologic agents administered during airway management range from highly desirable to life-threatening (e.g., paralysis, hypotension, or even anaphylaxis).[23] Descriptive information on the utilization of pharmacologic agents may provide indirect evidence of the perceived hemodynamic status and aspiration risk. In fact, specific neuromuscular blocking agents have been reported as an intervention to prevent aspiration in high-risk airway management.[24] Furthermore, detailed reporting of induction agents, including dosing data, allows the reader to better understand the conditions for intubation.[25] Knowledge of the induction agents used may also offer a potential explanation for hemodynamic changes.[26]

Primary Airway Device

Availability of routine medical record data on the primary airway management device has been as low as 3% of all assessed records.[6] Description of equipment used for airway management provides important information about the clinical approach in a given scenario and sets the basis for interpretation of clinical outcomes, including adverse events. For example, an episode of emesis has different potential for severe complications in an intubated patient and in a patient with a supraglottic airway. However, selection of the device for airway management can be a compromise between clinical indications and available resources. Device availability as an outcome is particularly relevant in the prehospital setting and was included as a core variable in the template for reporting data from prehospital advanced airway management proposed by Sollid and colleagues.[19]

Existing studies report both the airway management device used during the initial and during the successful attempt.[5,12,21] The reported rates of device use in studies of routine procedures provide descriptive information on the prevalent clinical practices and identify less commonly used equipment such as devices for noninvasive ventilation and lighted stylets as an emergency airway option.[12,21] The frequency and preventability of device malfunction have been reported.[27] The time to identification and correction of a malfunction or the need to use a backup device would also be of interest, but are seldom reported in the literature.

Procedural Outcomes

Airway management includes a series of decisions and practical steps that must be reported to present a complete clinical picture. The degree of success during each practical step and concurrent physical findings inform further management and represent valuable data for quality control and academic research. Protocols used to standardize airway management in clinical studies serve as an example of comprehensive reporting of airway procedures.[20] In clinical practice or simulated emergencies, adherence to practice standards has been measured using the ASA difficult airway algorithm—under revision at the time of this writing—as a gold standard.[28,29] A spectrum of airway management techniques has been reported based on the extent to which a technique can be described as invasive: from elective bag-mask ventilation to emergency surgical airway.[5,6] Airway management studies commonly report whether the airway was managed before or after induction of anesthesia, although in certain cases, such as intracranial procedures, intraoperative emergence and reinduction may be necessary.[30,31] Existing publications also frequently provide information on measures that are intended to reduce the risk of aspiration of gastric contents, including the rates of rapid sequence induction and cricoid pressure.[6,15]

Data on the use of specific airway management approaches are becoming increasingly available in the modern literature. An analysis of data from a Japanese trauma registry reported the rates of various initial approaches to airway management including nasal intubation, intubation with sedation without paralysis, and intubation without sedation.[21] When describing specific techniques some authors provide extensive details such as the use of lubricating gel[25] and time to endotracheal intubation in seconds.[32]

The procedural aspects of airway management are most commonly reported based on a relatively subjective categorization of airway management as "difficult" or "not difficult."[6] However, the extent of airway management complexity has also been quantified using dedicated scales such as the Intubation Difficulty Scale.[15,33] The causes of difficult airway management have been described in both general inpatient and trauma populations.[9,14] Still images and video files captured with videolaryngoscopes and newer camera-based flexible intubating systems can be used to quantify difficulty during intubation. A research group exploring the biomechanics of intubation used video image analysis to calculate the percentage of glottic opening visualized.[20] In another study comparing the use of a videolaryngoscope and a direct laryngoscope, the authors measured duration of intubation attempt.[16] One of the study conclusions was that in trauma patients the median duration of intubation with a videolaryngoscope was longer compared to direct laryngoscopy, with no difference in success rate. Such a finding has both clinical and organizational implications.

The ability to successfully secure the airway and achieve adequate oxygenation is undoubtedly a critical outcome. Success-related outcomes reported to date include both descriptions of technique used to identify successful airway management and the rate of successful attempts. For example, a prospective study of over 2000 prehospital intubations reported a success rate of 98.7%.[30] A number of techniques for visual confirmation of airway placement have been reported. These range from direct laryngoscopy to ultrasonographic measurement of the degree of LMA rotation.[13,34]

From a clinical perspective, it is important to know whether airway management required multiple attempts and if an alternative device had to be used. A research group assessing airway management by emergency physicians working on a prehospital helicopter service reported the frequency of a first-attempt intubation failure, overall failure, and utilization of techniques other than intubation.[12] In one study of trauma patients, the authors presented the perceived causes of failed intubation.[9] Data on the frequency of esophageal intubation are also available.[22]

Previous studies have extensively explored another key airway management outcome: safety. A National Audit Project carried out in the UK focused specifically on major complications of airway management in an inpatient setting.[5,14] In another study comparing the mechanics of intubation with a direct laryngoscope and a videolaryngoscope, the authors prospectively screened for complications of airway management: Patients were evaluated for six predefined adverse outcomes in the recovery room and on postoperative days 1, 3, and 7.[20] There are also published data on complications at the prehospital level.[12] A number of procedural aspects of airway management have been assessed as potential risk factors for complications, including the type of ventilation during induction of anesthesia, the induction agent, and endotracheal tube size.[35,36]

Emergency Surgical Airway

The emergency surgical airway is discussed extensively in the literature as a life-saving technique when noninvasive means to ensure adequate oxygenation were not successful. Large studies from Europe and North America have reported frequencies and types of emergency surgical airways.[8,14] For example, the rate of emergency surgical airways was 0.3% for trauma patients requiring an airway within 1 hour and 0.04% within 24 hours in a large trauma center in the United States.[9] Difficult anatomy was the most common cause of the need for surgical airway in the latter study. In an observational study from Japan, emergency department physicians proceeded with cricothyroidotomy as an initial airway management approach in 2.2% of trauma patients.[21]

Reports of success rates of emergency surgical airway suggest an alarmingly high failure rate of this last-resort technique. Based on the national audit data from the United Kingdom, 65% of cricothyroidotomies performed by anesthesiologists were unsuccessful, although most emergency surgical airway procedures were tracheostomies successfully carried out by surgeons.[5] A systematic review of literature on emergency cricothyroidotomy and tracheostomy reported the comparative success and complication rates.[37] Experience with surgical airway appears to be important; Stephens and colleagues reported no airway-related deaths in 31 urgent or emergent surgical airways over 10 years at a major trauma center.[9]

The authors of this chapter searched a 2012 NACOR data set for cases with Common Procedural Terminology (CPT) codes consistent with emergency surgical airway procedures. We identified 244 cases of reported emergency surgical airway reported by 85 practices in a sample of 4.9 million anesthesia records. We contacted half a dozen of these groups in an attempt to validate these cases and received responses from three practices: out of 10 cases with CPT codes of emergency surgical airway, only 3 required emergency surgical airway due to unsuccessful prior airway management attempt (unpublished data). It is likely when searching large administrative data sets that the very rare incidence of miscoding may be a significant confounder of the rate of very rare adverse events; confidence in the reliability of such findings will require confirmation from the individual medical records themselves. The role of the registry, therefore, becomes one of case finding for a subsequent more detailed review.

Mortality

Existing literature includes data on the frequency and causes of death related to airway management.[5] Survival until discharge in patients who underwent emergency surgical airway has also been documented.[9] One interventional study compared survival until discharge in patients who underwent airway management, based on the choice of equipment used.[16]

Team Structure

The success of airway management depends on the decisions and skills of the operator. The decision to request help is often seen as critical in difficult airway situations—percentages of clinical teams that did or did not call for help during an airway event have been reported.[5] The literature also includes assessments of whether the physician managing an airway event was expected to have appropriate expertise.[5] Some reports include considerable detail, such as the demographics of physicians managing the airway and the process measures reflecting technical and nontechnical skills.[38] More commonly, studies describe the level of training and clinical specialty of the clinicians involved in airway management and look for potential associations among these factors and the outcome.[16] The success of airway management and the frequency of complications have been used to compare performance of physicians with varying levels of experience or performance of physicians and nonphysicians.[25,39]

Quality Assessment

Quality assessment metrics reported in the literature include both process and outcome measures. For example, studies have reported associations between protocolization of care, implementation of an airway continuous quality improvement program, and clinical outcomes.[40,41] A systematic review of emergency surgical airway literature reported and classified procedure complications.[37] Frequency of suboptimal management in cases of death or brain damage and a semi-quantitative assessment of management as good, mixed, and poor were also reported in the National Audit Project in the UK.[5] Some study groups explored quality markers in high-risk patient groups such as obstructive sleep apnea patients undergoing surgery.[42] Existing literature reflects an increasing role of patient satisfaction as a quality measure—patient satisfaction scale and feedback postanesthesia have been reported.[25]

Levels of Outcome Reporting

The scale of data collection is likely to affect the quantity and quality of the collected data. For example, a chart review of individual patient records is likely to produce a larger number of variables with more values for each of the variables compared to an international registry that typically includes only a summary of the individual patient's data. Parallel documentation of data in different sections of an EMR allows for cross-checking of information, potentially increasing its reliability but also increasing methodologic confounding if the sources do not agree. As the number of patients in a sample increases, the total volume of data for each individual typically decreases. Such a relationship may be preserved even in the setting of increasing capacity for data collection and storage due to a parallel increase in the amount and complexity of collected data. For example, upgrading the hard drives in a data storage system can increase the storage capacity 10-fold, but adding video recordings to routinely collected patient data can increase the file size by several orders of magnitude.

Collection and analysis of airway management data at an institutional level allow for analysis of system performance while still offering the option for a detailed record review. For example, in one study the authors used an institutional trauma registry to identify the frequency and patterns of emergency intubations but referred to EMRs to elicit the clinical details of each case.[9]

Collection of data at a multi-institutional or national level provides a larger scale perspective on clinical practice. In a multicenter prospective study in Japan, the authors identified striking interinstitutional variation in the initial airway management approach and first-attempt success.[21] Such variation may have important implications for policy-making and is frequently targeted by national healthcare authorities. Indeed, the National Audit Project in the United Kingdom demonstrated that nearly 60% of adverse airway events were clustered in only 15% of the hospitals.

Collection of airway management data on an international and global scale may be complex but will improve generalizability and foster standardization of clinical and data collection practices. A prospective observational study of advanced airway management in helicopter emergency medical services relied on consistent reporting standards across six countries from around the globe.[12] The work carried out by the Cochrane Collaboration is another example of international collaboration with analysis of global data. The Cochrane Library (www.Cochranelibrary.com) includes multiple systematic reviews of literature reporting airway management in perioperative and critically ill patients.

The Concept of Difficult Airway Management

How then to characterize difficult airway management? As noted, this concept is very much in the eye of the beholder. The answer is to be as objective as possible and make full use of existing metrics with well-understood definitions. When no such standard exists, would-be authors or quality managers must impose their own definitions but should be transparent about how this is done. Table 52.1 lists variables for measuring airway management outcomes extracted from Table 52.2, reorganized on the basis of objectivity. Highly objective metrics should be sought whenever possible, as these will be more consistent across studies and centers, and less subject to "gaming" or intentional bias by clinicians who know they are being measured. The subjectivity

of many intermediate measures can be improved when needed—say for a research trial—by limiting the number of observers and protocolizing the means of collection. For example, thyromental distance will display significant interrater variability when documented in the medical record by a large group of clinicians using only a quick look but will be more consistent when recorded by a single research assistant instructed to always use a measuring tape. Similarly, events will be better captured by a dedicated observer working in real time, as opposed to a busy clinician after the fact. Even better is the use of video capture of airway management. Yeatts and colleagues compared DL to VAL in more than 500 seriously injured trauma patients using a single expert's review of video recordings, combined with automatically captured vital signs.[16] This approach enabled precise determination of personnel, number of attempts, time taken, equipment used, and variations in oxygen saturation, representing a best practice for future airway management studies.

Which metrics should be captured and reported depends on the purpose intended for the data. In general, more emphasis should be put on objective metrics, particularly those that can be automatically captured by electronic records or live video. When trying to define difficult airway management, it is less useful to provide a potentially confounded yes/no answer and more helpful to provide objective information about the patient's anatomy, the techniques used (including medications administered and equipment employed), the number of attempts required, and the outcomes achieved. These facts should be supplemented whenever possible with a written narrative that describes the course of airway management and the clinical decisions made.

The Future of Airway Management Measurement

An AIMS integrated in an institutional EMR offers enormous future potential for measuring results of airway management. The AIMS itself will passively and objectively integrate physiologic data from a dozen different monitors, including those of the ECG, pulse oximeter, blood pressure cuff (or arterial line), capnometer,

TABLE 52.1 Airway Management Metrics Organized on the Basis of Objectivity

Metric	Comment
Highly Objective	
Demographic data	Patient age, sex
Time of day	
Surgical case type	Defined by ICD-10 code
Body mass index	(or height and weight presented together)
CT or MRI calculated anatomic variables	
Abbreviated Injury Scale	… and the derived injury severity score; a highly consistent coding system for anatomic injuries
Glasgow Coma Scale	Well defined, but may vary over time in the same patient, and over different observers
Location of care	
Personnel present	Although who did what may not be clear, especially in training environments
Use of induction agents	… and dose and timing
Use of neuromuscular blocking agents	… and dose and timing
Endotracheal tube size and depth	

Continued

TABLE 52.1 Airway Management Metrics Organized on the Basis of Objectivity—cont'd

Metric	Comment
Data from physiologic monitors	(if automatically captured)
Neck motion	(if measured using fluoroscopy)
Initial intubating technique	
Successful intubating technique	
Initial use of cricoid pressure	
Initial use of manual in-line stabilization	(or presence of a cervical collar)
Use of adjuncts	Bougie, stylet, Magill forceps, tube exchangers, etc.
Need for surgical airway	
In-hospital mortality	
Cost of medications and equipment	
Hospital length of stay	
Intermediate	
ASA Physical Status	Well defined, but subjectively applied
Weight alone	Absent height, does not accurately describe the patient
Anthropomorphic variables	Subject to interrrater variation
Mallampati score	Well defined, but with interrater variability
Cormack-Lehane score	Well defined, but with interrater variability; better if captured on a video image
Comorbidities	ICD-10 describes them well, but they are often incompletely listed for individual patients, especially in anesthesia records
Depth of anesthesia or sedation	Can be inferred from medications given, but may change over the course of the procedure
Elective vs emergent status	Definitions vary; can be gamed
Data from physiologic monitors	(if recorded by the clinician in the medical record)
Number of attempts	Not precisely defined
Esophageal intubation	
Cardiac arrest	
30-day mortality	Confounded by patients lost to follow-up
Cost of hospital care and personnel	Multiple definitions; confounding between cost and payment
Subjective	
Preventability of adverse outcomes	
Indication for intubation	
History of difficult mask ventilation or intubation	
Patient anxiety	
Neck motion	(if recorded by an observer)
Quality of mask ventilation	
Laryngospasm	
Bronchospasm	
Hemodynamic instability	
Hypoxia	Multiple definitions; better if captured from automatic data
Aspiration	Better if radiographically defined
Sore throat	
Patient satisfaction	No established and validated metrics

TABLE 52.2 Examples of Airway Management Metrics Reported in the Literature

Outcome	Author, Year
Patient Characteristics	
Proportion of airway events in which patient characteristics were deemed contributing	Cook 2011
Demographic data	De Jong 2020
Anthropometric data	Hindman 2014
Presence of comorbidities	Gellerfors 2018
Mechanism of injury in trauma patients	Stephens 2009
Abbreviated Injury Scale	Yeatts 2013
Glasgow Coma Scale	Stephens 2009
American Society of Anesthesiologists Physical Status	Kim 2015
Indication for tracheal intubation	Sunde 2015
Anticipated difficult airway	McKeen 2011
History of difficult intubation Reliability of history of difficult intubation History of difficult mask ventilation Mouth opening Neck mobility	Rosenstock 2012
Thyromental distance Sternomental distance Interincisor distance Jaw forward subluxation distance Neck circumference Cervical offset distance	Hindman 2014
Mallampati score	De Jong 2020
Simplified Airway Risk Index	Rosenstock 2012
Patient agitation or anxiety	
Setting	
Prehospital vs hospital level	Gellerfors 2018
Aircraft	Sunde 2015
Facility type: academic vs community hospital	Nakao 2015
Hospital unit: shock and trauma center	Yeatts 2013
Hospital unit: emergency department	Choi 2015
Hospital unit: intensive care unit	Wang 2015
Perioperative area: operating room vs designated anesthetic room vs recovery area	Cook 2011
Utilization of general anesthesia	Inoue 2015
Timing with regard to working hours	Cook 2011
Emergency vs elective airway management Time of the day when airway management was attempted Time of the day when airway management was deemed difficult Seasonal variation in intubation frequency	Adams 2014
Data collection within 1 and 24 hours after arrival to trauma center	Stephens 2009
Physiologic Changes During Airway Management	
Plot of oxygen saturation over time	Yeatts 2013
Plot of end-tidal CO_2 over time	

Outcome	Author, Year
Definition of hypoxemia	Sakles 2019
Duration of desaturation	Rosenstock 2012
Blood pressure changes	Nakao 2015
Heart rate changes	Mort 2015
Peak airway pressure	Kim 2015
Laryngoscopy pressure and force Cervical spine intervertebral motion on fluoroscopy EEG-based monitoring of anesthetic depth: spectral entropy value	Hindman 2014
Cervical spine intervertebral motion during application of cricoid pressure	Prasarn 2016
Induction and Neuromuscular Blocking Agents	
Type of neuromuscular blocking agent used	Na 2015
Dose of neuromuscular blocking agent	Xue 2008
Frequency of adverse reactions to neuromuscular blocking agents	Reddy 2015
Type of induction agent used	De Jong 2020
Dose of induction agent used	Inoue 2015
Device Used for Airway Management	
Availability of routine medical record data on airway device used	McKeen 2011
Device used for initial attempt	Nakao 2015
Device used during successful attempt	Sunde 2015
Device malfunction Frequency of device malfunction Preventability of device malfunction	Kusumaphanyo 2009
Procedural Outcomes	
Protocol for airway management	De Jong 2020
Checklist for endotracheal intubation	Turner 2020
Adherence to practice standards	You-Ten 2015
Ventilation using mask vs supraglottic airway vs endotracheal tube	Cook 2011
Pre- or postinduction intubation	Gellerfors 2018
Sedation score	Rosenstock 2012
Intraoperative emergence and reinduction	Cai 2013
Frequency of utilization of rapid sequence induction	Choi 2015
Frequency of application of cricoid pressure	McKeen 2011
Changes in airway management plan after point-of-care gastric ultrasound	Alakkad 2015
Oral vs nasal intubation	Nakao 2015
Use of lubricant gel	Inoue 2015
Qualitative assessment of difficulty of airway management	McKeen 2011
Quantitative assessment of difficulty of airway management	Choi 2015
Difficult mask ventilation Difficult intubation	Norskov 2015

Continued

TABLE 52.2 Examples of Airway Management Metrics Reported in the Literature—cont'd

Outcome	Author, Year	Outcome	Author, Year
Cormack-Lehane grade	De Jong 2020	Frequency of complications in cricothyroidotomy and tracheostomy	Zasso 2020
Anesthesiologist-reported visualized percentage of glottic opening		Duration of emergency surgical airway procedure	
Visualized percentage of glottic opening based on video image analysis	Hindman 2014	Frequency of emergency surgical airway in cases of death due to difficult airway	Auroy 2009
Glottic view grade before and after external laryngeal manipulation	Kwak 2015	Type of complications in emergency surgical airway	Zasso 2020
Frequency of Magill forceps use		**Aspiration of Gastric Contents**	
Number of intubation attempts	Yeatts 2013	Frequency of intraoperative vomiting in children with unrestricted preoperative clear fluid intake	Andersson 2015
Duration of intubation attempt	Takeuchi 2017		
Ultrasound arytenoid grade of supraglottic airway position	Kim 2015	Frequency of suspected aspiration of gastric contents	
Presence of laryngeal mask airway rotation		Frequency of radiologically confirmed aspiration of gastric contents	
Flexible intubation scope grade of supraglottic airway position		Clinical outcomes in patient with aspiration of gastric contents	
Three-dimensional computed tomographic image of a supraglottic airway in situ		Frequency as an indication for intensive care unit admission	Cook 2011
Frequency of supraglottic airway repositioning		Frequency as a primary airway event in anesthesia	
Airway management success rate	Gellerfors 2018	Frequency as a complication of failed or difficult airway management	
Causes of failed intubation	Stephens 2009	Case fatality rate in intensive care unit admissions with aspiration of gastric contents	
Frequency of esophageal intubation	Jiang 2020		
Frequency of laryngospasm in pediatric patients	Oofuvong 2014	Timing with regard to induction and airway instrumentation	
Complications of airway management on postoperative days 1, 3, and 7	Hindman 2014	Occurrence during rapid sequence induction	
Objective assessment of voice after endotracheal intubation for surgery	Mehanna 2015	Type of airway used when aspiration of gastric contents occurred	
Self-reported Voice Handicap Index after endotracheal intubation for surgery		Frequency and cause of anesthesia-related death	Auroy 2009
Laryngoscopic findings before and after endotracheal intubation for surgery		**Mortality**	
Airway management complications recognized at prehospital level	Sunde 2015	Association of lethal outcomes with airway management	Cook 2011
Device used for endotracheal tube exchage	Mort 2015	Frequency of lethal outcomes in cases of general anesthesia	
Frequency of successful endotracheal tube exchange		Causes of airway-related mortality	Auroy 2009
Causes of unsuccessful endotracheal tube exchange		Survival to hospital discharge in patients who required emergency surgical airway	Stephens 2009
Model for assessing risk for first-attempt intubation failure	Sunde 2015	Survival to hospital discharge in patients with different devices used for airway management	Yeatts 2013
Emergency Surgical Airway		All-cause mortality in patients who underwent tracheal intubation	Norskov 2015
Type of emergency surgical airway	Cook 2011	**Structure of the Clinical Team**	
Frequency of emergency surgical airway utilization		Frequency of calling for help at the time of an airway event	Cook 2011a
Success rate of emergency surgical airway performed by anesthesiologists and surgeons		Management of the event by a physician not expected to have appropriate expertise	Cook 2011b
Rate of emergency surgical airway in trauma patients within 1 and 24 hours of arrival	Stephens 2009	Experience level and clinical specialty	Yeatts 2013
Causes of emergency surgical airway		First-pass success rate by experience level and clinical specialty	
Most common cause of emergency surgical airway			
Frequency of emergency surgical airway as an initial approach	Nakao 2015		

TABLE 52.2 Examples of Airway Management Metrics Reported in the Literature—cont'd

Outcome	Author, Year	Outcome	Author, Year
Demographic data for trainee physicians managing the airway	Gjeraa 2015	Frequency of airway-related critical events Causes attributed to critical events	Bolden 2020
Assessment of technical and nontechnical skills in anesthesiology trainees		Patient satisfaction scale and feedback postanesthesia	Inoue 2015
Frequency of sore throat or hoarseness after intubation by trainees and nontrainee physicians	Inoue 2015	**Cost**	
		Qualitative cost assessment of devices used for airway management	Slinn 2014
Success rate of airway management by paramedics and physicians	Garner 2020	Cost of supraglottic airway device per use	Eckelman 2012
Quality Assessment		Environmental effects of supraglottic airway devices	
Identification of inadequate practice and system failure	Auroy 2009	Cost of disposable airway equipment	Zaouter 2015
Frequency of suboptimal management in cases of death or brain damage	Cook 2011a	Hospital cost and charges in re-intubated patients	Menon 2012
Semi-quantitative assessment of management as good, mixed, and poor			

end-tidal gas analyzer, ventilator, and others. These data will be captured in the broader context of the EMR where they can be linked to meaningful patient outcomes, such as ventilator days, postoperative diagnostic codes, laboratory values, hospital length of stay, and disposition at the time of hospital discharge.

Although administrative data are frequently criticized for inaccuracy, this issue is rapidly improving as the incentives for accurate and complete coding continue to mount. The transition of US healthcare to ICD-10 coding (catching up with the rest of the world) will increase the specificity of coding and the ability to use these data for scientific and quality improvement purposes. Yet, as the authors' experience with NACOR illustrates, identification of rare outcomes in administrative data sets must be taken with a grain of salt: The most valid research in the next decade will use registries to find cases but will confirm them with review of individual medical records.

The future of airway management research may well depend on the present-day efforts of expert practitioners to define common data definitions and methods of collection. One example of this is the well-organized automated system proposed by Sollid and colleagues, which strikes a balance between academic rigor (the need for detail) and the practicality of data collection.[19] Another such example is evident in the work of Yeatts, which imposed a simple intervention—direct vs video-assisted laryngoscopy as the first approach to an emergent intubation—on a clinical information system capable of capturing real-time video of every event.[16]

The availability of big data will require innovation in analysis, including improved statistical methods for discriminating clinical from mathematic significance. Analyzing very large collections of patients and cases with traditional methods leads to almost universally "significant" results, many of which are clinically trivial. Bayesian analysis of large data sets with hundreds of variables may identify associations not previously appreciated: The nascent use of facial recognition software to predict difficult intubation is one such example.[8]

Advances in processing power may soon enable expert systems developed to provide real-time clinical alerts based on recognition of potentially dangerous patterns of medications and vital signs. At their simplest, such systems can display the institutional difficult airway algorithm at an opportune time, to remind clinicians of available options. At their most advanced, such systems will anticipate a crisis and alert the clinician in advance, to prevent a critical event from ever occurring.

While such improvements might reduce reliance on the technical skills of individual practitioners, there will be a corresponding increase in the need for a new breed of airway management expert, capable of integrating and interpreting large amounts of data from multiple disparate sources. No matter how finely tuned automated expert systems become in the future, there will always be situations that demand exceptions. Freeing the provider from routine decision-making will free cognitive capabilities that can be applied to ever more challenging patients and surgeries.

Conclusion

Airway management is an important function of anesthesia providers and has been the subject of scientific research and quality improvement efforts for many decades. The Information Age offers new tools for passive collection of big data that can be leveraged to further advance the science of airway management. Achieving this potential will require consensus on the right outcomes to measure, adoption of common definitions across multiple EMRs, and the availability of registries to collect the necessary information from multiple sites. The ideal measures will be meaningful to patients and practitioners and be as objective as possible. They will be based on data elements, such as vital signs, that can be automatically gathered without the need for practitioner energy or interpretation. As the bandwidth of healthcare information technology continues to increase, the potential to capture still images and video clips will provide objectivity to even the most challenging component of airway management data: the clinical narrative.

Selected References

5. Cook TM, Woodall N, Frerk C. Major complications of airway management in the UK: results of the Fourth National Audit Project of the Royal College of Anaesthetists and the Difficult Airway Society. Part 1: anaesthesia. *Br J Anaesth*. 2011;106(5):617-631.

9. Stephens CT, Kahntroff S, Dutton RP. The success of emergency endotracheal intubation in trauma patients: a 10-year experience at a major adult trauma referral center. *Anesth Analg.* 2009;109(3):866-872.

10. Nørskov AK, Rosenstock CV, Wetterslev J, Astrup G, Afshari A, Lundstrøm LH. Diagnostic accuracy of anaesthesiologists' prediction of difficult airway management in daily clinical practice: a cohort study of 188 064 patients registered in the Danish Anaesthesia Database. *Anaesthesia.* 2015;70(3):272-281.

15. Choi HJ, Kim YM, Oh YM, Kang HG, Yim HW, Jeong SH. GlideScope video laryngoscopy versus direct laryngoscopy in the emergency department: a propensity score-matched analysis. *BMJ Open.* 2015;5(5):e007884.

16. Yeatts DJ, Dutton RP, Hu PF, et al. Effect of video laryngoscopy on trauma patient survival: a randomized controlled trial. *J Trauma Acute Care Surg.* 2013;75(2):212-219.

22. Jiang J, Kang N, Li B, Wu AS, Xue FS. Comparison of adverse events between video and direct laryngoscopes for tracheal intubations in emergency department and ICU patients - a systematic review and meta-analysis. *Scand J Trauma Resusc Emerg Med.* 2020;28(1):10.

28. Apfelbaum JL, Hagberg CA, Caplan RA, et al. Practice guidelines for management of the difficult airway: an updated report by the American Society of Anesthesiologists Task Force on Management of the Difficult Airway. *Anesthesiology.* 2013;118(2):251-270.

30. Gellerfors M, Fevang E, Bäckman A, et al. Pre-hospital advanced airway management by anaesthetist and nurse anaesthetist critical care teams: a prospective observational study of 2028 pre-hospital tracheal intubations. *Br J Anaesth.* 2018;120(5):1103-1109.

33. Adnet F, Borron SW, Racine SX, et al. The intubation difficulty scale (IDS): proposal and evaluation of a new score characterizing the complexity of endotracheal intubation. *Anesthesiology.* 1997;87(6):1290-1297.

40. Turner JS, Bucca AW, Propst SL, et al. Association of checklist use in endotracheal intubation with clinically important outcomes: a systematic review and meta-analysis. *JAMA Netw Open.* 2020;3(7):e209278.

All references can be found online at eBooks.Health.Elsevier.com.

53

Role of the Airway Community

NARASIMHAN JAGANNATHAN AND ELLEN O'SULLIVAN

CHAPTER OUTLINE

KEY POINTS

- Airway societies exist to help patient care by improving the quality and safety of airway management practices, as well as disseminating educational and research-related activities through annual meetings (workshops, lectures) and educational forums.
- Given that there is still significant morbidity related to airway management, airway societies aim to improve patient care

- by advocating for airway techniques that remain safe for the patient.
- Use of social media and clinical forums will likely become even more prevalent for discussing the best airway management practices among society members.

Introduction

This chapter highlights the role and importance of various airway societies worldwide. These airway societies exist to help patient care by improving the quality and safety of airway management practices and disseminating educational and research-related activities through annual meetings (workshops, lectures) and educational forums. Three large airway societies currently exist: Society for Airway Management (SAM), Difficult Airway Society (DAS), and European Airway Management Society (EAMS). This chapter focuses on these societies and the benefits to clinicians and patients.

Individual Societies

Society for Airway Management (SAM)

This North American–based multidisciplinary society was established in 1995. Its membership includes physicians from all various specialties who deal with airway management, as well as nonphysicians involved in airway-related patient care, research, or product development. The majority of members of SAM are anesthesiologists and emergency physicians. The missions of SAM include (1) to associate and affiliate into one organization all physicians who are engaged in the practice of medicine dealing with airway management and nonphysicians who are involved in airway-related patient care, research, or airway-related product development, and (2) to advance the study of airway management, to contribute to the advancement of new airway-management techniques, encouraging research, education, teaching, and scientific advancement of airway management.

Difficult Airway Society (DAS)

DAS, like SAM, was established in 1995. This UK-based group's goal is to advance the public's understanding of airway management and is aimed at anaesthetists and critical care personnel. With nearly 3000 members, it is the world's largest and most active international airway management society. The aims of DAS are (1) to advance public education in the science and practice of the management of patients with difficult or unusual airway problems, by the conduct of courses, lectures, and demonstrations and by ensuring that due attention is paid to airway management techniques in the training curricula of medical and paramedical practitioners, and (2) to promote research and the development of new techniques in dealing with airway problems and to publish the useful results of that research. It has published a number of guidelines relating to various aspects of airway management which have been adopted worldwide. In conjunction with the Royal College of Anaesthetists DAS established the Airway Lead Network.

European Airway Management Society (EAMS)

This pan-European medical society founded in 2003 is also geared toward anaesthetists and critical care personnel.

Other Airway Societies

All India Difficult Airway Association (AIDAA)

AIDAA is an Indian-based professional forum of anesthesiologists, intensivists, physicians, and emergency medicine practitioners who are involved in the management of the airway. Its mission is to achieve the highest standards of professional competence in the art and science of difficult airway management through teaching and training, sharing of knowledge, liaison with national and international professional bodies, and multicenter research.

Confederación Latinoamericana de Sociedades de Anestesiología (CLASA)

CLASA is a Latin American society established in 1962 in Lima, Peru. Anesthesiology members are enrolled from 21 Latin American countries. Entrenamiento en Vía Aérea Latinoamérica (EVALa) is a subsection of CLASA and has scientific chapters, including one focused on airway management. EVALa was founded in 2011 and currently teaches in the 17 countries of Latin America. Invited professors and lecturers from Europe, Asia, and the United States have participated in teaching over 50 courses. Almost 5500 anesthesiology attendants have been trained by this organization.

International Airway Management Society (IAMS)

IAMS is a Chinese/American-based airway society. Its goal is promotion of education, training, and research on airway management and improvement of patient safety internationally. The International Airway Management Society (www.iamshq.com) was founded in 2016 by 75 directors from 17 countries and regions. The official language of IAMS is English. IAMS is managed by its board members and founding directors and is supported by its international members. The

IAMS is organized exclusively for scientific and educational purposes. IAMS promotes education, training, and research in airway management and patient safety through meetings, workshops, case discussion, research, academic exchange program funding, and assisted training centers. IAMS focuses on Asian countries and regions.

Airway Special Interest Group of the Australian & New Zealand College of Anaesthesiologists

This Airway Management Special Interest Group (SIG) was established in 2007 and has grown to nearly a thousand members within that time. The SIG comes under the umbrella of the Anaesthesia Continuing Education (ACE) section, a tripartite organization consisting of the Australian and New Zealand College of Anaesthetist (ANZCA), the Australian Society of Anaesthetists (ASA), and the New Zealand Society of Anaesthetists (NZSA). Its main objective is to promote safe airway management, science, and education across both nations. The 10 executive members are enthusiastic airway experts involved in all of these aspects, creating teaching and training materials, supporting the ANZCA library, and creating worldwide research. The SIG organizes regular education opportunities, workshops, and scientific meetings. Recently, the SIG executive developed the Australian Airway Leads Network, and there are now airway leads represented in multiple hospitals across every state.

Project for Universal Management of Airways (PUMA)

PUMA is an international and multidisciplinary working group of airway specialists that has been assembled to determine the key issues to be addressed by airway management guidelines. It is a nonprofit organization established to develop and deliver educational content that can be consistently applied to airway practitioners from all clinical backgrounds, independent of contextual factors such as indication, urgency, patient group, or intended airway device. PUMA published its first set of four guidelines in 2021, which are intended, as much as possible, to reflect the consensus of the existing published guidelines. The group is currently working on developing a globally accessible education program to facilitate translation of these guidelines into clinical practice.

Safe Airway Society

The Safe Airway Society is the interprofessional airway society for Australia and New Zealand. Established in 2019, its board and members represent both airway operators and airway assistants across a variety of areas involved in airway management, including prehospital, emergency medicine, anesthesia, intensive care, surgery, and rural general practice. The mission of the Safe Airway Society is to promote a collaborative approach, by practitioners from all these backgrounds, to achieving best airway management practices independent of discipline, role, or context. The society aims to create educational resources and to provide training and support research, with an emphasis on team performance and human factors in addition to technical skills.

Table 53.1 presents summary and contact information for these societies.

Common Goals of Airway Societies

Airway societies aim to advance the study of airway management by the following means: advocating for the advancement of new airway management techniques, encouraging research, education, teaching, and scientific advancement of airway management.

These societies exist to disseminate information concerning the importance of airway management to its members and to the public,

TABLE 53.1 Summary of Various Airway Societies Worldwide

Name of Airway Society	Composition of Membership	Website	Social Media Involvement	Newsletter	Online Forum	Annual Meeting (Time)
SAM	International; primarily North American; international chapters	http://www.samhq.com	Facebook & Twitter @samhqglobal	SAM Gazette, published quarterly	Yes	September
DAS	International; primarily from the United Kingdom	http://www.das.uk.com	Facebook & Twitter @dasairway	DAS Newsletter, published quarterly	Yes	November
EAMS	International; primarily European	http://www.eamshq.net	Facebook	Trends in Anaesthesia & Critical Care, the society's affiliated journal, published quarterly	Yes	March
CLASA	International; primarily South American countries	http://www.anestesia-clasa.org	Twitter @clasanews & Instagram	Yes	Yes	September
AIDAA	International; primarily Indian	http://aidaa.in/index.html	No	Yes	Yes	September/December
IAMS	International; primarily Chinese	Not established yet; society recently formed	No	No	No	Soon to be announced
PUMA	International	https://www.universalairway.org	Facebook & Twitter @UniversalAirway	No	No	No

to sponsor professional meetings or conferences, and to publish papers of scientific and cultural interest. For example, DAS is actively involved in training healthcare professionals in the safe and competent practice of advanced airway management. The group has produced various guidelines for airway management of patients undergoing anesthesia, and these guidelines, which are based on expert opinion, are very highly cited and a valuable resource worldwide for the care of patients.

Membership

Membership in any of these societies allows one to be involved in various committees, with the potential for advancement in the society leadership, including membership on the board of directors and executive positions, such as treasurer, secretary, vice-president, or president. Membership also includes receipt of the society's newsletter (*SAM Gazette*, *DAS Newsletter*, EAMS's *Trends in Anaesthesia & Critical Care*, the society's journal). These publications highlight the educational activities of these societies. They also convey important airway management strategies (e.g., new techniques, difficult airway scenarios). In addition, members of these societies benefit from the knowledge gained from attending and networking with experts at annual meetings. Table 53.2 summarizes potential advantages and benefits of airway society membership.

Annual Meetings

General Format

Annual meetings tend to be the highlight of these societies, as the educational value for the participant is immense. These educational venues often encourage a multidisciplinary approach for teaching airway management skills and often involve the following sessions:

1. Lectures and presentations in a variety of formats
   a. Plenary sessions
   b. Pro-con debates
   c. How do I do it?
   d. Expert panels
2. Hands-on workshops: Sessions allow participants to maintain and/or acquire skills with various airway devices, including devices that may rarely be utilized (e.g., use of cricothyroidotomy kits in a pig trachea model).

TABLE 53.2 Potential Benefits in Being a Member of an Airway Management Society

Type of Participation	Potential Benefits
Annual Meetings	Participation in high-quality lectures, workshops to acquire life-saving skills Networking with the experts face to face Presentation of one's research Involvement in various committees Improvement in clinical skill and decision-making in practice
Clinical Forums	Posting questions regarding difficult cases and receive quick feedback from airway enthusiasts/experts Improvement in clinical skill and decision-making in practice
Publications (newsletter, website journals)	Keeping abreast of new guidelines, publications, and expert opinions on airway management Improvement in clinical skill and decision-making in practice

3. Expert round table sessions: Group sessions in which 8 to 12 participants have a meaningful, intimate interaction with an instructor on a focused topic (e.g., how to set up a difficult airway service).

4. Guideline lectures: These major lectures disseminate expert guidelines for airway management. These guidelines are often presented by the key experts in airway management who are responsible for devising the guidelines, and the sessions allow participants to ask experts questions directly (e.g., about 2022 ASA difficult airway algorithm and 2021 DAS guidelines) for awake tracheal intubation in adults.

5. Poster and oral abstract presentations: These sessions allow participants to appreciate the current high-quality research endeavors occurring at various institutions. In society meetings, abstracts are often moderated by experts in the field, allowing for further one-on-one interaction. Additionally, the top 5 or 10 abstracts are often presented orally and are judged. This allows for appreciation of the efforts put forth by researchers and clinicians while highlighting their work in the large venue of an annual meeting. Furthermore, this format allows early exposure for trainees interested in airway management to be involved in presentations.

World Airway Management Meeting (WAMM) and Development of the World Alliance for Airway Management

For the first time in its 20-year history, both the SAM and the DAS combined their annual scientific meetings to produce an eclectic program of lectures, workshops, and social events for a world-class meeting in November 2015 in Dublin, Ireland. This meeting brought together over 1800 delegates and provided the opportunity for face-to-face meetings and collaboration between airway experts and airway enthusiasts from all over the world.

A second WAMM meeting was held in Amsterdam in November 2019 with 1804 attendees from 71 countries. A program of internationally renowned experts in the field of airway management was presented. The collaboration between SAM and DAS grew to include EAMS. This makes this the largest airway management meeting ever held worldwide.

Expert Opinions

Meaningful interaction among members of a society and other experts results from the face-to-face networking that occurs at annual meetings. This allows members to "pick the brains" of the experts and to learn airway management tips from them.

All the societies mentioned in this chapter engage their members, including board members, in active online forums. Participation in these forums allows participants to have the opportunity for real-time expert consults regarding airway management techniques and/or management of rare and/or difficult cases. These forums are accessed through the website of the respective societies and are a great benefit to being an active member.

Publications by Societies

The DAS has been involved in the creation of various clinical guidelines, which are then formally published on its website and/or in its journals. Examples include individualized guidelines for management of the obstetric, pediatric, and unanticipated difficult airways. The 2015 DAS guidelines for management of unanticipated difficult intubation were released during the WAMM 2015 meeting to increase awareness along with other new guidelines for the airway community. The DAS also provides these algorithms and simple cognitive aids through their website and apps available through Google Play and Apple (http://www.das.uk.com/guidelines/das_intubation_guidelines).

Another useful publication of the DAS is Airway Device Evaluation Project Team (ADEPT) guidelines, which establish a process by which an airway-management professional can lead a process of formal device/equipment evaluation.[1,2] Primarily established in the United Kingdom, with growing acceptance in the United States, these guidelines aim to allow widespread adoption of a professional standard to create an infrastructure by which required evidence can be obtained prior to airway equipment purchasing by clinicians and hospitals.

Additionally, the DAS website contains a patient information section. This resource allows for greater patient education and familiarity prior to a surgical procedure in order to help patients better understand the indications for certain techniques for airway management. This section contains simple and useful explanations, such as why airway management is needed for patients undergoing anesthesia and more complex details regarding why certain patients are candidates for an awake intubation.

SAM leadership has been influential in the development of both the ASA Difficult Airway Guidelines and Obstructive Sleep Apnea Guidelines. The new ASA Difficult Airway Guidelines were released in 2022[14]. Additionally, many SAM members perform clinical research in the field of airway management and are well published in this area, including peer-reviewed articles, book chapters, and books.

In 2019, SAM officially affiliated with *Anesthesia & Analgesia* (*A&A*), the official journal of the International Anesthesia Research Society. In 2020, this relationship matured to allow for a freestanding airway management section in *A&A* authored by SAM members. This affiliation has provided a venue for publishing and disseminating impactful airway management papers worldwide.

Impact on Patient Care: Patient Safety

General

As a clinician involved in airway management on a regular basis, the underlying goal remains being a patient advocate and improving airway management practices and safety. The societies presented in this chapter aim to disseminate knowledge of early advances in airway management by promoting and advocating techniques that are consistent with patient safety.

Strong and joint expert opinion is likely to impact clinical practice faster than publications regarding a technique that is likely to promote patient safety and outcome measures. A prime example of this is promotion of awake flexible scope intubation, which was particularly true with SAM's first president and founding member, Andranik Ovassapian. It is conceivable that early advocation of this practice potentially prevented major morbidity in patients with difficult airways. Likewise, the rapid and widespread use of videolaryngoscopy in patients with suspected difficult airways may be partially attributed to dissemination of anecdotal clinical experiences of airway experts prior to formal published guidelines. During the COVID-19 pandemic, consensus guidelines for safe airway management of patients with COVID-19[3,4] were published to encourage safe, accurate, and swift performance of tracheal intubation in patients with COVID-19.

The DAS extubation guidelines[5,6] are another prime example of expert opinions promoting patient care. These guidelines highlight the fact that tracheal extubation is a high-risk procedure, discuss potential problems arising during extubation and recovery, and promote a strategic, stepwise approach to extubation. They emphasize the importance of planning and preparation and include practical techniques for use in clinical practice and recommendations for postextubation care. In these scenarios, use of various devices and techniques were universally promoted by experts and likely implemented into clinical practice due to the early promotion by airway society expert members before they became officially published.

Airway Leads

The principal roles of Airway Leads (AWLs) are to enhance airway management throughout their organization, engaging other specialties and support groups with the single goal of improving standards of care wherever airways are managed.[7] The first Airway Leads Network was launched in the United Kingdom in 2011 by the Royal College of Anaesthetists and the DAS. It has since been adapted as a model for similar networks worldwide (e.g., Ireland, New Zealand). Coordinating dissemination of new knowledge, supervising the procurement of airway equipment, overseeing morbidity and mortality audits, and promoting practice guidelines throughout the hospital are vital components of the work of these individuals, thereby enhancing patient safety.

Adults

In 1990, the leading causes of respiratory-related complications were inadequate ventilation, esophageal intubation, and difficult intubation.[5] Although the rates of esophageal intubation have significantly decreased, difficult tracheal intubation remains a concern. This is because airway complications remain high on the list of categories in the American Society of Anesthesiologists (ASA) Closed Claims Database as a cause of permanent neurologic injury or mortality from inadequate oxygenation and ventilation.[8,9] The Fourth National Audit Project (NAP4) of the Royal College of Anesthetists and the DAS revealed that in the United Kingdom (1) most significant airway events occurred during elective surgery, (2) aspiration was the most frequent cause of airway-related mortality, and (3) many complications resulted from poor planning of primary and rescue techniques.[10]

Children

A multicenter study of children with difficult airways in 13 pediatric centres (Pediatric Difficult Intubation [PeDI] registry) demonstrated that greater than two direct laryngoscopy attempts in children with difficult tracheal intubation are associated with high failure rates and an increased incidence of severe complications.[11] This study was the first to confirm that airway management in a pediatric difficult airway population cared for by mostly pediatric anesthesiologists is associated with significant complication rates. In these children, tracheal intubation failed in 2% of cases, and 20% of children had at least one complication. The most common severe complication was hypoxemic cardiac arrest occurring in 2% of these children. The most common complication overall was transient hypoxemia (SpO_2 <85%). Additionally, the Pedi registry collaborative group subsequently

published on best practices for difficult airway management in children.[12,13]

In summary, large data have suggested that, although the incidence of death and brain damage from airway management during general anesthesia is low, there is still significant morbidity related to airway management. Therefore to reduce morbidity related to airway management, there is room for improvement in most cases that merits attention.

To facilitate more effective and safe management for the difficult airway and to reduce the likelihood of adverse outcomes, Airway Task Forces were formed by ASA and DAS. These airway societies have created airway guidelines and offer expert opinions that have served to reduce the number of adverse outcomes and improve the safety of airway management.

Social Media and Airway Management

Use of social media, such as Facebook and Twitter, are popular with members of these societies, as well as other airway enthusiasts. Like forums, these social networking sites allow real-time input and feedback during and after lectures/workshops.

Future Directions

Airway management societies have aimed to improve the quality of care in relatively underserved areas worldwide. For example, SAM has international chapters in Brazil and the Middle East. The society aims to expand its membership globally to spread the theme of improving airway management in areas outside the United States and United Kingdom by providing expert advice and education. DAS has an interest in supporting members in low-resource settings and has awarded international travel grants for this purpose and supported faculty delivering workshops in theses settings

Following the success of WAMM the three large airway management societies have formed an alliance that will be known as the World Alliance of Airway Management (WAAM). These are the objectives of WAAM:

- Provide a link between airway societies, special interest groups, airway fellowships, training centers, and airway-related charities
- Act as a central location for local, national, and international airway societies, guidelines, statements, airway-related topics, research projects, research opportunities, and grants
- Establish effective relationships with other organizations concerned with airway management
- Act as a central reference to industry partners involved in airway management
- Serve as an educational center for ongoing webinars and web-based educational activities
- Choose the location, administer, and coordinate with local teams/hosts for the quadrennial WAMM conference
- Strive to be an open-access global resource

Conclusion

Airway management societies have come a long way over the past several years. Their universal purpose and goal remain prevention of morbidity related to airway management by dissemination of patient safety guidelines. Educational endeavors, high-quality lectures, hands-on workshops, and a lively community of practitioners have aimed to teach and maintain the skills necessary for clinicians to take better care of the patients they serve.

Selected References

1. Pandit JJ, Popat MT, Cook TM, et al. The Difficult Airway Society "ADEPT" guidance on selecting airway devices: the basis of a strategy for equipment evaluation. *Anaesthesia.* 2011;66:726–737.
2. Difficult Airway Society. About ADEPT. Difficult Airway Society, Airway Device Evaluation Project Team (ADEPT); 2015. Available at https://www.das.uk.com/adept/about.
3. Cook TM, El-Boghdadly K, McGuire B, McNarry AF, Patel A, Higgs A. Consensus guidelines for managing the airway in patients with COVID-19: Guidelines from the Difficult Airway Society, the Association of Anaesthetists, the Intensive Care Society, the Faculty of Intensive Care Medicine, and the Royal College of Anaesthetists. *Anaesthesia.* 2020;75:785–799.
4. Matava CT, Kovatsis PG, Lee JK, et al. Pediatric Airway Management in COVID-19 Patients: Consensus Guidelines From the Society for Pediatric Anesthesia's Pediatric Difficult Intubation Collaborative and the Canadian Pediatric Anesthesia Society. *Anesth Analg.* 2020;131:61–73.
5. Difficult Airway Society Extubation Guidelines Group, Popat M, Mitchell V, et al. Difficult Airway Society Guidelines for the management of tracheal extubation. *Anaesthesia.* 2012;67:318–340.
6. Difficult Airway Society. DAS Extubation Guidelines. Difficult Airway Society; 2015. Available at https://das.uk.com/guidelines/das-extubation-guidelines1.
7. McNarry AF, M Cook T, Baker PA, O'Sullivan EP. The airway lead: opportunities to improve institutional and personal preparedness for airway management. *Br J Anaesth.* 2020;125(1):e22–e24.
8. Caplan RA, Posner KL, Ward RJ, et al. Adverse respiratory events in anesthesia: a closed claims analysis. *Anesthesiology.* 1990;72:828–833.
9. Joffe AM, Aziz MF, Posner KL, et al. Management of difficult tracheal intubation: a closed claims analysis. *Anesthesiology.* 2019;131:818–829.
10. Cook TM, Woodall N, Frerk C, et al. Major complications of airway management in the UK: results of the Fourth National Audit Project of the Royal College of Anaesthetists and the Difficult Airway Society. Part 1: anaesthesia. *Br J Anaesth.* 2011;106:617–631.
11. Fiadjoe JE, Nishisaki A, Jagannathan N, et al. Airway management complications in children with difficult tracheal intubation from the Pediatric Difficult Intubation (PeDI) registry: a prospective cohort analysis. *Lancet Respir Med.* 2016;4:37–48.
12. Burjek NE, Fiadjoe JE, Nishisaki, et al. Fiberoptic tracheal intubation through a supraglottic airway versus video laryngoscopy in children with difficult tracheal intubation: a multicenter analysis in the Pediatric Difficult Intubation Registry. *Anesthesiology.* 2017;127(3):432–440.
13. Garcia-Marcinkiewicz AG, Adams HD, et al. A retrospective analysis of neuromuscular blocking drug use and ventilation technique on complications in the Pediatric Difficult Intubation Registry using propensity score matching. *Anesth Analg.* 2020;131(2):469–479.

All references can be found online at eBooks.Health.Elsevier.com.

Index

Page numbers followed by "*f*" indicate figures, "*t*" indicate tables, and "*b*" indicate boxes.